GRIFFITH'S 5

MINUTE CLINICAL CONSULT 2000

MARK R. DAMBRO, MD, FAAFP

Forth Worth, Texas
Formerly Assistant Professor of Medicine
And Director of Medical Computing
Tucson, Arizona

Technical Editor:
Jo A. Griffith

Previous editor:
H. Winter Griffith, MD
Editions 1993, 1994

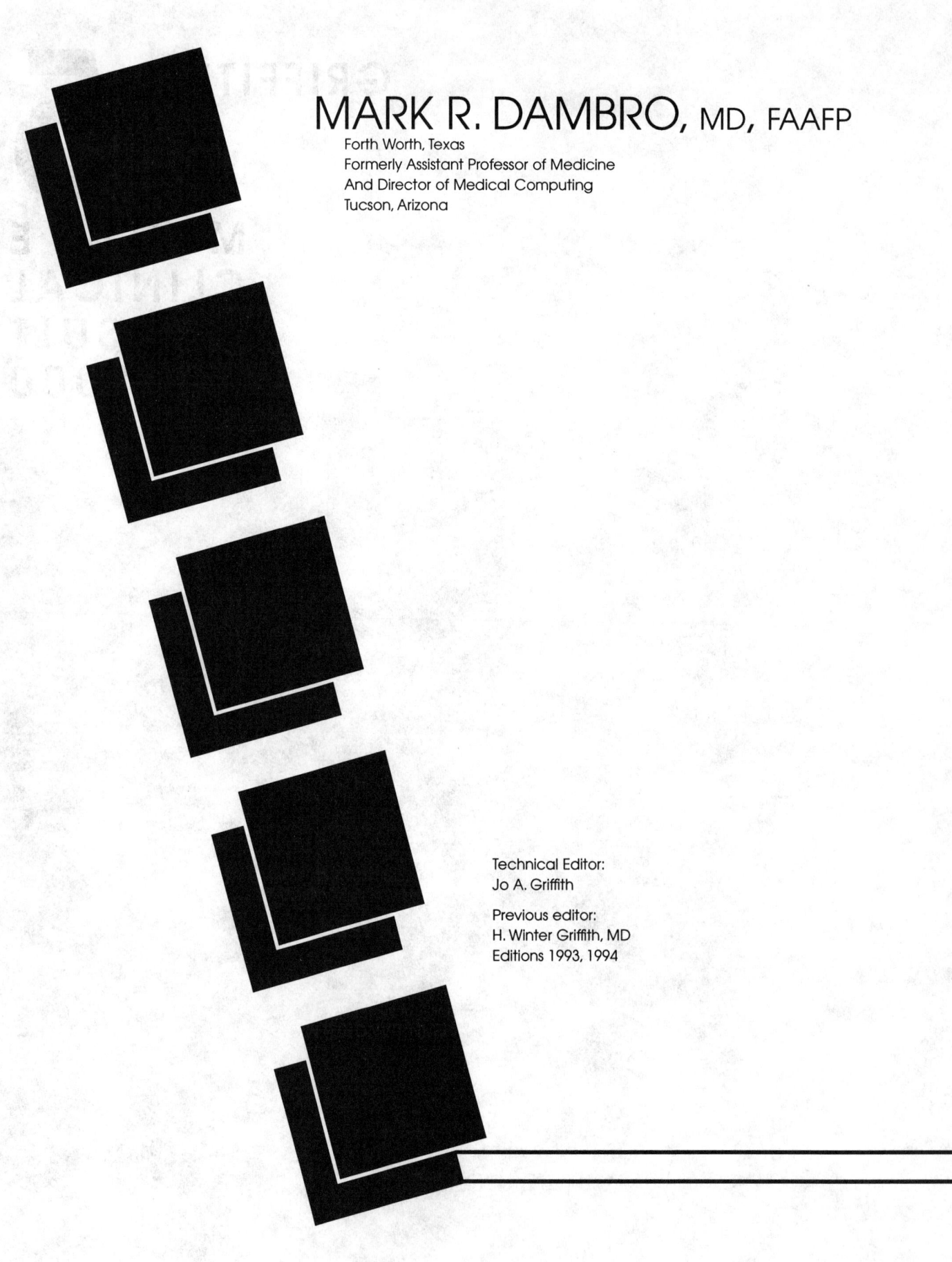

GRIFFITH'S 5

MINUTE CLINICAL CONSULT 2000

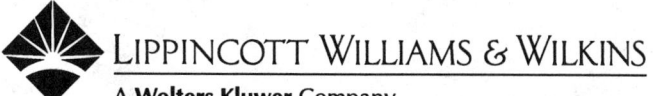

LIPPINCOTT WILLIAMS & WILKINS

A **Wolters Kluwer** Company

Philadelphia • Baltimore • New York • London
Buenos Aires • Hong Kong • Sydney • Tokyo

Acquisitions Editor: Richard Winters
Developmental Editor: Delois Patterson
Manufacturing Manager: Timothy Reynolds
Production Editor: Toni Ann Scaramuzzo
Printer: R.R. Donnelley, Crawfordsville

Printed in the United States of America

9 8 7 6 5 4 3 2

Care has been taken to confirm the accuracy of the information presented and to describe generally accepted practices. However, the authors, editors, and publisher are not responsible for errors or omissions or for any consequences from application of the information in this book and make no warranty, expressed or implied, with respect to the contents of the publication.

The authors, editors, and publisher have exerted every effort to ensure that drug selection and dosage set forth in this text are in accordance with current recommendations and practice at the time of publication. However, in view of ongoing research, changes in government regulations, and the constant flow of information relating to drug therapy and drug reactions, the reader is urged to check the package insert for each drug for any change in indications and dosage and for added warnings and precautions. This is particularly important when the recommended agent is a new or infrequently employed drug.

Some drugs and medical devices presented in this publication have Food and Drug Administration (FDA) clearance for limited use in restricted research settings. It is the responsibility of the health care provider to ascertain the FDA status of each drug or device planned for use in their clinical practice.

GRIFFITH'S *5 Minute Clinical Consult—2000* represents the eighth annual edition of quick medical reference for current medical diagnosis and treatment. These are the features:

SCOPE
Over one thousand topics arranged alphabetically and cross-indexed to synonyms of each. 593 expanded topics in a full format that contains enough detail to confirm the diagnosis and treat the problem. 424 short topics in a brief format.

CONTRIBUTING AUTHORS
Over 300 experienced clinicians writing on medical and surgical problems within their areas of interest and expertise. Authors make a final review of their topics just 3 months before the book is available in bookstores—insuring timeliness.

CONSULTANTS
Nearly 40 authorities in fields of general and specialty practice. Consultants review the topics for accuracy, currency, appropriateness, completeness, and safety. Medication entries and dosages reviewed by a Doctor of Pharmacy and contributing authors just prior to publication.

UPDATES
Annual. Assures inclusion of the most recent norms of practice and consensus of the majority of experts.

FORMAT
For the 593 major topics, a consistent, two-page, graphic, chart-like format, similar to the skeleton format presented below. The six major divisions and 36 information blocks cover the major aspects of each disorder.

BASICS	DIAGNOSIS	TREATMENT	MEDICATION	FOLLOW-UP	MISCELLANEOUS
• Description	• Differential	• General measures	• Drugs of choice	• Monitoring	• Associated conditions
• Genetics	• Laboratory	• Surgical measures	• Contraindications	• Prevention	• Age-related factors
• Prevalence	• Pathological findings	• Activity	• Precautions	• Complications	• Pregnancy
• Age	• Special tests	• Diet	• Interactions	• Prognosis	• Synonyms
• Signs and symptoms	• Imaging	• Patient education	• Alternate drugs		• ICD-9-CM
• Causes	• Diagnostics				• See also
• Risk factors					• Other notes
					• Abbreviations
					• References

Griffith's 5 Minute Clinical Consult aims to bring current, relevant data to:

- Busy practitioners who need to quickly refresh their memory of diagnostic or treatment alternatives
- Students who need a quick update on the basics (description, genetics, prevalence, signs and symptoms, etc.)
- Patients who want to review their particular diagnosis

To all these, and others, I hope the *5 Minute Clinical Consult* brings the kind of data they find useful. It has been and continues to be my desire that the database of information, collected and updated by so many clinicians, be easily accessible to its readers. Toward this end I strive to help all who share this goal to obtain and use the database for helping clinicians help their patients.

In addition to the book, a CD-ROM is available that includes the topics in a searchable format, with over 500 illustrations. Drs. Cowan and Miller have done an outstanding job of finding excellent examples of many of the topics. I hope you'll find these illustrations helpful.

In order to bring the data to even more people, the book's web site (http://www.5mcc.com), which initially contained the Table of Contents and summaries of each topic, continues to evolve. This year the reference citations for every topic will be available on the web site. And citations for a few lengthy topics that needed extra space will be available only on the web site. The web site has provided helpful information to many, and it is my hope that as it matures it will continue as a reliable source of reviewed, dependable clinical information. Renovations to the web site are underway to include more information, more links, and additional formats. Keep checking back for the latest.

The web site also delivers up-to-date information on the hand-held versions of the 5 Minute including Palm Pilot, Newton, Windows CE, and PDR. This year the 5 Minute has been made available in the smallest, lightest form yet, the Palm Pilot—a truly remarkable accomplishment. And a close second is the PDR, which makes available many references, including *Griffith's 5 Minute Clinical Consult*.

A Developer's Page helps bring the database to those who create the truly remarkable software and hardware devices that bring the 5 Minute to the clinician. Included are general comments regarding the database structure and a subset sample suitable for downloading and initial prototype work.

The book, CD-ROM, hand helds, and web site are a compilation of many people's efforts, including the contributing authors and the consultants who review the topics—each deserves a special thanks for their time. I'd especially like to also thank Mr. Richard Winters for his support; the staff at Lippincott Williams & Wilkins who have done so much to keep the book and concept of "The 5 Minute Consult" alive; my family for their patience and support; and finally, to Mrs. Jo Griffith whose hard work and persistent search for the elusive goal, perfection, has so improved the book.

Preface

I wish to make this work continuously responsive to the needs of its readers, and I thank those who have taken their time to write reviews and suggestions. I take your comments seriously and hope you will find many of them in this year's edition. As always, I invite you to express your wishes regarding chapters or changes you would like to appear in future editions. Send your comments and suggestions to:

Mark R. Dambro, MD
1650 W. Rosedale Street
Suite 307
Fort Worth, TX 76104

Email: mrdambo@5mcc.com

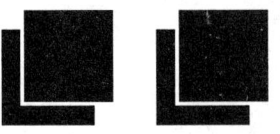

BOARD OF CONSULTANTS

CONTRIBUTING AUTHORS

STONEY A. ABERCROMBIE, MD
Professor, Family Medicine
Medical University of South Carolina
Anderson, SC

ABDULRAZAK ABYAD, MD, MPH, AGSF
Director, Abyad Medical Center
Coordinator, Ain WaZein Comprehensive Geriatric Program
Abyad Medical Center Ain WaZein Hospital
Tripoli, Lebanon

RODNEY D. ADAM, MD
Associate Professor of Medicine & Microbiology/Immunology
University of Arizona College of Medicine
Tucson, AZ

STEPHEN M. ADAMS, MD
Assistant Professor
Department of Family Medicine
University of Tennessee College of Medicine
Chattanooga Unit
Chattanooga, TN

ALAN ADELMAN, MD, MS
Department of Family and Community Medicine
Milton S. Hershey Medical Center
Hershey, PA

AUGUSTO AGUIRRE, MD
Associate Clinical Professor of Pathology
Ohio State University
Grant-Riverside Hospitals
Columbus, OH

RICHARD W. ALLINSON, MD
Senior Staff Physician
Scott & White Clinic, Waco
Waco, TX

EARL ROBERT G. ANG, MD
St. Francis Family Practice Residency Program
Lincolnwood, IL

VICENTE J. ARANO, MD
Private Practice
Yuca Valley Family Medial Associates
Yucca Valley, CA

HENRY ARGUINCHONA, MD
Physicians Clinic of Spokane
Spokane, WA

WATSON C. ARNOLD, MD
Director, Pediatric Nephrology
Cook Children's Medical Center
Fort Worth, TX

ROBERT L. ATMAR, MD
Department of Medicine
Baylor College of Medicine
Houston, TX

COLIN R. BAMFORD, MD
Department of Neurology
University of Arizona College of Medicine
Tucson, AZ

MUSTAFA BARUDI, MD
Assistant Professor of Pediatrics
Northeastern Ohio Universities College of Medicine
Tod Children's Hospital
Youngstown, OH

CHANDRAMOHAN BATRA, MD
Director, Women & Children's Services
East Kentucky Family Practice Residency Program
University of Kentucky
Hazard, KY

ROBERT P. BAUGHMAN, MD
Professor of Medicine
Pulmonary and Critical Care Medicine
University of Cincinnati Medical Center
Cincinnati, OH

KAY A. BAUMAN, MD, MPH
Professor
Department of Family Practice & Community Health
University of Hawaii School of Medicine
Mililani, HI

MARK T. BAYLEY, BA, MD, FRCPC
Medical Director
Acquired Brain Injury Program
Hamilton Health Sciences Corp.
Hamilton, Ontario   CANADA

KARIL BELLAH, MD
Cardiologist
Lawrence, KS

BRUCE G. BELLAMY, MD
Saint Luke's Medical
Clinton, MO

JAMES B. BENJAMIN, MD
Associate Professor of Surgery
University of Arizona College of Medicine
Tucson, AZ

PAUL J. BENKE, MD, PHD
University of Miami School of Medicine
Miami, FL

GEORGE R. BERGUS, MD
Associate Professor
Department of Family Practice
University of Iowa
Iowa City, IA

BRANDON I. BERMAN, MD
Grant Family Practice Residency
Columbus, OH

WILLIAM H. BILLICA, MD
Assistant Director
Family Practice Residency Program
Good Samaritan Medical Center
Phoenix, AZ

TIMOTHY L. BLACK, MD, FACS, FAAP
Medical Director of Trauma
Cook Children's Medical Center
Fort Worth, TX

BRUCE BLOCK, MD
Director, Primary Care Institute
UPMC - Shadyside Hospital
Pittsburgh, PA

MICHAEL BOESPFLUG, MD
Santa Clara Medical Clinic
Eugene, OR

JESS G. BOND, MD, MPH
Assistant Professor of Internal Medicine
Northeastern Ohio Universities College of Medicine
Akron, OH

PATRICIA BORMAN, MD
Faculty, Swedish Family Medicine
Clinical Instructor, University of Washington
Swedish Medical Center
Seattle, WA

MARJORIE A. BOWMAN, MD, MPA
Department of Family Practice & Community Medicine
University of Pennsylvania Health System
Philadelphia, PA

W. PAUL BOWMAN, MD
Medical Director, Hematology-Oncology
Cook Children's Medical Center
Fort Worth, TX

GEORGE R. BRADBURY, MD
Orthopedic Surgery
University City, MO

MARSHALL BRADSHAW, MD
Private Practice
Fort Worth, TX

ROBERT BURGOS, MD
Private Practice
Fort Worth, TX

JOHN R. BURK, MD
Private Practice
Fort Worth, TX

DAVID E. BURTNER, MD
Vice Chairman and Professor
Department of Family & Community Medicine
Mercer University School of Medicine
Macon, GA

ROGER CADY, MD
Director
Headache Care Center
Springfield, MO

CYNTHIA GAIL CARMICHAEL, MD
Staff Physician
North Richmond Center for Health
Berkley, CA

KEVIN CARMICHAEL, MD
Unit Chief
El Rio Special Immunology Associates
Tucson, AZ

TODD CARRAN, MD
Adjunct Assistant Professor of Clinical Family Medicine
University of Cincinnati
Cincinnati, OH

JOHN Z. CARTER, MD
Private Practice
Family Practice/Geriatrics
Tucson, AZ

L. PHILIP CARTER, MD
Western Neurological, Ltd.
Tucson, AZ

ROY R. CASIANO, MD
Professor
Department of Otolaryngology-Center for Sinus & Voice Disorders
University of Miami School of Medicine
Miami, FL

A. PETER CATINELLA, MD
Associate Professor and Vice Chairman
Department of Family & Preventive Medicine
University of Utah
Salt Lake City, UT

FRANK "CHIP" CELESTINO, MD
Associate Professor
Department of Family & Community Medicine
Wake Forest University Baptist Medical Center School of Medicine
Winston-Salem, NC

JASON CHAO, MD, MS
Associate Professor
Department of Family Medicine
Case Western Reserve University
Cleveland, OH

ROBERT A. CHENEY, MD
Associate Clinical Instructor
Orthopaedic Surgery
Albany Medical College
Albany, NY

ANTHONY W. CHOW, MD, FRCPC, FACP
Professor of Medicine
Division of Infectious Diseases
The University of British Columbia
Vancouver, British Columbia   CANADA

THOMAS W. CLARK, MS, MD
Private Practice
Newport News, VA

WILLIAM W. CLEVELAND, MD
Professor of Pediatrics
Chairman Emeritus
University of Miami
Miami, FL

RICHARD D. CLOVER, MD
Department of Family and Community Medicine
University of Louisville
Louisville, KY

RICHARD W. COHEN, MD
Resurgens Orthopaedics
Marietta, GA

RUSSELL G. COHEN, MD
Department of Surgery/Orthopedics
Tucson Orthopedic Institute
Tucson, AZ

JOHN J. COLEMAN, MD
Professor of Surgery
Director, Plastic Surgery
Indiana University Medical Center
Indianapolis, IN

JACK G. COPELAND, MD
Professor, Department of Surgery
Section of Cardiovascular and Thoracic Surgery
University of Arizona College of Medicine
Tucson, AZ

CAROL CORDY, MD
Family Physician
Residency Site Director
45th St. Clinic
Seattle, WA

ALAN J. CROPP, MD, FCCP
Associate Professor of Internal Medicine
Northeastern Ohio Universities College of Medicine
Youngstown, OH

PAUL T. CULLEN, MD
Director, Family Practice Residency Program
The Washington Hospital
Washington, PA

J. P. W. CUNNINGTON, MD, FRCPC
Associate Professor of Medicine
McMaster University
Hamilton, Ontario, CANADA

M. BEATRIZ CURRIER, MD
Department of Psychiatry
University of Miami School of Medicine
Miami, FL

JAMES E. DALEN, MD, MPH
Vice President for Health Sciences
Dean, College of Medicine
The University of Arizona
Tucson, AZ

MARK R. DAMBRO, MD, FAAFP
Private Practice
Fort Worth, TX

NANCY N. DAMBRO, MD
Cook Children's Medical Center
Fort Worth, TX

JERYL DANSKY, MD
Private Practice
Tucson, AZ

MARC DARR, MD
Associate Director
St. Joseph Hospital Family Practice Residency
Phoenix, AZ

MARK D. DARROW, MD
Associate Professor
Director Clinical Services Division
Department of Family Medicine
School of Medicine
East Carolina University
Greenville, NC

JANICE E. DAUGHERTY, MD
Associate Professor of Family Medicine
East Carolina University School of Medicine
Greenville, NC

BART DEMAERSCHALK, MD, FRCPC
Department of Clinical Neurological Sciences
The University of Western Ontario
London, Ontario   Canada

ROBERT DEMARCO, MD
Associate Professor of Clinical Internal Medicine
Northeastern Ohio Universities College of Medicine
Youngstown, OH

DAVID DEVLAMING, DDS
Private practice
Fort Worth, TX

EMIL S DICKSTEIN, MD, FACP
Associate Professor of Medicine
Northeastern Ohio Universities College of Medicine
Youngstown, OH

NUHAD D. DINNO, MD
Clinical Professor
Center on Human Development and Disability
Department of Pediatrics
University of Washington School of Medicine
Seattle, WA

J. HARLAN DIX, MD, FACP
Clinical Associate Professor
Northeastern Ohio Universities College of Medicine
Killbuck, OH

MICHEL J. DODARD, MD
Assistant Professor/Medical Director
Clinical Family Medicine & Community Health
Jefferson Reaves Sr. Health Center
Miami, FL

ROBERT DOLIN, MD
Department of Medicine
Kaiser Permanente
La Palma, CA

DAVID DONAHUE, MD
Private Practice
Fort Worth, TX

DAN DOSS, DDS
Private Practice
Fort Worth, TX

HELEN DRIEDIGER, RN, BA, BSW
Clinical Specialist
Acquired Brain Injury Program
Hamilton Health Sciences Corp.
Hamilton, Ontario   CANADA

S. SHEVAUN DUIKER, MD
Chair, Department of Family Medicine
The Children's Hospital
Denver, CO

BURRIS DUNCAN, MD
Professor
Department of Pediatrics
University of Arizona College of Medicine
Tucson, AZ

DONALD F. EIPPER, MD
Associate Professor, Internal Medicine
Northeastern Ohio Universities College of Medicine
Akron General Medical Center
Akron, OH

STEVEN EISENSTEIN, MD
Private Practice
The Family Doctors of Northbrook
Northbrook, IL

NANCY ELDER, MD, MSPH
Associate Professor
Oregon Health Sciences University
Portland, OR

GREG ELDERS, MD
Family Practice
Mountain Home, AR

JON A. ELIAS, MD
Assistant Professor of Clinical Family Medicine
Northeastern Ohio Universities College of Medicine
Assistant Director, Family Practice Residency Program
Barberton Citizens Hospital
Barberton, OH

PAMELA I. ELLSWORTH, MD
Pediatric Urology
Dartmouth-Hitchcock Medical Center
Lebanon, NH

BASSEM ELSAWY, MD
St. Francis Family Practice Residency Program
Lincolnwood, IL

KURT ELWARD, MD, MPH
Family Medicine of Albemarle
Clinical Assistant Professor, Department of Family Medicine
University of Virginia
Charlottesville, VA

JOSEPH G. EWING, MD
Assistant Professor of Family Practice
Family Practice Residency Program at Conroe
University of Texas Medical Branch, Galveston
Conroe, TX

ROBERT G. FANTE, MD
Advanced Oculoplastic Surgeons, PC
Denver, CO

ANDREW H. FENTON, MD, FACS
Assistant Professor of Surgery
Northeastern Ohio Universities College of Medicine
Akron General Medical Center
Akron, OH

MICHAEL FERREBEE, MD
Physician/Emergency Room
Stonewall Jackson Memorial Hospital
Morgantown, WV

SCOTT A. FIELDS, MD
Associate Professor
Family Medicine
Oregon Health Sciences University
Portland, OR

DOUGLAS P. FINE, MD
Professor and Chairman of Medicine
University of Oklahoma Health Sciences Center
Oklahoma City, OK

STANLEY FINEMAN, MD
Clinical Assistant Professor
Department of Pediatrics
Emory University School of Medicine
Marietta, GA

GENE S. FISCH, PHD
Research Scientist
Yale University School of Medicine
General Clinical Research Center
New Haven, CT

DANIEL B. FISHBEIN, MD
Associate Director for Science Division of International Health
Epidemiology Program Office
Centers for Disease Control
Atlanta, GA

JOSEPH A. FLORENCE, MD
Director, East Kentucky Family Practice Residency Program
University of Kentucky
Hazard, KY

GRANT C. FOWLER, MD
Associate Professor and Vice Chair of Family Practice Community
  Medicine
The University of Texas-Houston Medical School
Houston, TX

DAVID J. FRAMM, MD, FACC
Directory of Echocardiography
Mecklenburg Medical Group
Charlotte, NC

DAVID FRANK, MD
Medical Director
The Hetrick Center
Middletown, PA

WESLEY FURSTE, MD, FACS
Clinical Professor, Emeritus
Department of Surgery
Ohio State University
Columbus, OH

GREGORY G. GAAR, MD, FAAP, FACEP
Co-Medical Director
Florida Poison Information and Toxicology Resource Center
Tampa General Hospital
Tampa, FL

ERIC P. GALL, MD
Professor and Chairman
Department of Medicine
Finch University of Health Sciences
The Chicago Medical School
North Chicago, IL

JAMES M. GALLOWAY, MD, FACP, FACC
Director, Native American Cardiology Program
Clinical Assistant Professor, Public Health
University of Arizona College of Medicine
Tucson, AZ

LEONARD GANZ, MD
Electrophysiology Section
Cardiology Division
Allegheny General Hospital
Pittsburgh, PA

GALE GARDNER, MD, FACS
Clinical Professor
Department of Otolaryngology
University of Tennessee, Memphis
Memphis, TN

WILLIAM G. GARDNER, MD
Chairman, Department of Medicine
Akron General Medical Center
Akron, OH

MARK GERSTBERGER, DO
Family Health Center
Lakin, KS

JOHN P. GEYMAN, MD
Professor Emeritus of Family Medicine
University of Washington
Seattle, WA

JEFF RAY GIBSON, JR., MD
Department of Anesthesiology
Scott and White Clinic
Temple, TX

BRUCE C. GILLILAND, MD
Professor of Medicine and Laboratory Medicine
School of Medicine
University of Washington
Seattle, WA

MARSHALL GODWIN, MD
Hotel Dieu Family Medicine Center
Queen's University
Kingston, Ontario   CANADA

GARY A. GOFORTH, MD, MTMH
Associate Professor of Family Medicine
Medical University of South Carolina
_Program Director
Self Memorial Hospital Family
Practice Residency Program
Greenwood, SC

PAUL R. GORDON, MD
Department of Family & Community Medicine
University of Arizona College of Medicine
Tucson, AZ

R. SCOTT GORMAN, MD
Mayo Health Plan Arizona
Mayo Clinic Scottsdale
Scottsdale, AZ

MARK A. GRABER, MD
Associate Clinical Professor
Departments of Family Medicine & Surgery
The University of Iowa
Iowa City, IA

DAVID S. GRAY, MD
Sutter Medical Center
Family Practice Residency
University of California, San Francisco
Santa Rosa, CA

J. THOMAS GRAYSTON, MD
Professor, Department of Epidemiology
Dept of Epideniology
University of Washington
School of Public Health and Community Medicine
Seattle, WA

RONALD A. GREENFIELD, MD
Professor of Medicine & Chief, Infectious Diseases Section
University of Oklahoma Health Sciences Center
Oklahoma City, OK

DAVID A. GRIESEMER, MD
Division of Child Neurology
Department of Neurology and Pediatrics
Medical University of South Carolina
Charleston, SC

JOHN GUISTO, MD
Associate Professor of Clinical Surgery
Section of Emergency Medicine, Department of Surgery
University of Arizona College of Medicine
Tucson, AZ

VLADIMIR HACHINSKI, MD, DSC, FRCPC
Professor and Chair
Department of Clinical Neurological Sciences
The University of Western Ontario
London, Ontario   CANADA

DAVID E. HALL, MD
Clinical Associate Professor of Pediatrics
Emory University School of Medicine
Children's Medical Center of Atlanta at Scottish Rite
Atlanta, GA

HETTY B. HALL, MD
Iowa City, IA

R. BRUCE HALL, MD
Private Practice, Orthopedics
Southern Bone & Joint Specialists
Dothan, AL

LARRY W. HALVERSON, MD
Director, Cox Family Practice Residency Program
Cox Health Systems
Springfield, MO

CLYDE L. HARRIS, MD
Private Practice
Franklin, NC

IRWIN E. HARRIS, MD, MBA, MSHA, FACS
Orthopedic Oncology, Pediatric Orthopedics
Vice President of Medical Affairs
Good Samaritan Health Systems
Kearney, NE

FERN R. HAUCK, MD, MS
Associate Professor and Director of Research
Department of Family Medicine
Loyola University Chicago Stritch School of Medicine
Maywood, IL

STEVEN J. HAVENER, MD
Private Practice
Mission, TX

HARRY W. HAVERKOS, MD
Medical Officer
Food and Drug Administration
Rockville, MD

ADRIENNE HEADLEY, MD
Clinical Instructor
Family Medicine at Monument Square
New Brunswick, NJ

CATHRYN HEATH, MD
Assistant Professor of Family Medicine
UMDNJ Robert Wood Johnson Medical School
New Brunswick, NJ

DARELL E. HEISELMAN, DO, FCCM, FACP, FACC, FCCP
Chief, Critical Care Medicine, Akron General Medical Center
Professor, Northeastern Ohio Universities College of Medicine
Professor, Ohio University, Athens, Ohio
Akron, OH

THOMAS W. HEJKAL, MD, PHD
Assistant Professor
Department of Ophthalmology
University of Nebraska Medical Center
Omaha, NE

SCOTT T. HENDERSON, MD
Associate Professor of Family Practice
Family Practice Residency Program, Cheyenne
University of Wyoming
Cheyenne, WY

ERIC HENLEY, MD, MPH
Assistant Professor
Department of Family & Community Medicine
University of Illinois College of Medicine at Rockford
Rockford, IL

KEVIN M. HEPLER, MD, MBA
Medical Director
Office of Children, Youth, and Families
Department of Public Welfare, Commonwealth of PA
Harrisburg, PA

DOREEN L. HOCK, MD
Assistant Professor
UMDNJ/RWJ Medical School
St Peter's University Hospital
New Brunswick, NJ

BARTON L. HODES, MD
Professor
Department of Ophthalmology
University of Arizona College of Medicine
Tucson, AZ

IRA N. HOLLANDER, MD
Private Practice
Urology Clinics of North Texas
Fort Worth, TX

MICHAEL P. HOPKINS, MD
Chairperson, Department of Obstetrics & Gynecology
Akron General Medical Center
Professor, Northeastern Ohio Universities College of Medicine
Akron, OH

MARK HORATTAS, MD, FACS
Associate Professor
Department of Surgery
Northeastern Ohio Universities College of Medicine
Akron, OH

LAURENE L. HOWELL, MD
Associate Professor
Department of Otolaryngology
Oregon Health Sciences University
Portland, OR

DOUGLAS M. HOY, MD
Associate Clinical Professor
Department of Family Medicine
Medical College of Ohio
Bellevue, OH

DENNIS E. HUGHES, DO, FAAFP
Medical Director
Cox-Monett Emergency Department
Cox Health Systems
Cox Regional Services
Springfield , MO

WENDY HUMPHREY, MD
Clinical Professor of Obstetrics and Gynecology
Northeastern Ohio Universities College of Medicine
Naples, FL

JOHN J. HUTTER, JR., MD
Professor of Pediatrics
Chief, Pediatric Hematology/Oncology
University of Arizona College of Medicine
Tucson, AZ

FRANK L. IBER, MD
Department of Gastroenterology
Department of Veterans Affairs
Riverside, IL

CHARLES N. JACOBS, MD
Nephrologist
Waterville, ME

PHILIP E. JAFFE, MD
Chief, Gastroenterology
Cleveland Clinic - Florida
Naples Division
Naples, FL

PAUL J. JASTER, MD
Associate Director, Clinical Associate Professor
Smoky Hill Family Practice Residency Program
Salina, KS

ERIC L. JENISON, MD
Professor of Clinical Obstetrics & Gynecology
Director, Gyn-Oncology
Northeastern Ohio Universities College of Medicine
Akron General Medical Center
Aultman Hospital, Suma Health System
Akron, OH

CHARLES JENNINGS, MD, FACS
Urology Associates of Ohio, Inc.
Lima, OH

FURNIE W. JOHNSTON, MD
Private Practice
Dothan, AL

SMITH L. JOHNSTON, III, MD, MS
NASA Medical Officer/Flight Surgeon
Flight Medicine Clinic/SD26
NASA Johnson Space Center
Houston, TX

MICHAEL JONES, MD
Faculty Physician
St. Francis Family Practice Program
Evanston, IL

GRAHAM S. KAISER, DO
Michigan Medical, P.C.
Grand Rapids, MI

PAUL E. KAPLAN, MD
Professor & Vice Chairman
Department of Physical Medicine & Rehabilitation
Medical University of South Carolina
Charleston, SC

WAYNE J. KATON, MD
Professor of Psychiatry, Vice Chair
Department of Psychiatry, School of Medicine
University of Washington Medical School
Seattle, WA

RICK KELLERMAN, MD
Professor and Chair
Department of Family and Community Medicine
University of Kansas School of Medicine-Wichita
Wichita, KS

MICHAEL W. KELLY, PHARMD, MS
Clinical Assistant Professor
College of Pharmacy
University of Iowa
Iowa City, IA

ROBERT M. KERSHNER, MD, FACS
Clinical Professor, University of Utah Medical Center
Director, Orange Grove Center for Corrective Eye Surgery
Tucson, AZ

JEFFREY B. KESSLER, MD
St. Francis Family Practice Residency Program
Lincolnwood, IL

GEORGE E. KIKANO, MD
Vice Chairman
Department of Family Medicine
Case Western Reserve University
Cleveland, OH

JOHN KILBOURNE, MD
St. Francis Family Practice Residency Program
Lincolnwood, IL

SCOTT A. KINCAID, MD
Assistant Clinical Professor of Family Medicine
Medical College of Virginia, Richmond, VA
Radford, VA

MITCHELL S. KING, MD
Assistant Professor, Dept. of Family Medicine
Northwestern University Medical School
Chicago, IL

JEFFERY T. KIRCHNER, DO, FAAFP
Associate Director
Family Practice Residency Program
Lancaster General Hospital
Lancaster, PA

JULIENNE K. KIRK, PHARMD
Assistant Professor
Department of Family & Community Medicine
Wake Forest University Baptist Medical Center School of Medicine
Winston-Salem, NC

EVAN W. KLIGMAN, MD
Professor and Head, Department of Family Medicine
University of Iowa College of Medicine
Iowa City, IA

MARY E. KLINK, MD
Physicians Plus Medical Group
Medical Director, Sleep Disorders Program
Meriter Hospital
Madison, WI

SANDRA KNAUR, MSN, RN, C-ANP
Private Practice
Fort Worth, TX

AUBREY L. KNIGHT, MD
Director of Family Practice Education
Carilion Health Systems
Roanoke, VA

PETER KOZISEK, MD
Family Practice Residency of Idaho
Boise, ID

ALVIN LANGER, MD
Professor and Chairperson of Obstetrics & Gynecology
Associate Dean for Clinical Education
Northeastern Ohio Universities College of Medicine
Canton, OH

LARS C. LARSEN, MD
Professor
Department of Family Medicine
East Carolina University School of Medicine
Greenville, NC

RICHARD A. LARSON, MD
Professor of Medicine
Director, Leukemia Program
The University of Chicago Medical Center
Chicago, IL

MARK C. LEESON, MD, FACS
Professor of Orthopedic Surgery
Northeastern Ohio Universities College of Medicine
Akron, OH

GARY LEVINE, MD
Associate Professor, Department of Family Medicine
In-Patient Service Coordinator
East Carolina University School of Medicine
Greenville, NC

BARCEY T. LEVY, PHD, MD
Assistant Professor
Department of Family Medicine
University of Iowa
Iowa City, IA

RICHARD P. LEVY, MD
Professor of Internal Medicine
Northeastern Ohio Universities College of Medicine
Akron, OH

JAMES H. LEWIS, MD, FACP, FACG
Professor of Medicine
Division of Gastroenterology
Georgetown University Medical Center
Washington, DC

LEONARD S. LILLY, MD
Associate Professor of Medicine
Harvard Medical School
Brigham and Women's Hospital
Boston, MA

CAROL B. LINDSLEY, MD
Professor of Pediatrics
Director, Pediatric Rheumatology
University of Kansas School of Medicine
Kansas City, KS

JOHN M. LITTLE, MD
Chief Medical Officer and Medical Director, Companion Healthcare
Clinical Associate Professor
University of South Carolina
Columbia, SC

PHIL LOBSTEIN, MD
Private Practice
Fort Worth, TX

RICH LONDO, MD
Assistant Professor of Clinical Family Medicine
Department of Family and Community Medicine
University of Illinois College of Medicine
Associate Director, Rural Medical Education Program
Rockford, IL

Contributing Authors

DOROTHY LOWDER, RN
Holmes County Hospice
Killbuck, OH

EDGAR A. LUCUS, PHD, ACP
Private Practice
Fort Worth, TX

D. W. MACPHERSON, MD, MSC (CTM), FRCPC
Assistant Professor
Director, Regional Parasitology Laboratory
McMaster University/Hamilton Regional Laboratory Medicine Program
Hamilton, Ontario, CANADA

BARBARA A. MAJERONI, MD
Assistant Professor
Department of Family Medicine
State University of New York at Buffalo
Buffalo, NY

JONATHAN MAKS, MD
Internal Medicine Resident
Evanston Northwestern Healthcare
Evanston, IL

MOHAMMAD MALIK, MD
Chief Resident, Family Practice
St. Francis Hospital of Evanston
Evanston, IL

SYLVIA A. MAMBY, MD
Consultant
Division of Cardiovascular Diseases
Mayo Clinic, Scottsdale
Scottsdale, AZ

DANNEN D. MANNSCHRECK, MD
Assistant Director, Family Practice Residency Program
University of Illinois College of Medicine at Rockford
L.P. Johnson Family Health Center
Rockford, IL

ROBERT A. MARLOW, MD, MA
Associate Director/Director of Research
Family Practice Residency Program
Scottsdale Healthcare
Scottsdale, AZ

ANNA N. MAXEY, MD
Associate Director
Grant Family Practice Residency
Grant/Riverside Methodist Hospitals
Columbus, OH

SUSANA MAY, MD, MPH
Assistant Clinical Professor of Family Medicine
Department of Family Medicine
University of Miami School of Medicine
Tavernier, FL

SUMNER T. MCALLISTER, MD
Family Practice
Grant Family Practice Residency
Columbus, OH

PATRICK J. MCCARVILLE, MD
Private Practice
Valley, NE

ELIZABETH I MCCORD, MD, MS
Assistant Professor, Johnson City Family Practice Residency
East Tennessee State University
James H. Quillen College of Medicine
Johnson City, TN

K. PATRICIA MCGANN, MD, MSPH
Palo Alto Medical Foundation, Palo Alto, CA
Associate Professor of Clinical Medicine
Stanford University School of Medicine
Stanford, CA

DON MCHARD, MD
Staff Physician
Department of Family Practice
Cigna Healthcare of Arizona
Glendale, AZ

SEAN O. MCMENOMEY, MD
Department of Otolaryngology
Oregon Health Sciences University
Portland, OR

LEO C. MERCER, MD
Chief Executive Officer
Capital Coast Health
Wellington   South New Zealand

ERIC S. MILLER, MD, FABFP, FACOG
Clinical Assistant Professor
Director, Family Practice Residency OB/GYN Program at Shadyside
   Hospital
University of Pittsburgh Medical Center
Pittsburgh, PA

GARY M. MILLER, MD
Marietta Neurological Associates
Marietta, GA

JAMES P. MILLER, MD, FACS, FAAP
Pediatric Surgical Associates of Fort Worth
Fort Worth, TX

KARL E. MILLER, MD
Associate Professor
Department of Family Medicine
University of Tennessee College of Medicine
Chattanooga Unit
Chattanooga, TN

SANDRA MILLER, MD
Assistant Director, Residency
Family Practice Center
Good Samaritan Regional Medical Center
Phoenix, AZ

LARRY MILLIKAN, MD
Chairman, Department of Dermatology
Tulane University School of Medicine
New Orleans, LA

JEFFREY F. MINTEER, MD
Associate Director
Family Practice Residency Program
The Washington Hospital
Washington, PA

CHARLES D. MITCHELL, MD
Division of Immunology & Infectious Diseases
Department of Pediatrics
University of Miami School of Medicine
Miami, FL

REZA MOATTARI, MD
Associate Professor of Medicine and Head, Endocrinology Division
Northeastern Ohio Universities College of Medicine
Chief, Endocrinology Section, Akron General Hospital
Akron, OH

SUSAN LOUISA MONTAUK, MD
Professor of Clinical Family Medicine
Department of Family Medicine
University of Cincinnati College of Medicine
Cincinnati, OH

T. GLENDON MOODY, MD
Clinical Lecturer
Department of Ophthalmology
University of Arizona College of Medicine
Phoenix, AZ

BARBARA J. MORONT, MD
Program Director
St. Francis Family Practice Residency Program
Lincolnwood, IL

SAMUEL L. MOSCHELLA, MD, FACP
Clinical Professor Dermatology (Emeritus)
Harvard Medical School
Senior Consultant, Lahey Clinic
Burlington, MA

BRIAN J. MURRAY, MD
Clinical Professor and Asst. Vice Chancellor
Director, Student Health & Wellness Center
University of California at San Diego
La Jolla, CA

JAMES A. NARD, MD
Department of Pediatrics
Tod Children's Hospital
Youngstown, OH

JORY A. NATKIN, DO
Instructor, Department of Family Medicine
Northwestern University Medical School
Glenview, IL

DIANE NEDDENRIEP, MD
Pediatric Pulmonary Associates
Tucson, AZ

DONALD A. F. NELSON, MD
Director of Medical Informatics
Cedar Rapids Medical Education Foundation
Family Practice Center
Cedar Rapids, IA

JAMES C. NIEDERMAN, MD
Clinical Professor of Medicine and Epidemiology
Yale University School of Medicine
New Haven, CT

PETER T. NIEH, MD
Senior Staff
Department of Urology
Lahey Clinic Medical Center
Burlington, MA

ROBERT NOECKER, MD
Assistant Professor
Department of Ophthalmology
University of Arizona
Tucson, AZ

LAURA L. NOVAK, MD
Barberton Citizens Hospital
Barberton, OH

EDWIN J. OLSEN, MD, MBA
Department of Psychiatry
University of Miami School of Medicine
Miami, FL

TEJAL PARIKH, MD
Private Practice
Tucson, AZ

DOUGLAS S. PARKS, MD
Associate Professor
Family Practice Residency Program at Cheyenne
University of Wyoming
Cheyenne, WY

JOHN E. PERCHALSKI, MD, FAAFP
Private Practice
Van Wert, OH

BENITO B. PEREZ, MD
St. Francis Family Practice Residency Program
Lincolnwood, IL

JOHN R. PERSON, MD
Fallon Clinic
Worcester, MA

CLAUDIA A. PETERS, MD
Queen's Student Health Service
Queen's University
Kingston, Ontario, CANADA

DANA W. PETERSON, MD
Southwest Medical Associates
Albuquerque, NM

ELSIRA M. PINA, DO
Assistant Professor of Medicine
Pulmonary and Critical Care Medicine
University of Cincinnati Medical Center
Cincinnati, OH

GREGORY A. POLAND, MD
Professor
Department of Internal Medicine, Mayo Vaccine Research Group
The Mayo Clinic and Foundation
Rochester, MN

DAVID A. POPE, MD
Private Practice
Janesville, MN

DOUG POST, PHD
Assistant Professor
Rardin Family Practice Center
Columbus, OH

WILLIAM A. PRIMACK, MD
Professor of Pediatrics
University of Massachusetts Medical Center
Fallon Clinic
Auburn, MA

RONALD E PUST, MD
Director, Predoctoral Program
Department of Family and Community Medicine
University of Arizona
Tucson, AZ

JAMES K. RADIKE, MD
Infectious Disease Consultant
Stillwater, OK

KATHRYN REILLY, MD, MPH
Family Practice Residency Program
University of Oklahoma
Oklahoma City, OK

Contributing Authors

ANNE C. REITZ, MD
Resident, Family Practice
St. Francis Hospital of Evanston
Evanston, IL

RICK RICER, MD
Department of Family Medicine
University of Cincinnati College of Medicine
Cincinnati, OH

J. RANDALL RICHARD, MD
Professor of Clinical Family Medicine, Northeastern Ohio Universities
    College of Medicine
Associate Residency Director, Barberton Citizens Hospital
Barberton, OH

CHARLES W. RICKETSON, MD, FRCPC
Victoria General Hospital
Victoria, British Columbia   CANADA

MICHEL E. RIVLIN, MD
Department of Obstetrics & Gynecology
University of Mississippi Medical Center
Jackson, MS

TIMOTHY ROBINSON, DO
Private Practice
Bayside, NY

VANCE D. RODGERS, MD
Director, Inflammatory Bowel Disease Center
Scripps Clinic & Research Foundation
La Jolla, CA

DUANE C. ROE, MD
Associate Professor of Medicine
Northeastern Ohio Universities College of Medicine
Akron, OH

LEWIS C. ROSE, MD
Director, Family Health Center
Department of Family Practice
University of Texas Health Sciences Center at San Antonio
San Antonio, TX

BRUCE M. ROTHSCHILD, MD
Professor, Northeastern Ohio Universities College of Medicine
Director, Arthritis Center of Northeast Ohio
Youngstown, OH

JAMES H. RUDICK, MD, FACP
Assistant Professor of Internal Medicine
Northeastern Ohio Universities College of Medicine
Canton, OH

BARRY S. RUSSMAN, MD
Professor, Pediatrics and Neurology
Oregon Health Science University
Shriner Hospital for Children
Portland, OR

GLENN RUSSO, MD
Department of Dermatology
Tulane University Medical Center
New Orleans, LA

GREGORY W. RUTECKI, MD
Program Director Internal Medicine Residency
Associate Professor of Medicine
Evanston-Northwestern Healthcare
Northwestern University
Evanston, IL

RICHARD E. SAMPLINER, MD
Professor of Medicine
Chief of Gastroenterology Section
University of Arizona College of Medicine
Tucson, AZ

ARTHUR SANDERS, MD
Professor, Section of Emergency Medicine
Department of Surgery
University of Arizona College of Medicine
Tucson, AZ

DANIEL T. SCHELBLE, MD, FACEP
Chairman, Department of Emergency Medicine
Akron General Medical Center
Akron, OH

F. DAVID SCHNEIDER, MD, MSPH
Associate Professor, Department of Family Practice
Director of Medical Student Education
University of Texas Health Science Center at San Antonio
San Antonio, TX

ROBERT M. SCHULTZ, MD
Director, Pediatric Endocrinology
Scottish Rite Children's Medical Center
Atlanta, GA

WAYNE H. SCHWESINGER, MD
Head, Section of General Surgery
Department of Surgery
The University of Texas Health Science Center at San Antonio
San Antonio, TX

E. NAN SCOTT, PHD
Associate Professor
University of Oklahoma Health Sciences Center & Veterans
    Administration Medical Center
Oklahoma City, OK

ROBERT H. SCOTT, MD
Faculty
Family Practice Residency
Swedish Medical Center
Seattle, WA

DAVID P. SEALY, MD
Director, Sports Medicine
Associate Professor & Director, Resident Education
Self Memorial Hospital Family Medicine Residency
Greenwood, SC

WILLIAM V. SHARP, MD
Private Practice - Retired
Vero Beach, FL

MARK M. SHELTON, MD
Director, Infectious Diseases
Cook Children's Medical Center
Fort Worth, TX

ALBERT T. SHIU, MD, FACOG
Professor of Clinical Obstetrics and Gynecology
Director of Obstetrics and Gynecology Residency Program
Northeastern Ohio Universities College of Medicine
St. Elizabeth Health Center
Youngstown, OH

JOSEPH SHRUM, MD
Associate Professor of Dermatology
Department of Dermatology
Tulane University Medical Center
New Orleans, LA

GARY J. SILKO, MD
Director, Family Practice Residency Program
Saint Vincent Health Center
Erie, PA

RICHARD J. SIMENSEN, PHD
Research Scientist
Greenwood Genetic Center
Greenwood, SC

VIOLET SIWIK, MD
Medical Director
Department of Family and Community Medicine
University of Arizona
Tucson, AZ

LEONARD N. SLATER, MD
Professor of Medicine, Infectious Diseases Section
University of Oklahoma Health Sciences Center
& Veterans Affairs Medical Center
Oklahoma City, OK

ARTHUR R. SLAUGHTER, MD
Associate Director, Family Practice Education
Carilion Family Practice Residency Program
Roanoke, VA

ROBERT J. SLIMAN, MD
Associate Professor
Department of Internal Medicine
Northeastern Ohio Universities College of Medicine
Canton, OH

W. PAUL SLOMIANY, MD
Assistant Director
Family Practice Residency Program
Washington Hospital
Washington, PA

H. GRATIN SMITH, MD, FAAP
Director of Pediatric Education
Family Practice Residency Program
Self Memorial Hospital
Greenwood, SC

JAY W. SMITH, MD
Dean for Academic Affairs
University of Arizona College of Medicine
Tucson, AZ

MICHAEL J. SMITH, MD
Assistant Professor of Orthopedic Surgery
Northeastern Ohio Universities College of Medicine
Akron, OH

STANLEY G. SMITH, MA, MB, FCFPC
Centre Director
Southwest Middlesex Health Centre
Mt. Brydges, Ontario   CANADA

JOHN C. SMULIAN, MD, MPH
Assistant Professor of Obstetrics, Gynecology, and Reproductive
   Sciences
UMDNJ-Robert Wood Johnson Medical School
Saint Peter's University Hospital
New Brunswick, NJ

NANCY SNAPP, MD, MPH
Seattle, WA

GREGORY SNYDER, MD
Department of Family Medicine
State University of New York at Buffalo
Buffalo, NY

BECK SODERBERG, MD
Department of Family & Community Medicine
Lancaster General Hospital
Morgan hill, CA

VERA Y. SOONG, MD
Chairperson
Department of Dermatology
Lloyd Noland Hospital
Fairfield, AL

JOHN SPANGLER, MD, MPH
Assistant Professor
Department of Family and Community Medicine
Wake Forest University Baptist Medical Center School of Medicine
Winston-Salem, NC

NICHOLAS J. SPIRTOS, DO
Associate Professor
Director, Northeastern Ohio Fertility Center
Northeastern Ohio Universities College of Medicine & Summa Health
   System
Akron, OH

JEFFREY A. STEARNS, MD
Associate Professor
Family Medicine
University of Illinois College of Medicine
Rockford, IL

THOMAS R. STRIGLE, MD
Private Practice
Findlay Surgical Associates
Findlay, OH

DAVID H. STUBBS, MD, FACS
Department of Surgery Education
Iowa Methodist Medical Center
Des Moines, IA

GREGG W. SUITS, MD
Private Practice
Hillsboro, OR

SANDRA M. SULIK, MD
Assistant Professor of Family Medicine
St. Joseph's Family Practice Residency
SUNY Health Science Center
East Syracuse, NY

JACK L. SUMMERS, MD, PHD
Professor, Urology
Northeastern Ohio Universities College of Medicine
Chairman, Urology, Summa Health Systems
Akron, OH

GEOFFREY R. SWAIN, MD
Assistant Professor
Department of Family and Community Medicine
Medical College of Wisconsin
Associate Medical Director, City of Milwaukee Health Department
Milwaukee, WI

DAVID H. THOM, MD, PHD
Assistant Professor, Department of Medicine
Division of Family and Community MedicineStanford University School
   of Medicine
Palo Alto, CA

WILLIAM L. TOFFLER, MD
Professor
Department of Family Medicine
Oregon Health Sciences University
Portland, OR

Contributing Authors

MOSHE S. TOREM, MD, FAPA
Professor, Department of Psychiatry
Northeastern Ohio Universities College of Medicine
Chairman, Department of Psychiatry & Behavioral Sciences
Akron General Medical Center
Akron, OH

PETER P. TOTH, MD, PHD
Private Practice
Sullivan Clinic
Sarah Bush Lincoln Health System
Sullivan, IL

SHELDON M. TRAEGER, MD
Head, Intensive Care Service, Department of Internal Medicine
Summa Hospital System
Northeastern Ohio Universities College of Medicine
Akron, OH

MICHAEL TUTT
Assistant Clinical Professor
Department of Internal Medicine
Section of Rheumatology
University of Arizona College of Medicine
Tucson, AZ

FRANCISCO G. VALENCIA, MD
Section of Orthopedic Surgery
University of Arizona College of Medicine
Tucson, AZ

C. VAN DEVERE, MD
Associate Professor of Psychiatry
Northeastern Ohio Universities College of Medicine
Director, Pediatric Psychiatry at Children's Hospital Medical Center of
   Akron
Akron, OH

MICHAEL M. VAN NESS, MD
Department of Internal Medicine
Aultman Hospital
Canton, OH

BRUCE T. VANDERHOFF, MD
Associate Director
Grant Family Practice Residency
Columbus, OH

LISA VANTREASE, MD
Grant Family Practice Residency
Columbus, OH

V. VASUDEVIAH, BSC, MBBS
Consultant
Malleswaram, Bangalore   INDIA

RICHARD VIKEN, MD
Chairman, Department of Family Practice
The University of Texas Health Center at Tyler
Tyler, TX

CHRIS VINCENT, MD
Faculty
Family Practice Residency
Swedish Family Medicine
Seattle, WA

KENTON VOORHEES, MD
Assistant Clinical Professor
Medical Director Swedish Family Medicine Residency
Littleton, CO

KIMBERLE VORE, MD
Clinical Instructor
Washington Hospital
Washington, PA

GENE W. VOSKUHL, MD
Infectious Disease Section
University of Oklahoma Health Sciences Center
Oklahoma City, OK

NASIR WAHEED, MD
Division of Child Neurology
Department of Neurology and Pediatrics
Medical University of South Carolina
Charleston, SC

STANLEY WALLACH, MD
Department of Medicine, American College of Nutrition
Endocrine Division and Osteoporosis Center
Hospital for Joint Diseases/Orthopedic Institute
New York, NY

BRIDGET T. WALSH, DO
Department of Rheumatology
University of Arizona College of Medicine
Tucson, AZ

AMY Y. WANG, MD
Resident, Family Practice
St. Francis Hospital of Evanston
Evanston, IL

CHATRCHAI WATANAKUNAKORN, MD, FACP, FCCP
Professor of Internal Medicine
Northeastern Ohio Universities College of Medicine
Director, Infectious Disease Section, St. Elizabeth Health Center
Youngstown, OH

JOHN R. WATERSON, MD, PHD
Associate Professor of Pediatrics
Northeastern Ohio Universities College of Medicine
Akron, OH

KURT J. WEGNER, MD
Professor of Pediatrics
Neonatologist, Geneticist and Pediatric Consultant
Northeastern Ohio Universities College of Medicine
Tod Children's Hospital
Youngstown, OH

MARTIN E. WEINAND, MD
Associate Professor of Surgery
Division of Neurosurgery
University of Arizona College of Medicine
Tucson, AZ

BARRY D. WEISS, MD
Department of Family and Community Medicine
University of Arizona College of Medicine
Tucson, AZ

JEFFREY R. WELKO, MD
Director, Hyperbaric Oxygen Unit
Akron General Medical Center
Akron, OH

ROBERT L. WESTON, MD
Associate Clinical Professor, Division of International Health & Cross
   Cultural Medicine at UC, San Diego, School of Medicine
President, International Healthcare Division
International SOS Assistance, Inc.
Trevose, PA

GARY B. WILLIAMS, MD
Associate Professor of Surgery
Northeastern Ohio Universities College of Medicine
Akron, OH

FREMONT P. WIRTH, MD, FACS
Neurological Institute of Savannah
Savannah, GA

CHRISTOPHER M. WISE, MD
W. Robert Irby Associate Professor Medicine
Division of Rheumatology, Allergy & Immunology
Medical College of Virginia/Virginia Commonwealth University
Richmond, VA

JEFFREY D. WOLFREY, MD
Program Director, Family Practice Residency Program
Good Samaritan Hospital
Phoenix, AZ

DOUGLAS C. WOOLLEY, MD
Associate Professor
Family and Community Medicine
Kansas University School of Medicine - Wichita
Wichita, KS

MARK ERIC WORSHTIL, MD
Assistant Director
Family Practice Residency Program
Washington Hospital
Washington, PA

FRANCES WU, MD
Assistant Director
Somerset Family Practice Residency Program
Somerville, NJ

ALAYNE YATES, MD
Director, Division of Child Adolescent Psychiatry
John A. Burns School of Medicine
Kapiolani Medical Center
Honolulu, HI

WILLIAM F. YOUNG, JR., MD
Professor of Medicine, Division of Hypertension, Endocrinology &
  Metabolism
Mayo Clinic and Foundation
Rochester, MN

MICHAEL YOUTSEY, MD
Senior Internal Medicine Resident
Evanston Northwestern Healthcare
Evanston, IL

RICHARD KENT ZIMMERMAN, MD, MPH
Associate Professor, Departments of Family Medicine & Clinical
  Epidemiology & Health Services Administration
University of Pittsburgh
Pittsburgh, PA

CONTENTS

EXPANDED TOPICS

Contents

Contents

SHORT TOPICS

Contents

Contents

SKIN/EXOCRINE

Contents

NERVOUS

Contents

PULMONARY

Contents

CARDIOVASCULAR

Contents

ENDOCRINE/METABOLIC

Contents

▮ RENAL/UROLOGIC

HEMIC/LYMPHATIC/IMMUNOLOGIC

Contents

GASTROINTESTINAL

Contents

■ MUSCULOSKELETAL

REPRODUCTIVE

Contents

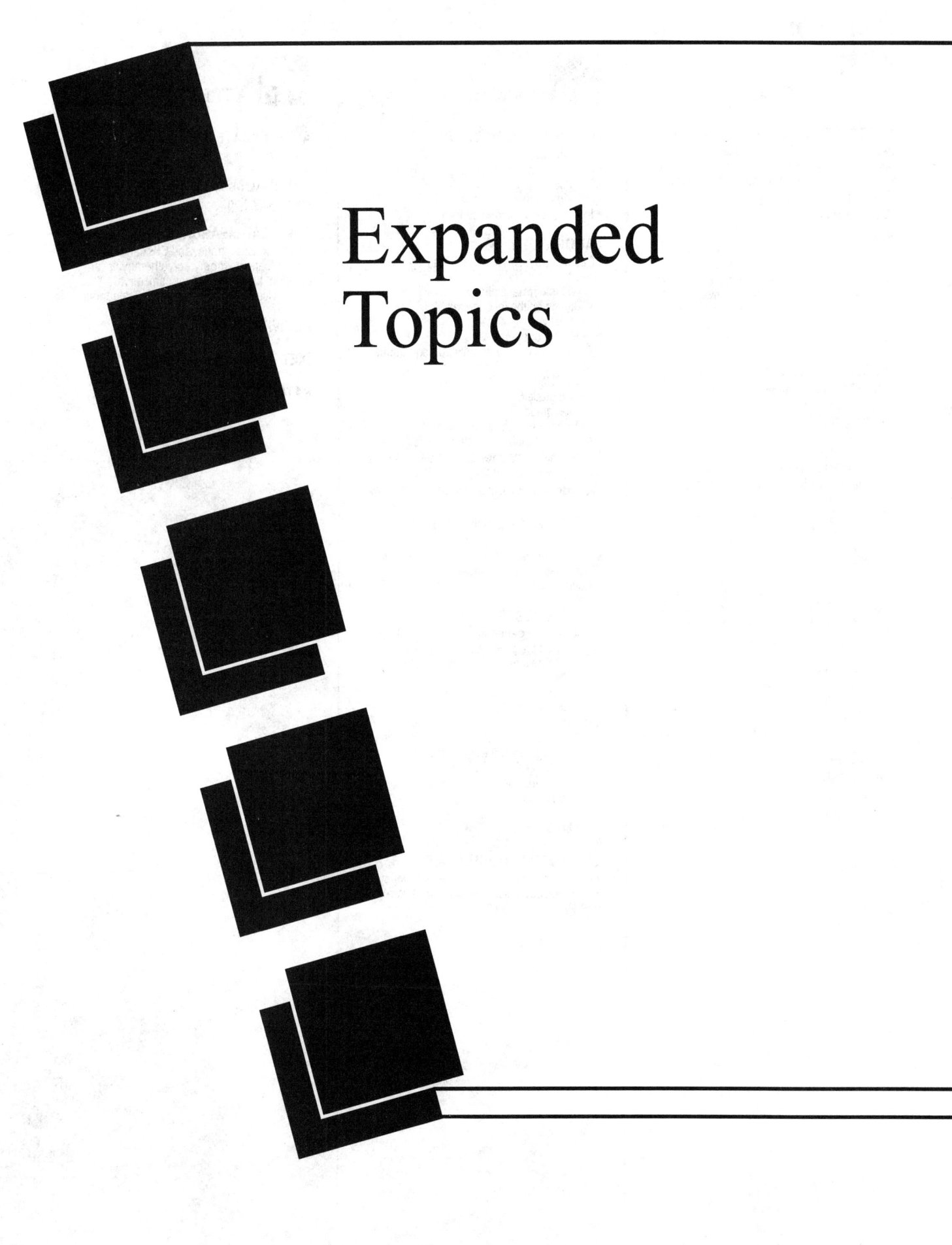

Expanded Topics

Abnormal Pap smear

BASICS

DESCRIPTION The abnormal Pap smear can range from benign cellular changes to suggestion of invasive cancer. The procedure is meant as a screen for cervical pathology.
System(s) affected: Reproductive
Genetics: N/A
Incidence/Prevalence in USA: SIL (squamous intraepithelial lesion) low grade ranges from 10-50% of all Pap smears. SIL High grade and invasive cancer is present on 4% of all Pap smears. Other reactive, reparative and ASCUS (atypical squamous cells of undeterminant significance) results are difficult to assess because of the lack of reporting mechanisms.
Predominant age: Can range from when a female becomes sexually active into the geriatric age group
Predominant sex: Female

SIGNS AND SYMPTOMS
- Frequently there are no symptoms
- Occasionally with have external genital HPV lesions
- Occasionally will have vaginal discharge related to STDs
- Rarely can have vaginal bleeding related to a malignant lesion

CAUSES Strong link to HPV infections virus types 6, 11, 16, 18, 31, 33 and 35. Viral types 16 and 18 are considered high risk viruses for cervical disease.

RISK FACTORS
- Multiple sexual partners
- Cigarette smoking
- Early age of intercourse
- Intercourse with a high risk male partner
- HPV infection
- Human immunodeficiency virus infection
- Immunosuppression

DIAGNOSIS

DIFFERENTIAL DIAGNOSIS
- Cervical SIL
- Acute or chronic cervicitis
- Vaginitis
- HPV infection
- Invasive cervical malignancy

LABORATORY
- Bethesda System for Reporting Pap Smear Results
  ◊ Within normal limits
  ◊ Benign epithelial changes
    - Infective
    - Reactive/reparative
  ◊ Epithelial cell abnormalities - squamous cells
    - ASCUS
    - Low grade SIL
    - High grade SIL
    - Squamous cell carcinoma
  ◊ Other glandular cell abnormalities
Drugs that may alter lab results: Surgical lubricant such as KY jelly
Disorders that may alter lab results: N/A

PATHOLOGICAL FINDINGS
- Atypical squamous or columnar cells
- Coarse nuclear material
- Increases nuclear diameter
- Koilocytosis

SPECIAL TESTS
- Colposcopy - generally recommended when any of these are present:
  ◊ Initial Pap smear shows high grade SIL or worse
  ◊ Two Pap smears at least 2 months apart, show ASCUS/CIN I or worse, and any intercurrent infection has been treated
  ◊ Any abnormal or suspicious lesions on the cervix or vagina seen with the naked eye
  ◊ Atypical endocervical cells
  ◊ ASCUS in which the pathologist suggests possible premalignant changes

IMAGING N/A

DIAGNOSTIC PROCEDURES
- Colposcopy with visually directed biopsy
- Loop electrosurgical excision procedure (LEEP)
- Cone biopsy
- Cervicography

TREATMENT

APPROPRIATE HEALTH CARE
Outpatient

GENERAL MEASURES Office evaluation and observation

SURGICAL MEASURES
- SIL Low, High grade, and CIS can be treated with outpatient surgery - cryotherapy, laser ablation, LEEP/LLETZ, or conization
- If cervical malignancy, see separate topic

ACTIVITY N/A

DIET No restrictions

PATIENT EDUCATION N/A

MEDICATIONS

DRUG(S) OF CHOICE
- Infective/reactive Pap smear
  ◊ Metronidazole 250 mg tid x 7 days
- Condyloma acuminata
  ◊ Cryotherapy
  ◊ Podophyllin
  ◊ Trichloroacetic acid (TCA)

Contraindications: N/A
Precautions: N/A
Significant possible interactions: N/A

ALTERNATIVE DRUGS N/A

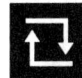 **FOLLOWUP**

PATIENT MONITORING
- Infective, reactive, reparative or ASCUS changes need repeat Pap smear in 4-6 months. If it persists, needs colposcopy. If it resolves, repeat Pap smear in 6 months and if it reoccurs follow-up with colposcopy.
- SIL low or high grade, invasive squamous or adenocarcinoma - colposcopy

PREVENTION/AVOIDANCE
- Delay first intercourse to age 20
- Monogamous relationship for both partners
- Smoking cessation
- Routine Pap smears
- Use barrier methods of birth control if nonmonogamous relationship

POSSIBLE COMPLICATIONS
- Minor abnormalities on Pap smears can mask more advanced lesions
- High grade SIL can progress to invasive cancer

EXPECTED COURSE/PROGNOSIS
- Generally excellent
- Less than half of the persistent infective, reactive, reparative or ASCUS Pap smears will have more advanced lesions
- Only a small percentage of SIL low grade will progress to more advanced lesion
- Lesions discovered early are very amenable to treatment with excellent results and few recurrences

 MISCELLANEOUS

ASSOCIATED CONDITIONS N/A

AGE-RELATED FACTORS
Pediatric: Very rare
Geriatric: Less frequent except in the unscreened population
Others: Abnormal Pap smears can occur at any age. The more advanced the abnormality, the more likely the patient is 25-45 years of age.

PREGNANCY SIL lesions can progress during pregnancy

SYNONYMS N/A

ICD-9-CM
795.0 Abnormal Cervical Pap smear
622.1 SIL low or High grade

SEE ALSO
- Condyloma acuminata
- Cervical dysplasia
- Cervical malignancy
- Trichomoniasis
- Vulvovaginitis, bacterial

OTHER NOTES N/A

ABBREVIATIONS
- HPV - human papilloma virus
- ASCUS - atypical squamous cells of undeterminant significance
- SIL - squamous intraepithelial lesion
- LEEP - loop electrosurgical excision procedure
- CIS - carcinoma in siitu
- LLETZ - large loop excision of transition zone

REFERENCES
- Lieu D. The Papanicolaou smear: its value and limitations. J Fam Pract 1996;42:391-99
- Gulde to Clinical Preventive Services: Report of the US Preventive Services Task Force, 2nd ed. Baltimore: Williams and Wilkins, 1996:105-17
- American College of Obstetricians and Gynecologists. Recommendations on frequency of Pap test screening. Committee opinion no. 152. Washington, DC: ACOG, 1995
- Shepherd JC, Fried RA. Preventing cervical cancer: the role of the Bethesda system. Am Fam Physician 1995;51:434-40
- The Bethesda System for reporting cervical/vaginal cytologic diagnoses: revised after the second National Cancer Institute Workshop, April 29-30, 1991. Acta Cytol 1993;37:115-24
Illustrations: N/A
Internet references: http://www.5mcc.com

Author(s)
Karl E. Miller, MD

Abortion, spontaneous

BASICS

DESCRIPTION Abortion is the separation of products of conception from the uterus prior to the potential for fetal survival outside the uterus. Gestationally, the point at which potential fetal viability exists has been the subject of much legal and scientific debate, and definitions vary from state to state; however, a "potentially viable" fetus generally weighs at least 500 grams and/or has a gestational age over 20 weeks.
• Spontaneous abortion: refers to expulsion of all (complete abortion) or part (incomplete abortion) of the products of conception from the uterus prior to the 20th completed week of gestation. The placenta, either in whole or in part, can be retained and leads to continuing vaginal bleeding (sometimes profuse). Abortion is "threatened" when vaginal bleeding occurs early in pregnancy, with or without uterine contractions, but without dilatation of the cervix, rupture of the membranes, or expulsion of products of conception. Cervical dilation, rupture of membranes or expulsion of products in the presence of vaginal bleeding portends "inevitable abortion." Differentiation between threatened and inevitable abortion is desirable since management differs.
• Missed abortion: Failed first trimester pregnancy but without the usual signs and symptoms such as bleeding or cramping. Term blighted ovum replaced with anembryonic gestation. Ultrasound findings of "empty sac."
• Induced abortion: refers to the evacuation of uterine contents/products of conception by either medical or surgical methodology
• Infected abortion: infection involving the products of conception and the maternal reproductive organs
• Septic abortion: dissemination of bacteria (and/or their toxins) into the maternal circulatory and organ system
• Habitual spontaneous abortion: three or more consecutive spontaneous abortions. Risk of another spontaneous abortion is approximately 25-30% with 70% rate of successful pregnancy in subsequent pregnancy.
System(s) affected: Reproductive, Endocrine/Metabolic
Genetics: Approximately 2/3 of first trimester spontaneous abortions have significant chromosomal anomalies with 1/2 of these being autosomal trisomies and the remainder being triploidy, tetraploidy, or 45X momosomies
Incidence/Prevalence in USA:
• Approximately 10-15% of all clinically recognized pregnancies end in spontaneous abortion
• Biochemical pregnancy manifests itself by the presence of ß-HCG in the blood 7-10 days after conception. When both clinical and biochemical pregnancies are considered, more than 50% of conceptions are spontaneous aborted.
Predominant age: Increases with advancing age, especially after 35 years of age. At age 40, the loss rate is 2 times that of age 20.
Predominant sex: Female only

SIGNS AND SYMPTOMS
• In a previously diagnosed intrauterine pregnancy
  ◊ Vaginal bleeding
  ◊ Uterine cramping
  ◊ Cervical dilation
  ◊ Ruptured membranes
  ◊ Passage of non-viable products of conception

CAUSES See Risk Factors

RISK FACTORS
• Chromosomal abnormalities
• Luteal phase defect
• Leiomyomas
• Incompetent cervix
• Infections
• Antifetal antibodies
• Autoimmune disease - phospholipid syndrome
• Alloimmune disease (shared paternal antigens)
• Drugs, chemicals, noxious agents (alcohol, smoking, caffeine)
• X-irradiation
• Contraceptive IUD

DIAGNOSIS

DIFFERENTIAL DIAGNOSIS
• Ectopic pregnancy: a potentially life-threatening complication, difficult to distinguish from threatened abortion. Transvaginal ultrasonography can identify intrauterine gestational sacs at 32 days of gestation (at serum HCG levels of 1500-2000 IU). The absence of transvaginal ultrasound evidence of an intrauterine gestation with serum HCG over 2000 IU/L should be considered an ectopic pregnancy until proven otherwise.
• Cervical polyps, neoplasias, and/or inflammatory conditions can cause vaginal bleeding. This bleeding is not usually associated with pain/cramping and is apparent on speculum exam.
• Hydatidiform mole pregnancy usually ends in abortion prior to the 20th week of pregnancy. Bloody discharge prior to abortion is common. An intrauterine grape-like appearing mass on the ultrasound is diagnostic (a "snow storm" appearance). Human chorionic gonadotropin (HCG) is often high.
• Membranous dysmenorrhea: characterized by bleeding, cramps and passage of endometrial casts can mimic spontaneous abortion. HCG is negative.
• HCG secreting ovarian tumor

LABORATORY
• Cultures - gonorrhea and chlamydia
• CBC
• Rh type
• Human chorionic gonadotropin (HCG)
• Serial ß-HCG measurements can assess viability of the pregnancy. Normal gestations have an approximate 67% increase over 2-day interval. Abnormal gestations do not rise appropriately, plateau, or decrease in level before the eighth week of gestation.
Drugs that may alter lab results: N/A

Disorders that may alter lab results: N/A

PATHOLOGICAL FINDINGS Products of conception, placental villi

SPECIAL TESTS Progesterone levels > 25 ng/mL are consistent with normal intrauterine pregnancy and are rarely seen in ectopic and/or non-viable pregnancy. A progesterone of < 5 ng/mL is an indicator of a nonviable intrauterine gestation or an ectopic pregnancy.

IMAGING
• Ultrasound examination for fetal viability and to rule out ectopic pregnancy
• Ultrasound imaging can be sensitive enough to confirm an intrauterine pregnancy in the fourth or fifth gestational week from last menstrual period

DIAGNOSTIC PROCEDURES
• Viable intrauterine pregnancy with fetal cardiac activity detected between 5-8 weeks from last menstrual period on transvaginal ultrasound
• Transvaginal ultrasound criteria for nonviable intrauterine gestation include:
  ◊ 5 mm fetal pole without cardiac activity, or
  ◊ 16 mm gestational sac without a fetal pole
• Fetal heart tones can be auscultated with doppler starting between 10-12 weeks gestation from last menstrual period for a viable pregnancy
• Consider a diagnosis of spontaneous abortion in a woman, of childbearing age, presenting with abnormal vaginal bleeding

TREATMENT

APPROPRIATE HEALTH CARE
Outpatient or inpatient, depending on severity of symptoms (bleeding or pain)

GENERAL MEASURES
• Explore any first trimester vaginal bleeding
• Serial quantitative ß-HCG determination and progesterone assay
• Transvaginal ultrasonography

SURGICAL MEASURES
• Inevitable or incomplete abortion: Dilatation and curettage (D&C) (usually suction)
• When completeness of an abortion is uncertain, a D&C for retained products should be performed

ACTIVITY If appropriate, bed rest; probably no effect on eventual outcome

DIET No special diet

PATIENT EDUCATION American College of Obstetricians & Gynecologists, 409 12th St., SW, Washington, DC 20090-6290 (800)762-2264, pamphlet #AP090

MEDICATIONS

DRUG(S) OF CHOICE
- Bleeding following uncomplicated D&C or spontaneous abortion usually controlled by:
  - ◊ Carboprost (Hemabate) 250 mcg IM
  - ◊ Oxytocin (Pitocin) 10 units IM, or IV
  - ◊ Methylergonovine (Methergine) 0.2 mg IM
- Analgesics if needed
- Rho(D) immune globulin if mother is Rh negative
- Progesterone, if deficiency confirmed prior to pregnancy

Contraindications: None

Precautions: Do not give methylergonovine IV. Refer to manufacturer's literature.

Significant possible interactions: Refer to manufacturer's literature

ALTERNATIVE DRUGS N/A

FOLLOWUP

PATIENT MONITORING
- Identification of products of conception within material expelled from the uterus or D&C specimen
- If abortion is complete, observe the patient for further bleeding
- Complete abortion usually indicated by decreased bleeding, closed cervix, intact or complete products of conception passed, and ultrasound findings of empty uterus and endometrial stripe. Follow HCG's weekly to zero to confirm complete evacuation of products of conception. Can take 2 weeks. If levels plateau, suspect retained products of conception or ectopic pregnancy.

PREVENTION/AVOIDANCE
- Any vaginal bleeding in intrauterine pregnancy is abnormal and should be considered a "threatened" abortion. In reality, vaginal bleeding in early pregnancy is common (occurring in up to 1/3 of pregnancies) and often the bleeding source eludes diagnosis.
- In habitual abortion, the abortus should be sent for karyotyping. Explore other causes of habitual abortion with the couple to determine the best therapy.
- Special care and attention for the patient who has a subsequent pregnancy

POSSIBLE COMPLICATIONS
- Complications of D&C include uterine perforation, infection and bleeding
- Possibly retained products of conception
- Depression and feelings of guilt (patient may need education and reassurance that she did not cause the miscarriage)

EXPECTED COURSE/PROGNOSIS
- If bleeding ceases, prognosis is excellent.
- Habitual abortion: prognosis is dependent on etiology. After a 2 consecutive abortions, most couples want some investigation of the problem. After 3 spontaneous abortions, evaluation is usually indicated. Prognosis is still excellent with up to 70% rate of success with subsequent pregnancy.

MISCELLANEOUS

ASSOCIATED CONDITIONS N/A

AGE-RELATED FACTORS
Pediatric: N/A
Geriatric: N/A
Others: N/A

PREGNANCY Confined to pregnancy

SYNONYMS
- Miscarriage
- Habitual abortion
- Recurrent abortion

ICD-9-CM
632 Missed abortion
629.9 Habitual abortion
634.92 Spontaneous abortion-complete
634.91 Spontaneous abortion-incomplete
640.03 Threatened abortion

SEE ALSO
- Ectopic pregnancy

OTHER NOTES N/A

ABBREVIATIONS N/A

REFERENCES
- Rempen A: Diagnosis and Viability of Early Pregnancy with Vaginal Sonography. J Ultras Med 1990; 9:711-716
- Daily CA, et al: The prognostic value of serum progesterone and quantitative ß-Human Chorionic Gonadotropin in early human pregnancy. Am J Obstet Gynecol 1994;171:380-384
- Ohno M, et al: A Cytogenic study of spontaneous abortion with direct analysis of chorionic villi. Obstet Gynecol 1991;77(3):394-398
- Benne H, Michael J: Abortion. In: Hacker & Moore (eds): Essentials of Obstetrics and Gynecology. 3rd ed. Philadelphia, WB Saunders Co., 1998
- Palmieri A, Moore G, et al: Ectopic pregnancy. In: Hacker & Moore (eds): Essentials of Obstetrics and Gynecology. 3rd ed. Philadelphia, WB Saunders Co., 1998
- Simpson JL: Fetal wastage. In: Gabbe S, Nieby J, et al (eds): Obstetrics: Normal & Problem Pregnancies. 3rd ed. New York, Churchill Livingstone, 1996
Illustrations: N/A
Internet references: http://www.5mcc.com

Author(s)
Wendy Humphrey, MD

Abruptio placentae

BASICS

DESCRIPTION Premature separation of otherwise normally implanted placenta. Sher's grades:
1: minimal or no bleeding; detected as retroplacental clot after delivery of viable fetus.
2: viable fetus with bleeding and tender irritable uterus.
3: type A with dead fetus and no coagulopathy; type B with dead fetus and coagulopathy (about 30% of grade 3's).
System(s) affected: Reproductive, Cardiovascular
Genetics: N/A
Incidence/Prevalence in USA:
• 1% of all deliveries
• 15% if one prior episode
• 25% if ≥ 2 prior episodes
Predominant age: All childbearing ages
Predominant sex: Female only

SIGNS AND SYMPTOMS
• Second or third trimester vaginal bleeding greater than one pad or tampon per hour
• Back pain, abdominal pain
• Uterine tenderness, hypertonia, or high frequency contractions
• Blood loss may be concealed; clinical signs of shock may occur with little vaginal bleeding
• Since blood volumes increase in pregnancy, volume lost may exceed 30% before signs of shock or hypovolemia. Vital signs may be preserved even with significant loss.
• Fetal distress or demise
• Idiopathic preterm labor with or without fetal distress

CAUSES
• Cocaine use and abuse
• Trauma of variable amounts; especially blunt abdominal trauma in which external signs of trauma may be incongruent with fetal injury (motor vehicle accidents or domestic violence)
• Sudden decompression of over-distended uterus as in hydramnios or twin gestation

RISK FACTORS
• Prior abruption
• Maternal smoking
• Severe small for gestational age birth
• Alcohol abuse
• Hypertension: pregnancy-induced and chronic
• Increased risk if hypertensive and parity > 3
• Preterm rupture of membranes, especially if bleeding occurs during observation interval
• Vaginal bleeding before spontaneous rupture of membranes

DIAGNOSIS

DIFFERENTIAL DIAGNOSIS Uterine rupture, placenta previa, vasa previa, marked bloody show, cervical and vaginal causes (e.g., chlamydia or gonorrhea with bloody, friable cervix), masses, other painful conditions (e.g., appendicitis, pyelonephritis), and labor.

LABORATORY
• Blood type, Rh, Coombs
• CBC with platelet count
• Prothrombin time (PT) , partial thromboplastin time (PTT), fibrinogen levels
• Cross match at least three units
Drugs that may alter lab results:
• Those affecting clotting parameters
• RhoD immune globulin less than 12 weeks prior may affect antibody test
Disorders that may alter lab results:
• Fibrinogen levels climb to 350-550 mg/dl (3.5-5.5 g/L) in third trimester and must fall to 100-150 mg/dl (1.0-1.5 g/L) before PTT will rise
• Fibrin split or degradation products are elevated in pregnancy so not very helpful in assessing disseminated intravascular coagulation (DIC)

PATHOLOGICAL FINDINGS
• Normocytic normochromic anemia with acute bleeding
• Elevated PT, PTT, fibrinogen levels below 100-150 mg/dl (1.0-1.5 g/L), platelets 20,000-50,000 if DIC active
• Positive Kleihauer-Betke reaction if fetal-maternal transfusion has occurred
• Positive antibody if RhoD isosensitization has occurred

SPECIAL TESTS
• Kleihauer-Betke for fetal-maternal transfusion
• Bedside clot test with red top tube of maternal blood with poor or non-clotting blood after 7-10 minutes indicating coagulopathy
• Apt test for fetal blood origin: mix vaginal blood with small amount tap water to cause hemolysis, centrifuge several minutes, mix pink hemoglobin containing supernatant with 1 cc 1% sodium hydroxide (NaOH) for each 5 cc supernatant, reading color in two minutes with fetal Hgb staying pink and adult turning yellow-brown
• Wright stain vaginal blood, observe for nucleated RBC's - usually of fetal origin
• Lecithin/sphingomyelin (L/S) ratio if delay of delivery is an option and length of pregnancy is preterm

IMAGING Although ultrasound may show sonolucent retroplacental clot, rounded placenta margin or thickened placenta, it is often not definitive - especially with posterior placement or mild abruption

DIAGNOSTIC PROCEDURES External uterine monitoring often shows elevated baseline pressure and frequent low amplitude contractions

TREATMENT

APPROPRIATE HEALTH CARE
Hospitalize until stable

GENERAL MEASURES
• History and physical exam with past medical history, allergies, prior ultrasounds this gestation, and time of last meal
• In general, severe abruption best managed by delivery of fetus
• Sher's grade 1 - usual labor protocol
• Sher's grade 2 - rapid delivery most often by cesarean section
• Sher's grade 3 - vaginal delivery preferable if mother stable
• In trauma monitor inpatient at least 4 hours for evidence of fetal insult, abruption, fetal-maternal transfusion
• Early aggressive restoration of maternal physiology to protect fetus and maternal organs from hypoperfusion/DIC
• Stabilize vitals, keep Hct >30, urine output >30 cc/hr
• Bedrest with external fetal and labor monitoring, if fetus is viable
• Large bore 16-18 gauge IV crystalloid infusion, central line placement only after coagulation status has been assessed
• Transfusions of whole blood may be necessary
• Follow hemoglobin/hematocrit (H/H) and coagulation status every 1-2 hours
• Place intrauterine pressure catheter (IUC) since fetal risk climbs with elevated pressure
• Role of amniotomy to prevent amniotic fluid embolism is debatable but will speed delivery
• Positioning on left side may enhance venous return and cardiac output
• Oxygen for all patients
• If trauma without compromise after observation or small abruption and preterm may observe outpatient encouraging reduction of risk factors

SURGICAL MEASURES May need cesarean section after maternal stabilization if fetus viable and situation urgent

ACTIVITY Bedrest until status defined

DIET NPO until status defined and cesarean section possibility ruled out

PATIENT EDUCATION Call physician or proceed to hospital whenever bleeding more than one pad occurs, or if severe uterine or back pain occurs
• Mayo Health; http://mayohealth.org/mayo/baby/htm/bab_3_6.htm#Placenta

MEDICATIONS

DRUG(S) OF CHOICE
- Oxygen
- Saline or Ringer's lactate
- Whole blood and packed RBC's to keep hematocrit > 30
- May use oxytocin (Pitocin) augmentation to speed delivery
- Tocolytics like terbutaline may be used in mild non-compromising preterm abruption
- Rho(D) immune globulin for RhoD negative mother if undelivered or indicated after delivery
- 300 mcg RhoD immune globulin/15 cc fetal blood transfused, if Kleihauer-Betke test returns positive
- Fresh frozen plasma and platelet transfusions for coagulopathy with cryoprecipitate and fibrinogen given if indicated

Contraindications: Tocolytics should be withheld in preterm labor until abruption ruled out and fetal status defined

Precautions:
- Suffusion of blood into myometrium with weakening may increase risk of uterine rupture with oxytocin (Pitocin) augmentation
- Cryoprecipitate and fibrinogen may represent greater transfusion infection transmission risk

Significant possible interactions: Refer to manufacturer's profile of each drug

ALTERNATIVE DRUGS   N/A

FOLLOWUP

PATIENT MONITORING
- If not delivered, monitor for intrauterine growth retardation (IUGR)
- See regularly and assess for preterm labor

PREVENTION/AVOIDANCE   Eliminate risk factors when possible

POSSIBLE COMPLICATIONS
- Infection transfusion risks: Hepatitis, cytomegalovirus infection, HIV and others
- Sensitization from blood product transfusion

EXPECTED COURSE/PROGNOSIS
- 0.5% to 1% fetal mortality and 30-50% perinatal mortality
- With trauma and abruption 1% maternal and 30-70% fetal mortality
- Labor typically more rapid but hypotonus from blood suffusion may occur

MISCELLANEOUS

ASSOCIATED CONDITIONS
- Preeclampsia and other forms of hypertension in pregnancy
- Hypertension
- Postpartum hemorrhage
- Maternal and fetal organ damage from hypoperfusion

AGE-RELATED FACTORS
Pediatric: N/A
Geriatric: N/A
Others: Multiparity, advanced maternal age - more at risk

PREGNANCY   This problem limited to pregnancy

SYNONYMS
- Placental abruption
- Premature separation of the placenta
- Couvelaire placenta

ICD-9-CM
641.2 Premature separation of placenta

SEE ALSO   Placenta previa

OTHER NOTES
- Increased pelvic blood flow of pregnancy may enhance blood loss
- Amniotic fluid embolism is rare but may present with DIC and severe respiratory distress
- Increased risk of fetal-maternal transfusion with trauma of anterior placenta location

ABBREVIATIONS   N/A

REFERENCES
- Kramer MS, et al: Etiologic determinants of abruptio placentae. Obstet Gynec 1997;89(2):221-226
- Cunningham PG, et al: Abruptio placentae. In: Cunningham FG, MacDonald PC, Gant NF (eds). Williams' Obstetrics. 20th Ed. 1997, Norwalk, CT, Appleton and Lange
Illustrations: N/A
Internet references: http://www.5mcc.com

Author(s)
Cathryn Heath, MD
Adrienne Headley, MD

Acetaminophen poisoning

BASICS

DESCRIPTION
• A disorder characterized by hepatic necrosis following large ingestions of acetaminophen. Symptoms may vary from initial nausea, vomiting, diaphoresis, and malaise to jaundice, confusion, somnolence, coma, and death. The clinical hallmark is the onset of symptoms within 24 hours of ingestion of acetaminophen-only or combination products.
• Acetaminophen poisoning is most often encountered following large single ingestions of acetaminophen-containing medications. However, poisoning also occurs following acute and chronic ingestions of lesser amounts in susceptible individuals including those who regularly abuse alcohol, are chronically malnourished, or take medications which affect hepatic metabolism of acetaminophen.
System(s) affected: Gastrointestinal, Renal/Urologic, Cardiovascular
Genetics: N/A
Incidence/Prevalence in USA:
• Over 115,000 ingestions of acetaminophen-containing medications reported by poison control centers in 1997
• 126 deaths in 1997, one in a child < 6
Predominant age:
• Occurs in children and adults at any age
• Approximately 43% of exposures are in children under 6 years
Predominant sex: No reported association

SIGNS AND SYMPTOMS
• Develop over the first 24 hours following large ingestions and may last as long as 8 days
• Severe symptoms indicate large ingestions or co-ingestants
• Fulminant hepatic failure occurs in less than 1% of adults and is very rare in children under 6 years
• Stage 1, first 24 hours
  ◊ Nausea
  ◊ Vomiting
  ◊ Diaphoresis
• Stage 2, 24-48 hours
  ◊ Right upper quadrant pain
  ◊ Typically less nausea, vomiting, diaphoresis, and malaise than in stage 1
• Stage 3, 72-96 hours
  ◊ Nausea, vomiting, malaise reappear
  ◊ Severe poisonings may result in jaundice, confusion, somnolence, and coma
• Stage 4, 7-8 days
  ◊ Resolution of clinical signs in survivors
• May develop gradually following long-term ingestion of smaller amounts of acetaminophen. Such patients may present in any stage 1-3 without a history of excessive acetaminophen ingestion.

CAUSES
Accidental or intentional ingestion of acetaminophen or combination medications containing acetaminophen

RISK FACTORS
• Age less than 6 years
• Concurrent oral poisoning with other substances
• Psychiatric illness
• History of previous toxic ingestions or suicide attempts
• Regular ingestion of large amounts of alcohol

DIAGNOSIS

DIFFERENTIAL DIAGNOSIS
• Consider presence of co-ingestants, especially alcohol
• Other ingested toxins which produce severe acute hepatic injury, including the mushroom Amanita phalloides and products containing yellow phosphorus or carbon tetrachloride

LABORATORY
• Plasma acetaminophen levels should be drawn on all patients 4 or more hours after ingestion (levels prior to 4 hours not helpful)
• At least one additional acetaminophen level drawn 4-6 hours after the first level is recommended if the ingested acetaminophen is an extended release product (e.g., Tylenol Extended Relief) or is not known to be an immediate release product
  ◊ If the second level is higher than the first level or is close to the "possible risk" level on the Rumack-Matthew nomogram, it may be prudent to obtain additional acetaminophen levels every 2 hours until the levels stabilize or decline
  ◊ If co-ingestants include drugs that slow gastrointestinal motility, an acetaminophen level drawn 4-6 hours after the second level may detect a late increase in serum acetaminophen concentration
• Screens for suspected co-ingestants (aspirin, iron, others) may be positive (especially when suicide is a possibility)
• With toxic ingestions, aspartate transaminase (AST; SGOT), alanine transaminase (ALT; SGPT), and bilirubin levels begin to rise in Stage 2 and peak in Stage 3. In severe poisonings, the PT will parallel these changes.
• AST levels over 1000 IU/L are consistent with the diagnosis and levels of 20,000 IU/L are not uncommon
• Laboratory abnormalities usually resolve by stage 4
• Renal function abnormalities are common in patients with hepatotoxicity
• Evidence of damage to the pancreas and heart may present following severe poisonings
Drugs that may alter lab results: None with clinically significant cross-reactivity with plasma acetaminophen assay
Disorders that may alter lab results: Diseases or toxic substances which damage the liver, particularly alcohol

PATHOLOGICAL FINDINGS
Centrilobular hepatic necrosis

SPECIAL TESTS N/A

IMAGING N/A

DIAGNOSTIC PROCEDURES None other than correlating plasma acetaminophen levels with the clinical presentation

TREATMENT

APPROPRIATE HEALTH CARE
• Contact a regional poison control center for management recommendations
• All patients should be evaluated at a health care facility
• Outpatient for non-toxic accidental ingestions
• Inpatient for toxic and intentional ingestions

GENERAL MEASURES
• The stomach of untreated patients should be emptied by ipecac or gastric lavage if within 4 hours of ingestion
• Gastric lavage is preferred in most situations
• Patients may receive (especially if ingestion is 100-150 mg/kg) ipecac at home if alert and unable to be evaluated within 1 hour of ingestion
• Activated charcoal should be used, but preferably not within 1 hour of administration of the antidote N-acetylcysteine (NAC)
• NAC should be given when plasma acetaminophen concentrations measured 4 or more hours after ingestion are in the "possible risk" or higher levels on the Rumack-Matthew nomogram. This corresponds to acetaminophen levels greater than 150 µg/mL (993 µmol/L), 75 µg/mL (497 µmol/L), and 40 µg/mL (265 µmol/L) at 4 hours, 8 hours, and 12 hours after ingestion, respectively.
• NAC therapy may be effective up to 36 hours or more after ingestion

SURGICAL MEASURES N/A

ACTIVITY Restricted if significant hepatic damage has occurred

DIET No special diet except with severe hepatic damage

PATIENT EDUCATION
• Education of parents/caregivers during well child visits
• Anticipatory guidance for caregivers, family, and cohabitants of potentially suicidal patients
• Patient brochure: Child Safety: How to keep your home safe for your baby. American Academy of Family Physicians, 8880 Ward Parkway, Kansas City, MO 64114-2797
• Education of patients taking long-term acetaminophen therapy

MEDICATIONS

DRUG(S) OF CHOICE
• Three classes of medicine:
  ◊ Ipecac syrup
  ◊ Activated charcoal
  ◊ Acetylcysteine (N-acetylcysteine, NAC, Mucomyst)
• At home:
  ◊ Ipecac syrup may be given (especially if ingestion is 100-150 mg/kg) if the patient is alert and unable to be evaluated at a health care facility within 1 hour
  ◊ Ipecac syrup: Age 6 months-1 year 5 mL; age 1-12 years 15 mL; age > 12 years 30 mL. Give with 240 mL of water when possible; may repeat in 30 minutes if emesis has not occurred.
• Emergency facility/hospital:
  ◊ Patients evaluated within 4 hours of ingestion should have their stomachs evacuated. Gastric lavage is the preferred method.
  ◊ Activated charcoal: 1 g/kg for initial dose; preferably not within 1 hour of NAC administration. Additional concurrent use during NAC therapy is controversial.
  ◊ Acetylcysteine: oral loading dose of 140 mg/kg, followed by 70 mg/kg every 4 hours for 17 additional doses. Whenever possible, NAC therapy should be initiated within 8 hours following the toxic ingestion.

Contraindications:
• Ipecac should not be given to patients with decreased responsiveness
• Medication allergies

Precautions:
• Aggressive ipecac therapy may result in prolonged vomiting, thereby interfering with NAC administration
• To avoid risks of decreased effectiveness and aspiration, activated charcoal should be given at least 30 minutes to 1 hour after ipecac and never before ipecac
• NAC may cause significant nausea and vomiting due to it's sulfur content; consider administration by nasogastric tube. Nausea can be treated with metoclopramide (Reglan, 0.5-1 mg/kg IV) or ondansetron (Zofran) 0.15 mg/kg IV, for age > 4 years; usually 4 mg/dose

Significant possible interactions:
Activated charcoal given within 1 hour of NAC may adsorb the NAC, thereby limiting its effectiveness

ALTERNATIVE DRUGS
• IV NAC outside US; in approved trials within US
• Oral racemethionine (methionine)

FOLLOWUP

PATIENT MONITORING
Psychiatric follow-up after intentional ingestions

PREVENTION/AVOIDANCE
• Parent/caregiver education essential
  ◊ Education during well child exams regarding poisoning prevention
  ◊ Ipecac syrup at home
  ◊ Emergency telephone numbers

POSSIBLE COMPLICATIONS
Rare following recovery from acute poisoning

EXPECTED COURSE/PROGNOSIS
• Complete recovery with early therapy
• Fewer than 1% of adult patients develop hepatic failure
• Hepatic failure is very rare in children under 6 years

MISCELLANEOUS

ASSOCIATED CONDITIONS N/A

AGE-RELATED FACTORS
Pediatric: Hepatic damage at toxic acetaminophen levels is decreased in children less than 6 years
Geriatric: Hepatic damage may be increased if taking hepatotoxic medications chronically
Others: N/A

PREGNANCY
• Increased incidence of spontaneous abortion, especially with overdose at early gestational age
• Incidence of spontaneous abortion or fetal death appears increased when NAC treatment is delayed

SYNONYMS
• Paracetamol poisoning

ICD-9-CM
965.4 poisoning by aromatic analgesics (acetaminophen)

SEE ALSO N/A

OTHER NOTES N/A

ABBREVIATIONS
NAC = N-acetylcysteine

REFERENCES
• Anker AL, Smilkstein MJ: Acetaminophen - concepts and controversies. Emerg Med Clin N Amer 1994;12:335-49
• Cetaruck EW, Dart RC, et al: Tylenol Extended Relief overdose. Ann Emerg Med 1997;30:104-108
• Lewis RK, Paloucek FP: Assessment and treatment of acetaminophen overdose. Clin Pharm 1991; l0:765-74
• Litovltz TL, Klein-Schwartz W, Dyer KS, Shannon M, Lee S, Powers M: 1997 Annual report of the American Association of Poison Control Centers Toxic Exposure Surveillance System. Am J Emerg Med 1998;16:443-97
Illustrations: N/A
Internet references: http://www.5mcc.com

Author(s)
Lars C. Larsen, MD

Acne rosacea

BASICS

DESCRIPTION Chronic skin eruption with flushing and dilation of small blood vessels in the face, especially nose and cheeks. Sometimes associated with ocular symptoms (ocular rosacea).
System(s) affected: Skin/Exocrine
Genetics: People of Northern European and Celtic background commonly afflicted
Incidence/Prevalence in USA: Common
Predominant age: 30-50
Predominant sex: Female > Male

SIGNS AND SYMPTOMS
• Skin flush - prominent at onset
• Redness - lower half of nose, sometimes whole nose, forehead, cheeks, chin
• Conjunctivae red - (sometimes)
• Erythema, dusky - (in advanced cases)
• Blood vessels in involved area collapse under pressure
• Acne lesions form papules, pustules, and nodules; comedones are rare
• Telangiectasia
• Rhinophyma (sometimes) more common in males

CAUSES
• No proven cause. Possibilities include:
  ◊ Thyroid and gonadal disturbance
  ◊ Alcohol, coffee, tea, spiced food overindulgence (unproven)
  ◊ Demodex follicular parasite (suspected)
  ◊ Exposure to cold, heat, hot drinks
  ◊ Emotional stress
  ◊ Dysfunction of the gastrointestinal tract

RISK FACTORS   N/A

DIAGNOSIS

DIFFERENTIAL DIAGNOSIS
• Drug eruptions (iodides and bromides)
• Granulomas of the skin
• Cutaneous lupus erythematosus
• Carcinoid syndrome
• Deep fungal infection
• Acne vulgaris
• Seborrheic dermatitis

LABORATORY   N/A
Drugs that may alter lab results: N/A
Disorders that may alter lab results: N/A

PATHOLOGICAL FINDINGS
• Inflammation around hypertrophied sebaceous glands, producing papules, pustules and cysts
• Absence of comedones and blocked ducts
• Vascular dilatation and dermal lymphocytic infiltrate

SPECIAL TESTS   N/A

IMAGING   N/A

DIAGNOSTIC PROCEDURES   N/A

TREATMENT

APPROPRIATE HEALTH CARE
Outpatient

GENERAL MEASURES
• Reassurance
• Treat psychological stress if present
• Avoid oil based cosmetics. Others are acceptable and may help women tolerate the symptoms.
• Electrodesiccation of permanently dilated blood vessels

SURGICAL MEASURES   Surgical treatment of rhinophyma

ACTIVITY   No restrictions. Support physical fitness.

DIET   Avoid any food or drink that causes facial flushing, e.g., hot drinks, spiced food, alcohol

PATIENT EDUCATION
• American Academy of Dermatology (708) 330-0230

MEDICATIONS

DRUG(S) OF CHOICE
- Low dose oral tetracycline 500-1000 mg/day
- Sulfur-containing local applications - alcohol-sulfur (Liquimat), sulfur (Fostril), resorcinol-sulfur (Rezamid), sulfacetamide-sulfur (Sulfacet-R)
- Topical steroids should not be used as they may aggravate rosacea
- Topical metronidazole 0.75% gel - apply each morning and at bedtime after cleansing skin; also available as a cream which may be better tolerated by some patients
- Topical erythromycin
- Topical clindamycin lotion preferred

Contraindications:
- Tetracycline: not for use in pregnancy or children < 8 years
- Isotretinoin: teratogenic; not for use in pregnancy or in women or reproductive age who are not using a reliable birth control method

Precautions:
- Tetracycline: may cause photosensitivity; sunscreen recommended

Significant possible interactions:
- Tetracycline: avoid concurrent administration with antacids, dairy products, or iron
- Broad-spectrum antibiotics: may reduce the effectiveness of oral contraceptives; barrier method recommended

ALTERNATIVE DRUGS
- For severe cases, isotretinoin orally for 4 months.

FOLLOWUP

PATIENT MONITORING
Occasional and as needed. Close follow-up for women using isotretinoin.

PREVENTION/AVOIDANCE
No preventive measure known

POSSIBLE COMPLICATIONS
- Rhinophyma (dilated follicles and thickened bulbous skin on nose), especially in men
- Conjunctivitis
- Blepharitis
- Keratitis

EXPECTED COURSE/PROGNOSIS
- Slowly progressive
- Subsides spontaneously (sometimes)

MISCELLANEOUS

ASSOCIATED CONDITIONS
- Seborrheic dermatitis of scalp and eyelids
- Keratitis with photophobia, lacrimation, visual disturbance
- Corneal lesions
- Blepharitis
- Uveitis

AGE-RELATED FACTORS
Pediatric: Unlikely in this age group
Geriatric: Uncommon after age 60
Others: N/A

PREGNANCY
Use of oral isotretinoin contraindicated

SYNONYMS
Rosacea

ICD-9-CM
695.3 rosacea

SEE ALSO
- Blepharitis
- Dermatitis, seborrheic
- Uveitis
- Lupus erythematosus, discoid
- Acne vulgaris

OTHER NOTES
N/A

ABBREVIATIONS
N/A

REFERENCES
- Fitzpatrick TB, et al, eds: Dermatology In General Medicine. 4th Ed. New York, McGraw-Hill, 1993
- Habif T: Clinical Dermatology. 3rd Ed. St. Louis, CV Mosby, 1996
Illustrations: 8 available on CD-ROM
Internet references: http://www.5mcc.com

Author(s)
John M. Little, MD

Acne vulgaris

BASICS

DESCRIPTION Acne is an androgenically stimulated, inflammatory disorder of the sebaceous glands, resulting in comedones, papules, inflammatory pustules and, occasionally, scarring
System(s) affected: Skin/Exocrine
Genetics:
• Approximately 50% of affected individuals have a family history of acne
• Higher prevalence in Caucasians
Incidence/Prevalence in USA: Virtually 100% of adolescents are affected to some degree. 15% will seek medical advice.
Predominant age: Early to late puberty, although some cases will persist into the third and fourth decade. Age 16, 100% affected; 25-34, 8% affected; 35-44, 3% affected
Predominant sex: Male = Female

SIGNS AND SYMPTOMS
• Closed comedones (whiteheads)
• Open comedones (blackheads)
• Nodules or papules
• Pustules, with or without redness and edema ("cysts")
• Scars - ice pick, atrophic macules, hypertrophic, depressed
• Lesions occur over the forehead, cheeks and nose, and may extend over the central chest and back
• Factors which influence symptomatology
  ◊ Sex: males - later onset, greater severity; females: earlier onset, lesser severity
  ◊ Seasonal variation - less severe in summer
  ◊ May be worse immediately prior to menses
• Grading system
  ◊ Grade 1: Comedonal - closed/open
  ◊ Grade 2: Papular > 25 lesions on face & trunk
  ◊ Grade 3: Pustular > 25 lesions, mild scarring
  ◊ Grade 4: Nodulocystic - inflammatory nodules and cysts, extensive scarring

CAUSES
• Overproduction of androgens
• Hyperresponsiveness of follicle/sebaceous gland to androgens
• Hypersensitivity to P. acnes & its metabolic products
• Pathophysiology
  ◊ Androgens stimulate sebum production & proliferation of keratinocytes in hair follicles
  ◊ Keratin plug obstructs the follicle opening, resulting in sebum accumulation and follicular distention
  ◊ Propionibacterium acnes, an anaerobe, colonizes & proliferates in the plugged follicle
  ◊ P. acnes hydrolyzes sebum triglycerides into free fatty acids, produces chemotactic factors and proinflammatory mediators, and activates complement, all of which result in inflammation of the follicle and surrounding dermis

RISK FACTORS
• Adolescence
• Male sex
• Androgenic steroids, e.g., steroid abuse, some birth control pills
• Oily cosmetics, including cleansing creams, moisturizers, oil-based foundations
• Rubbing or occluding the skin surface, as may occur with sports equipment (helmets and shoulder pads), holding the telephone or hands against the skin
• Drugs - iodides or bromides, lithium, phenytoins
• Systemic corticosteroids
• Virilization disorders
• Hot, humid climate

DIAGNOSIS

DIFFERENTIAL DIAGNOSIS
• Occupational exposure to tars, oils, grease
• Folliculitis
• Acne rosacea
• Perioral dermatitis
• Chloracne
• Acne cosmetica
• Steroid induced acne
• Folliculitis
• Pseudo-folliculitis barbae

LABORATORY N/A
Drugs that may alter lab results: N/A
Disorders that may alter lab results: N/A

PATHOLOGICAL FINDINGS
• Oiliness, thickening of the skin
• Hypertrophy of the sebaceous glands
• Perifolliculitis
• Scarring

SPECIAL TESTS Testosterone and its metabolites can be measured in those very rare cases when acne arises de novo in the previously unaffected adult

IMAGING N/A

DIAGNOSTIC PROCEDURES History and physical exam

TREATMENT

APPROPRIATE HEALTH CARE
Outpatient

GENERAL MEASURES
• Intralesional injection - of large cystic lesions with 0.05-0.3 mL of triamcinolone (Kenalog 2-4 mg/mL), use 30-gauge needle, slightly distend cyst
• Cleansing: gentle cleansing with a mild soap once or twice a day will control surface oiliness. More frequent washing will further irritate the skin and increase sebum production.

• Apply topical agents to both lesions and surrounding area of affected skin
• Oil-free sun screens: although UV light results in some improvement in untreated acne, it will react adversely with the medications used to treat acne. Long-term UV exposure causes permanent skin damage.
• Stress management: may be helpful if acne flares with stress

SURGICAL MEASURES
• Comedone extraction: use a comedone extractor or eye dropper opening, after incising the thin layer of epithelium directly over the comedone

ACTIVITY Full activity. Physical conditioning important.

DIET
• Counsel regarding good nutrition
• No special diet has been shown to diminish acne. Chocolate and fatty foods do not aggravate acne.

PATIENT EDUCATION
• It is important for the patient to know that there is no cure for acne, that treatment only controls the lesions
• Any treatment measure takes a minimum of 4 weeks to show results
• The topical agents can cause redness and drying of the skin and most people need encouragement to persist with these useful agents
• Picking at or popping lesions may increase inflammation and scarring
• For patient education materials favorably reviewed on this topic: American Academy of Dermatology, 930 N. Meacham Rd., P.O. Box 4014, Schaumberg, IL 60168-4014, (708)330-0230

MEDICATIONS

DRUG(S) OF CHOICE
• Comedonal acne
  ◊ Tretinoin (Retin-A): 0.025%, 0.05%, and 0.1% cream, 0.01% and 0.025% gel, 0.1% microemulsion, 0.05% solution, apply hs 30 minutes after after washing
    - Cream - better in cold/dry weather
    - Gel - more drying, better in hot/humid weather, better for chest/back
    - May cause an initial flare of lesions
  ◊ Adapalene (Differin): 0.1% gel, apply hs after washing
    - As effective and better tolerated than tretinoin
    - Side effects - erythema, dryness, scaling, pruritus
    - Pregnancy class C
  ◊ Azelaic acid (Azelex): 20% cream bid
    - Keratolytic, antibacterial, and anti-inflammatory
    - Reduces post-inflammatory hyperpigmentation in dark-skinned individuals
    - Side effects - erythema, dryness, scaling, hypopigmentation
    - Pregnancy class B

◊ Salicylic acid 0.5-2.0% hydroalcoholic
◊ Tazarotene (Tazorac): 0.1% gel, pregnancy class X
◊ Alpha-hydroxy acids, available OTC
• Mild Inflammatory acne
◊ Topical benzoyl peroxide 5% & 10% gel, apply hs
- Side effects - skin irritation, may bleach clothes
◊ Topical antibiotic
- Erythromycin (A/T/S, Emgel, Erycette, T-stat): 2% gel or solution, bid
- Clindamycin (Cleocin-T, Dalacin-T): 1% gel, solution, lotion, bid
- Metronidazole gel, once daily, used mostly for rosacea
- Azelaic acid (Azelex): 20% cream, bid; enhanced bactericidal effect and decreased risk of resistant P. acnes when used with zinc and benzoyl peroxide
- Benzoyl peroxide-erythromycin (Benzamycin): 5%/3% gel, bid; probably most effective topical antibiotic; needs to be refrigerated
- Tetracycline (Topicycline): 0.22% solution bid; may cause skin to fluoresce (black light in nightclubs)
• Inflammatory acne
◊ Topical tretinoin, and
◊ Topical antibiotic/benzoyl peroxide, or
◊ Systemic (oral) antibiotic
- Tetracycline: 500-1000 mg daily; begin at high dose, then taper in 2-4 wks if good response; avoid in children < 8 & pregnancy; side effects - photosensitivity, esophagitis
- Minocycline 50-200 mg daily; side effects - photosensitivity, urticaria, vertigo, autoimmune hepatitis, lupus-like syndrome
- Doxycycline 50-200 mg daily; side effects - photosensitivity
- Erythromycin: 500-1000 mg daily
- Trimethoprim-sulfamethoxazole (Bactrim-DS, Septra-DS) 160/800 mg, given once daily or bid
- Trimethoprim 300 mg bid
• Severe Inflammatory acne
◊ Isotretinoin (Accutane): 0.5-1.0 mg/kg day bid
- 60% cure rate
- Usually given for 12-20 weeks, total dose 120 mg/kg
- Side effects: cheilitis, arthralgias, tendinitis, hyperlipidemia, highly teratogenic (severe CNS & cardiovascular anomalies)
◊ Oral contraceptives (females)
- Most effective when estrogen component = 50 mg, and progestin component = norgestimate or desorgestrel

Contraindications:
• Allergy
• Severe hepatic dysfunction - all oral agents
• Tetracycline: not for use in pregnancy or children < 8 years
• Isotretinoin: teratogenic; not for use in pregnancy or in women or reproductive age who are not using a reliable birth control method.

Precautions:
• Tetracycline: may cause photosensitivity; sunscreen recommended.

Significant possible interactions:
• Tetracycline: avoid concurrent administration with antacids, dairy products, or iron.
• Erythromycin: astemizole; ECG abnormalities
• Broad-spectrum antibiotics: may reduce the effectiveness of oral contraceptives; barrier method recommended.

ALTERNATIVE DRUGS N/A

 FOLLOWUP

PATIENT MONITORING
• Monthly visits until adequate response is obtained
• Pre-treatment and monthly serum lipids, liver function tests, and pregnancy tests for patients on isotretinoin

PREVENTION/AVOIDANCE N/A

POSSIBLE COMPLICATIONS
• Acne conglobata - a severe confluent inflammatory acne with systemic symptoms
• Facial scarring
• Psychological scarring

EXPECTED COURSE/PROGNOSIS
Gradual improvement over time

 MISCELLANEOUS

ASSOCIATED CONDITIONS
• Acne fulminans - severe cystic acne with systemic symptoms, mostly in teenage boys
• Pyoderma faciale - explosive onset of purulent facial acne, mostly in young women
• Acne conglobata - large abscesses, cysts with sinus tracts, scarring, occurs with scalp cellulitis & hidradenitis suppurativa, mostly in young men
• Hidradenitis suppurativa - chronic suppurative lesions of the axilla, groin, perianal area, and scalp, mostly in women
• Acne excoriee des jeunes filles - mild acne with scaring and atrophy due to squeezing/picking lesions
• Acne mechanica - acne which occurs at sites of repeated mechanical trauma
• Acne aestivalis - summertime acne in women, may be due to Pityrosporum folliculitis or sunscreen use
• SAPHO syndrome - synovitis, acne, pustulosis, hyperostosis, osteitis
• PAPA syndrome - pyogenic sterile arthritis, pyoderma gangrenosum, cystic acne

AGE-RELATED FACTORS
Pediatric:
• Neonatal acne: mostly closed comedones, seen in 20% of newborns
• Infantile acne: inflammatory papules, beginning at 3-6 months of age, may be due to excessive androgens, increased risk for severe teenage acne vulgaris, treat with topical agents
• Age 1-7: acne is very rare and should prompt evaluation for hyperandrogenemia of adrenal or ovarian origin
Geriatric:
• Favre-Racouchot syndrome - comedones on face & head, due to sun exposure, peak incidence at age 60-80
Others: N/A

PREGNANCY
• May result in a flare, or remission, of acne
• Isotretinoin: causes severe fetal malformations; effective contraception should be ensured one month prior to and one month following isotretinoin therapy.
• Erythromycin can be used in pregnancy, would prefer topical agents when possible.

SYNONYMS N/A

ICD-9-CM 706.1 Other acne

SEE ALSO Acne rosacea

OTHER NOTES Acne is usually much more significant to the patient than it appears to the doctor; it subsides with time; is often an "entry ticket", frequently the adolescent also wants advice about life-style, contraception, physiology, etc.

ABBREVIATIONS N/A

REFERENCES
• Kaminer MS, Gilchrist BA: The many faces of acne. J of the Amer Acad of Dermatology;1995; 32(5), Part 3:S6-S14
• Adapalene for acne. The Medical Letter; 1997; Vol 39 (issue 995) 19-20
• Leyden JJ: Therapy for acne vulgaris. The NEJM 1997;336(16):1156-1162
• Mackrides PS, Shaughnessy AE: Azelaic acid therapy for acne. Amer Fam Phys 1996;54(8):2457-2459
• Thiboutot DM: Acne, an overview of clinical research findings. Dermatologic Clinics 1997;15(1):97-109
• Usatine RP, Quan MA, Strick RD: Acne vulgaris - a treatment update. Hospital Practice 1998; 111-127
• Webster G: Acne and rosacea. Medical Clinics of North America 1998; 82 (5): 1145-1154
• DeGroot HE, Friedlander SF: Update on acne. Current Opinion in Pediatrics 1998; 10: 381-386
Illustrations: 12 available on CD-ROM
Internet references: http://www.5mcc.com

Author(s)
Gary Levine, MD

Addison's disease

BASICS

DESCRIPTION Adrenal hypofunction from primary disease (partial or complete destruction) of the adrenal gland with inadequate secretion of glucocorticoids and mineralocorticoids. An autoimmune process is the most common cause (80% of the cases) followed by tuberculosis. AIDS is becoming a more frequent cause.
• Addison's disease (primary adrenocortical insufficiency) is differentiated from secondary (pituitary failure) and tertiary (hypothalamic failure) causes of adrenocortical insufficiency (see Differential Diagnosis)
• Addisonian (adrenal) crisis - acute complication of adrenal insufficiency (circulatory collapse, dehydration, hypotension, nausea, vomiting, hypoglycemia); usually precipitated by acute physiologic stressor such as surgery, illness, exacerbation of co-morbid process, acute withdrawal of long term corticosteroid therapy
System(s) affected: Endocrine/Metabolic
Genetics: Autoimmune adrenal insufficiency shows some hereditary disposition. Familial glucocorticoid insufficiency may have recessive pattern; adrenomyeloneuropathy is X-linked. Frequent association with other autoimmune disorders.
Incidence/Prevalence in USA:
Approximately 4:100,000
Predominant age: All ages; usually 3rd to 5th decade
Predominant sex: Females > Males (slight)

SIGNS AND SYMPTOMS
• Weakness, fatigue, tiredness
• Weight loss
• Dizziness; low blood pressure, orthostatic hypotension
• Increased pigmentation (extensor surfaces, hand creases, dental-gingival margins, buccal and vaginal mucosa, lips, areola, pressure points, scars; "tanning"; freckles; vitiligo)
• Anorexia; nausea; vomiting
• Chronic diarrhea
• Abdominal pain
• Decreased cold tolerance
• Salt craving
• Hair loss in females
• Depression

CAUSES
• Autoimmune adrenal insufficiency (~80%)
• Tuberculosis (~20%)
• Waterhouse-Friderichsen syndrome (disseminated adrenal infection and subsequent infarction; meningococcemia most common; Pseudomonas aeruginosa common in children; atypical pathogens, CMV, Cryptococcus, MAC in immunosuppressed and AIDS)
• Fungal disease (histoplasmosis, blastomycosis, coccidioidomycosis)
• Bilateral adrenal hemorrhage and infarction (anticoagulants; 50% are in therapeutic range at time of hemorrhage)
• Antiphospholipid syndrome
• Metastatic (lung, breast, kidney, colon), lymphoma, Kaposi's sarcoma (tumor must destroy 90% of gland to produce hypofunction)
• Drugs (ketoconazole, etomidate)

• Surgical adrenalectomy
• Radiation therapy
• Sarcoidosis
• Hemochromatosis
• Amyloidosis
• Adrenoleukodystrophy
• Adrenomyelodystrophy
• Polyglandular endocrine syndromes
• Congenital (enzyme defects; hypoplasia; familial glucocorticoid insufficiency)
• Idiopathic

RISK FACTORS
• Family history of autoimmune adrenal insufficiency. About 40% of patients have a first- or second-degree relative with one of the associated disorders.
• Taking steroids for prolonged periods, then experiencing severe infection, trauma or surgical procedures

DIAGNOSIS

DIFFERENTIAL DIAGNOSIS
• Secondary adrenocortical insufficiency
  ◊ Withdrawal of long-term corticosteroid use
  ◊ Sheehan's syndrome (postpartum necrosis of pituitary)
  ◊ Empty sella syndrome
  ◊ Surgical excision of pituitary
  ◊ Radiation to pituitary
  ◊ Pituitary adenomas, carcinomas (rare), craniopharyngiomas
  ◊ Infiltrative disorders of pituitary (sarcoidosis, hemochromatosis, amyloidosis, histiocytosis X)
  ◊ Megestrol
• Tertiary adrenocortical insufficiency
  ◊ Pituitary stalk transection
  ◊ Trauma
  ◊ Disruption of production of corticotropic releasing factor (CRF)
  ◊ Hypothalmic tumors
• Myopathies
• Other causes of hypoglycemia
• Syndrome of inappropriate antidiuretic hormone (SIADH)
• Heavy metal ingestion
• Severe nutritional deficiencies
• Sprue syndrome
• Hyperparathyroidism
• Neurofibromatosis
• Peutz-Jeghers syndrome
• Porphyria cutanea tarda
• Salt-losing nephritis
• Bronchogenic carcinoma
• Anorexia nervosa
• Other causes of hypoglycemia
• Depression
• Autoimmune polyglandular syndromes

LABORATORY
• Low serum sodium
• Elevated serum potassium
• Elevated BUN, creatinine
• Elevated serum calcium
• Hypoglycemia when fasted
• Metabolic acidosis
• Low cortisol level (between 8 and 9 a.m.)
• Elevated ACTH level
• Moderate neutropenia
• Eosinophilia
• Relative lymphocytosis
• Anemia
• Adrenal-cortex autoantibody (ACA/21)
Drugs that may alter lab results: Digitalis
Disorders that may alter lab results: Diabetes mellitus

PATHOLOGICAL FINDINGS Atrophic adrenals in autoimmune adrenalitis. Infiltrative and hemorrhagic disorders produce enlargement with destruction of entire gland.

SPECIAL TESTS
• Rapid ACTH stimulation test: Cosyntropin 0.25 mg IV, measure pre-injection and 60 minute post-injection cortisol levels. Patients with Addison's disease have low to normal values that do not rise
• Metapyrone test
• Insulin-induced hypoglycemia test
• CRH may help distinguish secondary from tertiary adrenal insufficiency
• Autoantibody tests
  ◊ 21-Hydroxylase (most specific)
  ◊ 17-Hydroxylase
  ◊ 17-alfa-Hydroxylase (may not be associated)

IMAGING
• Abdominal CT scan
  ◊ Small adrenal glands in autoimmune adrenalitis
  ◊ Enlarged adrenal glands in infiltrative and hemorrhagic disorders
• Abdominal x-ray: may show adrenal calcifications
• Chest x-ray: may show adrenal calcifications, small heart size, calcification of cartilage

DIAGNOSTIC PROCEDURES A work-up to determine the cause of Addison's disease. CT guided fine-needle biopsy of adrenal masses may be helpful.

TREATMENT

APPROPRIATE HEALTH CARE
• Outpatient
• Inpatient during adrenal crisis

GENERAL MEASURES
• Treatment for adrenal insufficiency is with glucocorticoid and mineralocorticoid replacement
  ◊ 5 S's of management of adrenal crisis: salt, sugar, steroids, support, search for precipitating illness
• Appropriate treatment for underlying cause (e.g., tuberculosis)

ACTIVITY As tolerated

DIET Arrange for a diet that maintains water, sodium and potassium balances

PATIENT EDUCATION
• For patient education materials favorably reviewed on this topic, contact: National Addison's Disease Foundation, 505 Northern Blvd., Suite 200, Great Neck, NY 11021, (516)487-4992
• Patient should wear or carry medical identification with information about the disease and the need for hydrocortisone or other replacement therapy
• Instruct patient in self-administering of parenteral hydrocortisone for emergency situations (e.g., traveling in remote areas away from medical help)

MEDICATIONS

DRUG(S) OF CHOICE
• For chronic adrenal insufficiency:
  ◊ Hydrocortisone 15-20 mg orally each morning upon arising and 10 mg at 4-5 each afternoon is usual dosage (dosage may vary and is usually less in children's),PLUS,
  ◊ Fludrocortisone 0.05-0.2 mg orally once/day
• Acute adrenal insufficiency
  ◊ Hydrocortisone hemisuccinate 100 mg IV followed by 10 mg/hr infusion
  ◊ IV glucose, saline, plasma expanders
• For acute illnesses (fever, stress, minor trauma)
  ◊ Double the patient's usual steroid dose
Contraindications: Refer to manufacturer's literature
Precautions:
• Patients with hepatic disease may need a reduced dose
• Elderly should have a slightly reduced dose
• Refer to manufacturer's literature for other precautions
Significant possible interactions: Refer to manufacturer's literature. Rifampin, phenytoin, and barbiturates may precipitate adrenal insufficiency in addisonian patients by inducing steroid-metabolizing liver enzymes

ALTERNATIVE DRUGS Prednisone 5 mg in AM and 2.5 mg at hs plus fludrocortisone

FOLLOWUP

PATIENT MONITORING
• Verify adequacy of therapy - normal blood pressure, serum electrolytes normal, normal plasma renin, improvement of appetite and strength, increase in heart size to normal, normal fasting blood glucose level
• Lifelong medical supervision for signs of continued adequate therapy and avoidance of overdose

PREVENTION/AVOIDANCE
• No preventive measures known for Addison's disease
• Prevention of complications
  ◊ Anticipate adrenal crisis and treat before symptoms begin
  ◊ If nausea and vomiting preclude oral therapy, patient should seek medical help to start parenteral therapy
  ◊ Elective surgical procedures require adjustment in steroid dose
  ◊ Prevent exposure to infections

POSSIBLE COMPLICATIONS
• Hyperpyrexia
• Psychotic reactions
• Complications from underlying disease
• Over- or under-steroid treatment
• Hyperkalemic paralysis (rare)
• Addisonian crisis

EXPECTED COURSE/PROGNOSIS
• Good outlook with appropriate treatment. With adequate replacement therapy, life expectancy approximates normal
• 100% lethal without treatment

MISCELLANEOUS

ASSOCIATED CONDITIONS
• Diabetes mellitus
• Grave's disease
• Hashimoto's thyroiditis
• Hypoparathyroidism
• Hypercalcemia
• Ovarian failure
• Pernicious anemia
• Myasthenia gravis
• Vitiligo
• Chronic moniliasis
• Sarcoidosis
• Sjögren's syndrome
• Chronic active hepatitis
• Schmidt's syndrome (multiple endocrine deficiency syndrome)
• Adrenoleukodystrophy

AGE-RELATED FACTORS
Pediatric:
• Hydrocortisone and fludrocortisone doses are lower than adults
• More difficult to diagnose
• Occurs in siblings
Geriatric: Acute adrenal crisis more likely
Others: N/A

PREGNANCY N/A

SYNONYMS
• Adrenocortical insufficiency
• Waterhouse-Friderichsen syndrome (adrenal crisis)
• Corticoadrenal insufficiency
• Primary adrenocortical insufficiency

ICD-9-CM
255.4 Corticoadrenal insufficiency

SEE ALSO
• Sjögren's syndrome

OTHER NOTES N/A

ABBREVIATIONS N/A

REFERENCES
• Dale DC, Federman DD, eds: Scientific American Medicine. New York, Scientific American, Inc., 1997
• Oelker W: Adrenal insufficiency. NEJM 1996;335(16):1206-1212
Illustrations: N/A
Internet references: http://www.5mcc.com

Author(s)
Rick Kellerman, MD
Mark Gerstberger, DO

Adenovirus infections

BASICS

DESCRIPTION   Usually self-limited febrile illnesses characterized by inflammation of conjunctivae and the respiratory tract. Adenovirus infections occur in epidemic and endemic situations.
• Common types
  ◊ Acute febrile respiratory illness (AFRI) affecting primarily children
  ◊ Acute respiratory disease (ARD) affecting adults
  ◊ Viral pneumonia affecting children and adults
  ◊ Acute pharyngoconjunctival fever (APC) affecting children, particularly after summer swimming
  ◊ Acute follicular conjunctivitis affecting all ages
  ◊ Epidemic keratoconjunctivitis (EKC) affecting adults
  ◊ Intestinal infections leading to enteritis, mesenteric adenitis and intussusception
System(s) affected: Pulmonary, Gastrointestinal, Renal/Urologic, Nervous, Hemic/Lymphatic/Immunologic, Musculoskeletal, Cardiovascular
Genetics: N/A
Incidence/Prevalence in USA: Very common infection, estimated at 2-5% of all respiratory infections. More common in infants and children.
Predominant age: All ages
Predominant sex: Male = Female

SIGNS AND SYMPTOMS
• Depends on type (see "Differential diagnosis")
In common with most respiratory forms:
• Headache
• Malaise
• Sore throat
• Cough
• Fever (moderate to high)
• Vomiting
• Diarrhea
• Mucosa exhibits patches of white exudate

CAUSES
• Adenovirus (DNA viruses 60-90 nm in size with 47 known serotypes; 3 types cause gastroenteritis); difficult to eliminate from skin and environmental surfaces
• Different serotypes have different epidemiologies
• Most common known pathogens are:
  ◊ Types 1, 2, 3, 5, 7 cause respiratory illness
  ◊ Type 3 causes pharyngoconjunctival fever
  ◊ Types 4, 7, 21 cause acute respiratory disease
  ◊ Several other types may cause epidemic keratoconjunctivitis

RISK FACTORS
• Large number of people gathered in a small area (military recruits, college students at the beginning of the school year, daycare centers, community swimming pools, etc.)
• Immunocompromised at risk for severe disease

DIAGNOSIS

DIFFERENTIAL DIAGNOSIS
Early diagnosis depends on clinical evaluation. The following are the primary characteristics of the major adenovirus infections:
• Acute febrile respiratory illness:
  ◊ Nonspecific cold-like symptoms, similar to other viral respiratory illnesses (fever, pharyngitis, tracheitis, bronchitis, pneumonitis)
  ◊ Mostly in children
  ◊ Incubation period 2 to 5 days
  ◊ May be pertussis-like syndrome rarely
• Acute respiratory disease:
  ◊ Malaise, fever, chills, headache, pharyngitis, hoarseness and dry cough
  ◊ Fever lasts 2 to 4 days
  ◊ Illness subsides in 10 to 14 days
• Viral pneumonia
  ◊ Sudden onset of high fever, rapid infection of upper and lower respiratory tracts, skin rash, diarrhea
  ◊ Occurs in children aged a few days up to 3 years
  ◊ Common; severe illness occurs in subset
• Acute pharyngoconjunctival fever
  ◊ Spiking fever lasting several days, headache, pharyngitis, conjunctivitis, rhinitis, cervical adenitis
  ◊ Conjunctivitis is usually unilateral
  ◊ Subsides in about 1 week
• Epidemic keratoconjunctivitis
  ◊ Usually unilateral onset of ocular redness and edema, periorbital edema, periorbital swelling, local discomfort suggestive of foreign body
  ◊ Lasts 3 or 4 weeks

LABORATORY
• Viral cultures from respiratory, ocular or fecal sources can establish diagnosis. Pharyngeal isolate suggests recent infection.
• Antigen detection in stool for enteric serotypes is available
• Serologic procedures such as complement fixation with a four fold rise in serum antibody titer identifies recent adenoviral infection
Drugs that may alter lab results: N/A
Disorders that may alter lab results: N/A

PATHOLOGICAL FINDINGS
• Varies with each virus, severe pneumonia may be reflected by extensive intranuclear inclusions
• Bronchiolitis obliterans may occur

SPECIAL TESTS   Cultures and serologic studies if appropriate

IMAGING   X-ray: bronchopneumonia in severe respiratory infections

DIAGNOSTIC PROCEDURES
• Biopsy (lung or other) may be needed in severe or unusual cases

TREATMENT

APPROPRIATE HEALTH CARE
Ambulatory except for severely ill infants or those with epidemic keratoconjunctivitis or infants with severe pneumonia. Contact and droplet precautions during a hospitalization are indicated.

GENERAL MEASURES   Treatment is supportive and symptomatic. Infections are usually benign and of short duration.

SURGICAL MEASURES   N/A

ACTIVITY   Rest during febrile phases

DIET   No special diet

PATIENT EDUCATION   Avoid aspirin in children. Give instructions for nasal spray, cough preparations, frequent hand washing.

MEDICATIONS

DRUG(S) OF CHOICE
• Acetaminophen, 10-15 mg/kg/dose, for analgesia (avoid aspirin)
• Topical corticosteroids for conjunctivitis (after consulting an ophthalmologist)
• Cough suppressants and/or expectorants
Contraindications: Refer to manufacturer's literature
Precautions: Refer to manufacturer's literature
Significant possible interactions: Refer to manufacturer's literature

ALTERNATIVE DRUGS N/A

FOLLOWUP

PATIENT MONITORING For severe infantile pneumonia and conjunctivitis: daily physical exam until well

PREVENTION/AVOIDANCE
• Live types 4 and 7 adenovirus vaccine orally in enteric coated capsule reduces incidence of acute respiratory disease
• Frequent hand washing among office personnel and family members

POSSIBLE COMPLICATIONS
• Few if any recognizable long-term problems

EXPECTED COURSE/PROGNOSIS
• Self-limited, usually without sequelae
• Severe illness and death in very young and in immunocompromised hosts

MISCELLANEOUS

ASSOCIATED CONDITIONS
• Hemorrhagic cystitis (can be caused by adenovirus)
• Viral enteritis
• Intussusception and mesenteric adenitis

AGE-RELATED FACTORS
Pediatric: Viral pneumonia in infants may be fatal
Geriatric: Complications more likely
Others: N/A

PREGNANCY No special precautions

SYNONYMS N/A

ICD-9-CM
079.0 Adenovirus infection in condition classified elsewhere
462 Pharyngitis
480.0 Pneumonia due to adenovirus

SEE ALSO
• Conjunctivitis
• Intussusception
• Pneumonia, viral

OTHER NOTES Conjunctivitis sometimes called "pink eye"

ABBREVIATIONS N/A

REFERENCES
• Mandell GL, et al, eds: Principles and Practice of Infectious Diseases. 5th Ed. New York, Churchill Livingstone, 1999
• Fields BN, Knipe DM, eds: Fundamental Virology. 3rd Ed. New York, Raven Press, 1995
Illustrations: N/A
Internet references: http://www.5mcc.com

Author(s)
Mark R. Dambro, MD, FAAFP

Alcoholism

BASICS

DESCRIPTION An illness characterized by significant physiologic, psychologic and/or social dysfunctions associated with persistent and excessive use of alcohol.
System(s) affected: Nervous, Gastrointestinal
Genetics: Twin and adoption studies support a genetic influence
Incidence/Prevalence in USA:
• 10% of men; 3.5% of women
• Lifetime prevalence for adults of 11.5-15.7%
Predominant age:
• All ages
• Highest prevalence of drinking problems is in the 18-29 age group. Subgroups of some age categories have higher prevalence rates.
Predominant sex: Males>Female (slightly)

SIGNS AND SYMPTOMS
• Behavioral
  ◊ Psychological and social dysfunction
  ◊ Marital problems (divorce or separation)
  ◊ Anxiety, depression, insomnia
  ◊ Social isolation or frequent moves
  ◊ Child or spouse abuse
  ◊ Alcohol-related arrests or legal problems (less likely in women)
  ◊ Preoccupation with recreational drinking
  ◊ Repeated attempts to stop or reduce drinking
  ◊ Loss of interest in non-drinking activities
  ◊ Employment problems (tardiness, absenteeism, decreased productivity, interpersonal problems at work, frequent job changes)
  ◊ Blackouts (not remembering what happened during drinking spells)
  ◊ Complaints by family members or friends about alcohol-related behavior
• Physical
  ◊ Gastrointestinal: anorexia, nausea, vomiting, abdominal pain, stigmata of chronic liver disease, peptic ulcer disease, pancreatitis, gastrointestinal malignancies
  ◊ Cardiovascular: modest hypertension, arrhythmias or palpitations (supraventricular), cardiomyopathy
  ◊ Respiratory: aspiration pneumonia, bronchitis and chronic pulmonary disease from associated cigarette smoking
  ◊ Genitourinary: impotence, menstrual irregularities, testicular atrophy
  ◊ Endocrine/metabolic: hypercholesterolemia, hypertriglyceridemia, cushingoid appearance, gynecomastia
  ◊ Dermatologic: signs of accidents and trauma, burns (esp. cigarette burns), bruises in various stages of healing, poor hygiene
  ◊ Musculoskeletal: old fractures and fractures in various stages of healing, myopathy
  ◊ Neurologic: cognitive deficits (e.g., mild impairment of recent memory), peripheral neuropathy, Wernicke-Korsakoff syndrome
  ◊ HEENT: plethoric facies, parotid hypertrophy, poor oral hygiene, head and neck malignancies

CAUSES
• Multifactorial including biological, psychological and sociocultural factors
• Possible biologic markers: brain neuro transmitters, cell membrane receptors, enzyme systems (monoamine oxidase and adenylate cyclase)
• No evidence for a characteristic personality predisposition

RISK FACTORS
• Alcohol use
• Use of other psychoactive drugs, including nicotine
• Family history of alcohol abuse
• Young, single male
• Heavy drinking - five or more drinks in one sitting, getting drunk at least once per week
• Peer group pressure
• Family or sociocultural background promoting intoxication; accepting it as a norm
• Increased accessibility of alcohol
• Adolescence (alcohol and drug use by peers or parents, delinquency, sociopathy in the parents, poor self-esteem, social non-conformity, and stressful life changes)

DIAGNOSIS

DIFFERENTIAL DIAGNOSIS N/A

LABORATORY
• Three laboratory findings diagnostic of alcoholism, others are only suggestive, and when present, indicate advanced alcoholism
• Blood alcohol concentration:
  ◊ > 100 mg/dL (22 mmol/L) during an office visit
  ◊ > 150 mg/dL (33 mmol/L) without obvious signs of intoxication
  ◊ > 300 mg/dL (65 mmol/L) at any time
• Suggestive - if increased:
  ◊ Gamma-glutamyl transferase (GGT)
  ◊ Alanine aminotransferase (ALT)
  ◊ Aspartate aminotransferase (AST)
  ◊ Alkaline phosphatase
  ◊ Lactate dehydrogenase (LDH)
  ◊ Bilirubin (total)
  ◊ Amylase
  ◊ Uric acid
  ◊ Triglycerides
  ◊ Cholesterol (total and high density lipoprotein fraction)
  ◊ Mean corpuscular volume
  ◊ Prothrombin time
• Suggestive - if decreased:
  ◊ Calcium
  ◊ Phosphorus
  ◊ Magnesium
  ◊ Blood urea nitrogen
  ◊ White blood cell count
  ◊ Platelet count
  ◊ Hematocrit
  ◊ Serum protein
  ◊ Coagulopathy
Drugs that may alter lab results: See manufacturer's profile for each drug patient takes

Disorders that may alter lab results:
Liver, heart, and kidney diseases

PATHOLOGICAL FINDINGS
• Liver: inflammation or fatty infiltration (alcoholic hepatitis), periportal fibrosis (alcoholic cirrhosis - occurs in only 20% of alcoholics)
• Gastric mucosa: inflammation, ulceration
• Pancreas: inflammation, liquefaction necrosis
• Intestine: flattening of villi, loss of enzymes
• Heart: interstitial fibrosis and myofibril atrophy (identical to other dilated cardiomyopathies)
• Immune system: depression of granulocyte production, lymphocyte proliferation response, and cell-mediated immunity
• Endocrine organs: elevated plasma cortisol levels, testicular atrophy, suppression of reproductive hormones in women
• Brain: cortical atrophy, enlarged ventricles

SPECIAL TESTS
• Psychological tests:
  ◊ Michigan Alcohol Screening Test (MAST): 25 item questionnaire, score > 5 indicates alcoholism, sensitivity 90%, specificity 74%
  ◊ Short MAST (SMAST): shortened version of the MAST, 13 questions, score > 3 indicates alcoholism, sensitivity 70%, specificity 74%
  ◊ CAGE: 4 questions, lower sensitivity and specificity, easily administered during a clinical interview, score > 2 suggests alcoholism
• Biologic tests:
  ◊ Mitochondrial AST-to-total AST ratio (investigational, limited availability, sensitivity 85-100%, specificity 81%)
  ◊ Acetate (investigational, limited availability, sensitivity 65%, specificity 92%)

IMAGING
• X-ray: multiple old rib fractures on chest x-ray suggests alcoholism
• CT scan, MRI of brain: cortical atrophy, structural lesions in the thalamic nucleus and basal forebrain

DIAGNOSTIC PROCEDURES Liver biopsy: for diagnosis of alcoholic hepatitis or cirrhosis

TREATMENT

APPROPRIATE HEALTH CARE
• Inpatient or outpatient depending on:
  ◊ Severity of alcoholism
  ◊ Risk of major alcohol withdrawal (delirium tremens)
  ◊ Patient's health
  ◊ Social situation
  ◊ In some cases, detoxification is done as an inpatient, with the remainder of treatment done as an outpatient

- Indications for inpatient alcohol detoxification:
  ◊ Symptoms or complications of major withdrawal, history of delirium tremens
  ◊ Failure to complete prior outpatient detoxification
  ◊ Associated medical problem requiring hospitalization
  ◊ Significant psychiatric symptoms
  ◊ Depressive symptoms, particularly suicidal ideation
  ◊ Lack of physician or other care provider during withdrawal
  ◊ Lack of clear commitment to complete abstinence from alcohol
  ◊ Inadequate social support network (family/friends)

GENERAL MEASURES
- Supportive, non-judgmental attitude helpful
- Addiction specialist consult helpful

SURGICAL MEASURES N/A

ACTIVITY Fully active as tolerated

DIET
- Well balanced (malnutrition common)
- Alcohol interferes with the metabolism of most vitamins
- Patients with alcoholic hepatitis or ketoacidosis may have specific vitamin deficiencies, particularly thiamine
- Other deficiencies include magnesium, phosphate and zinc

PATIENT EDUCATION Information, literature and emotional support (crisis hot line) available from local Alcoholics Anonymous

MEDICATIONS

DRUG(S) OF CHOICE
- For detoxification and management of alcohol withdrawal syndrome:
(dose depends on patient's alcohol tolerance)
  ◊ Chlordiazepoxide (Librium)
  ◊ Diazepam (Valium)
  ◊ Lorazepam: in severe liver disease
  ◊ Phenobarbital: used less often
- Detoxification adjunct: used, as adjuncts to benzodiazepines, in doses adequate to control withdrawal symptoms, suppress seizures and delirium tremens.
  ◊ Beta blockers (propranolol, atenolol): for persistent sinus tachycardia when other withdrawal signs are controlled
  ◊ Clonidine: relieves symptoms of autonomic hyperactivity (tremor, tachycardia, hypertension)
- To promote sobriety:
  ◊ Disulfiram: Contraindicated if patient in denial about alcoholism, is seeking a "quick fix", or if a serious medical condition or poor health status exists.
  ◊ Naltrexone: to reduce craving of alcohol
- Supplemental to all: thiamine 100 mg IV q day (e.g., 50 mg/liter of IV fluids), then 40 mg po daily

Contraindications: Patients who continue to drink while taking detox medications
Precautions:
- Use caution with severe liver disease, organic pain, organic brain syndromes
- Monitor for nystagmus, ataxia, excessive somnolence, slurred speech, other signs of intoxication
Significant Possible Interactions:
- Alcohol and benzodiazepines additive
- Other sedative hypnotics

ALTERNATIVE DRUGS N/A

FOLLOWUP

PATIENT MONITORING
- During detoxification: daily visits, if inpatient, frequent monitoring of vital signs
- Soon after patient completes treatment program: more frequent visits, e.g. weekly
- As patient more established in recovery: less frequent visits

PREVENTION/AVOIDANCE
- Preventive counseling of patients with a family history of alcoholism or other risk factors
- Anticipatory guidance for patients at increased risk due to life changes
- Public health and education measures

POSSIBLE COMPLICATIONS
- Relapse of drinking
- Wernicke-Korsakoff syndrome
- Neuropathy, dementia
- Increased susceptibility to infection
- Aseptic necrosis of the hip
- Malignancies (e.g., of gastrointestinal tract)
- Cirrhosis (women sooner than men)

EXPECTED COURSE/PROGNOSIS
- Chronic relapsing disease
- Untreated alcoholism is progressive and fatal

MISCELLANEOUS

ASSOCIATED CONDITIONS
- Nicotine addiction
- Women have associated reproductive tract disorders, history of sexual abuse or incest; concurrent prescription drug dependence.
- Variety of medical and psychiatric disorders:
  ◊ Depression
  ◊ Anxiety states
  ◊ Bipolar or manic-depressive disease
  ◊ Essential hypertension
  ◊ Peptic ulcer disease
  ◊ Viral gastroenteritis
  ◊ Ischemic heart disease
  ◊ Cholelithiasis
  ◊ Viral hepatitis
  ◊ Diabetes
  ◊ Pancreatitis
  ◊ Hyperlipidemia
  ◊ Solar skin damage

◊ Breast tumor
◊ Primary endocrine disorder
◊ Primary seizure disorder

AGE-RELATED FACTORS
Pediatric:
- Substance abuse (often multiple) has negative impact on normal maturation and development, attainment of social, educational and occupational skills
- Watch for depression, suicide thought or attempts, family disruption, disorderly behavior, violence or destruction of property, poor school or work performance, sexual promiscuity, social immaturity, lack of hobbies or interests, isolation, moodiness
Geriatric:
- Alcoholism often missed; signs and symptoms may be different or attributed to chronic medical problem or dementia
- More hidden due to social unacceptability: self-reports of alcohol consumption inaccurate
- Elderly more sensitive to alcohol effects
- Assessment tools standardized on younger populations often inappropriate
Others: N/A

PREGNANCY
- Alcohol is a morphologic and behavioral teratogen. Greatest teratogenic effect occurs during the early weeks of fetal development.
- Women should abstain when planning conception and throughout pregnancy

SYNONYMS N/A

ICD-9-CM
303 Alcohol dependence syndrome
303.90 Other and unspecified alcohol dependence; unspecified drinking behavior

SEE ALSO N/A

OTHER NOTES N/A

ABBREVIATIONS N/A

REFERENCES
- National Institute on Alcohol Abuse and Alcoholism. Seventh Special Report to the US Congress on Alcohol and Health. DHHS: Rockville, MD, 1990
3 additional references available at web site
Internet references: http://www.5mcc.com
Illustrations: 4 available on CD-ROM

Author(s)
David Frank, MD

Aldosteronism, primary

BASICS

DESCRIPTION The clinical syndrome of hypertension, hypokalemia, low plasma renin activity, and increased aldosterone secretion.
• Unilateral aldosterone-producing adenoma (APA) - cured with unilateral adrenalectomy
• Idiopathic hyperaldosteronism (IHA) due to bilateral zona glomerulosa hyperplasia - not cured with surgery. Chronic medical therapy is treatment of choice.
System(s) affected: Endocrine/Metabolic
Genetics: Unknown
Incidence/Prevalence in USA:
• 5-10% of the hypertensive population
Predominant age: Usually diagnosed third to sixth decades
Predominant sex: APA more common in women

SIGNS AND SYMPTOMS
• Usually asymptomatic
• Most patients are normokalemic
• Marked hypokalemia may be associated with muscle weakness and cramping, headaches, palpitations, polydipsia, polyuria, or nocturia
• Mild to severe hypertension
• Funduscopy - benign or grade 1-2
• Edema (rare)
• Hypokalemia (not required)
• Metabolic alkalosis
• Relative "hypernatremia"
• Impaired glucose tolerance
• Increased incidence of renal cysts

CAUSES
• Unilateral aldosterone-producing adrenal adenoma (APA)
• Idiopathic hyperaldosteronism (IHA)
• Aldosterone-producing adrenocortical carcinoma
• Other rare subtypes

RISK FACTORS N/A

DIAGNOSIS

DIFFERENTIAL DIAGNOSIS
• Diuretic use
• Renovascular hypertension
• Pheochromocytoma
• Renin-secreting tumor
• Malignant hypertension
• Congenital adrenal hyperplasia
• Deoxycorticosterone-producing tumor
• Exogenous mineralocorticoid
• High dose glucocorticoid therapy
• Apparent mineralocorticoid excess syndrome (congenital or acquired due to licorice ingestion)
• Liddle's syndrome

LABORATORY
• Hypokalemia with inappropriate kaliuresis
• Unsuppressible urine or plasma aldosterone levels
• Low ambulatory plasma renin activity
• High plasma aldosterone to renin ratio (> 20 in ng/dL [> 55 nmol/L] and ng/mL/h, respectively)
• Normal glucocorticoid excretion
Drugs that may alter lab results:
Spironolactone
Disorders that may alter lab results:
Malignant hypertension

PATHOLOGICAL FINDINGS Unilateral aldosterone-producing adrenal adenoma (APA), bilateral idiopathic adrenal hyperplasia (IHA), aldosterone-producing adrenocortical carcinoma

SPECIAL TESTS
• Aldosterone suppression test with either a high salt diet or saline infusion
• Posture study
• Spironolactone treatment trial
• Adrenal venous sampling (for aldosterone and cortisol)

IMAGING Adrenal computerized tomography (CT preferred over MRI). Use 3 mm cuts.

DIAGNOSTIC PROCEDURES Adrenal venous sampling

TREATMENT

APPROPRIATE HEALTH CARE
• Unilateral APA - unilateral adrenalectomy
• Bilateral IHA - chronic medical therapy

GENERAL MEASURES
• Unilateral APA - correct hypokalemia preoperatively with spironolactone
• Bilateral IHA - low sodium diet, regular isotonic exercise, maintenance of ideal body weight, tobacco avoidance, potassium-sparing agent, anti-hypertensive agent (e.g., calcium channel antagonist, ACE-inhibitor, low-dose thiazide diuretic)

SURGICAL MEASURES The treatment of choice for patients with an unilateral APA is adrenalectomy. Patients with bilateral IHA are treated medically.

ACTIVITY No limitations

DIET Low sodium

PATIENT EDUCATION N/A

MEDICATIONS

DRUG(S) OF CHOICE
• Potassium-sparing agent - spironolactone (Aldactone)or amiloride (Midamor)
• Antihypertensive agent - calcium channel antagonist, ACE-inhibitor, angiotensin-II receptor antagonist or low-dose thiazide diuretic
Contraindications: Potassium-sparing agent and ACE-inhibitors in renal failure, hyperkalemia, and pregnancy
Precautions: Monitor serum potassium closely after any adjustment in potassium replacement or potassium-sparing agent
Significant possible interactions: Lithium and diuretics, nonsteroidal anti-inflammatory agents with diuretics and ACE-inhibitors

ALTERNATIVE DRUGS   N/A

FOLLOWUP

PATIENT MONITORING
• Blood pressure checks
• Serum potassium check
• 24-hour urine aldosterone following surgery

PREVENTION/AVOIDANCE   N/A

POSSIBLE COMPLICATIONS   Cardiac
arrhythmia associated with severe hypokalemia

EXPECTED COURSE/PROGNOSIS
Surgical removal of an APA results in cure of hypertension in approximately 70% of cases. Hypertension does not resolve immediately post operatively, but rather over 1 to 4 months.

MISCELLANEOUS

ASSOCIATED CONDITIONS   Cystic
renal disease

AGE-RELATED FACTORS
Pediatric: Bilateral adrenal idiopathic hyperplasia is the most common form in children
Geriatric: N/A
Others: N/A

PREGNANCY   Treat hypertension with
agents proven to be safe during pregnancy; avoid spironolactone and ACE-inhibitors

SYNONYMS
• Conn's syndrome
• Hyperaldosteronism

ICD-9-CM
255.1 hyperaldosteronism

SEE ALSO
• Hypertension, essential
• Hypokalemia
• Liddle's syndrome

OTHER NOTES
• Who should be screened for primary aldosteronism?
1) All patients with hypertension and spontaneous hypokalemia
2) All patients with treatment-resistant hypertension

ABBREVIATIONS
APA = aldosterone-producing adenoma
IHA = idiopathic hyperaldosteronism

REFERENCES
• Young WF Jr, Stanton AW, Grant CS, et al: Primary aldosteronism: adrenal venous sampling. Surgery 1996;120:913-920
• Young WF Jr, Hogan MJ: Renin-independent hypermineralocorticoidism. Trends Endocrinol Metab 1994;5:97
• Weinberger MH, Fineberg NS: The diagnosis of primary aldosteronism and separation of the two major subtypes. Arch Int Med 1993;153:2125-2129
Illustrations: N/A
Internet references: http://www.5mcc.com

Author(s)
William F. Young, Jr., MD

Alopecia

BASICS

DESCRIPTION Absence of the hair from skin areas where it normally is present
• Telogen effluvium - diffuse hair loss that results in decreased hair density but does not progress to complete baldness
• Anagen effluvium - diffuse shedding of hairs, including growing hairs, that may progress to complete baldness
• Cicatricial alopecia - also known as scarring alopecia and characterized by slick, smooth scalp without any evidence of follicular openings of hair
• Androgenic alopecia - hair loss occurring in either sex, caused by stimulation of the hair roots by male hormones
• Alopecia areata - patchy, non-scarring hair loss
• Traction alopecia - patchy, initially non-scarring hair loss
• Tinea capitis - patches of hair broken off close to the scalp, with or without associated inflammation, caused by fungus infection
System(s) affected: Skin/Exocrine
Genetics: In Caucasians, androgenic alopecia follows a dominant trait with incomplete penetrance. The hereditary incidence is notable not only in men but also in women with a strong family history of baldness.
Incidence/Prevalence in USA: 50% of Caucasian males by 50 years of age have noticeable male-pattern baldness. 37% of postmenopausal females show some evidence of hair loss.
Predominant age: The incidence of androgenic alopecia increases with increasing age. Tinea capitis and traction alopecia are more common in children.
Predominant sex: Male > Female

SIGNS AND SYMPTOMS
• Hair loss
• Pruritus (in tinea capitis)
• Scaling of the scalp (in tinea capitis)
• Broken hairs (in tinea capitis and traction alopecia)
• Tapered hair at the borders of the patch of alopecia (in alopecia areata)
• Easily removable hairs at the periphery of the patch of alopecia (in alopecia areata)
• Inflammation (in tinea capitis)

CAUSES
• Telogen effluvium
  ◊ Postpartum
  ◊ Drugs (oral contraceptives, anticoagulants, retinoids, beta blockers, chemotherapeutic agents, interferon)
  ◊ Stress (physical or psychological)
  ◊ Hormonal (hypo- or hyperthyroidism, hypopituitarism)
  ◊ Nutritional (malnutrition, iron deficiency, zinc deficiency)
  ◊ Diffuse alopecia areata

• Anagen effluvium
  ◊ Mycosis fungoides
  ◊ X-ray treatment
  ◊ Drugs (chemotherapeutic agents, allopurinol, levodopa, bromocriptine)
  ◊ Poisoning (bismuth, arsenic, gold, boric acid, thallium)
• Cicatricial alopecia
  ◊ Congenital and developmental defects
  ◊ Infection (leprosy, syphilis, varicella-zoster, cutaneous leishmaniasis)
  ◊ Basal cell carcinoma
  ◊ Epidermal nevi
  ◊ Physical agents (acids and alkali, burns, freezing, radiodermatitis)
  ◊ Cicatricial pemphigoid
  ◊ Lichen planus
  ◊ Sarcoidosis
• Androgenic alopecia
  ◊ Adrenal hyperplasia
  ◊ Polycystic ovaries
  ◊ Ovarian hyperplasia
  ◊ Carcinoid
  ◊ Pituitary hyperplasia
  ◊ Drugs (testosterone, danazol, ACTH, anabolic steroids, progesterones)
• Alopecia areata
  ◊ Unknown, but possibly autoimmune
• Traction alopecia
  ◊ Trichotillomania (direct self-pulling of the hair)
  ◊ Tight rollers or braids
• Tinea capitis
  ◊ Microsporum species
  ◊ Trichophyton species

RISK FACTORS
• Positive family history of baldness
• Physical or psychological stress
• Pregnancy
• Poor nutrition

DIAGNOSIS

DIFFERENTIAL DIAGNOSIS Search for type of alopecia and then for possible reversible causes

LABORATORY
• Thyroid function tests
• Complete blood count (may reflect an underlying immunologic disorder)
• Free testosterone and dehydroepiandrosterone sulfate (DHEA-S) in women with androgenic alopecia
• Serum ferritin
• VDRL or RPR for syphilis
• Lymphocyte T and B cell number (sometimes low in patients with alopecia areata)
Drugs that may alter lab results:
• Antifungal drugs may make KOH examination falsely negative
• Thyroid drugs and iodine preparations (including topicals) will alter thyroid function tests
Disorders that may alter lab results: N/A

PATHOLOGICAL FINDINGS Scalp biopsy with routine microscopy and direct immunofluorescence will aid in the diagnosis of tinea capitis, diffuse alopecia areata, and the scarring alopecias due to lupus erythematosus, lichen planus, and sarcoidosis

SPECIAL TESTS
• Light hair-pull test (positive in alopecia areata)
• Direct microscopic examination of the hair shaft
• Potassium hydroxide (KOH) examination of the scale, if present (positive in tinea capitis)
• Fungal culture of the scale, if present

IMAGING N/A

DIAGNOSTIC PROCEDURES Scalp biopsy (sometimes)

TREATMENT

APPROPRIATE HEALTH CARE
Outpatient

GENERAL MEASURES
• Telogen effluvium - maximum shedding 3 months after the inciting event (medication, stress, nutritional deficiency) and recovery following correction of the cause. Rarely permanent baldness.
• Anagen effluvium - shedding begins days to a few weeks after the inciting event with recovery following correction of the cause. Rarely permanent baldness.
• Cicatricial alopecia - hair follicles are permanently damaged. Only effective treatment is surgical (graft transplantation, flap transplantation, or excision of the scarred area).
• Androgenic alopecia - by 12 months of using topical minoxidil, 39% of subjects reported moderate to marked hair growth. Other treatments for androgenic alopecia are surgical (hair transplantation, scalp reduction, transposition flap, and soft tissue expansion).
• Alopecia areata - usually the disease resolves within three years without treatment. Recurrences are, however, common.
• Traction alopecia - only with discontinuation of the hair pulling will the disorder resolve. Psychologic or psychiatric intervention may be necessary. Successful therapeutic approaches have included medications, behavior modification, and hypnosis.
• Tinea capitis - six to eight weeks of therapy are often necessary. Careful handwashing and laundering of headwear and towels.

SURGICAL MEASURES N/A

ACTIVITY Fully active

DIET No special diet

PATIENT EDUCATION National Alopecia Areata Foundation, 714 C Street, San Rafael, CA 94901

MEDICATIONS

DRUG(S) OF CHOICE
• Androgenic alopecia - topical minoxidil (Rogaine) 2%; finasteride (Propecia), 1 mg once daily
• Alopecia areata - high potency topical steroids, topical anthralin
• Tinea capitis - griseofulvin [ultramicrosize] 250-375 mg/day in adults, 5.5-7.3 mg/kg/day in children. Alternatively, ketoconazole 200 mg once daily. Treatment for 6-8 weeks.

Contraindications:
• Griseofulvin - pregnancy, porphyria, hepatocellular failure
• Ketoconazole and cisapride (Propulsid) should not be used together
• Itraconazole and cisapride should not be used together

Precautions:
• Topical minoxidil
◊ Burning and irritation of the eyes
◊ Salt and water retention
◊ Tachycardia
◊ Angina (rare)
• Topical steroids
◊ Local burning and stinging
◊ Pruritus
◊ Skin atrophy
◊ Telangiectasias
◊ Hypothalamic-pituitary-adrenal (HPA) suppression if high-potency steroids used for prolonged duration
• Griseofulvin
◊ Photosensitivity reaction
◊ Lupus-like syndrome
◊ Oral thrush
◊ Granulocytopenia
• Ketoconazole
◊ Anaphylaxis
◊ Hepatotoxicity
◊ Oligospermia
◊ Neuropsychiatric disturbances
◊ Gynecomastia
• Itraconazole
◊ Hepatotoxicity
◊ Nausea, vomiting
• Finasteride
◊ Not indicated for use in women
◊ Caution when there is liver disease

Significant possible interactions:
• Topical minoxidil-guanethidine: may potentiate orthostatic hypotension (rare)
• Griseofulvin-warfarin: decreased activity of warfarin
• Griseofulvin-barbiturates: depressed activity of griseofulvin
• Ketoconazole-warfarin: may enhance the activity of warfarin
• Ketoconazole-isoniazid, rifampin: decreased activity of ketoconazole
• Ketoconazole-phenytoin: may alter the metabolism of either drug
• Itraconazole-terfenadine: prolonged QT and ventricular arrhythmias
• Itraconazole-astemizole: prolonged QT and ventricular arrhythmias
• Itraconazole-cisapride: contraindicated
• Itraconazole-digoxin: may result in elevated levels of digoxin
• H2 blockers or antacids-ketoconazole: decreased absorption of ketoconazole. If concomitant therapy needed, give H2 blocker or antacids at least 2 hours after ketoconazole dose. Avoid using the proton pump inhibitor omeprazole for the same reason.

ALTERNATIVE DRUGS N/A

FOLLOWUP

PATIENT MONITORING With ketoconazole, monitor liver enzymes

PREVENTION/AVOIDANCE N/A

POSSIBLE COMPLICATIONS N/A

EXPECTED COURSE/PROGNOSIS
• Telogen effluvium - rarely permanent baldness
• Anagen effluvium - rarely permanent baldness
• Cicatricial alopecia - the hair follicles are permanently damaged
• Androgenic alopecia - depends on treatment
• Alopecia areata - recurrences are common
• Traction alopecia - depends on behavior modification
• Tinea capitis - usually complete recovery

MISCELLANEOUS

ASSOCIATED CONDITIONS Alopecia areata - Down syndrome, vitiligo, diabetes

AGE-RELATED FACTORS
Pediatric: Tinea capitis only common form of alopecia
Geriatric: Androgenic alopecia more common after 50
Others: N/A

PREGNANCY Post partum hair loss is due to altered physiology during pregnancy

SYNONYMS
• Androgenic alopecia

ICD-9-CM
704.00 alopecia, unspecified
704.01 alopecia areata
704.09 diseases of the hair and hair follicles
110.0 dermatophytosis of the scalp and beard

SEE ALSO
• Lichen planus
• Tinea capitis
• Syphilis
• Cutaneous T cell lymphoma
• Acrodermatitis enteropathica
• Werner's syndrome

OTHER NOTES N/A

ABBREVIATIONS
RPR = rapid plasma reagin
HPA = hypothalamic-pituitary axis

REFERENCES
• Rietschel RL: A simplified approach to the diagnosis of alopecia. Dermatol Clin 1996;14:691-695
• Whiting DA: Chronic telogen effluvium. Dermatol Clin 1996;14:723-731
• Fiedler VC, Alaiti S: Treatment of alopecia areata. Dermatol Clin 1996;14:733-738
• Habif TP: Hair diseases. Clinical Dermatology 1996:739-757
Illustrations: 14 available on CD-ROM
Internet references: http://www.5mcc.com

Author(s)
Aubrey L. Knight, MD

Altitude illness

BASICS

DESCRIPTION Altitude illness is a spectrum of medical problems ranging from mild discomfort to fatal illness that may occur on ascent to higher altitude. It can affect anyone, including the most experienced and fit individual, who ascends to more than about 8,000 feet (2438 m). Several factors appear to be important in adaptation to altitude: How long the ascent takes, how high, and length of stay. There is a great deal of variation between people and an individual's response may vary from ascent to ascent.
• Acute mountain sickness (AMS): Begins within 4 to 6 hours after arrival at altitude, rare below 8,000 feet (2438 m), and affects most above 10,000 (3048 m)
• High altitude pulmonary edema (HAPE): Abnormal accumulation of fluid in the lungs. Begins 24 to 96 hours after arrival at altitude. Rare below 8,000 (2438 m) feet but affects more than 10% of individuals above 14,500 feet (4420 m).
• High altitude cerebral edema (HACE): Indicates swelling of the. It is the least common but most severe of the high altitude illnesses since it can result in permanent injury or death. Occurs 48 to 72 hours after arrival at altitude. Rare below 12,000 feet (3656 m).
System(s) affected: Pulmonary, Cardiovascular, Nervous
Genetics: N/A
Incidence/Prevalence in USA: Unknown
Predominant age: Any age (young, well-conditioned climbers have a higher incidence of altitude illness, probably because they push themselves more)
Predominant sex: Male = Female

SIGNS AND SYMPTOMS
• AMS mild to moderately severe symptoms:
◊ Headache, plus at least one of the following:
◊ Lack of energy and appetite
◊ Mild nausea, vomiting or anorexia
◊ Dizziness
◊ Weakness
◊ Insomnia
• AMS severe symptoms:
◊ Increased headache
◊ Irritability
◊ Marked fatigue
◊ Shortness of breath with exercise
◊ Nausea and vomiting
◊ Irregular or periodic breathing at night (Cheyne-Stokes)
◊ Breathing apnea
• HAPE symptoms:
◊ Excessive shortness of breath on exertion
◊ Severe respiratory distress
◊ Shortness of breath at rest
◊ Dry cough and/or wheezing
◊ Heart rate and respiratory rate increased
◊ Marked periodic breathing present at night
◊ Gurgling breathing
◊ Frothy cough
◊ Wet crackling sounds in the lungs
◊ Confusion
◊ Coma

• HACE symptoms:
◊ Progressive headache that is unrelieved by mild pain relievers
◊ Lack of coordination (e.g., unable to perform a heel-to-toe walk)
◊ Confusion and bizarre behavior followed by unconsciousness
◊ Other symptoms of moderate AMS, such as dizziness, vomiting, and irritability, are usually present

CAUSES The physiology of altitude illness is still not completely understood. The fundamental problem results from the fact that with increasing altitude there is a progressive decrease in barometric pressure and a corresponding lower partial pressure of oxygen in inspired air, resulting in less oxygen delivery to the body.

RISK FACTORS
• In general, the faster the ascent and the higher, the more likely a person will experience symptoms of altitude illness
• Chronic illness
• Lack of conditioning

DIAGNOSIS

DIFFERENTIAL DIAGNOSIS
• Viral upper respiratory infection
• Gastroenteritis
• Pneumonia
• Other infections
• Cerebral vascular accident
• Ketoacidosis
• Pulmonary emboli
• Congestive heart failure

LABORATORY
• AMS: Laboratory studies are nonspecific and rarely required for diagnosis
• HAPE: WBC - often slightly elevated, erythrocyte sedimentation rate normal
• Arterial blood gas - may show hypoxia, hypocapnea, alkalosis
Drugs that may alter lab results: N/A
Disorders that may alter lab results: N/A

PATHOLOGICAL FINDINGS N/A

SPECIAL TESTS ECG may show only sinus tachycardia, possibly right heart strain

IMAGING Chest x-ray (in HAPE) shows Kerley's lines and a patchy distribution of edema

DIAGNOSTIC PROCEDURES N/A

TREATMENT

APPROPRIATE HEALTH CARE
Outpatient for mild cases, inpatient for severe cases

GENERAL MEASURES
• Therapy must be tailored to fit severity of disease and may be constrained by the environment
• Definitive treatment is to descend to a lower altitude. Dramatic improvement accompanies even modest reductions in altitude (as little as 1,000 feet [305 m]).
• Oxygen, given continuously at 1-2 liters per minute helps relieve symptoms. For severe symptoms, continuous oxygen should be administered and descent to a lower altitude is mandatory.
• AMS
◊ Stop ascent. Acclimatize at the same altitude; give acetazolamide 125 -250 mg orally two times a day, or descend 460 m (1500 ft) or more until symptoms resolved
• HAPE and HACE
◊ Patient must be treated by immediate evacuation to a lower altitude. Occasionally, however, foul weather, lack of transportation or long distances prevent immediate evacuation. In these cases, supportive measures, such as bedrest and oxygen, will help.
◊ Hyperbaric therapy is another effective and practical alternative when descent is not possible. A portable hyperbaric chamber, the "Gamow Bag," made of fabric and weighing only 8 pounds (3.6 kg) can be inflated to 2 pounds per square inch (13.8 kPa) using a foot pump. This is equivalent to a drop in altitude of about 5,000 feet (1524 m). Improvement is usually immediate after being placed in the hyperbaric chamber.
◊ If patient is hospitalized, rule out any other pulmonary disease first, provide adequate oxygen (possibly by intubation or positive end-expiratory pressure [PEEP]), bed rest, diuresis if needed and postural drainage

SURGICAL MEASURES N/A

ACTIVITY Rest until symptoms clear

DIET Increased intake of fluids, a light diet, and avoidance of alcohol

PATIENT EDUCATION See guidelines in Prevention/Avoidance

MEDICATIONS

DRUG(S) OF CHOICE
• Aspirin or codeine can be used to relieve the headache. Antibiotics, if infection is present.
• Both dexamethasone and acetazolamide have been used to treat patients with severe symptoms of AMS. Dosage of dexamethasone is 8 mg initially, followed by 4 mg every six hours by mouth. Doses of acetazolamide of up to 1.0 g/day may be required for effective treatment.
• Dexamethasone may be effective in mild cases of HAPE, but this has not been proven
• Diuretics have not been useful
• Corticosteroids should be given even though their effectiveness is questionable
Contraindications: Refer to manufacturer's profile of each drug
Precautions: Refer to manufacturer's profile of each drug
Significant possible interactions: Refer to manufacturer's profile of each drug

ALTERNATIVE DRUGS   N/A

FOLLOWUP

PATIENT MONITORING
• For mild cases, no follow-up needed
• For more severe cases, follow until symptoms subside
• If underlying cardiopulmonary or cardiovascular disease, follow as needed

PREVENTION/AVOIDANCE
• General guidelines
  ◊ Staged ascent: "Staging" is the process of remaining at an intermediate altitude (6600 to 9800 feet [2012 to 2988 m]) for a few days before attempting the ultimate altitude
  ◊ Conventional prescription for avoiding altitude illness is to allow one day to ascend and acclimatize each 1,000 feet (305 m) from elevations of 10,000 to 14,000 feet (3,048 to 4,267 m). Two days per 1,000 feet (305 m) at elevations above 14,000 feet (4267 m.
  ◊ Sleeping elevation - climber's maximum "climb high and sleep low" is a prudent practice for anyone going above 12,000 feet (3656 m)
  ◊ Adequate hydration - dehydration increases the likelihood of and worsens the symptoms of AMS
  ◊ Good physical conditioning
  ◊ Consider carrying a supply of oxygen
• Drug prophylaxis
  ◊ Acetazolamide (if patient has a history of problems at altitude and/or plans a rapid ascent to above 8,000 feet [2438 m] in a car or airplane). Dosage is usually 250 mg orally twice daily, starting 24 hours before ascent and continuing for two to three days while at altitude. Anyone with a known drug allergy to sulfa should avoid acetazolamide.
  ◊ Dexamethasone may significantly reduce the incidence and severity of acute mountain sickness. The dosage is 2 to 4 mg every six hours, begun the day of the ascent, continued for three days at the higher altitude, then tapered over five days. Adverse side effects are uncommon.

POSSIBLE COMPLICATIONS
• Without treatment, HACE can cause motor and sensory deficits, seizures and coma
• HAPE may progress to cyanosis and respiratory distress syndrome
• Patient may experience high altitude retinal hemorrhage (HARH) - can cause visual changes, but is usually asymptomatic

EXPECTED COURSE/PROGNOSIS
• Mild to moderate AMS resolves over 1-3 days. Patients may resume ascent once symptoms subside.
• HAPE and HACE patients can expect complete recovery, if there is no underlying disease. Should not resume ascent.
• Problems are more likely to recur in people who have had one or more attacks

MISCELLANEOUS

ASSOCIATED CONDITIONS   N/A

AGE-RELATED FACTORS
Pediatric: Children under 6 are more susceptible than adults
Geriatric: Elderly more likely to have chronic conditions (coronary artery disease, congestive heart failure, chronic obstructive pulmonary disease) that may be exacerbated at altitudes of 6000-8000 feet (1829-2438 m)
Others: Women in premenstrual phase are more vulnerable

PREGNANCY   N/A

SYNONYMS   Mountain sickness

ICD-9-CM
993.2 Other and unspecifiec effects of high altitude

SEE ALSO   N/A

OTHER NOTES   N/A

ABBREVIATIONS
• AMS = acute mountain sickness
• HACE = high altitude cerebral edema
• HAPE = high altitude pulmonary edema

REFERENCES
• Zell SC, Goodman PH: Acetazolamide and dexamethasone in the prevention of acute mountain sickness. West J Med 1988;148:541
• Johnson TS, Rock PB: Current concepts, acute mountain sickness. New Engl J Med 1988;319:841
Illustrations: N/A
Internet references: http://www.5mcc.com

Author(s)
Tejal Parikh, MD
Kevin Carmichael, MD

Alzheimer's disease

BASICS

DESCRIPTION A degenerative organic mental disease characterized by progressive intellectual deterioration and dementia; usually occurring after age 65. The diagnosis is made on clinical grounds after ruling out treatable disorders with similar characteristics. Long-term care cost to the nation is approximately $100 billion/year.
Usual course - progressive; chronic.
System(s) affected: Nervous
Genetics: Positive family history in 50% of cases. Markers on chromosomes: 1 and 14 (early onset disease); 12,19 (late onset); 21 (onset age 50-65).
Incidence/Prevalence in USA: 4 million cases/350 million people. 40% of those over age 85 are affected.
Predominant age: >60
Predominant sex: Female > Male (slightly)

SIGNS AND SYMPTOMS
• Acalculia
• Agnosia
• Anhedonia
• Anxiety
• Apathy
• Aphasia
• Apraxia
• Confabulation
• Delusions
• Dementia
• Depression
• Impaired abstraction
• Intellectual decline
• Loss of interest
• Occupational dysfunction
• Personality change
• Progressive cognitive impairment
• Recent memory loss (key finding)
• Restlessness
• Sleep disturbances
• Social withdrawal
• Visuospatial distortion
• Weight loss
• Late signs – seizures, myoclonus, extrapyramidal dysfunction, incontinence

CAUSES
• Unknown, but toxic beta-amyloid deposits in neuritic plaques and arteriolar walls appear critical to pathogenesis. Beta-amyloid precursor gene localized to chromosome 21.
• Unsubstantiated possibilities - slow virus, bacterial infection (*Chlamydia pneumoniae*), metals (aluminum), accelerated aging, autoimmune attack

RISK FACTORS
• Aging
• Head trauma
• Low education level
• Down syndrome
• Positive family history
• Inheritance of the E4 allele of apolipoprotein E gene on chromosome 19 (E4 is much less of a risk factor for African Americans and Hispanics)

DIAGNOSIS

DIFFERENTIAL DIAGNOSIS
• Vascular dementia
• Multi-infarct dementia
• Dementia associated with Parkinson's
• Normal pressure hydrocephalus
• Creutzfeldt-Jakob disease
• End-stage multiple sclerosis
• Brain tumor – primary or metastatic
• Subdural hematoma
• Progressive multifocal leukoencephalopathy
• Metabolic dementia (hypothyroidism)
• Drug reactions
• Alcoholism and other addictions
• Dementia pugilistica
• Subcortical dementias
• Depression (persistent diminished interest and pleasure, insomnia or hyposomnia, psychomotor retardation, feelings of hopelessness and helplessness, thoughts of death, decreased ability to concentrate)
• Toxicity from liver or kidney failure
• Vitamin and other nutritional deficiencies
• Vasculitis
• Lewy body disease
• Neurosyphilis

LABORATORY
• To help rule out other causes of dementia:
  ◊ CBC
  ◊ Chemistry panel
  ◊ Thyroid function studies
  ◊ Folate and B-12 levels
  ◊ VDRL
  ◊ Sedimentation rate
  ◊ HIV antibody (selected cases)
Drugs that may alter lab results: N/A
Disorders that may alter lab results: N/A

PATHOLOGICAL FINDINGS
• Gross - diffuse cerebral atrophy in association areas, hippocampus, amygdala and some subcortical nuclei
• Micro - pyramidal cell loss
• Micro - decreased cholinergic innervation (other neurotransmitters variably decreased)
• Micro - neuritic senile plaques
• Micro - degeneration of locus ceruleus and basal forebrain nuclei of Meynert
• Neurofibrillary tangles
• Amyloid angiopathy common

SPECIAL TESTS
• Cerebrospinal fluid (depending on circumstances and clinical information)
• Extensive neuropsychological battery - only needed if clinical picture is confusing

IMAGING
• Head CT/MRI - moderate cortical atrophy, ventricular enlargement - to rule out infarcts, subdural hematomas, normal pressure hydrocephalus, neoplasm
• MRI-based hippocampal volumetry, positron emission tomography (PET) and single photon emission computed tomography (SPECT) have not yet reached clinical reality as tools to distinguish early Alzheimer's disease from other dementias

DIAGNOSTIC PROCEDURES
• This is a clinical diagnosis - history, physical examination, tests (neurological and memory)
• More specific tests (CSF beta-amyloid, tau, AD7C levels; urinary AD7C; excessive pupillary dilatation to mydriatics) still investigational
• Testing for E4 allele of apolipoprotein E gene is available (but is not officially recommended) for assessing prognosis of early memory loss or predicting risk of dementia in patient's relatives

TREATMENT

APPROPRIATE HEALTH CARE
Outpatient, day care, assisted living center, nursing home (when necessary)

GENERAL MEASURES
• Supportive
• Optimize treatment of associated co-morbidities
• Exercises to reduce restlessness
• Occupational therapy
• Music therapy
• Continued cognitive challenge – shown to slow deterioration rate
• Analyze environment for safety and security
• Consider day care centers
• Assess needs of spouse/care giver
• Consider nursing home
• Referrals to:
  ◊ Visiting nurse
  ◊ Social worker
  ◊ Physical therapist
  ◊ Occupational therapist
  ◊ Lawyer
  ◊ Support groups for patient and family

SURGICAL MEASURES N/A

ACTIVITY To whatever extent possible

DIET No special diet

PATIENT EDUCATION
• Printed patient and family information available from: Alzheimer's Association, 919 N. Michigan Ave., Suite 1000, Chicago, IL, (312)335-8700, (800)272-3900
• Help family understand the progressive nature of the disease
• Arrange durable power of attorney
• Advance directives planning as early as possible

Alzheimer's disease

MEDICATIONS

DRUG(S) OF CHOICE
• No specific drug therapy available for halting disease. Clinical studies are ongoing.
• Use as few drugs as possible. Alzheimer's patients tolerate them poorly.
• No drugs are helpful for – wandering, restlessness, fidgeting, uncooperativeness, hoarding, irritability. Use behavioral techniques.
• For depression (which occurs in 1/3 of patients), use selective serotonin reuptake inhibitors or trazodone (Desyrel). Start with half the usual adult dose.
• For insomnia – can try trazodone 25-100 mg qhs, zolpidem (Ambien) 5 mg qhs or temazepam (Restoril) 7.5-15 mg qhs
• For moderate anxiety/restlessness – can try low dose, short-acting benzodiazepines, but efficacy unproven
• For severe aggressive agitation, especially if psychotic features present (delusions, hallucinations), use low dose butyrophenones or phenothiazines. Risperidone (Risperdal) 0.5 -1.0 mg bid and other newer atypical antipsychotic agents useful in this setting due to better side effect profile. Remember to attempt periodic dose reductions or discontinuation, especially in nursing home patient (see OBRA [Omnibus Reconciliation Act] 1987).
• Carbamazepine (Tegretol) 100 mg bid-tid, propranolol (Inderal) 10-40 mg bid-tid, trazodone 200 mg/day and valproic acid 250-1,500 mg/day also anecdotally reported in literature to help with severe aggressive agitation. SSRI's also being tried.
• For memory enhancement – donepezil (Aricept) 5-10 mg qd has supplanted tacrine (Cognex) as the agent of choice. Indicated in mild to moderate disease (Folstein's MMSE scores 10-24). 30-50% of patients will respond - average response is moving patient back up the slope of decline by 12 months. Unlike tacrine, no liver toxicity seen. Most common side effects are gastrointestinal disturbances.
• A recent study supported efficacy of selegiline 5 mg bid and/or vitamin E, 1000 IU bid in slowing progression of disease
• NSAIDs and estrogen replacement therapy are consistently related to lesser incidence and slower progression of Alzheimer's disease. No standards for routine use exist.
• Randomized clinical trials exploring efficacy of corticosteroids, NSAIDs, and estrogen are underway
• New cholinergic agonists and cholinesterase inhibitors are in phase 3 trials; revastigmine (Exelon) close to marketing in 1999

Contraindications:
• Avoid anticholinergic drugs, such as tricyclic antidepressants (TCA) and antihistamines
• Ginkgo biloba - avoid anticoagulants and aspirin

Precautions:
• Benzodiazepines may produce paradoxical excitation or daytime drowsiness
• Triazolam (Halcion) can produce confusion, memory loss and psychotic reactions in the elderly

Significant possible interactions:
• Antipsychotics: lithium may induce extrapyramidal symptoms and disorientation
• Benzodiazepines: increased serum phenytoin concentration. Cimetidine may increase the benzodiazepine concentration.
• Donepezil (Aricept): use with caution with anticholinergic medication or in patients with sick sinus syndrome or a history of peptic ulcers

ALTERNATIVE DRUGS
Ginkgo biloba, 40 mg tid has shown moderate efficacy

FOLLOWUP

PATIENT MONITORING
• As often as necessary to treat poor nutrition, medical complications, monitor drug use, provide support for family, assess need for placement
• Serial mental status testing helpful
• Monitor caregiver burnout

Manifestations of Alzheimer's disease by year

Problem with:	Onset (yrs)
Cognition	0 - 5
Financial mgt	1 - 5
Behavior	2 - 12
Self-bathing	4 - 7
Urinary continence	5 - 8
Death	8 - 12

PREVENTION/AVOIDANCE
• None known for patient
• Family members may seek genetic screening for presence of E4 allele of apolipoprotein E gene (kits already marketed), but such screening is not recommended

POSSIBLE COMPLICATIONS
• Behavioral - hostility, agitation, wandering, uncooperativeness
• Metabolic - infection, dehydration, drug toxicity, malnutrition
• Others - falls, "sundowning"
• Family or caregiver burnout
• Depression occurs in third of patients
• Suicide – in early stages, especially if depression present

EXPECTED COURSE/PROGNOSIS
Poor; 8-10 year average survival

MISCELLANEOUS

ASSOCIATED CONDITIONS
• Down syndrome
• Depression
• Insomnia

AGE-RELATED FACTORS
Pediatric: N/A
Geriatric: A frequent and serious problem in this age group
Others: N/A

PREGNANCY N/A

SYNONYMS
• Presenile dementia
• Senile dementia of the Alzheimer's type (SDAT)
• Primary degenerative dementia

ICD-9-CM
290.0 Senile dementia, uncomplicated
290.10 Presenile dementia, uncomplicated
331.0 Alzheimer's disease

SEE ALSO
• Dementia
• Creutzfeldt-Jakob disease
• Hypothyroidism, adult
• Alcoholism
• Depression
• Anemia, pernicious

OTHER NOTES N/A

ABBREVIATIONS
DAT = dementia of Alzheimer's type

REFERENCES
• Shadler M, Larson EB: What's new in Alzheimer's disease treatment. Postgrad Med 1999;105(1):109-118
• Sloan PD: Advances in the treatment of Alzheimer's disease. Amer Fam Phys 1998;58(7):1577-1586
• Adair JC: Is it Alzheimer's? Hosp Prac 1998;33(8):35-58
• Delagarza VW: New drugs for Alzheimer's disease. Amer Fam Phys 1998;58(5):1175-1182
• Cummings, et al: Alzheimer's disease. Neurology 1998;51(suppl):s2-s17
6 additional references available at web site
Internet references: http://www.5mcc.com
Illustrations: N/A

Author(s)
Frank "Chip" Celestino, MD

Amblyopia

BASICS

DESCRIPTION Amblyopia describes a reduction in visual acuity that cannot be corrected by eyeglasses or contact lenses in the absence of a structural or pathological abnormality of the eye.
System(s) affected: Nervous
Genetics: There is an increased incidence in children where one parent has a history of amblyopia
Incidence/Prevalence in USA:
Approximately 2-2.5% in the general population
Predominant age: May be present from birth or may be detected at any age
Predominant sex: Male = Female

SIGNS AND SYMPTOMS Preschool vision screening is advisable to detect a decrease in visual acuity in one eye

CAUSES
• Strabismic amblyopia is a loss of visual acuity in an individual due to suppression of the images in eye which turns out or in
• Anisometropic amblyopia is present when one eye has a significantly different refractive error than the fellow eye and leads to visual blurring
• Refractive amblyopia is due to uncorrected high refractive error resulting in visual blurring in either or both eyes
• Deprivation amblyopia (amblyopia ex anopsia) is due to relative complete visual deprivation in one eye that can be caused by a congenital abnormality such as a corneal scar or cataract

RISK FACTORS None identified

DIAGNOSIS

DIFFERENTIAL DIAGNOSIS The diagnosis of amblyopia can be confused with an organic lesion causing decreased visual acuity and this must always be excluded before the diagnosis of amblyopia is considered

LABORATORY N/A
Drugs that may alter lab results: N/A
Disorders that may alter lab results: N/A

PATHOLOGICAL FINDINGS N/A

SPECIAL TESTS Examination by an ophthalmologist to screen for unequal refractive error, outward turning, or inward turning of the eye (strabismic amblyopia) and proper vision testing of the eye under monocular conditions. A complete slit lamp and dilated funduscopic examination is necessary to exclude an organic cause for the decreased visual acuity.

IMAGING N/A

DIAGNOSTIC PROCEDURES N/A

TREATMENT

APPROPRIATE HEALTH CARE All children should have complete visual examinations prior to starting school with each eye tested individually. Those children from families with a known history of amblyopia or strabismus should have special exams by an ophthalmologist.

GENERAL MEASURES
• Correction of the underlying disorder should be instituted at the earliest opportunity
• Full refractive correction and/or patching of the stronger eye to encourage visual development of the amblyopic eye is warranted
• Amblyopia never corrects itself spontaneously and will always require treatment. Children do not outgrow amblyopia.
• Surgical correction of an abnormal eye position may also be required

SURGICAL MEASURES N/A

ACTIVITY No restrictions

DIET No special diet

PATIENT EDUCATION All parents should be made aware of the need to have their children's eyes examined prior to starting school

MEDICATIONS

DRUG(S) OF CHOICE N/A
Contraindications: N/A
Precautions: N/A
Significant possible interactions: N/A

ALTERNATIVE DRUGS N/A

FOLLOWUP

PATIENT MONITORING Once the diagnosis of amblyopia is made, the patient needs to be seen frequently at the discretion of the ophthalmologist until complete resolution of the problem occurs

PREVENTION/AVOIDANCE None

POSSIBLE COMPLICATIONS If there is failure to institute proper therapy early, permanent and profound visual loss can be expected

EXPECTED COURSE/PROGNOSIS
Amblyopia is a treatable condition in most cases if the diagnosis is made early. Patching therapy, eyeglasses, and surgical correction of abnormal eye positions can result in near normalcy of vision when instituted early. Visual development occurs during the first several years of life and amblyopia therapy can be effective until approximately age 12.

MISCELLANEOUS

ASSOCIATED CONDITIONS Amblyopia is more common in families with a history of unequal refractive errors, high uncorrected refractive errors, and strabismus

AGE-RELATED FACTORS
Pediatric: More commonly seen in the pediatric age group early in life
Geriatric: When seen in the geriatric population, the diagnosis has usually been made early in childhood
Others: N/A

PREGNANCY N/A

SYNONYMS Lazy eye

ICD-9-CM
368.0 Amblyopia ex anopsia

SEE ALSO
• Strabismus
• Refractive errors

OTHER NOTES
• Deficiency amblyopia: Also known as nutritional optic neuropathy or tobacco-alcohol amblyopia. Deficiencies of B1, B12, or riboflavine may be responsible. Treatment consists of balanced diet, vitamins, and avoidance of alcohol and tobacco.

ABBREVIATIONS N/A

REFERENCES
• Binocular Vision And Ocular Motility. In Ophthalmology Basic and Clinical Science Course. (American Academy of Ophthalmology)
• Harley RD: Pediatric Ophthalmology. Philadelphia, W.B. Saunders Co., 1983
Illustrations: N/A
Internet references: http://www.5mcc.com

Author(s)
Robert M. Kershner, MD, FACS

Amebiasis

BASICS

DESCRIPTION Amebiasis is caused by the intestinal protozoan, Entamoeba histolytica. Infection results from ingestion of fecally contaminated food, such as garden vegetables or by direct fecal-oral transmission. Most persons are asymptomatic or have minimal diarrheal symptoms. In a few patients, invasive intestinal or extraintestinal (e.g., liver, and less commonly kidney, bladder, male or female genitalia, skin, lung, brain) infection results. Amebic abscess of the liver may develop during the acute attack or 1-3 months later; symptoms may be abrupt or insidious.
Entamoeba histolytica has been divided into "pathogenic" and "nonpathogenic" strains. The pathogenic strains commonly cause invasive infection while the noninvasive strains cause only asymptomatic intestinal infection. More recently, the nonpathogenic strains have been assigned to a separate species, E. dispar. Unfortunately, the species cannot be distinguished in a routine clinical laboratory.
System(s) affected: Gastrointestinal, Renal/Urologic, Reproductive, Skin/Exocrine, Nervous
Genetics: N/A
Incidence/Prevalence in USA: Probably <1% overall, but much higher in some risk groups, such as areas with large immigrant populations
Predominant age: All
Predominant sex: Male > Female; probably because of greater occupational exposure

SIGNS AND SYMPTOMS
• Noninvasive infection (up to 99%)
  ◊ Asymptomatic (90%)
  ◊ Mild diarrhea
  ◊ Abdominal discomfort
• Invasive intestinal infection
  ◊ Abdominal pain and tenderness
  ◊ Rectal pain
  ◊ Diarrhea
  ◊ Bloody stools
  ◊ Fever (30%)
  ◊ Systemic toxicity
• Extraintestinal infection
  ◊ Fever
  ◊ Systemic toxicity
  ◊ RUQ abdominal pain and tenderness
  ◊ Nausea and vomiting
  ◊ Diarrhea (50%)
  ◊ Hematuria, dysuria, urinary frequency and urgency

CAUSES Infection is transmitted through contaminated food or water, or through person-to-person contact

RISK FACTORS
• Low socioeconomic status
• Institutional living
• Male homosexuality
• Invasive disease is more common in certain geographic locations, including some parts of Mexico, South Africa, and India

DIAGNOSIS

DIFFERENTIAL DIAGNOSIS
• Other infectious causes of colitis, including shigellosis, Campylobacter infection, pseudomembranous colitis, and occasionally salmonellosis or Yersinia infection
• Noninfectious causes of colitis include ulcerative colitis, Crohn's colitis and ischemic colitis
• Hepatic amebiasis must be distinguished from pyogenic liver abscess or superinfection of amebic abscess

LABORATORY
• Stool for ova and parasites (unfortunately, the sensitivity of this exam is poor). Diarrheal stool should be examined immediately for trophozoites in addition to fixed stool specimens (repeated as necessary). In invasive intestinal infection, stools are bloody, but fecal leukocytes are frequently absent.
• Serologic tests (especially indirect hemagglutination (IHA), positive in 85% of colitis patients and most patients with extraintestinal disease. Serologic tests should be done in patients with idiopathic inflammatory bowel disease to rule out amebiasis.
• In bladder infections – amoebae and/or cysts in urine
Drugs that may alter lab results: Many drugs interfere with stool exams
Disorders that may alter lab results: N/A

PATHOLOGICAL FINDINGS
• Colon biopsy
  ◊ Lysis of mucosal cells (flask ulcers)
  ◊ PAS-stained trophozoites
  ◊ Neutrophils at the periphery
• Liver biopsy
  ◊ Necrosis surrounded by a rim of trophozoites

SPECIAL TESTS N/A

IMAGING CT scan or ultrasound for hepatic infection

DIAGNOSTIC PROCEDURES
• Rectosigmoidoscopy with biopsy
• Needle aspirate of hepatic lesions may be needed to rule out pyogenic infection or superinfection

TREATMENT

APPROPRIATE HEALTH CARE
Outpatient

GENERAL MEASURES
• Fluids and nutrition
• Electrolyte management

SURGICAL MEASURES With severe amebic colitis, surgery may be necessary

ACTIVITY In accordance with illness of patient

DIET As tolerated

PATIENT EDUCATION Avoid conditions of re-exposure

MEDICATIONS

DRUG(S) OF CHOICE
• Noninvasive infection
  ◊ Diiodohydroxyquin [also called iodoquinol] 650 mg tid for 20 days
• Invasive infection
  ◊ Metronidazole (Flagyl) 750 mg tid for 5-10 days, followed by a 20 day course of diiodohydroxyquin to eliminate intestinal carriage

Contraindications:
• Diiodohydroxyquin - use cautiously in patients with thyroid diseases. Contraindicated in hepatic or renal dysfunction. May cause optic neuritis or peripheral neuropathy.
• Known allergy to given medication

Precautions: None of the agents are proven safe in pregnancy, but pregnant women with invasive disease should still be treated

Significant possible interactions:
• Metronidazole-ethanol: disulfiram reaction

ALTERNATIVE DRUGS
• Noninvasive infection
  ◊ Diloxanide 500 mg tid for 10 days
  ◊ Paromomycin 500 mg tid for 10 days
• Invasive infection
  ◊ Dehydroemetine [as effective as metronidazole, but cardiotoxic] 1-1.5 mg/kg/day IM for 5 days
  ◊ Chloroquine [less effective] 600 mg base/day for 2 days, then 200 mg/day for 2-3 weeks. Children 10 mg/kg/day up to maximum of 300 mg/day.
  ◊ Tinidazole 600-800 mg tid for 5 days (not available in US)

FOLLOWUP

PATIENT MONITORING
Patient signs and symptoms, stool for ova and parasite

PREVENTION/AVOIDANCE
Avoid risk factors when possible

POSSIBLE COMPLICATIONS
• Toxic megacolon with rupture
• Rupture of hepatic abscess which may perforate into subphrenic space, right pleural cavity or other nearby organs
• Bladder perforation, urethral strictures, vesicointestinal fistula

EXPECTED COURSE/PROGNOSIS
Untreated invasive amebiasis is frequently fatal. With treatment, improvement usually occurs within a few days. Some patients with amebic colitis have irritable bowel symptoms for weeks after successful treatment. Relapses possible.

MISCELLANEOUS

ASSOCIATED CONDITIONS N/A

AGE-RELATED FACTORS
Pediatric: More severe in neonates
Geriatric: More severe in elderly
Others: More severe in patients on corticosteroids and other immunocompromised patients

PREGNANCY
More severe in pregnancy. Most agents are avoided in pregnancy (especially first trimester) because of concerns of teratogenicity, but invasive disease must still be treated. Paromomycin is sometimes recommended for noninvasive disease because it is not absorbed. Infectious disease consultation should be obtained.

SYNONYMS
• Amebic colitis
• Amebic dysentery

ICD-9-CM
006.0 Acute amebic dysentery without mention of abscess
006.3 Amebic liver abscess
006.5 Amebic brain abscess
006.8 Amebic infection of other sites
006.9 Amebiasis, unspecified

SEE ALSO
• Diarrhea, acute
• Diarrhea, chronic

OTHER NOTES N/A

ABBREVIATIONS N/A

REFERENCES
• Fedorak RN, Rubinoff MJ: Basic Investigation of a Patient with Diarrhea. In: Field M. ed. Diarrheal Diseases. Elsevier Science Publishing Co., Inc., New York, 1991:191-218
• Bruckner DA: Amebiasis. Clin Microbiol Rev 1992;5:356-369
• Ravdin JI, Petri WA Jr: Entamoeba histolytica (amebiasis). In: Mandell GL, Douglas RG, Bennett JE, eds. Principles and Practice of Infectious Diseases. 4th Ed. New York, Churchill Livingstone Inc., 1995:2395-2408
Illustrations: N/A
Internet references: http://www.5mcc.com

Author(s)
Rodney D. Adam, MD

Amenorrhea

BASICS

DESCRIPTION The absence of menses.
• Primary amenorrhea - no menses by age 14 with absence of secondary sexual characteristics, or no menses by age 16 with normal secondary characteristics
• Secondary amenorrhea - the cessation of menses for three cycles or 6 months of amenorrhea
System(s) affected: Reproductive, Endocrine/Metabolic
Genetics: No known genetic pattern
Incidence/Prevalence in USA:
• Incidence of primary amenorrhea 0.3%
• Incidence of secondary amenorrhea 3.3%
Predominant age: Menarche to menopause
Predominant sex: Female only

SIGNS AND SYMPTOMS
• The absence of periods
• Galactorrhea
• Symptoms of hypothyroidism
• Symptoms of early pregnancy
• Signs of androgen excess
• Signs of estrogen deficiency

CAUSES
• Primary amenorrhea
 ◊ Imperforate hymen
 ◊ Agenesis of the uterus and upper 2/3 of the vagina (Müllerian agenesis)
 ◊ Turner's syndrome
 ◊ Constitutional delay
• Secondary amenorrhea
 ◊ Physiological - pregnancy, corpus luteal cyst, breast-feeding, menopause
 ◊ Suppression of the hypothalamic-pituitary axis - post pill amenorrhea, stress, intercurrent illness, weight loss, low body mass index
 ◊ Pituitary disease - ablation of the pituitary gland, Sheehan's syndrome, prolactinoma
 ◊ Uncontrolled endocrinopathies - diabetes, hypo- or hyperthyroidism
 ◊ Polycystic ovarian disease (PCOD), (Stein-Leventhal syndrome)
 ◊ Chemotherapy
 ◊ Pelvic irradiation
 ◊ Endometrial ablation (Asherman's syndrome)
 ◊ Drug therapy - systemic steroids, danazol, GRH-RH analogs, antipsychotics, OCP's
 ◊ Premature ovarian failure

RISK FACTORS
• Over-training (e.g., long-distance runner, ballet dancer)
• Eating disorders
• Psycho-social crisis

DIAGNOSIS

DIFFERENTIAL DIAGNOSIS Includes all of the causes listed above. The most common cause of secondary amenorrhea is early pregnancy.

LABORATORY
• Pregnancy test if negative, obtain:
 ◊ Serum prolactin
 ◊ FSH
 ◊ LH
 ◊ TSH
 ◊ Blood sugar
Drugs that may alter lab results: N/A
Disorders that may alter lab results: Pregnancy, menopause, hyperprolactinemia, ovarian suppression, endocrinopathy

PATHOLOGICAL FINDINGS Due to underlying disease

SPECIAL TESTS
• Progesterone challenge test - 10 mg of medroxyprogesterone acetate orally for 5 days
 ◊ If withdrawal bleeding occurs, amenorrhea most likely due to anovulation
 ◊ If no bleeding, evaluate estrogen status (FSH, LH)

IMAGING
• Ultrasound may show cysts undetectable on pelvic examination
• Radiologic evaluation of the sella turcica if prolactinomas suspected (elevated serum prolactin)

DIAGNOSTIC PROCEDURES
• Laparoscopy - diagnosis of the streak ovaries of Turner's syndrome, or polycystic ovarian disease
• Hysterosalpingogram - to rule out Asherman's syndrome

TREATMENT

APPROPRIATE HEALTH CARE
Outpatient

GENERAL MEASURES Definitive treatment depends on determining the cause of the amenorrhea. May not be necessary to treat all cases especially if just temporary amenorrhea.

SURGICAL MEASURES
• Hymenectomy, done as a day surgery, will be required for those whose primary amenorrhea is due to imperforate hymen
• Lysis at adhesions in Asherman's syndrome

ACTIVITY No restrictions

DIET Correct overweight or underweight by dietary management

PATIENT EDUCATION
• Consists of fully informing the patient of your findings, including the presence or absence of pregnancy, and of the underlying cause
• Specific educational resources can be utilized as necessary, e.g., prenatal classes, menopause support groups
• Specific information should be given about the expected duration of amenorrhea (temporary or permanent), effect on fertility, and the long-term sequelae of untreated amenorrhea (e.g., osteoporosis, vaginal dryness)
• Appropriate contraceptive advice should be given, as fertility returns before menses
• Additional support may be needed if the amenorrhea is associated with a reduction in, or loss of, fertility
• Society for Menstrual Cycle Research, 10559 N. 104th Place, Scottsdale, AZ 85258, (602)451-9731

MEDICATIONS

DRUG(S) OF CHOICE
• Progesterone replacement - medroxyprogesterone (Provera) 5 mg bid for 5 days, will result in a withdrawal bleed if the hypothalamo-pituitary-ovarian axis is intact and there is some endogenous estrogen production
• Estrogen replacement - conjugated estrogen, conjugated (Premarin) 0.625 mg for 25 days with progesterone added as above for the last 10 days will result in a withdrawal bleed if the uterus and lower genital tract are normal
• Use of hormonal therapies will not correct underlying problem. Other drugs might be required to treat specific conditions, e.g., bromocriptine for hyperprolactinemia.
• Use of hormonal replacement therapy is recommended after 6 months of amenorrhea (regardless of the primary cause) in order to reduce the risks of osteoporosis and hypercholesterolemia secondary to hypoestrogenism
• Calcium supplementation 1500 mg/day if cause is hypoestrogenism

Contraindications:
• Pregnancy
• Thromboembolic disease
• Previous myocardial infarct, cerebrovascular accident
• Estrogen-dependent malignancy
• Severe hepatic impairment or disease

Precautions:
• Diabetes
• Seizure disorder
• Migraine headache
• Smoker over 35

Significant possible interactions:
Barbiturates, phenytoin, rifampin, corticosteroids, theophyllines, tricyclics, oral anticoagulants (anticoagulant effect may be decreased)

ALTERNATIVE DRUGS
Use of oral contraceptives for hormonal replacement if patient has difficulty following above regimen

FOLLOWUP

PATIENT MONITORING
Depends on the cause, and the treatment chosen. If hormonal replacement is used, discontinuation after six months is advised, to assess spontaneous resumption of menses.

PREVENTION/AVOIDANCE
Maintenance of proper body mass index (BMI)

POSSIBLE COMPLICATIONS
• Estrogen deficiency symptoms, e.g., hot flushes, vaginal dryness
• Osteoporosis, in prolonged hypoestrogenic amenorrhea
• Increased risk of endometrial cancer in hyperestrogenism

EXPECTED COURSE/PROGNOSIS
Reflects the underlying cause. In secondary amenorrhea from hypothalamo-pituitary suppression, spontaneous resumption of menses with time (99% within 6 months) and correction of body mass index.

MISCELLANEOUS

ASSOCIATED CONDITIONS N/A

AGE-RELATED FACTORS
Pediatric: Primary amenorrhea commonly diagnosed in this group
Geriatric: N/A
Others: N/A

PREGNANCY One of the primary causes

SYNONYMS N/A

ICD-9-CM
626.0 Absence of menstruation

SEE ALSO
• Polycystic ovarian disease
• Diabetes mellitus, Type 1
• Diabetes mellitus, Type 2
• Hypothyroidism, adult
• Hyperthyroidism
• Osteoporosis

OTHER NOTES
• Use of hormonal replacement therapy is symptomatic and is discretionary if amenorrhea is temporary (e.g., hypothalamopituitary suppression)
• Patients who are amenorrheic and wish to become pregnant should not be given hormone replacement therapy, but should receive treatment for infertility based on specific cause
• Women less than age 30 with ovarian failure should have Karyotype analysis

ABBREVIATIONS N/A

REFERENCES
• Yen SSC, Jaffe RB, eds: Reproductive Endocrinology. 3rd Ed. Philadelphia, W.B. Saunders Co., 1991
• Speroff L, Glass R, Kase N, eds: Clinical Gynecology, Endocrinology and Infertility. 5th Ed. Baltimore, Williams & Wilkins, 1994
• Kiningham R, Apgar B, Schwenk T: Evaluation of amenorrhea, AM Fam Phys 1996;53:1185-1194
Illustrations: N/A
Internet references: http://www.5mcc.com

Author(s)
Barbara J. Moront, MD
Graham S. Kaiser, DO

Amyloidosis

BASICS

DESCRIPTION A disease characterized by increased deposition of amyloid fibrils in the tissues. Several different proteins may give rise to amyloid. These proteins are present due to their overproduction or decreased clearance. Their deposition may lead to compromise of vital organ function. The most common types of amyloidosis are:
• Primary amyloidosis: usually associated with the plasma cell disorders multiple myeloma and MGUS (monoclonal gammopathy of undetermined significance)
• Secondary amyloidosis: associated with several chronic inflammatory diseases such as rheumatoid arthritis, osteomyelitis, malaria, tuberculosis, leprosy and familial Mediterranean fever
• Familial (hereditary) amyloidosis may occur in almost every ethnic group
• Hemodialysis amyloidosis: associated with renal hemodialysis
System(s) affected: Endocrine/Metabolic, Cardiovascular, Pulmonary, Renal/Urologic, Musculoskeletal, Gastrointestinal, Nervous, Skin/Exocrine
Genetics: N/A
Incidence/Prevalence in USA:
• Primary amyloidosis: 5.1-12.8 per million person years
• Secondary amyloidosis: very rare
• Familial amyloidosis: 1 per million person years
Predominant age: 60-70
Predominant sex: Male > Female (2:1)

SIGNS AND SYMPTOMS

May be highly variable depending upon which organ system is affected and to what degree:
• Fatigue, weight loss, gastroparesis, pseudo-obstruction, malabsorption, diarrhea, macroglossia
• Peripheral neuropathy, carpal tunnel syndrome
• Ascites, hepatomegaly
• Dyspnea, interstitial lung disease, congestive heart failure, arrhythmia, sudden death
• Hilar adenopathy, mediastinal adenopathy
• Symmetrical polyarthritis, rubbery peri-articular soft tissue swelling
• Translucent/waxy skin papules, purpura (especially peri-orbital purpura), edema
• Renal failure, nephrotic syndrome
• Dementia (may play a role in development of Alzheimer's disease)

CAUSES

• Primary amyloidosis: The amyloid consists of immunoglobulin light chains (AL) which are overproduced in plasma disorders.
• Secondary amyloidosis: The amyloid consists of amyloid fibrillary protein (AA) formed from serum amyloid protein (SAA), which is overproduced in chronic inflammatory conditions
• Familial (hereditary) amyloidosis: The amyloid consists of abnormal transthyretin protein (ATTR) produced in the liver

• Hemodialysis amyloidosis: The amyloid consists of beta-2-microglobulin which is normally cleared by the kidney, but cannot be cleared by hemodialysis

RISK FACTORS

• Underlying plasma cell dyscrasia
• Underlying chronic inflammatory disease
• Familial Mediterranean fever
• Hemodialysis

DIAGNOSIS

DIFFERENTIAL DIAGNOSIS

• Peripheral neuropathy - diabetes mellitus, alcoholism, vitamin deficiencies
• Carpal tunnel syndrome - hypothyroidism, trauma, rheumatoid arthritis, etc.
• Restrictive cardiomyopathy: acute viral myocarditis, endomyocardial fibrosis, sarcoidosis, hemochromatosis
• Nephrotic syndrome - glomerulonephritis, renal vein thrombosis
• Renal failure - glomerulonephritis, obstructive uropathy, toxin or drug-induced, acute tubular necrosis
• Symmetric polyarthritis - rheumatoid arthritis, psoriatic arthritis, SLE
• Interstitial lung disease - connective tissue diseases, infectious, sarcoidosis, drug-induced, pneumoconiosis
• Demential - Alzheimer's disease and multi-infarct dementia

LABORATORY

• Anemia may be present
• Hypothyroidism may be present due to amyloidosis of the thyroid
• Renal insufficiency present in ~50%
• Proteinuria present in almost 80%
• In primary amyloidosis, an elevated monoclonal protein level will be found in the serum and/or urine
• In secondary amyloidosis, tests to assess the underlying inflammatory disease will be useful. In familial amyloidosis, an abnormal transthyretin protein may be isolated.
Drugs that may alter lab results: N/A
Disorders that may alter lab results: N/A

PATHOLOGICAL FINDINGS

• Demonstration of amyloid deposits in tissues
• With Congo red staining, amyloid produces a green birefringence under polarized light
• Electron microscopy is the definitive diagnostic tool

SPECIAL TESTS N/A

IMAGING Echocardiography (if cardiac involvement is suspected)

DIAGNOSTIC PROCEDURES

• Rectal biopsy (70% positive)
• Bone marrow biopsy (20% positive)
• Abdominal fat pad biopsy (up to 85% positive)
• Endomyocardial biopsy
• Renal biopsy

TREATMENT

APPROPRIATE HEALTH CARE
Outpatient except for serious complications (congestive heart failure, renal failure)

GENERAL MEASURES Change from hemodialysis to peritoneal dialysis, which clears beta-2-microglobulin, in those with hemodialysis amyloidosis

SURGICAL MEASURES
• Splenectomy may ameliorate this condition by decreasing the amount of amyloid produced
• Renal transplantation may improve the status of renal amyloidosis
• Liver transplantation may cure familial (hereditary) amyloidosis
• Other measures: Treatment of multiple myeloma with bone marrow transplantation is an option for some patients
• Pacemaker may be indicated in those with amyloid-induced conduction defects

ACTIVITY Fully active as tolerated

DIET
• Low protein, low salt for renal failure patients
• Low salt for congestive heart failure patients

PATIENT EDUCATION
• For more information:
  ◊ National Organization for Rare Disorders (NORD), Box 8923, New Fairfield, CT 06812
  ◊ National Institute of Diabetes, Digestive and Kidney Disorders Information Clearinghouse, Bldg 31, Rm 9A04, Bethesda, MD 20892
• For genetic information and counseling referrals:
  ◊ March of Dimes Birth Defects Foundation, 1275 Mamaroneck Ave., White Plains, NY 10605
  ◊ National Center for Education in Maternal and Child Health

MEDICATIONS

DRUG(S) OF CHOICE
• Primary amyloidosis
◊ Treatment of the underlying plasma cell disorder may or may not affect the outcome
◊ Melphalan and prednisone are among the drugs of choice for plasma cell disorders. Colchicine may slow the progression of amyloid deposition.
• Secondary amyloidosis
◊ Treatment of the underlying inflammatory process with disease-specific medications usually improves the outcome (i.e., isoniazid and rifampin for M. Tuberculosis, methotrexate for rheumatoid arthritis)
◊ Tacrine and donepezil have been approved for mild to moderate dementia caused by Alzheimer's disease
◊ Colchicine, 0.6 mg two or three times a day may improve familial Mediterranean fever
• Familial amyloidosis
◊ None
• Hemodialysis amyloidosis
◊ None
Contraindications: Refer to manufacturer's literature
Precautions:
• Colchicine - bone marrow depression, including agranulocytosis, pancytopenia, thrombocytopenia, or aplastic anemia, may occur with prolonged administration. Monitor CBC periodically. Counsel patient to report symptoms/signs of infection promptly (headache, sore throat, fever).
• Tacrine - significant liver function abnormalities in up to one quarter of patients. Monitor LFT's closely.
Significant possible interactions: Refer to manufacturer's literature

ALTERNATIVE DRUGS N/A

FOLLOWUP

PATIENT MONITORING
• Primary amyloidosis
◊ Regular testing of monoclonal protein levels to assess response to therapy
◊ Regular testing of renal function to assess response to therapy
• Secondary and hemodialysis amyloidosis
◊ Follow-up to assess control of the underlying disease process
◊ Regular testing of renal function to assess degree of impairment

PREVENTION/AVOIDANCE N/A

POSSIBLE COMPLICATIONS Despite
intervention, worsening renal failure, heart failure, arthropathy, interstitial lung disease, and neuropathy are common

EXPECTED COURSE/PROGNOSIS
• Primary amyloidosis
◊ The prognosis is dependent upon the underlying disease
◊ Once renal failure has developed, the prognosis is usually less than one year
◊ Congestive heart failure has a four month prognosis
◊ Overall prognosis is 12-14 months. Women have better survival chances than men.
• Secondary amyloidosis
◊ The prognosis is much better, depending upon the ability to control the underlying inflammatory process
• Familial and hemodialysis amyloidosis
◊ Highly variable
◊ Liver transplant may be curative

MISCELLANEOUS

ASSOCIATED CONDITIONS
• Amyloid may bind Factor X leading to bleeding problems

AGE-RELATED FACTORS
Pediatric: N/A
Geriatric: In general, older individuals do less well. Age may precipitate familial amyloidosis suggesting an age-related trigger.
Others: N/A

PREGNANCY No information available

SYNONYMS N/A

ICD-9-CM
277.3 amyloidosis

SEE ALSO N/A

OTHER NOTES N/A

ABBREVIATIONS N/A

REFERENCES
• Kyle RA, et al: Primary Systemic Amyloidosis: multivariate analysis for prognostic factors in 168 cases. Blood 1986;68(1):220-4
• Cohen AS, et al: Survival of patients with primary (AL) amyloidosis. Colchicine-treated cases from 1976-1983 compared with cases seen in previous years (1961-1973). Am J Med 1987;82(6):1182-90
• Fiter J, et al: Methotrexate treatment of amyloidosis secondary to rheumatoid arthritis. Clinical Review of Spain 1995;195(6):390-392
• Falk RH, et al: The systemic amyloidosis. NEJM 1997;337(13):898-909
Illustrations: 1 available on CD-ROM
Internet references: http://www.5mcc.com

Author(s)
R. Scott Gorman, MD

Amyotrophic lateral sclerosis

 BASICS

DESCRIPTION A degenerative disease (or group of diseases) which affects the upper and lower motor neurons.
• Amyotrophic lateral sclerosis: the term applied to the sporadic and most common form of the disease. Includes a number of overlapping syndromes such as pseudobulbar palsy, progressive bulbar palsy, progressive muscular atrophy and primary lateral sclerosis.
• Familial ALS: an autosomal dominant or recessive disease which is clinically similar to sporadic ALS but probably represents a distinct entity pathologically and biochemically.
• ALS-Parkinson-dementia complex of Guam: an ALS like syndrome, often, but not always, associated with Parkinson's syndrome and dementia, which is prevalent amongst the Chamorro Indians of Guam (very rare in the USA).
System(s) affected: Nervous
Genetics: Familial ALS
Incidence/Prevalence in USA:
0.4-1.76/100,000 incidence; 5 in 100,000 prevalence
Predominant age: Rare before age 40 years. Incidence increases with age.
Predominant sex: Male = Female

SIGNS AND SYMPTOMS
• Variable combinations of:
  ◊ Unexplained weight loss
  ◊ Focal wasting of muscle groups
  ◊ Limb weakness with variable symmetry and distribution
  ◊ Difficulty walking
  ◊ Difficulty swallowing
  ◊ Slurring of speech
  ◊ Inability to control affect
  ◊ Atrophy of muscle groups, initially in a myotomal distribution
  ◊ Fasciculations (other than calves)
  ◊ Hyperactive deep tendon reflexes (including jaw jerk)
  ◊ Spares cognitive, oculomotor, sensory and autonomic functions

CAUSES
• Sporadic ALS - degeneration of the upper and lower motor neurons with their respective axons. Cause is unknown.
• Familial ALS - a genetically transmitted degenerative disease. Gene locus has been localized to the long arm of chromosome 21 and encodes the enzyme superoxide dismutase (SOD1). At this writing, although activity is reduced, levels of superoxide dismutase have not yet been proven to be low.
• ALS-Parkinson-dementia complex of Guam - possible relationship to ingestion of the cycad nut or to some other environmental toxin

RISK FACTORS
• Age over 40
• Family history of ALS

 DIAGNOSIS

DIFFERENTIAL DIAGNOSIS
• Focal motor neuropathy
• Cervical spondylosis
• Lead intoxication
• Plasma cell dyscrasias
• Spinal muscular atrophy (adult form)
• Primary lateral sclerosis
• Familial spastic paraparesis
• Spinal multiple sclerosis
• Tropical spastic paraparesis

LABORATORY
• Anti GM1 autoantibodies in low titer commonly found
• Possibly reduced levels of nerve growth factor
• There is no simple reliable laboratory test available that confirms the diagnosis of ALS
Drugs that may alter lab results: N/A
Disorders that may alter lab results: N/A

PATHOLOGICAL FINDINGS
• Loss of Betz's cells in the motor cortex
• Atrophic or absent anterior horn cells of spinal cord
• Atrophic or absent neurons within the motor nuclei of the medulla and pons
• Degeneration of the lateral columns of the spinal cord
• Atrophy of the ventral roots
• Grouped atrophy of muscle (motor units)

SPECIAL TESTS N/A

IMAGING N/A

DIAGNOSTIC PROCEDURES
• Electromyography: denervation potentials (fibrillations, positive sharp waves) and often doublets are associated with prominent fasciculations (which suggest anterior horn cell dysfunction). Voluntary motor unit potentials have increased amplitude, long duration and/or polyphasia. The interference pattern is reduced for the force generated and individual motor units have a high rate of discharge.
• Muscle biopsy - will show groups of shrunken angulated muscle fibers (grouped atrophy) amid other groups of fibers with a uniform fiber type (fiber type grouping).

 TREATMENT

APPROPRIATE HEALTH CARE
• Outpatient initially, may ultimately need nursing home placement and/or hospice
• Supportive care for complicating emergencies (aspiration, respiratory failure). Use of a respirator is a major ethical dilemma and is usually not suggested.

GENERAL MEASURES Prosthetic devices, e.g., wheelchair, etc.

SURGICAL MEASURES N/A

ACTIVITY As tolerated

DIET Modify as tolerated. May need tube feedings.

PATIENT EDUCATION Printed material for patients (and reference lists for physicians) available from The Muscular Dystrophy Association, (520)529-2000, (800)572-1717

MEDICATIONS

DRUG(S) OF CHOICE Riluzole produces a slight prolongation in life expectancy
Contraindications: N/A
Precautions: N/A
Significant possible interactions: N/A

ALTERNATIVE DRUGS Therapeutic trials of the efficacy of anti-oxidants (vitamins E, C, and beta-carotene), nerve growth factor, gabapentin, myotrophin and thyrotropin releasing hormone are being undertaken. Preliminary reports are not encouraging.

FOLLOWUP

PATIENT MONITORING
• Initially every three months, frequency to be increased as need for symptomatic therapy develops
• Patients with a presumed diagnosis of ALS should have imaging of the cervical spine

PREVENTION/AVOIDANCE N/A

POSSIBLE COMPLICATIONS
• Aspiration pneumonia
• Decubitus ulcers
• Pulmonary embolism

EXPECTED COURSE/PROGNOSIS
• ALS usually terminates in death within five years
• Patients predominantly manifesting progressive muscular atrophy have a better prognosis
• There have been reports of spontaneous arrest of the disease

MISCELLANEOUS

ASSOCIATED CONDITIONS None

AGE-RELATED FACTORS
Pediatric: Infantile and juvenile spinal muscular atrophies are conditions which are distinct from amyotrophic lateral sclerosis clinically and pathologically
Geriatric: Symptoms of ALS may inappropriately be attributed to age
Others: N/A

PREGNANCY Pregnancy is uncommon among affected individuals. Pregnancy would be unwise in any individual suffering from a disease with so poor a prognosis. If pregnancy did occur, the only foreseeable difficulties would be related to weakness.

SYNONYMS
• Motor neuron disease
• Lou Gehrig's disease
• ALS

ICD-9-CM
335.2 motor neuron disease
335.20 amyotrophic lateral sclerosis

SEE ALSO N/A

OTHER NOTES Also referred to as Mill's variant (unilateral involvement)

ABBREVIATIONS N/A

REFERENCES
• Rowland LD, ed: Merritt's Textbook of Neurology. 9th Ed. Philadelphia, Williams & Wilkins, 1995
• Brown WF, Botton CF: Clinical Electromyography. 2nd Ed. Boston, Butterworth-Heinemann, 1993
Illustrations: N/A
Internet references: http://www.5mcc.com

Author(s)
Colin R. Bamford, MD

Anaerobic & necrotizing infections

BASICS

DESCRIPTION Gangrene is local death of soft tissues due to disease or injury and is associated with loss of blood supply. Anaerobic and necrotizing infections may be associated with gas.
System(s) affected: Skin/Exocrine, Cardiovascular
Genetics: N/A
Incidence/Prevalence in USA: Rare
Predominant age: Any
Predominant sex: Male = Female

SIGNS AND SYMPTOMS
• Local pain
• Foul odor
• Abnormally dark skin and tissues under skin (dark green to black)
• Crepitation (gas)
• Fever
• Rapid pulse
• Fulminant course leading to death without treatment

CAUSES
• Local injury
• Superimposed infection (surface or deep; local or distant)
• Pathologic conditions of large intestine
• Hematologic malignancies
• Severe neutropenia, related or not related to chemotherapy

RISK FACTORS
• Poor blood supply (arteriosclerosis)
• Old age
• Trauma
• Diabetes mellitus
• Malnutrition

DIAGNOSIS

DIFFERENTIAL DIAGNOSIS
• Deep infections with muscle involvement
  ◊ Gas gangrene
    - Gas gangrene resulting from soft tissue trauma with multiple aerobic and anaerobic organisms; synergistic necrotizing sepsis, synergistic necrotizing cellulitis; clostridial myositis; clostridial myonecrosis
    - Abdominal wall gas gangrene; postoperative clostridial sepsis of the abdominal wall; clostridial myonecrosis of the abdominal wall
    - Nontraumatic, metastatic, clostridial myonecrosis; metastatic clostridial myositis; metastatic gas gangrene; gas gangrene without a visible wound
      - Uterine clostridial infections
      - Gas gangrene of the heart
      - Gas gangrene of the brain
  ◊ Streptococcal myositis: anaerobic streptococcal myonecrosis; anaerobic streptococcal myositis
  ◊ Infected vascular gas gangrene; non-clostridial gas gangrene; non-clostridial myositis

• Superficial infections - with or without abscess
  ◊ Hemolytic streptococcal gangrene
  ◊ Acute, infectious staphylococcal gangrene
  ◊ Anaerobic cellulitis; crepitant phlegmon; clostridial cellulitis
  ◊ Necrotizing fasciitis due to multiple aerobic and anaerobic organisms; synergistic gangrene; non-clostridial anaerobic cellulitis; anaerobic cutaneous gangrene; perineal phlegmon; Fournier's gangrene. (Note: If there is extension to the tissues of the abdominal wall below the deep fascia, such as the anterior sheath of the rectus muscle, perineal phlegmon or Fournier's gangrene is a synergistic necrotizing sepsis rather than just a necrotizing fasciitis. These are similar infections but are in different locations.)
  ◊ Necrotizing fasciitis due to group A streptococcus (there may be very rapid extension to structures deep to the deep fascia)
  ◊ Panophthalmitis
• Simple clostridial contamination of wounds
• Infiltration or injection or aspiration of gas into wounds
  ◊ Wounds with gas not produced by bacteria
  ◊ Injection of gas into wounds
    - Therapy (e.g., hydrogen peroxide)
    - Pranksters' jokes
    - Malingerers
    - Psychiatric problems
  ◊ Aspiration and dissemination of air into wounds by muscular activity
  ◊ Subcutaneous emphysema related to air leak syndrome or trauma
• Gas in tissues after industrial accidents
  ◊ Magnesiogenous pneumagranuloma
• Gas in tissues after injections of chemicals
  ◊ Injection of drugs
  ◊ Accidental injection of a foreign agent, such as benzene
• Gas in tissues after laparoscopic examination and treatment

LABORATORY
• With severe gangrene, studies will reveal anemia and leukocytosis
• Gram smears for many possible organisms
• Daily serum creatine kinase determinations
Drugs that may alter lab results:
Antibiotics prior to culture
Disorders that may alter lab results: N/A

PATHOLOGICAL FINDINGS
• Necrosis of tissues with foul odor
• Sometimes, gas in tissues
• Microorganisms

SPECIAL TESTS
• Cultures and sensitivity tests for microorganisms reported to produce gas in human tissues:
  ◊ Gram-positive anaerobes: Cocci - Peptostreptococcus (anaerobic Streptococcus) (usually with group A Streptococcus [Streptococcus pyogenes, beta-hemolytic Streptococcus] or Staphylococcus aureus)
  ◊ Gram-positive anaerobes: Bacilli - Clostridium perfringens and other clostridia
  ◊ Gram-negative aerobes: Bacilli - Escherichia coli, Klebsiella pneumoniae, Enterobacter species, Proteus species (all usually in mixed infections)
  ◊ Gram-negative anaerobes: Bacilli - Bacteroides fragilis (usually with other gram-negative bacilli)

IMAGING Plain roentgenograms, gas in tissues; with MRI, edema

DIAGNOSTIC PROCEDURES
IMMEDIATE SURGICAL INTERVENTION with longitudinal incisions of skin, superficial fascia, deep fascia, and muscles to look for necrotic tissue and/or foreign bodies and with removal of necrotic tissue or foreign bodies. Daily repetition if indicated.

TREATMENT

APPROPRIATE HEALTH CARE
Hospital inpatient

GENERAL MEASURES
• Infectious disease consultation if possible
• Intravenous fluids with glucose, electrolytes, blood, vitamins
• Daily CBC and electrolytes in acute phase
• Prophylaxis for tetanus
• Hyperbaric oxygen: unclear therapeutic value; no delay of surgical intervention for hyperbaric oxygen therapy

SURGICAL MEASURES
• Surgical intervention for diagnosis and débridement of necrotic tissues; possibly daily
• Re-operation if possibility of spreading or unrecognized necrosis and/or foreign bodies (with abnormal daily CPK determination)
• Surgical repair for loss of skin and subcutaneous tissues

ACTIVITY Bedrest

DIET By mouth, as tolerated

PATIENT EDUCATION N/A

Anaerobic & necrotizing infections

MEDICATIONS

DRUG(S) OF CHOICE
• Initially broad spectrum, antibiotic regime; then specific antibiotic regime as determined by stained smears, cultures, and sensitivity tests with particular reference to the sensitivities of the hospital where the patient is being treated (although anaerobic organisms are difficult to culture and identify). Dosage will vary according to clinical circumstances; refer to manufacturer's literature and suggestions of infectious disease consultant. Important: don't delay treatment if smear, cultures and tests negative.

```
---------------------------------
Gram stain    Presumed organism
---------------------------------
+ cocci       Streptococcus
+ cocci       Staphylococcus
                aureus
+ bacilli     Clostridium spp
- bacilli     Bacteroides spp
- bacilli     Coliforms
---------------------------------
```

◊ Gram-positive cocci: penicillin G, nafcillin (Unipen), clindamycin (Cleocin), metronidazole (Flagyl), or cephalosporins
◊ Gram-positive bacilli: penicillin G, clindamycin, metronidazole or cephalosporins
◊ Gram-negative bacilli (Bacteroides): clindamycin, metronidazole, cefoxitin (Mefoxin) [many B. frag. are resistant], ticarcillin (Ticar) or mezlocillin (Mezlin)
◊ Gram-negative bacilli (Coliforms): gentamicin (Garamycin), tobramycin (Nebcin), amikacin (Amikin), cephalosporins, ampicillin, mezlocillin, or ticarcillin
• Intravenous calcium gluconate if extensive fat necrosis
Contraindications: Sensitivity to drugs
Precautions:
• Sedatives and analgesics (both before and after exploratory and therapeutic operations) may make recognition of spreading gangrene more difficult
• Repeated gram smears, culture and sensitivity tests for the best antibiotic(s)
Significant possible interactions: See manufacturer's profile of each drug.

ALTERNATIVE DRUGS As above

FOLLOWUP

PATIENT MONITORING
• Diligence required to RECOGNIZE SPREADING GANGRENE
• Monitor effective blood levels of prescribed antibiotics
• Electrolytes
• Nutrition
• CPK determinations daily for myonecrosis
• Progress notes in charts daily or as often as every 4 hours

PREVENTION/AVOIDANCE
• Avoidance of trauma
• Good care of skin
• Avoidance of tight orthopedic casts

POSSIBLE COMPLICATIONS
• Tissue and functional losses
• Amputation
• Death

EXPECTED COURSE/PROGNOSIS
• Fair if early diagnosis and treatment, and if gangrene arrested at an early stage
• Fatal without treatment and possibly with treatment
• Fair if large intestine disease is recognized and removed

MISCELLANEOUS

ASSOCIATED CONDITIONS
• Diabetes mellitus with impaired blood flow
• Altered immunocompetence: Depressed immunocompetence may require an alteration of treatment, especially with tumor treatments

AGE-RELATED FACTORS
Pediatric: N/A
Geriatric: Diseases of the aged with debility and poor blood supply
Others: N/A

PREGNANCY Treatment as for nonpregnant, but consider the pregnancy

SYNONYMS N/A

ICD-9-CM
785.4 Gangrene
040.0 Gas gangrene
136.9 Unspecified infectious and parasitic diseases
682.9 Cellulitis and abscess at unspecified site (phlegmon)

SEE ALSO
• Tetanus

OTHER NOTES
• Group A Streptococcus: "flesh eating bacterium"

ABBREVIATIONS
CBC = complete blood cell count
MRI = magnetic resonance imaging
CPK = serum creatinine phosphokinase

REFERENCES
• von Behring E, Kitasato S: Uber das Zustandelkommen der Diphtherie-Immunität und der Tetanus-Immunität bei Thieren. Dtsch Med Wochenschr 1890;16:1113
• Furste W, Lobe TE, Botros NM: Gangrenous soft tissue infections. Infections in Surgery 1985;4:837-878
• Furste W, Dolor MC, Rothstein LB, Vest CR: Carcinoma of the large intestine and nontraumatic metastatic clostridial myonecrosis. Diseases of Colon & Rectum 1986;29:899-904
• Furste W, Wheeler WL: Tetanus: a team disease. Curr Prob in Surg 1972;9:1-72
• Rice B: $15 million deep. Med Econ 1995;14:47-50
• Davies HD, McGeer A, Schwartz B, et al: Invasive group A streptococcal infections in Ontario, Canada. New Engl J Med 1996;335:547-554
• Golshani S, Simons AJ, Der R, et al: Necrotizing fasciitis following laparoscopic surgery. Surg Endosc 1996;10:751-754
• Holm SE: Invasive group A streptococcal infections. New Engl J Med 1996;335:590-591
• Tibbles PM, Edelsberg JS: Hyperbaric-oxygen therapy. New Engl J Med 1996;334:1642-1648
• Bury TF: Clostridial gas gangrene of the spleen presenting as pneumoperitoneum. Contemp Surg 1997;51:312-316
• Furste W: A golden opportunity, review of tetanus prophylaxis (1890-1998). J Trauma 1998;44:1110-1112
• Hagberg C, Radulescu A, Rex JH: Necrotizing fasciitis due to group A Streptococcus after an accidental needlestick injury. NEJM 1997;337:1699
• Larson CM, Bubrick MP, Jacobs DM, et al: Malignancy, mortality and medicosurgical management of Clostridium septicum infection. Surg 1995;118:592-598
• Lewis RT: Soft tissue infections. World J Surg 1998;22:146-151
• Sobolewski AP, Welling RE: Management of Fournier's gangrene. Surg Rounds 1997;20:285-287
• CDC: Nosocomial group A streptococcal infections associated with asymptomatic health-care workers-Maryland and California. MMWR 1999;48:163-166
• Stevens DL: The flesh eating bacterium: what's next? J Infect Dis 1999 179(suppl2):s366-74
• Kotrappa KS, Bansal RS, Amin NM: Necrotizong fasciitis. Am Fam Phys 1996;53(5):1691-7
Illustrations: N/A
Internet references: http://www.5mcc.com

Author(s)
Wesley Furste, MD, FACS
Augusto Aguirre, MD

Anaphylaxis

BASICS

DESCRIPTION
• An IgE mediated acute, systemic reaction following antigen exposure in a sensitized person.
• A non-IgE mediated idiopathic anaphylactoid reaction also may occur. Anaphylactoid reactions are clinically indistinguishable from anaphylaxis and are treated in the same manner.

System(s) affected: Pulmonary, Cardiovascular, Skin/Exocrine, Gastrointestinal, Endocrine/Metabolic, Hemic/Lymphatic/Immunologic

Genetics: Genetic predisposition for sensitization to certain antigens

Incidence/Prevalence in USA:
• Between 20,592 and 47,024 cases of idiopathic anaphylaxis occur per year (no identifiable cause)
• Drug-induced anaphylaxis in 1/2,700 hospitalized patients
• 0.3-0.7/100,000/yr anaphylaxis deaths

Predominant age: All ages

Predominant sex: Male = Female

SIGNS AND SYMPTOMS
• Pruritus, flushing, urticaria, angioedema
• Dyspnea, cough, rhonchi
• Rhinorrhea, bronchorrhea, wheezing
• Difficulty swallowing
• Nausea, vomiting, diarrhea, cramps, bloating
• Tachycardia, hypotension, shock, syncope
• Malaise, shivering
• Mydriasis

CAUSES
• IgE mediated mast cell degranulation
• Complement activation (C3a, C4a, C5a) by antigen-antibody complexes that contain complement fixing antibodies
• Other non-IgE dependent anaphylaxis-like syndromes may be caused by modulators of arachidonic acid metabolism, sulfiting agents, exercise induced anaphylaxis, and idiopathic recurrent anaphylaxis
• Some important causes of anaphylaxis are:
  ◊ Antimicrobials (e.g., penicillin)
  ◊ Blood products (especially in IgA deficient patients)
  ◊ Diagnostic chemicals (iodinated contrast media)
  ◊ Ethylene oxide gas (dialysis tubing, other sterilized products)
  ◊ Exercise
  ◊ Foods (e.g., peanuts, nuts, fish, crustaceans, mollusks, cow milk, eggs, soybean most common)
  ◊ Immunotherapy
  ◊ Insect stings (e.g., honeybees, wasps, kissing bugs, deer flies)
  ◊ Latex rubber (gloves, catheters)
  ◊ Macromolecules (e.g., chymopapain, insulin, dextran, glucocorticoid, protamine)
  ◊ Vaccines

RISK FACTORS
Previous anaphylaxis; history of atopy or asthma

DIAGNOSIS

DIFFERENTIAL DIAGNOSIS
• Anaphylactoid reactions: May occur after the first contact with substance, such as polymyxin, pentamidine, radiographic contrast media, aspirin
• Carcinoid syndrome
• Globus hystericus: may mimic pharyngeal edema.
• Hereditary angioedema: C1q esterase deficiency with painless, pruritus-free angioedema without urticaria, flushing or wheezing.
• Pheochromocytoma: Paradoxically, because of beta-2 stimulation, some patients have hypotensive attacks accompanied by tachycardia. Urticaria, angioedema, and wheezing absent.
• Pseudoanaphylactic reaction: After injection of procaine penicillin. Is a drug effect of procaine and not a penicillin allergy.
• Scombroid poisoning: From ingestion of dark meat fish (e.g., tuna, mackerel, mahi-mahi). Histamine-like mediator - symptoms include flushing, sweating, nausea, vomiting, diarrhea, headache, palpitations, dizziness, rash, swelling of face and tongue, respiratory distress, vasodilatory shock.
• Serum sickness: Occurs several days after exposure to inciting agent
• Systemic mastocytosis: Benign or malignant overgrowth of mast cells. Urticaria pigmentosa seen in benign form and the presence of reddish brown macular-papular cutaneous lesions which urticate after trauma - Darier's sign.
• Vasovagal reactions: Bradycardia and hypotension without tachycardia, flushing, urticaria, angioedema, pruritus, and wheezing
• Pulmonary embolism, foreign body aspiration, arrhythmia

LABORATORY
• Hypoxemia, hypercarbia, acidosis. Acidosis may cause apparent hyperkalemia by moving potassium extracellularly.
• Elevated serum and urine histamine (short-lived in circulation)
• Elevated serum tryptase, a mast cell enzyme marker for allergic and anaphylactic reactions. Peak level: 30-90 minutes after reaction onset.

Drugs that may alter lab results: Epinephrine and albuterol may cause apparent hypokalemia by shifting K+ intracellularly

Disorders that may alter lab results: N/A

PATHOLOGICAL FINDINGS   N/A

SPECIAL TESTS   N/A

IMAGING   N/A

DIAGNOSTIC PROCEDURES   N/A

TREATMENT

APPROPRIATE HEALTH CARE
• Outpatient: Patients with cutaneous angioedema, urticaria, and minimal bronchospasm may be released when symptoms and signs have cleared. Continue antihistamines (diphenhydramine/cimetidine) and oral steroids for 72 hours.
• Moderate-severe anaphylaxis, admit observation; may need ventilatory support.
• Allergist referral, if anaphylaxis cause unclear
• Patients with anaphylaxis from insect stings benefit from desensitization immunotherapy

GENERAL MEASURES
• Treatment depends on severity
• Maintain a patent airway - endotracheal intubation and assisted ventilation may be necessary; possibly tracheostomy
• Oxygen
• Tourniquet placed proximal to injected or stung site if possible, to occlude lymphatic and venous drainage (but not arterial flow)
• IV fluids (normal saline/lactated ringers) restores intravascular volume; avoid precipitating CHF
• Monitor vital signs

SURGICAL MEASURES   N/A

ACTIVITY
Bedrest until anaphylaxis clears and patient hemodynamically stable

DIET
Nothing until acute symptoms are controlled

PATIENT EDUCATION
• Printed patient information available from: Asthma & Allergy Foundation of America, 1717 Massachusetts Avenue, Suite 305, Washington, DC 20036,(800)7-Asthma or American Allergy Association, P.O. Box 7273, Menlo Park, CA 94026, (415)322-1663
• Medic-Alert type tags (Medic-Alert Foundation, Turlock, CA 95381-1009
• Avoid beta-blockers if possible
• Instruct patient in use of bee sting kit

MEDICATIONS

DRUG(S) OF CHOICE
• Epinephrine
  ◊ Less severe reaction: 0.3-0.5 mg (0.01 mg/kg in children)= (0.3-0.5 mL of a 1:1000 solution, 0.01 mL/kg in children), SQ q 20-30 minutes as needed up to 3 doses
  ◊ Life-threatening reactions: 0.5 mg (5 mL of a 1:10,000 solution)(for children: 0.05-0.1 mL/kg/dose) given IV slowly q 5-10 minutes as needed. If IV access not possible, endotracheal or intraosseous may be effective.
• Diphenhydramine, an H1 blocker 25-50 mg IV (IM or PO) immediately and then, q6h for 72 hours (children 1.25 mg/kg to 25 mg)

Anaphylaxis

• Cimetidine, an H2 blocker, 300 mg IV over 3-5 minutes (children 5-10 mg/kg/dose) and then 400 mg PO bid is helpful and may be more effective than diphenhydramine.
• Corticosteroids: No immediate effect and no good evidence that they prevent recurrence - can be administered if desired.
    ◊ Hydrocortisone sodium succinate 250-500 mg IV q 4-6 h (4-8 mg/kg for children), or
    ◊ Prednisone, 1 mg/kg in children, up to 60 mg, or
    ◊ Methylprednisolone 60-125 mg IV in adults. 1-2 mg/kg in children.
• Bronchodilator, if persistent bronchospasm
    ◊ Inhaled beta-2 agonists. Continuous nebulized albuterol of 10 mg/hr or 2.5 mg q 15-20 minutes is safe, effective and preferable to aminophylline as first line therapy.
• Laryngeal edema:
    ◊ Epinephrine 5 mL 1:1000 by nebulizer. More effective than racemic epinephrine and usually available.
• Persistent hypotension
    ◊ Dopamine 200 mg in 500 mL of dextrose in water given by infusion pump. Titrate to blood pressure (3-20 mcg/kg/min)
    ◊ Glucagon: May be beneficial for resistant hypotension caused by concurrent beta-blockade therapy 50 mcg/kg IV bolus over 1 minute, or alternatively, because of short half-life, can give as continuous infusion at 5-15 mcg/min
• Normal saline or Ringer's lactate: As necessary to maintain tissue perfusion
• Oral antihistamines and steroids for 72 hours

Contraindications:
Refer to manufacturer's literature
Precautions:
Refer to manufacturer's literature
Significant possible interactions: None

ALTERNATIVE DRUGS Several reports of tranexamic acid-1000 mg IV or sigma-aminocaproic acid for refractory anaphylaxis. Reserve for last resort in patient not responding to other therapy; these drugs not considered standard of care! Not to be used in pregnant women, or known vascular thrombosis.

FOLLOWUP

PATIENT MONITORING Follow vital signs closely during treatment and for several hours after anaphylaxis has resolved. Symptoms can recur for up to 72 hours.

PREVENTION/AVOIDANCE
• Avoid drugs, foods that cause the reaction
• Carry a pre-filled epinephrine syringe; avoid areas where insect exposure likely. Avoid wearing things that attract insects (e.g., perfumes, bright-colored clothing); avoid barefeet outdoors.
• Carry/wear medical alert ID about anaphylaxis-causing substance or event
• When radiologic contrast is unavoidable, use of low osmolar contrast agents (e.g., iothalamate) reduces risk of contrast reactions in those with previous contrast reaction to 3.1%; only 0.22% were considered severe. Stop beta-blockers before administering contrast materials; pre-treat with diphenhydramine (50 mg IV) and steroid (e.g., methylprednisolone 60 mg IV).
• Those with frequent (>6/year) episodes of idiopathic anaphylaxis should be treated prophylactically with prednisone 40-60 mg/day in a single a.m. dose, hydroxyzine-25 mg tid, and albuterol 2 mg po tid. The prednisone should be rapidly tapered to a qod regimen.
• Have latex-free kit (gloves, IVs, etc) available for treatment of latex allergic patients; some latex allergic patients will react to tropical fruits (e.g., kiwi, bananas) also avocados, chestnuts
• Avoid beta blockers

POSSIBLE COMPLICATIONS
Hypoxemia; cardiac arrest; death

EXPECTED COURSE/PROGNOSIS
• Good prognosis if treated immediately; worse outcome with a delay of >30 minutes in administration of epinephrine
• Of those with idiopathic anaphylaxis - 60% are free of anaphylactic episodes at 2.5 years; most others were steroid free with a decrease in the number of episodes

MISCELLANEOUS

ASSOCIATED CONDITIONS Asthma; atopy

AGE-RELATED FACTORS
Pediatric: N/A
Geriatric: Epinephrine may induce ischemia and myocardial infarction in those with cardiac disease; still the drug of choice. Be alert for anti-cholinergic and CNS side effects after giving diphenhydramine or cimetidine.
Others: N/A

PREGNANCY Epinephrine, other pressors may reduce placental blood flow; but may save life of mother and fetus

SYNONYMS
• Anaphylactoid reactions

ICD-9-CM
995.0 other anaphylactic shock
E947 other and unspecified drugs and medicinal substances
E947.9 unspecified drug or medicinal substance

SEE ALSO
• Food allergy
• Insect bites & stings
• Urticaria

OTHER NOTES
• Allergy to one species of legume (e.g., peanuts) or one type of seafood (e.g., shrimp) doesn't mean allergy to all products in that category. Skin testing is prudent.
• MMR vaccine can be safely administered to those with a history of egg allergy since most egg allergies are related to the albumin.
• Penicillin allergic patients can generally tolerate second and third generation cephalosporins as well as monobactams (e.g., aztreonam); generally will be allergic to carbapenems (e.g., imipenem) and first generation cephalosporins
• IgA deficient patients should have washed RBCs for transfusion
• Those allergic to seafood are not allergic to iodine-based radiocontrast. Shellfish allergy is protein related.

ABBREVIATIONS N/A

REFERENCES
• Tintinalli JE, et al: Emergency Medicine, A Comprehensive Study Guide. 4th Ed. New York McGraw-Hill, 1995
• Patterson R, Hogan MB, Yarnold PR, Harris KE: Idiopathic anaphylaxis: An attempt to estimate the incidence in the United States. Archives of Internal Medicine 1995;155(8):869-871
• Freeman TM: Allergy and Immunology. Anaphylaxis: Diagnosis and treatment. Primary Care; Clinics in Office Practice, 1998;25:809
• The Diagnosis and Management of Anaphylaxis. Joint Task Force on Practice Parameters, American Academy of Allergy, Asthma and Immunology, American College of Allergy, Asthma and Immunology, and the Joint Council of Allergy. Asthma and Immunology. Journal of Allergy and Clinical Immunology 1998;6(101)
6 additional references available at web site
Internet references: http://www.5mcc.com
Illustrations: N/A

Author(s)
Mark A. Graber, MD

Anemia, aplastic

 BASICS

DESCRIPTION An anemia in which the bone marrow fails to produce adequate numbers of peripheral blood elements. Usual course - insidious. Pure red cell aplasia is a related syndrome that is caused by a selective failure of the production of erythroid elements. It can be associated with thymomas. Constitutional (Fanconi's) anemia is associated with congenital anomalies.

System(s) affected:
Hemic/Lymphatic/Immunologic

Genetics:
• Genetic pattern undetermined in acquired
• Autosomal recessive in constitutional

Incidence/Prevalence in USA: Not very common

Predominant age:
• Constitutional - children and young adults
• Acquired - all ages

Predominant sex: Male = Female

SIGNS AND SYMPTOMS
• Dyspnea
• Ecchymoses, petechiae
• Fatigue, fever
• Hemorrhage, menorrhagia, occult stool blood, melena, epistaxis
• Pallor
• Palpitations
• Progressive weakness
• Retinal flame hemorrhages
• Systolic ejection murmur
• Weight loss
• Constitutional:
  ◊ Short stature
  ◊ Microcephaly
  ◊ Radius and thumb anomalies
  ◊ Renal anomalies
  ◊ Hypospadias
  ◊ Hyperpigmentation

CAUSES
• Idiopathic (about 50% of the cases)
• Injury to pluripotential stem cells
• Destruction of pluripotential stem cells
• Immunologic injury
• Toxic exposure, e.g., benzene, inorganic arsenic
• Infectious hepatitis
• Radiation exposure
• Drugs - especially antibiotics, anticonvulsants, gold
• Pregnancy (rare)
• Inherited (constitutional anemia)

RISK FACTORS
• Viral illness
• Toxin exposure
• Tumors of thymus (red cell aplasia)

 DIAGNOSIS

DIFFERENTIAL DIAGNOSIS
• Other causes of pancytopenia
• Myelodysplastic disorders
• Paroxysmal nocturnal hemoglobinuria
• Acute leukemia
• Hairy cell leukemia
• Systemic lupus erythematosus
• Disseminated infection
• Hypersplenism
• Transient erythroblastopenia of childhood

LABORATORY
• Pancytopenia
• Anemia
• Leukopenia
• Neutropenia
• Thrombocytopenia
• Increased bleeding time
• Decreased reticulocytes
• Increased serum iron secondary to transfusion
• Normal total iron binding capacity (TIBC)
• Borderline high mean corpuscular volume (MCV) > 104
• Hematuria
• Abnormal liver function tests (hepatitis)
• Increased fetal hemoglobin (Fanconi's)
• Increased chromosomal breaks under specialized conditions (constitutional anemia)
• Molecular determination of abnormal gene (Fanconi's)

Drugs that may alter lab results: N/A
Disorders that may alter lab results: N/A

PATHOLOGICAL FINDINGS
• Normochromic RBC
• Bone marrow:
  ◊ Increased iron stores
  ◊ Decreased cellularity (< 10%)
  ◊ Decreased megakaryocytes
  ◊ Decreased myelocytes
  ◊ Decreased erythroid precursors

SPECIAL TESTS
Chromosome breakage (constitutional anemia); fetal hemoglobin

IMAGING
• CT of thymus region if thymoma-associated RBC aplasia suspected
• Radiographs of radius and thumbs (constitutional anemia)
• Renal ultrasound (constitutional anemia)

DIAGNOSTIC PROCEDURES
Bone marrow biopsy

 TREATMENT

APPROPRIATE HEALTH CARE
Inpatient. Referral to an institution that has experience in treating these patients is recommended.

GENERAL MEASURES
• Vigorous supportive measures
• Oxygen therapy for severe anemia
• Good oral hygiene
• Avoid causative agents
• Human leukocyte antigen (HLA) testing on all patients and their immediate families
• Transfusion support (judiciously prescribed RBCs for severe anemia, consider leukocyte depleted units; platelets for severe thrombocytopenia; WBCs)
• Immunosuppressive therapy (cyclosporine, corticosteroids, antithymocyte globulin [ATG]) if no suitable donor
• Androgen therapy if less severe

SURGICAL MEASURES
• Bone marrow transplantation for patients with severe aplastic anemia and an HLA-identical donor. Upper age restrictions on transplantations varies among institutions that perform them.
• Unrelated donor transplants, if other therapy fails
• Thymectomy for thymoma

ACTIVITY Isolation procedures if neutropenic

DIET No special diet, but nutritious diet important to improve resistance to infection

PATIENT EDUCATION Printed patient information available from: Aplastic Anemia Foundation of America, P.O. Box 22689, Baltimore, MD 21203, (410)955-2803

MEDICATIONS

DRUG(S) OF CHOICE
• Antithymocyte globulin (ATG)
◊ It is a horse serum containing polyclonal antibodies against human T cells. Skin test patients to determine any hypersensitivity.
◊ Treatment for older patients and patients without a compatible donor
◊ Dosage is 10-20 mg/kg diluted in 500 mL saline, infused over 4-6 h for 8-14 consecutive days
◊ May be used as a single agent or in combination with corticosteroids
• Cyclosporine
◊ Dosage is 10 mg/kg initially, then taper to 5-10 mg/kg/day
◊ Monitor trough blood levels. Normal values for assays vary.
◊ 2-3 months trial may be necessary
• Cyclophosphamide; high dose [Blood 87:491,1996]
• Androgens
◊ Clinical trials inconclusive
◊ Useful for some patients lacking other options and less severe patients
◊ Oxymetholone - 1-2 mg/kg/day orally
◊ 2-3 month trial usually necessary to assess response
• Prednisone for pure red cell anemia
Note: Relapses may occur after initial response to immunosuppressive therapy
Contraindications: Refer to manufacturer's literature
Precautions: Refer to manufacturer's literature
Significant possible interactions: Refer to manufacturer's literature

ALTERNATIVE DRUGS   Prednisone and cyclophosphamide

FOLLOWUP

PATIENT MONITORING   Close monitoring for all treatments. Drugs and other forms of treatment have numerous and severe side effects.

PREVENTION/AVOIDANCE
• Avoid possible toxic agents
• Use safety measures when working with radiation

POSSIBLE COMPLICATIONS
• Hemorrhage
• Infection
• Transfusion hemosiderosis
• Transfusion hepatitis
• Heart failure
• Complications of therapy
• Development of acute leukemia
• Neoplasm may complicate constitutional anemia

EXPECTED COURSE/PROGNOSIS
Depending on age and treatment available - guardedly favorable

MISCELLANEOUS

ASSOCIATED CONDITIONS   N/A

AGE-RELATED FACTORS
Pediatric:
• Pure red cell anemia (Diamond-Blackfan) and constitutional anemia are seen more often in children
• Idiopathic aplastic anemia is more common in adolescents
• Secondary aplastic anemia seen in children exposed to ionizing radiation or treated with cytotoxic chemotherapeutic agents
Geriatric: The elderly are more exposed to large numbers of drugs and therefore more susceptible to secondary aplastic anemia
Others: N/A

PREGNANCY   Pregnancy may, rarely, be aassociated with aplastic anemia

SYNONYMS
• Hypoplastic anemia
• Panmyelophthisis
• Refractory anemia
• Aleukia hemorrhagica
• Toxic paralytic anemia

ICD-9-CM
284 Aplastic anemia

SEE ALSO
• Myelodysplastic syndromes (MDS)
• Systemic lupus erythematosus (SLE)
• Leukemia, hairy cell
• Paroxysmal nocturnal hemoglobinuria

OTHER NOTES   N/A

ABBREVIATIONS   N/A

REFERENCES
• Williams WJ, et al: Hematology. 4th Ed. New York, McGraw-Hill, 1990
• Lee GR, et al: Wintrobe's Clinical Hematology. 9th Ed. Philadelphia, Lea & Febiger, 1993
Illustrations: N/A
Internet references: http://www.5mcc.com

Author(s)
John J. Hutter, Jr., MD

Anemia, autoimmune hemolytic

BASICS

DESCRIPTION Acquired anemia induced by binding of autoantibodies and/or complement to the red cells
• Three main types
  ◊ Warm (37°C) antibody (80-90%)
  ◊ Cold reacting antibody (10%)
  ◊ Drug induced
System(s) affected:
Hemic/Lymphatic/Immunologic
Genetics: Unknown
Incidence/Prevalence in USA: 1/25,000 per year
Predominant age: < 50 years
Predominant sex: Female > Male

SIGNS AND SYMPTOMS
• Weakness
• Fatigue
• Exertional dyspnea
• Dizziness
• Palpitations
• Malaise
• Dyspnea
• Pallor
• Jaundice
• Splenomegaly
• Hepatomegaly
• Tachycardia
• Anemia (may be sudden and life threatening)

CAUSES
• Warm antibody
  ◊ Idiopathic (50%)
  ◊ Neoplasia (Leukemia, myeloma, lymphoma, thymoma)
  ◊ Collagen vascular disease
  ◊ Viral infection: e.g., hepatitis
• Cold antibody
  ◊ Idiopathic (50%)
  ◊ Infection (Mycoplasma, mononucleosis, viral)
  ◊ Neoplasia (lymphoma)
  ◊ Cold agglutinin disease
• Drug induced
  ◊ Methyldopa, quinidine, penicillin

RISK FACTORS   Listed with Causes

DIAGNOSIS

DIFFERENTIAL DIAGNOSIS Other hemolytic anemias

LABORATORY
• Direct Coombs' (antiglobulin test) - positive
• Anemia
• Increased mean corpuscular volume (MCV)
• Increased mean cell hemoglobin concentration (MCHC)
• Spherocytosis
• Poikilocytosis
• Anisocytosis
• Rouleaux
• Reticulocytosis
• Nucleated RBC
• Large polychromatophilic reticulocytes
• Hyperbilirubinemia
• Decreased haptoglobin
• Hemoglobinemia
Drugs that may alter lab results: N/A
Disorders that may alter lab results: N/A

PATHOLOGICAL FINDINGS
• Bone marrow hyperplasia
• Increased marrow hemosiderin

SPECIAL TESTS
• IgG antibody (warm)
• IgM antibody (cold)

IMAGING   N/A

DIAGNOSTIC PROCEDURES   N/A

TREATMENT

APPROPRIATE HEALTH CARE
Inpatient

GENERAL MEASURES
• Warm antibody
  ◊ Mild - conservative therapy
  ◊ Moderate - prednisone
  ◊ Severe - high dose prednisone, immunosuppressant, packed red cell transfusion (which is difficult to crossmatch - need special blood bank techniques; in emergency, use most compatible crossmatch)
• Cold antibody
  ◊ Supportive
  ◊ Avoid cold
  ◊ Red cell transfusion (which is difficult to crossmatch - need special blood bank techniques; in emergency, use most compatible crossmatch)
  ◊ Consider high dose prednisone
• Drug induced
  ◊ Stop the offending drug
• Plasmapheresis/exchange transfusion for severe life-threatening cases

SURGICAL MEASURES   Severe warm antibody - splenectomy

ACTIVITY   Rest until asymptomatic

DIET   No special diet

PATIENT EDUCATION   Griffith, H.W.: Instructions for Patients; Philadelphia, 1994 W.B. Saunders Co

MEDICATIONS

DRUG(S) OF CHOICE Glucocorticoids - prednisone 1-2 mg/kg each day in divided doses. May need to be adjusted downward if needed for long-term treatment.
Contraindications: Refer to manufacturer's literature
Precautions: Refer to manufacturer's literature
Significant possible interactions: Refer to manufacturer's literature

ALTERNATIVE DRUGS
• Immunosuppressive drugs (if prednisone and splenectomy do not cure)
  ◊ Azathioprine (Imuran) 125 mg/day for up to 6 months
• IV immune globulin (IVIG)

FOLLOWUP

PATIENT MONITORING Monitor carefully if transfusion essential

PREVENTION/AVOIDANCE No preventive measures known

POSSIBLE COMPLICATIONS
• Shock (severe anemia)
• Thromboembolism
• Thrombocytopenic purpura (Evans's syndrome)

EXPECTED COURSE/PROGNOSIS
• Good with appropriate treatment
• If secondary to an underlying disorder, the prognosis is determined by the course of the primary disease

MISCELLANEOUS

ASSOCIATED CONDITIONS
• Systemic lupus erythematosus
• Chronic lymphocytic anemia
• Diffuse lymphomas

AGE-RELATED FACTORS
Pediatric: May occur in pediatric age group
Geriatric: Unusual in this age group; rule out neoplasia
Others: N/A

PREGNANCY N/A

SYNONYMS N/A

ICD-9-CM
283.0 Autoimmune hemolytic anemias

SEE ALSO N/A

OTHER NOTES N/A

ABBREVIATIONS N/A

REFERENCES
• Hashimoto C: Autoimmune hemolytic anemia. Clinical reviews. Allergy Immunology 1998;16(3):285-295
• Rosenwasser LJ, Joseph BZ: Immunohematologic Disorders. JAMA 1992;268:2940-5
• Wheby MS, ed: Anemia. Medical Clinics of North America. Philadelphia, W.B. Saunders Co., 1992
Illustrations: N/A
Internet references: http://www.5mcc.com

Author(s)
Brian J. Murray, MD

Anemia, pernicious

BASICS

DESCRIPTION A disorder due to vitamin B12 deficiency. Pernicious anemia is invariably associated with atrophic gastritis and histamine-fast achlorhydria. Vitamin B12 cannot be absorbed in the terminal ileum without intrinsic factor (a secretion of the parietal cells of the gastric mucosa). Usual course - slowly progressive.
System(s) affected:
Hemic/Lymphatic/Immunologic,
Gastrointestinal, Nervous
Genetics: HLA-DR2; HLA-DR4. Present in the rare form of pernicious anemia that is hereditary. Endemic areas - northern Europe, including Scandinavia.
Incidence/Prevalence in USA: Unknown
Predominant age: Older adults (> 60 years)
Predominant sex: Male = Female

SIGNS AND SYMPTOMS
• Abnormal reflexes
• Anorexia; weight loss
• Ataxia
• Atrophic glossitis
• Babinski's sign - positive
• Confusion
• Congestive heart failure
• Dementia
• Depression
• Exertional dyspnea
• Extremity numbness
• Extremity paresthesias
• Hepatomegaly
• Pallor
• Palpitations
• Poor finger coordination
• Position sense - decreased
• Prematurely gray-haired
• Purpura
• Romberg's sign, positive
• Skin pigmentation increased
• Sore tongue
• Splenomegaly
• Tachycardia
• Tinnitus
• Vertigo
• Vibration sense - decreased
• Vitiligo
• Weakness

CAUSES
• Atrophic gastric mucosa
• Intrinsic factor deficiency
• Probable autoimmunity against gastric parietal cells
• Autoimmunity against intrinsic factor

RISK FACTORS
• Vegetarian diet, without B12 supplementation
• Gastrectomy
• Blind loop syndrome
• Fish-tapeworm infestation
• Malabsorption syndromes
• Drugs: oral calcium-chelating drugs, aminosalicylic acid, biguanides
• Chronic pancreatitis
• Alcoholism

DIAGNOSIS

DIFFERENTIAL DIAGNOSIS
• Folic acid deficiency
• Myelodysplasia
• Neurological disorders without B12 deficiency
• Liver dysfunction
• Hypothyroidism
• Hemolysis or bleeding
• Drug effects
• Alcoholism

LABORATORY
• Achlorhydria
• Anisocytosis
• Anti-intrinsic poikilocytosis factor antibody
• Anti-parietal cell antibody
• Direct hyperbilirubinemia
• Haptoglobin decreased
• Howell-Jolly bodies
• Hypergastrinemia
• Hypersegmented neutrophils
• LDH increased
• Leukopenia
• Macrocytic anemia
• Mean corpuscular volume - 110-140
• Pentagastrin stimulation - stomach pH > 6
• Peripheral blood smear - macro-ovalocytes
• Poikilocytes
• Serum ferritin increased
• Serum vitamin B12 level < 100 pg/mL (< 74 pmol/L)
• Thrombocytopenia
Drugs that may alter lab results: N/A
Disorders that may alter lab results:
• Falsely elevated MCV
  ◊ Cold agglutinins
  ◊ Hyperglycemia
  ◊ Marked hyperleukocytosis
• Falsely normal serum vitamin B12 level
  ◊ Myeloproliferative disorders
  ◊ Liver disease
• Falsely low serum B12 level
  ◊ Multiple myeloma
  ◊ Oral contraceptive intake
  ◊ Pregnancy
  ◊ Folate deficiency
  ◊ Transcobalamin I deficiency
  ◊ Recent isotope administration

PATHOLOGICAL FINDINGS
• Bone marrow - hypercellular, macrocytes, iron stores increased
• Nests of megaloblasts
• Giant metamyelocytes
• Macropolymorpholeukocytes
• Hypersegmented neutrophils
• Stomach - atrophic gastritis, goblet cells increased
• Parietal cell atrophy
• Chief cell atrophy
• Gastric cytology - cellular atypia
• Spinal cord - myelin degeneration of the dorsal and lateral tracts
• Peripheral nerve degeneration
• Degenerative changes of the posterior root ganglia

SPECIAL TESTS
• Schilling test plus intrinsic factor - normal vitamin B12 absorption
• Schilling test - decreased vitamin B12 absorption
• Gastric analysis - achlorhydria

IMAGING N/A:

DIAGNOSTIC PROCEDURES
• Bone marrow aspiration
• Detailed history and physical exam

TREATMENT

APPROPRIATE HEALTH CARE
Outpatient

GENERAL MEASURES
• Treatment must be continued for life
• Identification and treatment of the underlying disorder

SURGICAL MEASURES N/A

ACTIVITY Unlimited

DIET Emphasize meat, animal protein foods, legumes unless contraindicated

PATIENT EDUCATION Griffith, H.W.: Instructions for Patients, W.B. Saunders Co, Philadelphia (instructions to photocopy for patient)

MEDICATIONS

DRUG(S) OF CHOICE
• Parenteral Vitamin B12 (cyanocobalamin)
  ◊ 100 mcg subcutaneously for each dose
  ◊ Administer daily for the first week
  ◊ Administer weekly for one month
  ◊ Monthly injections for remainder of life
(patients may be taught to give self-injection)
Contraindications: None
Precautions: Do not give folic acid
supplements without vitamin B12 - may cause
fulminant neurological deficit
Significant possible interactions: N/A

ALTERNATIVE DRUGS None

FOLLOWUP

PATIENT MONITORING
• Monthly injections of vitamin B12
• Endoscopy every 5 years to rule out gastric
carcinoma

PREVENTION/AVOIDANCE Early
detection of anemia; workup of anemia

POSSIBLE COMPLICATIONS
• Hypokalemia may complicate first week of
treatment
• Central nervous system symptoms may be
permanent if patient is not treated in less than
six months after symptoms begin
• Gastric polyps
• Stomach cancer

EXPECTED COURSE/PROGNOSIS
Anemia reversible with parenteral vitamin B12;
neurologic effects not reversible with parenteral
vitamin B12

MISCELLANEOUS

ASSOCIATED CONDITIONS
• Autoimmune diseases including rheumatoid
arthritis, IgA deficiency
• Graves' disease
• Myxedema
• Iron deficiency
• Thyroiditis
• Vitiligo
• Idiopathic adrenocortical insufficiency
• Hypoparathyroidism
• Agammaglobulinemia
• Tropical sprue
• Celiac disease
• Crohn's disease
• Infiltrate disorders of the ileum and small
intestine

AGE-RELATED FACTORS
Pediatric:
• Juvenile pernicious anemia occurs in older
children and is the same in most respects as in
adults
• Congenital pernicious anemia - usually
evident before 3 years of age
Geriatric: More common in this age group and
often in association with other autoimmune
disorders, depression, and dementia
Others: N/A

PREGNANCY N/A

SYNONYMS
• Addison's anemia
• Megaloblastic anemia due to B12 deficiency

ICD-9-CM
281.0 pernicious anemia
281.1 other vitamin B12 anemia

SEE ALSO Tropical sprue

OTHER NOTES
• There is a 3-fold likelihood of developing
gastric carcinoma. Suggest endoscopy
approximately every 5 years even if
asymptomatic.
• Folic acid treatment in patients with
pernicious anemia is contraindicated

ABBREVIATIONS N/A

REFERENCES
• Bennett JC, Plum F, eds: Cecil Textbook of
Medicine. 20th Ed. Philadelphia, W.B.
Saunders Co., 1996
• Williams WJ, Beutler E, Erslev AJ, et al, eds:
Hematology. 4th Ed. New York, McGraw-Hill,
1990
• Munseys W, ed: The Medical Clinic of North
America 1992;76(3)
Illustrations: 1 available on CD-ROM
Internet references: http://www.5mcc.com

Author(s)
Abdulrazak Abyad, MD, MPH, AGSF

Anemia, sickle cell

BASICS

DESCRIPTION A chronic hemoglobinopathy transmitted genetically, marked by moderately severe chronic hemolytic anemia, periodic acute episodes of painful "crises," and increased susceptibility to intercurrent infections, especially S. pneumoniae. The heterozygous condition (Hb A/S) is called sickle cell trait and is usually asymptomatic, with no anemia.
System(s) affected:
Hemic/Lymphatic/Immunologic, Musculoskeletal
Genetics: Autosomal recessive, mostly in blacks. Homozygous presence of a variant hemoglobin, HbS or sickle hemoglobin. Heterozygous condition Hb A/S.
Incidence/Prevalence in USA:
Approximately 1/500 black Americans and 1/1000 Hispanics have sickle cell anemia; 10% black Americans have sickle trait
Predominant age: All ages
Predominant sex: Male = Female

SIGNS AND SYMPTOMS
• Often asymptomatic in early months of life
• After 6 months of age, earliest symptoms are pallor and symmetric, painful swelling of the hands and feet (hand-foot syndrome)
• Chronic hemolytic anemia
• Painful "crises" in bones, joints, abdomen, back, and viscera (account for 90% of all hospital admissions)
• Mild scleral icterus
• Increased susceptibility to infections, especially pneumococcal sepsis and Salmonella osteomyelitis
• Functional asplenia
• Delayed physical/sexual maturation, especially boys
• Many multi-system complications, especially in later childhood and adolescence
• Acute chest syndrome (clinical picture consistent with pneumonia and/or infection)

CAUSES
• At molecular level: Hb S is produced by substitution of valine for glutamic acid in the sixth amino acid position of the beta chains of the hemoglobin molecule. When deoxygenated, Hb S polymerizes and forms long rods that change RBC from biconcave to sickle shape.
• At cellular level: Sickle RBCs are inflexible; odd shape and cell rigidity cause increased blood viscosity, stasis, and mechanical obstruction of small arterioles and capillaries, leading to distal ischemia. Sickle RBCs are also more fragile than normal, leading to hemolytic destruction in blood and reticuloendothelial system.
• At clinical level: Chronic anemia; a variety of "crises"; infections
  ◊ Vaso-occlusive crisis ("painful crisis"): Most common; pain results from tissue necrosis secondary to vascular occlusion and tissue hypoxia. Progressive organ failure and acute tissue damage results from repeated vaso-occlusive episodes.
  ◊ Aplastic crisis: Temporary suppression of RBC production in bone marrow by severe infection
  ◊ Hyperhemolytic crisis: Accelerated hemolysis; increased RBC fragility/shortened life span
  ◊ Sequestration crisis: Splenic sequestration of blood (only in infants/young children)
  ◊ Susceptibility to infection: Impaired/absent splenic function; defect in the alternate pathway of complement activation

RISK FACTORS
• Vaso-occlusive crisis
  ◊ Hypoxia
  ◊ Dehydration
  ◊ Infection
  ◊ Fever
  ◊ Acidosis
  ◊ Cold
  ◊ Anesthesia
  ◊ Strenuous physical exercise
  ◊ Smoking
• Aplastic crisis
  ◊ Severe infections
  ◊ Human parvovirus B19 infection
  ◊ Folic acid deficiency
• Hyperhemolytic crisis
  ◊ Acute bacterial infections
  ◊ Exposure to oxidant drugs

DIAGNOSIS

DIFFERENTIAL DIAGNOSIS
• Anemia: Other hemoglobinopathies, e.g., Hb SC disease, Hb C disease, Sickle cell-beta thalassemia
• Painful crisis: Other causes of acute pain in bones, joints, and abdomen. Seek infection and other precipitating causes.

LABORATORY
• Hb electrophoresis: Hb S predominates, variable amount Hb F, no Hb A. (In sickle cell trait, both Hb S and A are present).
• Screening tests: Sodium metabisulfite reduction-test; "Sickledex" test
• Anemia; hemoglobin approximately 8 g/dL (1.24 mmol/L); RBC indices usually normal but mean corpuscular volume (MCV) > 75 µm3 (> 75 fL)
• Reticulocytosis of 10-20%
• Leukocytosis; bands normal in absence of infection
• Thrombocytosis
• Peripheral smear: few sickled RBC's, polychromasia, nucleated RBC's
• Serum bilirubin mildly elevated (2-4 mg/dL [34-68 µmol/L]); fecal/urinary urobilinogen high
• ESR low
• Serum LDH elevated
• Haptoglobin absent or very low
Drugs that may alter lab results: N/A
Disorders that may alter lab results:
• Infection
• Other anemias (e.g., iron deficiency)

PATHOLOGICAL FINDINGS
• Variable, dependent on tissue
• In moderate to severe cases, hyposplenism due to autosplenectomy is common
• Hypoxia/infarction in multiple organs

SPECIAL TESTS N/A

IMAGING
• Bone scan (to rule out osteomyelitis)
• CT/MRI (to rule out CVA)
• Chest x-ray: may show enlarged heart; diffuse alveolar infiltrates in acute chest syndrome

DIAGNOSTIC PROCEDURES N/A

TREATMENT

APPROPRIATE HEALTH CARE
• General health care maintenance on outpatient basis should include assessment of growth/development, regular immunizations, vision/hearing screening, and regular dental care
• Hospitalization required for most crises and complications

GENERAL MEASURES
• Infections/fever - prompt treatment with antibiotics
• Minimize factors that enhance sickling
• Painful crises - hydration (2 X maintenance fluids); analgesics (narcotic and non-narcotic); oxygen if hypoxic
• Transfusion needed with aplastic crises, severe complications (i.e., CVA), before surgery, and with recurrent debilitating painful crises
• Special immunizations:
  ◊ Influenza vaccine yearly starting at age 2
  ◊ Pneumococcal vaccine at age 2; booster at age 4
  ◊ Meningococcal vaccine after age 2; need for booster unknown

SURGICAL MEASURES Bone marrow transplantation is curative but availability is limited

ACTIVITY
• Bedrest with crises. Otherwise, activity level as tolerated.
• Activity may be somewhat limited because of chronic anemia and poor muscular development

DIET Well balanced diet with folic acid supplementation; avoid alcohol (leads to dehydration)

PATIENT EDUCATION
• Guidelines for prompt management of fever, infections, pain, and specific complications should be reviewed at each visit
• Stress importance of keeping well-hydrated
• Teach early recognition of possible complications, especially education about priapism
• Genetic counseling
• Avoidance of alcohol and smoking

MEDICATIONS

DRUG(S) OF CHOICE
• Painful crises (mild, outpatient): non-narcotic analgesics (ibuprofen, acetaminophen)
• Painful crises (severe, hospitalized): parenteral narcotics, e.g., morphine, meperidine (Demerol) on fixed schedule; (PCA pump may be useful way of delivering narcotics) gradually lower dose and replace with oral medication as soon as possible (acetaminophen-codeine, ibuprofen). Correct dehydration and acidosis.
• Corticosteroids (dexamethasone 0.3 mg/kg q 12 hours for 4 doses in children) have shown promise in reducing need for analgesia, oxygen, transfusions, and hospitalization in setting of painful crisis or chest syndrome
• Prevention of painful crisis:
    ◊ Hydroxyurea (Droxia) in adult patients with ≥ 3 crisis/year. Start with 15 mg/kg day single daily dose; titrate upward every 12 weeks if blood counts satisfactory. Increase in 5 mg/kg increments to maximum of 35 mg/kg/day. Reduces crisis and chest syndrome 50%; long term safety unknown. Contraindicated in pregnancy.
    ◊ Nitric oxide, arginine butyrate, clotrimazole, and combination of erythropoietin with hydroxyurea show promise.
• Priapism prevention - stilbestrol possibly helpful
• Infections: prior to culture results, give antibiotic that covers S. pneumoniae and H. influenzae.
• Prophylactic penicillin is indicated in all infants and children starting at 2 mos
    ◊ 2-6 mos 62.5 mg bid; 6 mos-3 yrs 125 mg bid; 3-5 yrs 250 mg bid
    ◊ If no pneumococcal infections and spleen functioning, stop prophylaxis at 6 years. If high risk remains, continue until puberty
    ◊ Alternative penicillin, benzathine IM regimen is 300,000 units a month ages 4 mos-3 yrs and 600,000 units monthly ages 3-5 yrs.
Contraindications: None
Precautions: Avoid high-dose estrogen oral contraceptives; consider Depo-Provera as alternate contraceptive
Significant possible interactions: None

ALTERNATIVE DRUGS
• Other NSAID's
• Folic acid supplements
    ◊ Recommended routinely by most authorities
    ◊ 0.1 mg/day from 0-6 mos; 0.25 mg/day from 6-12 mos; 0.5 mg/day from 1-2 yrs; 1 mg/day beyond age 2

FOLLOWUP

PATIENT MONITORING
• Frequency determined by number/severity of crises and complications
• Early recognition/early treatment of infections. Parents/patient should be instructed that temperature of 101° F (38.3°C) or above requires immediate medical attention.
• All febrile patients require cultures (blood/urine), chest x-ray, CBC/reticulocytes
• For patients who receive chronic transfusions - monitor for hepatitis and hemosiderosis

PREVENTION/AVOIDANCE
Avoid conditions that precipitate sickling (hypoxia, dehydration, cold, infection, fever, acidosis, anesthesia).

POSSIBLE COMPLICATIONS
• Bone infarct
• Aseptic necrosis of femoral head
• Cerebrovascular accidents with neurologic sequelae. In the 10% of patients who suffer these, transfusions q 3-4 weeks will reduce risk by 90%. With this therapy, most patients require iron chelation therapy.
• Cardiac enlargement
• Cholelithiasis/abnormal liver function
• Chronic leg ulcers
• Priapism
• Hematuria/hyposthenuria
• Retinopathy
• Acute chest syndrome (infection/infarction), leading to chronic pulmonary disease
• Infections (pneumonia, osteomyelitis, meningitis, pyelonephritis). Increased risk of sepsis with each.
• Hemosiderosis (2° to multiple transfusions)
• Decreased intellectual function - even without clinical stroke

EXPECTED COURSE/PROGNOSIS
Anemia is lifelong. In second decade, number of crises diminish but complications more frequent. Some patients die in childhood, of CVA or sepsis. Most patients live to early-mid adulthood; few live > 50 years. Common causes of death are infections, thrombosis, pulmonary emboli, or renal failure. Prognosis may be modified in future when gene therapy and/or messenger RNA repair become a reality

MISCELLANEOUS

ASSOCIATED CONDITIONS
Psychosocial effects of chronic illness, especially low self-esteem, depression, and dependency. May need counseling, tutoring, antidepressants and/or vocational training.

AGE-RELATED FACTORS
Pediatric:
• Sequestration crises and hand-foot syndrome seen only in infants/young children
• Functional asplenia in later childhood
• Adolescence/young adulthood:
    ◊ Frequency of complications and secondary organ/tissue damage increase with age; except for strokes which occur mostly in childhood
    ◊ Psychological complications, including body-image and sexual identity problems, interrupted schooling/career training, restriction of activities, stigma of chronic disease, low self-esteem, fear of future
Geriatric: N/A
Others: N/A

PREGNANCY
• Usually complicated and hazardous, especially 3rd trimester and delivery
• Complications include increased number/severity of crises, toxemia, infection, pulmonary infarction, phlebitis
• Fetal mortality 35-40%; abortions/stillbirths, prematurity
• Prophylactic partial exchange transfusion in 3rd trimester reduces maternal morbidity and fetal mortality

SYNONYMS
• Sickle cell disease
• Hb S disease

ICD-9-CM
282.60 Sickle cell anemia, unspecified

SEE ALSO   N/A

OTHER NOTES   N/A

ABBREVIATIONS   N/A

REFERENCES
• Serjeant GR: Sickle cell disease. 2 Ed. New York, Oxford University Press, 1992
• Committee on Genetics, American Academy of Pediatrics: Health supervision for children with sickle cell diseases and their families. Pediatr 1996;95(2):467-472
• Hillery CA: Potential therapeutic approaches for the treatment of vaso-occlusion in sickle cell disease. Curr Opin in Hematol 1998;5(2):151-155
• Okpala I: Management of crisis in sickle cell disease. Eur J Haematol 1998;60(1)1-6
• Ballas SK: Complications of sickle cell anemia in adults: guidelines for effective management. Clev Clin J Med;1999;66(1):48-58
• Reed W, Vachensky EP: New considerations in the treatment of sickle cell disease. Ann Rev Med 1998;49:461-474
• Davies HF: Oni L: Management of patients with sickle cell disease. BMJ 1997;315:656-660
• Bunn HF: Pathogenesis and treatment of sickle cell disease. NEJM 1997;337:762-767
• Serjeant GR: Sickle cell disease - a review. Lancet 1997;350::725-730
Illustrations: 1 available on CD-ROM
Internet references: http://www.5mcc.com

Author(s)
Frank "Chip" Celestino, MD

Aneurysm of the abdominal aorta

BASICS

DESCRIPTION A permanent localized (i.e., focal) dilatation of the abdominal aorta having at least a 50% increase in diameter compared to the expected diameter of the artery. The clinical presentation of aneurysms relates to location, size, type, and comorbid factors affecting the patient. The majority of aneurysms are asymptomatic. Some present with rupture, others with embolism or thrombosis. The management and indications for surgical repair is dictated by the natural history of the aneurysm, the type, the consequences of repair, and the general status of the patient. Types: infrarenal (90%) and thoracoabdominal.

System(s) affected: Cardiovascular
Genetics: Familial aggregations exist, but pathogenesis relates to interaction of genetics, environmental, and biochemical factors.
• Marfan's syndrome
• Ehlers-Danlos syndrome
Incidence/prevalence in USA:
• >15,000 deaths per year
• 10th leading cause of death in males over 55
• 2 to 5% of men > 60 years; 6% of men > 65; 11% of men > 75
• 4% of women > 65
Predominant age: Elderly
Predominant sex: Male > Female (4:1)

SIGNS AND SYMPTOMS Majority of patients with abdominal aortic aneurysm (AAA) are asymptomatic. Many are discovered during radiologic procedures performed for other reasons.
• Pulsatile epigastric mass
• Vague abdominal pain
  ◊ May radiate to the back of flank
• Encroachment by aneurysm
  ◊ Vertebral body erosion
  ◊ Gastric outlet obstruction
  ◊ Ureteral obstruction
• Lower extremity ischemia secondary to micro or macro embolization of mural thrombus
• The triad of shock, pulsatile mass, and abdominal pain should always suggest rupture of AAA:
  ◊ Shock may be absent if the rupture is contained
  ◊ Palpable pulsatile mass may be absent in up to 50% with rupture
  ◊ Pain may radiate to back or into groin
• Unusual presentations
  ◊ Primary aortoenteric fistula--erosion/rupture of AAA into duodenum
  ◊ Aortocaval fistula-- erosion/rupture of AAA into vena cava or left renal vein
  ◊ Inflammatory aneurysm--encasement of aneurysm by thick inflammatory rind associated with chronic abdominal pain, weight loss, and elevated ESR. Surrounding viscera are densely adherent.

CAUSES
• Atherosclerosis
• Dysfunctional connective tissue diseases (e.g., Marfan's)
• Genetic

RISK FACTORS
• Hypertension
• Nicotine

DIAGNOSIS

DIFFERENTIAL DIAGNOSIS
• Abdominal masses transmitting aortic pulse
• Other causes of abdominal pain (e.g., peptic ulcer disease)
• Other causes of back pain(e.g., arthritis, metastatic disease)

LABORATORY N/A
Drugs that may alter lab results: N/A
Disorders that may alter lab results: N/A

PATHOLOGICAL FINDINGS N/A

SPECIAL TESTS
• Evaluation for concomitant CAD
  ◊ Selective evaluation for CAD is appropriate prior to elective AAA repair:
  ◊ Mild, stable cardiac symptoms should have non invasive cardiac stress study
  ◊ Coronary revascularization should be performed when the CAD would merit intervention on its own

IMAGING N/A

DIAGNOSTIC PROCEDURES
• Ultrasonography. Preferred initial diagnostic tool in suspected AAA, but is not reliable for diagnosis of rupture.
• CT scans. Preferred preoperative study. Avoid contrast if patient has significant renal insufficiency. Diagnostic for inflammatory aneurysms.
• MRI. Similar to CT and avoids contrast. MR angiography may replace arteriograms.
• Aortography. Does not define outside dimensions of aneurysms. Indications for aortography:
  ◊ Associated renovascular hypertension
  ◊ Symptoms of visceral angina
  ◊ Significant iliofemoral occlusive disease
  ◊ Suprarenal involvement
  ◊ Peripheral aneurysms
  ◊ Horseshoe or pelvic kidney
  ◊ Prior colectomy

TREATMENT

APPROPRIATE HEALTH CARE
• The treatment of AAA is elective repair
• The prevention of RAAA is elective repair

GENERAL MEASURES
• Control hypertension
• Treat atherosclerotic risk factors

SURGICAL MEASURES
• Repair when:
  ◊ Rupture occurs
  ◊ Size over 4.5 cm (or > 6 cm in poor surgical risk patients)
  ◊ Expansion > 0.5 cm/6 months
  ◊ Symptoms occur
• Poor surgical risk patients:
  ◊ Class III - IV angina; LVEF < 30%; recent CHF or MI; severe valve disease
  ◊ Serum creatinine > 3 mg/dL
  ◊ PaO2 < 50 mmHg; FEV1< IL
  ◊ Cirrhosis with ascites
  ◊ Diffuse retroperitoneal fibrosis; hostile abdomen
  ◊ Physiologic age > chronological age
• Endovascular - experimental (phase 1 trials) alternative to operative repair
  ◊ Very limited application
  ◊ Technical complex
  ◊ Awaits further innovation and improved outcomes

ACTIVITY Ad lib

DIET Low fat

PATIENT EDUCATION N/A

MEDICATIONS

DRUG(S) OF CHOICE N/A
Contraindications: N/A
Precautions: N/A
Significant possible interactions: N/A

ALTERNATIVE DRUGS N/A

FOLLOWUP

PATIENT MONITORING
- Hypertension control
- Lipid control
- Peri-operative complications
  ◊ MI - 5%
  ◊ Renal failure - 6% chronic dialysis - 1%
  ◊ Pulmonary failure - 5-8%
  ◊ Ischemic colitis - 0.5-1%
  ◊ Wound infection - 2%
  ◊ Graft infection - < 0.5%
  ◊ Stroke - 0.5-1%
  ◊ Paraplegia - 0.2%
- Post-surgical monitoring
  ◊ Anastomotic aneurysms
  ◊ Graft infections
  ◊ Aortoenteric fistula
  ◊ Graft limb occlusion
  ◊ Additional aneurysms - thoracic, thoracoabdominal, femoral

PREVENTION/AVOIDANCE
- Screening not cost effective
- High risk groups & incidence
  ◊ Coronary disease: 5-9%
  ◊ Peripheral vascular disease: 10-15%
  ◊ First degree relative with AAA: 25%
  ◊ Obese patients > 65 yrs
  ◊ Presence of peripheral aneurysms

POSSIBLE COMPLICATIONS
- Rupture
- Associated dissection
- Thrombosis
- Embolization distally

EXPECTED COURSE/PROGNOSIS
- Usually expand over time (Laplace's Law: T=pr. Wall tension is directly related to blood pressure and the radius of the artery.) When wall tension exceeds wall tensile strength rupture occurs.
- 5 year rupture risk:

```
Diameter    Risk
---------------
  >7cm        75%
  6-7cm       35%
  5-6cm       25%
  0-5cm       low
---------------
```

- Mean expansion is 0.4 cm/year
- Rupture risk is increased by
  ◊ Diastolic hypertension
  ◊ Tobacco use
  ◊ Diameter > 6 cm
  ◊ COPD
  ◊ Familial history
- Ruptured aneurysms
  ◊ 80% die before receiving definitive care and 50% of the remaining die during their treatment or hospitalization

MISCELLANEOUS

ASSOCIATED CONDITIONS
- Marfan's syndrome
- Ehlers-Danlos syndrome

AGE-RELATED FACTORS
Pediatric: Etiology more likely infectious or collagen disorders
Geriatric: More common in this age group and may present atypically
Others: N/A

PREGNANCY N/A

SYNONYMS
- Aortic aneurysms

ICD-9-CM
441.0 Dissection of aorta (ruptured)
441.4 Abdominal aneurysm without mention of rupture

SEE ALSO
- Aortic dissection
- Marfan's syndrome
- Ehlers-Danlos syndrome
- Takayasu syndrome
- Giant cell arteritis
- Polyarteritis nodosa
- Turner's syndrome

OTHER NOTES N/A

ABBREVIATIONS
CAD = coronary artery disease
CHF = congestive heart failure
COPD = chronic obstructive pulmonary disease
LVEF = left ventricular ejection fraction
MI = myocardial infarction

REFERENCES
- Irvin TT: Abdominal pain: A surgical audit of 1190 emergency admissions. Brit J Surg 1989;76:1121
- Johnston W, et al: Suggested standards for reporting on arterial aneurysms. J Vasc Surg 1991;13:452
- Mason JJ, et al: The role of coronary angiography and coronary revascularization before non cardiac vascular surgery. JAMA 1995;273:1919
- Porter JM, ed: The Year Book of Vascular Surgery. New York, Mosby - Year Book, Inc. 1997
- Rutherford B, ed: Vascular Surgery. 14th Ed. Philadelphia, WB Saunders Co., 1995
- Szilagyi DE, et al: Contribution of abdominal aortic aneurysmectomy to prolongation of life. Ann Surg 1966;164:678
Illustrations: N/A
Internet references: http://www.5mcc.com

Author(s)
David H. Stubbs, MD, FACS

Angina

BASICS

DESCRIPTION Symptom complex resulting from mismatch of myocardial oxygen demand and supply
• Classic angina - a sense of choking or of pressure or heaviness deep to the precordium, usually brought on by exertion or anxiety and relieved by rest.
• Anginal equivalent - exertional dyspnea or exertional fatigue which results from myocardial ischemia and is relieved by rest or nitroglycerin
• Variant angina - also referred to as Prinzmetal's angina describes angina occurring at rest of in atypical patterns such as after exercise or nocturnally. Prinzmetal's angina is caused by coronary artery spasm and is associated with ECG changes (usually ST elevation) during symptoms
• Unstable angina - pain which is new or which is changed in character to become more frequent, more severe or both. Unstable angina portends myocardial infarction in a certain percentage of patients.
System(s) affected: Cardiovascular
Genetics: Coronary artery disease has genetic implications.
Incidence/Prevalence in USA: The presenting symptom of coronary artery disease in 38% of men and 61% of women.
Predominant age: Most common in middle age and older men; postmenopausal women
Predominant sex: Male > Female

SIGNS AND SYMPTOMS
• Precordial pressure or heaviness, radiating to the back, neck or arms, brought on by exercise, emotional stress, meals, cold air or smoking, and relieved by rest or nitrates
• Discomfort may radiate to neck, lower jaw, teeth, shoulders, inner aspects of the arms or back
• Discomfort may be described with a clinched fist over the sternum (Levine's sign)
• Dyspnea on exertion may present as the only symptom
• A choking sensation is a classic symptom

CAUSES
• Atherosclerosis of the coronary arteries
• Coronary artery spasm
• Thrombosis
• Aortic stenosis
• Hypertrophic cardiomyopathy
• Severe hypertension
• Aortic insufficiency
• Primary pulmonary hypertension

RISK FACTORS
• Family history of premature coronary artery disease (CAD)
• Hypercholesterolemia
• Hypertension
• Tobacco abuse
• Diabetes mellitus
• Male gender
• Advanced age

DIAGNOSIS

DIFFERENTIAL DIAGNOSIS
• Esophagitis
• Esophageal spasm
• Peptic ulcer
• Gastritis
• Cholecystitis
• Costochondritis
• Pericarditis
• Aortic dissection
• Pulmonary embolus
• Pulmonary hypertension
• Pneumothorax
• Radiculopathy
• Shoulder arthropathy
• Psychological - anxiety and panic disorders

LABORATORY
• Total cholesterol - frequently elevated
• HDL cholesterol - frequently reduced
• LDL cholesterol - frequently elevated
Drugs that may alter lab results: N/A
Disorders that may alter lab results: N/A

PATHOLOGICAL FINDINGS
Atherosclerosis of the coronary arteries

SPECIAL TESTS
• ECG - may show evidence of prior myocardial infarction. Other findings are nonspecific and tracings are frequently normal. Bundle branch block, Wolff-Parkinson-White syndrome or intraventricular conduction delay may make the ECG unreliable.
• Exercise stress testing

IMAGING
• Radionuclide scintigraphy
• Stress echocardiography
• Stress thallium
• Coronary angiography

DIAGNOSTIC PROCEDURES Rapid sequence MRI may show coronary artery artery calcification and thereby identify coronary artery disease. It does not identify obstructive coronary lesions however.

TREATMENT

APPROPRIATE HEALTH CARE The patient's symptoms should be brought under control medically. If symptoms are unstable, hospitalization is warranted.

GENERAL MEASURES
• Treatment goal - involves reducing myocardial oxygen demand or to increase oxygen supply
• Noninvasive testing is often indicated as a means of stratifying the patient's risk for an event that might seriously compromise myocardial function
• Quit smoking
• Minimize emotional stress

SURGICAL MEASURES Coronary artery bypass graft surgery, angioplasty, stent placement, atherectomy in selected cases

ACTIVITY
• As tolerated after consulting physician
• Exercise program after physician's approval

DIET Low fat, low cholesterol diet

PATIENT EDUCATION American Heart Association, 7320 Greenville Avenue, Dallas, TX 75231, (214)373-6300

Angina

MEDICATIONS

DRUG(S) OF CHOICE
• Aspirin, 325 mg qd for all patients with coronary disease in whom this medication is not contraindicated (i.e., warfarin usage)
• Beta-blockers: atenolol 25-100 mg qd, metoprolol 25-100 mg bid or propranolol 30-100 mg bid-tid. Beta-blockers are effective in reducing the heart rate and thereby decreasing oxygen consumption and reducing angina. Adjust doses according to the clinical response. Aim to maintain resting heart rate of 50-60 beats per minute. Side effects are frequent and include fatigue, impotence, exacerbation of peripheral vascular and obstructive pulmonary disease, depression.
• Nitroglycerin 0.3-0.6 mg sublingually is the most effective therapy for acute anginal episodes. The dose may be repeated 2-3 times over a 10-15 minute time period; if the patient does not experience relief he/she should be instructed to seek medical attention immediately.
• Nitrates: long acting nitrates (mononitrates or transdermal nitrates) should be used with allowance for drug free interval of 10-14 hours to prevent tolerance. Tachyphylaxis occurs rapidly. Act through preload reduction and coronary vasodilatation. Side effects which include headaches and hypotension, tend to clear with continued usage. A beta-blocker or calcium channel blocker should be used in conjunction with the nitrates during the drug free interval.
• Calcium antagonist: long acting formulations of verapamil 160-480 mg qd or diltiazem 90-360 mg qd or nifedipine 30-120 mg qd or amlodipine 5-20 mg qd are available. The various agents have their own individual side effects (i.e., verapamil - constipation; nifedipine - peripheral edema). Neither verapamil nor diltiazem should be used in patient with compromised ventricular function (left ventricular ejection fraction < 40%). (Short-acting types should be avoided.)
• HMC CoA reductase inhibitors (e.g., pravastatin, lovastatin, and others) should be started for hypercholesterolemia. These drugs recently have been shown to decrease incidence of symptomatic CAD, and to reduce both myocardial infarction and death from MI. The new statin drug atorvastatin is particularly effective in lowering total cholesterol, LDL and triglycerides.
• Heparin: intravenously in therapeutic doses should be initiated in patients hospitalized with unstable angina
• Combination therapy: especially nitrates plus calcium antagonists may be used. Triple therapy with addition of beta-blockers may be necessary. Combination therapies should be used with care to avoid impairment of LV function.

Contraindications:
• Sildenafil (Viagra) and nitrates should be avoided due to hypotension
Precautions: Refer to manufacturer's literature

Significant possible interactions:
• Beta-blockers and calcium channel blockers
  ◊ May combine to produce symptomatic heart block although either class of drug may act alone in producing this side effect
  ◊ Care must also be taken when combining these classes of drugs (beta-blockers and calcium channel blockers) in patients with even moderately compromised ventricular function
• Nitrates should not be used with sildenafil (Viagra)

ALTERNATIVE DRUGS
Lipid lowering drugs are often initiated in patients with unfavorable lipid profiles, whether symptomatic from CAD or not

FOLLOWUP

PATIENT MONITORING
• Depends on the frequency and severity of the complaints
• Hospitalization is indicated in patients diagnosed with unstable angina

PREVENTION/AVOIDANCE
• Discontinue tobacco, adherence to low fat/low cholesterol diet, regular aerobic exercise program
• Antilipidemics

POSSIBLE COMPLICATIONS
• Related to myocardial damage occurring during infarction
• Arrhythmia
• Cardiac arrest
• Congestive heart failure

EXPECTED COURSE/PROGNOSIS
• Variable and depending on the extent of coronary artery disease as well as left ventricular function
• Annual mortality is 3-4% overall

MISCELLANEOUS

ASSOCIATED CONDITIONS
• Hypercholesterolemia
• Claudication
• Mitral regurgitation
• Papillary muscle dysfunction
• Ventricular aneurysm
• Abdominal aortic aneurysm
• Hypertrophic subaortic stenosis
• Primary hyperthyroidism
• Pernicious anemia and other high output states

AGE-RELATED FACTORS
Pediatric: Suspect familial dyslipidemias in children presenting with manifestations of coronary artery disease
Geriatric: Patients may be very sensitive to the side effects of medications (i.e., beta-blockers - depression)
Others: N/A

PREGNANCY Other diagnosis should be excluded and the patient managed closely by an obstetrician and cardiologist as the metabolic demands of pregnancy will exacerbate symptoms and directly interfere with treatment

SYNONYMS
• Stenocardia
• Heberden's syndrome

ICD-9-CM
411.1 Angina, unstable
413 Angina pectoris
413.1 Prinzmetal's angina
413.9 Angina, unspecified

SEE ALSO N/A

OTHER NOTES N/A

ABBREVIATIONS N/A

REFERENCES
• Brandenburg RO, Fuster V, Giuliani ER, McGoon DC: Cardiology: Fundamentals and Practice, Chicago, Year Book Medical Publishers, 1987
• Braunwald E: Heart Disease: A Textbook of Cardiovascular Medicine. 4th Ed. Philadelphia, W.B. Saunders Co., 1992
Illustrations: N/A
Internet references: http://www.5mcc.com

Author(s)
Phil Lobstein, MD

Angioedema

BASICS

DESCRIPTION Rapid, localized edema of subcutaneous tissues up to several centimeters in diameter. Life threatening if larynx, pharynx is affected. Resolves in hours to days.
• Hereditary angioedema (HAE), type I: Recurrent episodes involving both skin and mucous membranes, without urticaria. 25% mortality. Many have abdominal pain from edema of intestinal mucosa. Due to hereditary deficiency of C1-esterase inhibitor (C1-INH).
• HAE, type II: Like type I, but has normal levels of non-functional C1-INH
• Acquired angioedema: Rare, in some patients with lymphoproliferative malignancies. Treatment of malignancy causes resolution of edema. Autoantibody inactivation or consumption of C1-INH.
• Vibratory angioedema: Rare. Local swelling in response to vibration. May be hereditary.
• Drug-induced angioedema:
   ◊ Immunologic hypersensitivity, as in penicillin reaction, or non-immunologic, as in aspirin or NSAID
   ◊ Angiotensin converting enzyme (ACE) inhibitor-induced angioedema has become the most common form of AE. non-immune; tendency to involve tongue, with life-threatening airway edema. Can't predict. May occur immediately, or many months after starting drug.
• Idiopathic angioedema: Acute or chronic
System(s) affected: Skin/Exocrine
Genetics: 2% of cases of angioedema are hereditary autosomal dominant
   ◊ 85% have CI-INH deficiency
   ◊ 15% have normal levels of defective CI-INH
Incidence/Prevalence in USA:
Approximately 1 in 5,000. Accompanies urticaria 50% of time.
Predominant age: All ages (idiopathic).
Predominant sex: Male = Female (idiopathic)

SIGNS AND SYMPTOMS
• Occurs alone or with urticaria
• May occur as part of generalized anaphylactic reaction, potentially fatal
• May occur anywhere on body; usually face, extremities, genitalia; often asymmetric (e.g., half of upper lip, one earlobe)
• Rapid onset, usually resolves spontaneously in < 72 hours
• Very little itching in comparison to urticaria. May have stinging or burning sensation.

CAUSES
• Allergic or non-allergic, mediated by release of histamine from mast cells in subcutaneous tissues
• Food allergy
   ◊ Allergy to peanuts and/or tree nuts a leading cause of severe (sometimes fatal) food-induced allergic reactions. Affects I% of the general population.
   ◊ Other foods that cause hives are chocolate, fish, tomatoes, eggs, fresh berries, milk. Also food additives and preservatives.

• ACE inhibitors (ACEI) are becoming among the most frequent causes, mostly within the first 3-4 weeks. However, first onset may be delayed years. ACEI-associated angioedema is not an allergic reaction. Failure to react to rechallenge with drug does not rule out a cause-effect relation between the ACEI and angioedema.
   ◊ Losartan (Cozaar) and valsartan (Diovan), both angiotensin 11 receptor blockers, also have caused angioedema
   ◊ Angioedema has occurred within 24 hours to 16 months after initiating losartan therapy.
• Helicobacter pylori has been increasingly associated with, and its eradication may stop, chronic urticaria
• Thyroid autoimmunity has been increasingly reported to be associated with angioedema. May be relieved by giving thyroid hormone.

RISK FACTORS Medications that cause allergic reactions, e.g., penicillin, aspirin. 0.2% of patients taking ACE inhibitors develop angioedema; some cases have proven fatal. Omeprazole and sertraline have also recently been implicated.

DIAGNOSIS

DIFFERENTIAL DIAGNOSIS
• Anaphylaxis
• Cellulitis
• Erysipelas
• Contact dermatitis
• Lymphedema
• Diffuse subcutaneous infiltrative process
• Localized edema

LABORATORY
• C4 assay (low in HAE). If C4 normal, do urticaria work-up.
• If C4 is low, do C1-INH assay (immunoreactive) for HAE type I, and C1-INH assay (functional) for HAE type II
• If not HAE, do neoplastic work-up to rule out acquired angioedema, vasculitis work-up (CBC, ANA, RA, ESR, skin biopsy) to rule out autoimmune disease
Drugs that may alter lab results:
Antihistamines, H2-blockers, tricyclic antidepressants
Disorders that may alter lab results: N/A

PATHOLOGICAL FINDINGS Edema, vasculitis and/or perivasculitis involving only subcutaneous tissues

SPECIAL TESTS N/A

IMAGING N/A

DIAGNOSTIC PROCEDURES Skin biopsy (correlates poorly with clinical picture)

TREATMENT

APPROPRIATE HEALTH CARE Ensure airway patency first! Protect airway if mouth, tongue, throat are involved. CPR and transport to emergency facility if necessary.

GENERAL MEASURES
• Avoidance of known triggers
• Cool, moist compresses to control itching

SURGICAL MEASURES N/A

ACTIVITY As desired. HAE patients should avoid violent exercise, trauma.

DIET Avoidance of known trigger foods.

PATIENT EDUCATION Educate HAE patient to provide history of disease to health care workers.

MEDICATIONS

DRUG(S) OF CHOICE
• First generation antihistamines for acute angioedema
   ◊ Older children and adults: hydroxyzine (Vistaril) or diphenhydramine (Benadryl), 25-50 mg q6h
   ◊ Children under six: diphenhydramine 12.5 mg (elixir) q6-8h (5 mg/kg/day)
• Second generation H1 blockers are more expensive, about as effective as older antihistamines, but are less sedating (14% of patients, still less than 1st generation drugs), because they do not cross the blood-brain barrier.
   ◊ Fexofenadine (Allegra) 60 mg bid
   ◊ Loratadine (Claritin) 10 mg daily
   ◊ Acrivastine (Semprex) 8 mg tid
   ◊ Cetirizine (Zyrtec)10 mg daily. More sedating than others in this class.
• HAE therapy:
   ◊ Intubation if airway threatened
   ◊ Epinephrine 1:1000, 0.2-0.3 mL IV or subcutaneous
   ◊ Fresh frozen plasma (only works 1-12 days; no long-term benefit. May transmit hepatitis B).
   ◊ C1-INH, not yet available in USA
   ◊ Attenuated androgen - danazol. For prevention (increases amount of active C1-INH in both types I and II). Give 200-600 mg daily for 1 month, then 5 days on, 5 days off. Ineffective in other forms of C1-INH deficiency. Side effects: headaches, weight gain, hematuria.

Contraindications:
• Danazol not for use in childhood, pregnancy.

Precautions:
• Drowsiness with first generation drugs.
• Second generation H1 blockers should be used with caution in pregnancy and the elderly.

Significant possible interactions: Refer to manufacturer's profile of each drug

ALTERNATIVE DRUGS
• Aminocaproic acid (epsilon-aminocaproic acid, EACA) was used before danazol available. Prevents activation of plasminogen and C1. Rarely can cause thrombophlebitis, embolism, myositis.
• Doxepin (Sinequan) effective for angioedema (10 to 25 mg at bedtime)

FOLLOWUP

PATIENT MONITORING
• Diagnostic work-up if symptoms severe, persistent or recurrent
• Protect airway if mouth, tongue, throat involved.

PREVENTION/AVOIDANCE
• If etiology known, avoidance
• Avoid ACE inhibitors in patients with history of angioedema

POSSIBLE COMPLICATIONS
Anaphylaxis, respiratory compromise

EXPECTED COURSE/PROGNOSIS
Most with idiopathic do well. Chronic forms dependent on nature of defect.

MISCELLANEOUS

ASSOCIATED CONDITIONS
• Urticaria
• Anaphylaxis

AGE-RELATED FACTORS
Pediatric: N/A
Geriatric: N/A
Others: N/A

PREGNANCY

SYNONYMS
• Angioneurotic edema
• Quincke's edema

ICD-9-CM
995.1 Angioneurotic edema
277.6 Other deficiencies of circulating enzymes (Hereditary angioedema)

SEE ALSO   Urticaria

OTHER NOTES   Same pathophysiology for urticaria and angioedema - localized anaphylaxis causes vasodilatation, vascular permeability of skin (urticaria) or subcutaneous tissue (angioedema)

ABBREVIATIONS
HAE = hereditary angioedema

REFERENCES
• Cooper KD: Urticaria and angioedema: Diagnosis and evaluation. J Am Acad Dermatol 1991;25:166
• Greaves M, Lawlor F: Angioedema: Manifestations and management. J Am Acad Dermatol 1991;25:155
• Monroe EW: Nonsedating H1 antihistamines in chronic urticaria. Ann Allergy 1993;71: 585-91
• van Rijnsoever EW, et al: Angioneurotic edema attributed to the use of losartan. Arch Intern Med 1998;158(18):2063-5
• Frye CB, Pettigrew TJ: Angioedema and photosensitive rash induced by valsartan. Pharmacotherapy 1998;18(4):866-8
• Kunschak M, et al: A randomized, controlled trial to study the efficacy and safety of C1 inhibitor concentrate in treating hereditary angioedema. Transfusion 1998;38(6):540-9
Illustrations: N/A
Internet references: http://www.5mcc.com

Author(s)
John E. Perchalski, MD, FAAFP

Animal bites

BASICS

DESCRIPTION Bite wounds to humans from dogs, cats, other animals including humans
System(s) affected: Endocrine/Metabolic, Skin/Exocrine, Hemic/Lymphatic/Immunologic, Nervous
Genetics: N/A
Incidence/Prevalence in USA:
• Dog bites: 1200/100,000
• Cat bites: 160/100,000
• Snake bites: 15/100,000 non-venomous bites and 3/100,000 venomous bites per year. Lifetime prevalence for animal bite 50,000/100,000.
• Dog bites are responsible for 1/3 million ER visits per year
Predominant age: All ages, but children more likely to be affected
Predominant sex: Male > Female

SIGNS AND SYMPTOMS
• Bite wounds can be tears, punctures, scratches, avulsions or crush injuries
• Dog bites (80-90% of bites)
  ◊ Hands are most commonly affected with up to 68% of bites
  ◊ The face is the site of injury in up to 29% of cases, the lower extremities in 10%, and involvement of the trunk is uncommon
• Cat bites (10% of bites)
  ◊ Predominantly involve the hands, followed by lower extremities, face and trunk
  ◊ Are more likely to become infected because of puncture type of wounds

CAUSES
• Most bite wounds are from a domestic pet known to the victim. Large dogs are the most common source.
• Human bites are often the result of one person striking another in the mouth with a clenched fist

RISK FACTORS
• Dog bites are more common in the early afternoon, especially during warm weather. Male dogs more likely to bite.
• Clenched fist injuries are frequently associated with the use of alcohol

DIAGNOSIS:

DIFFERENTIAL DIAGNOSIS The diagnosis is straight forward. What is of concern is judging the risk to the patient from the injury and resulting infection.

LABORATORY
• 85% of bite wounds will yield a positive culture, but culturing at time of injury is of little benefit
• Wound culture is essential in directing therapy of infected wounds. Some pathogens are slow growing so cultures should be kept for 7-10 days. Gram stain is sensitive but not specific for infecting organism.
• Dog bites - *Pasteurella multocida* is present in 25% of bites. *Streptococcus viridans*, *Staphylococcus aureus*, coagulase-negative Staphylococcus, *Bacteroides*, *C. canimorsus*, and *Fusobacterium* can also be found.
• Cat bites - *Pasteurella multocida* is present in 50% of bites. The wound is often contaminated by other mixed bacteria, including several species of both aerobic and anaerobic organisms.
• Human bites - Streptococcus species, *Staphylococcus aureus*, *Eikenella corrodens* and various anaerobic bacteria are common
• Other animal bites - scant information on the pathogens of these
Drugs that may alter lab results: Previous antibiotic therapy
Disorders that may alter lab results: N/A

PATHOLOGICAL FINDINGS N/A

SPECIAL TESTS N/A

IMAGING
• If bite wound is near a bone or joint, a plain radiograph is needed to check for bone injury and to use for comparison later if osteomyelitis is suspected
• In human bite wounds from clenched fist injuries, order plain film radiographs to check for metacarpal or phalanx fracture

DIAGNOSTIC PROCEDURES Surgical exploration might be needed to ascertain extent of injuries. Exploration should be performed on all serious hand wounds, especially clenched-fist injuries involving a joint.

TREATMENT

APPROPRIATE HEALTH CARE Outpatient setting unless patient has fulminant infection requiring systemic antibiotics, close observation, or surgery

GENERAL MEASURES Elevation of the injured extremity to prevent swelling. Contact the local health department and consult about the prevalence of rabies in the species of animal involved.

SURGICAL MEASURES
• Copious irrigation of the wound with normal saline via a catheter tip is needed to reduce risk of infection
• Devitalized tissue needs débridement
• Débridement of puncture wounds not advised
• Consider surgical closure if the wound is clean after irrigation and bite is less than 12 hours old. Puncture wounds should be left open.
• Delayed primary closure in 3-5 days is an option for infected wounds
• Splint hand if it is injured
• Human bite wounds on the hands should not be primarily closed due to the high risk of infection. Large, gaping wounds should be reapproximated with widely space sutures or steristrips.

ACTIVITY No restriction

DIET No special diet

PATIENT EDUCATION Discussion with parents at "well child checks" should include education on how to avoid animal bites

MEDICATIONS

DRUG(S) OF CHOICE
• Consider anti-rabies therapy
• Use tetanus toxoid in those previously immunized, but more than 5 years since their last dose
• Consider tetanus immune globulin (TIG) in patients without a full primary series of immunizations
• Prophylactic therapy if wound seen in first 12 hours:
◊ Dog, cat, human - amoxicillin-clavulanate 250-500 mg tid po; child 20-40 mg/kg/day po given tid
◊ Snake bite - if venomous, the patient needs rapid transport to facility capable of definitive evaluation. If an envenomation has occurred, the patient will need to receive antivenin unless envenomation was only minimal. Be sure patient is stable for transport; consider measuring and or treating coagulation and renal status along with any anaphylactic reactions before transport.
◊ Others - amoxicillin-clavulanate (Augmentin) potassium - dosage - adult 250-500 mg po tid; child 20-40 mg/kg/day given tid
• Established infection
◊ Once patient has developed a clinical infection, amoxicillin-clavulanate potassium (Augmentin) can be used pending culture reports
Contraindications: Do not use penicillin-derived antibiotics in those with penicillin allergy
Precautions: Prescribe dosage of antibiotics by body weight and renal function
Significant possible interactions: Antibiotics may decrease efficacy of oral contraceptives

ALTERNATIVE DRUGS
• Alternative therapy for penicillin allergic patients: (for prophylaxis or empiric treatment):
◊ Approximately 10% cross reactivity with cephalosporins in penicillin allergic patients
◊ Dog bite - doxycycline if patient is older than 9 years, and in women only if they are not pregnant or breast feeding. Ceftriaxone or erythromycin can also be used. Avoid cephalexin due to resistant strains of P. Multocida.
◊ Cat bite - as for dog bite
◊ Human bite - cefoxitin 80-160 mg/kg/day (up to 12 grams), given in 3 or 4 equally divided doses. Usual dose is 1-2 grams q 6-8 hours; doxycycline can also be used.

FOLLOWUP:

PATIENT MONITORING
• Patient should be rechecked in 24-48 hours if not infected at time of first encounter
• Daily followup is warranted with active infections
• If antibiotics are used for an active infection, the duration of therapy should be 7-14 days depending on the severity of the infection and the clinical response

PREVENTION/AVOIDANCE
Instruct children and adults about animal hazards. Education of dog owners about responsible dog ownership. Stronger enforcement of animal control laws.

POSSIBLE COMPLICATIONS
Complications from bites can include septic arthritis, osteomyelitis, extensive soft tissue injuries with scarring, sepsis, hemorrhage, death. Gas gangrene can take an exceedingly rapid course and should be treated very aggressively.

EXPECTED COURSE/PROGNOSIS
Wounds should steadily improve and close over by 7-10 days

MISCELLANEOUS

ASSOCIATED CONDITIONS N/A

AGE-RELATED FACTORS
Pediatric: Young children are more likely to have severe bites
Geriatric:
• Serious injury from any bite wound is more common in persons greater than 50 years old, those with wounds in the upper extremities or those with puncture wounds
• Increased risk of infection in those greater than 50 years old
Others: N/A

PREGNANCY No special precautions

SYNONYMS N/A

ICD-9-CM
879.8 open wound(s) of unspecified site(s) without mention of complications
882.0 hand, open wound (except fingers alone)
873.40 face, open wound, without mention of complications

SEE ALSO
• Rabies
• Snake Envenomations: Crotalidae
• Snake Envenomations: Elapidae
• Cellulitis
• Bartonella infections

OTHER NOTES Rabies: Contact your local health department for information about the risk of rabies

ABBREVIATIONS N/A

REFERENCES
• Wiggins ME, Akelman E, Weiss AC: The management of dog bite infections to the hand. Orthopedics 1994;17:617-623
• Griego RD, et al: Dog, cat and human bites: A review. J AM Acad Dermatol 1995;33:1019-1029
• Cummings P: Antibiotics to prevent infection in patients with dog bite wounds: A meta-analysis. Ann Emerg Med 1994;23:535-540
• Lewis KT, Stilles M: Management of Cat and dog bites. Am Fam Phys 1995;52:479-485
• Sacks JJ, et al: Fatal dog attacks 1989-1994. Pediatrics 1996;97:891-895
• Fleisher GR: The management of bite wounds. NEJM 1999;340;138-140
Illustrations: N/A
Internet references: http://www.5mcc.com

Author(s)
George R. Bergus, MD

Ankylosing spondylitis

BASICS

DESCRIPTION A chronic, usually progressive, condition in which inflammatory changes and new bone formation occurs at the attachment of tendons and ligaments to bone (enthesopathy)
• Sacroiliac joint involvement is the hallmark of ankylosing spondylitis with variable degrees of spinal involvement. However, 20-30% of patients also have larger peripheral joint involvement
System(s) affected: Musculoskeletal
Genetics: Familial clustering and higher than expected frequency of HLA-B27 tissue antigen
Incidence/Prevalence in USA:
• 0.5-5 per 1000 in white males
• Less common in women and Blacks
Predominant age:
• Usually symptoms begin in early twenties
• Onset of symptoms - rarely occurs after age 40
Predominant sex: Male > Female

SIGNS AND SYMPTOMS
• Subgluteal or low back pain and/or stiffness
• Insidious onset
• Onset usually in 3rd decade
• Duration greater than 3 months
• Morning stiffness
• Frequently awaken at night to "walk off" stiffness
• Improvement in stiffness with activity
• Increased symptoms with rest
• Pleuritic chest pain is often an early feature
• Thoracic and cervical spine complaints in advanced disease
• Hip, shoulder, or knee complaints
• Diminished range of motion in the lumbar spine in all three planes of motion
• Loss of lumbar lordosis
• Thoraco-cervical kyphosis (rarely occurs before ten years of symptoms)
• Aortic root dilatation (20%)
• Aortic regurgitation murmur (2%)
• Acute anterior uveitis (20-30%)
• Osteoporosis

CAUSES Unknown

RISK FACTORS
• HLA-B27
• Positive family history
• 10% risk of developing AS (Ankylosing Spondylitis) for HLA-B27 positive child of spondylitic parent

DIAGNOSIS

DIFFERENTIAL DIAGNOSIS
• Reiter's syndrome
• Psoriatic arthritis
• Diffuse idiopathic skeletal hypertrophy (DISH)
• Spondylitis associated with inflammatory bowel disease
• Rheumatoid arthritis

LABORATORY
• HLA-B27 tissue antigen is present in 90% of patients compared to 5-8% incidence in general population
• Erythrocyte sedimentation rate (ESR) is elevated in 80% of cases, but correlates poorly with disease activity and prognosis
• Absent rheumatoid factor
Drugs that may alter lab results: N/A
Disorders that may alter lab results: N/A

PATHOLOGICAL FINDINGS
• Erosive changes coupled with new bone formation at attachment of tendons and ligaments to bone resulting in ossification of periarticular soft-tissues
• Synovial changes are indistinguishable from rheumatoid arthritis. Erosion of articular cartilage is less severe than in rheumatoid arthritis.

SPECIAL TESTS
• Synovial fluid - mild leukocytosis, decreased viscosity
• Cerebrospinal fluid - increased protein
• EKG - conduction defects
• Measurement of respiratory excursion of chest wall - less than 5 cm maximal respiratory excursion of chest wall measured at fourth intercostal space. Less than 2.5 cm is virtually diagnostic of ankylosing spondylitis.
• Wright-Schober test for lumbar spine flexion is abnormal

IMAGING
• Sacroiliac joint early - sclerosis on both sides of joint not extending more than 1 cm from articular surface
• Sacroiliac joint late - ankylosis of sacroiliac joint
• Spine - "squaring" of vertebral bodies and ossification of annulus fibrosis giving appearance of "bamboo spine". Ankylosis of facet joints.
• Peripheral joint - symmetric erosive changes in larger joints. Pericapsular ossification, sclerosis, loss of joint space.

DIAGNOSTIC PROCEDURES
• Physical examination
• Radiographs - sacroiliac joint films, lumbar spine series

TREATMENT

APPROPRIATE HEALTH CARE
Outpatient

GENERAL MEASURES
• Posture training and range of motion exercises for spine are essential
• Firm bed
• Sleep in prone position or supine without a pillow
• Breathing exercises 2-3 times/day
• Swimming
• Physical therapy
• Stop smoking, if a smoker

SURGICAL MEASURES N/A

ACTIVITY Encourage active lifestyle

DIET No special diet

PATIENT EDUCATION
• For a listing of sources for patient education materials favorably reviewed on this topic, physicians may contact: American Academy of Family Physicians Foundation, P.O. Box 8418, Kansas City, MO 64114, (800)274-2237, ext. 4400

Ankylosing spondylitis

MEDICATIONS

DRUG(S) OF CHOICE
- Nonsteroidal anti-inflammatory drugs provide symptomatic relief
- Selection is empiric, but traditionally indomethacin, 50 mg tid or qid has been used
- Steroids and cytotoxic agents are not effective

Contraindications: See Precautions

Precautions:
- All patients on long term NSAID's should have renal function monitored
- NSAID's may aggravate peptic ulcer disease or cause gastritis
- Don't use NSAID's for patients with a bleeding diathesis or patients requiring anticoagulants

Significant possible interactions: Refer to manufacturer's profile of each drug

ALTERNATIVE DRUGS
Other NSAID's, such as sulindac, naproxen

FOLLOWUP

PATIENT MONITORING   Visits every six to twelve months to monitor posture and range of motion

PREVENTION/AVOIDANCE   N/A

POSSIBLE COMPLICATIONS
- Spine: Pseudarthrosis, cervical spine fracture (high mortality rate), C1-C2 subluxation, spondylodiscitis, cauda equina syndrome (rare)
- Peripheral joint ankylosis
- Pulmonary: Restrictive lung disease, diaphragmatic breathing, upper lobe fibrosis (rare)
- Cardiac: Conduction defects (20%), aortic insufficiency (2%)
- Uveitis

EXPECTED COURSE/PROGNOSIS
- Unpredictable course
- Prognosis good if mobility and upright posture maintained. Usually progressive disability.

MISCELLANEOUS

ASSOCIATED CONDITIONS
- Inflammatory bowel disease
- Uveitis
- Iritis

AGE-RELATED FACTORS
Pediatric: N/A
Geriatric: N/A
Others: N/A

PREGNANCY   N/A

SYNONYMS
- Rheumatoid spondylitis
- Marie-Strumpell disease

ICD-9-CM
720.0 ankylosing spondylitis

SEE ALSO
- Reiter's syndrome
- Crohn's disease
- Ulcerative colitis
- Arthritis, psoriatic
- Arthritis, rheumatoid (RA)

OTHER NOTES
Flexion contractures of the hip and ankylosis may be major contributors to poor posture. Hip arthroplasty should be strongly considered as it may restore upright posture. Heterotopic ossification may occur post operatively and appropriate prophylaxis should be considered.

ABBREVIATIONS   N/A

REFERENCES
- Calin A, ed: Spondyloarthropathies. New York, Grune & Stratton, 1983
- Calin A, Fries J: Ankylosing Spondylitis Discussions in Patient Management. Garden City, New York, Medical Examination Publishing Company, 1978

Illustrations: N/A

Internet references: http://www.5mcc.com

Author(s)
George R. Bradbury, MD
James B. Benjamin, MD

Anorectal abscess

 BASICS

DESCRIPTION Localized induration and fluctuance due to inflammation of the soft tissue near the rectum or anus. 80% are perianal, the remainder are intrasphincteric or supra-levator.
System(s) affected: Gastrointestinal, Skin/Exocrine
Genetics: No known genetic pattern
Incidence/Prevalence in USA: Common
Predominant age: All ages (most common in infants)
Predominant sex: Male > Female (4:1)

SIGNS AND SYMPTOMS
• Perirectal swelling for superficial abscesses
• Perirectal redness
• Perirectal tenderness
• Perirectal throbbing pain
• Fever and other toxic symptoms with deep abscesses
• If abscess is not accompanied by external swelling, digital exam will reveal a swollen tender mass
• Pain on defecation

CAUSES
• Bacterial invasion of the pararectal spaces, originating in an intersphincteric space which may begin with an abrasion or tear in lining of anal canal, rectum or perianal skin
• Organisms: usually mixed, E. coli, Proteus vulgaris, streptococci, staphylococci, bacteroides, pseudomonas aeruginosa

RISK FACTORS
• Inciting trauma
  ◊ Injections for internal hemorrhoids
  ◊ Enema tip abrasions
  ◊ Puncture wounds from eggshells or fish bones
  ◊ Foreign objects
  ◊ Prolapsed hemorrhoid
• Inflammatory bowel disease
• Chronic granulomatous disease
• Immunodeficiency disorders
• Hematologic malignancies (5-8% of these patients will have abscess at some time)

 DIAGNOSIS

DIFFERENTIAL DIAGNOSIS
• Carcinoma
• Retrorectal tumors
• Crohn's disease
• Primary lesions of syphilis
• Tuberculous ulceration

LABORATORY CBC - leukocytosis
Drugs that may alter lab results: N/A
Disorders that may alter lab results: N/A

PATHOLOGICAL FINDINGS
• Inflammation of anal mucosa
• Pus
• Inflammatory tissue

SPECIAL TESTS N/A

IMAGING Barium enema

DIAGNOSTIC PROCEDURES
Only indicated if diagnosis in doubt:
• Sigmoidoscopy - rule out unusual causes
• Proctoscopy - redness, induration of anus; tender mass

 TREATMENT

APPROPRIATE HEALTH CARE
• Outpatient surgery
• Inpatient surgery with IV antibiotics for supra-levator abscess or toxicity

GENERAL MEASURES N/A

SURGICAL MEASURES
• Perianal abscess
  ◊ Incise and drain abscess
  ◊ Local anesthetic frequently appropriate
  ◊ Pack wound with Iodoform gauze (24-48 hours)
• Ischiorectal abscess
  ◊ Incise and drain abscess
  ◊ General anesthetic usually required
  ◊ Pack wound with Iodoform gauze (removed gradually over several days)
  ◊ Fistulectomy may be done at same time in selected cases
• After surgery:
  ◊ Sitz baths q 2-4 hours
  ◊ Heating pad, heat lamp or warm compress as needed for pain
  ◊ Encourage moving legs as soon as possible
  ◊ Prevent constipation

ACTIVITY Resume work and normal activity as soon as possible

DIET Increase fiber and fluid intake

PATIENT EDUCATION
• Sitz bath instruction
• Diet instructions
• Dressing change instructions
• Stress length of time to heal
• Stress physical cleanliness
• Possible development of fistula-in-ano
• Stress stool regularity

Anorectal abscess

MEDICATIONS

DRUG(S) OF CHOICE
- Antibiotics - only for toxicity
- Stool softening laxatives

Contraindications: Refer to manufacturer's literature

Precautions: Refer to manufacturer's literature

Significant possible interactions: Refer to manufacturer's literature

ALTERNATIVE DRUGS N/A

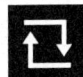

FOLLOWUP

PATIENT MONITORING
Routine postoperative care with attention to wound healing which should progress from the inside out

PREVENTION/AVOIDANCE
- Avoid constipation
- Don't use enemas
- Avoid rectal temperatures or medicines in immunocompromised patients

POSSIBLE COMPLICATIONS
- Possible anorectal fistula (in 25% of patients)
- Possible rectovaginal fistula
- Fecal incontinence due to rupture through sphincter muscle
- Recurrence of abscess if underlying cause not corrected

EXPECTED COURSE/PROGNOSIS
- Slow healing depending on extent of disease and concurrent illnesses, complete healing by 6 months if no complications
- Healing in infants may be complete in 1-3 weeks

MISCELLANEOUS

ASSOCIATED CONDITIONS
- Crohn's disease
- Other inflammatory disease such as appendicitis, salpingitis, diverticulitis
- Possibly perianal hidradenitis suppurativa, or HIV infection in patients with recurring perianal or ischiorectal abscesses

AGE-RELATED FACTORS
Pediatric: Common in first year of life
Geriatric: In elderly patients, a high pelvirectal abscess may cause no symptoms except lower abdominal pain and fever
Others: N/A

PREGNANCY N/A

SYNONYMS N/A

ICD-9-CM
566 Abscess of anal and rectal regions

SEE ALSO
- Anorectal fistula
- Crohn's disease

OTHER NOTES N/A

ABBREVIATIONS N/A

REFERENCES
- Schwartz SI, Shires GT, Spences FC, Storer EH: Principles of Surgery. 4th Ed. New York, McGraw-Hill Book Co., 1984
- Ashcraft KW, Holder TM: Pediatric Surgery. 2nd Ed. Philadelphia, W.B. Saunders Co., 1993
- Fazio VW: Anorectal Disorders. In Gastroenterology Clinics of North America. Philadelphia, W.B. Saunders Co., 1987
- Schouten WR, van Vroonhoven TJ: Treatment of anorectal abscess with or without primary fistulectomy. Results of a prospective randomized trial. Dis Colon Rectum 1991;34:60-3

Illustrations: N/A
Internet references: http://www.5mcc.com

Author(s)
Timothy L. Black, MD, FACS, FAAP

Anorectal fistula

BASICS

DESCRIPTION Inflammatory track with one opening in the anal canal and another in perianal skin. Fistulas occur spontaneously or secondary to perirectal abscess. Most fistulas originate in the anal crypts at the anorectal juncture.
- Goodsall's rule
  ◊ If external opening is anterior to an imaginary line drawn horizontally through anal canal, fistula usually runs directly into anal canal
  ◊ If external opening is posterior to line, the fistula usually curves to posterior midline of anal canal
  ◊ In children, track is usually straight
- Classification
  ◊ Intersphincteric
  ◊ Transsphincteric
  ◊ Suprasphincteric
  ◊ Extrasphincteric

System(s) affected: Gastrointestinal, Skin/Exocrine
Genetics: No known genetic pattern
Incidence/Prevalence in USA: Common
Predominant age: All ages
Predominant sex: Male = Female

SIGNS AND SYMPTOMS
- Constant or intermittent drainage or discharge
- Firm tender peri-anal lump
- External anal sphincter pain during and after defecation
- Spasm of external anal sphincter during and after defecation
- Anal bleeding
- Discoloration of skin surrounding the fistula
- Fistulous opening frequently granulose or scarred
- Possible fever

CAUSES
- Erosion of anal canal
- Extension from infection from a tear in lining in anal canal
- Infecting organism is commonly Escherichia coli

RISK FACTORS
- Injection of internal hemorrhoids, puncture wound from eggshells or fish bones, foreign objects, enema tip injuries
- Ruptured anal hematoma
- Prolapsed internal hemorrhoid
- Acute appendicitis, salpingitis, diverticulitis
- Inflammatory bowel disease (chronic ulcerative colitis, Crohn's disease)
- Previous perirectal abscess

DIAGNOSIS

DIFFERENTIAL DIAGNOSIS
- Pilonidal sinus
- Perianal abscess
- Urethroperineal fistulas
- Ischiorectal abscess
- Submucous or high muscular abscess
- Pelvirectal abscess (rare)
- Rule out: Crohn's disease; carcinoma; retrorectal tumors

LABORATORY CBC (usually not indicated)
Drugs that may alter lab results: N/A
Disorders that may alter lab results: N/A

PATHOLOGICAL FINDINGS
- Fistulous tract may be simple or multiple
- Fistulous tract has primary opening in anal crypt; secondary opening in anal skin, para-anal skin, perineal skin, or in rectal mucus membrane
- Anal sinus - opens in anal crypt
- Termination of sinus is blind and located in para-anal or pararectal tissue

SPECIAL TESTS N/A

IMAGING Lower GI series if inflammatory bowel disease suspected

DIAGNOSTIC PROCEDURES
- Proctoscopy
- Sigmoidoscopy
- Probe inserted into tract to determine its course (be careful not to create an artificial opening)

TREATMENT

APPROPRIATE HEALTH CARE
Outpatient surgery

GENERAL MEASURES Sitz baths 3-4 times per day until definitive surgery

SURGICAL MEASURES
- Fistulotomy - surgical incision of entire length of fistula (unroofing). Mucosal tract may be cauterized or curetted. Sphincterotomy.
- Fistulectomy - complete excision of tract is usually necessary. Sphincterotomy.
- General anesthesia or regional anesthesia usually required
- Postoperative - hot sitz baths
- Avoid constipation

ACTIVITY Resume work and normal activity as soon as possible

DIET Clear liquid diet until gastrointestinal function returns

PATIENT EDUCATION
- Stress peri-anal cleanliness
- Sitz baths

MEDICATIONS

DRUG(S) OF CHOICE
- Broad spectrum antibiotic if active infection
  ◊ Cephalexin (Keflex)
  ◊ Cefadroxil (Duricef)
  ◊ Ampicillin-sulbactam (Unasyn)
  ◊ Amoxicillin-clavulanate (Augmentin)
- Stool-softening laxative

Contraindications: Refer to manufacturer's literature

Precautions: Refer to manufacturer's literature

Significant possible interactions: Refer to manufacturer's literature

ALTERNATIVE DRUGS   N/A

FOLLOWUP

PATIENT MONITORING Frequent follow-up examinations following surgery to ensure complete healing and assess continence

PREVENTION/AVOIDANCE   N/A

POSSIBLE COMPLICATIONS
- Constipation (urge to defecate may be suppressed due to pain)
- Rectovaginal fistula
- Partial incontinence of fecal material if sphincter is divided
- Delayed wound healing
- Low grade carcinoma may develop in long-standing fistulas
- Recurrent anorectal fistula if fistula is incompletely opened or excised

EXPECTED COURSE/PROGNOSIS
- Surgical results usually excellent
- Postoperative healing requires 4-5 weeks for perianal fistulas; 12-16 weeks for deeper fistulas
- Postoperative healing may occur within 2-3 weeks in children

MISCELLANEOUS

ASSOCIATED CONDITIONS
- Possibly associated with penetrating injury, intestinal tuberculosis, ulcerative colitis
- Hidradenitis suppurativa
- Crohn's disease

AGE-RELATED FACTORS
Pediatric: Most common in infants. More frequent in males.
Geriatric: Constipation is a common complication
Others: N/A

PREGNANCY   N/A

SYNONYMS
- Fistula-in-ano
- Anal fistula

ICD-9-CM
565.1 Anal fistula

SEE ALSO
- Anorectal abscess
- Crohn's disease

OTHER NOTES   N/A

ABBREVIATIONS   N/A

REFERENCES
- Kirsner JB, Shorter G, eds: Diseases of the Colon, Rectum and Anal Canal. Baltimore, Williams & Wilkins, 1989
- Sleisenger MH, Fordtran JS, eds: Gastrointestinal Disease: Pathophysiology, Diagnosis, Management. 5th Ed. Philadelphia, W.B. Saunders Co., 1994
- Schwartz SI, Shires GT, Spences FC, Storer EH: Principles of Surgery. 4th Ed. New York, McGraw-Hill Book Co., 1984
- O'Neill JA, Rowe MI, Grosfeld JL, et al: Pediatric Surgery. 5th ed., St Louis, Mosby, 1998

Illustrations: N/A
Internet references: http://www.5mcc.com

Author(s)
Timothy L. Black, MD, FACS, FAAP

Anorexia nervosa

 BASICS

DESCRIPTION Anorexia (AN) always involves refusal to maintain a reasonable body weight. AN is divided into restricting and binge-eating/purging subtypes.
System(s) affected: Nervous, Endocrine/Metabolic, Gastrointestinal, Cardiovascular, Reproductive
Genetics: First degree female relatives contribute
Incidence/Prevalence in USA:
Approximately 1% of females; males comprise 5-10% of cases
Predominant age: Usually adolescents or young adults
Predominant sex: Female > Male

SIGNS AND SYMPTOMS
• Usually insidious in onset
• Onset may be stress related
• Deny seriousness of problem
• Claim to feel fat even when emaciated
• Preoccupation with body size, weight control
• Elaborate food preparation and eating rituals
• Extensive exercise, especially running or use of stair stepper
• Stress fractures
• Sexual disinterest; social isolation
• Cracked, dry skin, sparse scalp hair
• Fine, downy lanugo hair on extremities, face, and trunk
• Growth arrest
• Hypotension and bradycardia
• Hypothermia
• Peripheral edema
• Cognitive decline

CAUSES Unknown; thought to be largely emotional. Co-morbid major depression and/or dysthymia in 50-75% of patients. Obsessive-compulsive disorder in 10-13% of patients.

RISK FACTORS
• Perfectionistic personality, compulsivity
• Low self-esteem
• Achievement pressure; high self-expectations
• Acceptance of the culturally condoned ideal of slimness
• Ambivalence about dependence/independence
• Stress due to multiple responsibilities, tight schedules
• Weight dissatisfaction; perceived overweight
• Early puberty
• History of sexual abuse equivalent to other patient populations

 DIAGNOSIS

DIFFERENTIAL DIAGNOSIS Inanition due to physical disorder; brain tumor; bulimia; depressive disorders with loss of appetite; food phobia; conversion disorder; schizophrenic disorder; body dysmorphic disorder

LABORATORY
• Most findings are directly related to starvation, dehydration: no biological test is specific for anorexia. All findings may be within normal limits.
• Diminished plasma LH, FSH, T3, leptin
• Elevated growth hormone, cortisol, cholesterol, vasopressin
• Abnormal liver enzymes
• Diminished BUN, creatinine clearance
• Flat glucose tolerance curve, depressed fasting blood sugar
• Low resting metabolic rate
• Low CD4/CD8 ratio
• Electrolyte disturbance; prolonged QT interval
• Neutropenia with relative lymphocytosis
• Hypercarotenemia
• Low serum zinc
• Abnormal CT, MRI (ventricular enlargement)
Drugs that may alter lab results: N/A
Disorders that may alter lab results: N/A

PATHOLOGICAL FINDINGS All are directly related to starvation
• Arrested maturation
• Pathological fractures
• Cognitive deficits

SPECIAL TESTS Measure percent body fat

IMAGING Not indicated in most cases

DIAGNOSTIC PROCEDURES
• Psychological screening
• Symptom assessment scale (EAT, EDI, SCANS)

 TREATMENT

APPROPRIATE HEALTH CARE
• Hospitalize if weight less than 75% of normal for height and age; if marked orthostatic hypotension, bradycardia less than 40, tachycardia more than 100 or inability to sustain core body temperature of 98.6°, if patient is suicidal; or if there has been no response to outpatient therapy.
• Initial goal geared to weight restoration
• Partial hospitalization if patient more than 70% of ideal body weight, motivated and capable of interpersonal; relatedness

GENERAL MEASURES
• Inpatient:
  ◊ If possible admit to specialized eating disorders unit
  ◊ Initial bedrest with supervised meals may be necessary
  ◊ Stepwise gradual increase in calories consumed
  ◊ Stepwise increase in activity
  ◊ Involve patient in establishing target weight
  ◊ Weigh daily at first, then 3 x per week
  ◊ Achieve 1-2 pound (0.45-0.91 kg) per week weight gain
  ◊ Supportive therapy
  ◊ Behavioral approach to provide positive and negative reinforcement, plus feedback about progress and problems encountered
  ◊ Tube feeding only as last resort
• Outpatient:
  ◊ Build trust, treatment alliance
  ◊ Involve patient in establishing target weight
  ◊ Achieve gradual weight gain
  ◊ Weigh weekly at first, monthly when progress is evident
  ◊ Focus on overall indices of health, rather than weight gain alone
  ◊ Challenge fear of uncontrolled weight gain
  ◊ When initial weight gain achieved, consider cognitive-behavioral, educational-behavioral, individual
  ◊ Family therapy for adolescents; couples therapy for older patients
  ◊ Medicate for symptom relief
  ◊ When condition is chronic, goal may be to achieve a safe weight rather than a healthy weight

SURGICAL MEASURES N/A

ACTIVITY
• Monitor activity
• Stepwise increase as patient gains weight
• Focus on playful rather than goal oriented activities

DIET
• Goal is stabilization at a healthy weight on a balanced diet with normal eating pattern
• Diminished ruminations about calories, weight; increased enjoyment

PATIENT EDUCATION
• Provide information on nutrition, metabolic balance, natural history of the disorder
• Ask patient to keep a "food diary" listing feelings and foods eaten
• For patient education materials see Internet References

MEDICATIONS

DRUG(S) OF CHOICE
• Medications should not be used as sole or primary treatment of this disorder
• Fluoxetine (Prozac) 10-60 mg relieves symptoms and helps prevent relapse after weight gain
• Short term anxiolytic therapy for starved inpatients (oxazepam 15 mg or alprazolam 0.25 mg before meals) to lessen anxiety about weight gain
Contraindications: Refer to manufacturer's literature
Precautions: Starved patients are more sensitive to medication, likely to suffer dangerous or lethal side effects due to compromised cardiac, liver and kidney function; caution is indicated
Significant possible interactions: Refer to manufacturer's literature

ALTERNATIVE DRUGS
• Cyproheptadine (Periactin) 4 mg, increasing gradually if side effects permit, to 32 mg/day
• Cisapride (Propulsid) 10-20 mg before each meal and at bedtime for abdominal distension due to delayed gastric emptying
• Estrogen - estradiol 0.5-1 mg - does not enhance bone density in underweight patients, but may be used following weight gain
• Psyllium (Metamucil) preparations (1 tbs hs) to prevent constipation
• Therapeutic vitamin-mineral supplement

FOLLOWUP

PATIENT MONITORING
• Level of activity. Is the activity driven?
• Weigh weekly until stable, then monthly
• Depression, self-esteem, suicidal ideation
• Ruminations and rituals
• Repeat any abnormal lab values weekly or monthly

PREVENTION/AVOIDANCE
• Encourage rational attitude about weight
• Moderate overly high self-expectations
• Enhance self-esteem
• Diminish stress

POSSIBLE COMPLICATIONS
• Potassium depletion; cardiac arrhythmia; cardiac arrest in purging patients
• Nitrogen depletion, exhaustion, collapse
• Cardiomyopathy, congestive heart failure
• Delayed gastric emptying
• Necrotizing colitis
• Convulsions, peripheral neuropathy
• Osteoporosis, bone loss
• Too rapid initial weight gain can cause fluid retention and congestive heart failure
• Infertility, perinatal complications

EXPECTED COURSE/PROGNOSIS
• Highly variable; relapse common
• Poor prognosis when condition is chronic
• Mortality - twelve times that of controls
• Better outcome if patient hospitalized until weight in normal range
• Speed of weight gain does not predict treatment success
• Poor prognosis indicated by repeated hospitalization, failed treatment, initial low weight, vomiting, being married, poor maturation, disordered relationships
• Substance abuse may need to be treated first
• Patients often become depressed after they recover
• Early age of onset short duration indicates more favorable prognosis
• Many symptoms resolve spontaneously with weight gain
• Ruminations, rituals, social isolation, and abnormal attitudes toward food and the body often persist after weight gain
• Up to half will binge/purge eventually
• May need 200-400 more calories per day than anticipated in order to maintain weight

MISCELLANEOUS

ASSOCIATED CONDITIONS
• Major depression or dysthymia
• Social phobia
• Obsessive-compulsive disorder
• Other anxiety disorders
• Substance abuse disorder
• Borderline or avoidant personality disorder

AGE-RELATED FACTORS
Pediatric: Growth can be compromised in preadolescence and early adolescence
Geriatric: Difficult to diagnose in elderly
Others:
• High risk
◊ Ballet dancers, models, cheerleaders
◊ Athletes, especially runners, gymnasts, weight lifters, body builders, jockeys, divers, wrestlers, figure skaters, field hockey players
◊ Japanese, Caucasian

PREGNANCY   Unlikely due to amenorrhea

SYNONYMS   N/A

ICD-9-CM
307.1 anorexia nervosa

SEE ALSO
• Amenorrhea
• Osteoporosis
• Idiopathic edema

OTHER NOTES   N/A

ABBREVIATIONS   N/A

REFERENCES
• Yager J, et al: Practice Guidelines for the Eating Disorders. Am Psychiatric Association, 1999
• Brownell KD, Fairburn CB: Eating disorders and obesity: a comprehensive handbook. New York, Guilford Press, 1995
• Herzog DB, Nussbaum KM, Warmor AK: Comorbidity and outcome in eating disorders. Psychiatr Clin NA 1996;19:843-859
• Agras WS, Apple RF: Overcoming eating disorders (therapist's guide). The Psychological Corporation. San Antonio, Harcourt Brace & Co., 1998
• Davis C, et al: The role of physical activity in the development and maintenance of eating disorders. Psychol Med 1994;24:957-967
• Garner D, Garfinkel P (eds:) Handbook of Treatment for Eating Disorders. New York, Guilford Press, 1997
Illustrations: N/A
Internet references: http://www.5mcc.com

Author(s)
Alayne Yates, MD

Anxiety

BASICS

DESCRIPTION A common acute or chronic, fearful emotion with associated physical symptoms. DSM-IV-R recognizes the following sub types:
• Acute situational anxiety: Response to recent stressful event, usually transient symptoms
• Adjustment disorder with anxious mood: Persistent, maladaptive reaction following psychosocial stress and lasting up to six months
• Generalized anxiety disorder: Persistent underlying anxiety or adjustment disorder with anxious mood and significant symptoms of motor tension, autonomic hyperactivity and hypervigilance, lasting more than six months
• Panic disorder: Recurrent unexpected attacks with at least one attack (or more) associated with persistent concern about additional attacks, worries about implications of the attack (losing control, having a heart attack) or a significant change in behavior related to the attack; often leads to agoraphobia
• Post-traumatic stress disorder: Recurrent flashbacks or nightmares of catastrophic event by survivors, often associated with panic attacks and major depression
• Specific phobias: Intense recurrent fear of, and avoidance of, an object or situation
• Social phobia: Marked and persistent fear and avoidance of performance or social situations in which the person is exposed to unfamiliar people or scrutiny
• Obsessive-compulsive disorder: Persistent unwanted and disturbing thoughts and recurrent behavioral patterns (i.e., hand washing) which interfere with daily life
System(s) affected: Nervous
Genetics: Panic disorder - increased concordance in monozygotic versus dizygotic twins
Incidence/Prevalence in USA: 40 million (the most common psychiatric disorder in US)
• 12 month prevalence rate
  ◊ Panic disorder - female 3.2%, male 1.3%
  ◊ Obsessive compulsive disorder - female 2.6-3.1%, male 1.1-2.6%
  ◊ Agoraphobia - female 3.8%, male 1.7%
  ◊ Generalized anxiety disorder - female 4.3%, male 2.0%
  ◊ Social phobia - female 5.2%, male 3.8%
Predominant Age: Mainly adults, highest prevalence in 20 to 45 year age group
Predominant Sex: Female > Male (social phobia female 5.27:male 3.87)

SIGNS AND SYMPTOMS Patterns vary with subtype of anxiety; not all present in each case
• Unrealistic or excessive anxiety or worry
• Sense of impending doom
• Nervousness
• Instability
• Tachycardia; palpitations
• Systolic click murmur
• Hyperventilation, choking sensation
• Labile hypertension
• Sighing respiration
• Nausea or abdominal distress
• Paresthesias
• Diaphoresis
• Dizziness or syncope
• Flushing
• Muscle tension
• Tremulousness
• Restlessness
• Chest tightness, pressure (pseudoangina)
• Headache, backaches, muscle spasm

CAUSES
• Panic disorder, social phobia and obsessive compulsive disorder are associated with genetic factors
• Psychosocial stressors commonly trigger anxiety disorders and may provoke a genetic diathesis
• Mediated by abnormalities of neurotransmitter systems (serotonin, norepinephrine and gamma-aminobutyric acid [GABA])

RISK FACTORS
• Social and financial problems
• Medical illness
• Family history
• Lack of social support

DIAGNOSIS

DIFFERENTIAL DIAGNOSIS
• Cardiovascular:
  ◊ Ischemic heart disease
  ◊ Valvular heart disease
  ◊ Cardiomyopathies
  ◊ Myocarditis
  ◊ Arrhythmias
  ◊ Mitral valve prolapse (most symptomatic cases are associated with panic disorder)
• Respiratory:
  ◊ Asthma
  ◊ Emphysema
  ◊ Pulmonary embolism
  ◊ Hamman-Rich syndrome
  ◊ Scleroderma
• CNS:
  ◊ Transient cerebral insufficiency
  ◊ Psychomotor epilepsy
  ◊ Essential tremor
• Metabolic and Hormonal:
  ◊ Hyperthyroidism
  ◊ Pheochromocytoma
  ◊ Adrenal insufficiency
  ◊ Cushing's syndrome
  ◊ Hypokalemia, hypoglycemia
  ◊ Hyperparathyroidism
  ◊ Myasthenia gravis
• Nutritional:
  ◊ Thiamine, pyridoxine, or folate deficiency
  ◊ Iron deficiency anemia
• Intoxication:
  ◊ Caffeine
  ◊ Alcohol
  ◊ Cocaine
  ◊ Sympathomimetics
  ◊ Amphetamines
• Withdrawal:
  ◊ Alcohol
  ◊ Sedative-hypnotics
• Other:
  ◊ Depression
  ◊ Panic disorder is associated with several physical disorders, including
  (a) mitral valve prolapse (systolic click-murmur)
  (b) labile hypertension
  (c) migraine headaches
  (d) irritable bowel syndrome

LABORATORY
• Selective use of laboratory tests, (with minimal to more extensive workup depending on clinical picture). Laboratory tests often normal in anxiety disorders.
• CBC and urinalysis
• Sequential serial multiple analysis (SMA-12 panel)
• Thyroid function studies
Drugs that may alter lab results:
• SSRIs may raise serum levels of other medications such as coumadin
Disorders that may alter lab results: N/A

PATHOLOGICAL FINDINGS N/A

SPECIAL TESTS EEG, ECG, etc.

IMAGING Usually none; chest x-ray possibly

DIAGNOSTIC PROCEDURES
• Psychologic testing (e.g., Zung's anxiety self-assessment, Hamilton's anxiety scale)
• DSM-IV based interview

TREATMENT

APPROPRIATE HEALTH CARE
Outpatient

GENERAL MEASURES
• Should be based on careful workup and identification of etiology and subtype of anxiety disorders
• Adequate workup
• Identify co-existent substance abuse
• Counseling or psychotherapy along with medications
• Regular exercise program
• Biofeedback in selected cases
• Serial office visits
• Judicious reassurance after other medical disorders ruled out

SURGICAL MEASURES N/A

ACTIVITY Fully active

DIET No special diet

PATIENT EDUCATION
• For a listing of sources for patient education materials favorably reviewed on this topic, physicians may contact: American Academy of Family Physicians Foundation, P.O. Box 8418, Kansas City, MO 64114, (800)274-2237, ext. 4400
• National Institute of Mental Health (NIMH) - National Anxiety Awareness Program, 9000 Rockville Pike, Bethesda, MD 20892

Anxiety

MEDICATIONS

DRUG(S) OF CHOICE
CONDITIONS
• Acute situational anxiety:
  ◊ Short-term (up to 1 month) treatment with benzodiazepines
• Adjustment disorder with anxiety mood:
  ◊ Benzodiazepines
• Generalized anxiety disorder:
  ◊ Azapirones - e.g., buspirone
  ◊ SSRIs
• Panic disorder and social phobia:
  ◊ SSRIs
  ◊ TCAs - e.g., imipramine
• Obsessive-compulsive disorder:
  ◊ TCAs - e.g., clomipramine
  ◊ SSRIs also effective
DRUG DOSES
• SSRIs:
  ◊ Citalopram (Celexa) 10 mg q/day; increase by 10 mg q 7 days to maximum of 20-40 mg q/day
  ◊ Fluoxetine (Prozac) 10 mg; increase by 10 mg q 7 days to maximum daily dosage of 20-40 mg
  ◊ Paroxetine (Paxil) 10 mg; increase by 10 mg q 5 days
  ◊ Sertraline (Zoloft) 25 mg; increase by 25 mg q 5 days
  ◊ Venlafaxine (Effexor) 18.75 mg PO bid, increased by 18.75 mg every 5 days
• Benzodiazepines
  ◊ Alprazolam (Xanax) 0.25 mg bid-tid; increase by 0.25 mg if needed
  ◊ Clomipramine (Anafranil) 25 mg bid; increase gradually to maximum of 250 mg/day
  ◊ Clonazepam (Klonopin) 0.5 mg po tid, to maximum of 1.5-4.5 mg/day
  ◊ Diazepam (Valium) 2-5 mg bid; increase by 2 mg if needed
  ◊ Imipramine (Tofranil) 10-25 mg qhs; increase by 10-25 mg/day q 2 weeks to maximum of 300 mg/day (100 mg/day maximum in geriatric and adolescent patients)
  ◊ Lorazepam (Ativan) 0.5 mg bid-tid; increase by 0.5 mg if needed
• Azapirones
  ◊ Buspirone (BuSpar) 5 mg bid-tid; increase 5 mg q 2-3 days to maximum of 60 mg/day in divided doses
Contraindications:
• Benzodiazepines - 1st-trimester pregnancy, acute alcohol intoxication with depressed vital signs, acute angle-closure glaucoma, sleep apnea, history of personality disorder or substance abuse. Avoid long-term/prn use.
• Buspirone - concurrent MAO inhibitor use
• TCAs - acute myocardial infarction
Precautions:
• Benzodiazepines - advanced age, renal insufficiency, suicidal tendency, open-angle glaucoma. Sudden discontinuation increases risk of seizures, especially with alprazolam
• Benzodiazepines with short half-lives (e.g., alprazolam) increase potential for dependency and protracted withdrawal symptoms; extreme caution with severe panic disorder who are taking other CNS sedatives or who have a history of substance abuse/dependence

• Buspirone - hepatic and/or renal dysfunction. Buspirone will not protect against benzodiazepine withdrawal seizures; taper benzodiazepines.
• TCAs - advanced age, glaucoma, benign prostate hypertrophy, hyperthyroidism, cardiovascular disease, liver disease, urinary retention, MAO inhibitor treatment
Significant possible interactions:
• Benzodiazepines - cimetidine, ethanol, oral contraceptives, disulfiram, levodopa, rifampin
• Buspirone - MAO inhibitors
• TCAs - amphetamines, barbiturates, guanethidine, clonidine, epinephrine, ethanol, norepinephrine, MAO inhibitors, propoxyphene
• SSRIs - MAO inhibitors (may cause fatal serotonin syndrome [confusion, hyperthermia, etc.]), may raise serum levels of other medications

ALTERNATIVE DRUGS
• Generalized anxiety disorder: Short-term use of benzodiazepine or TCA's
• Panic disorder: Although TCAs or SSRIs are the drugs of choice for panic disorder, they are slow in onset of action (2-3 weeks). Benzodiazepines may be helpful for initial control of symptoms until the TCA's are effective. Also, 10-20% of patients with panic do not tolerate side effects of TCAs. High potency benzodiazepines (alprazolam, clonazepam, lorazepam) or MAO inhibitors are effective alternatives.
• Social phobia: Phenelzine - initial dose 15 mg bid, increase by 15 mg every week to a total dose of 45-90 mg. Benzodiazepines: clonazepam

FOLLOWUP

PATIENT MONITORING
• Follow-up by regular office visits
• Watch for and treat associated depression
• Monitor mental status on benzodiazepines and avoid drug dependence
• Monitor blood pressure, heart rate, anticholinergic side effects on TCAs
• Periodic serum levels, if indicated, for TCAs

PREVENTION/AVOIDANCE
Management of stress, to extent possible, relaxation techniques, meditation

POSSIBLE COMPLICATIONS
• Impaired social/occupational functioning
• Drug dependence (benzodiazepines)
• Cardiac arrhythmias (TCAs)

EXPECTED COURSE/PROGNOSIS
• With active treatment, excellent results can often be obtained, especially with short-term anxiety disorders, including panic disorder
• Obsessive-compulsive disorder, and post-traumatic stress disorder are more difficult to treat, often requiring longer-term psychotherapy and medication (combination treatment)

MISCELLANEOUS

ASSOCIATED CONDITIONS
• Depression (commonly)
• Agoraphobia
• Alcohol or substance abuse
• Somatoform disorders

AGE-RELATED FACTORS
Pediatric: Reduced dosage of medications in adolescent
Geriatric: Reduced dosage of medications
Others: N/A

PREGNANCY
• Benzodiazepines - contraindicated in first-trimester of pregnancy, and with caution later in pregnancy and during lactation. May cause lethargy and weight loss in nursing infants; avoid breast feeding if mother taking benzodiazepines chronically or in high doses.
• TCAs - some evidence of fetal risk, especially in first trimester
• SRIs - taper and discontinue, if possible, in first trimester; may be used later in pregnancy

SYNONYMS
• Hyperventilation syndrome
• Panic disorder

ICD-9-CM
300.0 anxiety states

SEE ALSO N/A

OTHER NOTES N/A

ABBREVIATIONS
DSM-IV-R = Diagnostic and Statistical Manual of Mental Disorders. 4th edition
TCA = tricyclic antidepressant
SSRI = selective serotonergic reuptake inhibitor

REFERENCES
• Katon W: Panic Disorder in the Medical Setting. Washington, D.C., American Psychiatric Press, 1991
• Landry MJ, Smith DE, et al: Benzodiazepine dependence and withdrawal: Identification and medical management. J Am Bd Fam Prac, 1992;5:167-171
• Lydiard RB, Brawman-Mintzor O, et al: Recent developments in the psychopharmacology of anxiety disorders. J Consulting Clin Psychology, 1996;64:660-668
• Roy-Byrne P, Stein M. Bystrisky A, Katon W: Pharmacotherapy of panic disorder. JA BFB 1998;11:282-90
3 additional references available at web site
Internet references: http://www.5mcc.com
Illustrations: N/A

Author(s)
Wayne J. Katon, MD
John P. Geyman, MD

Aortic dissection

BASICS

DESCRIPTION Intimal tear in the aorta propagated via hematoma formation causing further dissection and separation producing a false lumen in the arterial wall.
• The Debakey classification:
◊ Type I: Involves the aortic root, aortic arch, and the descending aorta
◊ Type II: Involves only the ascending aorta
◊ Type III: Involves only the distal aorta beyond the origin of the left subclavian artery
• Stanford classification:
◊ Type A: ascending and aortic arch
◊ Type B: descending aorta
System(s) affected: Cardiovascular
Genetics: Increased incidence among family members
Incidence/Prevalence in USA:
• 1 in 10,000 patients admitted to hospital; found 1 in 350 patients at autopsy
• 2000 new cases diagnosed annually
Predominant age: Dependent on etiology; Marfan's commonly present in the third and fourth decade; most common between the 6th and 8th decades
Predominant sex: Male > Female (3:1)

SIGNS AND SYMPTOMS
• Abrupt onset of tearing pain
• Shearing anterior chest pain which radiates to the interscapular region
• Back pain
• Syncope
• Symptoms of congestive heart failure
• Stroke
• Limb ischemia
• Abdominal pain
• Acute myocardial infarction/angina
• Spinal cord syndromes/deficits
• Hypotension or hypertension
• Wide pulse pressure
• Murmur of aortic insufficiency
• Features of tamponade
• Dullness in left lung base (effusion)
• Pulse deficits or asymmetry
• Fever

CAUSES
• Cystic medionecrosis
• Iatrogenic during arterial catheterization

RISK FACTORS
• Hypertension
• Pregnancy
• Chest trauma
• Cocaine use
• Cardiovascular surgery
• Age
• Marfan's syndrome
• Ehlers-Danlos syndrome

DIAGNOSIS

DIFFERENTIAL DIAGNOSIS
• Myocardial infarction
• Pulmonary embolism
• Pneumonia
• Pleurisy
• Pericarditis
• Pneumothorax
• Angina
• Acute pancreatitis
• Penetrating duodenal ulcer

LABORATORY No special studies required
Drugs that may alter lab results: N/A
Disorders that may alter lab results: N/A

PATHOLOGICAL FINDINGS
Approximately 60% of intimal tears occur in the proximal ascending aorta. The remainder are found between the origin of the left subclavian artery and ligamentum arteriosum, descending aorta (20%), aortic arch (10%), and the abdominal aorta. Although medionecrosis is found in normal aging aortas, it appears to be more extensive in patients who develop aortic dissection. Cystic medionecrosis is seen in patients with defects in elastin and connective tissue organization i.e., Marfan's, Ehlers-Danlos, etc. Death usually due to rupture and tamponade.

SPECIAL TESTS
• Electrocardiogram: LVH, nonspecific ST-T changes, electrical alternans with associated tamponade
• Echocardiogram: dilated aortic root, increased aortic posterior or anterior wall thickness, pericardial effusion, oscillating intimal flap

IMAGING Chest x-ray: widening of the superior mediastinum, left pleural effusion, haziness or enlargement of the aortic knob, double density of the descending aorta, irregular aortic contour, > 5 mm separation of intimal calcification from outer aortic contour, rightward displacement of the trachea, cardiomegaly.

DIAGNOSTIC PROCEDURES
[Sensitivity/Specificity indicated for each]
• CT chest - demonstration of two lumens with hematoma formation, detection of intimal flap, differential flow between two lumens, compression of true lumen by false lumen [88/100%]
• Spiral CT aortography may be more sensitive and specific.
• Aortogram - demonstration of two lumens, detection of intimal flap, compression of true lumen, ulcer-like projections of contrast, arterial compromise, altered flow patterns, aortic insufficiency (not as sensitive as previous thought) [88/94%]
• Transesophageal echocardiography (TEE) - test of choice for hemodynamically unstable patients [99/98%]
• MRI - if available and patient hemodynamically stable, test of choice for delineation of vascular anatomy

TREATMENT

APPROPRIATE HEALTH CARE
Admission to intensive care unit or transfer to operative suite

GENERAL MEASURES
• Treatment of choice - surgical for all ascending aortic dissections and medical for descending dissections without complications (Type III)
• Medical therapy is based on decreasing blood pressure and the "shearing" forces of myocardial contractility (dp/dt) to attempt to decrease intimal tear and hematoma propagation
• Arterial blood pressure monitoring is critical
• Careful observation for changes in mentation, neurological signs, or evidence of organ dysfunction
• A Foley catheter should be used to follow urine output
• Swan-Ganz catheterization may be very helpful to monitor cardiac performance and filling pressures during the use of vasoactive and cardiodepressive drugs
• Pain control may be difficult despite use of narcotics

SURGICAL MEASURES
• Surgical indications for Type III
◊ Increasing size of hematoma
◊ Impending rupture
◊ Inability to control pain
◊ Bleeding into pleural space
• Endovascular stents

ACTIVITY Bedrest

DIET NPO until surgical evaluation is complete and patient classified as medical therapy only

PATIENT EDUCATION Depending on etiology, emphasis must be placed on risk factors and recurrence of symptoms

MEDICATIONS

DRUG(S) OF CHOICE Propranolol in 0.5-1 mg IV doses every 5 minutes until the heart rate is 60-70 beats per minute plus nitroprusside titrated to reduce systolic blood pressure to 100-110 mm Hg (13.3-14.6 kPa)

Contraindications:
• Propranolol - in bronchial asthma, diabetes mellitus, Raynaud's disease, sinus bradycardia, A-V heart block greater than first degree, in presence of monoamine oxidase inhibitors, cardiogenic shock, congestive heart failure or right ventricular failure from pulmonary hypertension
• Nitroprusside - in treatment of compensatory hypertension, i.e., arteriovenous shunt, in patients with inadequate cerebral circulation, and for use during emergency surgery in moribund patients

Precautions:
• Use propranolol cautiously in patients with angina pectoris, cardiac failure, impaired renal or hepatic function, thyrotoxicosis, pre-excitation syndromes, diabetes, hypoglycemia or nonallergic bronchospasm. Propranolol may produce significant bradycardia, heart block or hypotension. Patients should not be suddenly withdrawn from beta blockers.
• Nitroprusside:
◊ May not lower blood pressure adequately, another agent may be required
◊ In patients with renal or hepatic insufficiency, may cause cyanide toxicity, through excessive production of serum thiocyanate. Confusion and hyperreflexia are the early signs of thiocyanate toxicity. Thiocyanate inhibits the uptake and binding of iodine, use caution in the presence of hypothyroidism. Check thiocyanate levels after 48 hours of nitroprusside use.
◊ Because of the rapid onset and potency, administration should be with the use of an infusion pump
◊ Methemoglobinemia may be seen rarely

Significant possible interactions:
• Propranolol with adenosine, albuterol, alfentanil, amiodarone, barbiturates, bromazepam, chlorothiazide, chlorpromazine, chlorpropamide, chlorprothixene, cimetidine, clonidine, dextroamphetamine, diazoxide, dihydroergotamine, diltiazem, disopyramide, tricyclic antidepressants, encainide, epinephrine, flecainide, fluvoxamine, furosemide, glipizide, halofenate, haloperidol, heparin, ibuprofen, indomethacin, insulin, isoniazid, isoproterenol, lidocaine, lidoflazine, methacholine, methyldopa, metoclopramide, naproxen, nifedipine, phenylpropanolamine, procainamide, quinidine, reserpine, rifampin, ritodrine, sulfonylureas, theophylline, thioridazine, tocainide, tubocurarine, verapamil, warfarin.
• Nitroprusside with clonidine and other antihypertensives to make their hypotensive effects cumulative

ALTERNATIVE DRUGS
• Labetalol, 10-20 mg IV bolus to a maximum of 300 mg total, then titrated to response with an infusion
• Trimethaphan, at an infusion rate of 1-2 mg/min
• Reserpine 0.5-2 mg intramuscularly every 4-8 hours. Onset of action is 1-3 hours.
• Methyldopa 250-500 mg every 6 hours. Unfortunately, it has a delayed onset of action of 4 to 6 hours and prolonged duration of 10 to 12 hours.

FOLLOWUP

PATIENT MONITORING
• Systolic blood pressure should be maintained at 120 mm Hg (16 kPa) or below as tolerated
• Routine chest x-rays and/or chest CT may be helpful in following the progress of any long-term medically treated patient
• Patients should have a one month follow-up visit, and then at three month intervals. During the follow-up, careful attention should be placed on signs and symptoms of aortic insufficiency, chest or back pain, and development of saccular aneurysms as displayed on chest roentgenogram.

PREVENTION/AVOIDANCE Long-term control of hypertension

POSSIBLE COMPLICATIONS
Redissection, localized saccular aneurysm, cardiac tamponade, aortic valvular insufficiency and progressive aortic enlargement

EXPECTED COURSE/PROGNOSIS
• Mortality of patients left untreated is: 33% in 24 hours, 60% in 2 weeks, approximately 90% in three months
• Hospital survival is estimated at approximately 70% in patients treated both medically and surgically
• Patients with ascending dissection treated early with surgery still have a mortality of 29-38%
• 10 year survival of all operated patients is 40%
• Redissection risk is 13% at 5 years; 23% at 10 years

MISCELLANEOUS

ASSOCIATED CONDITIONS
• Ehlers-Danlos syndrome
• Marfan's syndrome
• Aortic stenosis
• Coarctation of aorta
• Bicuspid valve
• Turner's syndrome
• Osteogenesis imperfecta
• Syphilis
• Relapsing polychondritis

AGE-RELATED FACTORS N/A
Pediatric: N/A
Geriatric: N/A
Others: N/A

PREGNANCY Aortic dissection may be associated with cystic medionecrosis of pregnancy and appears to have an increased associated risk with pregnancy. It is still unclear whether pregnancy itself is the originating factor or that it simply contributes to the worsening of an already pre-existing condition.

SYNONYMS
• Dissecting aneurysm

ICD-9-CM
441.0 Dissection of aorta (ruptured)

SEE ALSO
• Ehlers-Danlos syndrome
• Marfan's syndrome

OTHER NOTES N/A

ABBREVIATIONS N/A

REFERENCES
• Hirst AE Jr, Johns VJ Jr, Kim SW Jr: Dissecting aneurysm of the aorta: A review of 505 cases. Medicine 1958;37:217-219
• Rogers FB, et: Aortic dissection after trauma: Case report and review of literature. J Trauma 1996;41:906-908
• Pretre R, et al: Aortic dissection. Lancet. 1997;May17;349:1461-1464
• Lindsay JJ: Diagnosis and treatment of diseases of the aorta. Curr Probl Cardiol 1997;Oct 22(70) 485-542
• Cigarroa JE, Isselbacher EM, et al: Diagnostic imaging in the evaluation of suspected aortic dissection. N Eng J Med 1993;328(1):35-43
• Summer T, Fehska W, et al: Aortic dissection: a comparative study of diagnosis with spiral CT, multiplanar transesophageal echocardiography, and MR imaging. Radiology 1996; 199(2): 347-52
Illustrations: N/A
Internet references: http://www.5mcc.com

Author(s)
Darell E. Heiselman, DO, FCCM, FACP, FACC, FCCP

Aortic valvular stenosis

BASICS

DESCRIPTION An acquired or congenital obstruction to systolic left ventricular outflow across the aortic valve
System(s) affected: Cardiovascular
Genetics: N/A
Incidence/Prevalence in USA:
• Except for mitral regurgitation due to myocardial disease, valvular aortic stenosis is the most common fatal cardiac valve lesion
• Bicuspid aortic valve has a frequency of 400 per 100,000 live births
Predominant age:
• Age < 30 years - predominantly congenital
• Age 30 to 70 years - most commonly congenital or rheumatic
• Age > 70 years - most commonly degenerative calcification of the aortic valve
Predominant sex:
• Congenital bicuspid valves: Male > Female (4:1)
• Congenital unicuspid valves: Male > Female (3:1)

SIGNS AND SYMPTOMS
• Angina pectoris (most frequent symptom, occurring in 50-70% of patients with severe aortic stenosis)
• Near syncope
• Syncope (often exertional, occurs in 15-30% of patients with severe aortic stenosis)
• Exertional dyspnea
• Orthopnea
• Paroxysmal nocturnal dyspnea
• Palpitations
• Fatigue
• Neurologic events (transient ischemic attack or cerebrovascular accident) due to embolization
• Systolic crescendo-decrescendo murmur, usually best heard at the second right sternal border (may have associated thrill) and may radiate into the carotid arteries
• Ejection (early systolic) click
• Prolonged ejection time
• Delayed, small carotid upstroke
• Delayed/decreased intensity of A2
• Paradoxical splitting of S2
• Left ventricular heave
• A high pitched diastolic blow may be present at the left sternal border (associated aortic regurgitation)

CAUSES
• Congenital etiologies
  ◊ Unicuspid valve
  ◊ Bicuspid valve (not inherently stenotic, but becomes so as a result of 'wear and tear' thickening and calcification; a calcified bicuspid valve is the most common cause of isolated aortic stenosis in adults)
  ◊ Three cusped valve with fusion of commissures
  ◊ Hypoplastic annulus
• Acquired etiologies
  ◊ Rheumatic (or, rarely, other inflammatory disease)
  ◊ Degenerative calcific aortic stenosis in the elderly

RISK FACTORS History of rheumatic fever

DIAGNOSIS

DIFFERENTIAL DIAGNOSIS
• Mitral regurgitation, either primary or secondary to underlying coronary artery disease or dilated cardiomyopathy. Mitral regurgitation, however, is usually an apical, high frequency, pansystolic murmur, often radiating to the axilla.
• Hypertrophic obstructive cardiomyopathy. This murmur is also a systolic crescendo-decrescendo murmur, but is best heard at the left sternal border and may radiate into the axilla. However, this murmur characteristically is intensified by moving from squatting to standing position and/or Valsalva's maneuver, and lessened by changing from standing to squatting.
• Aortic supravalvular stenosis
• Discrete subaortic stenosis

LABORATORY N/A
Drugs that may alter lab results: N/A
Disorders that may alter lab results: N/A

PATHOLOGICAL FINDINGS
• Left ventricular hypertrophy
• Myocardial interstitial fibrosis
• Aortic valvular calcification in older patients
• 50% incidence of concomitant coronary artery disease

SPECIAL TESTS ECG: Left ventricular hypertrophy, often with associated ST segment depression, conduction defects, left atrial enlargement, ventricular arrhythmias

IMAGING
• Chest x-ray
  ◊ May be normal in compensated, isolated valvular aortic stenosis
  ◊ Cardiac hypertrophy early, later cardiomegaly
  ◊ Post stenotic dilatation of the ascending aorta
  ◊ Calcification of aortic valve cusps (may require fluoroscopy to visualize)

DIAGNOSTIC PROCEDURES
• Echocardiography:
  ◊ Aortic valve morphology, thickening, calcifications
  ◊ Decreased aortic valve excursion
  ◊ Planimetry of aortic valve area
  ◊ Left ventricular hypertrophy
  ◊ Left ventricular ejection fraction
  ◊ Chamber dimensions
  ◊ Presence or absence of wall motion abnormalities suggestive of coronary artery disease
• With Doppler echocardiography:
  ◊ Transvalvular gradient
  ◊ Valve area
  ◊ Diastolic function
  ◊ Associated aortic regurgitation
• Cardiac catheterization:
  ◊ Transvalvular gradient
  ◊ Valve area

◊ Left ventricle ejection fraction
◊ Concomitant coronary artery disease

TREATMENT

APPROPRIATE HEALTH CARE
Outpatient except for surgical intervention

GENERAL MEASURES
• Aortic stenosis is a progressive disease. The asymptomatic patient with non-critical aortic stenosis can be closely followed with appropriate evaluation.
• All patients with valvular aortic stenosis should receive endocarditis prophylaxis, prior to dental work or invasive procedures regardless of age, etiology or severity of the stenosis (as recommended by the American Heart Association in Circulation, 1997; 96: 358-366)
• Patients with a rheumatic etiology should receive (in addition to endocarditis prophylaxis prior to dental work or invasive procedures) rheumatic fever prophylaxis, especially if less than 35 years of age, or continue to be in close contact with young children

SURGICAL MEASURES
• Prompt aortic valve replacement is clearly indicated in patients with symptomatic aortic stenosis
• Consider aortic valve replacement in asymptomatic patients with critical aortic stenosis (aortic valve area < 0.8 cm2 or gradient > 50 mm Hg [> 6.6 kPa]) particularly if there is left ventricular dysfunction, increasing cardiomegaly, and clinical symptoms
• Surgical valve replacement consists of the removal of the stenotic, native valve and placement of a prosthetic mechanical or tissue valve
• Balloon angioplasty of stenotic aortic valves may be of benefit in the pediatric patient with congenital disease. Also feasible (although one must expect suboptimal results) in the elderly, debilitated patient who may not tolerate valve replacement.

ACTIVITY In known or suspected severe aortic stenosis, vigorous physical activity is contraindicated

DIET No restrictions except sodium restriction in presence of congestive heart failure

PATIENT EDUCATION
• Educate the patient about the symptoms of symptomatic aortic stenosis and to report these promptly should they occur
• If moderate or severe aortic stenosis is known or suspected, instruct the patient to avoid vigorous physical activity
• Instruct the patient when prophylactic antibiotics are needed for medical or dental procedures

MEDICATIONS

DRUG(S) OF CHOICE
• None for treatment. Prophylactic antibiotics when needed.
• The use of vasodilators, nitrates, calcium channel blockers, beta blockers as well as diuretics are potentially hazardous in aortic stenosis and should be used cautiously, if at all
Contraindications: N/A
Precautions: N/A
Significant possible interactions: N/A

ALTERNATIVE DRUGS   N/A

FOLLOWUP

PATIENT MONITORING
• Asymptomatic patients without critical aortic stenosis should be followed with a history and physical examination every 3-6 months
• An echocardiogram should be performed every 6-12 months to assess progression
• Advise the patient to immediately report any symptoms referable to the aortic stenosis

PREVENTION/AVOIDANCE
• Bacterial endocarditis prophylaxis
• Rheumatic fever prophylaxis, where indicated
• Avoidance of vigorous physical activity

POSSIBLE COMPLICATIONS
• Progressive stenosis
• Sudden death
• Congestive heart failure
• Angina
• Syncope
• Hemolytic anemia
• Infective endocarditis

EXPECTED COURSE/PROGNOSIS
• Mean life expectancy without intervention in patients with aortic stenosis is 5 years after the onset of exertional chest discomfort, 3 years after the onset of syncope, 2 years after the development of heart failure
• Sudden death occurs in 15 to 20% of patients with symptomatic aortic stenosis

MISCELLANEOUS

ASSOCIATED CONDITIONS
• Coronary artery disease is present in 50% of patients with aortic stenosis
• Aortic regurgitation (particularly seen in calcified bicuspid valves and rheumatic disease)
• Mitral valve disease (primarily in rheumatic heart disease)

AGE-RELATED FACTORS
Pediatric: N/A
Geriatric: Increased incidence of degenerative calcific aortic stenosis
Others: N/A

PREGNANCY   Severe critical aortic stenosis tolerates poorly the hemodynamic changes in pregnancy, labor and delivery. Pregnancy should be avoided with critical aortic stenosis.

SYNONYMS   N/A

ICD-9-CM
424.90 Endocarditis, valve unspecified, unspecified cause

SEE ALSO   N/A

OTHER NOTES   As the left ventricle is relatively noncompliant in aortic stenosis, atrial contraction is an important component of diastolic filling. The loss of this component with the onset of atrial fibrillation can cause acute clinical and hemodynamic deterioration.

ABBREVIATIONS   N/A

REFERENCES
• Brandenburg RO, et al: Cardiology: Fundamentals and Practice. New York, Year Book Publishers, 1987
• Dalen JE, Alpert JS: Valvular Heart Disease. 2nd Ed. New York, Little Brown & Co, 1987
• Hurst JW, et al: The Heart. 7th Ed. New York, McGraw-Hill, 1990
• Isselbacher KJ, et al, eds: Harrison's Principles of Internal Medicine. 13th Ed. New York, McGraw-Hill, 1994
Illustrations: N/A
Internet references: http://www.5mcc.com

Author(s)
James M. Galloway, MD, FACP, FACC

Appendicitis, acute

BASICS

DESCRIPTION Acute inflammation of the vermiform appendix
- First described by Fitz in 1886
- McBurney described the point of maximal tenderness

System(s) affected: Gastrointestinal

Genetics: Unknown.

Incidence/Prevalence in USA:
- 10/100,000
- Most common acute surgical condition of abdomen
- 1 in every 15 persons (7%) at some time in their life

Predominant age:
- Ages 10-30 - Male > Female (3:2)
- Over age 30 - Male = Female

Predominant sex: Slight male predominance

SIGNS AND SYMPTOMS
- Abdominal pain (100%) - periumbilical then right-lower-quadrant (RLQ). Pain lessened with flexion of thigh.
- Muscle guarding
- Anorexia (almost 100%)
- Nausea (90%)
- Vomiting (75%)-mild
- Obstipation
- Diarrhea-mild
- Sequence of symptom appearance (95%) - anorexia, then abdominal pain, then vomiting
- Slight temperature (one degree centigrade) elevation
- Slight tachycardia
- Patient frequently lies motionless with right thigh drawn up
- Maximal tenderness at "McBurney's point"
- Direct and referred RLQ tenderness
- Voluntary and involuntary guarding
- Cutaneous hyperesthesia at T10-12
- Rovsing's sign - RLQ pain with palpatory pressure in LLQ
- Psoas sign-pain with right thigh extension
- Obturator sign-pain with internal rotation of flexed right thigh
- Retrocecal appendix-flank tenderness in RLQ
- Pelvic appendix-local and suprapubic pain on rectal exam

CAUSES
- Obstruction of appendiceal lumen
  ◊ Fecaliths (most common)
  ◊ Lymphoid tissue hypertrophy
  ◊ Inspissated barium
  ◊ Vegetable, fruit seeds and other foreign bodies
  ◊ Intestinal worms (ascarids)
  ◊ Strictures

RISK FACTORS
- Adolescent males
- Familial tendency
- Intra-abdominal tumors

DIAGNOSIS

DIFFERENTIAL DIAGNOSIS
- Any cause of the "acute abdomen"
- 75% of erroneous diagnoses accounted for by acute mesenteric lymphadenitis, no organic pathologic condition, acute PID, twisted ovarian cyst, ruptured graafian follicle, acute gastroenteritis
- Also consider urologic causes, inflammatory bowel disease, colonic disorders, and other gynecologic diseases

LABORATORY
- Moderate leukocytosis - 10,000 to 18,000/mm3 in 75%
- Moderate polymorphonuclear predominance
- Urinalysis-elevated specific gravity, hematuria (sometimes), pyuria (sometimes), albuminuria (sometimes)

Drugs that may alter lab results:
- Antibiotics
- Steroids

Disorders that may alter lab results: N/A

PATHOLOGICAL FINDINGS
- Acute inflammation of the appendix
- Local vascular congestion
- Obstruction
- Gangrene
- Perforation with abscess (15-30%)

SPECIAL TESTS   N/A

IMAGING   (Used in differential diagnosis and to detect complications).
- KUB: gas-filled appendix; radiopaque fecalith; deformed cecum; fluid level; ileus; free air.
- Barium enema-non-filling appendix; RLQ mass effect
- Ultrasound-appendiceal inflammation; other pelvic pathology, such as inflammatory mass.
- CT scan for periappendiceal abscess

DIAGNOSTIC PROCEDURES
- Cornerstone of diagnosis is history and clinical findings
- Diagnostic laparoscopy - consider in young adult females
- Rectal and pelvic examinations
- Intensive in-hospital observation

TREATMENT

APPROPRIATE HEALTH CARE
- Inpatient surgery

GENERAL MEASURES
- Preoperative preparation
  ◊ Correction of fluid and electrolyte deficits
  ◊ Consider broad-spectrum antibiotic coverage

SURGICAL MEASURES
- Immediate appendectomy; open or laparoscopic
- Drainage of abscess, if present

ACTIVITY
- Early postoperative ambulation
- Return to full activity by 4 to 6 weeks postop

DIET Regular diet with return of bowel function, usually within 24 to 48 hours postop

PATIENT EDUCATION
- Restricted activity for 4 to 6 weeks postop
- Contact physician for development of postop anorexia, nausea, vomiting, abdominal pain, fever, or chills

MEDICATIONS

DRUG(S) OF CHOICE
• Uncomplicated acute appendicitis - one preoperative dose of broad spectrum antibiotic; cefoxitin (Mefoxin), cefotetan (Cefotan)
• Gangrenous or perforating appendicitis - broadened antibiotic coverage for aerobic and anaerobic enteric pathogens, dosage and choice of antibiotic should be adjusted based on intraoperative cultures. Continue antibiotics for 7 days postop or until patient becomes afebrile with normal white count. Pathogens usually sensitive to ampicillin, gentamicin, and clindamycin.
Contraindications: Documented allergy to specific antibiotic
Precautions: Adjust antibiotic dosages for elderly and renal failure patients
Significant possible interactions: Refer to manufacturer's literature for each drug

ALTERNATIVE DRUGS
• Metronidazole (Flagyl) - anaerobic coverage only
• Ampicillin-sulbactam (Unasyn)
• Ticarcillin-clavulanate (Timentin)

FOLLOWUP

PATIENT MONITORING
Routine visits at 2 and 6 weeks postoperatively

PREVENTION/AVOIDANCE   N/A

POSSIBLE COMPLICATIONS
• Wound infection
• Intra-abdominal abscess, sometimes diaphragmatic
• Fecal fistula
• Intestinal obstruction
• Incisional hernia
• Liver abscess (rare)
• Peritonitis with paralytic ileus

EXPECTED COURSE/PROGNOSIS
• Generally uncomplicated course in young adults with non-ruptured appendicitis.
• Factors increasing morbidity and mortality are extremes of age and appendiceal rupture.
• Morbidity rates:
  ◊ 3% with non-perforated appendicitis
  ◊ 47% with perforated appendicitis
• Mortality rates:
  ◊ 0.1% unruptured acute appendicitis
  ◊ 3% ruptured acute appendicitis
  ◊ 15% elderly patient with ruptured appendix

MISCELLANEOUS

ASSOCIATED CONDITIONS   N/A

AGE-RELATED FACTORS
Pediatric:
• Rare in infancy
• Decreased diagnostic accuracy
• Higher fever, more vomiting
• Rupture earlier
• Rupture rate: 15 to 50%
• May return to full activities earlier
Geriatric:
• Decreased diagnostic accuracy
• Rupture rate: 67 to 90%
• Patients over 60 years of age account for 50% of deaths from acute appendicitis
Others: N/A

PREGNANCY
• Most common extra-uterine surgical emergency
• 1 in 2000 pregnancies
• Difficult diagnosis
• Appendix displaced superolaterally by gravid uterus
• Fetal mortality rate: 2 to 8.5%

SYNONYMS   N/A

ICD-9-CM
540.0 appendicitis, with generalized peritonitis
540.9 appendicitis, without mention of peritonitis

SEE ALSO   N/A

OTHER NOTES
• In a non-surgical candidate, antibiotic therapy can be used - recurrence rate is too high to recommend as a primary therapy in other patients.

ABBREVIATIONS
KUB = kidney, ureter, bladder

REFERENCES
• Schwartz SI, ed: Principles of Surgery. 5th Ed. New York, McGraw-Hill, 1989
• Moody FG, ed: Surgical Treatment of Digestive Disease. 2nd Ed. Chicago, Year Book Medical Publishers, 1990
• Horattas MC, Guyton DP, Wu DA: Reappraisal of appendicitis in the elderly. American Journal of Surgery 1990;160:291-293
Illustrations: N/A
Internet references: http://www.5mcc.com

Author(s)
Andrew H. Fenton, MD, FACS
Thomas W. Clark, MS, MD

Arterial embolus & thrombosis

BASICS

DESCRIPTION
The acute loss of perfusion distal to an occlusion of a major artery due to an embolus which migrates to the point of occlusion or a clot intrinsic to the point of occlusion (thrombosis). Both are true emergencies. Following obstruction of an artery, a soft coagulum forms both proximally and distally in the areas of stagnant flow. As the clot extends, collateral pathways are involved and the process becomes self-propagating. Ultimately, the venous circulation can be involved. The extent of vascular compromise is critical and determines the "golden" period of four to six hours. After this time, the profound ischemia leads to cellular death and is irreversible.

System(s) affected: Cardiovascular, Hemic/Lymphatic/Immunologic
Genetics: Can be associated with inheritable hypercoagulable and premature atherosclerotic syndromes
Incidence/Prevalence in USA:
50-100/100,000 hospital admissions. A leading cause of death and limb loss in the elderly.
Predominant age: Elderly
Predominant sex: Male > Female

SIGNS AND SYMPTOMS
- To estimate occlusion location
  ◊ Symptoms typically start one joint below occlusion
  ◊ Palpable pulses are absent below an occlusion and are accentuated above
- The five "P's": Pain, Pulselessness, Pallor, Paresthesias, and Paralysis. If any one is present, frequent re-evaluations indicated. Proximal occlusions lead to a more rapid progression of findings. Occlusion at the aortic bifurcation can produce bilateral findings.
  ◊ Pain: Diffuse in distal area. If persists, crescendo in nature. Predominates as first symptom in embolism. Not alleviated by change of position.
  ◊ Pulselessness: Mandatory for the diagnosis of embolism or thrombosis. Pedal pulses subject to observer error. Always compare to the opposite limb.
  ◊ Pallor: Skin color pale early, cyanotic later. Check extremity temperature left to right and top to bottom. Look for signs of chronic ischemia - skin atrophy, loss of hair, thick nails.
  ◊ Paresthesia: Numbness early with thrombosis. Light touch first to be lost. Not reliable in diabetics. Loss of pain and pressure indicate advanced ischemia.
  ◊ Paralysis: Motor defect occurs after sensory and indicates profound ischemia
- Distribution of emboli
  ◊ Femoral artery 30%
  ◊ Iliac artery 15%
  ◊ Aortic bifurcation 10%
  ◊ Popliteal artery 10%
  ◊ Brachial 10%
  ◊ Mesenteric arteries 5%
  ◊ Renal 5%
  ◊ Cerebral - estimated 15-20%

CAUSES
- Emboli
  ◊ Cardiac
    - Atrial flutter/fibrillation
    - Valve disease
    - Myocardial infarction
    - Cardiomyopathy
    - Cardiac tumors
    - Endocarditis
  ◊ Aneurysms - cardiac, aortic, peripheral
  ◊ Paradoxical
- Thrombosis:
  ◊ Atherosclerotic occlusive disease
  ◊ Aortic and peripheral aneurysms - especially popliteal
  ◊ Hypercoagulable states
  ◊ Venous gangrene
  ◊ Drug abuse
  ◊ Heparin allergy
  ◊ Vascular bypass
- Trauma:
  ◊ Blunt
  ◊ Penetrating
  ◊ Vascular and cardiac interventional procedures

RISK FACTORS
- Drug abuse

DIAGNOSIS

DIFFERENTIAL DIAGNOSIS
Emboli vs thrombosis
- Emboli
  ◊ Myocardial diseases - myocardial infarction, arrhythmias - atrial fibrillation
  ◊ Aneurysms
  ◊ Pain as first symptom
- Thrombosis
  ◊ Absence of heart disease - arrhythmias/infarction
  ◊ Chronic vascular history
  ◊ Bilateral changes of chronic ischemia
  ◊ Numbness rather than pain as first symptom
  ◊ Vascular procedures - bypass/interventional
- Acute aortic dissection; chest or back pain
- Acute deep vein thrombosis; massive swelling and warm skin
- Low flow states

LABORATORY
- Acute diagnosis is by history and exam: Laboratory data is for preoperative evaluation, elucidation of etiology, or documentation of severity of ischemia.
  ◊ EKG
  ◊ Myocardial/muscle isoenzymes
  ◊ Coagulation parameters
  ◊ Blood pH/bicarbonate
  ◊ Urine myoglobin
  ◊ Electrolytes
Drugs that may alter lab results: N/A
Disorders that may alter lab results: N/A

PATHOLOGICAL FINDINGS N/A

SPECIAL TESTS
- Noninvasive - indirect:
  ◊ Doppler: presence or absence of flow
  ◊ A/ai (ankle/arm index): dorsal pedal/posterior tibial pressure divided by brachial pressure; a/ai > 0.30 favorable
- Noninvasive - direct
  ◊ Duplex imaging if time permits

IMAGING N/A

DIAGNOSTIC PROCEDURES
- Arteriography
  ◊ Rarely indicated preoperatively in threatened limb
  ◊ May help differentiate thrombosis from embolus in non-threatened limb
  ◊ Useful with occluded grafts

TREATMENT:

APPROPRIATE HEALTH CARE
Based on detailed exam, history, and Doppler exam. Triage determines appropriate therapy.
- Viable
  ◊ Mild ischemic pain
  ◊ Normal neurologic exam
  ◊ Capillary refill present
  ◊ Arterial signals present by Doppler in distal extremity
  ◊ A/ai > 0.30
- Threatened
  ◊ Ischemic pain
  ◊ Mild neurologic deficit
    - Weakness of dorsiflexion
    - Minimal sensory loss - light touch and/or vibratory
  ◊ No pulsatile flow by Doppler
  ◊ Venous flow present
- Major ischemic changes - irreversible
  ◊ Profound sensory loss
  ◊ Muscle paralysis
  ◊ Absent capillary refill
  ◊ Skin marbling
  ◊ Muscle rigor
  ◊ No arterial or venous signals by Doppler

GENERAL MEASURES
- Time is of the essence
- In the threatened category nothing should delay appropriate therapy
- Unless contraindicated, systemic heparinization to decrease clot propagation and prophylaxis against further emboli
- Resuscitation and stabilization of patient to extent permitted by time

- Viable - symptomatic
  - Heparin (see Medications)
  - Arteriography
  - Embolism
  - Surgical removal if acceptable operative risk, e.g., balloon embolectomy
  - Anticoagulation vs intraarterial urokinase if prohibitive risk
  ◊ Thrombosis
  - Trial of thrombolytics and correction of arterial defect if good risk
  - Anticoagulation if poor risk or thrombolytics contraindicated
- Threatened - salvageable
  ◊ Heparin (see Medications)
  ◊ Minimal delay to definitive therapy
  ◊ Arteriography
  ◊ Individualized thrombolysis and/or operative procedure (depending on extent of thrombosis and amenability for surgical removal)
  ◊ Thrombolysis to optimize alternatives
  ◊ Adjunctive operative therapy
  - Intraoperative lytic therapy
  - Bypass
  - Patch angioplasty
- Major ischemia - irreversible
  ◊ Arteriography usually not warranted
  ◊ Attempts at reperfusion contraindicated
  ◊ Anticoagulation
  ◊ Definitive amputation if possible

SURGICAL MEASURES See General Measures

ACTIVITY N/A

DIET N/A

PATIENT EDUCATION N/A

MEDICATIONS

DRUG(S) OF CHOICE
- Heparin
  ◊ 100 units/kg IV loading dose (approx 5,000-10,000 units)
  ◊ Continuous heparin infusion sufficient to double the PTT, generally 1000 to 1500 units/hour
Contraindications:
- Heparin:
  ◊ Allergy
  ◊ Bleeding diathesis
  ◊ Trauma (e.g., head injury)
  ◊ Hematuria/hemoptysis
  ◊ Acute aortic dissection
- Urokinase:
  ◊ Non-salvageable ischemia
  ◊ Recent MI
  ◊ Aneurysm
  ◊ Aortic dissection
  ◊ Stroke (CVA)
  ◊ Trauma
  ◊ Uncontrolled hypertension
  ◊ Recent operative procedure
Precautions: N/A
Significant possible interactions: N/A

ALTERNATIVE DRUGS
- Tissue plasminogen activator

FOLLOWUP

PATIENT MONITORING
- Post operative monitoring:
  ◊ Anticoagulation
  ◊ Establish brisk diuresis
  ◊ Continued resuscitation and diagnosis including echocardiography and other studies (see Causes and Risk Factors)
  ◊ Monitor perfusion stability
  ◊ Treat/eliminate causative factors

PREVENTION/AVOIDANCE
- Chronic anticoagulation in atrial arrhythmia
- Reduction of risk factors for atherosclerosis

POSSIBLE COMPLICATIONS
- Acidosis
- Myoglobinuria
- Hyperkalemia
- Recurrent occlusion
- Failure to remove clot/obstruction
- Compartment syndromes/reperfusion syndrome; delayed or instant
  ◊ Predisposing factors include: combined arterial injury, profound and prolonged ischemia, hypotension
  ◊ Occurs both in upper and lower extremities
  ◊ Clinical findings
  - Severe pain
  - Pain with passive muscle movement
  - Hypesthesias of nerves in compartment
  - Paralysis of nerves especially peroneal - foot drop
  - Tender, tense edema
  - Compartment pressure > 30-45 mm Hg
  ◊ Consequences of unrecognized compartment syndrome - acute
  - Amputation
  - Sepsis
  - Myoglobin renal failure
  - Shock
  - Multiple organ failure
  ◊ Delayed
  - Ischemic contracture
  - Infection
  - Causalgia
  - Gangrene
  ◊ Treatment
  - Fasciotomy

EXPECTED COURSE/PROGNOSIS
- 90% good outcome with prompt treatment
- Delayed/untreated associated with high mortality and limb loss
- 20-30% hospital mortality associated with causative factors

MISCELLANEOUS

ASSOCIATED CONDITIONS
- Acute mesenteric ischemia
- Renal infarction
- Carotid/CVA
- Multiple emboli
- Digital microembolization

AGE-RELATED FACTORS
Pediatric: Rare in children
Geriatric: Most common age affected
Others: N/A

PREGNANCY Rare

SYNONYMS N/A

ICD-9-CM
444.0 Arterial embolism and thrombosis of abdominal aorta
444.21 Arterial embolism and thrombosis of upper extremity
444.22 Arterial embolism and thrombosis of lower extremity
444.81 Arterial embolism and thrombosis of iliac artery
444.9 Arterial embolism and thrombosis of unspecified artery

SEE ALSO
- Complex regional pain syndrome

OTHER NOTES N/A

ABBREVIATIONS
A/ai = Ankle/arm index

REFERENCES
- Rutherford RB, Flannigan DP, Gupta SK, et al: Suggested standards of reports dealing with lower extremity ischemia. J Vasc Surg 1986;64:80-94
- Brewster DC, Chin AK, Fogarty TJ: Arterial Thrombosis. In: Rutherford RB, ed. Vascular Surgery. 3rd Ed. Philadelphia, W.B. Saunders Co., 1989
- Miller DC., Roon AJ, eds: Diagnosis and Management of Peripheral Vascular Diseases. Menlo Park, CA., Addison-Wesley Co., 1982
Illustrations: N/A
Internet references: http://www.5mcc.com

Author(s)
David H. Stubbs, MD, FACS

Arterial gas embolism

BASICS

DESCRIPTION Air released from an over-pressurized alveolus enters the pulmonary capillaries then travels through the arterial circulation causing occlusion of the cerebral and/or coronary circulation.
• Arterial gas embolism is the most serious and rapidly fatal of all SCUBA diving injuries and is second only to drowning as the leading cause of death associated with sport diving.
• Arterial gas embolism occurs on ascent and the time from alveolar rupture to the manifestation of symptoms is nearly always less than ten minutes.
System(s) affected: Cardiovascular, Nervous, Musculoskeletal
Genetics: N/A
Incidence/Prevalence in USA: It is estimated (based on injury/mortality reports collected by Divers Alert Network) to occur in approximately 4 per 100,000 sport divers per year.
Predominant age: Young adult
Predominant sex: Male > Female

SIGNS AND SYMPTOMS
• Group 1: Neurologic symptoms only. Divers presenting with neurologic symptoms but without impairment of spontaneous respirations and cardiac function. May be impossible to clinically distinguish from severe decompression sickness.
 ◊ Asymmetrical multiplegia or paralysis
 ◊ Tingling or numbness
 ◊ Blindness or other visual disturbances
 ◊ Deafness
 ◊ Vertigo
 ◊ Dizziness
 ◊ Headache
 ◊ Confusion
 ◊ Convulsions
 ◊ Aphasia
 ◊ Personality change; from subtle changes to unconsciousness
• Group 2: Loss of consciousness, apnea, and cardiac arrest or dysrhythmia. Divers presenting with both neurologic and cardiac impairments. All of the above signs and symptoms plus those below are possible.
 ◊ Dysrhythmias
 ◊ Cardiac arrest

CAUSES
• Group 1: Localized obstruction of cerebral blood flow by an embolus of air. Local capillary endothelial damage with vasogenic edema leading to a rise in intracranial pressure and ischemia.
• Group 2: This is thought to be due to localized obstruction of both cerebral and coronary blood flow by an embolus of air

RISK FACTORS
• History of a rapid ascent
• History of panic during dive
• History of holding breath while diving
• History of loss of consciousness (or with other noted symptoms) within seconds to minutes after or during a dive

DIAGNOSIS

DIFFERENTIAL DIAGNOSIS
Decompression sickness

LABORATORY
• Hematocrit - increased indicating volume depletion
• Urinalysis - increased specific gravity indicating volume depletion
Drugs that may alter lab results: N/A
Disorders that may alter lab results: N/A

PATHOLOGICAL FINDINGS N/A

SPECIAL TESTS
• ECG

IMAGING
• Chest x-ray to rule out pneumothorax

DIAGNOSTIC PROCEDURES N/A

TREATMENT

APPROPRIATE HEALTH CARE
• Hospital based hyperbaric chamber capable of performing a U.S. Navy Table 6A recompression (165 fsw).

GENERAL MEASURES
• Immediate transport to a suitable hyperbaric chamber for recompression as soon as possible; do not delay with nonessential procedures.
• Transport by aircraft is justifiable if it will save a significant amount of time (aircraft must fly at low altitudes or be capable of maintaining cabin pressure at about one atmosphere)
• Life-saving measures (CPR) must take precedence to sustain life
• Administration of high flow maximum concentration oxygen therapy by a tight fitting mask or by intubation and mechanical ventilation during transport
• Keep patient in recumbent position while maintaining airway
• Maintain hydration with IV fluids
• For assistance and advice in locating the nearest treatment chamber in your area (world-wide) call DIVERS ALERT NETWORK (DAN) at any hour (919) 684-8111

SURGICAL MEASURES N/A

ACTIVITY None until after treatment

DIET None until after treatment

PATIENT EDUCATION
• DIVERS ALERT NETWORK (DAN) Non-Emergency Information Line (Mon-Fri 9-5 EST) (919)684-2948; membership line (800)446-2671

MEDICATIONS

DRUG(S) OF CHOICE
• Oxygen
Contraindications: N/A
Precautions: N/A
Significant possible interactions: N/A

ALTERNATIVE DRUGS   None

FOLLOWUP

PATIENT MONITORING
• Frequent neurological checks in the acute pre-treatment and treatment phase
• Complete neurological assessment at one, three, six and twelve at months

PREVENTION/AVOIDANCE
• Strict adherence to diver safety protocols
• No diving after any dive injury or with any medical condition until evaluated and approved by a physician knowledgeable in diving medicine

POSSIBLE COMPLICATIONS
• Long term serious neurologic impairments
• Death

EXPECTED COURSE/PROGNOSIS
• Complete to partial resolution with adequate treatment

MISCELLANEOUS

ASSOCIATED CONDITIONS
• Pulmonary barotrauma leading to arterial gas embolism, can also cause pneumomediastinum, subcutaneous emphysema, pneumopericardium, pneumothorax, and pneumoperitoneum
• Always consider the possibility of decompression sickness in addition to arterial gas embolism in any SCUBA diver who has recently completed a dive

AGE-RELATED FACTORS
Pediatric: N/A
Geriatric: N/A
Others: N/A

PREGNANCY   N/A

SYNONYMS
• Gas embolism
• Air embolism

ICD-9-CM
958.0 Air embolism

SEE ALSO
• Decompression sickness

OTHER NOTES
• Any diver who has an onset of new symptom(s) or sign(s) after recently completing a SCUBA dive of any type, to any depth, for any period of time - serious consideration must be given as having sustained a dive related injury

ABBREVIATIONS
• DAN = Divers Alert Network
• AGE = arterial gas embolism

REFERENCES
• Shilling CW, ed: The Physicians Guide to Diving Medicine. New York, Plenum Press, 1984
• Strauss RH: Diving Medicine. Philadelphia, W.B. Saunders Co., 1976
Illustrations: N/A
Internet references: http://www.5mcc.com

Author(s)
Jess G. Bond, MD, MPH

Arteriosclerotic heart disease

BASICS

DESCRIPTION Arteriosclerosis is a group of diseases characterized by thickening and loss of elasticity of the arterial walls which progressively blocks the coronary arteries and their branches. Arteriosclerosis is the most common form of coronary arteriosclerosis. The process is chronic, occurring over many years, and is the most common cause of cardiovascular disability and death. Other forms of arteriosclerosis include arteriolosclerosis and medialcalcific stenosis, both of which are uncommon in the coronary vasculature.
System(s) affected: Cardiovascular
Genetics: Tendency is inheritable
Incidence/Prevalence in USA: Common. Causes 35% of deaths in men age 35-50. Death rate age 55-64 - 1:100.
Predominant age: Men 50-60, women 60-70, for peak clinical manifestations
Predominant sex: Male > Female

SIGNS AND SYMPTOMS
• Variable. May remain clinically asymptomatic even in advanced disease states, eg, silent ischemia.
• Clinical manifestations
  ◊ Substernal chest pain
  ◊ Exertional dyspnea
  ◊ Orthopnea
  ◊ Paroxysmal nocturnal dyspnea
  ◊ Cardiac arrhythmias
  ◊ Systolic murmur
  ◊ Cardiomegaly
  ◊ Pedal edema

CAUSES
• Atherosclerosis
• Narrowing of coronary arteries
• Embolism compromising coronary arteries at orifices
• Subintimal atheromas in large and medium vessels

RISK FACTORS
• Elevated low density lipoprotein (LDL)
• Decreased high density lipoprotein (HDL)
• Elevated triglycerides
• Smoking
• Family history of premature arteriosclerosis
• Obesity
• Hypertension
• Stress
• Sedentary life style
• Increasing age
• Male sex
• Postmenopausal female not on estrogen replacement therapy
• Diabetes mellitus

DIAGNOSIS

DIFFERENTIAL DIAGNOSIS N/A

LABORATORY
• Elevated triglycerides
• Elevated total cholesterol
• Elevated low density lipoproteins
• Decreased high density lipoproteins
• Elevated cholesterol/HDL ratio
Drugs that may alter lab results: N/A
Disorders that may alter lab results: N/A

PATHOLOGICAL FINDINGS
• Gross - narrowed coronary arteries
• Micro - cholesterol plaques on intima of coronary vessels
• Fibrotic subendothelial connective tissue of intima with plaque

SPECIAL TESTS
• ECG - variable. May be normal or may see ST segment elevation/depression and/or T wave inversion.
• Exercise stress test - positive

IMAGING
• Angiography - narrowed coronary arteries
• Echocardiography - wall motion abnormalities
• Pharmacologic stress tests (dobutamine, dipyridamole, adenosine) - positive
• Stress thallium test - positive

DIAGNOSTIC PROCEDURES N/A

TREATMENT

APPROPRIATE HEALTH CARE
• Outpatient for management of risk factors
• Inpatient for acute ischemic syndromes

GENERAL MEASURES
• Prevention of further progression of the disease
  ◊ Smoking cessation
  ◊ Treatment of hypercholesterolemia (diet, drugs)
  ◊ Increase high density lipoprotein (diet, exercise)
  ◊ Control of blood pressure
  ◊ Diabetes mellitus treated early and adequately
  ◊ Exercise
  ◊ Prophylactic aspirin
  ◊ Stress reduction
  ◊ Diet changes
  ◊ Weight loss
  ◊ Estrogen replacement therapy in postmenopausal women
• Treatment of complications
  ◊ Covered elsewhere under the individual topics (e.g., angina pectoris, myocardial infarction, heart failure, stroke, peripheral arterial occlusion, etc.)

SURGICAL MEASURES N/A

ACTIVITY Exercise may be helpful in preventing clinical coronary disease and useful for therapeutic measures

DIET
• Low-fat (20-30 grams of fat/day total intake)
• Weight-loss diet, if obesity a problem
• Increase soluble fiber

PATIENT EDUCATION For patient education materials favorably reviewed on this topic, contact: American Heart Association, 7320 Greenville Avenue, Dallas, TX 75231, (214)373-6300

MEDICATIONS

DRUG(S) OF CHOICE
- Aspirin, 160-325 mg/day, unless contraindicated
- Cholesterol-lowering agents
  ◊ Cholestyramine or colestipol, (bile acid sequestrants) 12-32 gm orally BID-QID
  ◊ Niacin 2-6 gm daily in divided doses (highly efficacious, but side effects restrict use)
  ◊ Gemfibrozil 600 mg bid
  ◊ Probucol 500 mg bid
  ◊ HMG-CoA reductase inhibitors (dose varies with product): atorvastatin (Lipitor), cerivastatin (Baycol), fluvastatin (Lescol), lovastatin (Mevacor), pravastatin (Pravachol), simvastatin (Zocor)

Contraindications: Refer to manufacturer's literature

Precautions: SR form of niacin may be linked to hepatotoxicity. Refer to manufacturer's literature.

Significant possible interactions: Refer to manufacturer's literature

ALTERNATIVE DRUGS
- Ticlopidine - antiplatelet activity

FOLLOWUP

PATIENT MONITORING
Monitor cholesterol, triglyceride levels, other preventive programs (weight loss, smoking cessation)

PREVENTION/AVOIDANCE
See General measures

POSSIBLE COMPLICATIONS
- Myocardial infarction
- Ventricular fibrillation
- Congestive heart failure
- Angina pectoris
- Sudden cardiac death

EXPECTED COURSE/PROGNOSIS
Guardedly favorable. Many risk factors can be modified.

MISCELLANEOUS

ASSOCIATED CONDITIONS
- Obesity
- Hypertension
- Diabetes
- Hypercholesterolemia

AGE-RELATED FACTORS
Pediatric: Preventive measures can begin early (proper nutrition, exercise, weight control, smoking deterrent programs, etc.)
Geriatric: Greatest incidence in this age group
Others: N/A

PREGNANCY
Rare in pregnant women

SYNONYMS
- Coronary artery disease (CAD)
- Coronary heart disease
- Coronary arteriosclerosis

ICD-9-CM
414.0 arteriosclerotic heart disease

SEE ALSO
- Angina
- Atherosclerosis
- Myocardial infarction

OTHER NOTES N/A

ABBREVIATIONS N/A

REFERENCES
- Hurst JW, et al: The Heart. 8th Ed. New York, McGraw-Hill, 1994
- Braunwald E. ed: Heart Disease: A Textbook of Cardiovascular Medicine. 4th Ed. Philadelphia, WB Saunders Co, 1992
- Goldman L, Braunwald E: Primary Cardiology. 1st Ed. Philadelphia, WB Saunders Co, 1998
Illustrations: N/A
Internet references: http://www.5mcc.com

Author(s)
Peter Kozisek, MD

Arthritis, infectious, bacterial

BASICS

DESCRIPTION   Invasion of joints by live micro-organisms or their fragments. One of the few curable causes of arthritis. May allow early recognition of systemic infection/disease.
System(s) affected: Musculoskeletal
Genetics: N/A
Incidence/Prevalence in USA:
• Neisserial:
  ◊ Responsible for 50% of infectious arthritis
  ◊ Arthritis occurs in 0.6% of the 3% of women with gonorrhea
  ◊ Arthritis occurs in 0.1% of the 0.7% of men with gonorrhea
  ◊ Arthritis occurs in 7% of individuals with N. meningitidis
• Non-Neisserial:
  ◊ Perhaps half as frequent as Neisserial
Predominant age:
• Neisserial:
  ◊ Especially 15-40, can occur at any age
• Non-Neisserial:
  ◊ 50% Prior to age 2: 27% Staphylococcus, 20% Streptococcus, 33% Haemophilus, and 13% other gram negative rods
  ◊ 70% Age 2-14: 34% Staphylococcus, 29% Streptococcus, 13% Haemophilus, and 13% other gram negative rods
  ◊ Adult: 34% Staphylococcus, 38% Streptococcus, 2% Haemophilus, and 26% other gram negative rods
Predominant sex:
• Neisserial: Female > Male (4:1)
• Non-Neisserial: Male > Female (2:1)
• Subacute bacterial endocarditis-related: Male = Female

SIGNS AND SYMPTOMS
• Predominantly monoarticular (90%). (Haemophilus may be pauciarticular and Mycoplasma often presents as a migratory polyarthritis).
• Limited joint use/motion (especially in children)
• Joint effusion, tenderness
• Joint warmth - present in less than 50%
• Joint redness- present in less than 50%
• Loss of joint motion
• Tenosynovitis
• Sudden flare of one or two joints in a patient with underlying joint disease
• Fever - in 90% at some time during the course of the infection
• Chills, malaise
• Cutaneous lesions
• Peripheral neuropathy
• Back pain - especially in subacute bacterial endocarditis (SBE)
• Hypertrophic osteoarthropathy - rare, secondary to endocarditis
• Fretfulness - especially in children
• Dermato-arthritis - usually pustular skin lesions in gonorrhea - usually petechial rash in meningococcemia
• Bacteremic phase - migratory polyarthritis, tenosynovitis, high fever, chills, pustules
• Localized phase - usually monoarticular, low grade fever (80%)

CAUSES
• Hematogenous invasion by microorganisms (80-90%)
• Contiguous spread (10-15%) from adjacent osteomyelitis in children
• Direct penetration of micro-organisms secondary to trauma or joint injection

RISK FACTORS
• Young patient with venereal exposure
• Concurrent extra-articular infection
• Prior arthritis in infected joint
• Trauma
• Joint puncture or surgery
• Prosthetic joint
• Prior antibiotic, corticosteroid, or immunosuppressive therapy
• Serious chronic illness (e.g., diabetes, liver disease, malignancy, primary immunodeficiency)
• Defective phagocytic mechanisms (e.g., chronic granulomatous disease)
• Intravenous drug abuse
• Travel/habitat history
• Sickle cell anemia

DIAGNOSIS

DIFFERENTIAL DIAGNOSIS
• Gout
• Pseudogout (calcium pyrophosphate deposition disease)
• Spondyloarthropathy (Reiter's syndrome, psoriatic arthritis, ankylosing spondylitis, the arthritis of inflammatory bowel disease)
• Juvenile rheumatoid arthritis
• Type IIa hyperlipoproteinemia
• Foreign body synovitis
• Rheumatoid arthritis
• Rheumatic fever
• AIDS
• Cellulitis
• Palindromic rheumatism
• Neuropathic arthropathy
• Lyme arthritis
• Sarcoidosis
• Granulomatous arthritis

LABORATORY
• Synovial fluid usually cloudy with > 50,000 WBC/HPF (high power field), but may have fewer white blood cells present or over 100,000. (Caveat - cell count must be performed within 1 hour of obtaining specimen to be valid).
• Synovial fluid white count can be recognized as elevated (in presence of trauma) if RBC:WBC ratio significantly less than 700
• Polymorphonuclear leukocytes usually predominate in synovial fluid
• Synovial fluid glucose often more than 40 mg/dL (2.22 mmol/L) less than in a simultaneously obtained serum glucose value (in fasting patient). However, arthrocentesis should not be delayed simply to obtain fasting synovial fluid glucose level.
• Westergren erythrocyte sedimentation rate - often elevated, but normal in 20%

• Rheumatoid factor positive in 50% - if endocarditis present and in viral arthritis
• Anti-techoic acid antibodies - with Staphylococcus infection
• Elevated peripheral white blood cell count (in 50-90%)
• Cryoglobulins
• Immune complexes
• Febrile agglutinins (to include Brucella and rickettsial-related titers)
• Antistreptolysin O (ASO) titer is usually normal, exclusive of streptococcal infections
• Depressed synovial fluid and occasionally depressed serum levels of complement
• Microscopic hematuria in subacute bacterial endocarditis (SBE)
• Presence of crystals (e.g., urate or calcium pyrophosphate) does not exclude infectious arthritis
Drugs that may alter lab results:
Antibiotics
Disorders that may alter lab results: N/A

PATHOLOGICAL FINDINGS   Synovial biopsy will reveal polymorphonuclear leukocytes and possibly the causative organism

SPECIAL TESTS
• Joint fluid - for gram stain (positive in 50%); culture (positive in 50-70%)
• Serum cidal level assessment of antibiotic adequacy is suggested with virulent organisms or therapeutic unresponsiveness (tenfold margin suggested)
• Blood, orifice, urine cultures. "Bedside culture" is recommended to enhance isolation of fastidious organisms.
• All cultures should be preserved and observed for at least 3 days and preferably 2 weeks. Observing synovial fluid cultures for at least 3 days allows isolation of fastidious organisms such as those of rat bite fever (Streptobacillus moniliformis and Spirillum minus).
• Neisserial infection generally requires use of special agars (e.g., chocolate or Thayer Martin) and relative anaerobic culturing conditions
• Countercurrent immunoelectrophoresis or complement fixation for specific bacterial antigens
• Polymerase chain reaction for specific bacterial DNA

IMAGING
• X-ray
  ◊ Soft tissue swelling
  ◊ Juxta-articular osteoporosis
  ◊ Radiolucent area (gas) in a joint space from gas forming organisms. (Caveat - may also occur normally as a "vacuum phenomenon").
  ◊ Effacement of the obturator fat pad (with hip involvement)
  ◊ X-ray changes are usually a late phenomenon
  ◊ Rarefaction of subchondral bone may occur as early as 2-7 days
  ◊ Joint space loss (secondary to cartilage destruction) may be seen as early as 4-10 days
  ◊ Erosions
  ◊ Joint destruction with ankylosis may occur as early as 2 weeks

- Other imaging techniques
  ◊ Technetium joint scans - reveal distribution of inflammation
  ◊ Gallium or Ceretec WBC scan-Indium scans - reveal inflammation as well as infection
  ◊ CT - to identify sequestration
  ◊ MRI - effusion, perhaps early cartilage damage, osteomyelitis

DIAGNOSTIC PROCEDURES
- Arthrocentesis with gram stain and culture - only positive in 50-70%. Must be done in all patients when possibility of infectious arthritis is considered. Arthrocentesis should probably be performed within 12 hours of suspicion.
- Arthrocentesis approach must avoid contaminated tissue (e.g., overlying cellulitis)

TREATMENT

APPROPRIATE HEALTH CARE
- Hospitalization for parenteral therapy
- Rarely an extremely compliant patient with a very sensitive organism might be treated as an outpatient

GENERAL MEASURES
- Repeat arthrocentesis to drain the joint, as fluid re-accumulates
- Avoid adding anti-inflammatory therapy so as not to compromise assessment of therapeutic response to antibiotic
- If a joint prosthesis is present in an infection, the infection is very difficult to eradicate, without removal of the prosthesis
- Treatment is continued for 1-2 weeks after total resolution of all signs of inflammation, 3-4 weeks for gram negative organisms, and 6-8 weeks if the joint was previously diseased (e.g., involved by arthritis)
- Intra-articular antibiotics are not required and may actually aggravate the arthritis

SURGICAL MEASURES
Arthrotomy indicated only if fluid accumulated is loculated and/or not amenable to needle drainage

ACTIVITY
Limit activity or splint the joint initially. Continuous passive motion may be used as an alternative approach.

DIET
No special diet

PATIENT EDUCATION
- Rothschild, B.: Diagnosing and treating infectious arthritis. Geriatric Consultant. 5:14-15, 1986
- Arthritis Foundation pamphlet

MEDICATIONS

DRUG(S) OF CHOICE
- Neisserial
  ◊ Ceftriaxone 1 gm IM or IV every day for 14 days (but at least 7 days after symptoms resolve)
  or
  ◊ Spectinomycin 2 gm IM every 12 hours for 10 days
- Non-Neisserial:
  ◊ Gram positive cocci in chains or clumps - nafcillin 150 mg/kg/day q 4-6 h IV/IM
  ◊ Gram positive diplococci - penicillin G 1.4 million units q6h
  ◊ Gram negative bacilli: In neonates - penicillin and gentamicin; in children age 6 months to 4 years - cefuroxime; in adult - penicillin or cephalosporin plus gentamicin, all at full dose. Add clindamycin, at full dose, in the presence of retroperitoneal or pelvic abscess.
  ◊ Gram negative pleomorphic organisms - clindamycin at full dose (clindamycin has gram negative activity only against anaerobes)
  ◊ No bacteria seen on smear - penicillin or cephalosporin plus gentamicin, all at full dose

Contraindications:
- Tetracycline: not for use in pregnancy or children < 8 years.

Precautions:
- Observe for allergic reactions/serum sickness
- Tetracycline: may cause photosensitivity; sunscreen recommended.

Significant possible interactions:
- Tetracycline: avoid concurrent administration with antacids, dairy products, or iron.
- Broad-spectrum antibiotics: may reduce the effectiveness of oral contraceptives; barrier method recommended.

ALTERNATIVE DRUGS
- Non-Neisserial
  ◊ In children age 6 months to 4 years - ampicillin [Chloramphenicol may be required to cover resistant Haemophilus]
  ◊ Infectious disease consult strongly advised to supplement rheumatologist input for Haemophilus infections
- Quinolones (e.g., ciprofloxacin)

FOLLOWUP

PATIENT MONITORING
- Recurrent arthrocentesis, as fluid re-accumulates - to verify sterilization of the joint and to verify reversion of inflammatory signs to normal
- If no definitive improvement within 48 hours, re-evaluate completely
- Complete blood count, liver and kidney function and urinalysis twice a week, while on antibiotics (perhaps with creatinine every other day when gentamicin used)
- Gentamycin levels
- It is essential to followup one week and a month after stopping antibiotics to detect any relapse

PREVENTION/AVOIDANCE
- Prophylaxis in presence of predisposing joint condition
- Condoms and discretion for STD protection

POSSIBLE COMPLICATIONS
- Death (9-33% in elderly, especially with gram negative organisms)
- Limited joint range of motion
- Flail or fused or dislocated joint
- Carpal tunnel syndrome
- Septic necrosis
- Sinus formation
- Ankylosis
- Osteomyelitis
- Postinfectious synovitis
- Shortening of the limb (in children)

EXPECTED COURSE/PROGNOSIS
- Early treatment should allow cure
- Delayed recognition/treatment complicated by morbidity and mortality

MISCELLANEOUS

ASSOCIATED CONDITIONS
- Systemic infection
- Infection elsewhere
- Immunodeficiency; immunosuppression
- Rheumatoid arthritis

AGE-RELATED FACTORS
Pediatric: N/A
Geriatric: N/A
Others: N/A

PREGNANCY N/A

SYNONYMS
- Suppurative arthritis
- Septic arthritis

ICD-9-CM
711.00 Pyogenic arthritis, site unspecified

SEE ALSO
- Reiter's syndrome
- Lyme disease

OTHER NOTES N/A

ABBREVIATIONS N/A

REFERENCES
- Kelly WW, Harris ED Jr, Rudd S, Sledge CB: Textbook of Rheumatology. Philadelphia, W.B. Saunders Co., 1997
- Garcia, Porrax, et al: The clinical spectrum of severe septic bursitis in Northwestern Spain. J Rheum 1999;26:663-667
- Berbari EF, et al: Risk factors for prosthetic joint infection. Clin Infect Dis 1998;27:1247-1254
- Wilkinson NZ, Kingsley GH, Jones HW, Sieper J, Braun J, Ward ME. The detection of DNA from a range of bacterial species in the joints of patients with a variety of arthritides using a nested, broad-range polymerase chain reaction. Rheumatology 1999;38:260-266.
3 additional references available at web site
Internet references: http://www.5mcc.com
Illustrations: N/A

Author(s)
Bruce M. Rothschild, MD

Arthritis, infectious, granulomatous

BASICS

DESCRIPTION Invasion of joints by live micro-organisms or their fragments. One of the few curable causes of arthritis. May allow early recognition of systemic infection/disease.
System(s) affected: Musculoskeletal
Genetics: N/A
Incidence/Prevalence in USA:
• One in three million
• Granulomatous arthritis occurs in 1-3% of patients with tuberculosis infections
Predominant age: Diffuse
Predominant sex:
• Male > Female (Brucella and mycobacterial)
• Female > Male (fungal)

SIGNS AND SYMPTOMS
• Predominantly monoarticular (90%). Fungal may present as a migratory polyarthritis.
• Joint tenderness
• Limited joint use/motion (especially in children)
• Joint effusion
• Joint warmth - present in less than 50%
• Joint redness - present in less than 50%
• Loss of joint motion
• Tenosynovitis
• Sudden flare of a single joint in a patient with underlying joint disease
• Fever - in 50% at some time during the course of the infection
• Chills
• Malaise
• Cutaneous lesions
• Peripheral neuropathy
• Back pain - especially in tuberculosis and brucellosis
• Hypertrophic osteoarthropathy
• Fretfulness - especially in children
• Doughy swelling, with minimal tenderness
• Dactylitis
• Diaphoresis
• Headache
• Hepatosplenomegaly
• Lymphadenopathy
• Erythema nodosum
• Iritis (with mycobacterial arthritis)

CAUSES
• Hematogenous invasion by microorganisms (80-90%)
• Contiguous spread (10-15%)
• Direct penetration of micro-organisms secondary to trauma

RISK FACTORS
• Concurrent acquired immunodeficiency disease
• Concurrent extra-articular infection
• Prior arthritis in infected joint
• Trauma
• Rheumatoid arthritis
• Joint puncture or surgery
• Prosthetic joint
• Prior antibiotic, corticosteroid, or immunosuppressive therapy
• Serious chronic illness (e.g., diabetes, liver disease, malignancy, primary immunodeficiency)

• Defective phagocytic mechanisms (e.g., chronic granulomatous disease)
• Intravenous drug abuse
• Exposure history (e.g., unpasteurized milk)
• Farmers, butchers, veterinarians
• Travel/habitat history
• Gardening, especially for sporotrichosis

DIAGNOSIS

DIFFERENTIAL DIAGNOSIS
• Gout
• Pseudogout (calcium pyrophosphate deposition disease)
• Spondyloarthropathy (Reiter's syndrome, psoriatic arthritis, ankylosing spondylitis, the arthritis of inflammatory bowel disease)
• Juvenile rheumatoid arthritis
• Type IIa hyperlipoproteinemia
• Foreign body synovitis
• Rheumatoid arthritis
• Rheumatic fever
• AIDS
• Cellulitis
• Palindromic rheumatism
• Neuropathic arthropathy
• Lyme arthritis
• Sarcoidosis
• Pyogenic arthritis

LABORATORY
• Synovial fluid usually cloudy with > 20,000 WBC/HPF, but may have fewer white blood cells present or over 100,000. (Caveat - cell count must be performed within 1 hour of obtaining specimen to be valid).
• Synovial fluid white count can be recognized as elevated (in presence of trauma) if RBC:WBC ratio significantly less than 700
• Polymorphonuclear leukocytes usually predominate in synovial fluid. (Granulomatous and viral arthritis may have a mononuclear cell predominance, but polymorphonuclear leukocytes usually predominate).
• Synovial fluid glucose often more than 40 mg/dL (2.22 mmol/L) less than in a simultaneously obtained serum glucose value (in fasting patient). However, arthrocentesis should not be delayed simply to obtain fasting synovial fluid glucose level.
• Synovial fluid eosinophilia may occasionally be seen in the healing phase of an infection, but parasitic (e.g., guinea-worm) infection must also be considered
• Westergren erythrocyte sedimentation - often elevated, but normal in 20%
• Rheumatoid factor positive in 50% - if endocarditis present
• Elevated peripheral white blood cell count
• Cryoglobulins
• Immune complexes
• Febrile agglutinins (to include Brucella and rickettsial related titers)
• Antistreptolysin O (ASO) titer is usually normal
• Depressed synovial fluid and occasionally serum levels of complement

• Presence of crystals in urine (e.g., urate or calcium pyrophosphate) does not exclude infectious arthritis
• Polymerase chain reaction for specific microorganisms
Drugs that may alter lab results: Insulin, antibiotics
Disorders that may alter lab results: Diabetes

PATHOLOGICAL FINDINGS Synovial biopsy may reveal granulomas and possibly the causative organism

SPECIAL TESTS
• Arthrocentesis - bacterial - for silver and acid fast stain and culture
• Arthrocentesis - mycobacterial - acid fast (positive in 20%); culture (positive in 80%)
• Drug sensitivity testing recommended
• Blood, urine cultures
• Sputum cultures
• Gastric lavage for acid fast - increases yield 7%
• Fungal blood cultures
• All cultures should be held for 2 weeks; acid-fast cultures for 6 weeks

IMAGING
• X-ray
  ◊ Soft tissue swelling
  ◊ Osteoporosis
  ◊ Effacement of the obturator fat pad (with hip involvement) or psoas shadow
  ◊ X-ray changes are usually a late phenomenon
  ◊ Rarefaction of subchondral bone
  ◊ Joint space loss
  ◊ Erosions
  ◊ Joint destruction with ankylosis
  ◊ Subchondral erosion with preservation of joint space is highly suggestive of granulomatous infection
• Other imaging techniques
  ◊ Technetium joint scans - reveal distribution of inflammation
  ◊ Gallium or Ceretec WBC scan-Indium scans - reveal inflammation as well as infection
  ◊ Computerized tomography - to identify sequestration
  ◊ Magnetic resonance imaging - perhaps early cartilage damage, osteomyelitis

DIAGNOSTIC PROCEDURES
• Arthrocentesis with gram, silver and acid fast stain, and culture. Must be done in all patients when possibility of infectious arthritis considered.
• Arthrocentesis approach must avoid contaminated tissue (e.g., overlying cellulitis)

TREATMENT

APPROPRIATE HEALTH CARE
• Fungal - initial hospitalization for parenteral therapy
• Mycobacterial - outpatient, once diagnosed
• Brucella - outpatient, once diagnosed

GENERAL MEASURES
• Repeat arthrocentesis to drain the joint, as fluid reaccumulates
• Avoid adding anti-inflammatory therapy so as not to compromise assessment of therapeutic response (to antibiotic)
• Infection associated with prosthetic joints may be difficult to eradicate without removal
• For Brucella or fungal infections, treatment is continued for 1-2 weeks after total resolution of all signs of inflammation, and 6-8 weeks if the joint was previously diseased (e.g., involved by arthritis)
• Anti-granulomatous therapy requires a long program (See Tuberculosis)
• Intra-articular antibiotics are not indicated
• Infectious disease consultation may be helpful

SURGICAL MEASURES
• Arthrotomy indicated only if fluid accumulated is loculated and/or not amenable to needle drainage

ACTIVITY
Limit/splint joint initially, while pursuing full passive range of motion. Continuous passive motion is an alternative approach.

DIET
As tolerated

PATIENT EDUCATION
• Rothschild, B.M.: Diagnosing and treating infectious arthritis. Geriatric Consultant, 5:14-15, 1986
• Arthritis Foundation
1314 Spring Street, NW
Atlanta, GA 30309
(404) 872-7100

MEDICATIONS

DRUG(S) OF CHOICE
• Medications based on sensitivity of organisms
• Mycobacterial: (use a combination of these three) isoniazid at 5 mg/kg, up to 300 mg po qd, rifampin at 10 mg/kg, up to 600 mg PO qd, and pyrazinamide at 15-30 mg/kg up to 2 gm/d. The latter is replaced after 2 months with ethambutol 15 mg/kg. Continue therapy for 9-24 months. Request infectious disease consultation.
• Brucella: tetracycline plus streptomycin or trimethoprim-sulfamethoxazole or rifampin (for dosage, see manufacturer's literature)
• Fungal infection: amphotericin B, ketoconazole, flucytosine (5-fluorocytosine) and even iodide, dependent upon organism

Contraindications:
• Tetracycline: not for use in pregnancy or children < 8 years.

Precautions:
• Observe for allergic reactions/serum sickness
• Tetracycline: may cause photosensitivity; sunscreen recommended.

Significant possible interactions:
• Tetracycline: avoid concurrent administration with antacids, dairy products, or iron.
• Ketaconazole - multiple drug interactions

ALTERNATIVE DRUGS
• See Tuberculosis

FOLLOWUP

PATIENT MONITORING
To verify sterilization of the joint and to verify reversion of inflammatory signs to normal
• Treatment of mycobacterial arthritis requires monthly complete blood count, liver and kidney function and urinalysis assessment
• It is essential to followup frequently after stopping antibiotics to detect relapse

PREVENTION/AVOIDANCE
Prophylaxis in presence of predisposing joint condition

POSSIBLE COMPLICATIONS
• Limited joint range of motion
• Flail or fused joint
• Carpal-tunnel syndrome
• Septic necrosis
• Sinus formation
• Ankylosis
• Joint dislocation
• Osteomyelitis
• Shortening of the limb (in children)

EXPECTED COURSE/PROGNOSIS
• Early initiation of treatment should allow cure
• Delayed recognition/treatment complicated by increased morbidity and mortality

MISCELLANEOUS

ASSOCIATED CONDITIONS
• Systemic infection
• Infection elsewhere
• Immunodeficiency - (medication)
• Immunosuppression

AGE-RELATED FACTORS
Pediatric: Infrequent
Geriatric:
• Grave in elderly
• Tuberculosis much more likely to occur
Others: N/A

PREGNANCY
N/A

SYNONYMS
• Fungal arthritis

ICD-9-CM
031.8 Mycobacterial arthritis
023.9 Brucellosis, unspecified
115.99 Fungal arthritis

SEE ALSO
• Brucellosis
• Atypical mycobacterial infection

OTHER NOTES
Infectious arthritis may be caused by many other organisms including bacterial (particularly neisseria), rickettsial, parasitic, fungal, and viral agents. Much of the information contained in this profile applies to these other organisms as well as to granulomatous infections.

ABBREVIATIONS
HPF = high power field

REFERENCES
• Rothschild BM: Infectious Arthritis. Fairlawn, CT, Clinical AV, 1982
• Gershwin ME, Robbins DL: Musculoskeletal Diseases of Children. New York, Grune & Stratton, 1983
• Rothschild BM, Martin L: Paleopathology: Disease in the Fossil Record. London, CRC Press, 1993
• Kelly WW, Harris ED Jr, Ruddy S, Sledge CB: Textbook of Rheumatology. Philadelphia, W.B. Saunders Co., 1997
• Rothschild BM, Rothschild C: Recognition of hypertrophic osteoarthropathy in skeletal remains. J Rheum 1998;25:2221-2228
Illustrations: N/A
Internet references: http://www.5mcc.com

Author(s)
Bruce M. Rothschild, MD

Arthritis, juvenile rheumatoid (JRA)

BASICS

DESCRIPTION Juvenile rheumatoid arthritis (JRA) is the most common form of chronic arthritis in children and a major cause of musculoskeletal disability. There are three subtypes of the disease, determined by the clinical characteristics occurring within the first six months of illness.
• Systemic (sys) JRA: occurs in 10-20% of affected children; usually characterized by a febrile onset and evanescent rash with multiple physical and laboratory abnormalities
• Polyarticular (poly) JRA: occurs in 30-40% of affected children; characterized by multiple (> 4) joint involvement and minimal systemic features
• Pauciarticular (pauci) JRA: occurs in 40-50% of affected children; characterized by ≤ 4 joints involved, usually larger joints; a risk for chronic uveitis in young girls and axial skeletal involvement in older boys
System(s) affected: Musculoskeletal, Hemic/Lymphatic/Immunologic
Genetics: HLA-B27 histocompatibility antigen associated with risk of evolving spondyloarthropathy in older boys with pauci JRA. Weaker HLA associations exist for other subtypes (HLA-DR5; HLA-DR8; HLA-DR4).
Incidence/Prevalence in USA: Prevalence approximately 1/1000 children; incidence 1/10,000 children
Predominant age: 1-4 years and 9-14 years
Predominant sex: Female > Male

SIGNS AND SYMPTOMS
• Systemic
  ◊ Arthralgias/arthritis
  ◊ Chest pain, pericardial friction rub
  ◊ Dyspnea
  ◊ Fatigue
  ◊ Fever
  ◊ Hepatosplenomegaly
  ◊ Lymphadenopathy
  ◊ Myalgias
  ◊ Rash
  ◊ Weight loss
• Polyarticular
  ◊ Arthralgia/arthritis
  ◊ Cold intolerance
  ◊ Difficulty writing
  ◊ Fatigue
  ◊ Growth retardation
  ◊ Hand weakness
  ◊ Limitation of motion
  ◊ Malaise
  ◊ Morning stiffness
  ◊ Rheumatoid nodules
  ◊ Synovial cysts
  ◊ Synovial thickening
  ◊ Weight loss
• Pauciarticular
  ◊ Abnormal gait
  ◊ Eye pain, redness
  ◊ Joint swelling
  ◊ Leg length abnormality
  ◊ Morning stiffness
  ◊ Photophobia

CAUSES Multifactorial including abnormal immune response, genetic predisposition and environmental triggers, possibly infectious

RISK FACTORS
• HLA-B27 in pauci JRA increases risk for development of spondyloarthropathy
• Rheumatoid factor positivity increases risk for severe arthritis in poly JRA
• ANA positivity increases risk for uveitis in pauci and poly JRA

DIAGNOSIS

DIFFERENTIAL DIAGNOSIS Other rheumatic diseases, especially SLE and dermatomyositis; atypical bacterial or viral infections; hemoglobinopathies; malignancy; vasculitis; rheumatic fever; Lyme disease; post-infectious arthritis; musculoskeletal developmental abnormalities; sympathetic dystrophy

LABORATORY
• WBC normal or markedly elevated (sys)
• Hb normal or low (especially sys)
• Platelet count normal or elevated
• ANA positive, 40% (poly or pauci)
• RF positive, 10-15% (usually polys)
• HLA-B27 positive, 70% in pauci boys
• Sedimentation rate (ESR) elevated in most patients with active disease; > 100 mL/hr (Westergren) in active systemic disease
Drugs that may alter lab results:
Anti-inflammatory therapy may alter CBC and ESR
Disorders that may alter lab results:
Hemoglobinopathies (ESR)

PATHOLOGICAL FINDINGS Synovium shows hyperplasia of synovial cells, hyperemia and infiltration of small lymphocytes and mononuclear cells

SPECIAL TESTS
• Echocardiography (pericarditis)
• Radionuclide scans (infection, malignancy)

IMAGING
• Early radiographic changes - soft tissue swelling, periosteal reaction, juxta-articular demineralization; later changes include joint space loss, articular surface erosions, subchondral cyst formation, sclerosis and joint fusion
• CT and MRI very helpful in delineating early erosions

DIAGNOSTIC PROCEDURES
• Joint fluid aspiration and analysis helpful in excluding infection
• Synovial biopsy occasionally indicated in persistent, atypical monoarthritis

TREATMENT

APPROPRIATE HEALTH CARE
• Outpatient care except for initial diagnostic workup of systemic JRA disease and complications for all subtypes
• Patients require regular (every 4 months in patients with pauciarticular disease) ophthalmic exams to uncover asymptomatic eye disease .

GENERAL MEASURES Physical therapy including daily home exercise program required for joints with limited motion; moist heat, sleeping bag or electric blanket to relieve morning stiffness

SURGICAL MEASURES Total hip replacement for severe disease may be needed

ACTIVITY
• Full activity as tolerated
• Regular school. May need modified physical education program.

DIET Regular diet with special attention to adequate calcium, iron, protein and caloric intake

PATIENT EDUCATION
• Ongoing education of patients and families needed with special attention to psychosocial needs, behavioral strategies for dealing with pain and noncompliance, and utilization of health care resources
• Printed and audio-visual information available from local Arthritis Foundation

MEDICATIONS

DRUG(S) OF CHOICE
• First-line:
◊ Nonsteroidal anti-inflammatory medications (NSAID's) adequate in approximately 60% of patients. Average of 2-3 trials needed to determine most effective drug for an individual patient; adequate duration of trial for given NSAID 4-6 weeks (if no adverse reaction). Drugs for children include:
  - Aspirin 75-90 mg/kg/d
  - Ibuprofen (Motrin, Advil, Nuprin) 30-50 mg/kg/d (usual dose is 40 mg/kg/d)
  - Naproxen (Naprosyn, Aleve) 10-20 mg/kg/d
  - Tolmetin sodium 15-30 mg/kg/d
• Second-line:
◊ 30-40% of patients ultimately require addition of disease-modifying antirheumatic drug (DMARD) e.g., gold, antimalarials, penicillamine, methotrexate
◊ Other agents - corticosteroids for serious cardiac involvement or unresponsive uveitis; IV immune globulin (IVIG) or cyclosporine in selected patients
Contraindications: Known allergies
Precautions: All (except salicyl salicylate) affect platelet adhesiveness and may worsen a bleeding diathesis. Use caution with all NSAID's in renal insufficiency and hypovolemic states.
Significant possible interactions: NSAID's may lower serum levels of digitalis and anticonvulsants, and blunt the effect of loop diuretics. NSAID's may increase serum methotrexate levels.

ALTERNATIVE DRUGS   Other NSAID's; analgesics for pain control

FOLLOWUP

PATIENT MONITORING
• Patients on NSAID's - CBC, urinalysis, minimum every 3-4 months
• Patients on aspirin and/or other salicylates - transaminase and salicylate levels, weekly for first month, then every 3-4 months
• Patients on gold - monthly CBC, urinalysis
• Patient on methotrexate - monthly liver function tests, CBC
• Ophthalmologic monitoring for antimalarials

PREVENTION/AVOIDANCE
• Avoid salicylate therapy during serious viral illness or following varicella exposure due to possible risk for Reye's syndrome
• No known preventive measures for JRA

POSSIBLE COMPLICATIONS
• Blindness
• Band keratopathy
• Glaucoma
• Short stature
• Debilitating joint disease
• Patient on NSAID's
  ◊ Peptic ulcer
  ◊ Gastrointestinal hemorrhage
  ◊ Rashes
  ◊ CNS reactions
  ◊ Renal disease
  ◊ Leukopenia
• Patient on DMARD's
  ◊ Bone marrow suppression
  ◊ Hepatitis
  ◊ Renal disease
  ◊ Dermatitis
  ◊ Mouth ulcers
  ◊ Retinal toxicity (antimalarials)

EXPECTED COURSE/PROGNOSIS
• 70-80% ultimately remit, but functional ability depends on adequacy of long-term therapy (disease control and maintaining muscle and joint function)
• Poorest prognosis in polyarticular patients with positive rheumatoid factor (RF); and in systemic juvenile arthritis

MISCELLANEOUS

ASSOCIATED CONDITIONS   Other autoimmune disorders

AGE-RELATED FACTORS
Pediatric: Behavioral and compliance problems frequent in toddlers and teenagers
Geriatric: N/A
Others: N/A

PREGNANCY   Unpredictable effect on disease activity

SYNONYMS
• Juvenile chronic arthritis
• Juvenile arthritis
• Still's disease

ICD-9-CM
714.30 Polyarticular juvenile rheumatoid arthritis, chronic
714.31 Polyarticular juvenile rheumatoid arthritis, acute
714.32 Pauciarticular onset JRA
714.33 Monoarticular onset JRA

SEE ALSO   N/A

OTHER NOTES   Treatment goal is to control active disease as well as extra-articular manifestations in order to maintain musculoskeletal function as normal as possible

ABBREVIATIONS
JRA = juvenile rheumatoid arthritis
RF = rheumatic factor
DMARD = disease modifying antirheumatic drug

REFERENCES
• Schaller JG: Juvenile Rheumatoid Arthritis. Pediatrics in Review 1980;2(6), 163-174
• Cassidy JT, Petty RE: The Textbook of Pediatric Rheumatology. 3rd Ed. New York, Churchill Livingstone, 1995
Illustrations: 1 available on CD-ROM
Internet references: http://www.5mcc.com

Author(s)
Carol B. Lindsley, MD

Arthritis, osteo

 BASICS

 DIAGNOSIS

 TREATMENT

BASICS

DESCRIPTION Osteoarthritis (OA) is the most common form of joint disease. Involves progressive loss of articular cartilage and reactive changes at joint margins and in subchondral bone.
• Primary
  ◊ Idiopathic
  ◊ Divided into subsets depending on clinical features
• Secondary
  ◊ Childhood anatomic abnormalities (e.g., congenital hip dysplasia, slipped femoral epiphyses)
  ◊ Inheritable metabolic disorders (e.g., alkaptonuria, Wilson's disease, hemochromatosis)
  ◊ Neuropathic arthropathy (Charcot's joints)
  ◊ Hemophilic arthropathy
  ◊ Acromegalic arthropathy
  ◊ Paget's disease
  ◊ Hyperparathyroidism
  ◊ Noninfectious inflammatory arthritis (e.g., rheumatoid arthritis, spondyloarthropathies)
  ◊ Gout, calcium pyrophosphate deposition disease (pseudogout)
  ◊ Septic or tuberculous arthritis
  ◊ Post-traumatic
System(s) affected: Musculoskeletal
Genetics: Unknown
Incidence/Prevalence in USA:
• Estimates of radiographic evidence of OA - range from 33% to almost 90% in those people over the age of 65
• Approximately 60 million patients at any one time
Predominant age:
• Over age 40 (for symptomatic disease)
• Leading cause of disability in those over age 65
Predominant sex: Male = Female

SIGNS AND SYMPTOMS
• Slowly developing joint pain
• Pain that follows use of a joint
• Stiffness (especially morning and after sitting) of less than 15 minutes duration
• Joint enlargement (e.g., Heberden's nodes of distal interphalangeal joints)
• Decreased range of motion
• Tenderness usually absent; may be associated with synovitis, with tenderness along joint margin
• Crepitation as late sign
• Local pain and stiffness with osteoarthritis of spine, with radicular pain (if there is compression of nerve roots)

CAUSES Biomechanical, biochemical, inflammatory, and immunological factors are all implicated in pathogenesis of osteoarthritis

RISK FACTORS
• Age over 50
• Obesity (weight bearing joints)
• Prolonged occupational or sports stress
• Injury to a joint

DIAGNOSIS

DIFFERENTIAL DIAGNOSIS
• Distinguish from other types of arthritis by absent systemic findings, minimal articular inflammation, and distribution of involved joints (e.g., distal and proximal interphalangeal joints, not wrist and metacarpophalangeal joints)
• In spine, distinguish from osteoporosis, metastatic disease, multiple myeloma, other bone disease

LABORATORY Not helpful (sedimentation rate not increased)
Drugs that may alter lab results: N/A
Disorders that may alter lab results: In secondary OA, the underlying disorder may have abnormal lab results, e.g., hemochromatosis - abnormal iron studies

PATHOLOGICAL FINDINGS
• Synovial fluid may have a slightly increased white blood cell count, predominantly mononuclear
• Calcium pyrophosphate dihydrate and/or apatite crystals may occasionally be seen in effusions and require polarized light microscopy or special techniques to see
• Subchondral bone trabecular microfractures
• Degradation response produced by release of proteolytic enzymes, collagenolytic enzymes, prostaglandins, and immune responses

SPECIAL TESTS N/A

IMAGING X-rays usually normal early; later often show narrowed joint space, osteophyte formation, subchondral bony sclerosis, and cyst formation. Erosions may occur on surface of distal interphalangeal (DIP) and proximal interphalangeal (PIP) joints when OA is associated with inflammation (erosive osteoarthritis).

DIAGNOSTIC PROCEDURES
• Joint aspiration
  ◊ May be helpful to distinguish between OA and chronic inflammatory arthritides
  ◊ OA - cell count usually < 500 cells/mm3, predominantly mononuclear
  ◊ Inflammatory - cell count usually > 2000 cells/mm3, predominantly neutrophils

TREATMENT

APPROPRIATE HEALTH CARE
Outpatient

GENERAL MEASURES
• Reassurance of absence of generalized systemic disease, with recognition of potential disability from osteoarthritis
• Weight reduction if obese
• General fitness program
• Heat (local, tub baths, etc.)
• Physical therapy to maintain or regain joint motion and muscle strength. Quadriceps strengthening exercises can relive pain and disability of the knee.
• Protect joints from overuse (e.g., cane, crutches, walker, neck collar, elastic knee support)

SURGICAL MEASURES Surgery may be indicated in advanced disease (e.g., osteotomy, debridement, removal of loose bodies, joint replacement)

ACTIVITY As active as tolerated

DIET No special diet

PATIENT EDUCATION
• For a listing of sources for patient education materials favorably reviewed on this topic, physicians may contact: American Academy of Family Physicians Foundation, P.O. Box 8418, Kansas City, MO 64114, (800)274-2237, ext. 4400
• Arthritis Foundation, PO Box 7669, Atlanta, GA 30357-0669; 800-283-7800

MEDICATIONS

DRUG(S) OF CHOICE
• Acetaminophen for relief of pain. If not effective, nonacetylated salicylates (e.g., salsalate, choline-magnesium salicylate), or low dose ibuprofen ≤ 1600 mg/d.
• Other NSAIDs can be used and have similar efficacy. Their prolonged use is associated with significant side effects, especially in the elderly. Since pain in osteoarthritis varies from day to day, brief course of a short acting NSAID are preferable.
• A new class of NSAID's referred to as cyclo-oxygenase-2 (COX-2) specific inhibitors have recently become available. They supposedly are less likely to cause stomach ulcers and they work as well as the nonspecific NSAID's in reducing arthritis inflammation and pain. They are currently much more expensive than then specific NSAID's and should be reserved for those patients who are at a higher risk for stomach ulcers.
• Opioid analgesics (e.g., codeine, oxycodone, propoxyphene) should be restricted for treatment of acute episodes of pain
Contraindications: NSAID's are contraindication if there is renal disease, congestive failure, hypertension, active peptic ulcer disease or previous hypersensitivity to a NSAID or aspirin (asthma, nasal polyps, urticaria/angioedema, hypotension)
Precautions:
• In patients with history of peptic ulcer disease, or risk factors for upper GI bleeding, acetaminophen is recommended. If a NSAID is necessary because of an inadequate response to acetaminophen, it should be given with misoprostol. Risk factors for upper GI bleeding are a previous history of bleeding or peptic ulcer, age 65, concomitant use of oral corticosteroids or anticoagulants. In these patients, the risk of stomach ulcers can be reduced by such drugs as misoprostol (Cytotec) and the proton pump inhibitors (eg, omeprazole and lansoprazole).
• Oral or parenteral adrenal corticosteroids are contraindicated
• Combinations of 2 or more NSAIDs are contraindicated because of increased risk of adverse reactions without concomitant improved efficacy
Significant possible interactions:
• NSAID's reduce effectiveness of ACE inhibitors and diuretics
• Aspirin and NSAID's may increase effects of anticoagulants
• Increased hypoglycemic effects of oral hypoglycemics with aspirin
• Avoid concomitant use of aspirin with NSAID's
• Salicylates reduce effectiveness of spironolactone (Aldactone) and uricosurics
• Corticosteroids and some antacids increase salicylate excretion, while ascorbic acid and ammonium chloride reduce salicylate excretion and may cause toxicity

ALTERNATIVE DRUGS
• Tailor drug to patient, and switch if response is not adequate
• Judicious use of intra-articular injections of corticosteroids for selected acute flare-ups of joints. No more than 3-4/year intra-articular corticosteroid injections up to a maximal total of 12 injections per joint. Intra-articular corticosteroid injections, if excessive, can accelerate joint deterioration.
• Non-acetylate salicylates - salsalates, e.g., magnesium salicylate, choline salicylate, provide anti-inflammatory action without significant antiplatelet effects; also have less GI toxicity
• Capsaicin cream - local application relieves pain - most effective in small joints of the hand. May cause a local burning.

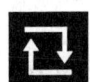
FOLLOWUP

PATIENT MONITORING
• Follow range of motion and functional status at regular intervals
• Watch for GI blood loss and follow cardiac, renal and mental status in older patients on NSAID's or ASA
• Periodic CBC, renal function tests, stool for occult blood

PREVENTION/AVOIDANCE Followup of secondary causes

POSSIBLE COMPLICATIONS
• Decompensated CHF, GI bleeding, decreased renal function on NSAID's or ASA
• Hypoglycemic reactions in diabetic patients taking aspirin (rare)
• Infection or accelerated cartilage loss with intra-articular corticosteroids

EXPECTED COURSE/PROGNOSIS
• Tends to be progressive
• Early in course, pain relieved by rest; later, pain may occur at rest and at night
• Joint effusions may occur, especially in knees
• Joint enlargement occurs later in course due to bony enlargement
• Osteophyte (spur) formation, especially at joint margins, as disease progresses
• Advanced stage with full thickness loss of cartilage down to bone

MISCELLANEOUS

ASSOCIATED CONDITIONS N/A

AGE-RELATED FACTORS
Pediatric: N/A
Geriatric:
• Prevalence increases with age
• Almost universal over 65 (by x-ray but not clinically)
Others: N/A

PREGNANCY ASA and NSAID's with some risk to fetus during pregnancy; compatible with breast feeding

SYNONYMS
• Osteoarthrosis
• Degenerative joint disease

ICD-9-CM 715.9 Osteoarthritis, unspecified whether generalized or localized

SEE ALSO N/A

OTHER NOTES Surgery may be indicated in advanced disease (for example joint replacement, fusion)

ABBREVIATIONS N/A

REFERENCES
• Mankin HJ, Brandt KD: Pathogenesis of osteoarthritis, In: Kelly WN, Harris ED, Ruddy S, Sledge CB, eds. Textbook of Rheumatology, 5th Ed, Philadelphia, W.B. Saunders Co., 1997,:1369-1382
• Solomon L: Clinical Features of Osteoarthritis. In: Kelly AN, Harris ED, Ruddy S, Sledge CB, eds: Textbook of Rheumatology, 5th Ed, Philadelphia, W.B. Saunders Co, 1997:1383-1393
• Brandt KD: Management of Osteoarthritis. In: Kelly WN, Harris ED, Ruddy S, Sledge CB, eds: Textbook of Rheurnatology, 5th Ed. Philadelphia, W.B, Saunders Co., 1997:1394-1403
• Golden BD, Abramson SB: Selective Cyclooxygenase-2 inhibitors. Rheumatic Dis Clin NA 1999;25(2):359-378
• Hochberg MC, Altman RD, Brandt KD: Guidelines for the medical management of osteoarthritis. Part 1. Osteoarthritis of the hip. Arthritis Rheum 1995;38:1535-1540
Illustrations: N/A
Internet references: http://www.5mcc.com

Author(s)
John P. Geyman, MD
Bruce C. Gilliland, MD

Arthritis, psoriatic

BASICS

DESCRIPTION Arthritis associated with psoriasis. Serologic tests for the rheumatoid factor are usually negative. Patients exhibit sausage-shaped digits and characteristic radiologic changes. Psoriatic arthropathy occurs in about 5% of individuals with psoriasis, especially those with psoriatic nail disease. There are several forms that have been described although the separation into these forms is not distinct. They are called by different descriptive terms by various authors.
• Forms of psoriatic arthropathy:
◊ Psoriatic nail disease and distal interphalangeal involvement (classic psoriatic arthritis). Characteristics - nail pitting, transverse depressions, subungual hyperkeratosis, distal interphalangeal arthritis.
◊ Arthritis mutilans - a destructive, resorptive arthropathy. Produces the so-called opera-glass hand.
◊ Symmetric polyarthropathy resembling rheumatoid arthritis - may be indistinguishable from RA and may represent coincidental rheumatoid arthritis in a patient who has psoriasis
◊ Asymmetric oligoarthropathy - little relationship between joint and skin activity; joints involved may be both large and small
◊ Psoriatic spondylitis - asymmetrical spondylitis and sacroiliitis
System(s) affected: Musculoskeletal, Skin/Exocrine
Genetics: HLA-B27 usually present in patients with spondylitis-type psoriatic arthropathy. Psoriasis itself is associated with HLA-B13, HLA-Bw17, HLA-Cw6, HLABw38, HLA-DR4 and HLA-DR7.
Incidence/Prevalence in USA: Uncommon, approximately 5% of individuals have psoriatic skin disease
Predominant age: Onset age 30-35
Predominant sex: Female > Male (slightly)

SIGNS AND SYMPTOMS
• Joint swelling, tenderness, warmth, restricted movement
• Distribution of arthritis dependent upon form of psoriatic arthritis
• Nail changes - pitting, transverse ridging, onycholysis, keratosis, yellowing and destruction of the entire nail
• Fever
• Malaise
• Psoriasis - variable severity
• Other symptoms applying characteristically to the several types of psoriatic arthropathy. See description.

CAUSES
• Unknown
• Probably genetically related

RISK FACTORS
• Psoriasis
• Positive family history

DIAGNOSIS

DIFFERENTIAL DIAGNOSIS
• Psoriasis
• Seropositive inflammatory polyarthritis
• Rheumatoid arthritis
• Osteoarthritis
• Gout
• Reiter's syndrome
• Ankylosing spondylitis

LABORATORY
• Serum rheumatoid factor - negative
• Elevated erythrocyte sedimentation rate
• Elevated uric acid
• Anemia
• HLA B27 - spondylitis
Drugs that may alter lab results: N/A
Disorders that may alter lab results: N/A

PATHOLOGICAL FINDINGS Synovitis (resembling rheumatoid arthritis)

SPECIAL TESTS N/A

IMAGING
• X-ray
◊ Gross destructive changes of isolated small joints
◊ Peripheral arthritis mutilans
◊ Erosions, ankylosis
◊ Extensive bone resorption to cause "opera-glass hand"
◊ Fluffy periostitis
◊ Atypical spondylitis with syndesmophyte formation
◊ Acro osteolysis, "pencil-in-cup" appearance
◊ Asymmetric sacroiliitis
◊ Absence of osteoporosis
• MRI is sensitive in detecting sacroiliitis, joint synovitis, erosions and enthesitis

DIAGNOSTIC PROCEDURES N/A

TREATMENT

APPROPRIATE HEALTH CARE
Outpatient

GENERAL MEASURES
• Immobilizing splints
• Isometric exercises and swimming later
• Paraffin baths or other heat therapy
• Protect affected joints
• Regular, moderate exposure to sun
• Psoriatic skin care

SURGICAL MEASURES N/A

ACTIVITY Encourage exercise (particularly swimming) to maintain strength and flexibility

DIET No special diet

PATIENT EDUCATION
• Stress non-contagious
• For a listing of sources for patient education materials favorably reviewed on this topic, physicians may contact: American Academy of Family Physicians Foundation, P.O. Box 8418, Kansas City, MO 64114, (800)274-2237, ext. 4400
• Arthritis Foundation, 1314 Spring Street N.W., Atlanta, GA 30309, (404)872-7100

MEDICATIONS

DRUG(S) OF CHOICE
• Several options available depending on involvement of skin and joints:
◊ Nonsteroidal anti-inflammatory drugs in usual doses. There is no evidence for superiority of any one NSAID in psoriatic arthritis.
◊ Local corticosteroid injection
◊ Low-dose systemic steroids, if necessary
◊ Low dose systemic corticosteroid may destabilize psoriasis
◊ Topical therapy including steroids for skin
◊ PUVA therapy may be helpful for skin lesions
• Others sometimes useful:
◊ Methotrexate, used only under specific guidelines and by someone experienced with its use.
◊ Gold salts
◊ Antimalarials (controversial)
◊ Sulfasalazine
◊ Immunosuppressives in resistant cases
◊ Cyclosporine in resistant cases
◊ Combination of MTX and Cyclosporin-A or sulfasalazine under the guidance of a rheumatologist
Contraindications:
• Antimalarials can provoke exfoliative dermatitis
• NSAID's may flare psoriasis
• Methotrexate contraindicated in HIV positive patients
Precautions: Phenylbutazone may cause bone marrow depression. NSAID's and ASA may cause gastritis and renal failure. Refer to manufacturer's literature.
Significant possible interactions: NSAID's may impair methotrexate excretion and cause methotrexate toxicity. Refer to manufacturer's literature.

ALTERNATIVE DRUGS   Etretinate
0.5-1.0 mg/kg/day in 2 divided doses (severe side effects, avoid during pregnancy since it is highly teratogenic) may be helpful for psoriasis

FOLLOWUP

PATIENT MONITORING   Frequent for
medication adjustment and encouragement

PREVENTION/AVOIDANCE   N/A

POSSIBLE COMPLICATIONS
• Chronicity
• Severe deforming arthritis (arthritis mutilans)
• Spondylitic form of arthritis with sacroiliitis and spinal involvement

EXPECTED COURSE/PROGNOSIS
• Course - acute, intermittent
• More favorable than rheumatoid arthritis (except for arthritis mutilans)
• Treatment of skin lesions can sometime improve arthritic symptoms
• Joint surgery is at least as successful as for rheumatoid arthritis; (RA) infectious complications are more common than RA

MISCELLANEOUS

ASSOCIATED CONDITIONS   Psoriasis

AGE-RELATED FACTORS
Pediatric: Not commonly seen in this age group
Geriatric: Arthritic symptoms worse
Others: N/A

PREGNANCY   N/A

SYNONYMS   Psoriasis, arthropathic

ICD-9-CM   696.0 Psoriatic arthropathy

SEE ALSO   N/A

OTHER NOTES
Pathogenesis: In contrast to the amiliorating affect of AIDS (HIV infection) on rheumatoid arthritis, AIDS is associated with more aggressive joint disease in psoriatic arthritis. Theoretically, then, CD4 cells, which seem to "drive" rheumatoid arthritis, are not involved in the pathogenesis of psoriatic arthritis.

ABBREVIATIONS   N/A

REFERENCES
• Kelley WN, Harris ED, Ruddy S, et al: Textbook of Rheumatology. 5th Ed. Philadelphia, W.B. Saunders, 1997
• Koopman WJ, eds: Arthritis and Allied Disorders. 13th Ed. Philadelphia, Lea & Febiger, 1997
• Salvarini, et al: Psoriatic arthritis. Curr Opin in Rheumatol 1998;10(4):299-305
• Kippel JH, Dippe PA, eds: Rheumatology. St. Louis, Mosby, 1994
Illustrations: N/A
Internet references: http://www.5mcc.com

Author(s)
Michael Tutt

Arthritis, rheumatoid (RA)

BASICS

DESCRIPTION A chronic systemic inflammatory disease of unknown etiology with a predilection for joint involvement. Articular inflammation may be remitting, but if continued usually results in joint damage and disability. Certain extra-articular manifestations are characteristic, including rheumatoid nodules, arteritis, neuropathy, scleritis, pericarditis, and splenomegaly.
System(s) affected: Musculoskeletal, Hemic/Lymphatic/Immunologic, Pulmonary, Cardiovascular, Nervous
Genetics: Seropositive RA aggregates in families. Genetic factors versus their interaction with environmental facilitators is unclear. HLA-DR4 is found in 70% of Caucasian seropositive patients compared to 25% of controls. Increased relative risk of 4-5 times for the DR4 positive person, although a minority are affected. African Americans tend not to exhibit this predilection.
Incidence/Prevalence in USA:
• 0.3-1.5%; women affected twice as often, but men and women have equal prevalence of erosive disease
• Prevalence in Native Americans is 3.5-5.3%
Predominant age: Third to sixth decades
Predominant sex:
• Female > Male (overall incidence and prevalence of articular manifestations)
• Male > Female (exhibit more systemic disease)

SIGNS AND SYMPTOMS
• Joints: most often involved are wrists, knees, elbows, shoulders, ankles, metatarsal-phalangeal and subtalar joints with swelling, joint heat, joint deformity, morning stiffness, pain on passive motion. Joint destruction occurs early; 70% show radiologic signs of damage within 3 years of onset.
• Systemic: fatigue, depression, malaise, anorexia, rheumatoid nodules, lymphadenopathy, splenomegaly, ocular disease, entrapment neuropathies
• Patients experience symptoms an average of 36 weeks before diagnosis

CAUSES Antibodies complexed with complement in the joint space result in inflammation.

RISK FACTORS
• HLA-DR4
• Family history
• Native American ethnicity
• Female gender, age 20-50 years

DIAGNOSIS

DIFFERENTIAL DIAGNOSIS
Sjögren's syndrome, sarcoidosis, poly-myositis, erosive osteoarthritis, seronegative polyarthritis, vasculitis, gout, pseudogout, inflammatory bowel disease, hypersensitivity reactions, Reiter's syndrome, Behçet's syndrome, psoriatic arthritis, systemic lupus erythematosus, Lyme disease, scleroderma, chronic infection, occult malignancy. Early clinical involvement of wrists speaks against osteoarthritis.

LABORATORY
• Hematocrit - mild anemia common
• ESR: usually elevated; helpful in following disease activity
• Rheumatoid factor: > 1:80 in 70-80% of patients with RA
  ◊ 20% will remain negative despite other signs of rheumatoid arthritis.
  ◊ RF tests are assays for IgM Ab
  ◊ RF is a poor screening tool with a positive predictive value (PPV) of only 20% in asymptomatic persons. In patients with rheumatologic symptoms, it's PPV = 80%.
  ◊ It is not useful to monitor the course of the illness
• ANA: present in 20-30%.
• Electrolytes, Cr, liver function, UA to assess organ comorbid states
• Synovial fluid
  ◊ Yellowish-white, turbid, poor viscosity
  ◊ "Mucin clot" poor due to degradation of hyaluric acid by lysosomal enzymes
  ◊ WBC increased (3500-50,000)
  ◊ CH50 is lower than serum
  ◊ Protein: approximately 4.2 g/dL (42 g/L)
  ◊ Serum-synovial glucose difference ≥ 30 mg/dL (≥ 1.67 mmol/L)
Drugs that may alter lab results: Prior treatment with immunosuppressives may "normalize" results
Disorders that may alter lab results: Numerous conditions can give positive RF results, including Sjögrens, mixed cryoglobulinemia, parasitic infections (eg, malaria), liver disease, endocarditis, and acute viral infections (eg, mononucleosis, influenza, rubella).

PATHOLOGICAL FINDINGS
• Synovial infiltration by lymphocytes, plasma cells, and macrophages
• Hypertrophy and hyperplasia of synovial lining cells
• Local production of "self-associating" IgG

SPECIAL TESTS None; biopsy of nodules is not indicated in diagnosis

IMAGING
• X-rays rarely necessary in diagnosis, but useful in following the progression of disease
• Arthrography: to define joint abnormalities or injury to a supporting structure
• Bone scan: if aseptic necrosis is suspected
• CT/MRI: useful in specific situations such as cervical spine symptoms

DIAGNOSTIC PROCEDURES
• American College of Rheumatology criteria: (5 of the 7 must be present. Numbers 1-4 must be continuous > 6 weeks.)
1. Morning stiffness > 1 hour's duration
2. Arthritis of at least three joint groups with soft tissue swelling or fluid
3. Swelling involving at least one of the following joint groups: proximal interphalangeal, metacarpophalangeal, or wrists
4. Symmetrical joint swelling
5. Subcutaneous nodules
6. Positive rheumatoid factor test
7. Radiographic changes consistent with RA

TREATMENT

APPROPRIATE HEALTH CARE
Primarily outpatient. Key elements are ongoing evaluation of disease activity and extent of synovitis, structural damage, and psycho/social functional status.

GENERAL MEASURES
• Intervene before joint damage occurs
• Emphasis on exercise and mobility; reduction of joint stress; general health care; education

SURGICAL MEASURES Possibly surgery for severe mechanical symptoms (consider long-term outcomes, risk/benefits, and cumulative effects of medical therapies on surgical decisions)

ACTIVITY
• Encourage full activity, but avoid heavy work and vigorous exercise during active phases due to risk of intensifying joint inflammation
• Hydrotherapy or water exercise is effective
• Exercise programs focusing on restoration of function. Isometric exercise is modality of choice in patients with active synovitis

DIET No special diet. Ingestion of certain foods may increase disease activity. Diets rich in omega-3 fatty acids (25 gm/day) may allow some patients to reduce NSAIDs dose.

PATIENT EDUCATION American Rheumatism Association (800)282-7023; Arthritis Foundation, 404-872-7100; www.arthritis.org

MEDICATIONS

DRUG(S) OF CHOICE
• "Pyramid of therapy" (beginning with anti-inflammatories and moving to disease modifying regimens) controversial. Stanford "rescue" - rapid escalation, selective combination, (followed by) unproven or experimental therapies involve NSAID and chloroquine or minocycline early on, then sulfasalazine. Early addition of MTX in moderate disease.
• Don't delay disease modifying agents (DMARDs) beyond 2 months, if patient has ongoing joint pain/morning stiffness, active synovitis, or persistent increase in ESR/CRP despite appropriate dose NSAIDs.

- Early disease or acute/chronic inflammation
  ◊ Aspirin or other NSAID
  ◊ Newer NSAIDs include the COX-2 inhibitors - celecoxib (Celebrex) and rofecoxib (Vioxx). These have the advantages of lessened risk of GI, renal and platelet injury; but are not necessarily more efficacious in anti-inflammatory effects.
- Prednisone 5-15 mg q day: Severe disease or to minimize disease activity while awaiting DMARDs to act, decrease activity for a short period of time, or control active disease when NSAIDs/DMARDs have failed. It is reasonable to try NSAIDs of different classes.
- Persistent disease activity (chronic synovitis, AM stiffness, increased ESR/CRP, extra-articular disease) - add DMARDs; HCQ or SSZ often chosen first. Once a second line agent's therapeutic level is reached, prednisone should be decreased slowly. Should only be used for short periods. Low dose maintenance therapy (eg, 5 mg qod) still controversial.
  ◊ Intraarticular steroid injections - use judiciously and as rarely as possible (due to long term effects)
  ◊ Antimalarials: hydroxychloroquine (HCQ, Plaquenil) 400 mg q hs for 2-3 months, then 200 mg/hs; 6 month trial usual
  ◊ Auranofin 6-10 mg/d po; reevaluate in 6 months or 1 gram total. Injectable gold: weekly for 22 weeks, then q 2-4 weeks
  ◊ Sulfasalazine (SSZ): 500 mg/d, increase to 2 g/d over one month; max: 2-3 g/day; 6 month trial
  ◊ Penicillamine (d-penicillamine): 250 mg/d, increasing slowly to 750-1000 mg/day; 9 month trial with 8-12 weeks at maximum dosage
  ◊ Azathioprine
  ◊ Methotrexate: 5-15 mg/wk po; 3-6 month trial - for steroid dependent disease or after other measures unsuccessful. MTX is the DMARD with most predictable benefit. Role in earlier disease debated; many recommend MTX in early stage disease
  ◊ Newer agents - leflunomide (Arava) inhibits a key enzyme needed for pyrimidine synthesis. Precise role in RA still unclear. 20 mg daily was comparable to sulfasalazine at 2 gm daily.

Contraindications: N/A

Precautions:
- Consider 1) misoprostol for patients on NSAIDs chronically, 2) folic acid (1-2 mg/d) for patients on MTX
- Avoid NSAID combinations

Significant possible interactions:
- NSAIDs:
  ◊ Antacids: reduce absorption
  ◊ Anticoagulants: increase bleeding risk
  ◊ Oral hypoglycemic agents (OHA): Aspirin, phenylbutazone, and oxyphenbutazone may potentiate the activity of OHA's; others currently available do not
  ◊ Antihypertensive/diuretics: NSAID's may attenuate the effect of diuretics, beta-blockers, hydralazine, prazosin, and ACE inhibitors
  ◊ Lithium: Elevation of plasma lithium levels may occur, especially with indomethacin and diclofenac
  ◊ Methotrexate: Salicylate inhibits the renal clearance of methotrexate, and toxic levels may occur
  ◊ Phenytoin: Phenylbutazone inhibits metabolism of phenytoin. Salicylates

increase the concentration of phenytoin.
  ◊ Probenecid: Inhibits renal clearance of several NSAID's

ALTERNATIVE DRUGS Combinations of methotrexate and cyclosporine, gold salts and prednisone, and methotrexate and hydroxychloroquine all may be useful for resistant disease. Use of methotrexate and either gold or SSZ is not currently supported by clinical trials.

FOLLOWUP

PATIENT MONITORING
- Discuss prognosis, treatment options (time and cost), adverse effects, lab and PE monitoring , patient preferences
- Duration of morning stiffness
- Time of onset of fatigue
- NSAID need/day
- Grip strength
- Number of joints that are tender or painful on passive range-of-motion
- Degree of swelling of affected joints
- Functional status assessment
- Progress of established disease on x-ray
- ESR - often best test of disease activity
- Other lab testing, depend on medications and disease progression

PREVENTION/AVOIDANCE
- Possible association of oral contraceptive use with decreased risk of RA

POSSIBLE COMPLICATIONS
- Erosive arthritis and joint destruction
- Skin vasculitis
- Pericarditis
- Intracardiac rheumatoid nodules causing valvular, conduction abnormalities
- Pleural, subpleural disease; interstitial fibrosis
- Mononeuritis multiplex, median nerve entrapment
- Sjögren's syndrome, scleral rheumatoid nodules
- Felty's syndrome

EXPECTED COURSE/PROGNOSIS
- Progressive decline in function has been the usual course; this may be altered significantly with proper medical, surgical, and physiotherapeutic interventions.
- Poor prognosis: early age at onset, high RF titer, high ESR, swelling of > 20 joints, extra-articular disease
- Complete remission defined as absence of: 1) symptoms of active inflammatory joint pain. 2) morning stiffness, 3) fatigue, 4) synovitis on physical exam, 5) progression of x-ray damage, 6) elevation of ESR

MISCELLANEOUS

ASSOCIATED CONDITIONS Sjögren's; Felty's

AGE-RELATED FACTORS
Pediatric: See Juvenile RA
Geriatric:
- Onset uncommon (20% of persons over age 60 with the disease)
- Despite improved treatment, expect increased contribution/interaction of other age-related comorbidities. Pericarditis, septic arthritis, Sjögren's syndrome more common.
- Less tolerance to medications; increased incidence of hydroxychloroquine- associated-maculopathy, D-penicillamine rash, and sulfasalazine induced nausea and vomiting. Toxicity from parenteral gold not age-related.
Others: N/A

PREGNANCY
- Use effective contraception when DMARDs given. Modify regimen if pregnancy or breast-feeding desired.
- Labor/delivery pose no serious problems, unless severe mechanical joint disease
- > 75% of RA patients improve during pregnancy (in spite of discontinuing medications, e.g., gold and methotrexate), but relapse in 6 months. Occasionally, first episodes occur during pregnancy.
- Fetal abnormalities not increased. Presence of Sjögren's syndrome and anti-Ro antibody associated (especially in mother's with lupus) with congenital complete heart block.

SYNONYMS N/A

ICD-9-CM
714.0 Rheumatoid arthritis
714.1 Felty's syndrome

SEE ALSO
- Arthritis, juvenile rheumatoid (JRA)
- Arthritis, osteo
- Sjögren's syndrome

OTHER NOTES
- Median life expectancy shortened 7 years in males, 3 years in females over 25 years. 50% of patients with RA cannot function in primary job within 10 years of onset
- Functional ability - As a restriction of normal activities
  ◊ Class I: None
  ◊ Class II: Moderate
  ◊ Class III: Marked restriction, inability to perform most of the patient's usual occupation or self-care
  ◊ Class IV: Incapacitation or confinement to a bed or wheelchair
- Functional ability tasks (Pincus, et al): To dress self; To get in and out of bed; To eat and drink with utensils; To walk outside on flat ground; To wash and dry entire body; To bend down & pick up clothing from floor; To turn regular faucets on and off; To get in and out of car

ABBREVIATIONS N/A

REFERENCES
5 additional references available at web site
Internet references: http://www.5mcc.com
Illustrations: 5 available on CD-ROM

Author(s)
Kurt Elward, MD, MPH

Artificial insemination

BASICS

DESCRIPTION   Artificial insemination is the placement of washed sperm into the female reproductive tract. Placement can be intracervical, intrauterine, intraperitoneal, or intrafollicular. Most common is intrauterine insemination (IUI). Sperm are washed to reduce antigenicity. Insemination can be with partner's sperm or therapeutic insemination with donor sperm (TID).
System(s) affected: Reproductive, Endocrine/Metabolic
Genetics: N/A
Incidence/Prevalence in USA: Varies, depending on etiology of infertility, i.e., male factor is responsible for approximately 35% of cases of infertility, and a cervical factor is responsible for approximately 10% of cases
Predominant age: Reproductive age women (18-45 years of age)
Predominant sex: Female only

SIGNS AND SYMPTOMS   Inability to conceive

CAUSES
• Indications for IUI include:
  ◊ Male factor infertility
   - Oligospermia
   - Asthenospermia
   - Hypospadias
   - Retrograde ejaculation
   - Coital dysfunction
  ◊ Female factors
   - Cervical mucous abnormalities
   - Poor postcoital test
  ◊ Unexplained infertility

RISK FACTORS
• Male factor 35%
• Cervical factor 10%

DIAGNOSIS

DIFFERENTIAL DIAGNOSIS
• Primary female cervical factor?
• Primary male factor?

LABORATORY
• Semen analysis
• Postcoital test
• Sperm antibody testing
Drugs that may alter lab results:
Clomiphene citrate (Clomid)
Disorders that may alter lab results:
• Abnormal pH of vagina or cervical mucus
• Bacterial infection semen/mucus

PATHOLOGICAL FINDINGS
• Chronic cervicitis
• Chronic prostatitis

SPECIAL TESTS
• Zona free hamster sperm penetration assay
• Bovine cervical mucus sperm penetration test

IMAGING   Hysterosalpingogram

DIAGNOSTIC PROCEDURES   Postcoital test

TREATMENT

APPROPRIATE HEALTH CARE
Outpatient

GENERAL MEASURES
• Intrauterine insemination should be closely timed with ovulation. Ovulation prediction kits detect the luteinizing hormone (LH) surge which precedes ovulation by 12-36 hours. Intrauterine insemination is performed the day of or the day after the LH surge.
• The volume of inseminate that can be transferred into the uterus is 0.25 to 0.5 mL. Small amounts are used to avoid cramping and flushing the oocyte out of the tube. The volume is also limited by space within the uterus.
• Intrauterine insemination is an office procedure. First, the position of the uterus is determined. A speculum is placed in the vagina and the cervix is visualized. The sample of washed sperm is placed into the uppermost portion of the uterine cavity using an insemination catheter with a disposable tuberculin syringe. Occasionally a tenaculum is needed on the anterior lip of the cervix to straighten the endocervical canal. Cervical dilatation or paracervical block is rarely required. The sample is injected slowly over 30-60 seconds.

SURGICAL MEASURES   N/A

ACTIVITY   No restrictions

DIET   No special diet

PATIENT EDUCATION   No vaginal lubricants or douching

MEDICATIONS

DRUG(S) OF CHOICE
• Clomiphene citrate (Clomid) or human menopausal gonadotropins - menotropins (Pergonal) may be used for controlled ovarian hyperstimulation and ovulation may be initiated by the administration of human chorionic gonadotropin (HCG), an LH-like molecule. Intrauterine insemination is performed 24-36 hours after HCG administration. Clomid predisposes to poor cervical mucus, which can adversely alter sperm/mucus interaction.
• Dosages:
◊ Clomiphene: 50 mg daily x 5 days to induce ovulation
◊ Menotropins (Pergonal): 75 IU FSH/75 IU LH IM daily x 12 days; then a single dose of chorionic gonadotropin 10,000 IU/day after last dose of menotropins

Contraindications:
• Uncontrolled thyroid and adrenal dysfunction
• An intracranial lesion
• High follicle-stimulating hormone (FSH) level indicating primary ovarian failure
• Abnormal bleeding of undetermined etiology
• Ovarian cysts of unknown origin
• Hypersensitivity
• Pregnancy

Precautions:
• Multiple births - Clomid 8%, Pergonal 25%
• Severe ovarian hyperstimulation (ascites, pleural effusion, dehydration, electrolyte imbalance, pain)
• Ovarian torsion

Significant possible interactions: N/A

ALTERNATIVE DRUGS
Estrogen in follicular phase of cycle to improve mucus

FOLLOWUP

PATIENT MONITORING
• Those patients on Clomid require a bimanual exam on a monthly basis
• Patients on Pergonal require serum estradiol measurements and pelvic sonography to monitor ovarian response

PREVENTION/AVOIDANCE   N/A

POSSIBLE COMPLICATIONS
• Uterine cramping
• Mild vasomotor symptoms
• Infection
• Theoretical but unproven risk is development of antisperm antibodies in response to increase exposure of the immune system to sperm antigens

EXPECTED COURSE/PROGNOSIS
• Virtually all pregnancies that result, occur within the first six treatment cycles. A 6 month treatment interval usually represents an adequate therapeutic trial.
• There is a documented increase in efficacy with combination of intrauterine insemination and controlled ovarian hyperstimulation (Pergonal)
• The highest success rates are seen with idiopathic or cervical factor problems
• The poorest outcome is with male factor
• Monthly fecundities of 14% have occurred with therapeutic inseminations utilizing fresh semen

MISCELLANEOUS

ASSOCIATED CONDITIONS   Causes of infertility

AGE-RELATED FACTORS
Pediatric: N/A
Geriatric: N/A
Others:
• Fecundity is inversely related to maternal age
• Contraindications to artificial insemination
◊ Infection (acute cervicitis, endometritis, acute prostatitis, epididymitis, salpingo-oophoritis)
◊ Pregnancy
◊ Unexplained uterine bleeding

PREGNANCY   N/A

SYNONYMS
• Therapeutic insemination
• Intrauterine insemination

ICD-9-CM
628.4 Female infertility of cervical or vaginal origin

SEE ALSO   N/A

OTHER NOTES   For donor insemination, only frozen semen is used and only after a 6 month period of "quarantine" to minimize danger of transmission of HIV

ABBREVIATIONS
LH = luteinizing hormone
HCG = human chorionic gonadotropin

REFERENCES
• Yen SSC, Jaffe RB, eds: Reproductive Endocrinology. 3rd Ed. Philadelphia, W.B. Saunders Co., 1991
• Berek JS, ed: Novak's Gynecology. 12th Ed. Williams & Wilkins, Baltimore, 1996
• Khamsi F, Lacanna I. Endman M, Wong J: Recent advances in assisted reproductive technologies. Endocrine 1998;9(1):15-25
Illustrations: N/A
Internet references: http://www.5mcc.com

Author(s)
Barbara A. Majeroni, MD

Asbestosis

BASICS

DESCRIPTION A chronic non-malignant lung disease caused by inhalation of asbestos, a hazardous dust found in a variety of work places. This disease persists in spite of substantial knowledge about its cause, and effective means of prevention. The disease typically occurs 10-15 years after initial exposure.
Asbestosis is a fibrotic interstitial lung disease caused by a cascade of responses to inhaled asbestos fibers. Pleural plaques and mesotheliomas can develop. It increases risk of tuberculosis and lung cancer in cigarette smokers.
System(s) affected: Pulmonary
Genetics: No known genetic pattern
Incidence/Prevalence in USA: There is no uniform surveillance or reporting of asbestosis. In the USA, less than 10 cases per 100,000 people are diagnosed annually; this probably represents an underestimate. 876 deaths reported from 1979 to 1992. Number of cases rising steadily. More than a million people have been exposed to significant levels of asbestos.
Predominant age: Middle age (40-75 years)
Predominant sex: Male > Female, due to exposure pattern

SIGNS AND SYMPTOMS
• No unique signs or symptoms
• Insidious onset
• Cough, dry or with sputum production
• Exercise intolerance
• Sexual dysfunction may be associated
• Basilar crackles
• Wheeze with forced exhalation
• Digital clubbing
• Cyanosis
• Right sided heart failure

CAUSES
• Diversity of settings for hazardous exposure
• Asbestos used in more than 3000 commercial products - production peaked in mid-1970s
• Risk to miners and millers of asbestos
• More people at risk in construction sites with unprotected use of asbestos, commonly for insulation
• Maintenance and removal of asbestos-containing material creates high levels
• Office workers, teachers, and students in buildings with asbestos in place have exposure orders of magnitude below those of construction workers, although societal concern has been high - actual health risk not considered significant

RISK FACTORS
• Cigarette smoking
• Asbestos maintenance and removal workers
• Construction workers
• Asbestos miners and millers
• Shipbuilders
• Textile workers
• Railroad workers

DIAGNOSIS

DIFFERENTIAL DIAGNOSIS Other pneumoconioses (siderosis, stannosis (due to inhalation of tin oxide), baritosis, coal worker's pneumoconiosis, silicosis, talcosis, shaver's disease)

LABORATORY
• Hypoxemia
• Bronchoalveolar lavage or biopsy - generally unnecessary in the clinical setting - research tools
Drugs that may alter lab results: N/A
Disorders that may alter lab results: N/A

PATHOLOGICAL FINDINGS
• Lung:
  ◊ Parietal pleural thickening
  ◊ Parietal pleural calcification
  ◊ Interstitial inflammation
  ◊ Interstitial fibrosis
  ◊ Alveolar wall fibrosis

SPECIAL TESTS
• Pulmonary function test:
  ◊ Not diagnostically specific
  ◊ Useful for following level of impairment
  ◊ Restrictive, mixed, or obstructive pattern
  ◊ Reduction in diffusing capacity to carbon monoxide can occur early, even when chest x-ray is normal

IMAGING
• Chest x-ray
  ◊ Primary diagnostic modality and screening tool - approximately 80% sensitive
  ◊ Diagnosis based on: credible history of exposure, delay from exposure to detection, and typical radiographic findings
  ◊ Irregular, linear opacities - start in bases at periphery, and spread upwards
  ◊ Circumscribed pleural plaques
  ◊ Rounded atelectasis (pseudotumor)
  ◊ Pleural thickening
  ◊ Classification scheme available through International Labour Office
• High resolution CT shows promise

DIAGNOSTIC PROCEDURES
Bronchoscopy - research tool

TREATMENT

APPROPRIATE HEALTH CARE
Outpatient

GENERAL MEASURES
• No effective treatment to reverse the course
• Early detection essential
• Approach directed at elimination of progression, amelioration of symptoms, reduction of risk of associated disorders
• Withdrawal from exposure
  ◊ Workers with no symptoms, and only CXR changes may make an informed choice to continue employment, with maximum environmental and personal protection
• Pneumococcal and influenza vaccines
• Chest physiotherapy
• Nutritional advice
• Home oxygen
• Graded exercise
• Stop smoking

SURGICAL MEASURES
• Whole lung lavage to remove retained dust is being investigated
• Lung transplantation for severe advanced cases

ACTIVITY Graded exercise

DIET High calorie, high protein with advanced disease

PATIENT EDUCATION Printed patient information available from: Asbestos Victims of America, P.O. Box 559, Capitola, CA 95010, (408)476-3646 or American Lung Association, 1740 Broadway, New York, NY 10019, (212)315-8700

MEDICATIONS

DRUG(S) OF CHOICE
• No specific pharmacologic treatment
• Oxygen
• Bronchodilators for pulmonary toilet
Contraindications: N/A
Precautions: N/A
Significant possible interactions: N/A

ALTERNATIVE DRUGS
• Antibiotics for respiratory infections
• Diuretics
• Treatment of congestive heart failure

FOLLOWUP

PATIENT MONITORING
• Chest x-rays
• Occasional pulmonary function tests
• Treat infections promptly

PREVENTION/AVOIDANCE
• Primary responsibility of employers
• Exposure control - substitution of safer material or adoption of control technologies
• Monitor workplace exposure
• During high exposure periods such as building repair - use of fit-tested personal respirators for workers
• WHO recommendations for regular health screening of exposed workers
  ◊ Chest x-ray at baseline
  ◊ For workers with less than 10 years since first exposure: chest x-ray every 3-5 years
  ◊ Longer than 10 years: chest x-ray every 1-2 years
  ◊ Longer than 20 years: chest x-ray annually
  ◊ All workers: annual respiratory symptom questionnaire, physical exam, and spirometry (alternatively can be done on CXR schedule)
• Reporting of new cases to health authorities

POSSIBLE COMPLICATIONS
• Cancers of the mesothelium of the lung
  ◊ Unrelated to tobacco use
• Lung cancer
  ◊ Risk increased in smokers by asbestos workers
• Gastrointestinal cancer risk may be increased
• Exudative pleural effusion
  ◊ Resolve with residual pleural thickening
• Hyaline plaques on parietal pleura can create pseudotumors
• Increased risk of tuberculosis in smokers

EXPECTED COURSE/PROGNOSIS
• Severity depends on duration of exposure and on intensity of exposure
• Lung disease irreversible
• Further increased lung cancer risk with smoking
• Increased risk for mesotheliomas
• Increased risk for tuberculosis

MISCELLANEOUS

ASSOCIATED CONDITIONS N/A

AGE-RELATED FACTORS
Pediatric: N/A
Geriatric: More likely to have terminal respiratory illness
Others: N/A

PREGNANCY N/A

SYNONYMS
• Asbestos pneumoconiosis

ICD-9-CM
501 asbestosis

SEE ALSO N/A

OTHER NOTES N/A

ABBREVIATIONS
CT = computed tomography
CXR = chest x-ray
WHO = World Health Organization

REFERENCES
• LaDou J, ed: Occupational Medicine. Norwalk, CT, Appleton and Lange, 1990
• Rosenstock L, Cullen MR: Clinical Occupational Medicine. Philadelphia, W.B. Saunders Co., 1986
• Wagner GR: Asbestosis and silicosis. Lancet 1997;349:1311-1315
• International Labour Office. Guidelines for the use of ILO international classification of radiographs of pneumoconioses, 1980
Illustrations: N/A
Internet references: http://www.5mcc.com

Author(s)
Nancy N. Dambro, MD

Ascites

BASICS

DESCRIPTION Effusion and accumulation of fluid in the abdominal cavity. Ascites may occur in any condition that causes generalized edema. In children, nephrotic syndrome and malignancy are the predominant causes. In adults, cirrhosis, heart failure, nephrotic syndrome and chronic peritonitis are most common.
System(s) affected:
Hemic/Lymphatic/Immunologic, Cardiovascular, Gastrointestinal, Renal/Urologic
Genetics: N/A
Incidence/Prevalence in USA: Determined by etiology
Predominant age: Determined by etiology
Predominant sex: Determined by etiology

SIGNS AND SYMPTOMS
- Abdominal pain
- Abdominal discomfort
- Abdominal distention
- Tight clothing
- Shortness of breath
- Anorexia
- Nausea
- Early satiety
- Pyrosis; heartburn
- Flank pain
- Weight gain
- Orthopnea
- Abdominal fluid wave
- Shifting dullness
- Penile edema
- Scrotal edema
- Umbilical herniation
- Pleural effusion
- Pedal edema
- Rales
- Tachycardia

CAUSES
- Peritoneal infection and inflammation:
  ◊ Tuberculosis
  ◊ Fungus disease
  ◊ Chronic bacterial (foreign body, fistula)
  ◊ Ruptured viscus
  ◊ Granulomatous peritonitis
  ◊ Filariasis
- Metabolic diseases
  ◊ Hypothyroidism
  ◊ Cirrhosis
  ◊ Prehepatic and posthepatic portal hypertension
  ◊ Myxedema
  ◊ Nephrogenous
  ◊ Marked hypoalbuminemia (< 2 gm/dL)
- Heart and hepatic congestion
  ◊ Congestive heart failure
  ◊ Constrictive pericarditis
  ◊ Tricuspid stenosis or insufficiency
- Traumatic
  ◊ Pancreatic fistula
  ◊ Biliary fistula
  ◊ Lymphatic fistula (chylous)
  ◊ Hemoperitoneum (trauma, ectopic pregnancy, tumor)
- Malignancy
  ◊ Peritoneal seeding - ovarian, colon, pancreas and others
  ◊ Lymphatic obstruction - leukemia, lymphoma

RISK FACTORS Those associated with possible causes

DIAGNOSIS

DIFFERENTIAL DIAGNOSIS
- Obesity
- Air and liquid in distended intestine
- Fluid type:
- Transudate
  ◊ Likely causes include: Congestive heart failure, constrictive pericarditis, cirrhosis, nephrotic syndrome, hypoalbuminemia
- Exudate
  ◊ Likely causes include: Neoplasm, tuberculosis, pancreatitis, myxedema, biliary pathology, Budd-Chiari syndrome

LABORATORY
- Ascitic fluid (must be sampled in all new onset, or new to treatment cases; obtain in all:
  ◊ Culture through inoculating blood culture bottles
  ◊ Total cell count < 500 mm3
  ◊ PMN < 200 mm3
  ◊ Albumin in both serum and ascites calculate. Serum - ascites < 1.1 gm indicates inflammation or exudate, > 1.1 gm indicates portal hypertension. Protein > 2.0 gm (some would suggest 2.5 gm) indicates exudate.
- Of use in specific circumstances
  ◊ Lactate dehydrogenase < 200 IU/L
  ◊ Amylase
  ◊ Acid fast or fungal cultures
  ◊ Cytology
  ◊ Triglycerides (with a serum test)
- In blood
  ◊ Creatinine < 1.4 mg/dL
  ◊ Electrolytes
- In urine - sodium levels in a single sample:
  ◊ < 10 mEq/L diuretic response unlikely
  ◊ 10-70 mEq/L diuretic response likely
  ◊ > 70 mEq/L diuretics unnecessary
Drugs that may alter lab results: Refer to laboratory test reference
Disorders that may alter lab results: Refer to laboratory test reference

PATHOLOGICAL FINDINGS N/A

SPECIAL TESTS Laparoscopy

IMAGING Sonography or CT scan

DIAGNOSTIC PROCEDURES
- Diagnostic paracentesis

TREATMENT

APPROPRIATE HEALTH CARE May be outpatient or inpatient depending on physical condition

GENERAL MEASURES
- For all patients
  ◊ Some sodium restriction required, must be most severe when urine sodium is very low
  ◊ Select a sodium restriction that patient can attain at home; treatment usually required 3-6 months
  ◊ Water restriction only necessary if sodium < 130 mEq/L
  ◊ Any persistent elevation of creatinine to > 2.5 mg/dL should lead to decreasing diuretic doses and therapeutic paracentesis
  ◊ Daily record of weight to monitor gains and losses
- For ascites with edema
  ◊ Salt restriction and diuretics usually effective
  ◊ Maximum weight loss of 5 lbs/day
  ◊ Weekly electrolytes on serum during rapid weight loss
- For ascites without edema
  ◊ Dietary restrictions and diuretics as above
  ◊ Maximum loss of 2 lbs/day
- Refractory ascites - ascites that is increasing despite maximal doses of spironolactone (300 mg/day) and furosemide (160-200 mg/day) and dietary sodium restriction OR progressive rise in creatinine to >2.0.
  ◊ Start paracentesis up to 10 L/session. Replace albumin IV for all removals > 5L at rate of 10 gm albumin for each liter >5 L removed. Continue diuretics at half previous dose.

SURGICAL MEASURES In chronic, refractory cases, consider peritoneovenous shunt or transjugular intrahepatic portal shunt (TIPS)

ACTIVITY Bedrest of benefit in heart failure and when leg edema is prominent, otherwise of limited value.

DIET Sodium restriction needed for several months; regulate on a diet that can be followed outside hospital

PATIENT EDUCATION Diet restrictions

MEDICATIONS

DRUG(S) OF CHOICE
• Diuretics are needed in nearly all patients
◊ Spironolactone 100-300 mg/day orally in one dose best for cirrhotic ascites; furosemide 40-120 mg/day orally best for all other etiologies. May use together.
◊ Dose should be sufficient to obtain net sodium loss in urine
◊ Spot sodium in mEq/L x estimated urine output (1 L if no information) should equal estimated dietary sodium. Increase diuretics daily until this is attained. Measure serum electrolytes before each dose change.
Contraindications: See manufacturer's literature
Precautions: In hospital, or when rapid diuresis, observe creatinine weekly. NSAIDs may worsen or initiate oliguria or azotemia. Potassium supplements are usually required when diuresis exceeds 1 lb/day.
Precautions: Observe patients closely for signs of volume depletion, encephalopathy and renal insufficiency. NSAIDs may worsen or initiate oliguria or azotemia.
Significant possible interactions: Avoid concomitant use of potassium supplements if spironolactone is used alone

ALTERNATIVE DRUGS   Other diuretics

FOLLOWUP

PATIENT MONITORING
• For ascites - changes in body weight and urinary sodium to measure response to therapy
• Monitoring as needed for other therapies
• Measure electrolytes whenever there is appreciable diuresis (>1 lb. loss of weight/day) weekly and at least monthly. Also measure after one week following any change in dose or type of diuretic.

PREVENTION/AVOIDANCE   Dependent upon etiology

POSSIBLE COMPLICATIONS
• Overly aggressive diuresis may lead to hypokalemia, worsening hepatic encephalopathy, intravascular volume depletion, azotemia, and possibly to renal failure and death
• Sympathetic pleural effusion
• Other complications as may be associated with cause of ascites

EXPECTED COURSE/PROGNOSIS
• Ascites is rarely life-threatening. Conservative therapy usually successful.
• Prognosis variable depending upon the underlying cause

MISCELLANEOUS

ASSOCIATED CONDITIONS   Listed in Causes

AGE-RELATED FACTORS
Pediatric: N/A
Geriatric: N/A
Others: N/A

PREGNANCY   N/A

SYNONYMS   N/A

ICD-9-CM
789.5 ascites

SEE ALSO
• Congestive heart failure
• Nephrotic syndrome
• Cirrhosis of the liver

OTHER NOTES   N/A

ABBREVIATIONS
NSAID = Non-steroid anti-inflammatory drug

REFERENCES   Runyon BA: Management of adult patients with ascites caused by cirrhosis. Hepatology 1998, 27:264-72
Illustrations: N/A
Internet references: http://www.5mcc.com

Author(s)
Frank L. Iber, MD

Aspergillosis

BASICS

DESCRIPTION
Disease caused by a ubiquitous mold that primarily involves the lungs. Disease frequently lethal in neutropenic and bone marrow transplant (BMT) patients. Syndromes include:
- Allergic aspergillosis
  ◊ Extrinsic allergic alveolitis - hypersensitivity pneumonitis in individuals repeatedly exposed to the fungus.
  ◊ Allergic bronchopulmonary aspergillosis (ABPA) - pulmonary infiltrates, mucous plugging; secondary to allergic reaction to fungus.
- Aspergillomas: "fungus ball" saprophytic colonization within pre-existing pulmonary cavities.
- Invasive aspergillosis: most common and severe in BMT and neutropenic patients. Also occurs with increased frequency in other immunocompromised persons, such as those with solid organ transplant or high dose corticosteroids; commonly fatal.

System(s) affected: Pulmonary, Nervous, Gastrointestinal, Musculoskeletal, Cardiovascular
Genetics: No known genetic pattern
Incidence/Prevalence in USA: Rare
Predominant Age: None
Predominant Sex: Male = Female

SIGNS AND SYMPTOMS
- Allergic - cough, wheezing, constitutional symptoms, plug expectoration
- Aspergillomas - hemoptysis; manifestations of underlying disease
- Invasive - fever, cough, rales, rhonchi; toxicity; CNS signs; GI bleeding

CAUSES
Aspergillus species in decreasing order of frequency: fumigatus, flavus, niger

RISK FACTORS
- Allergic - exposure, asthma
- Aspergillomas - COPD, bronchiectasis, TB, malignancy
- Invasive - neutropenia, corticosteroid therapy

DIAGNOSIS

DIFFERENTIAL DIAGNOSIS
- Allergic - other causes of asthma and hypersensitivity pneumonitis.
- Aspergillomas - neoplasm, TB
- Invasive - bacterial pneumonia, pulmonary hemorrhage, drug toxicity, malignancy; mucor (sinuses).

LABORATORY
- ABPA - eosinophilia, immediate skin reactivity to aspergillus antigen, precipitating–serum antibodies to aspergillus, elevated serum IgE concentrations.
- Invasive - sputum culture, cultures of bronchoalveolar lavage or bronchial washings; biopsy is definitive; blood cultures almost never positive

Drugs that may alter lab results: None
Disorders that may alter lab results: None

PATHOLOGICAL FINDINGS
Necrotizing pneumonia, hemorrhagic infarcts, blood vessel invasion; branching septate hyphae if organism seen microscopically

SPECIAL TESTS
- ABPA - immediate skin reactivity to aspergillus antigen, precipitating serum antibodies (precipitins) against aspergillus antigens, elevated serum IgE concentrations, elevated serum IgE and IgG antibodies specific to A. Fumigatus.
- Invasive - none

IMAGING
Chest x-ray - fleeting infiltrates (ABPA), round intracavity mass (aspergillomas); nodular or patchy infiltrates progressing to diffuse consolidation and cavitation (invasive)

DIAGNOSTIC PROCEDURES
Bronchoscopy, bronchial washings, bronchoalveolar lavage or transthoracic needle aspiration may be helpful in isolating organism in invasive disease; open lung biopsy is diagnostic but often not possible in severely ill, ventilated patients.

TREATMENT

APPROPRIATE HEALTH CARE
- Allergic - outpatient usually
- Aspergillomas - outpatient usually
- Invasive - inpatient

GENERAL MEASURES
- Allergic
  ◊ Extrinsic allergic alveolitis - drug therapy, exposure avoidance.
  ◊ ABPA - corticosteroids
- Aspergillomas - individualized therapy ranging from no therapy to surgical resection of cavities in cases of severe hemoptysis; systemic antifungal therapy is seldom useful
- Invasive - (prognosis tends to be poor) high dose intravenous antifungal therapy; treatment of underlying disease; ?adjunctive cytokine therapy to reverse neutropenia

SURGICAL MEASURES N/A

ACTIVITY As tolerated

DIET No special diet

PATIENT EDUCATION To specifics of individual circumstances.

MEDICATIONS

DRUG(S) OF CHOICE
- Allergic
  ◊ Extrinsic allergic alveolitis - bronchodilators, cromolyn, steroids
  ◊ ABPA - steroids
- Aspergillomas - none
- Invasive - high dose amphotericin B - up to 1 mg/kg/day. The lipid formulations of amphotericin may be useful if patients develop nephrotoxicity from amphotericin B.

Contraindications: Refer to manufacturers literature

Precautions: Amphotericin B can cause significant renal insufficiency and electrolyte abnormalities. Saline infusion at the time of amphotericin B administration may decrease the nephrotoxicity.

Significant possible interactions:
- Amphotericin B-other nephrotoxic drugs (aminoglycosides, cyclosporine, etc): accelerate development of renal insufficiency
- Amphotericin B-diuretics: accelerate electrolyte depletion
- Itraconazole-hepatically metabolized drugs: serum levels altered
- Itraconazole-gastric pH: normal, low pH is necessary for absorption

ALTERNATIVE DRUGS
Itraconazole is occasionally useful as an alternative agent

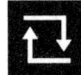
FOLLOWUP

PATIENT MONITORING
- Allergic
  ◊ Extrinsic allergic, alveolitis - spirometry
  ◊ ABPA - chest x-ray, IgE levels
- Aspergillomas - chest x-ray, symptoms
- Invasive - chest x-ray, CBC

PREVENTION/AVOIDANCE
- Allergic - avoid exposure
- Aspergillomas - treatment of underlying diseases, i.e., COPD, etc.

POSSIBLE COMPLICATIONS
- Allergic - bronchiectasis, pulmonary fibrosis, obstructive lung disease
- Aspergillomas - hemoptyses
- Invasive - metastatic infection of CNS, GI tract and other organs; death

EXPECTED COURSE/PROGNOSIS
- Allergic - with treatment prognosis is good; untreated can progress to severe fibrosis, COPD
- Aspergillomas - prognosis more related to underlying disease
- Invasive - poor prognosis

MISCELLANEOUS

ASSOCIATED CONDITIONS
- Allergic - asthma
- Aspergillomas - COPD, TB, pulmonary mycoses, silicosis, sarcoidosis, non-tuberculosis mycobacteria, ankylosing spondylitis, malignancy
- Invasive - neutropenia

AGE-RELATED FACTORS
Pediatric: N/A
Geriatric: N/A
Others:
- Allergic - Tends to occur in younger patients < 35.
- Aspergillomas - older patients with chronic lung disease
- Invasive - all ages

PREGNANCY   N/A

SYNONYMS
- Hypersensitivity pneumonitis
- Fungus ball

ICD-9-CM   117.3 aspergillosis

SEE ALSO   N/A

OTHER NOTES   N/A

ABBREVIATIONS   ABPA = allergic bronchopulmonary aspergillosis

REFERENCES
- Mandell GL, et al, eds: Principles and Practice of Infectious Diseases. 4th Ed. Churchill Livingstone, New York, 1995
- Denning DW: Invasive Aspergillosis. Clinical Infectious Diseases 1998;26:781-805
- Rosenberg M, Patterson R, Mintzer R, Cooper BJ, Roberts M, Harris KE: Clinical and immunologic criteria for the diagnosis of allergic bronchopulmonary aspergillosis. Ann Int Med 1977;86:405-414
- Denning DW, Stevens DA: Antifungal and surgical treatment of invasive aspergillosis: Review of 2,121 published cases. Rev Inf Dis 1990;12(6):1147-1201
Illustrations: 1 available on CD-ROM
Internet references: http://www.5mcc.com

Author(s)
Rodney D. Adam, MD

Asthma

BASICS

DESCRIPTION A disorder of the tracheobronchial tree characterized by mild to severe obstruction to airflow. Symptoms vary, generally episodic or paroxysmal, may be persistent. The clinical hallmark is wheezing, but cough may be the predominant symptom. Commonly misdiagnosed as recurrent pneumonia or chronic bronchitis.
• Acute symptoms are characterized by narrowing of large and small airways due to spasm of bronchial smooth muscle, edema and inflammation of the bronchial mucosa, and production of mucus
• Occurs in a setting in which asthma is likely and other, rarer conditions have been excluded
System(s) affected: Pulmonary
Genetics: Search for an asthma gene underway; there is a familial association of reactive airway disease (RAD), ectopic dermatitis, and allergic rhinitis
Incidence/Prevalence in USA:
• 10 million new cases each year, however, there is confusion due to lack of a uniform definition
• 7-19% of children
• A leading cause of missed school days - 7.5 million/year
Predominant age:
• 50% of cases are children under 10
• Young adult (16-40 years), but may occur at any age
Predominant sex:
• Children under 10: Male > Female
• Puberty: Male = Female
• Adult onset: Female > Male

SIGNS AND SYMPTOMS
Variation in pattern of symptoms; paroxysmal, constant, abnormal pulmonary function tests without symptoms
• Wheezing
• Cough
• Periodicity of symptoms
• Prolonged expiration
• Hyperresonance
• Decreased breath sounds
• Nocturnal attacks
• Pulsus paradoxus
• Cyanosis
• Tachycardia
• Accessory respiratory muscle use
• Flattened diaphragms
• Nasal polyp; seen in cystic fibrosis and aspirin sensitivity
• Clubbing is not seen in asthma
• Growth is usually normal

CAUSES
• Allergic factors
  ◊ Airborne pollens
  ◊ Molds
  ◊ House dust (mites)
  ◊ Animal dander
  ◊ Feather pillows
• Other factors
  ◊ Smoke and other pollutants
  ◊ Infections, especially viral
  ◊ Aspirin
  ◊ Exercise
  ◊ Sinusitis

◊ Gastroesophageal reflux
◊ Sleep (peak expiratory flow rate [PEFR] lowest at 4 am)
• Current research focuses on inflammatory response (including abnormal release of chemical mediators, eosinophil chemotactic factor, neutrophil chemotactic factor, and leukotrienes, etc.)

RISK FACTORS
• Positive family history
• Viral lower respiratory infection during infancy

DIAGNOSIS

DIFFERENTIAL DIAGNOSIS Foreign body aspiration - always consider; cystic fibrosis; viral respiratory infections (croup, bronchiolitis); epiglottitis; bronchopulmonary aspergillosis; tuberculosis; hyperventilation syndrome; mitral value prolapse; habit cough; recurrent pulmonary emboli; congestive heart failure; chronic obstructive pulmonary disease; hypersensitivity pneumonitis

LABORATORY
• CBC normal
• Nasal eosinophils
• Immunoglobulins
  ◊ Screen for immunodeficiency
  ◊ IgE elevated in allergic bronchopulmonary aspergillosis (ABPA)
• Sweat test in chronic childhood asthmatics
• Arterial blood gases in status asthmaticus
Drugs that may alter lab results: N/A
Disorders that may alter lab results: N/A

PATHOLOGICAL FINDINGS Smooth muscle hyperplasia; mucosal edema; thickened basement membrane; inflammatory response; hyperinflated lungs; mucus plugging; bronchiectasis is not seen except in association with ABPA; increased airway resistance; decreased airflow rates; ventilation-perfusion mismatching

SPECIAL TESTS
• Home monitoring of peak flow rates - report if drops below 70% of baseline
• Pulmonary function tests - reversible airway obstruction
• Allergy testing
• PPD yearly
• Exercise tolerance testing

IMAGING Chest x-ray (hyperinflation, atelectasis, airleak)

DIAGNOSTIC PROCEDURES
• Bronchoscopy: rarely indicated.
• Spirometry: decreased FEV1
• Chest x-ray: do at least one, but not necessary with each exacerbation

TREATMENT

APPROPRIATE HEALTH CARE
• Outpatient
• Inpatient for bronchospasm not relieved by beta-agonists and steroids

GENERAL MEASURES
• Eliminate irritants
• Education is essential
• Appropriate prophylactic management with anti-inflammatories such as inhaled steroids, cromolyn sodium
• Increase beta-agonists in response to symptoms
• Consider hyposensitization
• The following are NOT recommended: mist, large volumes of fluid, breathing exercises, IPPB

SURGICAL MEASURES N/A

ACTIVITY Early diagnosis and appropriate treatment facilitate unrestricted activity.

DIET No special diet

PATIENT EDUCATION
• American Lung Association, 1740 Broadway, New York, NY 10019, (212)315-8700
• Asthma and Allergy Foundation of America, Suite 305, Washington, DC 20036, (800)7-ASTHMA, (800)727-8462

MEDICATIONS

DRUG(S) OF CHOICE
• Six major classes of drugs are used:
  ◊ Cromoglycate and nedocromil
  ◊ Steroids (beclomethasone, fluticasone, prednisone, etc)
  ◊ Beta-agonists (albuterol, bitolterol, salmeterol, etc.)
  ◊ Methylxanthines (theophylline)
  ◊ Anticholinergics (atropine, ipratropium)
  ◊ Leukotriene modifiers
• Mild intermittant asthma: brief wheezing once or twice a week:
  ◊ Intermittent beta-agonist (MDI or nebulizer - albuterol, 2 puffs or 0.25-1.0 mL neb q2hr prn)
  ◊ Long acting beta-agonists [e.g., salmeterol (Serevent) 2 puffs bid]
  ◊ Oral beta-agonist or theophylline may be considered, but have more side effects
• Mild persistent asthma: symptoms > 2 times a week, but < 1 time a day; affects activity. Once daily medication - choose from:
  ◊ Cromolyn qid or nedocromil bid (2 puffs or 2 ml neb)
  ◊ Inhaled steroids (low doses)
  ◊ Consider zafirlukast or montelukast
  ◊ Consider oral theophylline (10-20 mg/kg/day); not preferred

- Moderate persistent asthma: weekly symptoms interfering with sleep or exercise, occasional ER visits, PEFR 60-80% of predicted, PEFR variability >30%
  ◊ Regular maintenance schedule
  ◊ Inhaled steroids (beclomethasone diproprionate) 400-800 µg/day.
  ◊ Consider cromolyn qid or nedocromil bid (2 puffs or 2 mL neb)
  ◊ If not controlled with moderate dose inhaled steroid (600 µg/day), consider addition of oral slow-release xanthines or inhaled ipratropium bromide
  ◊ Consider zafirlukast or montelukast
- Severe persistant asthma: frequent symptoms affecting activity, nocturnal symptoms, frequent hospitalizations, PEFR <60% predicted
  ◊ High dose inhaled steroids; some patients may need alternate day oral steroids
  ◊ Theophylline often useful, particularly for nighttime symptoms; therapeutic level 10-20 µg/mL (56-111 µmol/L)
  ◊ Consider zafirlukast or montelukast
  ◊ Consider cromolyn, ipratropium
- Acute exacerbation - outpatient management
  ◊ Inhaled beta-agonist (albuterol) to reverse airflow obstruction (1 mL albuterol neb)
  ◊ Look for increased work of breathing, air leak syndromes, atelectasis, lowered PEFR
  ◊ Short course of steroids, 2mg/kg po qam for 5-7 days
  ◊ IV aminophylline adds toxicity only
  ◊ Observe at least one hour
- Delivery systems
  ◊ Children under 2 - nebulizer or MDI with valved spacer and mask
  ◊ Children 2-4 years - MDI and valved spacer
  ◊ Over 5 years - MDI or powder inhaler
- Hospital management
  ◊ Steroids IV: methylprednisolone (Solu-Medrol) 2 mg/kg once, then 1 mg/kg IV q6h
  ◊ Frequent beta-agonist aerosols
  ◊ Ipratropium neb and/or aminophylline IV drip if not responding well
  ◊ Rarely: isoproterenol or terbutaline IV; mechanical ventilation

Contraindications:
- Sedatives, mucolytics
- Antibiotics are usually not necessary
- Avoid beta-adrenergic blocking drugs

Precautions: Concern regarding deleterious effects of chronic use of beta agonists. Use only when symptomatic (chronic asthma may necessitate chronic use). If using beta-agonist more than twice a week, should also be on anti-inflammatory.

Significant possible interactions:
Erythromycin and ciprofloxacin slow theophylline clearance and can increase levels 15-20%.

ALTERNATIVE DRUGS
- Ketotifen
- H1-antagonists
- Troleandomycin (TAO)
- methotrexate
- IV immune globulin (IVIG)
- Furosemide (Lasix)

FOLLOWUP

PATIENT MONITORING
- PEFR meter at home - record for trend; call if < 70% baseliine, ER if < 50% baseline
- pH and arterial blood gases
- Oximetry
- Electrolytes

PREVENTION/AVOIDANCE
- Co-management is essential
  ◊ Understand medication, inhalers, nebulizers, peak flow meters
  ◊ Monitor symptoms, peak flows
  ◊ Pre-arranged action plan for exacerbations
  ◊ Written guidelines
- Investigate and control triggering factors (pollutants, exercise, house-dust mite, molds, animal dander) if severe
- Annual influenza immunization
- Avoid aspirin
- Avoid sulfites (food additives)

POSSIBLE COMPLICATIONS
- Respiratory failure; mechanical ventilation
- Atelectasis in 25% of hospitalized patients
- Flaccid paralysis after exacerbation (self-limited)
- Death
- Air leak syndromes (pneumothorax, etc.)
- SIADH
- Altered theophylline metabolism

EXPECTED COURSE/PROGNOSIS
- Excellent, with attention to general health and use of medications to control symptoms
- Less than 50% of children with asthma "outgrow it"
- Mortality risk increases with:
  ◊ Greater than 3 emergency room visits/year
  ◊ Nocturnal symptoms
  ◊ History of ICU admission
  ◊ Mechanical ventilation
  ◊ Greater than 2 hospitalizations/year
  ◊ Steroid dependence (systemic use)
  ◊ History of syncope with asthma
  ◊ History of noncompliance
- Mortality rates are increasing
- If responsive to treatment is poor, review diagnosis and compliance prior to adding more potent therapy

MISCELLANEOUS

ASSOCIATED CONDITIONS
- Reflux esophagitis
- Sinusitis

AGE-RELATED FACTORS
Pediatric: 50% of new cases of asthma occur in children below 10 years
Geriatric: Unusual for initial episode to occur
Others: N/A

PREGNANCY
- About 50% of asthma patients have no changes, 25% seem to improve and 25% have worse symptoms
- Stress prevention
- Avoid medications with contraindications

SYNONYMS
- Bronchial asthma
- Reactive airway disease

ICD-9-CM
493.0 extrinsic asthma
493.1 intrinsic asthma
493.9 asthma, unspecified

SEE ALSO
- Cystic fibrosis
- Bronchitis, acute
- Immunodeficiency diseases
- Bronchiolitis
- Laryngotracheobronchitis
- Epiglottitis
- Congestive heart failure
- Chronic obstructive pulmonary disease & emphysema
- Hypersensitivity pneumonitis
- Tuberculosis

OTHER NOTES
Antihistamines are not contraindicated in asthma

ABBREVIATIONS
ABPA = allergic bronchopulmonary aspergillosis
PFT = pulmonary function test
RAD = reactive airway disease
TAO = toleandromycin
PEFR = peak expiratory flow
MDI = metered dose inhaler

REFERENCES
- Barnes PJ: A new approach to the treatment of asthma. New Engl J Med 1989;321:1517
- NHLBI Guidelines, 1997
- Rachelefsky G, Warner J: International Consensus on the Management of Pediatric Asthma. Ped Pulmon 1993;15:125-127
Illustrations: N/A
Internet references: http://www.5mcc.com

Author(s)
Nancy N. Dambro, MD

Atelectasis

BASICS

DESCRIPTION Atelectasis (lung collapse) is a portion of lung which is non-aerated, but otherwise normal. May be an asymptomatic finding on chest roentgenogram or associated with symptoms. Pulmonary blood flow to area of atelectasis is usually reduced, thereby limiting shunting and hypoxia. Diagnosis and therapy are directed at basic cause.
System(s) affected: Pulmonary, Cardiovascular
Genetics: Depends on basic condition e.g., cystic fibrosis, asthma, congenital heart disease, etc.
Incidence/Prevalence in USA: Common in general anesthesia and in intensive care with high inspired oxygen concentrations
Predominant age: All ages
Predominant sex: Male = Female

SIGNS AND SYMPTOMS
• Small atelectasis
 ◊ Commonly asymptomatic
 ◊ Produces no change in the overall clinical presentation
• Large atelectasis:
 ◊ Tachypnea
 ◊ Cough
 ◊ Hypoxia which resolves in some cases over 24-48 hours
 ◊ Dullness to percussion
 ◊ Absent breath sounds if airway is occluded
 ◊ Bronchial breathing if airway is patent
 ◊ Diminished chest expansion
 ◊ Tracheal or precordial impulse displacement
 ◊ Wheezing may be heard with focal obstruction

CAUSES
• Increased alveolar surface tension due to cardiogenic or non-cardiogenic pulmonary edema, primary surfactant deficiency, or infection
• Resorptive atelectasis due to airway obstruction from lumenal blockage (mucus, tumor, foreign body), airway wall abnormality (edema, tumor, bronchomalacia, deformation), or extrinsic airway compression (cardiac, vascular, tumor, adenopathy)
• Compression of the lung (lobar emphysema, cardiomegaly, tumor)
• Increased pleural pressure due to fluid or air in the pleural space (pneumothorax, effusion, empyema, hemothorax, chylothorax)
• Chest wall restriction due to skeletal deformity and/or muscular weakness (scoliosis, neuromuscular disease, phrenic nerve paralysis, anesthesia)

RISK FACTORS
• Varies with condition producing atelectasis
• Atelectasis following anesthesia is increased in smokers, obese individuals, and individuals with short, wide thoraces
• Asthma

DIAGNOSIS

DIFFERENTIAL DIAGNOSIS
• Atelectasis is not a specific diagnosis, but rather a result of disease or distorted anatomy. The differential is thus found under Causes.
• The roentgenographic differential includes pneumonia, fluid accumulation, lung hypoplasia, or tumor

LABORATORY N/A
Drugs that may alter lab results: N/A
Disorders that may alter lab results: N/A

PATHOLOGICAL FINDINGS
• Pathology varies with cause
• Obstructive atelectasis - non-aerated lung without inflammation or infiltration

SPECIAL TESTS N/A

IMAGING
• Chest roentgenography
 ◊ May demonstrate linear, round, or wedge shaped densities
 ◊ Right middle lobe and lingular atelectasis will obscure the ipsilateral heart border
 ◊ Lower lobe atelectasis will obscure the diaphragm
 ◊ Air bronchograms are usually absent in obstructive atelectasis
 ◊ Evidence of possible airway compression, pleural fluid or air should be sought
 ◊ Diffuse microatelectasis in surfactant deficiency may lead to a ground-glass appearance with striking air bronchograms
 ◊ Mediastinal structures and the diaphragm move toward the atelectatic region
 ◊ Adjacent lung may show compensatory hyperinflation

DIAGNOSTIC PROCEDURES
• Bronchoscopy to assess airway patency. (Bronchoscopy as therapy is controversial with the exception of foreign body or other structural causes).
• Echocardiography to assess cardiac status in cardiomegaly
• Chest CT or MRI to visualize airway and mediastinal structures
• Barium swallow to assess mediastinal vascular compression
• Other procedures vary with potential cause

TREATMENT

APPROPRIATE HEALTH CARE Varies with severity

GENERAL MEASURES
• Varies with severity and cause of atelectasis
• Ensure adequate oxygenation and humidification
• Chest physiotherapy with percussion and postural drainage. Consider adding treatments using new airway clearance techniques such as Positive Expiratory Pressure (PEP) mask.
• Incentive spirometry
• Positive pressure ventilation or continuous positive airway pressure in subjects with neuromuscular weakness

SURGICAL MEASURES N/A

ACTIVITY Encourage activity, mobilization as tolerated

DIET No special diet

PATIENT EDUCATION Encourage activity as appropriate. Instruct in basic cause and its therapy.

MEDICATIONS

DRUG(S) OF CHOICE
• Bronchodilator therapy (beta-agonist aerosol)
• Other therapies directed at basic cause -
antibiotics, foreign body removal, tumor
therapy, cardiac medication, steroids in
asthma
Contraindications: Refer to manufacturer's
literature
Precautions: Refer to manufacturer's
literature
Significant possible interactions: Refer to
manufacturer's literature

ALTERNATIVE DRUGS   N/A

FOLLOWUP

PATIENT MONITORING
• Varies with cause and patient status
• In simple atelectasis associated with asthma
or infection, monthly visits are adequate

PREVENTION/AVOIDANCE
• Avoidance of 100% inspired oxygen (which
can rapidly absorb causing atelectasis)
• Foreign body/aspiration precautions
• Postoperative mobilization and/or rotation
• Institute therapies such as chest
physiotherapy and incentive spirometry as
preventive maneuvers in at-risk patients

POSSIBLE COMPLICATIONS
• Infection with chronic lung damage is an
unlikely, but unfortunate complication
• Atelectasis is rarely life-threatening and
usually spontaneously resolves

EXPECTED COURSE/PROGNOSIS
• Resolution with medical therapy
• Surgical therapy needed only for certain
causes, or if chronic infection and
bronchiectasis supervene

MISCELLANEOUS

ASSOCIATED CONDITIONS   N/A

AGE-RELATED FACTORS   Very young
and very old patients with limited mobility at
greater risk
Pediatric: Congenital airway obstruction due
to mediastinal cysts, tumor, or vascular rings;
foreign body aspiration
Geriatric: Primary and secondary lung tumors
sometimes associated
Others: Asthma

PREGNANCY   Management is similar to
non-pregnant and varies with cause

SYNONYMS   Lung collapse

ICD-9-CM
518.0 Pulmonary collapse (atelectasis)

SEE ALSO
• Asthma
• Pneumonia, viral
• Pneumonia, bacterial
• Pneumonia, mycoplasma

OTHER NOTES
• Round atelectasis:
◊ A pleural based round density on chest
roentgenogram with a comet tail of vessel and
airway
◊ More common in patients with asbestos
exposure
◊ May mimic tumor, but can usually be
definitively diagnosed with imaging studies
thereby avoiding surgery

ABBREVIATIONS   N/A

REFERENCES
• Hazinski TH: Atelectasis. In: Chernick V, ed.
Kendig's Disorders of the Respiratory Tract in
Children. 5th Ed. Philadelphia, W.B. Saunders
Co., 1990
• Marini JJ, Pierson DJ, Hudson LD: Acute
lobar atelectasis: a prospective comparison of
fiberoptic bronchoscopy and respiratory
therapy. Am Rev Respir Dis 1971;119:971
• Rickstenste, Sventrik, et al: Effects of
periodic positive airway pressure by mask on
postoperative pulmonary function. Chest
1986;6:774-781
Illustrations: N/A
Internet references: http://www.5mcc.com

Author(s)
Nancy N. Dambro, MD

Atherosclerosis

BASICS

DESCRIPTION The common form of arteriosclerosis in which deposits of yellowish plaques (atheromas) containing cholesterol, lipoid material, and lipophages are formed within the intima and inner media of large and medium sized arteries.
System(s) affected: Cardiovascular
Genetics: Probable genetic link; many risk factors for atherosclerosis (lipid metabolism, hypertension, and diabetes) are clearly inheritable
Incidence/Prevalence in USA:
• Common, but declining steadily. The effects upon the brain, heart, kidneys, extremities and other vital organs form the leading cause of morbidity and mortality in the USA and most Western countries.
• Complications of atherosclerosis account for 1/2 of all deaths, and 1/3 of deaths in persons between ages 35-65
Predominant age: 35 and older
Predominant sex: Male > Female

SIGNS AND SYMPTOMS
• Characteristically silent until atheromas produce:
  ◊ Stenosis
  ◊ Thrombosis
  ◊ Aneurysm
  ◊ Embolus
• For lists of possible symptoms see the following titles elsewhere in this book:
  ◊ Essential hypertension
  ◊ Coronary arteriosclerosis
  ◊ Congestive heart failure
  ◊ Cerebrovascular accident
  ◊ Atrial arrhythmias
  ◊ Ventricular arrhythmias
  ◊ Renal failure, chronic
  ◊ Dissecting aneurysm
  ◊ Thrombosis and embolism, arterial

CAUSES
• Biochemical, physiologic, environmental factors that lead to thickening and occlusion of the lumen of arteries
• Aging (some degree of atherosclerosis is universal)
• One or more of the risk factors listed below

RISK FACTORS
• Hypertension
• Tobacco smoking
• Diabetes mellitus
• Obesity
• Male gender
• Physical inactivity
• Increasing age
• Family history of premature atherosclerosis
• Decreased high-density lipoprotein (HDL) cholesterol
• Increased low-density lipoprotein (LDL) cholesterol

DIAGNOSIS

DIFFERENTIAL DIAGNOSIS N/A

LABORATORY Associated with elevated serum cholesterol; elevated LDL and low HDL
Drugs that may alter lab results: N/A
Disorders that may alter lab results: N/A

PATHOLOGICAL FINDINGS
• Early changes (simple) potentially reversible
  ◊ Accumulation of lipid-laden cells in the intimal layer of the artery (usually monocytes/macrophages from circulating blood)
  ◊ Lipid streaks in aortas and coronary arteries
• Late changes (complicated) usually reversible
  ◊ Atheromatous plaques with necrosis, fibrosis, calcification
  ◊ Weakening of elastic lamellae
  ◊ Neovascularization
  ◊ Arterial obstruction
  ◊ Thrombosis

SPECIAL TESTS N/A

IMAGING Extensively calcified atherosclerotic plaques may be identified in major blood vessels on x-ray

DIAGNOSTIC PROCEDURES
• X-ray (often incidental finding)
• Associated with hypercholesterolemia; elevated LDL and low HDL
• Arterial doppler studies (carotid, renal)
• Angiography
• Ankle-brachial index (ABI)

TREATMENT

APPROPRIATE HEALTH CARE
Outpatient until complications occur; emphasis on prevention

GENERAL MEASURES
• For details see the following titles:
  ◊ Essential hypertension
  ◊ Congestive heart failure
  ◊ Cerebrovascular accident
  ◊ Renal failure, chronic
  ◊ Dissecting aneurysm
  ◊ Thrombosis & embolism, arterial

SURGICAL MEASURES N/A

ACTIVITY Encourage physical fitness

DIET
Recommended daily intake
• Initial diet; Step 1
  ◊ Total fat - < 30% of total calories; saturated fat < 10%
  ◊ Carbohydrates - 50-60% of total calories
  ◊ Protein - 10-20% of total calories
  ◊ Cholesterol - < 300 mg a day
  ◊ Total calories - amount required to achieve and maintain desirable weight
  ◊ Sodium - 1650-2400 mg
  ◊ Alcohol - < 30 g
• Initial diet; Step 2
  ◊ Total fat - < 30% of total calories; saturated fat < 7%
  ◊ Carbohydrates - 50-60% of total calories
  ◊ Protein - 10-20% of total calories
  ◊ Cholesterol - < 200 mg a day
  ◊ Total calories - amount required to achieve and maintain desirable weight
  ◊ Sodium - 1650-2400 mg
  ◊ Alcohol - < 30 g

PATIENT EDUCATION
• Crucial parts of preventing and treating atheroscleroses involve nutrition, fitness, and smoking cessation
• Extensive educational materials available from many agencies (e.g., American Heart Association, U.S. Government Printing Office, National Cholesterol Education Program). Use these to help teach patients how to avoid or eliminate risk factors.

MEDICATIONS

DRUG(S) OF CHOICE
- For details see the following titles:
  - ◊ Essential hypertension
  - ◊ Coronary arteriosclerosis
  - ◊ Congestive heart failure
  - ◊ Stroke
  - ◊ Atrial arrhythmias
  - ◊ Ventricular arrhythmias
  - ◊ Renal failure, chronic
  - ◊ Dissecting aneurysm
  - ◊ Thrombosis and embolism, arterial
  - ◊ Angina
  - ◊ Myocardial infarction
  - ◊ Arteriosclerotic heart disease

Contraindications: Refer to manufacturer's literature

Precautions: Refer to manufacturer's literature

Significant possible interactions: Refer to manufacturer's literature

ALTERNATIVE DRUGS   See specific titles

FOLLOWUP

PATIENT MONITORING   See specific titles

PREVENTION/AVOIDANCE   Eliminate risk factors - all or as many as possible

POSSIBLE COMPLICATIONS
- Coronary artery disease
- Renal failure
- Cerebrovascular accidents
- Dissecting or ruptured aneurysms
- Congestive heart failure
- Arterial thrombosis
- Gangrene
- Cardiac arrhythmias
- Sudden death

EXPECTED COURSE/PROGNOSIS
Avoiding risk factors has greatly decreased mortality rates in the past decade

MISCELLANEOUS

ASSOCIATED CONDITIONS
- Essential hypertension
- Coronary arteriosclerosis
- Congestive heart failure
- Cerebrovascular accident
- Atrial arrhythmias
- Ventricular arrhythmias
- Renal failure, chronic
- Aortic dissection
- Thrombosis and embolism, arterial

AGE-RELATED FACTORS
Pediatric: Fatty streaks and deposits in the intima of the aortas of all children begin as early as age 3 years
Geriatric: Atherosclerosis happens to all who live long enough. Its effects and complications can be minimized and/or delayed by avoiding all risk factors possible.
Others: N/A

PREGNANCY   N/A

SYNONYMS   N/A

ICD-9-CM
414.0 Coronary atherosclerosis

SEE ALSO
- Hypertension, essential
- Congestive heart failure
- Stroke (Brain attack)
- Renal failure, chronic
- Aortic dissection
- Arterial embolus & thrombosis

OTHER NOTES   N/A

ABBREVIATIONS   N/A

REFERENCES
- Hurst JW, et.al: The Heart. 7th Ed. New York, McGraw-Hill, 1990
- Hunninghake D, ed: Lipid disorders. Medical Clinics of North America. Vol. 78, No. 1, Jan., 1994
- Guidelines for cardiopulmonary resuscitation and emergency cardiac care. JAMA 1992;268(16)28
- Fauci AS, ed: Harrison's Principles of Internal medicine. 14th ed. New York, McGraw-Hill, 1998

Illustrations: 4 available on CD-ROM
Internet references: http://www.5mcc.com

Author(s)
Chandramohan Batra, MD

Atherosclerotic occlusive disease

 BASICS

DESCRIPTION A peripheral arterial disease can be acute or chronic. There is obstruction or narrowing of the lumen of the aorta and its major branches causing interruption of blood flow, usually to feet and legs. Involved arteries may include mesenteric and celiac arteries. Occlusions cause ischemia, discomfort, skin ulceration and gangrene.
System(s) affected: Cardiovascular
Genetics: Family history of early complications of atherosclerosis
Incidence/Prevalence in USA: Increases with age (parallels atherosclerosis)
Predominant age: Older adults
Predominant sex: Male > Female (2:1)

SIGNS AND SYMPTOMS
• Intermittent claudication - exercise induced pain that is relieved by rest is pathognomonic
• Site of occlusion determines site of pain
• Occlusion of abdominal aorta and/or iliac vessels produce claudication in the back, buttocks and hips
• Femoral obstruction causes pain in the calf
• The degree of occlusion determines the exercise tolerance and if severe enough produces pain at rest
• Pulses are diminished or absent
• The limb is cold and pale and typically develops dependent rubor
• Atrophic skin changes often result in shiny hairless skin

CAUSES
• Almost always a complication of atherosclerosis
• Mechanism of occlusion - embolus, thrombosis, fracture, or trauma

RISK FACTORS
• Smoking
• Hyperlipidemia
• Diabetes
• Hypertension
• Physical stress

 DIAGNOSIS

DIFFERENTIAL DIAGNOSIS
• Thromboangiitis obliterans (inflammatory disease primarily affecting young male smokers)
• Fibromuscular dysplasia of the peripheral vessels (rare)

LABORATORY N/A
Drugs that may alter lab results: N/A
Disorders that may alter lab results: N/A

PATHOLOGICAL FINDINGS
• Occluding mass in lumen of thrombosed artery
• Calcareous deposits in occluded vessel in medial coat with atheromas

SPECIAL TESTS Doppler ultrasound to compare systolic pressure in upper and lower limbs (ankle: brachial ratio should be higher than 0.95 at rest)

IMAGING Angiography for an individual who may be a candidate for surgery

DIAGNOSTIC PROCEDURES History and physical

 TREATMENT

APPROPRIATE HEALTH CARE
Outpatient for conservative management. Inpatient for surgery or more severe cases.

GENERAL MEASURES
• Smoking cessation
• Foot and limb care
• Graduated exercise program
• Weight control
• Pain management
• Cholesterol management
• Appropriate treatment of coexisting disease, i.e., diabetes
• Infection control
• Lifestyle modification

SURGICAL MEASURES
• Indications for surgery are ischemic pain at rest, or changes likely to lead to amputation, or intolerable symptoms
• The procedure depends upon site of lesion. Includes endarterectomy, bypass procedures, transluminal angioplasty, and amputation.
• Patients with aorto-iliac disease tend to have good surgical results to a disabling disorder
• Surgery should not be performed for femoral popliteal disease unless symptoms are very severe or disabling
• Bypass surgery for vessels distal to popliteal artery has little success
• Patch grafting
• Atherectomy
• Laser angioplasty
• Stents (wire plastic mesh to stretch and mold to the arterial wall to prevent re-occlusion)
• Amputation with failure of arterial reconstructive surgery or with development of gangrene, persistent infection, or intractable pain

ACTIVITY To the degree that symptoms permit

DIET
• Good diet control
• Lose weight, if overweight

PATIENT EDUCATION
• Educate patient regarding symptoms or signs that require early assessment by physician
• Teach careful foot care
• Avoid elevating or applying heat to affected parts
• Urge early ambulation after surgery
• Assist patient with a stop smoking program

MEDICATIONS

DRUG(S) OF CHOICE
• Vasodilator drugs are ineffective
• Pentoxifylline (Trental) for reducing blood viscosity and increasing red cell flexibility may help. Usual dose 400 mg tid.
• Aspirin to decrease platelet aggregation
Contraindications: In patients sensitive to xanthines
Precautions: Most adverse effects are gastrointestinal. Dizziness and headache are also common.
Significant possible interactions: Use cautiously in patients on oral coagulants. Monitor closely for bleeding complications.

ALTERNATIVE DRUGS Anticoagulants

FOLLOWUP

PATIENT MONITORING
• For acute phase with surgery, closely follow all aspects of postoperative recovery
• For mild chronic cases, follow patient at regular intervals, frequency dependent upon severity of symptoms
• Management/modification of risk factors

PREVENTION/AVOIDANCE
• Periodic health maintenance measures
• Healthy lifestyle including appropriate diet and adequate exercise
• Avoidance of smoking

POSSIBLE COMPLICATIONS
• Necrosis
• Gangrene
• Limb amputation

EXPECTED COURSE/PROGNOSIS
Course varies from slow progression with easily controlled symptoms to rapid deterioration with severe symptoms requiring surgical intervention

MISCELLANEOUS

ASSOCIATED CONDITIONS
• Atherosclerosis
• Arteriosclerosis obliterans
• Fibromuscular dysplasia
• Thromboangiitis obliterans
• Takayasu's arteritis
• Abdominal aortic coarctation
• Radiation injury
• Popliteal artery entrapment syndrome
• Popliteal cystic degeneration
• Arteritis

AGE-RELATED FACTORS
Pediatric: N/A
Geriatric: N/A
Others: N/A

PREGNANCY N/A

SYNONYMS
• Peripheral arterial disease
• Occlusive arterial disease

ICD-9-CM
444.22 Occlusion, arteries of extremities, lower
444.21 Occlusion, arteries of extremities, upper

SEE ALSO
• Arteriosclerosis obliterans

OTHER NOTES N/A

ABBREVIATIONS N/A

REFERENCES
• Marcus ML: The Coronary Circulation in Health and Disease. New York, McGraw-Hill, 1983
• Hurst JW, et al: The Heart. 7th Ed. New York, McGraw-Hill, 1990
• Braunwald E, ed: Heart Disease: A Textbook of Cardiovascular Medicine. 4th Ed. Philadelphia, W.B. Saunders Co., 1992
Illustrations: N/A
Internet references: http://www.5mcc.com

Author(s)
Stanley G. Smith, MA, MB, FCFPC

Atrial fibrillation

BASICS

DESCRIPTION Atrial fibrillation (AF) is a chronic or paroxysmal arrhythmia characterized by chaotic atrial electrical activity. The electrophysiologic mechanism is most likely multiple reentrant wavelets within the atria. Because the AV node is bombarded with nearly continuous atrial electrical impulses, the ventricular response is irregular and usually rapid (up to or exceeding 180 beats per minute). Symptoms vary from none to mild (palpitations, lightheadedness, fatigue, poor exercise capacity) to severe (angina, dyspnea, syncope), and are frequently more serious in patients with significant structural heart disease. In some patients with Wolff-Parkinson-White syndrome, AF may be extremely rapid and degenerate into ventricular fibrillation.
System(s) affected: Cardiovascular, Nervous
Genetics: No specific genetic pattern in most patients
Incidence/Prevalence in USA: Estimated at 1 per 1000 adults per year; estimated at 2-4% of adult population
Predominant age:
Prevalence increases with age:

Age	AF cases/1000
25-35	2-3
55-64	30-40
62-90	50-90

Predominant sex: Male > Female

SIGNS AND SYMPTOMS
- Irregular pulse
- Tachycardia
- Heart failure
- Hypotension
- Palpitations
- Lightheadedness
- Poor exercise capacity
- Fatigue
- Dyspnea
- Angina
- Near syncope/syncope
- Stroke
- Arterial embolization

CAUSES
- Hypertensive heart disease
- Valvular/rheumatic heart disease
- Coronary artery disease
- Acute myocardial infarction
- Pulmonary embolus
- Cardiomyopathy
- Congestive heart failure
- Infiltrative heart disease
- Pericarditis
- Intoxication/ingestion (e.g., ethanol in "Holiday Heart")
- Hyperthyroidism
- Postoperative state (especially cardiothoracic surgery)
- Sick sinus syndrome (tachycardia-bradycardia syndrome)
- Idiopathic (including "lone" atrial fibrillation)

RISK FACTORS
- Hypertension
- Diabetes mellitus
- Left ventricular hypertrophy
- Coronary artery disease
- Congestive heart failure
- Rheumatic heart disease

DIAGNOSIS

DIFFERENTIAL DIAGNOSIS
- Multifocal atrial tachycardia (MAT)
- Sinus tachycardia with frequent atrial premature beats
- Atrial flutter (see below)

LABORATORY
- ECG is diagnostic; low amplitude fibrillatory waves without clear P waves; irregularly irregular pattern of QRS complexes
- Holter monitor and event monitor helpful in diagnosing paroxysmal atrial fibrillation (PAF)
- Echocardiogram to assess for structural heart disease
- Thyroid function tests
Drugs that may alter lab results: N/A
Disorders that may alter lab results: N/A

PATHOLOGICAL FINDINGS
- Atrial dilatation
- Atrial injury (chronic or acute)
- Atrial thrombus, especially in atrial appendage
- Sclerosis/fibrosis of SA node
- Coronary artery disease, valvular/rheumatic disease, cardiomyopathy, pulmonary embolus, etc.

SPECIAL TESTS
- Ventilation-perfusion scan or pulmonary angiography if pulmonary embolus suspected
- Transesophageal echocardiography may be useful in detecting left atrial appendage thrombus and therefore risk of stroke with cardioversion

IMAGING
- Chest x-ray to screen for cardiopulmonary abnormalities
- Echocardiogram to assess for structural heart disease

DIAGNOSTIC PROCEDURES   As above

TREATMENT

APPROPRIATE HEALTH CARE
- Inpatient if significant symptoms, extremely rapid ventricular rate, initiating antiarrhythmic therapy, if AF triggered by acute process (acute myocardial infarction, congestive heart failure, pulmonary embolus, etc.)
- Outpatient management appropriate for many patients

GENERAL MEASURES
- Avoidance of potential triggers
  ◊ Avoid ethanol, caffeine, nicotine
  ◊ Management of underlying structural heart disease
- Prevention of complications
  ◊ Anticoagulation to reduce the risk of embolic complications
  ◊ Antibiotic prophylaxis if AF is due to valvular heart disease
- Therapy strategies (ongoing trials compare these two strategies)
  ◊ Ventricular rate control with AV nodal blocking agents
  ◊ Restore and maintain sinus rhythm with antiarrhythmic drugs

SURGICAL MEASURES
Nonpharmacological therapies
- Cardiac surgery (e.g., the "maze procedure") may be considered in severely symptomatic, medically refractory patients
- Permanent dual chamber pacing may reduce incidence of AF in patients with sick sinus syndrome
- Radiofrequency catheter ablation of AV node with permanent pacemaker implantation is a reasonable alternative in symptomatic medically refractory patients
- Radiofrequency catheter ablation procedures to prevent AF recurrence are investigational at present
- Implantable atrial defibrillators to detect and cardiovert paroxysms of AF are investigational at present

ACTIVITY
- As tolerated
- With medical management, minimal functional impairment in many patients

DIET As appropriate for underlying heart disease and other comorbidities

PATIENT EDUCATION
Printed material available from:
- Du Pont Pharmaceuticals, Wilmington, DE 19880-0026, (800)341-4004
- Krames Communications, 11100 Grundy Lane, San Bruno, CA 94066-9821; tel 800-333-3022
- Health Trend Publishing, PO Box 7390, Menlo Park, CA 94026; 800-747-1606

MEDICATIONS

DRUG(S) OF CHOICE
Note: Clinical risk factors for stroke include age > 65, diabetes, hypertension, history of prior stroke or transient ischemic attack (TIA), and prior history of congestive heart failure. Echocardiographic risk factors for stroke include left atrial enlargement, mitral regurgitation, and left ventricular dysfunction.
- Anticoagulation:
  ◊ Unless contraindications to anticoagulants exist, patients with AF with any of these risk factors should receive warfarin to maintain an international normalized ratio (INR) of 2.0-3.0

◊ Patients in whom warfarin is contraindicated should receive aspirin 325 mg/day. Aspirin 325 mg/day, is appropriate in low risk patients (e.g., age < 65 years with no risk factors for stroke). Data are fewer with paroxysmal AF, though treatment guidelines are the same for chronic AF.
• Debate exists as to whether control of the ventricular rate during AF or maintenance of sinus rhythm should be the objective of medical therapy. This is being evaluated in an ongoing multicenter clinical trial called AFFIRM.
• Control of ventricular rate
◊ Beta-blockers (propranolol, metoprolol, atenolol, nadolol, etc.)
◊ Non-dihydropyridine calcium channel blockers (diltiazem and verapamil). For example, diltiazem 10mg IV push, followed by 10mg/hr IV to control rate to approximately 100.
◊ Cardiac glycosides (digoxin). Frequently less effective than other agents in controlling the ventricular response.
• Conversion to/maintenance of sinus rhythm:
◊ Direct current (DC) cardioversion. Antiarrhythmic therapy for chemical cardioversion and maintenance of sinus rhythm following cardioversion carries a risk of pro-arrhythmia.
◊ Ibutilide, an intravenous type III agent, has been approved for chemical cardioversion of atrial fibrillation and flutter of short duration (less than 90 days)
◊ If the duration of AF is more than 24-48 hours or is unknown, patients should be treated with warfarin for at least 3 weeks before and 4 weeks after cardioversion. Transesophageal echocardiography to visualize left atrial thrombus has been proposed to expedite cardioversion.
◊ Chronic oral antiarrhythmic therapy to suppress AF recurrences
 - Type IA (procainamide, disopyramide, quinidine)
 - Type IC (flecainide, propafenone) only in patients with structurally normal hearts
 - Type III (sotalol, amiodarone)
• Acute therapy for hemodynamically compromised patients:
◊ Heparin for anticoagulation
◊ IV beta or calcium channel blocker for control of ventricular rate
◊ Pharmacologic and/or DC cardioversion:
Contraindications:
• Active bleeding precludes anticoagulation; risk of bleeding is a relative contraindication to long-term anticoagulation
• Warfarin is contraindicated in patients with prior history of warfarin skin necrosis
• Type IC drugs are contraindicated in patients with coronary artery disease and other forms of structural heart disease
• Type IA drugs and sotalol should not be used in patients with torsade de pointes history
Precautions:
• With type IA drugs, ibutilide and sotalol, the risk of torsade de pointes increases with the extent of QT interval prolongation (i.e., the QTc). In these patients, avoid other drugs that prolong the QT interval (phenothiazines, tricyclic antidepressants, terfenadine, astemizole, erythromycin, etc.). Avoid hypokalemia and hypomagnesemia. Torsade de pointes due to drug induced long QT syndrome is said to be "pause dependent" as

the risk increases with bradycardia, heart block, and sinus pauses.
• In many patients, adequate medical therapy of AF will cause bradycardia necessitating a permanent pacemaker.
Significant possible interactions:
• Quinidine increases digoxin levels
• Amiodarone increases digoxin levels and enhances effects of warfarin

ALTERNATIVE DRUGS N/A

FOLLOWUP

PATIENT MONITORING
• ECG/Holter monitor to assess maintenance of sinus rhythm, control of ventricular rate during AF
• Frequent PT to maintain INR at 2.0-3.0
• ECG to monitor QTc interval in patients on antiarrhythmic therapy

PREVENTION/AVOIDANCE
• Ethanol may trigger AF in some patients
• In cardiomyopathy/heart failure, hemodynamic decompensation may trigger AF

POSSIBLE COMPLICATIONS
• Embolic stroke
• Peripheral arterial embolization
• Significant complications of pharmacologic therapy (bradyarrhythmias and torsade de pointes)
• Bleeding with anticoagulation

EXPECTED COURSE/PROGNOSIS
• Stroke risk low with long-term anticoagulation
• AF increases the risk of cardiovascular morbidity and mortality, but long-term prognosis may be a function of underlying structural heart disease

MISCELLANEOUS

ASSOCIATED CONDITIONS
• Wolff-Parkinson-White syndrome
• Sick sinus syndrome
• Atrial flutter:
◊ A related arrhythmia with regular atrial electrical activity, typically at a rate of 250-350, manifested as sawtooth "flutter" waves on the ECG. 2:1 or 4:1 conduction through the AV node to the ventricle is usual, so the pulse is frequently regular.
◊ Many patients have both AF and atrial flutter
◊ Management for these closely related arrhythmias is similar, though atrial flutter is more difficult to control pharmacologically but more easily electrically cardioverted than AF

◊ Although atrial flutter alone may pose less of a risk of thromboembolism than AF, guidelines for anticoagulation of atrial flutter and AF are the same
◊ Radiofrequency catheter ablation to cure atrial flutter is becoming more widely applied

AGE-RELATED FACTORS
Pediatric: Though extremely uncommon in children with structurally normal hearts, AF may be seen in the setting of congenital heart disease and following surgical repair
Geriatric: Both the incidence of AF and the risk of stroke increase with age
Others: Young patients at lower risk for stroke. The risk of stroke is extremely low in young patients without structural heart disease, so called "lone atrial fibrillation."

PREGNANCY
• AF is unusual during pregnancy in the absence of structural heart disease (e.g., rheumatic mitral stenosis)
• Digoxin is safe during pregnancy; beta-blockers, procainamide, and quinidine are probably safe. There is limited information regarding calcium blockers.
• Risk of fetal hemorrhage makes anticoagulation problematic; moreover, warfarin causes fetal anomalies. SC heparin is probably the best choice if long-term anticoagulation is necessary.
• DC cardioversion does not seem to adversely affect the fetus

SYNONYMS
• AF; A Fib = atrial fibrillation

ICD-9-CM
427.3 Atrial fibrillation and flutter
427.31 Atrial fibrillation
427.32 Atrial flutter

SEE ALSO
• Atrial flutter
• Wolff-Parkinson-White syndrome

OTHER NOTES N/A

ABBREVIATIONS
• AF = atrial fibrillation
• CAF = chronic atrial fibrillation
• PAF = paroxysmal atrial fibrillation
• PT = prothrombin time
• INR = international normalized ratio

REFERENCES
• Prystowsky EN, Benson DW, Fuster V, et al: Management of patients with atrial fibrillation. Circulation 1996;93:1262-77
• The National Heart, Lung, and Blood Institute Working Group on Atrial Fibrillation. Atrial Fibrillation: Current Understandings and Research Imperatives. J Am Coll Cardiol 1993;22:1830-4
• Riley RD, Pritchell ELC: Pharmacologic management of atrial fibrillation. J Cardiovasc Electrophys 1997;8:818-829
Illustrations: 1 available on CD-ROM
Internet references: http://www.5mcc.com

Author(s)
Leonard Ganz, MD
Leonard S. Lilly, MD

Atrial septal defect (ASD)

BASICS

DESCRIPTION A defect or opening in the atrial septum allowing flow of blood between the two chambers. Shunting is typically left to right and occurs late in ventricular systole and early diastole. The degree of shunting depends on 1) the size of the defect, and 2) the relative compliance of the two ventricles. There can be minimal right to left shunting in early ventricular systole, especially during inspiration. Symptoms typically occur due to right ventricular and pulmonary vascular volume overload sometimes with resultant pulmonary hypertension.
Types:
• Ostium secundum - occurs in the region of the fossa ovalis (most common)
• Sinus venosus - occurs in the superior-posterior septum
• Ostium primum - occurs in the inferior portion of the septum (often involves mitral valve)
System(s) affected: Cardiovascular, Pulmonary
Genetics: Congenital, associated with multiple syndromes. rarely familial.
Incidence/Prevalence in USA: Accounts for 10% of congenital heart defects
Predominant age: Newborn, but may be diagnosed at any age
Predominant sex: Female > Male (2:1)

SIGNS AND SYMPTOMS
• Childhood symptoms - usually minimal. Can include failure to thrive and frequent pulmonary infections
• Adult symptoms - easy fatigability, dyspnea on exertion, heart failure (late)
• Signs vary according to extent of shunting and include:
• Right ventricular lift
• Palpable pulmonary artery pulse
• Fixed, widely-split S2
• Pulmonic flow murmur
• Low pitched diastolic murmur at left upper sternal border
• Cyanosis and clubbing
• Stroke due to paradoxical emboli

CAUSES Unknown

RISK FACTORS Congenital heart disease family history

DIAGNOSIS

DIFFERENTIAL DIAGNOSIS Other congenital heart disease

LABORATORY N/A
Drugs that may alter lab results: N/A
Disorders that may alter lab results: N/A

PATHOLOGICAL FINDINGS
• Gross defect in atrial septum
• Dilated right atrium
• Enlarged pulmonary artery

SPECIAL TESTS
• ECG findings:
  ◊ Ostium secundum - rightward axis, right ventricular hypertrophy, rSR' pattern
  ◊ Sinus venosus - leftward axis, inverted P wave in lead III
  ◊ Ostium primum - leftward axis
Note: All may be associated with PR prolongation

IMAGING
• X-ray - varying degrees of cardiac enlargement
• Cardiac catheterization (indicated in select patients) demonstrates right ventricle enlargement and location of the shunt
• Echocardiography

DIAGNOSTIC PROCEDURES
• Cardiac angiography
• Echo and Doppler
• Transesophageal echo in adults

TREATMENT

APPROPRIATE HEALTH CARE
Inpatient for work-up and when surgery is indicated

GENERAL MEASURES N/A

SURGICAL MEASURES
• Surgical repair (particularly when the pulmonary systemic flow ratio is ≥ 1.5:1)
• Surgical repair delayed until preschool age (2-4) except for large defects to be repaired earlier
• Small ASD - primary closure with umbrella-like patch via cardiac catheter is experimental
• Surgery if paradoxical emboli result in stroke

ACTIVITY As tolerated

DIET No special diet

PATIENT EDUCATION For patient education materials on this topic, contact: American Heart Association, 7320 Greenville Avenue, Dallas, TX 75231, (214)373-6300

MEDICATIONS

DRUG(S) OF CHOICE
• Antibiotic prophylaxis
• Anticoagulation if paradoxical emboli
Contraindications: N/A
Precautions: N/A
Significant possible interactions: N/A

ALTERNATIVE DRUGS N/A

FOLLOWUP

PATIENT MONITORING
• Until defect has closed
• Routine echocardiography followup

PREVENTION/AVOIDANCE
• Evaluation prior to pregnancy

POSSIBLE COMPLICATIONS
• Congestive heart failure
• Cyanosis
• Late-onset arrhythmias 10-20 years after surgery (5%)
• Stroke
• Pulmonary hypertension
• Eisenmenger's syndrome
• Infective endocarditis

EXPECTED COURSE/PROGNOSIS
• Course - chronic
• 50% mortality by age 50 in untreated patients
• Favorable in surgically treated symptomatic patients

MISCELLANEOUS

ASSOCIATED CONDITIONS
• Mitral stenosis
• Mitral regurgitation
• Anomalous pulmonary venous return
• Multiple congenital syndromes

AGE-RELATED FACTORS
Pediatric: Most frequently appears in this age group
Geriatric: Defects in older persons may still be closed surgically
Others: N/A

PREGNANCY
• Evaluation prior to pregnancy, since condition may worsen

SYNONYMS N/A

ICD-9-CM 429.71 Atrial septal acquired

SEE ALSO
• Ventricular septal defect (VSD)
• Patent ductus arteriosus
• Tetralogy of Fallot
• Pulmonic valvular stenosis
• Aortic valvular stenosis
• Coarctation of the aorta
• Transposition of the great vessels
• Complete atrioventricular (AV) canal
• Tricuspid atresia
• Truncus arteriosus

OTHER NOTES N/A

ABBREVIATIONS N/A

REFERENCES
• Friedman WF, Perloff JK: Congenital heart disease in infancy and childhood. In: Braunwald E, ed. Heart Disease. 4th Ed. Philadelphia, W.B. Saunders Co., 1992
• Hillis DL, Lange RA, Winniford MD, Page RL: Manual of Clinical Problems in Cardiology. New York, Little, Brown and Co., 1995
Illustrations: N/A
Internet references: http://www.5mcc.com

Author(s)
Karil Bellah, MD

Attention deficit hyperactivity disorder

BASICS

DESCRIPTION A behavior problem characterized by a short attention span, low frustration tolerance, impulsivity, distractibility, and usually, hyperactivity. This can result in poor school performance, difficulty in peer relationships, and parent/child conflict.
System(s) affected: Nervous
Genetics: Familial pattern
Incidence/Prevalence in USA: 5% of school aged children
Predominant age:
• Onset < 7 years old
• Lasts into adolescence and adulthood
• 50% meet diagnostic criteria by age 4
Predominant sex: Males > Females (5:1)

SIGNS AND SYMPTOMS
DSM-IV Criteria - 6 or more inattention criteria and/or 6 or more hyperactivity/impulsivity criteria
• Inattention
  ◊ Careless mistakes in tasks
  ◊ Difficulty sustaining attention
  ◊ Doesn't seem to listen
  ◊ Doesn't follow through or finish
  ◊ Difficulty organizing tasks
  ◊ Avoids tasks which require sustained mental effort
  ◊ Loses things
  ◊ Easily distracted
  ◊ Forgetful
• Hyperactivity/impulsivity
  ◊ Fidgets
  ◊ Difficulty remaining seated
  ◊ Runs or climbs excessively
  ◊ Difficulty playing quietly
  ◊ Acts as if "driven by a motor"
  ◊ Talks excessively
  ◊ Blurts out answers before question is complete
  ◊ Has difficulty awaiting turn
  ◊ Interrupts others

CAUSES Polyfactorial

RISK FACTORS
• Family history
• Co-morbid conditions (associated with, but not caused by)
  ◊ Learning disabilities
  ◊ Tourette's
  ◊ Mood disorders
  ◊ Oppositional defiant disorder
  ◊ Conduct disorder

DIAGNOSIS

DIFFERENTIAL DIAGNOSIS
• Refer to DSM IV-R (see References)
• Activity level appropriate for age
• Dysfunctional family situation
• Learning disability (dyslexia, etc.))
• Hearing/vision disorder
• Oppositional/defiant disorder (see DSM IV-R)
• Conduct disorder (see DSM IV-R)
• Lead poisoning
• Medication reaction (decongestant, antihistamine, theophylline, phenobarbital)
• Tourette's
• Pervasive developmental delay (autism)
• Hyperthyroidism (rare)
• Absence seizures (attention deficit only)

LABORATORY Rarely needed, can check lead level
Drugs that may alter lab results: N/A
Disorders that may alter lab results: N/A

PATHOLOGICAL FINDINGS
• "Soft" neurological signs - nonspecific (Romberg, mixed hand preference, etc.)
• Motor tics can be present (cough, noise, scratching)

SPECIAL TESTS
• Learning disability evaluation (mismatch of IQ and achievement) - usually by school
• Behavior rating scales to be completed by parents and teachers. Often repeated after therapy is started to gauge differences (e.g., Conner's scale, AcTERs scale).
• Good psychosocial evaluation of home environment
• Continuous Performance Tests - rapid fire computer test - high false negative
• See References

IMAGING Not needed

DIAGNOSTIC PROCEDURES Diagnosis is by DSM-IV criteria. (Do not need EEG unless symptoms highly suggestive of seizure disorder [e.g., absence seizures]).

TREATMENT

APPROPRIATE HEALTH CARE
Outpatient

GENERAL MEASURES
• Parent/school/patient education
• Work closely with teacher
• Avoid unproved therapies

SURGICAL MEASURES N/A

ACTIVITY
• Allow for increased activity in safe environment
• Often respond well to water play/bathtubs

DIET No dietary changes have been proven to help ADHD. Parents can experiment with non-harmful diets by eliminating:
• Sugar
• Dyes
• Additives

PATIENT EDUCATION
• Key points for parents:
  ◊ Strong emphasis on behavior therapy such as token systems
  ◊ Reinforce good behavior (with rewards and attention)
  ◊ Make eye contact with each request
  ◊ One task at a time
  ◊ Time out (brief) for problems
  ◊ Stop behavior before it escalates
  ◊ Find things child is good at and emphasize these
  ◊ Some families benefit from "anger training," "social training" and family therapy
  ◊ Educate parents to realistic expectations
  ◊ Awareness of child advocate groups and support groups
  ◊ Help to deal with negative feelings
• Key points for teachers:
  ◊ Short work sessions
  ◊ Clear rules
  ◊ Immediate consequences
  ◊ Reinforce good behavior
  ◊ Coordinate homework with parent with daily assignment notebook
  ◊ Have second set of books at home
• Support groups
  ◊ CHADD - Children and Adults with ADD, 499 NW 70th Ave, Suite 101, Plantation, FL 33317; 800-233-4050
  ◊ ADD Warehouse 300 NW 70th Ave, Suite 102, Plantation, FL 33317; 800-233-9273
  ◊ AD-IN - ADD Information Network, 475 Hillside Ave, Needham, MA 02174; 781-455-9895
  ◊ LDA - Learning Disabilities Association, 4156 Library Rd, Pittsburg, PA 15234

MEDICATIONS

DRUG(S) OF CHOICE
- Methylphenidate (Ritalin): 0.3-0.7 mg/kg/day up to 60 mg/day, lasts 3-4 hours, given am, noon, and ±4 pm, alter dose q week until effective. Ritalin SR - less effective
- Pemoline (Cylert): 18.75 mg-112.5 mg/day, long acting, alter dose q 2 weeks until effective, chewable tablets available
- Additional information:
  ◊ Many children need 4pm dose for homework and peer interactions
  ◊ Long acting drugs may be less effective, and should not be discontinued on weekends and short holidays
  ◊ End point is - improved grades, improved rating scales, acceptable family interactions, and improved peer interactions
  ◊ If not responding, check compliance and consider another diagnosis
  ◊ Methylphenidate has become a drug of abuse and should be monitored carefully - 20 mg nongeneric have highest street value
  ◊ Drug holidays should only be given if family/peer relationships aren't harmed
  ◊ Some children experience withdrawal (tearfulness, agitation) after a missed dose

Contraindications: N/A

Precautions: The manufacturer recommends:
- Don't crush sustained-release tablets
- Monitoring LFTs in pemoline every 3-6 months
- In coexisting Tourette's syndrome, methylphenidate may unmask tics
- May monitor CBC in methylphenidate

Significant possible interactions: N/A

ALTERNATIVE DRUGS
- Dextroamphetamine (Dexedrine) - 0.1-0.5 mg/kg/day, rarely used, indicated in age 3 and up, comes in elixir form
- Dextroamphetamine-amphetamine (Adderall) 2.5-20 mg q 4-6 hours. Longer acting; higher addiction potential
- Clonidine - helpful for motor tics - 4-5 µg/kg/day
- Tricyclics - useful if stimulants not working, or there is an accompanying mood disorder; not officially indicated, consider EKG to rule out conduction abnormalities (sudden death has been reported). Useful in older children when methylphenidate is less effective.
- Selective serotonin reuptake inhibitors (SSRIs) have not shown any clear benefit

FOLLOWUP

PATIENT MONITORING
- Parent/teacher rating scales (i.e., Conner's scale) initially, in 2 weeks, and regularly
- Office visits to monitor side effects and efficacy:
  ◊ Increased blood pressure
  ◊ Insomnia
  ◊ Headache
  ◊ Abdominal pain
  ◊ Poor growth
- Some physicians obtain look-alike placebo Ritalin from CIBA for blinded trials

PREVENTION/AVOIDANCE
- Children are at risk for: abuse, depression, social isolation
- Parents need regular support and advice
- Establish contact with teacher each school year

POSSIBLE COMPLICATIONS
- Medications can cause headaches, abdominal pain (take with meals), growth delay
- Untreated ADHD can lead to: failing school, parental abuse, social isolation, poor self esteem
- If appetite poor, offer food early am and late

EXPECTED COURSE/PROGNOSIS
- May last through school years and into adulthood (25%)
- It becomes easier to control with increasing age
- Encourage career choices which allow patient autonomy and mobility
- No increased incidence of delinquency unless other co-morbid features exist (e.g., conduct disorder)

MISCELLANEOUS

ASSOCIATED CONDITIONS   See Risk Factors

AGE-RELATED FACTORS
Pediatric: N/A
Geriatric: N/A
Others: N/A

PREGNANCY   Avoid stimulant medications in pregnancy

SYNONYMS
- Attention deficit disorder
- Hyperactivity

ICD-9-CM
314.0 Attention deficit disorder
314.01 ADD with hyperactivity

SEE ALSO   N/A

OTHER NOTES   N/A

ABBREVIATIONS
ADD = Attention Deficit Disorder
LFT = liver function test

REFERENCES
- Barkley RA: ADHD - A Handbook for Diagnosis and Treatment. 2nd Ed. New York, Guilford Press, 1998
- Behrman RE, Kliegman M, eds: Nelson Textbook of Pediatrics, Philadelphia, W.B. Saunders Co., 1994
- American Psychiatric Association: Diagnostic and Statistical Manual of Mental Disorders. 4th Ed, Revised. Washington, DC, American Psychiatric Association, 1994
- The Parents Guide to Attention Deficit Disorders, Hawthorne Education Services, Columbia, Missouri 65205, 1-314-874-1710
- Barkley RA: Defiant Children. 2nd Ed. New York, Guilford Press, 1997
- Barkley RA: Taking Charge of ADHD. New York, Guilford Press, 1995

Illustrations: N/A
Internet references: http://www.5mcc.com

Author(s)
Laura L. Novak, MD

Autism

BASICS

DESCRIPTION Autism is a pervasive developmental disorder of early childhood characterized by severe impairment in:
• Effective social skills
• Absent or impaired language development
• Repetitive and/or stereotyped activities and interests, especially inanimate objects

System(s) affected: Nervous

Genetics: High concordance in monozygotic twins, increased prevalence in siblings

Incidence/Prevalence in USA: 3-5 per 10,000 school age children

Predominant age: Onset prior to age 3, but generally abnormal development is apparent well before

Predominant sex: Male > Female (5:1)

SIGNS AND SYMPTOMS
• Impairment in social interaction:
◊ Inadequate or lack of use of multiple non-verbal behaviors, such as postures and facial expression
◊ Failure to develop appropriate peer relationships
◊ Lack of sharing interests and achievements
◊ Lack of social and/or emotional reciprocity
• Communication impairment:
◊ Delay or lack of development of spoken language without accompanying alternative modes of communication
◊ Impairment in initiating and sustaining conversation
◊ Idiosyncratic language with stereotyped or repetitive usage
◊ Lack of developmentally appropriate play, especially imitative
• Repetitive and stereotyped patterns of behavior:
◊ Abnormal preoccupations either in intensity or focus
◊ Inflexibility to non-functional activities
◊ Stereotyped or repetitive motor mannerisms
◊ Preoccupation with inanimate objects and their parts

CAUSES Unknown

RISK FACTORS Associated with increased risks during pregnancy, labor and delivery. Maternal rubella.

DIAGNOSIS

DIFFERENTIAL DIAGNOSIS
• Other mental and CNS disorders including:
◊ Schizophrenia
◊ Elective mutism
◊ Language disorder
◊ Mental retardation
◊ Stereotyped movement disorder
• Other pervasive developmental disorders including:
◊ Rett's disorder
◊ Childhood disintegrative disorder
◊ Asperger's disorder

LABORATORY N/A (other than to rule-out associated conditions)

Drugs that may alter lab results: N/A

Disorders that may alter lab results: N/A

PATHOLOGICAL FINDINGS N/A

SPECIAL TESTS
• Psychological testing using early childhood instruments, such as the Bailey or using non-verbal instruments, such as the Leiter
• Intellectual level needs to be established and monitored, as it is one of the best measures of prognosis
• EEG to rule-out brain damage and associated conditions. Autistic children have a markedly higher incidence of epilepsy which increases with age.

IMAGING Could be useful in ruling out associated conditions

DIAGNOSTIC PROCEDURES
• Developmental history
• Psychiatric examination
• Psychological testing
• Comprehensive language assessment

TREATMENT

APPROPRIATE HEALTH CARE
Comprehensive structured educational programming of a sustained and intensive design

GENERAL MEASURES Parent support groups and respite programs

SURGICAL MEASURES N/A

ACTIVITY As tolerated by the child

DIET No special diet

PATIENT EDUCATION
• The Autism Society of America, 8601 Georgia Ave., Suite 503, Silver Spring, MD 20910; 301-565-0433
• Atwood T: Asparger's Syndrome: A Guide for Parents, Jerrica Kingsley (publisher).

MEDICATIONS

DRUG(S) OF CHOICE None
Contraindications: N/A
Precautions: N/A
Significant possible interactions: N/A

ALTERNATIVE DRUGS
• Stimulant medications may be used to address concomitant symptoms of attention deficit disorder, such as impulsiveness, hyperactivity and inattention
• Fenfluramine, probably effects attentional symptoms as does other stimulants
• SSRI antidepressants, such as fluoxetine and sertraline have shown some help in reducing ritualistic behavior and improving moods
• Clomipramine (Anafranil), a tricyclic antidepressant, has been reported to decrease some forms of self-injurious behavior, obsessive/compulsive symptoms and compulsive, aggressive behavior
• Buspirone (BuSpar) has in some individuals reduced hyperactivity and stereotyped behavior
• Neuroleptics have been used with limited effectiveness
• Risperidone (Risperdal) in low doses has helped in some case reports

FOLLOWUP

PATIENT MONITORING
• Constant by caregivers. As indicated by physician, prescribed medical management.
• Intellectual and language testing every two years in childhood.

PREVENTION/AVOIDANCE   None known

POSSIBLE COMPLICATIONS   Increasing incidents of seizure disorders

EXPECTED COURSE/PROGNOSIS
• Prognosis is closely related to initial intellectual abilities with only 20% functioning above the mentally retarded level
• Communicative language development before age five is also associated with a better outcome
• The general expected course is for a life-long need of supervised structured care. Only 1-2% become independent.

MISCELLANEOUS

ASSOCIATED CONDITIONS
• Mental retardation
• Attention deficit/hyperactivity disorder
• Phenylketonuria, tuberous sclerosis, and fragile X syndrome

AGE-RELATED FACTORS
Pediatric: Onset seen only in children under three
Geriatric: N/A
Others: N/A

PREGNANCY   Increased risk of autism in complications of pregnancy, labor and delivery

SYNONYMS
• Early infantile autism
• Childhood autism
• Kanner's autism
• Pervasive developmental disorder

ICD-9-CM
299.0 Infantile autism

SEE ALSO
• Attention deficit hyperactivity disorder
• Mental retardation

OTHER NOTES
Refer also to Asparger's syndrome

ABBREVIATIONS   N/A

REFERENCES
• Volkmar FR, Cohen DJ: Autism: Current Concepts In: Volkmar FR, ed. Child and Adolescent Psychiatric Clinics of North American. Philadelphia, W.B. Saunders Co., 3;1:43-52, January, 1994
• Volkmar FR: Autism and the Pervasive Developmental Disorders. In: Lewis M, ed. Child and Adolescent Psychiatry; A Comprehensive Textbook. Baltimore, Williams and Wilkins, 1991
• Diagnostic and Statistical Manual of Mental Disorders. 4th Ed. American Psychiatric Association, Washington, D.C., 1994
Illustrations: N/A
Internet references: http://www.5mcc.com

Author(s)
C. Van Devere, MD

Balanitis

BASICS

DESCRIPTION
Balanitis: inflammation of glans penis
Posthitis: inflammation of the foreskin
System(s) affected:
Skin/Exocrine, Renal/Urologic
Genetics: N/A
Incidence/Prevalence in USA: N/A
Predominant age: Adult
Predominant sex: Male only

SIGNS AND SYMPTOMS
• Pain, penile
• Dysuria
• Drainage, site of infection
• Erythema
• Prepuce swelling
• Ulceration
• Plaques

CAUSES
• Allergic reaction (condom latex, contraceptive jelly)
• Fungal (Candida albicans) and bacterial infections (Borrelia vincentii, streptococci)
• Fixed drug eruption (sulfa, tetracycline, barbital)
• Plasma cell infiltration (Zoon's balanitis)
• Autodigestion by activated transplant exocrine enzymes

RISK FACTORS
• Presence of foreskin
• Oral antibiotics in male infants can predispose to Candida balanitis

DIAGNOSIS

DIFFERENTIAL DIAGNOSIS
• Leukoplakia
• Lichen planus
• Psoriasis
• Reiter's syndrome
• Lichen sclerosus et atrophicus
• Erythroplasia of Queyrat
• Balanitis Xerotica obliterans

LABORATORY
• Microbiology culture
• Wet mount
• Serology for syphilis
• Serum glucose
Drugs that may alter lab results: None
Disorders that may alter lab results: None

PATHOLOGICAL FINDINGS   Plasma cells infiltration with Zoon's balanitis

SPECIAL TESTS   Biopsy, if balanitis persistent

IMAGING   N/A

DIAGNOSTIC PROCEDURES   Biopsy, if persistent

TREATMENT

APPROPRIATE HEALTH CARE
Outpatient

GENERAL MEASURES
• Warm compresses or sitz baths
• Local hygiene

SURGICAL MEASURES   Consider circumcision as preventative measure

ACTIVITY   No limitations

DIET   No special diet

PATIENT EDUCATION
• Need for appropriate hygiene
• Avoidance of known allergens

Balanitis

MEDICATIONS

DRUG(S) OF CHOICE
• Fungal - clotrimazole (Lotrimin) 1% bid to affected area or nystatin (Mycostatin) bid to qid to affected area
• Bacterial - bacitracin qid to affected area or neomycin-polymyxin B-bacitracin (Neosporin) qid to affected area. If infection, cephalosporin or sulfa drug by mouth or injection.
• Dermatitis - topical steroids qid to affected area
• Zoon's balanitis - topical steroids qid
Contraindications: Refer to manufacturer's profile of each drug
Precautions: Refer to manufacturer's profile of each drug
Significant possible interactions: Refer to manufacturer's profile of each drug

ALTERNATIVE DRUGS N/A

FOLLOWUP

PATIENT MONITORING Every 1-2 weeks
until etiology has been established. Persistent balanitis may require biopsy to rule out malignancy.

PREVENTION/AVOIDANCE
• Proper hygiene and avoidance of allergens
• Circumcision

POSSIBLE COMPLICATIONS
• Meatal stenosis
• Premalignant changes from chronic irritations
• Urinary tract infections

EXPECTED COURSE/PROGNOSIS
With appropriate treatment it should resolve

MISCELLANEOUS

ASSOCIATED CONDITIONS Diabetes
mellitus

AGE-RELATED FACTORS
Pediatric: Oral antibiotics predispose infants to candida balanitis
Geriatric: Condom catheters can predispose to balanitis
Others: N/A

PREGNANCY N/A

SYNONYMS N/A

ICD-9-CM
607.1 balanitis
112.2 candida
099.8 venereal

SEE ALSO N/A

OTHER NOTES N/A

ABBREVIATIONS N/A

REFERENCES
• Gillenwater JY, Grayhack JT, Howard SS, Duckett JW: Adult and Pediatric Urology. 2nd Ed. Mosby Year Book, Philadelphia, 1991
• Zoon JJ: Balanoposthite chronique cireonscrite benigne à plasmacytes (contra èrythroplasie de Queyrat). Dermatologica 1952;105:1
• Tom WW, Munda R, First MR, et al: Autodigestion of the glans, penis and urethra by activated transplant pancreatic exocrine enzymes. Surgery 1987;102:99-101
Illustrations: 2 available on CD-ROM
Internet references: http://www.5mcc.com

Author(s)
James P. Miller, MD, FACS, FAAP
Timothy L. Black, MD, FACS, FAAP

Barotitis media

BASICS

DESCRIPTION Acute or chronic traumatic inflammation of the middle ear space secondary to the rapid development of a negative (or less commonly a positive) pressure differential between the surrounding atmosphere of the external canal and the middle ear compartments (tympanic cavity, eustachian tube, and mastoid air cells) This situation is brought about by the inability of the eustachian tube to adequately equilibrate the middle ear air pressure with the moment-to-moment changes in the environmental atmospheric pressures while descending or ascending in air (flight) and/or especially in water (diving). This causes the retraction or protraction of the tympanic membrane with subsequent inflammation and/or rupture. This also may cause asymmetric pressure stimulation of the inner ear and vestibular end-organ.
System(s) affected: Nervous
Genetics: N/A
Incidence/Prevalence in USA: The most common medical disorder experienced by SCUBA divers. Also highly prevalent among aircraft flight personnel (especially high-performance jet aircraft), passengers, and sky divers.
Predominant age: All ages
Predominant sex: Male = Female

SIGNS AND SYMPTOMS
• Abrupt in onset
• Otalgia (ear pain)
• Feeling of fullness in ear
• Conductive hearing loss
• Dizziness
• Tinnitus
• Vertigo
• Nausea and vomiting
• Transient facial paralysis
• With tympanic membrane rupture the ability to blow air and/or fluid out one's ear while performing a Valsalva maneuver or when sneezing
• Crying in children (which is their only means of autoinflation)

CAUSES
• Rapid descent or ascent with eustachian tube obstruction
  ◊ Eustachian tube lock
  ◊ Upper respiratory infections - sinusitis, rhinitis, tonsillitis, and adenoiditis
  ◊ Overzealous forceful Valsalva maneuver (in ascent with vestibular stimulation)
  ◊ Allergic rhinitis
  ◊ Non-allergic rhinitis with eosinophilia
  ◊ Obstructing nasal polyps
  ◊ Deviated nasal septum
  ◊ Congenital abnormalities of inner/middle ear (cleft palate)
  ◊ Nasopharyngeal tumors
• Rapid descent or ascent with external ear canal occlusion
  ◊ Otitis externa (swimmer's ear)
  ◊ Impacted cerumen
  ◊ Ear plugs

• Trauma to external and middle ear
  ◊ Activities involving external ear trauma - boxing, soccer, water skiing, accidents, etc.
  ◊ Overzealous use of cotton swab in cleaning ear canals

RISK FACTORS
• Participating in high risk activities without adequate eustachian tube autoinflation (Valsalva maneuver, swallowing) and/or with any of the listed causes of eustachian tube and external ear canal dysfunction:
• SCUBA diving
• Airplane flight
• Sky diving
• High altitude mountain travelers
• High altitude elevator rides
• Hyperbaric oxygen chamber therapy
• High impact sports
• Infants and young otologically healthy children have difficulty in dilating the eustachian tube (by swallowing) even at small pressure changes and therefore are at higher risk (especially with upper respiratory infection)

DIAGNOSIS

DIFFERENTIAL DIAGNOSIS
• Serous otitis media
• Acute and chronic otitis media
• External otitis
• Myringitis bullosa

LABORATORY N/A
Drugs that may alter lab results: N/A
Disorders that may alter lab results: N/A

PATHOLOGICAL FINDINGS
• Tympanic membrane retraction or protraction with hemotympanum or rupture
• Edema of mucosal lining and capillary engorgement with transudation of middle ear effusion
• Inner ear involvement with rupture of the round or oval windows and leakage of perilymph into the middle ear and perilymphatic fistula development

SPECIAL TESTS N/A

IMAGING Only to rule out suspected nasopharyngeal tumor or sinusitis

DIAGNOSTIC PROCEDURES
• Otoscopic exam
• Audiogram - conductive (middle ear) versus mixed (inner ear) loss
• Surgical exploration to rule out inner ear involvement if suspected

TREATMENT

APPROPRIATE HEALTH CARE
• Outpatient generally
• Inpatient for complicating emergencies, e.g., incapacitating pain requiring myringotomy, large tympanic perforation requiring tympanoplasty

GENERAL MEASURES
• Perform Valsalva method of eustachian tube autoinflation (patient inhales then closes nose with thumb and index finger on nasal alae, then exhales with mouth closed). This will equalize pressures, relieve pain, and restore hearing. This usually needs to be repeated several times during descent or ascent.
• Nasal decongestant spray with repeated applications
• Antihistamines
• If the suggested maneuvers are unsuccessful return to higher altitude if possible and repeat Valsalva
• If ear block occurs, then outpatient politzerization must be performed followed by systemic and oral decongestants
• If associated infection, treat with appropriate antibiotics

SURGICAL MEASURES N/A

ACTIVITY
• No flying or diving until complete resolution of all signs and symptoms and Valsalva maneuver can be performed
• In severe cases, bedrest

DIET Avoid food allergens that cause rhinitis

PATIENT EDUCATION
• Teach Valsalva maneuver
• Educate on how to create allergy-free environment
• Divers Alert Network of Duke University Medical Center, information line, (919) 684-2948

MEDICATIONS

DRUG(S) OF CHOICE
• Decongestants:
◊ 0.05% oxymetazoline (Afrin, Afrin 12-Hour) two initial sprays 5 minutes apart then q12h
◊ 0.05% phenylephrine (Neo-Synephrine) two initial sprays 5 minutes apart then q12h
◊ Pseudoephedrine (Sudafed 12-hour, Afrinol) 120 mg q12h po
◊ Phenylpropanolamine (Propagest) 25 mg q12h po
• Antihistamines for allergic component:
◊ Diphenhydramine (Benadryl) 25-50 mg q6h
◊ Loratadine (Claritin) 10 mg qday
◊ Fexofenadine (Allegra) 60 mg bid (60 mg qday in patients with decreased renal function)

Contraindications:
• Previous allergic reactions
• Hypertension
• Drowsiness
• Erythromycin and terfenadine or astemizole; cardiac toxicity.

Precautions:
• All medications must be used on the ground to rule out idiosyncratic reactions that could incapacitate in an airplane or underwater environment
• Elderly are more susceptible to drug side effects, especially with diphenhydramine

Significant possible interactions: Refer to manufacturer's profile of each drug. Terfenadine and astemizole have many possible interactions. Avoid with macrolide antibiotics, ketoconazole.

ALTERNATIVE DRUGS
Cetirizine (Zyrtec)

FOLLOWUP

PATIENT MONITORING
• Otoscopic until symptoms clear
• In severe cases, audiograms

PREVENTION/AVOIDANCE
• Avoid altitude changes with any risk factors for eustachian tube dysfunction
• Chewing gum while flying especially for children
• Use of recommended medications before the activity

POSSIBLE COMPLICATIONS
• Permanent hearing loss
• Ruptured tympanic membranes
• Serous otitis media

EXPECTED COURSE/PROGNOSIS
• Ear block - hours to days with complete resolution and return to flight or diving in days to weeks
• Tympanic rupture - weeks to months

MISCELLANEOUS

ASSOCIATED CONDITIONS
• Aerosinusitis
• Aerodontalgia
• Face mask squeeze
• Epistaxis
• Alternobaric vertigo
• Unequal caloric stimulation vertigo
• Anxiety - leading to panic attack
• Temporomandibular joint syndrome
• Inner ear cochlear damage and/or perilymph fistula

AGE-RELATED FACTORS
Pediatric: Healthy children have difficulty in dilating the eustachian tube (by swallowing) even at small pressure changes and therefore are at higher risk (especially with upper respiratory infection)
Geriatric: Drug side effects
Others: N/A

PREGNANCY Increased nasal congestion

SYNONYMS
• Aerotitis
• Otitic barotrauma
• Middle ear barotrauma
• Middle ear squeeze

ICD-9-CM
993.0 barotrauma, otic
993.1 barotrauma, sinus

SEE ALSO N/A

OTHER NOTES N/A

ABBREVIATIONS
SCUBA = self-contained underwater breathing apparatus

REFERENCES
• Paparella MM, Shumrick DA, et al, eds: Otolaryngology. 4th Ed. Philadelphia, W.B. Saunders Co., 1991
• Dehart R, ed: Fundamentals of Aerospace Medicine. Philadelphia, Lea & Febiger, 1985
Illustrations: N/A
Internet references: http://www.5mcc.com

Author(s)
Smith L. Johnston, III, MD, MS

Bartonella infections

BASICS

DESCRIPTION Bartonella infections cause manifestations in two broad categories:
• Localized skin lesions and prominent regional lymphadenitis, i.e., typical cat scratch disease (CSD). Atypical CSD manifestations often represent disseminated infection.
• Primary bacteremia, potential for persistent disseminated infection with localized inflammatory (and neovascular) lesions in a variety of organ systems and/or ongoing bacteremia.
System(s) affected: Nervous, Cardiovascular, Musculoskeletal, Pulmonary, Gastrointestinal, Skin/Exocrine, Hemic/Lymphatic/Immunologic
Genetics: No defined genetic predisposition
Incidence/Prevalence in USA:
• Non-B. bacilliformis infections:
  ◊ CSD: estimated 9.3/100,000 people (approximately 25,000 cases annually)
• Others, no incidence estimates
Predominant age:
• B. henselae infections:
  ◊ CSD: 55% in persons < 18 years old
  ◊ BA/BP, bacteremia, endocarditis, other syndromes: predominantly adults
Predominant sex: Non-B. bacilliformis infections: Male > Female

SIGNS AND SYMPTOMS
• Carrión's disease (the spectrum of B. bacilliformis infection)
  ◊ Oroya fever (acute bacteremia): abrupt onset 3 weeks after inoculation, morbid course; severe anemia due to bacterial invasion of erythrocytes, many complications
  ◊ Asymptomatic persistent bacteremia: <15% of Oroya fever survivors not treated with antibiotics
  ◊ Verruga peruana: crops of nodular angiomatous skin lesions months after Oroya fever; mucosal and internal lesions also; involute in months to years
• Typical CSD (89% of cases)
  ◊ 4-6 days after inoculation: 50-75% develop 2-3 mm macule at the trauma site; progresses to a papule or pustule
  ◊ Regional adenopathy 1-8 weeks post-inoculation; sole manifestation in up to 50%
  ◊ Nodes involved: 80% upper extremities, neck, head
  ◊ Suppuration of involved nodes: 15%.
  ◊ Malaise and/or fever: 30% of patients
  ◊ Spontaneous resolution: 2-4 months for majority
• Atypical CSD (11% of cases)
  ◊ Parinaud's oculoglandular syndrome: granulomatous conjunctivitis and ipsilateral preauricular lymphadenitis
  ◊ Neuroretinitis: usually unilateral; macular star exudate, papilledema, retinal nodules, angiomatous subretinal changes; self-limited, with return of visual acuity to near-baseline; concurrent B. henselae bacteremia found in some

  ◊ Encephalopathy: mild-profound changes of higher cortical functions; seizures; neurologic sequelae rare
  ◊ Other manifestations self-limited, sequelae rare: granulomatous hepatitis/splenitis, osteolysis, atypical pneumonitis, others
• Bacteremia due to non-B. bacilliformis species: short-term fatality uncommon
  ◊ B. quintana: (Eponyms: Trench fever, Wolhynia fever, shin-bone fever, quintan fever) Incubation days-weeks; sudden onset of fever, non-specific symptoms/signs; self-limited illness may be brief (4-5 days), prolonged (2-6 weeks), most commonly paroxysmal (3-5 episodes of 5 days duration).
  ◊ B. henselae: HIV-infected: insidious onset of fatigue, malaise, aches, weight loss, recurring fevers, headache; localizing findings uncommon. HIV-uninfected: abrupt onset of fever, may persist or become relapsing; myalgias, arthralgias, headache; localizing findings unusual; asymptomatic persistence can evolve.
• Endocarditis: fever, new or changed heart murmur
• Bacillary angiomatosis/peliosis (BA/BP): neovascular proliferation disorders
  ◊ BA: mostly immunocompromised hosts, e.g., HIV-infected; involves skin (crops of subcutaneous or dermal nodules, and/or skin-colored to purple papules; may ulcerate with serous or bloody drainage, and crusting), regional lymph nodes, internal organs; B. henselae and B. quintana both inculpated
  ◊ BP involves liver and spleen in HIV-infected and other immunosuppressed persons; can involve lymph nodes as well; nonspecific clinical manifestations
• Neurologic in HIV-infected: cognitive dysfunction, behavioral disturbances; may be mistaken for HIV-related or other dementia, psychiatric disease

CAUSES
• B. bacilliformis: Carrión's disease (limited to the Andes mountains)
• B. quintana: Trench fever, BA/BP, endocarditis
• B. henselae: Acute and persistent bacteremia, BA/BP complex, non-neovascular inflammation including endocarditis and CSD, neurologic manifestations
• B. elizabethae: Bacteremia with endocarditis (1 reported case)
• B. clarridgiae: CSD (1 reported case)

RISK FACTORS
• Vector exposure with cutaneous inoculation
  ◊ B. bacilliformis: Sandflies of the genus Lutzomyia (formerly Phlebotomus)
  ◊ B. quintana: Human body louse, possibly others as yet unidentified
  ◊ B. henselae: Domestic cat (especially scratch/bite from kitten < 1 year old), possibly cat fleas, possibly ticks
  ◊ B. elizabethae: unknown
• B. vinsonii: Bacteremia (one reported case)
• Cell-mediated immune dysfunction (a role in BA/BP, possibly endocarditis)
  ◊ HIV infection, especially with CD4+ lymphocyte count < 100/μL
  ◊ Chronic corticosteroid, azathioprine, cyclophosphamide, cyclosporine, ethanol

DIAGNOSIS

DIFFERENTIAL DIAGNOSIS
• Typical CSD: other causes of unilateral lymphadenopathy: Sporothrix schenckii, Pasturella species, Yersinia pestis, Francisella tularensis, mycobacteria, Erysipelothrix rhusiopathiae, staphylococci, streptococci, other agents associated injection drug use, lymphoma, metastatic malignancy
• Atypical CSD: other agents causing similar syndromes
• Non-bacilliformis Bartonella species bacteremia syndromes
  ◊ In immunocompromised, especially HIV-infected: Cryptococcus neoformans, Histoplasma capsulatum, Coccidioides immitis, Mycobacterium avium-complex
  ◊ After recent arthropod exposure: rickettsial infections, tularemia, plague, babesiosis, borreliosis (location-dependent).
  ◊ After cat/dog scratch/bite: Pasturella species infection
  ◊ Viral illnesses: influenza, infectious mononucleosis, acute hepatitis, etc.
• Endocarditis: other fastidious/slow-growing bacteria associated with endocarditis, e.g. species of Haemophilus, Actinobacillus, Cardiobacterium, Eikenella, Kingella, Coxiella
• BA/BP: Kaposi's sarcoma; pyogenic granuloma
• Neurologic in HIV-infected: other causes of encephalopathy, e.g., primary HIV-related, tertiary syphilis, cryptococcal meningitis, toxoplasmosis of brain, progressive multifocal leukoencephalopathy, alcohol or drug abuse

LABORATORY
• Non-bacilliformis Bartonella spp
  ◊ Blood cultures: lysis-centrifugation (Isolator) cultures plated on blood or chocolate agar, incubated at 35-37°C in 5% CO2 > 2 weeks; enriched broth media, e.g. Bactec, incubated at 35-37°C in 5% CO2 >2 weeks and subculture to agar if bacilli detected by periodic acridine orange staining.
  ◊ Tissue cultures: recovery from tissue homogenate plated on blood or chocolate agar may require >4 weeks
  ◊ 1st generation serologic tests available in reference labs
Drugs that may alter lab results:
Antibiotics: cultures falsely negative
Disorders that may alter lab results: N/A

PATHOLOGICAL FINDINGS
• Verruga peruana: neovascular proliferation, bacteria uncommonly identified
• CSD: stellate abscesses, mixed inflammatory infiltrates, granulomata, follicular hyperplasia of lymph nodes; bacilli in tissue demonstrable by silver impregnation stains (Warthin-Starry or Steiner) in about 1/3 cases
• Endocarditis: Warthin-Starry stained bacilli may be seen in vegetations

- BA/BP
  ◊ BA lesions: lobular proliferations of small blood vessels containing cuboidal endothelial cells interspersed with inflammatory cells, mostly neutrophils. Fibrillar- or granular-appearing amphophilic material often seen in interstitium hematoxylin and eosin stain. Warthin-Starry stain or electron microscopy demonstrate these to be clusters of bacilli.
  ◊ BP: involved organs contain blood-filled, partially endothelial cell-lined cystic structures and surrounding clumps of bacilli (identified by Warthin-Starry stain) in the midst of inflammatory cells.
- Neurologic in HIV-infected: little information

SPECIAL TESTS
- Skin testing reagents: not commercially available or standardized
- Co-incubation of tissue homogenates with cell culture lines to enhance culture recovery; PCR and immunohistochemical labeling for non-culture detection in tissue: currently remain research tools

IMAGING Ultrasonography or CT as indicated

DIAGNOSTIC PROCEDURES
- Biopsies for histology/culture of cutaneous nodules, lymph nodes, or internal organs as necessary
- Typical CSD; traditionally, diagnosis required 3 of 4 criteria fulfilled:
(1) Animal contact (usually cat or dog) resulting in a scratch, abrasion or ocular lesion
(2) Positive skin test with cat scratch antigen (not available commercially)
(3) Characteristic lymph node pathology
(4) Absence of evidence of other causes of lymphadenopathy
- Serologic testing preferable alternative to skin testing
- Atypical CSD: compatible syndrome, absence of other evident cause; positive skin or serologic testing
- Bacteremia: clinical suspicion; use of appropriate culture methods
- Endocarditis: compatible clinical syndrome, evidence of valve lesion (ultrasonographic or tissue), positive culture of blood or valve (or non-culture demonstration, e.g., immunohistochemistry, polymerase chain reaction [PCR])
- BA/BP: biopsy for definitive diagnosis; presumptive diagnosis by response to appropriate antibiotics
- Neurologic in HIV-infected: (1) compatible clinical syndrome plus elevated antibodies in CSF or detection in CSF by culture or PCR, (2) no other cause

TREATMENT

APPROPRIATE HEALTH CARE
- Outpatient for uncomplicated infection
- Initial hospitalization may be necessary for complications

GENERAL MEASURES
- CSD: symptom-specific supportive therapy, e.g., aspiration of suppurative lymph nodes to alleviate pain
- Other syndromes (perhaps including CSD-associated neuroretinitis and encephalopathy): antibiotic therapy

SURGICAL MEASURES N/A

ACTIVITY Fully active if uncomplicated

DIET No special diet

PATIENT EDUCATION N/A

MEDICATIONS

DRUG(S) OF CHOICE
- B. bacilliformis infection: chloramphenicol 500 mg po qid for 1 week
- For typical CSD: no proven response to many agents including erythromycin, doxycycline, penicillin, cephalosporins; anecdotal reports of efficacy of rifampin > ciprofloxacin > gentamicin > trimethoprim-sulfamethoxazole. One placebo-controlled trial of oral azithromycin found some efficacy for 5 day course.
  ◊ Azithromycin dose:
   - Adults and children > 45 kg: 500 mg on day 1, 250 mg daily on days 2-5
   - Children ≤ 45 kg: 10 mg/kg on day 1; 5 mg/kg daily on days 2-5
- Non-bacilliformis Bartonella infections including bacteremia without endocarditis, cutaneous BA + local lymph node involvement, CSD-associated neuroretinitis and encephalopathy, B. henselae-related neuro-psychiatric disorders in HIV-infected:
  ◊ Erythromycin 500-1000 mg po qid or doxycycline 100 mg po qid for 4 weeks in immunocompetent; 8-12 weeks in immunocompromised (rifampin may play adjunctive role)
- Endocarditis, visceral or bony involvement with BA/BP: Erythromycin 500-1000 mg qid or doxycycline 100 mg bid x 2-4 weeks parenteral; complete 8-12 weeks po

Contraindications: N/A

Precautions: N/A

Significant possible interactions: N/A

ALTERNATIVE DRUGS
- B. bacilliformis infection: tetracyclines
- Non-bacilliformis Bartonella infections: other tetracyclines, azithromycin, clarithromycin, chloramphenicol, ofloxacin, ciprofloxacin

FOLLOWUP

PATIENT MONITORING Relapse may occur in non-CSD syndromes if therapy is too brief, close follow-up after completion of antibiotics is warranted

PREVENTION/AVOIDANCE Avoid contact with potential vectors, especially young cats. If cat scratch or bite occurs, wash the wound promptly and thoroughly.

POSSIBLE COMPLICATIONS Relapse, especially in HIV infection

EXPECTED COURSE/PROGNOSIS
- CSD - spontaneous resolution usually in 2-4 months without specific therapy
- Other syndromes - with proper treatment, full resolution; if relapse, consider long-term suppressive antibiotics after retreatment

MISCELLANEOUS

ASSOCIATED CONDITIONS In advanced HIV infection, other opportunistic infections may be present

AGE-RELATED FACTORS
Pediatric: N/A
Geriatric: N/A
Others: N/A

PREGNANCY N/A

SYNONYMS N/A

ICD-9-CM
078.3 Cat scratch disease
083.1 Trench fever (B. quintana bacteremia)
083.8 Other Bartonella-related diagnoses, including BA/BP
088.0 B. bacilliformis infections (Oroya fever, verruga peruana)

SEE ALSO N/A

OTHER NOTES N/A

ABBREVIATIONS
CSD = Cat Scratch Disease
BA = Bacillary angiomatosis
BP = Bacillary peliosis
HIV = Human immunodeficiency virus

REFERENCES
- Bass LN, Vincent JM, Person DA: The expanding spectrum of Bartonella infections. Pediatr Infect Dis 1997;16:2-10, 163-179
- Spach DH, Koehler JE: Bartonella-associated infections. Infect Dis Clinics North Am 1988;12:137-155
Illustrations: 2 available on CD-ROM
Internet references: http://www.5mcc.com

Author(s)
Leonard N. Slater, MD

Basal cell carcinoma

BASICS

DESCRIPTION Malignant tumor of the skin originating from the basal cells of the epidermis and its appendages. Rarely metastasizes but capable of local tissue destruction.
System(s) affected: Skin/Exocrine
Genetics: More common in fair-skin blondes and redheads
Incidence/Prevalence in USA:
Approximately 400,000 cases/year
Predominant age: Generally > 40 but incidence is increasing in younger populations
Predominant sex: Males > Female (although incidence is increasing in females)

SIGNS AND SYMPTOMS
• Begins as a small, smooth surfaced, well defined nodule
• Color pink to red
• "Pearly" translucent border
• Telangiectatic vessels overlying
• May have varying degrees of melanin pigment
• As nodule enlarges, central ulceration and crusting occurs

CAUSES
• Sun exposure
• Inorganic arsenic exposure

RISK FACTORS
• Chronic sun exposure
• Light complexion
• Tendency to sunburn
• Male sex although increasing risk in women due to lifestyle changes e.g., suntan parlors, etc.

DIAGNOSIS

DIFFERENTIAL DIAGNOSIS Sebaceous hyperplasia, intradermal nevi (pigmented and non-pigmented), molluscum contagiosum

LABORATORY Pathologic examination required to confirm diagnosis
Drugs that may alter lab results: N/A
Disorders that may alter lab results: N/A

PATHOLOGICAL FINDINGS Nidus of basal cells extending into dermis. Characteristic cells resemble normal basal cells with large basophilic, oval nuclei. Rare mitoses. Tumor cells arranged in palisades at periphery.

SPECIAL TESTS N/A

IMAGING N/A

DIAGNOSTIC PROCEDURES Biopsy mandatory to confirm diagnosis

TREATMENT

APPROPRIATE HEALTH CARE
Outpatient unless extensive lesion

GENERAL MEASURES N/A

SURGICAL MEASURES
• Treatment selection varies with extent and location of lesion, tumor border distinctiveness
• High risk areas - inner canthus, nasolabial sulcus, philtrum, preauricular area, retroauricular sulcus, lip, temple
• Curettage and electrodesiccation - nodular lesion < l cm, in low risk area, if not deeply invasive. Requires specialized training and experience in surgical technique.
• Excision - useful for lesions in high risk areas, not as dependent on lesion size. Poor choice if multiple lesions. Requires appropriate training.
• Cryosurgery - reserved for small lesions in low risk area. Requires specialized training and equipment. May want pre- and post-treatment biopsies.
• Moh's surgery - the preferred microsurgically-controlled surgical treatment for lesions in high risk area, for recurrent lesion, if there is an aggressive growth pattern. Requires referral to appropriately trained dermatologic surgeon.
• Radiation - useful for patients who could not tolerate minor surgical procedures (e.g., elderly patients). Also may be used when preservation of local tissue important such as near lips and eyelids.

ACTIVITY No restrictions except to avoid overexposure to sun

DIET No special diet

PATIENT EDUCATION
• Teach patient appropriate sun avoidance techniques, sunscreens, etc.
• Skin self exam

MEDICATIONS

DRUG(S) OF CHOICE Topical antibiotics after excision for 24 to 48 hours (optional)
Contraindications: N/A
Precautions: N/A
Significant possible interactions: N/A

ALTERNATIVE DRUGS N/A

FOLLOWUP

PATIENT MONITORING Every month for 3 months, then twice yearly for 5 years, yearly thereafter

PREVENTION/AVOIDANCE
• Sunscreens
• Hats, long-sleeve shirts
• Avoid excessive tanning

POSSIBLE COMPLICATIONS
• Local recurrence and spread. Usually recurrences will appear within 5 years.
• Metastasis (rare)

EXPECTED COURSE/PROGNOSIS
• Proper treatment yields 90-95% cure
• Most recurrences happen within 5 years
• Development of new basal cell carcinomas. 36% of patients will develop a new lesion within 5 years.

MISCELLANEOUS

ASSOCIATED CONDITIONS
• Xeroderma pigmentosum
• Basal cell nevus syndrome

AGE-RELATED FACTORS
Pediatric: Rare in children
Geriatric: Greater frequency in geriatric patients
Others: N/A

PREGNANCY N/A

SYNONYMS
• Basal cell epithelioma
• Rodent ulcer

ICD-9-CM
173.3 Basal cell carcinoma, face
173.4 Basal cell carcinoma, scalp or neck
173.5 Basal cell carcinoma, trunk
173.6 Basal cell carcinoma, upper limb
173.7 Basal cell carcinoma, lower limb
173.9 Basal cell carcinoma, site unspecified

SEE ALSO N/A

OTHER NOTES N/A

ABBREVIATIONS N/A

REFERENCES
• Fitzpatrick TN, et al: Dermatology in General Medicine. New York, McGraw-Hill, 1987
• Friedman RJ, et al: Cancer of the Skin. Philadelphia, W.B. Saunders Co., 1991
Illustrations: 10 available on CD-ROM
Internet references: http://www.5mcc.com

Author(s)
John M. Little, MD

Behçet's syndrome

BASICS

DESCRIPTION Rare multisystem, chronic disease characterized by oral and genital mucocutaneous ulcerations, skin rashes, arthritis, thrombophlebitis, uveitis, colitis, and neurologic symptoms.
• Endemic in Japan and Northeastern Mediterranean region.

System(s) affected: Skin/Exocrine, Reproductive, Nervous, Renal/Urologic, Musculoskeletal

Genetics: One report in a mother and newborn (A. Fam, Ann Rheumatic Dis 1981;40:509-512). Very rarely familial.

Incidence/Prevalence in USA:
• 1/100,000
• In other countries, per 100,000
   ◊ Japan: 10
   ◊ Iran: 16-100
   ◊ Germany: 2
   ◊ Saudi Arabia: 20

Predominant age: 3rd to 4th decades

Predominant sex: Male > Female; as frequently to twice as often. Some studies suggest equal frequency.

SIGNS AND SYMPTOMS
• Aphthous stomatitis
• Genital ulcers - painful in the male, usually painless in the female
• Dermal - papulovesicular, erythema nodosum, pathergy, erythema multiforme, vasculitis, pyoderma
• Ocular - iritis, iridocyclitis, chorioretinitis, hypopyon, hemorrhage, papilledema, optic atrophy
• Morning stiffness - in 1/3
• Polyarthritis - self-limited and predominantly affecting lower extremities
• Thrombophlebitis - peripheral, pulmonary, cerebral, Budd Chiari syndrome
• Neurologic - cranial nerve palsy, hemiplegia, intracranial hypertension, meningomyelitis and recurrent meningitis, confusional state
• GI - aphthous ulcers, colitis, melena
• Pulmonary infiltrates - possibly related to thrombosis
• Myopathy/myositis - rare
• Peripheral gangrene - rare
• Epididymitis
• Glomerulonephritis - rare

CAUSES
• Unknown
   ◊ Classified as vasculopathy or autoimmune
   ◊ HLA-B5 alloantigen relationship
   ◊ Possible environmental toxin - heavy metals, pesticides
   ◊ Possibly English walnuts or Ginko nuts
   ◊ Fibrinolysis abnormality
   ◊ One report associated with HIV infection (C. Stein, J Rheumatol 1991;18,1427-8)

RISK FACTORS   See Causes

DIAGNOSIS

DIFFERENTIAL DIAGNOSIS
• Reiter's syndrome and other forms of spondyloarthropathy
• Inflammatory bowel disease (Crohn's disease and ulcerative colitis)
• Syphilis
• Erythema nodosum
• Aphthous stomatitis
• Herpes simplex
• Stevens-Johnson syndrome
• Vasculitis
• Multisystem disease
• Thrombophlebitis related to coagulation factor deficiency
• Mollaret's meningitis

LABORATORY
• Erythrocyte sedimentation rate elevation, but can be normal
• Immune complexes detected by Raji cell and C1q solid phase assays
• Cryoglobulin
• Hypergammaglobulinemia
• Circulating anticoagulation (rare)
• Anti-cardiolipin antibody (rare)
• Pathergy

Drugs that may alter lab results: N/A
Disorders that may alter lab results: N/A

PATHOLOGICAL FINDINGS
• May be no recognizable changes
• Mononuclear perivascular infiltration
• Mononuclear infiltrate in synovium
• Endothelial cell swelling
• Partial obliteration of vascular lumen
• Neutrophilic dermatitis (Sweet syndrome) rarely

SPECIAL TESTS
• None specific for Behçet's, but helpful in following disease course:
   ◊ Depression of plasma antithrombin III levels with active disease
   ◊ Increased fibrinolytic activity during attacks
   ◊ Anti-neutrophil cytoplasmic antigen antibodies, perinuclear variety
   ◊ Demyelinating antibodies in neuro-Behçet's syndrome
   ◊ Anti-cardiolipin antibodies, lupus anticoagulants
   ◊ Anti-endothelial antibodies
   ◊ Pathergy

IMAGING   N/A

DIAGNOSTIC PROCEDURES
• Careful history and physical and frequent reevaluation
• Synovial fluid - inflammatory effusion
• Arteriography - for aneurysms or thrombosis

TREATMENT

APPROPRIATE HEALTH CARE Usually outpatient. Inpatient usually required for neurologic complications

GENERAL MEASURES According to body system involved

SURGICAL MEASURES N/A

ACTIVITY   As tolerated

DIET   No special diet

PATIENT EDUCATION
• American Behçet's Association, 421 21st Avenue SW, Rochester, MN 55902, (507)281-3059

Behçet's syndrome

MEDICATIONS

DRUG(S) OF CHOICE
- Colchicine: 0.6 mg bid
- Topical ocular steroids
- Prednisone: 1 mg/kg for severe involvement, especially CNS
- Azathioprine: 2-3 mg/kg/day po
- Methotrexate: Use the lowest possible dose; perhaps 7.5 mg/week
- Cyclosporine: 1-4 mg/kg; but monitor LFT, magnesium, lipids q2 wks x 3 mo, then q mo
- Resistant cases may require
  ◊ Tacrolimus (FK 506) 0.09-0.15 mg/kg/day
  ◊ Thalidomide 300 mg/day
  ◊ Interferon alpha

Contraindications:
- Thalidomide contraindicated in pregnancy
- Refer to manufacturer's literature

Precautions:
- Refer to manufacturer's literature
- Absorption of drugs such as amitriptyline, diazepam, carbamazepine, phenytoin, and acetaminophen may be reduced

Significant possible interactions: Refer to manufacturer's literature

ALTERNATIVE DRUGS
- Levamisole - 100-150 mg two days per week
- Chlorambucil - but concern with respect to toxicity, especially its malignant potential
- Thalidomide
- Cyclophosphamide: 50-100 mg/day q am. Patient should drink 8-10 glasses of water/day and report any blood in the urine.

FOLLOWUP

PATIENT MONITORING
Dependent on severity of system involvement and medication monitoring

PREVENTION/AVOIDANCE
Avoid English walnuts

POSSIBLE COMPLICATIONS
- Death
- Blindness
- Paralysis
- Embolism/thrombosis - pulmonary, vena cava, peripheral
- Aneurysms
- Amyloidosis
- Thrombotic events, especially when anticardiolipin antibodies present

EXPECTED COURSE/PROGNOSIS
- Normal life expectancy, except with neurologic involvement
- Possible vision impairment

MISCELLANEOUS

ASSOCIATED CONDITIONS
- Amyloid
- Sweet syndrome

AGE-RELATED FACTORS
Pediatric: Rare
Geriatric: Rare
Others: N/A

PREGNANCY
- Thalidomide contraindicated in pregnancy
- Possible increase in thrombosis and fetal demise

SYNONYMS
- Mucocutaneous ocular syndrome
- Franceschetti-Valerio syndrome

ICD-9-CM
136.1 Behçet's syndrome

SEE ALSO
N/A

OTHER NOTES
N/A

ABBREVIATIONS
N/A

REFERENCES
- International diagnostic study group for Behçet's disease. Evaluation of ('classification') criteria in Behçet's disease - Towards internationally agreed criteria. Brit J Rheumatol 1992;31:299-308
- Mizushima Y: Behçet's disease. Curr Opin Rheumatol 1991;3:32-35
- Hashimoto T, Takeuchi A: Treatment of Behçet's disease. Curr Opin Rheumatol 1992;4:31-34
- Shimizu T, et al: Behcet disease. Semin Arthritis Rheum 1979; 8:223-260
- Chaleby K: Clin Chem 1987;33:1679-1681
- O'Duffy JD: Behcet's disease. Curr Opin Rheumatol 1994;6:39-43 (note: this is better than the more recent Curr Opin Rheumatol reviews)
- Hamuryudan V, et al: Systemic interferon alpha-2b treatment in Behcet syndrome. J Rheumatol 1994;21:1098-1100
- Kaklamon VG, Vaiopoulos G, Koklomonis PG. Behcet's disease. Semin Arth Rheum 1998;27:197=217
- Pacor ML, et al: Cyclosporin in Behçet's disease. J Rheumatol 1994;13:224-227
- Huong DL, et al: Arterial lesions in Behcet's disease. J Rheumatol 1995;22:2103-2113
- Akman-Demir G, et al: Seven year follow-up of neurologic involvment in Behcet syndrome. Arch Neurol 1996;53:691-768
- Gerber S, et al: Long-term MR follow-up of cerebral lesions in neuro-Behcet's disease. Neuroradiol 1996;38:761-768
- Kaklaman VG, et al: Behcet's disease. Semin in Arthritis Rheum 1998;27:197-217

Illustrations: 1 available on CD-ROM
Internet references: http://www.5mcc.com

Author(s)
Bruce M. Rothschild, MD

Bell's palsy

BASICS

DESCRIPTION Paralysis or weakness of the muscles supplied by the facial nerve, typically unilaterally, due to inflammation and swelling of the facial nerve within the facial canal
• Bell's palsy: Idiopathic
• Ramsay Hunt syndrome: Bell's palsy associated with vesicles within the outer ear canal or behind the ear, due to herpes zoster infection
• Facial diplegia: The simultaneous development of bilateral Bell's palsy is highly unusual and conditions such as Guillain-Barré syndrome and chronic meningitis should be considered as possible explanations.
System(s) affected: Nervous
Genetics: There is a familial tendency toward Bell's palsy
Incidence/Prevalence in USA: 25 in 100,000
Predominant age: Affects all ages. Most common in individuals over 30 years of age.
Predominant sex: Male = Female

SIGNS AND SYMPTOMS
• Sudden onset or onset over days
• Unilateral total or partial paralysis of the facial muscles
• Mild "numbness" on the affected side
• Ipsilateral inadequate tear production; ipsilateral tearing
• Ipsilateral loss of taste
• Ipsilateral ear ache

CAUSES
• Bell's palsy
  ◊ Inflammation of the facial nerve within the facial canal
    ◊ Exposure to cold
    ◊ Probably viral
• Ramsay-Hunt syndrome
  ◊ Herpes zoster
  ◊ Rarely herpes simplex

RISK FACTORS
• Age over 30
• Exposure to cold

DIAGNOSIS

DIFFERENTIAL DIAGNOSIS
• Neoplastic
  ◊ Carcinomatous meningitis
  ◊ Leukemic meningitis
  ◊ Tumors of the parotid gland
  ◊ Tumors of the base of the skull
• Infectious
  ◊ Chronic meningitis
  ◊ Bacterial meningitis
  ◊ Osteomyelitis of the base of the skull
  ◊ Otitis media
  ◊ Leprosy
• Other
  ◊ Sarcoidosis
  ◊ Melkersson-Rosenthal syndrome (facial paralysis with scrotal tongue)
  ◊ Head injury with fracture of the temporal bone
  ◊ Brainstem stroke (anterior-inferior cerebellar artery)
  ◊ Multiple sclerosis
  ◊ Guillain-Barré syndrome (can initially present as a very typical Bell's palsy)

LABORATORY
• CSF protein - mildly elevated in 1/3 of cases
• CSF cells - mildly elevated in 10% of cases, with a mononuclear cell predominance
Drugs that may alter lab results: N/A
Disorders that may alter lab results: N/A

PATHOLOGICAL FINDINGS
• Edema of the facial nerve
• Occasional hemorrhagic streaks
• Dilatation of the vasa nervorum
• Infiltration of mononuclear cells in some cases
• Atrophy of the facial nerve

SPECIAL TESTS
• Electromyography in the first three weeks after onset of the condition manifests a decreased or absent interference pattern on the affected side, which reflects a reduction or absence of function of the facial motor units. After three weeks, denervation potentials (fibrillations) are typically seen. Eventually, with recovery, low-amplitude, short-duration, polyphasic (nascent) motor units may appear in previously denervated areas. Recovery may be incomplete.
• Nerve conduction velocities may reveal absence or attenuation of the evoked potential, slowing of the conduction velocity or a normal conduction velocity and amplitude (variable due to varying severity and duration of condition)
• Blink reflex - the electrophysiological equivalent of the corneal reflex, should be abnormal in all cases

IMAGING
MRI to rule out posterior fossa lesions and intracanalicular 8th nerve tumors if clinical suspicion is high

DIAGNOSTIC PROCEDURES
Spinal tap may reveal an elevated protein or cell count, however, it is usually not necessary

TREATMENT

APPROPRIATE HEALTH CARE
Outpatient except for surgical decompression (very controversial and largely abandoned)

GENERAL MEASURES
• Close and patch ipsilateral eye
• Methylcellulose eye drops

SURGICAL MEASURES N/A

ACTIVITY
Fully active. Due to patching, use caution in activities requiring keen depth perception.

DIET No special diet

PATIENT EDUCATION
Explanation and reassurance when appropriate

MEDICATIONS

DRUG(S) OF CHOICE
• Corticosteroids: Prednisone 80 mg po qd for three days, then 60 mg po qd for three days, then 40 mg po qd for three days, then 20 mg po qd for three days, then discontinue use. Course of treatment to begin immediately after onset of Bell's palsy. There is little benefit in starting steroids after four days.
• Antiviral agents with activity against herpes group of viruses in Ramsay-Hunt syndrome and idiopathic Bell's palsy
Contraindications: Pre-existing infections including tuberculosis and systemic mycosis
Precautions: Use with discretion in pregnancy, peptic ulcer disease, and diabetes
Significant possible interactions: MMR, OPV, and other live vaccines

ALTERNATIVE DRUGS N/A

FOLLOWUP

PATIENT MONITORING
• Recheck monthly for six to twelve months
• Look for evidence of corneal abrasions. Expect early recovery.

PREVENTION/AVOIDANCE N/A

POSSIBLE COMPLICATIONS
• Unmasking of subclinical infection (such as tuberculosis) by steroid usage
• Steroid-induced psychological disturbances
• Steroid-induced avascular necrosis of hips, knees and/or shoulders
• Corneal abrasion and ulceration

EXPECTED COURSE/PROGNOSIS
Complete, partial or no recovery of function. Patients with partial denervation typically fully recover. Patients with total denervation usually partially recover, but may exhibit aberrant regeneration (e.g., crocodile tears) or hemifacial spasm as long term complications.

MISCELLANEOUS

ASSOCIATED CONDITIONS N/A

AGE-RELATED FACTORS
Pediatric: N/A
Geriatric: N/A
Others: N/A

PREGNANCY Use steroids cautiously in pregnancy. Consult with obstetrician.

SYNONYMS
• Idiopathic facial paralysis

ICD-9-CM 351.0 Bell's palsy

SEE ALSO
• Herpes simplex
• Herpes zoster

OTHER NOTES N/A

ABBREVIATIONS N/A

REFERENCES
• Dyck PJ, Thomas PK, et al, eds: Peripheral Neuropathy. 3rd Ed. Philadelphia, W.B. Saunders Co., 1993
• Murakemi S, et al. Bell palsy and herpes simplex virus: identification of viral DNA in endoneurial fluid and muscle. Ann Intern Med. 1996 Jan 1;124(1 Pt 1):27-30
Illustrations: N/A
Internet references: http://www.5mcc.com

Author(s)
Colin R. Bamford, MD

Bladder injury

BASICS

DESCRIPTION Due to its well protected location, bladder rupture is unusual. Injury most often secondary to penetrating or blunt trauma and classified as contusion, intraperitoneal or extraperitoneal rupture.
System(s) affected: Renal/Urologic
Genetics: N/A
Incidence/Prevalence in USA: N/A
Predominant Age: N/A
Predominant Sex: N/A

SIGNS AND SYMPTOMS
• Suprapubic pain
• Urinary retention
• Hematuria (94%)
• Muscle rigidity over lower abdomen
• No peritonitis

CAUSES
• Forceful blunt or penetrating blow to lower abdomen, particularly with a full bladder

RISK FACTORS
• Distended bladder at the time of trauma
• Congenital malformation of bladder
• Prior pelvic or bladder surgery
• Frequently associated with pelvic fractures

DIAGNOSIS

DIFFERENTIAL DIAGNOSIS
• Rupture of the urethra
• Rupture of abdominal viscus
• Pelvic fracture with hematoma

LABORATORY Hematuria on urinalysis
Drugs that may alter lab results: None
Disorders that may alter lab results: None

PATHOLOGICAL FINDINGS
• Jagged irregular tear in the bladder
• Perforation at the dome of bladder near urachus (blunt trauma)
• Extensive perivesicle hematoma

SPECIAL TESTS None

IMAGING
• Cystogram with drain out film
• Urethrogram

DIAGNOSTIC PROCEDURES
• Rarely is cystoscopy indicated

TREATMENT

APPROPRIATE HEALTH CARE
Inpatient

GENERAL MEASURES
• Extraperitoneal rupture, insert foley, admit, comfort care
• Antibacterial coverage, broad spectrum
• Anticholinergics for spasm
• Pain medication as required
• Catheter removal in 10-14 days

SURGICAL MEASURES
• Intraperitoneal rupture, immediate surgical repair
• Blunt trauma, contusion, comfort care
• Penetrating injury, exploration, surgical repair

ACTIVITY Full activity when associated injuries permit

DIET No special diet

PATIENT EDUCATION Printed material available from multiple sources

MEDICATIONS

DRUG(S) OF CHOICE
• Broad spectrum coverage, ciprofloxacin (Cipro) 500 mg bid
• Opium and belladonna suppositories q 6-8 hr prn spasms
• Oxybutynin (Ditropan) 5-10 mg tid for spasms
• Adequate pain control as required
Contraindications: Refer to manufacturer's profile of each drug
Precautions: Avoid quinolones (e.g., ciprofloxacin) in children
Significant possible interactions: Refer to manufacturer's profile of each drug

ALTERNATIVE DRUGS
• Other quinolones
• Other antispasmodics; e.g., flavoxate

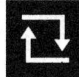

FOLLOWUP

PATIENT MONITORING
• Cystogram repeat in 7-10 days
• Remove catheter when bladder sealed
• Periodic check for infection and stricture formation

PREVENTION/AVOIDANCE
• Use seat belts
• Auto air bag

POSSIBLE COMPLICATIONS
• Infection
• Fistula formation (rare)
• Peritonitis (rare)

EXPECTED COURSE/PROGNOSIS
• Complete recovery
• Stricture (uncommon) - only long term complication

MISCELLANEOUS

ASSOCIATED CONDITIONS
• Frequently associated with pelvic fractures

AGE-RELATED FACTORS
Pediatric: Position of bladder makes intraperitoneal rupture more common
Geriatric: N/A
Others: N/A

PREGNANCY   N/A

SYNONYMS   N/A

ICD-9-CM
596.9 Unspecified disorder of bladder

SEE ALSO   N/A

OTHER NOTES   N/A

ABBREVIATIONS   N/A

REFERENCES   Walsh PC, Gittes RF, Perlmutter AD: 6th Ed. Campbell's Urology. Philadelphia, W.B. Saunders Co., 1992
Illustrations: N/A
Internet references: http://www.5mcc.com

Author(s)
Jack L. Summers, MD, PhD

Blastomycosis

BASICS

DESCRIPTION An uncommon, systemic, fungal infection with a broad range of manifestations including pulmonary, skin, bone and genitourinary involvement
System(s) affected: Skin/Exocrine, Pulmonary, Musculoskeletal, Renal/Urologic, Endocrine/Metabolic
Genetics: N/A
Incidence/Prevalence in USA: Ranges from 0.4-4 cases per 100,000 population per year. Higher prevalence in states bordering the Mississippi and Ohio Rivers. Sporadic cases occurring in other areas.
Predominant age: Adults, but 10-20% of cases occur in children
Predominant sex: Male > Female

SIGNS AND SYMPTOMS
- Acute infection
  ◊ Onset may be abrupt or insidious
  ◊ May be asymptomatic and self-limiting
  ◊ Incubation period 30-45 days
  ◊ Fever, chills, myalgias, arthralgias
  ◊ Cough initially nonproductive, then productive
  ◊ Hemoptysis (common)
  ◊ Erythema nodosum
- Pulmonary blastomycosis
  ◊ 60-90% of cases
  ◊ Three forms - acute, chronic, asymptomatic
  ◊ Cough - nonproductive to productive
  ◊ Hemoptysis
  ◊ Weight loss
  ◊ Pleuritic chest pain
  ◊ Pleural effusions - 10%
  ◊ Respiratory failure in small percentage
  ◊ Upper lobe fibronodular infiltrates - 50%
  ◊ Mass lesion - 30%
  ◊ Diffuse pulmonary infiltrates; cavitation (uncommon)
  ◊ Pleural thickening
- Cutaneous blastomycosis
  ◊ Most common extrapulmonary manifestation - 40-80%
  ◊ May occur with or without pulmonary disease
  ◊ Two types of lesions
  ◊ Verrucous lesions begin as small papulopustular lesions, slowly spread, become crusted, have sharp borders; central clearing with scar formation and depigmentation; microabscesses noted at periphery of lesion
  ◊ Ulcerative lesions (initially pustules) form shallow ulcers with raised edges and granulating base
  ◊ Mucosal lesions may occur
  ◊ Regional adenopathy (uncommon)
  ◊ Subcutaneous nodules - cold abscesses

- Skeletal blastomycosis
  ◊ 25-50% of extrapulmonary cases
  ◊ Long bones, vertebrae, ribs most commonly involved
  ◊ Well circumscribed osteolytic lesions
  ◊ May present with contiguous soft tissue abscesses and/or sinus tracts
  ◊ Paraspinous abscess may occur in vertebral disease
  ◊ Acute or chronic arthritis may result from extension of contiguous osteomyelitis
- Genitourinary blastomycosis
  ◊ Occurs in 10-30% of cases
  ◊ Involves prostate most commonly but also epididymis and testes
  ◊ Outflow obstruction
  ◊ Enlarged tender prostate
  ◊ Involvement of female genitalia uncommon and usually acquired through sexual contact
- Other
  ◊ Central nervous system involvement with acute or chronic meningitis, epidural or cerebral abscesses
  ◊ Liver, spleen, pericardium, thyroid, gastrointestinal tract, adrenal gland may each be involved

CAUSES
- Inhalation of spores of Blastomyces dermatitidis into lung with spread to other organ systems by lympho-hematogenous dissemination
- Primary inoculation of skin may rarely occur
- Female genital infection may result from sexual transmission
- Reactivation of previous infection may occur in immunocompromised patients including those with AIDS

RISK FACTORS
- Occupational or recreational exposure to soil containing spores of B. dermatitidis
- Residence in areas of increased disease prevalence
- Rarely associated with AIDS

DIAGNOSIS

DIFFERENTIAL DIAGNOSIS
- Pulmonary - acute bacterial pneumonia, tuberculosis, other fungal diseases, bacterial lung abscess, empyema, bronchogenic carcinoma
- Cutaneous - bacterial pyoderma, cutaneous mycobacterial infection, other cutaneous fungal infections (sporotrichosis, histoplasmosis, cryptococcosis), squamous cell carcinoma
- Bone - bacterial osteomyelitis, tuberculosis, neoplastic disease
- Genitourinary - bacterial prostatitis, prostate cancer, other fungal infections, tuberculosis

LABORATORY
- Culture of B. dermatitidis from tissue or body secretions on Sabouraud's or other enriched media
- Demonstration of yeast forms (5-15 micrometers in diameter, with refractile cell wall, broad-based budding and no capsule) in tissue or body secretions by wet mount or special stains
- Serologic tests include complement fixation, enzyme-linked immunoassay, immunodiffusion precipitin antibody tests. All have variable sensitivity and low specificity and are not helpful in diagnosis.
- Delayed hypersensitivity skin testing with blastomycin also has low sensitivity and specificity and not useful in diagnosis
Drugs that may alter lab results: N/A
Disorders that may alter lab results: Histoplasma cross-reacts with serologic tests for blastomycosis

PATHOLOGICAL FINDINGS
- Early inflammatory response with polymorphonuclear leukocytes followed by granuloma formation with lymphocytes and macrophages
- Granulomas do not show caseation necrosis
- Yeast is often found attached to or inside monocytes, macrophages and giant cells

SPECIAL TESTS
- Special staining of tissue with Gomori methenamine silver stain
- Periodic acid-Schiff's stain colors cell wall pink or red
- Mucicarmine stain helps differentiate from encapsulated Cryptococcus

IMAGING
- CT scan of head for CNS lesions
- CT scan of spine for vertebral lesions
- Bone scan for skeletal lesions
- Chest x-ray may show upper lobe fibronodular infiltrates, consolidation, diffuse alveolar infiltrates, mass lesions or pleural thickening

DIAGNOSTIC PROCEDURES
- Aspiration of abscess contents for wet mount and culture
- Needle or surgical biopsy of involved tissue

TREATMENT

APPROPRIATE HEALTH CARE
• Acute pulmonary blastomycosis may be treated with oral itraconazole as an outpatient
• Chronic blastomycosis, overwhelming pneumonia, or extrapulmonary disease should be treated initially with intravenous amphotericin B as a hospital patient

GENERAL MEASURES
• Systemic antifungal therapy is indicated for all cases of extrapulmonary blastomycosis
• Systemic antifungal therapy is indicated for all but the very mild or asymptomatic pulmonary cases in which a trial of observation may be appropriate

SURGICAL MEASURES
• Surgical débridement of bone lesions if there are areas of devitalized bone
• Surgical drainage of large cutaneous abscesses or pleural empyemas

ACTIVITY
No restrictions, once patient is released from hospital

DIET
No special dietary requirement

PATIENT EDUCATION
Counsel patient and family on potential adverse effects associated with antifungal therapy, duration of therapy required and potential for relapse or chronic infection

MEDICATIONS

DRUG(S) OF CHOICE
• Milder forms
  ◊ Itraconazole (Sporanox) 200 mg po twice daily for at least 6 months
• Severe forms
  ◊ Amphotericin B (Fungizone): 0.5-0.8 mg/kg IV over 4-6 hours daily for a cumulative dose of 1.5-2 gm
    - First dose of amphotericin B is given as a test dose of 1 mg in 200 mL dextrose 5% in sterile water intravenously over 2-4 hours
    - Dose is increased by 10 mg daily until a maintenance dose of 0.5 mg-0.8 mg per kg per day is reached. Slow escalation is not appropriate for severe blastomycosis. Full dose can be given on 1st or 2nd day of treatment.
    - Rigors can be prevented by pre-infusion dose of meperidine 50 mg
    - To reduce infusion-related fever, pre-infusion acetaminophen and diphenhydramine

Contraindications: Life threatening intolerance to amphotericin such as anaphylaxis

Precautions:
• Monitor for hypotension during the infusion
• Monitor renal function, serum sodium, potassium and magnesium, and CBC twice weekly during therapy
• Replace potassium and magnesium as indicated
• When serum creatinine rises to 1.6 mg/dL (141 μmol/L) or greater, dosage interval should be changed to 48 hours
• Watch for phlebitis at infusion site

Significant possible interactions: Avoid use of potentially nephrotoxic drugs such as aminoglycosides which may potentiate nephrotoxicity of amphotericin B

ALTERNATIVE DRUGS
Efficacy of alternate regimens not well established by controlled studies
• Fluconazole 400 mg daily for 6 months for non-life threatening blastomycosis
• Ketoconazole (Nizoral): 400-800 mg po daily for 6 months
• Hydroxystilbamidine isethionate useful in some patients

FOLLOWUP

PATIENT MONITORING
• Monitor closely during early therapy
• Frequency of followup depends on severity of disease
• Monitor serum electrolytes, creatinine and CBC twice weekly during amphotericin B therapy
• Post-therapy followup every 3 months for 2 years then twice yearly

PREVENTION/AVOIDANCE
• Unknown
• Condoms for sexual encounters

POSSIBLE COMPLICATIONS
Treatment-induced nephrotoxicity, electrolyte imbalance, anemia

EXPECTED COURSE/PROGNOSIS
• Cure in over 90% with appropriate therapy
• Relapse in less than 10% of cases
• Relapse rate higher with ketoconazole therapy
• Adverse reactions with amphotericin B are frequent and significant

MISCELLANEOUS

ASSOCIATED CONDITIONS N/A

AGE-RELATED FACTORS
Pediatric: Uncommon in children
Geriatric: Prognosis is worse in elderly patients with significant underlying pulmonary or renal disease
Others: N/A

PREGNANCY
Safety of amphotericin B and ketoconazole in pregnancy has not been established

SYNONYMS
North American blastomycosis

ICD-9-CM
116.0 Blastomycosis

SEE ALSO N/A

OTHER NOTES N/A

ABBREVIATIONS N/A

REFERENCES
• Mandell GL, ed: Principles and Practice of Infectious Diseases. 4th Ed. New York, Churchill Livingstone, 1995
• Bradsher RW: Blastomycosis. Infectious Disease Clinics of North America 1988:877
• Patel RG, et al: Clinical presentation, radiographic findings, and diagnostic methods of pulmonary blastomycosis: A Review of 100 consecutive cases. South Med J 1999;92:289-95
Illustrations: N/A
Internet references: http://www.5mcc.com

Author(s)
William G. Gardner, MD

Blepharitis

BASICS

DESCRIPTION An inflammatory reaction of the eyelid margin. It usually occurs as seborrheic (nonulcerative) or as staphylococcal (ulcerative) blepharitis. Both types may coexist.

System(s) affected: Skin/Exocrine

Genetics: N/A

Incidence/Prevalence in USA: Common (the most frequent ocular disease)

Predominant age: Adult

Predominant sex: Male = Female

SIGNS AND SYMPTOMS

- *Staphylococcus aureus* blepharitis
  ◊ Itching
  ◊ Lacrimation; tearing
  ◊ Burning
  ◊ Photophobia (light sensitivity)
  ◊ Usually worse in morning
  ◊ Recurrent stye (external hordeolum, or internal hordeolum)
  ◊ Recurrent chalazia (chronic inflammation of meibomian glands)
  ◊ Fine, epithelial keratitis, lower half of cornea
  ◊ Ulcerations at base of eyelashes
  ◊ Broken, sparse, misdirected eyelashes(trichiasis)
- Seborrheic blepharitis
  ◊ Lid margin erythema
  ◊ Dry flakes, oily secretions on lid margins and/or lashes
  ◊ Associated dandruff of scalp, eyebrows
  ◊ Sometimes nasolabial erythema, scaling
- Mixed blepharitis (seborrheic with associated Staph aureus)
  ◊ Most common type of blepharitis
  ◊ Symptoms and signs of both staph and seborrheic present

CAUSES

- Seborrheic
  ◊ Accelerated shedding of skin cells with associated sebaceous gland dysfunction
  ◊ P. ovale and P. orbiculare yeasts often colonize
  ◊ Oil and skin cells foster staph growth
- Staphylococcus
  ◊ Usually part of mixed blepharitis
  ◊ Colonization of Zeis glands of lid margin and meibomian glands posterior to lashes, with Staphylococcus aureus
  ◊ Impetigo contagiosa-staph
  ◊ Infectious eczematoid dermatitis-Staphylococcus is the hapten
  ◊ Staphylococcus scalded skin syndrome - entire body involved (in young children)
  ◊ Angular blepharitis-staph - most frequent bacteria involved
- Other types of blepharitis
  ◊ Contact dermatitis with or without secondary Staphylococcus infection
  ◊ Meibomian gland dysfunction

RISK FACTORS

- Candida
- Seborrheic dermatitis
- Acne rosacea
- Diabetes mellitus
- Immunocompromised state (AIDS, chemotherapy, etc.)

DIAGNOSIS

DIFFERENTIAL DIAGNOSIS

- Masquerade syndrome:
  ◊ Persistent inflammation and thickening of eyelid margin may indicate squamous cell, basal cell, or sebaceous cell carcinoma masquerading as "blepharitis"
  ◊ These carcinomas may also mimic styes or chalazions
  ◊ Sebaceous cell carcinoma has a 23% fatality rate (found in one study of eyelid sebaceous cell carcinomas). Up to one half of potentially fatal sebaceous cell carcinomas may resemble benign inflammatory diseases, particularly chalazions and chronic blepharoconjunctivitis.
  ◊ Any swelling or inflammation of eyelid which does not resolve promptly (within one month) with treatment, is suspect as a possible underlying carcinoma

LABORATORY N/A

Drugs that may alter lab results: N/A
Disorders that may alter lab results: N/A

PATHOLOGICAL FINDINGS Acute or chronic inflammatory cell types

SPECIAL TESTS

- Cultures in atypical blepharitis
- Biopsy in atypical cases that are suspect for carcinoma

IMAGING N/A

DIAGNOSTIC PROCEDURES See Special Tests

TREATMENT

APPROPRIATE HEALTH CARE
Outpatient

GENERAL MEASURES

- Mild seborrheic blepharitis (dry flakes, minimal inflammation) - apply eyelid margin scrubs with eyelid cleanser at least once daily
- If Staphylococcus likely, follow lid scrubs with application of bacitracin, or (second choice), erythromycin ophthalmic ointment, to eyelid margins, using cotton tipped applicator
- Clean lids and apply ointment nightly in mild cases, up to four times daily in severe cases
- Discontinue soft contact lenses until condition cleared
- Chronic recurrent blepharitis requires referral to ophthalmologist for evaluation as to whether patient should continue in lenses

SURGICAL MEASURES N/A

ACTIVITY No restrictions

DIET No restrictions

PATIENT EDUCATION

- Blepharitis "Fact Sheet" from American Academy of Ophthalmology (see References for ordering information)
- Advise patient that blepharitis is a chronic condition, prone to recurrence if hygiene (lid scrubs) are not maintained after antibiotic treatment is discontinued

MEDICATIONS

DRUG(S) OF CHOICE
• Topical treatment, if Staphylococcus likely, application of bacitracin, or (second choice), erythromycin ophthalmic ointment
• In some cases of Staphylococcus blepharitis (e.g., rosacea), systemic tetracycline 250 mg qid x several weeks, tapering to 250 mg daily for one to three months, or doxycycline 100 mg bid po. Alternative is oxacillin 250 mg qid for 1-2 weeks. Used for persistent (despite topical treatment) lid inflammation or recurrent meibomian styes.

Contraindications:
• Allergy to medication
• Tetracycline: not for use in pregnancy or children < 8 years

Precautions:
• Avoid medication containing neomycin, as it is sensitizing
• Tetracycline: may cause photosensitivity; sunscreen recommended

Significant possible interactions:
• Tetracycline: avoid concurrent administration with antacids, dairy products, or iron
• Broad-spectrum antibiotics: may reduce the effectiveness of oral contraceptives; barrier method recommended

ALTERNATIVE DRUGS
Quinolones may be helpful for persistent or recurrent Staphylococcal blepharitis

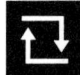
FOLLOWUP

PATIENT MONITORING   Every 2 months

PREVENTION/AVOIDANCE   Follow treatment guidelines

POSSIBLE COMPLICATIONS
• Hordeolum (stye)
• Scarring of eyelid margin
• Misdirection of eyelashes (trichiasis)
• Corneal infection

EXPECTED COURSE/PROGNOSIS
Long-term eyelid hygiene required to control

MISCELLANEOUS

ASSOCIATED CONDITIONS   See
diagnosis section above regarding blepharitis masquerade syndromes

AGE-RELATED FACTORS
Pediatric: N/A
Geriatric: N/A
Others: N/A

PREGNANCY   N/A

SYNONYMS   N/A

ICD-9-CM
373.00 Blepharitis

SEE ALSO   N/A

OTHER NOTES   N/A

ABBREVIATIONS   N/A

REFERENCES
• Tasman W, ed: Duane's Clinical Ophthalmology. Philadelphia, J.B. Lippincott Co., 1999
• Boniuk M, Zimmerman LE: Sebaceous carcinoma of the eyelid, eyebrow, caruncle, and orbit. Trans Am Acad Ophthalmol Otolaryngol 1968;72:619
• Rao NA, McLean IW, Zimmerman LE: Sebaceous carcinoma of the eyelids and caruncles: Correlation of clinicopathological features of prognosis. In: Jakobic FA, ed. Ocular and Adnexal Tumors. Birmingham, Aesculapius 1978:461
• American Academy of Ophthalmology, Department of Patient Education: Blepharitis Fact Sheet. San Francisco, American Academy of Ophthalmology. Available for order as tear-off pads, phone (415)-561-8500 to order or write AAO, P.O. Box 7424, San Francisco, CA 94120-7424
Illustrations: N/A
Internet references: http://www.5mcc.com

Author(s)
T. Glendon Moody, MD

Bone tumor, primary malignant

BASICS

DESCRIPTION
Primary malignant bone tumors are rare. Four types make up the majority.
• Malignant fibrous histiocytoma (MFH) - a pleomorphic sarcoma of storiform pattern without differentiation
• Osteosarcoma - similar to malignant fibrous histiocytoma with differentiation to osteoid production
• Chondrosarcoma - cellular cartilaginous lesion with abundant binucleate cells, myxoid areas, and pushing borders
• Ewing's sarcoma - small, blue-round cell neoplasm

System(s) affected: Musculoskeletal

Genetics:
• Ewing's sarcoma has 11/22 chromosomal translocation and EW5-FLI-1 fusion protein
• Osteosarcomas shows loss of retinoblastoma and p53 suppressor genes and amplification of the genes C-myc, mdm-2, SAS, and cyclin-dependent kinase

Incidence/Prevalence in USA:
Rare: 5000 bone and soft tissue sarcomas per year, a practicing orthopedic surgeon may see one primary malignant tumor of bone in every five years of practice. Ewing's sarcoma is less common in blacks.

Predominant age:
• MFH - teens and elderly
• Osteogenic sarcoma - teens and early twenties
• Chondrosarcoma - very young and very old
• Ewing's sarcoma - children, teens, and early twenties

Predominant sex: Male = Female

SIGNS AND SYMPTOMS
• Pain with weight bearing, at rest and at night
• Swelling
• Tenderness
• Fracture with minor trauma
• Minor injury may bring attention to lesion

CAUSES
• Generally unknown
• MFH often follows irradiation or arises in old bone infarct
• Osteosarcoma has association with loss of suppressor retinoblastoma and p53 genes
• Chondrosarcoma may arise in pre-existing enchondroma or exostosis

RISK FACTORS
• Multiple enchondromatosis (Ollier's disease)–chondrosarcoma
• Multiple hereditary exostosis–chondrosarcoma
• Previous irradiation, risk factor for MFH
• Previous history of bilateral retinoblastoma–osteosarcoma

DIAGNOSIS

DIFFERENTIAL DIAGNOSIS
• Solitary metastatic lesion or myeloma especially in the patient over age 40
• Lymphoma at any age
• Benign bone tumors and benign bone tumors that look aggressive (aneurysmal bone cyst, giant cell tumor, eosinophilic granuloma)
• Infection (osteomyelitis)
• Metabolic bone disease (osteopenia, Paget's, hyperparathyroidism)
• Synovial diseases (pigmented villonodular synovitis, synovial chondromatosis, degenerative or inflammatory synovitis)
• Myositis ossificans and repair reaction to trauma
• Avascular necrosis

LABORATORY
• Generally unhelpful
• 50% of osteosarcomas have an elevated alkaline phosphatase
• Ewing's sarcoma may be associated with an elevated ESR and LDH
• Acid phosphatase, prostatic specific antigen to exclude prostatic carcinoma
• Calcium, P04, alkaline phosphatase
• Thyroid function tests to exclude thyroid carcinoma
• Elevated ESR and WBC in osteomyelitis
• Serum protein electrophoresis and urine electrophoresis to exclude myeloma

Drugs that may alter lab results: N/A
Disorders that may alter lab results: N/A

PATHOLOGICAL FINDINGS
• Histology and special studies in combination with radiographic findings confirms the diagnosis
• PAS staining before and after glycogen digestion with diastase is useful in confirming the diagnosis in 80% of Ewing's sarcomas
• Electron microscopy: glycogen granules in Ewing's sarcoma; neurosecretory granules in neuroectodermal tumors; Birbeck bodies in histiocytosis-X

SPECIAL TESTS
• Open biopsy or needle biopsy. Needle biopsies may not provide enough tissue for frozen section, touch prep, permanent section, snap freezing, electron microscopy, cytogenetic and molecular studies, DNA indices, immunoperoxidase staining and immunophenotyping (lymphoma).
• Biopsy of associated soft tissue mass may lessen the risk of pathologic fracture
• Biopsy tract should to be excised in continuity with the tumor at the time of resection.

IMAGING
• Plain films provide the most important information regarding the nature of the lesion and guide further testing
• Bone scan - prior to biopsy, looking for other lesions
• CT scan for cortical destruction and internal calcification or ossification. Abdominal CT, MRI or renal ultrasound to exclude hypernephroma.
• MRI scan determines the extent of marrow involvement and associated soft tissue mass
• Chest x-ray and chest CT for metastatic disease.
• Mammogram to exclude breast carcinoma

DIAGNOSTIC PROCEDURES
• Rectal exam for prostatic nodules
• Laboratory studies for metabolic bone disease

TREATMENT

APPROPRIATE HEALTH CARE
Inpatient surgery

GENERAL MEASURES N/A

SURGICAL MEASURES
• Resection with adequate margin is required to minimize risk of local persistence
• For MFH and osteosarcoma, pre-resection neo-adjuvant chemotherapy treats micrometastatic disease immediately, allows time for ordering replacement prosthesis and bone graft, allows for an in vivo assessment of the chemotherapy responsiveness of the tumor, and may facilitate limb salvage by allowing a "safer" close margin
• Chondrosarcoma in the extremities should be treated exclusively by surgery unless it is of the mesenchymal or de-differentiated high grade variety
• Ewing's sarcoma was traditionally treated with chemotherapy and surgery was limited to those lesions that were extremely large, associated with pathologic fracture, or involved an expendable bone. Most Ewing's sarcoma lesions were irradiated. However, despite irradiation, local recurrence is common up to 25% in pelvic lesions. Therefore, surgery with limb salvage is increasingly accepted. A dramatic decrease in size in Ewing's sarcoma occurs after initial chemotherapy and a decision can then be made after restaging as to whether to irradiate or to resect the primary lesion.
• The treatment goal is to minimize local recurrence while preserving function. Limb salvage is employed whenever a safe margin can be obtained.

ACTIVITY
Varies with stage of disease and treatment

DIET No special diet

PATIENT EDUCATION
Refer to local branch of American Cancer Society for information and support groups

MEDICATIONS

DRUG(S) OF CHOICE
These drugs are administered according to specific protocols. Other protocols may be appropriate.
• MFH and osteosarcoma:
◊ Doxorubicin (Adriamycin)
◊ Intra-arterial and intravenous cisplatin
◊ High dose methotrexate with leucovorin rescue
◊ Ifosfamide [with mesna to protect against hemorrhagic cystitis]
◊ Cyclophosphamide (Cytoxan)
◊ Dactinomycin (actinomycin-D)
◊ Bleomycin
• Liposome-encapsulated muramyl tripeptide phosphatidylethanolamine (liposomal MTP-PE) immune modulating agent for osteosarcoma (under trial in CCSG and POG)
• Ewing's sarcoma:
◊ Cyclophosphamide
◊ Vincristine
◊ Actinomycin D
◊ Doxorubicin (Adriamycin)
◊ Ifosfamide
◊ Etoposide
Contraindications: Refer to manufacturer's literature
Precautions:
• Left ventricular dysfunction with Adriamycin. Cumulative dose > 450 mg/m2 increases risk. Follow with serial echocardiograms and/or MUGA scans when cumulative dose > 250 mg/m2.
• With high dose methotrexate, hydration, alkalinization of the urine, and close monitoring of plasma levels are needed
Significant possible interactions:
• Myelosuppression
• Renal tubular dysfunction with ifosfamide
• Renal and hepatic dysfunction and GI mucositis with methotrexate
• Nephrotoxicity and ototoxicity with cisplatin

ALTERNATIVE DRUGS
• Ondansetron (Zofran), dronabinol (Marinol), metoclopramide (Reglan), and others for nausea control
• Cyclosporin-A is used in clinical trials to reverse effect of multiple drug resistance gene (MDR-1) expression of P-glycoprotein in metastatic osteosarcomas (verapamil has toxicity)

FOLLOWUP

PATIENT MONITORING
• Patients who require adjuvant chemotherapy are treated after resection of the tumor with maintenance chemotherapy
• Blood counts for myelosuppression
• Serial echocardiograms when Adriamycin is being used. G-CSF often used to minimize neutropenia.

• Chest x-rays obtained every two months for the first year, every three months for the second year, and every four months in the third year
• CT scans of the lungs are initially repeated every six months during first two years
• Ewing's sarcoma may recur > 5 years after diagnosis

PREVENTION/AVOIDANCE None identified

POSSIBLE COMPLICATIONS
• Limb salvage with any primary malignant bone tumor is fraught with potential complications
• Micrometastatic disease may have occurred at the time of presentation and can appear at any time during the course of treatment or followup
• Local recurrence risk for osteosarcoma with limb salvage is about 10%
• There can be leg length discrepancy, infection, wound dehiscence, skin coverage problems, arterial and nerve injury, non-union of bone grafts, and mechanical loosening of prosthetic implants
• Thoracotomy and continued chemotherapy is often recommended for metastatic disease to the lung
• Ewing's sarcoma, metastatic to the lung, is quite diffuse and is less amenable to thoracotomy

EXPECTED COURSE/PROGNOSIS
• With amputation alone, 80% of patients with osteosarcoma had pulmonary metastatic disease by two years. With chemotherapy, the five year disease-free survival rate is 50-85%.
• Favorable prognostic factors for MFH and osteosarcoma include responsiveness to chemotherapy, distal portions of the extremities, small size, age over ten
• Most chondrosarcomas are of lower grade and have a low risk of metastatic spread and low incidence of local recurrence after adequate surgery
• MFH, osteosarcoma, and Ewing's sarcoma have an overall 50% survival with combined treatment modalities

MISCELLANEOUS

ASSOCIATED CONDITIONS
• A higher incidence of chondrosarcoma is seen in patients with multiple hereditary exostosis, multiple enchondromatosis (Ollier's disease) and patients with enchondromatosis and hemangiomatosis (Maffucci's syndrome)
• Patients with enchondromatosis more often die of GI malignancies than metastatic chondrosarcoma

AGE-RELATED FACTORS
Pediatric: N/A
Geriatric: N/A
Others: N/A

PREGNANCY
• Increased growth of musculoskeletal malignancies during pregnancy
• Soft tissue desmoid tumors have estrogen and progesterone receptors

SYNONYMS N/A

ICD-9-CM
170.9 Malignant neoplasm of bone and articular cartilage, site unspecified

SEE ALSO
• Osteitis deformans

OTHER NOTES
• Osteosarcoma variants like parosteal, periosteal, and intraosseous osteosarcoma are lower grade lesions with a more favorable prognosis, often not requiring chemotherapy. Other variants, post irradiation, and post-Paget's osteosarcoma metastasize early.
• Chordoma - rare malignant bone tumor that develops from the remnants of the primitive notochord. May be located in the sacrum or near the base of the skull. Usual course - slowly progressive; recurrent; cure possible.

ABBREVIATIONS
ESR = erythrocyte sedimentation rate
MUGA = nuclear multiple gated acquisition ventriculogram

REFERENCES
• Enneking WF: Musculoskeletal Tumor Surgery, Volumes I and II. New York, Churchill Livingstone, 1983
• Schajowicz F, McGuire MH: Diagnostic difficulties in skeletal pathology. Clinical orthopedics and Related Research 1991;240:281-310
• Womer RB: The cellular biology of bone tumors. Clinical orthopedics and Related Research 1991;262:12-21
• Simon MA: Limb salvage for osteosarcoma in the 1980's. Clinical orthopedics and Related Research 1991;270:264-270
• Velez-Yanguas, Warrier RP: The evolution of chemotherapeutic agents for the treatment of pediatric musculoskeletal malignancies, Orthopedic Clin NA 1996;27:545-549
Illustrations: N/A
Internet references: http://www.5mcc.com

Author(s)
Irwin E. Harris, MD, MBA, MSHA, FACS

Botulism

BASICS

DESCRIPTION An intoxication producing paralytic disease, caused by neurotoxins of *Clostridium botulinum*. The toxin prevents acetylcholine release at presynaptic membranes.
- Three forms exist:
  ◊ Foodborne botulism
  ◊ Infantile botulism
  ◊ Wound botulism

System(s) affected: Endocrine/Metabolic, Gastrointestinal, Nervous

Genetics: N/A

Incidence/Prevalence in USA:
- 0.034/100,000 with 75% the infantile form.
- Foodborne - 24 cases/yr
- Infantile - 71 cases/yr
- Wound botulism - 3 cases/yr

Predominant age:
- Foodborne - all ages
- Infantile mean age - 3 months
- Wound - usually young adult

Predominant sex:
- Foodborne and infantile - Male = Female
- Wound - Male > Female

SIGNS AND SYMPTOMS
- Foodborne
  ◊ Nonspecific findings early (nausea, vomiting, malaise, dizziness)
  ◊ Dry mouth
  ◊ Constipation, urinary retention
  ◊ Symmetric descending weakness or paralysis of motor and autonomic nerves, usually beginning with the cranial nerves
  ◊ Cranial nerve paralysis (ptosis; extraocular muscle paresis; fixed, dilated pupils; dysphagia)
  ◊ Postural hypotension
  ◊ Muscle weakness, respiratory paralysis
  ◊ Variable deep tendon reflexes
  ◊ Afebrile
  ◊ Progression over few days
- Infantile
  ◊ Constipation - early sign
  ◊ Loss of head control
  ◊ Loss of suck
  ◊ Loss of facial expression and verbalization
  ◊ Symmetric descending weakness and cranial nerve paresis similar to foodborne form
  ◊ Diminished or absent deep tendon reflexes
  ◊ Autonomic dysfunction
  ◊ Afebrile
  ◊ Usual progression over 2-5 days, can be as short as few hours
- Wound
  ◊ Onset 4-14 days post injury
  ◊ Findings similar to foodborne botulism
  ◊ May be febrile

CAUSES
- Ingestion of *C. botulinum* neurotoxins (A, B, and E most common)
- Foodborne usually from home-canned vegetables or prepared foods
- Infantile from ingestion of spores in environment or occasionally in honey
- Wound due to contamination with toxin-producing *C. botulinum*

RISK FACTORS
- Foodborne - ingestion of home-canned or prepared foods
- Infantile - ingestion of honey. Breast feeding (controversial)
- IV drug use (e.g., black tar heroin)

DIAGNOSIS

DIFFERENTIAL DIAGNOSIS
- Guillain-Barré syndrome
- Encephalitis
- Tick paralysis
- Myasthenia gravis
- Basilar artery stroke
- Congenital neuropathy or myopathy
- Sepsis
- Other poisonings (organophosphate, shellfish, Amanita mushrooms, atropine, aminoglycoside)

LABORATORY
- Routine tests including CSF exam normal
- Confirmation available at the CDC and some state laboratories

Drugs that may alter lab results: N/A

Disorders that may alter lab results: Underlying myoneural disease

PATHOLOGICAL FINDINGS
Nonspecific

SPECIAL TESTS
- Stool contains organism and toxin
- Serum toxin present in foodborne form

IMAGING N/A

DIAGNOSTIC PROCEDURES
Electromyogram (EMG) shows characteristic brief, low voltage compound motor-unit, small amplitude, overly abundant action potentials (BSAPs), incremental response to repetitive stimulation

TREATMENT

APPROPRIATE HEALTH CARE
Inpatient, with maximal monitoring capabilities, especially for respiratory failure

GENERAL MEASURES
- Meticulous airway management
- Physical therapy with range of motion exercise and assisted ambulation as tolerated
- Prevention of decubiti

SURGICAL MEASURES Wound excision débridement

ACTIVITY Bedrest initially

DIET
- Nasogastric feedings if needed
- Fluid restriction if inappropriate antidiuretic hormone (ADH) syndrome

PATIENT EDUCATION
- When preserving food at home, kill Clostridium botulinum spores by pressure cooking at 250°F (120°C) for 30 minutes
- Toxin can be destroyed by boiling for 10 minutes or cooking at 175°F (80°C) for 30 minutes
- Avoid honey in first year of life

Botulism

MEDICATIONS

DRUG(S) OF CHOICE
• Foodborne
  ◊ Antitoxin therapy with trivalent A-B-E antitoxin [available at CDC (404) 639-3670 or 639-2888], one vial IV and one vial IM, repeat IV in 2-4 hours if symptoms persist
  ◊ Penicillin therapy of unclear value
• Infantile
  ◊ Antitoxin therapy not needed
  ◊ Penicillin therapy of unclear value
  ◊ Enemas may assist in removal of toxin
• Wound
  ◊ Antitoxin therapy with trivalent A-B-E antitoxin (available at CDC (404) 639-3753 or 639-2888), one vial IV and one vial IM, repeat in 2-4 hours if persistent symptoms
Contraindications: Aminoglycosides - may potentiate paralysis
Precautions: Serum sickness or hypersensitivity reactions in 20% of antitoxin recipients
Significant possible interactions: N/A

ALTERNATIVE DRUGS N/A

FOLLOWUP

PATIENT MONITORING Cardiorespiratory monitoring during illness

PREVENTION/AVOIDANCE
• Avoid giving honey to infants
• Do not eat or taste food from bulging cans, or if food is off-smelling, discard it

POSSIBLE COMPLICATIONS
• Aspiration pneumonia
• Nosocomial infection
• Hypoxic tissue damage
• Death

EXPECTED COURSE/PROGNOSIS
• Foodborne and wound
  ◊ Mortality 25% (< 10% under 20 years of age), usually due to delayed diagnosis and respiratory failure
  ◊ Full recovery may require months
  ◊ Sequelae due to hypoxic insults
• Infantile
  ◊ Mortality < 1%
  ◊ Extended recovery period and sequelae as above

MISCELLANEOUS

ASSOCIATED CONDITIONS N/A

AGE-RELATED FACTORS
Pediatric: Avoid honey for first year
Geriatric: N/A
Others: N/A

PREGNANCY N/A

SYNONYMS
• Sausage poisoning
• Kerner's disease

ICD-9-CM
005.1 Botulism

SEE ALSO
• Food poisoning, bacterial
• Tick paralysis

OTHER NOTES Organism present in stools of 1-2% of healthy individuals

ABBREVIATIONS N/A

REFERENCES
• Shapiro RL, Hatheway C, Swerdlow DL. Botulism in the United States: a clinical and epidemiologic review. Ann Intern Med 1998 Aug 1;129(3):221-8
• Mandell G, Douglas R, Bennett J: Principles and Practice of Infectious Diseases. 4th Ed. New York, Churchill Livingstone, 1995
• Oski F, DeAngelis C, Feigin R, Warshaw J: Principles and Practice of Pediatrics. Philadelphia, J.B. Lippincott, 1990
Illustrations: N/A
Internet references: http://www.5mcc.com

Author(s)
Mark R. Dambro, MD, FAAFP

Brain abscess

 BASICS

DESCRIPTION
Single or multiple abscesses within the brain, usually occurring secondary to a focus of infection outside the central nervous system. May mimic brain tumor but evolves more rapidly (days to a few weeks). It starts as a cerebritis, becomes necrotic, and subsequently becomes encapsulated.

System(s) affected: Nervous
Genetics: No known genetic pattern
Incidence/Prevalence in USA: Infrequent
Predominant age: Median age 30-40
Predominant sex: Male > Female (2:1)

SIGNS AND SYMPTOMS
• Recent onset of headache becoming severe
• Nausea and vomiting
• Mental changes progressing to stupor and coma
• Afebrile or low-grade fever
• Neck stiffness
• Seizures
• Papilledema
• Focal neurological signs depending on location

CAUSES
• Direct extension from otitis, mastoiditis, sinusitis or dental infection
• Cranial osteomyelitis
• Penetrating skull trauma
• Prior craniotomy
• Bacteremia from lung abscess, pneumonia
• Bacterial endocarditis
• Fungal infection of the nasopharynx
• Toxoplasma gondii (in AIDS patients)
• Cyanotic congenital heart disease
• Intravenous drug use
• No source found in 20%
• Most common infective organisms - streptococci, staphylococci, enteric gram-negative bacilli and anaerobes (usually same as source of infection), Nocardia

RISK FACTORS
• AIDS
• Immunocompromised
• IV drug abuse

 DIAGNOSIS

DIFFERENTIAL DIAGNOSIS
• Brain tumors
• Stroke
• Resolving intracranial hemorrhage
• Subdural empyema
• Extradural abscess
• Encephalitis

LABORATORY
• WBC may be normal or mildly elevated
• Culture of abscess contents, predominant organisms include Toxoplasma (AIDS), Staphylococcus (trauma), aerobic or anaerobic bacteria, fungi (rare)
• Blood studies - mild polymorphonuclear leukocytosis, elevated sedimentation rate
Drugs that may alter lab results: Prior administration of antibiotics
Disorders that may alter lab results: N/A

PATHOLOGICAL FINDINGS
• Suppuration, liquification, encapsulation, depending on stage of evolution
• Fibrosis

SPECIAL TESTS
Surgical burr hole with aspiration to make a specific bacteriologic diagnosis

IMAGING
• CT or MRI are diagnostic methods of choice - findings are dependent on stages of the abscess
• Radionuclide 117 IN-labeled leukocytes may distinguish abscess from neoplasm

DIAGNOSTIC PROCEDURES
• History, physical exam
• Lumbar puncture often contraindicated
• Search for primary source of infection (chest x-ray, skull film for fracture, sinus films, etc.)

 TREATMENT

APPROPRIATE HEALTH CARE
Inpatient for close observation, diagnostic evaluation, and specialty consultation (neurology, neurosurgery, infectious disease)

GENERAL MEASURES
• Palliative and supportive
• Medical therapy
◊ For surgical inaccessible, multiple abscesses
◊ For abscesses in early cerebritis stage
◊ Therapy directed toward most likely organism
◊ Small (< 2.5 cm) abscess

SURGICAL MEASURES
• Surgical therapy
◊ Mandatory when neurologic deficits are severe or progressive
◊ Used when the abscess is in the posterior fossa
◊ Abscess drainage - (via needle) under stereotactic CT guidance through a burr hole under local anesthesia, is most rapid and effective method. May be repeated if needed.
◊ Craniotomy - if abscess is large or multilocular
◊ Abscess resulting from trauma

ACTIVITY
Bedrest until infection controlled and abscess evacuated or resolving, then up as tolerated

DIET
IV fluids if nausea and vomiting present

PATIENT EDUCATION
For patient education materials favorably reviewed on this topic, contact: Brain Research Foundation, 208 S. LaSalle Street, Suite 1426, Chicago, IL 60604, (312)782-4311

MEDICATIONS

DRUG(S) OF CHOICE
• Antibiotics according to organism if known
• If organism unknown, begin with penicillin G and metronidazole, or chloramphenicol (Chloromycetin), if metronidazole cannot be used
• Add oxacillin or nafcillin if trauma or IV drug user (use vancomycin in penicillin-sensitive patients)
• If gram-negative organism suspected (otic, GI, GU organ) add third-generation cephalosporin
• Abscess associated with HIV infection assumed to be due to Toxoplasma gondii - daily doses of sulfadiazine and pyrimethamine. (Therapy will be life-long in AIDS patients.)
• Anticonvulsants - phenytoin until abscess resolved or perhaps longer. Obtain anticonvulsant levels.
• Following surgical procedure - corticosteroids to reduce edema. Dexamethasone. Taper rapidly. Use usually limited to 1 week. Continue antibiotics for 6-8 weeks.
Contraindications: Sensitivity or allergy to any prescribed medications
Precautions:
• Sulfadiazine poorly water soluble. Patients must maintain adequate hydration or risk developing crystalluria.
• Decrease dosage of penicillins in patients with renal dysfunction
• Monitor serum levels of anticonvulsants
• Dose of pyrimethamine require for treatment of toxoplasmosis may approach toxic levels. Should observe for folic acid deficiency and treat with folinic acid (leucovorin) 5-15 mg (orally, IM, IV) if necessary
Significant possible interactions: Refer to manufacturer's literature

ALTERNATIVE DRUGS   N/A

FOLLOWUP

PATIENT MONITORING
• Postsurgical monitoring as needed
• Serial CT or MRI - to confirm progressive resolution, early detection and management of complications

PREVENTION/AVOIDANCE
• Adequate treatment of otitis media, mastoiditis, dental abscess, other predisposing factors
• Prophylactic antibiotics after compound skull fracture or penetrating head wound

POSSIBLE COMPLICATIONS
• Permanent neurological deficits
• Surgical complications
• Recurrent abscess
• Seizures

EXPECTED COURSE/PROGNOSIS
Survival > 80% with early diagnosis and treatment

MISCELLANEOUS

ASSOCIATED CONDITIONS
• AIDS
• Congenital heart disease

AGE-RELATED FACTORS
Pediatric:
• About one third of cases in pediatric age group. Rarely found in infants under 1 year of age.
• Cyanotic congenital heart disease frequently associated
Geriatric: Age does not affect outcome as much as abscess size and state of neurological dysfunction at presentation
Others: N/A

PREGNANCY   N/A

SYNONYMS   Cerebral abscess

ICD-9-CM   324.0 Intracranial abscess

SEE ALSO   N/A

OTHER NOTES   N/A

ABBREVIATIONS   N/A

REFERENCES
• Patel KS, Marks PV: Management of focal intracranial infections: Is medical treatment better than surgery? J Neuro Neurosurg Psychiatry 1990;53:472
• Maniglia AJ, Goodwin WJ, Arnold JE, et al: Intracranial abscesses secondary to nasal, sinus, and orbital infections in adults and children. Arch Otolaryngol Head Neck Surg 1989;115:1424
• Osenbach RK, Loftus CM: Diagnosis and Management of Brain Abscess. Neurosurgery Clinics of North America 1992;3:403-420
• Twomey CR: Brain diseases: An update. J Neuroscience Nursing 1992;24:34-39
• Adams RD, Victor M: Principles of Neurology. 5th Ed. New York, McGraw-Hill, 1993
• Rowland LD, ed: Merritt's Textbook of Neurology. 9th Ed. Baltimore, Williams & Wilkins, 1995
• Rakel RE, ed: Conn's Current Therapy. Philadelphia, W.B. Saunders Co., 1995
Illustrations: N/A
Internet references: http://www.5mcc.com

Author(s)
Peter Kozisek, MD

Brain injury - post acute care issues

BASICS

DESCRIPTION
Post acute severely brain injured patients with complex injuries, prolonged coma, initial GCS<9 who may have limited responses to environment, are often inconsistently able to communicate their needs and manage personal affairs, and frequently have motor deficits. These patients may reside in a long term care facility or at home with attendant care. Less severely injured individuals may have more evident cognitive and behavioral problems and less physical issues.
Management issues include:
• Changes in level of attention, arousal, cognition and behavior
• Neurogenic bladder and bowel
• Contractures and spasticity
• Heterotopic ossification
• Skin
• Respiratory
• Endocrine
System(s) affected: Nervous, Pulmonary, Skin/Exocrine, Endocrine/Metabolic, Musculoskeletal, Renal/Urologic, Reproductive
Genetics: N/A
Incidence/Prevalence in USA: N/A
Predominant age: Young adults
Predominant Sex: Male > Female

SIGNS AND SYMPTOMS
• Neurological
◊ Diminished arousal leads to limited responses and may be generalized (eg, decorticate posturing or focal such as eye blink or one limb voluntary movement)
◊ Cognitive impairment
◊ Disinhibited responses and behavior
◊ Impaired memory
◊ Anosagnosia (poor self-awareness)
◊ Focal motor deficits, eg, hemiparesis
◊ Cerebellar signs - ataxia, nystagmus, dysmetria, dysdiadochokinesis
◊ Cranial nerve palsies
◊ Hydrocephalus-triad of worse cognition, ataxia, incontinence
◊ Epilepsy - partial or generalized signs
• Urinary frequency and incontinence
• Bowel incontinence
• Spasticity
• Heterotopic ossification - erythema, pain or stiffness in soft tissue around joint
• Decubitus ulcers
• Decreased respiratory strength or poor cough
• Endocrine

CAUSES
MVA, assaults, sports injuries, falls

RISK FACTORS
See Brain injury, traumatic

DIAGNOSIS

DIFFERENTIAL DIAGNOSIS
A number of complications can create a change in functional level.
• Chronic infection (e.g., UTI)
• Depression
• Hypothyroidism, other endocrinopathy
• Hydrocephalus, hematoma
• Epilepsy
• Fractures
• Tracheal stricture

LABORATORY
• CBC, electrolytes, BUN, creatinine, calcium, albumin, vitamin B12, folate, TSH, alkaline phosphatase, AST, ALT, morning cortisol level, urine culture
• Culture, ova and parasites for diarrhea
• Calcium and alkaline phosphatase
• Skin culture
• Culture tracheal site
• Endocrine workup as indicated
Drugs that may alter lab results: N/A
Disorders that may alter lab results: N/A

PATHOLOGICAL FINDINGS
• Hydrocephalus with periventricular edema
• Joint contractures results in collagen cross linking: decreased range of motion
• Heterotopic ossification: disorganized osteoid calcification in soft tissue

SPECIAL TESTS
• Evoked potentials (auditory, visual and somatosensory)
• Behavioral assessment, neuropsychological testing and vocational assessment in the less severe
• Cognitive testing for orientation and arousal use Western Neuro Sensory Stimulation Profile (WNSS) or Galveston Orientation Amnesia Test (GOAT)
• EEG

IMAGING
• Bone scan: heterotopic ossification
• CT: hydrocephalus, atrophy, hematoma
• Video pharyngeal fluoroscopic swallowing study
• MRI

DIAGNOSTIC PROCEDURES
• Altered arousal - visual, auditory and somatosensory evoked potentials
• Neurogenic bladder- check post void residuals 3-4 times. If > 50cc or 20% of voided volume, urodynamics
• Ultrasound of bladder and kidney: urolithiasis and hydronephrosis
• Endoscopy: cause of dysphagia
• Contractures and spasticity: examination under anesthesia
• Respiratory and neurologic: sleep/oxygen saturation study, bronchoscopy for stricture

TREATMENT

APPROPRIATE HEALTH CARE
Outpatient; occasional inpatient care

GENERAL MEASURES
• Diminished level of arousal: identify best modality for communication, assess functional skills (proper seating, hand function), behavioral or neuropsychologist. Respiratory therapist (for those with tracheostomy), social work (to assist with family education and long term planning) and nursing
• Reduce sedatives
• Neurogenic bladder - treat UTI
◊ If post void residual < 50cc then trial of regular voiding routine q2hr
◊ If still incontinent add oxybutynin
◊ If still incontinent try condom catheter during the day; incontinent pads at night.
◊ If raised post void residuals or high pressure bladder or dyssynergic bladder on urodynamics then intermittent catheter q4-6h
• Neurogenic bowel - regular bowel routine
• Contractures and spasticity: stretching
◊ If no progress after 4 weeks consider serial casting or custom made orthotic
◊ Contractures > 45º consider tendon release
• Heterotopic ossification: stretch soft tissue to decrease maturation of osteoid, consider orthotics/splinting. Bone scan at baseline.
• Skin: q2hr turning, avoid seating in position of high shear on buttocks such as in bed at 45 degrees, observe for erythema around tube sites and rule out latex allergy
• Respiratory: night humidification if has a tracheotomy, may require suctioning
• Endocrine- monitor fluid balance
• Dental - assessment and dental x-rays

SURGICAL MEASURES
• Tendons releases; fundoplasty or gastrostomy; tracheostomy; ventriculoperitoneal or ventriculoatrial shunt

ACTIVITY
• As tolerated - outings in wheelchair can be beneficial - skin very sensitive to sun/wind - protect with clothing/golf umbrella clipped to chair
• Age appropriate activities related to premorbid interests yield best attention

DIET
• Consult with dietitian
• Ensure adequate hydration; 2-2.5L of water/day. More if outside or in hot weather.
• Bolus feeds preferred
• Upright and quiet activity for half an hour following feeds as aspiration can occur even with a g-tube

PATIENT EDUCATION
• For information and family support groups: http://www.tbinet.org/ or http://www.biausa.org/
• Families need support, advocacy, education, information - verbally and written (audio tape meetings), opportunities to have input regarding priorities, treatment plans and discuss limits of treatment for patient (advance directive)

MEDICATIONS

DRUG(S) OF CHOICE
Individualize pharmacotherapy
• Diminished arousal: Consider one of desipramine or amitriptyline 75-150 mg hs, methylphenidate (Ritalin) 20-40 mg/day in 2 divided doses, amantadine 50-200 mg bid, dextroamphetamine, bromocriptine, levodopa
• Agitation: treat epilepsy or depression otherwise, amitriptyline 75-150 mg hs, carbamazepine, valproic acid, lithium, propranolol, serotonin specific re-uptake inhibitor. Minimize use of haloperidol, antipsychotics and benzodiazepines as they worsen cognition. If necessary use antipsychotic with least cognitive side effects, eg, risperidone (Risperdal) or olanzapine (Zyprexa)
• Abulia and lack of initiation: amantadine, bromocriptine, methylphenidate, levodopa
• Epilepsy: if possible avoid phenytoin and phenobarbital - too sedating. Carbamazepine, valproic acid, gabapentin less sedating.
• Neurogenic bladder: oxybutynin 2.5 mg tid to 10 mg qid, if bladder pressures low and/or post void residuals low
• Bowel routine - stool softener such as docusate sodium (daily) combined with laxative (night before suppository), high fiber and suppository (every other day)to induce bowel movement
• Spasticity: all drugs may cause sedation; dantrolene 25-200 mg/day divided tid; or baclofen, benzodiazepines, clonidine. If focal spasticity consider botulinum toxin injection.
• Heterotopic ossification: indomethacin 25-50 mg tid. If severe, progressive or history of GI ulceration then etidronate (Didronel) 20 mg/kg for six months.
Contraindications: Refer to manufacturer's literature
Precautions: Refer to manufacturer's literature
Significant possible interactions: Refer to manufacturer's literature

ALTERNATIVE DRUGS N/A

FOLLOWUP

PATIENT MONITORING
• Patients make slow steady gains. Ongoing outcome assessments to determine progress (or not) in abilities and medication efficacy needed. These measures do not need to be sophisticated, for example: length of time able to hold head up or ability to respond to commands written or verbal. Modify program periodically to reflect outcome measures.
• Review medical status monthly

PREVENTION/AVOIDANCE
• Prevent further complications

POSSIBLE COMPLICATIONS
• Major affective disorder (depression, psychosis) in up to 50% of patients
• Family and caregiver burn out
• Substance abuse
• Social isolation
• May be a higher risk of dementia
• Latex allergy to g-tube, catheters
• Dental caries
• Osteoporosis
• Falls
• Aspiration pneumonia
• Pressure ulcers
• Heterotropic ossification
• Dysphagia, esophagitis
• Bladder incontinence
• Contractures/spasticity

EXPECTED COURSE/PROGNOSIS
• Most rapid return of neurological function is during first two years but some patients continue to improve slowly for 5-10 years as long as complications are prevented or managed appropriately.
• Highly variable (80% of individuals with severe injuries become independent in dressing and self-care at 1 year
• Negative prognostic factors:
  ◊ Age > 40
  ◊ Abnormal pupillary responses
  ◊ Prolonged coma i.e., GCS < 9 seven days after injury
  ◊ Abnormal evoked potentials
  ◊ Extraocular eye movement abnormalities

MISCELLANEOUS

ASSOCIATED CONDITIONS
• Psychosis
• Suicide attempts
• Substance abuse
• ADD

AGE-RELATED FACTORS
Pediatric: N/A
Geriatric: N/A
Others: N/A

PREGNANCY N/A

SYNONYMS N/A

ICD-9-CM
530.1 Esophagitis
750.6 Hiatus hernia
787.1 Heartburn
733.0 Osteoporosis
707.0 Decubitus ulcer
345.3 Grand mal status and status epilepticus

SEE ALSO
• Brain injury, traumatic
• Seizure disorders
• Sleep apnea, obstructive
• Stomatitis
• Stroke
• Stroke rehabilitation
• Osteoporosis
• Fecal impaction
• Hemorrhoids
• Constipation
• Dysphagia
• Gastroesophageal reflux disease
• Pressure ulcer

OTHER NOTES
• Paucity of research on this group of patients due to high number of variables, slow progress. However many people are misdiagnosed as being in a persistent vegetative state or locked in syndrome when voluntary responses can be elicited with thorough assessment
• No definitive research on optimum length of time for rehabilitation; slow and steady and over a lifetime appears most effective
• Rehabilitation program guidelines:
  ◊ Individualized: ideally using behavioral approach emphasizing reinforcement of task behavior
  ◊ Flexible: to account for patient's changing needs (eg, may have an infection that decreased their ability)
  ◊ Functional (based on practical activities): e.g., helping with self care activities also involves opportunity for range of motion exercises
  ◊ Consider patient's attention span and best time of day when planning
  ◊ Allow for as much control and choice as possible (eg, even if can only communicate with eye blinks can participate in choice of clothes to wear, music, preferred activity)
  ◊ Consistency and familiarity provide opportunities for learning
• Quality of life issues vital, e.g., comfort measures, sensory stimulation as tolerated, attention to spiritual and/or cultural needs, proper positioning
• For agitated behavior, consider consultation with behavioral psychologist to assist in design of program integrating medications and behavior therapy techniques. Minimize use of punishment and reinforce correct behavior. New technique known as Errorless Compliance Training may be helpful.

ABBREVIATIONS
GCS = Glasgow Coma Score

REFERENCES
13 additional references available at web site
Internet references: http://www.5mcc.com
Illustrations: N/A

Author(s)
Mark T. Bayley, BA, MD, FRCPC
Helen Driediger, RN, BA, BSW

Brain injury, traumatic

BASICS

DESCRIPTION Traumatic brain injury (TBI) is a principal cause of death and disability in young adults, at an estimated cost of $39 billion per year in the USA. Frequently related to rapid deceleration such as motor vehicle accidents, diving accidents. May also be due to blunt injury such as with a baseball bat, etc.
• TBI is a dynamic process with initial bleeding followed by secondary injury due to cerebral edema, continued intracranial bleeding, etc.
Predicting outcome initially is difficult and patients may improve for years.
• Consider child abuse in the proper circumstance.
• Categorize patients:
  ◊ Mild: Minimal trauma, no loss of consciousness (LOC) or amnesia, alert, oriented, normal GCS, non-focal exam. Vomiting once or twice may occur, especially in children. May have headache. No need for further imaging or intervention.
  ◊ Moderate: Evidence of intracranial injury, but non-focal exam. May have had transient loss of consciousness, amnesia, headache, evidence of basilar fracture (Raccoon eyes, Battle's sign, hemotympanum, CSF rhinorrhea). These patients should have a CT scan if practical and should be admitted for serial neurological exams.
  ◊ Severe: Continued LOC, focal exam, any decreased level of consciousness. These patients need CT and immediate neurosurgical consultation. Focal exam indicates the possibility of a space-occupying lesion that may need surgical correction. Admit to ICU.
System(s) affected: Nervous, Cardiovascular, Endocrine/Metabolic
Genetics: N/A
Incidence/Prevalence in USA: Incidence: 200/100,000; 500,000 hospitalizations and 75,000 deaths per year
Predominant age: 15-24
Predominant sex: Male > Female

SIGNS AND SYMPTOMS
Variable and dependent on degree of injury:
• Loss of consciousness (transient or persistent)
• External signs of head injury
• Headache
• Vomiting
• Amnesia
• Focal signs and symptoms
• Evidence for increased intracranial hypertension (elevated blood pressure, decreased pulse rate, slow or irregular breathing [Cushing's triad])
• Decorticate or decerebrate positioning (both a bad prognostic sign)
• Seizures
• Raccoon eyes, Battle's sign, hemotympanum
• CSF rhinorrhea (see Special tests)
• Unilateral dilated pupil in an alert patient is not a sign of impending herniation since such patients are always unconscious.

• Epidural hemorrhage from blunt trauma is generally acute, frequently with a "lucid interval" (initial loss of consciousness followed by recovery of consciousness then loss of consciousness secondary to the intracranial bleed).
• Subdural hemorrhage usually has a slower onset and may present weeks after the initial injury, especially in the elderly.

CAUSES
• Motor vehicle accident (50%)
• Falls
• Assault

RISK FACTORS
• Alcohol
• Prior head injury
• Contact sports

DIAGNOSIS

DIFFERENTIAL DIAGNOSIS Other causes of coma (e.g., drug overdose, infection, metabolic, vascular causes)

LABORATORY
• Patients may rapidly develop DIC; PT/INR, PTT, CBC (for decreased platelets), fibrin degradation products
• Drug and alcohol screening
Drugs that may alter lab results: N/A
Disorders that may alter lab results: N/A

PATHOLOGICAL FINDINGS
• Epidural, subdural or intraparenchymal hemorrhage
• Coup or contra-coup injury
• Evolving, diffuse axonal injury is a principle cause of neurologic sequelae with mild head trauma

SPECIAL TESTS
• Neuropsychometric testing when able
• CSF rhinorrhea contains glucose while nasal mucus does not. Check also for the double-halo sign: put a drop of bloody nasal discharge on filter paper. If it contains both CSF and blood, there will be two rings; a central ring followed by a paler ring.

IMAGING
• CT, C-spine as indicated
• Skull radiographs are not helpful in most cases, but can be done to document child abuse

DIAGNOSTIC PROCEDURES
Placement of intracranial pressure monitor when indicated, serial neurologic exams

TREATMENT

APPROPRIATE HEALTH CARE
Outpatient for mild, inpatient or ICU for more severe

GENERAL MEASURES
Acute management depends on severity of injury. Most patients need no interventions. [Note: There is very little evidence to support or refute the use of most of these measures (including hyperventilation and mannitol); further studies are in progress.]
• The immediate goal is to determine who needs further therapy, imaging studies (CT) and hospitalization, and to prevent further injury.
• All penetrating injury should be evaluated by a neurosurgeon.
• C-spine immobilization should be considered in all head trauma. Clear the cervical spine radiographically (AP, lateral showing all 7 cervical vertebrae and the C7/T1 interspace, obliques if indicated).
• ABCs (airway, breathing, circulation) take priority over head injury. Stabilization and prevention of mortality from other injuries is critical to insuring patient survival.
• For the severely injured patient:
  ◊ Immediate cardiopulmonary resuscitation, avoid hypotension or hypoxia. Head injury causes increased intracranial pressure secondary to edema and perfusion pressure must be maintained.
  ◊ Use normal saline for resuscitation fluid. If unable to obtain good IV access, can use 3% or 7% saline for resuscitation fluid (250cc boluses in adults). This does not seem to change mortality, however. Avoid lactated Ringer's which is slightly hypo-osmolar.
  ◊ Keep head of bed elevated at 30 degrees if possible
  ◊ Intubate and hyperventilate patients with significant injury to keep the PaCO2 at 25-30 mmHg. This reduces cerebral swelling. However, it also reduces brain circulation; the significance of this is not yet known. This recommendation may change.
  ◊ Start seizure prophylaxis (phenytoin) and continue for a week.
  ◊ Manage breakthrough seizures with lorazepam

SURGICAL MEASURES Dependent on neurological consult

ACTIVITY See ACTIVITY in topic Post-concussive syndrome for sports activity management.

DIET As tolerated

Brain injury, traumatic

PATIENT EDUCATION

- Brain Injury Association help-line: 1-800-444-6443
- Printed patient information: A Chance to Grow, 5034 Oliver Avenue North, Minneapolis, MN 55430, (612)521-2266
- Any patient discharged from your office or the ED should have instructions to watch for any changes in signs or symptoms that might indicate the need for further intervention (changing mental status, worsening headache, focal findings, etc.). Note that these instructions must be given to a competent surrogate who will observe the patient. If the patient deteriorates, it is not likely that he or she will be able to remember or act on any instructions.

MEDICATIONS

DRUG(S) OF CHOICE

- Acute management (do not hesitate to use morphine or benzodiazepines as indicated, but remember that they may alter the patient's mental status):
  ◊ Morphine 1-2 mg IV prn for pain control up to 15 mg or more per hour as needed
- Increased intracranial pressure:
  ◊ Mannitol 0.25-2 gm/kg given over 30-60 minutes. Only for use in patients with adequate renal function. For children, 0.25 -1 gm/kg over 30-60 minutes. Only one dose should be needed since these patients will require neurosurgical consultation.
- Furosemide 20-40 mg IV to promote diuresis and decrease CNS swelling
- Neither furosemide or mannitol should be given to the hypotensive patient
- Seizures: Seizure prophylaxis should be given using phenytoin
  ◊ Phenytoin (Dilantin) 15 mg/kg IV (1 mg/kg/min IV not to exceed 50 mg/min). Do not exceed 1 gm in adults. Monitor for QT prolongation and stop infusion if increases by > 50% (risk of torsades de pointes).
  ◊ Lorazepam (Ativan) 1-2 mg IV as needed for seizures for adults and 0.1 mg/kg in children. Higher doses may be needed and are OK as long as the patient is ventilated. Preferred over diazepam.
  ◊ Diazepam (Valium) 0.1-0.3 mg/kg IV (5-10 mg in adult, but may need 20-30 mg)
  ◊ Phenobarbital 15 mg/kg IV at 25-50 mg/min. May give IM.
- For paralysis:
  ◊ Vecuronium: 10 mg adults, followed by 2-5 mg IV as needed
  ◊ Pancuronium: 4 mg adults, and hourly as needed. Patient should be immediately intubated or airway should otherwise be controlled.
  ◊ Avoid succinylcholine which will increase ICP
- To prevent secondary injury from CNS arterial spasm:
  ◊ Nimodipine: after acute injury generally in consultation with neurosurgery or neurology
- Corticosteroids: there is no evidence to support their use in acute head injury and they may be detrimental. They should be given, however, if spinal cord injury is also present.

Contraindications: Neither furosemide nor mannitol should be given to the hypotensive patient. Make sure you can manage the airway before paralyzing the patient. Do not use morphine, benzodiazepines or phenobarbital unless you are prepared to manage the patient's airway.

Precautions: Refer to manufacturer's literature

Significant possible interactions: Phenobarbital, morphine and the benzodiazepines can have additive respiratory depression

ALTERNATIVE DRUGS Diuretics and IV beta-blockers (e.g. esmolol or labetalol) can be used to maintain the systolic pressure less than 170. Labetalol 5-10 mg IV until blood pressure is controlled. Nitroprusside may be helpful. Nitrates may increase intracranial pressure. Antibiotics (e.g., cefazolin) should be given if penetrating trauma is present. Prophylactic antibiotics are not useful in basilar skull fractures.

FOLLOWUP

PATIENT MONITORING

- Schedule regular followup
- Gradual return to work or school, even after mild to moderate head injury
- The post-concussion syndrome can follow mild head injury without loss of consciousness and includes headaches, dizziness, fatigue and subtle cognitive or affective changes. Most of these improve within 3 months.
- The most important element of mild TBI management, however, is recognizing the genuine organic basis for the patient's symptoms
- Proper counseling, symptomatic management and gradual return to normal activities is essential to prevent a post-traumatic neurosis which can become refractory to treatment

PREVENTION/AVOIDANCE

- Safety education
- Seat belts, bicycle and motorcycle helmets
- Protective headgear for contact sports

POSSIBLE COMPLICATIONS

- Delayed hematomas
- Chronic subdural hematoma, which may follow even "mild" head injury, especially in the elderly. Often present with headache, decreased mentation.
- Delayed hydrocephalus
- Emotional disturbances and psychiatric disorders resulting from head injury may be refractory to treatment
- Seizure disorders - in about 50% of penetrating head injuries, in about 20% of severe closed head injuries, and in < 5% of head injuries overall. Hematomas significantly increase risk of epilepsy.

EXPECTED COURSE/PROGNOSIS

- Gradual improvement for many
- 30-50% of severe head injuries may be fatal
- Prolonged coma may be followed by satisfactory outcome
- Following a significant acute injury, referral for rehabilitation is indicated. This includes involvement of the family in decision making and setting realistic goals for the patient and realistic expectations for the family. Some degree of improvement may continue for some time.

MISCELLANEOUS

ASSOCIATED CONDITIONS Alcohol and drug abuse

AGE-RELATED FACTORS
Pediatric: Outcome for children more positive, except in severe TBI
Geriatric:
- Poorer prognosis with increasing age
- Subdural hematomas are common after fall or blow; symptoms may be subtle
Others: None

PREGNANCY N/A

SYNONYMS
- Head injury
- Closed head injury

ICD-9-CM
800-804 Skull and facial fractures
850 Concussion
851 Cerebral laceration or contusion
852 Hematoma
854 Other cerebral injury of unspecified nature

SEE ALSO
- Seizure disorders
- Post-concussive syndrome
- Brain injury - post acute care issues

OTHER NOTES
- The GCS is not a linear scale. A level of 14 (normal being 15) puts the patient into the moderately severe injury category.

ABBREVIATIONS
GCS = Glasgow Coma Score
ICP = intracranial pressure

REFERENCES
5 additional references available at web site
Internet references: http://www.5mcc.com
Illustrations: N/A

Author(s)
Mark A. Graber, MD

Branchial cleft fistula

 BASICS

DESCRIPTION
A congenital, abnormal tract connecting the skin of neck with an internal structure, resulting from failure of closure of a branchial cleft.
• May involve branchial clefts I-IV
System(s) affected: Skin/Exocrine
Genetics: 10% have family history
Incidence/Prevalence in USA: Unknown
Predominant age: By definition are all present at birth although may remain unnoticed for some time. (Branchial cleft cysts may not present until later childhood.)
Predominant sex: Unknown

SIGNS AND SYMPTOMS
• Presence of tiny external opening usually on neck
• Spontaneous mucoid drainage
• External openings may also be marked by a skin tag or cartilage
• Infection may rarely be the presenting sign with erythema, swelling, pain, fever
• 10% are bilateral

CAUSES
• The 1st branchial cleft contributes to the tympanic cavity and eustachian tube. Related fistulae are very rare and tend to be infra- or retroauricular. (Preauricular cysts and sinuses are not thought to be of branchial cleft origin.)
• The 2nd branchial cleft forms the hyoid bone and tonsillar fossa. Related fistulae (most common variant) course between the internal and external carotid arteries. Internal opening usually at level of tonsillar fossa. External opening along anterior border of sternocleidomastoid muscle.
• 3rd and 4th branchial clefts form parathyroid glands, thymus and portions of thyroid (parafollicular cells). Fistulae are rare, those from 3rd cleft course lateral to carotid artery, both should have external ostia on lower anterior neck.

RISK FACTORS
Positive family history

 DIAGNOSIS

DIFFERENTIAL DIAGNOSIS
• External sinuses
• Cystic hygroma
• Dermoid cysts
• Lymphadenopathy

LABORATORY
Culture only if signs of infection
Drugs that may alter lab results: N/A
Disorders that may alter lab results: N/A

PATHOLOGICAL FINDINGS
Lined by stratified squamous epithelium, may contain hair follicles, sweat glands, sebaceous glands, cartilage. Some are lined by ciliated columnar epithelium.

SPECIAL TESTS
N/A

IMAGING
N/A

DIAGNOSTIC PROCEDURES
Sinogram or fistulogram may be done but is of little value

 TREATMENT

APPROPRIATE HEALTH CARE
• Surgical excision
• Outpatient status usually appropriate

GENERAL MEASURES
N/A

SURGICAL MEASURES
• Small transverse incision at external ostium with careful dissection of fistula
• Stepladder incisions may be needed
• End of fistula ligated flush with pharyngeal mucosa
• Drains are not used
• Antibiotics only for infection

ACTIVITY
N/A

DIET
N/A

PATIENT EDUCATION

MEDICATIONS

DRUG(S) OF CHOICE N/A
Contraindications: N/A
Precautions: N/A
Significant possible interactions: N/A

ALTERNATIVE DRUGS N/A

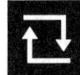
FOLLOWUP

PATIENT MONITORING
• Follow at weekly intervals, if infected, until resolution, than excision
• Postoperative visit at 2 weeks

PREVENTION/AVOIDANCE N/A

POSSIBLE COMPLICATIONS
• Facial nerve injury
• Infection
• Carotid artery injury
• Possible recurrence if any epithelium remains
• Neoplastic degeneration of branchial remnants (about 250 reported cases) if not resected

EXPECTED COURSE/PROGNOSIS
Good

MISCELLANEOUS

ASSOCIATED CONDITIONS Microtia and aural atresia occur with failure of development of 1st branchial cleft.

AGE-RELATED FACTORS
Pediatric: Almost all occur in pediatric age group
Geriatric: N/A
Others: N/A

PREGNANCY N/A

SYNONYMS N/A

ICD-9-CM
744.41 branchial cleft sinus or fistula

SEE ALSO N/A

OTHER NOTES Branchial cleft remnants, sinuses, cysts are also the result of failure of branchial cleft to complete its normal development

ABBREVIATIONS N/A

REFERENCES
• Ashcraft KW, Holder TM: Pediatric Surgery. 2nd Ed. Philadelphia, W.B. Saunders Co., 1993
• O'Neill JA, Rowe MI, Grosfeld JL, et al: Pediatric Surgery. 5th ed., St Louis, Mosby, 1998
Illustrations: N/A
Internet references: http://www.5mcc.com

Author(s)
Timothy L. Black, MD, FACS, FAAP

Breast abscess

BASICS

DESCRIPTION   Collection of pus usually localized. Can be associated with lactation or fistulous tracts secondary to squamous epithelial neoplasm or duct occlusion.
System(s) affected: Skin/Exocrine
Genetics: N/A
Incidence/Prevalence in USA: Common
Predominant age:
• Subareolar abscess - postmenopausal
• Puerperal abscess - premenopausal
Predominant sex: Female

SIGNS AND SYMPTOMS
• Tender breast lump, fluctuant, usually unilateral
• Erythema
• Draining pus
• Local edema
• Systemic malaise
• Fever
• Nipple and skin retraction
• Proximal lymphadenopathy

CAUSES
• Puerperal abscesses - blocked lactiferous duct
• Subareolar abscess - squamous epithelial neoplasm with keratin plugs or ductal extension with associated inflammation
• Peripheral abscess - stasis of the duct

RISK FACTORS
• Puerperal mastitis 5-11% go on to abscess
• Diabetes
• Rheumatoid arthritis
• Steroids
• Silicone/paraffin implants
• Lumpectomy with radiation
• Heavy cigarette smoking
• Nipple retraction

DIAGNOSIS

DIFFERENTIAL DIAGNOSIS
• Carcinoma (inflammatory)
• Tuberculosis (may be associated with HIV infection)
• Actinomycosis
• Typhoid
• Sarcoid
• Syphilis
• Hydatid cyst
• Sebaceous cyst

LABORATORY
• Leukocytosis
• Elevated sedimentation rate
• Culture and sensitivity of drainage to identify pathogen, usually staphylococci or streptococcus. Non-lactational abscess associated with anaerobic bacteria.
Drugs that may alter lab results: None
Disorders that may alter lab results: None

PATHOLOGICAL FINDINGS
• Squamous metaplasia of the ducts
• Intraductal hyperplasia
• Epithelial overgrowth
• Fat necrosis
• Duct ectasia

SPECIAL TESTS   None

IMAGING
• Ultrasound
• Mammogram - cannot exclude carcinoma

DIAGNOSTIC PROCEDURES
• Aspiration for culture
• Fine needle aspiration (FNA) not accurate to exclude carcinoma

TREATMENT

APPROPRIATE HEALTH CARE
Outpatient, unless systemically immunocompromised

GENERAL MEASURES
• Cold compresses
• Expression of milk

SURGICAL MEASURES
• Aspiration possibly under ultrasound guidance
• Incision and drainage with removal of loculations and biopsy of all non-puerperal abscesses to rule out carcinoma
• Open all fistulous tracts, especially in nonlactating abscesses

ACTIVITY   No restrictions

DIET   No restrictions

PATIENT EDUCATION
• Care of wound
• Breast feeding precautions

MEDICATIONS

DRUG(S) OF CHOICE
- Nonsteroidal anti-inflammatory agents
- Erythromycin 250-500 mg qid
- First generation, oral cephalosporin
  ◊ Cephalexin 500 mg bid
  ◊ Cefaclor 250 mg tid
- Amoxicillin-clavulanate (Augmentin) 250 mg tid
- Clindamycin 300 mg tid if anaerobes suspected

Contraindications: Allergy to antibiotic
Precautions: Refer to manufacturer's profile of each drug
Significant possible interactions: Refer to manufacturer's profile of each drug

ALTERNATIVE DRUGS   N/A

FOLLOWUP

PATIENT MONITORING   Assure resolution to exclude carcinoma

PREVENTION/AVOIDANCE
- Early treatment of mastitis with milk expression and cold compresses
- Early treatment with antibiotics

POSSIBLE COMPLICATIONS   Fistula

EXPECTED COURSE/PROGNOSIS
Good. Complete healing expected in 8 to 10 days, particularly if abscess can be incised and drained.

MISCELLANEOUS

ASSOCIATED CONDITIONS   N/A

AGE-RELATED FACTORS
Pediatric: N/A
Geriatric: N/A
Others: N/A

PREGNANCY   Most commonly associated with postpartum lactation

SYNONYMS
- Mammary abscess
- Peripheral breast abscess
- Subareolar abscess
- Puerperal abscess

ICD-9-CM
611.0 Acute, chronic, nonpuerperal
675.1 Puerperal, postpartum

SEE ALSO   N/A

OTHER NOTES   N/A

ABBREVIATIONS   N/A

REFERENCES
- Benson EA: Management of breast abscesses. World J Surg 1989;13:753-756
- Dixon JM: Periductal mastitis/duct ectasia. World J Surg 1989;13:715-720
- Ferrara JJ, et al: Non surgical management of breast infections in non-lactating women. Am Surg 1990;56:668-671
- Olsen CG, Gordon RE: Breast disorders in nursing mothers. Am Fam Physician 1990;41:1509-1515
- Smallwood JA: Benign breast disease. Baltimore, Urban & Schwarzenberg, 1990
- Maier WP, et al: Nonlactational breast infection. Amer Surg 1994;60:247-250
- Bundred NJ, Dover MS, et al: Breast abscess and cigarette smoking. Br Jour Surg 1992;79(1):58-59
- Karstoup S, et al: Acute puerperal breast abscess: US-guided drainage. Radiology 1993;188(3):807-809

Illustrations: N/A
Internet references: http://www.5mcc.com

Author(s)
Thomas R. Strigle, MD

Breast cancer

BASICS

DESCRIPTION Malignant neoplasm in the breast. Breast cancers are classified as noninvasive (in situ) or invasive (infiltrating) with approximately 70% of all breast cancers possessing a component of invasion.
System(s) affected: Skin/Exocrine, Pulmonary, Gastrointestinal, Musculoskeletal, Nervous
Genetics:
• Only 20% of patients have a significant family history of breast cancer. This predisposition tends to be autosomal dominant with maternal lineage.
• Recent studies have revealed families with breast cancer susceptibility genes including BRCA1 and BRCA2. Family history suggestive of breast cancer susceptibility genes include multiple first and second degree relatives with early breast cancer diagnosis and the presence of ovarian cancer. Approximately 1 in 400 U.S. women will carry a germ-line mutation for BRCA1. BRCA1 and BRCA2 carriers have a 50 - 85 % lifetime risk of breast cancer, ovarian cancer, or both. BRCA2 carriers have a higher risk of male breast cancer.
Incidence/Prevalence in USA:
• 1 in 8 women will develop breast cancer within a lifetime
• The American Cancer Society estimates that 175,000 new cases will be diagnosed in 1999 with 43,700 deaths (including 400 men)
Predominant age: 30-80 with peak age 45-65; 77% of cases occur in women > age 50
Predominant sex: Female > Male (1% occurs in male)

SIGNS AND SYMPTOMS
• Palpable mass (55%)
• Abnormal mammogram without a palpable mass (35%)
• Color changes
• Lymphedema (peau d'orange)
• Dimpling
• Nipple retraction
• Breast enlargement
• Axillary mass
• Bone pain (rare)

CAUSES Unknown

RISK FACTORS
• Increased breast cancer risk occurs in first degree relatives (relative risk [RR] = 2.3), with bilateral disease in premenopausal relatives (RR = 10.5), or bilateral disease in postmenopausal relatives (RR = 5.0)
• Increased hormone risks include early menarche, late menopause, nulliparity or first full term pregnancy after age 30
• Women with a prior history of breast cancer or previous breast biopsies revealing atypical changes are at increased risk (5-10 times) for subsequent cancer
• Inconclusive risk factors include exogenous estrogen use, high dietary fat, or high alcohol use

DIAGNOSIS

DIFFERENTIAL DIAGNOSIS
• Differential diagnosis is extensive
• Benign breast disorders such as abscesses, hematomas, or fibroadenomas
• Proliferative breast diseases such as fibrocystic changes, ductal and lobular hyperplasia, or sclerosing adenosis
• Malignant breast diseases including sarcomas, lymphomas, or metastatic disease to breast

LABORATORY Initial lab tests include CBC, LFTs, CXR, bilateral mammography +/- ultrasound, pathologic review of biopsy, estrogen and progesterone receptor determination, and S phase determination
Drugs that may alter lab results: N/A
Disorders that may alter lab results: N/A

PATHOLOGICAL FINDINGS
• Noninvasive cancers
  ◊ The percentage of non-invasive cancers diagnosed is increasing due to increased mammography screening
  ◊ Usually detected by abnormal mammogram
  ◊ Noninvasive cancers are of two types: Intraductal or intralobular. Intraductal cancers are subdivided by growth patterns: Micropapillary, cribriform, solid, or comedo. The comedo growth pattern is considered more aggressive.
• Invasive cancers
  ◊ Tend to present with a breast lump
  ◊ Subdivided into - not-otherwise-specified (50%), lobular (5%), Paget's disease (2%), and miscellaneous (metaplastic, neuroendocrine, or squamous cell carcinomas [1%])
  ◊ Patients with invasive histologies with medullary 6%, colloid 7%, tubular, papillary, and adenoid cystic carcinomas 2%, have improved survival

SPECIAL TESTS
• Bone scan should be performed if symptoms suggest bony metastasis, if alkaline phosphatase is elevated, or if widespread disease is suspected
• CT or US of the abdomen may be indicated if widespread or recurrent disease is suspected

IMAGING
• Mammography, which detects 80% of breast cancers, is the best technique for the detection of minimal (< 0.5 cm) breast cancer. The most common abnormality representing cancer is an irregular mass. Microcalcifications can occur as the only sign of malignancy in 35% of breast cancers.
• Ultrasound may confirm whether a suspicious lump is solid or cystic and help define its size and extent

DIAGNOSTIC PROCEDURES
• Tissue confirmation of the suspicious mass or abnormal mammogram is essential. Biopsy may be excisional or incisional depending upon the size and location of the abnormality.
• Biopsy of non-palpable lesions is achieved with needle localization
• Cytologic confirmation of a palpable abnormality may be obtained by fine needle aspiration

TREATMENT

APPROPRIATE HEALTH CARE
Patients are usually treated by a team consisting of a medical oncologist, a surgeon, and a radiation oncologist

GENERAL MEASURES
• Early breast cancer treatment (Stage 1/11)
  ◊ Lumpectomy (wide excision with breast conservation) and radiotherapy is the treatment of choice for early primary breast cancer.
  ◊ Axillary node dissection is indicated with all invasive tumors and large noninvasive ones. Identification and biopsy of sentinel nodes may soon be preferred over axillary dissection because of its lower morbity rate.
  ◊ Most women with primary breast cancer have subclinical metastases and many will have recurrence of disease despite apparently curative surgery and the use of radiotherapy.
• Treatment of locally advanced breast cancer (Stage 111)
  ◊ Usually multidisciplanary treatment consisting of mastectomy, axillary dissection, radiation, and chemotherapy +/- tamoxifen
  ◊ Preoperative chemotherapy or hormonal therapy often converts inoperable tumors to operable ones
• Treatment of advanced or recurrent disease (Stage IV)
  ◊ Surgical resection if possible; chemotherapy, radiation, hormonal therapy.

SURGICAL MEASURES See General Measures

ACTIVITY Minimal activity restrictions exist during treatment

DIET No proven relationship exists between breast cancer and diet

Breast cancer

PATIENT EDUCATION
• Instruct patients in monthly breast self-examination to detect lumps, skin or nipple changes and the importance of mammography
• For a listing of sources for patient education materials, physicians may contact: American Cancer Society and the National Cancer Institute

MEDICATIONS

DRUG(S) OF CHOICE
• Metastatic disease is considered incurable, but treatable with remissions occurring in 30-40% of patients
• The process of deciding when to use chemotherapy or hormonal therapy is complex and is dependent on tumor type, size, node status, hormone receptor status and other factors; practice guidelines are available
• Combination chemotherapy is preferred over single agents.
• Tamoxifen reduces the risk of recurrence and death for women of all ages; treatment should be continued for five years. It should be discontinued if tumor growth continues. It probably is not of benefit to women with estrogen receptor negative tumors.
Contraindications: Strict hematologic, renal, hepatic, and cardiac guidelines need to be followed for the administration of cytotoxic chemotherapy
Precautions: Monitoring for infection is important for patients receiving chemotherapy. Tamoxifen increases the patient's risk of developing endometrial cancer and interacts with warfarin, erythromycin, cyclosporin, nifedipine, and diltiazem.
Significant possible interactions: Drug interactions are common and depend on combinations used. Refer to manufacturer's literature.

ALTERNATIVE DRUGS   N/A

FOLLOWUP

PATIENT MONITORING
• Up to 60% of patients with invasive disease will relapse within five years despite initial therapy
• The status of the axillary lymph nodes is the most important indicator for disease relapse
• Surveillance for recurrent disease should include physical examination every 4 months for 2 years, every six months for 3 years, then yearly. Mammography and routine chemistries should be done annually. Women on tamoxifen should have annual pelvic exams.
• Workup of suspected recurrence should include CBC, LFTs, CXR, bone scan, CT of affected area, +/- biopsy

PREVENTION/AVOIDANCE
• Decreasing dietary fat or alcohol has not been shown to alter breast cancer risk
• The synthetic anti-estrogen, tamoxifen, may be a useful prophylactic agent in high risk women
• Mammography
   ◊ Screening for disease: US Preventive Services Task Force recommends mammography with or without clinical breast examination every 1-2 years for ages 50-69. American Cancer Society recommends mammography and a clinical breast examination every year after age 40. They also recommend clinical breast examination every 3 years for ages 20-39 and self-breast examination starting at age 20. ACOG and AMA recommend mammogram every 1-2 years and annual clinical breast examination starting at age 40 and then annual mammograms at age 50.
   ◊ Diagnostic mammography should be performed at the advice of the patient's physician
   ◊ In women ages 50-69, mammography screening can reduce mortality by 30%

POSSIBLE COMPLICATIONS
• Post-operative: lymphedema (< 5% in modified radical mastectomy), seromas, wound infection, and limited shoulder motion
• Chemotherapy: nausea, vomiting, alopecia, leukopenia, bladder irritation, stomatitis, fatigue, and menstrual abnormalities
• Tamoxifen: hot flushes, menstrual irregularities including menopause, vaginal discharge, hypercalcemia, skin rashes, and possible endometrial carcinoma
• Irradiation: skin reaction, fibrosis (1%), brachial plexopathy (1%), rib fracture (1%), arm edema, pulmonary fibrosis (1%), and rarely second breast malignancy.

EXPECTED COURSE/PROGNOSIS
• 5 year survival
   ◊ Stage 0 (noninvasive) 100%
   ◊ Stage I (2 cm, no spread) 98%
   ◊ Stage II (>2 cm, or spread to axillary lymph nodes) 76-88%
   ◊ Stage III (>5 cm or fixed nodes, metastatic disease to the skin, inflammatory changes, chest wall extension, or supraclavicular lymph nodes) 49-56%
   ◊ Stage IV (distant metastatic disease) 16%

MISCELLANEOUS

ASSOCIATED CONDITIONS   Organ disease at metastatic sites

AGE-RELATED FACTORS   Age-specific incidence of breast cancer increases sharply until menopause and continues to increase at a slower rate in the geriatric population
Pediatric: Breast cancer occurs rarely in children with the most common pathology being secretory carcinoma
Geriatric: There is a higher percentage of ER positive tumors (80%) in the geriatric population. This correlates with improved disease-free survival.
Others: N/A

PREGNANCY   Breast cancer occurs infrequently during pregnancy (2.8%). Delay in diagnosis is common, and most series report poorer survival related to advanced stage at diagnosis.

SYNONYMS   N/A

ICD-9-CM
174 Malignant neoplasm of female breast
175 Malignant neoplasm of male breast

SEE ALSO   N/A

OTHER NOTES   N/A

ABBREVIATIONS
• ER = estrogen receptor
• PgR = progesterone receptor

REFERENCES
• Hortobagyi G Treatment of breast cancer. N Engl J Med 1998;339(14):974-984
• Krag D, Weaver D, et al The sentinel node in breast cancer. N Engl J Med 1998;339(14):941-946
• Osborne C Tamoxifen in the treatment of breast cancer. N Engl J Med 1998;339(22):1609-1618.
• Update of the NCCN guidelines for the treatment of breast cancer. Oncology 1997; I I (I I A):199-220.
• US Preventive Services Task Force. Guide to Clinical Preventive Services. 2nd Ed. Baltimore, Williams & Wilkins, 1996
Illustrations: 1 available on CD-ROM
Internet references: http://www.5mcc.com

Author(s)
Stephen M. Adams, MD
Karl E. Miller, MD

Breast-feeding

BASICS

DESCRIPTION
• Advantages
◊ Fewer respiratory, gastrointestinal and otitis media infections
◊ Ideal food - easily digestible, nutrients well absorbed, less constipation
◊ Increased contact between mother and baby and, perhaps, added self-esteem for mother
◊ Economical, portable, easy to meet needs quickly
◊ Decreased incidence of allergies in childhood
◊ Decreased incidence of breast cancer in mother
◊ Mothers often like it more than bottle feeding
◊ More rapid and complete reversion of mother's pelvis and uterus to pre-puerperal state
• Contraindications
◊ HIV infection; active TB
◊ Hepatitis is not a contraindication
◊ Substances of abuse will pass into human milk; please see Reference on drugs in lactation
• Physiology
◊ Stimulation of areola causes secretion of oxytocin
◊ Oxytocin is responsible for let-down reflex when milk is ejected from cells into milk ducts
◊ Sucking stimulates secretion of prolactin which triggers milk production. Thus milk is made in response to nursing and increases supply.
• Technique
◊ Get in comfortable position, usually sitting or reclining with baby's head in crook of mother's arm (side-lying position often useful following C-section delivery)
◊ Bring baby to mother to decrease stress on back
◊ Baby's belly and mother's belly should face each other or touch (belly-to-belly)
◊ Initiate the rooting reflex by tickling baby's lips with nipple or finger. As baby's mouth opens wide, mother guides her nipple to back of her baby's mouth while pulling the baby closer. This will ensure that the baby's gums are sucking on the areola, not the nipple.
System(s) affected: Endocrine/Metabolic, Skin/Exocrine
Genetics: N/A
Incidence/Prevalence in USA: According to 1996 Healthy People 2000 Update, 59% of new mothers breastfed in the early postpartum period and 22% at 6 months (goal is 75% and 50%).
Predominant age: 16-45
Predominant sex: Female only

SIGNS AND SYMPTOMS N/A

CAUSES N/A

RISK FACTORS N/A

DIAGNOSIS

DIFFERENTIAL DIAGNOSIS N/A

LABORATORY N/A
Drugs that may alter lab results: N/A
Disorders that may alter lab results: N/A

PATHOLOGICAL FINDINGS N/A

SPECIAL TESTS N/A

IMAGING N/A

DIAGNOSTIC PROCEDURES N/A

TREATMENT

APPROPRIATE HEALTH CARE
Outpatient

GENERAL MEASURES See Patient Education

SURGICAL MEASURES N/A

ACTIVITY No restrictions

DIET
• Adequate calorie and protein intake while nursing. Drinking cow's milk is not necessary.
• Drink plenty of fluids
• Continue prenatal vitamins
• Fluoride supplement unnecessary

PATIENT EDUCATION
• Antepartum
◊ Regular promotion of advantages of breast-feeding
◊ Discuss woman's postpartum plans, i.e., if going to work. Emphasize possibility of nursing part-time after returning to work or nursing until weaning the week before returning to work
◊ Emphasize importance of breast-feeding only for first 3 weeks of life to allow adequate build up of sufficient milk supply. Substitution of a bottle feed can occur after this time and still allow for continued nursing.
◊ Counsel women on technique
• Natural history
◊ Colostrum present in breast at birth but may not be seen
◊ Milk will not come in before 3rd day postpartum
◊ Frequent nursing (at least 9 or more times/24 hours) will lead to milk coming in sooner and in greater quantities
◊ Allow baby to determine duration of each nursing; baby will lose weight the first few days and may not get back to birth weight until day 10
• Postpartum
◊ Immediate breast-feeding after the birth
◊ Rooming-in to encourage on-demand feeding
◊ Observation of a nursing session by experienced physician, nurse or lactation consultant
◊ Avoid formula or water supplementation
◊ Review expectations, techniques. Be very encouraging.
◊ See in office within a few days of discharge, especially if first-time nursing
• Signs of adequate nursing
◊ Breasts become hard before and soft after feeding
◊ 6 or more wet diapers in 24 hours
◊ Baby satisfied; appropriate weight gain (average one ounce/day in first few months)
◊ Growth spurts - anticipate these around 10 days, 6 weeks, 3 months, and 4-6 months. Baby will nurse more often at these times for several days. This will increase milk production to allow for further adequate growth.
◊ Supplemental baby vitamins are unnecessary unless the baby has very limited exposure to sun (then needs vitamin D)
• Weaning
◊ Breast milk alone is adequate food for first 6 months
◊ Solids may be introduced at 4-6 months
◊ For mothers going to work, start switching the baby to bottle feeding during the hours mother will be gone about a week ahead of time. Do this by dropping a breast-feed every few days and substituting pumped breast milk or formula, preferably given by another caregiver.
◊ To increase the likelihood that baby will take a bottle occasionally, introduce it at 3-4 weeks and give once or twice a week

Breast-feeding

MEDICATIONS

DRUG(S) OF CHOICE N/A
Contraindications: N/A
Precautions: N/A
Significant possible interactions: N/A

ALTERNATIVE DRUGS N/A

FOLLOWUP

PATIENT MONITORING See mother and baby within a few days of hospital discharge if she is a first-time breast-feeder

PREVENTION/AVOIDANCE N/A

POSSIBLE COMPLICATIONS
• Plugged ducts (mother is well except for)
◊ Sore lump in one or both breasts without fever
◊ Use moist hot packs on lump prior to and during nursing; more frequent nursing on affected side; ensure good technique
• Mastitis
◊ Sore lump in one or both breasts plus fever and/or redness on skin overlying lump
◊ Use moist hot packs on lump prior to and during nursing; more frequent nursing on affected side; antibiotics covering for Staph. aureus (the most common organism) for at least 7 days
◊ Patients can be quite ill with mastitis
◊ Other possible sources of fever should be ruled out - endometritis, pyelonephritis in particular. Mother should get increased rest, use acetaminophen (Tylenol) as necessary. Fever should resolve within 48 hours or consider changing antibiotics. Lump should also resolve. If it continues, an abscess may be present requiring surgical drainage.
• Milk supply inadequate
◊ Check weight gain
◊ Review signs of adequate supply; review technique, frequency and duration of nursing
◊ Check to see if mother has been supplementing, thereby decreasing her own milk production
• Sore nipples
◊ Check technique
◊ Baby should be taken off the breast by breaking the suction with a finger in the mouth
◊ Air-dry nipples after each nursing; no breast creams and do not wash nipples with soap and water; check for signs of thrush in baby and mother
• Engorgement
◊ Usually develops after milk first comes in (day 3 or 4)
◊ Signs are warm, hard, sore breasts
◊ To resolve, offer baby more frequent nursing; may have to hand express a little milk to soften areola enough to let baby latch on; nurse long enough to empty breasts; generally resolves within a day or two
• Flat or inverted nipples
◊ When stimulated, inverted nipples will retract inward, flat nipples remain flat; should check for this on initial prenatal physical
◊ Nipple shells, a doughnut-shaped insert, can be worn inside the bra during the last month of pregnancy to gently force the nipple through the center opening of the shell
◊ Babies can nurse successfully even if the shell does not correct the problem before birth. A lactation consultant or La Leche League member may be a good resource in this situation. Another source: J Human Lactation. 9(1):27-29, 1993.

EXPECTED COURSE/PROGNOSIS
Healthy baby

MISCELLANEOUS

ASSOCIATED CONDITIONS N/A

AGE-RELATED FACTORS N/A
Pediatric: N/A
Geriatric: N/A
Others: N/A

PREGNANCY N/A

SYNONYMS N/A

ICD-9-CM N/A

SEE ALSO N/A

OTHER NOTES N/A

ABBREVIATIONS N/A

REFERENCES
• Briggs GG, et al: Drugs in Pregnancy and lactation. 5th Ed. Baltimore, Williams & Wilkins, 1998
• Riordan J, Auerback K: Pocket Guide to Breast-feeding and Human Lactation. Jones and Bartlett, 1997
• Bedinghaus J, Melnikow J: promoting successful breast feeding skills. Am Fam Phys 1992;45:1309-1318
Illustrations: N/A
Internet references: http://www.5mcc.com

Author(s)
Eric Henley, MD, MPH

Breech birth

BASICS

DESCRIPTION At the time of delivery the fetal buttocks are the presenting part in the maternal pelvis
• Frank breech presentation - the fetal hips are flexed and the knees extended with the feet near the shoulders, accounting for 60-65% of breech presentations at term
• Incomplete breech presentation - one or both of the fetal hips are incompletely flexed, resulting in some part of the fetal lower extremity as the presenting part. Thus the terms single footling, double footling, knee presentation. Accounts for 25-35% of breech presentations.
• Complete breech - similar to frank breech except one or both knees are flexed rather than extended. Accounts for 5% of breech presentations.
System(s) affected: Reproductive
Genetics: Fetal anomalies including anencephaly, hydrocephalus, trisomy 21
Incidence/Prevalence in USA: 3-4% of singleton term deliveries and up to 15-30% of low birth weight infants (< 2500 grams)
Predominant age: N/A
Predominant sex: Female only

SIGNS AND SYMPTOMS
• Anus palpable on digital vaginal exam
• Leopold's maneuver reveals ballottable head in fundal region

CAUSES
Probably a combination of one or more of the risk factors listed below

RISK FACTORS
• Fetal anomalies including anencephaly, hydrocephalus, trisomy 21
• Uterine anomalies
• Uterine relaxation associated with great parity
• Uterine overdistension as in polyhydramnios or multiple gestation
• Placenta previa
• Placental implantation in cornual-fundal region
• Low birth weight or premature infant

DIAGNOSIS

DIFFERENTIAL DIAGNOSIS Diagnosis is made by vaginal exam and confirmed by ultrasound. Can be confused with face presentation on digital vaginal exam.

LABORATORY None
Drugs that may alter lab results: N/A
Disorders that may alter lab results: N/A

PATHOLOGICAL FINDINGS Congenital malformation among term breech infants: Overall incidence 9.0%

SPECIAL TESTS N/A

IMAGING
• Ultrasound - confirms presenting part
• X-ray - flat plate of abdomen and pelvimetry to determine extent of head flexion and pelvic measurements

DIAGNOSTIC PROCEDURES N/A

TREATMENT

APPROPRIATE HEALTH CARE
Inpatient for labor and delivery

GENERAL MEASURES N/A

SURGICAL MEASURES
• Breech delivery is accomplished either vaginally or by cesarean section
• When a patient presents in labor with the fetus in breech position, a decision about a trial of labor or immediate cesarean section must be made
• Obtain a flat plate of abdomen with pelvimetry and/or ultrasound to document fetal presentation, to check for fetal abnormalities, and to estimate fetal weight in deciding candidacy for vaginal delivery
• The selection criteria for vaginal delivery are fairly strict to reduce morbidity and mortality for both mother and infant
• Cesarean section is recommended in the following circumstances unless the fetus is too immature to survive:
  ◊ Large (> 3500 grams) or small (< 1500 grams) fetus, estimated by ultrasound or skilled observer
  ◊ Pelvic contraction or unfavorable pelvic shape (platypelloid and android)
  ◊ Hyperextended head
  ◊ Significant fetal heart rate abnormality
  ◊ Footling breech
  ◊ Severe fetal growth retardation
  ◊ Premature fetus greater than 26 weeks with mother in active labor
  ◊ Previous cesarean section
  ◊ Abnormal labor including failure to dilate, prolonged second stage, and failure of descent

• Cesarean section procedure:
  ◊ Prepare for cesarean section by starting IV fluids and obtaining blood type and screen, in all patients, in case needed for emergency
  ◊ A low transverse cesarean section may need to be extended vertically if there is difficulty with head entrapment
  ◊ General anesthesia with isoflurane can rapidly relax the uterus and allow delivery of an entrapped after-coming head
  ◊ Cord blood gases should be obtained following delivery
• Vaginal delivery procedures:
  ◊ The candidate for vaginal delivery needs to be attended by a birth attendant skilled in breech delivery, a scrubbed assistant, an anesthesiologist capable of rapid induction of general anesthesia, and an individual skilled in neonatal resuscitation
  ◊ Leave membranes intact as long as possible to prevent possible cord prolapse
  ◊ The patient should not push until fully dilated
  ◊ Cut large episiotomy to allow sufficient room for delivery
  ◊ The infant should not be touched before the umbilicus crosses the maternal perineum
  ◊ Traction prior to this point constitutes a complete breech extraction and is associated with higher risk of perinatal morbidity and mortality
  ◊ With the fetal back anterior, maintain downward traction while grasping the fetal hips until the scapula becomes visible
  ◊ Check for nuchal arm
  ◊ As one axilla becomes visible rotate the infant until the shoulders are oriented anteriorly and posteriorly allowing their delivery
  ◊ The fetal head is delivered in a face down position with either piper forceps or manual flexion of the head
  ◊ Cord blood gases should be obtained following delivery

ACTIVITY Bedrest during labor

DIET Nothing by mouth until delivery accomplished

PATIENT EDUCATION Come to the hospital at the first sign of labor

MEDICATIONS

DRUG(S) OF CHOICE None
Contraindications: N/A
Precautions: N/A
Significant possible interactions: N/A

ALTERNATIVE DRUGS N/A

FOLLOWUP

PATIENT MONITORING
• Continuous fetal heart rate monitoring should be done during labor and delivery
• Six weeks postpartum care is done as with other deliveries

PREVENTION/AVOIDANCE
• External version
  ◊ Conversion to vertex presentation can be attempted from 30-36 weeks gestation
  ◊ External version can cause abruption, premature rupture of membranes, and feto-maternal hemorrhage
  ◊ Should only be attempted with continuous fetal heart monitoring in the delivery suite where immediate cesarean section can be done
  ◊ Contraindications to external version include pelvic engagement of presenting part, placenta previa, previous uterine surgery, premature rupture of the membranes, or marked oligohydramnios

POSSIBLE COMPLICATIONS
• Trauma to head, soft tissue, brachial plexus and spinal cord - not always prevented by cesarean
• Asphyxia secondary to cord compression or prolapse

EXPECTED COURSE/PROGNOSIS
• Perinatal morbidity and mortality are much higher in breech births. A large proportion of the deaths are related to congenital abnormalities.
• In patients properly selected for vaginal delivery, potentially perinatal morbidity and mortality, and maternal morbidity are reduced
• For infants less than 1500 grams, there is a much higher rate of cerebral hemorrhage and perinatal death associated with vaginal compared to cesarean delivery

MISCELLANEOUS

ASSOCIATED CONDITIONS See Risk Factors

AGE-RELATED FACTORS
Pediatric: N/A
Geriatric: N/A
Others: N/A

PREGNANCY A problem of pregnancy

SYNONYMS N/A

ICD-9-CM
652.2 Breech presentation without mention of version
763.0 Breech delivery and extraction
763.4 Cesarean delivery

SEE ALSO
• Placenta previa
• Premature labor

OTHER NOTES Maneuvers of cesarean breech delivery are similar to vaginal breech extraction and can be associated with severe trauma to the infant

ABBREVIATIONS N/A

REFERENCES
• Cunningham FG, MacDonald PC, Gant NF, eds: Williams' Obstetrics. 19th Ed. Norwalk, CT, Appleton and Lange, 1993
• Gabbe S, Niebyl J, Simpson JL, eds: Obstetrics Normal and Problem Pregnancies 3rd ed. New York, NY, Churchill Livingstone Inc, 1996
• Scorza W: Intrapartum Management of Breech Presentation. Clinics in Pernat, Mar 1996;23(1):31-49
• Erkkola R: Controversies: Selective Vaginal Delivery for Breech Presentation, J Perinat Med, 24(1996):553-561
Illustrations: N/A
Internet references: http://www.5mcc.com

Author(s)
Kimberle Vore, MD

Bronchiectasis

BASICS

DESCRIPTION Chronic irreversible, abnormal dilatation of the bronchi, usually accompanied by infection and productive cough
System(s) affected: Pulmonary
Genetics: Associated with many conditions including some that are congenital or hereditary
Incidence/Prevalence in USA:
• No reliable figures available
• Less common than it once was, probably due to more effective treatment of childhood respiratory infections
Predominant age: Begins most often in early childhood, but symptoms may not appear until later in life
Predominant sex: Male = Female

SIGNS AND SYMPTOMS
• Cough
• Sputum - copious and purulent
• Hemoptysis
• Wheezing
• Coarse or moist crackles
• Cyanosis
• Digital clubbing
• Dyspnea
• Barrel chest
• Emaciation
• Fatigue
• Fever
• Recurrent pneumonia
• Tachycardia
• Tachypnea

CAUSES
• Alpha-1-antitrypsin deficiency
• Allergic bronchopulmonary aspergillosis
• Bronchial obstruction
• Cystic fibrosis
• Dyskinetic cilia syndromes
• Hypogammaglobulinemia
• Inhaling noxious chemicals
• Kartagener's syndrome (situs inversus, sinusitis, immotile spermatozoa, bronchiectasis)
• Necrotizing pulmonary infections
• Pulmonary abscess
• Severe lung infection in childhood (measles, adenovirus, influenza, pertussis, or bronchiolitis)
• Tuberculosis
• Congenital immunodeficiency syndromes
• Chronic aspiration
• Rheumatic diseases

RISK FACTORS
• Repeated bouts of pneumonia
• Any chronic respiratory illness
• Retained foreign body

DIAGNOSIS

DIFFERENTIAL DIAGNOSIS
• Chronic bronchitis
• Chronic obstructive pulmonary disease
• Cystic fibrosis
• Pulmonary tuberculosis
• Allergic bronchopulmonary aspergillosis

LABORATORY
• Positive sputum culture (yields H. influenzae, Streptococcus pneumoniae, staphylococcal, klebsiella, pseudomonas, or anaerobes)
• Hypoxemia
• Leukocytosis, usually
• Serum immunoglobulins - check for hypogammaglobulinemia, IgE level helpful
Drugs that may alter lab results: N/A
Disorders that may alter lab results: N/A

PATHOLOGICAL FINDINGS
• Bronchial dilation
• Inflamed bronchi
• Purulent bronchorrhea
• Necrosis of bronchial mucosa
• Peribronchial scarring

SPECIAL TESTS
• Sweat test
• Skin test for aspergillus
• Bronchoscopy useful in locating bleeding site and to exclude adenoma or foreign body
• Ciliary biopsy with electron microscopy (EM)
• Pulmonary function tests
• Sputum culture/sensitivity, AFB, fungus

IMAGING
• Bronchography
  ◊ For definitive diagnosis, to help determine extent, and if surgery contemplated
  ◊ Bronchial dilation, truncated
• Chest x-ray
  ◊ Can be normal
  ◊ Coarse lung markings - honeycomb/tram tracks
  ◊ Air-fluid level
  ◊ Cystic lesions
  ◊ Atelectasis
• CT scan
  ◊ Shows dilation of airways with signet rings
  ◊ High resolution scans best

DIAGNOSTIC PROCEDURES
• Fiberoptic bronchoscopy
  ◊ Recommended when disease is of recent onset or is unilateral
  ◊ May be combined with bronchography
  ◊ Obtain culture

TREATMENT

APPROPRIATE HEALTH CARE
Outpatient except for possible surgery

GENERAL MEASURES
• Airway clearance techniques
  ◊ Chest physical therapy
  ◊ Percussion
• Postural drainage
• Hydration
• Bronchial artery embolization may be lifesaving for massive pulmonary hemorrhage
• Avoid cigarette smoking
• Bronchoscopy may be required for extraction of mucus or mycelial plugs, or if physiotherapy has failed

SURGICAL MEASURES
Segmental pulmonary resection for localized disease or refractory hemoptysis

ACTIVITY
As fully active as possible

DIET
No restrictions

PATIENT EDUCATION
Printed patient information available from: American Lung Association, 1740 Broadway, New York, NY 10019, (212)315-8700

Bronchiectasis

MEDICATIONS

DRUG(S) OF CHOICE
• Bronchodilators
  ◊ Dependent on pulmonary function tests
  ◊ May be helpful for patients with associated asthma or aspergillosis
  ◊ Beta-adrenergic agonists (e.g., albuterol) given by metered dose inhaler with use of a spacer (reservoir device)
• Antibiotics
  ◊ Dependent on culture results, use at exacerbations
  ◊ Ampicillin: 250-500 mg orally q 6 hours (50 mg/kg/day in divided doses q 6-8 hours in children less than 20 kg)
or
  ◊ Trimethoprim-sulfamethoxazole: DS q12h
  ◊ Tetracycline: 250-500 mg orally q 6 hours
• Steroids
  ◊ Consider for patients with bronchopulmonary aspergillosis. IgE level guides steroid dosing.

Contraindications:
• Tetracycline: not for use in pregnancy or children < 8 years.

Precautions:
• Tetracycline: may cause photosensitivity; sunscreen recommended.

Significant possible interactions:
• Tetracycline: avoid concurrent administration with antacids, dairy products, or iron.
• Broad-spectrum antibiotics: may reduce the effectiveness of oral contraceptives; barrier method recommended.

ALTERNATIVE DRUGS
• For chronic persistent infection, long-term high dose of amoxicillin 3 g every 12 hours may be useful. It does not provide relief for everyone and has more side effects.
• Other broad-spectrum antimicrobials including anti-pseudomonals if required. Choice would depend on pathogen and susceptibility.
• Inhaled corticosteroids if reversible obstruction present
• Oxygen - if PO2 < 60 mm Hg
• Nicotine replacement, consider to aid smoking cessation

FOLLOWUP

PATIENT MONITORING
• Frequent followup for progress of illness, prevention of infection, smoking cessation, and to check on physiotherapy
• At some point in followup, need to discuss with patient the possibility of mechanical ventilation and cardiopulmonary resuscitation in the future. The patient, family and provider should determine if this type of treatment is appropriate.

PREVENTION/AVOIDANCE
• Treat all pneumonias adequately
• Immunizations for viral illnesses (i.e., influenza)
• Immunization for pneumococcal pneumonia
• Routine childhood immunizations, e.g., pertussis, measles, Hib
• Genetic counseling if inherited etiology

POSSIBLE COMPLICATIONS
• Recurrent pulmonary infections
• Pulmonary hypertension
• Secondary amyloidosis
• Cor pulmonale
• Brain abscess
• Massive hemoptysis
• Atelectasis
• Lung abscess

EXPECTED COURSE/PROGNOSIS
• Chronic. Surgery may be curative if disease localized.
• Average life expectancy - 55 years

MISCELLANEOUS

ASSOCIATED CONDITIONS
• Sinusitis
• Cor pulmonale
• Kartagener syndrome
• Cystic fibrosis

AGE-RELATED FACTORS
Pediatric: Cystic fibrosis and other congenital disorders
Geriatric: Elderly more likely to need hospitalization for treatment
Others: N/A

PREGNANCY N/A

SYNONYMS N/A

ICD-9-CM
494 bronchiectasis

SEE ALSO
• Aspergillosis
• Bronchiolitis obliterans & organizing pneumonia
• Cystic fibrosis
• Lung abscess
• Kartagener's syndrome

OTHER NOTES Conditions that may lead to bronchiectasis include severe pneumonia (especially measles, pertussis, adenoviral infections in children), necrotizing infections due to Klebsiella, staphylococci, influenza virus, fungi, mycobacteria, mycoplasma, bronchial obstruction from any cause (foreign body, carcinoma, enlarged mediastinal lymph nodes

ABBREVIATIONS N/A

REFERENCES
• Hardy KA: A review of airway clearance: New techniques, indications and recommendations. Respir Care 1994;39(5):440-445
• Lewiston NJ: Bronchiectasis in childhood. Pediatr Clin North Am 1984;31(4):865-878
• Marwah OS: Bronchiectasis: How to identify, treat and prevent. Postgrad Med 1995;97:149-159
Illustrations: N/A
Internet references: http://www.5mcc.com

Author(s)
Gregory Snyder, MD

Bronchiolitis

 BASICS

DESCRIPTION Inflammation of the bronchioles, usually seen in young children, occasionally in high-risk adults. May be seasonal (winter and spring) and often occurs in epidemics. Usual course: insidious; acute; progressive.
System(s) affected: Pulmonary
Genetics: N/A
Incidence/Prevalence in USA: Medical care provided to 1000-1500/100,000 annually. Estimated incidence is higher.
Predominant age: newborn-2 years (peak age 2-6 months)
Predominant sex: Male > Female

SIGNS AND SYMPTOMS
• Anorexia
• Cough
• Cyanosis
• Expiratory wheezing
• Apnea
• Fever
• Grunting
• Inspiratory crackles
• Intercostal retractions
• Irritability
• Noisy breathing
• Otitis media
• Pharyngitis
• Tachycardia
• Tachypnea
• Vomiting

CAUSES
• Respiratory syncytial virus
• Parainfluenza
• Adenovirus
• Rhinovirus
• Influenza virus
• Chlamydia
• Eye, nose, mouth inoculation
• Exposure to adult with URI
• Day care exposure (significant)
• Idiopathic (many adult cases)

RISK FACTORS
• Contact with infected person
• Children in day care environment
• Heart-lung transplantation patient
• Adults - exposure to toxic fumes, connective tissue disease

 DIAGNOSIS

DIFFERENTIAL DIAGNOSIS
• Asthma
• Vascular ring
• Lobar emphysema
• Foreign body
• Heart disease
• Pneumonia
• Reflux
• Aspiration
• Cystic fibrosis

LABORATORY
• Arterial blood gas - hypoxemia, hypercarbia, acidemia
• Respiratory viral culture - positive
• Respiratory viral antigens - positive
Drugs that may alter lab results: N/A
Disorders that may alter lab results: N/A

PATHOLOGICAL FINDINGS
• Abundant mucous exudate
• Mucosal - hyperemia, edema
• Submucosal lymphocytic infiltrate, monocytic infiltrate, plasmacytic infiltrate
• Small airway debris, fibrin, inflammatory exudate, fibrosis
• Peribronchiolar mononuclear infiltrate

SPECIAL TESTS
Infant pulmonary function studies - bronchodilator response

IMAGING
• Chest x-ray
  ◊ Focal atelectasis
  ◊ Air trapping
  ◊ Flattened diaphragm
  ◊ Increased anteroposterior diameter
  ◊ Peribronchial cuffing

DIAGNOSTIC PROCEDURES N/A

 TREATMENT

APPROPRIATE HEALTH CARE
• Most patients can be treated at home
• Inpatient indicated for patient with increased respiratory distress, cyanosis, and dehydration

GENERAL MEASURES
• Most critical phase is first 48-72 hours after onset. Treatment is usually symptomatic.
• Fluid at maintenance
• Mechanical ventilation in respiratory failure
• Isolation: contact; handwashing most important
• Antiviral agents for selected high-risk patients
• Cardio-respiratory monitoring
• Bronchodilators, especially inhaled
• Steroids may not change course - except in patients with reactive airway disease

SURGICAL MEASURES N/A

ACTIVITY
• Avoid exposure to crowds, viral illness for 2 months
• Avoid smoke

DIET
• Frequent small feedings of clear liquids
• If hospitalized, may require intravenous fluids

PATIENT EDUCATION Griffith: Instructions for Patients; Philadelphia, W.B. Saunders Co.

MEDICATIONS

DRUG(S) OF CHOICE
• Oxygen
• Albuterol: may be effective for acute symptoms.
• Epinephrine aerosols may be of benefit
• Ribavirin: For infants and children, an inhaled antiviral agent active against RSV, may be indicated in patients with underlying cardio-pulmonary disease, young age (< 6 weeks), or with severe RSV (elevated pCO2; require mechanical ventilation - use with caution via ventilator). Nebulize via small particle aerosol generator (SPAG). Use of ribavirin has decreased in recent years, secondary to lack of significant clinical efficacy.
Contraindications: Refer to manufacturer's literature
Precautions: None
Significant possible interactions: None

ALTERNATIVE DRUGS
• Antibiotics only if secondary bacterial infection present (rare)
• Corticosteroids do not change course, unless infant has reactive airway disease. In adults corticosteroids may be helpful.

FOLLOWUP

PATIENT MONITORING
• If patient is receiving home care, follow daily by telephone for 2-4 days
• For hospitalized patient, monitor as needed depending on severity of infection. Bronchiolitis can be associated with apnea.

PREVENTION/AVOIDANCE
• Hand washing
• Contact isolation of infected babies
• Persons with colds should keep contacts with infants to a minimum
• Palivizumab (Synagis), a monoclonal product, can be used for prevention in high-risk patients (young prematures and patients with moderately severe BPD up to 2 years old). Administer monthly (November thru March) 15 mg/kg IM. Single use vial of 100 mg.
• RSV immune globulin, a human blood product, can also be used in at-risk patients. Monthly infusions of 750 mg/kg, November thru March, in a controlled setting. Avoid fluid overload. Vial is 50 mg/mL; infuse at 1.5 to 6mL/kg/hr; monitor oximeter and vital signs.
• Both of these medications are quite expensive.

POSSIBLE COMPLICATIONS
• Bacterial superinfection
• Viral obliterative bronchiolitis
• Apnea
• Respiratory failure
• Death
• Increased incidence of RAD

EXPECTED COURSE/PROGNOSIS
• In most cases, recovery is complete within 7-10 days
• Mortality statistics differ, but probably under 1%
• High-risk infants (BPD, CHD) may have prolonged course

MISCELLANEOUS

ASSOCIATED CONDITIONS
• Common cold
• Conjunctivitis
• Pharyngitis
• Otitis media
• Diarrhea

AGE-RELATED FACTORS
Pediatric: Most common in infants
Geriatric: N/A
Others: N/A

PREGNANCY N/A

SYNONYMS N/A

ICD-9-CM
466.1 acute bronchiolitis

SEE ALSO N/A

OTHER NOTES N/A

ABBREVIATIONS
BPD = bronchopulmonary dysplasia
CHD = congenital heart disease
RAD = reactive airway disease
SPAG = small particle aerosol generator

REFERENCES
• Mandell GL, ed: Principles and Practice of Infectious Diseases. 4th Ed. New York, Churchill Livingstone, 1995
• Fields BN, et al, eds: Virology. 2nd Ed. New York, Raven Press, 1990
Illustrations: N/A
Internet references: http://www.5mcc.com

Author(s)
Nancy N. Dambro, MD

Bronchiolitis obliterans & organizing pneumonia

BASICS

DESCRIPTION This is a specific reaction of lung tissue to a variety of injuries. The lungs show a pattern of multiple patchy pneumonia. These are seen on chest x-ray as patchy alveolar or ground glass opacifications with or without interstitial infiltrates and may have air bronchograms as well.
System(s) affected: Pulmonary
Genetics: N/A
Incidence/Prevalence in USA: Uncommon
Predominant age: Reported cases range age 0-70, mean age 50's
Predominant sex: N/A

SIGNS AND SYMPTOMS
- Most cases present with a flu-like illness that lasts 4-10 weeks or longer. Most have been treated with antibiotics without success.
- Fever
- Dry cough
- Weight loss
- Dyspnea may be severe
- Crackles and perhaps squeaks over involved area
- Fatigue

CAUSES Idiopathic. A complex response to a variety of injuries, such as toxic inhalation; post mycoplasma, viral and bacterial infection; aspiration; immunologic factors.

RISK FACTORS
- AIDS
- Immunocompromised patients, including transplant patients

DIAGNOSIS

DIFFERENTIAL DIAGNOSIS
- Usual interstitial pneumonitis (UIP)
- Noninfectious diseases
- Tuberculosis
- Sarcoidosis
- Histoplasmosis
- Berylliosis
- Goodpasture's syndrome
- Neoplasm
- Polyarteritis nodosa
- Systemic lupus erythematosus
- Wegener's granulomatosis
- Sjögren's syndrome
- Chronic eosinophilic pneumonia
- Cryptogenic bronchiolitis

LABORATORY
- Leukocytosis with a normal differential
- Elevated ESR, usually quite elevated
- Negative cultures
- Negative serology for mycoplasma, Coxiella, Legionella, psittacosis, and fungus
- Negative viral studies
Drugs that may alter lab results: N/A
Disorders that may alter lab results: N/A

PATHOLOGICAL FINDINGS
- Intraluminal fibrosis of distal airspaces is the major pathologic feature
- Fibroblasts and plugs of inflammatory cells and loose connective tissue fill these distal airways
- The inflammatory cells are mainly lymphocytes and plasma cells
- Interstitial fibrosis is present
- The plugs of edematous granulation tissue in the terminal and respiratory bronchioles and alveolar ducts do not cause permanent damage

SPECIAL TESTS
- Pulmonary function shows a restrictive/obstructive pattern
- Flow-volume loop shows terminal airway obstruction
- Chest x-ray may show patchy alveolar opacities often in the mid or upper lung area. A ground glass pattern that may have air bronchograms.
- V/Q scan: matched patchy defects

IMAGING
- Chest x-ray - often appears more normal than the physical examination
- CT scans more accurately define the distribution and extent of the patchy alveolar opacities with areas of hyperlucency

DIAGNOSTIC PROCEDURES
- Open lung biopsy
- Transbronchial biopsy
- It may be well to use a trial of steroids as a diagnostic trial, though not all would agree
- If a diagnostic trial is successful, be prepared to treat the patient for at least a year

TREATMENT

APPROPRIATE HEALTH CARE
Inpatient

GENERAL MEASURES
- Monitor blood gases or pulse oximetry
- Oxygen as necessary

SURGICAL MEASURES N/A

ACTIVITY As tolerated

DIET No special diet

PATIENT EDUCATION Followup is especially important. Relapse is common. Treatment is prolonged. If medication tapered too rapidly, relapse may well occur.

Bronchiolitis obliterans & organizing pneumonia

MEDICATIONS

DRUG(S) OF CHOICE
• Prednisone
  ◊ 60 mg daily for 1-3 months
  ◊ Then tapered over a few weeks to 20 mg (this dose may later be given as alternate day therapy). Increase length of taper for patients on long-term therapy to avoid precipitating Addisonian crisis.
  ◊ Treatment may be needed for one year or more

Contraindications: Refer to manufacturer's literature

Precautions: Be aware of the patient's Mantoux status and history of peptic ulcer disease. Long-term steroid associated with significant adverse effects including Cushing's syndrome, fluid retention, osteoporosis, hyperkalemia, poor wound healing.

Significant possible interactions: Refer to manufacturer's literature

ALTERNATIVE DRUGS
• Steroids other than prednisone may be used
• One paper reported the use of erythromycin 600 mg/day for 3-4 months after initial control with prednisone
• Antimicrobials if original infection is persistent. Choice depends on the pathogen.

FOLLOWUP

PATIENT MONITORING
• Frequent visits, weekly initially
• Emphasize the need to continue the prednisone because of the chance of relapse
• Monitor the lung disease and the side effects of prednisone therapy (Mantoux, monthly CBC, funduscopic exam every 3-6 months)

PREVENTION/AVOIDANCE Except for prevention of relapse, none known

POSSIBLE COMPLICATIONS
• Bronchiectasis
• Death, but with proper treatment, recovery is usually complete without permanent sequelae

EXPECTED COURSE/PROGNOSIS
Complete recovery but individual case management is mandatory

MISCELLANEOUS

ASSOCIATED CONDITIONS
• Drug-induced pneumonitis
  ◊ Paraquat poisoning
  ◊ Amiodarone toxicity
  ◊ Acebutolol toxicity
  ◊ Freebase cocaine pulmonary toxicity
  ◊ Overdose of L-tryptophan
  ◊ Though most were treated with antibiotics only penicillamine and sulfasalazine have been implicated
• Infections
  ◊ Chronic infectious pneumonia
  ◊ Malaria
• Immuno-compromise
  ◊ Bone marrow transplantation
• Connective tissue diseases
  ◊ Rheumatic lung
  ◊ Sjogren's syndrome
  ◊ Polymyositis
  ◊ Scleroderma
  ◊ Essential mixed cryoglobulinemia
• Miscellaneous
  ◊ Cystic fibrosis
  ◊ Bronchopulmonary dysplasia
  ◊ Renal failure
  ◊ Congestive heart failure
  ◊ Adult respiratory distress syndrome
  ◊ Chronic eosinophilic pneumonia
  ◊ Hypersensitivity pneumonitis
  ◊ Histiocytosis X
  ◊ Sarcoidosis
  ◊ Pneumoconioses
  ◊ Radiation pneumonitis

AGE-RELATED FACTORS
Pediatric: Rare, but has been reported after viral pneumonia (adenovirus influenza). Characteristics include delayed recovery, persistent cough, crackles or wheezing after pneumonia. The laboratory findings are generally not helpful. Imaging shows: V/Qm matched defects; HRCT, bronchiectasis, bronchogram, pruned tree appearance. Diagnosis confirmed by biopsy. Treatment includes steroids - 1 mg/kg/24 hrs for one month, followed by weaning over several months.
Geriatric: Not common
Others: Apparently only seen in adults

PREGNANCY N/A

SYNONYMS
• Intraluminal fibrosis of distal airways
• Idiopathic BOOP
• Cryptogenic organizing pneumonia (COP)
• Obliterative bronchiolitis

ICD-9-CM
491.8 Other chronic bronchitis

SEE ALSO
• Sjögren's syndrome

OTHER NOTES This disease behaves differently than bronchiolitis obliterans (BO). BOOP is a restrictive problem, BO is an obstructive problem. BO causes permanent lung damage and BOOP is completely reversible.

ABBREVIATIONS
V/Q = ventilation-perfusion ratio
HRCT = high resolution computed tomography

REFERENCES
• Cordier JF, Loire R, Brune J: Idiopathic Bronchiolitis Obliterans Organizing Pneumonia. Chest 1989;96:999-1004
• Mueller NL, Staples CA, Miller RR: Bronchiolitis Obliterans Organizing Pneumonia: CT features in 14 patients. AJR 1990;154:983-987
• Epler GR, Colby TV, et al: Bronchiolitis Obliterans Organizing Pneumonia. N Eng J Med 1985;312:152-158
• Hardy KA, Schidlow D, Zaeri N: Obliterative Bronchiolitis in Children. CHEST 1988;93:460-466
• St John RC, Dorinsky PM: Cryptogenic bronchiolitis. Clin Chest Med 1993;14(4): 667-75
• Lynch DA: Imaging of small airways diseases. Clin Chest Med 1993;14(4):623-34
Illustrations: N/A
Internet references: http://www.5mcc.com

Author(s)
David A. Pope, MD

MEDICATIONS

DRUG(S) OF CHOICE Nonsteroidal anti-inflammatory agents such as ibuprofen 400 mg three or four times a day or naproxen sodium 500 mg twice a day will provide significant relief of symptoms in many patients
Contraindications: Gastrointestinal intolerance
Precautions: Gastrointestinal side effects of NSAIDs may preclude their use in selected patients
Significant possible interactions: Refer to manufacturer's literature

ALTERNATIVE DRUGS Other NSAIDs

FOLLOWUP

PATIENT MONITORING
• Patients treated with wrist splints or other palliative measures such as cortisone injections will require followup in the ensuing 4 to 12 weeks to assess the success of treatment modalities
• Patients treated surgically rarely experience recurrence of the disorder. Routine followup once healing of the incision has occurred is not necessary.

PREVENTION/AVOIDANCE Take a break once an hour when doing repetitive work involving hands

POSSIBLE COMPLICATIONS
• Post-op infection (rare)
• Injury to recurrent branch of the nerve

EXPECTED COURSE/PROGNOSIS
Untreated the condition can be expected to lead to numbness and weakness in the hand with atrophy of hand muscles and permanent loss function of the extremity

MISCELLANEOUS

ASSOCIATED CONDITIONS
• Diabetes
• Obesity
• Pregnancy

AGE-RELATED FACTORS
Pediatric: N/A
Geriatric: N/A
Others: N/A

PREGNANCY May occur in pregnancy

SYNONYMS N/A

ICD-9-CM
354.0 Carpal tunnel syndrome

SEE ALSO
• Acromegaly
• Arthritis, rheumatoid (RA)
• Hypoparathyroidism
• Systemic lupus erythematosus (SLE)
• Scleroderma

OTHER NOTES N/A

ABBREVIATIONS N/A

REFERENCES
• Joynt RJ, ed: Clinical Neurology. Vol. 4. Philadelphia, J.B. Lippincott Co, 1990
• Seddon H: Surgical Disorders of the Peripheral Nerves. Baltimore, Williams and Wilkins Co., 1972
Illustrations: N/A
Internet references: http://www.5mcc.com

Author(s)
Fremont P. Wirth, MD, FACS

Cataract

BASICS

DESCRIPTION Any opacity of the lens, either localized or generalized. Single largest cause of blindness in the world, blinding an estimated 17 million people.
• Types include:
◊ Age-related ("senile") - over 90%
◊ Congenital - 1/250 newborns, 10-38% of childhood blindness
◊ Toxic/nutritional
◊ Systemic disease associated e.g., myotonic dystrophy, atopic dermatitis
◊ Metabolic - diabetes (accelerated sorbitol pathway), hypocalcemia, Wilson's disease
◊ "Complicated" - secondary to associated eye disease, e.g., uveitis (juvenile rheumatoid arthritis, sarcoid, etc.). Also secondary to occult tumor (melanoma, retinoblastoma).
◊ Trauma - heat (infrared), electrical shock, radiation, concussion, perforating eye injuries, intraocular foreign body

System(s) affected: Nervous

Genetics:
• Age related cataract has no clear pattern
• Congenital sometimes associated, e.g., heredofamilial systemic disorders (Laurence-Moon-Biedl syndrome), chromosomal disorders (Down syndrome)

Incidence/Prevalence in USA:
• 5% of age 52-62
• 46% of age 75-85 have significant vision loss (20/30 or worse)
• 92% of age 75-85 have some cataract changes

Predominant Age: Depends on type of cataract

Predominant Sex: Male = Female

SIGNS AND SYMPTOMS
• Age-related cataract:
◊ Blurred vision, distortion or "ghosting" of images
◊ Problems with visual acuity in bright light or night driving (glare)
◊ Falls or accidents
◊ Injuries (e.g., hip fracture)
◊ Signs on eye examination: A lens opacity consistent with the symptoms
• Congenital:
◊ Lens opacity present at birth or within three months after birth
• Often asymptomatic or parents notice child's visual inattention or strabismus (lazy eye)
◊ Leukocoria (white pupil reflex), strabismus, nystagmus, associated syndrome signs (as in Down or rubella syndromes)
◊ Visual acuity tests abnormal for one or both eyes
◊ Note: Must always rule out ocular tumor. Early diagnosis and treatment of retinoblastoma may be lifesaving.
• Other types of cataract:
◊ May present with decreased visual acuity complaint
◊ Appropriate history or signs to help in diagnosis

CAUSES
• Age-related cataract:
◊ Continual addition of layers of lens fibers throughout life creates hard, dehydrated lens nucleus which impairs vision (nuclear cataract)
◊ Aging alters biochemical and osmotic balance required for lens clarity, outer lens layers hydrate and become opaque, affecting vision
• Congenital:
◊ Usually obscure
◊ Drugs (corticosteroids in first trimester, sulfonamides, etc.)
◊ Metabolic - diabetes in mother, galactosemia in fetus
◊ Intrauterine infection - first trimester (rubella, herpes, mumps)
◊ Maternal malnutrition
• Other cataract types:
◊ Have in common that a biochemical/osmotic imbalance disrupts lens clarity
◊ Local changes in lens protein distribution lead to light scattering manifest as lens opacity

RISK FACTORS
• Aging
• Patient with one of the predisposing diseases

DIAGNOSIS

DIFFERENTIAL DIAGNOSIS
• An opaque appearing eye may be due to surface opacities of the cornea (scarring), lens opacities, tumor, retinal detachment, gliotic retinal scar. Biomicroscopic examination (slit lamp) or careful ophthalmoscopic exam should provide diagnosis. A visual acuity worse than 20/30, not easily correctable by glasses, and explainable by the degree of cataract noted on examination makes the diagnosis.
• In the elderly, visual impairment often due to multiple factors, e.g., cataract and macular degeneration both contributing to visual loss
• Age-related cataract - significant if symptoms and ophthalmic exam support cataract as major cause of vision impairment
• Congenital - lens opacity in absence of other ocular pathology such as tumor, nerve glioma, retinopathy of prematurity may be consistent with the visual loss. May cause severe amblyopia.
• Note: No cataract produces an afferent pupillary reaction defect (Marcus Gunn pupil). Abnormal pupillary reactions mandate further evaluation for other pathology.

LABORATORY N/A
Drugs that may alter lab results: N/A
Disorders that may alter lab results: N/A

PATHOLOGICAL FINDINGS Consistent with lens changes found in the type of cataract

SPECIAL TESTS
• Visual quality assessment: Glare testing, contrast sensitivity are sometimes indicated. (Hyperglycemic state as in poor diabetic control creates osmotic change within lens and may alter measurement of visual acuity and refractive state.)
• Retinal/macular function assessment: Potential acuity meter testing, fluorescein retinal angiography sometimes required

IMAGING N/A

DIAGNOSTIC PROCEDURES Noted above in special testing

TREATMENT

APPROPRIATE HEALTH CARE
Outpatient or inpatient surgery

GENERAL MEASURES
• Age-related cataract
◊ Since significant cataract may develop gradually, patient may not be aware of how it has changed his/her lifestyle. Physician may note a significant cataract and patient reports "no problems." Thus the evaluation requires physician/patient exchange of information.
◊ Pre-surgical evaluation - by the primary care physician includes physical exam, lab work (CBC, electrolytes, ECG). Patients on anticoagulants may need to temporarily discontinue one week before surgery if possible. Not always necessary, so need to discuss with ophthalmologist.

SURGICAL MEASURES

• Age-related cataract

◊ Surgical removal of the cataract - indicated if visual impairment producing symptoms distressing to the patient, or interfering with lifestyle or occupation, or posing risk of fall or injury

◊ Since significant cataract may develop gradually, patient may not be aware of how it has changed his/her lifestyle. Physician may note a significant cataract and patient reports "no problems." Thus the evaluation requires physician/patient exchange of information.

◊ Surgical technique - cataracts are not removed by laser. Most surgical techniques include implantation of a plastic intraocular lens immediately following cataract extraction.

◊ Anesthesia - usually local, with anesthesiologist monitoring vital signs

◊ Pre-surgical evaluation - by the primary care physician includes physical exam, lab work (CBC, electrolytes, ECG). Patients on anticoagulants may need to temporarily discontinue one week before surgery if possible. Not always necessary, so need to discuss with ophthalmologist.

◊ Postoperative care - usually protective eye shield as directed, topical antibiotic and steroid ophthalmic medications. Avoid lifting, bending over for a few weeks.

• Congenital cataract

◊ Treatment is surgical removal of cataract. Newborn may need surgery within days to reduce risk of severe amblyopia. Use of implant lenses controversial.

◊ Postoperative care - long-term patching program for good eye to combat amblyopia. Refractive correction of operative eye, with multiple repeat examinations. Very difficult challenge for physician and parents.

ACTIVITY See above

DIET N/A

PATIENT EDUCATION See above

MEDICATIONS

DRUG(S) OF CHOICE There is no medication at present to prevent or slow the progression of cataracts
Contraindications: N/A
Precautions: N/A
Significant possible interactions: N/A

ALTERNATIVE DRUGS N/A

FOLLOWUP

PATIENT MONITORING

• As cataract progresses, the ophthalmologist may change spectacle correction to maintain vision. When this is no longer practical or successful, surgery is recommended.
• Following surgery, spectacle correction may be required to maximize visual acuity for the patient's need. Usually measured several weeks after surgery.

PREVENTION/AVOIDANCE

• Use of ultraviolet protecting glasses in sunny climates may slow progression of cataract, but this is not proven by controlled studies to date
• Antioxidants (vitamins C, E, etc.) theoretically beneficial, but not proven

POSSIBLE COMPLICATIONS Blindness

EXPECTED COURSE/PROGNOSIS

• Ocular prognosis good after cataract removal if no prior ocular disease.
• In congenital cataracts prognosis is often poor because of the high risk of amblyopia.

MISCELLANEOUS

ASSOCIATED CONDITIONS
• Diabetes
• Ocular diseases

AGE-RELATED FACTORS
Pediatric: See information on congenital cataracts
Geriatric: 92% of people over age 75 have cataracts
Others: N/A

PREGNANCY See information on congenital cataracts (e.g., rubella syndrome)

SYNONYMS N/A

ICD-9-CM
366.19 Age-related cataract
743.30 Congenital cataract

SEE ALSO N/A

OTHER NOTES If patient has cataract and symptoms do not seem to support recommended surgery, a second opinion by another ophthalmologist may be indicated

ABBREVIATIONS N/A

REFERENCES
• Tasman W, ed: Duane's Ophthalmology. Philadelphia, J.B. Lippincott Co., 1999
Illustrations: N/A
Internet references: http://www.5mcc.com

Author(s)
T. Glendon Moody, MD

Celiac disease

BASICS

DESCRIPTION A chronic diarrheal disease characterized by intestinal malabsorption of virtually all nutrients and precipitated by eating gluten-containing foods.
System(s) affected: Gastrointestinal
Genetics: See Risk factors
Incidence/Prevalence in USA: 50-75 in 100,000
Predominant age: Two incidence peaks, age 1 and 60's
Predominant sex: Female > Male (3:2)

SIGNS AND SYMPTOMS
• Diarrhea
• Steatorrhea
• Muscle cramps
• Vertigo
• Nervousness
• Weight loss
• Failure to thrive
• Weakness
• Lassitude
• Fatigue
• Large appetite
• Abdominal distention
• Explosive flatulence
• Abdominal pain, nausea, vomiting are rare

CAUSES Sensitivity to gluten, specifically gliadin fraction

RISK FACTORS
• First order relatives - 10% incidence
• 71% in monozygotic twins

DIAGNOSIS

DIFFERENTIAL DIAGNOSIS Rule out short bowel syndrome, pancreatic insufficiency, Crohn's disease, Whipple's disease, hypogammaglobulinemia, tropical sprue, lymphoma, acquired immune deficiency syndrome, acute enteritis, giardiasis, eosinophilic gastroenteritis

LABORATORY
• Positive anti-gliadin IgA and IgG
• Positive anti-reticulum and anti-endomycial antibodies
• 72 hour fecal fat showing greater than 7% fat malabsorption
• D-xylose test showing malabsorption of this sugar
• Decreased calcium
• Decreased prothrombin time
• Decreased neutral fats
• Decreased cholesterol
• Decreased vitamin A
• Decreased vitamin B12
• Decreased vitamin C
• Decreased folic acid
• Decreased iron
• Decreased total protein
• Anemia
Drugs that may alter lab results: N/A
Disorders that may alter lab results: N/A

PATHOLOGICAL FINDINGS Small bowel biopsy - flattened villi, hyperplasia and lengthening of crypts, infiltration of plasma cells and lymphocytes in lamina propria

SPECIAL TESTS Endoscopy

IMAGING Upper GI series showing flocculation of barium, edema and flattening of mucosal folds

DIAGNOSTIC PROCEDURES Biopsy of the duodenal mucosa with repeat endoscopy and normal biopsy on a gluten-free diet is necessary before a firm diagnosis can be made.

TREATMENT

APPROPRIATE HEALTH CARE
Outpatient

GENERAL MEASURES Removal of gluten from the diet. Rice, corn and soybean flour are safe, palatable substitutes.

SURGICAL MEASURES N/A

ACTIVITY No restrictions

DIET Removal of gluten - wheat, rye, barley and those with gluten additives

PATIENT EDUCATION
• Clinical dietician
• Copy of gluten-free diet
• Possible lay self-help group
• American Celiac Society, 45 Gifford Avenue, Jersey City, NJ 07304, (201)432-1207.
• Gluten Intolerance Group (206) 325-6980

Celiac disease

 MEDICATIONS

DRUG(S) OF CHOICE
• Usually none
• Prednisone, 40-60 mg/day po in cases of refractory sprue
Contraindications: History of tuberculosis, fungus or herpes infections
Precautions: Use with caution in congestive heart failure, diabetes, peptic ulcer, myasthenia gravis
Significant possible interactions: Diuretics taken concomitantly may lead to potassium depletion

ALTERNATIVE DRUGS
May require supplemental calcium, calcium carbonate, 500 mg po bid, and vitamin D (ergocalciferol) 10-100 mcg/day; in severe malabsorption, up to 2.5 mg/day may be required

 FOLLOWUP

PATIENT MONITORING
Repeat endoscopy after 6-8 weeks on a gluten-free diet (in selected cases)

PREVENTION/AVOIDANCE
Avoid all gluten containing products

POSSIBLE COMPLICATIONS
• Malignancy - less than 10% of patients (50% of which are small bowel lymphoma)
• Refractory sprue - may respond to prednisone 40-60 mg/day po
• Chronic ulcerative jejunoileitis - associated with multiple ulcers, intestinal bleeding, strictures, perforation, obstruction, peritonitis - 7% mortality
• Osteoporosis secondary to decreased vitamin D and calcium absorption
• Dehydration
• Electrolyte depletion
• Death (rare)

EXPECTED COURSE/PROGNOSIS
Good with correct diagnosis and adherence to gluten free diet. Feel better in seven days. All symptoms usually disappear in four to six weeks. It is unknown whether strict dietary adherence decreases cancer risk.

 MISCELLANEOUS

ASSOCIATED CONDITIONS
• May have secondary lactase deficiency
• Extraintestinal manifestation may include marked decrease in bone density
• Dermatitis herpetiformis

AGE-RELATED FACTORS
Pediatric: Children reaching adolescence may outgrow intolerance to wheat but should be cautioned to watch for signs of recurrence in middle age
Geriatric: N/A
Others: N/A

PREGNANCY
No significant effect

SYNONYMS
• Sprue
• Gluten enteropathy
• Celiac sprue

ICD-9-CM
579.0 Celiac disease

SEE ALSO
N/A

OTHER NOTES
N/A

ABBREVIATIONS
N/A

REFERENCES
• McClave S: Celiac and Tropical Sprue. In: Chobanian SJ, Van Ness MM, eds. A Manual of Clinical Problems in Gastroenterology. 2nd Ed. Boston, Little-Brown, 1993
• Stenson WF: Gastrointestinal Diseases. In: Orland MJ, Saltman RJ, eds. A Manual of Medical Therapeutics. 25th Ed. Boston, Little-Brown, 1986
• Trier JS: Celiac Sprue. In: Sleisenger MH, Fordtran JS, eds. Gastrointestinal Disease. 4th Ed. Philadelphia, W.B. Saunders Co., 1988
Illustrations: N/A
Internet references: http://www.5mcc.com

Author(s)
Michael M. Van Ness, MD

Cellulitis

BASICS

DESCRIPTION An acute, spreading infection of the dermis and subcutaneous tissue. Several entities are recognized:
• Cellulitis of the extremities - characterized by an expanding, red, swollen, tender or painful plaque with an indefinite border that may cover a wide area
• Recurrent cellulitis of the leg after saphenous venectomy - patients have an acute onset of swelling, erythema of the legs arising months to years after coronary artery bypass. (Surgery using lower extremity veins for by-pass grafts.)
• Dissecting cellulitis of the scalp - recurrent painful, fluctuant dermal and subcutaneous nodules
• Facial cellulitis in adults - a rare event. Patients usually develop pharyngitis, followed by high fever, rapidly progressive anterior neck swelling, tenderness and erythema associated with dysphagia
• Facial cellulitis in children - potentially serious. Swelling and erythema of the cheek develop rapidly, usually unilateral.
• Perianal cellulitis - bright perianal erythema extending from the anal verge approximately 2 to 3 cm onto the surrounding perianal skin
• Pseudomonas cellulitis - may be a localized phenomenon or it may occur during pseudomonas septicemia
System(s) affected: Skin/Exocrine
Genetics: No known genetic pattern
Incidence/Prevalence in USA: Unknown
Predominant age:
• Perianal cellulitis - principally in children
• Facial cellulitis - in adults, usually older than 50 years. In children, between 6 months and three years.
Predominant sex: Male = Female (perianal cellulitis more common in boys)

SIGNS AND SYMPTOMS
• General
  ◊ Local tenderness
  ◊ Pain
  ◊ Erythema
  ◊ Malaise
  ◊ Fever, chills
  ◊ Involved area is red, hot, and swollen
  ◊ Borders of the area are not elevated and not demarcated
  ◊ Regional lymphadenopathy is common
• Recurrent cellulitis
  ◊ Same as above
  ◊ Edema
  ◊ High fever, chills and toxicity
• Dissecting cellulitis of the scalp
  ◊ Purulent drainage from burrowing interconnecting abscesses
• Facial cellulitis in adults
  ◊ Malaise
  ◊ Anorexia
  ◊ Vomiting
  ◊ Itching
  ◊ Burning
  ◊ Dysplasia
  ◊ Anterior neck swelling
• Facial cellulitis in children
  ◊ Irritability
  ◊ Upper respiratory tract infection symptoms

• Perianal cellulitis
  ◊ Intense perianal erythema
  ◊ Pain on defecation
  ◊ Blood streaked stools
  ◊ Perianal pruritis

CAUSES
• By site
  ◊ Cellulitis of the extremities: *Group A streptococcus, Staphylococcus aureus*
  ◊ Recurrent cellulitis of the leg: Non-group A beta hemolytic Streptococci (group C,G,B)
  ◊ Dissecting cellulitis of the scalp: *Staphylococcus aureus*
  ◊ Facial cellulitis in adults: *H. influenzae* type B
  ◊ Facial cellulitis in children: *H. influenzae* type B, over 3 years with portal of entry: staphylococcal and streptococcal
  ◊ Synergetic necrotizing cellulitis: Mixed aerobic-anaerobic flora
  ◊ Intravenous drug use: *Staphylococcus aureus*, Streptococci, Enterobacteriaceae, Pseudomonas, Fungi
  ◊ Synergetic necrotizing cellulitis: Mixed aerobic-anaerobic flora
• Specific diseases
  ◊ Diabetes mellitus: *Staphylococcus aureus*, Streptococci, Enterobacteriaceae, Anaerobes
  ◊ Human bites: Eikenella corrodens
  ◊ Animal bites (cat and dog): Staphylococci, *Pasteurella multocida*
• Patient groups
  ◊ Neonates: *Group B streptococcus*
  ◊ Immunocompromised
    - Bacteria (Serratia, Proteus and other Enterobacteriaceae)
    - Fungi (*Cryptococcus neoformans*)
    - Atypical mycobacterium
  ◊ Children with nephrotic syndrome: *E. coli*
  ◊ Environmental and occupational exposures
    - *Erysipelothrix rhusiopathiae*
    - *Vibrio species*
    - *Aeromonas hydrophilia*
• Rare causes
  ◊ Anaerobic
  ◊ *Clostridium perfringens* (gas forming cellulitis)
  ◊ Tuberculosis
  ◊ Syphilitic gumma
  ◊ Fungal: Mucormycosis, Aspergillosis

RISK FACTORS
• General
  ◊ Previous trauma (laceration, puncture, human or animal bite)
  ◊ Underlying skin lesion (furuncle, ulcer)
  ◊ Surgical wound
  ◊ Recurrent cellulitis
  ◊ Post coronary artery bypass in patients whose saphenous veins have been removed
  ◊ Lower extremity lymphedema secondary to a) radical pelvic surgery b) radiation therapy c) neoplastic involvement of pelvic lymph nodes
  ◊ Mastectomy
  ◊ Diabetes mellitus
  ◊ Intravenous drug use
  ◊ Immunocompromised host
  ◊ Burns
  ◊ Environmental and occupational factors

DIAGNOSIS

DIFFERENTIAL DIAGNOSIS
• Perianal cellulitis
  ◊ Candida intertrigo
  ◊ Psoriasis
  ◊ Pin worm infection
  ◊ Inflammatory bowel disease
  ◊ Behavioral problem
  ◊ Child abuse
• Others
  ◊ Acute gout
  ◊ Fasciitis/myositis
  ◊ Mycotic aneurysm
  ◊ Ruptured Baker's cyst
  ◊ Thrombophlebitis
  ◊ Osteomyelitis
  ◊ Herpetic whitlow
  ◊ Cutaneous diphtheria
  ◊ Pseudogout

LABORATORY
• Aspirates from the point of maximum inflammation. Yield a 45% positive culture rate as compared to a 5% from leading edge culture.
• Blood cultures - potential pathogens isolated in 25% of patients
• Mild leucocytosis with a left shift
• A mildly elevated sedimentation rate
• CBC
Drugs that may alter lab results: Previous antibiotic therapy may alter the results
Disorders that may alter lab results: N/A

PATHOLOGICAL FINDINGS Biopsy of skin shows marked infiltration of the dermis with eosinophils and inflammatory changes

SPECIAL TESTS
• Serial serological testing with antistreptolysin O, anti-deoxyribonuclease B, and anti hyaluronidase tests may be successful in diagnosing cellulitis caused by group A, C, or G hemolytic streptococci
• Sinus drainage and culture of aspirate

IMAGING
• Gas forming cellulitis
  ◊ Plain x-rays show gas bubbles in the soft tissue
  ◊ CT shows gas and myonecrosis

DIAGNOSTIC PROCEDURES
• Skin biopsy
• Lumbar puncture should be considered for all children with H. influenzae type B cellulitis

TREATMENT

APPROPRIATE HEALTH CARE
Outpatient for mild cases, inpatient for severe infections

GENERAL MEASURES
• Immobilization and elevation of the involved limb to reduce swelling may be needed in *H. influenzae type B*
• Sterile saline dressings to decrease local pain
• Moist heat to localize the infection
• Cool Burrow's compresses for pain relief

SURGICAL MEASURES
• Debridement for gas/purulent collections
• Intubation or tracheotomy may be needed for cellulitis of the head or neck
• Wide filleting incision in necrotizing cellulitis

ACTIVITY   Ambulatory in mild infection; bedrest in severe infection

DIET   Regular diet

PATIENT EDUCATION
• Good skin hygiene
• Avoid skin traumas
• Report early skin changes to physician

MEDICATIONS

DRUG(S) OF CHOICE
Treat 10-30 days. Guided by culture results whenever possible.
• Mild early suspected streptococcal etiology: Aqueous penicillin G, 600,000 U, then IM procaine penicillin at 600,000 U q8-12 hrs
• Staphylococcal infection or no clues to etiology: penicillinase-resistant penicillin (e.g., oxacillin 0.5-1.0 g po q6 hrs)
• Severe infection: penicillinase-resistant penicillin (e.g., nafcillin 1.0-1.5 g IV q4 hrs)
• Gram negative bacillus as possible etiology: aminoglycoside (gentamicin) plus a semisynthetic penicillin
• Rapidly progressive cellulitis after a fresh water injury: penicillinase-resistant penicillin plus gentamicin or chloramphenicol
• Human bites: amoxicillin-clavulanate (Augmentin)
• Animal bites (cellulitis at the saphenous site): penicillin or nafcillin, in high dosage, IV for 7 days before switching to oral therapy
• Facial cellulitis in adults and children: (H. influenza B) cefotaxime IV
• Gas forming cellulitis: Aqueous penicillin G 10-20 million U/day IV
• Diabetes mellitus: Cefoxitin or if toxic, clindamycin and gentamicin
• Intravenous drug abuse: Vancomycin and gentamicin
• Compromised hosts: clindamycin and gentamicin
• Burn patients: vancomycin and gentamicin

Contraindications:
• Allergies to the antibiotic
Precautions: Renal failure, other organ failure
Significant possible interactions: Refer to manufacturer's literature

ALTERNATIVE DRUGS
• Mild infection
  ◊ Penicillin allergy: erythromycin, 500 mg po q6 hrs
• Severe infection
  ◊ Vancomycin 1.0-1.5 g/day IV
  ◊ Human bite and animal bites: IV cefoxitin
• Gas forming cellulitis
  ◊ Metronidazole 500 mg IV q6h
  ◊ Clindamycin 600 mg IV q8h

FOLLOWUP

PATIENT MONITORING
• A blood culture at the end of treatment to ensure cure
• Repeat needle aspirate culture
• Repeat blood count if patient was toxic
• Repeat lumbar puncture in case of meningitis

PREVENTION/AVOIDANCE
• Treatment of tinea pedis with antifungal (such as clotrimazole) will prevent recurrent cellulitis of the legs in patients who have had coronary bypass
• Avoid trauma
• Avoid swimming in fresh water or salt water in the presence of skin abrasion
• Avoid human or animal bite
• Support stocking with peripheral edema
• Good skin hygiene
• For recurrent cellulitis - prophylactic penicillin G (250-500 mg po bid)
• H. influenzae cellulitis - rifampin prophylaxis for entire family of index case or in day-care classroom in which one or two children exposed. Dosage: 20 mg/kg/day (maximum: 600 mg/day) for 4 days.

POSSIBLE COMPLICATIONS
• Bacteremia
• Local abscesses
• Super infection with gram negative organisms
• Lymphangitis especially in recurrent cellulitis
• Thrombophlebitis of lower extremities in older patients
• Dissecting cellulitis of the scalp - scarring; alopecia
• Facial cellulitis in children - meningitis in 8% of patients
• Gas forming cellulitis - gangrene; amputation; 25% mortality

EXPECTED COURSE/PROGNOSIS
With adequate antibiotic treatment, outlook is good

MISCELLANEOUS

ASSOCIATED CONDITIONS
• Facial cellulitis in children
  ◊ Upper respiratory tract infection
  ◊ Unilateral or bilateral otitis media in 68% of patients
  ◊ Meningitis in 8% of patients
• Perianal cellulitis
  ◊ Pharyngitis may precede the infection
• Frontal sinus in adult
  ◊ Subacute bacterial endocarditis
  ◊ Scarlet fever
  ◊ Vaccinia
  ◊ Herpes simplex
  ◊ Herpes zoster

AGE-RELATED FACTORS
Pediatric: N/A
Geriatric: In cellulitis of lower extremities, patients are more prone to develop thrombophlebitis
Others: N/A

PREGNANCY   N/A

SYNONYMS   N/A

ICD-9-CM
682.9 Cellulitis

SEE ALSO
• Cellulitis, periorbital & orbital
• Erysipelas
• Animal bites
• Thrombophlebitis, superficial

OTHER NOTES   N/A

ABBREVIATIONS   N/A

REFERENCES
• Habif T: Clinical Dermatology. 3rd Ed. St. Louis, CV Mosby, 1996
• Mandell GL, ed: Principles and Practice of Infectious Diseases. 4th Ed. New York, Churchill Livingstone, 1995
Illustrations: 18 available on CD-ROM
Internet references: http://www.5mcc.com

Author(s)
Abdulrazak Abyad, MD, MPH, AGSF

Cellulitis, periorbital & orbital

BASICS

DESCRIPTION An acute, spreading infection of the dermis and subcutaneous tissue. Several entities are recognized. Cellulitis around the eyes is a potentially dangerous periorbital and orbital infection.
System(s) affected: Skin/Exocrine, Nervous
Genetics: No known genetic pattern
Incidence/Prevalence in USA: Unknown
Predominant age: N/A
Predominant sex: Male = Female

SIGNS AND SYMPTOMS
• Lid edema
• Rhinorrhea
• Orbital pain, tenderness
• Headache
• Conjunctival hyperemia
• Chemosis
• Ptosis
• Limitation to occular motion
• Increase intraocular pressure
• Disease in corneal sensation
• Congestion of retinal veins
• Chorioretinal stria
• Gangrene and sloughing of lids

CAUSES
• Cellulitis around the eye in adult
  ◊ *Staphylococcus aureus* most common
  ◊ *Streptococcus pyogenes*
  ◊ *Streptococcus pneumonia*
  ◊ Mixed infection
• Cellulitis around the eye in children less than five years
  ◊ *H. influenzae* most common

RISK FACTORS
• Trauma
• Chronic sinusitis (anaerobic)
• Acute sinusitis (aerobic)
• Retained orbital foreign bodies
• Puncture wound
• Surgical procedure: Exploration of orbital tumor, retinal detachment procedure, strabismus operation
• Acute dacryocystitis
• Dental or intracranial infection
• Bacteremia

DIAGNOSIS

DIFFERENTIAL DIAGNOSIS
• Retro-orbital cellulitis/abscess

LABORATORY
• Aspiration of fluid from the orbit is contraindicated
• Blood culture more likely to be positive in children < 5 years
• Culture of discharge from nasal mucosa, nasopharynx and conjunctiva
Drugs that may alter lab results: Previous antibiotic therapy
Disorders that may alter lab results: N/A

PATHOLOGICAL FINDINGS N/A

SPECIAL TESTS Serial serological testing with antistreptolysin O, anti-deoxyribonuclease B, and anti hyaluronidase tests may be successful in diagnosing cellulitis caused by group A, C, or G hemolytic streptococci

IMAGING
• B-scan ultrasound
• Plain orbital and sinus films
• Computed tomography (CT) is the most accurate and provides the most important information
• Magnetic resonance imaging is the imaging modality of choice in diagnosing suspected cases of cavernous sinus thrombosis

DIAGNOSTIC PROCEDURES
• Skin biopsy
• Lumbar puncture should be considered for all children with H. influenzae type B cellulitis

TREATMENT

APPROPRIATE HEALTH CARE
Outpatient for mild cases, inpatient for severe infections

GENERAL MEASURES N/A

SURGICAL MEASURES
• Surgical debridement and/or drainage is needed if abscess develops or if clinical situation deteriorates despite adequate therapy in 24-48 hours or if visual acuity decreases
• In orbital mucormycosis, surgical debridement of devitalized tissue is extremely important

ACTIVITY
• Ambulatory in mild infection
• Bedrest in severe infection

DIET Regular diet

PATIENT EDUCATION
• Good skin hygiene
• Avoid skin traumas
• Report early skin changes to health professional

Cellulitis, periorbital & orbital

MEDICATIONS

DRUG(S) OF CHOICE
• In adults, nafcillin or oxacillin 1.5 g every 4 hours
• In children, ampicillin 200 mg/kg/day in divided doses intravenously plus nafcillin or oxacillin (100 mg/kg/day)
• Sinus decongestion - nasal sprays, oral decongestants, oral antihistamines
Contraindications:
• Allergies to the antibiotic
• Previous history of allergy to the drug
Precautions: Renal failure, other organ failure
Significant possible interactions: Refer to manufacturer's literature

ALTERNATIVE DRUGS
• In adults, cefotaxime or clindamycin or chloramphenicol or vancomycin
• In children, if H. influenzae resistant to ampicillin - third generation cephalosporin, cefotaxime or chloramphenicol
• In immunocompromised - piperacillin and gentamicin

FOLLOWUP

PATIENT MONITORING Repeat imaging in patients with orbital cellulitis

PREVENTION/AVOIDANCE
• Avoid trauma
• Avoid swimming in fresh water or salt water in the presence of skin abrasion
• In H. influenzae cellulitis - rifampin prophylaxis for the entire family of an index case. Rifampin prophylaxis in day-care classroom in which one or two children exposed. Dosage - 20 mg/kg/24 h (maximum of 600 mg a day) for 4 days.

POSSIBLE COMPLICATIONS
• Osteomyelitis
• Strabismus
• Afferent pupillary defect
• Chronic draining sinus
• Scarred upper eyelid
• Profound visual loss
• Blindness
• Ophthalmoplegia
• Cavernous sinus thrombosis
• Meningitis
• Intracranial abscess
• Acute infarction of retina and choroid

EXPECTED COURSE/PROGNOSIS
With adequate antibiotic treatment, outlook is good

MISCELLANEOUS

ASSOCIATED CONDITIONS Sinusitis ethmoiditis in children in 84% of patients

AGE-RELATED FACTORS
Pediatric: Newborn may acquire orbital cellulitis secondary to intrauterine infection
Geriatric: N/A
Others: N/A

PREGNANCY N/A

SYNONYMS N/A

ICD-9-CM
376.01 Orbital cellulitis

SEE ALSO
• Cellulitis
• Erysipelas
• Animal bites
• Thrombophlebitis, superficial

OTHER NOTES N/A

ABBREVIATIONS N/A

REFERENCES
• Habif T: Clinical Dermatology. 3rd Ed. St. Louis, CV Mosby, 1996
• Mandell GL, ed: Principles and Practice of Infectious Diseases. 4th Ed. New York, Churchill Livingstone, 1995
Illustrations: N/A
Internet references: http://www.5mcc.com

Author(s)
Abdulrazak Abyad, MD, MPH, AGSF

Cerebral palsy

BASICS

DESCRIPTION A term used to describe a group of patients with a non-progressive disorder of movement or posture that is a result of a central nervous system abnormality that occurred prenatally, perinatally, or during the first three years of life
System(s) affected: Nervous
Genetics: Although familial cases have been described, this is not considered a genetic disease
Incidence/Prevalence in USA: 2.1 per 1,000 live births
Predominant age: Because of the definition, this problem is restricted to life. The disease is lifelong, although changes occur as the patient matures.
Predominant sex: Male = Female

SIGNS AND SYMPTOMS
By subtypes
• Spastic
  ◊ Associated and significant spasticity
  ◊ Contractures
  ◊ Mental retardation
  ◊ Aphonia
  ◊ Seizures
• Athetotic
  ◊ Usually normal intelligence
  ◊ Choreiform movements
  ◊ Muscular hypertrophy
• Ataxic
  ◊ Clumsy disposition
  ◊ Normal intelligence
  ◊ Some are highly talkative (cocktail party syndrome)
• Spastic diplegia
  ◊ Spares upper extremities
  ◊ Spastic (scissor gait)
  ◊ Normal intelligence

CAUSES
• 70% of the time, neither causes nor risk factors can be identified
• In utero infections, malformations, chromosomal abnormalities and strokes are causes

RISK FACTORS
• Prematurity
• Hypoxic ischemia
• Encephalopathy in the perinatal period
• Seizures in the perinatal period
• Interventricular hemorrhage in the perinatal period
• In utero infections
• Meningitis/encephalitis postnatally
• Child abuse

DIAGNOSIS

DIFFERENTIAL DIAGNOSIS Children with muscle disease will appear floppy; however, the most common cause of the floppy baby syndrome is cerebral palsy

LABORATORY
• Laboratory data is not required to make the diagnosis.
• Other tests may help exclude Tay-Sachs metachromatic leukodystrophy, mucopolysaccharidosis
Drugs that may alter lab results: None
Disorders that may alter lab results: None

PATHOLOGICAL FINDINGS Central nervous system abnormalities: CT and MRI might show abnormalities of the brain including cysts, cerebral atrophy, calcification, tumors, malformation, strokes, etc.

SPECIAL TESTS Urine amino acid screening

IMAGING N/A

DIAGNOSTIC PROCEDURES
• History and careful physical exam
• EEG

TREATMENT

APPROPRIATE HEALTH CARE
Outpatient

GENERAL MEASURES
• Physical therapy, occupational therapy, orthosis, adaptive equipment
• Medications by mouth usually not very successful; side effects occur before beneficial effects are present
• Alter muscle tone, assuming that the abnormal tone is adversely affecting function, by:
  ◊ Injection of botulinum toxin into the abnormal muscles
  ◊ Rhizotomy
  ◊ Continuous infusion of intrathecal baclofen

SURGICAL MEASURES Tendon transfers, release of contractures, rhizotomy to decrease spasticity

ACTIVITY Full activity depending upon the patient's dysfunction

DIET Normal diet, although constipation is frequent and stool softeners might be considered

PATIENT EDUCATION
• It is very important to educate the patient and parents about the child's disabilities as well as prognosis; mental retardation seen in 20-25% of patients with cerebral palsy.
• United Cerebral Palsy Associations, 7 Penn Plaza, Suite 804, New York, NY 10001, (800)USA-1UCP

MEDICATIONS

DRUG(S) OF CHOICE
• Medications to decrease spasticity (e.g., diazepam, dantrolene sodium and baclofen)
• Botulinum toxin (Botox) type A also to decrease spasticity
• Baclofen delivered intrathecally is of value
• Medications for epilepsy might have to be used

Contraindications: Refer to manufacturer's literature
Precautions: Refer to manufacturer's literature
Significant possible interactions: Refer to manufacturer's literature

ALTERNATIVE DRUGS   Other centrally acting muscle relaxants

FOLLOWUP

PATIENT MONITORING   Followup visits
are important - to determine the development of contractures and to determine the presence of associated problems including epilepsy, learning disabilities, strabismus, hearing loss and mental retardation.

PREVENTION/AVOIDANCE   N/A

POSSIBLE COMPLICATIONS   Chronicity
with permanent disability

EXPECTED COURSE/PROGNOSIS
• The patient should improve in function with time
• Muscle tone may change for the worse during adolescence (does not mean that the disease is progressive)

MISCELLANEOUS

ASSOCIATED CONDITIONS
• Epilepsy
• Learning disabilities
• Mental retardation
• Behavioral problems
• Strabismus
• Hearing loss

AGE-RELATED FACTORS
Pediatric: Contractures will increase as a result of growth associated with asymmetrical muscle tone and strength. Scoliosis may develop as a result.
Geriatric: N/A
Others: N/A

PREGNANCY   N/A

SYNONYMS
• Little disease
• Cerebral diplegia
• Infantile cerebral paralysis

ICD-9-CM
343.9 Infantile cerebral palsy, unspecified

SEE ALSO   N/A

OTHER NOTES   N/A

ABBREVIATIONS   N/A

REFERENCES   Russman BS, Gage JR:
Cerebral Palsy. Current Problems in Pediatrics 1989;19(2):65-111
Illustrations: N/A
Internet references: http://www.5mcc.com

Author(s)
Barry S. Russman, MD

Cervical dysplasia

BASICS

DESCRIPTION Pre-invasive neoplastic epithelial changes in the transformation zone of the uterine cervix often associate with human papillomavirus infections
• Mild dysplasia (CIN I or SIL low grade) - cellular changes are limited to the lower one-third of the squamous epithelium
• Moderate dysplasia (CIN II or SIL high grade) - cellular changes are limited to the lower two-thirds of the squamous epithelium
• Severe dysplasia (CIN III or SIL high grade or carcinoma in situ) - cellular changes involves the full thickness of the squamous epithelium
System(s) affected: Reproductive
Genetics: N/A
Incidence/Prevalence in USA: Difficult to assess due to wide variability in false negative Pap smear reporting and uneven distribution of qualified colposcopists. Prevalence 3,600/100,000 at age 27-28.
Predominant age: The median age for carcinoma in situ is 28 years. Earlier lesions can be expected at younger ages
Predominant sex: Female only

SIGNS AND SYMPTOMS
• Frequently none
• Occasionally there is association with condyloma acuminatum in the vulva, vagina, or anus
• Occasionally there are co-existing sexually transmitted diseases in the lower reproductive tract, e.g., chlamydia, gonorrhea

CAUSES Strong linkage with infections by human papilloma viruses types 6, 11, 16, 18, 31, 33, and 35. Other types of the same virus have also been implicated.

RISK FACTORS
• Multiparity and pregnancy before age 20 years
• Multiple sexual partners
• Early age in first sexual intercourse
• Condyloma acuminatum infection elsewhere in the body
• Cigarette smoking
• Prostitution
• Lower socio-economic status

DIAGNOSIS

DIFFERENTIAL DIAGNOSIS
• Invasive carcinoma of the cervix
• Condyloma acuminatum

LABORATORY
• Pap smear
Drugs that may alter lab results:
• Surgical lubricants e.g., K-Y Jelly
Disorders that may alter lab results: N/A

PATHOLOGICAL FINDINGS
• Clumping of the nuclear chromatin material
• Reversal of the nuclear/cytoplasmic ratio
• Koilocytosis
• Hyperchromasia

SPECIAL TESTS
• Viral DNA hybridization (Virapap) and others
• Colposcopy
• PAPNET system to review negative Pap smears
• CYTYC 2000 thin prep Pap test (replacement of current Pap preparations)

IMAGING N/A

DIAGNOSTIC PROCEDURES
• Papanicolaou smear
• Colposcopy and directed cervical biopsies
• Cone biopsy (by cold knife, laser, or loop excision)
• Endocervical curettage
• Loop electrosurgical excision procedure (LEEP)
• Cervicography
• Speculoscopy
• Use of HPV DNA typing to select certain cases with borderline abnormalities, e.g., atypical squamous cells of undetermined significance (ASCUS), for closer followup and colposcopy

TREATMENT

APPROPRIATE HEALTH CARE
Outpatient

GENERAL MEASURES Office evaluation and observation

SURGICAL MEASURES Outpatient surgery - cryotherapy, laser ablative or excisional cone, cold knife cone, electro-surgical loop excision of transformation zone

ACTIVITY Four weeks of pelvic rest after cone biopsy

DIET No restriction

PATIENT EDUCATION See Followup section

MEDICATIONS

DRUG(S) OF CHOICE
• Treatment is primarily surgical
• Fluorouracil (Efudex) once or twice daily as 5% vaginal cream supplemental therapy
Contraindications: Hypersensitivity to 5-fluorouracil
Precautions:
• If hand is used in application of 5-fluorouracil, wash hand immediately afterwards
• Avoid contact of 5-fluorouracil with eyes, nose, or mouth
Significant possible interactions: N/A

ALTERNATIVE DRUGS   N/A

FOLLOWUP

PATIENT MONITORING   Repeat Pap smears every 4 months during the first year after cone excision for severe dysplasia, every 6 months thereafter. For lesser lesions, repeat Pap smear yearly. Probe endocervical canal to assure patency.

PREVENTION/AVOIDANCE
• Monogamy of both sexual partners
• Use of condom during coitus if unable to practice monogamy
• Abstain from smoking
• Emphasize importance of yearly Pap smears for patients
• Ability to obtain skilled colposcopy service as needed
• Patient education (individually or by community services) to emphasize the need for Pap smear
• Educate medical care providers to make patient referrals for the screening service unless they provide it themselves

POSSIBLE COMPLICATIONS
• Some severe dysplasia will progress to invasive carcinoma of the cervix
• Possible complications following cone biopsy of the cervix:
  ◊ Hemorrhage
  ◊ Infection
  ◊ Cervical stenosis
  ◊ Cervical incompetence
  ◊ Infertility
  ◊ Incomplete excision of dysplastic tissue
  ◊ Recurrence

EXPECTED COURSE/PROGNOSIS
• Generally excellent
• Persistence of dysplasia can occur due to incomplete excision
• Recurrence of dysplasia can occur due to inability to eradicate the human papilloma virus in the patient's body or prevent new infections

MISCELLANEOUS

ASSOCIATED CONDITIONS
• Condyloma acuminatum
• Carcinoma of the cervix

AGE-RELATED FACTORS
Pediatric: Very rare
Geriatric: Less frequent
Others: This is usually a problem for the women in the reproductive age group. The median age is 28 years for severe dysplasia. For lesser lesions, the median ages tend to be much lower.

PREGNANCY
• Dysplasia may progress during pregnancy
• It is important to determine the severity of dysplasia and to exclude the presence of invasive carcinoma during pregnancy
• Dysplasia does not require definitive treatment during pregnancy
• Dysplasia by itself is not an indication for cesarean section

SYNONYMS   N/A

ICD-9-CM   622.1 Dysplasia of cervix (uteri)

SEE ALSO
• Abnormal Pap smear
• Condyloma acuminata
• Cervical malignancy

OTHER NOTES   Squamous intraepithelial lesion (SIL) is in reference to Pap smear only

ABBREVIATIONS
• CIN = cervical intraepithelial neoplasia (CIN)
• SIL = squamous intraepithelial lesion (SIL)

REFERENCES
• Koss LG: Reducing the error rate in Papanicolaou smears. The Female Patient 1994;19:6
• Sherman ME, et al: PAPNET analysis of reportedly negative smears preceding the diagnosis of high grade intraepithelial lesion or carcinoma. Modern Pathol 19947(5):578-581
• Disaia PJ, Creasman WT: Clinical Gynecologic Oncology. 4th Ed. St. Louis, The C.V. Mosby Co., 1993
• Wright TC, Richart RM, Ferencz A: Electrosurgery for HPV-related diseases of the lower genital tract. New York, Arthur Vision, Inc. & Biovision, Inc., 1992
• Kurman RJ, ed: Blaustein's Pathology Of The Female Genital Tract. 3rd Ed. New York, Springer-Verlag, 1987
• Novak ER, Woodruff JD: Novak's Gynecologic and Obstetric Pathology With Clinical and Endocrine Relations. 8th Ed. Philadelphia, W.B. Saunders Company, 1979
• Herbst AL, Mishel DR, Stenchever MA, Drogemueller W: Comprehensive Gynecology. 2nd Ed. St. Louis, C.V. Mosby Co., 1992
• Richart R, Jones HW III, Reid R: Classification and Interpretation of Pap smears. ACOG Update 1993;18;10:1-10
• Korn AP: Management of abnormal cervical/vaginal Pap smears. Medscape Women's Health 1996;1(3)
• Update: National Breast and Cervical Cancer Early Detection Program MMWR 1996;45(23):484-487
• BlockBB, Branham RA: Efforts to improve the follow-up of abnormal Papaniculaou test results. J of Am Board of Fam Prac 1998;11:1
Illustrations: N/A
Internet references: http://www.5mcc.com

Author(s)
Albert T. Shiu, MD, FACOG

Cervical hyperextension injuries

BASICS

DESCRIPTION Result from upward or backward injury to frontal head, jaw, and face. May involve:
• Soft tissues of neck - "whiplash"
• Vertebral structures - fractures, dislocations, ligamentous tears, and disc disruption
• Spinal cord - acute central cord syndrome (CCS) secondary to cord compression or vascular insult
System(s) affected: Musculoskeletal, Nervous
Genetics: Related to predisposing factors like ankylosing spondylitis associated with HLA-B27
Incidence/prevalence in USA: About 1/4 of spinal injuries caused by hyperextension
Predominant age: Trauma and sports injuries most common in young adults, average age 29.4 years; CCS most common among elderly, average age 53 years
Predominant sex: Male > Female

SIGNS AND SYMPTOMS
• Neck pain, stiffness and tenderness
• Headaches
• Paresthesia
• Numbness
• Shoulder pain, spasms and tenderness; range of motion limitation; radicular signs
• Classically, with forehead, face, or jaw abrasion, laceration, or contusion
• CCS
  ◊ Typically distal upper extremity (UE) weakness or paralysis worse than proximal UE, worse than lower extremity
  ◊ Variable sensory changes and sphincter disturbances
  ◊ Horner's syndrome if C8-T11 involved

CAUSES
• Trauma
  ◊ Mostly vehicular accidents
  ◊ Sports injuries
  ◊ Falls
  ◊ Assaults

RISK FACTORS
Present in 65% of CCS
• Spinal stenosis
  ◊ Congenital
  ◊ Acquired - prior trauma, spondylosis
• Spinal rigidity
  ◊ Klippel-Feil syndrome
  ◊ Ankylosing spondylitis

DIAGNOSIS

DIFFERENTIAL DIAGNOSIS
• Herniated discs
• Arthritis
• Radiculopathy
• Myelopathy
• For CCS
  ◊ Bell's cruciate palsy
  ◊ Bilateral brachial plexus injuries

LABORATORY N/A
Drugs that may alter lab results: N/A
Disorders that may alter lab results: N/A

PATHOLOGICAL FINDINGS
• Whiplash - based on animal experiments
  ◊ Muscle tears of the longus colli and sternocleidomastoid
  ◊ Injuries to anterior longitudinal ligament
  ◊ Intervertebral discs and vertebral body endplates
  ◊ Retropharyngeal hematoma, rarely
• CCS
  ◊ Traditionally reported as central gray matter injury with hemorrhage
  ◊ Recent reports show predominantly white matter injury with involvement of the lateral column, particularly, corticospinal tracts ◊ Pathologic hallmark - diffuse axonal disruption
  ◊ With more severe injuries, central hemorrhage is seen

SPECIAL TESTS See Imaging

IMAGING
• Plain c-spine films still main initial diagnostic tool
  ◊ Static - c-spine series; findings of slight extension, prevertebral swelling from anterior longitudinal ligament disruption
  ◊ Dynamic - flexion/extension, only if asymptomatic neck and no neurologic deficits or change in level of consciousness
• CT scan or tomograms - better delineation of fractures, spinal canal status
• CT myelogram - alternative to MRI, show cutoffs of thecal sac and nerve sleeve
• MRI - diagnostic procedure of choice in CCS; show ligament and disc injuries, vertebral body endplate fractures, disc-endplate disruption

DIAGNOSTIC PROCEDURES
Discussed in other sections; care needs to be taken to avoid overlooking subtle hyperextension injuries

TREATMENT:

APPROPRIATE HEALTH CARE
Outpatient or inpatients as required by injury

GENERAL MEASURES
• Whiplash; depending on severity
  ◊ Activity restriction
  ◊ Soft to rigid collar
  ◊ Medicines - analgesics, muscle relaxants, anti-inflammatory
  ◊ Post resolution of spasms, repeat flexion/extension lateral c-spine to confirm stability
• CCS
  ◊ See Medications
  ◊ If no instability, bed rest with soft collar for 4-6 weeks followed by mobilization with collar for another 4-6 weeks
• Fractures; stability determined by usual radiologic criteria; surgical decompression and stabilization is indicated:
  ◊ In patients with incomplete spinal cord injuries and spinal canal compromise from bone, disc, subluxation, or hematoma
  ◊ In those who deteriorate or do not improve on conservative therapy
• Hangman's fracture - traumatic spondylolisthesis of the axis is a fracture through the C2 pedicles, often with subluxation of C2 over C3
  ◊ Usually stable, managed with orthosis, SOMI (sternal-occipital-mental orthosis)
  ◊ Unstable if C2 subluxation over C3 is over 50% of C3
  ◊ If excessive angulation of C2 over C3
  ◊ Treated with halo vest immobilization for 8-14 weeks when lateral films in flexion and extension again done
  ◊ If stable, rigid collar for additional 8-12 weeks
• Odontoid fracture - treated according to type
  ◊ I - through apex, may be unstable and require surgical fusion
  ◊ II - at base of neck, usually unstable; nonunion rates up to 30% on immobilization alone, especially if displacement more than 5 mm in patients more than 7 years old
  ◊ III - through C2 body, usually stable; immobilized in halo for 8-14 weeks, rigid collar for 8-14 weeks, then mobilization
• C3-C7 hyperextension fractures
  ◊ If stable, rigid collar for 8-14 weeks then mobilization
  ◊ If unstable, halo brace; serial lat c-spine films from supine to upright; if still unstable, surgical stabilization
  ◊ Post-op, followup x-rays until trabeculation across fracture site or interbody fusion achieved

SURGICAL MEASURES
• CCS
◊ In acute cases, surgery is associated with deterioration and increased complications, and therefore contraindicated
◊ Surgery may be indicated in patient who is improving and then deteriorates
◊ Otherwise, surgical decompression and stabilization performed only when neurologic function has reached a plateau or maximum recovery
◊ Fractures: See General Measures

ACTIVITY   Rest and immobilization until pain is controlled; followed by gradual mobilization, and rehabilitation exercises if needed

DIET   No special diet

PATIENT EDUCATION   For patient instruction on prevention: THINK FIRST Foundation, 22 S. Washington St., Park Ridge, IL 60068, (708)692-2740

MEDICATIONS

DRUG(S) OF CHOICE   CCS - methylprednisolone 30 mg/kg IV over 1 hour followed by 5.4 mg/kg IV per hour for 23 hours should be started within 8 hours of injury. It has been proven to improve neurologic outcome, motor and sensory function at 6 months and 1 year after incomplete spinal cord injury.
Contraindications: N/A
Precautions: N/A
Significant possible interactions: N/A

ALTERNATIVE DRUGS   N/A

FOLLOWUP

PATIENT MONITORING
• Patients seen and checked with x-rays every 3-4 weeks for about 3 months, when bone healing is usually adequate
• Halo then replaced with rigid collar for next 3 months or rigid collar replaced with soft collar for comfort

PREVENTION/AVOIDANCE   Wearing seat belts; using proper equipment when participating in sports activities

POSSIBLE COMPLICATIONS
• Persistent symptoms
• Nonunion of fractures
• Persistent instability requiring another procedure
• Reactions and infection related to orthosis

EXPECTED COURSE/PROGNOSIS
Most important prognostic factor is the initial neurologic status
• Whiplash - most patients recover well, mild symptoms resolving within 6 months
◊ On the average, more severe injuries without disc involvement resolve in 21 months
◊ 30 months for those with degenerative changes
◊ At 2 years, 42% complete recovery, 15% mild discomfort, 43% significant discomfort affecting work
• CCS
◊ Most patients recover motor strength within 2 weeks
◊ Younger patients have better prognosis
◊ Leg, bowel, and bladder function return first
◊ Return of arm strength follows, then that of hand
◊ However, upper extremities recover less well, and fine finger movements is usually not regained completely
◊ With cord contusion but no hematomyelia, 50% recover enough strength and sensation to ambulate independently although usually with spasticity
• Fracture-dislocation
◊ Hangman's fracture - 93-100% fusion rate after 8-14 weeks external immobilization
◊ Odontoid fracture - type III, 90% fusion with immobilization

MISCELLANEOUS

ASSOCIATED CONDITIONS   N/A

AGE-RELATED FACTORS
Pediatric: N/A
Geriatric: N/A
Others: N/A

PREGNANCY   N/A

SYNONYMS   N/A

ICD-9-CM
952.0 Spinal cord injury without evidence of spinal bone injury, cervical

SEE ALSO   N/A

OTHER NOTES   N/A

ABBREVIATIONS   N/A

REFERENCES
• Greenberg MS: Handbook of Neurosurgery. Florida, Greenberg Graphics, Inc., 1994
• Larson SJ: Hyperextension, hyperflexion, and torsion injuries of the spine. In Youman's Neurological Surgery. 3rd Ed, Philadelphia, W.B. Saunders Co., 1990:2392-2402
• McSwain NE, Martinez JA, Timberlake GA: Cervical Spine Trauma: Evaluation and Acute Management. New York, Thieme Medical Publishers, Inc.,1989
• Pitts LH, Wagner FC Jr: Craniospinal Trauma, New York, Thieme Medical Publishers, Inc., 1990
• Sonntag VKH, Francis PM: Controversies in spinal cord syndromes. In: Grafin SR, Northru BE, eds. Surgery For Spinal Cord Injuries. New York, Raven Press, 1993:15-30
• Wagner FC: Injuries to the cervical spine and spinal cord. In Youman's Neurological Surgery. 3rd Ed. Philadelphia, W.B. Saunders Co., 1990:2378-2391
Illustrations: N/A
Internet references: http://www.5mcc.com

Author(s)
Martin E. Weinand, MD

Cervical malignancy

BASICS

DESCRIPTION Invasive cancer of the uterine cervix commonly involves the vagina, parametria and the pelvic side-walls. In advanced cases, the cancer may invade the bladder, rectum, or other pelvic sites.
System(s) affected: Reproductive
Genetics: Not an inherited disease
Incidence/Prevalence in USA: In 1997, there were 14,500 new cases, and 4,800 deaths due to the disease
Predominant age: Greater than 25% of all cervical cancer cases occur in women 65 years or older. 40-50% of women dying from cervical cancer are over 65 years of age.
Predominant sex: Female only

SIGNS AND SYMPTOMS
• Abnormal vaginal bleeding
• Post-coital vaginal bleeding
• Pelvic pain, leg pain, back pain
• Dyspareunia
• Hematuria
• Rectal bleeding
• Foul vaginal discharge
• Cervical ulcer, crater, or fungating mass
• Extension of the cervical mass into upper vagina and/or parametria, with induration, nodularity, and fixation to surrounding tissue

CAUSES Unknown. There is a strong association with genital infection by the oncogenic strains of human papilloma virus (HPV) in 90% of cases.

RISK FACTORS
• Multiple sexual partners
• Male partner with multiple sexual partners
• Male partner who has had a partner with cervical carcinoma
• Early onset of first sexual intercourse
• Current or previous HPV infections, eg, condyloma acuminatum, cervical intraepithelial neoplasia
• History of sexually transmitted diseases
• Smoker
• Immunosuppression from drugs or HIV infection
• Diethylstilbestrol (DES) offspring

DIAGNOSIS

DIFFERENTIAL DIAGNOSIS
• Marked cervicitis and erosion
• Cervical polyp
• Cervical condyloma
• Metastasis from endometrial carcinoma or gestational trophoblastic disease
• Cervical pregnancy

LABORATORY
• For initial diagnosis: Papanicolaou smear and cervical biopsies
• Complete blood count
• BUN, creatinine
Drugs that may alter lab results: Vaginal lubricants may obscure Pap smears
Disorders that may alter lab results: Vaginitis or excessive vaginal bleeding may obscure Pap smears

PATHOLOGICAL FINDINGS
• Invasive squamous cell carcinoma is the major cell type
• Invasive adenocarcinoma is becoming increasingly evident
• Other cell types are also present in the minority

SPECIAL TESTS
• Colposcopy, if indicated
• Endocervical curettage
• Cervical conization, if indicated
• Liver function tests
• Cystoscopy
• Sigmoidoscopy

IMAGING
• Computed tomographic scans of the abdomen and pelvis, if needed, for detection of lymph node metastasis, and for evaluation of planned radiation therapy
• Lymphangiogram, if needed, for detection of pelvic and para-aortic lymph node metastasis
• Chest x-ray
• Excretory pyelogram

DIAGNOSTIC PROCEDURES Cervical conization can resolve the question of early invasion, and if present, can determine the depth of invasion, and the presence of lymphatic and vascular involvement

TREATMENT

APPROPRIATE HEALTH CARE
According to the depth of invasion and clinical staging

GENERAL MEASURES
• Improve the patient's nutritional state, correct any anemia and treat any vaginal and/or pelvic infections
• Chemotherapy has been used extensively as adjuvant therapy to metastatic disease

SURGICAL MEASURES
• Stage 1a1 (lesions with less than 3 mm invasion from basement membrane): cervical conization with total hysterectomy later when patient's family is completed; otherwise total hysterectomy by either the abdominal or vaginal route.
• Stage 1a2 (lesions with greater than 3 mm but less than 5 mm invasion from the basement membrane) and for stages 1b1, 1b2, 2a: patient has the option of radical hysterectomy, bilateral pelvic lymphadenectomy, and para-aortic nodes sampling; or primary radiation with brachytherapy and teletherapy
• Stage 4A (lesions limited to central metastasis to the bladder and/or rectum): pelvic exenteration may be feasible
• Radiation measures
  ◊ Stages 1a2 or higher, the following techniques have been used:
    - Brachytherapy with intracavitory radium or cesium or interstitial cessium needles to treat the central tumor sites, and
    - Teletherapy with external megavoltage radiation to treat tumor metastasis in the pelvic walls
• For localized persistent or recurrent disease, radiation therapy or pelvic exenteration as appropriate

ACTIVITY As tolerated

DIET As appropriate

PATIENT EDUCATION American Cancer Society, 1599 Clifton Rd., Atlanta, GA 30329, (404)320-3333

Cervical malignancy

MEDICATIONS

DRUG(S) OF CHOICE
• Cisplatin, hydroxyurea, and fluorouracil have been used as adjuvant sensitizer to radiation therapy
• Cisplatin/carboplatin, etoposide (VP-16), ifosfamide, bleomycin have been used as adjuvant therapy for recurrent, metastatic disease
Contraindications: Refer to manufacturer's profile of each drug.
Precautions: Refer to manufacturer's profile of each drug
Significant possible interactions: Refer to manufacturer's profile of each drug

ALTERNATIVE DRUGS
• Ondansetron (Zofran), dronabinol (Marinol), metoclopramide (Reglan), and others for nausea control

FOLLOWUP

PATIENT MONITORING
• With completion of definitive therapy. each patient is evaluated with physical/pelvic examinations and Pap smear at the following intervals:
    ◊ Every 3 months for 1-2 years
    ◊ Every 6 months until the 5th year
    ◊ Yearly thereafter
• The three most common signs of cancer recurrence are: unexplained weight loss, leg edema, and pelvic or thigh pain

PREVENTION/AVOIDANCE
• Stop smoking
• Avoid sexually transmitted diseases
• Regular Pap smears and pelvic exams; appropriate interval for Pap smear (reference: 1988 American College of Obstetricians and Gynecologists and American Cancer Society):
    ◊ All women who are or who have been sexually active, or who have reached age 18, should undergo an annual Pap test and pelvic examination.
    ◊ After a woman has had three or more consecutive satisfactory annual examinations with normal findings, the Pap smear may be performed less frequently at the discretion of her physician

POSSIBLE COMPLICATIONS
• Hemorrhage
• Pelvic infection
• Bladder dysfunction
• Genito-urinary fistula
• Ureteral obstruction with renal failure
• Bowel obstruction
• Lymphocyst
• Pulmonary embolism
• Loss of ovarian function from radiotherapy or indication for bilateral oophorectomy

EXPECTED COURSE/PROGNOSIS
After commonly accepted surgical and radiation treatments.

```
Stage    5 yr survival
--------------------------------
  1        80%
  2        65%
  3        30%
  4        15%
```

MISCELLANEOUS

ASSOCIATED CONDITIONS
• Condyloma acuminatum
• Preinvasive/invasive lesions of the vulva and vagina

AGE-RELATED FACTORS
Pediatric: N/A
Geriatric: Since more than half the invasive cancer cases are seen in the over 65 age group, efforts should be concentrated in expanding the availability of Pap smear screening to the geriatric population
Others: Selection of surgical therapy in younger women with early stages of cancer provides ovarian conservation

PREGNANCY Generally, the choice of treatment is dependent on the length of gestation, the patient's wish to continue pregnancy to attainment of fetal lung maturity, and the treating physician's comfort level in delaying definitive therapy. If treatment is delayed, the patient must receive close follow-up care with its frequency dependent upon the severity of the disease. Selection of the mode of therapy is based upon clinical staging as noted previously.

SYNONYMS
• Cancer of the uterine cervix
• Cervical cancer
• Cervical carcinoma

ICD-9-CM
180.0 Malignant neoplasm of cervix uteri

SEE ALSO
• Abnormal Pap smear

OTHER NOTES N/A

ABBREVIATIONS N/A

REFERENCES
• McMeekin DS, McGonigle KH, Vasilev SA. Cervical cancer prevention: towards cost effective screening. Medscape Women's Health 12-2-1997
• Parke SL, Tong T, Bolden S, et al. Cancer statistics, 1997. Ca-A cancer Jour for Clinicians 1997;47(1):5-27
• National Cancer Institute: Cancer Statistics Review 1973-1987. Bethesda, NCI Publication No. (NIH)90-2789, 1990
Illustrations: N/A
Internet references: http://www.5mcc.com

Author(s)
Albert T. Shiu, MD, FACOG

Cervical polyps

BASICS

DESCRIPTION Pedunculated masses, usually single, which vary in size from a few millimeters to 3 centimeters and protrude from the cervix; may bleed
System(s) affected: Reproductive
Genetics: N/A
Incidence/Prevalence in USA: Common
Predominant age: Most often ages 30-50
Predominant sex: Female only

SIGNS AND SYMPTOMS
• Painless
• Intermenstrual bleeding (slight)
• May cause post-coital spotting

CAUSES
• Unknown for most
• Secondary reaction to cervical infection, erosion, or ulceration

RISK FACTORS   None known

DIAGNOSIS

DIFFERENTIAL DIAGNOSIS
• Prolapsed submucous myoma
• Other causes of intermenstrual bleeding

LABORATORY   N/A
Drugs that may alter lab results: N/A
Disorders that may alter lab results: N/A

PATHOLOGICAL FINDINGS
• Benign hyperplastic endocervical epithelium often with large number of blood vessels
• Size may be increased by edema and inflammation

SPECIAL TESTS
• Diagnosis usually made by pelvic examination
• Perform Pap smear prior to treatment

IMAGING   N/A

DIAGNOSTIC PROCEDURES
Characteristic appearance noted at time of pelvic examination

TREATMENT

APPROPRIATE HEALTH CARE
Outpatient usually. Very large polyps may require removal in operating room.

GENERAL MEASURES   N/A

SURGICAL MEASURES
• Simple surgical excision in office with snare, electrocautery, or liquid nitrogen, control bleeding with silver nitrate
• No douching following excision

ACTIVITY   Avoid sexual intercourse until postoperative followup

DIET   General diet

PATIENT EDUCATION   Routine care instructions

MEDICATIONS

DRUG(S) OF CHOICE None
Contraindications: N/A
Precautions: N/A
Significant possible interactions: N/A

ALTERNATIVE DRUGS N/A

FOLLOWUP

PATIENT MONITORING Recheck at routine appointments, 1 and 6 weeks following surgical excision

PREVENTION/AVOIDANCE None known

POSSIBLE COMPLICATIONS
• Bleeding and mild pain with removal
• Spotting for 1 or 2 days

EXPECTED COURSE/PROGNOSIS
Almost always benign. Very rare incidence of dysplasia in polyp. Very rare possibility of malignancy arising.

MISCELLANEOUS

ASSOCIATED CONDITIONS None

AGE-RELATED FACTORS
Pediatric: Very rare
Geriatric: Rare
Others: N/A

PREGNANCY Delay removal until postpartum

SYNONYMS N/A

ICD-9-CM
622.7 Mucous polyp of cervix

SEE ALSO N/A

OTHER NOTES N/A

ABBREVIATIONS N/A

REFERENCES
• Danforth DM, Scott JR, et al, eds: Obstetric and Gynecology. 6th Ed. Philadelphia, J.B. Lippincott, 1990
• Novak ER, et al, eds: Novak's, Textbook of Gynecology. 11th Ed. Baltimore, Williams & Wilkins, 1988
Illustrations: N/A
Internet references: http://www.5mcc.com

Author(s)
Mark Eric Worshtil, MD

Cervical spine injury

BASICS

DESCRIPTION
Though an over-simplification, it is best to classify injuries as flexion, extension, compression, or unknown
- Flexion injuries
  ◊ Anterior subluxation - best seen on lateral view of cervical spine as a kyphotic angulation at the point of ligamentous injury. Widening of spinous process at the point of injury may occur.
  ◊ Facet dislocation - unstable injury, especially when bilateral. Anterior displacement of vertebra (50% of its width) usually indicates bilateral facet dislocation.
  ◊ Compression fractures - usually associated with disruption of the posterior ligament complex and therefore unstable
  ◊ Clay-shovelers fracture - avulsion fracture of C7-C6 or T1 spinous process with intact posterior ligaments and therefore stable
- Extension injuries
  ◊ Hangman's fracture - fracture of the pars interarticularis of the axis. It accounts for 10-15% of fractures.
  ◊ Laminar fracture - difficult to see. Usually in older people who have spondylosis.
  ◊ Fracture posterior arch atlas - usually stable when an isolated injury
  ◊ Fracture dislocations - may resemble a flexion injury since the vertebral body is propelled forward and therefore appears as a flexion subluxation
- Compression
  ◊ Jefferson's fracture - a fracture of the arches of C1, best seen on the open mouth view as displacement of C1 lateral masses
  ◊ Burst fracture - seen on the AP radiograph as a vertical fracture of the body and on the lateral as a commutation of the body with varying degrees of retropulsion of the body
- Unknown mechanisms
  ◊ Odontoid fractures - best seen on the AP view, but lateral views may show a tilt or displacement

System(s) affected: Musculoskeletal, Nervous

Genetics: N/A

Incidence/Prevalence in USA: Cervical injuries account for twelve thousand deaths in the U.S. each year. One-half of these are from motor vehicular accidents.

Predominant age: Most common in ages 16-25

Predominant sex: Male > Female

SIGNS AND SYMPTOMS
- Pain, stiffness, and/or tenderness in an alert patient. If none of these are present the incidence of cervical spine injury is only 1-2%, provided the patient is alert and without alcohol or drug intake. (A lateral cervical spine x-ray should be taken routinely in all severe trauma).
- Head and/or facial trauma/lacerations in patients with altered consciousness

CAUSES
Trauma

RISK FACTORS
- Motor vehicle accidents
- Diving accidents

DIAGNOSIS

DIFFERENTIAL DIAGNOSIS
- Joint, muscle or ligament inflammation
- Paresthesias
- Arthritis
- Cervical disk protrusion
- Cervical spondylosis

LABORATORY
N/A
Drugs that may alter lab results: N/A
Disorders that may alter lab results: N/A

PATHOLOGICAL FINDINGS
N/A

SPECIAL TESTS
Tomograms may be obtained to visualize otherwise obscure fractures, but even these are usually inferior to imaging by CT. MRI is superior in evaluating soft tissue injury.

IMAGING
- The use of CT and MRI scanning has greatly facilitated diagnosis of obscure cervical injuries. The CT may be a little better in some bone injuries, especially in the foramen, while the MRI has the edge with soft tissue evaluation. Both are superior to any previous method.
- X-ray - a lateral view of the cervical spine is only 80-85% accurate in picking up abnormalities. Adding an AP and open mouth odontoid view will increase the accuracy of screening to 90-95%. However, in the presence of pain, tenderness, and/or stiffness, the use of a CT or MRI scan should be considered since 5-10% of cases will have normal radiographs even with a significant cervical injury.
- X-rays vary with the type of injury, but a few salient features to be observed are:
  ◊ Soft-tissue swelling on the lateral view of greater than 5 mm when measured from the inferior border of C3 to the trachea indicates a severe injury (except children)
  ◊ Widely divergent spinous processes on the lateral view indicates rupture of ligaments
  ◊ Abnormal widening of either a complete interspace or a portion of the anterior or posterior interspace on lateral view (compare with interspaces above and below)
  ◊ Malrotation of the spinous processes on the AP view (they should form a straight line)
  ◊ Inequality of the space on either side of the odontoid on open mouth views

DIAGNOSTIC PROCEDURES
N/A

TREATMENT

APPROPRIATE HEALTH CARE
- Transportation
  ◊ A carefully applied rigid collar supplemented by sand bags on either side of the head on a rigid backboard is probably the safest method
  ◊ Oxygen should be given to all patients with injury to the spinal cord. (Patients with high cord lesions die of asphyxiation so assisted ventilation may be needed).
  ◊ 50% of serious cervical injuries will have associated head, chest, abdominal or major extremity injuries in association. Give first aid to these patients maintaining the "ABC" principle of airway, breathing, and circulation.
  ◊ Military antishock garment (MASG) can be used in cases of shock
  ◊ Start an intravenous line if it can be done rapidly. Otherwise, this should not be done as valuable time may be wasted. The principle of "load and go" in cases of ambulance or "swoop and scoop" in the case of helicopters is a good one if an acute care center is close at hand.
- Hospital
  ◊ Prior to dealing with the cervical injury, attention should be directed towards the ABC's (airway, breathing, circulation)
  ◊ Arterial oxygen should be measured immediately since oxygenation of an injured spinal cord helps prevent further damage and aids in recovery. If the oxygen partial pressure (pO2) is less than 70 mm of mercury, or the cervical lesion is above C5, intubation is indicated. If the patient is breathing, blind nasal intubation can be tried; otherwise the oral approach with a laryngoscope is necessary. Both require careful technique with avoidance of neck extension. If this cannot be done with ease or if there are severe facial injuries, a cricothyroidotomy should be done.
  ◊ A nasogastric (NG) tube should always be inserted to prevent vomiting, aspiration. It also prevents gastric dilatation with lung compression and difficult breathing.
  ◊ In most cases, volume replacement is best accomplished through the femoral route. The subclavian approach risks pneumothorax and further oxygenation problems.
  ◊ If a pneumothorax is present, a chest tube should always be inserted (first confirmed by x-ray). Needle aspiration is indicated only as a temporary measure to relieve symptoms in a tension pneumothorax prior to insertion of the tube.
  ◊ In all cord injuries, abdominal and chest CT scan should be done to rule out a severe intra-abdominal injury. This procedure is highly accurate while all physical findings and symptoms are unreliable. (The NG tube and an indwelling Foley catheter should be done prior to the scans.)

GENERAL MEASURES

• Spinal shock occurs in 25-40% of spinal cord injuries. It is characterized by systolic hypotension and bradycardia. The cause is loss of distal sympathetic tone.
• Head injuries alone do not cause hypotension but can cause hypertension
• Because patients with cervical trauma may sustain other significant injuries, systolic hypotension may be from blood loss and/or spinal shock. Remember that several liters of blood can be lost from a head or perineal wound.
• Shock other than from volume loss or spinal shock can come from pericardial tamponade, tension pneumothorax, or cardiac contusion

SURGICAL MEASURES
Surgical management as needed for type of injury

ACTIVITY N/A

DIET N/A

PATIENT EDUCATION N/A

MEDICATIONS

DRUG(S) OF CHOICE

• Methylprednisolone
  ◊ If given within 8 hours after the injury, has been shown to not only minimize further injury, but to improve both motor function and sensation for up to six months. This steroid apparently prevents lipid hydrolysis and subsequent destruction of the cell membrane.
  ◊ Initial dose: 30 mg/kg over a 15 minute period. Then 45 minutes later, 5.4 mg/kg/hr for the next 23 hours. See Bracken 1990, N Engl J Med 322:1405-1411.

Contraindications: None

Precautions: Intravenous cimetidine (Tagamet) 300 mg q6h or ranitidine (Zantac) 50 mg q8h can be given if a history of ulcer is present. In cases of multiple injuries this is a good way to prevent stress ulcer.

Significant possible interactions: None

ALTERNATIVE DRUGS

• Naloxone, nimodipine and thyrotropin releasing hormones have been tried with equivocal results. Tests are underway using chemotherapeutic drugs, but these await the outcome of several studies.
• Other H2 receptor antagonists

FOLLOWUP

PATIENT MONITORING Critical care facilities must be available initially and later physical and occupational therapy units with special skills in spinal cord injuries

PREVENTION/AVOIDANCE N/A

POSSIBLE COMPLICATIONS
• Paresthesia
• Muscle weakness
• Reflex loss
• Sensory loss
• Radiculopathy

EXPECTED COURSE/PROGNOSIS In cases of significant cord injuries, the prognosis is guarded. Development of newer orthopedic devices can stabilize the spine and allow early mobilization, but do not help to reverse neurological damage if present.

MISCELLANEOUS

ASSOCIATED CONDITIONS N/A

AGE-RELATED FACTORS
Pediatric: N/A
Geriatric: N/A
Others: N/A

PREGNANCY N/A

SYNONYMS Cervical fracture, dislocation

ICD-9-CM 952.0 Cervical spinal cord injury

SEE ALSO N/A

OTHER NOTES N/A

ABBREVIATIONS N/A

REFERENCES

• Torg JS, Sennett B, et al: Axial loading injuries to middle cervical spine segment. An analysis and classification of 25 cases. American Journal of Sports Medicine 1991:19(1):6-20
• Soderstrom CA, Brumback RJ: Orthopedic Clinics of North America 1986;17(1):3-13
• Bracken MB, et al: Efficacy of methylprednisolone in acute spinal cord Injury; JAMA 1984;251:45-52
• Bracken MB, et al: A randomized control trial of methylprednisolone or naloxone in the treatment of acute spinal cord injury. Results of the second acute spinal cord Injury study. N Engl J Med 1990;322:1405-1411
• Jacobs B: Cervical Fractures and Dislocations, Clinical Orthopedics 1975;109:18
Illustrations: N/A
Internet references: http://www.5mcc.com

Author(s)
Furnie W. Johnston, MD
R. Bruce Hall, MD

Cervical spondylosis

BASICS

DESCRIPTION Degenerative changes in the cervical vertebra and/or disk with spur formation and subsequent impingement of neural elements in a narrow cervical canal
System(s) affected: Musculoskeletal
Genetics: N/A
Incidence/Prevalence in USA: 30-40% of the population above age 40 years
Predominant age: Above 40 the incidence increases with each passing decade
Predominant sex: Male > Female (3:2)

SIGNS AND SYMPTOMS
• Pain in the posterior neck often associated with radiation into the arms
• Scapular pain
• Pain in the arms is almost always on the outer aspect of the arm at least to elbow level (coronary heart pain is almost always on the inner aspect of the arm)
• Radicular pain into the arms or scapular area may be present without neck pain
• Dysphagia may develop with large anterior osteophytes
• Weakness of extremities - upper and/or lower
• Bladder or bowel incontinence in severe cases
• If an osteophyte develops on a neurocentral joint and extends laterally, it can encroach on the vertebral artery and may cause dizziness, vertigo, tinnitus or interorbital blurring of vision. Symptoms are exacerbated by extremes of movement and even minor neck trauma.
• Loss of neck extension (common)
• Lateral flexion of the cervical spine is limited in the erect position, but greatly increased on lying down. (Functional disorders are not improved by lying down.)
• Long tract signs may develop in severe cases with positive Babinski
• Tenderness of biceps and pectoralis major in C5-6 segment disease
• Triceps tenderness in C6-7 segment disease

CAUSES Degenerative changes with osteophytes and disk space narrowing

RISK FACTORS N/A

DIAGNOSIS

DIFFERENTIAL DIAGNOSIS
• Cervical disk disease (the two often co-exist)
• Pancoast tumor of lung
• Rheumatoid arthritis
• Neurological disorders such as multiple sclerosis

LABORATORY N/A
Drugs that may alter lab results: N/A
Disorders that may alter lab results: N/A

PATHOLOGICAL FINDINGS N/A

SPECIAL TESTS N/A

IMAGING
• X-rays of cervical spine, AP, lateral open mouth odontoid and both oblique views should be obtained. Osteophytes and/or joint space narrowing will be evident.
• CT or MRI scans are quite valuable in cases where surgery is contemplated or the diagnosis is in doubt. It is not indicated in the great majority of cases as a careful history and physical examination coupled with routine cervical spine x-rays will make the diagnosis. The decision as to which is better, the CT scan or MRI, is controversial. The MRI depicts cord changes, enlargement, compression, or atrophy better. While the CT, especially in conjunction with myelography, shows the bony changes, especially in foramina involvement. MRI has the obvious advantage of not requiring a myelogram. Postoperatively, the MRI is excellent in evaluation of patients who have failed to obtain relief from surgery or have developed new symptoms. If this does not demonstrate a cause, then a CT scan with contrast can be obtained.

DIAGNOSTIC PROCEDURES N/A

TREATMENT

APPROPRIATE HEALTH CARE
Outpatient for conservative treatment, inpatient if surgery indicated

GENERAL MEASURES
• Acute phase - moist heat, gentle massage and temporary immobilization with a cervical collar that holds the neck in slight flexion. Intermittent cervical traction may be helpful, but the line of pull should be such that the neck is slightly flexed. Ultrasonic treatments, especially combined with gentle muscle stimulation (US-MS) for 15-20 minutes daily or bid may be helpful in the acute phase.
• Chronic - no treatment necessary except for non-narcotic analgesics for symptoms. Any type of activity or work which causes strain of the neck should be avoided.

SURGICAL MEASURES
• Indications: Severe pain unresponsive to conservative measures, significant or progression of neurologic deficits, long tract signs, vertebral artery syndrome
• Most common surgery is anterior interbody fusion with excision of disk and any accessible osteophytes

ACTIVITY Any activity which does not cause symptoms should be encouraged as the disease is chronic. Needless restrictions can make the patient a medical invalid.

DIET No special diet

PATIENT EDUCATION
• Personally instruct (or have a therapist instruct) in the proper use of orthopedic appliances. Cervical collars should produce a slight flexion of the neck as should traction. Avoid extension in all situations.
• Instruct patient in home traction to relieve symptoms; instruct patient in home exercise routine to relieve spasm and discomfort
• Instruct patients to report any weaknesses, eye symptoms, bladder or bowel incontinence immediately

MEDICATIONS

DRUG(S) OF CHOICE
• Acetaminophen (Tylenol) 500 mg qid is the safest regimen. Studies have shown it to be at least as effective as NSAID's.
• NSAID's - aspirin 1.0 gm qid is effective in many cases. If this fails, any of the other NSAID's are used with all having about the same success rate. Piroxicam 10 mg daily, tolmetin 600 mg tid are some examples. If aspirin therapy is used, salicylate levels should be obtained; therapeutic range is 10-30 mg/dL (0.724-2.17 mmol/L). Enteric-coated aspirin may be helpful to minimize GI upset.
• Cortisone should not be used in long term management. Occasional injections of trigger zones with 40 mg methylprednisolone (Depo-Medrol) may be used, but this should be saved for severe exacerbations.
• Trigger point injection of lidocaine 1%, injected into the "hot areas", especially in the scapular area. Often as effective in relieving symptoms alone as when combined with methylprednisolone
Contraindications: NSAID's, except aspirin, should not be used in patients with chronic liver disease. Use with caution in cases of ulcers. If NSAID's are used, misoprostol (Cytotec) 200 µg qid should be given concomitantly.
Precautions: Patients on long term NSAID's should be monitored with liver studies 6-8 weeks after initial treatment and then every 3-4 months
Significant possible interactions: Refer to manufacturer's profile of each drug

ALTERNATIVE DRUGS   Listed in Drug(s) of Choice

FOLLOWUP

PATIENT MONITORING   Patients should be seen in 3-4 weeks for evaluation of neurologic status. If this has not changed follow at intervals of 3-6 months, depending on severity of symptoms.

PREVENTION/AVOIDANCE   The midcervical spine is the area usually involved in spondylosis. This portion will develop a flexion deformity causing extension of the upper spine as the body tries to keep the head erect. Avoid any extension strain such as a "spinal manipulation," extension during intubation for a general anesthesia, or cervical strain from auto accidents, especially rear-end collisions. These can cause a basilar artery thrombosis or thrombosis of the posterior inferior cerebellar artery with a subsequent Wallenberg's syndrome. Dysphagia, pain and temperature loss to the same side of the face and opposite side of the body, nystagmus and Horner's syndrome are present in Wallenberg's syndrome.

POSSIBLE COMPLICATIONS   Loss of motion, especially extension, may require adjustments to certain occupations to prevent uncommonly significant muscle loss and instability of gait, bladder or bowel function

EXPECTED COURSE/PROGNOSIS
Fortunately, the prognosis is for a benign course in the overwhelming majority of cases, though for most of their lives patients will be plagued by pain which exacerbates often with no known cause

MISCELLANEOUS

ASSOCIATED CONDITIONS   Cervical disk disease

AGE-RELATED FACTORS
Pediatric: N/A
Geriatric: N/A
Others: N/A

PREGNANCY   As in the case of rheumatoid arthritis, the symptoms often improve but occasionally are made worse

SYNONYMS
• Cervical arthritis
• Cervical myelopathy
• Cervical osteophyte

ICD-9-CM
722.4 Degeneration of cervical intervertebral disc
721.0 Cervical spondylosis without mention of myelopathy
721.1 Cervical spondylosis with myelopathy

SEE ALSO   N/A

OTHER NOTES   N/A

ABBREVIATIONS
US-MS = ultrasonic treatment with muscle stimulation

REFERENCES
• McNab I: Cervical Spondylosis: Clinical Orthopedics 1975;109:69-77
• Clifton AG, et al: Identifiable causes for poor outcome in surgery for cervical spondylosis. Neuroradiology 1990;177(2):313-325
• Karnaze MG, et al: Comparison of MR and CT myelography in imaging the cervical and thoracic spine. American Journal of Roentgenography 1988;150(2):397-403
Illustrations: N/A
Internet references: http://www.5mcc.com

Author(s)
Furnie W. Johnston, MD
R. Bruce Hall, MD

Cervicitis

BASICS

DESCRIPTION An inflammation of the uterine cervix. Infectious cervicitis may be caused by Chlamydia trachomatis, Neisseria gonorrhoeae, herpes simplex or Trichomonas vaginalis.
• Chronic cervicitis is characterized by inflammation of the cervix without an identified pathogen
System(s) affected: Reproductive
Genetics: N/A
Incidence/Prevalence in USA:
• Gonorrhea 166/100,000
• Chlamydia 290/100,000 women
• Trichomonas 1200/100,000
• Gonorrhea 2% of sexually active women under age 30
• Chlamydia 5-35% of women
• Trichomonas 5-25%
Predominant age: Infectious cervicitis is most common in adolescents, but can be seen in women of any age
Predominant sex: Female only

SIGNS AND SYMPTOMS
• Mucopurulent (yellow) discharge from the cervix
• Cervical erosion or erythema
• Easily induced endocervical mucosal bleeding
• Tenderness of cervix
• Postcoital bleeding
• Frequently asymptomatic

CAUSES
• Chlamydia trachomatis
• Neisseria gonorrhoeae
• Herpes simplex virus
• Trichomonas vaginalis
• Cause of chronic cervicitis unknown

RISK FACTORS
• Multiple sexual partners
• History of sexually transmitted disease
• Postpartum period

DIAGNOSIS

DIFFERENTIAL DIAGNOSIS
• Vaginal infections with Candida albicans or Trichomonas vaginalis extending onto the cervix
• Carcinoma of the cervix

LABORATORY
• Endocervical gram stain, more than 10 WBC's per high power field (hpf) suggests cervicitis
• Cervical cultures for C. trachomatis, N. gonorrhoeae
• Enzyme assays (Chlamydiazyme and others) sometimes used to screen for chlamydia
• Polymerase chain reaction (PCR) and ligase chain reaction (LCR) more sensitive than cultures for Chlamydia. LCR can be used with urine.
• Wet mount for Trichomonas vaginalis
• If ulcerations present, culture for herpes simplex virus
• Venereal Disease Research Laboratory (VDRL) or rapid plasma reagin (RPR) to rule out concurrent syphilis
Drugs that may alter lab results: Recent antibiotic treatment
Disorders that may alter lab results: N/A

PATHOLOGICAL FINDINGS
Inflammatory changes on Pap smear

SPECIAL TESTS   N/A

IMAGING   N/A

DIAGNOSTIC PROCEDURES
Colposcopy is indicated in chronic inflammation, with biopsy of suspicious areas

TREATMENT

APPROPRIATE HEALTH CARE
Outpatient treatment

GENERAL MEASURES   Chronic cervicitis with negative cultures and biopsies may be treated with cryosurgery

SURGICAL MEASURES   N/A

ACTIVITY   Full activity

DIET   No special diet

PATIENT EDUCATION
• Advise patient to use condoms consistently
• If infectious etiology, advise patient to inform her partners

Cervicitis

MEDICATIONS

DRUG(S) OF CHOICE
• If infectious cervicitis suspected, treat without awaiting culture results. Ceftriaxone (Rocephin) 125 mg IM single dose; followed by either doxycycline (Vibramycin) 100 mg po bid for 7 days or azithromycin (Zithromax) 1 g single dose
• For Trichomonas, metronidazole (Flagyl) 2 g single dose
• For herpes, acyclovir (Zovirax) 200 mg po 5 times daily (or 400 mg tid) for 7 days
• Chronic cervicitis associated with postmenopausal vaginal atrophic changes may respond to topical estrogen creams

Contraindications:
• Doxycycline should not be used in pregnant or nursing mothers
• Metronidazole contraindicated in first trimester of pregnancy

Precautions: Doxycycline should not be taken with milk, antacids, or iron containing preparations

Significant possible interactions:
Doxycycline - warfarin (Coumadin) and oral contraceptives may have their effectiveness reduced

ALTERNATIVE DRUGS
• Any of the following can be substituted for ceftriaxone:
  ◊ Cefixime 400 mg po once
  ◊ Ofloxacin 400 mg po once
  ◊ Spectinomycin 2 g IM once
• Erythromycin base or stearate 500 mg po qid, or erythromycin ethylsuccinate 800 mg po qid can be substituted for doxycycline
• Ofloxacin (Floxin) 300 mg po bid x 7 days
• Grepafloxacin (Raxar) 400 mg qd x 7 days

FOLLOWUP

PATIENT MONITORING
• Repeat cultures after treatment for chlamydia or gonorrhea are indicated in pregnant or high risk patients
• Annual Pap smears in sexually active patients screen for chronic cervicitis

PREVENTION/AVOIDANCE
Patients with more than one sexual partner should be advised to use condoms at every encounter

POSSIBLE COMPLICATIONS
• Cervicitis with C. trachomatis or N. gonorrhoeae is associated with an 8-10% risk of subsequent pelvic inflammatory disease
• Moderate to severe inflammation is associated with condyloma acuminatum and cervical carcinoma

EXPECTED COURSE/PROGNOSIS
• Infectious cervicitis usually responds to systemic antibiotics
• Chronic cervicitis may be resistant to treatment, and should be monitored closely for cervical dysplasia

MISCELLANEOUS

ASSOCIATED CONDITIONS
Patients with infectious cervicitis should be screened for other sexually transmitted diseases, syphilis, trichomonas, and possibly human immunodeficiency virus (HIV)

AGE-RELATED FACTORS
Pediatric: Infectious cervicitis in children should lead to investigation for possible sexual abuse
Geriatric:
• Chronic cervicitis in postmenopausal women may be related to lack of estrogen
• The possibility of infectious cervicitis should not be overlooked, as many geriatric patients remain sexually active
Others: Adolescents remain a high-risk group for sexually transmitted diseases

PREGNANCY
Screen all pregnant women for infectious cervicitis because of the risk of transmission to the fetus

SYNONYMS
Mucopurulent cervicitis

ICD-9-CM
616.0 cervicitis
098.15 acute gonococcal cervicitis
079.8 chlamydia infection

SEE ALSO
• Chlamydial sexually transmitted diseases
• Gonococcal infections
• Trichomoniasis
• Cervicitis, ectropion & true erosion
• Cervical dysplasia

OTHER NOTES
The presence of Trichomonas does not rule out other concurrent infection

ABBREVIATIONS
N/A

REFERENCES
• Sweet RL: The enigmatic cervix. Dermatologic Clinics 1998;16(4):739-745)
• MMWR 1998;47:53-69
• Clinical Chemistry 1996;42:809-812
• Danforth DN, Scott JR, eds: Obstetrics and Gynecology. 7th Ed. Philadelphia, Lippincott, 1994
• The Medical Letter, 1995;37:117-122
• Obstet Gynecol 1997;89:556-560
• Med Clin N Am 1995;79:1277-1280
Illustrations: N/A
Internet references: http://www.5mcc.com

Author(s)
Barbara A. Majeroni, MD

Cervicitis, ectropion & true erosion

BASICS

DESCRIPTION
• Cervicitis - inflammatory changes due to infections
• Ectropion - eversion of the cervix in pregnancy
• True erosion - abrupt loss of overlying vaginal epithelium due to trauma, e.g., forceful insertion of vaginal speculum in patient with atrophic mucosa

System(s) affected: Reproductive
Genetics: N/A
Incidence/Prevalence in USA:
• Cervicitis - very common in sexually active women
• Ectropion - with oral contraceptive use; very common in pregnant women
• True erosion - occasionally seen in postmenopausal women

Predominant Age: Sexually active women
Predominant Sex: Female only

SIGNS AND SYMPTOMS
• Cervicitis - metrorrhagia, post-coital bleeding, vaginal discharge
• Ectropion - red cervix due to color of the columnar epithelium
• True erosion - vaginal bleeding, sharply defined ulcers of cervix

CAUSES
• Cervicitis - Chlamydia trachomatis, Trichomonas vaginalis
• Ectropion - hormonal changes with oral contraceptive use (especially with progesterone) or during pregnancy,
• True erosion - injury to atrophic epithelium due to estrogen deficiency in menopause

RISK FACTORS
• Cervicitis - sexual contact with infected partner(s), recurrence due to inadequate therapy
• Ectropion - pregnancy
• True erosion - estrogen deficiency, trauma

DIAGNOSIS

DIFFERENTIAL DIAGNOSIS
• Cervical dysplasia
• Carcinoma of the cervix

LABORATORY
• Saline and potassium hydroxide preparation of cervical/vaginal smears
• Chlamydiazyme or chlamydia cell culture, gonorrhea culture
• Papanicolaou (Pap) smear of the cervix
• Chlamydia DNA probe

Drugs that may alter lab results: N/A
Disorders that may alter lab results: N/A

PATHOLOGICAL FINDINGS
• Cervicitis - acute and chronic inflammatory changes, presence of infective organisms
• Ectropion - none/squamous metaplasia
• True erosion - sharply defined ulcer borders, loss of epithelium

SPECIAL TESTS None

IMAGING None

DIAGNOSTIC PROCEDURES
Colposcopy

TREATMENT

APPROPRIATE HEALTH CARE
Outpatient

GENERAL MEASURES N/A

SURGICAL MEASURES N/A

ACTIVITY No restrictions

DIET No special diet

PATIENT EDUCATION Provide printed material about sexually transmitted diseases and about estrogen deficiency and estrogen replacement therapy

MEDICATIONS

DRUG(S) OF CHOICE
• Trichomoniasis - metronidazole 500 mg bid for 7 days or 2 g once or 1 g bid for 2 doses
• Chlamydial infection - for non-pregnant women, doxycycline 100 mg bid po for 7 days; for pregnant women, erythromycin base 500 mg qid po for 7 days, or erythromycin ethylsuccinate 800 mg qid for 7 days
• Ectropion - none
• True erosion - estrogen, conjugated vaginal cream daily for 2 weeks, follow by estrogen replacement therapy

Contraindications:
• Metronidazole - first trimester of pregnancy
• Doxycycline - pregnancy or lactation
• Estrogen - see extended list of contraindications to estrogen use in standard texts

Precautions:
• Metronidazole - possible fetal harm if used in first trimester of pregnancy, disulfiram reaction with alcohol
• Doxycycline - possible fetal harm if used during pregnancy, staining of the infant's teeth if used during breast-feeding, allergy, photosensitization
• Erythromycin - nausea or vomiting
• Estrogens - history of estrogen dependent neoplasms, history of thromboembolic diseases, see extended list of contraindications to estrogen therapy in standard texts

Significant possible interactions:
• Metronidazole and alcohol
• Doxycycline and dairy products, iron preparations, warfarin, and oral contraceptives (use backup contraceptive method)
• Erythromycin with terfenadine (Seldane) or astemizole - may increase latter's levels with subsequent ECG changes
• Erythromycin and theophylline (elevated theophylline level)
• Estrogen - N/A

ALTERNATIVE DRUGS
• Metronidazole - sulfanilamide-aminacrine-allantoin cream (AVC cream)
• Doxycycline - erythromycin or azithromycin
• Erythromycin - clindamycin
• Estrogen - lubricant, same as that used for vaginal speculum
• Azithromycin 1 g for one dose only (pregnancy category B)
• Ofloxacin 300 mg bid x 7 days
• Amoxicillin-clavulanate (Augmentin) 250 mg po q8h for 7 days

FOLLOWUP

PATIENT MONITORING
• Trichomoniasis - repeat vaginal smear until infection is cleared
• Chlamydial infection - repeat chlamydial culture post antibiotic therapy
• Estrogen deficiency - re-examine in one month to confirm healing

PREVENTION/AVOIDANCE
• Trichomoniasis or chlamydial infection - treatment of sexual partners and use of condom during coitus
• Estrogen deficiency - estrogen replacement therapy

POSSIBLE COMPLICATIONS N/A

EXPECTED COURSE/PROGNOSIS
• Cervicitis - excellent healing once infection is eradicated
• Ectropion - spontaneous regression postpartum, cessation or oral contraceptive use
• True erosion - spontaneous healing

MISCELLANEOUS

ASSOCIATED CONDITIONS
• Gonorrhea
• Bacterial vaginosis

AGE-RELATED FACTORS
Pediatric: N/A
Geriatric: Menopause
Others: N/A

PREGNANCY
• Ectropion
• Azithromycin should be used with caution
• Doxycycline should not be used in pregnancy

SYNONYMS N/A

ICD-9-CM
616.0 Cervicitis and endocervicitis

SEE ALSO N/A

OTHER NOTES N/A

ABBREVIATIONS N/A

REFERENCES
• Disaia PJ, Creasman WT: Clinical Gynecologic Oncology. 3rd Ed. St. Louis, The C.V. Mosby Company, 1989
• Herbst AL, Mishell DR, Stenchever MA, Droegemueller W: Comprehensive Gynecology. 2nd Ed. St. Louis, The C.V. Mosby Co., 1992
• Kurman RJ, ed: Blaustein's Pathology Of The Female Genital Tract. 3rd Ed. New York, Springer-Verlag, 1987
• Novak ER, Woodruff JD: Novak's Gynecologic and Obstetric Pathology With Clinical and Endocrine Relations. 8th Ed. Philadelphia, W.B. Saunders Company, 1979
• Lebhere TB: In: Hacker NF, Moore JG, eds. Essentials Obstetrics and Gynecology. 2nd Ed. Philadelphia, W.B. Saunders Co., 1992
Illustrations: N/A
Internet references: http://www.5mcc.com

Author(s)
Albert T. Shiu, MD, FACOG

Chancroid

BASICS

DESCRIPTION A sexually transmitted disease characterized by painful genital ulcerations and inflammatory inguinal adenopathy. It is uncommon in the United States but found worldwide. Chancroid is endemic in developing countries.
System(s) affected: Reproductive, Skin/Exocrine
Genetics: N/A
Incidence/Prevalence in USA:
Approximately 1,000 cases annually (1993, 1994, 1995 - CDC data). Actual numbers felt to be greater due to underreporting of cases.
Predominant age: Teenagers and adults
Predominant sex: Male > Female

SIGNS AND SYMPTOMS
• Tender genital papule that ulcerates after 24 hours
• Irregular edged, painful ulcer(s)
• Ulcers may be 1 mm to 5 cm in size
• Ulcers may occur on the shaft of the penis, glans and meatus in men
• Ulcers in women most commonly occur in labia majora but also seen in labia minora, perineum, thigh, and cervix
• Painful inguinal adenopathy with abscess (bubo) formation in 30% of patients
• Atypical presentations include folliculitis and foreskin abscess

CAUSES Haemophilus ducreyi (gram negative bacterium)

RISK FACTORS
• Multiple sexual partners
• Uncircumcised males
• Prostitutes often are carriers

DIAGNOSIS

DIFFERENTIAL DIAGNOSIS
• Syphilis
• Herpes Simplex Virus (HSV 1 and 2)
• Lymphogranuloma venereum (LGV)
• Granuloma inguinale

LABORATORY Serologic testing for antibody with ELISA technique. Gram stain; culture of organism on Mueller-Hinton agar with incorporated vancomycin. Polymerase chain reaction (PCR) where available.
Drugs that may alter lab results: Previous antibiotics
Disorders that may alter lab results:
None expected

PATHOLOGICAL FINDINGS "School of fish" pattern on gram stain

SPECIAL TESTS N/A

IMAGING N/A

DIAGNOSTIC PROCEDURES
• Gram stain and culture of ulcer exudate
• Aspiration of inguinal bubo (lymph node)
• Dark-field examinations of exudate to rule out Treponema pallidum

TREATMENT

APPROPRIATE HEALTH CARE
Outpatient treatment

GENERAL MEASURES
• Saline or Burow's solution soaks to ulcers
• Aspiration of buboes if greater than 5 cm

SURGICAL MEASURES N/A

ACTIVITY Refrain from sexual intercourse until genital lesions fully resolved

DIET N/A

PATIENT EDUCATION
• Sexual counseling
• Use of condoms
• Local wound care
• Treatment of all sexual partners with same regimen as index case

MEDICATIONS

DRUG(S) OF CHOICE
• Azithromycin 1 gm po single dose (more expensive than other treatments)
• Ceftriaxone 250 mg IM single dose
• Ciprofloxacin 500 mg po bid for 3 days or other quinolone
• Erythromycin base 500 mg qid x 7 days
Contraindications:
• Allergy to the medication
• Ciprofloxacin in pregnancy and lactation, and patients less than age 18
Precautions: Refer to manufacturer's profile of each drug
Significant possible interactions: Refer to manufacturer's profile of each drug

ALTERNATIVE DRUGS   N/A

FOLLOWUP

PATIENT MONITORING
• Patient followed until all clinical signs of infection resolved
• Should see symptomatic improvement within 3 days and objective improvement by day 7
• Baseline syphilis serology and at 3 months
• HIV testing at 3 months post-treatment

PREVENTION/AVOIDANCE   Avoidance of sexual activity until ulcers resolved

POSSIBLE COMPLICATIONS
• Phimosis
• Balanoposthitis
• Rupture of buboes with fistula formation and scarring

EXPECTED COURSE/PROGNOSIS
• Full clinical resolution with appropriate treatment
• 5% relapse after treatment
• Primary infection is not believed to provide immunity

MISCELLANEOUS

ASSOCIATED CONDITIONS
• Syphilis - concurrently in 10% of patients (per new CDC data)
• HSV or HIV infection

AGE-RELATED FACTORS   N/A
Pediatric: N/A
Geriatric: N/A
Others: HIV disease may affect treatment response

PREGNANCY   Maternal to infant transmission has not been reported

SYNONYMS
• Soft chancre
• Ulcus molle

ICD-9-CM
099.O Chancroid

SEE ALSO
• Syphilis

OTHER NOTES   Chancroid has been shown to be an established risk factor for acquisition of HIV infection

ABBREVIATIONS   N/A

REFERENCES
• U.S. Department of Health and Human Services, Centers for Disease Control and Prevention: Sexually transmitted diseases treatment guideline. Morbidity and Mortality Weekly Report. MMWR 1998;47(RR-1):1-115
• Schulte JM, Schmid G: Recommendations for treatment of chancroid. Clin Infect Dis 1995;20(Suppl 1):539-546
• Trees DL, Morse SA: Chancroid and haemophilus ducreyi: an update. Clin Microbiol Rev 1995;8(3):357-375
Illustrations: N/A
Internet references: http://www.5mcc.com

Author(s)
Jeffery T. Kirchner, DO, FAAFP

Chickenpox

BASICS

DESCRIPTION A common, highly contagious, childhood exanthem characterized by the development of typical crops of vesicles on the skin and mucous membranes.
• The virus is spread by respiratory droplets or direct contact with vesicles or indirectly through freshly soiled articles
• Outbreaks tend to occur from January to May
• The usual incubation period is 14-16 days (range 11-21). Patients are infectious from 24 hours before appearance of the rash until the final lesions have crusted. Most people acquire chickenpox during childhood and develop long immunity.
System(s) affected: Skin/Exocrine, Nervous
Genetics: No known genetic pattern
Incidence/Prevalence in USA: Common
Predominant age: Peak incidence 5-9 years, but may occur at any age
Predominant Sex: Male = Female

SIGNS AND SYMPTOMS
• Prodromal symptoms - fever, malaise, anorexia, mild headache
• Characteristic rash - crops of "teardrop" vesicles on erythematous bases
• Lesions erupt in successive crops
• Progress from macule to papule to vesicle, then begin to crust
• Rash present in various stages of development
• Pruritic
• Usually begins on trunk, then spreads to face and scalp
• Minimal involvement of the extremities
• Lesions may be present on mucous membranes, oral and vaginal

CAUSES
• Human (alpha) herpesvirus 3 (varicella-zoster virus, V-Z virus), a member of the Herpesvirus group; a double-stranded DNA virus. (Reservoir: humans.)

RISK FACTORS
• No prior history of varicella
• Immunosuppressed (especially children with leukemia/lymphoma in remission or on high-dose corticosteroids)

DIAGNOSIS

DIFFERENTIAL DIAGNOSIS
• Herpes simplex
• Herpes zoster
• Impetigo
• Coxsackievirus infection
• Papular urticaria
• Scabies
• Dermatitis herpetiformis
• Drug rash
• Rickettsialpox

LABORATORY
• Leukocyte count may be normal, low, or mildly increased
• Marked leukocytosis is suggestive of secondary infection
• Multinucleated giant cells on Tzanck smear from scrapings of vesicles
• Isolated virus from human tissue culture
Drugs that may alter lab results: N/A
Disorders that may alter lab results:
• Herpes zoster
• Herpes simplex

PATHOLOGICAL FINDINGS
• Skin lesions histologically identical to herpes simplex virus
• In fatal cases intranuclear inclusions can be found in the endothelium of blood vessels and most organs

SPECIAL TESTS
For complicated cases and epidemiologic studies:
• Visualization of the virus by EM
• Serologic testing by FAMA or ELISA
• Detection of viral DNA by PCR

IMAGING N/A

DIAGNOSTIC PROCEDURES N/A

TREATMENT

APPROPRIATE HEALTH CARE
Outpatient except for complicating emergencies

GENERAL MEASURES
• Supportive/symptomatic treatment
• Good hygiene to avoid secondary infection

SURGICAL MEASURES N/A

ACTIVITY As tolerated. Children may return to school when lesions have scabbed over, temperature is normal and sense of well-being has returned.

DIET No special diet

PATIENT EDUCATION Griffith: Instructions for Patients; Philadelphia, 1994, W.B. Saunders Co.

MEDICATIONS

DRUG(S) OF CHOICE
• Antipyretics for fever
• Avoid aspirin because of its link to Reye's syndrome
• Local and/or systemic antipruritic agents for itching
• In immunocompromised host, then varicella-zoster immune globulin (VZIG) available for passive immunization. VZIG must be given within 96 hours after exposure to be beneficial. After 4th day postexposure, wait for rash to develop then give acyclovir 500 mg/m2/day intravenously every 8 hours for 7 days.
• Acyclovir - decreases duration of fever and shortens time of viral shedding. Recommended for adolescents, adults and high-risk patients. Most beneficial if initiated early in the disease ($\leq$ 24 hours).
◊ 2-16 yr: 20 mg/kg/dose (max. 800 mg/dose), qid for 5 days
◊ Adults: 800 mg, 5 times daily.
Contraindications: Hypersensitivity to the drug
Precautions: Possible renal insufficiency with acyclovir
Significant possible interactions: Concurrent administration of probenecid increases half-life. Increased effect with zidovudine (drowsiness, lethargy)

ALTERNATIVE DRUGS
• Famciclovir
• Valacyclovir
• Vidarabine
• Interferon

FOLLOWUP

PATIENT MONITORING
Usually none in mild cases. If complications occur, intensive supportive care may be required.

PREVENTION/AVOIDANCE
• Exposed, susceptible individuals considered infectious for 21 days
• Isolation of hospitalized patients
• Passive immunization with ZIG, VZIG, or the intravenous formulation of ZIP. Both ZIG and VZIG should be given within 96 hours (preferably within 72 hours) of exposure to ensure efficacy. ZIP can be given somewhat later. Recommended for persons exposed to chickenpox or shingles within 96 hours who are immunocompromised, $\geq$15 years old without prior history of chickenpox, newborns of mothers with onset of chickenpox < 5 days before delivery or < 2 days after delivery. Exposure criteria: continued household contact, prolonged face-to-face contact (same room), or indoor playmate > 1 hour.

• Varicella-Virus vaccine (Varivax) - a live attenuated vaccine approved by the FDA and recommended by ACIP for immunization of healthy individuals, 12 months and above, who have not had chickenpox. Duration of immunity is unknown
◊ 12m-12y: single dose 0.5 mL SC. Cumulative efficacy 70-90%
◊ 13y and above: two 0.5 mL SC doses 4-8 weeks apart. Efficacy 70%.
◊ Has been shown to prevent or significantly reduce the severity of varicella if given within 72 hours and possibly up to 5 days, postexposure in several studies.
◊ Maybe considered for a subset of HIV positive children in CDC Class I with CD4 > 25%
• Vaccine recipients should avoid contact with immunocompromised people, and pregnant women who have never had chickenpox and their newborns, for up to 6 weeks after vaccination

POSSIBLE COMPLICATIONS
• Secondary bacterial infection - cellulitis, abscess, erysipelas, sepsis, septic arthritis/osteomyelitis, staphylococcal pyomyositis
• Pneumonia (20-30% of adults with chickenpox have lung involvement)
• Encephalitis (the most common CNS complication)
• Reye's syndrome
• Purpura
• Lymphadenitis
• Nephritis

EXPECTED COURSE/PROGNOSIS
• In the healthy child, chickenpox is rarely a serious disease and recovery is complete
• Confers long immunity
• Second attack rare, but subclinical infection common
• Infection latent and may recur years later as herpes zoster in adults (and sometimes in children)
• Fatalities rarely occur from complications

MISCELLANEOUS

ASSOCIATED CONDITIONS
N/A

AGE-RELATED FACTORS
Pediatric:
• Neonates born to mothers who develop chickenpox 5 days before or 2 days after delivery are at risk for serious disease. Must give VZIG.
• Varicella bullosa seen mainly in children under two. Lesions appear as bullae instead of vesicles. Clinical course unchanged.
• Case-fatality (in USA) 2/100,000
• Most common cause of death: septic complications and encephalitis

Geriatric:
• Infection more severe than in children
• Latent varicella infection may reactivate and cause the exanthem shingles or zoster
• Case-fatality 30/100,000
• Most common cause of death: primary viral pneumonia
Others: N/A

PREGNANCY
Risk of transplacental infection following maternal infection is 25%. Congenital malformations are seen in 5% when the fetus is infected during the 1st or 2nd trimester. There is an increased morbidity for women infected during pregnancy (e.g., pneumonia)

SYNONYMS
• Varicella

ICD-9-CM
052.9 Varicella without mention of complication

SEE ALSO
• Immunizations
• Herpes Zoster

OTHER NOTES
N/A

ABBREVIATIONS
ACIP = Advisory Committee on Immunization Practices
FAMA = flourescent antibody to membrane antigen
ZIG = zoster immune globulin
ZIP = zoster immune plasma
DNA = deoxyribonucleic acid
EM = electron microscopy
PCR = polymerase chain reaction
VZIG = varicella-zoster immune globulin

REFERENCES
• Mandell GL, ed: Principles and Practice of Infectious Diseases. 4th Ed. New York, Churchill Livingstone, 1995
• Benenson, AS, ed: Control of Communicable Diseases Manual. 16th ed. Baltimore, United Book Press, Inc, 1995.
• Fauci AS, ed: Harrison's Principles of Internal medicine. 14th ed. New York, McGraw-Hill, 1998
Illustrations: 6 available on CD-ROM
Internet references: http://www.5mcc.com

Author(s)
Vicente J. Arano, MD

Child abuse

BASICS

DESCRIPTION
• Emotional abuse: sustained, repetitive, inappropriate emotional response to the child's experience of emotion and its accompanying expressive behavior
• Psychological abuse: sustained, repetitive, inappropriate behavior which damages or substantially reduces the creative and developmental potential of crucially important mental faculties and mental processes of a child
• Physical abuse: injury to a child caused by a caretaker for no apparent reason including reaction to unwanted behavior. The use of an instrument on any part of the body is abuse, i.e., belt.
• Sexual abuse: any contact or interaction between a child and another person in which the child is sexually exploited for the gratification or profit of the perpetrator. Offenders can be juveniles.
• Neglect: occurs when those responsible for meeting the basic needs of a child fail to do so, either acute or chronic
System(s) affected: Nervous, Reproductive, Endocrine/Metabolic, Musculoskeletal, Gastrointestinal, Skin/Exocrine
Genetics: N/A
Incidence/Prevalence in USA: More than 1 million per year; extremely difficult to estimate
Predominant age: 7 years old
Predominant sex: Male = Female

SIGNS AND SYMPTOMS
• Non-specific symptoms of abuse
  ◊ Behavior regression
  ◊ Anxiety, depression
  ◊ Sleep disturbances, night terrors
  ◊ Increased sex play
  ◊ School problems
  ◊ Self-destructive behaviors
• Physical abuse
  ◊ May be no physical signs
  ◊ Skin markings (lacerations, burns, ecchymoses, linear contusions)
  ◊ Contusions with definite shapes (coat hangers, belt buckles)
  ◊ Circular contusions on trunks or limbs (finger pressure points)
  ◊ Bites
  ◊ Cigarette burns on palms, extremities
  ◊ Immersion injuries with clearly demarcated lines
  ◊ Oral trauma (torn frenulum, loose teeth)
  ◊ Ear trauma (ear pulling)
  ◊ Eye trauma (hyphema, hemorrhage)
  ◊ Abdominal blunt trauma
  ◊ Fractures
  ◊ Head trauma
• Sexual abuse
  ◊ Unequivocal abnormalities are found in a small number of children (2-8%)
  ◊ Abuse often consists of fondling, rubbing and other contacts not likely to produce detectable injuries
  ◊ Unexplained vaginal injuries or bleeding
  ◊ Pregnancy
  ◊ Sexually transmitted diseases
  ◊ Sexual promiscuity/prostitution
  ◊ Erythema and increased vascularity of the perihymenal tissues
  ◊ Increased friability of the posterior fourchette
  ◊ Hymenal attenuation and asymmetry, lacerations, especially if hymenal margin is altered
  ◊ Perianal lacerations, scars and fissures, circumferential edema (Tyre sign), delta-shaped abrasion
  ◊ May be no physical signs
• Neglect
  ◊ May be small, scrawny, dirty, with rashes
  ◊ Fearful or too trusting
  ◊ Clinging to or avoiding mother
  ◊ Flat or balding occiput
  ◊ Abnormal development or growth parameters

CAUSES   Not well-defined

RISK FACTORS   May be many, but poverty (5 times greater risk), parental substance abuse, lower educational status, maternal history of abuse and negative maternal attitude toward pregnancy appear to be strongly associated, history of parent(s) having been abused, mentally ill parent, parental isolation, presence of domestic violence

DIAGNOSIS

DIFFERENTIAL DIAGNOSIS
• Physical trauma
  ◊ Accidental injury
  ◊ Bleeding disorders (e.g., classic hemophilia)
  ◊ Metabolic diseases (e.g., vitamin K deficiency)
  ◊ Congenital (type I Ehlers-Danlos syndrome)
  ◊ Salicylate toxicity
  ◊ Conditions with skin manifestations: Mongolian spots, Schönlein-Henoch purpura, purpura fulminans of meningococcemia, erythema multiforme, hypersensitivity vasculitis, platelet aggregation disorders, disseminated intravascular coagulation (DIC), phytophotodermatitis, car seat burns, staphylococcal scalded skin syndrome, chicken pox, impetigo, osteogenesis imperfecta, congenital syphilis
• Neglect
  ◊ Endocrinopathies (e.g., diabetes mellitus, diabetes insipidus, thyroid disorders, adrenal problems, pituitary problems)
  ◊ Constitutional
  ◊ GI (clefts, chalasia, gastroesophageal reflux, celiac disease, inflammatory bowel disease)
  ◊ Cystic fibrosis
  ◊ Liver disease
  ◊ Renal tubular acidosis
  ◊ CNS abnormalities
• Skeletal trauma
  ◊ Obstetrical trauma
  ◊ Prematurity
  ◊ Nutritional - metabolic defects (scurvy, rickets, mucolipidosis II, secondary hyperparathyroidism)
  ◊ Infection (congenital syphilis, osteomyelitis)
  ◊ Osteogenesis imperfecta
  ◊ Infantile cortical hyperostosis
  ◊ Leukemia
  ◊ Histiocytosis X
  ◊ Metastatic neuroblastoma

LABORATORY
• Urinalysis, urine culture and sensitivity
• CBC
• Electrolytes, creatinine, BUN, glucose
• May add PT, PTT, bleeding time, platelet count, factor XIII, urine toxicology screen
Drugs that may alter lab results: N/A
Disorders that may alter lab results: See Differential Diagnosis

PATHOLOGICAL FINDINGS
• Spiral fractures in non-ambulatory patients
• Chip fractures or bucket-handle fractures (classic for abuse)
• Epiphyseal - metaphyseal rib fractures in infants
• Rupture of liver and spleen in abdominal blunt trauma
• Retinal hemorrhages in shaken baby syndrome
• Abnormalities strongly suggesting sexual abuse include: Recent or healed lacerations of the hymen and vaginal mucosa, procto-episiotomy, bite marks
• The presence of sperm is a definitive finding of child abuse

SPECIAL TESTS
• Sexual abuse
  ◊ Wet mount for motile sperm and one fixed for cytopathology exam for sperm
  ◊ Tests for gonorrhea, chlamydia
  ◊ Serum pregnancy tests
  ◊ Rapid plasma reagin (RPR)
  ◊ Consider HIV testing (repeat in 6 months)
  ◊ Acid phosphatase test of secretions for sperm
  ◊ If the assault occurred within 72 hours of the examination, samples should be collected for the forensic laboratory (contact police investigator for proper protocol)
• Neglect
  ◊ Stool exam
  ◊ Calorie count
  ◊ Purified protein derivative (PPD) and anergy panel
  ◊ Sweat test
  ◊ Lead and zinc protoporphyrin levels

IMAGING
• Photographs
• Chest x-ray, skeletal survey (skull frontal and lateral, lateral thoracolumbar spine, frontal upper extremities to include shoulder girdle and hands, frontal lower extremities to include lower lumbar spine, pelvis and feet)
• In some hospitals a standard set of x-rays called a SNAT (suspected non-accidental trauma) series is defined
• Possible bone scan

DIAGNOSTIC PROCEDURES   Consider photocolposcopy in sexual abuse

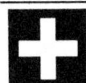

TREATMENT

APPROPRIATE HEALTH CARE
• Acute episodes, especially of sexual abuse, are often best managed in an emergency room equipped for collecting forensic specimens and maintaining "chain of evidence"
• Hospital admission for children with moderate to severe injuries, unstable neurologic or cardiovascular exams and those with acute psychological trauma
• If not hospitalized, a child should be sent to another relative or arrange for foster care if the suspected abuser lives with the child
• Counseling is imperative
• Mandatory reporting to Child Protective Authorities
• Counseling for entire family

GENERAL MEASURES
• After initial evaluation, consider referral to sexual assault center
• Always explain what the physical exam will involve and why certain procedures are necessary
• Examine child in a quiet, comfortable setting and allow child to choose who will be in the room
• To examine female genitalia, use dorsolithotomy position for older girls and the "frog leg" position for younger girls
• Examine anus of all young children in prone knee-chest position

SURGICAL MEASURES   As clinically indicated

ACTIVITY   As clinically indicated

DIET   As clinically indicated

PATIENT EDUCATION   Counsel family not to use negative terms such as "ruined," "violated," or "dirty" in reference to the child. The child's emotional reaction to abuse will be profoundly influenced by the responses of adult caretakers.

MEDICATIONS

DRUG(S) OF CHOICE   Antibiotics as indicated for treatment of documented sexually-transmitted disease
Contraindications: Refer to manufacturer's profile of each drug
Precautions: Refer to manufacturer's profile of each drug
Significant possible interactions: Refer to manufacturer's profile of each drug

ALTERNATIVE DRUGS   Other postcoital contraceptive drugs

FOLLOWUP

PATIENT MONITORING   Patient must be referred to the appropriate state protective services and followed as closely as clinically and psychologically indicated

PREVENTION/AVOIDANCE   Early detection of and intervention in dysfunctional families whenever possible

POSSIBLE COMPLICATIONS   Long-term physical and psychological damage

EXPECTED COURSE/PROGNOSIS
Without intervention, child abuse is a recurrent and escalating phenomenon

MISCELLANEOUS

ASSOCIATED CONDITIONS
• Failure-to-thrive
• Shortfalls in development
• Poor school performance
• Poor social skills
• Psychological illnesses

AGE-RELATED FACTORS
Pediatric: N/A
Geriatric: N/A
Others: N/A

PREGNANCY   Use of ethinyl estradiol and norgestrel (Ovral) reduces rate of pregnancy after rape to under 2% which is one-third the rate that would be expected without intervention. It is thought to work by making the uterine lining inhospitable to implantation and must be considered an abortifacient in this setting.

SYNONYMS
• Battered child syndrome
• SNAT

ICD-9-CM
995.50 Child abuse, unspecified

SEE ALSO   N/A

OTHER NOTES   When documenting an examination on an allegedly or suspected abused child, especially in cases of possible sexual abuse, never record "findings not consistent with abuse" or "no evidence of abuse." Simply record findings and note that the findings neither exclude nor confirm allegations of abuse. The absence of physical findings does not indicate the child's history is incorrect.

ABBREVIATIONS
SNAT = suspected non-accidental trauma

REFERENCES
• Reece RM, ed: Pediatric Clinics of North America, Vol 37, No. 4. Philadelphia, W.B. Saunders Co, August 1990
• Rosenstein BJ, Fosarelli PD: Pediatric Pearls. Yearbook Medical Publishers, Inc, 1989:330-334
• Flaherty EG, Weiss H: Medical Evaluation of Abused and Neglected Children. American Journal of Diseases of Children 1990;144
• Muram D: Child Sexual Abuse. Obstetrics and Gynecology Clinics of North America 1992;19(1)
• Child Abuse and Neglect Statistical Fact Sheet. National Clearinghouse on Child Abuse Information, 1996
• Gibbons M, Vincent EC: Childhood Sexual Abuse. Amer Fam Phys 1994;49:125-136
• O'Hagan KP: Emotional and psychological abuse: Problems of definition. Child Abuse and Neglect 1995;19:4
Illustrations: 3 available on CD-ROM
Internet references: http://www.5mcc.com

Author(s)
Sumner T. McAllister, MD
Bruce T. Vanderhoff, MD

Chlamydia pneumoniae

BASICS

DESCRIPTION Chlamydia pneumoniae, an obligate intracellular bacteria, has been established as an important cause of adult respiratory disease including pneumonia, bronchitis, sinusitis and pharyngitis. There is no animal reservoir.
System(s) affected: Pulmonary
Genetics: No known genetic predisposition
Incidence/Prevalence in USA: Estimated incidence of 100 to 200 cases of pneumonia/100,000/year. Accounts for 6 to 12% of pneumonias and 3 to 6% of bronchitis cases. Studies to date have included relatively few geographic areas. Numbers do not necessarily apply to all areas. Incidence of subclinical infection much greater.
Predominant age: Uncommon in children under 5 years. Pneumonia more common in elderly.
Predominant sex: Male > Female (10-25% more)

SIGNS AND SYMPTOMS
• 70% to 90% of infections are mild or subclinical
• Onset often gradual with delayed presentation
• Sore throat and hoarseness may precede cough by a week or more, giving biphasic appearance to illness
• Cough (often prominent with scant sputum)
• Fever (usually early in illness)
• Sore throat
• Rhinitis
• Headache
• Malaise
• Hoarseness
• Sinus congestion
• Rales, rhonchi or wheezing
• Pharyngeal erythema
• Sinus tenderness

CAUSES Infection with C. pneumoniae

RISK FACTORS Outbreaks have occurred among groups of military recruits, university students, students and nursing home residents. Incubation period is approximately 30 days. Sporadic cases often have no apparent source of exposure. No known animal hosts.

DIAGNOSIS

DIFFERENTIAL DIAGNOSIS Consider other common bacterial respiratory pathogens, including Streptococcus, Bordetella, Hemophilus, Klebsiella, Mycoplasma and Legionella species

LABORATORY
• Leukocyte count usually normal or low
• Sedimentation rate often moderately elevated
• Sputum usually negative by gram stain and routine culture
Drugs that may alter lab results: Early treatment with tetracycline may blunt IgG antibody response
Disorders that may alter lab results: None known

PATHOLOGICAL FINDINGS Not usually available

SPECIAL TESTS
• Most easily cultured in HL or HEp2 cells
• Complement fixation (CF) serology for Chlamydia widely available but cannot distinguish C. pneumoniae infection from C. psittaci
• Microimmunofluorescence (MIF) test, which is specific for C. pneumoniae, is available at some research institutions or commercially (from American Medical Laboratories, MRL Diagnostics)
• Every effort should be made to obtain paired sera. The convalescent sera should be obtained 3 weeks after disease onset.
• Four-fold antibody rise diagnostic of acute infection
• Presence of IgM antibody ($\geq$ 1:16) or of high IgG antibody titers ($\geq$ 1:512) by MIF suggests a recent or acute infection
• Polymerase chain reaction (PCR) from pharyngeal swab or bronchoalveolar lavage specimen

IMAGING
• Chest radiograph may be abnormal even in clinically mild disease
• Variable radiographic abnormalities include unilateral and bilateral infiltrates and pleural effusions. Single, subsegmental infiltrate is common.

DIAGNOSTIC PROCEDURES Definite diagnosis requires positive serology or culture

TREATMENT

APPROPRIATE HEALTH CARE
• Usually outpatient
• Patients with severe pneumonia or coexisting illness may require hospitalization

GENERAL MEASURES No specific general measures

SURGICAL MEASURES N/A

ACTIVITY Usually reduced during illness

DIET No special diet

PATIENT EDUCATION
• Griffith HW: Instructions for Patients; Philadelphia, W.B. Saunders Co.
• For a listing of sources for patient education materials favorably reviewed on this topic, physicians may contact: American Academy of Family Physicians Foundation, P.O. Box 8418, Kansas City, MO 64114, (800)274-2237, ext. 4400

Chlamydia pneumoniae

MEDICATIONS

DRUG(S) OF CHOICE
• Azithromycin (Zithromax) 500 mg on day 1, then 250 mg a day on days 2 through 5
or
• Clarithromycin (Biaxin) 500 mg po every 12 hours for 10-14 days
or
• Tetracycline 500 mg po qid for at least 14 days
or
• Doxycycline 100 mg po q 12 hours for at least 14 days

Contraindications:
• Tetracycline not for use in pregnancy or children < 8 years.

Precautions: Tetracycline may cause photosensitivity; sunscreen recommended.

Significant possible interactions:
• Tetracyclines may increase the anticoagulant effect of warfarin
• Broad-spectrum antibiotics may reduce the effectiveness of oral contraceptives; barrier method recommended.

ALTERNATIVE DRUGS
• Erythromycin base 250-500 mg qid for 14-21 days
• Beta-lactam (penicillin based) antibiotics and sulfisoxazole not effective

FOLLOWUP

PATIENT MONITORING
Weekly until well, for response to treatment and resolution of radiographic abnormalities

PREVENTION/AVOIDANCE
• Transmission presumably via respiratory secretions. Avoid infected persons.
• Hand washing

POSSIBLE COMPLICATIONS
• Reactive airway disease
• Erythema nodosum
• Otitis media
• Endocarditis
• Myocarditis
• Pericarditis
• Sarcoidosis
• Meningitis
• Reactive arthritis
• Mild bacterial infection
• Associated with atherosclerotic disease (causal relationship is unknown)

EXPECTED COURSE/PROGNOSIS
• Resolution of cough and malaise often requires several weeks or longer
• Chronic bronchospastic disease has been reported following acute infection
• Persistent or relapsed symptoms may respond to second course of antibiotics

MISCELLANEOUS

ASSOCIATED CONDITIONS
• Chronic obstructive pulmonary disease
• HIV infection
• Cystic fibrosis

AGE-RELATED FACTORS
Pediatric: Usually milder disease in children
Geriatric: Usually more severe in older adults
Others: None known

PREGNANCY
• No known special risks
• Tetracyclines contraindicated

SYNONYMS
• TWAR

ICD-9-CM
078.89 Chlamydia pneumoniae

SEE ALSO
• Pneumonia, Mycoplasma
• Psittacosis

OTHER NOTES
• No significant seasonal variation
• Most cases occur sporadically, though intrafamilial spread also occurs
• Infection in debilitated or hospitalized patients can be severe
• Reinfection is possible
• Individuals have been reported who are persistently culture positive despite antibiotic treatment
• Country-wide epidemics of C. pneumoniae infections have been documented in the Scandinavian countries
• Found in atherosclerotic plaque in coronary arteries, carotid arteries and the aorta. Also associated with MI and stroke in seroepidemiologic studies. Role in atherogenesis in humans not established. Clinical significance not known.

ABBREVIATIONS   N/A

REFERENCES
• Kauppinen M, Saikku P: Pneumonia due to Chlamydia pneumoniae: prevalence, clinical features, diagnosis and treatment. Clin Infect Dis 1995;21:s244-252
• Grayston JT: Chlamydia pneumoniae (TWAR). In: Mandel GI, Bennett JE, Dolin R (eds): Principles and Practices of Infectious Disease. 4th ed. New York, Churchill Livingstone, 1995:1696-1701
Illustrations: N/A
Internet references: http://www.5mcc.com

Author(s)
David H. Thom, MD, PhD
J. Thomas Grayston, MD

Chlamydial sexually transmitted diseases

BASICS

DESCRIPTION The most common STD in USA is caused by Chlamydia trachomatis serovars D-K. Among the smallest prokaryotic organisms, these obligate intracellular, membrane bound organisms cause disease that is often asymptomatic to non-specific in presentation. It is difficult to diagnose both clinically, in the lab, and difficult to provide screening. The infection has serious sequelae and its transmission is difficult to control.

System(s) affected: Reproductive
Genetics: Unknown
Incidence/Prevalence in USA:
• Males 3-5% general medical population, 15-20% STD clinics
• Females 3-5% general medical population, 20% STD clinics
Predominant age: 15-25
Predominant sex: Male = Female

SIGNS AND SYMPTOMS The majority of women infected with Chlamydia trachomatis are asymptomatic, historical variables are typically not predictive of risk. Chlamydia trachomatis has a tropism for columnar or transitional epithelium with subsequent extension to the cervix, uterus, fallopian tubes and peritoneum in females, and epididymis in males, as well as rectal epithelial cells.
• Males
  ◊ Urethritis
  ◊ Epididymitis
  ◊ Proctitis
  ◊ Reiter's syndrome
• Females
  ◊ Cervicitis - typically mucopurulent
  ◊ Urethral syndrome
  ◊ Bartholinitis
  ◊ Endometritis
  ◊ Salpingitis/pelvic inflammatory disease (PID)
  ◊ Fitz-Hugh-Curtis perihepatitis syndrome
• Infants
  ◊ Conjunctivitis
  ◊ Pneumonitis
  ◊ Carriage-pharynx/GI tract

CAUSES Chlamydia trachomatis serovars D-K

RISK FACTORS
• Sexual promiscuity
• Lower socioeconomic groups
• Prevalence correlates inversely with age

DIAGNOSIS

DIFFERENTIAL DIAGNOSIS
• Neisseria gonorrhea
  ◊ Urethritis
  ◊ Proctitis
  ◊ Epididymitis
  ◊ Cervicitis
  ◊ PID
  ◊ Bartholin's abscess
  ◊ Perihepatitis
• Ureaplasma urealyticum
  ◊ Urethritis, epididymitis
  ◊ Reiter's disease
  ◊ PID
• Chlamydia trachomatis (Serovars LI-3)
  ◊ Lymphogranuloma venereum
  ◊ Proctitis

LABORATORY
• Chlamydial culture - costly, requires 3-7 days, 70-90% sensitive
• Antigen detection - sensitivity 50-90+%
• Monoclonal antibody direct immunofluorescence, requires experienced lab technician
• ELISA determination of eluded chlamydial antigens
Drugs that may alter lab results: N/A
Disorders that may alter lab results: N/A

PATHOLOGICAL FINDINGS N/A

SPECIAL TESTS Polymerase chain reaction test is available. Highly sensitive and specific.

IMAGING N/A

DIAGNOSTIC PROCEDURES
• Specimen collection: cell scrapings (obtain with cytology brush) rather than inflammatory discharge will improve yield since this is an epithelial cell disease
• Transport media is imperative: sucrose-phosphate media supplemented with gentamicin, vancomycin, and nystatin

TREATMENT

APPROPRIATE HEALTH CARE
Outpatient care for virtually all problems

GENERAL MEASURES
• All patients should be evaluated for syphilis and gonorrhea by appropriate Gram stains, cultures and serology.
• Empirical therapies may be indicated
• Offer HIV counseling and testing
• Evaluation and treatment of sex partners - institute empirical treatment of women who are sex partners of men with non-gonococcal urethritis is recommended. Partners of women with mucopurulent cervicitis or salpingitis should also be empirically treated. Since Chlamydial co-infection occurs with gonorrheal disease, anti-chlamydial therapy should be instituted concomitantly.

SURGICAL MEASURES N/A

ACTIVITY Sexual abstention pending elucidation and treatment of underlying infection

DIET N/A

PATIENT EDUCATION
• Risk-reduction counseling
• Safe sex practices, such as barrier protection
• Serious sequelae of Chlamydial disease i.e., tubal infertility
• Stress need to finish entire course of antibiotics
• For a listing of sources for patient education materials favorably reviewed on this topic, physicians may contact: American Academy of Family Physicians Foundation, P.O. Box 8418, Kansas City, MO 64114, (800)274-2237, ext. 4400

MEDICATIONS

DRUG(S) OF CHOICE
• Urethritis, cervicitis, sexual partners of infected persons
◊ Doxycycline - 100 mg po bid x 7 days
◊ Azithromycin - 1 gm orally in a single dose
◊ Pregnant women - erythromycin base, 250 mg po qid x 14 days
• Chlamydial syndromes.
◊ Epididymitis - tetracycline, doxycycline, erythromycin for 10-14 days as above.
◊ Pelvic inflammatory disease - doxycycline for 10-14 days to cover the chlamydial component of PID (gonorrhea and anaerobic organisms must be treated as well; see CDC recommendations: ceftriaxone 250 mg IM once, cefoxitin, other 3rd generation cephalosporin, or a quinolone), erythromycin for 10-14 days may be needed in pregnant or tetracycline intolerant females to treat chlamydial component.
Contraindications:
• Tetracycline: not for use in pregnancy or children < 8 years.
Precautions:
• Tetracycline: may cause photosensitivity; sunscreen recommended.
Significant possible interactions:
• Tetracycline: avoid concurrent administration with antacids, dairy products, or iron.
• Broad-spectrum antibiotics: may reduce the effectiveness of oral contraceptives; barrier method recommended.
• Erythromycin: terfenadine (Seldane); ECG abnormalities

ALTERNATIVE DRUGS
• Erythromycin base - 500 po qid x 7 days
• Ofloxacin - 300 mg po bid x 7 days (contraindicated in pregnancy)

FOLLOWUP

PATIENT MONITORING
• Test of cure is not routine, although it is reasonable to retest women weeks to months after treatment
• Sexual partners need to be evaluated and treated empirically if necessary, to prevent passing the disease back and forth between partners. Partnerships with community health departments should be fostered.
• Non-resolution or recurrence of symptoms must be immediately reported to the physician
• Severe cases of urethritis/cervicitis as well as the chlamydial syndromes should be seen in followup after completion of therapy
• Up to 25% of asymptomatic patients screened for chlamydia may not return for treatment post-chlamydia culture results. Strategies must be developed to insure treatment can be instituted.

PREVENTION/AVOIDANCE
Target populations, where prevalence of disease is > 5%, that should be screened for Chlamydia trachomatis:
• Women with mucopurulent cervicitis
• Sexually active women < 20 years of age
• Women 20-24 years of age who meet either of the following criteria or women > 24 years of age who meet both criteria:
◊ Inconsistent use of barrier contraception
◊ New or more than one sex partner during the prior 3 months
• Patients attending the following clinics:
◊ Adolescent clinics and family planning clinics - all adolescents < 25 years of age
◊ STD clinics
◊ Abortion clinics
◊ Detention center clinics
◊ Prenatal clinics - third trimester testing so that treatment can be administered predelivery
• Women and men with anorectal pain, tenesmus, rectal discharge
• Men with testicular pain with or without urethral discharge

POSSIBLE COMPLICATIONS
Enhances transmission of HIV
• Males
◊ Transient oligospermia
◊ Post epididymitis urethral stricture (rare)
• Females
◊ Tubal infertility
◊ Tubal pregnancy
◊ Chronic pelvic pain

EXPECTED COURSE/PROGNOSIS
Prognosis good with early and compliant therapy. However, due to the asymptomatic nature of early disease and the population affected, symptomatic PID still accounts annually for 2.5 million outpatient visits and more than one quarter million hospitalizations.

MISCELLANEOUS

ASSOCIATED CONDITIONS
• Pelvic inflammatory disease, epididymitis, cervicitis, urethritis
• Other diseases caused by other chlamydial species:
◊ Psittacosis - Chlamydia psittaci
◊ Pneumonia - Chlamydia pneumoniae - Chlamydia trachomatis (infants)
◊ Lymphogranuloma venereum - Chlamydia trachomatis serovars L1-L3
◊ Trachoma - Chlamydia trachomatis serovars A-C

AGE-RELATED FACTORS
Pediatric: N/A
Geriatric: N/A
Others: Prevalence inversely proportional to age after onset of sexual activity

PREGNANCY
Perinatal acquisition may result in neonatal pneumonia and/or conjunctivitis. Tetracycline and ofloxacin contraindicated in pregnancy. Erythromycin should be used in this situation.

SYNONYMS N/A

ICD-9-CM
615 Inflammatory diseases of uterus, except cervix
616 Inflammatory diseases of cervix, vagina, and vulva

SEE ALSO
• Pelvic inflammatory disease (PID)
• Epididymitis
• Cervicitis
• Urethritis
• HIV infection & AIDS
• Gonococcal infections
• Syphilis

OTHER NOTES N/A

ABBREVIATIONS
• STD = sexually transmitted disease
• PID = pelvic inflammatory disease
• HIV = human immunodeficiency virus
• CBD = common bile duct

REFERENCES
• Stamm WE, Holmes K, et al: Chlamydia trachomatis Infections in the Adult. In: Sexually Transmitted Diseases. 2nd Ed. New York, McGraw-Hill, 1990
• Centers for Disease Control and Prevention: Sexually transmitted disease treatment guidelines. MMWR 1993.42 (no. RR-14): 50-52
• Hook EW III, et al: Use of cell culture and a rapid diagnostic assay for Chlamydia trachomatis screening. JAMA 1995;272(11):867
• Heath C, Heath J: Chlamydia trachomatis infection update. Am Fam Phys 1995;52:1455-1461
Illustrations: N/A
Internet references: http://www.5mcc.com

Author(s)
Henry Arguinchona, MD

Cholangitis

BASICS

DESCRIPTION Bacterial inflammation of the bile duct system that is associated with obstructive biliary duct pathology. May be acute or chronic.
System(s) affected: Gastrointestinal
Genetics: N/A
Incidence/Prevalence in USA: N/A
Predominant age: 55-70 years, rare in children, more common in adults
Predominant sex: Female > Male

SIGNS AND SYMPTOMS
May have only one or two symptoms, and the abdominal exam may be unrevealing
• Right upper quadrant pain (RUQ), not severe
• Jaundice
• Chills and fever
• Shock
• CNS depression

CAUSES
• Biliary tract obstruction from:
  ◊ Stones
  ◊ Tumor (pancreatic, CBD, ampulla, metastatic)
  ◊ Benign strictures (postsurgical, PSC)
  ◊ Parasites (Ascaris)
  ◊ Pancreatitis
  ◊ Blood clots
• Reflux of small bowel bacteria
  ◊ Choledochoenterostomy
  ◊ "Sump syndrome"
• Other
  ◊ Cholecystitis
  ◊ Bacteriemia
  ◊ Surgical, radiographic, endoscopic manipulation

RISK FACTORS
• Cholelithiasis
• Endoscopic or surgical manipulation
• Foreign bodies, such as parasites

DIAGNOSIS

DIFFERENTIAL DIAGNOSIS
• Acute cholecystitis - pain and tenderness are invariably present. (May be very difficult to distinguish between cholangitis and acute cholecystitis).
• Pyogenic liver abscess
• Hepatitis
• Acute pancreatitis
• Perforated duodenal ulcer
• Pelvic inflammatory disease with peritonitis
• Kidney stones

LABORATORY
• Increasing WBC with left shift
• Hyperbilirubinemia - in 90%
• Alkaline phosphatase - increasing in 90%
• Positive blood culture - in 50% (gram negative aerobes, and some anaerobes)
Drugs that may alter lab results: N/A
Disorders that may alter lab results: N/A

PATHOLOGICAL FINDINGS In acute toxic disease, pus under pressure in the common bile duct

SPECIAL TESTS
• Need to delineate underlying biliary tract abnormality
• Cholangiography is definitive test
• Percutaneous transhepatic cholangiography (PTC) or endoscopic retrograde cholangiopancreatography (ERCP)

IMAGING Ultrasound will diagnose gallbladder stones and common bile duct size, but will demonstrate common bile duct calculi in less than 15%

DIAGNOSTIC PROCEDURES N/A

TREATMENT

APPROPRIATE HEALTH CARE
Inpatient

GENERAL MEASURES Control sepsis, then evaluate with cholangiography and treat underlying biliary tract pathology

SURGICAL MEASURES
• Patients who do not respond to antibiotics and supportive care require emergency decompression of the biliary duct system. This may be accomplished by surgery, endoscopy, or transhepatic cholangiography.
• In case of obstruction secondary to stones, endoscopic papillotomy and stone extraction will drain the duct and may be definitive treatment of the underlying cause and is shown to reduce mortality

ACTIVITY As tolerated

DIET Nothing by mouth until acute phase is terminated

PATIENT EDUCATION For patient education materials favorably reviewed on this topic, contact: National Digestive Diseases Information Clearinghouse, Box NDDIC, Bethesda, MD 20892, (301)468-6344

Cholangitis

MEDICATIONS

DRUG(S) OF CHOICE
• Antibiotic regimen should cover gram negative aerobes, enterococci, and anaerobes.
  ◊ Ampicillin 1 gm q6h IV (substitute ciprofloxacin in penicillin allergic patient) +
  ◊ Aminoglycoside (e.g., tobramycin, amikacin is an alternative but is expensive) +
  ◊ Metronidazole 500 mg q8h IV
Contraindications: Refer to manufacturer's profile of each drug
Precautions: Renal toxicity of aminoglycoside therapy; check peak and trough levels
Significant possible interactions: Refer to manufacturer's profile of each drug

ALTERNATIVE DRUGS N/A

FOLLOWUP

PATIENT MONITORING Requires careful monitoring of hemodynamic parameters

PREVENTION/AVOIDANCE
Cholangiography when indicated at time of cholecystectomy with endoscopic, radiographic, or surgical clearance of retained CBD stones

POSSIBLE COMPLICATIONS
• Most serious is hepatic abscess
• Sepsis
• Secondary sclerosing cholangitis

EXPECTED COURSE/PROGNOSIS
• Acute cholangitis - good
• Acute toxic cholangitis - mortality high

MISCELLANEOUS

ASSOCIATED CONDITIONS
• Choledocholithiasis
• Malignant tumors
• Benign strictures
• Biliary-enteric anastamosis
• Invasive procedures
• Foreign bodies
• Parasites
• Secondary sclerosing cholangitis

AGE-RELATED FACTORS
Pediatric: N/A
Geriatric: N/A
Others: N/A

PREGNANCY N/A

SYNONYMS N/A

ICD-9-CM 576.1 Cholangitis

SEE ALSO Cholelithiasis

OTHER NOTES N/A

ABBREVIATIONS N/A

REFERENCES
• Nahrwold DL: Cholangitis. In: Sabiston DC, ed. Textbook of Surgery. 13th Ed. Philadelphia, W.B. Saunders Co., 1986
• Boeg JH, Way LW: Acute Cholangitis. Ann Surg 1980;191:264
• Pitt HA, Longmire WP Jr: Suppurative Cholangitis. In: Hardy JM, ed. Critical Surgical Illness. 2nd Ed. Philadelphia, W.B. Saunders Co., 1980
Illustrations: N/A
Internet references: http://www.5mcc.com

Author(s)
Leo C. Mercer, MD

Cholecystitis

BASICS

DESCRIPTION
Inflammation of the gallbladder occurring acutely or chronically, often secondary to previously asymptomatic gallstones.
System(s) affected: Gastrointestinal
Genetics: Increased prevalence in Native Americans and Caucasians, less prevalent in African Americans
Incidence/Prevalence in USA:
• Steady increase with age, varies in different ethnic groups. Percentage with gallstones (approximately half will develop symptoms over their lifetime):
◊ By age 30, 30% of Native Americans
◊ By age 60, 80% of Native Americans
◊ By age 60, 30% of Caucasians
◊ By age 60, 20% of African Americans
Predominant age: 5th and 6th decade
Predominant sex: Female > Male (2:1)

SIGNS AND SYMPTOMS
• Asymptomatic. 5-10% become symptomatic each year.
• Acute cholecystitis
◊ Abdominal pain - sudden onset, intense, in epigastrium or right upper quadrant, radiates to shoulder or back. Pathognomonic feature is "biliary colic" a pain rising over 2-3 minutes to a plateau of intensity that is maintained for > 20 minutes.
◊ Nausea and vomiting
◊ Recurrent attacks following meals by 1-6 hours, lasting > 12 hours until recovered, usually < 3 days
◊ Elevated temperature - mild to moderate
◊ Local tenderness, rarely diffuse
◊ Murphy's sign - inspiratory arrest elicited when palpating right upper quadrant while asking the patient for deep inhalation
◊ Palpable gall bladder - 5% of cases
• Common duct stone
◊ Jaundice in 50%
◊ Biliary colic 60%
◊ Fever and chills 30%
◊ Pruritus 10%
◊ Loose bowel movements, light color
◊ Mild to marked hepatomegaly > 80%
◊ Tenderness infrequent
◊ Palpable gall bladder 10%
◊ Gallstone ileus (rare)
◊ Gallstone > 3 cm fistulizes into bowel and obstructs at ileocecal area
◊ Antecedent pain, often over weeks with non-biliary colic
◊ Abdominal distension, mild tenderness
◊ Air in biliary passages on plain x-ray
◊ Intestinal obstruction at level of terminal ileum
• Pancreatitis
◊ Pain over upper abdomen
◊ Nausea and vomiting
• Empyema
◊ Phlegmon of obstructed gall bladder
◊ Insidious weight loss, mild wasting
◊ Gradual onset of occult infection signs, fever, anorexia
◊ Mass usually present
◊ Tenderness usually absent

• Chronic cholecystitis
◊ Associated with gallstones, often asymptomatic; 20% become symptomatic over 15-20 years
◊ Mild dyspepsia following fatty meals

CAUSES
• Gallstones in 90-95% of cases. May obstruct the cystic duct, leading to acute cholecystitis; obstruction of the common bile duct, causing jaundice, or obstruction of the pancreatic duct, causing pancreatitis.
• Gallbladder sludge, a viscous material, insoluble in bile, that layers on sonogram, and occasionally produces cholecystitis, common duct obstruction or pancreatitis. Occurs in most pregnant women, most total parenteral nutrition, and most patients with rapid weight loss
• Acalculous cholecystitis in 5% of cases. Associated with severe stressful situations including cardiac surgery, multiple trauma. May be associated with ischemic damage to the gallbladder wall.
• Bacteria. Usually do not initiate the inflammation but important in the complications of empyema and ascending cholangitis. In emphysematous cholecystitis, Clostridia are probably responsible for both initiation and complications.
• Neoplasms and strictures of common bile duct. Usually associated with cholangitis and pancreatitis.
• Ischemia - in patients with diabetes, but uncommon
• Torsion - lost fixation of gallbladder, uncommon

RISK FACTORS
• Cardiac surgery
• Trauma
• Biliary parasites
• Gallstones (see topic Cholelithiasis)
• Rapid weight loss
• Prolonged parenteral alimentation
• Pregnancy

DIAGNOSIS

DIFFERENTIAL DIAGNOSIS
Acute pancreatitis, ulcer, diverticulitis, pyelonephritis, pneumonitis, hepatic abscess, hepatic tumors, Irritable bowel disease, non-ulcer dyspepsia

LABORATORY
• Acute cholecystitis
◊ Leukocytosis - 12,000-15,000
◊ Liver tests usually abnormal; ALT, AST slightly elevated, alkaline phosphatase, GGT elevated with common duct obstruction

• Common duct stone
◊ High bilirubin in 50%, in 100% after 10 days
◊ Elevated alkaline phosphatase and gamma glutamyl transpeptidase (GGT) in 85%
◊ Positive blood culture in 15%
◊ Barely abnormal ALT, AST
◊ Elevated fasting bile salts
◊ Elevated WBC if infection
◊ Serum amylase may be elevated. If > 1000 units, concomitant pancreatitis should be considered.
Drugs that may alter lab results:
• Steroids
• Immunosuppressive drugs. These may mask leukocytosis and early signs of inflammation.
Disorders that may alter lab results:
• Old age, malnutrition
• Lymphoma, other immunocompromised states

PATHOLOGICAL FINDINGS   N/A

SPECIAL TESTS
99mTc Imino diacetic acid (HIDA) scan - highly sensitive (97%) for diagnosis of acute cholecystitis. HIDA derivatives are taken up by hepatocytes and excreted in bile and concentrated in gallbladder. Failure to see gallbladder in 1 hour is highly suspicious for acute cholecystitis. Usually abnormal in acalculous cholecystitis.

IMAGING
• Plain radiographs (upright)
◊ 20% of gallstones are radio-opaque
◊ Air cholangiogram if there is gallbladder-gut fistula
◊ Emphysematous cholecystitis - air in the gallbladder wall or in lumen
• Ultrasonography
◊ Best technique to diagnose gallstones (high sensitivity - 95%, and specificity - 98%)
◊ Best noninvasive imaging technique to diagnose acute cholecystitis. Findings include thick gall bladder wall (> 3 mm), gallbladder distension, sludge in lumen, pericholecystic fluid.
• CT scan
◊ No advantage over ultrasonography in gallstone/acute cholecystitis diagnosis
◊ Better than ultrasonography to detect enlargement of pancreas. Helpful in the diagnosis of abscess formation. Shows thickened gall bladder wall in cancer.
◊ Better than US for dilated common bile duct

DIAGNOSTIC PROCEDURES
• Ultrasound or CT scan often diagnostic
• Tc HIDA test during acute pain
• Endoscopic retrograde cholangiopancreatography (ERCP) - to see status of biliary and pancreatic ducts
• Percutaneous transhepatic cholangiography test (PTC) - gives more information about intrahepatic biliary system
• Laparotomy - if unable to make diagnosis by less invasive means

Cholecystitis

TREATMENT

APPROPRIATE HEALTH CARE
• Outpatient for patients with mild symptoms
• Inpatient - patients with biliary colic lasting for more than 6 hours and showing toxicity, jaundice, rigors, or requiring narcotics for pain
• Ascending cholangitis is a surgical emergency. If laparotomy is inappropriate, drainage can be obtained by ERCP or transhepatic cholangiography.
• Direct drainage of gallbladder by invasive radiologist occasionally required

GENERAL MEASURES
NPO, IV fluids, nasogastric suction

SURGICAL MEASURES
• Surgery (cholecystectomy) is the appropriate treatment for symptomatic cholecystitis. Best performed by laparoscopy if available, but a standard laparotomy is acceptable. Mortality rate - 0.1% in age <50 years and 0.8% age > 50.
• If there is jaundice, exploration of the common bile duct is essential at open laparotomy, or by a separate ERCP. Mortality rate for laparotomy is 0.1% < 50 years and 0.8% > 50 years. In acute cholecystitis - early cholecystectomy is the general practice rather than delayed interval cholecystectomy (delay only if surgery is contraindicated)
• Laparoscopic cholecystostomy - rapidly replacing alternative surgical drainage procedure. If the patient is a poor risk, drainage of the gallbladder or biliary passages can be achieved by radiological or endoscopic techniques. This will allow control of infection and jaundice for several weeks or months.
• Dissolution therapy - infrequently used if laparoscopic cholecystectomy can be performed. Ursodeoxycholic acid (Actigall) in 10 mg/kg is the drug of choice. To be effective there must be a functioning gallbladder on oral cholecystography. Stones must be free of calcium. Many small stones have best prognosis to dissolve. An alternative drug is chenodeoxycholic acid (Chenodiol) 12-15 mg/kg/day.
• Other indications for emergency surgery include - toxic patient, doubtful diagnosis, perforation or abscess

ACTIVITY
As tolerated by the patient

DIET
• NPO during acute cholecystitis
• Fatty meals precipitate mild attacks. Avoid if possible.

PATIENT EDUCATION
National Digestive Diseases Information Clearinghouse, Box NDDIC, Bethesda, MD 20892, (301) 468-6344

MEDICATIONS

DRUG(S) OF CHOICE
• Mild attack
  ◊ Diclofenac 75 mg IV may abort early attack
  ◊ Ampicillin 4-6 gm/day or cefazolin (Ancef) 2-4 gm/day
• Severe attack - gentamicin 3-5 mg/kg/day and clindamycin 1.8-2.7 gm/day. A penicillin could be added if needed.
• The formation of gallstones during rapid weight loss after bariatric surgery or severe diets is prevented by ursodiol (ursodeoxycholic acid) 10 mg/kg/day
• Formation of gallstones in prolonged parenteral alimentation is prevented by daily feeding of 100 kcal or daily injection of cholecystokinin
Contraindications: Hypersensitivity reactions
Precautions:
• Nephrotoxicity, ototoxicity with aminoglycosides
• Adjust the dose according to creatinine clearance
Significant possible interactions: Refer to manufacturer's profile of each drug

ALTERNATIVE DRUGS
For acute cholecystitis - 3rd generation cephalosporins

FOLLOWUP

PATIENT MONITORING
Post cholecystectomy - follow through postoperative period

PREVENTION/AVOIDANCE
• Avoid risk factors when possible
• During rapid weight loss following bariatric surgery or very low calorie diets, ursodeoxycholic acid (ursodiol) 10 mg/kg/day
• During total parenteral alimentation for more than one month, daily ingestion of 100 kcal, or injection of cholecystokinin

POSSIBLE COMPLICATIONS
Occur in about 5% cases of acute cholecystitis and include - perforation, abscess formation, fistula formation (intestine, colon, cutaneous), gangrene, empyema, cholangitis, hepatitis, pancreatitis, gallstone ileus, carcinoma

EXPECTED COURSE/PROGNOSIS
• In general the prognosis is good for gallbladder disease. Those who die during acute episodes are mainly due to other conditions, especially coronary artery disease.
• Symptomatic gallstones usually have recurrent symptoms in 3 to 6 months indicating need for future action
• After cholecystectomy, stones may recur in bile ducts

MISCELLANEOUS

ASSOCIATED CONDITIONS
• Pancreatitis
• Hemolytic anemias such as sickle cell disease, spherocytosis
• Cirrhosis, hypersplenism

AGE-RELATED FACTORS
Pediatric: N/A
Geriatric: Sometimes difficult to diagnose; complications more likely; cholecystectomy mortality rate higher
Others: N/A

PREGNANCY   N/A

SYNONYMS   N/A

ICD-9-CM
574.0 Calculus of gallbladder with acute cholecystitis
574.1 Calculus of gallbladder with other cholecystitis
575.0 Acute cholecystitis
575.1 Other cholecystitis (without mention of calculus)

SEE ALSO
• Cholelithiasis
• Cholangitis
• Choledocholithiasis
• Adenocarcinoma of the gallbladder
• Jaundice

OTHER NOTES
Lithotripsy - can be used in patients with chronic cholecystitis. Contraindications - stones greater than 25 mm, more than 3 stones, calcified stones, bile duct stones, poor general condition. Largely replaced by laparoscopic cholecystectomy.

ABBREVIATIONS   N/A

REFERENCES
• Ko CW, Sekijima JH, Lee SP: Biliary sludge. Ann of Int Med 1999;130:301-311
6 additional references available at web site
Internet references: http://www.5mcc.com
Illustrations: N/A

Author(s)
Frank L. Iber, MD

Choledocholithiasis

BASICS

DESCRIPTION Stones in common bile duct (usually composed of cholesterol) that migrate from the gallbladder. Calcium bilirubinate stones may form de novo.
System(s) affected: Gastrointestinal
Genetics: N/A
Incidence/Prevalence in USA: 10-15% of patients with gallbladder stones discovered at time of cholecystectomy
Predominant age: Incidence increases with age
Predominant sex: Female > Male

SIGNS AND SYMPTOMS
• May be asymptomatic
• Biliary colic
• Common bile duct obstruction
• Cholangitis
• Pancreatitis
• Pain can't be differentiated from pain arising from gallbladder
• Epigastric pain
• Abdominal tenderness
• Pain unrelieved by antacids
• Anorexia, vomiting
• Dark urine
• Light colored feces
• Right upper quadrant tenderness
• Palpable gallbladder

CAUSES
• Increased biliary cholesterol secretion
• Chronic hemolytic states
• Hepatobiliary parasitism
• Duct stricture

RISK FACTORS
• Cholelithiasis
• Obesity
• Cirrhosis
• Chronic hemolysis
• Prior cholecystectomy

DIAGNOSIS

DIFFERENTIAL DIAGNOSIS
• Biliary stricture
• Narrowed biliary - enteric anastomosis
• Sclerosing cholangitis
• Sphincter of Oddi dysfunction
• Biliary parasites
• Papillary stenosis
• Blood clots

LABORATORY
• Increasing WBC
• Increasing alkaline phosphatase
• Hypercholesterolemia (when associated with chronic cholestasis)
• Increased transaminases
• Hyperbilirubinemia
Drugs that may alter lab results: N/A
Disorders that may alter lab results: N/A

PATHOLOGICAL FINDINGS
• Dilated bile ducts
• Bile plugging
• Small bile duct proliferation
• Cholesterol gallstones

SPECIAL TESTS Nuclear medicine (PIPIDA), endoscopic retrograde cholangiopancreatography (ERCP), percutaneous transhepatic cholangiography (PTC)

IMAGING
• Intraoperative cholangiography - common bile duct filling defects
• Nuclear medicine cholescintigraphy
• Endoscopic cholangiography or PTC - common bile duct filling defects
• Endoscopic ultrasonography - can likely detect stones, but no therapeutic capability

DIAGNOSTIC PROCEDURES
• Ultrasound will reveal gallbladder stones - not reliable for common bile duct stones, but may reveal ductal dilatation over 75% of the time
• ERCP will visualize the common bile duct and other portions of the upper gastrointestinal tract and will allow for papillotomy plus stone extraction in majority of cases.

TREATMENT

APPROPRIATE HEALTH CARE
Inpatient

GENERAL MEASURES N/A

SURGICAL MEASURES
• In the elderly, ERCP and papillotomy with stone removal may prevent or delay the need for cholecystectomy
• Identification and removal of stones in the course of cholecystectomy
• If the gallbladder has been previously removed, ERCP, papillotomy plus stone extraction

ACTIVITY As tolerated

DIET Low fat may be helpful

PATIENT EDUCATION National Digestive Diseases Information Clearinghouse, Box NDDIC, Bethesda, MD 20892, (301)468-6344

Choledocholithiasis

MEDICATIONS

DRUG(S) OF CHOICE Antibiotics to treat gram negative aerobes and anaerobes. Selection based on culture and sensitivities. One useful specific regimen, for example: Cefoxitin, 2 grams intravenously perioperatively.
Contraindications: Refer to manufacturer's profile of each drug
Precautions: Refer to manufacturer's profile of each drug
Significant possible interactions: Refer to manufacturer's profile of each drug

ALTERNATIVE DRUGS N/A

FOLLOWUP

PATIENT MONITORING Routine postoperative care

PREVENTION/AVOIDANCE
• Operative cholangiography at time of cholecystectomy to identify common bile duct stones and then duct exploration or endoscopic sphincterotomy for their removal
• T-tube cholangiogram before removal of tube after operative bile duct exploration

POSSIBLE COMPLICATIONS
• Cholangitis - most frequent (60%)
• Bile duct obstruction
• Pancreatitis
• Biliary enteric fistula
• Hemobilia

EXPECTED COURSE/PROGNOSIS
Good prognosis if treated

MISCELLANEOUS

ASSOCIATED CONDITIONS
• Cholecystitis
• Cholangitis
• Periampullary diverticula

AGE-RELATED FACTORS
Pediatric: N/A
Geriatric: Prognosis guarded
Others: N/A

PREGNANCY Cholestasis of pregnancy may lead to choledocholithiasis

SYNONYMS
• Common bile duct stone
• Common bile duct calculi

ICD-9-CM
547.3 Calculus of bile duct with acute cholecystitis
574.5 Calculus of bile duct without mention of cholecystitis

SEE ALSO
• Cholangitis
• Cholecystitis
• Cholelithiasis
• Adenocarcinoma of the gallbladder
• Jaundice

OTHER NOTES N/A

ABBREVIATIONS
• ERCP = endoscopic retrograde cholangiopancreatography
• PTC = percutaneous transhepatic cholangiography

REFERENCES
• Nahrwold DL: The Biliary System. In: Sabisto DC, ed. Textbook of Surgery. Philadelphia, W.B. Saunders, 1986
• Jordan GL Jr: Choledocholithiasis. Curr Prob Surg 1982;19:723
Illustrations: N/A
Internet references: http://www.5mcc.com

Author(s)
Leo C. Mercer, MD

Cholelithiasis

BASICS

DESCRIPTION Cholesterol or pigmented stones formed and contained in the gallbladder
System(s) affected: Gastrointestinal
Genetics: N/A
Incidence/Prevalence in USA: 8-10% of population. Increased incidence in American Indians and Hispanics.
Predominant age: Increases with age - peak at sixth decade
Predominant sex: Female > Male (2:1)

SIGNS AND SYMPTOMS
• Mostly asymptomatic. 5-10% become symptomatic each year. Over lifetime, less than half of patients with gallstones develop symptoms.
• Episodic right upper quadrant or epigastric pain radiating to back (biliary colic)
• Nausea
• Vomiting
• Fatty food intolerance (not proven)
• Indigestion

CAUSES
• Production of bile supersaturated with cholesterol
• Decrease in bile content of either phospholipids or bile acids
• Biliary stasis
• Hemolytic diseases
• Biliary infection

RISK FACTORS
• Short gut syndrome
• Inflammatory bowel disease
• Multiparity
• Long term total parenteral nutrition
• Cirrhosis (for pigment stones)
• Hemolytic disorders - hereditary spherocytosis, sickle cell anemia
• Prosthetic cardiac valves
• Biliary parasites
• Rapid weight loss
• Childhood malignancy
• Native American descent
• Diabetes (for complications)
• Female gender

DIAGNOSIS

DIFFERENTIAL DIAGNOSIS
• Peptic ulcer
• Hepatitis, pancreatitis
• Coronary artery disease
• Appendicitis
• Pneumonia
• Gallbladder cancer
• Renal stones
• Blood clots
• Stricture
• Gallbladder polyps
• Biliary sludge

LABORATORY   None
Drugs that may alter lab results: N/A
Disorders that may alter lab results: N/A

PATHOLOGICAL FINDINGS   Gallstones

SPECIAL TESTS   Hepatobiliary radionuclide scan

IMAGING
• Ultrasound (best technique to diagnose gallstones)
• Oral cholecystogram
• CT scan (no advantage over ultrasound)

DIAGNOSTIC PROCEDURES   N/A

TREATMENT

APPROPRIATE HEALTH CARE
Inpatient for surgical procedures

GENERAL MEASURES
• Treat only symptomatic gallstones
• Advise patient of presence of stones
• Observe asymptomatic stones
• Oral dissolution - only if surgery option not available (less than 25% of all patients eligible)

SURGICAL MEASURES
• Laparoscopic cholecystectomy
• Open cholecystectomy
• Direct contact dissolution - only for a small subset of patients - high recurrence rate
• Extracorporeal shock wave lithotripsy - role of this modality unclear and currently under study - not FDA approved
• Percutaneous cholecystostomy in high risk patients

ACTIVITY   N/A

DIET   Low fat diet may be helpful

PATIENT EDUCATION
• National Digestive Diseases Information Clearinghouse, Box NDDIC, Bethesda, MD 20892, (301)468-6344

Cholelithiasis

MEDICATIONS

DRUG(S) OF CHOICE
• Analgesic for symptom relief
• Ursodiol (ursodeoxycholic acid, Actigall) 8-10 mg/kg/day bid-tid - for up to two years - oral dissolution
• Chenodiol (Chenix) 250 mg bid for 2 weeks; then increase by 250 mg increments until a dose of 13-16 mg/kg daily is reached or intolerance develops - oral dissolution
• Methyl tert-butyl ether - contact dissolution

Contraindications:
• Known allergy
• Acute cholecystitis - dissolution agents
• Severe abnormal liver function tests
• Non-functioning gallbladder
• Calcified (radiopaque) stones - relative
• Multiple stones
• Stones greater than 2 cm
• Stones that don't float on oral cholecystogram

Precautions:
• Monitor liver enzymes - may rise in up to 30% of patients
• Monitor serum cholesterol
• Methyl tert-butyl ether should only be used by one experienced with this contact dissolution method
• Observe for severe diarrhea

Significant possible interactions: N/A

ALTERNATIVE DRUGS
NSAID's may have a role in pain relief since prostaglandins are important in the development of pain
Note:
• Oral dissolution only effective for radiolucent (cholesterol) stones
• Ursodiol probably preferred over chenodiol as it has a lower incidence of adverse effects

FOLLOWUP

PATIENT MONITORING
• Medical attention if asymptomatic stones become symptomatic
• Patients on oral dissolution agents should be followed with liver enzymes, serum cholesterol and imaging studies

PREVENTION/AVOIDANCE
Use of ursodiol (Actigall) with rapid weight loss prevents stone formation

POSSIBLE COMPLICATIONS
• Acute cholecystitis (90-95% secondary to gallstones)
• Gallstone pancreatitis
• Acute cholangitis
• Common bile duct stones with obstructive jaundice
• Gallstone ileus
• Liver abscess
• Biliary-enteric fistula
• Peritonitis
• Gallbladder cancer

EXPECTED COURSE/PROGNOSIS
• Less than half of patients with gallstones will become symptomatic
• Cholecystectomy - mortality 0.5% elective, 3-5% emergency, morbidity less than 10% elective, 30-40% emergency
• 10-15% will have associated choledocholithiasis
• After cholecystostomy, stones may recur in bile duct

MISCELLANEOUS

ASSOCIATED CONDITIONS
90% of gallbladder carcinomas have gallstones

AGE-RELATED FACTORS
Pediatric:
• Uncommon before 10 years of age
• Associated with blood dyscrasia
Geriatric:
• Incidence increases with age
• Age alone should not alter therapy plan
Others: N/A

PREGNANCY
Attempt conservative therapy but surgery if indicated

SYNONYMS
Gallstones

ICD-9-CM
574.0 Calculus of gallbladder with acute cholecystitis
574.1 Calculus of gallbladder with other cholecystitis
574.2 Calculus of gallbladder without mention of cholecystitis
575.0 Acute cholecystitis
575.1 Other cholecystitis (without mention of calculus)

SEE ALSO
• Cholangitis
• Choledocholithiasis
• Cholecystitis
• Adenocarcinoma of the gallbladder
• Jaundice

OTHER NOTES
Laparoscopic cholecystectomy has become most frequently used procedure. (Lithotripsy can be considered in rare circumstances.)

ABBREVIATIONS
N/A

REFERENCES
• Hardy JD, ed: Hardy's Textbook of Surgery. 2nd Ed. Philadelphia, J.B. Lippincott, 1988
• Pitt HA, ed: The Surgical Clinics of North America. Vol. 70, No. 6. Philadelphia, W.B. Saunders, Dec, 1990
Illustrations: N/A
Internet references: http://www.5mcc.com

Author(s)
Gary B. Williams, MD

Cholera

BASICS

DESCRIPTION An acute infectious disease caused by Vibrio cholerae (El Tor type is responsible for current epidemic, the other type, classic, is found only in Bangladesh). (New serotype now in Bangladesh, India (0139). Important because of lack of efficacy of standard vaccine.) Characteristics include severe diarrhea with extreme fluid and electrolyte depletion, and vomiting, muscle cramps and prostration. Usual course: acute; chronic; relapsing.
• Clinical course is 3-5 days, and in the early stages a severely affected patient can lose one liter of fluid per hour
• Endemic areas: India; Southeast Asia; Africa; Middle East; Southern Europe; Oceania; South and Central America
System(s) affected: Gastrointestinal
Genetics: N/A
Incidence/Prevalence in USA: 0.01 cases/100,000. The few cases in the U.S. have been in returning travelers or associated with food brought into the country illicitly.
Predominant age: All ages
Predominant sex: Male = Female

SIGNS AND SYMPTOMS
• Abdominal discomfort
• Anorexia
• Anuria
• Apathy
• Cholera gravis
• Cyanosis
• Decreased skin turgor
• Dehydration
• Diarrhea, painless
• Distant heart sounds
• Diuresis, sudden
• Dysrhythmias
• Fever
• Hypotension
• Hypothermia
• Hypovolemic shock
• Increased or decreased bowel sounds
• Lethargy
• Listlessness
• Malaise
• Non-tender abdomen
• Oliguria
• Rice-water diarrhea
• Seizures
• Sunken eyes
• Tachycardia
• Thirst
• Vomiting
• Washerwoman's fingers
• Weak peripheral pulses
• Weakness

CAUSES
• Enterotoxin elaborated by gram-negative
• Vibrio cholera (O-group 1)
• Human host
• Contaminated food
• Contaminated water
• Contaminated shellfish

RISK FACTORS
• Traveling or living in epidemic areas
• Exposure to contaminated food or water
• Person-to-person transmission (rare)
• In endemic areas, children under age 5
• Attack more severe in blood group O as compared to AB
• Individual with low gastric acid secretion
• Gastrectomy
• Individuals on acid-suppressing medications

DIAGNOSIS

DIFFERENTIAL DIAGNOSIS Other causes of severe diarrhea and dehydration (e.g., Shigella, E. coli, viruses)

LABORATORY
• Stool culture - on selective media (thiosulfate citrate bile salts sucrose [TCBS])
• Typed antisera specific agglutination
• Dark field microscopy - characteristic vibrio motility in stool
• Increased vibriocidal antibodies in unimmunized individual
• Laboratory abnormalities of severe dehydration:
  ◊ Acidemia
  ◊ Acidosis
  ◊ Hypokalemia
  ◊ Hyponatremia
  ◊ Hypochloremia
  ◊ Hypoglycemia
  ◊ Increased specific gravity
  ◊ Polycythemia
  ◊ Mild neutrophilic leukocytosis
Drugs that may alter lab results: N/A
Disorders that may alter lab results: N/A

PATHOLOGICAL FINDINGS
• Electron microscopy - organism adherent to mucosa
• Intact mucosa
• Increased cellularity of lamina propria
• Increased cellularity of mucosa
• Vascular congestion
• Lymphoid hyperplasia of Peyer's patches
• Lymphoid hyperplasia of mesenteric lymph nodes
• Lymphoid hyperplasia of spleen
• Cerebral edema
• Acute tubular necrosis
• Vacuolar hypokalemic nephropathy
• Pulmonary edema
• Hyaline membranes
• Bronchopneumonia
• Focal myocardial damage
• Lipid-depleted adrenals
• Tubularization of zona fasciculata

SPECIAL TESTS   N/A

IMAGING
• Abdominal film - ileus
• Chest x-ray - microcardia

DIAGNOSTIC PROCEDURES   Physical examination and medical history that includes recent travel

TREATMENT

APPROPRIATE HEALTH CARE
Outpatient for mild cases, inpatient for moderate or severe cases

GENERAL MEASURES
• Determination of the amount of fluid loss (may compare patient's previous weight to current weight)
• Rehydration therapy. Oral for mild to moderate cases. Patients with severe dehydration may require intravenous replacement.

SURGICAL MEASURES   N/A

ACTIVITY   Bedrest until symptoms resolved and strength returns

DIET   Small, frequent meals when vomiting stops and appetite returns

PATIENT EDUCATION
• Centers for Disease Control. Traveler's Information Hotline: (404)332-4559 (available 24 hours via a touch-tone telephone).
• International Association for Medical Assistance to Travelers, 417 Center St., Lewiston, NY 14092, (716)754-4883

Cholera

MEDICATIONS

DRUG(S) OF CHOICE
• Oral rehydration therapy
For mild disease:
◊ Oral rehydration solution (ORS) commercial brands available (Pedialyte, Rehydralyte, Resol, Ricelyte) or
◊ ORS formula from World Health Organization (WHO) - per liter:
- Sodium chloride 3.5 grams
- Potassium chloride 1.5 grams
- Glucose 20 grams
- Trisodium citrate 2.9 grams
• Parenteral rehydration
Severely dehydrated patients
◊ IV rehydration (Ringer's lactate) is followed by oral or nasogastric administration of glucose or sucrose-electrolyte solution
• Antibiotics
◊ For older children and adults - doxycycline (Vibramycin) - 300 mg once or 100 mg bid for 3 days or tetracycline 50 mg/kg/day for 3 days
◊ For young children - trimethoprim-sulfamethoxazole (SMX-TMP, Bactrim, Septra) 8 mg/kg trimethoprim plus 40 mg/kg sulfamethoxazole per day, divided q12h. This dosage is equivalent to 1 mL/kg of SMX/TMP suspension. Alternatively, furazolidone (Furoxone) 5-10 mg/kg/day divided q6h for 3 days.
◊ In pregnancy - furazolidone 100 mg qid x 7-10 days.
Contraindications:
• Tetracycline: not for use in pregnancy or children < 8 years.
• Furazolidone and alcohol may cause disulfiram-like reaction.
Precautions:
• Tetracycline: may cause photosensitivity; sunscreen recommended.
Significant possible interactions:
• Tetracycline: avoid concurrent administration with antacids, dairy products, or iron.

ALTERNATIVE DRUGS N/A

FOLLOWUP

PATIENT MONITORING Follow patient until symptoms resolved

PREVENTION/AVOIDANCE
• Water purification
• Careful food selection, e.g., no unpeeled raw fruits or vegetables, no raw or undercooked seafood
• Enteric precautions
• Tetracycline for contacts
• Natural infection confers long-lasting immunity
• Prophylactic vaccine
◊ 50% effective for 3 to 6 months
◊ Not recommended unless required by destination country, and if so, a single dose is sufficient
◊ Concomitant administration with yellow fever vaccine may result in reduced vaccine response to yellow fever
◊ Invariably associated with local side effects
◊ Systemic side effects of fever and malaise
◊ A new vaccine shows promise, but still in the testing stage

POSSIBLE COMPLICATIONS
• Hypovolemic shock
• Chronic biliary infection
• Up to 50% mortality with untreated shock
• Intermittent stool shedding

EXPECTED COURSE/PROGNOSIS
• Prompt oral or IV treatment can be lifesaving
• Appropriate disposal of human waste
• Antibiotic treatment reduces duration and infectivity of disease
• Mortality less than 1% with appropriate supportive care
• Increased mortality with untreated hypovolemic shock

MISCELLANEOUS

ASSOCIATED CONDITIONS Increased risk of disease with gastric achlorhydria

AGE-RELATED FACTORS
Pediatric:
• Breast-feeding is protective against cholera
• Vaccine not recommended for children less than 6 months
Geriatric: N/A
Others: N/A

PREGNANCY N/A

SYNONYMS
• Asiatic cholera
• Epidemic cholera
• Rice water diarrhea
• Cholera gravis

ICD-9-CM 001.9 Cholera, unspecified

SEE ALSO
• Oral rehydration
• Diarrhea, acute

OTHER NOTES Centers for Disease Control does not expect a major outbreak of cholera in the U.S., but it has issued a "Cholera Preparedness Plan," outlining steps for proper surveillance, treatment, laboratory diagnosis, investigation of outbreaks, and public education

ABBREVIATIONS N/A

REFERENCES
• Mandell GL, ed: Principles and Practice of Infectious Diseases. 4th Ed. New York, Churchill Livingstone, 1995
• Warren KS, Mahmoud AA, eds: Tropical and Geographical Medicine. New York, McGraw-Hill, 1990
• Dhiman BR, Greenough CB III, eds: Cholera. New York, Plenum Medical Book Co., 1992
Illustrations: N/A
Internet references: http://www.5mcc.com

Author(s)
Abdulrazak Abyad, MD, MPH, AGSF

Chronic fatigue syndrome

BASICS

DESCRIPTION Chronic fatigue syndrome (CFS) is characterized primarily by profound fatigue, in association with multiple systemic and neuropsychiatric symptoms, lasting at least 6 months. The fatigue must have a new or definite onset (i.e., not lifelong), is not relieved by rest, and results in a substantial reduction in previous activities (occupation, education, social, and personal).
System(s) affected: Endocrine/Metabolic, Musculoskeletal
Genetics: N/A
Incidence/Prevalence in USA: 10/100,000
Predominant age: Young adult
Predominant sex: Female > Male (slightly)

SIGNS AND SYMPTOMS
- Fatigue (100%)
- Ability to date onset of illness (100%)
- Unexplained general muscle weakness (90%)
- Arthralgias (90%)
- Forgetfulness (90%)
- Inability to concentrate (90%)
- Emotional lability (90%)
- Myalgias (90%)
- Confusion (90%)
- Mood swings (90%)
- Low-grade fever (37.5-38.6°C) (85%)
- Irritability (85%)
- Prolonged fatigue lasting 24 hours after exercise (80%)
- Depression (80%)
- Headaches (76%)
- Photophobia (76%)
- Difficulty sleeping (76%)
- Allergies (70%)
- Vertigo (40%)
- Adenopathy (40%)
- Shortness of breath (33%)
- Chest pain (33%)
- Nausea (33%)
- Weight loss (30%)
- Hot flushes (30%)
- Palpitations (30%)
- Painful lymph nodes (30%)
- Gastrointestinal complaints (30%)
- Night sweats (25%)
- Weight gain (15%)
- Rash (15%)

CAUSES
Unknown. Multiple immunologic abnormalities suggestive of viral reactivation syndrome have been reported. Attention has been to viruses (EBV, HHV-6, enteroviruses), possibly in concert, possibly with environmental factors. No infectious agent has been implicated in the syndrome.

RISK FACTORS Unknown

DIAGNOSIS

DIFFERENTIAL DIAGNOSIS
- Malignancies
- Autoimmune disease
- Localized infection (occult abscess, etc.)
- Chronic or subacute bacterial disease (endocarditis)
- Lyme disease
- Fungal disease (histoplasmosis, coccidioidomycosis)
- Parasitic disease (amebiasis, giardiasis, helminths)
- HIV related disease
- Psychiatric disorders
  ◊ Drug dependency or abuse (including prescription drugs)
  ◊ Depression
  ◊ Hypochondriasis
  ◊ Anxiety disorders
  ◊ Somatization disorder
- Chronic inflammatory disease (sarcoidosis, Wegener's granulomatosis)
- Known chronic viral disease (chronic hepatitis)
- Neuromuscular disease (multiple sclerosis, myasthenia gravis)
- Endocrine disorder (hypothyroidism, Addison's, Cushing's, diabetes mellitus)
- Iatrogenic (as from medication side effects)
- Toxic agent exposure
- Other known or defined systemic disease (chronic pulmonary, cardiac, hepatic, renal, or hematologic disease)
- Physiologic (inadequate or disrupted sleep, menopause, etc.)

LABORATORY
- Initial lab studies
  ◊ Chemistry panel
  ◊ CBC
  ◊ Urinalysis
  ◊ Thyroid function
- Additional studies
  ◊ ESR
  ◊ ANA
  ◊ VDRL
  ◊ Rheumatoid factor
  ◊ Purified protein derivative
  ◊ Serum cortisol
  ◊ HIV
  ◊ Immunoglobulin
  ◊ Epstein-Barr serology
Drugs that may alter lab results: N/A
Disorders that may alter lab results: N/A

PATHOLOGICAL FINDINGS N/A

SPECIAL TESTS None. Diagnosis of exclusion. History, physical exam normal.

IMAGING Experimental at present

DIAGNOSTIC PROCEDURES
To establish the diagnosis - 2 major criteria and at least 6 symptoms plus at least 2 physical signs; or at least 8 symptoms
- Major criteria:
  ◊ New onset fatigue lasting longer than 6 months with a 50% reduction in activity
  ◊ No other medical or psychiatric conditions that could cause symptoms
- Symptoms:
  ◊ Low grade fever
  ◊ Sore throat
  ◊ Painful cervical or axillary adenopathy
  ◊ Generalized muscle weakness
  ◊ Myalgias
  ◊ Headaches
  ◊ Migratory arthralgias
  ◊ Sleep disturbances (hypersomnia or insomnia)
  ◊ Neuropsychological complaints (one or more of: photophobia, visual scotomas, forgetfulness, irritability, confusion, difficulty concentrating, depression)
- Physical signs:
  ◊ Low grade fever (37.5-38.6°C)
  ◊ Pharyngitis (nonexudative)
  ◊ Cervical or axillary adenopathy

TREATMENT

APPROPRIATE HEALTH CARE
Outpatient

GENERAL MEASURES
- Because the cause of CFS is unknown and no specific therapy has shown consistent results, mainstay of therapy is supportive care
- A program of moderate exercise (with rest periods during exacerbations of the disease), a healthy diet, stress reduction, and support groups or counseling is likely to be beneficial and while not necessarily curative will help the patient cope with their disease
- Alternative therapies (chiropractic, homeopathy, acupuncture, enforced rest, guided image hypnosis) helpful for some; may be worth trying
- Psychiatric symptoms often prominent but generally felt secondary rather than causative, but symptom treatment beneficial

SURGICAL MEASURES N/A

ACTIVITY As tolerated, but strenuous exercise tends to exacerbate symptoms in most

DIET Rich in vitamins and minerals

PATIENT EDUCATION
- Support groups available. Contact CFS Association, 3521 Broadway, Suite 222, Kansas City, MO 64111, (816)931-4777
- CFIDS Association. P.O. Box 220398, Charlotte, NC 28222-0398
- International Chronic Fatigue Syndrome Society. P.O. Box 230108, Portland, OR 97223

MEDICATIONS

DRUG(S) OF CHOICE
• None
• Ampligen, essential fatty acid therapy, IV immune globulin, vitamin B12, and bovine liver extract (LEFAC) are used experimentally.
• Supportive therapy directed toward symptoms with NSAID's, antidepressants including fluoxetine, buspirone, and others.
Contraindications: Refer to manufacturer's literature
Precautions: Refer to manufacturer's literature
Significant possible interactions: Refer to manufacturer's literature

ALTERNATIVE DRUGS N/A

FOLLOWUP

PATIENT MONITORING No consensus.
Periodic re-evaluation appropriate for support, symptom relief, assessment for other cause.

PREVENTION/AVOIDANCE Unknown

POSSIBLE COMPLICATIONS
• Depression
• Socio-economic problems

EXPECTED COURSE/PROGNOSIS
• Indolent; waxes and wanes
• Generally very slow improvement over months or years

MISCELLANEOUS

ASSOCIATED CONDITIONS
• Fibromyalgia (70% reported to meet criteria)
• Depression
• Hypochrondriasis

AGE-RELATED FACTORS
Pediatric: Reported in children
Geriatric: Reported in elderly
Others: N/A

PREGNANCY No information

SYNONYMS
• CFS
• Chronic Epstein-Barr syndrome
• Yuppie flu

ICD-9-CM
300.5 neurasthenia

SEE ALSO
• Epstein-Barr virus infections
• Depression
• Fibromyalgia

OTHER NOTES Controversial topic, data often conflicting

ABBREVIATIONS
CFS = chronic fatigue syndrome

REFERENCES
• Holmes GP, Kaplan JE, et al: Chronic Fatigue Syndrome: A Working Case Definition. Annals of Internal Medicine 1988;108, 387-389
• Klimas NG, et al: Immunologic Abnormalities in Chronic Fatigue Syndrome. J. Clinical Microbiology 1990;28(6),1403-1410
• English T: Skeptical of Skeptics. JAMA 1991;265(8):964,
• An information packet, for health care providers, is available from the CDC's Viral Diseases Division (404)639-1338
• Deale A, Chalder T, Wessely S. Illness beliefs and treatment outcome in chronic fatigue syndrome. J Psychsom Res 1998;45:77-83
• Jason LA, Melrose H, et al. Managing chronic fatigue syndrome: Overview and case study. AAOHN J 1999;47:(1)17-21
• Wessely S. The epidemiology of chronic fatigue syndrome. Epidemiol Psychiatr Soc 1998;7(1):10-24
• Taylor RR, Jason LA. Psychiatric Aspects of chronic fatigue syndrome. Psychiatr Times 16:(7)1-7.
• Friedberg F, Jason LA. Understanding chronic fatigue syndrome: An empirical guide to assessment and treatment. Am Psychological Assoc 1998 - Washington, DC
Illustrations: N/A
Internet references: http://www.5mcc.com

Author(s)
Moshe S. Torem, MD, FAPA

Chronic obstructive pulmonary disease & emphysema

BASICS

DESCRIPTION Chronic obstructive pulmonary disease encompasses several diffuse pulmonary diseases including chronic bronchitis, asthma, cystic fibrosis, bronchiectasis, and emphysema. The term usually refers to a mixture of chronic bronchitis and emphysema.
• Chronic bronchitis is defined clinically by increased mucus production and recurrent cough present on most days for at least three months during at least two consecutive years.
• Emphysema is the destruction of interalveolar septa. The disease occurs in the distal or terminal airways and involves both airways and lung parenchyma.
System(s) affected: Pulmonary
Genetics:
• Chronic bronchitis is not a genetic disorder although some studies have hinted at a predisposition for development of this condition.
• A rare form of emphysema, antiprotease deficiency (due to alpha 1-antitrypsin deficiency), is an inherited disorder that is an expression of two autosomal codominant alleles.
Incidence/Prevalence in USA:
• 10-20% of adults; more than 60,000 deaths/year
• 8 million people have chronic bronchitis; 2 million people have emphysema
Predominant age: Over 40 years
Predominant sex: Male > Female

SIGNS AND SYMPTOMS
• Chronic bronchitis
  ◊ Cough
  ◊ Sputum production
  ◊ Frequent infections
  ◊ Intermittent dyspnea
  ◊ Pedal edema
  ◊ Plethora
  ◊ Cyanosis
  ◊ Wheezing
  ◊ Weight gain
  ◊ Diminished breath sounds
• Emphysema
  ◊ Minimal cough
  ◊ Scant sputum
  ◊ Dyspnea
  ◊ Often significant weight loss
  ◊ Occasional infections
  ◊ Barrel chest
  ◊ Minimal wheezing
  ◊ Use of accessory muscles of respiration
  ◊ Pursed lip breathing
  ◊ Cyanosis is slight or absent
  ◊ Breath sounds very diminished

CAUSES
• Cigarette smoking
• Air pollution
• Antiprotease deficiency
• Occupational exposure (i.e., firefighters)
• Infection possibly (viral)

RISK FACTORS
• Passive smoking (especially adults whose parents smoked)
• Severe viral pneumonia early in life
• Aging
• Ethyl alcohol (EtOH) consumption
• Airway hyperactivity

DIAGNOSIS

DIFFERENTIAL DIAGNOSIS Acute bronchitis, asthma, bronchiectasis, bronchogenic carcinoma, acute viral infection, normal aging of lungs, occupational asthma, chronic pulmonary embolism, sleep apnea, primary alveolar hypoventilation, chronic sinusitis

LABORATORY
• Chronic bronchitis
  ◊ Hypercapnia
  ◊ Polycythemia
  ◊ Hypoxia can be moderate to severe
• Emphysema
  ◊ Normal serum hemoglobin or polycythemia
  ◊ Normal PaCO2; unless FEV1 < 1 L/sec, then can be elevated
  ◊ Mild hypoxia
Drugs that may alter lab results:
Sedatives including alcohol
Disorders that may alter lab results:
Obesity, concurrent restrictive lung dysfunction, primary pulmonary hypertension, acute infections, anemia, pulmonary embolism sleep apnea, congestive heart failure

PATHOLOGICAL FINDINGS
• Chronic bronchitis
  ◊ Bronchial mucous gland enlargement
  ◊ Increased number of secretory cells in surface epithelium
  ◊ Thickened small airways from edema and inflammation
  ◊ Smooth muscle hyperplasia
  ◊ Mucus plugging
  ◊ Bacterial colonization of airways
• Emphysema
  ◊ Entire lung affected
  ◊ Bronchi usually clear of secretions
  ◊ Anthracotic pigment
  ◊ Alveoli enlarged with loss of septa
  ◊ Cartilage atrophy
  ◊ Bullae

SPECIAL TESTS
• Pulmonary function testing
  ◊ Decreased FEV1 with concomitant reduction in FEV1/FVC ratio
  ◊ Poor or absent reversibility to bronchodilators
  ◊ FVC may be normal or reduced
  ◊ Normal or increased total lung capacity
  ◊ Increased residual volume
  ◊ Diffusing capacity is normal or reduced
• Nocturnal oximetry

IMAGING
• Chronic bronchitis chest x-ray shows increased bronchovascular markings and cardiomegaly
• Emphysema chest x-ray shows small heart, hyperinflation, flat diaphragms and possibly bullous changes

DIAGNOSTIC PROCEDURES
• Pulmonary function tests
• ABGs
• Chest x-ray

TREATMENT

APPROPRIATE HEALTH CARE
• Outpatient treatment is usually adequate. However, hospitalization may be required for exacerbation, infection, or diagnostic procedures (i.e., transbronchial lung biopsy).
• Acute respiratory failure may require an intensive care unit and possibly a mechanical ventilator to support the patient

GENERAL MEASURES
• Smoking cessation
• Aggressive treatment of infections
• Treat any reversible bronchospasm
• Reduction of secretions through good pulmonary hygiene
• Cor pulmonale may necessitate use of home oxygen
• Pulmonary rehabilitation
• Appropriate vaccinations
• Adequate hydration

SURGICAL MEASURES
• Lung reduction surgery (selected cases)
• Lung transplantation (selected cases)

ACTIVITY As tolerated. Full activity should be encouraged.

DIET A well balanced, high protein diet is suggested. Low carbohydrates may benefit those with hypercarbia.

PATIENT EDUCATION
• Printed material is available from the National Jewish Hospital in Denver, Colorado. The local branch of the American Lung Association also has educational material.
• Coach patients in pulmonary rehabilitation

Chronic obstructive pulmonary disease & emphysema

MEDICATIONS

DRUG(S) OF CHOICE
• Theophylline - (Theo-Dur, Slo-bid, Unidur, Uniphyl) 400 mg/day. Increase by 100-200 mg in one to two weeks if necessary.
• Sympathomimetics - e.g., metaproterenol (Alupent), albuterol (Proventil, Ventolin), pirbuterol (Maxair), terbutaline (Brethaire). 1-2 puffs from the metered dose inhaler every 4-6 hrs. May be increased to every 3 hrs. Use of spacer device (aerochamber, inspirease) may be beneficial. (Up to 4 puffs recommended by some.) Long acting sympathomimetics - salmeterol (Serevent) to be considered.
• Anticholinergics - ipratropium (Atrovent). Two puffs (36 μg) 4 times daily. May take additional inhalations not to exceed 12 in 24 hrs.
• Corticosteroids - prednisone (Deltasone). Given orally 7.5-15 mg/day. Most useful in bronchitis with some reversibility.

Contraindications:
• Theophylline - hypersensitivity
• Sympathomimetics - cardiac arrhythmias associated with tachycardia; hypersensitivity
• Anticholinergics - hypersensitivity to atropine or its derivatives
• Corticosteroids - systemic fungal infections; hypersensitivity

Precautions:
• Theophylline - reduce dosage in patients with impaired renal or liver function; age over 55; CHF. Therapeutic drug level is 5-15 μg/mL (55.5-111 μmol).
• Rifampin - may cause a decrease in theophylline levels by increasing theophylline metabolism. Monitor serum theophylline level.
• Sympathomimetics - excessive use may be dangerous. May need to reduce dose in patients with cardiovascular disease, hypertension, hyperthyroidism, diabetes or convulsive disorders.
• Anticholinergics - narrow angle glaucoma, prostatic hypertrophy, bladder-neck obstruction
• Corticosteroids - may mask infection or predispose to infection, especially fungal; subcapsular cataracts; glaucoma; adrenocortical insufficiency; psychic derangements; gastrointestinal bleeding; diabetes mellitus, reactivation of tuberculosis

Significant possible interactions:
• Theophylline - lithium carbonate; propranolol; erythromycin; cimetidine; ranitidine; rifampin; ciprofloxacin
Addition of cimetidine, ciprofloxacin, or erythromycin will decrease theophylline clearance causing theophylline levels to rise. Careful monitoring of serum theophylline levels is warranted. (Note: cimetidine is now an OTC drug.)
• Sympathomimetics - other sympathomimetics, monoamine oxidase inhibitors or tricyclic antidepressants
• Anticholinergics - refer to manufacturer's profile
• Corticosteroids - NSAID's (indomethacin), aspirin, synthetic thyroid hormone

ALTERNATIVE DRUGS
• Theophylline may be given orally, intravenously or by rectal suppository
• Sympathomimetics may be given as aerosolized solution (albuterol, metaproterenol [Metaprel], isoetharine) when mixed with saline; orally (Alupent, Proventil, Brethine, Ventolin) or subcutaneously (terbutaline)
• Anticholinergics - atropine sulfate, glycopyrrolate. Ipratropium (Atrovent) now available in aerosolized solution and may be mixed with albuterol.
• Corticosteroids may be given intravenously (hydrocortisone, methylprednisolone) or inhaled (beclomethasone, flunisolide, triamcinolone acetonide)
• Home oxygen

FOLLOWUP

PATIENT MONITORING
• Severe or unstable patients should be seen monthly
• When stable, may be seen biannually
• Check theophylline level with each dose adjustment until the desired level (or result) is achieved, then check every 6-12 months
• With home oxygen, check arterial blood gasses yearly or with any change in condition. Monitor oxygen saturation (pulse oximetry) more frequently.
• Some patients only desaturate at night thereby only needing nocturnal oxygen
• Avoid travel at high altitude. Air travel with oxygen requires pre-arrangement.

PREVENTION/AVOIDANCE
Avoidance of smoking is the most important preventive measure. Passive smoke also has been shown to be harmful.

POSSIBLE COMPLICATIONS
• Infection is common
• Cor pulmonale, secondary polycythemia, bullous lung disease, acute or chronic respiratory failure, pulmonary hypertension, malnutrition

EXPECTED COURSE/PROGNOSIS
• The patient's age and post-bronchodilator forced expiratory volume (FEV1) are the most important predictors of prognosis. Young age and FEV1 > 50% predicted have a good prognosis. Older patients with more severe lung disease do worse.
• Supplemental oxygen, when indicated, has been shown to increase survival
• Smoking cessation is also important for an improved prognosis
• Malnutrition, cor pulmonale, hypercapnia and pulse > 100 indicate a poor prognosis

MISCELLANEOUS

ASSOCIATED CONDITIONS
• Lung cancer
• Coronary artery disease
• Peptic ulcer disease
• Chronic sinusitis
• Malnutrition
• Laryngeal carcinoma

AGE-RELATED FACTORS
Pediatric: Repeated childhood respiratory illnesses make COPD a greater risk
Geriatric: Relative risk is 1.2 to 2.3 times greater than in younger person
Others: Unusual under age 25 unless antiprotease deficiency is present. Incidence increases as age approaches 60.

PREGNANCY N/A

SYNONYMS
• Bronchitis
• COLD (Chronic obstructive lung disease)
• OAD (Obstructive airways disease)
• COPD

ICD-9-CM
496 COPD
492.8 Emphysema

SEE ALSO
• Asthma
• Bronchitis, acute

OTHER NOTES
• Albuterol is also known as salbutamol
• Other important considerations for treatment include adequate hydration, supplemental oxygen, antibiotics when indicated, mucolytic agents, pulmonary rehabilitation, good pulmonary hygiene

ABBREVIATIONS
FVC = forced vital capacity
FEV1 = forced expiratory volume at 1 second
COPD = chronic obstructive pulmonary disease
ABG = arterial blood gases

REFERENCES
Fishman A: Pulmonary Diseases and Disorders. 2nd Ed. New York, McGraw-Hill Book Co., 1988
Illustrations: N/A
Internet references: http://www.5mcc.com

Author(s)
Alan J. Cropp, MD, FCCP

Cirrhosis of the liver

BASICS

DESCRIPTION Histologically cirrhosis is defined by the presence of fibrosis with regenerative nodules. Clinically cirrhosis presents with evidence of portal hypertension, i.e. ascites, variceal bleeding, hepatic encephalopathy.
System(s) affected: Gastrointestinal, Cardiovascular, Endocrine/Metabolic
Genetics: For hereditary hemochromatosis HFe gene mutation C282Y; for Wilson's disease mutation on chromosome 13
Incidence/Prevalence in USA: Accounts for over 30,000 deaths per year
Predominant age: Etiology dependent
Predominant sex: Etiology dependent

SIGNS AND SYMPTOMS
• The onset of the disease is often insidious with:
  ◊ Fatigue
  ◊ Anorexia
  ◊ Nausea
  ◊ Abdominal discomfort and distention
  ◊ Weakness and malaise
• Signs and symptoms that are related to cirrhosis are those of complications:
  ◊ Hematemesis
  ◊ Encephalopathy
  ◊ Jaundice
  ◊ Hepatomegaly
  ◊ Splenomegaly
  ◊ Abdominal collateral circulation
  ◊ Ascites
  ◊ Gynecomastia
  ◊ Testicular atrophy
  ◊ Asterixis (liver flap)
  ◊ Palmar erythema
  ◊ Spider angiomas

CAUSES
• Alcoholic cirrhosis
• Chronic viral hepatitis, B (with/without D), C
• Wilson's disease
• Hemochromatosis
• Alpha 1-antitrypsin deficiency
• Cystic fibrosis
• Autoimmune chronic hepatitis with cirrhosis
• Primary biliary cirrhosis
• Secondary biliary cirrhosis
• Primary sclerosing cholangitis
• Cardiac cirrhosis
• Drug induced (other than alcohol)
• Nonalcoholic steatohepatitis (NASH)
• Inherited causes that may be present in infancy and childhood:
  ◊ Glycogen storage disease
  ◊ Galactosemia
  ◊ Fructose intolerance
  ◊ Tyrosinemia
  ◊ Acid cholesterol ester hydrolase deficiency

RISK FACTORS
• Alcohol use
• Hepatotoxic drugs
• Excessive iron ingestion

DIAGNOSIS

DIFFERENTIAL DIAGNOSIS
• Depends on presentation
• Ascites - increased right heart pressure, hepatic vein thrombosis, peritoneal infection or malignancy, pancreatic disease, thyroid disease, lymphatic obstruction
• Other causes of UGI bleeding
• Other metabolic encephalopathies - renal, cardiopulmonary, drug.

LABORATORY
• Recognition of liver injury - elevated AST, elevated ALT; elevated alkaline phosphatase. Note: All liver injury tests may be normal.
• Functional impairment of the liver - elevated bilirubin, decreased albumin, elevated globulin, prolonged prothrombin time
• Etiologic screen for liver disease
  ◊ Ceruloplasmin (Wilson's disease)
  ◊ Iron, iron binding capacity, ferritin (hemochromatosis)
  ◊ Alpha fetoprotein (hepatocellular cancer)
  ◊ HBsAg (hepatitis B)
  ◊ Anti-HCV (hepatitis C)
  ◊ HCV RNA by PCR to confirm activity
  ◊ ANA (autoimmune hepatitis)
  ◊ Anti-smooth muscle antibody (autoimmune hepatitis)
  ◊ Anti-mitochondrial antibody (AMA) (primary biliary cirrhosis)
  ◊ Alpha 1-antitrypsin (deficiency)
  ◊ Serum protein electrophoresis (SPEP) - increased IgG with any liver disease; increased IgM with primary biliary cirrhosis (PBC)
Drugs that may alter lab results: N/A
Disorders that may alter lab results: N/A

PATHOLOGICAL FINDINGS
• Fibrosis and regenerative nodules; specific findings/patterns may indicate etiology
• Quantitative liver chemistry for iron, copper
• Special stains for iron, copper, bilirubin, collagen, alpha 1-antitrypsin, hepatitis B

SPECIAL TESTS
• Laparoscopic liver biopsy to reduce sampling error
• Cholangiography by endoscopy and MRI to rule out common duct obstruction and recognize sclerosing cholangitis
• Doppler ultrasound to indicate direction of flow in and patency of the portal and hepatic veins
• Visceral angiography to determine vascular anatomy, patency and collaterals
• Esophagogastroduodenoscopy to assess varices

IMAGING
• Ultrasound good for detecting bile duct dilatation and space occupying lesions. Cannot make diagnosis of cirrhosis based on ultrasound alone.
• CT, if ultrasound technically inadequate

DIAGNOSTIC PROCEDURES
• A liver biopsy establishes the diagnosis of cirrhosis
• Patterns of injury as well as special stains may identify a precise etiology such as alcoholic liver disease, hemochromatosis, alpha 1-antitrypsin deficiency, hepatitis B, primary biliary cirrhosis
• Level of activity determined

TREATMENT

APPROPRIATE HEALTH CARE
Outpatient except for complicating emergencies:
• GI bleeding
• Hepatic encephalopathy
• Spontaneous bacterial peritonitis
• Unexplained decompensation
• Renal failure

GENERAL MEASURES
• Treatment designed to remove or alleviate underlying cause of cirrhosis, prevent further liver damage and prevent complications
• Phlebotomy for hemochromatosis
• Therapies involve drug treatment, dietary restrictions, rest, other supportive measures. Adequate protein intake for liver regeneration.

SURGICAL MEASURES
• Interventional
  ◊ Possible procedures for portal hypertension include - splenorenal or portacaval anastomosis, transjugular intrahepatic portal-systemic shunt
  ◊ Transplantation - in suitable candidate (substance free, motivated and adherent). Evaluate prior to major decompensation.

ACTIVITY
Maintain as active as possible. With peripheral edema, leg elevation necessary.

DIET
• Adequate protein (1 gm/kg) and generous calories to help regenerate the liver
• In the presence of hepatic encephalopathy protein restriction is necessary
• In the presence of ascites salt restriction is necessary (2 gm or less/day)
• In the presence of hyponatremia (Na < 130 mEq [< 130 mmol]) fluid restriction is necessary (< 1 L)
• No alcohol

PATIENT EDUCATION
• Pamphlets are available through: American Liver Foundation, (800)223-0179
• Additional material: National Digestive Diseases Information Clearinghouse, Box NDDIC, Bethesda, MD 20892, (301)468-6344

Cirrhosis of the liver

MEDICATIONS

DRUG(S) OF CHOICE
• Large esophageal varices seen at endoscopy prior to clinical bleeding - nonselective beta blocker at a dose to decrease the resting pulse by 25%
• Ascites: spironolactone 100 mg up to 400 mg every day as a single dose. Takes three days before onset of action. Add furosemide 40-160 mg/day if needed. Loop diuretics may produce a rapid diuresis and subsequent intravascular volume depletion.
• Encephalopathy: lactulose (Cholac) 15-30 mL/day to produce 2-3 soft stools per day
• Spontaneous bacterial peritonitis (SBP): cefotaxime alone as initial treatment; norfloxacin 400 mg/day or trimethoprim-sulfamethoxazole decreases risk for subsequent development of SBP after treatment
• Specific drug based on etiology
   ◊ Wilson's disease: penicillamine, 125-250 mg qid (give on empty stomach to avoid inactivation by metal binding)
   ◊ Autoimmune chronic hepatitis: corticosteroids with or without azathioprine
   ◊ Chronic hepatitis B: interferon
   ◊ Hepatitis C: interferon and ribavirin
   ◊ PBC: ursodiol (ursodeoxycholic acid), 12-15 mg/kg/day in a bid dose
Contraindications: Refer to manufacturer's literature
Precautions: Refer to manufacturer's literature
Significant possible interactions: Refer to manufacturer's literature

ALTERNATIVE DRUGS
Ursodiol (ursodeoxycholic acid) for cholestatic disease

FOLLOWUP

PATIENT MONITORING
• In a stable patient - yearly battery of liver tests. After 10 years, consider alpha-fetoprotein and imaging to detect hepatocellular carcinoma.
• In an unstable patient - tests may be repeated at weekly intervals
• Have patient monitor weight and maintain a daily diary

PREVENTION/AVOIDANCE
• Limit use of alcohol and other liver toxins
• No sharing of syringes
• Safer sex
• Screening of family members when a genetic disease is recognized
• Influenza and pneumococcal vaccines for cirrhosis patients exposed to crowds
• Hepatitis A and B vaccines
• Liver test surveillance while on hepatotoxic drugs (e.g., INH)

POSSIBLE COMPLICATIONS
• Ascites
• Jaundice
• Coagulopathy
• Hepatic encephalopathy
• Bleeding esophageal varices
• Liver failure
• Carcinoma of the liver (uncommon)
• Susceptibility to infections
• Spontaneous bacterial peritonitis
• Renal failure

EXPECTED COURSE/PROGNOSIS
A function of ongoing hepatic injury as well as residual hepatic reserve. If a treatable cause is identified and intervention results in cessation of liver destruction, then the prognosis may be good.

MISCELLANEOUS

ASSOCIATED CONDITIONS
• Hepatitis
• Diseases and defects of the bile ducts
• Cystic fibrosis
• Heart failure
• Hepatocellular cancer

AGE-RELATED FACTORS
Pediatric: N/A
Geriatric: Cirrhosis is one of the leading causes of death for people over age 65
Others: N/A

PREGNANCY
Cirrhosis may decompensate during pregnancy. Higher rates of spontaneous abortion, premature birth and perinatal death.

SYNONYMS
N/A

ICD-9-CM
571.2 Alcoholic cirrhosis of liver
571.5 Cirrhosis of liver without mention of alcohol

SEE ALSO
N/A

OTHER NOTES
N/A

ABBREVIATIONS
PBC = Primary biliary cirrhosis
UGI = upper gastrointestinal
ANA = anti-nuclear antibody

REFERENCES
• Sampliner RE: The recognition of early liver disease. Hospital Practice 1989;53-56
• Schiff ER, Sorrell MF, Maddrey WC, eds: Diseases of the Liver. Philadelphia, Lippincott Williams & Wilkins, 1999
• Runyon BA: Care of patients with ascites. NEJM 1994;330:337-342
Illustrations: N/A
Internet references: http://www.5mcc.com

Author(s)
Richard E. Sampliner, MD

Claudication

BASICS

DESCRIPTION The feeling of muscle fatigue after a period of minimal exercise of an extremity. The feeling may progress to a cramp-like pain, usually in the calf muscles. It is always relieved by resting the extremity. It can be reproduced by undergoing a similar exercise pattern. It may occur in the arms, but is more common in the legs, calf > thigh.

System(s) affected: Cardiovascular, Musculoskeletal
Genetics: N/A
Incidence/Prevalence in USA: Common
Predominant age: Common in males > 55, females > 60
Predominant sex: Male > Female (4:1)

SIGNS AND SYMPTOMS
• May start gradually or suddenly
• Unable to walk distances
• Pain varies from muscle tiredness to a frank cramp in muscle group involved
• May be a loss of hair on toes
• Foot may show rubor on dependency
• Pedal pulses absent
• Popliteal pulse absent
• With thigh claudication, femoral pulse absent
• Absent pulses in the distal extremity, secondary to more proximal arterial occlusion. The occlusion is usually from an arterial plaque.

CAUSES
• Lower extremity claudication - blockage of superficial femoral artery, secondary to arteriosclerosis in 95% of cases
• Other causes of arterial blocks - embolus, popliteal entrapment, adventitious cystic disease of popliteal artery, thromboangiitis obliterans
• Thigh and hip claudication - blockage of aortic and iliac vessels
• Upper extremity claudication - similar blocks of subclavian, axillary, and brachial artery

RISK FACTORS
• Smoking
• Diabetes
• Hypertension
• Hyperlipidemia
• Obesity
• Preexisting heart disease

DIAGNOSIS

DIFFERENTIAL DIAGNOSIS
• Pseudoclaudication, sometimes secondary to some form of spinal stenosis, usually impinging on the cauda equina portion of the spinal cord. The pain in the legs is characteristically relieved by squatting or sitting. The latter relieves tension on spinal nerve roots.
• Osteoarthritis of hips and knees sometimes can be confused with claudication, but pain starts immediately on weight bearing.

LABORATORY N/A
Drugs that may alter lab results: None
Disorders that may alter lab results:
Arterial calcinosis, often found in diabetics, will cause a falsely high ankle/arm index

PATHOLOGICAL FINDINGS N/A

SPECIAL TESTS
• Noninvasive vascular tests - pulse volume recordings. Measurement of blood pressure in the arm compared to pedal arterial pressures before and after exercise establish the diagnosis as well as the severity of occlusion. The patient with one to two block claudication will have an ankle/arm index of 0.7-0.4 with 1.0 being normal. If below 0.4, there is a major threat of losing part of the leg if left untreated. Pseudoclaudication does not affect the pulses in the extremity.

IMAGING
• Duplex ultrasound
• Intra-arterial arteriography

DIAGNOSTIC PROCEDURES
• Arteriography - when surgical correction is anticipated
• Noninvasive vascular tests

TREATMENT

APPROPRIATE HEALTH CARE
Outpatient, except for severe cases or advanced disease

GENERAL MEASURES
• Conservative measures: stop smoking, initiate walking and exercise program, control of hyperlipidemia
• Reduce risk factors

SURGICAL MEASURES
• Surgical treatment with bypass of arterial obstruction may be appropriate in selected cases
• Angioplasty

ACTIVITY Ambulatory

DIET None

PATIENT EDUCATION Prevention methods

MEDICATIONS

DRUG(S) OF CHOICE
• Aspirin - to reduce platelet aggregation: low dose 80 mg/day
• Pentoxifylline (Trental) - to decrease internal configuration of red cells - 400 mg bid-tid. Administer for at least 6-8 weeks to determine if therapy is effective.
Contraindications: Refer to manufacturer's literature
Precautions: Try to reduce risk factors first
Significant possible interactions: Refer to manufacturer's literature

ALTERNATIVE DRUGS
• Ticlopidine
• Vasodilators
• Calcium channel blockers
• Anticoagulants

FOLLOWUP

PATIENT MONITORING
Peripheral non-invasive vascular studies every 6 months

PREVENTION/AVOIDANCE
• Institute walking program of 4-5 miles
• Avoid smoking

POSSIBLE COMPLICATIONS
Only 10% of people without diabetes will progress to some amputation of the involved extremity

EXPECTED COURSE/PROGNOSIS
Gradual improvement in walking distance or progression of problem to gangrene, rest pain and/or tissue necrosis

MISCELLANEOUS

ASSOCIATED CONDITIONS
Other manifestations of arteriosclerotic vascular disease - history of myocardial infarction(s), carotid disease, renal vascular hypertension

AGE-RELATED FACTORS
Pediatric: N/A
Geriatric: More common with advancing age
Others: N/A

PREGNANCY
N/A

SYNONYMS
N/A

ICD-9-CM
443.9 Peripheral vascular disease, unspecified (intermittent claudication)

SEE ALSO
• Thromboangiitis obliterans (Buerger's disease)

OTHER NOTES
N/A

ABBREVIATIONS
N/A

REFERENCES
Rutherford RB, ed: Vascular Surgery. 4th Ed. Philadelphia, WB Saunders Co, 1995
Illustrations: N/A
Internet references: http://www.5mcc.com

Author(s)
William V. Sharp, MD

Coarctation of the aorta

BASICS

DESCRIPTION A constriction (discrete or of varying lengths) of the aorta usually located just distal to the left subclavian artery at the junction of the ligamentum arteriosum
System(s) affected: Cardiovascular
Genetics: No Mendelian inheritance, but common in Turner's syndrome
Incidence/Prevalence in USA: 64/100,000 under 1 year of age
Predominant age: Usually diagnosed in infancy
Predominant sex: Male > Female (1.7:1)

SIGNS AND SYMPTOMS
• Headaches
• Exertional leg fatigue and pain
• Prominent neck pulsations
• Epistaxis
• Hypertension
• Pulse disparity
• Delayed, weak, or absent pulse
• Prominent left ventricular impulse
• Murmur (aortic stenosis or insufficiency, ventricular septal defect, rarely mitral valve)
• S4 systolic ejection click
• Bruit (coarctation, collaterals, patent ductus arteriosus)
• Cyanosis, rarely
• In infancy may also have heart failure, failure to thrive, irritability, tachypnea, and dyspnea
• Extensive collaterals develop from branches of the subclavian, internal mammary, superior intercostal, and axillary arteries

CAUSES Congenital: Takayasu's arteritis, Turner's syndrome, multiple left-sided obstruction

RISK FACTORS
• Turner's syndrome
• Congenital left heart abnormalities

DIAGNOSIS

DIFFERENTIAL DIAGNOSIS
• Takayasu's arteritis
• Neurofibromatosis
• Pseudocoarctation (with or without hypertension, peripheral vascular disease)

LABORATORY N/A
Drugs that may alter lab results: N/A
Disorders that may alter lab results: N/A

PATHOLOGICAL FINDINGS
• Segmental tubular hypoplasia
• Discrete obstruction with medial thickening
• Distal aneurysm

SPECIAL TESTS
• Doppler examination of pulses reveals disparity
• Electrocardiogram may show left ventricular hypertrophy
• Blood pressures - all 4 extremities

IMAGING
• Chest x-ray may show rib notching, "3" sign, rarely cardiomegaly
• Echocardiography for coarctation and coexisting cardiac anomalies
• Transesophageal echocardiography
• Magnetic resonance imaging (MRI)

DIAGNOSTIC PROCEDURES Cardiac catheterization and angiography: post-stenotic dilation

TREATMENT

APPROPRIATE HEALTH CARE
Inpatient surgery

GENERAL MEASURES N/A

SURGICAL MEASURES
• Surgical correction or balloon angioplasty can be done in infancy if urgently needed. Best results when performed age 1-2 years.
• Surgery should be done in childhood and adulthood as soon as coarctation diagnosed to prevent late complications
• Three common surgical procedures for correction of coarctation include (1) end-to-end anastomosis, (2) patch aortoplasty (insertion of dacron patch), and, (3) subclavian flap procedure
• Balloon angioplasty of coarctation offers good results for primary treatment and for post-operative re-stenosis

ACTIVITY Exercise may exacerbate hypertension, but normal activity recommended after correction

DIET No special diet

PATIENT EDUCATION
• Discuss post-coarctation syndrome
• For patient education materials favorably reviewed on this topic, contact: American Heart Association, 7320 Greenville Avenue, Dallas, TX 75231, (214)373-6300

Coarctation of the aorta

 MEDICATIONS

DRUG(S) OF CHOICE
• Alprostadil (prostaglandin E1), patency of ductus arteriosus
• Antibiotic prophylaxis (for dental and/or invasive procedures) for life (even after correction)
• Antihypertensives if needed
• Preload and afterload reduction if heart failure develops
Contraindications: Refer to manufacturer's profile of each drug
Precautions:
• Lowering upper extremity blood pressure may cause hypoperfusion of lower extremities
• Lowering blood pressure not advised in pregnancy unless emergency
Significant possible interactions: Refer to manufacturer's profile of each drug

ALTERNATIVE DRUGS N/A

 FOLLOWUP

PATIENT MONITORING Frequent post-operative followup for evidence of re-stenosis (check for hypertension and pulse disparities) and late complications

PREVENTION/AVOIDANCE Patients should be encouraged to have normal lifestyles and activities after coarctation correction

POSSIBLE COMPLICATIONS
• Most common with late or no correction
• Heart failure
• Aneurysm of circle of Willis, rupture possible
• Hypertension
• Rupture or dissection of aortic aneurysm
• Endarteritis or endocarditis (need antibiotic prophylaxis)
• Aortic valve disease (stenosis or insufficiency)
• Post coarctectomy syndrome: recurrence, hypertension, atherosclerotic heart disease, aneurysm at site of coarctectomy, progressive aortic stenosis and/or regurgitation

EXPECTED COURSE/PROGNOSIS
• Depends on age of repair and presence of other cardiac abnormalities
• Residual or restenosis (6-33%)
• Subsequent cardiac surgery (11%)
• Hypertension (25%)
• Survival after surgery: 10 years (91%), 20 years (84%), 30 years (72%)
• Uncorrected, 80% mortality before age 50

 MISCELLANEOUS

ASSOCIATED CONDITIONS
• Bicuspid aortic valve (85%)
• Patent ductus arteriosus (65%)
• Ventricular septal defect (30-35%)
• Aortic stenosis and/or insufficiency
• Subvalvular aortic stenosis
• Mitral valve abnormalities (common)
• Transposition of great vessels or double outlet right ventricle
• Aneurysm of circle of Willis

AGE-RELATED FACTORS Greater risk of complications if correction is delayed beyond early childhood. Often diagnosis is delayed.
Pediatric: N/A
Geriatric: N/A
Others: N/A

PREGNANCY Uncorrected (or restenosis) coarctation carries high risk of aortic rupture or dissection and cerebral hemorrhage (aneurysm of circle of Willis rupture), but lower risk of pre-eclampsia than other forms of hypertension

SYNONYMS N/A

ICD-9-CM
747.1 Coarctation of aorta

SEE ALSO N/A

OTHER NOTES N/A

ABBREVIATIONS N/A

REFERENCES
• Hurst JW, et al: The Heart. 7th Ed. New York, McGraw-Hill, 1990
• Adams FH, Emmanouilides GC, Riemenschneider TA: Moss' Heart Disease in Infants, Children and Adolescents. 4th Ed. Baltimore, Williams & Wilkins, 1989
• Braunwalk E: Heart Disease. 4th Ed. Philadelphia, WB Saunders Co, 1992.
Illustrations: N/A
Internet references: http://www.5mcc.com

Author(s)
Karil Bellah, MD

Coccidioidomycosis

BASICS

DESCRIPTION Pulmonary fungal infection endemic to the Southwest USA. Can become progressive and involve extrapulmonary sites, including bone, CNS, and skin. Known as the "great imitator." Incubation period is 1 to 4 weeks after exposure.
System(s) affected: Pulmonary, Nervous, Musculoskeletal, Skin/Exocrine, Endocrine/Metabolic
Genetics: Unknown
Incidence/Prevalence in USA: 100,000 cases per year. (0.5% extrapulmonary)
Predominant age: All ages
Predominant sex: Male = Female

SIGNS AND SYMPTOMS
- Anorexia
- Arthralgias
- Chest pain
- Chills
- Confusion
- Cough, dry or productive
- Cyanosis
- Dyspnea
- Erythema nodosum
- Fatigue
- Fever
- Headache
- Hepatomegaly
- Hydrocephalus
- Hyperreflexia
- Malaise
- Night sweats
- Pleural friction rub
- Rash
- Sore throat
- Splenomegaly
- Tachycardia
- Tenosynovitis
- Toxic erythema
- Weight loss
- Note: Over half of cases are subclinical

CAUSES Coccidioides immitis, a soil fungus especially adapted to arid conditions. Liberated spores are inhaled when soil is disturbed: digging, construction sites, archaeological sites, dust storms, spelunking (exploring caves). Soil that lines rodent burrows is worst.

RISK FACTORS
- Certain groups are more prone to dissemination: immunocompromised hosts, pregnant women, African-Americans, Filipinos.
- CNS involvement more common in young white males
- Immunosuppression. Previously infected patients can experience relapse years later through the mechanism of cell-mediated immune deficiency.
- Diabetes mellitus
- AIDS

DIAGNOSIS

DIFFERENTIAL DIAGNOSIS
- Pneumonia, all etiologies
- Lung carcinoma
- Sarcoidosis
- Histoplasmosis, other fungi
- Lung abscess
- TB
- Lymphoma
- Meningitis
- Plus all other causes of cough, fever, fatigue
- Old granulomas can be mistaken for tumors

LABORATORY
- Skin test turns positive at 3 weeks to 3 months; may remain positive indefinitely; applying skin test will not interfere with serologies
- Serology - precipitin antibodies (IgM) rise within 2 weeks and disappear after 2 months; complement fixation antibodies (IgG) rise at 1-3 months; patients with mild symptoms may never develop detectable serology
- Culture of sputum, wound exudate, joint aspirate; unlikely to grow fungus in urine, blood, pleural fluid
Drugs that may alter lab results: Steroids may alter ability to react to skin testing
Disorders that may alter lab results: N/A

PATHOLOGICAL FINDINGS Fungal elements, spherules

SPECIAL TESTS Biopsy of affected tissue, e.g., lung nodule, skin lesion

IMAGING Chest x-ray findings include - normal, infiltrate(s), nodule(s), cavity, adenopathy mediastinal or hilar, pleural effusion

DIAGNOSTIC PROCEDURES If unable to establish diagnosis from skin testing and serologies - bronchoscopy, fine-needle biopsy, open lung biopsy, pleural biopsy, bone/skin/node biopsy

TREATMENT

APPROPRIATE HEALTH CARE
- Outpatient except in very severe cases
- Recommend referral to pulmonary or infectious disease specialist if drug treatment becomes imperative. Consider such treatment if IgG titers > 1:16, if disease persists without improvement over 6 weeks, or if skin test remains negative in the face of positive serology.

GENERAL MEASURES
- Cool mist humidifier for dry cough or sore throat
- Rest
- Supportive therapy

SURGICAL MEASURES N/A

ACTIVITY As tolerated

DIET No special diet

PATIENT EDUCATION For patient education materials favorably reviewed on this topic, contact: American Lung Association, 1740 Broadway, New York, NY 10019, (212)315-8700

MEDICATIONS

DRUG(S) OF CHOICE
• In mild cases, treat for symptomatic relief of cough with antitussives plus treat pleuritic pain with nonsteroidal anti-inflammatory agents
• For persistent, progressive, or disseminated disease the following drugs are indicated. However, dosing, whom to treat, and length of treatment is controversial.
  ◊ Amphotericin B: 0.5-1.0 mg/kg with a total cumulative dose of 2-4 gm
  ◊ Ketoconazole: 200-400 mg/day
  ◊ Fluconazole: 200-400 mg/day.
Fluconazole is also the treatment of choice for coccimeningitis with a usual dose of 800 mg/day.
Contraindications: Avoid steroids
Precautions: Amphotericin is highly nephrotoxic.
Significant possible interactions:
• Ketoconazole-H2 blockers: decrease absorption of ketoconazole (ketoconazole requires an acidic pH for absorption).
• Azole antifungals-terfenadine (Seldane) or astemizole (Hismanal): QT prolongation and ventricular arrhythmias

ALTERNATIVE DRUGS N/A

FOLLOWUP

PATIENT MONITORING
• If skin test and serology are negative but index of suspicion is high, repeat every 2 weeks. With positive serologies, follow titers every 2 weeks until titers are dropping and patient has clinical improvement or resolution.
• Follow abnormal chest x-rays until findings are resolved or scarring process is complete

PREVENTION/AVOIDANCE
• Not contagious between host and contacts
• Cultures in lab are highly contagious via inhalation and lab personnel must be very cautious when handling specimens
• High risk populations (see Risk factors) should consider avoiding high risk activities, such as construction, archaeological digs, etc.)

POSSIBLE COMPLICATIONS
• Severe cases are fatal, especially if associated with meningitis. Can cause destruction of pulmonary tissue due to scarring, cavities, etc.
• Hemoptysis

EXPECTED COURSE/PROGNOSIS
• Most cases are self-limited, resolve within a few months. Progressive and disseminated disease can be difficult to eradicate.
• Prognosis poor if weak cell mediated immunity response or high IgG
• Relapse of extrapulmonary or disseminated disease is common.

MISCELLANEOUS

ASSOCIATED CONDITIONS N/A

AGE-RELATED FACTORS
Pediatric: N/A
Geriatric: N/A
Others: N/A

PREGNANCY Increased risk for dissemination, especially if contracted late in gestation

SYNONYMS
• Cocci
• Desert fever
• Posada-Wernicke disease
• Valley fever
• San Joaquin fever

ICD-9-CM
114.9 Coccidiomycosis, unspecified

SEE ALSO N/A

OTHER NOTES Travel history is essential when working up any pulmonary infection not responding to normal measures

ABBREVIATIONS N/A

REFERENCES
• Isselbacher KJ, et al, eds: Harrison's Principles of Internal Medicine. 13th Ed. New York, McGraw-Hill, 1994
• Hedges E, Miller S: Coccidiomycosis: Office diagnosis and treatment. Amer Fam Phys 1990
Illustrations: N/A
Internet references: http://www.5mcc.com

Author(s)
Sandra Miller, MD

Colic, infantile

BASICS

DESCRIPTION Colic is an incompletely understood state of excessive crying seen in young infants who are otherwise well. A working definition - abnormal crying that lasts > 3 hours/day for at least 3 times/week.
System(s) affected: Gastrointestinal, Nervous
Genetics: N/A
Incidence/Prevalence in USA:
10,000/100,000 in some reports, as high as 25,000/100,000 in others
Predominant Age: 3 weeks of age to 3 months of age
Predominant Sex: Male = Female

SIGNS AND SYMPTOMS
• Rhythmic crying, paroxysmal
• No consolability
• Fist clenching
• Back arching
• Drawing up of infant's legs
• Excessive flatus

CAUSES
• Poorly understood
• Small percentage related to milk allergy

RISK FACTORS Physiologic predisposition in infant

DIAGNOSIS

DIFFERENTIAL DIAGNOSIS
• Any organic cause for excessive crying in infants (i.e. meningitis, sepsis, strangulated hernia, occult fracture)
• Entirely a clinical diagnosis

LABORATORY N/A
Drugs that may alter lab results: N/A
Disorders that may alter lab results: N/A

PATHOLOGICAL FINDINGS N/A

SPECIAL TESTS N/A

IMAGING N/A

DIAGNOSTIC PROCEDURES N/A

TREATMENT

APPROPRIATE HEALTH CARE
Outpatient management

GENERAL MEASURES
• Handling of the colicky infant in a calm and non-stimulating manner should be demonstrated
• Use of pacifier
• Use of gentle rhythmic motion (i.e., car rides)
• Use of music

SURGICAL MEASURES N/A

ACTIVITY N/A

DIET Removal of cow's milk from diet for a one week trial

PATIENT EDUCATION American Academy of Pediatrics, 141 Northwest Point Blvd., P.O. Box 927, Elk Grove Village, IL 60009-0927, (800)433-9016

MEDICATIONS

DRUG(S) OF CHOICE Simethicone may be useful in some cases
Contraindications: N/A
Precautions: N/A
Significant possible interactions: N/A

ALTERNATIVE DRUGS N/A

FOLLOWUP

PATIENT MONITORING Frequent outpatient visits as needed for parental reassurance and education

PREVENTION/AVOIDANCE N/A

POSSIBLE COMPLICATIONS N/A

EXPECTED COURSE/PROGNOSIS
• Usually subsides by 3 months of age
• Prognosis not sufficiently investigated

MISCELLANEOUS

ASSOCIATED CONDITIONS N/A

AGE-RELATED FACTORS
Pediatric: A problem of infancy
Geriatric: N/A
Others: N/A

PREGNANCY N/A
Others: N/A

SYNONYMS N/A

ICD-9-CM 789.0 abdominal pain

SEE ALSO N/A

OTHER NOTES N/A

ABBREVIATIONS N/A

REFERENCES Behrman RE, Kleigman RM: Nelson Textbook of Pediatrics. Philadelphia, WB Saunders Co, 1993
Illustrations: N/A
Internet references: http://www.5mcc.com

Author(s)
Jeryl Dansky, MD

Colorectal malignancy

BASICS

DESCRIPTION A malignant neoplasm arising from the luminal surface of the colon, rectum or anus.
- Adenocarcinoma - by far, most common histologic form, usually arising from benign adenoma. Unequally distributed, with 38% in proximal colon and 62% in distal colon or rectum.
- Carcinoid - uncommon, arising from enterochromaffin cells. Usually located in appendix or rectum; not likely to metastasize unless larger than 2 cm in diameter.
- Squamous cell carcinoma - uncommon form; located in the anal canal. Also called epidermoid or cloacogenic.
- Melanoma - rare; usually presents as pigmented lesion adjacent to dentate line

System(s) affected: Gastrointestinal

Genetics:
- Hereditary autosomal dominant in 5-10%; first-degree relative in 20%
- Ras oncogene mutations seen in 40-50% of adenocarcinoma; alterations of suppressor genes also seen in 75%, especially involving chromosomes 17,18

Incidence/Prevalence in USA: 155,000 new cases/year

Predominant age: Adenocarcinoma usually occurs in individuals > age 50 years with peak incidence in the seventh decade

Predominant sex: Male = Female

SIGNS AND SYMPTOMS
- Vary with location
- Early lesions are frequently asymptomatic
- Right-sided adenocarcinoma
  ◊ Anemia
  ◊ Pain and/or mass in right lower quadrant
  ◊ Occult blood in stool
  ◊ Change in appearance of stool (infrequent)
- Left-sided adenocarcinoma
  ◊ Change in bowel habits (may be constipation or diarrhea)
  ◊ Reduced caliber of stool
  ◊ Red blood mixed in stool
- Rectal adenocarcinoma
  ◊ Bright red rectal bleeding
  ◊ Tenesmus
  ◊ Mass on digital exam
- Carcinoid
  ◊ Often incidental finding
  ◊ Appendicitis-like if located in appendix
  ◊ Rectal bleeding
  ◊ Crampy abdominal pain
  ◊ Carcinoid syndrome; occurs with metastases to liver; includes facial flushing, abdominal cramps, diarrhea
- Squamous cell carcinoma
  ◊ Painful defecation
  ◊ Rectal bleeding
  ◊ Mass or ulcer in anal canal
  ◊ Non-healing anal fissure

CAUSES
- Undetermined; both genetic and environmental factors may contribute
- Environmental - high dietary animal fat, low dietary fiber

RISK FACTORS
- Adenocarcinoma
  ◊ Two-thirds of patients are over 50 years old
  ◊ Pancolonic ulcerative colitis, (2% per year after 10 years active disease)
  ◊ Familial polyposis (100%)
  ◊ Hereditary nonpolyposis colorectal cancer (family history)
  ◊ Benign adenomas (tubular 3%; villous 9-12%)
  ◊ Coexisting (synchronous) colon cancer (5%)
  ◊ Previous (metachronous) colon cancer (2-5%)
- Carcinoid
  ◊ Multiple endocrine adenopathy (MEA), rare
  ◊ Other organs with carcinoid (small bowel, bronchial)
- Squamous cell carcinoma
  ◊ Bowen's disease
  ◊ Paget's disease

DIAGNOSIS

DIFFERENTIAL DIAGNOSIS
- Strictures (ischemic, Crohn's, diverticulosis)
- Other neoplasms (prostatic carcinoma, lipoma, leiomyoma, sarcoma, others)
- Infectious/inflammatory lesions (ameboma, tuberculoma, hemorrhoids)
- Extrinsic masses (abscesses, cysts/pseudocysts, phlegmons)

LABORATORY
- Positive fecal occult blood test
- Anemia
- Urinary 5-hydroxyindoleacetic acid (5-HIAA); elevated in carcinoid
- Elevated plasma carcinoembryonic antigen (CEA)

Drugs that may alter lab results:
- Aspirin-containing medications and nonsteroidal anti-inflammatory drugs - positive fecal occult blood test
- Smoking - increased carcinoembryonic antigen

Disorders that may alter lab results:
- Peptic ulcer disease, ulcerative colitis, hemorrhoids, benign polyps - positive fecal occult blood test
- Renal failure - increased carcinoembryonic antigen

PATHOLOGICAL FINDINGS
- Adenocarcinoma
  ◊ May appear as ulcerated, polypoid, or fungating mass. May extend to local structures or metastasize by blood, lymphatics; staging of tumor reflects level of penetration.
  ◊ Duke's Stage A - mucosal involvement with or without submucosal extension
  ◊ Duke's Stage B1 - to muscularis propria but not through serosa
  ◊ Duke's Stage B2 - extends beyond serosa
  ◊ Duke's Stage C - regional nodes involved
  ◊ Duke's Stage D - distant metastases (liver, lung)
- Carcinoid
  ◊ Tend to be multicentric
  ◊ Metastasize by blood, lymphatics
- Squamous cell carcinoma
  ◊ Most are ulcerative but may vary greatly in size
  ◊ Metastasize to inguinal lymphatics

SPECIAL TESTS Carcinoembryonic antigen - usually elevated with bulky tumor or metastases

IMAGING
- Barium enema (air-contrast preferred) - may not be necessary if colonoscopy is complete and provides adequate diagnostic information
- Computed tomography - sometimes used to determine extent of pelvic or liver involvement; not usually necessary
- Transrectal ultrasound - may be useful in defining extent of involvement by small rectal lesions

DIAGNOSTIC PROCEDURES
- Anoscopy - useful for anal canal visualization, biopsies
- Proctoscopy/flexible sigmoidoscopy with biopsy - used for distal lesions when complementary barium enema available for proximal colon
- Colonoscopy with biopsy - for primary diagnosis, screening of high-risk patients and post-resection surveillance

TREATMENT

APPROPRIATE HEALTH CARE
Inpatient

GENERAL MEASURES N/A

SURGICAL MEASURES
• Surgical procedures - radical resection of tumor with wide margins; includes segments of normal colon, mesentery, lymph nodes
• Right hemicolectomy for proximal tumors
• Left hemicolectomy for descending colon cancers
• Sigmoid colectomy for sigmoid cancers
• Abdominoperineal resection with colostomy for cancers of distal rectum (within 5-7 cm of dentate line)
• Preoperative or postoperative radiotherapy and chemotherapy: May improve outcome when used for rectal carcinoma
• For carcinoma of anus - combined chemotherapy (5-fluorouracil and mitomycin C) and radiotherapy. Convert to abdominoperineal resection for residual or recurrent tumor.

ACTIVITY Usually normal; may be slightly modified for patient with stoma

DIET Usually normal; avoidance of gas-producing foods may be helpful in ostomates (cabbage, beans, onions, alcoholic beverages)

PATIENT EDUCATION
• American Cancer Society
• National Cancer Institute, Dept. of Health And Human Services, Public Inquiries Section, Office of Cancer Communications, Building 31, Room 101-18, 9000 Rockville Pike, Bethesda, MD 20892, (301)496-5583,

 MEDICATIONS

DRUG(S) OF CHOICE
• Steroids, somatostatin or methysergide may ameliorate symptoms of carcinoid syndrome
• Stage C adenocarcinoma - fluorouracil (5-FU) plus levamisole
Contraindications: Peptic ulcer disease (steroids)
Precautions: Refer to manufacturer's literature
Significant possible interactions: Refer to manufacturer's literature

ALTERNATIVE DRUGS N/A

 FOLLOWUP

PATIENT MONITORING
• Adenocarcinoma (after remainder of colon is cleared of all lesions)
  ◊ Colonoscopy - repeat 1year; then every 3 years
  ◊ Carcinoembryonic antigen test, liver chemistries, fecal occult blood test - every 3 months for 2 years; then every 6 months for 3 years; then annually
• Carcinoid:
  ◊ 5-HIAA every 6 months x 2 years, then annually
• Squamous cell carcinoma:
  ◊ Clinical evaluation every 4 months x 1 year, then annually
  ◊ Biopsy suspicious areas in anus, groin

PREVENTION/AVOIDANCE Colonic polyps should be removed, examined microscopically. If benign, surveillance colonoscopy should be performed every 3 years.

POSSIBLE COMPLICATIONS
• Following resections:
  ◊ Mortality 5-10%
  ◊ Wound infection 5-15%
  ◊ Anastomotic stricture/leak/abscess 2-5%
  ◊ Pneumonia 5-10%
  ◊ Urinary tract infection 5-20%
• During chemotherapy or radiation therapy:
  ◊ Stomatitis
  ◊ Proctitis/diarrhea
  ◊ Temporary loss of hair

EXPECTED COURSE/PROGNOSIS
• Adenocarcinoma: Overall 5-year survival is 55% but relates to tumor stage in individual patients
  ◊ Duke's A - 95%
  ◊ Duke's B1 - 85-90%
  ◊ Duke's B2 - 60-70%
  ◊ Duke's C - 15-25%
  ◊ Duke's D - 5%
• Carcinoid:
  ◊ Overall 5-year survival is 65%
  ◊ Relates to tumor stage as in adenocarcinoma
• Squamous cell carcinoma:
  ◊ Overall 5-year survival is 79%

 MISCELLANEOUS

ASSOCIATED CONDITIONS Colonic carcinoid - multiple endocrine neoplasia types I, II

AGE-RELATED FACTORS
Pediatric: Adenocarcinoma of colon occurs rarely in children; prognosis is very poor
Geriatric: Coexistence of medical illness may complicate postoperative course
Others: N/A

PREGNANCY N/A

SYNONYMS N/A

ICD-9-CM
154.0 Malignant neoplasm of rectosigmoid junction

SEE ALSO N/A

OTHER NOTES N/A

ABBREVIATIONS N/A

REFERENCES
• Engstrom PF: NCCN colorectal cancer practice guidelines. Oncology 1997;10:140-175
• Craanen ME, Blok P, Offerhaus GT, Tygat GN: Recent developments in hereditary nonpolyposis colorectal cancer. Scand J Gastroenterol 1996;31(suppl 218):92-97
• Winawer SJ, Fletcher RH, Miller L, et al: Colorectal cancer screening: clinical guidelines and rationale. Gastroenterology 1997;112:594-642
• Jessup JM, McGinnis LS, Steele GD, et al: The national cancer data base report on colon cancer. Cancer 1996;78:;918-926
Illustrations: N/A
Internet references: http://www.5mcc.com

Author(s)
Wayne H. Schwesinger, MD

Common cold

BASICS

DESCRIPTION Inflammation of the nasal passages due to any number of respiratory viruses. Usually not serious; vast majority are self-treated.
System(s) affected: Pulmonary
Genetics: American Indians and Eskimos at higher risk than other ethnic groups and have more frequent complications such as otitis media; individuals with certain alpha-1-antitrypsin genotypes may be unusually susceptible to the common cold.
Incidence/prevalence in USA: Preschool children 6-10 colds/yr; kindergarten 12/yr; schoolchildren 7/yr; adolescents/adults 2-4/yr. National Ambulatory Survey: 31 episodes/100 persons/year (counting only colds that lead to medical attention or at least one day of restricted activity).
Predominant age: Children > adults
Predominant sex: Male = Female

SIGNS AND SYMPTOMS
• Nasal stuffiness and/or obstruction (80-100%)
• Sneezing (50-70%)
• Scratchy throat (50%)
• Cough (40%)
• Hoarseness (30%)
• Malaise (20-25%)
• Headache (25%)
• Fever > 100°F/37.7°C (0-1%)

CAUSES
• Usually due to one of 200 virus strains from six virus families; many strains present within the same geographic region or family
  ◊ Rhinovirus (> 200 serotypes)
  ◊ Influenza A, B, C viruses
  ◊ Parainfluenza viruses
  ◊ Respiratory syncytial viruses
  ◊ Coronaviruses
  ◊ Adenoviruses
  ◊ Certain ECHO viruses
• In 40% cases, no agent can be identified

RISK FACTORS
• Exposure to infected individuals
• Touching one's nose or conjunctiva with contaminated fingers

DIAGNOSIS

DIFFERENTIAL DIAGNOSIS
• Mumps
• Rubeola
• Allergic rhinitis
• Cytomegalovirus
• Epstein-Barr virus
• Mycoplasma pneumonia
• Influenza – systemic symptoms including myalgias, malaise, severe headache and ocular symptoms overshadow the respiratory complaints

LABORATORY
• CBC if symptoms persist for more than 10 days or with fever > 100°F (37.8°C)
• Nasal smear for eosinophilia may be useful in select individuals
Drugs that may alter lab results: N/A
Disorders that may alter lab results: N/A

PATHOLOGICAL FINDINGS
• Rhinovirus infects the ciliated epithelium lining the nose. Edema and hyperemia of nasal mucous membranes results.
• Exudation of serous and mucinous fluid containing immunoglobulins
• Histology: edema of subepithelial connective tissue, and a scanty cellular infiltrate containing neutrophils, plasma cells, lymphocytes, and eosinophils
• Rhinovirus causes a "non-destructive" inflammation of the mucous membranes, in contrast to influenza and parainfluenza which denude epithelium to the basement membrane

SPECIAL TESTS
In some centers, rapid antigen tests for various respiratory viruses are available for patients requiring hospitalization or for research purposes

IMAGING
Not indicated unless there is concern for bacterial superinfection of the sinuses, supraglottic region, trachea, or lungs

DIAGNOSTIC PROCEDURES
In rare cases, may want to attempt to culture virus from nasal washings or identify by ELISA or RIA methods

TREATMENT

APPROPRIATE HEALTH CARE
Outpatient self-care

GENERAL MEASURES
• Rest, fluids, and symptomatic measures
• Reassure that usual course is 6-10 days
• Humidify inspired air
• Discontinue tobacco and alcohol products (if not already done)
• In infants, clear nasal passages with a bulb syringe, position mattress at 45°, use saline nasal drops

SURGICAL MEASURES N/A

ACTIVITY
Up as tolerated with increased rest in the first few days

DIET
Encourage fluids

PATIENT EDUCATION
• Reassure that colds are ubiquitous and a normal part of human existence
• Spread is primarily via hand-to-hand transmission of virus contaminated nasal secretions; persons with colds touch their nose and eyes and then touch others
• Small-particle aerosols released in talking, coughing, and sneezing do not travel very far and contain only a low concentration of rhinovirus
• Rhinovirus survives for hours on the hands and hard surfaces, but does not survive long on porous surfaces such as tissues
• Individual susceptibility to colds, depends in large part, on pre-existing antibody levels
• Serum immunity lasts for years, but most individuals gain little protection against future colds due, in part, to the large number of viral serotypes and the antigenic drift that occurs over time in some viral types (rhinovirus, influenza)
• Educate about the expected course and symptomatic measures
• Advise patients to contact you if they develop dyspnea, productive cough, temperature > 102°F (38.9°C), or shaking chills

MEDICATIONS

DRUG(S) OF CHOICE
No cure or practical preventive measure documented. Medications targeting a particular symptom reduce the likelihood of adverse systemic effects
• Topical decongestants (sympathomimetics) reduce edema and swelling of the nasal mucosa, promote drainage, and reduce nasal airflow resistance. Preferred over oral because of minimal systemic effects. Sprays preferred over drops in ages > 6.
  ◊ oxymetazoline
    - Adults and children ages 6-12: 0.05% solution, 2 or 3 sprays in each nostril bid
    - Children ages 2-6: 0.025% solution, 2 or 3 drops in each nostril bid
    - Rebound congestion (rhinitis medicamentosa) unlikely if used < 5 days
• Topical anticholinergics. Control rhinorrhea but do not relieve nasal congestion or sneezing
  ◊ Ipratropium: Adults and children >11: 0.06% solution, 2 sprays to each nostril TID for 4 days
• Oral decongestants (sympathomimetics) Advantages over topical decongestants: longer duration of action, lack of local irritation and no risk of rhinitis medicamentosa
  ◊ Pseudoephedrine
    - Adults: 60 mg q4-6h (120 mg sustained release q12h)
    - Children ages 6-12: 30 mg q4-6h
    - Children 2-5: 15 mg q4-6h
• Antihistamines. Histamine does not play a significant role in the common cold, but are safe and effective in alleviating sneezing and rhinorrhea. Their perceived benefit may come from anticholinergic effects, drying nasal and pharyngeal secretions and sedative effects promoting rest.
• Chlorpheniramine
  ◊ Adults: 4 mg q4-6h (or 8 mg tid, 12 mg bid)
  ◊ Children ages 6-12: 2 mg q4-6h
  ◊ Children ages 2-6: 1 mg q4-6h

- Cough suppressants. Cough most likely due to irritation of tracheobronchial receptors by post-nasal drip and may therefore benefit from decongestants. If nonproductive or interferes with sleep or normal activities, a cough suppressant is indicated. Codeine and dextromethorphan exhibit comparable efficacy. Adverse effects: drowsiness and GI upset.
  ◊ Codeine
    - Adults: 10-20 mg q4-6h
    - Children ages 6-12: 5-10 mg q4-6h
    - Children ages 2-6: 2.5-5 mg q4-6h
  ◊ Dextromethorphan
    - Adults: 10-30 mg q4-8h
    - Children ages 6-12: 15 mg q6-8h
    - Children ages 2-6: 2.5-7.5 mg q4-8h
- Expectorants. Though commonly employed, efficacy not proven
  ◊ guaifenesin
    - Adults: 100-400 mg q4h
    - Children ages 6-12: 100-200 mg q4h
    - Children ages 2-5: 50-100 mg q4h

Contraindications:
- Oral decongestants-monoamine oxidase inhibitors or selegiline

Precautions:
- Oral decongestants
  ◊ Affect all vascular beds and may increase blood pressure. They are cardiac stimulants and may result in arrhythmias. They may increase glucose levels in individuals with glucose intolerance or diabetes mellitus.
  ◊ Other adverse effects include headache, nervousness, sleeplessness, and dizziness
  ◊ Should be used with caution in patients taking guanethidine
- Antihistamines
  ◊ Nasal blockage and sinus congestion may worsen
- Cough suppressants
  ◊ Misuse and dependence can occur with codeine, but dextromethorphan abuse by adolescents is reported
- Expectorants
  ◊ Liquid preparations may contain high concentrations of alcohol
  ◊ Nausea, vomiting or abdominal pain are common adverse effects

Significant possible interactions: See manufacturer's literature

ALTERNATIVE DRUGS
- Many mouthwashes, gargles and lozenges are promoted to relieve the pain of sore throat. The demulcent effects of hard candy, gargling with warm saline, and products with anesthetics (e.g., benzocaine or phenol), may provide pain relief.
- Aromatic oils (e.g., menthol, camphor, eucalyptus), when applied topically or taken in a lozenge, produce a sensation of increased airflow in the absence of a significant change in airflow resistance.
- Antibacterials are of no value
- Antivirals
  ◊ Interferon. Prevents viral invasion of mucosa to prevent colds; side effects include nasal irritation or bleeding in about 10% of patients; may be useful in groups that have close contact
  ◊ Zinc chloride. Prevents viral replication in vitro, but efficacy of lozenges unproven

- Vitamin C (ascorbic acid)
  ◊ No preventative effects and only a modest (average 23%) reduction in the severity and duration of symptoms.
  ◊ Precipitation of urate, oxalate, or cystine stones has been seen, and urine glucose monitoring may be inaccurate in individuals taking large doses
  ◊ Interferes with stool guiaic testing

FOLLOWUP

PATIENT MONITORING Patients should contact their physician if they develop fever associated with systemic symptoms, difficulty breathing, dyspnea, and/or purulent drainage

PREVENTION/AVOIDANCE Frequent hand washing and avoiding touching the face may help prevent colds

POSSIBLE COMPLICATIONS
- Lower respiratory tract infection
- Bronchial hyperreactivity
- May lead to decompensation in patients with asthma and chronic lung disease
- Otitis media (2% of colds)
- Acute sinusitis (0.5% of colds)
- Pneumonia
- Rhinitis medicamentosa

EXPECTED COURSE/PROGNOSIS
Complete recovery expected within 3-10 days

MISCELLANEOUS

ASSOCIATED CONDITIONS
- Pharyngitis
- Sinusitis
- Bronchitis
- Bronchiolitis
- Pneumonia
- Croup
- Asthma

AGE-RELATED FACTORS
Pediatric:
- Medications are likely to produce adverse effects or toxicity in young children
- Incidence of colds is highest
Geriatric: Medications commonly produce adverse effects in the elderly
Others: N/A

PREGNANCY
- Decongestants: no clear association between drug use and congenital defects
- Antihistamines: no clear association between drug use and congenital defects
- Codeine: indiscriminate use during pregnancy may pose a risk to the fetus

SYNONYMS
- URI
- Upper respiratory infection

ICD-9-CM
460 Acute nasopharyngitis (common cold)

SEE ALSO
- Pharyngitis
- Mumps
- Measles, rubeola
- Rhinitis, allergic
- Cytomegalovirus inclusion disease
- Epstein-Barr virus infections
- Pneumonia, mycoplasma
- Influenza

OTHER NOTES N/A

ABBREVIATIONS
- ELISA = enzyme linked immunosorbent assay
- RIA = radioimmunoassay
- URI = upper respiratory infection

REFERENCES
- Bryant BG, Lombardi TP: Cold, cough and allergy products. In: Covington CR, Lawson LC, Young LL, eds. Handbook of Nonprescription Drugs.10th Ed. Washington, D.C, American Pharmaceutical Association, 1993:89-115
- Gadomski A: Rational use of over-the-counter medications in young children. JAMA 1994;272:1063-1064
- Hemila H: Does vitamin C alleviate the symptoms of the common cold?-a review of current evidence. Scandinavian Journal of Infectious Diseases 1994;26(1):1-6
- Hendeles L: Efficacy and safety of antihistamines and expectorants in nonprescription cough and cold preparations. Pharmacotherapy 1993;13(2):154-158
- Hendeles L: Selecting a decongestant. Pharmacotherapy 1993;13(6 Pt2):129S-134S
- Hendley JO, Gwaltney JM Jr: Mechanisms of transmission of rhinovirus infections. Epidemiologic Reviews 1988;10:243-258
- Lowenstein SR, Parrino TA: Management of the common cold. Advances in Internal Medicine 1987;32:207-233
- Saroea HG: Common colds: Causes, potential cures, and treatment. Canadian Family Physician 1993;39:2215-2216, 2219-2220
- Smith MB, Feldman W: Over-the-counter cold medications. A critical review of clinical trials between 1950 and 1991. JAMA 1993;269(17):2258-2263
- Tyrrell DA: A view from the common cold unit. Antiviral Research 1992;18(2):105-125
Illustrations: N/A
Internet references: http://www.5mcc.com

Author(s)
Barcey T. Levy, PhD, MD
Michael W. Kelly, PharmD, MS

Complete atrioventricular (AV) canal

BASICS

DESCRIPTION The central atrioventricular (AV) portion of the cardiac septum and the contiguous mitral and tricuspid valves are abnormal, allowing for an unobstructed atrioventricular canal. Children with Down syndrome and this anomaly rapidly progress to pulmonary vascular obstructive disease (within 3 to 6 months).
• Rastelli classification:
  ◊ Type A: Common anterior AV valve leaflet is divided and attached to the crest of the ventricular septum by chordae
  ◊ Type B: Common anterior AV valve leaflet is divided and chordae tendineae from the midportions of the divided anterior leaflet are attached to the right ventricular medial papillary muscle
  ◊ Type C: Common anterior AV valve leaflet is undivided and not attached to the ventricular septum (free-floating leaflet)
System(s) affected: Cardiovascular
Genetics: No known genetic pattern
Incidence/Prevalence in USA: 1 in 250,000 live births; type A being the most common
Predominant age: Congenital, present at birth
Predominant sex: Female > Male

SIGNS AND SYMPTOMS
• Pulmonary congestion
• Congestive heart failure
• Low systemic arterial blood oxygen saturation
• Tachycardia
• Poor feeding
• Growth failure
• Mitral regurgitation
• Pulmonary vascular obstructive disease, and cyanosis (30% in the first 2-3 years)

CAUSES Defective development of the endocardial cushions

RISK FACTORS Unknown

DIAGNOSIS

DIFFERENTIAL DIAGNOSIS
• Atrial septal defect
• Ventricular septal defect
• Incomplete or intermediate AV canal
• Patent ductus arteriosus
• Mitral valve prolapse
• Secondary mitral regurgitation
• Pulmonary vascular obstructive disease
• Anomalous pulmonary venous return

LABORATORY Arterial blood gas
Drugs that may alter lab results: N/A
Disorders that may alter lab results: N/A

PATHOLOGICAL FINDINGS Low oxygen saturation in the arterial blood gas

SPECIAL TESTS
• Cardiac 2-D echo-Doppler showing anatomic defect, increased pulmonary pressures, mitral regurgitation, tricuspid regurgitation, right and left atrial and ventricular enlargements
• ECG - superior QRS axis, right ventricular hypertrophy (RVH), left ventricular hypertrophy (LVH), possibly peaked P waves

IMAGING
• Cardiac angiogram demonstrating AV canal and mitral and tricuspid regurgitation, left and right atrial and ventricular enlargement
• Chest x-ray showing increased pulmonary vasculature, left and right atrial and ventricular enlargement
• MRI offers excellent imaging of crux

DIAGNOSTIC PROCEDURES
• Pulmonary artery catheter showing prominent "V" waves, elevated pulmonary capillary wedge pressures, right atrial "step-up" in oxygen saturations
• Angiography

TREATMENT

APPROPRIATE HEALTH CARE Medical management (digoxin, diuretics, afterload reducers) either as an inpatient or an outpatient, dependent upon the patient's condition

GENERAL MEASURES Provide general treatment for congestive heart failure

SURGICAL MEASURES If pulmonary edema, growth failure and congestive heart failure is refractory in spite of optimal medical therapy, reparative surgery should be pursued as early as possible. Repair should be especially early in children with Down syndrome (approximately 3 months). Repair should be performed before 2 years of age to avoid the continued progression of pulmonary vascular obstructive disease. Patients more than 2 years of age can undergo repair if the pulmonary vascular resistance (PVR) does not exceed 8-10 units-meters squared. At a minimum, surgical correction includes closure of the interatrial and interventricular septal defects and suspension of the medial aspects of the left and right AV valve leaflets. Pulmonary artery banding might still be a possibility.

ACTIVITY As tolerated

DIET High calorie, low salt

PATIENT EDUCATION Instruct regarding travel to altitudes and plane travel causing potential hypoxia

MEDICATIONS

DRUG(S) OF CHOICE Digoxin, ACE inhibitors or isosorbide dinitrate plus hydralazine, furosemide, potassium supplementation
• Doses for term infants
  ◊ Digoxin - oral 30 µg/kg (digitalizing), then 10 µg/kg/24 hrs. Adjust to maintain levels within therapeutic range - 0.5-2.0 ng/mL (0.64-2.6 nmol/L)
  ◊ Captopril - 0.05-0.1 mg/kg/dose tid-qid
  ◊ Isosorbide dinitrate - refer to manufacturer's literature
  ◊ Hydralazine - 0.75-3.0 mg/kg/dose, increase as needed to maximum of 6 mg/kg/dose
  ◊ Furosemide - oral 2 mg/kg, increase as needed to maximum of 6 mg/kg
  ◊ Potassium - supplement patients who require furosemide. Maintenance dose is 2-3 mEq/kg/24 hours.
Contraindications: Profound systemic hypotension, worsening hypoxia and V/Q mismatch with treatment
Precautions: Refer to manufacturer's literature
Significant possible interactions: Refer to manufacturer's literature

ALTERNATIVE DRUGS Dobutamine or amrinone drips

FOLLOWUP

PATIENT MONITORING
• As indicated by clinical intervention and disease progression
• Serial measurements of arterial oxygen content
• Serial measurements of pulmonary vascular resistance

PREVENTION/AVOIDANCE Avoid
hypoxic embarrassment in environments of low oxygen tension

POSSIBLE COMPLICATIONS
• Refractive hypoxia secondary to progressive pulmonary vascular obstructive disease
• Cyanosis
• Polycythemia
• Growth failure
• Congestive heart failure/pulmonary edema
• Complications of surgery:
  ◊ Residual ventricular septal defect
  ◊ Residual left ventricular to right atrial shunting
  ◊ Complete AV block

EXPECTED COURSE/PROGNOSIS
• PVR less than 5:
  ◊ If undergoing reparative surgery, are at risk for an approximate 10% surgical mortality
  ◊ The majority of those surviving realize complete relief of their symptoms and will need no further treatment
• PVR between 5-13 undergoing surgery:
  ◊ Perioperative mortality approaches 33%
  ◊ Survivors realize functional class I or II (New York Heart Association [NYHA] classification)
• PVR greater than 5 who do not or can not undergo surgical intervention:
  ◊ Deterioration is progressive with death ranging from 2-16 years of age

MISCELLANEOUS

ASSOCIATED CONDITIONS
• Down syndrome. Very high percentage have complete atrioventricular canal lesions.
• Tetralogy of Fallot
• Unbalanced canal with left or right dominance

AGE-RELATED FACTORS
Pediatric: Surgical intervention before age 2 or before marked increase in PVR occurs
Geriatric: N/A
Others: N/A

PREGNANCY N/A

SYNONYMS N/A

ICD-9-CM 745.69 Endocardial cushion defects, other

SEE ALSO
• Atrial septal defect (ASD)

OTHER NOTES N/A

ABBREVIATIONS
AVC = atrioventricular canal
PVR = pulmonary vascular resistance
V/Q = ventilation-perfusion ratio

REFERENCES
• Brandenburg RO, Fuster V, Giuliani ER, McGoon DC: Cardiology: Fundamentals and Practice. Chicago, Year Book Medical Publishers, 1987
• Braunwald E, ed: Heart Disease: A Textbook of Cardiovascular Medicine. 4th Ed. Philadelphia, WB Saunders Co, 1992
Illustrations: N/A
Internet references: http://www.5mcc.com

Author(s)
David J. Framm, MD, FACC

Complex regional pain syndrome

 BASICS

DESCRIPTION
Pain syndrome following injury to bone and soft tissue. Pathogenesis is obscure.
• Type I - reflex sympathetic dystrophy
• Type II - causalgia . Type II is caused by a demonstrable nerve injury.
System(s) affected: Nervous
Genetics: No known genetic pattern
Incidence/Prevalence in USA: Unknown
Predominant age: No predominant age
Predominant sex: Male > Female

SIGNS AND SYMPTOMS
• Deep aching pain
• Burning pain with superimposed lancinating pain
• Hyperesthesia
• Hyperalgesia
• Pain from a non-noxious stimulus
• Pain most likely in palm or sole, aggravated by minimal physical stimulus such as friction or heat
• Skin - discolored, edematous, cold, hyperesthetic, smooth, glossy
• Stiff joints
• Nails curved and brittle
• Hyperhidrosis

CAUSES
Other than known nerve injury (type II or causalgia), there is no known definitive pathogenesis

RISK FACTORS
Trauma

 DIAGNOSIS

DIFFERENTIAL DIAGNOSIS
Rule out infection, hypertrophic scar, bone fragments, neuroma, central nervous system tumor or syrinx

LABORATORY
N/A
Drugs that may alter lab results: N/A
Disorders that may alter lab results: N/A

PATHOLOGICAL FINDINGS
• Partial or complete damage to afferent nerve pathways and probably reorganized central pain pathways
• Most common nerves involved are median and sciatic
• Atrophy in affected muscles
• Incomplete nerve plexus lesion

SPECIAL TESTS
N/A

IMAGING
Bone scan (3 phase)

DIAGNOSTIC PROCEDURES
None

 TREATMENT

APPROPRIATE HEALTH CARE
Outpatient, except for operative procedures or intravenous sympathetic nerve blockade

GENERAL MEASURES
• Treatment is empirical
• Anesthetic blockade (chemical or surgical) of sympathetic nerve function (transient relief suggests that chemical or surgical sympathectomy will be helpful)
• Intravenous regional sympathetic block with guanethidine or reserpine by pain specialist or anesthetist
• Physical therapy (essential during all phases of treatment)
• Transcutaneous electric nerve stimulation (controversial)
• Inject myofacial painful trigger points
• Briskly rub the affected part several times per day
• Acupuncture can be tried
• Hypnosis
• Relaxation training (alternate muscle relaxing and contracting)
• Biofeedback
• Discourage maladaptive behaviors
• Refer the patient to a specialty pain clinic in difficult cases

SURGICAL MEASURES
Sympathectomy sometimes necessary

ACTIVITY
Maintain as high a level of physical and intellectual activity as possible

DIET
No special diet

PATIENT EDUCATION
• Stress staying active physically
• Careful instructions about any prescribed medications

Complex regional pain syndrome

MEDICATIONS

DRUG(S) OF CHOICE
• No single drug or combination of drugs has produced consistent results; early therapy is beneficial.
◊ Prazosin, 1-8 mg orally in divided doses
◊ Phenoxybenzamine 40-120 mg daily, orally in divided doses. The initial dose should not exceed 10 mg.
◊ Nifedipine 10-30 mg tid
◊ Prednisone 60-80 mg/day orally, tapered over 2-4 weeks
◊ Tricyclic antidepressants (see manufacturers recommended dose)
• Anticonvulsants. (Require serum drug level monitoring, except for clonazepam. Doses must be individualized.):
◊ Carbamazepine 200-1000 mg/day orally
◊ Phenytoin 100-300 mg/day orally
◊ Clonazepam 1-10 mg/day orally
◊ Valproic acid 750-2250 mg/day orally, maximum of 60 mg/kg
• Skeletal muscle relaxant:
◊ Baclofen 10-40 mg/day orally - may act synergistically with carbamazepine and phenytoin
Contraindications: Refer to manufacturer's literature
Precautions: Refer to manufacturer's literature
Significant possible interactions: There are many with this group of drugs. Refer to manufacturer's literature.

ALTERNATIVE DRUGS
• Narcotics - only after all non-opioid therapies are exhausted
• Other alpha-adrenergic blockers or dihydropyridine calcium channel blockers may be tried though experience with them is limited

FOLLOWUP

PATIENT MONITORING
• Watch carefully for adverse reactions to medications
• Several different forms of therapy may need to be tried

PREVENTION/AVOIDANCE
• Mobilization following injury
• Avoidance of nerve damage during surgical procedures
• Splinting of an injured extremity for adequate period of time
• Adequate analgesics during recovery from injuries

POSSIBLE COMPLICATIONS
• Drug mishaps
• Joint contractures
• Contralateral spread of symptoms

EXPECTED COURSE/PROGNOSIS
• Course - variable; chronic; remitting
• Outlook only satisfactory, may need attempts at several treatment modalities. No one form of therapy is superior to others. Failure to respond to one form does not mitigate against success with another.
• Those patients receiving work compensation for an injury or secondary gain from family or friends are in a separate category and may never get well

MISCELLANEOUS

ASSOCIATED CONDITIONS
• Serious injury to bone and soft tissue
• Herpes zoster

AGE-RELATED FACTORS
Pediatric: N/A
Geriatric: Painful perception is frequently worse in older patients. Start with smaller than usual doses of drugs.
Others: N/A

PREGNANCY Many of the useful drugs are contraindicated in pregnancy

SYNONYMS
• Traumatic erythromelalgia
• Weir-Mitchell causalgia
• Causalgia
• Reflex sympathetic dystrophy
• Posttraumatic neuralgia
• Sympathetically maintained pain

ICD-9-CM
337.21 Complex regional pain of upper limb, type I (reflex sympathetic dystrophy)
337.22 Complex regional pain of lower limb, type I (reflex sympathetic dystrophy)
354.4 Complex regional pain of upper limb, type II (causalgia)
355.71 Complex regional pain of lower limb, type II (causalgia)

SEE ALSO
• Herpes zoster
• Arterial embolus & thrombosis

OTHER NOTES
• Postherpetic neuralgia is a result of partial or complete damage to afferent nerve pathways
• Pain occurring in dermatomes as a sequela of herpes zoster

ABBREVIATIONS N/A

REFERENCES
• Adams RD, et al, eds: Principals of Neurology. 6th Ed. New York, McGraw-Hill, 1997
Pittman DM, Miles JB: Complex regional pain syndrome. Am Fam Phys 1997;56(9):2265-2270
• Kasdan ML, Johnson AL: Reflex sympathetic dystrophy. Occupational Med 1998;13(3):521-531
Illustrations: N/A
Internet references: http://www.5mcc.com

Author(s)
Dennis E. Hughes, DO, FAAFP

Condyloma acuminata

BASICS

DESCRIPTION Condyloma acuminata are soft, skin colored, fleshy warts that are caused by the HPV (human papilloma virus). There are at least 70 known types of HPV and types 6, 11, 16, 18, 31, 33, 35 have been associated with condyloma acuminata. The disease is highly contagious, can appear singly or in groups, small or large. They appear in the vagina, on the cervix, around the external genitalia and rectum, in the urethra, anus, also conjunctival, nasal, oral and laryngeal warts and occasionally, the throat. The incubation period may be from 1-6 months.
System(s) affected: Skin/Exocrine, Reproductive
Genetics: N/A
Incidence/Prevalence in USA: Minimum of 10-20% of sexually active women may be infected with HPV. Studies in men suggest a similar prevalence.
Predominant Age: 15-30 years of age
Predominant Sex: Male = Female

SIGNS AND SYMPTOMS
• Tumors, soft, sessile
• Surface smooth to very rough
• Multiple fingerlike projections
• Perianal condylomata acuminatum usually rough and cauliflower-like
• Penile lesions often smooth and papular
• Penile lesions often occur in groups of three or four
• Male sites - frenulum, corona, glans, prepuce, meatus, shaft, scrotum
• Female sites - labia, clitoris, periurethral area, perineum, vagina, cervix (flat lesions)
• Pruritis
• Irritation
• Bleeding (result of trauma)
• Perianal area (both sexes)
• Subclinical HPV infection
• May be detected by Pap test

CAUSES Human papillomaviruses. These are circular double-stranded DNA molecules. There are over 70 HPV subtypes. The cause of common venereal warts are types 6 and 11. Cervical dysplasia and carcinoma in situ are likely caused by types 16, 18, 31, 33, and 35.

RISK FACTORS
• Young adult
• Sexually active
• Not using condoms
• Possibly subclinical infection
• Young age of commencing sexual activity
• Cigarette smoking
• Poor hygiene
• Pregnancy
• Caucasian
• History of genital warts

DIAGNOSIS

DIFFERENTIAL DIAGNOSIS
• Condyloma lata (flat warts of syphilis)
• Lichen planus
• Normal sebaceous glands
• Seborrheic keratosis
• Molluscum contagiosum
• Keratomas
• Scabies
• Crohn's disease
• Skin tags
• Melanocytic nevi
• Vulvar intraepithelial neoplasia
• Boschke-Lowenstein tumor

LABORATORY Serologic test for syphilis - negative
Drugs that may alter lab results: N/A
Disorders that may alter lab results: N/A

PATHOLOGICAL FINDINGS
• Possible cervical dysplasia in females
• Benign
• Well organized basal layer
• Underlying infiltration of lymphocytes
• Plasma cells
• Hyperplastic epithelial changes
• Basement membrane intact
• Sometimes difficult to differentiate from squamous cell carcinoma

SPECIAL TESTS Acetowhitening: Subclinical lesions can be visualized by wrapping the penis with gauze soaked with 5% acetic acid for 5 minutes. Using a ten X hand lens or colposcope, warts appear as tiny white papules. A shiny white appearance of the skin represents foci of epithelial hyperplasia (subclinical infection). Not highly specific, low positive predictive value.

IMAGING N/A

DIAGNOSTIC PROCEDURES
• Biopsy with highly specialized identification techniques (not clinically useful)
• Colposcopy, androscopy, anoscopy, Pap smear

TREATMENT

APPROPRIATE HEALTH CARE
Outpatient

GENERAL MEASURES
• May resolve on their own
• Treatment determined by location and size of warts
• Small warts may be treated with topical applications
• Cryotherapy
• Change therapy if no improvement after 3 treatments, no complete clearance after 6 treatments, or therapy exceeding manufacturer's recommendations

SURGICAL MEASURES
• Larger warts require laser treatment or electrocoagulation
• Surgical excision for large warts

ACTIVITY No restrictions

DIET No special diet

PATIENT EDUCATION
• Explain preventive measures and chronic nature of the infection
• Numerous pamphlets on HPV, STD prevention, condom use
• Emphasize need for women to get regular Pap smears

Condyloma acuminata

MEDICATIONS

DRUG(S) OF CHOICE
- Imiquimod (Aldara) 5% cream applied overnight 3 times weekly until warts clear for up to 16 weeks
- Cryotherapy - liquid nitrogen is applied to warts in 5-10 second bursts. Usually requires 2-3 weekly sessions.
- Podophyllin in tincture of Benzoin. Apply directly to warts. Leave on for 1-4 hours, then wash off. Repeat treatment every 7 days until gone
- or
- Podofilox (Condylox) - for external warts. Apply to external warts every 12 hours (allowing to dry) for 3 consecutive days. May repeat after 4 days.

Contraindications:
- Podophyllin - do not use during pregnancy or on oral, cervical, urethral or perianal warts. Can use on small number of vaginal warts with careful drying after application.
- Cryotherapy - cryoglobulinemia

Precautions:
- Podophyllin - to minimize local and systemic reactions, wash treated areas 1-4 hours after application and use ointments to protect surrounding skin from contact with podophyllin
- Cryotherapy - none
- Electrocautery - don't use in patient with pacemaker

Significant Possible Interactions: N/A

ALTERNATIVE DRUGS
- External (penile and perianal)
  ◊ Podophyllin
  ◊ Podofilox (Condylox) self-treatment
  ◊ Trichloroacetic acid (TCA) - apply weekly
  ◊ Electrocautery, laser, intralesional interferon
- Urethral meatus
  ◊ Laser
  ◊ Podophyllin
  ◊ Topical fluorouracil
- Anal
  ◊ Trichloracetic acid (TCA) - apply weekly
  ◊ Topical fluorouracil
- Oral
  ◊ Electrocautery
  ◊ Surgery
  ◊ Laser

FOLLOWUP

PATIENT MONITORING
- Every 2 weeks for treatment until clear
- Pap test every 1 year for indefinite period
- Biopsy for persistent warts
- Monitor sex partners

PREVENTION/AVOIDANCE
- Use of condoms by infected men
- Use of condoms by male sexual partners of individuals who have been treated for HPV infection
- Abstinence by women until treatment completed
- Circumcision may prevent recurrence in some men

POSSIBLE COMPLICATIONS
- Cervical dysplasia
- Carcinoma - cervical (squamous or adenocarcinoma) penile or rectal
- Male urethral obstruction

EXPECTED COURSE/PROGNOSIS
- Warts clear with treatment or spontaneous regression
- Recurrence is common with all forms of therapy (30-70%)
- Asymptomatic infection persists indefinitely

MISCELLANEOUS

ASSOCIATED CONDITIONS
- 90% of cervical cancer contains evidence of HPV infection
- Gonorrhea
- Syphilis
- AIDS
- Chlamydia
- Other sexually transmitted disease

AGE-RELATED FACTORS
Young adults, infants and children
Pediatric: N/A
Geriatric: N/A
Others:
- Venereal warts are increasing in an ever younger population. A recent study of 487 college women showed an infection rate of 48%.
- Increased size and number in immunocompromised states

PREGNANCY
- Warts often grow larger in pregnancy and regress spontaneously after delivery. Use cryotherapy.
- HPV can be transmitted to infant at time of delivery and cause laryngeal papillomas

SYNONYMS
- Genital warts
- Venereal warts
- Papilloma acuminatum

ICD-9-CM
078.1 Condyloma acuminatum
078.11 Warts, condyloma

SEE ALSO
- Abnormal Pap smear

OTHER NOTES   N/A

ABBREVIATIONS   N/A

REFERENCES
- Fitzpatrick TB, et al: Color Atlas and Synopsis of Clinical Dermatology. New York, McGraw-Hill, 1992
- Beutner KR, Wiley DJ, et al: Genital warts and their treatment. Clin Infect Dis 1999;28(suppl1):537-56
- Edwards L: Imiquimod in clinical practice. Australia J Dermatol 1998;39(suppl1)s14-16

Illustrations: 2 available on CD-ROM

Internet references: http://www.5mcc.com

Author(s)
Barbara J. Moront, MD
Earl Robert G. Ang, MD
Bassem Elsawy, MD

Congenital megacolon

BASICS

DESCRIPTION Congenital disease of the colon, characterized by functional obstruction and accumulation of feces and massive dilatation of colon

System(s) affected: Gastrointestinal, Nervous

Genetics: Familial 50 times base rate. Sometimes associated with Down syndrome.

Incidence/Prevalence in USA: 1 in 2000 to 5000 births (Caucasians 91%, Blacks 8%, Oriental 0.5%)

Predominant age: Infancy

Predominant sex:
• Males > Females for short segment (8:2)
• Males > Females for long segment (5:4)

SIGNS AND SYMPTOMS
• Stools in pellets or ribbons with pasty consistency
• Early infancy:
  ◊ Onset early in infancy, newborn fails to pass meconium in 24 to 48 hours after birth
  ◊ Obstipation
  ◊ Marked enlargement and distention of abdomen
  ◊ Colonic peristalsis visible
  ◊ Vomiting
  ◊ Palpable fecal mass
  ◊ Growth retardation (possible)
• Older infants:
  ◊ Failure to thrive
  ◊ Anorexia
  ◊ Lack of physiologic urge to defecate
  ◊ Empty rectum on digital examination
  ◊ Palpable colon
  ◊ Visible peristalsis
  ◊ Hypoalbuminemia

CAUSES Congenital absence of Auerbach's and Meissener's autonomic plexuses in bowel wall - usually limited to the colon

RISK FACTORS
• Family history of Hirschsprung's disease
• Offspring risk if parent has short segment - 2%; if parent has long segment - up to 50%
• Sibling risk if male affected - female has 0.6% risk (short segment)
• Sibling risk if female affected - male has 18% risk (long segment)

DIAGNOSIS

DIFFERENTIAL DIAGNOSIS
• Megacolon, secondary (to Chagas' disease)
• Megacolon, acquired, functional
• Functional constipation
• Hypoganglionosis
• Meconium plug syndrome
• Small left colon syndrome
• Meconium ileus

LABORATORY Electrolytes, albumin, CBC, urinalysis, thyroid function

Drugs that may alter lab results: N/A

Disorders that may alter lab results: N/A

PATHOLOGICAL FINDINGS
• Congenital absence of Auerbach's and Meissner's autonomic plexuses in myenteric plexus of colon wall
• Obstruction may begin at anus, and may extend proximally to involve varying portions of the colon or terminal ileum
• Enormous dilatation and hypertrophy of all layers of involved colon
• Rectosigmoid aganglionosis
• Submucosal hypertrophied nerve bundles

SPECIAL TESTS
• Proctoscopy: Ampulla empty of feces
• Biopsy: Absence of ganglia in wall of narrowed rectum
• Ano-rectal manometry

IMAGING
• X-ray - barium enema shows:
  ◊ Large ovoid mass mottled by small, irregular gas shadows
  ◊ Dilatation of sigmoid colon above narrowed distal sigmoid or rectum
  ◊ Narrowed portion rippled or segmented
  ◊ Fluid levels within bowel
  ◊ Diaphragm elevated

DIAGNOSTIC PROCEDURES
• Suction aspiration biopsy of bowel wall
• Barium enema
• Proctosigmoidoscopy
• Large bowel wall biopsy
• Laparoscopy: Normal proximal colon dilatation
• Ano-rectal manometry: Internal sphincter relaxation failure

TREATMENT

APPROPRIATE HEALTH CARE Early work-up (ambulatory or hospital). Inpatient for surgery.

GENERAL MEASURES
• Treatment may be symptomatic or definitive
• May need emergency correction of fluid and electrolyte imbalance
• Removal of fecal accumulation - retention enemas of 3-4 ounces (90-120 mL) of mineral oil followed by repeated colonic irrigations with isotonic saline solution. Avoid use of other solutions, e.g., water, soapsuds enemas.

SURGICAL MEASURES Surgery (inpatient) for colostomy at site in the colon proximal to aganglionic segment or resection of the aganglionic segment or bypass of the segment. Endorectal pull-through techniques may be utilized.

ACTIVITY No restrictions

DIET
• Dictated by stage of disease
• Diet will not control the obstipation of Hirschsprung's
• Postoperative diet - standard for age

PATIENT EDUCATION
• After surgery instruct parents to detect and report dehydration, decreased urinary output, sunken eyes, poor skin turgor, vomiting, fever
• Encourage bonding with parents by having parents participate in child's care as much as possible
• Request enterotomy therapist to teach family

MEDICATIONS

DRUG(S) OF CHOICE
• None recommended for treatment
• Preliminary to surgery: Bowel prep with neomycin or nystatin
Contraindications: N/A
Precautions: N/A
Significant possible interactions: N/A

ALTERNATIVE DRUGS
• Metronidazole (Flagyl) for bowel preparation

FOLLOWUP

PATIENT MONITORING Closely until recuperated fully from surgical intervention

PREVENTION/AVOIDANCE N/A

POSSIBLE COMPLICATIONS
• Toxic enterocolitis, possibly fatal
• Bleeding and/or perforation

EXPECTED COURSE/PROGNOSIS
Guardedly favorable with surgery prior to onset of complications

MISCELLANEOUS

ASSOCIATED CONDITIONS
• Chagas' disease (secondary aganglionic megacolon may be a late complication of Chagas')
• Megacolon, acquired, functional usually begins in 3rd or 4th year of life
• Down syndrome
• Septal defects
• Tetralogy of Fallot
• Dandy-Walker syndrome
• Associated with anomalies 22% of the time, especially neurological, cardiovascular, urological, gastrointestinal

AGE-RELATED FACTORS
Pediatric: Occasionally infants have only mild or intermittent constipation with intervening bouts of diarrhea. These cases may not be diagnosed until later in infancy.
Geriatric: N/A
Others: N/A

PREGNANCY N/A

SYNONYMS
• Aganglionic megacolon
• Hirschsprung's disease
• Zer-Wilson's disease (total colonic aganglionosis)

ICD-9-CM
751.3 Hirschsprung's disease

SEE ALSO
• Constipation

OTHER NOTES Diagnosis must be made as early as possible to prevent toxic enterocolitis

ABBREVIATIONS N/A

REFERENCES
• Ryan ET, et al: J Ped Surg 1992;1:76-81
• Walsh K, et al, eds: Pediatric Surgery. New York, Yearbook Medical Publishers, 1986
• Eastwood GL, Avunduk C, eds: Manual of Gastroenterology. Boston, Little, Brown, 1988
• Barakat AY, ed: Renal Disease in Children: Clinical Evaluation & Diagnosis. New York, Springer-Verlag, 1990
Illustrations: N/A
Internet references: http://www.5mcc.com

Author(s)
James A. Nard, MD

Congestive heart failure

BASICS

DESCRIPTION Congestive heart failure (CHF) is the principal complication of heart disease. It is a pathophysiologic state produced by an abnormality in cardiac pump function (either transient or prolonged). The heart is unable to transport blood in a sufficient flow to meet metabolic needs. CHF occurs at some time in most cases of severe heart disease.
• This produces a variety of clinical circumstances from acute left ventricular dysfunction (due to tachyarrhythmia, bradyarrhythmia, and acute myocardial infarction) to chronic left ventricular dysfunction (due to chronic volume/pressure overload as seen in valvular heart disease)
• Two physiologic components explain most of the clinical findings of CHF - most patients have findings consistent with both mechanisms:
  ◊ an inotropic abnormality resulting in diminished systolic emptying (systolic failure)
  ◊ a compliance abnormality in which the ability of the ventricles to accept blood is impaired (diastolic failure).
System(s) affected: Cardiovascular, Pulmonary
Genetics: N/A
Incidence/Prevalence in USA:
• Most common inpatient diagnosis for patients over 65
Predominant age: Varies by etiology of heart disease
Predominant sex:
• Male > Female - ages 40-75
• Male = Female - ages 75 and over

SIGNS AND SYMPTOMS
• Early and mild impairment:
  ◊ Basilar rales
  ◊ Positive hepatojugular reflux
  ◊ Faint S3 gallop
  ◊ Nocturia
  ◊ Dyspnea on exertion-cardinal sign of left heart failure
  ◊ Deteriorating exercise capacity
  ◊ Fatigue
  ◊ Difficulty breathing
  ◊ Weakness
  ◊ Tachypnea with mild exertion
• Moderate impairment:
  ◊ Nocturnal nonproductive cough
  ◊ Orthopnea
  ◊ Paroxysmal nocturnal dyspnea
  ◊ Wheezing, especially nocturnal in absence of history of asthma or infection (cardiac asthma)
  ◊ Anorexia
  ◊ Fullness to dull pain in RUQ
  ◊ Tachypnea at rest
  ◊ Anxiety
  ◊ Hepatomegaly with tenderness to palpation
  ◊ Cool extremities due to peripheral vasoconstriction
  ◊ Prominent rales over bases
  ◊ Right pleural effusion
  ◊ Edema
  ◊ Gallop rhythm

◊ Diastolic hypertension
◊ Elevated jugular venous pressure
◊ Cardiomegaly
• Severe impairment:
  ◊ Cerebral dysfunction
  ◊ Abdominal bloating (ascites)
  ◊ Cyanosis
  ◊ Hypotension
  ◊ Pulsus alternans
  ◊ Anasarca
  ◊ Frothy and/or pink sputum
  ◊ Increased P2
  ◊ Cardiac cachexia
  ◊ Cheyne-Stokes respirations

CAUSES
• Myocardial infarction
• Cardiomyopathy
  ◊ Alcoholic
  ◊ Viral
  ◊ Long-standing hypertension
  ◊ Drugs (e.g., cyclosporine)
• Valvular abnormalities
  ◊ Aortic stenosis or regurgitation
  ◊ Rheumatic heart disease (mitral and aortic valvular disease)
• Volume overload
• Cardiac depressants; negative inotropes (e.g., beta blockers)
• Arrhythmias, eg, atrial fibrillation
• High output states
  ◊ Hyperthyroidism
  ◊ Beriberi heart disease

RISK FACTORS
• Iatrogenic inappropriate reduction of intensity of therapy
• Inappropriate Na+ and/or fluid excess
• Patient non-compliance
• Intercurrent arrhythmia, eg, atrial fibrillation
• Administration of drug with negative inotropic effects
• Inappropriate physical, emotional, or environmental stress
• Thyrotoxicosis, pregnancy, or any condition associated with increased metabolic demand

DIAGNOSIS

DIFFERENTIAL DIAGNOSIS
• Nephrotic syndrome: excluded by absence of history of asymptomatic edema, proteinuria in nephrotic range, and history of renal disease
• Cirrhosis: excluded by absence of stigmata of liver disease, and history of liver disease and its risk factors
• Left heart failure: findings of pulmonary congestion and diminished cardiac output appearing in patients with myocardial infarction, aortic and mitral valve disease, and hypertensive disease
• Right heart failure: findings of systemic vascular congestion (edema, ascites) appear in patients with cor pulmonale, tricuspid insufficiency, and most commonly in patients with uncorrected prolonged left heart failure
• Venous occlusive disease with subsequent peripheral edema

LABORATORY
• Lab findings - early and mild to moderate in severity
  ◊ Respiratory alkalosis
  ◊ Mild azotemia
  ◊ Decreased erythrocyte sedimentation rate
  ◊ Proteinuria (usually less than 1 gm/24 h that clears with treatment)
• Lab findings - severe
  ◊ Increased creatinine
  ◊ Hyperbilirubinemia in severe cases
  ◊ Dilutional hyponatremia with treatment in severe cases
Drugs that may alter lab results: N/A
Disorders that may alter lab results: N/A

PATHOLOGICAL FINDINGS
• Early and acute
  ◊ Firm lungs with microscopic revealing engorged capillaries with thickening of the alveolar septa with extravasation of red cells and edema fluid
  ◊ Liver is engorged, firm, and fluid-filled. Microscopic - reveals dilated central hepatic veins and sinusoids.
• Late and chronic
  ◊ Hemosiderin deposits in lungs
  ◊ "Nutmeg" liver with centrilobular necrosis
  ◊ Occasionally hemorrhagic nonbacterial enterocolitis with hemorrhagic necrosis secondary to mesenteric vasoconstriction

SPECIAL TESTS   N/A

IMAGING
• X-ray - mild changes: pulmonary artery wedge pressure = 18-23 mm Hg (2.4-3.1 kPa)
  ◊ Increased heart size
  ◊ Increased blood flow to the upper lobes
  ◊ Equalization of flow between the upper and lower lobes
• X-ray - moderate severe pulmonary artery wedge pressure = 20-25 mm Hg (2.7-3.3 kPa)
  ◊ Interstitial edema
  ◊ Kerley's B lines
  ◊ Perivascular edema
  ◊ Subpleural effusions
• X-ray - severe changes: pulmonary artery wedge pressure > 25 mm Hg (> 3.3 kPa)
  ◊ Alveolar edema
  ◊ Butterfly pattern of pulmonary edema

DIAGNOSTIC PROCEDURES
• Echocardiographic studies
• Cardiac catheterization, both right and left, for full diagnosis and prognosis

TREATMENT

APPROPRIATE HEALTH CARE
Inpatient when severe

GENERAL MEASURES
• Immediate treatment of the heart failure
• Search for underlying correctable conditions
• Eliminate contributing factors when possible
• Supplemental oxygen
• Antiembolism stockings
• Fluid and sodium restriction. Education about this is imperative for long term control. Daily weights guide overall therapy.
• Identify and control underlying correctable conditions (e.g., acute MI, valvular disease, hyperthyroidism, but most commonly inadvertent salt and/or fluid overload)

SURGICAL MEASURES
• Heart valve surgery - possibly, if defective heart valve is responsible; mitral valve repair especially helpful if mitral regurgitation is aggravating CHF
• Cardiac transplantation - to be considered in patients (age < 55) without other disqualifying medical problems, who are developing CHF unresponsive to other therapeutic maneuvers, and who are felt to have a life expectancy of less than a year

ACTIVITY
• During severe stage, bed rest with elevation of head of bed and anti-embolism stockings to help control leg edema
• Gradual increase in activity with walking will help increase strength

DIET
• Sodium restriction (initially 4 gm sodium qd)
• Weight reduction diet if appropriate
• Low fat diet to retard coronary artery disease
• Appropriate fluid restriction

PATIENT EDUCATION
• Printed patient information available from:
  ◊ American Heart Association, 7320 Greenville Avenue, Dallas, TX 75231, (214)373-6300
  ◊ American College of Cardiology, 911 Old Georgetown Road, Bethesda, MD 20814, (301) 897-5400

MEDICATIONS

DRUG(S) OF CHOICE
Diuretics, usually in combination with digitalis are used to initiate therapy. ACE inhibitors have become a mainstay of therapy. For acute pulmonary edema, IV morphine remains cornerstone of therapy.

• Digoxin
  ◊ Improves contractility, slows ventricular rate in atrial fibrillation
  ◊ May be harmful in acute MI, hypertrophic cardiomyopathy
  ◊ Loading dose should be sufficient to have early beneficial effect, especially in atrial fibrillation with a rapid rate, e.g., 0.5-1.0 mg IV/po, then another 1.0-1.5 mg in divided doses q4-6h
• Diuretics
  ◊ Furosemide (Lasix): IV or po, depending on severity of pulmonary congestion. May require continuous drip
  ◊ Metolazone (Zaroxolyn): excellent addition when furosemide does not seem to be sufficient
  ◊ Spironolactone: when used carefully, to avoid hyperkalemia. May be proper addition to difficult chronic cases.
• ACE Inhibitors
  ◊ Used to decrease afterload
  ◊ Improve general symptomatology and overall exercise capacity
• Beta blockers
  ◊ Carvedilol (Coreg) 3.125 mg po bid for 2 weeks, then 6.25 mg bid for 2 weeks, increased to maximum 25 mg bid for class I to III CHF
  ◊ Bisoprolol (Zebeta) 5-20 mg/day: in CIBIS-II study significantly decreases all-cause mortality and sudden death ("treatment effects were independent of the severity or cause of heart failure")
• Vasodilators
  ◊ IV nitroglycerin may be of short-term benefit to decrease preload, afterload, and systemic resistance.
  ◊ Oral medications, e.g., hydralazine, prazosin, and Isosorbide dinitrate demonstrate tachyphylaxis
Contraindications: Refer to manufacturer's literature
Precautions: ACE inhibitors may produce hypotension on first use in volume depleted patients. Beta blockers may produce profound hypotension.
Significant possible interactions: Refer to manufacturer's literature

ALTERNATIVE DRUGS
• Sympathomimetic amines. Can be used in severe CHF unresponsive to above measures
  ◊ Dopamine and dobutamine have been successful for short periods in treatment
  ◊ Dobutamine can be used on an intermittent outpatient basis with intermittent infusion. However, in spite of possibly improving quality of life, reduces long-term survival.

FOLLOWUP

PATIENT MONITORING
• Variable depending on clinical circumstances. Initially every 2-3 weeks after patient stabilized.
• Closely follow - history and physical findings, chest x-ray, electrolytes, BUN, and creatinine

PREVENTION/AVOIDANCE Treatment of underlying disorders when possible

POSSIBLE COMPLICATIONS
• Electrolyte disturbance
• Atrial and ventricular arrhythmias
• Mesenteric insufficiency
• Protein enteropathy
• Digitalis intoxication

EXPECTED COURSE/PROGNOSIS
• Result of initial treatment is usually good, whatever the cause
• Long-term prognosis variable. Mortality rates range from 10% with mild symptoms to 50% with advanced, progressive symptoms.

MISCELLANEOUS

ASSOCIATED CONDITIONS See Causes

AGE-RELATED FACTORS
Pediatric: Usually associated with congenital heart disease
Geriatric: Medications may need dosage adjustment
Others: N/A

PREGNANCY If occurs, will require special care

SYNONYMS
• Heart failure
• Dropsy
• Circulatory failure
• Cardiac failure

ICD-9-CM
428.0 Congestive heart failure

SEE ALSO N/A

OTHER NOTES N/A

ABBREVIATIONS
CCF = congestive cardiac failure

REFERENCES
• Braunwald E, ed: Heart Disease: A Textbook of Cardiovascular Medicine. 4th Ed. Philadelphia, W.B. Saunders Co., 1992
• Harvey AM: The Principles and Practice of Medicine. 22nd Ed. Norwalk, CT, Appleton & Lange, 1988
• The Cardiac Insufficiency Bisoprolol Study II. Lancet 1999;353:9-13
Illustrations: 8 available on CD-ROM
Internet references: http://www.5mcc.com

Author(s)
Phil Lobstein, MD

Conjunctivitis

BASICS

DESCRIPTION Inflammation of palpebral and/or bulbar conjunctiva. Pink eye refers to non-Neisseria bacterial conjunctivitis.
System(s) affected: Nervous, Skin/Exocrine
Genetics: N/A
Incidence/Prevalence in USA: Unknown, but common
Predominant age: Depends on cause
Predominant sex: Male = Female

SIGNS AND SYMPTOMS
• General
  ◊ Conjunctival hyperemia
  ◊ Burning
  ◊ Foreign body sensation
  ◊ Pruritus
  ◊ Lacrimation
  ◊ Exudation and matting
  ◊ Chemosis
  ◊ Pseudoptosis
  ◊ Preauricular adenopathy
  ◊ Tarsal plate papillary hypertrophy
  ◊ Tarsal plate lymphoid follicles
  ◊ Pseudomembranous and membranes
  ◊ Photosensitivity
  ◊ Decreased acuity if there is complicating ulcer or keratitis
  ◊ Granulomas (rare)
• Bacterial
  ◊ Minimal pruritus
  ◊ Moderate tearing
  ◊ Profuse exudate, particularly Neisseria species
  ◊ Usually unilateral (or initially unilateral)
  ◊ Small tarsal plate papillae
  ◊ Neisseria species may cause chemosis
  ◊ Gram and Giemsa stain: Polymorphonuclear neutrophils (PMN's) and bacteria (gram negative intracellular diplococci with Neisseria species)
• Viral
  ◊ Minimal pruritus
  ◊ Profuse tearing
  ◊ Minimal exudate
  ◊ Often bilateral
  ◊ Preauricular adenopathy common
  ◊ Subconjunctival hemorrhage (acute hemorrhagic conjunctivitis)
  ◊ Associated viral systemic symptom (fever, myalgia, etc.)
  ◊ Tarsal plate follicles
  ◊ Pharyngeal follicles if associated pharyngitis
  ◊ Gram and Giemsa stain: Mononuclear cells (lymphocytes)
  ◊ Rare chemosis except with epidemic keratoconjunctivitis
  ◊ Subepithelial corneal opacities with epidemic keratoconjunctivitis
  ◊ Diffuse punctate corneal fluorescein uptake or dendrites with herpes simplex
  ◊ Typical zoster rash along ophthalmic branch of trigeminal nerve with varicella-zoster blepharoconjunctivitis
  ◊ Typical measles rash, Koplik's spots, etc. with measles
• Chlamydial
  ◊ Minimal pruritus
  ◊ Moderate to profuse tearing
  ◊ Profuse exudate (sometimes modest)
  ◊ Often bilateral
  ◊ Small tarsal plate papillae
  ◊ Tarsal plate follicles present
  ◊ Gram and Giemsa stain: PMN's, plasma cells, inclusion bodies, in trachoma large palely staining lymphoblastic cells
  ◊ Inclusion conjunctivitis commonly has preauricular adenopathy and large tarsal plate papillae and follicles. Occasionally associated genitourinary symptoms in young adults or history of bilateral conjunctivitis unresponsive to topical antibiotics.
  ◊ Lymphogranuloma venereum is rare and non-follicular (mostly granulomatous conjunctival) with large preauricular node (visible bubo)
  ◊ Trachoma rare in the USA (except American Indians of Southwest) and has 4 clinical stages
• Allergic
  ◊ Severe pruritus
  ◊ Moderate tearing
  ◊ No exudate
  ◊ Bilateral
  ◊ Chemosis very common
  ◊ Tarsal papillae
  ◊ Gram and Giemsa's stain: Eosinophils and basophils
  ◊ Allergic rhinoconjunctivitis has associated sneezing, rhinitis but if not of sufficient duration will not develop papillae
  ◊ Vernal conjunctivitis is recurrent in warm weather associated with large "cobblestone" papillae in those with history of atopic allergy
  ◊ Giant papillary conjunctivitis has similar appearance to vernal conjunctivitis with less pruritis and is seen in soft (and occasionally hard) contact lens use
• Chemical or irritative
  ◊ Tarsal follicles with conjunctivitis of topical medications
  ◊ Tearing and exudation depends on toxicity of chemical
  ◊ Chemosis common in post therapeutic irrigation
  ◊ Gram and Giemsa stain: PMN's if tissue necrosis

CAUSES
• Bacterial
  ◊ *Staphylococcus aureus*
  ◊ *Streptococcus pneumoniae*
  ◊ *Haemophilus influenzae*
  ◊ *Neisseria gonorrhoeae*
  ◊ *Neisseria meningitidis*
  ◊ Rarely other Streptococcal sp., pseudomonas, *Branhamella catarrhalis*, Coliforms, Klebsiella, Proteus, *Corynebacterium diphtheriae, Mycobacterium tuberculosis, Treponema pallidum*
• Viral
  ◊ Adenoviruses types 3, 4, 7 (pharyngitis with conjunctivitis)
  ◊ Adenoviruses types 8 and 19 (epidemic keratoconjunctivitis)
  ◊ Adenovirus 11, Coxsackie A24, enterovirus 70 (acute hemorrhagic conjunctivitis)
  ◊ *Herpes simplex* (primary and recurrent)
  ◊ Coxsackievirus type A28
  ◊ Molluscum contagiosum
  ◊ Varicella
  ◊ *Herpes zoster*
  ◊ Measles virus
• Chlamydial
  ◊ *Chlamydia trachomatis* (trachoma)
  ◊ *Chlamydia oculogenitalis* (inclusion conjunctivitis)
  ◊ *Chlamydia lymphogranulomatis* (lymphogranuloma venereum)
• Allergic
  ◊ Rhinoconjunctivitis (hay fever) - humoral
  ◊ Vernal conjunctivitis
  ◊ Giant papillary conjunctivitis
  ◊ Delayed (cellular)
  ◊ Autoimmune (Sjögren's, pemphigoid, Wegener's granulomatosis)
• Chemical or irritative
  ◊ Topical medication
  ◊ Home/industrial chemicals
  ◊ Wind
  ◊ Smoke
  ◊ Ultraviolet light
• Other
  ◊ Rickettsial, fungal, parasitic, tuberculosis, syphilis, Kawasaki disease
  ◊ Thyroid disease, gout, carcinoid, sarcoidosis, psoriasis, Stevens-Johnson syndrome, Ligneous conjunctivitis, Reiter's syndrome

RISK FACTORS
Numerous, including trauma from wind, cold and heat, chemicals and foreign body

DIAGNOSIS

DIFFERENTIAL DIAGNOSIS
• Uveitis (iritis, iridocyclitis, choroiditis)
• Acute glaucoma
• Corneal disease or foreign body
• Canalicular obstruction (canaliculitis, dacryocystitis)
• Scleritis and episcleritis

LABORATORY
• Culture from conjunctiva
• Gram and Giemsa stain of the discharge or scrapings
Drugs that may alter lab results: N/A
Disorders that may alter lab results: N/A

PATHOLOGICAL FINDINGS N/A

SPECIAL TESTS
• Cultivation on HeLa cells and neutralization tests for epidemic keratoconjunctivitis
• Bovin fixation and Papanicolaou stain for multinucleated giant cells of herpes simplex conjunctivitis. Also available, viral culture and immunofluorescence test for Herpes simplex.
• Immunofluorescent antibody tests for chlamydia serology
• Frei test for lymphogranuloma venereum

IMAGING N/A

DIAGNOSTIC PROCEDURES
• Culture of exudate
• Smear and stain of exudate

TREATMENT

APPROPRIATE HEALTH CARE
Outpatient

GENERAL MEASURES
• Record acuity
• Fluorescein staining to detect ulcer, keratitis
• No patch
• See Medications
• Culture
• No topical steroids
• Ophthalmologic referral if ulcer, keratitis, suspected herpes or worsens after 24 hours of treatment
• Compresses - warm if infective, cold if allergic or irritative
• Remove purulent material and debris (may require frequent irrigation)
• Giant papillary allergic conjunctivitis requires discontinuing use of contact lenses

SURGICAL MEASURES   N/A

ACTIVITY   No restrictions

DIET   No restrictions

PATIENT EDUCATION
• Transmission route of infecting agent if contagious
• Demonstrate eye drop techniques
• Demonstrate ointment techniques

MEDICATIONS

DRUG(S) OF CHOICE
• Bacterial
  ◊ 0.3% tobramycin or gentamicin. As drops (1-2 gtts) instilled every 4 hours while awake for 5 days, as ointment qid.
  ◊ 10% sodium sulfacetamide. As drops (1-2 gtts) instilled every 4 hours while awake for 5 days, as ointment qid and hs (stings).
  ◊ Erythromycin ophthalmic ointment qid
  ◊ Systemic treatment for Neisseria species as other sites usually involved. Some authorities (with ophthalmology consult) add topical erythromycin.
• Viral
  ◊ Trifluridine 1% drops, 1 drop every 2 hours while awake, maximum 9 drops a day
  ◊ Acyclovir oral and topical for herpetic (wide range of doses, consult drug reference)
  ◊ Topical antibiotics to prevent bacterial superinfection or if diagnosis is in doubt
• Chlamydial
  ◊ Oral doxycycline 100 mg bid (3 weeks) for inclusion conjunctivitis
• Allergic
  ◊ Topical vasoconstrictor and/or antihistamine combination such as naphazoline 0.05% or antazoline (Albalon-A, Vasocon-A) 0.5%
  ◊ Oral antihistamine

◊ Topical cromolyn (Opticrom) 2%, 4% qid starting 2 weeks before season. (Opticrom no longer imported into the U.S. Available in Canada, UK, and Europe in 2% solution.)

Contraindications:
• Tetracycline: not for use in pregnancy or children < 8 years.

Precautions:
• Tetracycline: may cause photosensitivity; sunscreen recommended.
• Vasoconstrictors make the eye appear less severely affected
• Avoid contamination of medication bottles by touching lids

Significant possible interactions:
• Tetracycline: avoid concurrent administration with antacids, dairy products, or iron.

ALTERNATIVE DRUGS
• Bacterial
  ◊ Polymyxin-gramicidin
  ◊ Neomycin-polymyxin B-bacitracin (Neosporin); 15% of people have hypersensitivity reaction to neomycin
  ◊ Chloramphenicol - warning, slight hematological risk
  ◊ Ciprofloxacin
  ◊ Framycetin
  ◊ Norfloxacin
• Chlamydial
  ◊ Oral tetracycline or erythromycin (3 weeks) for inclusion conjunctivitis. Some authorities recommend topical tetracycline or erythromycin in addition.
• Allergic
  ◊ Numerous topical vasoconstrictors and antihistamines
  ◊ Numerous oral antihistamines

FOLLOWUP

PATIENT MONITORING   Referral if worse in 24 hours

PREVENTION/AVOIDANCE
• Avoid listed causes when possible
• Wash hands frequently

POSSIBLE COMPLICATIONS
• Bacterial
  ◊ Chronic marginal blepharitis
  ◊ Conjunctival scar if membrane developed
  ◊ Corneal ulcer or perforation
  ◊ Hypopyon
  ◊ Rare portal of entry for meningococcus
• Viral
  ◊ Corneal scars with herpes simplex
  ◊ Corneal scars, lid scars, entropion, misdirected lashes with Varicella-zoster
  ◊ Bacterial superinfection
• Chlamydial
  ◊ Clinical trachoma (not with inclusion conjunctivitis)
• Allergic, chemical and others
  ◊ Bacterial superinfection

EXPECTED COURSE/PROGNOSIS
• Bacterial
  ◊ 10-14 days without treatment
  ◊ 2-4 days with treatment
• Viral
  ◊ 10 days for pharyngitis with conjunctivitis
  ◊ 3-4 weeks for epidemic keratoconjunctivitis
  ◊ 2-3 weeks for herpes simplex
• Chlamydial
  ◊ 3-9 months for untreated inclusion conjunctivitis
  ◊ 3-5 weeks for trachoma with treatment

MISCELLANEOUS

ASSOCIATED CONDITIONS   N/A

AGE-RELATED FACTORS
Pediatric: Neonatal conjunctivitis may be toxic, bacterial (genital tract bacteria or nosocomial) or chlamydial
Geriatric: More likely to have diseases or problems listed in Causes
Others: N/A

PREGNANCY   N/A

SYNONYMS   Pink eye

ICD-9-CM
077.99 Viral conjunctivitis
372.50 Conjunctival degeneration, unspecified
372.14 Other chronic allergic conjunctivitis

SEE ALSO
• Rhinitis, allergic
• Vernal keratoconjunctivitis
• Sjögren's syndrome

OTHER NOTES   N/A

ABBREVIATIONS
PMN = polymorphonuclear neutrophils

REFERENCES
• Rosen P, Barkin R: Emergency Medicine. 3rd Ed. St. Louis, Mosby, 1992
• Howes R: Emergency Clinics of North America 1988;6(I)
Illustrations: 1 available on CD-ROM
Internet references: http://www.5mcc.com

Author(s)
Charles W. Ricketson, MD, FRCPC

Constipation

BASICS

DESCRIPTION
A combination of changes in the frequency, size, consistency, and ease of stool passage, which leads to an overall decrease in volume of bowel movements. Very subjective, each individual has their own threshold level.

System(s) affected: Gastrointestinal

Genetics: Unknown (the condition may be familial)

Incidence/Prevalence in USA:
- Higher at extremes of life, i.e., among infants/children and the elderly
- Common; affects a majority of persons during their lifetimes

Predominant age: All ages can be affected; more frequent at the extremes of life (infancy and old age)

Predominant Sex: Female > Male

SIGNS AND SYMPTOMS
- Less frequency of stooling than the patient perceives as "normal" (normal is 3-5 times/week)
- Harder stool than "normal"
- Smaller stools than normal (average < 35 grams/day is abnormal)
- Impaction of stool secondary to hardness
- Inspissated stool
- Lack of consistent urgency to stool
- Difficulty expelling feces from the rectum
- Painful evacuation of feces
- Lingering sense of incomplete emptying of the bowel
- Abdominal fullness or a feeling of malaise secondary to inadequate bowel evacuation
- Tenesmus

CAUSES
- Electrolyte abnormalities
  ◊ Hypercalcemia
  ◊ Hypokalemia
- Hormonal abnormalities
  ◊ Hypothyroidism
  ◊ Diabetes
- Congenital impediments, e.g., aganglionic megacolon (Hirschsprung's disease) or excessively elongate, redundant, capacious bowel (dolichocolon)
- Congenital or acquired neuromuscular bowel impairment ("pseudo-obstruction")
- Concomitant illness, injury, or debility
- Mechanical bowel impediment (obstruction or ileus, due to any cause)
- Inadequate fluid intake
- Side-effect of drugs (e.g., anticholinergic agents, opiates)
- Chronic abuse of laxatives or cathartics
- Psychiatric, cultural, emotional, environmental factors
- Painful fecal evacuation from anal disease (e.g., fissures)

RISK FACTORS
- Extremes of life (very young and very old)
- Neurosis
- Polypharmacy
- Sedentary life style or condition

DIAGNOSIS

DIFFERENTIAL DIAGNOSIS
- Congenital
  ◊ Hirschsprung's
  ◊ Hypoganglionosis
  ◊ Congenital dilation of the colon
  ◊ Small left colon syndrome
- Meconium ileus
- "Normal" stooling with anxious patient or parent
- Illnesses predisposing to constipation
  ◊ Dehydration
  ◊ Hypothyroidism
  ◊ Hypokalemia
  ◊ Hypercalcemia
- Other causes of abdominal pain

LABORATORY
- Only necessary when other disorders are being considered
  ◊ CBC to detect anemia that may indicate colorectal neoplasm
  ◊ Thyroid functions
  ◊ Electrolytes, glucose, calcium

Drugs that may alter lab results: N/A
Disorders that may alter lab results: N/A

PATHOLOGICAL FINDINGS
- None in common, "functional" constipation
- Paucity or absence of intramural enteric ganglia in certain cases of congenital or acquired megacolon
- Neuromuscular abnormalities in certain cases of "pseudo-obstruction"

SPECIAL TESTS
- In selected cases of long-standing constipation, timed measure of passage of ingested stool markers may help discern differing impediments
- Anorectal motility in patients with suspected Hirschsprung's or anorectal motility disorders

IMAGING
- Plain (KUB) film of the abdomen may help to discern the extent and nature of the problem
- Barium enema or barium swallow with small bowel follow through looking for anatomical defects (mass lesions, ileus)
- Cineradiography of passage of barium, instilled in, then expelled from the rectosigmoid segment ("defecography"), may help define evacuation disorders in selected cases

DIAGNOSTIC PROCEDURES
- Digital rectal exam to rule out a rectal mass, check for blood in the stool, and define stool consistency
- Sigmoidoscopy or colonoscopy is seldom required, unless needed to define an abnormality discovered by barium enema or when there is evidence of iron deficiency anemia or blood in the stool

TREATMENT

APPROPRIATE HEALTH CARE
Outpatient usually, except when investigation discloses an underlying lesion or obstruction that requires hospitalization

GENERAL MEASURES
- Attempt to eliminate medications that may cause or worsen constipation
- Increase fluid intake
- Modify diet
- Enemas if other methods fail

SURGICAL MEASURES N/A

ACTIVITY Encourage exercise

DIET
- If no anatomic abnormalities, increase fiber to approximately 15 gm/day (bran, fruit, green vegetables, and whole grain cereals and breads)
- Encourage liberal intake of fluids

PATIENT EDUCATION
- Define constipation and normal variations
- Occasional mild constipation is normal
- Instruction in consistent "bowel training" i.e., allowing adequate time for bowel evacuation in a quiet, unhurried environment; instruction in facilitating posture on commode, e.g., thighs flexed toward abdomen
- Parents sometimes needs more treatment/advice than the constipated child

Constipation

MEDICATIONS

DRUG(S) OF CHOICE
• Hydrophilic colloids (bulk-forming agents; not really drugs)
◊ Psyllium (Konsyl, Metamucil, Perdiem)
◊ Methylcellulose (Citrucel)
◊ Polycarbophil (Mitrolan, Fibercon)
• Osmotic laxatives - appropriate for short-term use. The usual dose is 15 mL to 30 mL once or twice a day.
◊ Milk of magnesia 15-30 mL bid
◊ Magnesium citrate 15-30 mL bid
◊ Phosphate of soda 15-30 mL bid
◊ Lactulose (Chronulac) 15-30 mL bid
◊ Sorbitol 15-30 mL bid
◊ Alumina-magnesium (Maalox, Mylanta)
◊ Polyethylene glycol (MiraLax) 17 g in 8 oz of water q day
• Stool softeners
◊ Docusate sodium (Colace) 100 mg bid
Contraindications:
• Any impediment to bowel transit, such as an obstructing lesion or ileus. Osmotic laxatives may result in overdistension or bowel perforation
• Any acute intra-abdominal inflammatory condition
• Renal and heart failure are relative contraindications
Precautions: Advise patient against chronic use of irritant and osmotic laxatives
Significant possible interactions:
• Magnesium containing laxatives
◊ Bind tetracyclines preventing their absorption
◊ Reduce the effectiveness of digitalis and phenothiazines
◊ Sodium polystyrene sulfonate (Kayexalate) bind and prevent neutralization of bicarbonate, leading to systemic alkalosis, which may be severe

ALTERNATIVE DRUGS
• Lubricants (e.g., mineral oil) are unpalatable to many patients, subject to leakage, and impose the risk of aspiration
• Emollient suppositories are useful, if at all, in allaying anorectal soreness
• Irritant cathartics (stimulants)
◊ Ricinoleic acid or castor oil (Neoloid); 30-60 mL/day
◊ Phenolphthalein (Ex-Lax, Modane)
◊ Bisacodyl (Dulcolax); 2-3 tabs swallowed whole or 1 suppository bid
• Motor and secretory properties
◊ Anthraquinones-senna (Senokot); 1-2 cap or 15-30 mL qhs
• Enemas (avoid soap suds - may lead to colitis)
◊ Phospho soda (Fleets)
• Suppositories
◊ Osmotic: sodium phosphate
◊ Lubricant: glycerin
◊ Stimulatory: bisacodyl
• Prokinetic agents

FOLLOWUP

PATIENT MONITORING What seems to be simple, "functional" constipation, if it persists, should be further investigated for a possible "organic" cause

PREVENTION/AVOIDANCE Because for some patients a tendency to constipation is habitual, instruction in proper diet, bowel training, and use of bulk-forming supplements must be reinforced

POSSIBLE COMPLICATIONS
• Acquired megacolon: in severe, long-standing cases
• Cathartic colon: repeated laxative abuse
• Fluid and electrolyte depletion: laxative abuse
• Rectal ulceration ("stercoral ulcer") related to recurrent fecal impaction

EXPECTED COURSE/PROGNOSIS
Constipation that is only occasional, brief, and responsive to simple measures is harmless. That which is habitual can be a lifelong nuisance.

MISCELLANEOUS

ASSOCIATED CONDITIONS Debility, either general, as in the aged, or that imposed by specific, underlying illness

AGE-RELATED FACTORS
Pediatric: Consider Hirschsprung's disease
Geriatric:
• Elderly persons, who have enjoyed regular bowel action throughout their lives, seldom suffer constipation due to age alone
• Persons with a lifelong tendency to constipation often encounter increasing difficulty with advancing age
• There is an increased incidence of colorectal neoplasms with age that may be associated with constipation.
Others: N/A

PREGNANCY Women with a tendency to constipation may find the condition more troublesome in the third trimester and require dietary adjustment and supplements

SYNONYMS
• Costive bowel
• Locked bowels

ICD-9-CM
564.0 constipation
564.7 megacolon, other than Hirschsprung's
564.8 Other specified functional disorders of intestine (includes atony of colon)
751.3 Hirschsprung's disease and other congenital functional disorders of colon

SEE ALSO
• Congenital megacolon
• Encopresis

OTHER NOTES
Obstipation refers to intractable constipation

ABBREVIATIONS N/A

REFERENCES
• Rogers AI: Constipation In: Berk JE, Haubrich WS, eds. Gastrointestinal Symptoms: Clinical Interpretation. Philadelphia, B.C. Decker Inc., 1991
• Haubrich WS: Constipation. In: Berk JE, et al, eds. Bockus Gastroenterology. 4th Ed. Philadelphia, W.B. Saunders Co., 1985
• Devroede G: Constipation. In: Sleisenger MH, Fordtran JS, eds. Gastrointestinal Disease. 4th Ed. Philadelphia, W.B. Saunders Co., 1989
• Wald A: Approach to the patient with constipation. In: Yamada T, ed. Textbook of Gastroenterology. Vol. I. Philadelphia, J.B. Lippincott Co., 1991
• Nunez M, Robinson B: Management of Constipation in the Older Patient. J Florida MA 1991;78:12, 829-831
• Leonard-Jones JE: Clinical Management of Constipation, Pharmacology 1993;47(suppl1):216-223
• Goroll AH, May LA, Mulley AG: Approach to the Patient with Constipation. In Primary Care Medicine, Lippincott, 1987
Illustrations: N/A
Internet references: http://www.5mcc.com

Author(s)
David Frank, MD

Contraception

BASICS

DESCRIPTION Variety of practices designed to prevent pregnancy, to prevent implantation, to be spermicidal or to prevent sperm from reaching egg. Natural family planning aims to avoid coitus at the time of expected ovulation. The most effective is permanent sterilization, either tubal sterilization in the female (by electrocautery, loops, clips, or ligation and excision) or vasectomy in the male. Neither should be considered reversible, but either may be reversed under certain circumstances.
• Reversible methods and approximate pregnancy rates during first year of use (preg/100 women/year):
◊ Implantable contraceptive (Norplant) - 0.05
◊ Injectable contraceptive (Depo-Provera) - 0.3
◊ Oral contraceptives (the pill) - 5
◊ Intrauterine device (IUD) - 2
◊ Condom (rubber) - 12
◊ Diaphragm - 18
◊ Periodic abstinence - 20
◊ Spermicides alone - 21
◊ Female condom - 25
System(s) affected: Reproductive
Genetics: N/A
Incidence/Prevalence in USA:
• About two-thirds of women at risk for unwanted pregnancies use contraception
• Among individuals of reproductive age having regular coitus:
◊ Tubal sterilization 27%
◊ Vasectomy 12%
◊ Oral contraceptives 27%
◊ Condoms 21%
◊ Diaphragm 3.5%
◊ Intrauterine device 1.2%
◊ Natural family planning 2%
◊ Foam 0.6%
◊ Implantable contraceptive (Norplant) - N/A
◊ Injectable contraceptive (Depo-Provera) - 2.5
• In 1994, 3 million unintended pregnancies in the U.S.
Predominant age:
• Female - 11-52 years
• Male - any age after puberty
Predominant sex: Female. However, condom or vasectomy are the common male methods.

SIGNS AND SYMPTOMS N/A

CAUSES N/A

RISK FACTORS
• For pregnancy
◊ Any woman who is ovulating and having intercourse with a fertile male
◊ Young adolescents
◊ Socioeconomic factors - less access to medical care, or have limited knowledge about reproduction

DIAGNOSIS

DIFFERENTIAL DIAGNOSIS N/A

LABORATORY
• Female
◊ Cervical cytology
◊ Cultures for gonorrhea and Chlamydia
◊ Blood lipids, blood sugar
◊ Pregnancy test (if hormonal contraception is not initiated at time of menses)
• Male
◊ None except routine pre-operative studies prior to vasectomy
◊ Semen analysis after vasectomy; aspermia will require up to 15 ejaculations
Drugs that may alter lab results: N/A
Disorders that may alter lab results: N/A

PATHOLOGICAL FINDINGS N/A

SPECIAL TESTS N/A

IMAGING N/A

DIAGNOSTIC PROCEDURES N/A

TREATMENT

APPROPRIATE HEALTH CARE
Outpatient

GENERAL MEASURES
Non-drug methods
• Latex condom. Instruct on proper use.
• IUD. Insert at menses to rule out pregnancy. Contraindicated in nulliparity or multiple sexual partners (because of the risk of PID). Not advisable in patients with heavy menses.
◊ Progestasert (change annually)
◊ Paragard (change every 10 years)
• Diaphragm
◊ Use largest size which can be inserted without discomfort or distortion
◊ Refit after childbirth or if weight changes by more than 10%
◊ Contraindicated in significant uterine prolapse
• Female condom (Reality); OTC
• Periodic abstinence
◊ Regular cycles and accurate record of menstrual cycles for at least 12 months prior to use
◊ Fertile period calculated as shortest cycle minus 18 days to longest cycle minus 11 days
◊ Added effectiveness attained by observing cervical mucus (for disappearance of abundant clear mucus) and by observing basal temperature rise of about 1° for 3 days. Both indicate ovulation.
• Permanent sterilization
◊ Tubal sterilization in the female - sometimes performed as an office procedure
◊ Vasectomy in the male (almost always an office procedure)

SURGICAL MEASURES N/A

ACTIVITY N/A

DIET N/A

PATIENT EDUCATION
• Condoms. Use water-based lubricants. Add spermicide to increase effectiveness
• IUD. Check string periodically
• Diaphragm
◊ Before inserting, place one tablespoon of spermicidal gel or cream into the dome of diaphragm and line entire rim of the diaphragm with it
◊ Insert the diaphragm and check for proper placement
◊ Leave in for at least 8 hours after coitus - then remove and clean according to directions. Check for holes.
◊ If another act of coitus occurs before 8 hours, insert additional spermicidal gel or cream into vagina without displacing the diaphragm
• Female condom
◊ Use new condom for each sex act
◊ Insert properly so that inner ring is well into vagina and outer ring lies against vulva. Make sure that penis enters inside the sheath.
◊ Remove condom after intercourse being careful not to spill semen
• Oral contraception
◊ Take pill daily at approximately same time
◊ If a pill is missed, take two the following day but use an additional method of protection, such as a barrier method, until next period
◊ If two periods are missed, check for pregnancy. Do not stop pills if a period is missed.
• Medroxyprogesterone (Depo-Provera): return every 3 months for injection
• Norplant: replace after 5 years. Requires surgical insertion and removal.
• Printed materials available from ACOG (1-800-673-8444)
• Be aware of emergency contraceptive options and when to utilize

MEDICATIONS

DRUG(S) OF CHOICE
• Oral contraceptives
◊ Use sub-50 microgram estrogen dose to minimize side effects and risks (current pills contain 20, 30, or 35 mcg)
◊ Triphasics contain less total progestogen and therefore are less likely to affect lipid profile adversely
◊ All current pills contain ethinyl estradiol or mestranol as the estrogen. Newer formulations vary the amount of estrogen or give 5 days of estrogen alone during the usual placebo week.

◊ The progestogen varies between manufacturers - all are derivatives of testosterone and slight differences in the molecule produce different biological effects. Newer progestogens are less androgenic and therefore should have less adverse effects on lipoproteins. However, there is concern about an increased risk of stroke with pills containing desogestrel, e.g., desogestrel-ethinyl estradiol (Desogen, Orthocept). Low dose progestogen-only pills have high pregnancy rates; avoid them except in lactating women.

◊ Avoid generics because of uncertain or fluctuating dosage in each batch of pills.

◊ Eliminate side effects by trial and error
- Spermicides
  - ◊ All contain nonoxynol-9 (a surfactant)
  - ◊ Choice depends upon user preferences. Foam or creams are preferable since they disperse well.
- Implantable contraceptive - levonorgestrel (Norplant)
  - ◊ 6 silastic tubes implanted into the upper arm by physician
  - ◊ Effective for up to 5 years; after implantation do not require an active role by the patient
- Injectable contraceptive; medroxyprogesterone acetate (Depo-Provera)
  - ◊ 150 mg IM q 3 months
  - ◊ Contraceptive levels persist for up to 4 months (giving a 2-4 week margin of safety)
- Emergency Contraception (EC). Contraceptive methods which rely on changes to endometrial implantation receptivity and do not interfere with an established pregnancy.
  - ◊ ethinyl estradiol-norgestrel (Preven, Ovral) with 0.05mg + 0.25 mg respectively; these trade name products contain half the required dose for EC, so give 2 tabs and repeat in 12 hours. Give the first dose within 72 hours after intercourse, at a time which makes the second dose convenient. Other OCPs can be used and are effective (e.g., Triphasil: use 4 yellow pills per dose, which supplies .12mg estradiol + .5 mg of levogorgestrel). Nausea and vomiting are the primary side effects; consider pre-treatment with meclizine 2 hours before each dose.
  - ◊ Copper T IUD can be inserted within 5 days of intercourse
  - ◊ Progestin-only pills. Effective and avoids some of the side effects of the estrogen-containing regimens, but difficult to take [norgestrel (Ovrette); take 20 yellow pills and repeat in 12 hours]

Contraindications:
- Implantable or injectable contraceptives
  - ◊ Active liver disease
  - ◊ Thrombophlebitis
  - ◊ Pregnancy
  - ◊ Unexplained, abnormal, uterine bleeding
  - ◊ Cholestatic jaundice
  - ◊ Hyperlipidemia
- Oral contraceptives
  - ◊ Same as implantable contraception plus noncompliance and estrogen dependent malignancies
  - ◊ Relative contraindications are uterine leiomyomata, hypertension, insulin-requiring diabetes mellitus, and migraine headaches

Precautions: Refer to manufacturer's literature

Significant possible interactions:
- When these drugs needed, add a barrier method (or rarely, use a 50 mcg estrogen pill)
  - ◊ Phenytoin (Dilantin) - induces microsomal liver enzymes causing accelerated metabolism of hormones.
  - ◊ Antibiotics - decreased enterohepatic circulation. Rifampin may also increase metabolism of oral contraceptives.

ALTERNATIVE DRUGS N/A

FOLLOWUP

PATIENT MONITORING
- Annual pelvic exam and Pap smear
- Whenever side effects or problems occur
- Check for presence of IUD 1 month after insertion. If string is not found, use pelvic ultrasound to locate.
- Oral contraceptive users: 3 months after starting for hypertension; then annually

PREVENTION/AVOIDANCE N/A

POSSIBLE COMPLICATIONS
- Oral contraceptives, serious
  - ◊ Thromboembolism - stop method and treat the disorder. Do not resume oral contraception.
  - ◊ Hypertension - stop method; do not resume
  - ◊ MI - main risk in smokers, after age 35. Avoid in such patients.
- Oral contraceptives, minor
  - ◊ Nausea/vomiting - take after eating
  - ◊ Breakthrough bleeding - usually self-limited after 3 months. If not, change pill.
  - ◊ Amenorrhea - rule out pregnancy, then either change to a different pill or add conjugated estrogen 0.3 mg for the first 10 days of pill package
  - ◊ Cyclic weight gain - use smallest dose of estrogen available
  - ◊ Breast tenderness - rare with low dose pill
  - ◊ Depression - rare with low dose pill
  - ◊ Chloasma - stop pill or cover with makeup
  - ◊ Acne or hirsutism - change to a less androgenic progestogen
  - ◊ Cholestatic jaundice - stop pill; do not restart
  - ◊ Weight gain throughout cycle - use triphasic pill to minimize dose of progestogen or use newer progestogen
- Implantable contraceptive (Norplant)
  - ◊ Amenorrhea - about 33% (if it persists for 2 months, rule out pregnancy)
  - ◊ Irregular bleeding - about 33%
  Note: Both are self-limited after about a year - inform patient of side effects before choosing this method
- Injectable contraceptive (Depo-Provera)
  - ◊ Irregular bleeding during first few months
  - ◊ Not readily reversible
  - ◊ Amenorrhea - common after 1 year of use
  - ◊ Weight gain
- IUD
  - ◊ PID or salpingitis - remove IUD and start antibiotics
  - ◊ Heavy bleeding and cramps - remove IUD

EXPECTED COURSE/PROGNOSIS
- Pregnancy may occur with any method
  - ◊ After permanent sterilization - pregnancy indicates failure of the procedure and need for reoperation; evaluate for tubal implantation.
  - ◊ If IUD, remove the device if string visible. If string not seen, leave in place and account for device postpartum; slight increased risk of spontaneous abortion.
  - ◊ If oral contraceptive - stop pill. No expected increase birth defect rate; very slight chance of virilization in female fetus.
  - ◊ If implantable contraceptive - remove implants

MISCELLANEOUS

ASSOCIATED CONDITIONS N/A

AGE-RELATED FACTORS
Pediatric: Use of estrogen prior to pubertal growth spurt may lead to a reduction in ultimate height due to epiphyseal closure
Geriatric: For estrogen replacement therapy, avoid high dose oral contraceptives
Others: Healthy non-smokers may use oral contraceptives until age 50. When stopped, observe for menopause signs. Use other contraceptive method during this period.

PREGNANCY See above

SYNONYMS
- Birth control
- Family planning

ICD-9-CM N/A

SEE ALSO N/A

OTHER NOTES
- Benefit: decrease in the amount of menstrual flow and some protection against ovarian and endometrial cancer
- Breast cancer relationship uncertain; some suggest slight risk increase in certain groups

ABBREVIATIONS
PID = pelvic inflammatory disease
EC = emergency contraception

REFERENCES
- Speroff L, Glass RH, Kase NG: Clinical Gynecologic Endocrinology and Infertility. 5th Ed. Baltimore, Williams & Wilkins, 1994
- Trussel J, Stewart F. Dialogues in Contraception, University of Southern California, Fall 1998, Volume 5, Number 6
- Grimes DA, Wallach M (eds): Modern Contraception. Totawa, NJ, Emron, 1997
Illustrations: N/A
Internet references: http://www.5mcc.com

Author(s)
Alvin Langer, MD

Cor pulmonale

BASICS

DESCRIPTION Right ventricular enlargement/dysfunction and failure caused by pulmonary hypertension (increased right ventricular afterload) secondary to diseases of the lung, thorax, and pulmonary vasculature.
• Acute cor pulmonale: acute dilatation or overload of the right ventricle secondary to massive pulmonary embolism
• Chronic cor pulmonale: hypertrophy and dilatation of the right ventricle resulting from diseases of the pulmonary parenchyma and/or pulmonary vasculature (most commonly COPD)
System(s) affected: Cardiovascular, Pulmonary, Renal/Urologic
Genetics: No known genetic pattern
Incidence/Prevalence in USA: 5-10% of adult heart diseases
Predominant age: >45
Predominant sex: Male > Female

SIGNS AND SYMPTOMS
• Acute cor pulmonale:
  ◊ Severe dyspnea
  ◊ Pallor
  ◊ Diaphoresis
  ◊ Jugular venous distention with inspiration (Kussmaul's sign)
  ◊ Systolic murmur loudest at left sternal border (tricuspid regurgitation)
  ◊ Distended, tender, pulsatile liver
  ◊ S3 gallop
  ◊ Hypoxemia
  ◊ Cardiovascular collapse because of right ventricle's low output state
• Chronic cor pulmonale:
  ◊ Tachypnea/shortness of breath not relieved by sitting upright
  ◊ Productive or nonproductive cough
  ◊ Chest pain secondary to pulmonary artery root dilatation and right ventricular ischemia
  ◊ Hepatomegaly
  ◊ Peripheral edema
  ◊ Cyanosis
  ◊ Right ventricular systolic heave
  ◊ Pulmonary ejection click
  ◊ S3 gallop that increases with inspiration
  ◊ Jugular venous distention with prominent a- and v-waves
  ◊ Systolic murmur of tricuspid regurgitation
  ◊ Diastolic murmur of pulmonary regurgitation
  ◊ Right ventricular failure (indicated by increased venous pressure, edema, hepatojugular reflux, worsening tricuspid regurgitation, right ventricular pulsus alternans, development of S3 and S4).

CAUSES
• Disease affecting pulmonary air spaces
  ◊ Diffuse interstitial lung diseases: idiopathic pulmonary fibrosis, radiation induced fibrosis
  ◊ Pulmonary resection
  ◊ Chronic obstructive pulmonary diseases (chronic bronchitis, emphysema, asthma)

◊ Granulomatous and connective tissue diseases: sarcoidosis, rheumatoid arthritis, systemic lupus erythematosis, eosinophilic granuloma, mixed connective tissue disease
  ◊ Bronchiectasis
  ◊ Cystic fibrosis
  ◊ Malignant infiltration
  ◊ Chronic hypoxia at high altitude
  ◊ Congenital structural defects
• Diseases affecting the pulmonary vasculature
  ◊ Primary pulmonary hypertension
  ◊ Pulmonary embolism
  ◊ Tumor embolism
  ◊ Amniotic fluid embolism
  ◊ Schistosomiasis
  ◊ Sickle cell disease
  ◊ Pulmonary vascular disease secondary to systemic illness
  ◊ Granulomatous pulmonary arteritis
  ◊ Chronic liver disease
  ◊ Intravenous drug abuse
• Diseases affecting thoracic cage function
  ◊ Obesity
  ◊ Kyphoscoliosis
  ◊ Neuromuscular diseases
  ◊ Sleep apnea
  ◊ Pleural fibrosis
  ◊ Idiopathic hypoventilation

RISK FACTORS
• Tobacco abuse
• Living at high altitudes
• Industrial exposures

DIAGNOSIS

DIFFERENTIAL DIAGNOSIS
• Primary disease of the left side of the heart
• Congenital heart disease with left-to-right shunting

LABORATORY
• Acute cor pulmonale: ventilation/perfusion mismatch with hypoxia and hypocarbia
• Chronic cor pulmonale: pulmonary function testing shows airflow obstruction with reduced pO2 and possibly elevated hematocrit
Drugs that may alter lab results: N/A
Disorders that may alter lab results: N/A

PATHOLOGICAL FINDINGS
• Evidence of underlying etiology
• Dilated, hypertrophic right ventricle

SPECIAL TESTS
ECG: often normal, but findings can include:
• RVH: most common in primary pulmonary hypertension. Indicated by clockwise rotation of electrical axis, right axis deviation, and P pulmonale (increased P wave amplitude in II, III, and AVF)
• Right-sided heart failure suggested by:
  ◊ R/S in V1>1
  ◊ R/S in V6<1
  ◊ R wave in V1>5mm
  ◊ P wave in II>2.5 mm, consistent with right atrial enlargement
• Transient changes with hypoxia (arterial O2 saturation <85% and mean pulmonary arterial pressure >25 mm Hg) which may include:
  ◊ Rightward mean QRS axis (shift of 30° or

more from former position)
  ◊ Biphasic, flattened, or inverted T waves in the precordial leads
  ◊ ST segment depression in II, III and aVF
  ◊ Incomplete or complete (rare) right bundle-branch block

IMAGING
• Chest x-ray:
  ◊ Heart size may be normal in mild to moderate disease
  ◊ There may be counter-clockwise cardiac rotation and loss of aortic knob prominence with severe disease
  ◊ In the PA view, the left heart border is mostly comprised of the right ventricle
  ◊ Pulmonary hypertension gives rise to dilatation of the pulmonary trunk and hilar vessels
• Echocardiography estimates right ventricular dimensions, right atrial pressure, systolic pulmonary artery pressure, and the severity of tricuspid regurgitation. In patients with chronic cor pulmonale secondary to COPD, there may also be late diastolic LV filling secondary to RV pressure/volume overload-induced structural distortion of the left ventricale.
• Thallium-201 myocardial scintigraphy and MRI can be used to diagnose right ventricular hypertrophy

DIAGNOSTIC PROCEDURES
Right heart catheterization for quantitation of ventricular and pulmonary pressures and exclusion of congenital heart disease as etiology of right heart failure. Lung biopsy also helpful in discriminating among granulomatous and collagen-vascular diseases.

TREATMENT

APPROPRIATE HEALTH CARE
• Acute cor pulmonale: ICU setting
• Chronic cor pulmonale: outpatient

GENERAL MEASURES
• Vigorous antibiotic treatment of acute respiratory tract infections
• Avoidance of airway irritants (eg, tobacco smoke), sedatives and tranquilizers
• Treatment of underlying pulmonary disease, for example:
  ◊ Chronic obstructive pulmonary disease
    - Bronchodilators to relieve obstruction
    - Supplemental oxygen to correct hypoxia and acidemia
    - Vasodilators, diuretics and phlebotomy (when HCT 55-60%) are possibly useful
    - Digoxin with concomitant left ventricular failure
  ◊ Ventilatory abnormalities, eg, sleep apnea
    - CPAP (continuous positive airway pressure) or BiPAP (biphasic positive airway pressure)
    - Progestins
    - Tracheostomy
• Acute or chronic thromboembolic disease
  ◊ Appropriate anticoagulation and hemodynamic support

SURGICAL MEASURES N/A

ACTIVITY As tolerated

DIET Moderate salt restriction

PATIENT EDUCATION
• Signs of COPD exacerbation
• Sudden unilateral swelling of lower extremity in patient with hypercoagulability
• Diet restrictions
• Signs of edema to watch for
• Stress the need for adequate rest
• Referral to social service agency for home care help (oxygen, suctioning, etc)
• Report any signs of infections to physician
• Avoid use of nonprescription medications, especially sedatives

MEDICATIONS

DRUG(S) OF CHOICE
• Oxygen: Maintain arterial oxygen over 60 mm Hg (>8.0 kPa), if possible. Oxygen reduces pulmonary vascular resistance and improve myocardial dynamics by increasing tissue oxygen content. Excess oxygen depresses respiratory drive in patients with carbon dioxide retention.
• Theophylline: Bronchodilator, increases right ventricular ejection fraction (RVEF), and decreases pulmonary and systemic vascular resistance.
• Beta-adrenergic agonists: During acute, short-term administration, terbutaline beneficial probably by increasing RVEF and lowering pulmonary vascular resistance.
• Bronchodilators: (e.g., ipratropium, metaproterenol, albuterol) used every six hours and more often if necessary in order to maintain airway patency and arterial oxygen saturations
• Diuretics: (e.g., furosemide) for the relief of peripheral edema, combinations of furosemide and spironolactone (Aldactone) for ascites.
• Vasodilators: (e.g., hydralazine, nifedipine, diltiazem, prazosin) may be tried if conventional measures (oxygen and bronchodilators) fail. Success with these agents can only be accurately assessed with invasive monitoring. Benefit is obtained if the following criteria are met:
   ◊ There is a reduction in pulmonary vascular resistance by 20%
   ◊ Cardiac output increases or remains unchanged
   ◊ Pulmonary artery pressure decreases or remains unchanged
   ◊ Systemic vascular resistance does not drop significantly.
Consistent with the latter, monitor for systemic hypotension during initiation of therapy.

Contraindications: Sedatives and respiratory depressants should be avoided
Precautions: Diuretics-electrolytes should be monitored as excessive loss of potassium and chloride may result in profound metabolic alkalosis further impairing respiratory drive.
Significant possible interactions: Refer to manufacturer's literature

ALTERNATIVE DRUGS
• Digoxin: Controversial in the treatment of cor pulmonale. Although digoxin increases right heart contractility, it also induces pulmonary vasoconstriction, which may exacerbate right heart failure. Consequently, digoxin should only be used in cor pulmonale patients with concomitant left ventricular failure. Because of hypoxia and diuretic use in many of these patients, dangerous arrhythmias may develop.

FOLLOWUP

PATIENT MONITORING Dependent on the severity of the underlying disease, the extent of right heart failure, and medications in use

PREVENTION/AVOIDANCE Discontinue tobacco use, limit exposure to inhalational irritants and allergens

POSSIBLE COMPLICATIONS N/A

EXPECTED COURSE/PROGNOSIS
• Depends on underlying disease and degree of pulmonary hypertension. 50,000 deaths per year in US from acute pulmonary embolism. In more chronic forms of cor pulmonale, there is a 10-50% 5 year mortality which improves with supplemental oxygen. In COPD with cor pulmonale, 3 year mortality can approach 60%.
• The development of an S1S2S3 on EKG, an alveolar-arterial gradient >48 mm Hg during oxygen therapy, and right atrial overload are all predictors of poor prognosis when chronic cor pulmonale is secondary to COPD

MISCELLANEOUS

ASSOCIATED CONDITIONS Left heart failure

AGE-RELATED FACTORS
Pediatric: N/A
Geriatric: Metabolism of sedatives and narcotics may be slow, thus the respiratory drive of these patients may be affected for prolonged periods
Others: N/A

PREGNANCY Cardiology consultation indicated as the consequences of increased demand for placental perfusion may be severe

SYNONYMS N/A

ICD-9-CM
416.9 Cor pulmonale, chronic
415.0 Cor pulmonale, acute

SEE ALSO
• Congestive heart failure
• Cystic fibrosis
• Obesity
• Bronchiectasis

OTHER NOTES N/A

ABBREVIATIONS N/A

REFERENCES
• Brandenburg RO, Fuster V, Giuliani ER, McGoon DC: Cardiology: Fundamentals and Practice. Chicago, Year Book Medical Publishers, 1987
• Braunwald E: Cor Pulmonale. In: Fauci AS, et al, eds: Harrison's Principles of Internal Medicine.14th ed. new York, McGraw Hill, 1998:1324-1328
• Wiedemann HP, Matthay RA: Cor Pulmonale. In: Braunwald E, ed: Heart Disease: A Textbook of Cardiovascular Disease. 5th ed. Philadelphia, WD Saunders Co, 1997:1604-1625
• Incalzi RA, et al: Elwctrocardiographic chronic cor pulmonale: a negative prognostic finding in chronic obstructive pulmonary disease. Circulation 1999;99:1600-1605
• Tutar E, et al: Echocardiographic evaluation of left ventricular diastolic function in chronic cor pulmonale. Am J Cardiol 1999;83:1414-1417
Illustrations: N/A
Internet references: http://www.5mcc.com

Author(s)
Peter P. Toth, MD, PhD

Corneal ulceration

BASICS

DESCRIPTION Corneal ulcers represent an infection of the cornea by bacteria, virus or fungi as a result of breakdown in the protective epithelial barrier. If left untreated, corneal ulcers can result in blindness. Ulcerations may be central or marginal.
System(s) affected: Nervous
Genetics: None
Incidence/Prevalence in USA: Common
Predominant age: None
Predominant sex: Male = Female

SIGNS AND SYMPTOMS
• Eyelid and conjunctiva become inflammed
• Mucopurulent discharge
• The corneal epithelium will be absent with underlying ulceration and infiltration of the corneal stroma with leukocytes
• Foreign body sensation
• Blurred vision
• Light sensitivity
• Pain

CAUSES
• Corneal ulcers are predisposed by the presence of an entry to the external eye. Dry eye, burns, abrasion, contact lenses, inappropriate use of topical anesthetics, antibiotics, or anti-viral drops, immunosuppressant drugs, diabetes, immunodeficiency.
• Causative agents for foreign entry:
  ◊ Gram positive organisms (staphylococci, streptococci, and bacilli)
  ◊ Anaerobes (cocci, bacilli)
  ◊ Gram negative organisms (diplococcus, rods, and anaerobes)
  ◊ Pseudomonas
  ◊ Viruses such as herpes

RISK FACTORS
• Any abrasive injury
• Contact lenses (especially soft lenses)
• Chronic topical steroid use

DIAGNOSIS

DIFFERENTIAL DIAGNOSIS Identify infecting organisms

LABORATORY Culture the ulcer
Drugs that may alter lab results: Pretreatment with topical antibiotics or corticosteroids may delay diagnosis
Disorders that may alter lab results: N/A

PATHOLOGICAL FINDINGS Scrapings for Gram's and Giemsa's stain may demonstrate bacteria, yeast, or intranuclear inclusions which may aid in the diagnosis

SPECIAL TESTS N/A

IMAGING N/A

DIAGNOSTIC PROCEDURES Scrapings of the corneal ulcer may be necessary to identify the underlying organism. The sample should be plated onto the culture media directly.

TREATMENT

APPROPRIATE HEALTH CARE
• Outpatient or inpatient for severe ulcer or noncompliant patient
• All cases of corneal ulceration should be promptly referred to an ophthalmologist

GENERAL MEASURES
• Aggressive topical antibiotic treatment directed toward the causative agent should be instituted immediately while culture studies are pending
• Supplemental topical cycloplegia reduces the inflammation and aids in patient comfort
• Bandaging the eye should be avoided and topical steroids should never be used. Daily evaluation is necessary and prompt consultation with an ophthalmologist or corneal specialist is advised.

SURGICAL MEASURES N/A

ACTIVITY Reduced, until vision returns to normal and healing is complete

DIET No special diet

PATIENT EDUCATION Prevention of abrasions and proper handling of contact lenses can prevent recurrence of corneal ulcers

MEDICATIONS

DRUG(S) OF CHOICE
• Sulfacetamide 10% suspension (bacteriostatic) is only good for low grade conjunctival infections
• Topical gentamicin and tobramycin are effective against Pseudomonas, Enterobacter, Klebsiella, and aerobic gram negative organisms, while cephalosporins (e.g., cefazolin 50 mg/mL) may be effective against many gram negative organisms. The combination aminoglycoside and cephalosporin may be the most appropriate initial therapy.
• Topical quinolones, e.g., ciprofloxacin (Ciloxan) 0.3%, also ofloxacin (Ocuflox) 0.3%. These may be treatment of choice for Pseudomonas infections.
• Fungal keratitis needs to be treated with parenteral amphotericin B for candida and aspergillus; clotrimazole, miconazole, econazole, and ketoconazole may also be required

Contraindications: Refer to manufacturer's profile of each drug
Precautions: Refer to manufacturer's profile of each drug
Significant possible interactions: Refer to manufacturer's profile of each drug

ALTERNATIVE DRUGS   N/A

FOLLOWUP

PATIENT MONITORING   The patient should be monitored at least daily

PREVENTION/AVOIDANCE   Avoid corneal abrasion or injury and improper contact lens handling

POSSIBLE COMPLICATIONS   Scarring of the cornea and loss of vision

EXPECTED COURSE/PROGNOSIS
• Corneal ulcerations should improve daily and heal with appropriate therapy
• If healing does not occur or the ulcer extends, then consideration should be given to an alternative diagnosis and treatment

MISCELLANEOUS

ASSOCIATED CONDITIONS   Chronic ulcerations may be associated with neurotrophic keratitis due to lack of fifth nerve innervation of the cornea. Individuals with thyroid disease, diabetes, immunosuppressive conditions are particularly at risk.

AGE-RELATED FACTORS
Pediatric: N/A
Geriatric: Ring ulceration more common
Others: N/A

PREGNANCY   N/A

SYNONYMS   N/A

ICD-9-CM   370.0 Corneal ulcer

SEE ALSO   N/A

OTHER NOTES   N/A

ABBREVIATIONS   N/A

REFERENCES   None
Illustrations: N/A
Internet references: http://www.5mcc.com

Author(s)
Robert M. Kershner, MD, FACS

Costochondritis

BASICS

DESCRIPTION Anterior chest wall pain associated with pain and tenderness of the costochondral and costosternal regions.
System(s) affected: Musculoskeletal
Genetics: Unknown
Incidence/Prevalence in USA: 10% of chest pain complaints. 15-20% of teenagers with chest pain.
Predominant age: 20-40
Predominant sex: Female

SIGNS AND SYMPTOMS
• Insidious onset
• Pain usually sharp in nature, sometimes pleuritic
• Pain involves multiple locations, the second through fifth costal cartilage most often involved
• Pain worse with movement and breathing
• Heat often provides relief of pain
• Chest tightness is often associated with the pain
• Pain sometimes radiates into arm
• Non-suppurative edema and tenderness at rib articulations
• Redness and warmth at sites of tenderness

CAUSES
• Not fully understood
• Trauma
• Overuse

RISK FACTORS
• Unusual physical activity or overuse
• Recent upper respiratory infection

DIAGNOSIS

DIFFERENTIAL DIAGNOSIS
• Cardiac
  ◊ Coronary artery disease
  ◊ Aortic aneurysm
  ◊ Mitral valve prolapse
  ◊ Pericarditis
  ◊ Myocarditis
• Gastrointestinal
  ◊ Gastroesophageal reflux
  ◊ Peptic esophagitis
  ◊ Esophageal spasm
  ◊ Gastritis
• Musculoskeletal
  ◊ Fibromyalgia
  ◊ Slipping rib syndrome - involves the lower ribs
  ◊ Costovertebral arthritis
  ◊ Painful xiphoid syndrome
  ◊ Rib trauma with swelling
  ◊ Thoracic disk compression
  ◊ Ankylosing spondylitis
  ◊ Epidemic myalgia
  ◊ Precordial catch syndrome
• Psychogenic
  ◊ Anxiety disorder
  ◊ Panic attacks
  ◊ Hyperventilation
• Respiratory
  ◊ Asthma
  ◊ Pneumonia
  ◊ Chronic cough
  ◊ Pneumothorax
• Other
  ◊ Herpes zoster
  ◊ Spinal tumor
  ◊ Metastatic cancer
  ◊ Substance abuse (cocaine)

LABORATORY The diagnosis of costochondritis is based on a complete and thorough history and physical examination. Laboratory exams should only be utilized if there is concern regarding other elements of the differential diagnosis. Erythrocyte sedimentation rate inconsistently elevated.
Drugs that may alter lab results: N/A
Disorders that may alter lab results: N/A

PATHOLOGICAL FINDINGS
Costochondral joint inflammation

SPECIAL TESTS None indicated for the diagnosis of costochondritis

IMAGING No imaging is indicated for the diagnosis of costochondritis. Chest x-ray normal.

DIAGNOSTIC PROCEDURES None

TREATMENT

APPROPRIATE HEALTH CARE
Outpatient therapy

GENERAL MEASURES Patient reassurance. Rest and heat.

SURGICAL MEASURES N/A

ACTIVITY As tolerated

DIET Regular

PATIENT EDUCATION Educate the patient in regards to the self-limited nature of the illness. Instruct patient on proper physical activity regimens to avoid overuse syndromes. Also stress the importance of avoiding sudden, significant changes in activity.

Costochondritis

MEDICATIONS

DRUG(S) OF CHOICE Nonsteroidal anti-inflammatory drugs (NSAID's) such as aspirin, ibuprofen (Advil, Motrin), naproxen (Anaprox, Naprosyn, Aleve) or diclofenac (Voltaren). Other analgesics may be used as needed.

Contraindications:
• History of anaphylaxis to aspirin
• Peptic ulcer disease
• Renal insufficiency

Precautions:
• Peptic ulcers may occur with chronic use of nonsteroidal anti-inflammatory drugs
• Acute interstitial nephritis
• Drug accumulation with renal insufficiency
• Liver function abnormalities in up to 15% of patients

Significant possible interactions:
• NSAID's
   ◊ Albumin-bound drugs - displacement of either drug
   ◊ Warfarin - increased prothrombin time. Monitor prothrombin times closely and adjust warfarin dosage as needed. Monitor lithium levels and adjust lithium dosage as needed. May need to increase lithium dosage when non-steroidal anti-inflammatory drugs have been discontinued.
   ◊ Lithium - increased lithium plasma level
   ◊ Furosemide - decreased natriuretic effect and increased risk of acute renal failure secondary to decreased renal blood flow
   ◊ Propranolol - decreased anti-hypertensive effect

ALTERNATIVE DRUGS Acetaminophen

FOLLOWUP

PATIENT MONITORING Followup in one week

PREVENTION/AVOIDANCE Avoid activity which increases the pain

POSSIBLE COMPLICATIONS
Incomplete attention to differential diagnosis or inappropriate interventions in a desire to ensure that a more life-threatening diagnosis is not missed

EXPECTED COURSE/PROGNOSIS
• Self-limited illness, although sometimes chronic
• Often recurs

MISCELLANEOUS

ASSOCIATED CONDITIONS Upper respiratory infections

AGE-RELATED FACTORS
Pediatric: Special attention should be paid to psychogenic chest pain with children who perceive family discord
Geriatric: Often present with multiple problems capable of causing chest pain, making a thorough history and physical exam imperative.
Others: N/A

PREGNANCY Unknown

SYNONYMS
• Costosternal syndrome
• Parasternal chondrodynia
• Anterior chest wall syndrome
• Tietze's disease
• Tietze's syndrome
• Chondrocostal junction syndrome

ICD-9-CM
733.6 Tietze's disease (costochondritis)

SEE ALSO N/A

OTHER NOTES N/A

ABBREVIATIONS N/A

REFERENCES
• A report from ASPN: An exploratory report of chest pain in primary care. J Am Board Fam Prac 1990, 3:143-150
• Klinkman MS, Stevens D, Gorenflaw DW: Episodes of care for chest pain: A preliminary report. From MIRNET, J Fam Practice 1994;38(4):345-52
• Disla E, Rhim HR, Reddy A, Karten I, Taranta A: Costochondritis. a prospective analysis in an emergency department setting. Archives Int Med 1994:154(21):2466-2469
• Mukamel M, Kornreich L, Horev G, Zaharia A, Mimoun M: Tietze's syndrome in children. J Ped 1997;131(5):774-775
• Klinkman MS, Stevens D, Gorenflow DU: Episodes of cure for chest pain: a preliminary report from MIRNET. Michigan Research Network. J Fam Prac 1994;38(4):345-352
Illustrations: N/A
Internet references: http://www.5mcc.com

Author(s)
Scott A. Fields, MD

Crohn's disease

BASICS

DESCRIPTION An idiopathic inflammatory disease of the small intestine (60%), the colon (20%) or both; involving all of the layers of the bowel, but most commonly involving the terminal ileum. It is a slowly progressive and recurrent disease with prominent involvement of multiple regions of the intestine with normal sections in between.

System(s) affected: Gastrointestinal

Genetics: 15% of patients have first-degree relatives with inflammatory bowel disease. Family members develop the disease with similar patterns and similar age of onset.

Incidence/Prevalence in USA:
• More common in Caucasians than African-Americans or Asians
• More common in Jews
• 20-100/100,000 prevalence

Predominant Age:
• Most cases 15-25 age of onset
• Second smaller peak in ages 55-65

Predominant Sex: Female > Male (slightly)

SIGNS AND SYMPTOMS
• All forms of Crohn's
  ◊ Diarrhea occurs in most patients
  ◊ Abdominal pain in two-thirds
  ◊ Weight loss
  ◊ Abdominal tenderness often less than expected, in view of symptoms
  ◊ Abdominal mass (occasionally)
  ◊ Fistula - perirectal, bladder, skin, vagina
  ◊ Extraluminal disease (10%) skin, iritis, arthritis, sclerosing cholangitis
• Small bowel disease only
  ◊ Diarrhea prominent, including nocturnal
  ◊ Vague abdominal pain frequent. Only half of patients with abdominal pain have associated tenderness, not relieved with evacuation and often aggravated by food.
  ◊ Intestinal obstruction in 1/3. Cramping abdominal pain precedes for months.
  ◊ Bleeding in 20%, rarely massive
  ◊ Perianal disease, including fistulae
  ◊ Internal fistulae
  ◊ Arthritis 5%
• Colon disease only
  ◊ Diarrhea prominent, including nocturnal
  ◊ Hematochezia
  ◊ Abdominal pain in 1/2, often relieved by stooling
  ◊ Perianal disease in 40%, fistulae
  ◊ Weight loss prominent
  ◊ Megacolon occurs in about 10%
  ◊ Arthritis in 20%
  ◊ Intestinal obstruction occasional
• Colon and small bowel disease
  ◊ Intestinal obstruction much more common
  ◊ Arthritis 5%

CAUSES
• Idiopathic
• Aggravated by bacterial infection
• Aggravated by inflammatory cascade
• Aggravated by smoking cessation

RISK FACTORS
• More cigarette smokers than expected

DIAGNOSIS

DIFFERENTIAL DIAGNOSIS
• Colon disease
  ◊ Ulcerative colitis
  ◊ Ischemic colitis (older age group)
  ◊ Enteric pathogens: Amebiasis, Tuberculosis, Yersinia, Campylobacter, Gonorrhea, Clostridium difficile toxin, Shigella, Salmonella, LGV and non-LGV Chlamydia, Fungi(e.g., actinomycosis)
  ◊ Malignancy: Lymphoma, adenocarcinoma
  ◊ Caustic enemas (e.g., H2O2)
• Small bowel disease
  ◊ Enteric pathogens: Tuberculosis, Yersinia, Campylobacter, LGV and non-LGV Chlamydia, Fungi (e.g., actinomycosis), Chlamydial pelvic inflammation in women
  ◊ Lymphoma
  ◊ Drugs (e.g., NSAID's)
  ◊ Eosinophilic gastroenteritis

LABORATORY
• Elevated sedimentation rate
• Anemia common
• Albumin decreased in severe cases
• Serum electrolytes imbalance
• Specific nutrient deficiency: B12, fat soluble vitamins, folate

Drugs that may alter lab results: Sulfa drugs may lower folate after years of administration

Disorders that may alter lab results: All tests are non-specific, similar degrees of disease from other causes produce similar changes

PATHOLOGICAL FINDINGS
• Involvement of all layers of gut wall with inflammation in > 95% cases at least focal areas
• Skip areas in 80% (a normal segment between two involved segments)
• Granuloma in 15%
• Fat hypertrophy following mesenteric vessels in 50% of small bowel disease

SPECIAL TESTS Colonoscopy is most helpful. The colon is not uniformly involved. The typical lesion is nodular with undermined pus filled mucosal ulcers. Strictures commonly present, occasionally preventing passage of the endoscope. The terminal ileum often has aphthous ulcers and may have nodularity. Small bowel proximal to an anastamosis is a very common site of recurrence.

IMAGING
• Barium x-rays - enema and small bowel
  ◊ Loss of smooth mucosa, undermined ulcers prominent
  ◊ Narrowed lumen in most involved segments of small bowel
  ◊ Fistulae from involved segment to other bowel loops, bladder, vagina or external
  ◊ Skip areas, multiple lesions common
  ◊ Failure to reflux into ileum on barium enema (not specific)
  ◊ Ulcers undermining mucosa
  ◊ Small bowel ulcerated wall
  ◊ Narrowed lumen
  ◊ Fistula to other parts of intestine

• Plain x-rays
  ◊ Intestinal obstruction
  ◊ Toxic patient with colon disease, toxic megacolon
  ◊ Evaluation of arthritis
  ◊ Sacroiliitis
• CT Scans
  ◊ Define thickening of bowel wall if lumen not narrowed
  ◊ Define abscess cavities and fistulae
  ◊ Identify extensive perirectal disease

DIAGNOSTIC PROCEDURES
• Ileoscopy and enteroscopy
• The constellation of barium-identified distribution of lesions, endoscopic findings, and biopsies usually establish the diagnosis
• Biopsies of mucosa in involved areas usually compatible with diagnosis, but not diagnostic. Helps rule out other causes.

TREATMENT

APPROPRIATE HEALTH CARE
• Outpatient customary, inpatient for complications or special treatments
• Progressive disease - average patient requires surgery each 4-7 years

GENERAL MEASURES
• Attention to maintaining weight and nutrition
• Monitor severe cases for fat malabsorption
• Perirectal disease, sitz baths, soap and water after stooling, surgical drainage of perirectal abscesses, surgical treatment of recurrent fistulae if medical management fails
• Extracolonic disease (uveitis, arthritis, dermatitis, sclerosing cholangitis) managed as other diseases in that special area
• Folate supplements often needed

SURGICAL MEASURES
• Indications for surgery:
  ◊ Severe recurrent hemorrhage
  ◊ Inability to thrive
  ◊ Abscess
  ◊ Total or recurrent intestinal obstruction
  ◊ Toxic megacolon or extensive disease
  ◊ Symptomatic fistulae other than rectal
  ◊ Failure of ostomy to function after ≥1 year

ACTIVITY Full activity as tolerated

DIET
• Usually no restrictions
• If fat malabsorption, diminish fat in diet
• If strictures or recurrent obstruction, avoid highly fibrous substances
• If diarrhea prominent, increase dietary fiber (sometimes recommended), decrease fat

Crohn's disease

PATIENT EDUCATION An important part of management. Crohn's and Colitis Foundation of America Inc, 11th floor, Park Ave South, NY 10016, Phone (800)343-3637. Joining local chapters recommended.

MEDICATIONS

DRUG(S) OF CHOICE
• Maintenance therapy
◊ Usually with mesalamine (5-aminosalicylic acid, Asacol, Claversal, Rowasa), methotrexate, or azathioprine (Imuran) prolongs remission and delays additional surgery
◊ Inducing a remission usually depends on prednisone or mesalamine enemas for rectal symptoms because the response is rapid
◊ Several delivery forms of mesalamine exist; each targets a different portion of the intestine. Select form appropriate to patient.
• Bringing acute exacerbations or complications under control
◊ Prednisone 20 to 40 mg/day. Response in 1-3 weeks, taper after 4-6 weeks.
◊ Sulfasalazine, or 5-aminosalicylic acid derivative. Increase dose each 4 days from 0.5 gm bid to 1 gm qid if tolerated. Response in 4 to 6 weeks.
• Rectal and left sided colon disease
◊ Mesalamine enema (5-aminosalicylic acid, 5-ASA, Rowasa) 2 gm 2-3 times daily
◊ Hydrocortisone (Cortenema) enema 2-3 times daily or suppositories for proctitis
• Predominantly perirectal disease with fistulae
◊ Metronidazole (Flagyl) 250 mg tid for max of 8 weeks
• Colon disease in sulfasalazine intolerant patient
◊ Mesalamine (5-ASA) preparations, enteric-coated: Asacol (800 mg tid), Claversal, Rowasa controlled release
◊ Olsalazine (Dipentum) 1 gm/day in two divided doses, increase up to maximum of 2 gm/day.
• Ileal disease
◊ Oral or IV steroids
◊ Mesalamine (Asacol)
◊ Nicotine patches or gum are occasionally used to relieve cramping symptoms or diarrhea
Contraindications: Allergy to prescribed drugs
Precautions:
• Sulfasalazine may not be tolerated by the stomach at necessary dose since it frequently causes nausea, vomiting, and other gastrointestinal distress
• Allergies common
• Male sterility problem with chronic use
• Watch for thrombocytopenia and pancytopenia
Significant possible interactions: Folic acid supplements needed with mesalamine. Refer to manufacturer's profile of each drug.

ALTERNATIVE DRUGS
• Sulfasalazine least costly and well tolerated in 90% of patients. Similar effectiveness but better tolerance with the 5-aminosalicylic acid compounds.
• Metronidazole produces severe peripheral neuritis after months of treatment. Other antibiotics similar in action may be used.
• Antibiotics
• Azathioprine (Imuran), mercaptopurine (6-mercaptopurine), methotrexate
• Refractive cases may respond to 6 week courses of cyclosporine or infliximab (Remicade), particularly useful to heal fistulae.

FOLLOWUP

PATIENT MONITORING
• Regular assessment (each 3-6 months if patient is stable) of symptoms, particularly status of weight, pain, diarrhea, hemoglobin and sedimentation rate
• Regular calculation of an activity index based upon:
1) loose stools/day, 2) pain, 3) general well being, 4) systemic manifestations, 5) use of antidiarrheal, 6) presence of abdominal mass, 7) hematocrit, 8) change in body weight. Highly useful in following patients and making decisions to increase or diminish medications and/or hospitalize.
• Endoscopy and further images if there are changes in symptoms and signs
• Check liver tests yearly
• Check vitamin B12 level in those with ileal disease or ileal resection
• Check folate level in all on 5-aminosalicylate, use supplements in all

PREVENTION/AVOIDANCE
• Ongoing care with available physician
• Consultant for review; long term advice

POSSIBLE COMPLICATIONS
• Progression nearly certain - both expansion of old lesions and new lesions occur
• Recurrence after operation nearly certain, usually occurs in gut segment most proximal to anastomoses
• Fistulae occur about 15% of patients; perirectal, cutaneous, enterovaginal, enterovesicular are all seen
• Extraluminal disease occurs in 10% with skin, uveal tract, joint, and biliary tract disease most common. All fairly specific in pattern; do not parallel activity of the luminal disease.
• Extensive colon disease associated with increased risk of adenocarcinoma
• Colon perforation and massive bleeding
• Toxic megacolon

EXPECTED COURSE/PROGNOSIS
• Average patient has surgery each 7 years; >4 surgeries, expect short-bowel syndrome
• Expect disease to recur
• Majority will have normal life (work, children, full activities); overall life is shortened

MISCELLANEOUS

ASSOCIATED CONDITIONS
• Viral gastroenteritis may be more devastating
• Arthritis of two types - similar to rheumatoid and spondylitis
• Variety of skin lesions, erythema nodosum, non-specific rashes, pyoderma gangrenosum
• Uveal tract disease rare but related
• Sclerosing cholangitis in about 10%, manifest from mild liver test abnormalities including pericholangitis on biopsy to full syndrome

AGE-RELATED FACTORS
Pediatric: Rare
Geriatric: N/A
Others: Occurs at any age

PREGNANCY
• Reversible male sterility after long time on sulfasalazine - folate defers
• No contraindications to pregnancy

SYNONYMS
• Granulomatous colitis
• Regional enteritis
• Regional ileitis
• Regional colitis
• Regional ileocolitis

ICD-9-CM
555.0 Regional enteritis, small intestine
555.1 Regional enteritis, large intestine
555.9 Regional enteritis, unspecified site

SEE ALSO
• Ulcerative colitis
• Diarrhea, acute
• Diarrhea, chronic
• Intestinal parasites
• Short-bowel syndrome
• Celiac disease

OTHER NOTES N/A

ABBREVIATIONS N/A

REFERENCES
• Hanauer SB, Cohen RD, Becker RV, 3rd, Larson LR, Vreeland MG: Advances in the management of Crohn's disease: economic and clinical potential of infliximab. Clinical Therapeutics 1998;20:1009-1028
• Winter AM, Hanauer SB: Medical management of perianal Crohn's disease. Semin in Gastrointest Dis 1998;9:10-14
7 additional references available at web site
Internet references: http://www.5mcc.com
Illustrations: 5 available on CD-ROM

Author(s)
Frank L. Iber, MD

Cryptococcosis

 BASICS

DESCRIPTION Cryptococcus neoformans is a fungus which rarely causes disease in hosts with normal immune function. Cryptococcal meningitis is one of the more common AIDS-defining infections in HIV seropositive persons.
System(s) affected: Nervous, Pulmonary, Skin/Exocrine, Endocrine/Metabolic
Genetics: N/A
Incidence/Prevalence in USA: Accounts for 5-8% of opportunistic infections in AIDS patients. Incidence has been decreasing in recent years.
Predominant age: Generally adults
Predominant sex: Male > Female (reflects HIV prevalence)

SIGNS AND SYMPTOMS
• Cryptococcal meningitis
◊ Often insidious onset with subtle findings
◊ Frontal or temporal headache (80-95% of patients)
◊ Fever (60-80% of patients)
◊ Impaired mentation
◊ Seizures or focal neurologic signs (less common)
◊ Meningismus may be absent (80% of patients)
◊ Deaths within first few weeks of diagnosis is often related to increases intracranial pressure
• Pulmonary cryptococcus
◊ May be asymptomatic
◊ Cough
◊ Shortness of breath
◊ Fever
◊ Hemoptysis
◊ Frequently disseminates in immunosuppressed patients
• Disseminated cryptococcus
◊ Painless skin nodules (5-10% of patients). May occur as erythematous papules, vesicles, macules, or ulcers.
◊ The heart, bone, kidney, adrenals, eyes, prostate and lymph nodes may harbor infection with symptoms referable to affected organ

CAUSES The cryptococcus fungus is ubiquitous. Person to person transmission is rare.

RISK FACTORS Immunosuppression which results in reactivation of latent infection (usually foci in lungs). Rarely, invasive infection may occur in normal hosts.

 DIAGNOSIS

DIFFERENTIAL DIAGNOSIS
• In CNS disease - toxoplasmosis, lymphoma, AIDS dementia complex, progressive multifocal leukoencephalopathy, herpes encephalitis, other fungal disease
• In pulmonary disease - tuberculosis, pneumocystis, histoplasmosis, coccidioidomycosis, Kaposi's sarcoma, lymphoma
• In disseminated disease - tuberculosis, histoplasmosis, lymphoma, coccidioidomycosis

LABORATORY
• Serum cryptococcal antigen (if positive, search for dissemination)
• CSF cryptococcal antigen (positive in 95% of culture-proven positive cases)
• India ink preparation of CSF (50% positive in non-AIDS patients; 80% (bronchoalveolar lavage) positive in AIDS patients)
• Culture of CSF, sputum, blood, urine
Drugs that may alter lab results: N/A
Disorders that may alter lab results: In presence of rheumatoid factor, false positive latex agglutination tests have occurred

PATHOLOGICAL FINDINGS
Inflammation, granuloma formation (may caseate and cavitate), basilar meningitis with mucoid exudate

SPECIAL TESTS Lumbar puncture in cryptococcal meningitis: Imperative to check opening pressure initially (may repeat if clinical deterioration) significantly increased intracranial pressure associated with poor prognosis. In non-AIDS patients - elevated opening pressure, elevated CSF protein, decreased glucose and lymphocytic pleocytosis. In AIDS patients - abnormal CSF findings in 40% of patients. high opening pressure > 200 mm water in 70% of patients.

IMAGING
• In cryptococcal meningitis - CT of brain is negative unless focal cryptococcomas present
• In pulmonary cryptococcosis - chest x-ray may show infiltrates, nodules, mass lesions (with rare cavitation), miliary spread, hilar adenopathy (10%), pleural effusions (less than 5%)

DIAGNOSTIC PROCEDURES Biopsies of skin lesions may be diagnostic

 TREATMENT

APPROPRIATE HEALTH CARE
Inpatient; outpatient for mild cases

GENERAL MEASURES N/A

SURGICAL MEASURES N/A

ACTIVITY As tolerated

DIET As tolerated

PATIENT EDUCATION Life-long antifungal medication required for suppression. In severely immune deficient patients, consider prophylaxis with fluconazole.

MEDICATIONS

DRUG(S) OF CHOICE
• Amphotericin B at 0.7 mg/kg/day IV plus flucytosine 100 mg/kg/day until patient is clinically improving (2-3 weeks); followed by
• Fluconazole (Diflucan) or itraconazole (Sporanox) 400 mg/day (oral or intravenous) until a total of 8 weeks of primary therapy has been completed
Contraindications: Refer to manufacturer's profile of each drug
Precautions: With amphotericin B - permanent renal impairment may occur, hypokalemia, hypomagnesemia; during infusion - fever, chills, headache - pretreat with diphenhydramine, acetaminophen to decrease fever and chill. Add heparin 500 U and hydrocortisone 50 mg to IV amphotericin B to decrease phlebitis.
Significant possible interactions: Refer to manufacturer's literature

ALTERNATIVE DRUGS
• For patients with elevated intracranial pressure - aggressive management with daily lumbar punctures; lumbar drains or acetazolamide is indicated
• Liposomal amphotericin treatment is being studied but is not recommended at this time
• Combination fluconazole plus flucytosine is being studied (may be useful in patients intolerant or nonresponsive to amphotericin B)

FOLLOWUP

PATIENT MONITORING
• Monitor clinical status and repeat LP if indicated
• Foci in the prostate may be difficult to eliminate

PREVENTION/AVOIDANCE
• Without lifelong suppression, relapse is common (50% in AIDS patients within one year)
• Fluconazole 200 mg po daily
• Avoid bird roosts
• Primary prophylaxis with fluconazole (100-200 mg/day or tiw) in selected patients with CD4 < 50 decreases the incidence of cryptococcosis, however, no change in mortality is seen. Cost; possible drug resistance; and drug interactions should be considered.

POSSIBLE COMPLICATIONS
• Cryptococcal infections are fatal unless treated
• Increased intracranial pressure

EXPECTED COURSE/PROGNOSIS
• Fatal without treatment
• No statistics available on survival

MISCELLANEOUS

ASSOCIATED CONDITIONS
• HIV infection
• AIDS

AGE-RELATED FACTORS
Pediatric: N/A
Geriatric: N/A
Others: N/A

PREGNANCY
Amphotericin contraindicated in pregnancy except when treating cryptococcal meningitis

SYNONYMS
Torulosis

ICD-9-CM
117.5 Cryptococcosis

SEE ALSO
• HIV infection & AIDS

OTHER NOTES
N/A

ABBREVIATIONS
CSF = cerebrospinal fluid
AIDS = acquired immunodeficiency syndrome

REFERENCES
• Mitchell TG, Perfect JR. Cryptococcosis in the era of AIDS - 100 years after the discovery of Cryptococcus neoformans. Clin Microbiol Rev 1998;8:51-548
• Aberg JA, Powderly WG. Cryptococcosis. In: Cohen PT, Sande MA, Volberdig PA (eds). AIDS Knowledge Base. On the Internet
• Van der Horst CM, Saag MS, Cloud GA, et al. Treatment of cryptococcal meningitis associated with the acquired immunodeficiency syndrome. NEJM 1997;337:15-21
• Haubrich RM, et al: High dose fluconazole for treatment of cryptococcal disease in patients with human immunodeficiency virus infection. J Infect Dis 1994;170:238-44
Illustrations: 2 available on CD-ROM
Internet references: http://www.5mcc.com

Author(s)
Cynthia Gail Carmichael, MD

Cryptorchidism

BASICS

DESCRIPTION Incomplete or improper descent of one or both testicles. Normally, descent is in the 7th to 8th month of gestation. The cryptorchid testis may be palpable or non-palpable.
• Ectopic testes: Lies outside the normal path of descent. It may be located within the perineum, above the symphysis pubis, along the medial thigh or on the contralateral side.
• Incomplete descent: The testis lies along the normal path of descent but hasn't reached the scrotum
• Intra-abdominal: The testis has not moved into the inguinal canal due to lack of development of the processus vaginalis and gubernaculum
• Gliding testis: Seen in boys with a patent processus vaginalis and gubernaculum. The testis may be present in the canal or intra-abdominally
• Iatrogenic: A testis that was previously located in the scrotum, but after a hernia repair or some other surgery has become trapped in the scar
System(s) affected: Reproductive
Genetics: Occurrence of undescended testes in siblings as well as fathers suggests a genetic etiology
Incidence/Prevalence in USA: 3% of full-term and 33% of premature newborn males
Predominant age: Premature newborns
Predominant sex: Male only

SIGNS AND SYMPTOMS One or both testicles in a site other than the scrotum. May be an isolated defect or associated with other congenital anomalies.

CAUSES
• Not fully known
• May involve alterations in mechanical factors (gubernaculum, length of vas deferens and testicular vessels, groin anatomy, epididymis, cremasteric muscles, and abdominal pressure), hormonal factors (gonadotropin, testosterone, dihydrotestosterone, and Müllerian inhibiting substance), and neural factors (ilioinguinal nerve and genitofemoral nerve)

RISK FACTORS Family history of cryptorchidism. Some have noted the following to be associated with an increased risk of cryptorchidism: firstborn child, c-section delivery, toxemia of pregnancy, hypospadias, congenital subluxation of hip, low birth weight and prematurity.

DIAGNOSIS

DIFFERENTIAL DIAGNOSIS
• Retractile testis (hypermobile testis): A normally descended testis that ascends into the inguinal canal because of an active cremasteric reflex
• Atrophic testis: May occur as a result of neonatal torsion

LABORATORY N/A
Drugs that may alter lab results: N/A
Disorders that may alter lab results: N/A

PATHOLOGICAL FINDINGS Higher incidence of carcinoma in undescended testis and alterations in spermatogenesis

SPECIAL TESTS N/A

IMAGING Ultrasonography is able to detect testicles in the inguinal canal and pubic region in 70% of cases, but is only able to detect 20% of intra-abdominal testicles. CT scan findings in children are inconsistent.

DIAGNOSTIC PROCEDURES
• Physical exam
◊ Performed with child in sitting, standing and squatting positions with warm hands
◊ A Valsalva maneuver and applied pressure to lower abdomen may help identify the testes, especially a gliding testis
◊ Failure to palpate a testis after repeated exams suggests an intra-abdominal or atrophic testis
◊ An enlarged contralateral testis in the presence of a non-palpable testis suggests testicular atrophy/absence
◊ Laparoscopy is useful in the child with impalpable cryptorchidism to accurately confirm testicular absence or presence and to determine the feasibility of performing a standard orchiopexy

TREATMENT

APPROPRIATE HEALTH CARE
Outpatient until surgery performed

GENERAL MEASURES
• Rule out retractile testis
• Most testicles will descend by age 6 months, if they are going to descend
• Administration of chorionic gonadotropin - may cause testicular descent in some boys. Reports of efficacy are inconsistent.

SURGICAL MEASURES
• Reasons to consider: Avoids torsion, averts trauma, decreases but does not eliminate risk of malignancy, and prevents further alterations in spermatogenesis
• Orchiopexy should be performed by age 1. Alterations in germ cell count in the cryptorchid testis have been identified by age 2.

ACTIVITY No restrictions

DIET No special diet

PATIENT EDUCATION Discuss with parents about causes, available treatments, and possible effects on patient's reproductive potential

Cryptorchidism

MEDICATIONS

DRUG(S) OF CHOICE The International Health Foundation recommendations for HCG therapy is biweekly injections of 250 IU for infants, 500 IU for children up to 6 years of age and 1000 IU for those 6 years of age and older, for a total of 5 weeks

Contraindications: Contraindicated in patients with a clinically apparent inguinal hernia, those with a history of previous ipsilateral groin surgery or in ectopic testicles. Also refer to manufacturer's literature.

Precautions: May induce precocious puberty - discontinue drug, effects should reverse in 4 weeks. Premature epiphyseal closure.

Significant possible interactions: Refer to manufacturer's literature

ALTERNATIVE DRUGS N/A

FOLLOWUP

PATIENT MONITORING
Patients should be followed after surgery to evaluate testicular growth and when older be taught testicular self-examination

PREVENTION/AVOIDANCE No
preventive measures known

POSSIBLE COMPLICATIONS
• Progressive failure of spermatogenesis, if left untreated. Even with orchiopexy, the fertility rate is still reduced, especially with bilateral undescended testicles. Spermatogenesis related to duration of cryptorchidism and the location of the testis. Abnormalities have also been identified in the contralateral descended testis, although less severe
• Higher risk (20-46 times) of testicular cancer (risk may remain despite orchiopexy)
• Hernia development (25%)

EXPECTED COURSE/PROGNOSIS
• Disorder usually corrected with medical or surgical therapy, however; possible lifelong consequences
• If testicle is absent or orchiectomy required, may consider placement of testicular prothesis

MISCELLANEOUS

ASSOCIATED CONDITIONS
• Inguinal hernia
• Hemiscrotum
• Hydrocele
• Abnormalities of vas deferens and epididymis
• Klinefelter's syndrome
• Hypogonadotropic hypogonadism
• Germinal cell aplasia
• Mullerian inhibiting factor deficiency
• 5 alpha-reductase deficiency
• True hermaphrodite
• Prune belly syndrome
• Meningomyelocele
• Hypospadias
• Wilm's tumor

AGE-RELATED FACTORS
Pediatric: This problem is usually detectable at birth or soon thereafter. If surgery is to be the treatment, it should be performed during the first year of life.
Geriatric: N/A
Others: Puberty: If unilateral cryptorchidism is discovered at or after puberty, usual treatment is orchiectomy

PREGNANCY N/A

SYNONYMS
• Undescended testes

ICD-9-CM
752.5 Undescended testicle

SEE ALSO
• Hydrocele
• Meningomyelocele
• Wilms' tumor

OTHER NOTES N/A

ABBREVIATIONS
IU = international units

REFERENCES
• Cendron M, Keating MA, Huff DS, et al: Cryptorchidism, Orchidopexy and Infertility: Critical Long-Term Retrospective Analysis. J Urol 1989;142:559-62
• Gill B, Kagan S: Cryptorchidism current concepts. Pediatr Clin NA 1997;44(5):1211-1227
• Merguerian PA, Mevorach RA, et al: Laparoscopy for the evaluation and management of the nonpalpable testis. Urology 1998;51(5A suppl):3-6
• Rogers E, Teahan S, et al: The role of orchiectomy in the management of postpubertal cryptorchidism. J Urol 1998;159:851-854
• Hjertkvist M, Dauber JE, Bergh A: Cryptorchidism: a registry-based study in Sweden on some factors of some possible etiological importance. J Epidemiol Community Health1989;146:324
• Merguerian PA, Ellsworth P: Current Management of Cryptorchidism. In: Rous SN, ed. Urology Annual. Vol. 7. New York, WW Norton & Co, 1993:287-308
Illustrations: N/A
Internet references: http://www.5mcc.com

Author(s)
Pamela I. Ellsworth, MD
William A. Primack, MD

Cushing's disease and syndrome

BASICS

DESCRIPTION Clinical abnormalities associated with chronic exposure to excessive amounts of cortisol (the major adrenocorticoid). The most frequent cause is prolonged use of exogenous glucocorticoids.
System(s) affected: Endocrine/Metabolic, Musculoskeletal, Skin/Exocrine, Cardiovascular
Genetics:
• Multiple endocrine neoplasia type I
• Carney complex
Incidence/Prevalence in USA: Uncommon
Predominant age: All ages
Predominant sex: Females > Males

SIGNS AND SYMPTOMS
• Moon face (facial adiposity)
• Increased adipose tissue in neck and trunk
• Central weight gain
• Emotional lability
• Hypertension
• Osteoporosis
• Purple striae on the skin
• Diabetes or glucose intolerance with fasting hyperglycemia and/or glycosuria
• Muscle weakness due to loss of muscle mass from increased catabolism
• Skeletal growth retardation in children
• Easy bruising
• Hirsutism

CAUSES
• Exogenous glucocorticoids and/or ACTH
• Endogenous ACTH-dependent hypercortisolism
  ◊ ACTH-secreting pituitary tumor
  ◊ Ectopic ACTH production (e.g., small-cell carcinoma of lung, bronchial carcinoid)
• Endogenous ACTH-independent hypercortisolism
  ◊ Adrenal adenoma
  ◊ Adrenal carcinoma
  ◊ Macro/micro nodular hyperplasia

RISK FACTORS
• Any medical problem requiring prolonged use of corticosteroids
• Pituitary tumor
• Adrenal mass
• Neuroendocrine tumor (e.g., bronchial carcinoid)

DIAGNOSIS

DIFFERENTIAL DIAGNOSIS
• Obesity, diabetes mellitus, hypertension
• Adrenogenital syndrome
• Hypercortisolism secondary to alcoholism (pseudo-Cushing's)

LABORATORY
• 24 hour urinary cortisol
• Plasma cortisol (am and pm)
• Plasma ACTH concentration
• Glycosuria (possible)
• Neutrophilia
• Lymphopenia
• Hyperglycemia
• Hyperlipidemia
• Hypokalemia
• Dynamic endocrine testing (e.g., dexamethasone suppression test)
Drugs that may alter lab results: Refer to lab test or drug reference
Disorders that may alter lab results: Refer to lab test reference

PATHOLOGICAL FINDINGS
• Hyalinization of basophilic cells (anterior pituitary) - Crooke's cell changes
• Muscular atrophy
• Nephrosclerosis

SPECIAL TESTS If ACTH-dependent, inferior petrosal sinus sampling for ACTH

IMAGING
• Chest films
• X-rays of the lumbar spine - osteoporosis is common
• If pituitary tumor suspected - pituitary MRI scan
• If adrenal disease suspected -abdominal CT scan
• If ectopic ACTH-secretion suspected - chest CT scan

DIAGNOSTIC PROCEDURES Not all tests indicated for every case. Choice of diagnostic procedure dependent on circumstances and judgment.

TREATMENT

APPROPRIATE HEALTH CARE
Inpatient for surgical procedures

GENERAL MEASURES
• Depends on etiology. Surgery is the treatment of choice; persistent disease may require - radiation, drug therapy, or surgery
• Medical treatment with adrenocortical inhibitors
  ◊ Has not been too successful
  ◊ Should be used when other methods fail
  ◊ In consultation with a clinician having experience in their use

SURGICAL MEASURES
• Primary hypersecretion of ACTH
  ◊ Transsphenoidal microsurgery. Bilateral adrenalectomy as an adjunct for patients not cured.
• Adrenocortical tumors
  ◊ Surgical removal when possible
  ◊ If adrenocortical carcinoma, prognosis is poor
• Ectopic ACTH production
  ◊ Removal of the neoplastic tissue
  ◊ Metastatic spread makes surgical cure unlikely/impossible
  ◊ Bilateral adrenalectomy

ACTIVITY Determined by patient's symptoms and form of treatment used

DIET
• Potassium supplements
• High protein diet

PATIENT EDUCATION
• National Adrenal Disease Foundation (NADF), 505 Northern Blvd, Great Neck, NY 11021; 516-407-4992; e-mail: nadf@aol.com
• Instructions on drug therapy, diet, activity
• Early treatment of infections
• Monitor weight daily
• Emotional lability prevention

MEDICATIONS

DRUG(S) OF CHOICE
All of the below listed medications are equally efficacious for depression. Selection is based on side effects profile.
• Polycyclic (mostly tricyclic [TCA's]) antidepressants with sedating properties (also have anticholinergic properties, potential for fatal overdose):
◊ Amoxapine (Asendin) 50-400 mg/day in divided doses. Maximum hs dose 300 mg
◊ Amitriptyline (Elavil, Endep) 150-300 mg/day qhs
◊ Maprotiline (Ludiomil) 75-225 mg/day. Useful with associated anxiety.
◊ Mirtazapine (Remeron) 15-45 mg/day at hs
◊ Nortriptyline (Pamelor, Aventyl) 75-150 mg/day qhs (a metabolite of amitriptyline)
◊ Doxepin (Adapin, Sinequan) 150-300 mg/day qhs
◊ Trimipramine (Surmontil) 75-250 mg/day qhs
◊ Trazodone (Desyrel) 150-300 mg/day qhs
• Polycyclic antidepressants with activating properties (also have anticholinergic properties, insomnia, anxiety, potentially fatal overdose):
◊ Imipramine (Tofranil, Tipramine) 150-300 mg/day
◊ Desipramine (Norpramin, Pertofrane) 150-300 mg/day
◊ Protriptyline (Vivactil) 30-60 mg/day
• Selective serotonin reuptake inhibitors (can cause insomnia, anxiety, appetite suppression; overdose less likely to be fatal):
◊ Fluoxetine (Prozac) 20 mg/day q am
◊ Nefazodone (Serzone) 300-600 mg/day in divided doses. Start at 100 mg bid.
◊ Sertraline (Zoloft) 50-100 mg/day q am
◊ Paroxetine (Paxil) 10-30 mg/day q am
• Others:
◊ Venlafaxine (Effexor) 75-100 mg/day in divided doses. Increases effective serotonin and norepinephrine; can cause insomnia, anxiety, anorexia).
◊ Bupropion (Wellbutrin) 100-450 mg/day in divided doses (catecholamine reuptake inhibitor)
Contraindications: Refer to manufacturer's profile of each drug
Precautions:
• Decrease beginning dose by half for children and elderly
• Fluoxetine, sertraline, paroxetine best given in the morning
• Polycyclic antidepressant prescriptions should initially be written for small total amounts to prevent suicide (TCA's fatal with doses > 1-1.5 gm in adults)
• TCA's may produce arrhythmias and lower seizure threshold
• Venlafaxine - allow approximately two weeks washout of other medications before instituting therapy with venlafaxine
Significant possible interactions:
• Refer to manufacturer's profile of each drug
• Avoid nonprescription drugs containing pseudoephedrine, phenylephrine, or phenylpropanolamine (cold medicines)

ALTERNATIVE DRUGS
• Clomipramine (Anafranil) 100-250 mg/day (although primarily used to treat obsessive-compulsive disorder)
• Fluvoxamine (Luvox) 100-300 mg/day in divided doses. Indicated for obsessive-compulsive disorder.
• MAO inhibitors - significant drug and food interactions limit their use, but can be useful in refractory cases
• Hypericum perforatum (St. John's Wort) maybe useful in mild depression, avoid simultaneous use of SSRI's or MAO inhibitors

FOLLOWUP

PATIENT MONITORING
• See patient within 2 weeks after starting medication. The patient will probably not feel greatly improved at this visit.
• During followup visits evaluate side effects, dosage and effectiveness of the medication
• Follow about every 2 weeks until improvement begins. If treatment is adequate, the depression should improve within 4 weeks of initiating treatment.
• Follow every 3 months thereafter
• Explain to the patient that the treatment must continue even after improvement
• Plan to treat at least 6 months to 2 years. Longer in patients with family history of depression and the very young.

PREVENTION/AVOIDANCE See
Causes and Risk factors

POSSIBLE COMPLICATIONS
• Suicide
• Failure to improve

EXPECTED COURSE/PROGNOSIS
This is one of the most rewarding conditions to treat because, once you find the right drug and the right dose, you can almost guarantee the patient that he or she will improve

MISCELLANEOUS

ASSOCIATED CONDITIONS
• Manic depression (bipolar)
• Schizophrenia
• Schizo-affective disorders
• Psycho-physiological disorders
• Physical disorders
• Cyclothymic and grief reactions
• Alcoholism

AGE-RELATED FACTORS
Pediatric: Depression occurs in children
Geriatric: More common in elderly and difficult to precisely diagnose. Depression frequently coexists with dementia or delirium.
Others: N/A

PREGNANCY Caution in using
psychoactive medications in pregnancy. Rely on psychotherapy and support groups until pregnancy is completed.

SYNONYMS Unipolar affective disorder

ICD-9-CM
311 Depressive disorder, not elsewhere classified
296.2 Major depressive disorder, single episode
296.3 Major depressive disorder, recurrent episode

SEE ALSO
• Obsessive compulsive disorder

OTHER NOTES
• Depression is the fourth most common reason to visit the family physician
• Like so many other medical illnesses with psychological symptoms, family, doctors and patients tend to try to overlook this condition because they feel they should be able to control it themselves
• Attention deficit syndromes are being treated with antidepressants. They may be more effective than methylphenidate (Ritalin) or amphetamines.

ABBREVIATIONS
OBS = organic brain syndrome
TCA = tricyclic antidepressant
TSH = thyroid stimulating hormone

REFERENCES
• Diagnosis and Treatment (Quick reference guide for Physicians) AHCPR publication 93-0552
• Shererer SL, Adams GK: Nonpharmacologic aids in the treatment of depression. Amer Fam Phys;1993(2)
Illustrations: N/A
Internet references: http://www.5mcc.com

Author(s)
Dannen D. Mannschreck, MD

Dermatitis, atopic

BASICS

DESCRIPTION Chronic pruritic eczematous condition affecting characteristic sites. Associated with family history of atopy (asthma, allergic rhinitis, atopic dermatitis).
System(s) affected: Skin/Exocrine
Genetics: Genetic predisposition - family history positive in two-thirds of cases
Incidence/Prevalence in USA: Common; incidence 7-24/1000
Predominant age: Mainly childhood disease. Affects 5% of all children, usually appearing in the first year of life and gradually subsiding over subsequent years.
Predominant sex: Male = Female (females tend to have somewhat worse prognosis)

SIGNS AND SYMPTOMS
• Pruritus is the most common symptom
• Distribution of lesions
  ◊ Infants - trunk, face, and extensor surfaces
  ◊ Children - antecubital and popliteal fossae
  ◊ Adults - face, neck, upper chest, and genital areas
  ◊ In adults with limited distribution of lesions a history of childhood eczema is a clue to diagnosis
• Morphology of lesions
  ◊ Infants - erythema and papules; may develop oozing, crusting vesicles
  ◊ Children and adults - lichenification and scaling are typical with chronic eczema
  ◊ Family history of atopic dermatitis may be more useful than morphology in making the diagnosis
• Associated features
  ◊ Facial erythema, mild to moderate
  ◊ Perioral pallor
  ◊ Infraorbital fold (Dennie's sign/Morgan line)
  ◊ Dry skin
  ◊ Increased palmar linear markings
  ◊ Pityriasis alba (hypopigmented asymptomatic areas on face and shoulders)
  ◊ Keratosis pilaris

CAUSES Unknown. Genetically determined, non-allergic disease.

RISK FACTORS
• Skin infections
• Emotional stress
• Irritating clothes and chemicals
• Excessively hot or cold climate
• Food allergy in children (controversial)
• Exposure to tobacco smoke

DIAGNOSIS

DIFFERENTIAL DIAGNOSIS
• Photosensitivity rashes
• Contact dermatitis (especially if only the face is involved)
• Scabies
• Seborrheic dermatitis (especially in infants)
• Psoriasis or lichen simplex chronicus if only localized disease is present in adults
• Rare conditions of infancy: histiocytosis X, Wiskott-Aldrich syndrome, ataxia-telangiectasia syndrome
• Ichthyosis vulgaris

LABORATORY Serum IgE levels are frequently elevated
Drugs that may alter lab results: N/A
Disorders that may alter lab results: N/A

PATHOLOGICAL FINDINGS Epidermis is thickened and hyperkeratotic. Dermis shows perivascular inflammation.

SPECIAL TESTS None

IMAGING None

DIAGNOSTIC PROCEDURES Skin biopsy shows nonspecific eczematous changes. (Biopsy is rarely required since diagnosis is made on clinical grounds.)

TREATMENT

APPROPRIATE HEALTH CARE Generally outpatient, using topical corticosteroids

GENERAL MEASURES
• Decrease stress if possible
• Avoid agents that may cause irritation (e.g., wool, perfumes)
• Minimize sweating
• Lukewarm (not hot) baths
• Minimize use of soap (superfatted soaps best)
• Frequent systemic lubrication with oil baths, moisturizers, etc. (use oil after soaking)
• Sun exposure may be helpful
• Humidify the house
• Avoid excessive contact with water

SURGICAL MEASURES N/A

ACTIVITY No restrictions

DIET There is controversy regarding the role of food allergies and exacerbations of atopic dermatitis. The most common suspicious foods are eggs, milk, wheat and peanuts. Consider elimination diets (e.g., for 3-4 weeks) and food challenges. Also consider delaying introduction of the common suspicious foods until an infant is 6 months old.

PATIENT EDUCATION
• Goal is control, not cure (although many patients will outgrow their disease)
• See also Epstein, E.: Common Skin Disorders. 4th Ed. Medical Economics, 1994

Dermatitis, atopic

MEDICATIONS

DRUG(S) OF CHOICE
• Topical steroids achieve good control in 90% of patients
• In infants and children, use 0.5-1% topical hydrocortisone creams or ointments
• In adults, may use higher potency (over 1%) topical corticosteroids in areas other than face and skin folds
• Use short courses of higher potency corticosteroids for flares, then return to the lowest potency (creams preferred) that will control dermatitis
Contraindications: None
Precautions: Beware that chronic potent fluorinated corticosteroids use may cause striae or atrophy, especially in children. High potency topical corticosteroids may produce systemic effects if used for prolonged periods.
Significant possible interactions: None

ALTERNATIVE DRUGS
• Coal tar, e.g., tar-oil baths, topical tar at bedtime, etc.
• Antihistamines for pruritus (e.g., hydroxyzine, 10-25 mg at bedtime and prn)
• Plastic occlusion - in combination with topical medication, this promotes absorption
• For stubborn localized eczema, may use intralesional steroids
• For severe atopic dermatitis, consider systemic steroids for 1-2 weeks, e.g., prednisone 2 mg/day po (max 80 mg) initially, tapered over 7-14 days.
• Topical tricyclic doxepin as a 5% cream may decrease pruritus
• Evening primrose oil, includes high content of fatty acids, believed to decrease prostaglandin synthesis, believed to promote conversion of linoleic acid to omega-6 fatty acid

FOLLOWUP

PATIENT MONITORING   Individualize, depending on severity of disease

PREVENTION/AVOIDANCE
• Smallpox vaccine should be avoided because of risk of eczema herpeticum (see Possible Complications)

POSSIBLE COMPLICATIONS
• Cataracts are more common in patients with atopic dermatitis
• Skin infections (usually *Staphylococcus aureus*); sometimes subclinical
• Eczema herpeticum - generalized vesiculopustular eruption caused by infection with herpes simplex or vaccinia virus. Patients are acutely ill and require hospitalization.
• Atrophy and/or striae if fluorinated corticosteroids are used on face or skin folds
• Systemic absorption may occur if large areas of skin are treated, particularly if high-potency medications and occlusion are combined

EXPECTED COURSE/PROGNOSIS
• Chronic disease that tends to burn out with age. 90% of patients have spontaneous resolution by puberty.
• Some adults may continue to have localized eczema, e.g., chronic hand or foot dermatitis, eyelid dermatitis, or lichen simplex chronicus

MISCELLANEOUS

ASSOCIATED CONDITIONS
• Asthma
• Allergic rhinitis
• Hyper-IgE syndrome (Job's syndrome) which is characterized by atopic dermatitis, elevated IgE, recurrent pyodermas, and decreased chemotaxis of mononuclear cells

AGE-RELATED FACTORS
Pediatric: More frequent
Geriatric: Relatively rare
Others: N/A

PREGNANCY   N/A

SYNONYMS
• Eczema
• Disseminated neurodermatitis
• Atopic eczema
• Atopic neurodermatitis
• Constitutional dermatitis
• Besnier's prurigo

ICD-9-CM
691.8 Other atopic dermatitis and related conditions

SEE ALSO   N/A

OTHER NOTES   If very resistant to treatment, search for a coexisting contact dermatitis

ABBREVIATIONS   N/A

REFERENCES
• Habif T: Clinical Dermatology. 3rd Ed. St. Louis, CV Mosby, 1996
• Behrman RE, et al, eds: Nelson Textbook of Pediatrics. 15th ed. Philadelphia, 1996
• Landow K: Atopic dermatitis. Current concepts support old theories and spur new ones. Postgrad Med 1997;101(3):101-117
Illustrations: 10 available on CD-ROM
Internet references: http://www.5mcc.com

Author(s)
Dennis E. Hughes, DO, FAAFP

Dermatitis, contact

BASICS

DESCRIPTION The cutaneous reaction to an external substance
• Primary irritant dermatitis is due to direct injury of the skin. It affects individuals exposed to specific irritants and generally produces discomfort immediately after exposure.
• Allergic contact dermatitis (ACD) affects only individuals previously sensitized to the contactant. It represents a delayed hypersensitivity reaction, requiring several hours for the cascade of cellular immunity to be completed to manifest itself.
System(s) affected: Skin/Exocrine
Genetics: Increased frequency of ACD in families with allergies
Incidence/Prevalence in USA: N/A
Predominant age: All ages
Predominant sex: Male = Female. Variations due to differences in exposure to offending agents as well as normal cutaneous variations between male and female (eccrine and sebaceous gland function and hair distribution).

SIGNS AND SYMPTOMS
• Acute
  ◊ Papules, vesicles, bullae with surrounding erythema
    ◊ Crusting and oozing may be present
    ◊ Pruritus
• Chronic
  ◊ Erythematous base
  ◊ Thickening with lichenification
  ◊ Scaling
  ◊ Fissuring
• Distribution
  ◊ Where epidermis is thinner (eyelids, genitalia)
  ◊ Areas of contact with offending agent (e.g., nail polish)
  ◊ Palms and soles more resistant
  ◊ Deeper skinfolds spared
  ◊ Linear arrays of lesions
  ◊ Lesions with sharp borders and sharp angles - pathognomonic

CAUSES
• Plants
  ◊ Rhus-urushiol (poison ivy, oak, sumac)
  ◊ Primary contact - plant (roots/stems/leaves)
  ◊ Secondary contact - clothes/fingernails (not blister fluid)
• Chemicals
  ◊ Nickel - jewelry, zippers, hooks, watches
  ◊ Potassium dichromate - tanning agent in leather
  ◊ Paraphenylenediamine - hair dyes, fur dyes, industrial chemicals
  ◊ Turpentine - cleaning agents, polishes, waxes
  ◊ Soaps, detergents

• Topical medicines
  ◊ Neomycin - topical antibiotics
  ◊ Thimerosal (Merthiolate) - preservative in topical medications
  ◊ Anesthetics - benzocaine
  ◊ Parabens - preservative in topical medications
  ◊ Formalin - cosmetics, shampoos, nail enamel

RISK FACTORS
• Occupation
• Hobbies
• Travel
• Cosmetics
• Jewelry

DIAGNOSIS

DIFFERENTIAL DIAGNOSIS
• Based on clinical impression - appearance, periodicity, localization
• Groups of vesicles - herpes simplex
• Diffuse bullous or vesicular lesions - bullous pemphigoid
• Photo-distribution - phototoxic/allergic reaction to systemic allergen
• Eyelids - seborrheic dermatitis
• Scaly eczematous lesions - atopic dermatitis, nummular eczema, lichen simplex chronicus, stasis dermatitis, xerosis

LABORATORY N/A
Drugs that may alter lab results: N/A
Disorders that may alter lab results: N/A

PATHOLOGICAL FINDINGS
• Intercellular edema
• Bullae

SPECIAL TESTS Patch tests for allergic contact dermatitis (systemic corticosteroids or recent, aggressive use of topical steroids may alter results)

IMAGING N/A

DIAGNOSTIC PROCEDURES Patch test

TREATMENT

APPROPRIATE HEALTH CARE
Outpatient

GENERAL MEASURES
• Removal of offending agent
• Topical soaks with cool tap water, Burow's solution (1:40 dilution), or saline (1 tsp/pint water), or silver nitrate solution (25.5%)
• Lukewarm water baths - antipruritic
• Aveeno (oatmeal) baths
• Chronic - emollients (white petrolatum, Eucerin)

SURGICAL MEASURES N/A

ACTIVITY Stay active, but avoid overheating

DIET No special diet

PATIENT EDUCATION
• Avoidance of irritating substance
• Cleaning of secondary sources (nails, clothes)
• Fallacy of blister fluid spreading disease

MEDICATIONS

DRUG(S) OF CHOICE
• Topical
  ◊ Shake lotion of zinc oxide, talc, menthol 0.25%, phenol 0.5%
  ◊ Corticosteroids: high potency steroids, fluocinonide (Lidex) 0.05% ointment 3-4 times daily. Caution regarding face/skinfolds - use lower potency steroids and avoid prolonged usage.
  ◊ Calamine lotion
  ◊ Topical antibiotics for secondary infection (bacitracin, gentamicin, erythromycin)
• Systemic
  ◊ Antihistamine: hydroxyzine 25-50 mg qid, diphenhydramine 25-50 mg qid
  ◊ Corticosteroids: prednisone. Taper starting at 60-80 mg/d, tapered over 10-14 days.
  ◊ Antibiotics: erythromycin 250 mg qid if secondarily infected

Contraindications: N/A

Precautions:
• Drowsiness from antihistamines
• Local skin effects: atrophy, stria, telangiectasia from prolonged use of potent topical steroids

Significant possible interactions: N/A

ALTERNATIVE DRUGS
Other topical antibiotics depending on organisms and sensitivity

FOLLOWUP

PATIENT MONITORING
• As necessary for recurrence
• Patch testing for etiology after resolved

PREVENTION/AVOIDANCE
Avoid causative agents. Use of protective gloves (with cotton lining) may be helpful.

POSSIBLE COMPLICATIONS
• Generalized eruption secondary to autosensitization
• Secondary bacterial infection

EXPECTED COURSE/PROGNOSIS
Self-limited, benign

MISCELLANEOUS

ASSOCIATED CONDITIONS N/A

AGE-RELATED FACTORS
Pediatric: Younger individuals - increased incidence of positive patch testing due to better delayed hypersensitivity reactions
Geriatric: Increased incidence of irritant dermatitis secondary to skin dryness
Others: N/A

PREGNANCY Usual cautions with medications

SYNONYMS Dermatitis Venenata

ICD-9-CM
692 Contact dermatitis and other eczema
692.9 Unspecified cause

SEE ALSO N/A

OTHER NOTES N/A

ABBREVIATIONS
ACD = allergic contact dermatitis

REFERENCES
• Bondi E, Jegasothy B, Lazarus G: Dermatology, Diagnosis and Therapy. Norwalk, CT, Appleton & Lange, 1991
• Abel E, Farber E: Scientific American Inc., New York, 1985
Illustrations: 32 available on CD-ROM
Internet references: http://www.5mcc.com

Author(s)
Jeffrey A. Stearns, MD

Dermatitis, diaper

 BASICS

DESCRIPTION Diaper dermatitis is a rash occurring under the covered area of a diaper. The rash may be an irritant contact dermatitis, candidiasis, atopic dermatitis or seborrheic dermatitis.
System(s) affected: Skin/Exocrine
Genetics: N/A
Incidence/Prevalence in USA: Common
Predominant age: Infants
Predominant sex: Male = Female

SIGNS AND SYMPTOMS
• Irritant contact diaper dermatitis
  ◊ Prominent rash on buttocks and pubic skin
  ◊ Creases of skin are relatively spared
  ◊ Rash is dusky red and shiny
  ◊ Skin seems chapped
  ◊ Weeping, crusting, and excoriations are not prominent
• Candidiasis diaper rash
  ◊ Initial involvement of creases with rapid extension
  ◊ Color: bright red
  ◊ Accompanying edema
  ◊ Isolated satellite papules and pustules at margins of inflammatory plaques
  ◊ Excoriations are prominent
  ◊ Positive KOH preparation
  ◊ Positive cultures
• Atopic diaper dermatitis
  ◊ Distribution spares creases
  ◊ Genitalia frequently involved
  ◊ Itch-scratch cycle with excoriations are prominent
  ◊ Child scratches vigorously at night
  ◊ Weeping, crusting, excoriations sometimes present; secondary bacterial infection can occur
• Seborrheic diaper dermatitis
  ◊ Dusky-red patches and plaques deep within skin creases
  ◊ Non-intertriginous skin is relatively spared
  ◊ Weeping, crusting, excoriations - not prominent
  ◊ Other sites of seborrheic dermatitis are frequently present: retroauricular, axillary folds, scalp

CAUSES Irritation to skin from prolonged contact with urine or feces

RISK FACTORS
• Infrequent diaper changes
• Waterproof diapers
• Improper laundering
• Family history of dermatitis
• Hot, humid weather
• Recent treatment with oral antibiotics
• Diarrhea

 DIAGNOSIS

DIFFERENTIAL DIAGNOSIS
• Contact dermatitis
• Seborrheic dermatitis
• Candidiasis
• Atopic dermatitis
• Acrodermatitis enteropathica
• Letterer-Siwe disease
• Congenital syphilis

LABORATORY Culture will reveal candida, if present
Drugs that may alter lab results: N/A
Disorders that may alter lab results: N/A

PATHOLOGICAL FINDINGS Varying inflammation is the most prominent finding

SPECIAL TESTS
• KOH preparation
• Culture pustules if present

IMAGING N/A

DIAGNOSTIC PROCEDURES
• Culture lesions
• KOH preparation

 TREATMENT

APPROPRIATE HEALTH CARE
Outpatient

GENERAL MEASURES
• Expose the buttocks to air as much as possible
• Don't use waterproof pants during treatment - day or night. They keep skin wet and subject to rash or infection.
• Change diapers frequently - even at night if the rash is extensive
• Super absorbable diapers beneficial
• Discontinue using baby lotion, powder, ointment or baby oil (except zinc oxide)
• Zinc oxide ointment to the rash at the earliest sign of diaper rash, and 2 or 3 times a day thereafter (apply to clean, thoroughly dry skin)
• Use mild soap and pat dry

SURGICAL MEASURES N/A

ACTIVITY Protect from overheating

DIET No special diet

PATIENT EDUCATION N/A

MEDICATIONS

DRUG(S) OF CHOICE
• If candidiasis suspected or diaper rash persistent, use antifungal such as miconazole nitrate 2% cream, miconazole powder, econazole (Spectazole), clotrimazole (Lotrimin), or ketoconazole (Nizoral) cream, at each diaper change.
• If inflammation is prominent, consider very low potency steroid cream, such as hydrocortisone 0.5-1% tid along with an antifungal cream or and combination product such as clioquinol-hydrocortisone (Vioform-Hydrocortisone) cream
• If a secondary bacterial infection is suspected, use an anti-Staphylococcal oral antibiotic or mupirocin (Bactroban) ointment topically

Contraindications: N/A

Precautions: Avoid high or moderate potency steroids often found in combination steroid-antifungal mixtures

Significant possible interactions: N/A

ALTERNATIVE DRUGS N/A

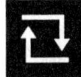
FOLLOWUP

PATIENT MONITORING Recheck weekly until clear, then at times of recurrence

PREVENTION/AVOIDANCE See General Measures

POSSIBLE COMPLICATIONS
• Secondary bacterial infection
• Secondary yeast infection

EXPECTED COURSE/PROGNOSIS
Quick complete clearing with appropriate treatment

MISCELLANEOUS

ASSOCIATED CONDITIONS
• Contact (allergic or irritant) dermatitis
• Seborrheic dermatitis
• Psoriasis
• Candidiasis
• Atopic dermatitis

AGE-RELATED FACTORS
Pediatric: Problem most common in this age group
Geriatric: Incontinence
Others: N/A

PREGNANCY N/A

SYNONYMS
• Diaper rash

ICD-9-CM
691.0 Diaper or napkin rash

SEE ALSO
• Dermatitis, contact
• Candidiasis
• Dermatitis, atopic
• Psoriasis

OTHER NOTES Two or more types of diaper dermatitis can exist concomitantly. If so, treat each accordingly.

ABBREVIATIONS N/A

REFERENCES
• Janniger CK, Thomas I: Diaper Dermatitis: An approach to prevention employing effective diaper care. Cutis 1993;52:153-55
• Habif T: Clinical Dermatology. 3rd Ed. St. Louis, CV Mosby, 1996
• Dershewitz R (ed): Ambulatory Pediatric Care. 3rd ed. Philadelphia, Lippincott-Raven, 1999
Illustrations: N/A
Internet references: http://www.5mcc.com

Author(s)
Dennis E. Hughes, DO, FAAFP

Dermatitis, exfoliative

BASICS

DESCRIPTION A generalized scaling eruption of the skin, either idiopathic in nature or secondary to underlying cutaneous or systemic disease
System(s) affected: Skin/Exocrine
Genetics: No known genetic pattern
Incidence/Prevalence in USA: Rare; estimated 1% of hospitalizations for skin disease
Predominant Age: 75% of patients are over age 40
Predominant sex: Male > Female (2:1)

SIGNS AND SYMPTOMS
• Fine generalized scales with mild erythema and lichenification of skin
• With acute onset and in early stages of exudative dermatitis, may have thin epidermis, erythema, and exudation with subsequent development of crusting
• Initial distribution is that of any underlying cutaneous disease, Subsequently, as exfoliative dermatitis further develops, this distribution is lost and the scaling is generalized.
• With no underlying cutaneous disease, the distribution initially favors the genital region, trunk, and head before generalizing
• Sensation of skin tightness
• Nail dystrophy
• Hair loss, with alopecia in up to 25%
• Pruritus
• Fever in 40-50%
• Chills
• Malaise/weakness
• Mucous membranes spared
• Anemia (both microcytic and macrocytic) in up to 65%
• Eosinophilia
• Nontender generalized lymphadenopathy
• Steatorrhea
• Hepatomegaly in 20-35%
• Splenomegaly when underlying lymphoma/leukemia present
• Gynecomastia
• Hypoproteinemia
• Dehydration
• High output cardiac failure
• Tachycardia
• Lymphadenopathy in 60% or more

CAUSES
• Idiopathic in up to 19% of cases
• 80% may occur in response to one of the following:
  ◊ Atopic dermatitis
  ◊ Colon carcinoma
  ◊ Contact dermatitis (10%)
  ◊ Drug eruptions (14%)
  ◊ Fungal disease with id reaction
  ◊ HIV infection
  ◊ Ichthyosiform dermatoses
  ◊ Leukemia
  ◊ Lichen planus
  ◊ Lung carcinoma
  ◊ Lymphoma - 15% of cases overall and 35-50% of patients over age 40
  ◊ Medications - sulfonamides and sulfones, penicillins, cephalosporins, anticonvulsants, NSAID's, codeine, heavy metals, INH, quinidine, captopril, iodine, antimalarials, Phenothiazines, methotrexate
  ◊ Multiple myeloma
  ◊ Mycosis fungoides
  ◊ Pemphigus foliaceus
  ◊ Photosensitivity reaction
  ◊ Pityriasis rosea
  ◊ Pityriasis rubra pilaris
  ◊ Psoriasis
  ◊ Pyoderma with id reaction
  ◊ Reiter's syndrome
  ◊ Scabies
  ◊ Seborrheic dermatitis
  ◊ Sézary syndrome
  ◊ Staphylococcal scalded skin syndrome
  ◊ Stasis dermatitis
  ◊ Systemic lupus erythematosus
  ◊ Toxic epidermal necrolysis

RISK FACTORS
• Underlying diseases as noted above
• Male sex
• Age greater than 40

DIAGNOSIS

DIFFERENTIAL DIAGNOSIS Acutely eczematous dermatoses such as contact dermatitis and drug eruptions should be considered

LABORATORY None diagnostic. May have elevated WBC with eosinophilia, anemia, elevated ESR, decreased albumin and electrolyte abnormalities
Drugs that may alter lab results: N/A
Disorders that may alter lab results: N/A

PATHOLOGICAL FINDINGS May have characteristics of the underlying cutaneous disease. Other changes are nonspecific: Hyperkeratosis, parakeratosis, acanthosis in the epidermis; and edema, vasodilation, perivascular infiltrates with lymphocytes, histiocytes, and eosinophils in the dermis.

SPECIAL TESTS None

IMAGING Chest x-ray and other imaging procedures as indicated to investigate any underlying disease process

DIAGNOSTIC PROCEDURES
• Careful history and physical exam
• Skin biopsy; lymph node biopsy and bone marrow biopsy as indicated to investigate an underlying disease process

TREATMENT

APPROPRIATE HEALTH CARE
Outpatient except in those cases with complications of secondary infection, dehydration, or heart failure

GENERAL MEASURES
• Withdrawal of any implicated medications or treatment of any identified underlying infection/disease
• Protection from development of hypothermia
• Cool colloid baths with oatmeal (Aveeno) - 1 cup in 10 inches [25.4 cm] water
• Local moisturizing ointments/lotions

SURGICAL MEASURES N/A

ACTIVITY As tolerated

DIET
• High protein. Increased fluid intake should be encouraged in those with more extensive skin involvement.
• Watch for folate iron deficiency in chronic cases

PATIENT EDUCATION
• Patients should avoid any identified etiologic agents
• Patients with underlying diseases that have caused exfoliative dermatitis can be educated regarding symptomatic treatment of the dermatitis and be advised that successful treatment of the underlying disease will usually also be successful for the exfoliative dermatitis
• Protection against hypothermia and dehydration and identification of signs of infection should be part of the education process
• Advise those patients, without an identified cause for the exfoliative dermatitis, that many cases spontaneously remit (exact number uncertain) and that medical therapy to control symptoms can be provided
• American Academy of Dermatology (708)330-0230

MEDICATIONS

DRUG(S) OF CHOICE
• Systemic corticosteroids initial dosage equivalent to prednisone 40 mg/day with increases in dosage by 20 mg/day if there is no response after 3-4 days at a given dose. Subsequently, dosage should be tapered to control symptoms.
• In addition, treatment specific to any underlying infection or disease should be provided
Contraindications: Psoriasis as the underlying cause of the exfoliative dermatitis
Precautions:
• Atopic dermatitis and seborrheic dermatitis as underlying causes
• Avoid coal tar treatment except with psoriasis, and then only use after 24-48 hours of hydration therapy
Significant possible interactions: Refer to manufacturer's literature

ALTERNATIVE DRUGS
• Antihistamines can be useful for pruritus and topical steroids can be used for more localized disease
• When psoriasis is the underlying cause, methotrexate, etretinate, phototherapy, or other treatments specific to this disease should be provided
• Photochemotherapy may be useful therapy for treating exfoliative dermatitis associated with mycosis fungoides
• Isotretinoin has been used when pityriasis rubra pilaris is the underlying cause
• Antibiotic or antifungal therapy as indicated for superinfection

 ## FOLLOWUP

PATIENT MONITORING Patients should be monitored for response to therapy, development of complications, and for adverse effects related to therapy

PREVENTION/AVOIDANCE Known or suspected etiologic agents should be avoided

POSSIBLE COMPLICATIONS
• Infection
• Hypothermia
• Dehydration/electrolyte disturbances
• Heart failure
• Bacterial/fungal superinfection

EXPECTED COURSE/PROGNOSIS
• In patients with an identified underlying cause, the course and prognosis will parallel the primary disease
• For patients with idiopathic exfoliative dermatitis, the prognosis is poor with frequent recurrences or chronic symptoms requiring chronic steroid therapy

 ## MISCELLANEOUS

ASSOCIATED CONDITIONS Any of the infections or diseases listed under causes

AGE-RELATED FACTORS
Pediatric: Less common, but may occur, associated with atopic dermatitis medications or the inherited dermatoses
Geriatric: N/A
Others: N/A

PREGNANCY N/A

SYNONYMS
• Erythroderma
• Pityriasis rubra

ICD-9-CM 695.89 Other specified erythematous conditions, other

SEE ALSO N/A

OTHER NOTES N/A

ABBREVIATIONS N/A

REFERENCES
• Fitzpatrick TB, et al, eds: Dermatology In General Medicine. 4th Ed. New York, McGraw-Hill, 1993
• Moschella SL, Hurley HJ: Dermatology. 3rd Ed. Philadelphia, W.B. Saunders Co., 1992
• Domonkos AN, Arnold HL, Odom RB: Andrews' Diseases of the Skin. 8th Ed. Philadelphia, W.B. Saunders Co., 1990
• Sauer GC: Manual of Skin Diseases. 7th Ed. Philadelphia, J.B. Lippincott Co., 1996
Illustrations: 4 available on CD-ROM
Internet references: http://www.5mcc.com

Author(s)
Mitchell S. King, MD

Dermatitis, herpetiformis

BASICS

DESCRIPTION Dermatitis herpetiformis is an intensely pruritic papulovesicular disease on extensor skin surfaces
System(s) affected: Skin/Exocrine
Genetics: High incidence of HLA B8/Dw3
Incidence/Prevalence in USA: Uncommon. Prevalence not known and most likely varies with the race and ethnicity of the population studied.
Predominant age: 15-60, mean age of onset is in the fourth decade
Predominant sex: Male > Female (1.5:1)

SIGNS AND SYMPTOMS
• Symmetrical intensely pruritic, papulovesicular eruption
• Elbows and extensor forearms are the most common site of involvement
• Buttocks, knees, upper back, posterior neck and scalp also frequent
• Oral lesions in 33%
• Secondary excoriations may be prominent
• Burning or stinging feeling may be prominent

CAUSES Unknown

RISK FACTORS
• Gluten-sensitive enteropathy
• Family history of dermatitis herpetiformis

DIAGNOSIS

DIFFERENTIAL DIAGNOSIS
• Scabies
• Erythema multiforme
• Bullous pemphigoid
• Transient acantholytic dermatosis
• Subcorneal pustular dermatosis
• Erythema elevatum diutinum
• Papular urticaria
• Eczema
• Tinea corporis
• Excoriations

LABORATORY Abnormal thyroid function tests in 32%
Drugs that may alter lab results:
• Thyroid
• Steroids
Disorders that may alter lab results: N/A

PATHOLOGICAL FINDINGS
• Papillary dermal neutrophilic microabscesses
• Subepidermal vesicles

SPECIAL TESTS Direct immunofluorescence reveals granular IgA deposition in the dermal papilla

IMAGING Thyroid scan if indicated by physical exam

DIAGNOSTIC PROCEDURES Skin biopsy

TREATMENT

APPROPRIATE HEALTH CARE
Outpatient

GENERAL MEASURES No special measures

SURGICAL MEASURES N/A

ACTIVITY Fully active

DIET Clinical improvement occurs with gluten-free diet

PATIENT EDUCATION Contact American Academy of Dermatology, 930 N. Meacham Rd., P.O. Box 4014, Schaumber, IL 60168-4014, (708)330-0230

MEDICATIONS

DRUG(S) OF CHOICE Dapsone 50 mg per day will usually improve symptoms within 24 to 48 hours in adults. Average maintenance dose is 100 to 200 mg per day.
Contraindications: See manufacturer's profile of each drug
Precautions:
• Side effects of dapsone include:
  ◊ Hemolytic anemia
  ◊ Methemoglobinemia
  ◊ Toxic hepatitis
  ◊ Cholestatic jaundice
  ◊ Hypoalbuminemia
  ◊ Sensory and motor neuropathy
  ◊ Psychosis
  ◊ Infectious mononucleosis syndrome with fever and lymphadenopathy
  ◊ Agranulocytosis
  ◊ Aplastic anemia
  ◊ Exfoliative dermatitis
  ◊ Erythema multiforme
  ◊ Erythema nodosum
  ◊ Urticaria
  ◊ Dapsone is secreted in breast milk and will produce hemolytic anemia in infants
  ◊ Dapsone will produce a severe hemolytic anemia in patients with glucose-6-phosphate dehydrogenase (G6PD) deficiency
Significant possible interactions: See manufacturer's profile of each drug

ALTERNATIVE DRUGS
• Sulfapyridine; colchicine; prednisone

FOLLOWUP

PATIENT MONITORING
• Baseline CBC and liver function studies should be obtained
• G6PD should be quantified in Asians, blacks and those of southern Mediterranean descent
• CBC should be checked weekly for first month, monthly for the next five months and semi-annually thereafter
• Chemistry profile should be checked every six months
• Patient should be made aware of potential hemolytic anemia and the blue-gray discoloration associated with methemoglobinemia

PREVENTION/AVOIDANCE N/A

POSSIBLE COMPLICATIONS N/A

EXPECTED COURSE/PROGNOSIS
• Patients respond dramatically to dapsone
• Strict adherence to a gluten-free diet will produce improvement of clinical symptoms and a decrease in dapsone requirement in the majority of patients
• Occasional new lesions (2-3 per week) are to be expected and are not an indication for altering daily dosage

MISCELLANEOUS

ASSOCIATED CONDITIONS
• Gluten-sensitive enteropathy
• Hyperthyroidism
• Hypothyroidism
• Thyroid nodules
• Multi-nodular goiter
• Thyroid carcinoma
• Pernicious anemia
• Gastrointestinal lymphoma
• Glomerulopathy
• Immunologic disorders including systemic lupus erythematosus, Addison's disease, rheumatoid arthritis, ulcerative colitis, Raynaud's phenomenon, atopy, Sjögren's syndrome, vitiligo, and dermatomyositis have been reported to be associated with dermatitis herpetiformis

AGE-RELATED FACTORS
Pediatric: Dapsone dose must be adjusted
Geriatric: N/A
Others: N/A

PREGNANCY Data is inconclusive but suggests that dapsone is safe during pregnancy. It is recommended that adherence to a strict gluten-free diet, preferably for 6-12 months before conception be instituted in the hope of eliminating the need for dapsone during pregnancy.

SYNONYMS Duhring's disease

ICD-9-CM
694.0 Dermatitis herpetiformis

SEE ALSO
• Sjögren's syndrome

OTHER NOTES N/A

ABBREVIATIONS N/A

REFERENCES
• Zone JJ: Prob. in Derm. Vol. 3, No. 1:6-11
• Hall RP: The pathogenesis of herpetiformis: Recent advances. J. Am Acad. Derm 1987;16:1129-44
• Hall RP: Dermatitis herpetiformis. J Invest Dermatol 1992;99:873
Illustrations: N/A
Internet references: http://www.5mcc.com

Author(s)
Vera Y. Soong, MD

Dermatitis, seborrheic

BASICS

DESCRIPTION Chronic, superficial, inflammatory condition affecting hairy regions of the body, especially scalp, eyebrows, and face. Mechanism of disease unknown.
System(s) affected: Skin/Exocrine
Genetics: Positive family history common
Incidence/Prevalence in USA: Common
Predominant age: Infancy, adolescence, and adulthood
Predominant sex: Male = Female

SIGNS AND SYMPTOMS
• Infants
◊ Cradle cap - greasy scaling of scalp, sometimes with associated mild erythema
◊ Diaper and/or axillary rash
◊ Onset typically about age one month
◊ Usually resolves by age 8-12 months
• Adults
◊ Red, greasy, scaling rash in most locations, consisting of patches and plaques with indistinct margins
◊ Red, smooth, glazed appearance in skin folds
◊ Minimal pruritus
◊ Chronic waxing and waning course
◊ Bilateral and symmetrical
◊ Most commonly located in hairy skin areas with numerous sebaceous glands, e.g., scalp and scalp margins, eyebrows and eyelid margins, nasolabial folds, ears and retroauricular folds, presternal area and mid-upper back

CAUSES
• Skin surface yeasts may be a contributing factor
• Genetic and environmental factors also contribute to disease, i.e., disease flares are common with any stress or illness
• Disease also seems to parallel increased sebaceous gland activity in infancy and adolescence or as a result of some acnegenic drugs

RISK FACTORS
• Parkinson's disease
• AIDS (disease severity correlated with progression of immune deficiency)
• Emotional stress

DIAGNOSIS

DIFFERENTIAL DIAGNOSIS
• Atopic dermatitis - (distinction may be difficult in infants)
• Psoriasis - usually knees, elbows, nails will be involved. Scalp psoriasis will be more sharply demarcated than seborrhea, with crusted, infiltrated plaques rather than mild scaling and erythema.
• Candida
• Tinea cruris or capitis - suspect these when usual medications fail, or if there is hair loss
• Eczema of auricle or otitis externa
• Rosacea
• Discoid lupus erythematosus
• Histiocytosis X - may appear as seborrheic type eruption. Consider biopsy if usual therapies fail and especially if petechiae are noted.
• Dandruff (scalp only, noninflammatory)

LABORATORY N/A
Drugs that may alter lab results: N/A
Disorders that may alter lab results: N/A

PATHOLOGICAL FINDINGS
Nonspecific changes of eczematous dermatitis. (Biopsy unnecessary unless there is a suspicion of histiocytosis X).

SPECIAL TESTS N/A

IMAGING N/A

DIAGNOSTIC PROCEDURES N/A

TREATMENT

APPROPRIATE HEALTH CARE
Outpatient

GENERAL MEASURES
• Increase frequency of shampooing
• Sunlight in moderate doses may be helpful

SURGICAL MEASURES N/A

ACTIVITY Full activity

DIET No special diet

PATIENT EDUCATION Goal of treatment is control, rather than cure, of disease. Seborrheic dermatitis does not cause hair loss.

MEDICATIONS

DRUG(S) OF CHOICE
• Cradle cap:
  ◊ Frequent shampooing with a mild, non-medicated shampoo
  ◊ Remove thick scale by applying warm olive or mineral oil and then wash off several hours later with Dawn dishwashing detergent and a soft bristle toothbrush
  ◊ May use a coal tar shampoo or ketoconazole (Nizoral) shampoo if the non-medicated shampoo is ineffective
• Adults:
  ◊ Wash off all affected areas with antiseborrheic shampoos. Start with over-the-counter brands (Tegrin, Selsun Blue) and increase to more potent preparations (containing coal tar, sulfur, selenium or salicylic acid) if no improvement is noted.
  ◊ For dense scalp scaling, 10% Liquor Carbonic Detergens (LCD) in Nivea Oil may be used at bedtime, covering the head with a shower cap. This should be done nightly for 1-3 weeks.
  ◊ Ketoconazole (Nizoral) cream may be used to clear scales in other areas, followed by application of steroids to reduce inflammation. Begin with 1% hydrocortisone and advance to more potent (fluorinated) steroid preparations as needed. Avoid continuous use of the more potent steroids to reduce the risk of skin atrophy or systemic absorption (especially in infants and children).
  ◊ Once controlled, washing with zinc soaps or selenium lotion with periodic use of steroid cream will help maintain remission
• For secondary infections: Short course of erythromycin or dicloxacillin

Contraindications: None

Precautions: Fluorinated corticosteroids and higher concentrations of hydrocortisone (e.g., 2.5%) may cause atrophy or striae if used on the face or on skin folds

Significant possible interactions: None

ALTERNATIVE DRUGS   N/A

FOLLOWUP

PATIENT MONITORING   Every 2 to 12 weeks as necessary, depending on disease severity and degree of patient sophistication

PREVENTION/AVOIDANCE   N/A

POSSIBLE COMPLICATIONS
• Skin atrophy or striae possible from fluorinated corticosteroids, especially if used on the face
• Glaucoma - can result from use of fluorinated steroids around the eyes
• Photosensitivity - occasionally caused by tars
• Herpes keratitis - rare complication of herpes simplex. Instruct patient to stop eyelid steroids if herpes simplex develops.

EXPECTED COURSE/PROGNOSIS
• In infants, seborrheic dermatitis usually remits after 6 to 8 months
• In adults, seborrheic dermatitis is usually chronic and unpredictable, with exacerbations and remissions. Disease is usually easily controlled with shampoos and topical steroids.

MISCELLANEOUS

ASSOCIATED CONDITIONS   Parkinson's disease, AIDS (disease severity correlated with progression of immune deficiency)

AGE-RELATED FACTORS
Pediatric: Common in infants
Geriatric: N/A
Others: N/A

PREGNANCY   N/A

SYNONYMS
• Seborrhea
• Cradle cap

ICD-9-CM
690.1 Seborrheic dermatitis

SEE ALSO
• Dermatitis, atopic
• Tinea capitis
• Tinea cruris

OTHER NOTES   N/A

ABBREVIATIONS   N/A

REFERENCES
• Janniger CK, Schwartz, RA: Seborrheic Dermatitis. American Family Physician 1995;52:149-155
• Hay RJ, Graham-Brown RAC: Dandruff and seborrhoeic dermatitis: causes and management. Clinical & Experimental Dermatology 1997;22:3-6
• Habif T: Clinical Dermatology. 3rd Ed. St Louis, CV Mosby, 1996
• Dershewitz R (ed): Ambulatory Pediatric Care. 3rd ed. Philadelphia, Lippincott-Raven, 1999
Illustrations: 3 available on CD-ROM
Internet references: http://www.5mcc.com

Author(s)
Dennis E. Hughes, DO, FAAFP

Dermatitis, stasis

BASICS

DESCRIPTION Chronic, noninflammatory edema of the lower leg accompanied by cycle of scratching, excoriations, weeping, crusting, and inflammation
System(s) affected: Skin/Exocrine
Genetics: Familial link probable
Incidence/Prevalence in USA: Common in patients over 50 years of age
Predominant age: Adult, geriatric
Predominant sex: Female > Male

SIGNS AND SYMPTOMS
• Violaceous (sometimes brown), erythematous colored lesions - due to deoxygenation of venous blood (postinflammatory hyperpigmentation)
• Distribution - medial aspect of ankle with frequent extension onto the foot and lower leg
• Noninflammatory edema precedes the skin eruption
• Stasis ulcers (frequently accompanies stasis dermatitis) secondary to cuts, bruises, excoriations to the weakened skin around the ankle
• Mild pruritus, pain (if ulcer present)

CAUSES
• Continuous presence of edema in ankles, usually present because of venous valve incompetency (varicose veins)
• Trauma to edematous, eczematized skin

RISK FACTORS
• Atopy
• Superimposition of itch-scratch cycle
• Trauma
• Previous deep vein thrombosis
• Previous pregnancy
• Prolonged medical illness
• Obesity
• Secondary infection
• Low-protein diet
• Old age

DIAGNOSIS

DIFFERENTIAL DIAGNOSIS
• Other eczematous diseases such as:
  ◊ Atopic dermatitis
  ◊ Contact dermatitis (due to topical agents used to self-treat)
  ◊ Neurodermatitis

LABORATORY Culture stasis ulcers if you decide to use antibiotics (use of antibiotics topically or systemically is controversial)
Drugs that may alter lab results: N/A
Disorders that may alter lab results: N/A

PATHOLOGICAL FINDINGS Chronic inflammation

SPECIAL TESTS Culture ulcer base or prurient crusted areas to determine whether secondary infection is present

IMAGING N/A

DIAGNOSTIC PROCEDURES N/A

TREATMENT

APPROPRIATE HEALTH CARE
• Outpatient
• Inpatient for vein stripping or skin grafts

GENERAL MEASURES
• Reduce edema:
  ◊ Leg elevation - heels higher than knees, knees higher than hips
• Elastic bandage wraps - Ace bandages or Unna's paste boot (zinc gelatin) if lesions are dry or compression stockings (Jobst or non-fitted type)
  ◊ Diuretic therapy
• Treat infection:
  ◊ S. aureus or beta-hemolytic streptococcus, treat with oral antibiotics
  ◊ Gram-negative colonization, treat with topical antimicrobial agents (e.g., benzoyl peroxide, acetic acid, silver nitrate, or Hibiclens) or broad-spectrum topical antibiotics (e.g., neomycin or Polysporin)
• Debride the ulcer base of necrotic tissue

SURGICAL MEASURES N/A

ACTIVITY
• Avoid standing still
• Stay active
• Elevate foot of bed unless contraindicated

DIET No special diet. Lose weight, if overweight.

PATIENT EDUCATION
• Stress staying active to keep circulation and leg muscles in good condition. Walking is ideal.
• Keeping legs elevated while sitting or lying
• Don't wear girdles, garters, or pantyhose with tight elastic tops
• Don't scratch
• Elevate foot of bed with 2-4 inch blocks

MEDICATIONS

DRUG(S) OF CHOICE
• 5% aluminum acetate solution (Burow's) wet dressings and cooling pastes
• Topical triamcinolone 0.1% (Kenalog, Aristocort) cream/ointment tid or topical betamethasone
• Betamethasone valerate 0.1% (Valisone) cream/ointment/solution tid
• Topical antipruritic - pramoxine, camphor, menthol, doxepin

Contraindications: N/A

Precautions: Refer to manufacturer's literature

Significant possible interactions: N/A

ALTERNATIVE DRUGS
• Consider antibiotics on basis of culture results of exudate from ulcer craters
• Lubricants when dermatitis is quiescent
• Antipruritic medications

FOLLOWUP

PATIENT MONITORING If Unna's boot is used - cut off and reapply boot once a week (restricts edema and prevents scratching)

PREVENTION/AVOIDANCE
• Avoid recurrence of edema with compression stockings
• Topical lubricants twice daily to prevent fissuring and itching

POSSIBLE COMPLICATIONS
• Secondary bacterial infection
• Deep vein thrombus
• Bleeding at dermatitis sites
• Squamous cell carcinoma in edges of long standing stasis ulcers
• Scarring, which in turn leads to further compromise to blood flow and increased likelihood of minor trauma

EXPECTED COURSE/PROGNOSIS
Chronic course with intermittent exacerbations and remissions

MISCELLANEOUS

ASSOCIATED CONDITIONS
• Varicose veins
• Other eczematous disease

AGE-RELATED FACTORS
Pediatric: N/A
Geriatric: Common in this age group
Others: N/A

PREGNANCY N/A

SYNONYMS
• Gravitational eczema
• Varicose eczema
• Venous dermatitis

ICD-9-CM 454.1 Stasis dermatitis

SEE ALSO Varicose veins

OTHER NOTES N/A

ABBREVIATIONS N/A

REFERENCES
• Prystowsky JH, Cohen PR: Venous stasis ulcers. In: Sams WM Jr, Lynch PR, eds. Principles and Practices of Dermatology. New York, Churchill Livingstone, 1990
• Fitzpatrick TB, et al, eds: Dermatology In General Medicine, 3rd Ed. New York, McGraw-Hill, 1987
• Sauer GC: Manual of Skin Diseases. 6th Ed. Philadelphia, J.B. Lippincott, 1991
Illustrations: 9 available on CD-ROM
Internet references: http://www.5mcc.com

Author(s)
Joseph A. Florence, MD

Diabetes insipidus

BASICS

DESCRIPTION Defective regulation of water balance secondary to decreased secretion of, or failure of response to, vasopressin
• Inadequate secretion of vasopressin may be due to loss of or malfunction of the neurosecretory neurons that make up the neurohypophysis (posterior pituitary)
• Insensitivity to vasopressin - a disorder of renal tubular function resulting in inability to respond to vasopressin in absorption of water
• Excessive water intake - (primary polydipsia) usually of functional origin
System(s) affected: Endocrine/Metabolic
Genetics: Familial cases of vasopressin deficiency have been reported (commonly autosomal dominant) but the disease is usually isolated, and often secondary to other disorders.
• Nephrogenic diabetes insipidus (insensitivity to vasopressin)- usually inherited (sex linked recessive), expressed in males, rarely in females
Incidence/Prevalence in USA: N/A
Predominant age:
• Vasopressin deficiency may occur at any age including infancy and childhood
• Nephrogenic diabetes insipidus is usually manifest in infancy
Predominant sex: Nephrogenic diabetes insipidus is encountered in males with rare exception, reflecting its X-linked recessive mode of inheritance

SIGNS AND SYMPTOMS
• Thirst/polydipsia
• Polyuria
• Nocturia
• Dehydration
• Headache
• Visual disturbance

CAUSES
• Inadequate secretion of vasopressin: a variety of pathological lesions may produce damage including tumors (craniopharyngioma, lymphoma, metastasis); infections (meningitis, encephalitis), trauma, granulomas (sarcoid, histiocytosis), or vascular disorders. Some are idiopathic or familial.
• Excessive water intake (psychogenic)
• Insensitivity to vasopressin: genetic defect in resorption of water in renal tubule (collecting ducts)
• Drugs: Lithium, demeclocycline, and methoxyflurane may produce nephrogenic diabetes insipidus

RISK FACTORS N/A

DIAGNOSIS

DIFFERENTIAL DIAGNOSIS
• Diabetes mellitus and other causes of polydipsia and polyuria
• Increased solute load for excretion as occurs with high salt intake
• Psychogenic polydipsia (ultimately impairs vasopressin secretion)
• Nephrogenic diabetes insipidus (differentiate from vasopressin deficiency by clinical trial of desmopressin [DDAVP])

LABORATORY
• Hypernatremia (presenting manifestation, particularly in infants and children)
• Inability to concentrate urine (measure by osmolality, rather than specific gravity)
• Urinary glucose (to rule out diabetes mellitus)
• Plasma vasopressin or urinary vasopressin following osmotic stimulus, such as fluid restriction or administration of hypertonic saline
Drugs that may alter lab results: Lithium, demeclocycline and methoxyflurane may produce vasopressin insensitivity
Disorders that may alter lab results: Hypokalemia and hypercalcemia alter ability to concentrate urine

PATHOLOGICAL FINDINGS
Degeneration and death of neurosecretory neurons in the neurohypophysis

SPECIAL TESTS
• Testing ability to concentrate urine in face of water deprivation should be done by measuring urine and plasma osmolality before and after a six hour period of thirst. This should be done during the day. It is not wise to do overnight thirst tests, particularly in children.
• The most valuable measurements are the urine/plasma osmolal ratio and plasma vasopressin concentrations. The results are sometimes difficult to interpret since low ratios may be found in patients with primary polydipsia. If results support the diagnosis, desmopressin should be administered to test renal concentrating ability.

IMAGING If the diagnosis of diabetes insipidus is made, appropriate studies for cause including imaging of the brain must be performed

DIAGNOSTIC PROCEDURES Fluid deprivation to concentrate urine

TREATMENT

APPROPRIATE HEALTH CARE Initial diagnosis and management may require hospitalization. Continuing care is provided on an outpatient basis with self-medication.

GENERAL MEASURES
• Control fluid balance and prevent dehydration
• Check weight daily
• Provide good skin and mouth care

SURGICAL MEASURES N/A

ACTIVITY Not restricted

DIET Normal with free access to fluids except that young infants with nephrogenic diabetes insipidus may benefit from low solute formula

PATIENT EDUCATION
• Administration and dosage of intranasal desmopressin
• Importance of having access to fluids as thirst dictates
• Wear a medical identification neck tag or bracelet

MEDICATIONS

DRUG(S) OF CHOICE
• Central (vasopressin deficient) diabetes insipidus - desmopressin (DDAVP) (a derivative of vasopressin) given intranasally two times daily in dosage necessary to control polyuria or polydipsia usually (10-25 µg) or 2-4 µg parenterally in 2 divided doses
• Nephrogenic diabetes insipidus - thiazide diuretics
Contraindications: Desmopressin should be used with caution in the immediate postoperative period for intracranial lesions because of possible cerebral edema
Precautions: Overdose of desmopressin may produce water intoxication in patients with excessive water intake
Significant possible interactions: See manufacturer's profile of each drug

ALTERNATIVE DRUGS
• Chlorpropamide (Diabinese) 250-500 mg/day reduces polyuria and polydipsia
• Clofibrate (Atromid-S) at a maximum dose of 1 gm tid also has an antidiuretic effect
• Hydrochlorothiazide 50 mg/day
Note: The effects of these alternate drugs are not as predictable as desmopressin

FOLLOWUP

PATIENT MONITORING
• Requires regular followup at intervals of 2-3 weeks initially and 3-4 months later
• Adjustment of treatment based on the urine and electrolyte concentrations and patient's symptoms

PREVENTION/AVOIDANCE
Avoid situations of marked increase in water loss. Take fluids as dictated by thirst with no water restriction.

POSSIBLE COMPLICATIONS
• Dilatation of urinary tract has been observed (probably secondary to large volume of urine)
• Complications of primary disease (tumor histiocytosis, etc.) should be anticipated
• In nephrogenic diabetes, there is an associated retardation of mental development in some patients (cause undetermined)
• Subnormal growth rate

EXPECTED COURSE/PROGNOSIS
• Condition is usually permanent, although an occasional case following trauma or tumor goes into permanent remission
• Prognosis of diabetes insipidus per se is good depending on underlying disorder
• Without treatment, dehydration can lead to confusion, stupor and coma

MISCELLANEOUS

ASSOCIATED CONDITIONS
• Infection (e.g., encephalitis, tuberculosis, syphilis)
• Tumors
• Xanthomatosis
• Pyelonephritis
• Renal amyloidosis
• Potassium depletion
• Sjögren's syndrome
• Sickle cell anemia
• Chronic hypercalcemia
• Wolfram syndrome (DIDMOAD)

AGE-RELATED FACTORS
Pediatric: Nephrogenic diabetes insipidus is usually manifest in infancy
Geriatric: N/A
Others: N/A

PREGNANCY N/A

SYNONYMS N/A

ICD-9-CM
253.5 Diabetes insipidus

SEE ALSO
• Sjögren's syndrome

OTHER NOTES N/A

ABBREVIATIONS
• DI = diabetes insipidus
• DIDMOAD = diabetes insipidus, diabetes mellitus, optic atrophy and deafness

REFERENCES Robertson G: Posterior Pituitary Hormones. In: Felig P, Baxter JD, Broadus AE, Frohman LA, eds. Endocrinology and Metabolism. New York, McGraw-Hill, 1995:385
Illustrations: N/A
Internet references: http://www.5mcc.com

Author(s)
William W. Cleveland, MD

Diabetes mellitus, Type 1

BASICS

DESCRIPTION
A chronic disease caused by pancreatic insufficiency (deficiency) of insulin production, resulting in hyperglycemia and end-organ complications such as accelerated atherosclerosis, neuropathy, nephropathy, and retinopathy. Features include:
- Patients insulinopenic and require insulin
- Prone to ketosis
- Usually of rapid onset
- Nutritional status - normal or thin
- Disease lability
- Response to oral drugs uncommon
- Seasonability: January-April are peak onset periods (children less than 6 years old have greater degree of seasonability)

System(s) affected: Endocrine/Metabolic

Genetics:
- Mode of genetic expression not clear
- Genes located on major histocompatibility complex on chromosome 6
- HLA DR3 and DR4 are individually associated with increased risk factor of 4; if carrying both susceptibility genes, relative risk factor increases to 12
- HLA B8 and B15 also associated with increased risk

Incidence/Prevalence in USA: Incidence of 15/100,000/ year. Racial predilection for Caucasian. African-Americans have lowest overall incidence.

Predominant age: Mean age of onset 8-12 years, peaking in adolescence; onset about 1.5 years earlier in girls than boys. Rapid decline in incidence after adolescence.

Predominant sex: Male = Female

SIGNS AND SYMPTOMS
- Polyuria and polydipsia
- Polyphagia is classic, but not common
- Anorexia is commonly observed
- Weight loss (usually from 10-30%, and often almost devoid of body fat at time of diagnosis)
- Increased fatigue
- Decreased energy levels and lethargy
- Muscle cramps
- Irritability and emotional lability
- Vision changes, such as blurriness
- Altered school and work performance
- Headaches
- Anxiety attacks
- Chest pain and occasional difficult breathing
- Abdominal discomfort and pain
- Nausea
- Diarrhea or constipation

CAUSES
- The inherited defect causes an alteration in immunologic integrity, placing the beta cell at special risk for inflammatory damage. The mechanism of damage is autoimmune.
- Environmental factors include:
  ◊ Viruses (such as mumps, Coxsackie, CMV, and hepatitis viruses)
  ◊ Dietary factors - breast feeding may provide a degree of protection against the disease while diets high in dairy products are associated with increased risk
  ◊ Possible risk in diets high in nitrosamines
  ◊ Environmental toxins
  ◊ Emotional and physical stress

RISK FACTORS
- Certain HLA types (see above)
- Presence of a specific 64K protein which may be responsible for antibody formation
- Increased risk when either insulin-dependent or non-insulin dependent diabetes present in any first-degree relatives

DIAGNOSIS

DIFFERENTIAL DIAGNOSIS
- Benign renal glycosuria
- Glucose intolerance
- Type II (non-insulin-dependent) diabetes mellitus - a small number of children might have MODY (maturity-onset diabetes of the young)
- Infantile-onset diabetes mellitus
- Secondary diabetes
  ◊ Pancreatic disease (pancreatitis, cystic fibrosis)
  ◊ Hormonal disorders (pheochromocytoma, multiple endocrine adenomatosis)
  ◊ Inborn errors of metabolism (glycogen storage disease, Type I)
  ◊ Genetic disorders with insulin resistance (acanthosis nigricans)
  ◊ Hereditary neuromuscular disease
  ◊ Progeroid syndromes
  ◊ Obesity (Prader-Willi syndrome)
  ◊ Cytogenetic syndromes (trisomy 21, Klinefelter's and Turner's syndromes)
  ◊ Drug or chemical-induced glucose intolerance (see list below)
  ◊ Acute poisonings (salicylate poisoning can be associated with hyperglycemia and glycosuria, and may mimic diabetic ketoacidosis)

LABORATORY
- Blood glucose
- Electrolytes
- Venous pH
- U/A for glucose and ketones
- CBC (WBC may be elevated)
- Hemoglobin Alc level
- C-peptide insulin level
- Islet-cell antibodies
- T4 and thyroid antibodies

Drugs that may alter lab results:
- The following may cause hyperglycemia (particularly in patients prone to diabetes)
  ◊ Hormones: glucagon, glucocorticoids, growth hormone, epinephrine, estrogen and progesterone (oral contraceptives), thyroid preparations
  ◊ Drugs: thiazide diuretics, furosemide, acetazolamide, diazoxide, beta-blockers, alpha-agonists, calcium channel blockers, phenytoin, phenobarbital sodium, nicotinic acid, cyclophosphamide, l-asparaginase, epinephrine-like drugs (decongestants and diet pills), nonsteroidal anti-inflammatory agents, nicotine, caffeine, sugar-containing syrups, fish oils

Disorders that may alter lab results: See Differential Diagnosis

PATHOLOGICAL FINDINGS
Inflammatory changes with lymphocytic infiltration around the Islets of Langerhans, or islet cell destruction

SPECIAL TESTS
- Oral glucose tolerance test (possibly with insulin levels, if diagnosis is questionable)
- Intravenous glucose test (for possible early detection of subclinical diabetes)
- Consider HLA-typing

IMAGING   None indicated

DIAGNOSTIC PROCEDURES   N/A

TREATMENT

APPROPRIATE HEALTH CARE
- Initial care: inpatient stabilization versus outpatient management, preferably in a diabetes unit where a team approach is used
- If in diabetic ketoacidosis (DKA): initially IV fluids and IV insulin until stable, then restore electrolyte and acid-base balance, correct hyperglycemia, prevent hypoglycemia and hypokalemia, risk of cerebral edema
- Remaining health care is done by the family at home. Encourage the child to do as much self-care as possible.

GENERAL MEASURES
- Overall "control" of carbohydrate metabolism for the very young child:
  ◊ Normoglycemia (adjusted for age) "tight" control with striving for blood glucose levels in range of 80-150 mg/dL (4.4-8.3 mmol/L) all the time, might be dangerous (risk of repeated hypoglycemia)
  ◊ Hemoglobin Alc level as close to the normal (nondiabetic) range as possible
- Overall good health
  ◊ Asymptomatic
  ◊ Normal appearance
  ◊ Try to keep lipid profile normal
- Normal growth and development
  ◊ Reach optimal height for genetic potential
  ◊ Appropriate and timely pubertal maturation
  ◊ Coping psychosocial development: Normal school or work attendance and performance. Normal future goals and career plans.
- Prevent acute complications
  ◊ Hypoglycemic insulin reactions
  ◊ Ketoacidosis
- Delay or prevent chronic complications

SURGICAL MEASURES   N/A

ACTIVITY
- All normal activities, including full participation in sports activities
- Regular, rather than periodic, aerobic exercise is preferable

DIET Appropriate diabetes exchange (ADA) diet for age (carbohydrate-50%, protein-20%, fat-30%)

PATIENT EDUCATION
• Complete initial education and ongoing education for patient and family. Team approach is ideal, if available
• For a listing of sources, physicians may contact: American Academy of Family Physicians Foundation, P.O. Box 8418, Kansas City, MO 64114, (800)274-2237, ext. 4400

MEDICATIONS

DRUG(S) OF CHOICE
• Insulin (Humulin, Humalog, Velosulin, Lente) [U-100]
◊ Source: Human (Humulin) or pure pork
◊ Types: NPH, Lente, Regular, Ultralente, 70/30 premixture, Humalog (very quick acting insulin, starts working immediately, no wait before eating) - in many patients may replace regular insulin
• Insulin regimens (given subcutaneously)
◊ 2 dose: NPH/Lente and Regular often in a 2:1 ratio before breakfast and before supper). AM dose usually 1/2 to 2/3 of total daily insulin dose.
◊ 3 dose: NPH/Lente and regular before breakfast; supper dose of regular; and bedtime dose of NPH/Lente (this regimen may prevent the dawn or Somogyi phenomenon)
◊ 4 dose: Humalog or regular insulin before breakfast, lunch, and supper, and NPH/Lente at bedtime
◊ Insulin pump (external) therapy: in select patients, giving basal hourly insulin, 50% of total daily needs; pre-meal boluses, before 3 meals and bedtime snack; all insulin given is Humalog or Velosulin
Contraindications: None
Precautions: Avoid hypoglycemia, the dawn phenomenon, and Somogyi syndrome (rebound hyperglycemia)
Significant possible interactions:
• Beta-blockers may mask symptoms of hypoglycemia and delay return to normoglycemia

ALTERNATIVE DRUGS
• Oral hypoglycemics usually not indicated in Type I diabetes (unless an obese patient, who may have MODY; or a combination of Type 1 and Type 2)
• Immunosuppressants
◊ Cyclosporine: reduces rate of autoimmune beta cell destruction, must be started in initial weeks after the diagnosis of diabetes is made (studies: at 1 year, 20% of cyclosporine - treated patients on no insulin, compared to 12-15% of placebo controls; after 1 year, progressive decline in beta cell function and loss of remission. Toxic side effects include renal disease, hypertension, lymphoma formation.
◊ Other interventional drugs being studied - azathioprine, steroids, nicotinamide

FOLLOWUP

PATIENT MONITORING
• Initially, frequent outpatient followup visits till stable; every 2-3 months thereafter. Monitor height, weight, sexual maturation.
• Daily home blood glucose monitoring with home blood glucose meter (One-Touch, Accuchek, Glucometer, Exactech, Answer, Elite, Precision QID, Advantage, Fasttake, Sure-Step, Complete, etc.) 3-4 times daily, with adjustment/supplementation of insulin dose based on blood glucose levels
• Periodic (about every 3 months) measurement of hemoglobin A1c to assess overall glycemic control
• Yearly measurement of serum lipids and thyroid function
• Regular review and update of dietary management. Adjust for increased caloric needs for age, level of physical activity, pubertal growth spurt, changes in weight.

PREVENTION/AVOIDANCE   None known

POSSIBLE COMPLICATIONS
• Microvascular disease (retinopathy, nephropathy, neuropathy)
• Hyperlipidemia
• Macrovascular disease (coronary and cerebral artery disease)
• Foot problems
• Hypoglycemia
• Diabetic ketoacidosis
• Excessive weight gain
• Psychologic problems related to chronic disease

EXPECTED COURSE/PROGNOSIS
• Initial remission or "honeymoon" phase with decreased insulin needs and easier overall control, usually lasts 3-6 months and rarely beyond a year
• Progression to "total diabetes" when endogenous insulin is insignificant; usually is gradual, but a major stress or illness may bring it on more acutely
• Current prognosis
◊ Increasing longevity and "quality of life" with careful blood glucose monitoring and improvement in insulin delivery regimens and systems
◊ At this time, probable reduced life expectancy, but this has improved dramatically over the past 20 years
◊ Continue to be optimistic about advances in understanding diabetes that may prevent or minimize complications

MISCELLANEOUS

ASSOCIATED CONDITIONS
• Other autoimmune diseases such as hypothyroidism and Addison's Disease (screening regularly for hypothyroidism particularly important in females, who have a much higher incidence of this already)
• Diabetes mellitus can also be seen as part of multiple endocrine adenomatosis

AGE-RELATED FACTORS
Pediatric: More prevalent in this age. Over the past 10 years, a larger percentage of very young children (less than 5 years of age) present with diabetes.
Geriatric: N/A
Others: N/A

PREGNANCY
• At the time of embryogenesis, hyperglycemia increases the incidence of congenital malformations. Hence, tight control of blood sugar before conception is important.
• Safe pregnancy possible, with vaginal delivery of a term baby.

SYNONYMS
• Childhood diabetes
• Brittle diabetes

ICD-9-CM
250.xx Diabetes mellitus (4th and 5th digits should be specified)
250.01 Diabetes mellitus without complications, juvenile type

SEE ALSO
• Diabetic ketoacidosis (DKA)
• Diabetes mellitus, Type 2

OTHER NOTES   N/A

ABBREVIATIONS
MODY = maturity-onset diabetes of the young

REFERENCES
• Travis L, et al: Diabetes Mellitus in Children and Adolescents. Philadelphia, WB Saunders Co, 1987
• Pediatric and Adolescent Endocrinology. Pediatric Clinics of North America, Volume 34, Number 4, W.B. Saunders Co., August 1987
• Lebovitz HE, ed: Therapy for Diabetes Mellitus and Related Disorders. American Diabetes Association, Inc., 1991
• Clark CM, et al: Prevention and treatment of the complications of diabetes mellitus. New Engl J Med 1995;332(18):1210-1217
Illustrations: N/A
Internet references: http://www.5mcc.com

Author(s)
Robert M. Schultz, MD

Diabetes mellitus, Type 2

BASICS

DESCRIPTION Non-ketosis prone hyperglycemia and glucose intolerance due to defects in insulin secretion and peripheral insulin action. Accounts for 80% of diabetic cases.

System(s) affected: Endocrine/Metabolic, Nervous, Renal/Urologic, Cardiovascular

Genetics: Strong polygenic familial susceptibility. Concordance is nearly complete in identical twins.

Incidence/Prevalence in USA:
• Incidence:
  ◊ 300/100,000 (males 230/100,000, females 340/100,000)
• Prevalence:
  ◊ 5,000/100,000
  ◊ More common in some groups such as Pima Indians with 35% prevalence

Predominant age: Typically occurs after age 40

Predominant sex: Female > Male in Caucasian populations

SIGNS AND SYMPTOMS
• Related to hyperglycemia and complications including nephropathy, neuropathy, and retinopathy
• Polyuria
• Polydipsia
• Polyphagia
• Weight loss
• Weakness
• Fatigue
• Frequent infections

CAUSES Genetic factors and obesity are important

RISK FACTORS
• Family history
• Gestational diabetes
• Obesity

DIAGNOSIS

DIFFERENTIAL DIAGNOSIS
• Type 1 diabetes mellitus
• Other specific types of diabetes mellitus
  ◊ Genetic defects of B-cell function
  ◊ Genetic defects in insulin action
  ◊ Diseases of exocrine pancreas
  ◊ Endocrinopathies
  ◊ Drug or chemical induced
  ◊ Infections
  ◊ Immune mediated
  ◊ Genetic syndromes sometimes associated with diabetes
• Gestational diabetes mellitus

LABORATORY
Criteria for diagnosis
• Symptoms of diabetes (polyuria, polydipsia, weight loss) plus casual (random) plasma glucose ≥ 200 mg/dL (11.1 mmol/L)
or
• Fasting plasma glucose ≥ 126 mg/dL (7.0 mmol/L) on 2 occasions
or
• 2 hour plasma glucose ≥ 200 mg/dL (11.1 mmol/L) during OGTT with 75 g glucose load

Drugs that may alter lab results:
• Pentamidine
• Nicotinic acid
• Glucocorticoids
• Thyroid hormone
• Diazoxide
• Beta adrenergic agonists
• Thiazides
• Dilantin
• Alpha-interferon

Disorders that may alter lab results: See Differential Diagnosis

PATHOLOGICAL FINDINGS   N/A

SPECIAL TESTS
• Glucose tolerance test usually not necessary, except when diagnosing gestational diabetes
• Hemoglobin A1C not recommended for diagnosis, but helpful in management

IMAGING   N/A

DIAGNOSTIC PROCEDURES   N/A

TREATMENT

APPROPRIATE HEALTH CARE Regular outpatient follow-up except for complicating emergencies such as severe hyperglycemia, hyperosmolar coma, and severe infections

GENERAL MEASURES
• Home monitoring of blood glucose
• Regular examination for complications: retinopathy, neuropathy, nephropathy

SURGICAL MEASURES   N/A

ACTIVITY Regular aerobic exercise can improve glucose tolerance and decrease medication requirements

DIET
• American Diabetes Association (ADA) provides dietary recommendations for NIDDM. The emphasis is on achieving glucose, lipid, and blood pressure goals. Mild caloric restriction is recommended to achieve mild to moderate weight loss (5-10 kg).
• Food choices are similar to Dietary Guidelines for Americans and the Food Guide Pyramid:
  ◊ 10-20% of calories from protein
  ◊ < 10% of calories each from saturated and polyunsaturated fat
  ◊ Remainder of calories from monounsaturated fat and carbohydrates, depending on individual patient factors
  ◊ Sugar is not specifically prohibited

PATIENT EDUCATION
• Education is critical for patients with NIDDM. Include information on the disease, medication treatment, self-monitoring, foot care, physical activity and diet management
• Support groups and classes certified by the ADA are recommended
• The ADA has prepared numerous patient education materials (430 North Michigan Ave. Chicago, IL 60611 or contact local ADA affiliate listed in white pages of telephone directory)

Diabetes mellitus, Type 2

MEDICATIONS

DRUG(S) OF CHOICE
• First generation oral agents (avoid in elderly and renal failure):
◊ Tolbutamide 500-3000 mg/d in 2-3 doses
◊ Tolazamide 100-1000 mg/d in 1-2 doses
◊ Chlorpropamide 100-500 mg/d in 1 dose
• Second generation oral agents:
◊ Glyburide (Diabeta, Micronase) 1.25-20 mg/d in 1-2 doses (1st 10 mg in AM)
◊ Glipizide (Glucotrol) 2.5-40 mg/d in 1-2 doses (1st 20 mg in AM)
◊ Glipizide extended release tablets 5-20 mg/day in one dose
Note: All oral agents may be taken with meals except glipizide which should be taken 30 minutes before meals
• Insulin - lispro, regular, NPH, Lente, Ultralente in 1 or preferably 2-3 injections per day
• Oral agents + insulin useful occasionally. Some clinicians add an evening dose of intermediate acting insulin when oral agents fail to control blood glucose levels (e.g., fasting plasma glucose >180 or hemoglobin A1c > 1.5% above normal range). When 2 doses of insulin are required to control glucose levels, oral agents are probably best discontinued.
Contraindications:
• To oral agents: Insulin dependent diabetes mellitus, ketotic patient, pregnancy, history of allergy
• Use caution in liver or renal disease and acute infection or stress
Precautions:
• Warn patients of signs of hypo- and hyperglycemia
• Home glucose monitoring (1-4 times/day) recommended for most patients taking insulin
Significant possible interactions:
• Drugs which potentiate oral hypoglycemics, e.g., salicylates, clofibrate, warfarin (Coumadin), chloramphenicol, ethanol
• Beta-blockers may mask symptoms of hypoglycemia and delay return to normoglycemia

ALTERNATIVE DRUGS
• Glimepiride (Amaryl): as monotherapy or in combination with insulin. Begin 1-2 mg q AM and increase by 1-2 mg each week to maximum 8 mg q AM. Usual dose range 1-4 mg.
• Repaglinide (Prandin): 0.5-2 mg before meals qid
• Troglitazone (Rezulin): Begin 200 mg q day, increasing each 2 weeks to maximum 600 mg q day in patients on insulin with poor glycemic control despite doses over 30 U/day, or rosiglitazone (Avandia) 2-4 mg qd or bid. May be used with metformin. Monitor periodic liver enzymes. [Note: Troglitazone has been associated with severe hepatotoxicity. Check serum transaminase levels q month for first year.]

• Metformin (Glucophage): 500-850 mg bid-tid; can be used concurrently with a sulfonylurea to improve control/overcomes insulin resistance. Avoid metformin (in situations which increase risk for lactic acidosis): renal insufficiency, radiocontrast agents, surgery or acute illnesses such as liver disease, cardiogenic shock, pancreatitis or hypoxia. Use caution in CHF, alcohol abuse, elderly or with tetracycline.
• Alpha-glucosidase inhibitor - Acarbose (Precose): 25-100 mg tid or miglitol (Glyset) 25-100 mg tid at beginning of meals to decrease postprandial glucose peaks. Avoid use in renal insufficiency, inflammatory bowel disease, colonic ulceration or partial bowel obstruction.

FOLLOWUP

PATIENT MONITORING
• Frequency of followup depends on compliance and degree of metabolic control. Every two to four months is typical.
• Review of symptoms and home blood glucose levels
• Hemoglobin A1c
• Funduscopy
• Cardiopulmonary exam
• Foot exam for ulcers, arterial insufficiency, neuropathy
• After five years, perform yearly: Ophthalmologist exam, monitor for proteinuria and renal insufficiency

PREVENTION/AVOIDANCE Avoidance of weight gain and obesity and maintenance of regular physical activity may prevent or delay NIDDM

POSSIBLE COMPLICATIONS
• Appear to be due to effects of diabetes mellitus on arterial walls in one form or another
• Peripheral neuropathy
• Proliferative retinopathy
• Nephropathy and chronic renal failure
• Atherosclerotic cardiovascular and peripheral vascular disease
• Hyperosmolar coma
• Gangrene of extremities
• Blindness
• Glaucoma
• Cataracts
• Skin ulceration
• Charcot joints

EXPECTED COURSE/PROGNOSIS
• Maintenance of normal blood sugar levels may delay or prevent complications of diabetes
• In susceptible individuals, complications begin to appear 10-15 years after onset, but can be present at time of diagnosis since disease may go undetected for years

MISCELLANEOUS

ASSOCIATED CONDITIONS
• Hypertension is common (strict control may retard renal complications)
• Hyperlipidemia
• Impotence

AGE-RELATED FACTORS
Pediatric: Occasional cases of nonketosis-prone diabetes mellitus have been seen in children
Geriatric: Common in the elderly and is a significant contributing factor to blindness, renal failure, and lower limb amputations
Others: Generally diagnosed after age 40

PREGNANCY Diabetes can cause significant maternal complications and fetal wasting. Intensive management has improved the outcome dramatically.

SYNONYMS
• Adult onset diabetes mellitus
• Nonketotic diabetes mellitus
• NIDDM

ICD-9-CM
250.xx Diabetes mellitus (4th and 5th digits should be specified)
250.02 Diabetes mellitus without complications, adult-onset type

SEE ALSO
• Diabetes mellitus, Type 1
• Diabetic ketoacidosis (DKA)

OTHER NOTES N/A

ABBREVIATIONS
NIDDM = Non-insulin dependent diabetes mellitus
ADA = American Diabetic Association

REFERENCES
• Report of the Expert Committee on the diagnosis and classification of diabetes mellitus. Diabetes 1997;20:1183-1197
• Purnell JQ, Hirsch IB: New oral therapies for type 2 diabetes. Am Fam Phys 1997;56:1835-1842
• American Diabetes Association clinical practice recommendations 1997. Diabetes Care 1997;20(S1): S1-S70
Illustrations: N/A
Internet references: http://www.5mcc.com

Author(s)
David S. Gray, MD

Diabetic ketoacidosis (DKA)

BASICS

DESCRIPTION A true medical emergency secondary to absolute or relative insulin deficiency characterized by hyperglycemia, ketonemia, metabolic acidosis, and electrolyte depletion
System(s) affected: Endocrine/Metabolic
Genetics: N/A
Incidence/Prevalence in USA: 46 episodes/10,000 diabetic patients; 2 per 100 patient years of type 1 DM
Predominant age: 0-19 years of age
Predominant sex: Male = Female

SIGNS AND SYMPTOMS
- Polyuria
- Polydipsia
- Generalized weakness
- Malaise/lethargy
- Nocturia
- Nausea/vomiting
- Abdominal pain and tenderness
- Decreased bowel sounds
- Decreased perspiration
- Hypotension
- Hypothermia
- Decreased reflexes
- Coma
- Confusion
- Tachycardia
- Tachypnea
- Fever +/-
- Breath fruity, with acetone smell
- Dry mucous membranes
- Anorexia or increased appetite

CAUSES
- Insulin dependent diabetes mellitus (20-30% in newly diagnosed diabetics)
- Infarction (myocardial) 5-7%
- Infection (30-40%) usually respiratory or urinary
- Idiopathic (20-30%)
- Medication non-compliance
- CVA
- Trauma
- Surgery
- Emotional stress

RISK FACTORS
- Any condition that leads to an absolute or relative insulin deficiency
- History of corticosteroid therapy

DIAGNOSIS

DIFFERENTIAL DIAGNOSIS
- Hyperosmolar non-ketotic coma
- Alcoholic ketoacidosis
- Lactic acidosis
- Acute hypoglycemic coma
- Uremia

LABORATORY
- Blood sugar elevated (usually 250-800 mg/dL [13.88-44.4 mmol/L] range)
- Serum ketosis
- Urine ketosis
- Glycosuria
- Hyponatremia
- Hyperamylasemia
- Hypertriglyceridemia
- Hypercholesterolemia
- Increased BUN
- $HCO3 < 15$ (< 15 mmol/L)
- Decreased calculated total body K+
- Metabolic acidosis on ABGs
- Increased serum osmolality
- Increased anion gap

Drugs that may alter lab results: N/A
Disorders that may alter lab results:
- With concomitant lactic acidosis, acetoacetate production may be inhibited in presence of high levels of beta hydroxybutyrate. The nitroprusside reaction, which measures only acetoacetate, may not be strongly positive.
- A very low serum sodium (< 110 mmol/L) suggests an artifact due to severe hypertriglyceridemia
- Severe acidosis gives artificially high K+ level
- Markedly increased serum ketones may cross react and cause a falsely high serum creatinine

PATHOLOGICAL FINDINGS N/A

SPECIAL TESTS
- ECG (especially if MI suspected). May also assist in evaluation of K+ status. Usually shows sinus tachycardia.
- Urine and blood cultures

IMAGING Chest x-ray to rule out pulmonary infection

DIAGNOSTIC PROCEDURES N/A

TREATMENT

APPROPRIATE HEALTH CARE
- Inpatient intensive care. This is a life threatening emergency.
- Goals are to increase rate of glucose utilization by insulin-dependent tissues, to reverse ketonemia and acidosis, and to correct the depletion of water and electrolytes.

GENERAL MEASURES
- IV Fluids adults: 1000 mL over first hour, then 500 mL/hr (approximately 7 mL/kg/hr) x 4 hrs or until dehydration improves, then 250 mL/hour (3.5 mL/kg/hr). Switch to D5 in 1/2 NS when serum glucose < 300 mg/dL (16.65 mmol/l). Expect to give 4-8 L/ first 24 hrs. (Some do not recommend initial IV bolus).
- Pediatric maintenance requirements: 100 mL/kg for first 10 kg, 50 mL/kg for second 10 kg and 20 mL/kg thereafter. Fluid deficit: (Multiply patient's body weight by percentage dehydration). Replace maintenance and deficit evenly over 48 hours.

SURGICAL MEASURES N/A

ACTIVITY Bedrest

DIET Nothing by mouth initially. Advance to pre-ketotic diet when nausea and vomiting are controlled.

PATIENT EDUCATION
- For prevention, careful control of blood glucose (usually HgA1c 7%)
- Monitor glucose carefully during periods of stress, infection, trauma etc.

MEDICATIONS

DRUG(S) OF CHOICE
- Insulin - initiate infusion at 0.1U/kg/hr
- Potassium phosphate or Potassium chloride
- Sodium bicarbonate, rarely

Contraindications:
- No demonstrable clinical benefit from bicarbonate with a pH > 7.0.
- Hold K+ if > 5.5 (> 5.5 mmol/L)

Precautions:
- Double insulin if no response in serum glucose over first 2 hours
- Must continue insulin until serum bicarbonate and anion gap normalize
- Add dextrose to IV fluid when blood sugar < 300 mg/dL (16.65 mmol/L)
- If using bicarbonate, add 50 mg NaHCO3 to 1L 1/2 NS and give over 2 hours
- Delay K+ administration in patients with inadequate urine output or evidence of diabetic nephropathy
- If blood sugar does not fall by approximately 75 mg % q2h, increase insulin rate
- Taper IV insulin and start NPH/Reg insulin after acidosis clears and patient is eating

Significant possible interactions: For each 0.1 unit of pH, serum K+ will change by approximately 0.6 mEq (0.6 mmol/L) K in the opposite direction

ALTERNATIVE DRUGS N/A

FOLLOWUP

PATIENT MONITORING
- Monitor mental status, vital signs, urine output q 30-60 minutes until improved, then q2-4 h x 24 hrs
- Blood sugar q 1 hr until < 300 mg/dL (16.65 mmol/L), then q2-6h
- K+, HCO3, Na+, anion gap, q 2 hrs
- Phosphate, Ca++, Mg++, q4-6h

PREVENTION/AVOIDANCE
- Monitor glucose closely during stressful situations
- Careful insulin control

POSSIBLE COMPLICATIONS
- Cerebral edema
- Pulmonary edema
- Venous thrombosis
- Hypokalemia
- Myocardial infarction
- Acute gastric dilatation
- Late hypoglycemia
- Erosive gastritis
- Infection
- Respiratory distress
- Hypophosphatemia
- Mucormycosis

EXPECTED COURSE/PROGNOSIS
- DKA accounts for 14% of all hospital admissions for diabetes and for 16% of all diabetic related fatalities
- Overall mortality of 5-15%
- In children < 10 years old, DKA causes 70% diabetes related fatalities

MISCELLANEOUS

ASSOCIATED CONDITIONS Look for complications of chronic diabetes (nephropathy, neuropathy, retinopathy, etc.)

AGE-RELATED FACTORS
Pediatric:
- Occasionally children or adolescents with DKA exhibit marked mental deterioration, including development of coma 4-6 hrs after therapy has begun. Mortality is high.
  ◊ Diagnose by CT scan (cerebral edema)
  ◊ Treat with IV bolus of 1 gram mannitol/kg in 20% solution
  ◊ If no response, hyperventilation to a pCO2 of 28 mm Hg

Geriatric: Must be careful with renal status or congestive heart failure

Others: N/A

PREGNANCY Risk of fetal death with DKA during pregnancy is nearly 50%

SYNONYMS N/A

ICD-9-CM
250.1 Diabetes with ketoacidosis

SEE ALSO
- Diabetes mellitus, Type 1

OTHER NOTES N/A

ABBREVIATIONS
NS = normal saline
ABG = arterial blood gases
D5 = 5% dextrose

REFERENCES
- Isselbacher KJ, et al, eds: Harrison's Principles of Internal Medicine. 13th Ed. New York, McGraw-Hill, 1994
- Bennett JC, Plum F, eds: Cecil Textbook of Medicine. 20th Ed. Philadelphia, W.B. Saunders Co., 1996
- Bell DS, et al: Diabetic ketoacidosis: Why early detection and aggressive treatment are crucial. Postgrad Med 1997;101(9):193-200

Illustrations: N/A

Internet references: http://www.5mcc.com

Author(s)
Stoney A. Abercrombie, MD

Diarrhea, acute

BASICS

DESCRIPTION Diarrhea of abrupt onset in a healthy individual is most often related to an infectious process. A variety of symptoms are often observed, including frequent passage of loose or watery stools, fever, chills, anorexia, vomiting and malaise.
• Acute viral diarrhea - the most common form, usually occurs for 1-3 days, and is self-limited. It causes changes in the small intestine cell morphology such as villous shortening and an increase in the number of crypt cells.
• Bacterial diarrhea - may be suspected if there is a history of a similar and simultaneous illness in individuals who have shared contaminated food with the patient. Diarrhea developing within 12 hours of the meal is most likely due to ingestion of a preformed toxin.
• Protozoal infections - such as Giardia lamblia cause prolonged, watery diarrhea that often afflicts travelers returning from endemic areas where the water supply has been contaminated.
• Traveler's diarrhea - typically begins three to seven days after arrival in a foreign location and is generally quite acute
System(s) affected: Gastrointestinal, Endocrine/Metabolic
Genetics: N/A
Incidence/Prevalence in USA: N/A
Predominant age: All ages
Predominant sex: N/A

SIGNS AND SYMPTOMS
• Loose liquidy stools +/- blood or mucus
• Fever
• Abdominal pain and distension
• Headache
• Anorexia
• Malaise
• Vomiting
• Myalgia
• With Giardia - cramping, pale-greasy stools, fatigue, weight loss, chronicity

CAUSES
• Bacterial
  ◊ E. coli
  ◊ Salmonella
  ◊ Shigella
  ◊ Campylobacter jejuni
  ◊ Vibrio parahaemolyticus
  ◊ Vibrio cholerae
  ◊ Yersinia enterocolitica
• Viral
  ◊ Rotavirus
  ◊ Norwalk virus
• Parasitic
  ◊ Giardia lamblia
  ◊ Cryptosporidium
  ◊ Entamoeba histolytica

RISK FACTORS
• Individual from an industrialized country visiting a developing country
• Immunocompromised host

DIAGNOSIS

DIFFERENTIAL DIAGNOSIS
• Ulcerative colitis
• Crohn's disease
• Drugs (cholinergic agents, magnesium-containing antacids)
• Pseudomembranous colitis secondary to antibiotic use
• Diverticulitis
• Spastic (irritable) colon
• Fecal impaction
• Malabsorption
• Zollinger-Ellison syndrome
• Ischemic bowel
• Gastrinoma

LABORATORY
• CBC - increased WBC with a left shift may indicate an infectious process; decreased hemoglobin/hematocrit may indicate anemia from blood loss
• Serum electrolytes - increased sodium from dehydration, decreased potassium from diarrhea
• BUN, creatinine - elevated in dehydration
• pH - hyperchloremic acidosis
• Stool sample - occult blood (present in IBD, bowel ischemia, bacterial infections), fecal leukocytes (present in diarrhea caused by Salmonella, Campylobacter, Yersinia), bacterial culture and sensitivity (for Salmonella, Yersinia, Shigella, Campylobacter), ova and parasites, C. difficile toxin, Ziehl-Neelsen stain (for Cryptosporidium)
Drugs that may alter lab results: N/A
Disorders that may alter lab results: N/A

PATHOLOGICAL FINDINGS
• Viral diarrhea - changes in small intestine cell morphology that include villous shortening, increased number of crypt cells and increased cellularity of the lamina propria
• Bacterial diarrhea - bacterial invasion of colonic wall leads to mucosal hyperemia, edema and leukocytic infiltration

SPECIAL TESTS N/A

IMAGING Abdominal x-rays (flat plate and upright) are indicated in patients with abdominal pain or evidence of obstruction to rule out toxic megacolon and bowel ischemia

DIAGNOSTIC PROCEDURES
Sigmoidoscopy indicated in patients with bloody diarrhea or suspected pseudomembranous or ulcerative colitis

TREATMENT

APPROPRIATE HEALTH CARE
Outpatient except for complicating emergencies (dehydration)

GENERAL MEASURES
• Replacement of lost fluid and electrolytes
• Clear liquids such as tea, broth, carbonated beverages (without caffeine) and rehydration fluids (e.g., Gatorade) to replace lost fluid
• Packets of rehydration salts (one packet to be diluted in one quart of water); drink until thirst is quenched; will help in replacing lost electrolytes. Treatment of choice for pediatric patients.

SURGICAL MEASURES N/A

ACTIVITY Bedrest

DIET
• During periods of active diarrhea, avoid coffee, alcohol, dairy products, most fruits, vegetables, red meats, and heavily seasoned foods
• After 12 hours with no diarrhea, begin by eating clear soup, salted crackers, dry toast or bread, and sherbet
• As stooling rate decreases, slowly add to diet, rice, baked potato, and chicken soup with rice or noodles
• As stool begins to retain shape, add to diet baked fish, poultry, applesauce, and bananas

PATIENT EDUCATION See guidelines in Prevention/Avoidance

MEDICATIONS

DRUG(S) OF CHOICE
• Loperamide, 4 mg followed by 2 mg capsule after each unformed stool, or bismuth subsalicylate, 30 mL every half hour until 8 doses, may be helpful in mild diarrhea
• If diarrhea persists and a bacterial or parasitic organism is identified, antibiotic therapy should be started:
◊ Giardia: metronidazole 250 mg tid for 5-10 days
◊ E. histolytica: metronidazole 500-750 mg tid for 10 days
◊ Shigella: trimethoprim-sulfamethoxazole 160 mg and 800 mg, respectively, bid for five days, or ciprofloxacin (Cipro) 500 mg bid for 10 days
◊ Campylobacter: erythromycin 250 mg qid for 5 days or ciprofloxacin (Cipro) 500 mg bid for 7 days
◊ C. difficile: metronidazole 250 mg tid for 10-14 days
◊ Traveler's diarrhea: trimethoprim-sulfamethoxazole one double strength tablet bid for 3 days or ciprofloxacin (Cipro) 500 mg bid for 3 days

Contraindications:
• Antibiotics are contraindicated in Salmonella infections unless caused by S. typhosa or the patient is septic
• Avoid alcoholic beverages with metronidazole due to possibility of disulfiram reaction

Precautions:
• Antiperistaltic agents (e.g., loperamide) should be used with caution in patients suspected of having infectious diarrhea or antibiotic associated colitis
• Doxycycline, sulfamethoxazole-trimethoprim, ciprofloxacin - may cause photosensitivity. Use sunscreen.

Significant possible interactions:
• Salicylate absorption from bismuth subsalicylate can cause toxicity in patients already taking aspirin containing compounds and may alter anticoagulation control in patients taking coumadin
• Ciprofloxacin and erythromycin increase theophylline levels

ALTERNATIVE DRUGS
• Doxycycline 100 mg bid for 3 days
• Diphenoxylate-atropine in nonpregnant adults
• Tinidazole or secnidazole for E. histolytica
• Vancomycin for C. difficile infections

FOLLOWUP

PATIENT MONITORING   If diarrhea
continues for three to five days with or without blood or mucus then consult physician

PREVENTION/AVOIDANCE
• Frequent oversights during foreign travel include brushing teeth with contaminated water, ingesting ice cubes, or eating cold salads or meats
• Avoid uncooked or undercooked seafood or meat, buffet meals left out for several hours, or food served by street vendors

POSSIBLE COMPLICATIONS
• Dehydration
• Sepsis
• Shock
• Anemia

EXPECTED COURSE/PROGNOSIS   A
common problem that is rarely life-threatening if attention is given to maintaining adequate hydration

MISCELLANEOUS

ASSOCIATED CONDITIONS
• Diabetes mellitus
• Ileal resection
• Gastrectomy
• Hyperthyroidism

AGE-RELATED FACTORS
Pediatric:
• Rotavirus is a common cause of viral diarrhea in the winter months and is accompanied with vomiting
• Other etiologies include overfeeding, medications, cystic fibrosis and malabsorption
Geriatric: Watery diarrhea in elderly patient with chronic constipation may be caused by fecal impaction or obstructing neoplasm
Others: N/A

PREGNANCY   Avoid dehydration since this
may lead to preterm labor

SYNONYMS   N/A

ICD-9-CM
005.9 Food poisoning, unspecified
558.2 Toxic gastroenteritis and colitis
558.9 Unspecific noninfectious gastroenteritis and colitis

SEE ALSO
• Cholera
• Botulism
• Food poisoning, bacterial

OTHER NOTES   N/A

ABBREVIATIONS
IBD = inflammatory bowel disease

REFERENCES
• Hirschhorn N, Greenough WB: Progress in oral rehydration therapy. Scientific American 1991;264:5
• Dupont HL, Edelman R: Infectious diarrhea: From E.Coli to Vibrio. Patient Care, May 30,1991
Illustrations: N/A
Internet references: http://www.5mcc.com

Author(s)
Tejal Parikh, MD

Diarrhea, chronic

BASICS

DESCRIPTION Healthy adults have daily stool weights < 200 grams (7 oz). Stool weights in excess are abnormal and if > 3 weeks are considered chronic. Causes include: inflammatory diarrhea, osmotic diarrhea (malabsorption), secretory diarrhea (endogenous and exogenous), and intestinal dysmotility.
System(s) affected: Gastrointestinal
Genetics:
• Celiac sprue and inflammatory bowel disease may be familial
• Lactose intolerance - increased incidence in certain geographic regions
Incidence/Prevalence in USA:
• Unknown, but felt to be underdiagnosed, especially in celiac sprue
• Inflammatory bowel disease probably underdiagnosed because many patients don't seek therapy
Predominant age: Determined by certain illnesses
Predominant Sex: Female > Male

SIGNS AND SYMPTOMS
• Frequent loose stools, fever, abdominal pain, weight loss, tenesmus, flatus, bulky stools plus
  ◊ Inflammatory: blood (must rule out colonic neoplasm), anemia, abdominal pain
  ◊ Osmotic: steatorrhea, azotorrhea, weight loss, improves with fasting
  ◊ Secretory: large volumes, persists with fasting
  ◊ Altered intestinal motility: alternating diarrhea and constipation, passage of mucus and incomplete evacuation, bloating, anxiety, depression (not noctural)
  ◊ Factitious: peripheral edema, weakness, nausea, noctural, hypokalemia

CAUSES
• Inflammatory diarrhea
  ◊ Inflammatory bowel disease (ulcerative colitis and Crohn's disease)
  ◊ Radiation entercolitis
  ◊ Eosinophilic gastroenteritis
  ◊ Hypersensitivity, e.g, food allergy
  ◊ AIDS - mucosal and submucosal inflammation with possible impairment in absorption and excessive secretion
• Infectious
  ◊ Parasites (e.g., *Giardia, Isospora*)
  ◊ Helminths (e.g., *Strongyloides*)
  ◊ Bacterial (e.g., *Mycobacterium avium intracellulare, Clostridium difficile*)

• Osmotic diarrhea
  ◊ Pancreatic insufficiency (e.g, alcohol-induced, cystic fibrosis)
    ◊ Bacterial overgrowth
    ◊ Celiac disease
    ◊ Thyrotoxicosis
    ◊ Lactase deficiency
    ◊ Whipple's disease
    ◊ Abetalipoproteinemia
    ◊ Post-surgical (short gut, PUD surgery)
    ◊ Drugs: colchicine, neomycin, and para-aminosalicylic acid, antacids with magnesium, nondigestible intraluminal solute that exerts an osmotic force increasing the intraluminal fluid overwhelming the colonic mucosal absorptive capacities
• Secretory diarrhea (endogenous)
  ◊ Carcinoid syndrome
  ◊ Zollinger-Ellison syndrome
  ◊ Vasoactive intestinal peptide-secreting pancreatic adenomas
  ◊ Medullary carcinoma of thyroid
  ◊ Villous adenoma of rectum
  ◊ Microscopic colitis
  ◊ Choleraic diarrhea - excessive secretion of electrolytes
  ◊ Diabetic
  ◊ Alcohol-induced
• Secretory (exogenous)
  ◊ Factitious
  ◊ Laxatives (phenolphthalein, cascara , senna, aloe)
  ◊ Medications (cholinergics, ACE inhibitors, cholchicine, theophyllines, thyroid)
  ◊ Toxins (arsenic, mushrooms, insecticides, alcohol)
• Altered intestinal motility (most common in clincial practice)
  ◊ Irritable bowel syndrome (most common in young females)
  ◊ Fecal impaction
  ◊ Neurologic diseases
  ◊ Diabetes - increased transit and possible bacterial overgrowth

RISK FACTORS
• Inflammatory: AIDS, infections, radiation, family history
• Osmotic: infectious, abdominal surgery including cholecystectomy, resection gastric and small bowel, vagotomy, chronic alcohol abuse, Sorbitol, fructose, gluten
• Secretory: distal ileal surgery
• Altered intestinal motility: diabetes, fecal impaction or neurological diseases
• Factitious: laxative use

DIAGNOSIS

DIFFERENTIAL DIAGNOSIS
• Functional disorder
• Inflammatory bowel disease: look for systemic illness or extra-intestinal manifestations (arthritis, pyoderma gangrenosum, erythema nodosum, uveitis or vasculitis); consider Crohn's or ulcerative colitis
• Factitious: psychiatric disease or history of
• Irritable bowel syndrome: alternating diarrhea and constipation, psychiatric overtones
• Tropical sprue
• TB enteritis
• Chronic radiation enterocolitis
• Colonic neoplasm
• Diverticular disease

LABORATORY
• Stool ova and parasites
• Stool leukocytes
• Stool fat, osmolality, and occult blood
• Stool for *C. difficile* toxin
• Serum electrolytes and CBC
• Serum iron studies, vitamin B12, folate, vitamin D, PT, blood chemistry for albumin and cholesterol, serum carotene
• D-xylose absorption test
• Biopsies with esophagogastroduodenoscopy (EGD) or colonoscopy when performed
• Inflammatory diarrhea: blood or leukocytes in stool, hypoproteinemia (hypoalbuminemia and hypoglobulinemia)
• Factitious: hypokalemia
Drugs that may alter lab results: Screen for laxative abuse, e.g., phenolphthalein
Disorders that may alter lab results: Unspecified noninfectious gastroenteritis; psychiatric behavior in factitious diarrhea may contaminate stool study

PATHOLOGICAL FINDINGS
• When present, findings are those of the associated or underlying disease
• None seen in functional disorder

SPECIAL TESTS
• Inflammatory: colonic biopsies
• Fecal fat stool collections: 48-72 hours
• Breath test for labeled CO2 to assess fat, carbohydrate, and bile salt malabsorption
• Blood and urine hormone levels in endocrine diseases

IMAGING Barium enema, KUB

DIAGNOSTIC PROCEDURES
• Thorough history and physical exam helpful
• Colonoscopy for inflammatory lesions and associated occult blood in stool or with iron deficiency
• If barium enema is negative and diarrhea persists, biopsies are required (to rule out microscopic colitis in which the mucosa may appear normal). UGI evaluation with small bowel biopsies for malabsorption evaluation
• Melanosis coli suggests cathartic abuse

TREATMENT

APPROPRIATE HEALTH CARE
Unless electrolyte abnormality, deconditioning or hypotensive, outpatient therapy is adequate

GENERAL MEASURES
Fluids with electrolyte supplementation

SURGICAL MEASURES
• For villous adenomas, hormone producing tumors, and refractory ulcerative colitis

ACTIVITY
Restricted only for the debilitated patient

DIET
• Abstain from gluten products, sorbitol, lactose-containing products, food allergens
• In IBS, may need to add dietary fiber (bulking agents) (e.g. 20-30 grams of supplemental fiber per day)

PATIENT EDUCATION
• Explain in simple terms of bowel physiology
• Reassure that normal frequency varies widely
• Dietary consult when appropriate
• Restrict colon stimulants

MEDICATIONS

DRUG(S) OF CHOICE
• Efforts to increase stool consistency may be undertaken using psyllium or other hydrophilic agents
• In secretory diarrhea, opiates may help
• Diphenoxylate-atropine (Lomotil) 5-20 mg daily or loperamide (Imodium) 4-16 mg daily; given in doses calculated and timed according to the patient's individual needs. These agents may be contraindicated in infectious diarrheas because of possible organism enhancement of tissue.
• Kaolin-pectin (Kapectolin, Donnagel) 2-16 tablespoons daily, divided and timed according to individual need
• Specific agents include:
  ◊ Octreotide (Sandostatin) a analogue of somatostatin used in carcinoid syndrome and severe fluid loss in AIDs patients
  ◊ Omeprazole: an H-K-ATPase inhibitor for use in Zollinger-Ellison syndrome
  ◊ Indomethacin: prostaglandin inhibitor used in medullary carcinoma of the thyroid and villous adenomas (rare)
  ◊ H1 and H2 receptor antagonists combination for systemic mastocytosis
  ◊ Cholestyramine (Questran) for bile salt malabsorption and certain post-surgical patients
  ◊ Lactase (Lactaid, Lactrase) for lactose intolerance

Contraindications: Any impediment to bowel transit, obstruction, ileus
Precautions: Excessive treatment may lead to obstipation
Significant possible interactions: N/A

ALTERNATIVE DRUGS
• Anti-cholinergics and anti-spasmotics in irritable bowel syndrome
• Steroids and azulfadine derivitives in inflammatory bowel disease
• Clonidine in diabetes mellitus diarrhea

FOLLOWUP

PATIENT MONITORING
If diarrhea persists, further evaluation recommended

PREVENTION/AVOIDANCE
Refrain from dietary or pharmacological agents that may precipitate a diarrhea event

POSSIBLE COMPLICATIONS
• Fluid and electrolyte abnormalities
• Malnutrition
• Anemia
• Sepsis
• Cachexia

EXPECTED COURSE/PROGNOSIS
Variable, from a short (factitious and altered intestinal motility) and treatable course, to a chronic illness (e.g., Crohn's, ulcerative colitis, etc.)

MISCELLANEOUS

ASSOCIATED CONDITIONS
• Immune-complex mediated extra-intestinal complications of inflammatory bowel disease
  ◊ Arthritis
  ◊ Uveitis
  ◊ Pyoderma gangrenosum
  ◊ Nephritis

AGE-RELATED FACTORS
Pediatric: Diarrhea secondary to dietary products, e.g., fructose and apple juice
Geriatric: Patients with life-long diarrhea may suffer increasing difficulty with advanced age
Others: N/A

PREGNANCY
N/A

SYNONYMS
• Loose bowels
• The runs

ICD-9-CM
005.9 Food poisoning, unspecified
558.2 Toxic gastroenteritis and colitis
558.9 Unspecific noninfectious gastroenteritis and colitis

SEE ALSO
• Crohn's disease
• Cryptococcosis
• Diarrhea, acute
• Giardiasis
• Irritable bowel syndrome
• Uveitis
• Ulcerative colitis

OTHER NOTES
N/A

ABBREVIATIONS
IBD = inflammatory bowel disease
IBS = irritable bowel syndrome

REFERENCES
• Spiro HM: Diarrhea Diseases. In: Spiro HM, ed. Clinical Gastroenterology. 4th Ed. New York, McGraw-Hill, Inc., 1993:356-358
• Krejs GJ: Diarrhea. In: Wyngaarden JB, Smith HL, eds. Cecil Textbook of Medicine. 19th Ed. Philadelphia, W.B. Saunders Co., 1992:680-687
• Freidman LS, Isselbacher KJ: Chronic Diarrhea. In: Braunwald E, Isselbacher KJ, et al, eds. Harrison's Principles of Internal Medicine. 13th Ed. New York, McGraw-Hill, Inc., 1994:216-219.
• Fine KD, Krejs GJ, Fordtran JS: Diarrhea. In: Sleisenger MH, Fordtran JS, eds. Gastrointestinal Disease. 5th Ed. Philadelphia, W.B. Saunders Co., 1994:1043-1072
• Powell D. Approach to the patient with diarrhea in Yamada, Textbook of Gastroenterology, 1998
Illustrations: N/A
Internet references: http://www.5mcc.com

Author(s)
Robert Burgos, MD

Digitalis toxicity

BASICS

DESCRIPTION A condition that may result from digitalis overdosage, hypokalemia, advanced degenerative heart disease with conduction disturbances, or a combination of factors. Toxicity may develop even when serum levels are within normal range. Usual course - acute; chronic.
System(s) affected: Cardiovascular, Nervous, Gastrointestinal
Genetics: No known genetic pattern
Incidence/Prevalence in USA: Occurs in 5-23% of patients sometime during therapy
Predominant age: Middle age to elderly (40-75 years)
Predominant sex: Male = Female

SIGNS AND SYMPTOMS
- Abdominal pain
- Anorexia
- Bilateral central scotomata
- Bizarre mental symptoms in elderly patients
- Blurred vision
- Bradycardia
- Confusion
- Delirium
- Depression
- Diarrhea
- Disorientation
- Drowsiness
- Fatigue
- Hallucinations
- Halos around lights
- Headache
- Hypotension
- Impaired color vision
- Irregular pulse
- Lethargy
- Loss of visual acuity
- Mydriasis
- Nausea
- Neuralgia
- Nightmares
- Personality changes
- Photophobia
- Restlessness
- Vertigo
- Vomiting
- Weakness

CAUSES
- Alkalosis
- Amiodirone
- Broad spectrum antibiotics
- Cor pulmonale
- Diltiazem
- Hemodialysis
- Hypernatremia
- Hypokalemia
- Hypomagnesemia
- Hypothyroidism
- Macrolides
- Myocarditis
- Overdosage
- Poisoning with plants containing cardiac glycosides, such as oleander, foxglove
- Procaine
- Quinidine
- Reserpine
- Spironolactone
- Steroids

RISK FACTORS
- Anoxia
- Catecholamines
- Decompensating heart failure
- Diuretics
- Hypercalcemia
- Myocardial infarction
- Recent cardiac surgery
- Renal failure
- Suicide attempt

DIAGNOSIS

DIFFERENTIAL DIAGNOSIS
- Heart block
- Renal disease
- Other causes of life-threatening arrhythmia

LABORATORY
- Eosinophilia
- Increased digitalis level, especially if ≥ 4 ng/mL (≥ 5.1 nmol/L). Digoxin levels may not correlate with amount taken in acute ingestion.
- Potassium - hyperkalemia with acute ingestion; hypokalemia with chronic ingestion of excess or chronic renal failure
Drugs that may alter lab results: Any digitalis drug
Disorders that may alter lab results: Many cardiac abnormalities

PATHOLOGICAL FINDINGS N/A

SPECIAL TESTS
- EKG (Note that no arrhythmia is unique to digitalis toxicity, thus any sudden change in cardiac rhythm suggests possible toxicity)
  ◊ Accelerated junctional rhythms
  ◊ Atrial flutter
  ◊ Atrial premature contractions
  ◊ Atrial tachycardia with AV block
  ◊ Bidirectional tachycardia
  ◊ Bundle branch block
  ◊ Junctional premature beats
  ◊ Sinus bradycardia
  ◊ Sinus bradycardia with junctional tachycardia
  ◊ Ventricular fibrillation
  ◊ Ventricular premature contractions
  ◊ Wenckebach's block with junctional premature beats
  ◊ P-R changes
  ◊ Q-T changes

IMAGING N/A

DIAGNOSTIC PROCEDURES N/A

TREATMENT

APPROPRIATE HEALTH CARE
Inpatient - coronary care unit

GENERAL MEASURES
- Maintain airways
- Continuous cardiac monitoring
- Discontinue digitalis
- Check serum electrolytes; maintain potassium in high-normal range. Treat hyperkalemia (K >5.5) with NaHCO3 (1 mEq/kg) glucose (0.5 g/kg), and insulin 0.1 U/kg. Do not use calcium as it may worsen ventricular arrhythmias.
- Correct calcium and magnesium abnormalities
- Avoid quinidine, which may increase serum digoxin levels by displacing digoxin from its binding sites and by decreasing renal and nonrenal excretion
- Avoid beta-adrenergic blocking drugs and isoproterenol
- Procainamide may be used
- If the patient is hemodynamically stable with primarily enhanced vagal activity (1st or 2nd degree AV block) and if the peak digitalis effect has been reached, no acute therapy is required
- Must monitor for 24 hours after ingestion

SURGICAL MEASURES N/A

ACTIVITY Bedrest with monitoring

DIET Low salt, low fat

PATIENT EDUCATION Griffith, H.W.: Instructions for Patients; Philadelphia, W.B. Saunders Co.

Digitalis toxicity

MEDICATIONS

DRUG(S) OF CHOICE
• Fluid plus electrolyte therapy
• Correct acidosis
• Digoxin Immune Fab (Digibind)
 ◊ Indicated for treatment of severe, life-threatening arrhythmias due to digoxin or digitoxin overdosage
 ◊ Obtain a digoxin level before administration - be aware that the digoxin level may be falsely high if measured < 6 hours after ingestion
 ◊ Do not draw another digoxin level for 4 days after digoxin antibody (Digibind) administration since drug's half-life is up to 20 hours in patients with normal renal function
 ◊ For adults and children ingesting an unknown amount of digoxin, administer 10 vials of digoxin Immune Fab in 50 mL of NS IV over 30 minutes. However, if there is a life-threatening arrhythmia, give as bolus. Observe response and administer an additional 10 vials if clinically indicated. Watch for volume overload in children.
 ◊ For toxicity during chronic therapy: Adults, 15 vials digoxin Immune Fab in 50 mL NSS IV over 30 minutes; children, < 20 kg, 1 vial should suffice
• For ventricular arrhythmias use
 ◊ Lidocaine 50 to 100 mg IV (for ventricular arrhythmias), repeated in 3-5 minutes if needed, up to a total of 300 mg. Give no more than 300 mg in 1 hour. One protocol calls for an initial bolus of lidocaine followed by 20-50 mcg/kg/min infusion for maintenance.
 ◊ Phenytoin - 100 mg q 3-5 minures up to 1000 mg
 ◊ Magnesium
 ◊ Digoxin Immune Fab (Digibind)
• Treat bradycardia and heart block with atropine 0.5-2 mg IV. There is a controversy as to whether pacing should be done as it is associated with a high complication rate in digoxin intoxicated patients and should be used for those to whom Fab is ineffective.
Contraindications: Refer to manufacturer's literature
Precautions: Refer to manufacturer's literature
Significant possible interactions: Refer to manufacturer's literature

ALTERNATIVE DRUGS
• Phenytoin as alternative to lidocaine - 100 mg q 3-5 minutes up to 1000 mg
• Consider atropine, cholestyramine

FOLLOWUP

PATIENT MONITORING
• Close EKG monitoring, potassium and digitalis levels throughout total treatment
• Monitor kidney function

PREVENTION/AVOIDANCE
• Store digitalis safely
• Monitor for toxicity
• Fluid plus electrolyte therapy according to need as determined by periodic studies, particularly of potassium level
• If there is a documentable recent exposure, consider gastric decontamination by lavage and administer activated charcoal
• Symptomatic overdose patients might best be managed by a poison control center or toxicologist
• Educate regarding potential for drug interactions
• Onset of vague symptoms should raise suspicion of toxicity
• Be aware of illnesses that predispose to toxicity such as heart failure and dehydration

POSSIBLE COMPLICATIONS
• Death
• Conduction defects
• Life threatening rhythm disturbances

EXPECTED COURSE/PROGNOSIS
Recovery likely if patient survives 24 hours

MISCELLANEOUS

ASSOCIATED CONDITIONS
• Chronic heart failure
• Acute pulmonary edema

AGE-RELATED FACTORS
Pediatric: N/A
Geriatric: Morbidity and mortality greater
Others: N/A

PREGNANCY   N/A

SYNONYMS   N/A

ICD-9-CM   972.1 poisoning by cardiotonic glycosides

SEE ALSO   Ventricular tachycardia (VT)

OTHER NOTES   N/A

ABBREVIATIONS
NS = normal saline

REFERENCES
• Carter BL, et al: Monitoring digoxin therapy in two long-term facilities. J Am Geriatr Soc 1981;29:263
• Beller GA, et al: Digitalis intoxication: a prospective clinical study with serum level correlations. N Engl J Med 1971;284:989
• Duhme DW, et al: Reduction of digoxin toxicity associated with measurement of serum levels. Ann Int Med 1974;80:516
• Marcus FI: Diagnosing digitalis intoxication. Hospital Med 1990;7:75
• Burroughs Wellcome Co: Digibind product information. Research Triangle Park, NC., 1991
• Borron SW, et al: Advances in the management of digoxin toxicity in the older patient. Drugs and Aging 1997;10:18-33
• Cauffield JS, et al: The serum digoxin concentration. 10 questions to ask. Amer Fam Phys 1997;56(2):495-503
• Olson K, et al: Poisoning and Drug Overdose. Norwalk, CT, Appleton & Lange, 1994:124-125
Illustrations: N/A
Internet references: http://www.5mcc.com

Author(s)
Lisa Vantrease, MD
Bruce T. Vanderhoff, MD

Diphtheria

BASICS

DESCRIPTION Acute respiratory tract infection caused by Corynebacterium diphtheriae, usually producing a membranous pharyngitis
• Incubation period 2 to 5 days. Infection usually occurs in fall and winter in temperate regions. In the tropics, seasonal trends are less distinct.
• Transmission by respiratory route from infected person or carrier. Humans are the only reservoir.
• Several forms occur:
 ◊ Membranous pharyngotonsillar diphtheria - the membrane is gray, adheres to the pharynx and is surrounded by erythema. The underlying mucosa bleeds when the membrane is removed.
 ◊ Nasal diphtheria - unilateral discharge
 ◊ Obstructive laryngotracheitis - complication when membrane descends into larynx or bronchial tree. When it breaks up in young children, total obstruction of the airway may occur.
 ◊ Cutaneous diphtheria - punched-out ulcer covered by gray membrane (particularly in tropics and among homeless). Peaks August to October in southern United States.
System(s) affected: Pulmonary, Skin/Exocrine, Cardiovascular, Nervous
Genetics: N/A
Incidence/Prevalence in USA: 1.6 in 100,000,000 for non-cutaneous form
Predominant age: Children less than 15 and poorly immunized adults. Diphtheria is a rare condition in the U.S. today. Recent outbreaks have occurred in the new independent states of the former Soviet Union.
Predominant sex: Male = Female

SIGNS AND SYMPTOMS
• Membranous pharyngotonsillar diphtheria:
 ◊ Initially, white to yellow membrane which is easily removed
 ◊ Adherent, whitish-gray, leathery membrane on tonsils or pharynx
 ◊ Removing membrane causes bleeding of mucosa
 ◊ Injected pharynx
 ◊ Membrane may become black due to hemorrhage
 ◊ Sore throat
 ◊ Cervical adenopathy with swelling
 ◊ Malaise and prostration
 ◊ Enlarged, tender cervical and submandibular lymph nodes
 ◊ May progress to edematous, swollen neck (bull neck)
 ◊ Paralysis of soft palate
 ◊ Low grade fever of 37.8-38.8°C (100-100.9°F)
 ◊ Thrombocytopenia and purpura
• Nasal diphtheria:
 ◊ Serosanguineous or seropurulent discharge and excoriations
 ◊ Often discharge is unilateral
 ◊ Often chronic, mild course

• Obstructive laryngotracheitis:
 ◊ Hoarseness
 ◊ Croupy cough
 ◊ Progresses to dyspnea and stridor
 ◊ Labored breathing
 ◊ Thick speech
• Cutaneous diphtheria:
 ◊ On skin, conjunctiva, vulva, vagina, penis
 ◊ Primary cutaneous diphtheria - starts as tender pustule on lower extremity and becomes deep, round, punched-out ulcer covered by grayish membrane
 ◊ Secondary infection of preexisting wound - purulent exudate, partial membrane

CAUSES Corynebacterium diphtheriae

RISK FACTORS
• Crowded living conditions
• Inadequate immunization. In the USA, 22-62% of people age 18 to 39 years and 41-84% of people over 60 years of age lack protective levels of antibody.
• Lower socioeconomic status
• Native Americans
• Alcoholism
• Travelers - outbreaks have occurred in the Ukraine and Russia

DIAGNOSIS

DIFFERENTIAL DIAGNOSIS
• Bacterial pharyngitis including group A streptococcus
• Viral pharyngitis
• Mononucleosis
• Oral syphilis
• Candidiasis
• Vincent's angina
• Acute epiglottitis

LABORATORY
• Gram-positive rods in the pathognomonic Chinese character configuration
• Moderate leukocytosis
• Thrombocytopenia
• Transient albuminuria
• Methylene-blue stains can assist in a presumptive diagnosis in experienced hands
• Culture from nose and throat beneath membrane and have plated on special media; inform lab that diphtheria is suspected
• Should test for toxigenicity of strain
Drugs that may alter lab results: If an antibiotic was used, then 5 or more days may be required for the culture to grow on Loeffler's medium
Disorders that may alter lab results: N/A

PATHOLOGICAL FINDINGS
• Pleomorphic gram-positive rods
• Necrotic epithelium
• Hyaline degeneration

SPECIAL TESTS
• Serial ECG's and cardiac enzymes to detect myocarditis
• Delayed peripheral nerve conduction velocities
• Culture on Loeffler's or tellurite medium is positive in 8 to 12 hours if not previously treated with an antibiotic. Laboratory must be alerted to use one of the special media.

IMAGING N/A

DIAGNOSTIC PROCEDURES
• Culture throat or lesions
• Smear of exudate for gram stain

TREATMENT

APPROPRIATE HEALTH CARE
• Inpatient, initially hospitalized in unit which can monitor cardiac and respiratory status. (Must act on presumptive diagnosis because therapy cannot wait for culture confirmation).
• Isolation until cultures on two consecutive days are negative. The first culture must be taken at least 24 hours after the cessation of antibiotic therapy.

GENERAL MEASURES
• Have intubation or tracheostomy readily available. For laryngeal disease, laryngoscopy is desirable. Intubation or tracheostomy should be considered early for laryngeal disease.
• Avoid hypnotics and sedatives while monitoring respiratory status
• Physical therapy in convalescence for range of motion exercises to prevent contractions

SURGICAL MEASURES N/A

ACTIVITY Rest (for at least 3 weeks until risk of developing myocarditis has passed)

DIET Liquid to soft as tolerated

PATIENT EDUCATION Explain aspects of illness and complications

MEDICATIONS

DRUG(S) OF CHOICE
Both antitoxin and antibiotics are needed for non-cutaneous diphtheria
• Diphtheria antitoxin, equine: Use 20,000 to 40,000 units of antitoxin for laryngeal or pharyngeal disease of less than 48 hours duration, 40,000 to 60,000 units for nasopharyngeal lesions, 80,000 to 120,000 units for extensive disease of 3 or more days duration or swelling of the neck (bull neck). Administer antitoxin by IV infusion over 60 minutes and/or by intramuscular injection. Some experts recommend treating cutaneous disease with 20,000 to 40,000 units of antitoxin while others doubt its value when there are no signs of systemic disease. Antitoxin is obtained from the CDC.
• Erythromycin parenterally or orally, 40-50 mg/kg/day; maximum of 2 grams/day for 14 days

Contraindications: See Precautions

Precautions:
• Equine antitoxin: 7% of patients are sensitive to equine antitoxin and need desensitization. Always test for hypersensitivity to antitoxin prior to its administration.
◊ First, a drop of 1:100 dilution of antitoxin is placed on a scratch on the forearm. If negative, an interdermal skin test is done with 1:1000 dilution (0.02 mL).
◊ A positive reaction is the development of urticaria within 20 minutes of injection
◊ If no reaction, then repeat test with a 1:100 dilution. If person has a negative history for animal allergy, has not previously received animal serum and had a negative scratch test, then 1:100 dilution may be used initially.

Significant possible interactions: N/A

ALTERNATIVE DRUGS
• Penicillin G intramuscularly, 100,000 to 150,000 units/kg/day in four divided doses up to 600,000 units per day
• DL-carnitine 100 mg/kg/day given bid po in children for 4 days in myocarditis (experimental)

FOLLOWUP

PATIENT MONITORING
• ECG, cardiac enzymes and respiratory status. Serial ECG 2-3 times per week for 4-6 weeks to detect myocarditis.
• Elimination of the organism should be documented by three negative cultures at least 24 hours apart. The first culture should be at least 24 hours after the completion of antimicrobial therapy.
• During convalescence, patients should be immunized against diphtheria because infection does not necessarily confer immunity

PREVENTION/AVOIDANCE
• Prevention is by immunization:
◊ Children 6 weeks up to 7 years of age should receive doses at 2, 4, 6 and 15-18 months of age with 0.5 mL of DTaP vaccine IM If the pertussis component is contraindicated then pediatric DT should be used. A booster dose should be given at 4-6 years of age and again at age 11-12 or 14-16 years
◊ Unimmunized persons 7 years of age or older should receive two doses of Adult Td 4-8 weeks apart with a third dose 6-12 months later. 0.5 mL of Td should be given IM.
◊ Subsequently, booster doses with Td should be given every 10 years to all individuals without a contraindication. An alternative strategy after the booster at age 11-12 or 14-16 years is a single adult booster at 50 years of age.
◊ Immunized individuals may develop diphtheria but their course is milder; immunization protects against the toxin, not infection or microbial carriage in the nose, pharynx or skin
◊ Disinfect all articles in contact with patient
◊ Close contacts should be cultured and given antibiotic prophylaxis regardless of immunization status. Previously immunized contacts should receive a booster of diphtheria toxoid. Unimmunized contacts should begin the series. Erythromycin prophylaxis for 7 days.

POSSIBLE COMPLICATIONS
• Myocarditis (in 10-25%) may occur early
• Cranial and peripheral neuropathy (2-6 weeks after onset)
• ECG abnormalities in two-thirds of patients, including: bundle branch block, tachycardia, atrial or ventricular fibrillation, extrasystoles
• Right sided heart failure
• Local paralysis of soft palate and posterior pharynx demonstrated by regurgitation of fluids through the nares
• Peripheral and cranial neuropathy affecting primarily motor nerve functions. Motor dysfunction starts proximally and extends distally. Usually slowly resolves.
• Guillain-Barré-like syndrome

EXPECTED COURSE/PROGNOSIS
• < 5% mortality rate
• Prognosis guarded until recovery
• 5-10% persistance in nasopharynx in convelescing patients

MISCELLANEOUS

ASSOCIATED CONDITIONS N/A

AGE-RELATED FACTORS
Pediatric: N/A
Geriatric: N/A
Others: N/A

PREGNANCY N/A

SYNONYMS N/A

ICD-9-CM
032 Diphtheria
032.0 Faucial diphtheria
032.1 Nasopharyngeal diphtheria
032.2 Anterior nasal diphtheria
032.3 Laryngeal diphtheria
032.8 Other specified diphtheria
032.81 Conjunctival diphtheria
032.82 Diphtheritic myocarditis
032.83 Diphtheritic peritonitis
032.84 Diphtheritic cystitis
032.85 Cutaneous diphtheria
032.89 Other
032.9 Diphtheria, unspecified

SEE ALSO N/A

OTHER NOTES N/A

ABBREVIATIONS N/A

REFERENCES
• Rakel RE, ed: Conn's Current Therapy 1998. Philadelphia, WB Saunders Co, 1998
• Red Book Report of the Committee on Infectious Diseases, 1997. Elk Grove Village, American Academy of Pediatrics, 1997
• Advisory Committee on Immunization Practices
Illustrations: N/A
Internet references: http://www.5mcc.com

Author(s)
Richard Kent Zimmerman, MD, MPH
Gregory A. Poland, MD

Disseminated intravascular coagulation (DIC)

BASICS

DESCRIPTION Generation of fibrin in the blood and consumption of procoagulants and platelets occurring in complications of obstetrics, (e.g., abruptio placenta), infection (especially gram-negative), malignancy and other severe illnesses

System(s) affected:
Hemic/Lymphatic/Immunologic

Genetics: Homozygous protein C or protein S deficiency

Incidence/Prevalence in USA: Unknown

Predominant age: None

Predominant sex: Male = Female

SIGNS AND SYMPTOMS
- Epistaxis
- Gingival bleeding
- Mucosal bleeding
- Hemoptysis
- Hematemesis
- Metrorrhagia
- Cough
- Dyspnea
- Confusion
- Disorientation
- Stool blood
- Hematuria
- Oliguria
- Fever
- Skin petechiae
- Purpura
- Ecchymosis
- Skin hemorrhagic necrosis
- Localized rales
- Tachypnea
- Pleural friction rub
- Retinal hemorrhages
- Anuria
- Thrombosis
- Stupor
- Peripheral cyanosis

CAUSES
- Coagulation disorder due to widespread activation of clotting mechanism
- Obstetric complications
- Infection
- Neoplasms
- Intravascular hemolysis
- Vascular disorders; thrombosis
- Snake bite
- Massive tissue injury
- Trauma
- Hypoxia
- Liver disease
- Infant and adult RDS
- Purpura fulminans
- Thermal injury

RISK FACTORS
- Pregnancy
- Prostatic surgery
- Head injury
- Inflammatory states

DIAGNOSIS

DIFFERENTIAL DIAGNOSIS
- Massive hepatic necrosis
- Vitamin K deficiency
- Thrombocytopenic purpura
- Hemolytic-uremic syndrome
- Primary fibrinolysis

LABORATORY
- Thrombocytopenia
- Increased partial thromboplastin time
- Increased prothrombin time
- Increased thrombin time
- Decreased fibrinogen
- Increased fibrin degradation product (FDP)
- Decreased antithrombin III
- Positive D-Dimer assay
- Increased bleeding time
- Schizocytosis
- Anemia
- Leukocytosis
- Increased lactate dehydrogenase (LDH)
- Increased BUN
- Decreased factor V
- Decreased or increased factor VIII
- Decreased factor X
- Decreased factor XIII
- Hemoglobinemia
- Hematuria
- Guaiac-positive stools
- Decreased protein C

Drugs that may alter lab results: N/A
Disorders that may alter lab results: N/A

PATHOLOGICAL FINDINGS N/A

SPECIAL TESTS N/A

IMAGING Chest x-ray: Bilateral perihilar soft density

DIAGNOSTIC PROCEDURES N/A

TREATMENT

APPROPRIATE HEALTH CARE
Inpatient

GENERAL MEASURES
- Treat underlying condition e.g., evacuation of uterus in abruptio placenta. Broad-spectrum antibiotics for gram-negative sepsis.
- Replacement of blood loss
- Platelet concentrates
- Fresh frozen plasma
- Cryoprecipitate
- Antithrombin III concentrate

SURGICAL MEASURES N/A

ACTIVITY As tolerated

DIET No special diet

PATIENT EDUCATION Griffith, H.W.: Instructions for Patients; Philadelphia, W.B. Saunders Co.

Disseminated intravascular coagulation (DIC)

MEDICATIONS

DRUG(S) OF CHOICE
• Anticoagulants (heparin) if clinical findings suggest developing thrombotic complications, but never after head injury
• Broad-spectrum antibiotics for sepsis
Contraindications:
• Head injury
• Hemorrhagic stroke
Precautions: Refer to manufacturer's literature
Significant possible interactions: Refer to manufacturer's literature

ALTERNATIVE DRUGS For DIC associated with metastatic prostatic carcinoma, consider heparin, aminocaproic acid (Amicar). Do not use fibrinolytic inhibitors (Amicor) unless severe fibrinolysis is documented.

FOLLOWUP

PATIENT MONITORING Closely until much improved

PREVENTION/AVOIDANCE No preventive measures known

POSSIBLE COMPLICATIONS
• Acute renal failure
• Shock
• Cardiac tamponade
• Hemothorax
• Intracerebral hematoma
• Gangrene and loss of digits

EXPECTED COURSE/PROGNOSIS
Related to severity of cause of DIC

MISCELLANEOUS

ASSOCIATED CONDITIONS
Thromboembolic phenomena associated with venous thrombosis, thrombotic vegetations on the aortic heart valve, arterial emboli, neonatal purpura fulminans (homozygous protein C or protein S deficiency)

AGE-RELATED FACTORS
Pediatric: Neonatal purpura fulminans associated with DIC and protein C or protein S deficiency (homozygous)
Geriatric: N/A
Others: N/A

PREGNANCY N/A

SYNONYMS
• Consumptive coagulopathy
• Defibrination syndrome
• DIC

ICD-9-CM
286.6 Defibrination syndrome

SEE ALSO N/A

OTHER NOTES N/A

ABBREVIATIONS
RDS = respiratory distress syndrome
FDP = fibrin degradation products

REFERENCES
• Isselbacher KJ, et al, eds: Harrison's Principles of Internal Medicine. 13th Ed. New York, McGraw-Hill, 1994
• Stites DP, Stobo JD, Wells JV, eds: Basic and Clinical Immunology. 8th Ed. New York, Appleton & Lange, 1994
Illustrations: 2 available on CD-ROM
Internet references: http://www.5mcc.com

Author(s)
Stanley G. Smith, MA, MB, FCFPC

Dissociative disorders

BASICS

DESCRIPTION A sudden change in state of consciousness, identity, motor behavior, thoughts, feelings and perception of external reality to such an extent that these functions do not operate congruently. Many pathologic symptoms can be found, but the patient experiences dysphoria, suffering, and maladaptive functioning. Disorders include:
• Dissociative amnesia
• Dissociative fugue
• Dissociative identity disorder
• Depersonalization disorder
• Dissociative disorder not otherwise specified (NOS). Authors may include somnambulism (sleep-walking disorder), conversion reactions, pseudo-epilepsy and (in some cultures) a variety of possession syndromes.
System(s) affected: Nervous
Genetics: N/A
Incidence/Prevalence in USA: 8-10% of the general psychiatrically ill. As many as 70% of young adults report short periods of dissociative experiences that are self-limiting and resolve spontaneously.
Predominant age: Adolescents and young to middle age adults; rare as a new illness in elderly. If untreated, may linger from childhood into adult and old age.
Predominant sex: Female > Male (2:1)

SIGNS AND SYMPTOMS
All disorders share:
• Symptoms cause significant distress or impairment in social, occupational, or other important areas of functioning
• Symptoms are not due to the direct physiological effects of a substance (e.g., drug of abuse, a medication) or a general medical condition (e.g., temporal lobe epilepsy)
• Dissociative amnesia:
  ◊ One or more episodes of inability to recall important personal information that is too extensive to be explained by ordinary forgetfulness
  ◊ Not occurring during another psychiatric illness and not due to effects of chemical substance (drug abuse or medication)
  ◊ Not due to a neurological or other medical condition (e.g., head trauma)
• Dissociative fugue:
  ◊ Sudden unexpected travel away from home or one's customary place of work with an inability to recall one's past
  ◊ Confusion about personal identity or assumption of a new identity (partial or complete)
  ◊ Above symptoms do not occur exclusively during course of dissociative identity disorder
  ◊ Symptoms cause significant distress or impairment in social, occupational, or other important areas of functioning with activities of daily living
• Dissociative identity disorder:
  ◊ Presence of two or more distinct identities or personality states (each with its own relatively enduring pattern of perceiving, relating to, and thinking about environment and self).

◊ At least two of these identities or personality states recurrently take control of the person's behavior
◊ Inability to recall important personal information (too extensive to be explained by ordinary forgetfulness)
◊ Reports of time distortion, lapses and discontinuities
◊ Experiencing voices from inside one's head
◊ Chronic headaches
◊ History of severe emotional or physical abuse as a child
◊ Referring to self as "he/she," "we," "us"
◊ Eating disorders
◊ Flashbacks
◊ Feelings of derealization
◊ Feelings of depersonalization
◊ Amnesia about important childhood events
◊ Personal objects and belongings that cannot be accounted for
◊ Disowning unrecalled behaviors
◊ Different handwriting styles
◊ Different signatures and names found in personal diary
◊ Sudden mood changes
◊ Sudden behavioral changes, i.e., from adult to young child
◊ Episodes of déjà vu
◊ Feeling controlled by "another person" from within
◊ Self-inflicted violence such as wrist cutting
• Depersonalization disorder:
  ◊ Persistent or recurrent experiences of feeling detached from, and as if one is an outside observer of one's mental processes or body (e.g., feeling like one is in a dream)
  ◊ During the depersonalization experience, reality testing remains intact
  ◊ The depersonalization experience does not occur exclusively during the course of another mental disorder, such as schizophrenia, panic disorder, acute stress disorder or another dissociative disorder
• Dissociative disorder NOS: Predominant feature is a dissociative symptom (i.e., a disruption in the usually integrated functions of consciousness, memory, identity, or perception of the environment) that does not meet the criteria for any specific dissociative disorder. Examples:
  ◊ Clinical presentations similar to dissociative identity disorder that fail to meet the full criteria for this disorder. Examples include a) there are not two or more distinct personality states or b) amnesia for important personal information does not occur
  ◊ Derealization unaccompanied by depersonalization in adults
  ◊ States of dissociation that occur in individuals who have been subjected to periods of prolonged and intense coercive persuasion (e.g., brainwashing, thought reform, or indoctrination while captive)
  ◊ Dissociative trance disorder: Single or episodic disturbances in the state of consciousness, identity, or memory that are indigenous to particular locations and cultures. Dissociative trance involves narrowing of awareness of immediate surroundings or stereotyped behaviors or movements that are experienced as being beyond one's control.

◊ Possession trance: Involves replacement of the customary sense of personality identity, attributed to the influence of a spirit, power, and associated with stereotyped "involuntary" movements or amnesia.
◊ Loss of consciousness, stupor, or coma not attributed to a general medical condition
◊ Ganser syndrome: The giving of approximate answers to questions (e.g., "2 plus 2 equals 5") when not associated with dissociative amnesia or dissociative fugue

CAUSES
• Physical, emotional, verbal, or sexual abuse in childhood
• Sudden and severe trauma or threat to one's psychological or physical integrity
• Sudden and unexpected exposure to watching others being killed or severely injured (as in an industrial or car accident)
• A preponderance of coping with trauma and internal or inter-personal conflicts by the use of dissociation
• Psychological/social support to cope with the trauma/abuse was not available

RISK FACTORS
• Exposure to neglect, abuse and trauma in one's childhood
• Tendency to cope with life stresses by excessively using an escape mechanism of day dreaming and/or dissociation

DIAGNOSIS

DIFFERENTIAL DIAGNOSIS
• Other mental/CNS disorder: Schizophrenia, depression, anxiety disorder, mania, obsessive/compulsive disorder, identity disorder, phobic disorders, eating disorders
• Other: Extreme sensory deprivation, epilepsy; early phases of dementia, encephalitis, head trauma, migraine, cerebral vascular disease, brain tumors
• Endocrinopathy: Hypoglycemia, hypothyroidism, hyperthyroidism
• Miscellaneous: Huntington's disease, carbon monoxide poisoning, mescaline intoxication, botulism, hyperventilation
• Obstructive sleep apnea, nocturnal myoclonus

LABORATORY Toxicology screening may be helpful
Drugs that may alter lab results: Lithium carbonate may produce hypothyroidism
Disorders that may alter lab results:
Patients (especially those with dissociative identity disorder) may present with medical oddities such as fast healing of broken bones, radiographs resembling brain atrophy, brain infarcts, lupus, or abnormal pulmonary function tests.
A variety of symptoms (including blurred vision, nausea and vomiting, rapid heart beat, palpitation, extreme bradycardia, urinary frequency and urgency, extreme changes in levels of blood glucose) may lead to erroneous diagnosis

PATHOLOGICAL FINDINGS N/A

SPECIAL TESTS EEG to rule out epilepsy and sleep disorders. Polysomnogram to rule out sleep apnea.

IMAGING CT scan and MRI of the head to rule out multiple infarct dementia, brain tumors, and some forms of encephalopathy

DIAGNOSTIC PROCEDURES
• Neuro-psychological testing is helpful in ruling out learning disabilities and cognitive deficits due to early dementia or borderline mental retardation
• Psychological testing helps identify specific psychiatric disorders, personality structure and dynamics
• Dissociation scales help assess the tendency to dissociate in daily living activities
• Sodium amytal interviews (narcoanalysis) and special interviews under hypnosis are useful in selected cases
• Clinician reviews patient's diary for handwriting and signature changes.

TREATMENT

APPROPRIATE HEALTH CARE
• Outpatient, individual psychotherapy
• At times of crisis: intensive hospital-based treatment (as a protection for patients with suicidal or homicidal impulses, and/or self-inflicted violence)
• Use inpatient care to verify diagnosis with special tests and begin treatment program that continues on outpatient basis
• Note: Treatment emphasis on progress in the adaptive functions with daily living activities, symptom alleviation, ego strengthening, prevent regressions

GENERAL MEASURES
• Individual psychotherapy plus behavior modification, narcoanalysis and narcosynthesis, hypnoanalysis and hypnotherapy
• Adjuncts: support groups, group therapy, expressive art therapy, occupational and recreational therapy
• Bibliotherapy and graphotherapy are useful

SURGICAL MEASURES N/A

ACTIVITY Based on patient's condition

DIET N/A

PATIENT EDUCATION
• Self-hypnosis, relaxation exercises and guided imagery
• Encourage patients to read about their condition and be inspired by others who have been diagnosed, treated, and recovered, e.g., "A Mind of My Own" by Chris Sizemore, published by W. Morrow, New York, 1989

MEDICATIONS

DRUG(S) OF CHOICE
No medications are specifically curative. The following have been helpful:
• Antidepressants: depression
• Benzodiazepines: anxiety and insomnia
• Propranolol 80-400 mg/day: flashbacks and other dissociative symptoms
• Neuroleptics (in low doses): self-abusive behavior. Thioridazine 10-200 mg/day; haloperidol 2-10 mg/day; chlorprothixene 3-200 mg/day, and perphenazine 4-22 mg/day or risperidone 1-4 mg/day.
• In severe agitation, droperidol 1-5 mg IM is effective in producing calm sleep and stopping agitation
• Mood swings, in dissociative disorders, do not respond to the use of lithium carbonate, carbamazepine or valproic acid unless patient has co-morbid bipolar disorder
Contraindications: N/A
Precautions:
• Abuse potential of short-acting benzodiazepines
• Overdose/suicide potential with TCA's
• Very low doses of neuroleptics can be used without producing tardive dyskinesia (try to avoid higher doses).
Significant possible interactions: Avoid MAO inhibitors with TCA's or SSRI's

ALTERNATIVE DRUGS
• Buspirone for anxiety 30-80 mg/day
• Clomipramine, 75-200 mg/day or fluvoxamine 100-300 mg/day for obsessive-compulsive symptoms

FOLLOWUP

PATIENT MONITORING
• Outpatients: 1-4 hrs of psychotherapy per week to avoid hospitalization
• Inpatients: more intensive treatment, e.g. daily psychotherapy

PREVENTION/AVOIDANCE
• Child abuse prevention via parent education and community agency intervention
• Crisis intervention following individual trauma or disasters for prevention of chronic morbidity/disability

POSSIBLE COMPLICATIONS Self-inflicted violence; suicide attempts; substance abuse and chemical dependency

EXPECTED COURSE/PROGNOSIS
• Natural history ranges from spontaneous improvement, in cases of dissociative amnesia, dissociative fugue, and depersonalization disorder, to acute and chronic morbidity in others

• Without treatment, dissociative identity disorder patient may have a healthy functioning facade, with episodes of depression, confusion, mood swings, etc. With age, intensity/frequency of dissociative experiences may decrease and crystallize around 1-2 major personality states.
• Effective treatment produces partial or full recovery for many patients

MISCELLANEOUS

ASSOCIATED CONDITIONS See Causes

AGE-RELATED FACTORS
Pediatric: Suspect abuse or neglect
Geriatric: Decrease in dissociative disorders. Medication side effects more likely.
Others: N/A

PREGNANCY N/A

SYNONYMS
• Hysterical neurosis, dissociative type
• Ganser's syndrome

ICD-9-CM
300.15 Dissociative disorder or reaction
301.50 Histrionic personality disorder

SEE ALSO N/A

OTHER NOTES N/A

ABBREVIATIONS N/A

REFERENCES
• Michelson LK, Ray WJ, eds: Handbook of Dissociation. New York, Plenum Press, 1996
• Torem MS: Medications in the treatment of dissociative identity disorder. Spira JL, ed. In: Treating Dissociative Identity Disorder. San Francisco, CA, 1996:99-132
• Steinberg M: Handbook for the assessment of dissociation, a clinical guide. American Psychiatric Press, 1995
• Kirsh I, Lynn SJ: Dissociation theories of hypnosis. Psychological Bulletin, 1998;123:100-115
• Spiegel D: Trauma, dissociation, and memory. Anals New York Academy of Sciences, 1997;821:225-237
• Chu JA, et al. Memories of childhood abuse; dissociation, amnesia, and corroboration. Am J Psychiatry 1999;156:749-755
• Spitzer C, et al. Dissociative experiences and psychopathology in conversion disorders. J of Psychsomatic Research 1999;46:291-294
• Lipsarer T, el al. Visual distortions and dissociation. J of Nerv and Ment Disease 1999; 187:109-112
5 additional references available at web site
Internet references: http://www.5mcc.com
Illustrations: N/A

Author(s)
Moshe S. Torem, MD, FAPA

Diverticular disease

 BASICS

DESCRIPTION Diverticulosis of the colon and its varied clinical consequences. Diverticuli develop in people in countries eating a low fiber diet and are much more prevalent in western societies.
• Diverticula of colon: Herniation of the colon mucosa through the muscular layer, usually at the site of a perforating artery, lying between two layers of serosa in the mesentery. They are more common in the sigmoid and distal colon and increase in numbers with age.
• Diverticulitis: An abscess or peridiverticular inflammation initiated by the rupture of a mucosal microscopic abscess into the mesentery. Such infection may progress, fistulize into the genitourinary system, obstruct, or spontaneously resolve. Develops in about 5% of subjects with diverticulosis each year. Over a lifetime about half of patients with diverticulosis develop inflammation.
System(s) affected: Gastrointestinal
Genetics: No known genetic pattern
Incidence/Prevalence in USA:
• 2200-3000/100,000 (diverticulitis)
• Up to 20% in general population but increases progressively with age reaching up to 40%-50% in 6th-8th decade
Predominant age: Rare below 40 years, most common in 6th-8th decade
Predominant sex: Male = Female

SIGNS AND SYMPTOMS
• Diverticulosis
 ◊ Only 10-25% of subjects harboring diverticula will develop symptoms (possibly related to coexistent irritable bowel disease)
 ◊ Pain - due to tension in colonic wall, mostly in left lower quadrant, worse after eating, some relief following bowel movement or passage of flatus
 ◊ Diarrhea or constipation
 ◊ Palpable mass in left iliac fossa - firm, tender
 ◊ Abdomen may be distended and tympanitic
 ◊ Absent signs of peritoneal inflammation
 ◊ Melena, hematochezia if diverticula bleed
• Diverticulitis
 ◊ Pain - acute onset, mostly localized in left lower quadrant. Prominently associated with tenderness in same region.
 ◊ Fever with chills as severity increases
 ◊ Anorexia, nausea, vomiting
 ◊ Constipation or diarrhea
 ◊ Rebound tenderness, involuntary guarding, board-like rigidity
 ◊ Palpable mass - tender, firm, fixed
 ◊ Abdomen distended and tympanitic
 ◊ Bowel sounds depressed or could be exaggerated if obstruction ensues
 ◊ Dysuria, frequency if bladder involved
 ◊ Pneumaturia, fecaluria if colovesical fistula develops
 ◊ Rectal exam may reveal tenderness, induration, mass in the cul-de-sac
 ◊ Enterocutaneous, enterovaginal, and perirectal fistulae may be initial manifestation

CAUSES
• Causes are speculative/not clearly proven
• Defects in colonic motility and increased intraluminal pressure, partially brought about by too little fecal volume
• Colonic segmentation - nonpropulsive contractions producing isolated segments or little chambers with high pressure in them
• Low fiber diet - increases segmentation and causes higher intraluminal pressure
• Defects in colonic wall strength
• Cause of bleeding unclear, not related to diverticulitis. Right sided diverticula, though less common, account for 50% of all bleeding from diverticula.

RISK FACTORS
• Age over 40
• Low residue diet
• Previous diverticulitis
• Number of diverticuli in the colon

 DIAGNOSIS

DIFFERENTIAL DIAGNOSIS
• Irritable bowel syndrome
• Lactose intolerance
• Carcinoma of distal colon
• Ulcerative colitis, Crohn's disease
• Angiodysplasia (for rectal bleed)
• Ischemic or infectious colitis
• Appendicitis
• Other gynecologic and urologic disorders

LABORATORY
• WBC count normal in diverticulosis, elevated with immature polymorphs in diverticulitis
• Hemoglobin low if bleeding is a symptom
• Sedimentation rate elevated in diverticulitis
• Urine analysis may reveal WBC's, RBC's, pus cells in fistula formation
• Urine culture - persistent infection in colovesical fistula
• Blood culture - positive in diverticulitis with generalized peritonitis
Drugs that may alter lab results:
• Steroids
• Other immunosuppressive drugs
Disorders that may alter lab results:
• Elderly patient
• Lymphomas, other immunocompromised states
• Severe malnutrition

PATHOLOGICAL FINDINGS
• Prediverticular state - myochosis (thickening of circular layer of muscle, shortening of tenia, restriction of lumen)
• Multiple diverticula - spastic colon diverticulosis, simple massed diverticulosis, right sided diverticulosis
• Solitary diverticulum - giant sigmoid diverticulum
• Diverticulitis - inflammation, necrosis, perforation
• Diverticulitis - earliest stage, rupture of a mucosal abscess into mesentery. Does not start with obstruction of the neck as does appendicitis.

SPECIAL TESTS
• 99mTc labeled RBC scan for bleeding (rarely used) and/or angiography
• Gallium or indium labeled leukocytes to localize abscess (rarely used)

IMAGING
• Plain film abdomen supine and upright - useful in peritonitis and perforation
• Barium enema - best means for diagnosis of diverticulosis. Less useful in diagnosis of diverticulitis.
• Diverticuli may be seen on endoscopy, but less sensitive than Barium enema.
• CT scan with or without rectal contrast - diagnostic for abscess, fistula, size and location of inflammatory mass
• Angiography - diagnostic as well as therapeutic in diverticular bleeding
• Fistulograms
• Spiral CT scan with bolus of IV contrast dye may demonstrate bleeding

DIAGNOSTIC PROCEDURES
• Colonoscopy and flexible sigmoidoscopy - helpful in diagnosis of diverticulosis and extremely valuable in differential diagnosis to prove or rule out cancer. Ulcerative or ischemic colitis can uniformly be diagnosed by these modalities.
• Cystoscopy - in colovesical fistula

 TREATMENT

APPROPRIATE HEALTH CARE
• Diverticulosis - outpatient with fiber supplements to soften stools
• Outpatient diverticulitis (pain, tenderness, leukocytosis, but no toxicity or peritoneal signs)
• About 2% subjects require hospitalization for toxicity, septicemia, peritonitis or failure to resolve in a few days. About half of these will require surgery.
• Toxic patients require hospitalization and intravenous antibiotics at least until response

GENERAL MEASURES
• IV fluids, analgesics, nasogastric suction
• Indications for surgery - severe diverticulitis, perforation, abscess, fistula, severe diverticular bleeding (requiring more than 2,000 mL of blood in 24 hours), recurrent episodes

SURGICAL MEASURES
• Usual indication related to diverticulitis. Multiple attacks in 2 years, unhealing fistulae, abscess or toxicity may lead to surgery.
• Large pus collections are usually drained radiologically and when resolved, the most involved segment of the colon resected

ACTIVITY Fully active in diverticulosis, restricted activity in diverticulitis

DIET
• NPO during acute diverticulitis, progress to fluids, then to high fiber as normal bowel function returns
• All patients with diverticula should increase dietary fiber to high level through foods, and/or fiber supplement if appropriate

PATIENT EDUCATION
• Importance of high fiber diet and recognizing the symptoms of complications at early stage
• Additional material from:
National Digestive Diseases Information Clearinghouse, Box NDDIC, Bethesda, MD 20892, (301)468-6344

MEDICATIONS

DRUG(S) OF CHOICE
• Diverticulosis
◊ Pain syndromes may be treated with antispasmodics - hyoscyamine (Levsin) 0.125 mg or 2 each 4 hours; buspirone (BuSpar) 15-30 mg/day; or meperidine (Demerol) 100-150 mg/day along with high fiber diet
◊ Constipation and diarrhea, manage as indicated for irritable bowel disease
• Diverticulitis
◊ Oral treatment for mild disease - metronidazole (Flagyl) 250-500 mg q 8 hours and amoxicillin 500 mg q 8 hours combination, or ciprofloxacin 500 mg bid. Expect response within 3 days. Continue oral therapy for one week.
◊ More severe cases in hospital - gentamicin 3-5 mg/kg/day plus clindamycin 1.8-2.7 gm/day along with analgesic. Aminoglycoside dose varies with creatinine clearance.
• Diverticular bleeding
◊ Vasopressin 0.2-0.3 units/minute through selective intra-arterial catheter. Used when bleeding demonstrated at angiography.
Contraindications: Hypersensitivity reaction
Precautions:
• Avoid morphine and other opiates except for Demerol
• Watch for renal toxicity and ototoxicity with aminoglycosides
Significant possible interactions: Refer to manufacturer's profile of each drug

ALTERNATIVE DRUGS Tobramycin and metronidazole, 3rd generation cephalosporins

FOLLOWUP

PATIENT MONITORING
• Some physicians would not do any invasive studies; others have recommended repeat barium enema every 3 years if symptoms infrequent or absent, or following corrective surgery
• Colonoscopy, if needed based on above results

PREVENTION/AVOIDANCE High fiber diet, psyllium, agar, methylcellulose

POSSIBLE COMPLICATIONS
• Hemorrhage
• Perforation
• Peritonitis
• Bowel obstruction
• Abscess - paracolic, subhepatic, subphrenic
• Fistula - colovesical, colovaginal, colocutaneous

EXPECTED COURSE/PROGNOSIS
• Prognosis is good with early detection and treatment of the complications
• Of those with a first episode of diverticulitis who are successfully managed medically, up to 67% will not have subsequent attacks requiring hospitalization; 33% will recur. Two or three recurrences in 1-2 years is an indication to electively remove the involved segment of colon.
• Of those with diverticular bleeding, up to 20% will rebleed in a period of months to years

MISCELLANEOUS

ASSOCIATED CONDITIONS Often occurs in conjunction with spastic colon

AGE-RELATED FACTORS
Pediatric:
• Very rare
• When present, it is more aggressive and recurrent in young age
Geriatric:
• More common
• May sometimes be difficult to diagnose
Others: N/A

PREGNANCY Differentiate from ectopic pregnancy

SYNONYMS N/A

ICD-9-CM
562.10 Diverticulosis of colon without mention of diverticulitis
562.11 Diverticulitis of colon

SEE ALSO Irritable bowel syndrome

OTHER NOTES N/A

ABBREVIATIONS N/A

REFERENCES
• Ferzoco LB, Raptopoulos V, Silen W: Acute diverticulitis. NEJM 1998;338:1521-1526
Illustrations: N/A
Internet references: http://www.5mcc.com

Author(s)
Frank L. Iber, MD

Down syndrome

BASICS

DESCRIPTION
A common form of mental retardation whose cause is unknown. All patients have extra chromosome 21 material; chromosome non-disjunction usually occurs in female meiosis. The syndrome occurs in all races with equal frequency.
• Trisomy 21: 90% of patients, an extra chromosome 21 is found in all cells
• Translocation 21: 5% of patients, extra chromosome 21q material is translocated to another chromosome, usually 13 or 15. For the 5% of translocation trisomies, 2/3 are new, 1/3 have a parental carrier.
• Mosaic 21: 5% of patients, 2 or more cell populations found, usually normal and trisomy 21. Clinical manifestations milder.
System(s) affected: Nervous, Cardiovascular, Skin/Exocrine
Genetics: As above. Extra chromosome comes from mother in > 90% of the cases.
Incidence/Prevalence in USA: 1 in 1000 births
Predominant age: Most identified at birth. Life-span shortened.
Predominant sex: Male = Female

SIGNS AND SYMPTOMS
• Infants and children
  ◊ Brachycephaly (100%)
  ◊ Hypotonia (80%)
  ◊ Posterior 3rd fontanel
  ◊ Small ears, +/- superior ear folds, +/- low set ears
  ◊ Mongoloid slant, eyes (90%)
  ◊ Epicanthic folds (90%)
  ◊ Brushfield's (speckled) spots of iris (50%)
  ◊ Esotropia (50%)
  ◊ Depressed nasal bridge
  ◊ Enlarged tongue (75%)
  ◊ Small chin
  ◊ Short neck
  ◊ Cardiac murmur (50%)
  ◊ Abnormal dermatoglyphics, including single palmar crease, distal palmar triradius, and absence of plantar whorl (ball of foot)
  ◊ Developmental delay, which may not be apparent in 1st year
  ◊ Mild-moderate instability of neck at C1-C2
  ◊ Most findings milder, but brachycephaly remains
  ◊ Patients are retarded (IQ = 40-45) but usually personable and cooperative
  ◊ Most adults can care for their personal needs. Some have jobs, but all require a sheltered environment.
  ◊ A small percent of patients have some autistic features. A small percent of patients are non-verbal.

CAUSES
• Genetic - unequal chromosome division
• Genetic - translocation (5% of cases)

RISK FACTORS
• Increases with mother's age:
  ◊ 1/2000, age 20
  ◊ 1/200, age 35
  ◊ 1/100, age 37
  ◊ 1/20, age 45

DIAGNOSIS

DIFFERENTIAL DIAGNOSIS
• Minor familial anomalies such as Mongoloid slant, epicanthic folds and depressed nasal bridge, particularly in a child with hypotonia
• The presence of a whorl on the ball of the foot usually indicates a normal child

LABORATORY
A chromosome test is definitive and should always be done because of the chance of translocation
Drugs that may alter lab results: N/A
Disorders that may alter lab results: N/A

PATHOLOGICAL FINDINGS
Alzheimer's plaques found in 100% of brains after age 20

SPECIAL TESTS   N/A

IMAGING
Abdominal ultrasound for urinary tract anomalies in children with pyuria or fevers of unknown origin

DIAGNOSTIC PROCEDURES
• Cardiac echo in all children. A VSD/endocardial cushion defect may not be apparent at birth.
• X-ray of neck for minor trauma, or there is neck pain, long tract symptoms or breathing problems
• Thyroid resting for children with poor weight gain, constipation

TREATMENT

APPROPRIATE HEALTH CARE
• Genetic evaluation and counseling
• Cardiac evaluation and ECG
• Appropriate pediatric health care

GENERAL MEASURES
• Parents can usually adapt to a special child
• Most important is to address parental fears and treat the infant normally
• Infant stimulation programs recommended, but definitive proof of effectiveness is lacking

SURGICAL MEASURES   N/A

ACTIVITY
• Fully active unless heart disease
• A controlled environment is needed for older children and adults

DIET
No special diet. Programs suggesting megavitamin therapy have been disproved.

PATIENT EDUCATION
• National Down Syndrome Congress (800)232-NDSC
• Down syndrome Usenet list serv: listserv@vm1.nodak.edu
• Down syndrome information and counseling is available: http://www.nas.com/downsyn

Down syndrome

MEDICATIONS

DRUG(S) OF CHOICE N/A
Contraindications: N/A
Precautions: N/A
Significant possible interactions: N/A

ALTERNATIVE DRUGS Current enthusiasm for "neural enhancers", e.g., piracetam, a GABA analog, not proven, but under study

FOLLOWUP

PATIENT MONITORING
• 1 or 2 subsequent genetic visits to complete counseling and a visit at 1-2 years
• Follow cardiac status carefully
• Thyroid and possibly cardiac investigation if growth rate decreased

PREVENTION/AVOIDANCE
• Prenatal chorion villus biopsy at 9-10 weeks and amniocentesis at 13-15 weeks
• A low screening maternal serum alpha-fetoprotein (MSAFP, and abdominal triple screen at 14-16 weeks gestation finds 50-60% of cases
• Prenatal testing recommended for all pregnant females over 35, but this only impacts 25% of cases
• Recurrence:
  ◊ 1% for trisomy 21 if child has trisomy 21
  ◊ Is one-fifth to one-sixth for parents with a balanced translocation
  ◊ If the parental translocation is 21:21 (45,t (21:21)), the recurrence is 100%
  ◊ Increased recurrence in families with mosaic Down syndrome is not clear, but prenatal testing is recommended

POSSIBLE COMPLICATIONS
• Bowel obstruction (fistula, intestinal anomalies [10%])
• Hirschsprung's disease (3%)
• Thyroid disease (hypo-and hyperthyroidism 5-8%)
• Leukemia (0.5%)
• Congenital heart disease (50%) especially endocardial cushion defect, ventricular septal defect
• Alzheimer's disease
• Seizures (3-4%)

EXPECTED COURSE/PROGNOSIS
• Development is normal in the first year in about one-third of cases and mildly delayed in the rest
• Development slows after age 1 and language and cognition are moderately delayed
• The outcome and longevity may be dependent on congenital heart disease
• Some adult individuals can work in protected situations; a few largely independent
• Intestinal complications and congenital heart disease may be of immediate concern
• Hypothyroid disease occurs after 6 months when found, and diminished growth is the principal sign
• Clinical Alzheimer's disease in 1/3 of patients after age 35
• There is premature aging. Most patients die at 50-60, earlier if there is heart disease.

MISCELLANEOUS

ASSOCIATED CONDITIONS N/A

AGE-RELATED FACTORS
Pediatric: N/A
Geriatric: Seldom survive to geriatric age
Others: N/A

PREGNANCY Pregnancy is possible in patients with Down syndrome. The risk for Down syndrome in an infant is 50%.

SYNONYMS
• Trisomy 21
• Trisomy G
• Down's syndrome

ICD-9-CM
758.0 Down syndrome

SEE ALSO N/A

OTHER NOTES Mongolism is a term no longer used

ABBREVIATIONS N/A

REFERENCES
• Behrman RE, Kliegman RM, eds: Nelson Textbook of Pediatrics. 14th Ed. Philadelphia, W.B. Saunders Co., 1992
• Smith D: Recognizable Patterns of Human Malformation. 4th Ed. Philadelphia, W.B. Saunders Co., 1988
Illustrations: N/A
Internet references: http://www.5mcc.com

Author(s)
Paul J. Benke, MD, PhD

Dumping syndrome

 BASICS

DESCRIPTION Gastrointestinal symptoms resulting from rapid gastric emptying. Usually occurs following gastric surgery (gastrectomy, vagotomy, pyloroplasty).
System(s) affected: Gastrointestinal
Genetics: N/A
Incidence/Prevalence in USA: After vagotomy: 0.9% of proximal gastric vagotomy; 10-22% truncal vagotomy
Predominant age: Middle age to elderly
Predominant sex: Male = Female

SIGNS AND SYMPTOMS
Most common to least common:
• Abdominal discomfort, pain
• Diarrhea (postprandial)
• Bloating
• Nausea
• Palpitations
• Diaphoresis
• Weight loss
• Flushing
• Lightheadedness
• Confusion and syncope

CAUSES Multifactorial including:
• Rapid delivery of hyperosmolar material into intestine
• Supraphysiologic release of various peptides/vasoactive mediators
• Reactive hypoglycemia

RISK FACTORS Surgical drainage procedures, particularly gastrectomy; anti-ulcer surgery

 DIAGNOSIS

DIFFERENTIAL DIAGNOSIS
• Mechanical obstruction
• Gastroenteric fistula
• Celiac sprue
• Crohn's disease
• Pancreatic exocrine insufficiency
• Neuroendocrine tumors (e.g., carcinoid)

LABORATORY
• Postprandial hypoglycemia
• Anemia
• Hypoalbuminemia
Drugs that may alter lab results: Insulin
Disorders that may alter lab results: Diabetes mellitus

PATHOLOGICAL FINDINGS N/A

SPECIAL TESTS N/A

IMAGING
• Upper GI series - barium rapidly emptying from stomach
• Nuclear medicine gastric emptying study
• Endoscopy (exclude mechanical obstruction)

DIAGNOSTIC PROCEDURES N/A

 TREATMENT

APPROPRIATE HEALTH CARE
Outpatient except in rare circumstances

GENERAL MEASURES Dietary and medical management

SURGICAL MEASURES Surgery only if dietary and medical management unsuccessful and symptoms debilitating; variable results

ACTIVITY
• No restrictions
• Lying down after eating or when symptoms occur

DIET
• Low carbohydrate
• Frequent small meals with minimal liquid
• Drink fluids between meals only
• High protein diet
• Adequate caloric intake

PATIENT EDUCATION National Digestive Diseases Information Clearinghouse, Box NDDIC, Bethesda, MD 20892, (301)468-6344

MEDICATIONS

DRUG(S) OF CHOICE
• Octreotide (Sandostatin) 200-400 mcg/day subcutaneous, given in divided doses q8h. Can be very expensive.
• Pectin/guar gum
Contraindications:
• Hypersensitivity
Precautions: N/A
Significant possible interactions: Refer to manufacturer's literature

ALTERNATIVE DRUGS
Anticholinergics. Results generally disappointing.

FOLLOWUP

PATIENT MONITORING Follow to be sure of adequate nutrition

PREVENTION/AVOIDANCE
• Eating frequent, small, dry meals that contain no refined carbohydrates
• Restrict fluids to between meals

POSSIBLE COMPLICATIONS
• Hypoglycemia
• Malnutrition
• Electrolyte disturbances including hypokalemia

EXPECTED COURSE/PROGNOSIS
Favorable

MISCELLANEOUS

ASSOCIATED CONDITIONS
• Peptic ulcer disease
• Reactive hypoglycemia
• Gastrectomy/vagotomy

AGE-RELATED FACTORS
Pediatric: N/A
Geriatric: N/A
Others: N/A

PREGNANCY N/A

SYNONYMS Early postgastrectomy syndrome

ICD-9-CM
564.2 Postgastric surgery syndromes

SEE ALSO
• Peptic ulcer disease
• Diarrhea, chronic
• Hypoglycemia, nondiabetic

OTHER NOTES N/A

ABBREVIATIONS N/A

REFERENCES
• Sleisenger MH, Fordtran JS, eds: Gastrointestinal Disease: Pathophysiology, Diagnosis, Management. 5th Ed. Philadelphia, W.B. Saunders Co., 1994
• Spiro HW, ed: Clinical Gastroenterology. 4th Ed. New York, McGraw-Hill, 1993
Illustrations: N/A
Internet references: http://www.5mcc.com

Author(s)
Philip E. Jaffe, MD

Dupuytren's contracture

BASICS

DESCRIPTION Contracture of the palmar fascia due to fibrous proliferation resulting in flexion deformities and loss of function. Similar change may rarely occur in plantar fascia. It usually appears simultaneously.

System(s) affected: Musculoskeletal

Genetics:
• Autosomal dominant with variable penetrance
• 10% of patients have a positive family history

Incidence/Prevalence in USA:
• Unknown
• Norway - 9% males and 3% females

Predominant age: 50

Predominant sex: Male > Female (ranges from 2:1 to 10:1)

SIGNS AND SYMPTOMS
• Unilateral or bilateral (50%)
• Right hand more frequent
• Ring finger more frequent
• Ulnar digits more affected than radial
• Mild pain early
• Later painless plaques or nodules in palmar fascia
• Extends into a cord-like band in the palmar fascia
• Skin adheres to fascia and becomes puckered
• Nodules can be palpated under the skin
• Digital fascia becomes involved as disease progresses
• Web space contractures
• Dupuytren's diathesis can involve plantar (Ledderhose's - 10%) and penile (Peyronie's - 2%) fascia
• Knuckle pads

CAUSES
• Unknown
• Ischemia to the fascia with oxygen free radical formation
• Possibly related to release of angiogenic basic fibroblast growth factor
• Related to microhemorrhage and release of growth factors

RISK FACTORS
• Smoking (mean 16 pack-years, odds ratio 2.8)
• Alcohol intake
• Increasing age
• Male/Caucasian
• Diabetes mellitus (one-third affected, increases with time, usually mild; middle and ring finger involved)
• Epilepsy
• Chronic illness (e.g., pulmonary tuberculosis, liver disease)
• Hypercholesterolemia
• Liver disease
• HIV infection

DIAGNOSIS

DIFFERENTIAL DIAGNOSIS
• Early for callosity
• Tendon abnormalities
• Camptodactyly - early teens tight facial bands ulnar side of small finger

LABORATORY N/A
Drugs that may alter lab results: N/A
Disorders that may alter lab results: N/A

PATHOLOGICAL FINDINGS
• Myofibroblasts
• First stage (proliferative) - increased myofibroblasts
• Second stage (residual) - dense fibroblast network
• Third stage (involutional) - myofibroblasts disappear

SPECIAL TESTS N/A

IMAGING MR can assess cellularity of lesions which correlate with higher recurrence after surgery

DIAGNOSTIC PROCEDURES N/A

TREATMENT

APPROPRIATE HEALTH CARE
• Outpatient monitoring and physical therapy
• Inpatient if surgery indicated

GENERAL MEASURES
• Steroid injection for acute tender nodule
• Physiotherapy is ineffective alone
• Isolated involvement of palmar fascia can be followed
• Metacarpo-phalangeal (MP) joint involvement can be followed if flexion contracture is < 30 degrees

SURGICAL MEASURES
• Surgery - selective fascial ray release
  ◊ Indications: Any involvement of the proximal interphalangeal (PIP) joints. Hueston's table-top test, if positive, consider surgery (when the palm is placed on a flat surface, the digits can not be simultaneously placed fully on the same surface as the palm because of flexion contractures).
  ◊ May require skin grafts for wound closure with severe cutaneous shrinkage
  ◊ 80% have full range of movement if operated on early
  ◊ Continuous elongation technique is useful to prepare a severely contracted PIP joint for surgery. The digit can frequently be completely extended, however, will relapse if surgery not performed.
  ◊ Amputation of little finger, if severe and deforming

ACTIVITY
• No restrictions
• Physical therapy after surgery - started 3-5 days postsurgery (passive and active exercises, posterior dynamic extension splints)

DIET No special diet

PATIENT EDUCATION
• Avoid risk factors especially with a strong family history
• Regular follow-up by physician every 6 months-1 year

MEDICATIONS

DRUG(S) OF CHOICE Steroid injection for an acute tender nodule, painful knuckle pad
Contraindications: N/A
Precautions: N/A
Significant possible interactions: N/A

ALTERNATIVE DRUGS Topical high-potency steroids - case report of improvement with clobetasol 0.1% bid and hs for 2-4 weeks

FOLLOWUP

PATIENT MONITORING Follow patient in early stages of disease

PREVENTION/AVOIDANCE None known. Avoid risk factors when possible.

POSSIBLE COMPLICATIONS
• Postsurgery development of reflex sympathetic dystrophy
• Postoperative recurrence or extension 46-80%
• Postoperative hand edema and skin necrosis
• Digital infarction

EXPECTED COURSE/PROGNOSIS
• Unpredictable, but usually slowly progressive
• Patients likely to have aggressive disease (one or more) < 40 at onset, knuckle pads, positive family history, bilateral disease involving radial side of hand
• Reports of clinical regression with continuous passive skeletal traction in extension and under a skin graft
• Recurrence rate after surgery is 10-34%
• Prognosis better for MP joint vs PIP joint after surgery

MISCELLANEOUS

ASSOCIATED CONDITIONS
• Alcoholism
• Epilepsy
• Diabetes mellitus
• Chronic lung disease
• Occupational hand trauma (vibration white finger)
• Shoulder-hand syndrome
• Status post myocardial infarction
• Hypercholesterolemia

AGE-RELATED FACTORS
Pediatric: N/A
Geriatric: Primarily in this age group
Others: N/A

PREGNANCY N/A

SYNONYMS N/A

ICD-9-CM
728.6 Contracture of palmar fascia (Dupuytren's)

SEE ALSO N/A

OTHER NOTES N/A

ABBREVIATIONS
MP = metacarpo-phalangeal
PIP = proximal interphalangeal

REFERENCES
• Attali P, Ink O, et al: Dupuytren's Contracture, Alcohol Consumption and Chronic Liver Disease. In Arch Intern Med 1987;147:1065-1067
• Hill N, Hurst L: Dupuytren's Contracture. Hand Clinics 1989;5(3):349-357
• Way LW: Current Surgical Diagnosis & Treatment. 8th Ed. Los Altos, CA, Lange, 1989
• Hueston JT: Repression of Dupuytren's contracture. J of Hand Surg 1992;17(4):453-457
• McFarlane RM: The current status of Dupuytren's disease. J of Hand Surg 1995;8(3):181-184
Illustrations: N/A
Internet references: http://www.5mcc.com

Author(s)
Jeffrey F. Minteer, MD

Dysfunctional uterine bleeding (DUB)

BASICS

DESCRIPTION Abnormal uterine bleeding, usually associated with anovulatory cycles, in the absence of other detectable organic lesions. This unit will deal only with women of reproductive age. Three major categories are:
• Estrogen breakthrough bleeding
• Estrogen withdrawal bleeding
• Progestin breakthrough bleeding

System(s) affected: Reproductive, Endocrine/Metabolic

Genetics: Unclear; tendency to have familial characteristics

Incidence/Prevalence in USA: Exact numbers not available, widespread prevalence, without specific geographic variation

Predominant age: 12-45

Predominant sex: Female only

SIGNS AND SYMPTOMS
• Uterine bleeding:
  ◊ Unrelated to menses
  ◊ In excess of normal menstrual flow
  ◊ Occurring in an irregular pattern
  ◊ Rarely painful
• Absence of:
  ◊ Other systemic symptoms
  ◊ Unusual bleeding from other areas
  ◊ Urinary or gastrointestinal irregularities
  ◊ Sustained aspirin or anticoagulant use
  ◊ Use of hormonal preparations
  ◊ Evidence of thyroid disease
  ◊ Galactorrhea
  ◊ Pregnancy (especially ectopic)
  ◊ Evidence for reproductive tract malignancy

CAUSES
• After Eisenberg:
  ◊ Midcycle spotting - caused by a decrease in estrogen at midcycle following ovulation
  ◊ Frequent menses - due to short follicular phase as a result of inappropriate feedback at pituitary/hypothalamic level
  ◊ Deficiency of luteal phase - associated with premenstrual spotting or polymenorrhea when luteal phase is suddenly shortened by prematurely decreased progesterone; due to corpus luteum insufficiency
  ◊ Prolonged corpus luteum activity - caused by persistent progesterone production - results in prolonged cycles or protracted episodes of bleeding
  ◊ Anovulation - production of estrogen unaccompanied by cyclic surges of leuteinizing hormone (LH) or secretion of progesterone from the corpus luteum. 90% of all DUB is anovulatory. Usually seen at extremes of reproductive life.
  ◊ Other - uterine lesions, leiomyomata, polyps, carcinoma, vaginal infection, foreign body, ectopic pregnancy, hydatid mole, endocrine dysfunction (especially thyroid), blood dyscrasias

RISK FACTORS Listed with Causes

DIAGNOSIS

DIFFERENTIAL DIAGNOSIS
• Advanced liver disease
• Anabolic steroids
• Hematological disease (von Willebrand's, leukemia, thrombocytopenia)
• Hormonal imbalance
• Iatrogenic causes
• Intrauterine devices
• Medications (oral contraceptives, corticosteroids, hypothalamic depressants, anticholinergics, digitalis, anticoagulants
• Pregnancy (ectopic, incomplete miscarriage
• Thyroid disease
• Trauma
• Uterine cancer
• Uterine leiomyomas

LABORATORY
• Rarely necessary unless clinical picture suggests other endocrine or hematological disease, or if patient is perimenopausal
• Consider thyroid function tests, CBC, PT, PTT, workup for hirsutism, HCG (to rule out pregnancy and/or hydatid mole), prolactin (pituitary dysfunction)

Drugs that may alter lab results: N/A
Disorders that may alter lab results: N/A

PATHOLOGICAL FINDINGS Variable, depending on the disease process present. Pathological review of endometrial sampling specimens is mandatory in all patients.

SPECIAL TESTS Basal body temperature to document anovulation

IMAGING
• Ultrasound may be helpful in identifying ovarian cysts and uterine tumors
• Transvaginal ultrasound (TVUS) recently developed and may be useful in many circumstances. Consider TVUS if you suspect pregnancy, anatomic problems, polycystic ovarian syndrome. The ultrasonographer should have a great deal of experience with the technique.

DIAGNOSTIC PROCEDURES
• Careful history of bleeding, with graphic display of cycles often helpful
• Pelvic examination
• Pap smear
• Endometrial biopsy in selected patients:
  ◊ All patients over 35 years of age
  ◊ Obese patients
  ◊ Patients with diabetes mellitus
  ◊ Patients with hypertension
  ◊ Patients with suspected polycystic ovary syndrome
• Dilatation and curettage in those who have higher risk for endometrial hyperplasia and carcinoma (consider D&C more strongly over endometrial biopsy if the suspected diagnosis is endometritis, atypical hyperplasia, or carcinoma):
  ◊ Heavy, uncontrolled bleeding
  ◊ Histological examination is necessary, but biopsy is contraindicated
  ◊ Medical curettage fails

TREATMENT

APPROPRIATE HEALTH CARE Almost always outpatient; may need hospitalization for profuse bleeding and hemodynamic instability

GENERAL MEASURES See Medications

SURGICAL MEASURES
• Acute (profuse bleeding, hemodynamic instability):
  ◊ Dilatation and curettage
  ◊ Hysterectomy in selected (rare) cases
• Nonacute:
  ◊ Hysterectomy in selected patients if medical therapy fails
  ◊ Endometrial ablation in selected patients if medical therapy fails

ACTIVITY As tolerated

DIET Normal; include adequate iron

PATIENT EDUCATION
• Thorough yet easily comprehended explanation of diagnostic approach and plan of treatment is important. Many questions regarding fertility, cancer, and infectious disease.
• Discuss ways for patient to avoid prolonged stress or emotional turmoil
• American College of Obstetricians & Gynecologists (ACOG), 409 12th St., SW, Washington, DC 20024-2188, (800)762-ACOG

Dysfunctional uterine bleeding (DUB)

MEDICATIONS

DRUG(S) OF CHOICE
• Acute (heavy bleeding, unstable):
◊ Conjugated equine estrogens (25 mg intravenously) every 4 hours for a maximum of six doses
◊ When bleeding has stopped, induce shedding of the endometrium with 10 mg medroxyprogesterone qd for 10-13 days, or with oral contraceptive medication containing 35 mcg of ethinyl estradiol or equivalent
◊ Correct anemia with supplemental iron therapy
• Nonacute:
◊ Progestin: Medroxyprogesterone acetate 10 mg each day for 10-13 days
◊ Estrogen and progesterone (if bleeding when seen or bleeding continues with progesterone or with OCP's): Add 1.25 mg conjugated estrogens daily for days 1-25
◊ Oral contraceptives: Any preparation is usually adequate; initial therapy is one pill qid for 5-7 days. After withdrawal bleeding, may begin normal regimen, usually for at least 3 months or give medroxyprogesterone, 10 mg every day for 10 days every 30 days to regulate menses. Can add estrogen, conjugated (Premarin), 1.25 mg daily for 7 days during and in addition to regimen in order to stop intermenstrual bleeding.
◊ Prostaglandin synthetase inhibitors (e.g., naproxen sodium, mefenamic acid): Can decrease amount of blood loss
◊ Gonadotropin-releasing hormone agonists (induce hypoestrogenism and amenorrhea): Leuprolide acetate, nafarelin, goserelin
◊ Correct anemia with supplemental iron therapy

Contraindications: Therapy should not be instituted until a reasonable attempt at diagnosis has been made, and other causes of uterine bleeding have been considered. "Blind" hormonal therapy is ill-advised and potentially dangerous.

Precautions: Absence of withdrawal bleeding requires workup. Estrogens should not be administered to perimenopausal women or those at risk for endometrial cancer until endometrial hyperplasia and carcinoma have been excluded. Failure of a particular regimen should prompt thorough review of the diagnostic pathway before further steps are taken.

Significant possible interactions: Refer to manufacturer's profile of each drug

ALTERNATIVE DRUGS
• Progesterone:
◊ 100 mg IM progesterone in oil (an alternate to oral methylprogesterone). This works well for active bleeding. Not appropriate for cyclic therapy.
◊ Vaginal suppositories due to leakage and uncertain amount of effective medication should not be used
◊ "Natural" progesterone lozenges (sublingual/oral) have not be adequately studied for use with DUB and have questionable safety.
• Danazol [unlabeled use]: 200-400 mg/day. Much more expensive and may cause masculinization. Usually reserved for women planning to undergo endometrial ablation soon.

FOLLOWUP

PATIENT MONITORING
All women treated for DUB with estrogens should maintain a menstrual calendar to document the pattern of bleeding abnormalities and their relation to therapy

PREVENTION/AVOIDANCE   N/A

POSSIBLE COMPLICATIONS
• Anemia
• Adenocarcinoma of the uterus if prolonged unopposed estrogen stimulation in women with intact uterus
• Significant side effects of individual preparations. See manufacturer's printed information.

EXPECTED COURSE/PROGNOSIS
• Varies with pathophysiologic process
• In young women, most anovulatory cycles can be treated confidently and successfully with physiologically sound therapeutic regimens, without surgical intervention

MISCELLANEOUS

ASSOCIATED CONDITIONS   Listed with Causes

AGE-RELATED FACTORS
Pediatric: N/A
Geriatric: Uterine bleeding in a postmenopausal female must be pursued as if there were carcinoma or other significant pathology present
Others: Early postpubertal females and those in their later reproductive years most often affected

PREGNANCY   May confuse with ectopic pregnancy, hydatidiform mole

SYNONYMS   N/A

ICD-9-CM
626.8 Disorders of menstruation and other abnormal bleeding from female genital tract, other

SEE ALSO
• Ectopic pregnancy
• Dysmenorrhea
• Menorrhagia

OTHER NOTES   If DUB cannot be controlled with medical treatment, options besides hysterectomy are available. Among these are the ND:YAG laser or electrocautery of the endometrium with a ball-end resectoscope.

ABBREVIATIONS   N/A

REFERENCES
• Anderson ABM, Haynes PJ, Guilleband J, Turnbull AC: Reduction of menstrual blood loss by prostaglandin synthetase inhibitors. Lancet 1976;1:774
• DeVore GR, Owens O, Kase N: Use of intravenous Premarin in the treatment of dysfunctional uterine bleeding - a double-blind randomized control study. Obstet Gynecol 1982;59:285
• Speroff L, Glass RH, Kase NG, eds: Clinical Gynecologic Endocrinology and Infertility. 5th Ed. Baltimore, Williams and Wilkins, 1994
• Cowan BD, Morrison JC: Management of abnormal genital bleeding in girls and women. N Engl J Med 1991;324:1710
• Apgar BS. Dysmenorrhea and dysfunctional uterine bleeding. Primary Care; Clinics in Office Practice. 1997:24: 161-178
• Goldfarb HA: A review of 35 endometrial ablations using ND:YASG laser for recurrent menorrhagia. Obstet Gynecol Clin 1990;79 (5pt1):833-835
Illustrations: N/A
Internet references: http://www.5mcc.com

Author(s)
Kurt Elward, MD, MPH

Dyshidrosis

 BASICS

 DIAGNOSIS

 TREATMENT

DESCRIPTION
• Dyshidrotic eczema: Recurrent vesicular eruption primarily of the palms, soles and interdigital areas. The term pompholyx (Greek "bubble") is generally reserved for the cases of deep-seated pruritic vesicles (the so-called "sago grain" appearance). Generally associated with, but not caused by, hyperhidrosis.
• Lamellar dyshidrosis: A fine spreading exfoliation of the superficial epidermis in the same distribution as described above. Hyperhidrosis may or may not be associated.
System(s) affected: Skin/Exocrine
Genetics: N/A
Incidence/Prevalence in USA: 20/100,000
Predominant age: Usually < age 40
Predominant sex: Male = Female

SIGNS AND SYMPTOMS
• Dyshidrotic eczema
  ◊ Small superficial vesicles of the palms and soles and between the fingers and toes
  ◊ Scaling, fissures and lichenification may follow vesicle formation
  ◊ Burning and itching are common
  ◊ Bilateral and frequently symmetrical lesions
  ◊ Vesicles may sometimes coalesce to form larger vesicles or even bullae
  ◊ Vesicles may rupture leading to a fine scaling similar to tinea
• Lamellar dyshidrosis
  ◊ Small white macules which spread peripherally
  ◊ Central area begins to scale
  ◊ Desquamation of the horny layer of the skin that continues to spread

CAUSES
• Exact cause is not known
• May represent an id reaction especially to a dermatophyte infection, atopic reaction, reaction to allergens
• Stress may play a role since dyshidrosis is more frequent in anxious individuals, and those with psychosocial stress
• Hyperhidrosis is not a cause, but is often associated with the disease

RISK FACTORS
• Atopic dermatitis
• Contact dermatitis
• Dermatophytosis
• Bacterial infections
• Foods
• Drugs, such as aspirin or other salicylates

DIFFERENTIAL DIAGNOSIS
• Tinea manuum or pedis
• Id reaction
• Contact dermatitis
• Atopic dermatitis
• Drug reaction
• Dermatophytid
• Pustular psoriasis
• Seborrheic dermatitis
• Acrodermatitis continua
• Pustular bacterid

LABORATORY N/A
Drugs that may alter lab results: N/A
Disorders that may alter lab results: N/A

PATHOLOGICAL FINDINGS
• Dyshidrotic eczema: Reveals fine 1-2 mm spongiotic vesicles intraepidermally. Sweat ducts are not involved.
• Lamellar dyshidrosis: Exfoliation of the horny layer of the epidermis

SPECIAL TESTS N/A

IMAGING N/A

DIAGNOSTIC PROCEDURES
• Diagnosis is usually based on clinical exam
• Skin biopsy

APPROPRIATE HEALTH CARE
Outpatient

GENERAL MEASURES
• Avoidance of possible causative factors (see Risk factors)
• Though hyperhidrosis is not a cause, excessive sweating may increase pruritus and burning
• Moisturizers will give symptomatic relief of dry scaly lesions
• If feet involved:
  ◊ Wear shoes with leather soles rather than rubber (e.g., sneakers)
  ◊ Wear socks made of cotton instead of synthetic materials
  ◊ Remove shoes and socks whenever possible to allow sweat evaporation and to apply lubricants

SURGICAL MEASURES N/A

ACTIVITY
• Avoid, when possible, stress or excessive sweating (may be psychological or thermal sweating)
• Avoid excess detergents and water

DIET No restrictions

PATIENT EDUCATION
• Instructions on self-care, complications and avoidance
• Explain the association between stress and dyshidrosis and suggest counseling if appropriate

MEDICATIONS

DRUG(S) OF CHOICE
Remove stool impaction: (before starting maintenance treatment program)
• Give 1 ounce of mineral oil the first day
• On the next day, give 1-3 enemas till clear; this may need to be repeated on 1-2 subsequent days
   ◊ First give an oil retention enema
   ◊ Follow the oil retention enema with hypophosphate enemas, e.g., sodium phosphate (Fleet's) 1 ounce (28.4 gm) per 20 pounds (9.1 kg) of body weight, or
   ◊ Normal saline enemas - 2 tsp table salt per quart (946 mL) of warm water and give 2 ounces (60 mL) per year of age to a maximum of 16 ounces (480 mL)
   ◊ A bisacodyl (Dulcolax) suppository can be inserted to assist the evacuation
• Alternative: give an oral solution of polyethylene glycol (Colyte, Nulytely) at 20 mL/kg/hr for 4 hours on 2 consecutive days. Nulytely is a newer, equally effective and more palatable preparation.
• Maintenance treatment
   ◊ Up to 6 months or more to keep stool slippery or soft, and for child to develop regular bowel habit
   ◊ Give mineral oil (at least 2 tablespoons each day) mixed with cold orange juice to help it go down
   ◊ Fiber or other hydrophilic agents may be used to soften the stool - lactulose, methylcellulose (Citrucel), psyllium (Metamucil, Perdiem), polycarbophil (Mitrolan), malt soup extract (Maltsupex) and fiber wafers; adjust dose to keep the stool soft.
   ◊ Multivitamins must be given between mineral oil doses to ensure absorption of the fat soluble vitamins (A,D,E,K)
Contraindications: Refer to manufacturer's profile of each drug
Precautions: Avoid bedtime doses of mineral oil to decrease risk of aspiration
Significant possible interactions: Refer to manufacturer's profile of each drug

ALTERNATIVE DRUGS
• Cisapride (Propulsid) has been effective for some children

FOLLOWUP

PATIENT MONITORING
• Continue the maintenance treatment program for at least 6 months and maybe for as long as 1-2 years
• Visits every 4-10 weeks for support and to ensure compliance
• Telephone availability to prevent problems and adjust doses
• Redevelopment of impaction must be removed as above
• Counseling and/or referral for associated psychosocial issues

PREVENTION/AVOIDANCE
• Optimal feeding practices
• Normal bowel function and recommendations for bowel training
• Early detection of problems
• Use of dark Karo syrup and fiber for hard stools
• Prompt treatment of perianal dermatitis to avoid painful defecation
• Look for signs of relapse which include large caliber stools, decrease in frequency of defecation, soiling

POSSIBLE COMPLICATIONS
• Excessive enemas or suppositories may cause colitis
• Perianal dermatitis
• Anal fissure

EXPECTED COURSE/PROGNOSIS
• Usually responds well though relapses may occur
• Children with psychosocial or emotional problems which preceded the encopresis are more recalcitrant to treatment

MISCELLANEOUS

ASSOCIATED CONDITIONS
• Perianal dermatitis
• Urinary tract infections
• Sexual abuse in boys

AGE-RELATED FACTORS
Pediatric: N/A
Geriatric: N/A
Others: N/A

PREGNANCY N/A

SYNONYMS
Soiling

ICD-9-CM
787.6 Incontinence of feces

SEE ALSO Constipation

OTHER NOTES N/A

ABBREVIATIONS N/A

REFERENCES
• Hatch TF: Encopresis and constipation in children. Pediatric Clinics of N Am 1988;35(2):257-78
• Schmitt BD: Soiling with constipation. Parent handout in Clinical Reference Systems, Ltd., 1989
• Olness K, McParland F, Piper L: Biofeedback: A new modality in the management of children with fecal soiling. J Pediatrics 1980;96:505-509
• Iwata G, Iwai N, Nagashima M, Fukata R: New biofeedback therapy in children with encopresis. Europ J Pediatr Surg 1995;5:231-234
• Nurko S, Garcia-Aranda JA, Guerrero VY, Worona LB. Treatment of intractable constipation in children: experience with cisapride. J Pediatr Gastro Nutr 1996;22:38-44
• Van der Plas, Benninga MA, Buller HA, Bossuyt PM, Akkermans LM, Redekop WK, Taminiau JA. Biofeedback training in treatment of childhood constipation: a randomised controlled trial. Lancet 1996;348(9030):776-780
• Loening-Bauche V. Biofeedback training in children with functional constipation. A critical review. Digestive Dis Sciences 1996;41:65-71.
Illustrations: N/A
Internet references: http://www.5mcc.com

Author(s)
Burris Duncan, MD

Endocarditis, infective (part 1)

BASICS

DESCRIPTION A disease resulting from infection primarily of the valvular endocardium and occasionally the mural endocardium
• Acute endocarditis: Aggressive course, usually caused by more virulent organisms, such as *Staphylococcus aureus, group B streptococcus*, may not have underlying valve lesion
• Subacute endocarditis: Indolent course, usually caused by *alpha-hemolytic streptococci, enterococci* (usually in setting of underlying structural valve disease)
• Endocarditis in intravenous drug abusers: Commonly involves the tricuspid valve. *Staphylococcus aureus* is the most common infecting organism.
• Early prosthetic valve endocarditis: Occurs within 60 days of valve implantation. Staphylococci, gram-negative bacilli and Candida are common infecting organisms.
• Late prosthetic valve endocarditis: Occurs 60 days or longer after valve implantation. *Staphylococcus epidermidis, alpha-hemolytic streptococci* and *enterococci* are common infecting organisms.
System(s) affected: Cardiovascular
Genetics: Unknown
Incidence/Prevalence in USA:
1.7-4.2/100,000; 0.32-1.3/1000 hospital admissions
Predominant age: All ages
Predominant sex: Male > Female (slightly)

SIGNS AND SYMPTOMS
• Fever, may be high, low or absent. May be only symptom in prosthetic valve endocarditis.
• Night sweats, chilly sensation
• Malaise, myalgia, joint pain
• Back pain, may be severe
• Anorexia, weight loss
• Stiff neck
• Delirium, headache
• Paralysis, hemiparesis, aphasia
• Numbness, muscle weakness
• Cold extremity with pain
• Bloody urine, may be gross or microscopic
• Bloody sputum, from septic pulmonary emboli
• Petechiae
• Conjunctival hemorrhage
• Hemorrhagic or necrotic pustule
• Pain of finger tip, or toe tip (subjective symptom of Osler node)
• Chest pain, shortness of breath, cough
• Pallor
• Roth spot
• Osler node
• Janeway lesion
• Heart murmur, may be absent
• Neck vein distention
• Gallops
• Rales
• Cardiac arrhythmia
• Pericardial rub
• Pleural friction rub
• Splenomegaly

CAUSES
• Staphylococcus aureus is a causative organism in all types of endocarditis, especially acute endocarditis and endocarditis seen in IV drug abusers
• Acute endocarditis
  ◊ *Staphylococcus aureus*
  ◊ Streptococcus groups A, B, C, G
  ◊ *Haemophilus influenzae*
  ◊ *Haemophilus parainfluenzae*
  ◊ *Streptococcus pneumoniae*
  ◊ *Staphylococcus lugdunensis*
  ◊ *Enterococcus species*
  ◊ *Neisseria gonorrhoeae*
• Subacute endocarditis
  ◊ *Alpha-hemolytic streptococci* (*viridans streptococci*)
  ◊ *Streptococcus bovis*
  ◊ *Enterococcus species* (*E. faecalis, E. faecium, E. durans*)
  ◊ *Haemophilus aphrophilus* and *H. paraphrophilus*
  ◊ *Actinobacillus actinomycetemcomitans*
  ◊ *Cardiobacterium hominis*
  ◊ *Eikenella corrodens*
  ◊ *Kingella kingae*
  ◊ *Staphylococcus aureus*
• Endocarditis in intravenous drug-abusers
  ◊ *Staphylococcus aureus*
  ◊ *Pseudomonas aeruginosa*
  ◊ *Burkholderia cepacia*
  ◊ Other gram-negative bacilli
  ◊ *Enterococcus species*
  ◊ Candida species
• Early prosthetic valve endocarditis
  ◊ *Staphylococcus aureus*
  ◊ *Staphylococcus epidermidis*
  ◊ Gram-negative bacilli
  ◊ Candida species
  ◊ Aspergillus species
• Late prosthetic valve endocarditis
  ◊ *Alpha-hemolytic streptococci* (*viridans streptococci*)
  ◊ Enterococcus species
  ◊ *Staphylococcus epidermidis*
  ◊ Candida species
  ◊ Aspergillus species
• Culture-negative endocarditis
  ◊ 5-10%
  ◊ Patients on antibiotics
  ◊ *Bartonella quintana* (homeless people)
  ◊ *Bartonella henselae* (cat owners)
  ◊ Brucella
  ◊ Fungi
  ◊ *Coxiella burnetii* (Q fever)
  ◊ *Chlamydia trachomatis*
  ◊ *Chlamydia psittaci*

RISK FACTORS
• Conditions predisposed to development of endocarditis
  ◊ Prosthetic cardiac valves, including bioprosthetic and homograft valves
  ◊ Previous bacterial endocarditis, even in the absence of heart disease
  ◊ Most congenital cardiac malformations
  ◊ Rheumatic and other acquired valvular dysfunction, even after valvular surgery
  ◊ Hypertrophic cardiomyopathy
  ◊ Mitral valve prolapse with valvular regurgitation
  ◊ Indwelling intravascular devices
• Dental or surgical procedures that may cause transient bacteremia leading to endocarditis in susceptible hosts
  ◊ Dental procedures known to produce gingival irritation, including professional cleaning
  ◊ Tonsillectomy and/or adenoidectomy
  ◊ Surgical operations that involve intestinal or respiratory mucosa
  ◊ Bronchoscopy with a rigid bronchoscope
  ◊ Sclerotherapy for esophageal varices
  ◊ Esophageal dilatation
  ◊ Gallbladder surgery
  ◊ Cystoscopy
  ◊ Urethral dilatation
  ◊ Urethral catheterization if urinary tract infection is present
  ◊ Urinary tract surgery if urinary tract infection is present
  ◊ Prostatic surgery
  ◊ Incision and drainage of infected tissue
  ◊ Vaginal hysterectomy
  ◊ Vaginal delivery in the presence of infection

DIAGNOSIS

DIFFERENTIAL DIAGNOSIS
• Brain abscess
• Cerebral embolus especially in a young person
• Cerebral hemorrhage with fever
• Connective tissue diseases
• Fever of unknown origin
• Glomerulonephritis
• Intra-abdominal infections
• Meningitis
• Myocardial infarction
• Osteomyelitis
• Pericarditis
• Purulent meningitis
• Rheumatic fever
• Salmonellosis
• Tuberculosis
• Septic pulmonary infarcts

LABORATORY
• Positive blood cultures taken at different times
• 2-dimensional echocardiography, not always positive for vegetations (transesophageal echocardiography has high sensitivity)
• Leukocytosis in acute endocarditis
• Anemia in subacute endocarditis
• Elevated erythrocyte sedimentation rate
• Decreased C3, C4, CH50 in subacute endocarditis
• Hematuria, microscopic or macroscopic
• Rheumatoid factor in subacute endocarditis
• Serologies for Chlamydia, Q fever (Coxiella) and Bartonella may be useful in "culture-negative" endocarditis
Drugs that may alter lab results:
Antibiotics may make blood cultures falsely negative
Disorders that may alter lab results:
• Endocarditis caused by fungi, Chlamydia trachomatis, Chlamydia psittaci, Coxiella burnetii, Bartonella species may be associated with negative blood cultures
• Prolonged incubation of blood cultures is needed in endocarditis caused by fastidious organisms, e.g., HACEK organisms (Haemophilus species, Actinobacillus actinomycetemcomitans, Cardiobacterium hominis, Eikenella corrodens, Kingella species), Brucella species

PATHOLOGICAL FINDINGS
• Vegetations on the affected endocardium are composed of platelets, fibrin and colonies of micro-organisms. Destruction of valvular endocardium, perforation of valve leaflets, rupture of chordae tendineae, abscesses of myocardium, rupture of sinus of Valsalva, pericarditis may occur.
• Emboli and/or infarction may be found in different body organs. Abscesses and micro-abscesses may be found in different organs. Kidneys may show embolic and/or immune-complex glomerulonephritis.

SPECIAL TESTS   N/A

IMAGING
• Pulmonary ventilation perfusion scan may be useful in right-sided endocarditis
• Computerized axial tomographic scan may be useful in locating abscesses

DIAGNOSTIC PROCEDURES
• Transesophageal echocardiography may be useful, especially in prosthetic or bioprosthetic valve endocarditis
• Cardiac catheterization may be indicated to ascertain the degree of valvular damage
• Aortic root injection may be useful when aortic root abscess or rupture of sinus of Valsalva is suspected

• Duke criteria for diagnosis of infective endocarditis
   ◊ 2 major criteria, or
   ◊ 1 major and 3 minor criteria, or
   ◊ 5 minor criteria
• Major criteria
   ◊ Positive blood culture
   - Typical microorganism for infective endocarditis from 2 separate blood cultures: Viridans streptococci,† Streptococcus bovis, HACEK†† group, or community acquired Staphylococcus aureus or enterococci, in the absence of a primary focus, or
   - Persistently positive blood culture. Defined as recovery of a microorganism consistent with infective endocarditis from: blood cultures drawn more than 12 hours apart, or all of 3 or a majority of 4 or more separate blood cultures, with first and last drawn at least 1 hour apart
• Evidence of endocardial involvement
   ◊ Positive echocardiogram: (a) oscillating intracardiac mass, on valve or supporting structures, or in the path of regurgitant jets, or on implanted material, in the absence of an alternative anatomic explanation, or (b) abscess, or (c) new partial dehiscence of prosthetic valve
   ◊ New valvular regurgitation (increase or change in pre-existing murmur not sufficient)
• Minor criteria
   ◊ Predisposition: predisposing heart condition or intravenous drug use
   ◊ Fever ≥ 38.0°C (100.4°F)
   ◊ Vascular phenomena: major arterial emboli, septic pulmonary infarcts, mycotic aneurysm, intracranial hemorrhage, conjunctival hemorrhage, Janeway lesions
   ◊ Immunologic phenomena: glomerulonephritis, Osler's nodes, Roth spots, rheumatoid factor
   ◊ Microbiologic evidence: positive blood culture, but not meeting major criterion as noted previously††† or serologic evidence of active infection with organism consistent with infective endocarditis
   ◊ Echocardiogram: consistent with infective endocarditis but not meeting major criterion as previous noted

---

† Including nutritional variant strains
†† HACEK = Haemophilus spp, Actinobacillus actinomycetemcomitans, Cardiobacterium hominis, Eikenella spp, Kingella kingae
††† Excluding single positive cultures for coagulase-negative staphylococci and organisms that do not cause endocarditis

Endocarditis, infective (part 2)

TREATMENT

APPROPRIATE HEALTH CARE
• Initial hospitalized care
• Intensive care may be needed in critically ill patients
• Outpatient home intravenous antibiotic therapy may be utilized in selected patients who are stable and reliable

GENERAL MEASURES
• Treatment for congestive heart failure if it occurs
• Oxygen treatment may be indicated
• Hemodialysis may be used in patients who develop renal failure

SURGICAL MEASURES
• Cardiac surgery to replace infected valve may be performed before antibiotic treatment course is completed when:
  ◊ There is evidence of congestive heart failure due to valve incompetence,
  or
  ◊ Multiple major systemic emboli have occurred,
  or
  ◊ The infection is caused by resistant organisms, e.g., fungus, Pseudomonas aeruginosa,
  or
  ◊ There is dehiscence of infected prosthetic valve,
  or
  ◊ There is relapse of prosthetic valve endocarditis,
  or
  ◊ There is persistent bacteremia despite antibiotic treatment

ACTIVITY
• Bedrest is indicated initially
• Ambulation when clinically improved

DIET No special diet

PATIENT EDUCATION
• Instruct patient regarding importance of dental hygiene
• Emphasize to patient that it is important to take antibiotic prophylaxis when undergoing certain dental/surgical procedures
• Give the patient an AHA wallet card listing antibiotic regimens for prophylaxis. Obtain the AHA wallet card, 78-1005 (CP), from local chapters of American Heart Association.

MEDICATIONS

DRUG(S) OF CHOICE
• Endocarditis due to penicillin-susceptible viridans streptococci and Streptococcus bovis: Aqueous crystalline penicillin G 10-20 million U/24 h IV in 4-6 equally divided doses, plus gentamicin [see Other Notes] for 2 weeks (6 weeks for prosthetic valve endocarditis). In patients with native valve endocarditis: Those older than 65 years of age, those with impairment of the eighth nerve or of renal function, or those with central nervous system involvement, use aqueous crystalline penicillin G only, in the same dosage alone for 4 weeks.
• Endocarditis due to enterococci: Aqueous crystalline penicillin G 20-40 million U/24 h in 6 equally divided doses, plus gentamicin (see Other Notes) for 4-6 weeks (6 weeks for prosthetic valve endocarditis). Test the enterococcal strain in vitro for high-level resistance to gentamicin and streptomycin (minimal inhibitory concentration [MIC] > 2000 µg/mL). Use streptomycin, 1 gm IM every 24 hours, instead of gentamicin if there is high-level resistance to gentamicin and not to streptomycin.
• Endocarditis of native valve due to Staphylococcus: Oxacillin or nafcillin 2 g IV every 4 h for 6 weeks. For the first 3-5 days, gentamicin (see Other Notes) may be added.
• Prosthetic valve endocarditis due to staphylococci: Vancomycin 15 mg/kg (usual dose 1 g) IV infused over 1 h every 12 h, plus rifampin 300 mg po every 8 h, both for 6 weeks, plus gentamicin (see Other Notes) for the first 2 weeks
• Endocarditis due to HACEK organisms (Haemophilus species, Actinobacillus actinomycetemcomitans, Cardiobacterium hominis, Eikenella corrodens, Kingella kingae) - ceftriaxone 2 gm IM or IV every 24 h for 4 weeks

Contraindications: For patients who are allergic to penicillin, use alternative drugs

Precautions:
• In patients with renal impairment, dosage adjustment should be made for penicillin G, gentamicin, cefazolin, vancomycin
• Rapid infusion of vancomycin (less than one hour) may cause "red-neck syndrome", an intense redness or rash over the upper half of the body. This is due to histamine release and not an allergic reaction. It will disappear when the rate of infusion is reduced.

Significant possible interactions:
• The combination of vancomycin and gentamicin may cause increased incidence of renal toxicity
• Rifampin may increase the requirement for coumarin oral anticoagulant and oral hypoglycemic agents

ALTERNATIVE DRUGS
• For patients who are allergic to penicillin
  ◊ Endocarditis due to penicillin-susceptible viridans streptococci and Streptococcus bovis: ceftriaxone 2 g IM or IV once daily for 4 weeks or ceftriaxone 2 g IV plus gentamicin 3 mg/kg once daily for 2 weeks (not to be used in patients with immediate type hypersensitivity to penicillin), or vancomycin 15 mg/kg (usual dose 1 g) IV infused over 1 h every 12 h for 4 weeks (6 weeks for prosthetic valve endocarditis)
  ◊ Endocarditis due to enterococci: Desensitization to penicillin should be considered. Vancomycin 15 mg/kg (usual dose 1 g) IV infused over 1 h every 12 h, plus gentamicin (see Other Notes) for 4-6 weeks (6 weeks for prosthetic valve endocarditis).
  ◊ Endocarditis of native valve due to Staphylococcus: Cefazolin 2 gm IV every 8 h (not to be used in patients with immediate-type hypersensitivity to penicillin), or vancomycin 15 mg/kg (usual dose 1 g) IV infused over 1 h every 12 h, for 6 weeks

FOLLOWUP

PATIENT MONITORING
• Gentamicin blood levels should be performed if used for more than 5 days, and in patients with renal dysfunction. Peak gentamicin level should be around 3 µg/mL and trough less than 1 µg/mL.
• Vancomycin blood levels should be performed in patients with renal dysfunction. Desired peak level is 30-45 mcg/mL and trough less than 10 mcg/mL.
• Twice weekly BUN and serum creatinine should be performed while the patient is receiving gentamicin
• Consider audiometry baseline and follow-up during long-term aminoglycoside therapy

PREVENTION/AVOIDANCE
• Dental caries should be treated while the patient is being treated for endocarditis
• Patients should maintain good oral hygiene
• Antibiotic prophylaxis should be given to the patient who is undergoing dental or surgical procedures that may cause transient bacteremia
• Standard antibiotic regimen for dental/oral/upper respiratory tract procedures: (May be used in patients with prosthetic valves)
◊ Amoxicillin 2 g orally one h before procedure
◊ For patients who are allergic to penicillin: clindamycin 600 mg orally 1 h before a procedure
• Alternate antibiotic regimens for dental/oral/upper respiratory tract procedures
◊ For patients unable to take oral medications: Ampicillin 2.0 g IV (or IM) 30 minutes before procedure
◊ For patients who are allergic to penicillin: Clindamycin 600 mg IV 30 minutes before a procedure
• Standard antibiotic regimen for genitourinary/gastrointestinal procedures
◊ Ampicillin 2.0 g IV (or IM) plus gentamicin 1.5 mg/kg IV (or IM) (not to exceed 120 mg) 30 minutes before procedure
◊ For patients who are allergic to penicillin: vancomycin 1.0 g IV infused over one hour plus gentamicin 1.5 mg/kg IV (or IM) (not to exceed 120 mg); complete infusion 30 minutes before procedure
• Alternate oral regimen for moderate-risk patients undergoing genitourinary/gastrointestinal procedures
◊ Amoxicillin 2.0 g orally one hour before procedure or ampicillin 2 g IV (or IM) 30 minutes before procedure
◊ For patients who are allergic to penicillin: vancomycin 1.0 g IV infused over 1 hour; complete infusion 30 minutes before procedure

POSSIBLE COMPLICATIONS
• Congestive heart failure
• Ruptured valve cusp
• Sinus of Valsalva aneurysm
• Aortic root abscesses
• Myocardial abscesses
• Myocardial infarction
• Pericarditis
• Cardiac arrhythmia
• Meningitis
• Cerebral emboli
• Brain abscesses
• Ruptured mycotic aneurysm
• Septic pulmonary infarcts
• Splenic infarcts
• Arterial emboli and infarcts
• Arthritis
• Myositis
• Glomerulonephritis
• Acute renal failure
• Mesenteric infarct

EXPECTED COURSE/PROGNOSIS
• In staphylococcal endocarditis, fever and positive blood cultures may persist up to 10 days after appropriate treatment started
• In streptococcal endocarditis, there should be clinical response within 48 hours of antibiotic treatment and blood cultures should be negative soon after antibiotic treatment is started
• Prognosis depends largely on the possible complications

MISCELLANEOUS

ASSOCIATED CONDITIONS Most patients who have tricuspid valve endocarditis are intravenous drug abusers or have indwelling IV lines

AGE-RELATED FACTORS
Pediatric: N/A
Geriatric: Prognosis is worse in elderly people
Others: N/A

PREGNANCY Gentamicin should be used with caution; avoid use if possible

SYNONYMS
• Bacterial endocarditis
• Infectious endocarditis
• Subacute bacterial endocarditis
• Subacute infective endocarditis
• Acute bacterial endocarditis
• Acute infective endocarditis

ICD-9-CM
421.0 Endocarditis/ABE
421.9 Endocarditis/SBE
996.61 Prosthetic valve endocarditis or infection

SEE ALSO
• Bartonella infections
• Brucellosis

OTHER NOTES
• Gentamicin dosing: 3 mg/kg/day in divided doses every 8-12 hours, depending on renal function and results of peak/trough measures.

ABBREVIATIONS
IE = Infective endocarditis
ABE = Acute bacterial endocarditis
SBE = Subacute bacterial endocarditis

REFERENCES
• Watanakunakorn C, Burkert T: Infective endocarditis at a large community teaching hospital, 1980-1990. A review of 210 episodes. Medicine 1993;72:90-102
• Watanakunakorn C: Staphylococcus aureus endocarditis at a community teaching hospital, 1980 to 1991. An analysis of 106 cases. Arch Inter Med 1994;154:2330-2335
• Wilson WR, Karchner AW, Dajani AS, et al: Antibiotic treatment of adults with infective endocarditis due to streptococci, enterococci, staphylococci, and HACEK microorganisms. JAMA 1995;274:1706-1713
• Durack DT, Lukes AS, Bright DK, et al: New criteria for diagnosis of infective endocarditis: Utilization of specific echogradiographic findings. Am Jour Med 1994;96:200-209
• Dajani AS, Taubert KA, Wilson W, et al: Prevention of bacterial endocarditis. Recommendations by the American Heart Association. JAMA 1997;277:1794-1801
• Sexton DJ, Tenenbaum MJ, Wilson WR, et al: Ceftriaxone once daily for four weeks compared with ceftriaxone plus gentamicin once daily for two weeks for treatment of endocarditis due to penicillin-susceptable streptococci. Clin Infect Dis 1998;27:1470-1474
Illustrations: 2 available on CD-ROM
Internet references: http://www.5mcc.com

Author(s)
Chatrchai Watanakunakorn, MD, FACP, FCCP

Endometriosis

BASICS

DESCRIPTION Heterotopic islands of uterine mucosa (endometrium) found in many locations.
• Pelvic sites - peritoneal surfaces (bladder, cul-de-sac, pelvic side walls, broad ligaments, uterosacral ligaments, fallopian tubes, and uterus), lymph nodes, ovaries, bowel
• Distant sites - vagina, cervix, abdominal wall, arm, leg, pleura, lung, diaphragm, kidneys, spleen, gallbladder, nasal mucous membranes, spinal canal, stomach, breast
System(s) affected: Reproductive
Genetics: N/A
Incidence/Prevalence in USA:
8-30/100,000; may be as high as 50% in women of reproductive age (probable range 8-30%)
Predominant age: Women of reproductive age
Predominant Sex: Female only

SIGNS AND SYMPTOMS
• Infertility (30-40% of patients with endometriosis)
• Dyspareunia
• Dysmenorrhea
• Dyschezia
• Chronic pelvic pain
• Premenstrual spotting
• Spontaneous abortion
• Luteinized unruptured follicle syndrome

CAUSES
• Retrograde menstruation (Sampson's theory)
• Lymphatic/vascular metastases (Halban's theory)
• Direct implantation
• Coelomic metaplasia (coelomic epithelium undergoes metaplasia forming functioning endometrium)

RISK FACTORS
• Hereditary/genetic predisposition
• Personality traits (achieving, egocentric, overanxious, perfectionist, intelligent, underweight - but validity of these observations lacking)
• Delayed childbearing
• Luteinized unruptured follicle syndrome (granulosa/theca cells undergo luteinization but actual follicular rupture fails to occur, thereby predisposing to limited progesterone secretion into peritoneal cavity thus allowing refluxed endometrial cells to implant and proliferate)

DIAGNOSIS

DIFFERENTIAL DIAGNOSIS Differential diagnosis of pelvic pain include all causes of acute abdomen including complications of intrauterine pregnancy and extrauterine, urinary tract infection, irritable bowel syndrome, ulcerative colitis, Crohn's disease, pelvic adhesions, acute salpingitis, ruptured ovarian cyst, and other conditions

LABORATORY No special value, but CA-125 levels may be elevated
Drugs that may alter lab results: N/A
Disorders that may alter lab results: N/A

PATHOLOGICAL FINDINGS Biopsy of endometriotic lesions usually demonstrate both endometrial glands and stroma

SPECIAL TESTS CA-125

IMAGING
• Vaginal/abdominal ultrasound (identify only endometriomas of ovaries)
• MRI for pelvic masses (endometriomas)
• Hysterosalpingography for tubal occlusion proximally or distally and periadnexal adhesions

DIAGNOSTIC PROCEDURES
Laparoscopy

TREATMENT

APPROPRIATE HEALTH CARE
Diagnose and treat "early" to prevent sequelae such as infertility and pelvic pain

GENERAL MEASURES N/A

SURGICAL MEASURES
• At the time of laparoscopy, attempt laser vaporization or fulguration of implants, drainage/resection of ovarian endometriomas, and lysis of pelvic adhesions
• Consider uterosacral ligament laser vaporization/fulguration for presacral neurectomy for severe pelvic pain or dysmenorrhea. Microsurgery or in-vitro fertilization (IVF) or gamete intrafallopian tube transfer (GIFT) may be necessary when laparoscopic surgery followed by superovulation induction with human menopausal gonadotropins (Pergonal, Humegon), pure follicle-stimulating hormone (Follistim, Fertinex, Gonal-F) and artificial intrauterine insemination have failed to achieve pregnancy.

ACTIVITY Activity may be limited depending upon severity of pelvic pain

DIET No special diet

PATIENT EDUCATION
• Prevention of disease difficult but may be maintained in quiescent state with oral contraceptive agents
• Printed materials available from The American Fertility Society, 2140 11th Ave South, Suite 200, Birmingham, AL 35205-2800, (205)933-8494

Endometriosis

MEDICATIONS

DRUG(S) OF CHOICE
• Gonadotropin-releasing hormone (GnRH) agonists such as
◊ Nafarelin (Synarel) intranasal 400 µg/day divided as 2 inhalations/day, one in each nostril. If patient continues with menses after 2 months of treatment, dose may be increased to 800 µg
◊ Leuprolide acetate (Lupron, Depo-Lupron) 0.5-1.0 mg/day or 3.75-7.5 mg/month, respectively
◊ Goserelin (Zoladex) implant 3.6 mg subcutaneously every 4 weeks for 6 months
• Maintenance:
◊ 6-9 months of therapy followed by "active" attempts at pregnancy or maintenance therapy with oral contraceptive agents
◊ Calcium supplementation 1000-1500 mg/day is recommended when using GnRH analog therapy to prevent calcium loss as women become severely hypoestrogenic
Contraindications: Any contraindication to the drug itself or of hypoestrogenemia
Precautions:
• Calcium loss secondary to hypoestrogenemia
• Hot flashes secondary to hypoestrogenemia
• Paresthesias of face and upper extremities
• Contraception measures should be used by sexually active women since ovulation may not be suppressed even if menses cease
Significant possible interactions: Refer to manufacturer's literature

ALTERNATIVE DRUGS
• Danazol (Danocrine) 400-800 mg/day for 6-9 months
• Medroxyprogesterone (Provera) 30 mg/day for 6-9 months
• Megestrol (Megace) 40 mg/day for 6-9 months
• "Continuous" oral contraceptives, e.g., ethinyl estradiol-norgestrel (Lo/Ovral, Ovral) until childbearing is desired

FOLLOWUP

PATIENT MONITORING
• Monitor serum estradiol levels until less than 10 pg/mL (37 pmol/L) when using GnRH analogs
• Monitor patient's pain response with history and physical exams every 8-12 weeks
• Monitor size of ovarian endometriomas with ultrasound every 8-12 weeks
• May need additional surgery depending upon patient's fertility and/or pelvic pain

PREVENTION/AVOIDANCE
• Pregnancy seems to have a temporary ameliorating effect upon the course of the disease
• Endometriosis is generally a recurring disorder that may persist even into early menopause

POSSIBLE COMPLICATIONS
• Infertility/subfertility
• Sterility
• Chronic pelvic pain
• Total abdominal hysterectomy and bilateral salpingo-oophorectomy

EXPECTED COURSE/PROGNOSIS
• Pregnancy should occur, but depends upon the severity of the disease
• Signs and symptoms generally regress with the onset of the menopause, but can usually be controlled during the reproductive years

MISCELLANEOUS

ASSOCIATED CONDITIONS
• Pelvic endometriosis is rarely associated with endometrioid carcinoma of the ovary
• Hematuria with bladder involvement
• Rectal bleeding with bowel involvement
• Hemoptysis with lung involvement

AGE-RELATED FACTORS
Pediatric: N/A
Geriatric: Endometriosis may persist even during early menopause and may be exacerbated with estrogen replacement therapy
Others:
• Endometriosis of the intramural portion of the fallopian tube may cause isthmic proximal tubal obstruction and infertility
• Infertility may not only be related to anatomical disruption of pelvic structures but to liberation of peritoneal macrophages which can predispose to gamete phagocytosis
• Immune disorders such as production of anti-endometrial antibodies can also be associated with reproductive dysfunction

PREGNANCY Refer to board certified reproductive endocrinologist or gynecologist with expertise in infertility

SYNONYMS Endometriosis externa

ICD-9-CM
617.1 Endometriosis of uterus
617.3 Endometriosis of pelvic peritoneum

SEE ALSO
• Appendicitis, acute
• Ectopic pregnancy

OTHER NOTES Educate female patients of reproductive age as to the signs and symptoms of pelvic endometriosis

ABBREVIATIONS N/A

REFERENCES Speroff L, Glass RH, Kase NG: Endometriosis and Infertility. In: Brown CL, ed. Clinical Gynecologic Endocrinology and Infertility. 5th Ed. Baltimore, Williams & Wilkins, 1994
Illustrations: N/A
Internet references: http://www.5mcc.com

Author(s)
Nicholas J. Spirtos, DO

Enuresis

BASICS

DESCRIPTION
Involuntary urination
- Nocturnal enuresis: involuntary urination during sleep more than once a month in girls over 5 and in boys over 6 years of age
- Day-time enuresis: involuntary urination during waking hours
- Primary enuresis: the child who has never been completely continent for an extended (3-6 month) period
- Secondary enuresis: the return of the involuntary loss of urinary control after an extended period of urinary continence.

System(s) affected: Renal/Urologic, Nervous

Genetics: In some families, there appears to be an inheritance which follows an autosomal dominant pattern with a penetrance of 90% and the marker has been identified on chromosome 13q

Incidence/Prevalence in USA:
Approximately 10% of children

Predominant age: Occurs in 40% of three year olds, 10% of six year olds, 3% of 12 year olds, and 1% of 18 year olds

Predominant sex: Male > Female

SIGNS AND SYMPTOMS
- Important historical information includes age, primary or secondary incontinence, nocturnal or diurnal or both, voiding pattern (intermittently continent or wet all the time), any delay in developmental milestones, toilet training techniques
- Inability to keep from urinating while asleep at least once per month
- Diurnal enuresis may be associated with frequency, dysuria, or activities that cause an increase in intra-abdominal pressure
- Some children may be withdrawn and shy and some may show aggressive behaviors; both may be secondary to the enuresis and not primary behaviors
- Stress factors such as intrafamilial discord, significant life events, psychosocial or emotional problems may be present

CAUSES
- Primary enuresis
  ◊ Some enuretic children lack a normal increase in nocturnal ADH secretion resulting in an amount of urine which exceeds the bladder capacity
  ◊ Nocturnal enuresis alone rarely has a psychiatric, neurologic or anatomic basis (reduced bladder capacity is usually functional, not anatomic)
  ◊ Reduced bladder capacity (normal capacity is 2 oz at birth and increases 1 oz per year of age up to 12 oz) and/or frequent uninhibited contractions (maturational lag or persistent infantile pattern)
  ◊ Recent reports suggest enuretic children have a lower morning level of vasopressin
  ◊ Some suggestion that food allergies may influence bladder capacity
  ◊ Spinal cord malformations are rarely found
  ◊ Most patients are deep sleepers or have a high arousal threshold
  ◊ Sleep apnea has been associated with primary nocturnal enuresis

- Secondary enuresis and/or diurnal enuresis
  ◊ Bacteriuria
  ◊ Inability to concentrate urine due to insufficient anti-diuretic hormone or to renal tubular defect
  ◊ Glucosuria
  ◊ Pelvic mass such as pregnancy
  ◊ Spinal cord malformations are still rare but a careful examination of the lower back for signs of spinal dysrhaphia and a thorough neurologic examination of lower extremities and genital area is mandatory

RISK FACTORS
- History of one parent having been enuretic gives 44% occurrence rate in offspring
- History of both parents having been enuretic gives a 77% occurrence rate in their offspring
- First born child

DIAGNOSIS

DIFFERENTIAL DIAGNOSIS
- Diabetes insipidus
- Diabetes mellitus
- Renal tubular defects
- Spinal cord malformations or tumors; particularly suggestive in the case of secondary enuresis and with diurnal enuresis

LABORATORY
- Urinalysis including specific gravity, glucose, protein, microscopic exam
- Urine culture
- Tests for pregnancy if history indicates

Drugs that may alter lab results: N/A
Disorders that may alter lab results: N/A

PATHOLOGICAL FINDINGS
Usually none

SPECIAL TESTS
Estimation of bladder size: Have the child hold urine until the urge is unbearable. Then measure urine in a measuring cup.

IMAGING
- Renal ultrasound, intravenous pyelogram, or voiding cystourethrogram are necessary only if urinary tract infections are associated with the enuresis
- Historical information and/or abnormal physical findings may suggest the need for spinal x-rays or imaging studies of the cord

DIAGNOSTIC PROCEDURES
Observation of the child's urinary stream for caliber and projectile force may be helpful

TREATMENT

APPROPRIATE HEALTH CARE
Outpatient

GENERAL MEASURES
- Anticipatory guidance relative to toilet training beginning by 18 months
- Counseling and behavior modification
- Treatments which are free from side effects can be started when child is toilet trained
- Secondary or diurnal enuresis needs more investigation and other treatments appropriate to the identified etiology
- Encourage daytime fluids and encourage less frequent urination to help increase bladder size
- Discourage any fluids during the 2 hours prior to bedtime
- Protect the bed from urine by covering the mattress with plastic, have the child wear extra thick underwear (not diapers), and put a towel on the bed in the area of the child's bottom
- Encourage the child to take responsibility for the problem
- Encourage the child to get up to urinate during the night but parents should not awaken the child to urinate
- When enuresis occurs, the child should rinse pajamas and underwear and the towel
- Do not punish the child for wet nights, but act sympathetically
- Heap praise on the child for dry nights. A calendar for gold stars or happy faces can be used as an incentive.
- Bladder stretching exercises may be helpful
- Self-awakening or hypnotherapy programs may be helpful
- Bed-wetting alarms have the greatest rate of success (70%) and the lowest rate of relapse (30%)

SURGICAL MEASURES
N/A

ACTIVITY
No restrictions

DIET
No fluids for 2 hours prior to bedtime

PATIENT EDUCATION
- Inform parents and the patient that most children overcome the problem between ages 6 and 10, and in only a very few cases does the problem persist beyond 16 years of age
- Since enuresis is self-limiting, potential harmful treatments should be avoided

MEDICATIONS

DRUG(S) OF CHOICE
• Tricyclic antidepressants - such as imipramine, 1-2 mg/kg q hs to maximum of 50 mg, or desipramine. Initial success is offset by a high relapse rate resulting in an overall success rate after withdrawal of only 40%.
• Desmopressin (DDAVP): An analogue of vasopressin, used in children over 6 years of age has a high success rate and a high relapse rate when discontinued. Initial dose is 20 mcg intranasally qhs, maximum of 40 mcg (or 600 mcg po qhs)
• Oxybutynin (Ditropan) has be used alone and in combination with desmopressin with fair results
Contraindications: Refer to manufacturer's profile of each drug
Precautions:
• Imipramine can cause arrhythmias or conduction blocks. Obtain an ECG prior to starting this drug.
• Imipramine is one of the leading causes of childhood drug-related deaths in the US; usually from accidental overdose
• DDAVP has been associated with hyponatremia (and seizures) due to water intoxication. Prevent this problem by limiting fluids.
Significant possible interactions: Refer to manufacturer's profile of each drug

ALTERNATIVE DRUGS N/A

FOLLOWUP

PATIENT MONITORING Frequent visits are necessary for support and encouragement

PREVENTION/AVOIDANCE No preventive measures known

POSSIBLE COMPLICATIONS Urinary tract infection

EXPECTED COURSE/PROGNOSIS
• Self-limiting problem
• By age 4-5 years, only 12% of children will not have complete urinary control. These 12% convert to complete control at a rate of 15% per year. By puberty, only 2-3% have not achieved complete control.

MISCELLANEOUS

ASSOCIATED CONDITIONS
• Psychosocial problems
• Institutionalization
• Attention-deficit hyperactivity disorder

AGE-RELATED FACTORS
Pediatric: N/A
Geriatric: N/A
Others: N/A

PREGNANCY N/A

SYNONYMS
• Bed-wetting
• Primary nocturnal enuresis

ICD-9-CM
307.6 Enuresis
788.30 Urinary incontinence, unspecified (enuresis)

SEE ALSO N/A

OTHER NOTES N/A

ABBREVIATIONS N/A

REFERENCES
• McLorie GA, Husmann DA: Incontinence and enuresis. Pediatr Clinics of N Am 1987;34:1159-1174
• Rutherford A: Enuresis: its diagnosis and management. A general practice perspective. Aust Fam Phys 1988;17(9):749-754
• Starfield: Enuresis: its pathogenesis and management. Clin Pediatr 1972;11(6):343-350
• Stenberg A, Lackgren G: Desmopressin tablets in the treatment of severe nocturnal enuresis in adolescents. Pediatr 1994;94(6):841-846
• Willie S, Aili M, Harris A, Aronson S: Plasma and urinary levels of vasopressin in enuretic and non-enuretic children. Scandinavian Jour Urology & Nephrology 1994;28(2):119-122
• Willie S: Primary nocturnal enuresis in children. Scandinavian Jour Urology & Nephrology Suppl 1994;156:1-48
• Eiberg H, Berendt I, Mohr J: Assignment of dominant inherited nocturnal enuresis to chromosome13q. Nature Genetics 1995;75:354-434
• Mark SD, Frank JD: Nocturnal enuresis. Brit Jour Urology 1995;75:427-434
• Schmitt BD. Nocturnal enuresis. Pediatr in Review 1997;18:183-190
• Ulferb J, Thuman R. A non-urologic cause of nocturia and enuresis-obstructive sleep apnea syndrome (OSAS). Scandinavian J Urology & Nephrology 1996;30:135-137
• Neveus T, Lackgren G, Stenberg A, Tuvemo T, Hetta J. Sleep and night-time behavior of enuretics and non-enuretics. Brit J Urology 1998;81(suppl 3):67-71
• Skoog SJ, Stokes A, Turner KL. Oral desmopressin: a randomized double-blind placebo controlled study of the effectiveness in children with primary nocturnal enuresis. J Urology 1997;158:1035-1040
• Caione P, Arena F, Biraghi M, et al. Nocturnal enuresis and daytime wetting; a multicentric trial with oxybutynin and desmopressin. Europ Urology 1997;31:459-463
• Robson WL, Norgaard JP, Leung Ak. Hyponatremia in patients with nocturnal enuresis treated with DDAVP. Europ J Pediatr 1996;155:959-962
• Moilanen I, Tirkkonen T, Jarvelin MR, Linna SI, et al. A follow-up of enuresis from childhood to adolescence. Brit J Urology 1998;81(suppl 3):94-97
Illustrations: N/A
Internet references: http://www.5mcc.com

Author(s)
Burris Duncan, MD

Eosinophilic pneumonias

BASICS

DESCRIPTION Eosinophilic pneumonias are characterized by eosinophilic lung infiltrates with or without peripheral blood eosinophilia. They are classified as acute or chronic and can be either idiopathic or secondary to other causes.
• Included are:
◊ Löffler's syndrome (simple pulmonary eosinophilia)
◊ Allergic bronchopulmonary aspergillosis (ABPA)
◊ Drug-induced pulmonary eosinophilia
◊ Tropical pulmonary eosinophilia
◊ Chronic or prolonged pulmonary eosinophilia
◊ The hypereosinophilic syndrome
◊ Churg-Strauss syndrome (polyarteritis nodosa) or allergic angiitis
System(s) affected: Pulmonary
Genetics: No known genetic pattern
Incidence/Prevalence in USA: Rare
Predominant age: Any age
Predominant sex: Male = Female (male in 4th decade; female in 6th decade)

SIGNS AND SYMPTOMS
• Low grade fever
• Symptoms may be mild or life-threatening
• Cough
• Chills
• Hypoxia
• Hepatomegaly
• Dyspnea
• Wheezing
• Anorexia
• Decreased localized breath sounds
• Mucoid sputum
• Tachycardia

CAUSES
• Idiopathic (though hypersensitivity suspected) in one third of cases
• Drugs/toxins (penicillin, nitrofurantoin, isoniazid, chlorpropamide, sulfonamides, antituberculosis therapy (PAS), gold, aspirin, hydralazine)
• Tropical
◊ Parasites
◊ Toxocara larvae
◊ Filariae
◊ Nematodes (Strongyloides, Ascaris, Ancylostoma
• Aspergillus fumigatus (asthmatic pulmonary eosinophilia)
• Systemic vasculitis

RISK FACTORS
• Patients with chronic disorders, e.g., asthma, cystic fibrosis
• Living or traveling in certain geographical areas, e.g., India, Ceylon, Burma, Malaysia, Indonesia, tropical Africa, South America, South Pacific

DIAGNOSIS

DIFFERENTIAL DIAGNOSIS
• Tuberculosis
• Sarcoidosis
• Hodgkin's disease
• Other lymphoproliferative disorders
• Eosinophilic granuloma of the lung
• Desquamative interstitial pneumonitis
• Hypereosinophilic syndrome
• Wegener's granulomatosis

LABORATORY
• Findings determined by etiology
• Leukocytosis
• Eosinophilia in peripheral blood
• A. fumigatus found in sputum
• Positive filarial complement fixation
• Elevated IgE levels
• Increased WBC
• Elevated ESR
• Stool examination for parasites
Drugs that may alter lab results: N/A
Disorders that may alter lab results: N/A

PATHOLOGICAL FINDINGS
• Lung
◊ Alveolar eosinophilic filling
◊ Septal eosinophilic infiltration
◊ Septal plasma cell infiltration

SPECIAL TESTS
• Bronchoscopy with broncho alveolar lavage
• Lung biopsy when diagnosis uncertain or clinical course is severe (rare)
• Pulmonary function studies

IMAGING High resolution chest CT, chest x-ray - migratory infiltrates, small pleural effusion; transient infiltrates; interstitial opacities

DIAGNOSTIC PROCEDURES History and physical exam with particular emphasis on drug intake, recent travel to tropical areas, and systemic symptoms

TREATMENT

APPROPRIATE HEALTH CARE Outpatient for milder cases. More severe cases may require inpatient care.

GENERAL MEASURES
• Evaluate for secondary causes
• Mild cases may require no specific therapy
• Coughing and deep breathing exercises to clear secretions
• Discontinuing offending drug
• Treatment of underlying parasite infestation

SURGICAL MEASURES N/A

ACTIVITY As tolerated.

DIET High calorie, high protein, soft diet

PATIENT EDUCATION Information about activity, diet, symptoms of recurrence

MEDICATIONS

DRUG(S) OF CHOICE
• Corticosteroid therapy. In chronic pulmonary eosinophilia, 20-40 mg prednisone daily. In Churg-Strauss syndrome may require large doses e.g., 40-60 mg of prednisone daily. Withdrawal should be possible after recovery. In chronic conditions, treatment should continue for 6-12 months.
• Treat asthma, if present
• Piperazine for Ascaris infestation
• Diethylcarbamazine [available only from the manufacturer] 6-8 mg/kg orally in 3 divided doses a day for 10-14 days for tropical pulmonary eosinophilia
• Appropriate vermifuges for helminthic infections
Contraindications: Refer to manufacturer's literature
Precautions: Refer to manufacturer's literature
Significant possible interactions: Refer to manufacturer's literature

ALTERNATIVE DRUGS   In Churg-Strauss syndrome, cases resistant to corticosteroid therapy, adding azathioprine or cyclophosphamide may be helpful

FOLLOWUP

PATIENT MONITORING   Physical examinations and chest x-rays until resolved

PREVENTION/AVOIDANCE   None

POSSIBLE COMPLICATIONS
• Some patients may show evidence of small airways dysfunction
• Delay in treatment of tropical pulmonary eosinophilia may result in irreversible pulmonary fibrosis

EXPECTED COURSE/PROGNOSIS
• Excellent in the milder forms
• Corticosteroid therapy is dramatically effective in more severe cases
• Relapse is rare

MISCELLANEOUS

ASSOCIATED CONDITIONS
• Asthma
• Hypersensitivity pneumonitis
• Wegener's granulomatosis

AGE-RELATED FACTORS
Pediatric: N/A
Geriatric: More morbidity, probably due to decreased lung capacity and likelihood of concomitant diseases
Others: N/A

PREGNANCY   N/A

SYNONYMS
• Löffler's syndrome
• Pulmonary infiltrates with eosinophilia syndrome (PIE)

ICD-9-CM
518.3 eosinophilic pneumonia

SEE ALSO
• Aspergillosis
• Hodgkin's disease
• Roundworms, tissue
• Sarcoidosis
• Tuberculosis
• Wegener's granulomatosis

OTHER NOTES   N/A

ABBREVIATIONS   N/A

REFERENCES
• Idiopathic eosinophilic pneumonias: Acute and chronic. In Kelly NW (ed): Textbook of Internal Medicine. New York, Lippincott-Raven, 1997
Illustrations: N/A
Internet references: http://www.5mcc.com

Author(s)
George E. Kikano, MD

Epididymitis

BASICS

DESCRIPTION Inflammation of the epididymis resulting in scrotal pain, swelling and induration of the posterior-lying epididymis, and eventual scrotal wall edema, involvement of the adjacent testicle, and hydrocele formation
System(s) affected: Reproductive
Genetics: N/A
Incidence/Prevalence in USA: Common
Predominant age: Usually younger sexually active men or older men with urinary infection, but may also rarely occur in prepubertal boys
Predominant sex: Male only

SIGNS AND SYMPTOMS
• Scrotal pain, sometimes extending to the groin region, may begin relatively acutely over several hours
• Urethral discharge or symptoms of urinary tract infection, such as frequency of urination, dysuria, cloudy urine, or hematuria
• Initially, only the posterior-lying epididymis, usually the lowermost tail section, will be very tender and indurated
• Elevation of the testes/epididymis improves the discomfort
• Entire hemiscrotum becomes swollen, the testis becomes indistinguishable from the epididymis, the scrotal wall becomes thick and indurated, and reactive hydrocele may occur
• Fever and chills occur with severe infection and abscess formation

CAUSES
• Younger than age 35
  ◊ Usually chlamydia or *Neisseria gonorrhea*
  ◊ Look for serous urethral discharge (chlamydia) or purulent discharge (gonorrhea)
• Older than age 35
  ◊ Coliform bacteria usually, but sometimes Staphylococcus aureus or epidermidis
  ◊ Often associated with distal urinary tract obstruction
  ◊ Tuberculosis, if sterile pyuria and nodularity of vas deferens
  ◊ Sterile urine reflux after transurethral prostatectomy
  ◊ Granulomatous reaction following bacillus Calmette-Guerin (BCG) intravesical therapy for superficial bladder cancer
• Prepubertal boys
  ◊ Usually coliform bacteria
  ◊ Evaluate for underlying congenital abnormalities, such as vesicoureteral reflux or ectopic ureter
• At any age
  ◊ Amiodarone, an antiarrhythmic agent, may cause a non-infectious epididymitis, that resolves with decreasing the drug dose

RISK FACTORS
• Urinary tract infection, particularly prostatitis
• Indwelling urethral catheter
• Urethral instrumentation or transurethral surgery
• Urethral stricture

DIAGNOSIS

DIFFERENTIAL DIAGNOSIS
• Epididymal congestion following vasectomy
• Testicular torsion
• Torsion of appendix testis
• Mumps orchitis
• Testicular tumor
• Testicular trauma
• Epididymal cyst
• Spermatocele
• Hydrocele
• Varicocele

LABORATORY Pyuria on urinalysis, leukocytosis, gram stain urethral discharge
Drugs that may alter lab results: N/A
Disorders that may alter lab results: N/A

PATHOLOGICAL FINDINGS
• Gross and microabscesses
• Organisms reach the epididymis through the lumen of the vas deferens
• Interstitial congestion
• Fibrous scarring

SPECIAL TESTS N/A

IMAGING Ultrasound of scrotum, radionuclide scan

DIAGNOSTIC PROCEDURES Scrotal exploration or aspiration of epididymis (rarely performed)

TREATMENT

APPROPRIATE HEALTH CARE
• Outpatient, usually
• Inpatient, if septic or if surgery is scheduled

GENERAL MEASURES
• Scrotal elevation
• Ice pack
• Spermatic cord block with local anesthesia in severe cases

SURGICAL MEASURES
• Aspiration of hydrocele to assist examination of scrotal contents and relieve discomfort
• Vasostomy to drain infected material
• Scrotal exploration, if uncertain whether this is epididymitis or testicular torsion
• Drainage of abscesses, epididymectomy, or epididymo-orchiectomy in severe cases not responding to antibiotics

ACTIVITY Bedrest for minimum of 1-2 days

DIET No restrictions, but force fluids

PATIENT EDUCATION
• Limit activity, immobilize scrotal contents
• Stress completing course of antibiotics, even when asymptomatic

MEDICATIONS

DRUG(S) OF CHOICE
• Younger than age 35 for chlamydia
◊ Doxycycline 100 mg po bid for 10 days
or
◊ Tetracycline 500 mg po qid for 10 days
• Older men with bacteriuria
◊ Trimethoprim-sulfamethoxazole (Bactrim, Septra) double strength po bid for 10-14 days
◊ Ciprofloxacin (Cipro) 500 mg po bid x 10-14 days
◊ Levofloxacin (Levaquin) 250 mg po q day x 10-14 days
◊ Norfloxacin (Noroxin) 400 mg po bid x 10-14 days
• Analgesia
◊ Nonsteroidal anti-inflammatory drug (e.g., naproxen or ibuprofen) for mild to moderate pain
◊ Acetaminophen-codeine or oxycodone-acetaminophen for moderate to severe pain
• Septic or toxic patient
◊ Third generation cephalosporin (ceftriaxone 1-2 gm IV/IM every 24 hours)
◊ Aminoglycoside (gentamicin 1 mg/kg IV/IM every 8 hours, adjusted for renal function) after a loading dose of 2 mg/kg
Contraindications: None
Precautions: Refer to manufacturer's profile of each drug
Significant possible interactions: Refer to manufacturer's profile of each drug

ALTERNATIVE DRUGS
• Other aminoglycosides or third generation cephalosporin depending on specific pathogen
• Add rifampin (rifampicin) or vancomycin as required

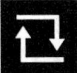
FOLLOWUP

PATIENT MONITORING   Office visits until all signs of infection have cleared

PREVENTION/AVOIDANCE
• Vasectomy or vasoligation during transurethral surgery
• Antibiotic prophylaxis for urethral manipulation
• Early treatment of prostatitis
• Avoid vigorous rectal examination with acute prostatitis

POSSIBLE COMPLICATIONS
• Recurrent epididymitis
• Infertility
• Fournier's gangrene (necrotizing synergistic infection)

EXPECTED COURSE/PROGNOSIS
• Pain improves within 1-3 days, but induration may take several weeks/months to completely resolve
• If bilateral involvement, sterility may result

MISCELLANEOUS

ASSOCIATED CONDITIONS
• Prostatitis
• Urethritis

AGE-RELATED FACTORS
Pediatric:
• Bacteremia from Haemophilus influenzae infection may produce acute epididymitis
• In adolescent males, must rule out acute testicular torsion
Geriatric: Diabetic patients with sensory neuropathy may have little pain despite severe infection/abscess
Others: N/A

PREGNANCY   N/A

SYNONYMS
Epididymo-orchitis

ICD-9-CM
604 Orchitis and epididymitis

SEE ALSO   N/A

OTHER NOTES
• Syphilis, brucellosis, blastomycosis, coccidioidomycosis, and cryptococcosis are rare causes of epididymitis
• Non-bacterial epididymitis and epididymo-orchitis are not rare. Cause is not clear, but may be secondary to retrograde extravasation.

ABBREVIATIONS   N/A

REFERENCES   Berger RE: Acute epididymitis. Semin Urol 1991;9:28
Illustrations: N/A
Internet references: http://www.5mcc.com

Author(s)
Peter T. Nieh, MD

Epiglottitis

BASICS

DESCRIPTION Acute inflammation of the supraglottic structures with inflammation of the epiglottis, vallecula, aryepiglottic folds and arytenoids
System(s) affected: Pulmonary
Genetics: N/A
Incidence/Prevalence in USA: Incidence has decreased dramatically since the introduction of the Haemophilus b vaccine
Predominant age:
• 3-7 years most common, though any age can be affected
• Generally older than typical croup patient
• Infrequent in adults
Predominant sex: Male = Female

SIGNS AND SYMPTOMS
• Sudden onset and fulminating course
• Fever
• Dysphagia, drooling
• Sore throat
• Cervical adenopathy
• Respiratory distress
• "Tripod" position (sitting propped up on hands with head forward and tongue out)
• Muffled voice/cry (vs. hoarseness in croup)
• Minimal cough (vs. barky cough in croup)
• Toxic appearance/shock (occasionally, due to associated septicemia)
• Stridor softer and less prominent than croup
• Usually no history of prodromal upper respiratory infection (vs. positive history in croup)
• Bacteremia
• Hypoxia. A late symptom usually not present unless totally obstructed.

CAUSES
• Haemophilus influenzae in children
• Haemophilus influenzae and Group A Streptococcus in adults

RISK FACTORS   N/A

DIAGNOSIS

DIFFERENTIAL DIAGNOSIS
• Viral croup (laryngotracheobronchitis)
• Sepsis
• Aspirated foreign body
• Bacterial tracheitis (pseudomembranous croup)
• Peritonsillar abscess
• Retropharyngeal abscess
• Diphtheria in an unimmunized patient

LABORATORY
• Blood culture (positive in over 90%). See under Diagnostic Procedures - should not visualize/swab epiglottis except in controlled environment, i.e., operating room. Blood tests also contraindicated until airway secured.
• Epiglottic swab culture (positive in 70%)
Drugs that may alter lab results: N/A
Disorders that may alter lab results: N/A

PATHOLOGICAL FINDINGS   N/A

SPECIAL TESTS   N/A

IMAGING
• Neck radiographs are contraindicated if epiglottitis is suspected, due to danger of sudden complete airway obstruction
• Chest radiographs are indicated for endotracheal tube placement. Pneumonia can occur as a complication.

DIAGNOSTIC PROCEDURES
• Visualization of epiglottis with tongue depressor is contraindicated due to danger of sudden complete airway obstruction
• Controlled visualization of epiglottis at intubation in operating room is diagnostic
• Lumbar puncture is indicated if there is clinical suspicion of meningitis
• In adult, indirect laryngoscopy is generally safe

TREATMENT

APPROPRIATE HEALTH CARE
Hospitalize during acute illness

GENERAL MEASURES
• Each institution should have emergency protocol involving a team of emergency room physicians, pediatricians, anesthesiologists, surgeons, pediatric intensivists, and pediatric ICU nurses (principles are similar for pediatric and adult patients)
• Call anesthesiologist to bedside
• Have equipment for intubation and needle cricothyrotomy or percutaneous tracheostomy at bedside
• Notify OR
• Notify pediatric surgery or ENT for standby in OR in case tracheostomy becomes necessary
• Keep patient quiet, calm, sitting up (in parent's arms)
• Avoid venipuncture, blood gases, oxygen masks, intravenous lines, injections, monitors, and radiographs
• Avoid sedation
• Avoid racemic epinephrine
• Avoid examining the pharynx
• Transport patient and parent together to OR in a wheelchair
• Intubate all patients, preferably in OR under controlled circumstances by experienced anesthesiologist with surgery or ENT on standby for emergency tracheostomy
• Tracheostomy not indicated unless intubation unsuccessful
• Tape airway securely in place and use a bite block if indicated
• Splint elbows and restrain arms to avoid self-extubation
• Use humidity in a tent and avoid T-piece (traction increases risk of accidental extubation)
• CPAP, mechanical ventilation, and sedation usually unnecessary
• Pay attention to supervision and pulmonary toilet/suctioning to minimize risk of endotracheal tube plugs

SURGICAL MEASURES   See General Measures

ACTIVITY   N/A

DIET   IV fluid initially, then nasogastric feedings while intubated

PATIENT EDUCATION   Reassurance about treatment and outcome

Epiglottitis

MEDICATIONS

DRUG(S) OF CHOICE Cefotaxime 100 mg/kg/day divided q 6 hours IV or ceftriaxone 75 mg/kg/day divided q 12 hours IV. Start promptly after blood and epiglottic cultures are obtained.
Contraindications: Refer to manufacturer's profile
Precautions: Refer to manufacturer's profile
Significant possible interactions: Refer to manufacturer's profile

ALTERNATIVE DRUGS
• Ampicillin 100 mg/kg/day divided q 6 hours IV and chloramphenicol 100 mg/kg/day divided q 6 hours. Follow levels. May stop chloramphenicol only if H. influenzae B sensitive to ampicillin.
• Steroids and racemic epinephrine of no benefit
• Antipyretics if necessary

FOLLOWUP

PATIENT MONITORING
• Serial exams to detect secondary foci of infection
• Follow swallowing ability and presence of an air leak around endo/nasotracheal tube
• Followup laryngoscopy prior to extubation (advocated by some)
• Observe in ICU for 24 hours following extubation

PREVENTION/AVOIDANCE
• H. influenzae vaccine is effective though not 100% protective
• Rifampin prophylaxis (20 mg/kg once daily for 4 days, maximum daily dose 600 mg) for all household and day care contacts. Family and close contacts may be asymptomatic carriers of H. influenza

POSSIBLE COMPLICATIONS
• Pneumonia, meningitis, cervical adenitis, septic arthritis, pericarditis, cellulitis (rare)
• Septic shock (in about 1%)
• Pneumothorax, pneumomediastinum (very rare)
• Death from asphyxia

EXPECTED COURSE/PROGNOSIS
• Most can be extubated after 24 to 48 hours
• Morbidity and mortality is low with appropriate intervention

MISCELLANEOUS

ASSOCIATED CONDITIONS N/A

AGE-RELATED FACTORS
Pediatric: N/A
Geriatric: N/A
Others: N/A

PREGNANCY N/A

SYNONYMS Supraglottitis

ICD-9-CM
464.30 Acute Epiglottitis without mention of obstruction
464.31 Acute Epiglottitis with mention of obstruction

SEE ALSO N/A

OTHER NOTES N/A

ABBREVIATIONS N/A

REFERENCES
• Gerber AC, Pfenningerm J: Acute epiglottitis: Management during intubation and hospitalization. Intensive Care Med 1986;12:407-411
• Vernon DD, Ashok PS: Acute epiglottitis in children: A conservative approach to diagnosis and management. Crit Care Med 1986;14:23-25
• Blanc VF, Duquenne P, Charest J: Acute epiglottitis: An overview. Acta Anaesthesial Belg 1986;37:171-178
Illustrations: N/A
Internet references: http://www.5mcc.com

Author(s)
Diane Neddenriep, MD

Epistaxis

BASICS

DESCRIPTION Hemorrhage from nostril, nasal cavity or nasopharynx
• Anterior bleed: Originates from anterior nasal cavity, usually Little's area (Kiesselbach's plexus) on septum just above posterior end of nasal vestibule. Second most common is anterior end of inferior turbinate.
• Posterior bleed: Originates from posterior nasal cavity or nasopharynx usually under the posterior half of the inferior turbinate or the roof of the nasal cavity
System(s) affected: Pulmonary
Genetics: N/A
Incidence/Prevalence in USA: Unknown
Predominant age: Less than 10 years and over 50 years
Predominant sex: Male = Female

SIGNS AND SYMPTOMS Usually nostril hemorrhage, however cases of posterior bleed may be asymptomatic or present with hemoptysis, nausea, hematemesis or melena

CAUSES
• Idiopathic (most common)
• Traumatic/blunt - nose picking (epistaxis digitorum), low humidity, foreign body
• Infection - upper respiratory, acute/chronic rhinitis, acute/chronic sinusitis
• Vascular abnormalities - sclerotic vessels of age, hereditary hemorrhagic telangiectasia, arteriovenous malformation
• Neoplasm
• Hypertension (usually in combination with another cause)
• Coagulopathy - hereditary (e.g., hemophilia), therapeutic or adverse effect of drugs, blood dyscrasias, leukemias, thrombocytopenia or platelet dysfunction
• Septal perforation
• Septal deviation (one side is overexposed to dry air)
• Bleeding originating in a sinus (fracture, tumor)
• Endometriosis (nasal ectopic endometrium)

RISK FACTORS Included in Causes

DIAGNOSIS

DIFFERENTIAL DIAGNOSIS Epistaxis is a symptom or a sign, not a disease. Less than 10% are caused by neoplasm or coagulopathy.

LABORATORY CBC, crossmatch for hypovolemic shock or anemia
Drugs that may alter lab results: N/A
Disorders that may alter lab results: N/A

PATHOLOGICAL FINDINGS N/A

SPECIAL TESTS As indicated for unusual causes

IMAGING Sinus films (rarely)

DIAGNOSTIC PROCEDURES
Angiography (rarely)

TREATMENT

APPROPRIATE HEALTH CARE
• Outpatient (usually). Inpatient for severe hemorrhage.
• Elderly patient with posterior bleeds and balloon or packing usually requires admission

GENERAL MEASURES
• Resuscitation as indicated
• Sedation, analgesic, antihypertensive or anticoagulant reversal as needed
• Patient should be gowned and sitting, if stable. Gown, gloves, and eye protection for examiner.
• Attempt to locate bleeding site using headlamp, suction, nasal speculum and help of assistant. Clear nasal cavity of blood with suction, forceps withdrawal of clot or patient blowing nose. If bleeding has stopped, rub suspicious areas with wet cotton tipped applicator to identify site. Diffuse ooze or multiple sites suggests systemic cause. In cases of posterior bleed try to identify as either roof or low posterior site since each has different arterial supply (will be important if arterial ligation is necessary).
• Locating the bleeding site may be difficult if patient presents with bilateral bleed. Usually there is only one bleeding site and the blood appears on the other because of (1) septal perforation, (2) obstruction of the affected side by pinching or packing or (3) there is a posterior bleed and blood passes behind the nasal septum. Clues are the side on which bleeding started and a careful examination using suction, headlamp and speculum.

• Anterior bleed:
◊ Place pledget soaked in vasoconstrictor and local anesthetic in cavity and pinch nostril for several minutes to stop bleeding by direct pressure
◊ Remove pledget and visualize vessel. Cauterize with silver nitrate stick directly on vessel with firm pressure for 30 seconds.
◊ Alternative chemical cautery includes bead of chromic acid or 25% trichloracetic acid. Larger vessels respond better to thermal cautery or bipolar electrocautery. Avoid indiscriminate cauterization of a large area.
◊ If unsuccessful, apply second dose of anesthetic and place anterior pack using 1/2 x 72 inch ribbon gauze impregnated with petroleum jelly (Vaseline). Use bayonet forceps and nasal speculum to insert in folding layers as far back as possible. Press each layer firmly down on the last in one continuous strip with the folded ends alternating front and back. The average nasal cavity will accommodate the full length if properly placed. Tape 2x2 gauze over nostril as drip catch and to prevent packing end from falling out of nostril.
• Posterior bleed:
◊ Traditional posterior packing as described in ENT texts has been replaced by various balloon systems. However it is very effective if balloon systems fail to control bleeding.
◊ Balloon systems include single large balloon with or without central tube for airway. They usually come in 3 or 4 sizes and right or left. Other systems provide a small (10 cc) posterior balloon and larger (30 cc) anterior balloon. After local anesthesia, the tube is placed in the affected nostril and is passed to the nasopharynx as one would a nasogastric tube. Then inflate the posterior balloon with air or water (see manufacturer's directions) and pull forward to press upon the posterior area. Then inflate the anterior balloon (see note under Complications) . A very effective method uses a 10 to 14 Fr Foley catheter. Place tip of Foley through the nostril to nasopharynx or upper oropharynx. Visualize through mouth avoiding placement in hypopharynx. Inflate balloon 7 to 15 cc. Pull forward until balloon wedges in posterior passage. Have assistant maintain gentle traction and place catheter along mid-section of lateral wall of nasal cavity. Insert anterior pack described above. Maintain catheter traction and stretch slightly. Place umbilical cord clamp on catheter across nostril against anterior pack so that elasticity of catheter compresses balloon against anterior pack. Protect facial skin from clamp by padding with 2x2 gauze. Drape rest of catheter over ear and tape in place.
• Intractable bleed:
◊ Bilateral packing is sometimes required to achieve adequate compression
◊ Bleeding from roof may be controlled by placing double balloon system with small anterior pack placed above anterior balloon. Inflation then raises pack to place pressure on roof.
◊ Intractable bleed will require surgical arterial ligation (ideally after visual identification of bleeding site to define appropriate arterial supply). Alternative is angiographic selective arterial embolization.

Epistaxis

SURGICAL MEASURES
• Arterial ligation for intractable bleeding

ACTIVITY
Bedrest with head at 45 to 90 degrees

DIET
No alcohol or hot liquids

PATIENT EDUCATION
Demonstrate proper pinching pressure techniques

MEDICATIONS

DRUG(S) OF CHOICE
• Vasoconstrictor: Cocaine 4%, phenylephrine 0.25%, xylometazoline 0.1%, epinephrine l:1000
• Anesthetic: Cocaine 4%, lidocaine laryngeal spray, lidocaine jelly 2%, lidocaine solution 4%, lidocaine viscous 2%
• Some experts suggest systemic antibiotics and decongestants to prevent sinusitis with packs or balloons
• Consider iron supplementation for patients with considerable blood loss

Contraindications: Allergy to any component

Precautions:
• Hypertension, coronary artery disease with epinephrine
• Large doses of cocaine in children

Significant possible interactions: Refer to manufacturer's profile of each drug

ALTERNATIVE DRUGS
Numerous other topical anesthetics and vasoconstrictors

FOLLOWUP

PATIENT MONITORING
Hemodynamics and blood loss as indicated. Packs or balloons removed in 24 to 36 hours.

PREVENTION/AVOIDANCE
Liberal application of petroleum jelly (Vaseline) to nostril to prevent drying and picking. Humidification at night. Cut fingernails.

POSSIBLE COMPLICATIONS
• Sinusitis
• Double balloon systems tend to migrate posteriorly, if anterior balloon breaks, patient may obstruct airway with migrated posterior balloon. Prevent by placing umbilical cord clamp across end of tubing at nostril after inflation.
• Septal hematoma or abscess from excessive trauma during packing
• Septal perforation secondary to aggressive cauterization
• External nasal deformity secondary to pressure necrosis from the anterior component of posterior packing
• Mucosal pressure necrosis secondary to high balloon inflation pressures
• Cocaine, lidocaine toxicity
• Vasovagal episode during packing

EXPECTED COURSE/PROGNOSIS
Good results with proper treatment

MISCELLANEOUS

ASSOCIATED CONDITIONS
In the elderly - hypertension, atherosclerosis and conditions that decrease platelets and clotting functions

AGE-RELATED FACTORS
Pediatric: More likely anterior bleed
Geriatric: More likely posterior bleed
Others: N/A

PREGNANCY
N/A

SYNONYMS
Nosebleed

ICD-9-CM
784.7 Epistaxis

SEE ALSO
N/A

OTHER NOTES
N/A

ABBREVIATIONS
N/A

REFERENCES
• Votey R, Dudley JP: Emergency ear, nose and throat procedures. Emerg. Clin. NA 1989;7(1)117-154
• Perretta LJ, et al: Emergency evaluation and management of epistaxis. Emerg. Clin. NA 1987;5(2)265-277
• Wong, Jafek: Pediatric Otorhinolaryngology. Appleton-Century-Crofts,1989
Illustrations: N/A
Internet references: http://www.5mcc.com

Author(s)
Charles W. Ricketson, MD, FRCPC

Epstein-Barr virus infections

BASICS

DESCRIPTION EBV is tropic for B lymphocytes which apparently are infected in the oropharynx through salivary exchange; infected B cells then circulate in the blood and are distributed to the bone marrow and lymphoreticular system. The virus can also be found in infected epithelial cells of the buccal mucosa, salivary glands, tongue and endocervix. Within the oropharynx both parotid ductal epithelium and pharyngeal squamous epithelial cells harbor EBV DNA and are sites of viral replication and release. This suggests that chronic epithelial replication brings about continuous reinfection of B lymphoid cells. Immune T cell responses to latently infected B cells account for the clinical findings.
• Epstein-Barr virus (EBV) infections acquired early in life are asymptomatic or associated with non-specific symptoms suggesting an upper respiratory infection.
System(s) affected:
Hemic/Lymphatic/Immunologic
Genetics: N/A
Incidence/Prevalence in USA:
• Incidence is about 60/100,000 persons
• College students: 5,000/100,000 persons
• Worldwide in distribution, but clinical IM is observed predominantly in countries with advanced socio-hygienic conditions
Predominant Age:
• Older children, adolescents and young adults
• By young adult life, 60-90% of persons are antibody positive
Predominant Sex: Male = Female

SIGNS AND SYMPTOMS
• May begin abruptly or insidiously
• In adults, the temperature may rise to 103°F (39.4°C) and gradually falls over a variable period of 7-10 days; in severe cases temperature elevations of 104-105° F (40.0-40.6°C) may persist for 2 weeks
• Children usually have a low-grade fever or may be afebrile
• Diffuse hyperemia and hyperplasia of oropharyngeal lymphoid tissue
• Gelatinous, grayish-white exudative tonsillitis persists for 7-10 days in 50%
• Petechiae develop at the border of the hard and soft palates in 33%
• Tender lymphadenopathy (cervical nodes are most commonly enlarged)
• Axillary, epitrochlear, popliteal, inguinal, mediastinal and mesenteric nodes may also be affected
• Lymph node enlargement subsides over days or weeks
• Splenomegaly in 50%
• Abnormal hepatic enzymes in 80% of patients for several weeks after onset. Hepatomegaly in 15-20%.
• Pneumonitis
• Chest pain (myocarditis and pericarditis)
• Hilar adenopathy may be observed in IM cases having extensive lymphoid hyperplasia
• Neurologic (rare)
  ◊ Aseptic meningitis
  ◊ Bell's palsy
  ◊ Meningoencephalitis
  ◊ Guillain-Barré syndrome

  ◊ Transverse myelitis
  ◊ Cerebellar ataxia
  ◊ Acute psychosis
• Hematologic (rare)
  ◊ Thrombocytopenia, slight to moderate, early in illness
  ◊ Hemolytic anemia with marked neutropenia during early weeks of disease
  ◊ Aplastic anemia
  ◊ Agammaglobulinemia
• Skin manifestations (3-16%)
  ◊ Erythematous macular or maculopapular rash
  ◊ Petechial and purpuric exanthems have been reported
  ◊ Rash location - trunk and upper arms; occasionally the face and forearms involved
  ◊ Urticarial lesions on the abdomen, arms, legs

CAUSES The Epstein-Barr virus, a member of the herpesvirus (DNA virus) group.

RISK FACTORS
• Age
• Socio-hygienic level
• Geographic location

DIAGNOSIS

DIFFERENTIAL DIAGNOSIS
• Streptococcal pharyngitis and tonsillitis
• Diphtheria
• Blood dyscrasias
• Rubella
• Measles
• Viral hepatitis
• Cytomegalovirus
• Toxoplasmosis

LABORATORY
• Lymphocytes and atypical lymphocytes
  ◊ Increased numbers of lymphocytes and atypical lymphocytes (may be up to 70% of leukocytes) in peripheral blood.
  ◊ In the first week after onset of illness, the white blood cell count is normal or moderately decreased. By the second week, lymphocytosis develops with more than 10% atypical lymphocytes. Such cells vary in size and shape with indented, oval or horseshoe-shaped nuclei and basophilic, vacuolated, foamy cytoplasm.
  ◊ During early illness, atypical lymphocytes are B cells transformed by EBV; later, the atypical cells are primarily T cells having immunoregulatory function
• Antibodies
  ◊ Heterophil antibodies in 80-90% of adults.
  ◊ The responsible heterophile antibody is an IgM response which appears during the first or second week of illness and persists for 3-6 months. Sheep cell agglutinins are not specific for IM and may occur in other conditions including serum sickness, infectious hepatitis, rubella, leukemia and Hodgkin's disease; low titers may also be found in normal healthy individuals.
  ◊ Differential absorption techniques distinguish these agglutinins from IM-associated heterophile antibodies. In general, the agglutinin titer is higher in IM than in other disorders; an unabsorbed heterophile

titer greater than 1:128 and 1:40 or higher after absorption is significant.
• Specific antibodies to EBV-associated antigens
  ◊ Develop regularly in IM
  ◊ Viral capsid (VCA)-specific IgM and IgG are present early in illness; VCA-IgM responses disappear after several months whereas VCA-IgG antibodies persist for life.
  ◊ Antibodies to EBV early antigen (EA) complexes, associated with viral replication, are present in 70-80% of patients during acute disease and usually disappear after 6 months
  ◊ Antibodies to the EBV nuclear antigen complex (EBNA) appear slowly and develop 1-6 months after onset of illness
Drugs that may alter lab results: N/A
Disorders that may alter lab results:
Atypical lymphocytes are not specific for Epstein-Barr infections and may be present in other clinical conditions including rubella, infectious hepatitis, allergic rhinitis, asthma and primary atypical pneumonia. In IM, increased numbers of atypical forms are present in peripheral blood whereas in other disorders the quantitative percentage is usually less.

PATHOLOGICAL FINDINGS
• Widespread focal and perivascular aggregates of mononuclear cells are found throughout the body
• Mononuclear infiltrations involve lymph nodes, tonsils, spleen, lungs, liver, heart, kidneys, adrenal glands, skin and central nervous system
• Bone marrow hyperplasia develops regularly and small granulomas may be present; these are non-specific and have no prognostic significance
• A polyclonal B cell proliferative response is characteristic of IM. Relatively few circulating lymphocytes are infected by EBV and represent less than 0.1% of circulating mononuclear cells in acute illness.

SPECIAL TESTS   N/A

IMAGING   Ultrasound, splenomegaly

DIAGNOSTIC PROCEDURES   See under Laboratory

TREATMENT

APPROPRIATE HEALTH CARE
Outpatient usually

GENERAL MEASURES
• The treatment is chiefly supportive
• During acute stage, rest in bed

SURGICAL MEASURES
• With profound thrombocytopenia, refractory to corticosteroid therapy, splenectomy may be necessary.

ACTIVITY
• Decided on an individual basis during convalescence
• Excess exertion, heavy lifting and participation in contact sports are prohibited during acute illness and also in the presence of splenomegaly. Rupture of the spleen may be fatal if not recognized and requires blood transfusion, treatment for shock, and splenectomy.

DIET
• Maintain adequate fluid intake
• Low fat, high carbohydrate diet
• Avoid alcohol for 6-8 months

PATIENT EDUCATION Reassurance and support

MEDICATIONS

DRUG(S) OF CHOICE
• Antimicrobial agents (usually a penicillin) if throat culture is positive for Group A, beta-hemolytic streptococci. Avoid ampicillin because of rash that occurs with ampicillin in mononucleosis.
• Aspirin and warm saline gargles for the pain of pharyngeal involvement and enlarged lymph nodes
• Codeine or meperidine, for unrelieved pain
• Corticosteroids
 ◊ With severe pharyngo-tonsillitis with oropharyngeal edema and airway encroachment, a short course of corticosteroids may be utilized. Prednisone or its equivalent is used. Start with an initial dosage of 10-15 mg qid for 2 days. Decrease by 5 mg daily so that steroid treatment is discontinued in approximately 10 days.
 ◊ Considered for patients with marked toxicity or major complications (e.g., hemolytic anemia, thrombocytopenic purpura, neurologic sequelae, myocarditis, pericarditis and severe generalized dermatologic lesions).
Contraindications: Steroids not recommended for mild, uncomplicated IM
Precautions: Refer to manufacturer's literature
Significant Possible Interactions: Refer to manufacturer's literature

ALTERNATIVE DRUGS N/A

FOLLOWUP

PATIENT MONITORING
• Avoid contact sports, heavy lifting, and excess exertion until the spleen and liver have returned to normal size.
• Eliminate alcohol or exposure to other hepatotoxic drugs until liver function studies return to normal
• Monitor patients closely during the first 2-3 weeks after onset of symptoms. Thereafter follow until symptoms subside.
• Rarely, laboratory results resolve more slowly and symptoms (malaise, fatigue, intermittent sore throat, lymphadenopathy) may persist for several months

PREVENTION/AVOIDANCE N/A

POSSIBLE COMPLICATIONS
• Airway obstruction
• Hematologic or neurologic complications
• Toxemia
• Splenic rupture (rare)
• Hypersensitivity rash
 ◊ Develops 7-10 days after initiation of ampicillin (or its analogues and other penicillins like methicillin) treatment; this generalized erythematous maculopapular eruption occurs mainly over the trunk and extremities, including palms and soles. Rash persists for a week; desquamation may continue for several days

EXPECTED COURSE/PROGNOSIS
• IM usually mild or moderate severity
• Acute symptoms 2-3 weeks with full recovery in 4-8 weeks

MISCELLANEOUS

ASSOCIATED CONDITIONS
• Infectious mononucleosis (IM): the symptomatic primary EBV infection seen in otherwise healthy older children, adolescents and young adults. Clinical features are variable in severity and duration; in children the disease is generally mild, whereas in adults it is more severe and protracted. The incubation period is 30-50 days.
• X-linked lymphoproliferative syndrome (Duncan's disease)
• Lymphoproliferative syndromes due to EBV infections in transplant patients
• Lymphomas (B cell lymphoblastic, T cell)
• Lymphocytic interstitial pneumonitis
• Hairy leukoplakia of the tongue and central nervous system lymphomas in AIDS patients
• Burkitt's lymphoma
• Nasopharyngeal carcinoma
• Parotid carcinoma
• Hodgkin's disease

AGE-RELATED FACTORS
Pediatric:
• Infection during infancy and childhood usually subclinical and inapparent
• Clinical IM more common in older children and young adults
Geriatric: Heterophile positive IM has been reported in an elderly patient 5 weeks following blood transfusion
Others: N/A

PREGNANCY One large prospective study of pregnant women failed to demonstrate evidence of any intrauterine EBV infection. However, rare birth defects considered to be due to congenital EBV infection have been reported; such defects include cataracts, hypotonia, cryptorchidism and micrognathia.

SYNONYMS N/A

ICD-9-CM 075 Infectious mononucleosis

SEE ALSO N/A

OTHER NOTES N/A

ABBREVIATIONS
IM = infectious mononucleosis
EBNA = Epstein-Barr nuclear antigen

REFERENCES
• Niederman JC, McCollum RW, Henle G, Henle W: Infectious mononucleosis: clinical manifestations in relation to EB virus antibodies. JAMA 1968;203:205-208
• Miller G, Niederman JC, Andrews LL: Prolonged oropharyngeal excretion of Epstein-Barr virus after infectious mononucleosis. New Engl J Med 1973;288:229-232
• Rickinson AB, Yao QY, Wallace LE: The Epstein-Barr virus as a model of virus-host interactions. Br Med Bull 1985;41:75-79
• Miller G, Katz BZ, Niederman JC: Some recent developments in the molecular epidemiology of Epstein-Barr virus infection. Yale J Biol Med 1986;60:307-316
• Straus SE, Tosato G, Meier J. Epstein-Barr virus infections: biology, pathogenesis, and management. Ann Int Med 1993;118(1):45-58
Illustrations: N/A
Internet references: http://www.5mcc.com

Author(s)
James C. Niederman, MD

Erectile dysfunction

BASICS

DESCRIPTION Dissatisfaction with size, rigidity, or duration of erection. Male sexual dysfunction encompasses an even larger group of complaints and disorders of arousal, desire, orgasm, sensation, and relationship. Transient periods of impotence occur in about half of adult males and are not considered dysfunctional.
System(s) affected: Reproductive, Nervous, Cardiovascular, Renal/Urologic
Genetics: Rarely related to chromosomal disorders
Incidence/Prevalence in USA: Erectile failure involves about 10% of men, but is underreported by patients
Predominant Age:
• Patients with psychologic, gender, and primary organic problems often present themselves for help between adolescence and the third decade
• Patients with relationship problems, but concerned mainly about physical problems, tend to seek care in the sixth decade
• Most patients with physical problems are in the seventh and eighth decade, but rarely seek help
Predominant Sex: Male only

SIGNS AND SYMPTOMS
• Reduction of erectile size and rigidity
• Inability to maintain erection
• Inability to achieve erection
• Reduced body hair
• Thyromegaly
• Gynecomastia
• Testicular atrophy or absence
• Deformed penis
• Peripheral vascular disease
• Neuropathy

CAUSES
• Endocrine
• Neurologic
• Vascular
• Medication
• Psychological
• Structural

RISK FACTORS
• Prior pelvic surgery
• Medication use
• Risk factors for disorders listed in Causes

DIAGNOSIS

DIFFERENTIAL DIAGNOSIS
• Endocrine
  ◊ Low or high thyroxine
  ◊ Low testosterone
  ◊ High prolactin
  ◊ Diabetes
  ◊ High estrogen effect
  ◊ Renal failure
  ◊ Zinc deficiency
• Neurological
  ◊ Central
  ◊ Spinal
  ◊ Peripheral
• Vascular
  ◊ Arterial insufficiency
  ◊ Cavernosal insufficiency
  ◊ Venous insufficiency
• Medication
  ◊ Many types, e.g., beta-blockers, thiazides
• Psychological
  ◊ Depression
  ◊ Schizophrenia
  ◊ Relationship disorders
  ◊ Personality disorders
  ◊ Anxiety
• Structural
  ◊ Microphallus
  ◊ Chordee and Peyronie's disease
  ◊ Cavernosal scarring
  ◊ Phimosis
  ◊ Hypospadias
  ◊ Postsurgical sequelae

LABORATORY
• CBC
• Glucose
• K+
• Na+
• Albumin
• BUN/creatinine
• TSH
• Prolactin
• Testosterone
Drugs that may alter lab results: N/A
Disorders that may alter lab results: N/A

PATHOLOGICAL FINDINGS Most men over age 55 will have some test abnormality or risk factor, but it is not necessarily the cause of the patient's impotence

SPECIAL TESTS
• 24 hour urine zinc
• Dorsal nerve somatosensory evoked potentials
• Sacral evoked response
• Penile-brachial blood pressures
• Aortogram
• Selective pudendal angiogram
• Dynamic cavernosography
• Nocturnal penile tumescence (NPT) testing
• Penile blood pressure

IMAGING Doppler, angiogram, cavernosogram

DIAGNOSTIC PROCEDURES Response to papaverine or alprostadil injection

TREATMENT

APPROPRIATE HEALTH CARE Since erectile dysfunction is multifactorial, evaluation by a generalist in an outpatient setting

GENERAL MEASURES
• Early use of penile implants is now discouraged because of success with vacuum erectile devices, sensate focus therapy, injection therapy and oral therapy
• Improve partner communication
• Reduce performance pressure
• Use sensate focus therapy
• Try vacuum erectile device or oral therapy
• Use of psychiatrists, psychologists, sex therapists, vascular surgeons, urologists, endocrinologists, neurologists, plastic surgeons, etc., often necessary for refractory cases

SURGICAL MEASURES N/A

ACTIVITY No restrictions

DIET Control diabetes if present

PATIENT EDUCATION The New Male Sexuality by Bernie Zilbergeld, Ph.D., Bantam Books, 1992; and problem-specific handouts

Erectile dysfunction

MEDICATIONS

DRUG(S) OF CHOICE
• If hypogonadism present, testosterone cypionate 200 mg IM every two weeks
• If hyperprolactinemia present, bromocriptine 2.5 mg bid up to 40 mg/day
• To induce erection
◊ Intracavernous injection of a solution containing phentolamine 0.5-1.0 mg and papaverine 30 mg per mL, starting with 0.1 mL
or
◊ Alprostadil (Caverject) 10-20 μg/mL; inject into the dorsolateral aspect of proximal third of the penis. Do not exceed 60 mg dose. Do not use more than 3 times a week or more than once in 24 hours. Patient to notify physician if erection lasts > 6 hours for immediate attention.
◊ Alprostadil (Muse) urethral suppository 125 mg, 250 mg, 500 mg, and 1000 mg pellets. Maximum of 2 uses in 24 hours.
◊ Sildenafil (Viagra) 25 mg, 50 mg, or 100 mg tablets. 50 mg 1 hr before desired erection. May be effective in 30 minutes and up to 4 hours after dosage. Older patients or those with renal or hepatic disease need half the dose of others with similar blood levels. Side effects: headache, flushing, indigestion, visual changes.

Contraindications:
• Injections should be avoided in patients with bleeding disorders, patients with sickle cell disease or trait, and in patients with penile deformities.
• Avoid use in patients with known allergies to constituents

Precautions:
• With testosterone, watch for urinary retention, acne, sodium retention and gynecomastia
• With bromocriptine, watch for self-limited nausea, vomiting
• With injection therapy, watch for priapism, fibrosis, hypotension and nausea
• With urethral suppositories, watch for penile pain and irritation, as well as testicular pain. No reports yet of priapism.
• Lowered blood pressure is common with sildenafil; NTG should not be given in tandem with this drug.

Significant possible interactions: N/A

ALTERNATIVE DRUGS
Use vacuum erection device before injections

FOLLOWUP

PATIENT MONITORING
Meet with patient and, if possible, his partner, as required by cause, therapy, and response

PREVENTION/AVOIDANCE
Since erectile dysfunction is multifactorial, referral to a sex therapist or couples therapist may help to speed recovery and prevent future problems

POSSIBLE COMPLICATIONS
Specific to therapy

EXPECTED COURSE/PROGNOSIS
• Given that the majority of patients have unspecified causes of their erectile disorders, vacuum erection device, injection or suppository therapy with alprostadil, oral sildenafil and penile implant have improved the outlook greatly
• Expect 20% failure rate of vacuum erection device, high drop-out rate from injection therapy, and a 10-30% non-use rate for penile implants
• Spontaneous cure rate is about 15%
• Studies indicate a response rate of 40-60% for urethral alprostadil compared to 85-90% for the injection
• Sildenafil works in about 70% of persons at maximum dose

MISCELLANEOUS

ASSOCIATED CONDITIONS N/A

AGE-RELATED FACTORS
Pediatric: N/A
Geriatric: Aging alone is not a cause of impotence
Others: N/A

PREGNANCY N/A

SYNONYMS Impotence

ICD-9-CM
302 Sexual disorders
302.7 Psychosocial dysfunction
302.70 Psychosocial dysfunc nos
302.71 Inhibited sexual desire
302.72 Inhibited sex excitement
302.79 Psychosocial dysfunc nec
302.8 Psychosocial dis nec
302.89 Psychosexual dis nec
302.9 Psychosexual dis nos
V41.7 Sexual function problem
607.84 Impotence, organic origin

SEE ALSO
• Priapism

OTHER NOTES N/A

ABBREVIATIONS N/A

REFERENCES
• Montague D: Disorders of Male Sexual Dysfunction. Boca Raton, Year Book Medical Publishers, 1988
• Wagner G, Green R: Impotence. New York, Plenum Press, 1981
• Segraves RT, Schoenberg HW: Diagnosis and Treatment of Erectile Disturbances. New York, Plenum Medical Book Company, 1985
• Block B: Erectile Dysfunction Decision Support System. Chapel Hill, Health Sciences Consortium, 1995
• Eardley I: New oral therapies for the treatment of erectile dysfunction. [Review] [45 refs]. Brit J of Urology 1998:81(I):122-7
• Evans C: The use of penile prostheses in the treatment of impotence. [Review] [25 refs]. Brit J of Urology 1998:81(4):591-8
• Gingell JC: New developments in self-injection therapy for erectile dysfunction. [Review] [33 refs]. Brit J of Urology 1998:81(4):599-603
• Oakley N, Moore KT: Vacuum devices in erectile dysfunction: indications and efficacy. [Review] [90 refs]. Brit J of Urology 1998:82(5):673-81
• Korenman S. New insights into erectile dysfunction: a practical approach. Am J Med 1998;105 (2):13 5-144
Illustrations: N/A
Internet references: http://www.5mcc.com

Author(s)
Bruce Block, MD

Erysipelas

BASICS

DESCRIPTION Bacterial cellulitis involving the superficial skin and lymphatics usually due to group A streptococcus. Usually acute, but a chronic recurrent form also exists.
System(s) affected: Skin/Exocrine
Genetics: N/A
Incidence/Prevalence in USA: Unknown
Predominant age: Usually infants and adults over 40. Greatest in elderly (> 75 years).
Predominant sex: Male = Female

SIGNS AND SYMPTOMS
• Prodrome of malaise, fever and chills
• Headache, vomiting are prominent
• Arthralgias
• Pruritus
• Skin discomfort
• Vesicles
• Facial redness
• Acute onset of erythema
• Begins as erythematous patch
• Sharply demarcated raised border
• Center of lesion defervesces as periphery spreads
• Desquamation and vesicle formation can occur
• Face is the most common area involved, especially nose and ears
• Chronic form may recur hours to years after initial episode
• Chronic form usually recurs at site of the previous infection
• Fever is usually the differentiating factor among similar skin manifestations

CAUSES
Group A beta-hemolytic streptococcus primarily; occasionally other strep groups or staph

RISK FACTORS
• Operative wounds
• Fissured skin (especially at the nose and ears)
• Any inflamed skin
• Traumatic wounds/abrasions
• Leg ulcers/stasis dermatitis
• Chronic diseases (diabetes, malnutrition, nephrotic syndrome)
• Immunocompromised or debilitated individual

DIAGNOSIS

DIFFERENTIAL DIAGNOSIS
• Erysipeloid (little toxicity)
• Contact dermatitis (no fever)
• Angioneurotic edema (no fever)
• Scarlet fever (usually more widespread without edema)
• Lupus (of the face, less fever, positive antinuclear antibodies)
• Polychondritis (of the ear)
• Dermatophytid
• Tuberculoid leprosy

LABORATORY
• Leukocytosis (usually > 15,000)
• Strep may be cultured from exudate or from non-involved sites
• Antistreptolysin (ASO), streptozyme, anti-DNAse may be helpful
• Blood culture (< 5% positive)
Drugs that may alter lab results: N/A
Disorders that may alter lab results: N/A

PATHOLOGICAL FINDINGS
• Edema
• Vasodilation and enlarged lymphatics
• Infiltration of polymorphonuclear leukocytes, lymphocytes and other inflammatory cells
• Endothelial cell swelling
• Gram positive cocci

SPECIAL TESTS   N/A

IMAGING   N/A

DIAGNOSTIC PROCEDURES   None

TREATMENT

APPROPRIATE HEALTH CARE
Outpatient

GENERAL MEASURES
• Symptomatic treatment of aches and fever
• Adequate fluid intake
• Local treatment with cold compresses

SURGICAL MEASURES   N/A

ACTIVITY   Bedrest with activity based on severity of illness

DIET   No special diet

PATIENT EDUCATION   Importance of completing medication regimen prescribed

TREATMENT

APPROPRIATE HEALTH CARE
Outpatient. May be inpatient for biopsy or surgery.

GENERAL MEASURES
• Evaluate to be certain there is no malignancy by means of imaging and diagnostic procedures
• Pain rarely severe or disabling
• Frequently resolves spontaneously
• Reassure patient there is no malignancy
• Cold compresses may be helpful
• Well fitting, supportive brassiere (worn night and day)

SURGICAL MEASURES
Possibly excision (under local anesthesia) of benign fibroadenoma or phyllode tumors, and fat necrosis lesions

ACTIVITY
No restrictions. Avoid activities that may cause trauma to the breasts.

DIET
Abstention from methylxanthines (coffee, tea, chocolate)

PATIENT EDUCATION
• American College of Obstetricians & Gynecologists, 409 12th St., SW, Washington, DC 20024-2188, (800)762-ACOG
• Booklet on Breast Self Examination from Primary care and Care and Cancer, 17 Prospect St., Huntington, NY 11743, (516)424-8900
• National Cancer Institute, (800)4-CANCER
• American Cancer Society; http://www3.cancer.org/cancerinfo/documents/bbreast.asp?ct=5

MEDICATIONS

DRUG(S) OF CHOICE
• For cyclical pain and swelling unresponsive to general measures - oral contraceptives have been shown to decrease the risk of fibrocystic breast disease; spironolactone (Aldactone) 10 mg bid premenstrually may be helpful or vitamin A 150,000 IU daily for 3 months; vitamin E 300-600 IU a day for 3 months
• For more severe disease - danazol (Danocrine) 100-200 mg per day or bromocriptine 2.5 mg bid for 3 months may be useful, but side effects and expense limit their usefulness
Contraindications: Refer to manufacturer's literature
Precautions: Refer to manufacturer's literature
Significant possible interactions: Refer to manufacturer's literature

ALTERNATIVE DRUGS
N/A

FOLLOWUP

PATIENT MONITORING
• Patients with fibrocystic change may have an increased risk of malignancy
• If there is no atypia on biopsy the risk is only minimally increased
• Patients need to be assessed with clinical examination, radiological studies, and, sometimes, biopsy to be certain a given lump is not malignant
• Followup times are variable depending on the clinical situation. A young patient in whom physiological nodularity is suspected should be observed through one menstrual cycle.
• Mammograms should be obtained at age 35, at least every 1-2 years after age 40, and yearly after age 50
• Ultrasound is useful to differentiate cysts from solid lesions, but is not used for screening
• Aspiration cytology is useful for diagnosis of cysts and solid lesions. The false positive rate ranges from 0-5.8%, and the false negative rate from 1.7-22%.
• When physical examination, mammography, and needle aspiration are used in combination, detection rates for breast cancer range from 93-100%

PREVENTION/AVOIDANCE
Avoiding caffeine may reduce breast pain

POSSIBLE COMPLICATIONS
• Fibrocystic change can make physical examination and mammograms difficult to interpret
• Atypical hyperplasia may lead to cancer

EXPECTED COURSE/PROGNOSIS
Benign, chronic, recurring, intermittent

MISCELLANEOUS

ASSOCIATED CONDITIONS
Breast carcinoma

AGE-RELATED FACTORS
Pediatric: Biopsy in children should be avoided since a developing breast bud may be inadvertently removed
Geriatric: Not as common in this age group
Others: Prophylactic mastectomy for pain is rarely indicated since many patients have underlying psychiatric problems

PREGNANCY
N/A

SYNONYMS
• Chronic cystic mastitis
• Adenosis
• Benign breast disease
• Mammary dysplasia
• Fibrocystic disease

ICD-9-CM
610.1 diffuse cystic mastopathy

SEE ALSO
N/A

OTHER NOTES
N/A

ABBREVIATIONS
N/A

REFERENCES
• Rohan TE, Miller AB: A cohort study of oral contraceptive use and risk of benign breast disease. Int J Cancer 1999;82(2):191-6
• Rosenfeld JA: Women's Health in Primary Care. Baltimore, Williams & Wilkins, 1997
Illustrations: N/A
Internet references: http://www.5mcc.com

Author(s)
Cathryn Heath, MD
John C. Smulian, MD, MPH

Fibromyalgia

 BASICS

DESCRIPTION Extremely common pain phenomenon occurring in a defined pattern, reproduced by pressure on "trigger points"
System(s) affected: Musculoskeletal
Genetics: N/A
Incidence/Prevalence in USA: 3 in 100
Predominant age: 18-70
Predominant sex: Female > Male

SIGNS AND SYMPTOMS
• Pressure manually applied to specific sites, referred to as "trigger points" reproduce the patient's symptoms:
  ◊ Temporalis - above the ear
  ◊ Anterior to tragus of ear
  ◊ Scalenus capitis
  ◊ Sternocleidomastoid
  ◊ Low anterior neck
  ◊ Pectoralis minor
  ◊ Manubriosternal
  ◊ Anterior and posterior axillary folds
  ◊ Trapezius ridge
  ◊ Upper rhomboids
  ◊ Lower rhomboids
  ◊ Iliac crest
  ◊ Mid-buttocks
  ◊ Mid-rectus femoris
  ◊ Mid-vastus lateralis
  ◊ Quadriceps insertion - at the patella
  ◊ Humeral epicondyles (many investigators would diagnose fibromyalgia, while some prefer epicondylitis) and negative tenderness at "neutral sites" (e.g., scapula, glabella)
• Other signs and symptoms
  ◊ Typically insidious in onset
  ◊ Pain is increased in the morning, with weather changes, anxiety, stress
  ◊ Pain improved by mild physical activity or vacations (stress-relieving situations)
Non-restorative sleep, with early morning awakening in an unrefreshed state.
  ◊ Abnormal non-rapid eye movement (non-REM) stage IV sleep
  ◊ Generalized fatigue or tiredness
  ◊ Anxiety
  ◊ Chronic headache
  ◊ Irritable bowel syndrome
  ◊ Subjective, non-confirmable complaints of swelling or numbness, not associated with objective neurologic findings
  ◊ Depression
  ◊ Reduced physical endurance
  ◊ Decreased social interaction

CAUSES
• Loss of non-REM stage IV sleep
• Stress
• Trauma

RISK FACTORS
• Sleep disturbance
• Trauma
• Depression
• Weather changes

 DIAGNOSIS

DIFFERENTIAL DIAGNOSIS
• Hypothyroidism
• Psychogenic rheumatism
• Muscle strain/sprain
• Muscle disease
• Polymyalgia rheumatica
• Temporal arteritis

LABORATORY
• Normal Westergren erythrocyte sedimentation rate
• Normal creatine phosphokinase and aldolase
• Normal TSH, T3 resin uptake and T4
• Normal complete blood count, renal and liver function
Drugs that may alter lab results: Steroids
Disorders that may alter lab results: N/A

PATHOLOGICAL FINDINGS None

SPECIAL TESTS Thermography
(controversial)

IMAGING N/A

DIAGNOSTIC PROCEDURES The
clinical history and physical examination

 TREATMENT

APPROPRIATE HEALTH CARE
Outpatient

GENERAL MEASURES Electroprobe,
electrical stimulation (but not TENS), ultrasound, hot packs, conditioning, increasing social interactions and general conditioning exercises

SURGICAL MEASURES N/A

ACTIVITY Fully active. However, the pain
of fibrositis may be so distracting as to reduce attentiveness, predisposing to error and accident.

DIET No restrictions

PATIENT EDUCATION
• Printed material: Rothschild, B.: Diagnosing and treating fibrositis and fibromyalgia. Geriatric Consultant, 9(5/6):26-28, 1990
• Your personal guide to living with fibromyalgia. Arthritis Foundation, Atlanta, 1997

MEDICATIONS

DRUG(S) OF CHOICE
• Sleep restorative without interfering with stage IV sleep:
Reinforce discontinuation if paradoxical effect, memory loss, thought process changes, or behavior changes.
◊ Zolpidem (Ambien) 5 mg po hs prn, increased to 10 mg
◊ Temazepam (Restoril) 15 mg po hs prn, increased to 30 mg
◊ Flurazepam (Dalmane) 15 mg po hs prn, increased to 30 mg (note: Significant "hangover" potential secondary to long half-life)
◊ Triazolam (Halcion) 0.125 mg po hs prn increased gradually to 0.5 mg (use is controversial)
◊ Lidocaine 1% injectable 1/2 cc to trigger points
◊ Amitriptyline (Elavil) 10 mg 2 po hs prn, increased gradually to 50 mg (of lesser efficacy)
◊ Cyclobenzaprine (Flexeril) 10 mg tid prn (of lesser efficacy)
• Nonsteroidal anti-inflammatory drugs (NSAIDs) may provide non-narcotic symptomatic pain relief (of lesser efficacy)
Contraindications: Drug allergy, suicide potential
Precautions:
• NSAID's - refer to manufacturer's literature
• Others - observe for grogginess or aberrant behavior, discontinue if it occurs. Psychological and/or physical dependence may occur. However, if the patient is nonfunctional without them, long-term use is reasonable.
Significant possible interactions:
• NSAID's - refer to manufacturer's literature
• Others - digoxin, phenytoin, MAO inhibitors

ALTERNATIVE DRUGS   Trazodone
(Desyrel) 50 mg po hs prn

FOLLOWUP

PATIENT MONITORING
• For efficacy at 2-4 weeks
• For medication side effects every 3-6 months

PREVENTION/AVOIDANCE
• Adequate sleep
• General conditioning exercises

POSSIBLE COMPLICATIONS
• Chronicity
• Fibromyalgia is allegedly a greater source of work loss and dysfunction than rheumatoid arthritis

EXPECTED COURSE/PROGNOSIS
• With resolution of sleep disturbance, may resolve totally
• Aggressive physical therapy is critical in those who do not respond
• Approximately 5% do not respond to any form of therapeutic intervention. Hypnosis may be attempted in that group.

MISCELLANEOUS

ASSOCIATED CONDITIONS   So common almost any disease can be associated with it

AGE-RELATED FACTORS
Pediatric: Uncommon
Geriatric: Common; polypharmacy may be part of the problem
Others: N/A

PREGNANCY   Limits therapeutic approach to physical therapy modalities

SYNONYMS
• Fibrositis
• Myofascial pain syndrome

ICD-9-CM
729.1 Fibromyositis

SEE ALSO
• Irritable bowel syndrome
• Chronic fatigue syndrome

OTHER NOTES   Perhaps the most common cause of neck or back pain in this patient population and most common rheumatologic problem in general

ABBREVIATIONS   N/A

REFERENCES
• Rothschild BM: Fibromyalgia: An explanation for the aches and pains of the 90's. Comprehensive Therapy 1991;17(6):9-14
• Rothschild BM: Diagnosing and treating fibrositis and fibromyalgia. Geriatric Consultant 1990;9(5/6):26-28
• Vu J, Rothschild BM: Retrospective assessment of fibromyalgia therapeusis. Comprehensive Therapy, 1994;20:545-549
• Yunus M, Masi AT, Calabro JJ, Miller KA, Feigenbaum SL: Primary fibromyalgia (fibrositis): Clinical study of 50 patients with matched normal controls. Semin Arthritis Rheum 1981;11:151-171
• Wolfe F, Smythe HA, Yunus MB, Bennett RM, et al: The American College of Rheumatology criteria for the classification of fibromyalgia. Arthritis Rheum 1990;33:160-172
• Siceloff E, et al: Variability of fibromyalgia-like symptoms. Comp Ther, Cin Press
Illustrations: N/A
Internet references: http://www.5mcc.com

Author(s)
Bruce M. Rothschild, MD

Folliculitis

BASICS

DESCRIPTION Inflammation of hair follicles, often in clusters, often due to local infection or chemical irritation or associated with underlying disease. May be superficial or deep.
System(s) affected: Skin/Exocrine
Genetics: No known genetic pattern
Incidence/Prevalence in USA: Common (no statistics available)
Predominant age: All ages
Predominant sex: Male > Female

SIGNS AND SYMPTOMS
• Characteristic lesions are small yellow or gray pustules surrounded by erythema and pierced by a hair. Common folliculitis can appear on any part of the body. Sycosis barbae is folliculitis of the beard area of the shaved face, particularly common in black men. Hot tub folliculitis occurs in the bathing suit area. Eosinophilic pustular folliculitis (EPF) occurs mainly on the trunk of HIV positive patients, but can occur in atopic children sensitive to skin fungi, and as Ofuji's disease in non-HIV patients, especially in Japan.
• Lesions are commonly grouped
• Eosinophilic folliculitis is often very pruritic, but other folliculitides are only mildly pruritic, or not at all
• Patients who are not HIV positive are usually afebrile and without systemic symptoms

CAUSES
• Staphylococcus aureus
• Pseudomonas aeruginosa in hot-tub folliculitis
• Gram negative bacteria in patients on long term antibiotics
• Candida albicans in patients on immunosuppressants or long term antibiotic therapy
• Dermatophyte fungi - uncommon
• Occasionally herpes simplex 1, herpes zoster, molluscum contagiosum virus
• Plastic occlusive dressings

RISK FACTORS
• Abrasion
• Injury
• Nearby surgical wounds or draining abscesses
• Tight clothing (jeans folliculitis)
• Poor hygiene
• Exposure to hydrocarbons
• Use of hot tubs or saunas
• Immunodeficiency
• Diabetes mellitus
• Lithium therapy
• Wax epilation

DIAGNOSIS

DIFFERENTIAL DIAGNOSIS
• Keratosis pilaris (follicular papules on the extensor surfaces of extremities in atopic individuals)
• Contact dermatitis
• Tinea
• Acne
• Pustular miliaria (10)
• Flat warts
• Molluscum contagiosum
• Scabies
• Perioral dermatitis
• Diaper dermatitis

LABORATORY
• Gram stain - look for bacteria or eosinophils
• KOH preparation - looking for budding yeast or hyphae
• Culture of pus
• Fasting blood sugar
• HIV status
Drugs that may alter lab results: N/A
Disorders that may alter lab results: N/A

PATHOLOGICAL FINDINGS
• For common or hot tub folliculitis - suppurative inflammation of hair follicles
• For eosinophilic pustular folliculitis there is a perifollicular and perivascular infiltrate in which eosinophils exceed the numbers of neutrophils

SPECIAL TESTS N/A

IMAGING N/A

DIAGNOSTIC PROCEDURES Biopsy if diagnosis is in doubt or in cases resistant to treatment

TREATMENT

APPROPRIATE HEALTH CARE
Outpatient

GENERAL MEASURES
• Cleanse areas bid with antibacterial soap (e.g. Dial)
• Shampoo daily with Selsun Blue for scalp lesions
• Apply moist heat to pustules to encourage them to drain
• For shaved areas:
  ◊ Try electric razor instead of blade, and sterilize electric razor cutting parts with alcohol for 30 minutes daily.
  ◊ Or change blade of sharp razor daily
  ◊ Allow hair to grow.
• Avoid wax epilatories if they cause a rash.
• Avoid skin oils or greasy ointments
• Avoid topical oils

SURGICAL MEASURES N/A

ACTIVITY Full

DIET No special diet

PATIENT EDUCATION As listed above under General measures

MEDICATIONS

DRUG(S) OF CHOICE
- Staphylococcal folliculitis,
  ◊ Dicloxacillin 250 mg qid
  ◊ Erythromycin 250 mg qid
  ◊ Cephalosporin
- Pseudomonas folliculitis
  ◊ Usually self limited, no antibiotic indicated
  ◊ If severe or persistent adults can use ciprofloxacin 500 mg or ofloxacin 400 mg bid for 10 days
- Eosinophilic pustular folliculitis
  ◊ No local causative organism, no specific antibiotic
  ◊ Non-HIV related EPF often responds to oral indomethacin
  ◊ For EPF in HIV positive patients isotretinoin therapy appears to be promising

Contraindications:
- History of hypersensitivity to the drug
- Quinolone antibiotics are contraindicated in pregnancy and for children
- Indomethacin is contraindicated in patients who have had a peptic ulcer

Precautions: Refer to manufacturers literature

Significant possible interactions:
- Ciprofloxacin and ofloxacin - antacids, sucralfate, oral anticoagulants, theophylline, caffeine, probenecid
- Erythromycin - theophylline, oral anticoagulants, carbamazepine, corticosteroids, digoxin, ergot alkaloids, cyclosporine, phenytoin, terfenadine, astemizole

ALTERNATIVE DRUGS
- Mupirocin (Bactroban) topical therapy to affected area tid
- First generation cephalosporins for Staph. aureus
- For pseudomonas, third generation cephalosporins, aminoglycosides, or ticarcillin

FOLLOWUP

PATIENT MONITORING
- One return visit in two weeks if symptoms abate
- Resistant cases should be followed every two weeks until cleared

PREVENTION/AVOIDANCE
- Good personal hygiene; avoid sharing a towel or washcloth
- Discard any dressings carefully
- Avoid causative factors
- Find and treat family members or friends who may be a source of reinfection

POSSIBLE COMPLICATIONS
May progress to become furuncles or abscesses

EXPECTED COURSE/PROGNOSIS
- Usually resolves with treatment
- May recur in staph carriers. Mucopirocin may be required on nares of patient to treat carrier state. Family carriers may also require treatment.
- äResistant or severe cases may warrant testing for diabetes mellitus or immunodeficiency

MISCELLANEOUS

ASSOCIATED CONDITIONS
- Diabetes mellitus
- Immunodeficiency

AGE-RELATED FACTORS
Pediatric: N/A
Geriatric: N/A
Others: N/A

PREGNANCY
Pruritic folliculitis of pregnancy is a rare disorder that resolves spontaneously after delivery

SYNONYMS Sycosis

ICD-9-CM 704.8 other specified diseases of hair and hair follicles

SEE ALSO N/A

OTHER NOTES N/A

ABBREVIATIONS
EPF = eosinophilic pustular folliculitis

REFERENCES
- Fitzpatrick TB, et al: Color Atlas & Synopsis of Clinical Dermatology. 2nd Ed. New York, McGraw Hill, 1992
- Majors MJ, et al: HIV-related eosinophilic folliculitis: a panel discussion Seminars in Cutaneous Medicine and Surgery 1997;16(3):219-223
- Saunders Electronic Atlas of Dermatology. Philadelphia, WB Saunders Co, 1996
- Schmidt A: Malassezia furfur; a fungus belonging to the physiological skin flora and its relevance in skin disorders. Cutis 1997;59(1):21-24
- Abdel-Razek M, et al: Pityrosporon, (Malassezia) folliculitis in Saudi Arabia - diagnosis and therapeutic trials. Clinical & Experimental Dermatology 1995;20(5):406-409
- Wakelin SH, et al: Lithium-induced follicular hyperkeratosis. Clinical & Experimental Dermatology 1996;21(4):296-298
- Mimouni-Bloch A, et al: Severe folliculitis with keloid scars induced by wax epiliation in adolescents. Cutis 1997;59(1):41-42
- Fushimi M, et al: Eosinophilic pustular folliculitis effectively treated with recombinant interferon-gamma: suppression of mRNA expression of interleukin 5 in peripheral blood mononuclear cells British Journal of Dermatology 1996;134(4):766-772
- Calleen J, et al: Color Atlas of Dermatology. Philadelphia, WB Saunders Co, 1993
- Teraki Y: Ofuji's disease and cytokines: Remission of eosinophilic pustular folliculitis associated with increase serum concentrations of interferon gamma. Dermatology. 192(1): 16-18
- Otley CC, et al: Isotretinoin treatment of human immunodeficiency virus-associated eosinophilic folliculitis. Results of an open pilot trial. Archives of Dermatology 1995;131(9):1047-1050

Illustrations: N/A
Internet references: http://www.5mcc.com

Author(s)
Lewis C. Rose, MD

Food allergy

BASICS

DESCRIPTION Food allergy is a hypersensitivity reaction which is caused by certain foods. Adverse reactions after food ingestion may be caused by immunologic mechanisms, such as the classic IgE allergic response, or by non-immunologic mediated mechanisms.

System(s) affected:
Hemic/Lymphatic/Immunologic, Gastrointestinal, Skin/Exocrine, Pulmonary, Nervous

Genetics: In family members with a history of food hypersensitivity, the probability of food allergy in subsequent siblings may be as high as 50%

Incidence/Prevalence in USA:
• The incidence of IgE mediated food allergy has been estimated to range from 1-7% of the population
• In children up to 4 years of age the incidence is between 8-16%
• Only about 3-4% of children over 4 years of age have persisting food allergy. Therefore, it is frequently a transient phenomena.

Predominant age: All ages, but more common in infants and children

Predominant sex: Male > Female (2:1)

SIGNS AND SYMPTOMS
• Gastrointestinal (system usually affected)
  ◊ More common: Nausea, vomiting, diarrhea, abdominal pain, occult bleeding, flatulence, bloating
  ◊ Less common: Malabsorption, protein losing enteropathy, eosinophil-gastroenteritis, and colitis
• Dermatologic
  ◊ More common: Urticaria/angioedema, atopic dermatitis, pallor or flushing
  ◊ Less common: Contact rashes
• Respiratory
  ◊ More common: Allergic rhinitis, asthma and bronchospasm, cough, serous otitis media
  ◊ Less common: Pulmonary infiltrates (Heiner's syndrome), pulmonary hemosiderosis
• Neurologic
  ◊ Less common: Hyperkinesis, tension-fatigue syndrome, migraine headaches, syncope
• Other symptoms:
  ◊ Systemic anaphylaxis, vasculitis
  ◊ Suspected manifestations include enuresis, proteinuria and arthropathy
  ◊ Growth retardation

CAUSES
• Any food or ingested substance can cause allergic reactions. Most commonly implicated foods include cow's milk, egg whites, wheat, soy, peanut, fish, tree nuts (walnut and pecan), shellfish, melons, sesame seeds, sunflower seeds, chocolate.
• Several food dyes and additives can elicit allergic-like reactions

RISK FACTORS
• Persons with allergic or atopic predisposition are at increased risk of hypersensitivity reaction to foods
• Family members with a history of food hypersensitivity

DIAGNOSIS

DIFFERENTIAL DIAGNOSIS
• A careful history is necessary to document a temporal relationship with the manifestations of suspected food hypersensitivity
• The gastrointestinal, dermatologic, respiratory, neurologic or other systemic manifestations may mimic a variety of clinical entities

LABORATORY
• Eosinophilia in either blood or tissue suggests atopy
• Epicutaneous (prick or puncture) allergy skin tests are useful in documenting IgE mediated immunologic hypersensitivity. In most clinical situations, the allergy skin tests are good for screening. An oral challenge should be completed to accurately determine the clinical hypersensitivity. The overall agreement between allergy skin testing and oral food challenge is approximately 60% (i.e., a positive skin test showing a positive challenge reaction to a particular food).
• Radioallergosorbent (RAST) test can also detect specific IgE antibodies to offending foods. In certain laboratories, the RAST test was almost as accurate as a skin test in predicting positive oral challenges.
• Leukocyte histamine release and assays for circulating immune complexes are predominantly research procedures and are of limited use in clinical practices. Assays for IgG and IgG 4 subclass antibodies are commercially available. There are no convincing data that these tests are reliable for the diagnosis of food allergy.
• The provocative injection and sublingual provocative tests are both highly controversial and have been proven to be useless for the diagnosis of food allergy
• The leukocytotoxic assay is an unproven diagnostic procedure and is not useful for the diagnosis of allergy

Drugs that may alter lab results: N/A
Disorders that may alter lab results: N/A

PATHOLOGICAL FINDINGS Acute and chronic rectal inflammation

SPECIAL TESTS Stool exam, mucus, eosinophilia

IMAGING Upper GI series for gastric antral inflammation, in rare cases

DIAGNOSTIC PROCEDURES
• Elimination and challenge test
  ◊ The best procedure for confirming food allergy
  ◊ First, the suspected food is eliminated from the diet for 1-2 weeks
  ◊ The patient's symptoms are monitored. If the patient's symptoms disappear or substantially improve, an oral challenge with the suspected food should be performed under medical supervision.
  ◊ Optimally, this challenge should be performed in a double-blind, placebo controlled manner
  ◊ Most allergic reactions will occur within 30 minutes to 2 hours after the challenge, although late reactions have also been described, which may occur from 12-24 hours

TREATMENT

APPROPRIATE HEALTH CARE
Outpatient

GENERAL MEASURES
• Avoidance of the offending food is the most effective mode of treatment for patients with food allergies
• Those patients with exquisite and severe allergy hypersensitivity to a food should be more cautious in their avoidance of that food. They should carry epinephrine for self-administration in the event that the offending food is ingested unknowingly, and a subsequent immediate reaction develops.
• Immunotherapy or hyposensitization with food extracts by various routes, including subcutaneous immunotherapy or sublingual neutralization are not recommended since the success with these methods have not been proven in controlled scientific studies

SURGICAL MEASURES N/A

ACTIVITY No restrictions

DIET As determined by tests

PATIENT EDUCATION
• Patients should be counselled by a dietician to be sure that they maintain a nutritionally sound diet, in spite of avoiding those foods to which patient is sensitive
• Patient support - Food Allergy Network, 4744 Holly Ave., Fairfax, VA 22030-5647, 703-691-3179

MEDICATIONS

DRUG(S) OF CHOICE
• Symptomatic treatment, e.g., antihistamine
• The use of cromolyn has been suggested, but is not practical for use in most patients with food allergy
• Recent studies have suggested the use of ketotifen, which is a mast cell stabilizer. This drug is not available in the United States.
Contraindications: N/A
Precautions: N/A
Significant possible interactions: N/A

ALTERNATIVE DRUGS N/A

FOLLOWUP

PATIENT MONITORING As needed

PREVENTION/AVOIDANCE Avoidance of offending food

POSSIBLE COMPLICATIONS
• Anaphylaxis
• Angioedema
• Bronchial asthma
• Enterocolitis
• Eczematoid lesions

EXPECTED COURSE/PROGNOSIS
• Most infants will outgrow their food hypersensitivity by 2-4 years. It may be possible to reintroduce the offending food cautiously into the diet (particularly helpful when the food is one that is difficult to avoid).
• Adults with food hypersensitivity (particularly to milk, fish, shellfish or nuts) tend to maintain their allergy for many years

MISCELLANEOUS

ASSOCIATED CONDITIONS N/A

AGE-RELATED FACTORS
Pediatric: N/A
Geriatric: N/A
Others: N/A

PREGNANCY N/A

SYNONYMS
• Allergic bowel disease
• Dietary protein sensitivity syndrome

ICD-9-CM
693.1 Dermatitis due to food taken internally
692.5 Contact dermatitis and other eczema due to food in contact with the skin
995.60 Anaphylactic shock or reaction due to food

SEE ALSO
• Celiac disease
• Irritable bowel syndrome
• Pyloric stenosis
• Epiglottitis

OTHER NOTES N/A

ABBREVIATIONS N/A

REFERENCES
• Sampson HA: Food Allergy. JAMA, 1997;278:1888-94
• Chandra RK, ed: Food Allergy. Clin Rev Allergy/Immu 1995;13:291-376
• Metcalf DD, et al, eds: Food Allergy, Adverse Reactions to Foods and Food Additives. New York, Blackwell Scientific, 1991
Illustrations: N/A
Internet references: http://www.5mcc.com

Author(s)
Stanley Fineman, MD

Food poisoning, bacterial

BASICS

DESCRIPTION A variety of related illnesses resulting from ingestion of food contaminated with bacteria capable of causing disease. The illness may be produced by bacterial infection itself (salmonellosis, shigellosis) or by toxins produced by the bacteria (Staphylococcus aureus, Clostridium perfringens, Bacillus cereus).
System(s) affected: Gastrointestinal
Genetics: N/A
Incidence/Prevalence in USA: Poor reporting overall. Estimated 6.3 million cases/year. 1 in 10 Americans with foodborne diarrhea/year. Approximate incidence is 2,500/100,000. Most commonly reported cause in the US is *C. jejuni*.
Predominant age: All ages
Predominant sex: Male = Female

SIGNS AND SYMPTOMS
Suspect when multiple persons become ill after eating the same meal. Timing and type of clinical presentation can aid in establishing etiology.
• Nausea, vomiting 1-8 hours after meal (S. aureus, B. cereus)
• Cramps, diarrhea 8-16 hours after meal (C. perfringens, B. cereus)
• Fever, cramps, diarrhea 18-72 hours after meal (*Campylobacter jejuni, Yersinia enterocolitica, E. coli, Vibrio parahaemolyticus*, Shigella and Salmonella species)
• Bloody diarrhea without fever 3-5 days after meal (verotoxigenic E. coli, occasionally *C. jejuni*)
• Pseudoappendicitis (Y. enterocolitica)
• Sepsis, meningitis (Listeria monocytogenes, Shigella and Salmonella species)
• Occasional metastatic foci of infection (arthritis, *L. monocytogenes, Salmonella*, etc.)

CAUSES
• *S. aureus* (preformed enterotoxin)
• *B. cereus* (preformed enterotoxin)
• *C. perfringens* (enterotoxin elaborated in gut)
• *C. jejuni* (tissue invasion)
• *Y. enterocolitica* (tissue invasion)
• *E. coli* (enterotoxigenic, verotoxigenic [hemorrhagic], and tissue invasive forms), including *E. coli* O157:H7
• *V. parahaemolyticus* (toxin elaboration, possibly invasion)
• *Shigella species* (tissue invasion)
• *Salmonella species* (tissue invasion), including Salmonella serotype Typhimurium Definitive Type 104.
• *L. monocytogenes* (tissue invasion)

RISK FACTORS
Ingestion of:
• High protein foods: egg salad, cream-filled pastries, poultry, ham - S. aureus
• Cereals, fried rice, dried foods and herbs, meats, vegetables - B. cereus
• Meats, gravies, dried foods, vegetables - C. perfringens
• Under-cooked poultry, meat, raw dairy products - C. jejuni
• Under-cooked pork, other meat and dairy products - Y. enterocolitica
• Raw vegetables and other foods, contaminated water - E. coli
• Raw and cooked seafood - V. parahaemolyticus
• Raw vegetables, egg salads, contaminated water - Shigella
• Under-cooked eggs, poultry, dairy products, meat - Salmonella
• Under-cooked meat, dairy products, and many other foods - L. monocytogenes

DIAGNOSIS

DIFFERENTIAL DIAGNOSIS
• Infectious gastroenteritis of any kind
• Inflammatory bowel disease
• Appendicitis and other acute surgical abdominal processes
• Hepatitis

LABORATORY Culture of stool most reliable. Laboratory must be specifically notified of diagnostic considerations for most pathogens except Salmonella and Shigella.
Drugs that may alter lab results: Prior or concomitant antibiotic therapy may eliminate pathogen from stool
Disorders that may alter lab results: N/A

PATHOLOGICAL FINDINGS Only present in invasive or colitic syndromes

SPECIAL TESTS Sigmoidoscopy (occasionally needed)

IMAGING N/A

DIAGNOSTIC PROCEDURES
• Stool culture
• Epidemiologic investigation
• Culture of suspected food source if available

TREATMENT

APPROPRIATE HEALTH CARE Usually outpatient management sufficient. Hospitalization for septicemias or focal infections, severe electrolyte imbalance or dehydration.

GENERAL MEASURES
• Most are self-limited syndromes and do not require specific therapy
• Oral solutions for rehydration. Intravenous fluid and electrolyte replacement if necessary for more severe dehydration (particularly in the elderly).
• For infants, rehydration products (e.g., Pedialyte) provides adequate fluid and electrolyte replacement. Don't use for more than 1 to 2 days without clinical reassessment of nutritional needs.

SURGICAL MEASURES N/A

ACTIVITY Bedrest for comfort if needed during the acute phase

DIET Eliminate contaminated food. Bland diet during recovery. Nothing by mouth, if needed, for excessive vomiting or diarrhea.

PATIENT EDUCATION
• Avoidance of raw or under-cooked foods
• Proper food storage and preparation techniques such as refrigeration
• Instruction on prevention if patient traveling to foreign countries
• Avoid anti-diarrheal drugs in most cases

MEDICATIONS

DRUG(S) OF CHOICE For septicemias and focal infections, systemic antibiotic therapy may be indicated (e.g., ampicillin plus aminoglycoside for listeriosis)
• Shigella: trimethoprim-sulfamethoxazole 160 mg and 800 mg, respectively, bid for five days, or ciprofloxacin (Cipro) 500 mg bid for 10 days
• Campylobacter: erythromycin 250 mg qid for 5 days or ciprofloxacin (Cipro) 500 mg bid for 7 days
• Traveler's diarrhea: trimethoprim-sulfamethoxazole one double strength tablet bid for 3 days or ciprofloxacin (Cipro) 500 mg bid for 3 days
Contraindications:
• Avoid antiperistaltic agents in colitic (bloody diarrhea) syndromes since they may increase the chance of dissemination
• Antiemetics may be given but are usually unnecessary
Precautions: N/A
Significant possible interactions: Digoxin toxicity with electrolyte imbalance, exacerbation of diuretic effects

ALTERNATIVE DRUGS N/A

FOLLOWUP

PATIENT MONITORING Individualized based on degree of dehydration and electrolyte imbalance, or signs of sepsis. Serious disturbances require hospitalization, frequent vital signs, strict recording of input and output with appropriate fluid replacement.

PREVENTION/AVOIDANCE
• No ingestion of raw seafood, meats, or poultry
• Avoid any unpasteurized dairy products
• Clean thoroughly any food preparation area in contact with causative items
• Ensure proper cooling of any prepared foods not immediately consumed

POSSIBLE COMPLICATIONS
• Cardiovascular collapse
• Arrhythmias from electrolyte disturbance
• Septicemias or other metastatic infections
• Hypoglycemic seizures or coma

EXPECTED COURSE/PROGNOSIS
• Resolution of signs and symptoms over a few days in most cases
• Chronic sequelae include Guillian-Barre syndrome, reactive arthritis

MISCELLANEOUS

ASSOCIATED CONDITIONS N/A

AGE-RELATED FACTORS
Pediatric:
• Day care center outbreaks may occur. Perhaps at higher risk of complications from antiperistaltic drugs.
• Newborns and infants are a high risk for mortality and complications
• Shigellosis is a rare cause of chronic vaginal discharge in young girls
Geriatric:
• Nursing home outbreaks may occur
• Significant cause of mortality
Others: N/A

PREGNANCY Perinatal salmonellosis, listeriosis, and campylobacteriosis may secondarily infect newborn with severe consequences of sepsis and meningitis

SYNONYMS N/A

ICD-9-CM
003.0 Salmonella gastroenteritis
004.0 Shigella dysenteriae
004.9 Shigellosis, unspecified
005.0 Staphylococcal food poisoning
005.1 Botulism
005.9 Food poisoning, unspecified
008.0 Escherichia coli intestinal infection

SEE ALSO
• Diarrhea, acute
• Eosinophilic gastroenteritis
• Intestinal parasites
• Salmonella infection
• Typhoid fever
• Brucellosis
• Botulism
• Dehydration
• Hypokalemia
• Appendicitis, acute
• Guillain-Barre syndrome

OTHER NOTES
• *C. jejuni* antimicrobial therapy resistance is increasing

ABBREVIATIONS N/A

REFERENCES
• Mandell GL, Douglas RG Jr, Bennett JE: Principles and Practice of Infectious Diseases. 4th Ed. New York, Churchill Livingstone, 1995
• Roberts D: Sources of infection: Food. Lancet 1990;336:859
• Altekruse SF, Stern NJ, Fields PE, Swerdlow DL. Campylobacter jejuni--an emerging foodborne pathogen. Emerg Infect Dis 1999 Jan-Feb;5(1)28-35
Illustrations: N/A
Internet references: http://www.5mcc.com

Author(s)
Mark R. Dambro, MD, FAAFP

Fragile X syndrome

BASICS

DESCRIPTION Fragile X syndrome is the most common known inheritable cause of mental retardation. As a result, it is the most common form of familial mental retardation. This condition received its name from the cytogenetic "fragile site" which is seen on the long arm of the X chromosome (Xq27.3). It is associated with abnormal increase in CGG repeats in the untranslated region of the FMR-1 gene in both carriers and affected individuals. Affected individuals also exhibit hypermethylation at the fragile site.

System(s) affected: Nervous, Reproductive, Musculoskeletal

Genetics:
• The pattern of inheritance is X-linked, however, this condition is seen in both sexes. Males usually more severely affected than females.
• The specific factors controlling the expression of genes at the fragile X site are not fully understood
• 80% of males with the fragile X chromosome will be affected with moderate to severe mental retardation, with 20% unaffected and defined as transmitting males
• Only one third of the female carriers will have mental retardation, and their degree of handicap usually is less severe. Females may demonstrate emotional problems.

Incidence/Prevalence in USA: Affected males = 1/1250 and transmitting males 1/5000 which gives an overall male prevalence of 1/1000. Affected females = 1/2000 and an overall female carrier rate of 1/700. Based on these estimates, 1/850 people carry the fragile X chromosome.

Predominant age: Life-long condition

Predominant sex: Males usually more severely affected, but females demonstrate a higher carrier rate

SIGNS AND SYMPTOMS
• The signs and symptoms seen in the "classic" case of fragile X syndrome may be diagnostic; however, the clinical presentation is extremely varied, is age-dependent, and sex-influenced. Blacks are also less likely to show the characteristic features.
• Early childhood:
  ◊ Global developmental delay with speech and language severely affected
  ◊ Overgrowth
  ◊ Autistic-like behaviors
• Postpubertal males (affected)
  ◊ Mental retardation (100%)
  ◊ Connective tissue dysplasia
  ◊ Characteristic physical features
  - Macro-orchidism (95%)
  - Long, thin face (60-65%)
  - Prominent jaw (60-65%)
  - Large ears (> 7.0 cm) (60-65%)
  - Midface hypoplasia (50-60%)
  - Prominent forehead (40%)
  - Large, fleshy hands (30%)
  - Unusual dermatoglyphics

CAUSES Transmission of affected X chromosome

RISK FACTORS
• Transmitting males are intellectually normal and pass the affected chromosome to all of their daughters, the latter who may have affected sons
• Affected females transmit the affected chromosome to their offspring on a 50/50 chance basis

DIAGNOSIS

DIFFERENTIAL DIAGNOSIS
• Fragile X syndrome should be considered in patients (male or female) with mental retardation of unknown etiology
• Many male children will present primarily with speech delay or overgrowth and may have been misdiagnosed as having cerebral gigantism (Soto) syndrome
• Males or females with significant learning disabilities with speech and language deficits
• Familial pattern of MR
• Pervasive developmental disorder
• Significant learning disability
• FRAXE - cytogenetically positive/DNA negative
• Autism

LABORATORY Molecular genetic testing (DNA) is the diagnostic test of choice. Molecular studies can identify full mutations, mosaic patterns, and premutations thereby identifying affected carriers among normal relatives.

Drugs that may alter lab results: N/A
Disorders that may alter lab results: N/A

PATHOLOGICAL FINDINGS N/A

SPECIAL TESTS Affected patients are in need of educational and psychological evaluation for the development of learning programs

IMAGING N/A

DIAGNOSTIC PROCEDURES N/A

TREATMENT

APPROPRIATE HEALTH CARE
Affected individuals will usually require life-long adult supervision and should be referred to the local mental retardation board for case management

GENERAL MEASURES Early detection allows initiation of pre-school intervention programs

SURGICAL MEASURES N/A

ACTIVITY Full activity

DIET No special diet

PATIENT EDUCATION
• The patient and the family should receive genetic evaluation and counseling
• Patient and family could contact: The National Fragile X Foundation, (800)688-8765
• National Fragile X Advocate 800-434-0322

Fragile X syndrome

MEDICATIONS

DRUG(S) OF CHOICE Folic acid 20 mg qd, has been reported anecdotally to improve behavior and attention span in prepubertal males. No statistical benefit has been observed in children or adults during double-blind studies.
Contraindications: N/A
Precautions: N/A
Significant possible interactions: N/A

ALTERNATIVE DRUGS N/A

FOLLOWUP

PATIENT MONITORING General health maintenance

PREVENTION/AVOIDANCE Genetic counseling and evaluation of at-risk family members and pregnancies. Prenatal diagnosis is available.

POSSIBLE COMPLICATIONS Learning and/or behavioral problems (which are more frequent among female patients)

EXPECTED COURSE/PROGNOSIS
• Males with a full mutation may require life-long adult supervision
• Among affected males and females, life-span is generally not affected
• Among males, intellect manifests early plateauing which causes a decline in IQ scores
• Females are less affected but may have mild to moderate mental retardation
• Approximately 1/3 of affected females manifest learning disabilities

MISCELLANEOUS

ASSOCIATED CONDITIONS
• Speech and language problems
• Developmental delay
• Mental retardation
• Maladaptive behavior
• Attention deficit disorder/hyperactivity disorder (ADHD)
   ◊ Is found with greater frequency among individuals with neuropsychological dysfunction
   ◊ Treatment for ADHD among the mentally retarded is not unlike that for the "normal" population
   ◊ Data indicate overuse of psychoactive substances to aid caretakers

AGE-RELATED FACTORS
Pediatric: N/A
Geriatric: N/A
Others: N/A

PREGNANCY Patient and family should receive genetic evaluation and counseling as prenatal diagnosis is available

SYNONYMS
• Martin-Bell syndrome
• Marker X syndrome
• X-linked mental retardation

ICD-9-CM
758.9 Conditions due to anomaly of unspecified chromosome

SEE ALSO
• Down syndrome
• Mental retardation
• Attention deficit hyperactivity disorder
• Autism

OTHER NOTES Extensive family history is mandatory

ABBREVIATIONS ADHD = attention deficit disorder/hyperactivity disorder

REFERENCES
• Simensen RJ, Rogers RC: Fragile X Syndrome. Amer Fam Phys 1989;39(5):185-193
• Special Issue: X-Linked Mental Retardation. American Journal of Medical Genetics 1996;64:1&2
• Hagerman RJ, Cronister A: Fragile X Syndrome: Diagnosis, Treatment and Research. Baltimore, Johns Hopkins University, 1996
Illustrations: N/A
Internet references: http://www.5mcc.com

Author(s)
Richard J. Simensen, PhD
Gene S. Fisch, PhD

Frostbite

BASICS

DESCRIPTION A localized complication of exposure to cold, resulting in diminished blood flow to the affected part (especially hands, face or feet). Dehydration, enzymatic destruction and ultimately cell death occurs. In severe cases, deep tissue freezing may occur with damage to underlying blood vessels, muscles and nerve tissue.
System(s) affected: Endocrine/Metabolic, Skin/Exocrine
Genetics: N/A
Incidence/Prevalence in USA:
Approximately 4,800/year
Predominant age: All ages
Predominant sex: Male = Female

SIGNS AND SYMPTOMS
• Injured area first appears cold, hard, white and is anesthetic to touch. Progresses to blotchy-red, swollen and painful regions after rewarming.
• Loss of cutaneous sensation
• Numbness
• Throbbing pain
• Paresthesia
• Excessive sweating
• Joint pain
• Pallor
• Subcutaneous edema
• Hyperemia
• Blistering
• Blue discoloration
• Skin necrosis
• Gangrene

CAUSES
• Prolonged exposure to cold
• Refreezing thawed extremities

RISK FACTORS
• Impaired cerebral function
• Under the effects of alcohol or drug abuse
• Underlying psychiatric disturbance
• Ambient temperature less than 0°F (-17.8°C)
• Smoker
• Elderly
• Raynaud's phenomenon

DIAGNOSIS

DIFFERENTIAL DIAGNOSIS Frostnip - superficial damp cold injury

LABORATORY
• Hemoconcentration
• Decreased hepatic function
Drugs that may alter lab results: N/A
Disorders that may alter lab results: N/A

PATHOLOGICAL FINDINGS
• Ice crystallization in the intravascular extracellular space
• Atrophy
• Fibroblastic proliferation
• Skin necrosis

SPECIAL TESTS ECG - bradycardia, atrial fibrillation, atrial flutter, ventricular fibrillation, diffuse T wave inversion

IMAGING N/A

DIAGNOSTIC PROCEDURES
Consider Doppler studies

TREATMENT

APPROPRIATE HEALTH CARE
Outpatient or inpatient, depending on severity

GENERAL MEASURES
• Emergency measures for patient without pulse or respiration. Such measures may include CPR and internal warming with warm IV's and warm oxygen (see hypothermia)
• Prevent refreezing. May be necessary to keep frostbitten part frozen until patient can be transported to a care facility.
• Treat for hypothermia
• Cautious rewarming. May immerse frozen body part for several minutes in water no hotter than 40-42°C (104-107°F).
• Keep patient dry. If conscious, give warm fluids with high sugar content.
• Amputation not to be considered until it is definite that tissues are dead. May take about 3 weeks to know if the tissue is permanently injured.
• Prevention of infection, once treatment begins
• Ongoing whirlpool therapy for cleansing and debridement
• Prevention of damage to other body parts

SURGICAL MEASURES N/A

ACTIVITY
• As tolerated, protect injured body parts
• Initiate physical therapy once healing progresses sufficiently

DIET
• As tolerated
• Warm oral fluids

PATIENT EDUCATION
• Local library
• Exposure protection
• Early signs and symptoms of frostbite

MEDICATIONS

DRUG(S) OF CHOICE
• Warm IV fluids via central venous pressure (CVP) line
• Heated oxygen
• For myxedema coma - Levothyroxine 500 µg IV plus 300 mg hydrocortisone
• Tetanus toxoid
• For severe pain - analgesics or narcotics
• Antibiotics may be required for infection
• Maintenance - gastric lavage, peritoneal dialysis, hemodialysis, and mediastinal lavage if needed (using warmed fluids)
Contraindications: Refer to manufacturer's profile of each drug
Precautions: Refer to manufacturer's profile of each drug
Significant possible interactions: Refer to manufacturer's profile of each drug

ALTERNATIVE DRUGS Consider nifedipine or pentoxifylline

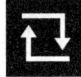
FOLLOWUP

PATIENT MONITORING
• Preferably electronic probe for temperature monitoring (rectal or vascular)
• Followup for physical therapy progress, infection, other complications

PREVENTION/AVOIDANCE
• Dress in layers with appropriate cold weather gear. Cover exposed areas and extremities appropriately.
• Proper preparation for trips to cold climates. Avoid alcohol.

POSSIBLE COMPLICATIONS
• Hyperglycemia
• Acidosis
• Refractory arrhythmias
• Tissue loss. Distal parts of an extremity may undergo spontaneous amputation.
• Gangrene
• Death

EXPECTED COURSE/PROGNOSIS
• Anesthesia and bullae may occur
• The affected areas will heal or mummify without surgery. The process may take 6-12 months for healing. Patient may be sensitive to cold and experience burning and tingling.

MISCELLANEOUS

ASSOCIATED CONDITIONS Alcohol and/or drug abuse

AGE-RELATED FACTORS
Pediatric: Loss of epithelial growth centers
Geriatric:
• Associated disease states increase mortality
• Periarticular osteoporosis complicates
• More prone to hypothermia
Others: N/A

PREGNANCY Acidosis

SYNONYMS
• Dermatitis congelationis
• Frostnip
• Environmental injuries

ICD-9-CM
991.1 Frostbite of hand

SEE ALSO
• Hypothermia

OTHER NOTES N/A

ABBREVIATIONS N/A

REFERENCES
• Rakel RE, ed: Textbook of Family Practice. 5th Ed. Philadelphia, W.B. Saunders Co., 1995
• Berkow R, et al, eds: Merck Manual. 16th Ed. Rahway, NJ, Merck Sharp & Dohme, 1992
• Kelly KJ, Glaeser P, Rice TB, Wendelberger KJ: Profound accidental hypothermia and freeze injury of the extremities in a child. In Critical Care Medicine. Baltimore, Williams & Wilkins, 1990
• Urschel JD: Frostbite: Predisposing factors and predictors of poor outcome. In Trauma. Baltimore, Williams & Wilkins, 1990
• Mills WF, et al: Cold Injury: A Collection of Papers. Alaska Med 1993;35(1)
Illustrations: N/A
Internet references: http://www.5mcc.com

Author(s)
Timothy Robinson, DO

Frozen shoulder

BASICS

DESCRIPTION Adhesive capsulitis which restricts shoulder motion in all directions. The disorder may complicate other inflammatory shoulder disorders.
System(s) affected: Musculoskeletal
Genetics: N/A
Incidence/Prevalence in USA: Unknown
Predominant age: Middle aged and elderly
Predominant sex: Female > Male

SIGNS AND SYMPTOMS
• Decreased range of motion in all directions
• Diffuse shoulder tenderness

CAUSES
• Alteration in the axillary fold of the shoulder capsule
• Chronic bursitis
• Trauma
• Chronic bicepital tendonitis
• Chronic rotator cuff tear

RISK FACTORS
• Sedentary workers
• Immobilization
• Diabetes
• Peripheral vascular disease
• Cervical degenerative disc disease

DIAGNOSIS

DIFFERENTIAL DIAGNOSIS
• Infection
• Degenerative arthritis
• Pancoast's tumor
• Chronic posterior dislocation
• Cervical degenerative disc disease

LABORATORY N/A
Drugs that may alter lab results: N/A
Disorders that may alter lab results: N/A

PATHOLOGICAL FINDINGS
Morphologic changes of fibrosis and fibroplasia with or without inflammation

SPECIAL TESTS N/A

IMAGING
• Routine radiographs of shoulder, cervical spine
• Arthrogram (if used) - decreased redundancy in axillary folds and obliteration of the space in axillary region
• MRI - to evaluate rotator cuff

DIAGNOSTIC PROCEDURES N/A

TREATMENT

APPROPRIATE HEALTH CARE
Outpatient

GENERAL MEASURES
• Prophylactic physiotherapy
• Application of heat or ice
• Gentle passive and active assisted range-of-motion to tolerance

SURGICAL MEASURES
• Passive manipulation under general anesthesia and injection of steroids (controversial)
• Operative arthroscopy

ACTIVITY No restrictions except excessive weight. Passive exercise of the shoulder. Avoid forceful manipulation of the shoulder joint during exercises.

DIET No restrictions

PATIENT EDUCATION Techniques for passive active exercise

MEDICATIONS

DRUG(S) OF CHOICE
• NSAID's: ibuprofen 200-800 mg tid; naproxen 375-500 mg bid
Contraindications: Refer to manufacturer's literature
Precautions: Refer to manufacturer's literature
Significant possible interactions: Refer to manufacturer's literature

ALTERNATIVE DRUGS
• Corticosteroid injections (controversial)

FOLLOWUP

PATIENT MONITORING As needed

PREVENTION/AVOIDANCE Stretching, both active and passive

POSSIBLE COMPLICATIONS N/A

EXPECTED COURSE/PROGNOSIS
Persistence in exercise program shows improvement in motion and decreased pain over 6-18 weeks

MISCELLANEOUS

ASSOCIATED CONDITIONS N/A

AGE-RELATED FACTORS
Pediatric: N/A
Geriatric: N/A
Others: N/A

PREGNANCY N/A

SYNONYMS Adhesive capsulitis

ICD-9-CM
726.0 Adhesive capsulitis of shoulder

SEE ALSO N/A

OTHER NOTES N/A

ABBREVIATIONS N/A

REFERENCES
• Rakel RE, ed: Textbook of Family Practice, 5th Ed. Philadelphia, W.B. Saunders Co., 1995
• Parker RD, et al: Frozen Shoulder Part I, Orthopedics 1989;12(6)
Illustrations: N/A
Internet references: http://www.5mcc.com

Author(s)
Richard W. Cohen, MD

Furunculosis

BASICS

DESCRIPTION Acute abscess of a hair follicle due to infection by Staphylococcus aureus. Spreads away from hair follicle into surrounding dermis.
System(s) affected: Skin/Exocrine
Genetics: Unknown
Incidence/Prevalence in USA:
• Uncommon in children unless immunodeficiency state present (i.e., can appear in young girls with hyperimmunoglobulin E-Staphylococcal syndrome [Job's syndrome])
• Increase in frequency after puberty
Predominant age: Adolescents and young adults. Uncommon in young children unless immunodeficiency state present (i.e., can appear in young girls with hyperimmunoglobulin E-staphylococcal syndrome [Job's syndrome]).
Predominant sex: Males = Females

SIGNS AND SYMPTOMS
• Painful erythematous papules/nodules (1-5 cm) with central pustulation
• Located only in hirsute sites of body, especially areas prone to friction or minor trauma (i.e., underneath belt, anterior thighs)
• May be singular or multiple
• No fever or systemic symptoms
• Tender red perifollicular swelling, terminating in discharge of pus and necrotic plug
• Pus usually drains spontaneously

CAUSES Pathogenic strain of
Staphylococcus aureus

RISK FACTORS
• Carriage of pathogenic strain of Staphylococcus in nares, skin, axilla, and perineum
• Rarely, polymorphonuclear leukocyte defect or hyperimmunoglobulin-E/Staphylococcus abscess syndrome
• Diabetes mellitus, malnutrition, alcoholism
• Primary immunodeficiency disease (chronic granulomatous disease, Chediak-Higashi syndrome, C3 deficiency, C3 hypercatabolism, transient hypogammaglobulinemia of infancy, immunodeficiency with thymoma, Wiskott-Aldrich syndrome)
• Secondary immunodeficiency (leukemia, leukopenia, neutropenia, therapeutic immunosuppression)

DIAGNOSIS

DIFFERENTIAL DIAGNOSIS
• Folliculitis
• Pseudofolliculitis
• Carbuncles
• Ruptured epidermal cyst
• Hidradenitis suppurativa

LABORATORY Culture of abscess material
Drugs that may alter lab results:
Antibiotics
Disorders that may alter lab results: N/A

PATHOLOGICAL FINDINGS
Histopathologically - perifollicular necrosis containing fibrinoid material and neutrophils. At deep end of necrotic plug, in subcutaneous tissue, is a large abscess with a gram stain positive for small collections of staph aureus.

SPECIAL TESTS None except for immunoglobulin levels in rare cases

IMAGING N/A

DIAGNOSTIC PROCEDURES Culture of abscess material

TREATMENT

APPROPRIATE HEALTH CARE
Outpatient

GENERAL MEASURES
• Moist, warm compresses (provides comfort, encourages localization/pointing/drainage) 30 minutes, 4 times a day
• If pointing or large, incise and drain
• Consider packing to promote drainage
• Routine culture not necessary for localized abscess in non-diabetic patients with normal immune system
• Systemic antibiotics usually unnecessary, unless extensive surrounding cellulitis or fever
• If recurrent, problem usually related to chronic skin carriage of particular strain of Staphylococcus in nares or on skin. Treatment goals are to 1) decrease or eliminate pathogenic strain or 2) in very difficult cases, implant less aggressive strain.
• Suppression of pathogenic strain
  ◊ Culture nares, skin, axilla, perineum
  ◊ Begin therapeutic antibiotic doses
  ◊ Wash entire body and fingernails (with nailbrush) daily for 1-3 weeks with povidone-iodine (Betadine), hisachlorophene (Hibiclens), or Phisohex soap (all can cause dry skin)
  ◊ After shower ointments
  ◊ Sanitary practices - change towels, washcloths and sheets daily; clean shaving instruments; avoid nose-picking; change wound dressings frequently
• Replacement of pathogenic strain with nonpathogenic strain (502A bacterial interference)
  ◊ Culture nose and lesions to document pathogenic strain
  ◊ Culture family members if disease involves them
  ◊ Treat patient and infected household members with antibiotics
  ◊ Discontinue topical/oral antibiotics 48 hours then inoculate anterior nares with Staphylococcus aureus 502A (stock bacteria) (tilt head back, swab each anterior nares with 2 soaked cotton swabs of culture while patient sniffs material into nares and nasopharynx)
  ◊ Followup 1 month later; repeat process if abscesses not controlled

SURGICAL MEASURES N/A

ACTIVITY Avoid contact sports (i.e., wrestling) if active lesions. Otherwise no restrictions.

DIET Unrestricted

PATIENT EDUCATION Refer to: Habif T: Clinical Dermatology. 3rd Ed. St. Louis, CV Mosby, 1996

MEDICATIONS

DRUG(S) OF CHOICE
• If abscesses multiple, if lesions have marked surrounding inflammation, or if immunocompromised
   ◊ Obtain culture and place on antibiotics for at least 14 days
   ◊ Cloxacillin (Tegopen) or dicloxacillin (Dynapen, Pathocil) 250 mg qid, or
   ◊ Erythromycin (E-mycin, PCE) 250-500 tid
• Suppression of pathogenic strain
   ◊ Dicloxacillin or cloxacillin 250 mg qid x 21 days
   ◊ Erythromycin 250-500 mg tid (if penicillin allergic) x 21 days
   ◊ If above fails - begin 1-3 month course of antibiotics. May need to add rifampin 600 mg q day x 10 days
   ◊ After showering - bacitracin ointment or mupirocin to both anterior nares with cotton swab tid-qid x > 14 days
• Replacement of pathogenic strain
   ◊ Treat patient and infected household members with dicloxacillin 250 mg qid or if child/infant with 50 mg/kg/day qid x 7-10 days
Contraindications:
• Cloxacillin and dicloxacillin - penicillin allergy
• Erythromycin, mupirocin - hypersensitivity
Precautions:
• Cloxacillin and dicloxacillin - anaphylactic reaction
• Erythromycin - cautious use in patients with impaired hepatic function; GI side effects especially abdominal cramping; pregnancy category B. Increased cardiac toxicity with terfenadine (Seldane), astemizole
Significant possible interactions:
Erythromycin - increases theophylline and carbamazepine levels; decreases warfarin clearance

ALTERNATIVE DRUGS
• Resistant strains of Staph. aureus: first generation cephalosporins, clindamycin, ciprofloxacin + rifampin (rifampicin), Trimethoprim-sulfamethoxazole (cotrimoxazole) + rifampicin
• If known or suspected impaired neutrophil function (i.e., impaired chemotaxis, phagocytosis, superoxide generation), add vitamin C 500 mg/day for 30 days (prevents oxidation of neutrophils)
• If fail with antibiotic regimens
   ◊ May try oral pentoxifylline 400 mg tid for 2-6 months
   ◊ Contraindications - recent cerebral and/or retinal hemorrhage; intolerance to methylxanthines (i.e., caffeine, theophylline)
   ◊ Precautions - prolonged prothrombin time and/or bleeding; if on warfarin, frequent monitoring of prothrombin time

FOLLOWUP

PATIENT MONITORING
Instruct patient to see physician if compresses unsuccessful

PREVENTION/AVOIDANCE
Patient education regarding self care (see General Measures section. Treatment and prevention are interrelated.)

POSSIBLE COMPLICATIONS
• Scarring
• Bacteremia
• Metastatic seeding (i.e., septal/valve defect, arthritic joint)

EXPECTED COURSE/PROGNOSIS
• Self-limited (usually drains pus spontaneously and will heal with or without scarring within several days)
• Recurrent/chronic lasting for months or years

MISCELLANEOUS

ASSOCIATED CONDITIONS
• Usually normal immune system
• Diabetes mellitus
• Polymorphonuclear leukocyte defect (rare)
• Hyperimmunoglobulin-E/staphylococcal abscess syndrome (rare)
• See Risk Factors for others

AGE-RELATED FACTORS
Pediatric: N/A
Geriatric: N/A
Others: Most common after puberty. Clusters have been reported in teenagers living in crowded quarters.

PREGNANCY   N/A

SYNONYMS
• Boils

ICD-9-CM
680.9 Carbuncle and furuncle, unspecified site

SEE ALSO
• Folliculitis
• Hidradenitis suppurativa

OTHER NOTES
• If abscess culture grows gram negative bacteria or fungus then consider polymorphonuclear neutrophil (PMN) leukocyte function defect
• Hydradenitis suppurativa is a particular form of furunculosis
• Can order Staphylococcus aureus 502A from American Type Culture Collection, Rockville, Md.

ABBREVIATIONS   N/A

REFERENCES
• Sams WM Jr, Lynch P: Principles and Practice of Dermatology. New York, Churchill Livingstone, 1990
• du Vivier A: Dermatology in Practice. Philadelphia, J.B. Lippincott Co., 1990
• Habif T: Clinical Dermatology. 3rd Ed. St. Louis, CV Mosby, 1996
• Levy R, Schlaeffer F: Successful treatment of a patient with recurrent furunculosis by vitamin C. International J of Dermatology 1993;32(11):832-834
• Wahba-Yahav AV: Intractable chronic furunculosis: Prevention of recurrence with pentoxifylline. Acta Dermato-Venereologica 1992;72(6):461-462
Illustrations: 4 available on CD-ROM
Internet references: http://www.5mcc.com

Author(s)
W. Paul Slomiany, MD

Galactorrhea

BASICS

DESCRIPTION Milky nipple discharge not associated with gestation. Galactorrhea does not include serous, purulent or bloody nipple discharge. Most cases are associated with hyperprolactinemia either from over production or loss of inhibitory regulation by dopamine.
System(s) affected: Endocrine/Metabolic, Reproductive, Nervous
Genetics: N/A
Incidence/Prevalence in USA: 1-50% of non-pregnant reproductive age women
Predominant age: 15-50 (reproductive)
Predominant sex: Males are rarely affected

SIGNS AND SYMPTOMS
Bilateral milky nipple discharge, other findings vary with causes
• Hypogonadism from hyperprolactinemia
  ◊ Oligomenorrhea, amenorrhea
  ◊ Inadequate luteal phase, anovulation, infertility
  ◊ Decreased libido (especially in affected males)
• Mass effects from pituitary enlargement
  ◊ Headache, cranial neuropathies
  ◊ Bitemporal hemianopsia, amaurosis, scotomata
• Signs/symptoms of associated conditions
  ◊ Adrenal insufficiency, acromegaly, hypothyroidism, chest wall conditions

CAUSES
• Pituitary gland overproduction
  ◊ Prolactinoma, acromegaly, empty sella, lymphocytic hypophysitis
• Hypothalamic region dysregulation
  ◊ Craniopharyngiomas, meningiomas, dysgerminomas, tumors, sarcoid, irradiation, vascular insult, stalk disruption or dissection
• Medications that suppress dopamine
  ◊ Phenothiazines, SSRI's, TCAD's, butyrophenones, cimetidine, ranitidine, reserpine, alpha methyl-dopa, verapamil, estrogens, isoniazid, opioids, stimulants, neuroleptics, metaclopromide
• Chest wall conditions
  ◊ Zoster, fibrocystic breast disease, surgical or other trauma
• Post surgical condition especially oophorectomy
• Other causes
  ◊ Primary hypothyroidism, cirrhosis, Cushing's disease, ectopic prolactin secretion, renal failure, sarcoid, lupus, multiple sclerosis, polycystic ovary syndrome
• Physiologic with pregnancy or up to 6 month after stopping lactation
  ◊ Chiari-Frommel - idiopathic galactorrhea more than six month postpartum
• Idiopathic - normal prolactin levels

RISK FACTORS N/A

DIAGNOSIS

DIFFERENTIAL DIAGNOSIS
• Primary hypothyroidism
• Non-milky nipple discharge
  ◊ Intraductile papilloma, fibrocystic disease
• Purulent breast discharge
  ◊ Mastitis, breast abscess, impetigo, eczema
• Bloody breast discharge - think malignancy

LABORATORY
• Confirm microscopic of secretions is lipoid
• Check prolactin level and thyroid functions
• Check pregnancy test, liver and renal functions
• Consider FSH/LH if amenorrheic
• Consider growth hormone levels if acromegaly suspected
• Check adrenal steroids if signs of Cushing's disease
Drugs that may alter lab results: See medications that can cause hyperprolactinemia
Disorders that may alter lab results: See disorders listed under Causes

PATHOLOGICAL FINDINGS None
unless pituitary resection required, gland can have woody fibrosis is patient took bromocriptine (Parlodel) for very long

SPECIAL TESTS Formal visual field testing if pituitary adenoma suspected, progesterone withdrawal bleed if amenorrheic

IMAGING Pituitary MRI (CT, coned-down views or tomograms are substandard)

DIAGNOSTIC PROCEDURES No additional

TREATMENT

APPROPRIATE HEALTH CARE
• Out patient care unless pituitary resection required
• Bromocriptine patients need good hydration

GENERAL MEASURES
• Treat underlying cause if possible
• Treat to manage symptoms, reduce patient anxiety, restore fertility
• Reduce tumor size or prevent progression to prevent neurologic sequelae
• If microadenoma "watchful waiting" can be appropriate as 95% to do not enlarge
• Treat asymptomatic tumors if >10 mm
• Discontinue offending medications

SURGICAL MEASURES
• Macroadenomas need surgery if medical management does not halt growth, if any neurologic symptoms, if >10 mm, or patient cannot tolerate medications
  ◊ Transphenoidal pituitary resection
  ◊ 50% recurrence after surgery
• Radiation is an alternate therapy
  ◊ 20-30% success rate
  ◊ 50% risk of panhypopituitarism after radiation
• In some research centers gamma knife is being tried

ACTIVITY No restrictions

DIET No restrictions

PATIENT EDUCATION
• Warn about symptoms of mass enlargement in pituitary
• Discuss treatment rationale and risks of treating or not
• Patient education material available from: Pituitary Tumor Network Assoc., 16350 Ventura Blvd. #231, Encino, CA 91436: (805) 499-9973

MEDICATIONS

DRUG(S) OF CHOICE The dopamine antagonist bromocriptine (Parlodel) works to reduce prolactin levels and shrink tumor size. Therapy is suppressive not curative. Start low 1.25 mg at night with a snack and increase to 2.5 mg tid. Doses as high as 30 mg/day may be required for tumor regression. 10 -15% are resistant so try alternates.
Contraindications: Uncontrolled hypertension, sensitivity to ergot alkaloids, preeclampsia
Precautions:
• Nausea, vomiting, drowsiness are common
• Orthostasis, lightheadedness or syncope
• Hypertension, seizures, acute psychosis, digital vasospasm are rare
• Long term treatment can cause woody fibrosis of the pituitary gland
Significant possible interactions:
Phenothiazines, butyrophenones, other drugs listed under Causes

ALTERNATIVE DRUGS
• Other forms of bromocriptine - intravaginal, sustained release, intramuscular
• Pergolide (Permax) 0.05 - 0.15 mg once daily
• Cabergoline (Dostinex) 0.25 - 1.0 mg twice a week
• Quinagolide, Metorgolide marketed in Europe

FOLLOWUP

PATIENT MONITORING
• Varies with cause, check prolactin levels every six weeks until normalized, then every 6-12 months
• Monitor visual fields and MRI at least yearly, if clinical course is stable, then every 2-5 years

PREVENTION/AVOIDANCE Keep medication causes in mind

POSSIBLE COMPLICATIONS
• Depends on underlying cause
• If enlarging pituitary adenoma risk of permanent visual field loss
• Panhypopituitarism can complication radiation or surgical therapy.
• Osteoporosis if amenorrhea persists without estrogen replacement

EXPECTED COURSE/PROGNOSIS
• Depends on underlying cause
• Symptoms recur after discontinuation of medication
• Surgery can have 50% recurrence
• Prolactinomas less than 10 mm can resolve spontaneously

MISCELLANEOUS

ASSOCIATED CONDITIONS See Causes

AGE-RELATED FACTORS
Pediatric: N/A
Geriatric: N/A
Others: N/A

PREGNANCY Adenomas can grow rapidly during pregnancy. The majority of galactorrhea during pregnancy is physiologic.

SYNONYMS
• Disordered lactation
• Nipple discharge

ICD-9-CM
676.6 Galactorrhea

SEE ALSO
• Hyperprolactinemia
• Pituitary basophilic or chromophobe adenoma

OTHER NOTES Can occur in males, 20% of patients with MEN-1 have prolactinomas

ABBREVIATIONS
SSRI = selective seratonin reuptake inhibitors
MAOI = monoamine oxidase inhibitors
TCAD = tricyclic antidepressants
FSH = follicle stimulating hormone
LH = leutinizing hormone

REFERENCES
• Molitch ME: Advances in pituitary tumor therapy, medical treatment of prolactinomas. Endocrinology and Metabolism Clinics 1999;28(1):144-69
• Yazigi RA, Quintero CH, Salameh WA: Prolactin disorders. Fertility and Sterility 1997;67(2):215-25
• Haney AF: Galactorrhea. Current Therapy in Endocrinology and Metabolism 1997;6:393-6
• Katznelson L, Klibanski A: Prolactinomas. Cancer Treatment Research 1997;89:41-55
• Taber SW: The Clinical Challenge of nipple discharge. Kentucky Medical Assn J 1996;94(9):387-92
Illustrations: N/A
Internet references: http://www.5mcc.com

Author(s)
Patricia Borman, MD

Gastric malignancy

BASICS

DESCRIPTION Gastric malignancy may occur anywhere in the stomach. Over the last 20 years the incidence of adenocarcinoma of the proximal stomach and the gastroesophageal junction has risen while the incidence of distal cancers has remained unchanged or decreased slightly. Infiltration to lymph nodes, omentum, lungs and liver is rapid. Uncommon in U.S. natives.

System(s) affected: Gastrointestinal

Genetics:
- 2 to 4 times more common in first degree relatives
- More common in people with blood group A

Incidence/Prevalence in USA: 7/100,000; 21,900 new cases per year

Predominant age: Over 55 (2/3 over age 65)

Predominant sex: Male > Female (1.7:1)

SIGNS AND SYMPTOMS
- Chronic non-colicky abdominal pain (especially in epigastrium) ranging from postprandial fullness to severe steady pain
- Anorexia
- Pain unrelieved by antacids
- Pain exacerbated by food
- Pain relieved by fasting
- Dysphagia
- Nausea and vomiting
- Constipation
- Early satiety
- Weight loss

CAUSES Unknown. Probably arises from a non-specific mucosal injury. H. pylori may trigger carcinogenesis by causing chronic atropic gastritis and intestinal metaplasia. Probable association with food preservatives (e.g., nitrates, sulfites).

RISK FACTORS
- Diet rich in additives (smoked, pickled or salted foods; highly spiced oriental foods)
- Achlorhydria
- Atrophic gastritis/intestinal metaplasia
- Pernicious anemia
- Prior gastric resection
- Smoking/tobacco abuse
- Ethnic background: Hispanic, Japanese, Chilean, Costa Rican. First or second generation Japanese, Chilean or Costa Rican in the United States.
- Polyps or dysplasia anywhere in alimentary canal
- Helicobacter pylori infection
- Familial polyposis
- Barrett's esophagus
- Low consumption of fruits and vegetables
- Individuals with blood group A

DIAGNOSIS

DIFFERENTIAL DIAGNOSIS
- Gastric lymphoma
- Peptic ulcer with or without hemorrhage
- Eosinophilic gastroenteritis
- Giant hypertrophic gastritis (Ménétrier's disease)
- Carcinoma of the colon
- Functional dyspepsia
- Carcinoma of body or tail of the pancreas
- Angiodysplasia of the colon
- GI sarcoidosis
- Small intestinal lymphoma
- Crohn's disease

LABORATORY
- Positive stool guaiac for blood
- Hemoglobin less than 12 g/dL (1.86 mmol/L)
- Hematocrit less than 35 (0.35)
- Albumin less than 3 g/dL (30 g/L)

Drugs that may alter lab results: N/A

Disorders that may alter lab results: Pernicious anemia may cause a false positive pentagastrin test

PATHOLOGICAL FINDINGS
- Adenocarcinomas 85% (types: intestinal and diffuse [linitis plastica])
- Gastric lymphomas 12-14%
- Gastric sarcomas 1-3%

SPECIAL TESTS Pentagastrin test - stomach pH less than 6

IMAGING Double contrast upper GI study - barium filling defect, endoscopy, endoscopic ultrasound, CT scan

DIAGNOSTIC PROCEDURES Upper endoscopy for direct visualization, cytology and biopsy, endoscopic ultrasound is most accurate preoperative staging tool

TREATMENT

APPROPRIATE HEALTH CARE
Inpatient

GENERAL MEASURES
- Surgical excision of the tumor with resection of the local lymph nodes offers the only chance for cure. Even patients who are not felt to have a curable lesion should be offered an attempt at surgical reduction of the tumor since it offers the best form of palliation and improves the likelihood of benefit if chemotherapy and/or radiation therapy is administered. Exception is early (superficial) gastric cancer where nonsurgical ablation (usually endoscopic) may be curative. Gastric cardia tumors may be effectively palliated by nonsurgical means.
- Radiation therapy is of little benefit due to the radioresistancy of gastric tumors and the high doses of radiation required. It does have use in the palliation of pain.

SURGICAL MEASURES
- Radical subtotal gastrectomy with gastrojejunostomy or gastroduodenostomy is the usual treatment of choice. A large part of the stomach along with the greater and lesser omentum is removed en bloc. At times a splenectomy and distal pancreatectomy are also performed. Direct extensions are also excised.
- Total gastrectomy is indicated only if necessary to remove the local lesion
- Local excision for palliation of incurable lesion by resection of bleeding area or area of obstruction

ACTIVITY Adjusted to patient's ability

DIET Dependent on the surgical procedure. Supplemental feedings or total parenteral nutrition (TPN) may be necessary to ensure adequate caloric intake.

PATIENT EDUCATION
- Contact local American Cancer Society
- Cancer Research Institute Helpbook: What to Do If Cancer Strikes. FDR Station, Box 5199, New York, NY 10150-5199

MEDICATIONS

DRUG(S) OF CHOICE
• Chemotherapy has little activity in the treatment of gastric malignancy. Multiple combinations have been tried. The following combinations may offer some palliation or possible prolongation of life:
◊ Fluorouracil
◊ Fluorouracil + leucovorin
◊ Fluorouracil + doxorubicin ± methotrexate
◊ Fluorouracil + doxorubicin + mitomycin
◊ Etoposide + fluorouracil + cisplatin
◊ Etoposide + cisplatin ± doxorubicin
◊ Etoposide + leucovorin + fluorouracil
◊ Fluorouracil + epirubicin + carmustine
Note: Dosing of these agents is patient specific; refer to Drug Evaluations Annual. American Medical Association or other sources

Contraindications:
• 5-fluorouracil: Poor nutritional state, depressed bone marrow function, serious infections, major surgery in last month
• Doxorubicin: Preexisting myelosuppression, impaired cardiac function
• Mitomycin-C: Platelet count less than 75,000/mm3, leukocyte count less than 3000/mm3, serum creatinine greater than 1.7 mg/dL (150 µmol/L), coagulation disorders, serious infections

Precautions:
• Myelosuppression can occur with any of these agents
• Fluorouracil: Stomatitis, gastrointestinal injury, alopecia
• Doxorubicin: Stomatitis, gastrointestinal injury, alopecia, cardiac toxicity
• Mitomycin-C: Renal toxicity, hypercalcemia, gastrointestinal injury, cardiac toxicity
• Etoposide: Peripheral neuropathy, mucositis, hepatic damage
• Methotrexate: Stomatitis, mucositis, gastrointestinal damage, pulmonary infiltrates and fibrosis
• Epirubicin: cardiac toxicity
• Cisplatin: Ototoxicity, renal tubular damage, hypomagnesemia, hypokalemia, hypocalcemia, hemorrhagic cystitis

Significant possible interactions:
• Cisplatin: Aminoglycosides may potentiate nephrotoxicity and ototoxicity
• Loop diuretics may potentiate ototoxicity

ALTERNATIVE DRUGS
• Ondansetron (Zofran), dronabinol (Marinol), metoclopramide (Reglan), and others for nausea control

FOLLOWUP

PATIENT MONITORING
Routine, frequent followup is necessary to monitor disease state, assess treatments, monitor for recurrence/metastasis, and assess nutritional status

PREVENTION/AVOIDANCE
• Insufficient data to establish that screening would decrease mortality in US population
• Screening may be of benefit in high prevalence areas

POSSIBLE COMPLICATIONS
• Metastatic disease (especially hepatic, cerebral and pulmonary)
• Anemia (especially pernicious)
• Pyloric stenosis

EXPECTED COURSE/PROGNOSIS
• The prognosis for gastric carcinoma is not optimistic. Since most lesions do not produce symptoms until late in their course, gastric carcinomas are usually advanced at the time of diagnosis. Surgery offers the only chance for a cure.
• Overall 5 year relative survival rate 19% (if local disease 57%, regional spread 19%, distant spread 2%)
• Early gastric cancers are usually detected as incidental findings or when screening endoscopy is performed in endemic areas. Five year survival rate is > 40% depending on specific staging and tumor differentiation.
• Primary gastric lymphoma more treatable than adenocarcinoma of the stomach. 5 year survival rate of 40% - 60% with subtotal gastrectomy followed by combination chemotherapy.

MISCELLANEOUS

ASSOCIATED CONDITIONS
• Predisposed by giant hypertrophic gastritis (Ménétrier's disease)
• Predisposed by intestinal metaplasia of the stomach
• Atrophic gastritis
• H. pylori

AGE-RELATED FACTORS
Pediatric: Rare
Geriatric: Prevalence greater
Others: N/A

PREGNANCY
Gastric cancer is rarely diagnosed in pregnancy. Prognosis is poor if diagnosed.

SYNONYMS
Linitis plastica

ICD-9-CM
151 Malignant neoplasm of stomach
150.0 Malignant neoplasm of stomach, cardia
151.1 Malignant neoplasm of stomach, pylorus
151.2 Malignant neoplasm of stomach, pyloric antrum
151.3 Malignant neoplasm of stomach, fundus of stomach
151.4 Malignant neoplasm of stomach, body of stomach
151.5 Malignant neoplasm of stomach, lesser curvature, unspecified
151.6 Malignant neoplasm of stomach, greater curvature, unspecified
151.8 Malignant neoplasm of stomach, other specified sites of stomach
151.9 Malignant neoplasm of stomach, unspecified

SEE ALSO
Esophageal tumors

OTHER NOTES
• Patients in lower socioeconomic classes are at greater risk of developing gastric tumors
• Migrants from high incidence areas (such as Iceland, Chile or Japan) to low incidence areas maintain an increased risk while their offspring have an occurrence rate that corresponds to the new location

ABBREVIATIONS
N/A

REFERENCES
• Fauci AS, et al, eds. Harrison's Principles of Internal Medicine. 14th ed. New York, McGraw-Hill, 1998
• Sawyers JL: Gastric carcinoma. Curr Prob Surg 1995;32:105-178
• Fuchs CS, Mayer RJ: Gastric carcinoma. NEJM 1995;333:32-41
Illustrations: N/A
Internet references: http://www.5mcc.com

Author(s)
Scott T. Henderson, MD

Gastritis

BASICS

DESCRIPTION Inflammatory reaction in the stomach; typically involves the mucosa, seldom the full thickness of the stomach wall
• Patchy erythema of gastric mucosa: a common endoscopic finding; usually insignificant
• Erosive gastritis: a reaction to mucosal injury by a noxious chemical agent, e.g., drugs (especially NSAID's) or alcohol
• Reflux gastritis: a reaction to protracted reflux exposure to bile and pancreatic juice, usually associated with a defective pylorus; typically limited to the prepyloric antrum
• Hemorrhagic gastritis (stress ulceration): a reaction to hemodynamic disorder, viz., hypovolemia or hypoxia (as in shock). Also, very common in intensive care units (ICU).
• Infectious gastritis: commonly associated with Helicobacter pylori (possibly causative, maybe opportunistic); viral infection, usually as a component of systemic infection, is common; significant infection by other specific microbes is rare
• Gastric mucosal atrophy, sometimes called atrophic gastritis: frequent, in varying degrees, in the elderly; invariable in primary (pernicious) anemia
System(s) affected: Gastrointestinal
Genetics: Unknown (except, probably, for gastric mucosa atrophy)
Incidence/Prevalence in USA: N/A
Predominant age: All ages; an estimated 60% of persons older than 60 years harbor H. pylori in their gastric mucosa, but in only a small fraction is this significant
Predominant sex: Male = Female

SIGNS AND SYMPTOMS
• Nondescript epigastric distress, often aggravated by eating
• Anorexia
• Nausea, with or without vomiting
• Significant bleeding is unusual except in hemorrhagic gastritis
• Hiccups

CAUSES
• Alcohol
• Aspirin and other nonsteroidal anti-inflammatory drugs
• Bile reflux
• Pancreatic enzyme reflux
• Stress (hypovolemia or hypoxia)
• Radiation
• Staphylococcus aureus exotoxins
• Bacterial infection (eg: Helicobacter pylori)
• Viral infection
• Pernicious anemia
• Gastric mucosal atrophy
• Portal hypertension gastropathy

RISK FACTORS
• Age over 60
• Exposure to potentially noxious drugs or chemical agents
• Hypovolemia, hypoxia (shock)
• Candidal autoimmune

DIAGNOSIS

DIFFERENTIAL DIAGNOSIS
• Functional gastrointestinal disorder
• Peptic ulcer disease
• Linitis plastica
• Viral gastroenteritis
• Pancreatic disease
• Gastric cancer (elderly)

LABORATORY Usually unremarkable, except when blood loss results in anemia
Drugs that may alter lab results:
Antibiotics or omeprazole may affect urea breath test for H. pylori
Disorders that may alter lab results: N/A

PATHOLOGICAL FINDINGS Acute or chronic inflammatory infiltrate in gastric mucosa, often with distortion or erosion of adjacent epithelium. Presence of H. pylori may be confirmed.

SPECIAL TESTS
• 13C-urea breath test for H. pylori (not widely available)
• Serologic test available for H. pylori (office and clinical laboratory), inexpensive
• Gastric acid analysis may be abnormal but is not a reliable indicator of gastritis

IMAGING Nuclear scintigraphy not done clinically

DIAGNOSTIC PROCEDURES
Gastroscopy, usually with biopsy, is essential for a precise diagnosis

TREATMENT

APPROPRIATE HEALTH CARE
Outpatient, except for severe hemorrhagic gastritis

GENERAL MEASURES
• No specific therapy for gastritis (with the exception of H. pylori infection)
• Parenteral fluid and electrolyte supplements required if vomiting prevents food intake
• Consider discontinuing NSAIDs or adding misoprostol

SURGICAL MEASURES N/A

ACTIVITY Usually no restriction

DIET Restriction, if any, depends on severity of symptoms (e.g., light, soft diet); avoid caffeine

PATIENT EDUCATION
• Explanation, reassurance
• Smoking cessation

Gastritis

MEDICATIONS

DRUG(S) OF CHOICE
• Antacids - best given in liquid form, 30 mL 1 hour after meals and at bedtime; useful mainly as an emollient
• H2 receptor antagonists e.g., cimetidine (Tagamet) - "priming" dose of 300 mg IV, then a steady infusion of 37.5-75 mg per hour, dissolved in the running fluid. Patients less severely ill - oral cimetidine 300 mg q6h (or ranitidine [Zantac] or famotidine [Pepcid] or nizatidine [Axid]). Not shown to be clearly superior to antacids.
• Sucralfate (Carafate) 1 g q4-6h on an empty stomach. Rationale uncertain, but empirically helpful.
• Prostaglandins, e.g., misoprostol (Cytotec), can help allay gastric mucosal injury, suggested dosage of 100-200 µg qid
• To eradicate H. pylori:
  ◊ "Triple therapy" is advised – bismuth (as Pepto-Bismol) 30 mL liquid or 2 tablets qid for 4 weeks plus metronidazole 250 mg qid for the first week, plus tetracycline 250 mg qid or amoxicillin 250 mg tid for 2-4 weeks
  or
  ◊ "Dual therapy" with omeprazole 20 mg bid plus amoxicillin 500 mg qid for 2 weeks
  ◊ Short course therapy with 1 week of metronidazole, omeprazole, and clarithromycin bid - 90% effective
Contraindications: Hypersensitivity to the drug(s)
Precautions:
• If bismuth is prescribed, warn patient of black stools
• Refer to manufacturer's profile of each drug
Significant possible interactions: Refer to manufacturer's profile of each drug

ALTERNATIVE DRUGS N/A

FOLLOWUP

PATIENT MONITORING Gastroscopy should be repeated after 6 weeks if gastritis has been severe or if symptomatic response to treatment has not been achieved

PREVENTION/AVOIDANCE
• Patients should be warned of known or potentially injurious drugs or chemical agents
• Patients liable to hypovolemia or hypoxia (especially patients confined to an intensive care ward) should receive prophylactic therapy

POSSIBLE COMPLICATIONS Bleeding from extensive mucosal erosion or ulceration

EXPECTED COURSE/PROGNOSIS
• Most cases clear spontaneously when the cause has been identified and allayed
• Recurrence of H. pylori infection may require a repeated course of treatment

MISCELLANEOUS

ASSOCIATED CONDITIONS
• Gastric or duodenal peptic ulcer
• Primary (pernicious) anemia
• Portal hypertension

AGE-RELATED FACTORS
Pediatric: Gastritis rarely occurs in infants or children
Geriatric: Persons over 60 often harbor apparently harmless H. pylori infection
Others: N/A

PREGNANCY N/A

SYNONYMS
• Erosive gastritis
• Reflux gastritis
• Hemorrhagic gastritis
• Acute gastritis

ICD-9-CM
535.5 Gastritis and gastroduodenitis, unspecified

SEE ALSO N/A

OTHER NOTES N/A

ABBREVIATIONS
NSAID's = nonsteroidal anti-inflammatory drugs

REFERENCES
• Richardson CT: Gastritis. In: Wyngaarden JB, Smith LH Jr, eds. Cecil Textbook of Medicine. Philadelphia, W.B. Saunders Co., 1988:689-692
• Graham DY, Malaty HM, Evans G, et al: Epidemiology of Helicobacter pylori in an asymptomatic population in the US. Gastroenterology 1991;100:1495-1501
• Zinner MJ, Rypins EB, Martin LR, et al: Misoprostol versus antacid titration for preventing stress ulcers in postoperative surgical ICU patients. Ann Surg 1989;210:590-595
• Cutler AP: Testing for Helicobacter pylori in clinical practice. Am J Med 1996;100:355-415
• Ofman JJ, et al: Management strategies for Helicobacter pylori seropositive patients with dyspepsia: clinical and economic consequences. Ann Inter Med 1997;126:280-291
Illustrations: N/A
Internet references: http://www.5mcc.com

Author(s)
Douglas M. Hoy, MD

Gastroesophageal reflux disease

BASICS

DESCRIPTION Reflux of gastroduodenal contents into the esophagus with or without esophageal inflammation
System(s) affected: Gastrointestinal
Genetics: N/A
Incidence/Prevalence in USA: 65% of adults have suffered heartburn; 24% have had symptoms for > 10 years. 17% of adults use indigestion aids at least once weekly, only 24% of sufferers have consulted a physician. Children affected 1/300-1000. 30-80% of pregnant women report heartburn.
Predominant age: All ages
Predominant sex: Male = Female

SIGNS AND SYMPTOMS
- Heartburn (pyrosis) 70-85%
- Regurgitation 60%
- Dysphagia (possible stricture) 15-20%
- Angina-like chest pain 33%
- Bronchospasm (asthma) 15-20%
- Laryngitis (dysphonia)
- Chronic cough
- Globus sensation
- Loss of dental enamel
- In infants: Recurrent emesis, failure to thrive, apnea syndrome

CAUSES
- Inappropriate relaxation of lower esophageal sphincter (LES) (idiopathic, food- or drug-related)
- Familial clustering of GERD has been described suggesting a possible genetic basis
- Pregnancy (progestational hormones cause decreased LES pressure)
- Scleroderma (reduced esophageal motility and incompetent LES)
- Chalasia of infancy
- Delayed gastric emptying (impaired acid clearance)
- Acid hypersecretion (e.g., Zollinger-Ellison syndrome)
- Heller's myotomy for achalasia (30% develop reflux)

RISK FACTORS
- Foods that lower LES pressure (high-fat content, yellow onions, chocolate, peppermint)
- Foods that irritate esophageal mucosa (citrus fruits, spicy tomato drinks)
- Hiatal hernia - acid trapping
- Cigarette smoking; excessive alcohol; coffee
- Medications that lower LES pressure (e.g., theophylline, anticholinergics, progesterone, calcium channel blockers (nifedipine, verapamil), alpha adrenergic agents, diazepam, meperidine
- Indwelling nasogastric tube
- Chest trauma
- In children: Down syndrome, mental retardation, cerebral palsy, repaired tracheoesophageal fistula
- Eradication of H. pylori infection (resulting in increased acid production, loss of acid buffering, etc.) - remains controversial

DIAGNOSIS

DIFFERENTIAL DIAGNOSIS
- Infectious esophagitis (candida, herpes, HIV, cytomegalovirus)
- Chemical esophagitis (lye ingestion)
- Radiation injury
- Crohn's disease of esophagus
- Angina pectoris
- Esophageal carcinoma
- Pill-induced esophagitis (e.g., doxycycline, ascorbic acid, quinidine, potassium chloride, bisphosphonates, etc.)
- Achalasia
- Ulcer disease

LABORATORY N/A
Drugs that may alter lab results: N/A
Disorders that may alter lab results: N/A

PATHOLOGICAL FINDINGS
- Acute inflammation (especially eosinophils)
- Hyperplasia (thickening) of the basal zone of the epithelium seen in 85%
- Lengthening of vascular channels within vascular papillae so that they approach the luminal surface
- Barrett's epithelial change - gastric columnar epithelium (intestinal metaplasia) migrates upward into the distal esophagus; may be associated with strictures and peptic ulceration; dysplasia and malignant transformation

SPECIAL TESTS
- Esophageal pH monitoring (antacids, H2 blockers, proton pump inhibitors and other antisecretory agents can give false negative pH monitoring)
- Esophageal manometry (anticholinergics, theophylline, calcium channel blockers, meperidine, diazepam may give falsely low LES pressure on manometry)
- Acid perfusion (Bernstein) test
- Gastric analysis (exclude gastric hypersecretion)

IMAGING
- Barium swallow: Presence of a sliding hiatal hernia appears to be a predictor of reflux esophagitis; mucosal irregularity due to inflammation and edema; prominent longitudinal folds, erosions, ulcers; smoothly tapered strictures; pseudodiverticula
- Radionuclide scintigraphy

DIAGNOSTIC PROCEDURES
Endoscopy:

Grade	Finding	% Patients with grade
0	Normal	20-40
I	Erythema, friability	20-30
II	Isolated round or linear erosions	20-30
III	Confluent erosions, exudate	5-10
IV	Deep ulceration, stricture/stenosis	5

- Barrett's change suspected when salmon colored mucosa extends > 2 cm above normal squamocolumnar junction (in up to 10%).
- Mucosal biopsy

- Cytology for Barrett's dysplasia (flow cytometry useful adjunct when available)
- Metoclopramide or cisapride may give falsely negative gastric emptying results
- Empiric trial of proton pump inhibitor compares well to pH monitoring as a diagnostic tool in reflux-induced symptoms

TREATMENT

APPROPRIATE HEALTH CARE
- Outpatient diagnosis (typical heartburn history has a positive predictive value of > 80% and warrants empiric therapy in absence of alarm symptoms)
- Inpatient if surgery indicated

GENERAL MEASURES
- Elevate head of bed, avoid lying down directly after meals; avoid stooping, bending, tight-fitting garments
- Avoid drugs causing decreased LES pressure
- Weight loss
- Avoid voluntary eructation
- Stepped therapy
  ◊ Phase I: lifestyle and diet modifications plus antacids or OTC H2 blockers
  ◊ Phase II: H2 blockers in prescription doses; proton pump inhibitors increasingly used as initial therapy of uncomplicated heartburn
  ◊ Phase III: (1) high-dose H2 blocker or proton pump inhibitor (e.g., omeprazole or lansoprazole) or (2) H2 blockers or proton pump inhibitor plus cisapride
  ◊ Phase IV: surgery

SURGICAL MEASURES Phase IV of stepped therapy (see General Measures)

ACTIVITY Full activity

DIET Avoid chocolate, peppermint, onions, high-fat foods, alcohol, tobacco, coffee, citrus juices

PATIENT EDUCATION Digestive Diseases Clearinghouse, Suite 600, 1555 Wilson Blvd., Rosslyn, VA 22209, (212)685-3440

MEDICATIONS

DRUG(S) OF CHOICE
- Mild to moderate disease: H2 blockers in equipotent oral doses, e.g., cimetidine (Tagamet) 800 mg bid or 400 mg qid or ranitidine (Zantac) 150 bid or famotidine (Pepcid) 20 mg bid or nizatidine (Axid) 150 mg bid or cisapride (Propulsid) 10-20 mg qid or 20 mg bid (before meals and at bedtime). Proton pump inhibitors (eg, omeprazole 20 mg/d newly indicated for initial treatment of heartburn symptoms.

• Erosive esophagitis: Omeprazole (Prilosec) 20 mg qd or lansoprazole (Prevacid) 30 mg qd, or higher dose H2 receptor antagonist (e.g., ranitidine 150 mg qid or famotidine 40 mg bid) with or without cisapride for up to 12 weeks
• Severe disease (refractory to initial therapy): Omeprazole (Prilosec) 20-40 mg daily or lansoprazole (Prevacid) 30 mg qd; or higher-dose H2 blockers (e.g., ranitidine 150 mg qid)
Contraindications: Known hypersensitivity to H2 blockers, omeprazole, lansoprazole, cisapride
Precautions:
• Dose reduction of H2 blockers for renal failure
• Avoid cimetidine when potentially interacting drugs are co-administered (or closely monitor prothrombin time or serum theophylline levels, etc.)
• Cisapride should be used with caution with antifungal imidazole agents (e.g., ketoconazole, fluconazole, etc.) and erythromycin as prolonged QT intervals may occur
Significant possible interactions:
• Cimetidine interacts with > 60 drugs (e.g., theophylline, warfarin, phenytoin, lidocaine). Refer to manufacturer's profile.
• Omeprazole
  ◊ May prolong the elimination of diazepam, warfarin and phenytoin
  ◊ Prolonged PPI use associated with hypergastrinemia and potential for carcinoid tumors of the stomach (experimental data)
• Sedative effects of alcohol or benzodiazepines may be accelerated by cisapride
• Avoid anticholinergics with cisapride

ALTERNATIVE DRUGS
• Antacids; alginates e.g., alumina-magnesium (Gaviscon)
• Metoclopramide (Reglan) 5-10 mg before meals used adjunctively with H2 blockers (neuropsychiatric side effects in 30% limits its usefulness)
• Bethanechol (Urecholine) adjunct with H2 blocker (cholinergic side effects)

FOLLOWUP

PATIENT MONITORING Follow symptomatically; repeat endoscopy at 6-12 weeks for poor symptomatic response; annual endoscopy and biopsy for Barrett's esophagus (to detect dysplasia)

PREVENTION/AVOIDANCE
• Long-term maintenance therapy with H2 blockers or proton pump inhibitors along with lifestyle and diet modifications to prevent symptomatic relapse
• Peptic strictures may require periodic dilatation (although frequency of dilatation is reduced by PPI maintenance)
• Omeprazole 20 mg daily or lansoprazole 15 mg daily, effective (both approved for chronic maintenance in severe GERD)
• Antireflux surgery should be considered for patients with severe disease in lieu of chronic drug therapy (laparoscopic approach

increasingly being used)
• Every other year endoscopy, biopsy and cytology to detect dysplasia in Barrett's epithelium (more frequently if dysplasia present)

POSSIBLE COMPLICATIONS
• Peptic stricture (10-15%)
• Hemorrhage (3%)
• Barrett's esophagus (10%)
• Pulmonary or ear, nose, throat complications (5-10%)
• Noncardiac chest pain
• Adenocarcinoma from Barrett's epithelium

EXPECTED COURSE/PROGNOSIS
• Majority of patients respond well to antisecretory or prokinetic therapy. Overall healing rate at ≤ 12 weeks for PPIs is 84% vs H2 blockers 52%. Speed of healing is 12% per week for PPI vs 6% per week for H2 blockers. Complete freedom from heartburn is 77% for PPI vs 48% for H2 blockers.
• Symptoms and esophageal inflammation often return promptly when treatment withdrawn
• Relapse prevention therapy with H2 blockers/proton pump inhibitor often requires the full healing dose be maintained
• Antireflux surgery (e.g., fundoplication) for complications or "refractory" disease; excellent short-term results but long-term followup is relatively limited
• Regression of Barrett's epithelium does not routinely occur despite aggressive medical or surgical therapy
• Cost effectiveness of long-term maintenance therapy has been shown for PPIs and H2 blockers (PPI more cost effective than high dose H2 blockers)

MISCELLANEOUS

ASSOCIATED CONDITIONS
• Reflux-induced asthma
• Pulmonary aspiration
• Chronic cough/throat clearing
• Loss of dental enamel
• Halitosis
• Laryngitis
• Globus sensation
• Vocal cord granulomas

AGE-RELATED FACTORS
Pediatric:
• Reflux symptoms usually resolve by 18 mo
• Vomiting, weight loss, failure to thrive more common than heartburn
• Positional treatment = use of infant seat for 2-3 hours after meals; thickened feedings
• Drug treatment = antacids or liquid H2 blockers (e.g., Zantac syrup)
• Surgery for severe symptoms (apnea, choking, persistent vomiting) successful in 85-95%
Geriatric: Complications more likely
Others: N/A

PREGNANCY
• Heartburn (when first experienced): 52% 1st trimester, 24% 2nd trimester, 9% 3rd trimester
• Tends to recur in subsequent pregnancies
• Symptomatic therapy includes multiple small meals, avoid lying down for 2-3 hours after meals, elevating the head of the bed at night
• Antacids or H2 blockers are probably safe in the 2nd trimester

SYNONYMS
• Reflux esophagitis
• Peptic esophagitis
• Barrett's esophagus
• Symptomatic hiatal hernia

ICD-9-CM
530.1 Esophagitis
750.6 Hiatal hernia
787.1 Heartburn

SEE ALSO
• Peptic ulcer disease
• Esophageal tumors

OTHER NOTES Alkaline (bile) reflux accounts for up to 15% of Barrett's esophagus and severe esophagitis; promotility agent or surgery may be required in this setting

ABBREVIATIONS
• LES = lower esophageal sphincter
• GER = gastroesophageal reflux
• GERD = gastroesophageal reflux disease
• PPI = proton pump inhibitor

REFERENCES
• DeVault KR, Castell DO: Updated guidelines for the diagnosis and treatment of gastroesophageal reflux disease. Am J Gastroenterol 1999;94:1434-42
• Labenz J: Does helicobacter pylori affect the management of GERD: Am J Gastroenterol 1999;94:867-868
• Gotley DC, Smithers BM, Rhodes M, et al: Laparoscopic Nissen fundoplication-200 consecutive cases. Gut 1996;38:487-491
• Kahrilas PJ: Gastroesophageal reflux disease. JAMA 1996;276:983-986
• Chiba N, DeGara CJ, et al: Speed of healing and symptoms relief in grade III to IV gastroesophageal reflux disease; a meta analysis. Gastroenterol 1997;112:11798-1810
• Harris RA, et al: Proton pump inhibitors or histamine-2 receptor antagonists for the prevention of erosive reflux esophagitis; a cost-effective analysis. Am J Gastroenterol 1997;92:2179-2187
• Katz D, et al: The development of dysplasia and adenocarcinoma during endoscopic surveillance of Barrett's esophagus. Am J Gastroenterol 1998;93:536-541
• Trudgill NJ, et al: Familial clustering of reflux symptoms. Am J Gastroenterol 1999:94:1172-1178
1 additional references available at web site
Internet references: http://www.5mcc.com
Illustrations: N/A

Author(s)
James H. Lewis, MD, FACP, FACG

Giant cell arteritis

 BASICS

DESCRIPTION
A systemic granulomatous, predominantly, large vessel arteritis, most commonly affecting the branches of the cranial arteries, (but may involve other aortic branches), seen primarily in the elderly. Frequently associated with polymyalgia rheumatica (PMR).

System(s) affected:
Hemic/Lymphatic/Immunologic, Cardiovascular

Genetics: May be important, several family clusters have been identified

Incidence/Prevalence in USA: More common in northern latitudes (15-30/ 100,000 person over 50/year) vs. southern latitudes (less than 2/100,000 in some series). Primarily Caucasian, Northern European descent.

Predominant age: 60 years or older (very rare under 50). Incidence increases with age.

Predominant sex: Female > Male (2:1)

SIGNS AND SYMPTOMS
• Onset may be abrupt or insidious over months
• Local
  ◊ Headache (usually unilateral temporal, may be generalized or occipital) seen in 2/3 of patients
  ◊ Jaw/tongue "claudication" upon mastication (fairly specific)
  ◊ Visual disturbances early - amaurosis fugax, scotoma, diplopia); late - ischemic optic neuritis, blindness
  ◊ Scalp tenderness
  ◊ Swollen, red temporal artery
  ◊ Decreased temporal artery pulse (may be increased early)
  ◊ Sore throat, cough (10%)
  ◊ Neurologic manifestations - TIA, stroke, peripheral neuropathy, mononeuritis multiplex (3%)
• Systemic
  ◊ Polymyalgia rheumatica - seen in 40-60%
  ◊ Fever (low grade) - 15% with FUO
  ◊ Fatigue/malaise
  ◊ Weight loss/anorexia
  ◊ Arthralgias, myalgias, arthritis

CAUSES
• Etiology unknown
• Possibly immunologic mechanism

RISK FACTORS
• Age over 50
• Presence of polymyalgia rheumatica

 DIAGNOSIS

DIFFERENTIAL DIAGNOSIS
• Cerebral vasculitides
• Other causes of headache (tumor, sinusitis, cervical or temporomandibular joint arthritis)
• Cerebral vascular insufficiency
• Other connective tissue disease
• Retinal detachment or other causes of loss of vision
• Septic arteritis

LABORATORY
• ESR (Westergren) usually greater than 50 (may be over 100)
• ESR may be normal in 10% of patients
• Elevated alkaline phosphatase over 1.5 x normal (unusual)
• Elevated aspartate aminotransferase (AST) over 1.5 x normal (unusual)
• Anemia - mild to moderate, normochromic/normocytic
• Mild leukocytosis
• Mild thrombocytosis

Drugs that may alter lab results:
Prednisone

Disorders that may alter lab results:
• Tumor, infarction, serum protein abnormalities all raise the ESR.

PATHOLOGICAL FINDINGS
• Inflammatory infiltrate (either mononuclear cells or granulomas with giant multinucleated cells) seen in the intima and media of large vessels with resultant disruption of the internal elastic lamina. Lesions may be isolated (i.e., skip lesions)
• Biopsy may not show evidence of active arteritis. However, changes of healing arteritis or vasculitis supports the diagnosis of GCA. If clinically active disease (headache, jaw claudication, elevated ESR), treat as GCA and use high dose steroids.

SPECIAL TESTS
• Temporal artery biopsy

IMAGING
Temporal arteriography (in selected cases)

DIAGNOSTIC PROCEDURES
• Temporal artery biopsy
  ◊ Minimum 2.5 cm segment of vessel with serial sections
  ◊ Within 96 hours of starting steroids
  ◊ If negative, must consider biopsy of contralateral artery (may increase yield up to 10-14%)

 TREATMENT

APPROPRIATE HEALTH CARE
• Inpatient (or outpatient surgery) initially for temporal artery biopsy. Outpatient subsequently.
• If there is a high index of suspicion, immediately institute corticosteroid therapy while arranging temporal artery biopsy

GENERAL MEASURES
N/A

SURGICAL MEASURES
• Temporal artery biopsy

ACTIVITY
Ambulatory ad lib

DIET
• Appropriate salt restriction
• Adequate calcium intake (1500 mg/day)
• Watch serum glucose

PATIENT EDUCATION
• Precautions regarding steroid use, especially osteoporosis
• Exacerbation of disease with medication dose adjustment
• Adrenal suppression - patients should get medical alert bracelet or neck tag

MEDICATIONS

DRUG(S) OF CHOICE
• Prednisone - early:
◊ 60 mg prednisone/d; divided dose initially, then single morning dose (never use every other day steroids)
◊ Begin slow taper after 6 weeks if asymptomatic and ESR decreased (occasionally patient may not normalize ESR)
• Prednisone - taper:
◊ Taper initially by 5 mg every 2 weeks to dose of 25 mg. Then slow taper by 2.5 mg decrements every 2-4 weeks to a dose of 10-15 mg if above guidelines are met. (Must be individualized).
◊ Continue 10-15 mg daily for several months-year, with periodic attempts to taper (i.e., every 3-6 months) by 1 or 2 mg
◊ Use symptoms and ESR to help guide taper
◊ Average time to disease remission 3-4 years, range 1-10 years

Contraindications:
• Systemic fungal infections, although physician must evaluate risks and benefits.
• Relative contraindications: Avoid, if possible, in patients with congestive heart failure, diabetes mellitus, systemic fungal or bacterial infection (must treat infection concurrently if steroids are necessary).

Precautions:
• Long term steroid use
◊ Associated with several potentially severe adverse effects, including: Increased susceptibility to infection, glucose intolerance, adrenal suppression, muscle wasting, osteoporosis, peptic ulcer disease, sodium and water retention, cataracts, avascular necrosis, GI bleeding, psychosis, weight gain
◊ Use lowest possible dose for shortest duration
◊ Upon discontinuing, if the patient has received long-term therapy, taper slowly to avoid Addisonian crisis. May need temporary stress dose steroids for surgical procedures, accidents or severe infections.

Significant possible interactions: Refer to manufacturer's literature

ALTERNATIVE DRUGS Cytotoxic
agents only if patient cannot use steroids (brittle diabetes mellitus, severe osteoporosis, congestive heart failure, etc.) or fails to respond to steroids

FOLLOWUP

PATIENT MONITORING
• ESR - repeat at monthly intervals initially and while tapering, then every 3 months
• Follow visual/constitutional symptoms monthly initially, then as needed

PREVENTION/AVOIDANCE   N/A

POSSIBLE COMPLICATIONS
• Complications related to steroids
• Exacerbation of disease during therapy or taper

EXPECTED COURSE/PROGNOSIS
• With early treatment, resolution of symptoms and preservation of vision
• Average length of disease 3-4 years
• With no treatment, high risks of blindness and stroke
• Occasionally ESR elevation not related to GCA activity and cannot be used to monitor and/or adjust treatment

MISCELLANEOUS

ASSOCIATED CONDITIONS
Polymyalgia rheumatica

AGE-RELATED FACTORS
Pediatric: Does not occur in this age group
Geriatric: Incidence increases with age (twice as common in patients over 80 as it is in 50-59 age group)
Others: N/A

PREGNANCY   N/A

SYNONYMS
• Temporal cell arteritis

ICD-9-CM   446.5 giant cell arteritis

SEE ALSO
• Polymyalgia rheumatica
• Fibromyalgia
• Polymyositis/dermatomyositis
• Depression
• Headache, tension
• Headache, cluster

OTHER NOTES   Westergren ESR is
preferable. If other ESR used (i.e., Wintrobe or ZSR) then cannot use the listed guidelines for abnormalities.

ABBREVIATIONS
GCA = Giant cell arteritis
TA = temporal arteritis

REFERENCES
• Hunder GG: Giant Cell Arteritis and Polymyalgia Rheumatica. In: Kelly WN, Harris ED, Ruddy S, Sledge CB, eds. Textbook of Rheumatology. 4th Ed. p1123-1132, Philadelphia, W.B. Saunders Co., 1997
• Hunder GG, et al: The American College of Rheumatology 1990 Criteria for the Classification of Giant Cell Arteritis. In Arthritis Rheum 1990;33:1122-1128
Illustrations: N/A
Internet references: http://www.5mcc.com

Author(s)
Bridget T. Walsh, DO
Eric P. Gall, MD

Giardiasis

BASICS

DESCRIPTION Intestinal infection caused by the protozoan parasite, Giardia lamblia. Infection results from ingestion of the cysts that excyst into trophozoites which colonize the small intestine and cause the symptoms. The cycle is continued when the trophozoites encyst in the small intestine and water, food, or hands are contaminated by feces of the infected person. Most infections result from fecal-oral transmission or ingestion of contaminated water, less commonly from contaminated food.
System(s) affected: Gastrointestinal
Genetics: N/A
Incidence/Prevalence in USA: 5% of patients with stools submitted for ova and parasite exams. Overall prevalence is lower and variable.
Predominant age: All ages, but most common in early childhood
Predominant sex: Slightly more common in males

SIGNS AND SYMPTOMS
• Approximately 25-50% of infected persons are symptomatic
• Chronic diarrhea (lasting more than 5-7 days and frequently weeks)
• Abdominal bloating
• Flatulence
• Loose, greasy, foul-smelling stools
• Weight loss
• Nausea
• Lactose intolerance

CAUSES Protozoan parasite (Giardia lamblia) infection acquired through fecal-oral transmission or ingestion of contaminated water, less commonly from contaminated food

RISK FACTORS
• Day care centers
• Male homosexuality
• Wilderness camping

DIAGNOSIS

DIFFERENTIAL DIAGNOSIS
• Includes other etiologies of small intestinal diarrhea
• Infectious causes include cryptosporidiosis, isosporiasis, cyclosporiosis
• Other causes of malabsorption includes celiac sprue, tropical sprue, bacterial overgrowth syndromes, Crohn's ileitis
• Irritable bowel is suspected when diarrhea is not accompanied by weight loss

LABORATORY
• Stool for ova and parasites, repeated 3 times if necessary. Cysts are seen in fixed or fresh stools and occasionally, trophozoites are found in fresh diarrheal stools.
• Fluorescent antibody and ELISA tests of fecal specimens are available
Drugs that may alter lab results: A number of drugs interfere with stool exams
Disorders that may alter lab results: N/A

PATHOLOGICAL FINDINGS Intestinal biopsy shows flattened, mild lymphocytic infiltration and trophozoites on the surface.

SPECIAL TESTS String test (Enterotest). A gelatin capsule on a string is swallowed and left in the duodenum for several hours or overnight.

IMAGING N/A

DIAGNOSTIC PROCEDURES
Esophagogastroduodenoscopy with biopsy and sample of small intestinal fluid.

TREATMENT

APPROPRIATE HEALTH CARE
Outpatient for mild cases, inpatient if symptoms are severe

GENERAL MEASURES
• Medical therapy for all infected individuals
• Fluid replacement if dehydrated

SURGICAL MEASURES N/A

ACTIVITY As tolerated

DIET Good nutrition, low lactose, low fat

PATIENT EDUCATION Avoidance of risk factors

Giardiasis

MEDICATIONS

DRUG(S) OF CHOICE
• Metronidazole (Flagyl) 250 mg tid for 5-7 days

Contraindications: Relatively contraindicated in pregnancy, especially first trimester

Precautions:
• Rare toxic psychosis with quinacrine
• Theoretical risk of carcinogenesis with metronidazole

Significant possible interactions: Occasional disulfiram reaction with metronidazole

ALTERNATIVE DRUGS
• Furazolidone 8 mg/kg/day tid for 10 days (slightly less effective, but commonly used in pediatrics because it is well tolerated)
• Paromomycin (Humatin), a nonabsorbable aminoglycoside which is probably less effective, but commonly recommended in pregnancy because of theoretical risk of teratogenicity of other agents
• Tinidazole is effective when given as a single dose. It is the treatment of choice in much of Europe, but is not available in the US.
• Quinacrine 100 mg tid for 5-7 days. Was the treatment of choice for giardiasis, but is no longer available commercially in the US.
• Albendazole 400 mg daily for 5 days. Antihelminthic drug which is as effective as metronidazole and better tolerated.

FOLLOWUP

PATIENT MONITORING
Symptoms, weight, stool exams

PREVENTION/AVOIDANCE
Good hand washing when caring for diapered children, water purification when camping

POSSIBLE COMPLICATIONS
Those of malabsorption and weight loss

EXPECTED COURSE/PROGNOSIS
Untreated giardiasis lasts for weeks. Patients usually (90%) respond to treatment within a few days and most of the non-responders or relapses respond to a second course with the same or a different agent.

MISCELLANEOUS

ASSOCIATED CONDITIONS
Hypogammaglobulinemia and possibly IgA deficiency. The diarrhea is more severe and prolonged in these patients.

AGE-RELATED FACTORS
Pediatric: Most common in early childhood
Geriatric: N/A
Others: N/A

PREGNANCY
Concern for potential teratogenicity of medications. Consult infectious disease specialist or gastroenterologist for symptomatic disease.

SYNONYMS
N/A

ICD-9-CM
007.1 Giardiasis

SEE ALSO
N/A

OTHER NOTES
G. lamblia is also called G. duodenalis, G. intestinalis

ABBREVIATIONS
N/A

REFERENCES
• Fedorak RN, Rubinoff MJ: Basic Investigation of a Patient with Diarrhea. In: Field M, ed. Diarrheal Diseases. New York, Elsevier Science Publishing Co., Inc., 1991
• Adam R.D: The Biology of Giardia spp. Microbiol, Rev 1991;55:706-732
• Hill DR: Giardia lamblia. In: Mandel GL, Douglas RG, Bennett JE, eds. Principles and Practice of Infectious Diseases. 4th Ed. New York, Churchill Livingstone, 1995
• Ortega I, Adam RD: Giardia: overview and update. Clinical Infectious Dis, 25:545-549, 1997

Illustrations: N/A
Internet references: http://www.5mcc.com

Author(s)
Rodney D. Adam, MD

Gilbert's disease

BASICS

DESCRIPTION Mild chronic or intermittent unconjugated hyperbilirubinemia (not due to hemolysis) with otherwise normal liver function
System(s) affected:
Hemic/Lymphatic/Immunologic
Genetics: A gene defect resulting in reduced bilirubin UDP-glucuronosyltransferase-1 appears to be necessary but not sufficient for Gilbert's syndrome.
Incidence/Prevalence in USA: About 7% of the population
Predominant age: Present from birth, but most often presents in the second or third decade of life; heterozygous for single abnormal gene
Predominant sex: Male > Female (2-7:1)

SIGNS AND SYMPTOMS No significant symptoms have been attributed to this disorder, although a variety of nonspecific symptoms have been described. There are no abnormal physical findings other than occasional mild jaundice

CAUSES The hyperbilirubinemia results from impaired hepatic bilirubin clearance (approximately 30% of normal). Hepatic bilirubin conjugation (glucuronidation) is reduced, though this is likely not the only defect.

RISK FACTORS None

DIAGNOSIS

DIFFERENTIAL DIAGNOSIS Hemolysis, ineffective erythropoiesis (megaloblastic anemias, certain porphyrias, thalassemia major, sideroblastic anemia, severe lead poisoning, congenital dyserythropoietic anemias), cirrhosis, chronic persistent hepatitis, pancreatitis or biliary tract disease

LABORATORY
• Bilirubin: less than 6 mg/dL (103 µmol/L) and usually less than 3 mg/dL (51 µmol/L), virtually all unconjugated (indirect)
• CBC with peripheral smear is normal
• Reticulocyte count is normal
• Liver function tests (SGOT, SGPT, alkaline phosphatase, GGT) are normal
• Fasting and postprandial serum bile acids are normal
• Up to 60% of patients have clinically insignificant mild hemolysis which frequently can only be detected with sophisticated red cell survival studies
Drugs that may alter lab results: Bilirubin level may be raised by nicotinic acid and lowered by phenobarbital
Disorders that may alter lab results: Bilirubin levels increase during fasting, and may increase during a febrile illness

PATHOLOGICAL FINDINGS None

SPECIAL TESTS None

IMAGING N/A

DIAGNOSTIC PROCEDURES
• A liver biopsy is not usually needed to exclude other diagnoses
• Some clinicians recommend confirming the diagnosis by reducing daily caloric intake to 400 kcal for 48 hours, which results in a two to threefold increase in unconjugated bilirubin

TREATMENT

APPROPRIATE HEALTH CARE
Outpatient. The most important treatment is to make a positive diagnosis of Gilbert's disease to reassure the patient and prevent further unnecessary procedures

GENERAL MEASURES None

SURGICAL MEASURES N/A

ACTIVITY Full activity

DIET Normal

PATIENT EDUCATION Reassure the patient that the condition is benign with no known sequelae

MEDICATIONS

DRUG(S) OF CHOICE N/A
Contraindications: N/A
Precautions: N/A
Significant possible interactions: N/A

ALTERNATIVE DRUGS N/A

FOLLOWUP

PATIENT MONITORING If history, physical examination, and laboratory tests are normal, see the patient on two or three further occasions during the ensuing 12 to 18 months. If the patient develops no symptoms, reticulocytosis or new liver function abnormalities, make the diagnosis of Gilbert's disease.

PREVENTION/AVOIDANCE N/A

POSSIBLE COMPLICATIONS No known complications

EXPECTED COURSE/PROGNOSIS
The disorder is benign with an excellent prognosis

MISCELLANEOUS

ASSOCIATED CONDITIONS Gilbert's disease may be part of a spectrum of hereditary disorders which includes types I and II Crigler-Najjar syndrome

AGE-RELATED FACTORS
Pediatric: It is rare for the disorder to be diagnosed before puberty
Geriatric: N/A
Others: N/A

PREGNANCY The relative fasting that may occur with morning sickness can elevate the bilirubin level

SYNONYMS Gilbert's syndrome

ICD-9-CM
277.4 Disorders of bilirubin excretion

SEE ALSO
• Crigler-Najjar syndrome

OTHER NOTES N/A

ABBREVIATIONS N/A

REFERENCES
• Okolicsanyi L, Fevery J, Billing B, et al: How should mild, isolated unconjugated hyperbilirubinemia be investigated? Sem Liver Dis 1983;3(1):36-41
• Watson KJR, Gollan JL: Gilbert's syndrome. Bailliere's Clin Gastroenterol 1989;3(2):337-55
• Bosma PJ, Choudhury JR, Bakker C, et al: The genetic basis of the reduced expression of bilirubin UDP-glucuronosyltransferase-1 in Gilbert's syndrome. NEJM 1995;333:1171-5
Illustrations: N/A
Internet references: http://www.5mcc.com

Author(s)
Robert A. Marlow, MD, MA

Gingivitis

BASICS

DESCRIPTION Inflammation of the gingiva, one of the forms of significant oral infections
• Others forms of oral infection:
◊ Periodontitis - progression of gingivitis to connective tissue and alveolar bone
◊ Vincent's angina (trench mouth, necrotizing ulcerative gingivitis, fusospirochetosis) - fusiform bacillus or spirochete infection
◊ Glossitis - inflammation of the tongue (see separate title on this subject)
System(s) affected: Gastrointestinal
Genetics: No known genetic pattern
Incidence/Prevalence in USA: Pandemic, 90% of the population affected
Predominant age: Mostly adult
Predominant sex: Male = Female

SIGNS AND SYMPTOMS
• Mouth odor (bad breath)
• Gum swelling (painless)
• Gum redness
• Change of normal gum contours
• Gum bleeding when flossing or brushing
• Edema of interdental papillae
• Narrow band of bright red inflamed gum surrounding neck of tooth
• Vincent's angina - ulcers, fever, malaise, regional lymphadenopathy, pain

CAUSES
• Noncontagious
• Inadequate plaque removal
• Blood dyscrasias
• Reaction to oral contraceptives
• Vincent's - fusiform bacillus or spirochete infection
• Allergic reactions
• Endocrine disturbances, i.e., pregnancy, menses
• Chronic debilitating disease

RISK FACTORS
• Diabetes mellitus
• Malocclusion
• Poor dental hygiene
• Mouth breathing
• Faulty dental restoration
• HIV positive
• Pregnancy

DIAGNOSIS

DIFFERENTIAL DIAGNOSIS
• Acute necrotizing ulcerative gingivitis (Vincent's disease)
• Afunctional gingivitis
• Chronic desquamative gingivitis
• Diabetic gingivitis
• Diphenylhydantoin gingivitis
• Hormonal gingivitis
• Leukemic gingivitis
• Pregnancy gingivitis
• Pericoronitis
• HIV

LABORATORY Smear to identify causative agent
Drugs that may alter lab results: N/A
Disorders that may alter lab results: N/A

PATHOLOGICAL FINDINGS
• Acute or chronic inflammation
• Broken crepuscular epithelium
• Hyperemic capillaries
• Polymorphonuclear infiltration
• Papillary projections in subepithelial tissue
• Fibroblasts

SPECIAL TESTS N/A

IMAGING N/A

DIAGNOSTIC PROCEDURES N/A

TREATMENT

APPROPRIATE HEALTH CARE
Outpatient

GENERAL MEASURES
• Remove irritating factors (plaque, calculus, faulty dentures)
• Good oral hygiene
• Regular dental check-ups
• No smoking
• Warm saline rinses twice daily
• Prophylaxis by dental hygienist

SURGICAL MEASURES N/A

ACTIVITY No restrictions

DIET Assure adequate vitamins and minerals

PATIENT EDUCATION Printed patient information available from: American Dental Association, 211 E. Chicago Avenue, Chicago, IL 60611, (800)621-8099

MEDICATIONS

DRUG(S) OF CHOICE
• Antibiotics indicated only for acute necrotizing ulcerative gingivitis (Vincent's angina)
• Antibiotics, e.g., penicillin V, pediatric dose 25-50 mg/kg/day divided q6h; adult dose 250-500 mg q6h, or
• Erythromycin - pediatric dose 30-40 mg/kg/day divided q6h; adult dose 250 mg q6h
• Topical corticosteroids e.g., triamcinolone in orabase)
Contraindications: Allergy to antibiotics
Precautions: Erythromycin frequently causes significant gastrointestinal upsets
Significant possible interactions: Refer to manufacturer's literature

ALTERNATIVE DRUGS   Other antibiotics according to culture or smear

FOLLOWUP

PATIENT MONITORING   Until clear

PREVENTION/AVOIDANCE
• Good oral hygiene, daily brushing and flossing
• Cleaning by a dentist or hygienist every 6 months or sooner

POSSIBLE COMPLICATIONS   Severe periodontal disease

EXPECTED COURSE/PROGNOSIS
• Usual course - acute; relapsing; intermittent; chronic
• Prognosis - generally favorable, responds well to appropriate treatment

MISCELLANEOUS

ASSOCIATED CONDITIONS
• Periodontitis
• Glossitis

AGE-RELATED FACTORS
Pediatric: Mild cases common in children and usually requires no treatment
Geriatric: More frequent in this age group (due more to lifelong accumulation, rather than increased susceptibility)
Others: N/A

PREGNANCY   Characteristics - hyperplasia, pedunculated gingival growths, pyogenic granuloma

SYNONYMS   Denture sore mouth

ICD-9-CM   523.1 Chronic gingivitis

SEE ALSO   Glossitis

OTHER NOTES   N/A

ABBREVIATIONS   N/A

REFERENCES   Berkow, R., et al. (eds.): Merck Manual, 16th Ed. Rahway, NJ, Merck Sharp & Dohme, 1992
Illustrations: 1 available on CD-ROM
Internet references: http://www.5mcc.com

Author(s)
David deVlaming, DDS

Glaucoma, chronic open-angle

BASICS

DESCRIPTION A precise definition of "glaucoma" is difficult to find. It is believed (although not without controversy) that sufficiently high intraocular pressure will result in damage to the optic nerve and ultimately loss of visual field and visual acuity. Glaucoma is a disease of pressure; adequate lowering of intraocular pressure almost always stops optic nerve damage.
• In chronic open-angle glaucoma, aqueous secretion by the ciliary body is normal, and its flow between the lens and the iris through the pupil into the anterior chamber is normal; however, the trabecular meshwork does not permit adequately rapid egress of aqueous with a resultant pressure elevation
System(s) affected: Nervous
Genetics: N/A
Incidence/Prevalence in USA: Glaucoma affects approximately 4% of the population above the age of 40, with over 90% of these glaucomas being COAG
Predominant age: Over age 40, but can occur at any age.
Predominant sex: Male = Female

SIGNS AND SYMPTOMS None, until far advanced; then, gradual painless visual loss

CAUSES
• Impaired outflow through the trabecular meshwork (most common)
• Obstruction to the outflow from Schlemm's canal and the aqueous veins created by elevated orbital venous pressure (as in AV malformations, orbital congestion due to thyroid disease, etc.)
• Too much aqueous secretion (extremely rare)

RISK FACTORS
• Positive family history
• Diabetes mellitus
• African-American ancestry

DIAGNOSIS

DIFFERENTIAL DIAGNOSIS
• Vascular occlusive disease
• Severe anemia
• Hemodynamic crisis in past
• Cerebral neoplasia

LABORATORY N/A
Drugs that may alter lab results: N/A
Disorders that may alter lab results: N/A

PATHOLOGICAL FINDINGS
Ophthalmoscopic - optic nerve head damage

SPECIAL TESTS N/A

IMAGING N/A

DIAGNOSTIC PROCEDURES
• IOP recording - elevated
• Visual field testing - loss
• Characteristic optic nerve damage

TREATMENT

APPROPRIATE HEALTH CARE
Outpatient

GENERAL MEASURES
• Treatment of COAG is directed at lowering the intraocular pressure so that a healthy IOP to optic nerve perfusion pressure gradient is restored
• The disease cannot be cured. Control can be obtained by decreasing the rate of aqueous secretion, by increasing the rate of aqueous outflow, or by a combination of the two.
• Usually medical therapy is able to lower the IOP sufficiently to protect the optic nerve from progressive damage and ultimate visual field damage and visual loss
• Early detection and adequate treatment can prevent visual loss in virtually every case.

SURGICAL MEASURES
• When medical therapy not successful, laser or conventional surgery (trabeculectomy) is indicated.

ACTIVITY No limitations

DIET No special diet

PATIENT EDUCATION
• Necessity for periodic IOP checks and eye exams
• For patient education materials favorably reviewed on this topic, contact:
  ◊ Foundation for Glaucoma Research, 490 Post Street, Suite 830, San Francisco, CA 94102, (415)986-3162
  ◊ American Academy of Ophthalmology, 655 Beach Street, San Francisco, CA 94109, (415)561-8500

MEDICATIONS

DRUG(S) OF CHOICE
Medications can be used singly or in combination to achieve the desired reduction of IOP. Begin with a single agent, then add a 2nd or 3rd in a stepwise fashion.
• Topicals to reduce aqueous secretion
◊ Beta-adrenergic blocking agents (timolol, betaxolol, levobunolol, carteolol, metipranolol)
◊ Adrenergic agents (epinephrine and dipivefrin, the "pro-drug" of epinephrine; apraclonidine; brimonidine)
◊ Carbonic anhydrase inhibitors (dorzolamide)
• Topicals to increase aqueous humor outflow (cholinergic agents)
◊ Direct-acting cholinergic agents (pilocarpine, carbamylcholine) "fool" the eye into believing that acetylcholine has been administered
◊ Indirect acting cholinergic agents (physostigmine, demecarium bromide, echothiophate iodide, and isoflurophate [DFP]) are all cholinesterase inhibitors
• Prostaglandin analog [latanoprost (Xalatan)]
• Systemics to reduce aqueous secretion
◊ Acetazolamide (Diamox)
◊ Dichlorphenamide [sulfonamide]
◊ Methazolamide [sulfonamide]

Contraindications:
• The non-selective beta-adrenergic blocking agents (timolol, levobunolol, carteolol, metipranolol) are relatively contraindicated for patients with asthma/obstructive airway disease
• Carbonic-anhydrase inhibitors are contraindicated with history of sensitivity to sulfonamides

Precautions:
• Sympathomimetic agents - used with caution in patients with cardiovascular disease
• Carbonic anhydrase inhibitors - used with caution in patients with a history of nephrolithiasis, myeloproliferative disorders, respiratory acidosis, severely compromised lung capacity, diabetes mellitus, hepatic disease (especially cirrhosis), history of sulfonamide sensitivity
• Beta-adrenergic blocking agents are contraindicated in patients with a history of asthma/COPD, and must be used with caution with patients with marginal cardiac output, bradycardia, and patients using calcium channel blockers.

Significant possible interactions:
• Cholinesterase inhibitors - with the administration of general anesthesia. Should a depolarizing agent such as succinylcholine be used for intubation, these patients will not be able to metabolize this agent and will be respirator-dependent until the systemic activity of cholinesterase is restored, i.e., 3 weeks. Deaths have been reported from this unfortunate complication.
• Carbonic anhydrase inhibitors - may decrease excretion of some drugs (e.g., amphetamines, procainamide, quinidine, tricyclic antidepressants). May potentiate salicylate toxicity secondary to systemic acidosis.
• Beta-adrenergic antagonists have been associated with death in patients also on calcium channel blockers

ALTERNATIVE DRUGS N/A

FOLLOWUP

PATIENT MONITORING
• Every 3-4 months for life
• Chronic carbonic anhydrase inhibitor therapy requires periodic monitoring of the blood count for evidence of reduction in the hemoglobin, hematocrit, and white blood cell count as well as K+ wasting

PREVENTION/AVOIDANCE N/A

POSSIBLE COMPLICATIONS N/A

EXPECTED COURSE/PROGNOSIS
• Lifetime IOP control
• Excellent visual prognosis, unless diagnosis delayed until disorder far advanced or in end-stages

MISCELLANEOUS

ASSOCIATED CONDITIONS Diabetes mellitus

AGE-RELATED FACTORS
Pediatric: N/A
Geriatric: N/A
Others: N/A

PREGNANCY N/A

SYNONYMS Chronic simple glaucoma

ICD-9-CM
365.11 Primary open angle glaucoma
377.14 Glaucomatous atrophy (cupping) of optic disc

SEE ALSO N/A

OTHER NOTES N/A

ABBREVIATIONS
COAG = chronic open-angle glaucoma
IOP = intraocular pressure

REFERENCES Hoskins HD, Kass M, eds: Becker-Shaffer's Diagnosis and Therapy of the Glaucomas. 6th Ed. St. Louis, C.V. Mosby, 1989
Illustrations: N/A
Internet references: http://www.5mcc.com

Author(s)
Barton L. Hodes, MD

Glaucoma, primary angle-closure

BASICS

DESCRIPTION Primary angle-closure glaucoma results from obstruction of aqueous humor outflow through the trabecular meshwork by peripheral iris apposition to the cornea which causes a consequent elevation in intraocular pressure (IOP). The underlying mechanism is pupillary block, in which aqueous egress through the pupil is limited causing forward iris displacement. Angle-closure glaucoma can occur in subacute, acute, and chronic forms and is associated with an anatomically narrow anterior chamber angle; the angle comprises the peripheral iris, anterior ciliary body, trabecular meshwork, and peripheral cornea and can only be observed with a special examination technique called gonioscopy. In its acute form, primary angle-closure glaucoma is an ophthalmic emergency with a natural history of severe visual loss.
System(s) affected: Nervous
Genetics: Polygenic inheritance; first degree relatives have a 2-5% lifetime risk
Incidence/Prevalence in USA:
• 100 cases/100,000 population
• 500/100,000 (Blacks and Asians more common than Caucasians)
Predominant Age: 55-70
Predominant Sex: Female > Male

SIGNS AND SYMPTOMS
• Subacute
  ◊ Dull ache in or around one eye
  ◊ Mildly blurred vision
  ◊ Symptoms occur when watching TV or movies in dark room, reading, or when fatigued. Relieved by sleep or rest.
  ◊ Normal intraocular pressure (10-23 mmHg)
  ◊ Shallow anterior chamber
  ◊ Iris bombé
  ◊ Intermittent peripheral anterior synechiae
  ◊ Enlarged pupil
• Acute
  ◊ Ocular pain
  ◊ Blurred vision
  ◊ Lacrimation
  ◊ Halos around lights
  ◊ Frontal headache
  ◊ Nausea and vomiting
  ◊ Symptoms likely to occur with times of emotional stress and with activities as for subacute form
  ◊ Elevated intraocular pressure (usually 40-80 mm Hg)
  ◊ Corneal microcystic edema
  ◊ Lid edema, conjunctival hyperemia, and circumcorneal injection
  ◊ Fixed mid-dilated pupil, often oval
  ◊ Shallow anterior chamber often with inflammatory reaction
• Chronic
  ◊ May have symptoms of subacute form or may be asymptomatic
  ◊ Multiple peripheral anterior synechiae
  ◊ Normal or elevated intraocular pressure
  ◊ Increased cup to disc ratio
  ◊ Normal pupil

CAUSES Predisposing ocular anatomy

RISK FACTORS
• Small cornea
• Hyperopia
• Shallow anterior chamber
• Eskimo ancestry
• Female sex
• Use of antidepressants or other drugs with cholinergic inhibition
• Cataract
• Iris and ciliary body cysts

DIAGNOSIS

DIFFERENTIAL DIAGNOSIS
• Neovascular glaucoma
• Absolute glaucoma
• Malignant glaucoma
• Plateau iris syndrome
• Miotic induced glaucoma
• Phacomorphic glaucoma
• Anterior uveitis

LABORATORY None
Drugs that may alter lab results: N/A
Disorders that may alter lab results: N/A

PATHOLOGICAL FINDINGS
• Corneal stromal and epithelial edema
• Endothelial cell loss
• Iris stromal necrosis
• Anterior subcapsular cataract (glaukomflecken)
• Optic disc congestion, cupping
• Optic nerve atrophy

SPECIAL TESTS Gonioscopy

IMAGING N/A

DIAGNOSTIC PROCEDURES Careful ophthalmic examination including indentation gonioscopy and tonometry

TREATMENT

APPROPRIATE HEALTH CARE
• For acute form - inpatient admission from office or emergency room
• Other forms - outpatient
• Ophthalmology consultation

GENERAL MEASURES
• For acute form
  ◊ Intravenous access for administering medications is helpful, antiemetics may be necessary
  ◊ Definitive treatment is laser iridotomy once the attack is broken, intraocular pressure has normalized, and intraocular inflammation has subsided

SURGICAL MEASURES
• Peripheral iridectomy
• Argon or Nd:YAG laser iridotomy (procedure of choice for subacute and chronic forms)
• Argon laser gonioplasty

ACTIVITY For acute form - bedrest until attack subsides

DIET Usual for patient

PATIENT EDUCATION
• Usually patients need bilateral treatment since second eye is at risk for same disease process
• For patient education materials favorably reviewed on this topic, contact:
  ◊ Foundation for Glaucoma Research, 490 Post Street, Suite 830, San Francisco, CA 94102, (415)986-3162
  ◊ American Academy of Ophthalmology, 655 Beach Street, San Francisco, CA 94109, (415)561-8500

MEDICATIONS

DRUG(S) OF CHOICE
• For acute form: (a combination of the following)
◊ Hyperosmotic agents - oral 50% glycerin 0.1-1.5 g/kg or oral isosorbide dinitrate 1.5-2.0 g/kg, and/or intravenous mannitol 20% 1-2 g/kg over 45 minutes
◊ Carbonic anhydrase inhibition - acetazolamide (Diamox) 500 mg IV plus 500 mg po, then 250 mg po q6h prn; dorzolamide 2% eyedrops q8h.
Note: Use of the intravenous and oral agents above is sometimes necessary prior to the use of eye drops in order to lower the IOP enough to permit intraocular penetration.
◊ Beta-blockers - timolol (Timoptic) 0.5% q12h or levobunolol (Betagan) 0.5% q12h or betaxolol (Betoptic) 0.5% q12h
◊ Miotics - pilocarpine 2-4% one dose. In complicated cases with multiple mechanisms, miotics may paradoxically worsen the condition. Hence, they must be used with caution. See Contraindications.
◊ Corticosteroid - prednisolone acetate (Pred Forte) 1% q4-6h
◊ Other - apraclonidine (Iopidine) 0.5% or 1% q8h; also, latanoprost (Xalatan) 0.005% q24h
• For subacute and chronic forms:
◊ Treatment is surgical
Contraindications: With history of recent intraocular surgery, possibility of malignant glaucoma is increased and miotics may be contraindicated
Precautions:
• Timolol, levobunolol, and betaxolol, use with caution in patients with chronic heart failure or chronic obstructive pulmonary disease
• Mannitol, use with caution in patients with chronic heart failure or renal failure
• Acetazolamide, use with caution in patients with history of nephrolithiasis or metabolic acidosis
Significant possible interactions:
Acetazolamide may accelerate potassium loss and metabolic acidosis in patients on other diuretics

ALTERNATIVE DRUGS As above

FOLLOWUP

PATIENT MONITORING
• Subacute and chronic forms, check tonometry and gonioscopy initially every 3 months after laser iridotomy, follow visual fields every 6-12 months
• Acute form, discharge after laser iridotomy and intraocular pressure are controlled and follow as with the chronic form
• Consider frequent serum electrolytes while on mannitol
• Semi-annual CBC while on acetazolamide

PREVENTION/AVOIDANCE
Prophylactic laser treatment of second eye

POSSIBLE COMPLICATIONS
• Chronic corneal edema
• Corneal fibrosis and vascularization
• Iris atrophy
• Cataract
• Lens subluxation
• Optic atrophy
• Malignant glaucoma
• Central retinal vein occlusion

EXPECTED COURSE/PROGNOSIS
• Varies with delay of patient presentation and severity of attack
• Preceding chronic angle-closure may have caused optic atrophy
• Recurrence is quite rare following peripheral iridotomy or iridectomy and implies a rare variant known as the iris plateau syndrome

MISCELLANEOUS

ASSOCIATED CONDITIONS
• Cataract
• Microphthalmos
• Hyperopia

AGE-RELATED FACTORS
Pediatric: Rare
Geriatric: Secondary angle closure glaucoma can be caused by many common eye conditions in the elderly including cataract, ocular surgery and diabetes
Others: N/A

PREGNANCY N/A

SYNONYMS
• Acute glaucoma
• Narrow angle glaucoma

ICD-9-CM
365.20 Primary angle-closure glaucoma, unspecified
365.02 Borderline glaucoma, anatomical narrow angle

SEE ALSO Glaucoma, chronic open-angle

OTHER NOTES
• Medications (higher risk) that may exacerbate angle-closure glaucoma:
◊ Systemic or topical anticholinergics
◊ Topical sympathomimetics
◊ Antihistamines
◊ Phenothiazines
◊ Antidepressants
• Medications (lower risk) that may exacerbate angle-closure glaucoma:
◊ Benzodiazepine
◊ Carbonic anhydrase inhibitors
◊ CNS stimulants (including cocaine)
◊ MAO inhibitors
◊ Systemic sympathomimetics
◊ Theophylline
◊ Vasodilators

ABBREVIATIONS
NAG = narrow angle glaucoma

REFERENCES
• Ritch R, Shields MB, Krupin T: The Glaucomas. St. Louis, C.V. Mosby, 1989
• Fraunfelder FT, Roy FH: Current Ocular Therapy 3. 3rd Ed. Philadelphia, W.B. Saunders Co., 1990
Illustrations: N/A
Internet references: http://www.5mcc.com

Author(s)
Robert G. Fante, MD

Glomerulonephritis, acute

BASICS

DESCRIPTION
An immunologic response to an infection (usually streptococcal) which damages the renal glomeruli. It can be initiated by other bacterial and viral infections. This is an immune complex, hypocomplementemic glomerulonephritis. Most common in children. Characterized by diffuse inflammatory changes in the glomeruli and clinically by the abrupt onset of hematuria with red blood cell casts, and mild proteinuria. Accompanied in many cases by hypertension, edema, and azotemia.

System(s) affected: Renal/Urologic
Genetics: No known genetic pattern
Incidence/Prevalence in USA:
20/100,000/year (1-2% of pyodermas and 8% of streptococcal infections in children; occurs with impetigo in the late summer and with streptococcal pharyngitis in the winter)
Predominant age:
• 60% of cases in children 2-12 years old
• Only 10% older than 40 years of age
Predominant sex: Male > Female (60:40)

SIGNS AND SYMPTOMS
• Classic findings of acute nephritis
  ◊ Hematuria (100%)
  ◊ Oligoanuria (52%)
  ◊ Edema (85%)
  ◊ Hypertension (82%)
  ◊ Hypocomplementemia (C3) (83%)
  ◊ Gross hematuria (30%), tea-colored urine
  ◊ Edema of face and eyes in the am and feet and ankles in the afternoons and evenings
  ◊ Fever (rare)
• Other signs and symptoms
  ◊ Pharyngitis
  ◊ Respiratory infection
  ◊ Scarlet fever
  ◊ Dark urine
  ◊ Weight gain
  ◊ Abdominal pain
  ◊ Anorexia
  ◊ Back pain
  ◊ Pallor
  ◊ Impetigo

CAUSES
• Follows group A beta-hemolytic streptococcus infection
• "Nephritogenic" strains of strep - groups 1, 4, 11, 12, 49 "Red Lake", 55, 60
• Unusual to have a second attack - protective immunity to nephritogenic antigen
• Cases of "postinfective" glomerulonephritis have also been reported from pneumococcus, staphylococcus, meningococcus, chickenpox, and hepatitis
• Streptococcal infection precedes renal lesions by 1-3 weeks
• Pharyngitis precedes renal lesions by 1-2 weeks (types 1, 2, 4, 12)
• Impetigo - (types 49, 55, 57) usually precedes throat or otitis media infection by 2-4 weeks

RISK FACTORS
• 15% occurrence rate after infection with nephritogenic strain
• Endemic with cyclic epidemics
• Subclinical cases 20 times more common
• Streptococcal infection (e.g., scarlet fever or erysipelas) can be associated with rheumatic fever or acute glomerulonephritis, rarely both

DIAGNOSIS

DIFFERENTIAL DIAGNOSIS
• Membranoproliferative glomerulonephritis
• Other postinfective glomerulonephritis
• Systemic lupus erythematosus
• IgA nephropathy
• Anaphylactoid purpura
• Rapidly progressive glomerulonephritis

LABORATORY
• Streptococcal tests (Streptozyme) that include many antigens are most sensitive (+ or -) for screening but not quantitative
• Antistreptolysin O (ASO) - quantitative titer. Increased in 60-80% of cases. Increase begins 1-3 weeks, is highest 3-5 weeks, normal in 6 months. ASO titer is unrelated to severity, duration or prognosis of renal disease.
• Red blood cells casts on urinalysis:
  ◊ destroyed by centrifugation
  ◊ disintegrate in urine, particularly alkaline urine
• Characteristically, red blood cells from glomerular bleeding are distorted while those from lower urinary tract have normal morphology
• U/P creatinine > 40, decreased renin
• Culture throat and skin lesions for streptococcus
• C3 and C4 complements are best for evaluation
• Streptozyme
• Hypertriglyceridemia
• Proteinuria
• Decreased glomerular filtration rate
• Uremia
• Increased serum creatinine
• Anemia
• ANA to rule out systemic lupus erythematosus
Drugs that may alter lab results: N/A
Disorders that may alter lab results: N/A

PATHOLOGICAL FINDINGS
• On renal biopsy
  ◊ Diffuse proliferative and exudative glomerulonephritis
  ◊ Electron microscopy - subepithelial deposits
  ◊ Immunofluorescence - C3 in almost all cases, some with IgG and IgM

SPECIAL TESTS N/A

IMAGING
X-rays and/or ultrasound are not necessary to make the diagnosis

DIAGNOSTIC PROCEDURES
• If progressive, consider renal biopsy. Biopsy usually not indicated.

TREATMENT

APPROPRIATE HEALTH CARE
• Most patients can be safely followed as outpatients
• Inpatient usually until blood pressure and creatinine normalized and edema begins to recede

GENERAL MEASURES
• Decrease salt: no-added salt diet until edema and hypertension clear
• Decrease fluids to insensible losses plus 2/3 of the urine output until diuresis
• Control hypertension with diuretics
• Dialysis: peritoneal dialysis or hemodialysis for symptomatic azotemia, unresponsive hyperkalemia, intractable acidosis, diuretic resistant pulmonary edema

SURGICAL MEASURES N/A

ACTIVITY
Can return to full activity after clinically improved. May have increased hematuria after exercise for up to two years.

DIET
• "No-added" salt diet until edema, hypertension, and azotemia clear
• Restrict protein in presence of azotemia and metabolic acidosis
• Avoid high potassium foods

PATIENT EDUCATION
National Kidney Foundation, 30 E. 33rd Street, Suite 1100, New York, NY 10016, (212)889-2210

Glomerulonephritis, acute

MEDICATIONS

DRUG(S) OF CHOICE
• Hyperkalemia
◊ No potassium in IV fluids until hyperkalemia resolves
◊ Sodium polystyrene sulfonate (Kayexalate) resin: 1 gm/kg in 10% sorbitol, pr or po
◊ If acidosis present, treat as indicated below
◊ Hypocalcemia with symptomatic hyperkalemia: 0.5 cc/kg 10% calcium gluconate IV over 30 minutes
◊ Hypocalcemia with asymptomatic hyperkalemia: oral calcium carbonate (Tums) 1-2 gm calcium/day. (Tums have 650 mg calcium/tablet)
• Pulmonary edema
◊ Oxygen
◊ Furosemide (Lasix)
◊ Digitalization is not effective
• Peripheral edema
◊ Furosemide 1-2 mg/kg/dose given bid-tid po or IV
◊ Treatment with diuretics decreases the duration and severity of edema and hypertension
• Acidosis
◊ Sodium bicarbonate 1-2 mEq/kg/dose (1-2 mmol/kg/dose) IV over 30 minutes to correct acidosis
• Strep infection
◊ Give penicillin for 10 days (po if possible)
◊ Erythromycin in penicillin allergic patients
• Hypertension
◊ Control with diuretics (furosemide 0.5-1 mg/kg IV or 2 mg/kg po bid or tid) and vasodilators (hydralazine [Apresoline] 0.25-1.0 mg/kg qid or nifedipine 0.25 mg/kg po prn or qid)
Contraindications: Refer to manufacturer's literature
Precautions: Refer to manufacturer's literature
Significant possible interactions: Refer to manufacturer's literature

ALTERNATIVE DRUGS   N/A

FOLLOWUP

PATIENT MONITORING
• Depends on severity of disease
• Urinalysis at 2, 4 and 8 weeks and 4, 6 and 12 months
• Stop followup when urinalysis is normal
• Monitor blood pressure each visit
• Monitor serum creatinine at 2, 6, and 12 months
• C3 complement should be normal by 6 weeks

PREVENTION/AVOIDANCE   Treat streptococcal infections aggressively

POSSIBLE COMPLICATIONS
• Hypertensive retinopathy
• Hypertensive encephalopathy
• Rapidly progressive glomerulonephritis
• Abnormal urinalysis may persist for years (microhematuria)
• Chronic renal failure (rare)
• Nephrotic syndrome (approximately 10%)
• Marked decline in glomerular filtration rate (rare)

EXPECTED COURSE/PROGNOSIS
• Usually self-limited to 2-3 weeks
• Immediate mortality < 0.5%
• Long-term: excellent in children; almost all patients recover completely.
• May have more morbidity in adults or in those with pre-existing renal lesions
• Microscopic hematuria may persist for 24 months (or longer with complete recovery)
• Proteinuria persists for up to 3 months
• Symptoms can be exacerbated by a intercurrent illness but rarely after 12 months
• Urine may be darker (microscopic hematuria) after strenuous exercise

MISCELLANEOUS

ASSOCIATED CONDITIONS   N/A

AGE-RELATED FACTORS
Pediatric: Common in children ages 2-16
Geriatric: N/A
Others: N/A

PREGNANCY   N/A

SYNONYMS
• Acute nephritic syndrome
• Postinfectious glomerulonephritis
• Acute post-streptococcal glomerulonephritis

ICD-9-CM
580 Glomerulonephritis, acute

SEE ALSO
• Glomerulonephritis, membranous
• Hyperkalemia
• Renal failure, acute (ARF)
• Hypocalcemia
• Hypertensive emergencies

OTHER NOTES   N/A

ABBREVIATIONS   N/A

REFERENCES
• Brenner B, Rector F: The Kidney. 5th Ed. Philadelphia, W.B. Saunders Co., 1995
• Holliday M., Barratt T, Avner E: Pediatric Nephrology. 3rd Ed. Baltimore, Williams & Wilkins, 1993
Illustrations: N/A
Internet references: http://www.5mcc.com

Author(s)
Watson C. Arnold, MD

Glossitis

BASICS

DESCRIPTION Acute or chronic inflammation of the tongue either as a primary disease or symptom of systemic disease
System(s) affected: Gastrointestinal
Genetics: N/A
Incidence/Prevalence in USA: Common
Predominant age: All ages
Predominant sex: Male > Female

SIGNS AND SYMPTOMS
• Reddened tip and edges of tongue (with pellagra, anemia, excess smoking)
• Fiery red, swollen, ulcerated tongue (pellagra)
• Tongue smooth and pale (anemias)
• Ulcers (herpetic or aphthous lesions, streptococcal infection, erythema multiforme, pemphigus)
• White patches (candidiasis, syphilis, leukoplakia, lichen planus, mouth breathing)
• Denuded smooth areas (geographic tongue)
• Painful tongue (anemia, pellagra, viral)
• Hairy tongue (follows antibiotic therapy, fever or excessive use of mouthwashes with peroxide)
• Tenderness, pain, swelling of the tongue (infections or trauma)
• Burning, painful tongue (candidiasis, anemia, diabetes, malignancies)
• Non-painful solitary ulcerations (malignancy)
• Painful combination of ulcers, nodules, linear fissures (herpetic geometric glossitis in HIV)
• Malignancy - painless red and/or white lesions

CAUSES
• Systemic:
  ◊ Malnutrition with avitaminosis (e.g., B group)
  ◊ Anemia (pernicious, iron deficiency)
  ◊ Skin diseases (e.g., lichen planus, erythema multiforme, aphthous lesions, Behçet's syndrome, pemphigus vulgaris, syphilis)
  ◊ HIV (candidiasis, HSV, loss of papillae)
  ◊ Lansoprazole plus clarithromycin, amoxicillin, metronidazole (for treatment of H. Pylori in PUD)
• Local:
  ◊ Infections (viral, candidiasis, tuberculosis, streptococcal)
  ◊ Trauma (ill-fitting dentures, burns, convulsive seizures)
  ◊ Primary irritants (alcohol, tobacco, hot foods, spices, excessive peppermint, citrus)
  ◊ Sensitization (chemical irritants, e.g., dyes, mouth wash, toothpaste, systemic drugs)
  ◊ Malignancy

RISK FACTORS
• Low socioeconomic status
• Poor nutrition
• Dentures
• Smoking, smokeless tobacco
• Alcoholism
• Anxiety, stress
• Depression
• Advancing age
• Immunocompromised state

DIAGNOSIS

DIFFERENTIAL DIAGNOSIS
• Systemic:
  ◊ Avitaminosis (particularly B group, e.g., pellagra)
  ◊ Anemia (pernicious, iron deficiency)
  ◊ Skin diseases (e.g., lichen planus, erythema multiforme, aphthous lesions, Behçet's syndrome, pemphigus vulgaris, syphilis)
  ◊ HIV
• Local:
  ◊ Infections (viral, candidiasis, tuberculosis, streptococcal)
  ◊ Trauma (ill-fitting dentures, burns, convulsive seizures)
  ◊ Primary irritants: alcohol, tobacco, hot foods, spices
  ◊ Sensitization (chemical irritants, e.g., dyes, mouth wash, toothpaste, systemic drugs)
  ◊ Malignancy (95% are squamous cell)
  ◊ Geographic tongue (also known as migratory glossitis) - benign, but recurrent

LABORATORY
• CBC
• Serologic tests for syphilis
• Chemical profile
• Tests for vitamin B12 deficiency
• Postprandial glucose
• Smear and culture lesions when indicated
Drugs that may alter lab results: N/A
Disorders that may alter lab results: N/A

PATHOLOGICAL FINDINGS Varies
according to underlying causes

SPECIAL TESTS
• Biopsy solitary lesions that do not respond to treatment in one week
• 10% KOH scrapings for suspected candidiasis

IMAGING N/A

DIAGNOSTIC PROCEDURES
• Biopsy
• KOH scrapings

TREATMENT

APPROPRIATE HEALTH CARE
Outpatient

GENERAL MEASURES
• Avoid any possible sensitizing irritants or agents
• Specific therapy for oral infections (see Medications)
• Local treatment (see Medications)
• Analgesics when needed
• Request dental evaluation
• Scrupulous oral hygiene

SURGICAL MEASURES N/A

ACTIVITY No restrictions unless there is a systemic infection

DIET Bland or liquid diet

PATIENT EDUCATION Griffith:
Instructions for Patients; Philadelphia, W.B. Saunders Co. 5th ed., 1994

Glossitis

MEDICATIONS

DRUG(S) OF CHOICE
- For candidiasis:
  ◊ Nystatin oral suspension 400,000 units (4 mL) to 600,000 units qid for 10 days as an oral rinse, then swallowed
- For oral infections:
  ◊ Oral penicillin V
  ◊ Multivitamins (vitamin B-complex, vitamin E)
  ◊ Iron (if deficient)
- Local treatment:
  ◊ Mouth rinse with 2% lidocaine viscous, 1 tablespoon before each meal and every 3 hours if needed for pain
  ◊ Mouth wash of 1/2 teaspoon sodium bicarbonate in 8 oz (240 mL) warm water qid
  ◊ Mouth rinse with carbamide peroxide (Gly-Oxide) 10% 0.5 mL or 10 drops qid (expectorate after use) for irritation, aphthous ulcers
  ◊ Triamcinolone (Kenalog) in dental paste (Orabase): Compound triamcinolone 0.1% in emollient dental paste applied to specific lesions, especially aphthous ulcers
  ◊ 50/50 mixture of kaolin-pectin and diphenhydramine (Benadryl) as mouth rinse (coats and topically anesthetizes)

Contraindications: Refer to manufacturer's literature

Precautions: Depressed gag reflex with lidocaine viscous. Decreased sensitivity to hot/cold liquids.

Significant possible interactions: Refer to manufacturer's literature

ALTERNATIVE DRUGS
- For candidiasis:
  ◊ Clotrimazole - 10 mg oral lozenges 5 times a day for 10 days
  or
  ◊ Ketoconazole - one 200 mg tablet (for children 1/4 tablet) orally once a day

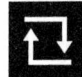

FOLLOWUP

PATIENT MONITORING
- Re-visits periodically when needed until healing occurs
- If lesions do not heal, biopsy is indicated

PREVENTION/AVOIDANCE
- Evaluation of nutritional status including B-vitamin deficiencies, anemias
- Cessation of tobacco use (including "smokeless")
- Assess for irritation from teeth, dentures

POSSIBLE COMPLICATIONS
- Lymphadenopathy
- Chronicity

EXPECTED COURSE/PROGNOSIS
- Prompt improvement when cause can be identified and treated
- Aphthous ulcers, erythema multiforme and hairy tongue often recur

MISCELLANEOUS

ASSOCIATED CONDITIONS
- Diabetes mellitus
- HIV infection

AGE-RELATED FACTORS
Pediatric: Median rhomboid glossitis is a developmental lesion causing a rhomboid-shaped, smooth, reddish, nodular area on the dorsal surface of the back portion of the middle third of the tongue. This type of glossitis is innocuous and requires no treatment.
Geriatric: Many patients with glossitis are postmenopausal or elderly
Others: N/A

PREGNANCY N/A

SYNONYMS N/A

ICD-9-CM 529 Glossitis

SEE ALSO
- HIV infection & AIDS
- Vitamin deficiency
- Candidiasis

OTHER NOTES Some symptoms of glossitis have no organic cause. Treat symptoms and reassure regarding malignancy.

ABBREVIATIONS N/A

REFERENCES
- Scully C, et al: Oral manifestations of HIV-infection and their management: More common lesions. Oral Surg, Oral Med & Oral Path 1991;71:158-166
- Cohen PR, et al: Geometric glossitis. Southern Med Jour 1995;88(12):1231-1235
- Kretzschmar JL, Kretzschmar DP: Common oral conditions. Amer Fam Phys 1996;54(1):225-234
- Grecos S: Glossitis, stomatitis, and black tongue with lansoprazole plus clarithromycin, etc. Annals of Pharmacother 1997;31(12):1548
- Drezner DA, Schaffer SR: Geographic tongue: Otolaryngology-Head and Neck Surgery 1997;117(3):291
Illustrations: 1 available on CD-ROM
Internet references: http://www.5mcc.com

Author(s)
J. Randall Richard, MD

Gonococcal infections

BASICS

DESCRIPTION Gonorrhea is a purulent inflammation of mucous membrane surfaces caused by a sexually transmitted microorganism, Neisseria gonorrhoeae. Virtually any mucous membrane can be infected. Occasionally the organism may become blood-borne causing a syndrome comprised of combinations of any of the following features: Fever, skin lesions, arthralgias/tenosynovitis, and septic arthritis.
• Hematogenous dissemination may also lead to endocarditis, or rarely, meningitis
• In women, salpingitis, local extension from the endocervical canal to the fallopian tubes is common. The ovaries may be involved with abscess formation. The entire complex of upper genital tract infection in women is referred to as pelvic inflammatory disease (PID).
• In men, the epididymis may become infected with extension to the testicle
• An asymptomatic carrier state can occur in both sexes
System(s) affected: Reproductive, Musculoskeletal, Nervous, Cardiovascular, Skin/Exocrine
Genetics: Individuals with congenital deficiency of the late components of the complement cascade (C 7,8,9) are prone to develop dissemination of local gonococcal infections
Incidence/Prevalence in USA: 600,000 new infections annually; approximately 240/100,000
Predominant age: 15-29
Predominant sex: Male > Female (symptomatic disease)

SIGNS AND SYMPTOMS
• Adolescent and adult males:
◊ Scant to copious purulent urethral discharge (98%)
◊ Dysuria (98%)
◊ Testicular pain (1%)
◊ Asymptomatic urethral infection (incidence of about 1%)
◊ Urethral stricture
• Adolescent and adult females without PID:
◊ Asymptomatic cervical infection (approximately 20%)
◊ Endocervical discharge (on pelvic exam) (96%)
◊ Vaginal discharge
◊ Dysuria
◊ Bartholin's gland abscess
• Adolescent and adult females with PID:
◊ Dysmenorrhea
◊ Metromenorrhagia
◊ Lower abdominal pain and tenderness
◊ Fever
◊ Cervical traction tenderness
◊ Palpable, tender fallopian tubes and/or ovaries
◊ Abdominal rebound tenderness
◊ Infertility
◊ Chronic pelvic pain

• Either sex, if receptive partner in anal intromission:
◊ Rectal discharge: purulent or bloody
◊ Tenesmus
◊ Rectal burning or itching
◊ Asymptomatic rectal infection
• Either sex, other syndromes:
◊ Pharyngeal infection - asymptomatic infection (98%), sore throat, exudative pharyngitis (< 1%)
◊ Eye infection (rare) - purulent discharge, conjunctivitis, chemosis, eyelid edema, corneal ulceration
◊ Disseminated syndromes - fever; chills; arthralgias (small joints); synovial sheath tenderness and swelling (hands and/or feet); painful skin lesions (pustular, red, tender); septic arthritis (usually asymmetric, polyarticular, and mainly involving elbows, knees and more distal joints; manifested by joint pain, swelling, erythema, and induration)
◊ Endocarditis - rapid cardiac valve destruction, high fevers
◊ Meningitis - meningeal signs, headache, skin lesions, fever, altered mental status
• Infants and children
◊ Eye infection (rare - because of routine ocular prophylaxis in the USA)
◊ Pneumonia (of the newborn) - fever, infiltrate on chest x-ray
◊ Vulvovaginitis - vaginal discharge
◊ Rectal infection
◊ Pharyngeal infection
◊ Meningitis
◊ Other forms of disseminated infection - fever, chills, arthralgias, synovial sheath tenderness and swelling, skin lesions, septic arthritis, endocarditis

CAUSES Neisseria gonorrhoeae (gonococcus)

RISK FACTORS
• Sexual exposure to an infected individual without barrier protection (condom)
• Multiple sexual partners
• Infant - passage through the infected birth canal of the mother
• Children - sexual abuse by infected individual
• Auto-inoculation (finger to eye)
• For PID - use of intrauterine devices

DIAGNOSIS

DIFFERENTIAL DIAGNOSIS
• Chlamydia infections (may mimic all aspects of gonococcal infections except disseminated syndromes)
• Urinary tract infections
• Vaginitis caused by other infectious agents (yeast, trichomonas, bacterial vaginosis)

LABORATORY
• Gram stain of exudate from infected mucosal surface
• Demonstration of pairs or clumps of Gram-negative kidney-shaped diplococci associated with the cytoplasm of polymorphonuclear leukocytes. The adjacent surfaces are slightly concave.
• Sensitivity of urethral smear in symptomatic male ≥95%
• Sensitivity of endocervical smear in infected woman = 40-60%
• DNA probes (not approved for use in children): sensitivity 92->99% dependent upon population; specificity >97%
• Culture of exudate on selective medium (Thayer-Martin or Martin-Lewis, containing antibiotics to inhibit other microorganisms). Demonstration of typical organisms by Gram-stain morphology and growth on selective media constitutes a "presumptive" diagnosis of gonococcal infection. Culture should always be done in suspected cases of infection in children.
• Sensitivity of blood culture in disseminated disease - 50%
• Sensitivity of joint fluid culture in septic arthritis - 50%
Drugs that may alter lab results: Prior administration of even small amounts of many antibiotics may render a culture falsely negative
Disorders that may alter lab results: N/A

PATHOLOGICAL FINDINGS
• Exudate of polymorphonuclear leukocytes is typical
• In PID - loss of ciliated columnar epithelium from the fallopian tubes. Tubes, pelvic mesentery, and ovaries may be bound together with dense fibrosis and abscess formation.

SPECIAL TESTS
• Confirmation of the isolate as the gonococcus by standard sugar fermentation tests, enzymatic tests or DNA probes. Important in medicolegal situations such as rape or child abuse since other Neisseria, which are normal inhabitants of mucosal surfaces, may look like gonococcus on Gram-stained smear.
• Testing for antimicrobial susceptibility. ß-lactamase production and chromosomally mediated resistance to penicillin and/or tetracycline are becoming more common. Although routine ß-lactamase testing of N. gonorrhoeae has been recommended by the U.S. Public Health Service, the need for such testing is questionable if current therapy guidelines are observed.

IMAGING Pelvic ultrasound or CT scan may demonstrate thick, dilated fallopian tubes or abscess formation

DIAGNOSTIC PROCEDURES
• Culdocentesis may demonstrate free purulent exudate, and provide material for gram staining and culture
• Gram staining material from unroofed skin lesions may show typical organisms

TREATMENT

APPROPRIATE HEALTH CARE
• Outpatient for uncomplicated infection, with contact notification and contact treatment
• Hospitalize for:
  ◊ Hematogenously disseminated infection
  ◊ Pneumonia or eye infection in infants
  ◊ PID: if unable to take oral medications, significant tubo-ovarian abscess, or patient is pregnant

GENERAL MEASURES
• Abstain from sexual activity until after full treatment, plus testing and treatment of partner(s)
• DNA probe testing for chlamydia
• Serologic test for syphilis
• Encourage testing for HIV infection

SURGICAL MEASURES N/A

ACTIVITY Fully active for uncomplicated disease

DIET No special diet

PATIENT EDUCATION
• Discuss sexually transmitted diseases and methods of prevention
• Discuss HIV infection and risks; encourage patient and partner(s) to be tested

MEDICATIONS

DRUG(S) OF CHOICE
• Treatment of adults:
  ◊ Uncomplicated N. gonorrhoeae infection of urethra, cervix, rectum, and/or pharynx: Initial single dose of ceftriaxone 125 mg IM or cefixime 400 mg po or ofloxacin 400 mg po or ciprofloxacin 500 mg po plus an agent with activity against chlamydia, e.g., doxycycline 100 mg po bid x 7 days or azithromycin 1.0 g po as a single dose
Note: In pregnancy, ceftriaxone is the treatment of choice. Erythromycin 500 mg po qid x 7 days is an alternative anti-chlamydia agent for use in pregnancy. In the absence of pregnancy, ofloxacin 300 mg po bid x 7 days is another alternative anti-chlamydia therapy. Alternative parenteral agents for therapy of gonococcal infections include other 3rd generation cephalosporins and spectinomycin.
  ◊ PID: outpatients regimens (see citations for treatment of hospitalized patients)
    - Regimen A: Ofloxacin 400 mg po bid x 14 days plus clindamycin 450 mg po qid x 14 days or metronidazole 500 mg po bid x 14 days
    - Regimen B: Cefoxitin 2g IM + probenecid 1g po or ceftriaxone 250 mg IM plus doxycycline 100 mg po bid x 14 days

• Disseminated infections in adults
  ◊ Bacteremia and dermatitis-arthritis complex: ceftriaxone 1g IV daily. With clinical improvement, complete of 7-10 days of therapy with cefixime 400 mg po bid, ciprofloxacin 500 mg po bid, or other agents to which the infecting organism has been proven fully susceptible.
  ◊ Meningitis: Ceftriaxone 1-2g IV q 12 hours for 10-14 days
  ◊ Endocarditis: Ceftriaxone 1-2g IV q 12 hours for 4 weeks
Note: Parenteral penicillin G can be used to treat disseminated infection if full susceptibility is documented. Other third generation cephalosporins also can be substituted for ceftriaxone for parenteral therapy; spectinomycin 2 g IM q12hr is an alternative to initial ß-lactamase; IV ofloxacin or ciprofloxacin are also alternatives.
• Treatment of infants and children < 45 kg: (patients >45 kg should receive full adult dose)
  ◊ Uncomplicated genital, pharyngeal, rectal, or conjunctival infection and infants born to mothers with untreated gonorrhea
    - Ceftriaxone 125 mg IM in single dose. Alternative is spectinomycin 40 mg/kg up to 2 g as single IM dose.
  ◊ Disseminated infections: ceftriaxone 50 mg/kg IV or IM daily
    - 7 days for bacteremia or dermatitis/arthritis complex
    - 10-14 days for meningitis
    - 28 days for endocarditis
  ◊ Ophthalmic neonatorum prophylaxis: single application of:
    - 1% silver nitrate aqueous solution, or
    - 0.5% erythromycin ophthalmic ointment, or
    - 1% tetracycline ophthalmic ointment
Contraindications: Fluoroquinolones and tetracyclines such as doxycycline are contraindicated in pregnancy
Precautions: Refer to manufacturer's profile of each drug
Significant possible interactions: Refer to manufacturer's profile of each drug

ALTERNATIVE DRUGS If organisms not penicillin-resistant, use IV penicillin G. (Note: Some penicillin resistance is now due to penicillinase production.) Oral ampicillin or amoxicillin plus probenecid may be substituted for cephalosporins in uncomplicated disease, also after lab confirms absence of penicillin-resistance. Spectinomycin is an alternative if ß-lactam agents, fluoroquinolones cannot be used.

FOLLOWUP

PATIENT MONITORING Retesting to document cure is not necessary if one of the recommended regimens is used unless symptoms persist or there is concern about poor compliance with therapy

PREVENTION/AVOIDANCE
• Condoms offer partial protection
• Sexual contacts should be treated

POSSIBLE COMPLICATIONS
• Urethral stricture in men
• Infertility in women
• Corneal scarring after eye infections
• Destruction of joint articular surfaces
• Destruction of cardiac valves
• Death from CHF or meningitis

EXPECTED COURSE/PROGNOSIS
With adequate, early therapy complete cure and return to normal function is the rule

MISCELLANEOUS

ASSOCIATED CONDITIONS Other sexually transmitted infections (chlamydia, syphilis, HIV, hepatitis B, herpes) and vaginal infections

AGE-RELATED FACTORS
Pediatric: N/A
Geriatric: N/A
Others: N/A

PREGNANCY PID may lead to fetal loss, or premature labor and delivery

SYNONYMS
• GC
• Clap

ICD-9-CM
098 Gonococcal infections
098.0 Acute, lower genitourinary tract
614.9 Unspecified inflammatory disease of female pelvic organs and tissue

SEE ALSO
• Chlamydial sexually transmitted diseases
• Pelvic inflammatory disease (PID)
• Syphilis

OTHER NOTES N/A

ABBREVIATIONS
• GC = gonococcal
• PID = pelvic inflammatory disease

REFERENCES
• Centers for Disease Control and Prevention (CDC). 1998 Guidelines for treatment of sexually transmitted diseases. Morbidity Mortality Weekly report 1998;47(RR-1):1-118
• Handsfield HH, Sparling FR: Neisseria gonorrhoeae. In: Mandell GL, Bennett JE, Dolin R, eds. Principles and Practice of Infectious Diseases, 4th Ed. New York, Churchill Livingstone, 1995:1409-1926
Illustrations: 1 available on CD-ROM
Internet references: http://www.5mcc.com

Author(s)
Leonard N. Slater, MD

Gout

BASICS

DESCRIPTION Inflammatory reaction to urate crystals in joints, bones and subcutaneous structures. Initially, a hyperacute arthritis which may progress to a chronic arthritis. Rarely it may present as a chronic arthritis. Recognition of the crystals in fluid is pathognomonic.
• Primary gout - the most common: underexcretion or overproduction of uric acid
• Secondary gout - related to myeloproliferative diseases or their treatment, therapeutic regimens producing hyperuricemia, renal failure, renal tubular disorders, lead poisoning, hyperproliferative skin disorders, enzymatic defects (e.g., deficient hypoxanthine guanine phosphoribosyltransferase, glycogen storage diseases)
System(s) affected: Musculoskeletal, Endocrine/Metabolic, Renal/Urologic
Genetics: N/A
Incidence/Prevalence in USA: 100/100,000. Under age 18: rare; age 18-44: 3; age 45-64: 21; age over 65: 35
Predominant age: 30-60
Predominant sex: Male > Female (20:1)

SIGNS AND SYMPTOMS
• Hyperacute onset (within 24 hours) of severe pain, swelling, redness, and warmth in one or two joints (75% are monoarticular)
• Soft tissue redness, swelling, warmth
• Exquisite tenderness
• Propensity for first MTP joint, symptomatic in 50% of initial attacks; eventually in 75%
• Acute untreated attacks last 2-21 days
• Attack may be isolated, more often repetitive, 2nd attack may not occur for years
• Recurrent attacks last longer and occur more frequently with each recurrence
• Intracritical period - absence of inflammation (until the chronic or tophaceous phase occurs)
• Rarely polyarticular - proximal interphalangeal, distal interphalangeal, metacarpal phalangeal, wrist, knee, ankle, midtarsal joints, heel
• Migratory polyarthritis is a rare presentation
• 50% of untreated patients develop a chronic arthritis within 3-42 years
• Inflammatory synovial effusion
• Subcutaneous or intraosseous nodules (20%), referred to as tophi - may affect ears (antihelix), extensor aspects of peripheral joints (e.g., olecranon), rarely fingertips, cornea, aorta, spine or even intracranial
• Subcutaneous nodules may have a creamy (urate) discharge
• Fever, chills
• Carpal tunnel syndrome
• Kidney stones

CAUSES
• Hyperuricemia
• Dietary excess (e.g., anchovies, sardines, sweetbreads, kidney, liver and meat extracts)
• Inborn errors of metabolism
• Lead poisoning (Saturnine gout from moonshine)
• Kidney disease
• Hemoproliferative disorders

RISK FACTORS
• Ethanol ingestion
• Family history
• Polynesian extraction (e.g., Samoan gout)
• Medications - aminophylline, caffeine, corticosteroids, cytotoxic drugs (cyclosporine), diazepam, diphenhydramine, diuretics, L-dopa, dopamine, epinephrine, ethambutol, methaqualone, alpha-methyl dopa, nicotinic acid, probenecid (low dose), pyrazinamide, salicylates (< 10/dL blood levels), sulfinpyrazone (low dose), vitamins B12 and C.
• Diuretics may be responsible for 20% of secondary gout
• Ketosis
• Surgery or trauma
• Obesity (50%)
• Hypertension (50%)
• Vascular disease
• Diabetes
• Renal failure
• Hypothyroidism
• Hyperparathyroidism; hypoparathyroidism
• Hyperlipidemia types II, IV, V
• Paget's disease
• Hyperproliferative skin disorders (e.g., psoriasis)
• Lymphoproliferative disorders
• Calcium pyrophosphate deposition disease
• Sarcoidosis
• Hemolytic anemia
• Hemoglobinopathies
• Pernicious anemia
• Radiation treatment
• Type I glycogen storage disease
• Down syndrome
• Gut sterilization by antibiotics

DIAGNOSIS

DIFFERENTIAL DIAGNOSIS Infectious arthritis, pseudogout (calcium pyrophosphate deposition disease), type IIa hyperproteinemia, amyloidosis, multicentric reticulohistiocytosis, hyperparathyroidism, spondyloarthropathy, rheumatoid arthritis (rarely)

LABORATORY
• WBC usually elevated with left shift during acute attacks
• ESR usually elevated during acute attacks
• Hyperuricemia may be present, although not diagnostic
Drugs that may alter lab results:
• Intra-articular steroids - many have inherent birefringence, which will cause confusion on synovial fluid analysis
• Hyperuricemia - induced by drugs that reduce effective circulating blood volume (induced by low dose aspirin, probenecid or sulfinpyrazone)
• Cyclosporine - induced renal insufficiency
Disorders that may alter lab results:
Alcoholism, sarcoidosis, lead poisoning, kidney failure, psoriasis, hemoglobinopathy

PATHOLOGICAL FINDINGS
• Urate crystals in synovial membrane (98% of specimens processed entirely anhydrously [urate is water soluble])
• Tophus in 29% of individuals with untreated gout of 5 years duration, in 74% of individuals with untreated gout of 40 years duration

SPECIAL TESTS
• Synovial fluid white blood cell count is usually inflammatory (10,000-70,000 cells/dL), but may have as few as 1,000 WBC/dL
• Wet mounts of synovial fluid reveal negatively birefringent urate crystals on polarizing exam
• Gout crystals may be identified in asymptomatic joints

IMAGING
• X-ray is usually normal in the first year of uncontrolled disease.
• X-ray in chronic gout reveals "punched-out" erosions (lytic areas) often with periosteum overgrowing the erosion ("overhanging edge" sign). This is highly suggestive, but may also be caused by amyloidosis, type IIa hyperlipoproteinemia, and by multicentric reticulohistiocytosis.
• X-ray erosions with preservation of joint space is similarly characteristic. X-ray rarely reveals intraosseous lytic areas (tophi).
• Bone scan reveals increased nuclide concentration at affected sites

DIAGNOSTIC PROCEDURES
• Arthrocentesis with polarizing optical examination
• Biopsy of synovial membrane or subcutaneous nodule, processing the specimen anhydrously (urate is water soluble) and examining with polarizing optics

TREATMENT

APPROPRIATE HEALTH CARE
Outpatient, except for consideration of associated joint infection or for therapeutic unresponsiveness

GENERAL MEASURES
• Control the acute attack of gout
• Addressing the underlying cause

SURGICAL MEASURES N/A

ACTIVITY Affected joint(s) at rest until hyperacute phase is controlled

DIET Reduce ingestion of fat, alcoholic beverages, sardines, anchovies, liver, sweetbreads

PATIENT EDUCATION
• Arthritis Foundation pamphlet on gout
• Rothschild, BM.: Hyperuricemia in the elderly. Geriatric Consultant, 4:14-16, 31, 1985.

Gout

MEDICATIONS

DRUG(S) OF CHOICE
- Acute attack
  - ◊ A NSAID at full dosage for 2-5 days
  - ◊ When acute attack is controlled, reduce dose by 1/4 - 1/2
- Chronic treatment
  - ◊ Initiate when acute attack controlled (unless kidneys at risk because of unusual uric acid load)
  - ◊ Generally not pursued unless recurrent attacks or evidence of tophaceous or renal disease
  - ◊ Any contributing medication regimens are first altered and any predisposing medical conditions/habits addressed
  - ◊ Patient is tested for uric acid excretion (<600 mg/day while on purine free diet or <800 mg/day on unrestricted diet implies hypoexcretor)
    - Hypoexcretor: probenecid is initiated at 500 mg qd and increased by 500 mg at monthly intervals, until the uric acid is lowered to normal range or at least 2 mg/dL (0.12 mmol/L) less than the levels during which attacks are noted. (Maximum dose 2-3 g/day.) Urinary alkalinization and recommendation of ingestion of copious amounts of fluid are adjunctive.
    - Hyperexcretor, tophaceous or renal disease are present: allopurinol, initiated at 100 mg qd and increased by 100 mg weekly, to a maximum of 600 mg per day.

Contraindications:
- NSAIDs:
  - ◊ Peptic ulcer disease
  - ◊ Psychosis
  - ◊ Severe headache
  - ◊ Pregnancy
  - ◊ Concomitant anticoagulant use
  - ◊ Presence of a blood dyscrasia
- Probenecid:
  - ◊ Uric acid overproduction
  - ◊ Uric acid stones
  - ◊ Renal impairment
  - ◊ Concomitant salicylates
- Allopurinol:
  - ◊ Bone marrow suppression
  - ◊ Liver disease
  - ◊ Concomitant cytotoxic drugs
  - ◊ Diuretics may require increased amount of allopurinol

Precautions:
- Probenecid and allopurinol may predispose to acute gouty attacks. Use low dose NSAID for 6-24 mos to reduce risk.
- Reduce NSAID dosage in presence of renal or liver disease
- Reduce cytotoxic drug dose in presence of allopurinol
- With allopurinol risk of skin rash

Significant possible interactions:
- NSAIDs:
  - ◊ Anticoagulants
  - ◊ Anti-diabetic agents
  - ◊ Anticonvulsants
  - ◊ Lithium
- Probenecid:
  - ◊ Antibiotics
  - ◊ Antidiabetic agents
  - ◊ Thiopental
  - ◊ Ketamine
  - ◊ NSAID's
  - ◊ Lorazepam
  - ◊ Rifampin
  - ◊ Antagonized by pyrazinamide, salicylates
- Allopurinol:
  - ◊ Mercaptopurine (requires reduction of chemotherapy dose to 1/3 of usual dose)
  - ◊ Azathioprine
  - ◊ Methotrexate
  - ◊ Possibly cyclophosphamide
  - ◊ Anticoagulants
  - ◊ Antidiabetic agents

ALTERNATIVE DRUGS
- Related to control of the acute attack:
  - ◊ Colchicine, a controversial toxic agent which must be taken within 24 hours of onset of the acute attack to be effective; IV preferred 2 mg, followed by 1 mg q6h for 2 doses; do not repeat in less than 3 days
  - ◊ Intra-articular long-acting (depot) corticosteroid (if infection definitely ruled out)
- Related to control of the underlying hyperuricemia in the hypoexcretor:
  - ◊ Sulfinpyrazone, initiated at 400 mg qd
  - ◊ ACTH 40-80 IU IM

FOLLOWUP

PATIENT MONITORING
- Related to medicinal control of the acute attack and suppressing attacks:
  - ◊ Adjusting therapeutic regimen if no significant clinical response to therapy within 3 days of its initiation.
  - ◊ CBC, renal and hepatic blood testing and urinalysis at 1 wk, 6 wks and every 3 months
- Related to control of the underlying hyperuricemia:
  - ◊ CBC, uric acid level, renal and hepatic blood testing, and urinalysis at monthly intervals (with dosage/regimen modification) until desired serum uric acid level achieved

PREVENTION/AVOIDANCE
Avoidance of exacerbating medications/diets/habits

POSSIBLE COMPLICATIONS
- Increased susceptibility to infection
- Urate nephropathy
- Uric acid nephropathy
- Renal stones
- Nerve/spinal cord impingement
- Recognition of urate crystals does not preclude concomitant infectious arthritis

EXPECTED COURSE/PROGNOSIS
- With early treatment, total control
- If recurrent attacks, successful uric acid adjustment (requiring lifelong use of uricosuric or allopurinol medication) usually effective
- During the first 6-24 months of uricosuric or allopurinol therapy, acute gout may occur

MISCELLANEOUS

ASSOCIATED CONDITIONS
- Myeloproliferative disorders
- Lymphoproliferative disorders
- Ethanolism
- Hyperlipidemia
- Obesity
- Hypertension
- Diabetes
- Lesch-Nyhan syndrome - chorea, spasticity, self-mutilation in childhood

AGE-RELATED FACTORS
Pediatric: Onset in this age group identifies gout secondary to an inborn error of metabolism or underlying disease process
Geriatric: Usually related to medications
Others: N/A

PREGNANCY
Usual pregnancy precautions

SYNONYMS
N/A

ICD-9-CM
274.0 Gouty arthropathy
274.1 Gouty nephropathy
274.11 Uric acid nephrolithiasis
274.81 Gouty tophi of ear
984.9 Toxic effect of unspecified lead compound

SEE ALSO
- Alcoholism
- Anemia, sickle cell

OTHER NOTES
N/A

ABBREVIATIONS
MP = metatarsal phalangeal
NSAID = nonsteroidal anti-inflammatory drug

REFERENCES
- Yu TF: Gout. In: Katz W, ed. Diagnosis and Management of Rheumatic Diseases. Philadelphia, J.B. Lippincott, 1988
- Kelley WN, Harris ED Jr, Ruddy S, Sledge CB: Textbook of Rheumatology. Philadelphia, W.B. Saunders Co., 1997
- Rothschild BM: Crystalline Arthritis: Gout. Fairlawn, CT, Clinical AV, 1982
- Rothschild BM, Heathcote GM: Characterization of gout in a skeletal population sample. Amer J Phys Anthrol 1995;98:529-525
- Vazquez-Mellado J, et al: Intradermal topic in gout. J Rheum 1997;26:136-140
Illustrations: 2 available on CD-ROM
Internet references: http://www.5mcc.com

Author(s)
Bruce M. Rothschild, MD

Granuloma annulare

BASICS

DESCRIPTION Chronic, self-limited inflammation of the skin exhibited by annularly arranged papules
• Localized granuloma annulare: the more common form consists of a solitary group of flesh colored papules that gradually involute centrally to form circles or semi-circles
• Disseminated granuloma annulare: occurs less often (approximately 15%) and consists of widespread lesions with the same characteristics as the localized type
System(s) affected: Skin/Exocrine
Genetics: Not specified, although a familial incidence has been noted among siblings, twins, and successive generations
Incidence/Prevalence in USA: N/A
Predominant age:
• Localized granuloma annulare: children and young adults
• Disseminated granuloma annulare: younger than age 10 or older than 40 years
Predominant sex: Females > Males (2:1)

SIGNS AND SYMPTOMS
• Papular, circular or semi-circular lesions
• Papules usually found on dorsal surface of hands, fingers, feet, extensor aspects of arms and legs, trunk
• Subcutaneous nodules seen on palms, legs, buttocks, scalp
• Papules can perforate
• Lesions may be pruritic on rare occasions, but usually asymptomatic

CAUSES   Unknown

RISK FACTORS
• Diabetes mellitus
• Positive family history
• Rheumatoid arthritis

DIAGNOSIS

DIFFERENTIAL DIAGNOSIS
• Papular lesions
  ◊ Necrobiosis lipoidica
  ◊ Cutaneous amyloidosis
  ◊ Annular elastolytic granuloma
  ◊ Papular sarcoid
  ◊ Lichen planus
  ◊ Tinea
  ◊ Tuberculoid (TT) or borderline tuberculoid (BT) leprosy
  ◊ Erythema migrans
  ◊ Verruca plana
  ◊ Majocchi granuloma
  ◊ Appendageal hamartomas, e.g., eruptive syringomata
• Subcutaneous nodules
  ◊ Rheumatoid nodules

LABORATORY   If disseminated form, check blood sugar. Also rheumatoid factor if symptoms of RA present.
Drugs that may alter lab results: N/A
Disorders that may alter lab results: N/A

PATHOLOGICAL FINDINGS   Palisading granuloma with histiocytes and epithelial cells surrounding a central zone of altered collagen in the mid to upper dermis

SPECIAL TESTS   N/A

IMAGING   N/A

DIAGNOSTIC PROCEDURES
• Inspection of skin usually reveals diagnosis
• Skin scraping to rule out fungi can be done
• If diagnosis is in doubt, skin biopsy can be performed

TREATMENT

APPROPRIATE HEALTH CARE
Outpatient

GENERAL MEASURES   Treatment is not always satisfactory.

SURGICAL MEASURES   N/A

ACTIVITY   Full activity

DIET   American Diabetic Association guidelines when associated with diabetes

PATIENT EDUCATION   If patient has disseminated form, papules may be accentuated by sun exposure

Granuloma annulare

MEDICATIONS

DRUG(S) OF CHOICE
• Localized form - intralesional triamcinolone acetonide, 5-10 mg/mL injected into the elevated border only. A 30 gauge needle is used. May be repeated at monthly intervals.
• Topical steroids with occlusion or incorporated in tape are occasionally useful for localized form
• Disseminated form - dapsone 100 mg qd or bid; PUVA or REPUVA

Contraindications: Dapsone should not be given to patients with G6PD deficiency
Precautions: See manufacturer's profile of each drug
Significant possible interactions: See manufacturer's profile of each drug

ALTERNATIVE DRUGS
• Superficial lesions of the localized form may respond to cryotherapy with liquid nitrogen, but atrophy is possible
• For disseminated form isotretinoin 80 mg qd is used in refractive cases
• Niacin 1.5 gm qd or potassium iodide is recommended by some

FOLLOWUP

PATIENT MONITORING Depends on nature of treatment; generally two week intervals while undergoing treatment

PREVENTION/AVOIDANCE Avoid sun-exposure in patients with disseminated form if association with light

POSSIBLE COMPLICATIONS None

EXPECTED COURSE/PROGNOSIS
• Lesions disappear without scarring in 75% of patients in two years
• 40% of patients experience recurrences, often at the original site

MISCELLANEOUS

ASSOCIATED CONDITIONS
• Diabetes mellitus is mainly associated with disseminated granuloma annulare but the frequency is unknown. Likewise, some patients with rheumatoid arthritis have developed granuloma annulare.
• Can be associated with other granulomatous disease, such as, necrobiosis lipoidica, rheumatoid nodules and sarcoidosis

AGE-RELATED FACTORS
Pediatric: N/A
Geriatric: Disseminated form is more common in older patients
Others: N/A

PREGNANCY N/A

SYNONYMS N/A

ICD-9-CM
695.89 Other specified erythematous conditions, other

SEE ALSO
• Diabetes mellitus, Type 1
• Diabetes mellitus, Type 2
• Arthritis, rheumatoid (RA)
• Sarcoidosis

OTHER NOTES N/A

ABBREVIATIONS N/A

REFERENCES
• Habif T: Clinical Dermatology. 3rd Ed. St Louis, Mosby, 1996
• Goldstein B, Goldstein A: Practical Dermatology. 2nd Ed. St Louis, Mosby, 1997
• Freedberg IM, et al: Fitzpatrick's Dermatology in General Medicine, 5th ed. New York, McGraw Hill, 1999.
Illustrations: 6 available on CD-ROM
Internet references: http://www.5mcc.com

Author(s)
Gary J. Silko, MD

Granuloma, pyogenic

BASICS

DESCRIPTION Benign, solitary mass that involves exposed areas such as distal extremities and face as well as the oral cavity (most frequently the gingiva)
System(s) affected: Skin/Exocrine, Gastrointestinal
Genetics: N/A
Incidence/Prevalence in USA: Unknown
Predominant age: Any, most frequently children and second to fifth decades
Predominant sex: Slight predilection for females

SIGNS AND SYMPTOMS
• Sessile or pedunculated
• Granular, smooth or slightly nodular
• Soft
• May be ulcerated, bleeding easily
• Red, purple, or brown in color
• Ranges from a few millimeters to 2-3 centimeters in diameter

CAUSES
• Thought to be an over-reaction to minor trauma
• May be related to hormonal changes in pregnancy

RISK FACTORS
• Pregnancy
• Intraoral trauma or surgery

DIAGNOSIS

DIFFERENTIAL DIAGNOSIS
• Peripheral ossifying granuloma
• Giant cell granuloma
• Odontogenic fibroma
• Kaposi's sarcoma
• Malignant melanoma
• Angiolymphoid hyperplasia with eosinophilia
• Metastatic carcinoma
• IN AIDS patients, bacillary angiomatosis, deep mycoses

LABORATORY N/A
Drugs that may alter lab results: N/A
Disorders that may alter lab results: N/A

PATHOLOGICAL FINDINGS
• Micro-small, endothelial lined vascular spaces
• Micro- loose or dense connective tissue stroma
• Micro- acute and chronic inflammatory cells
• Micro- no true granuloma formation
• Micro- abundant mitotic activity

SPECIAL TESTS N/A

IMAGING N/A

DIAGNOSTIC PROCEDURES
Excisional biopsy

TREATMENT

APPROPRIATE HEALTH CARE
Outpatient

GENERAL MEASURES
• Occasional spontaneous resolution
• Good oral hygiene

SURGICAL MEASURES
• Surgical excision of lesion (with cleaning of adjacent teeth if lesion is gingival)
• May recur if inadequately excised

ACTIVITY As tolerated

DIET As tolerated

PATIENT EDUCATION Patient should avoid trauma to the area following excision

MEDICATIONS

DRUG(S) OF CHOICE None
Contraindications: N/A
Precautions: N/A
Significant possible interactions: N/A

ALTERNATIVE DRUGS N/A

FOLLOWUP:

PATIENT MONITORING As needed

PREVENTION/AVOIDANCE Good oral hygiene

POSSIBLE COMPLICATIONS
Recurrence. After removal or destruction of a solitary lesion, multiple satellite lesions can form around the original treatment site.

EXPECTED COURSE/PROGNOSIS
Complete resolution expected with adequate excision.

MISCELLANEOUS

ASSOCIATED CONDITIONS N/A

AGE-RELATED FACTORS N/A
Pediatric: N/A
Geriatric: N/A
Others: N/A

PREGNANCY Lesion also occurs in pregnant women, and is known as "pregnancy tumor"

SYNONYMS
• Pregnancy tumor
• Granuloma gravidum

ICD-9-CM
686.1 Pyogenic granuloma
522.6 Maxillary alveolar ridge
528.9 Oral mucosa

SEE ALSO N/A

OTHER NOTES N/A

ABBREVIATIONS N/A

REFERENCES
• Wood NK, Goaz PW: Differential Diagnosis of Oral Lesions. St. Louis, C.V. Mosby, 1985
• Ash MM: Oral Pathology. Philadelphia, Lea & Febiger, 1986
Illustrations: 3 available on CD-ROM
Internet references: http://www.5mcc.com

Author(s)
Laurene L. Howell, MD
Gregg W. Suits, MD

Guillain-Barre syndrome

BASICS

DESCRIPTION A group of demyelinating diseases causing acute progressive weakness, usually an ascending paralysis. 30% have respiratory paralysis requiring mechanical ventilation, but complete or substantial recovery is the rule.
System(s) affected: Nervous
Genetics: Not directly genetically inherited. presumed to be individual's idiosyncratic response to preceding infection, which may have a genetic basis
Incidence/Prevalence in USA:
0.6-1.9/100,000, non-seasonal, non-epidemic
Predominant age: All ages
Predominant sex: Male > Female (1.5:1)

SIGNS AND SYMPTOMS
• Acute, progressive weakness of all 4 limbs, symmetric and usually ascending
• Areflexia associated with the muscle weakness
• Pain common, especially back, legs, and extremities, may be severe, not predictive of disease course
• Gait disorder common in all age groups: the most common presentation of disease
• Dysesthesias, paresthesias (often perioral), pain in band distribution, decreased position and vibratory sensation common
• Autonomic neuropathy (50%) with hypo- and hypertension, labile BP, arrhythmias (atrial and ventricular), ileus, and/or urinary retention
• Respiratory muscle paralysis 30% in untreated disease. Neck muscle weakness, dysphagia, shoulder weakness predictors of impending respiratory failure.
• Cranial nerve involvement 50%: usually facial weakness, 10-20% ocular involvement
• Important variants
 ◊ Miller-Fisher syndrome (5%): ataxia, ophthalmoplegia, and areflexia
 ◊ Bulbar variant: dysphagia, dysarthria, drooling with descending weakness
 ◊ AMAN (acute motor axonal neuropathy): pure motor involvement, previous Campylobacter jejuni infection, axonal injury, poorer prognosis for recovery
 ◊ AMSAN (acute motor-sensory axonal neuropathy): both motor and sensory involvement, otherwise similar to AMAN
 ◊ Other variants: only lower extremity weakness; pharyngeal-cervical-brachial muscle weakness; pure sensory forms. Upper extremity weakness may occur before lower extremity weakness; proximal reflexes may be lost before distal. Cranial nerves frequently involved.

CAUSES
• Autoimmune destruction of myelin and/or axon
• Upper respiratory or diarrheal illness within previous 1-3 weeks in 50-70%, including Campylobacter jejuni (30-40%), CMV (13%), EBV (10%), Mycoplasma pneumoniae (5%), HIV
• Vaccinations: swine flu (but not other influenza vaccine) and rabies
• Malignancies (lymphoma, especially Hodgkin's)
• Surgery

• Drugs: gold, penicillamine, streptokinase, captopril, danazol, IV heroin, IV gangliosides

RISK FACTORS Antecedent infection, especially C. jejuni, which has more severe course and higher residual disability (AMAN)

DIAGNOSIS

DIFFERENTIAL DIAGNOSIS
• Brain disease: strokes, encephalitis
• Spinal cord syndromes: transverse myelitis, cord compression, cauda equina syndrome; HIV, Lyme disease, sarcoid meningoradiculitis
• Motor neuron: polio
• Muscle disease: toxic myopathy, myositis, metabolic myopathies including hypokalemic periodic paralysis, polymyositis, critical illness polyneuropathy
• Neuromuscular junction: myasthenia gravis, Eaton-Lambert, toxins (botulism, organophosphates), hypermagnesemia
• Peripheral nerve: tick paralysis, diphtheria, porphyria, neurotoxins (heavy meals, shellfish poisoning e.g. ciguatoxin and saxitoxin, glue sniffing), metabolic (hypophosphatemia), drugs (cholesterol lowering agents, chemotherapeutics, nitrofurantoin, others), SLE and polymyositis and PAN
• Psychiatric: hysteria

LABORATORY
• CSF: elevated protein with normal cell count and pressure. Protein normal 50% cases in first week of illness becoming elevated within 3 weeks.
• Blood: CBC, electrolytes, liver and renal function studies; SLE and PAN screen; HIV testing; if appropriate Lyme disease and sarcoidosis testing
• Urine: acute intermittent porphyria
• Imaging: MRI spinal cord if any evidence cord lesion or myelopathy
• Other: consider heavy metal testing; review medications (e.g. chemotherapeutics, nitrofurantoin, megavitamins especially pyridoxine); if previous diarrheal illness consider C. jejuni antibodies
Drugs that may alter lab results: N/A
Disorders that may alter lab results: N/A

PATHOLOGICAL FINDINGS Multifocal inflammatory cell infiltration of peripheral nerves with patchy demyelination and/or axonal degeneration

SPECIAL TESTS N/A

IMAGING To exclude other causes, especially spinal cord lesions/cord compression

DIAGNOSTIC PROCEDURES
• Nerve conduction studies: Evidence of multifocal demyelination (decreased amplitude, prolonged distal latencies, decreased CMAP, F-wave abnormal, and asymmetry conduction block) in motor and sensory nerves. Important to test several different nerves. May be normal early in disease.
• Lumbar puncture: elevated protein with normal cell count

TREATMENT

APPROPRIATE HEALTH CARE
• Hospitalization with monitoring of respiratory function and elective intubation for impending respiratory failure
• IVIG/plasmapharesis for all patients too weak to walk, rapid progression, or poor prognostic indicators
• Intensive care monitoring for dysautonomia and arrhythmias as indicated

GENERAL MEASURES
• Serial measurements FVC and oximetry with intubation for respiratory distress or FVC<20 mL/kg (<1L in adults). FVC best measurement (oximetry/ABGs normal until respiratory failure has occurred; peak flow measures air flow resistance not respiratory muscle strength).
• Intubation for difficulty swallowing/aspiration from bulbar palsy
• Cardiac monitoring for arrhythmias: tachyarrhythmias usually do not require treatment; bradyarrhythmias - atropine; sinus arrest and complete heart block - temporary pacemaker
• Hypertension: often does not need treatment. Small doses beta blockers if needed. Avoid vasodilators including calcium channel blockers (may precipitate hypotension).
• Hypotension: Trendelenburg position and volume expansion (IV fluids)
• Pain common, can be severe and recalcitrant: analgesics including opioids; TCAs, carbamazepine, TENS for neuropathic pain
• Constipation/ileus from autonomic neuropathy: laxatives, enemas, cisapride (Propulsid)
• Urinary retention from autonomic neuropathy: catheterization
• Prevent complications of immobilization, e.g. pneumonia, decubitus ulcers, DVT/PE, contractures
• Depression: frequent reminders that recovery is the rule; antidepressants

SURGICAL MEASURES Tracheostomy for prolonged intubation

ACTIVITY No limitation. Prevent contractures and assist with weakness.

DIET No special diet. Enteral feedings if intubated.

PATIENT EDUCATION Important to stress expectation of full/significant recovery

Guillain-Barre syndrome

MEDICATIONS

DRUG(S) OF CHOICE
• IV immune globulin (IVIG) and plasma exchange equally effective, shorten duration and severity of disease. IVIG preferred (more available, fewer side effects).
  ◊ IVIG: 2 g/kg x 2-4 days OR 400 mg/kg/day x 5 consecutive days
  ◊ Plasmapharesis/plasma exchange: 200-250 mL/kg in 3-5 sessions over 8-13 d
• Steroids not effective and possibly deleterious
• Beta-blockers for significant hypertension
• Analgesics for pain

Contraindications: IVIG in IgA deficiency

Precautions:
• IVIG: risk of anaphylaxis (IgA deficiency), acute renal failure, and hepatitis C
• Plasmapharesis: hypotension, autonomic instability, sepsis

Significant possible interactions: N/A

ALTERNATIVE DRUGS
No advantage to using both IVIG and plasmapharesis over using either one by itself

FOLLOWUP

PATIENT MONITORING Physical rehabilitation to regain muscle strength

PREVENTION/AVOIDANCE N/A

POSSIBLE COMPLICATIONS
• Paralysis, permanent weakness
• Respiratory failure, mechanical ventilation
• Hypotension, hypertension, labile BP
• Cardiac arrhythmias
• Ileus
• Urinary retention
• Aspiration, pneumonia, sepsis
• DVT, PE
• Psychiatric problems including depression

EXPECTED COURSE/PROGNOSIS
• 3 phases of illness:
  ◊ Initial progression phase 24 hours - 3 weeks, usually 10-14 d: highest risk of death and complications during this phase
  ◊ Plateau phase same approximate duration as initial phase
  ◊ Recovery phase generally 1-6 months, up to 2 years. No further improvement after 2 years.
• 2-5% mortality (most often from dysautonomia or complications), 50% complete recovery, 50% some residual disability with 5% severe permanent disability. Relapses may occur both before and after recovery.
• Poor prognostic signs:
  ◊ Rapid progression to severe disease (<7d)
  ◊ Mechanical ventilation
  ◊ Nerve conduction studies: CMAP <10% or mean distal motor amplitude <20%
  ◊ AMAN (see Differential Diagnosis)
  ◊ Preceding C. jejuni infection
  ◊ Age over 60 years

MISCELLANEOUS

ASSOCIATED CONDITIONS Chronic inflammatory demyelinating polyneuropathy (CIDP)

AGE-RELATED FACTORS
Pediatric: Disease tends to be milder
Geriatric: Worse prognosis >60 years
Others: N/A

PREGNANCY No data

SYNONYMS
• Acute inflammatory demyelinating polyradiculopathy
• GBS
• Landry-Guillain-Barre-Strohl syndrome
• Acute inflammatory neuropathy
• Acute idiopathic polyneuritis
• Acute immune mediated polyneuritis (AIMP)
• Landry's ascending paralysis
• Acute segmentally demyelinating polyradiculoneuropathy

ICD-9-CM
357.0 Acute infective polyneuritis

SEE ALSO
• Amyotropic lateral sclerosis
• Arsenic poisoning
• Botulism
• Diphtheria
• Lead poisoning
• Poliomyelitis
• Spinal cord compression
• Thallium poisoning

OTHER NOTES N/A

ABBREVIATIONS
GBS = Guillain-Barre syndrome
AMAN = acute motor axonal neuropathy
AMSAN = acute motor-sensory axonal neuropathy
CMAP = compound muscle action potential
CIDN = chronic inflammatory demyelinating neuropathy
DVT = deep venous thrombosis
PE = pulmonary embolism
IVIG = intravenous immunoglobulin
IgA = immunoglobulin A
SLE = systemic lupus erythematosus
PAN = polyarteritis nodosa
CMV = cytomegalovirus
EBV = Ebstein-Barr virus
HIV = human immunodeficiency virus

REFERENCES
• Rowland: Merritt's Textbook of Neurology 9th ed, Chapter 100 Acquired Neuropathies: 657-660. Williams and Wilkins, 1995
• Evans O, Vedanarayanan V: Guillain-Barre Syndrome. Pediatrics in Review 1997;18(1):10-17
• Pascuzzi R, Fleck J: Acute Periph Neuropathy in Adults. Neurol Clinics 1997;15(3): 529-548
• Bella I, Chad D: Neuromuscular Disorders and Acute Respiratory Failure. Neurol Clinics 1998; 6(2):391-417
• Trojaborg W: Acute and chronic neuropathies: new aspects of Guillain-Barre. Electroencephalogr Clinc Neurophysiol 1998;107(5):303-16.
Illustrations: N/A
Internet references: http://www.5mcc.com

Author(s)
Hetty B. Hall, MD

Gynecomastia

BASICS

DESCRIPTION A benign glandular enlargement of the male breast that is generally bilateral (may be asymmetric, or rarely, unilateral)
• Type I: Benign adolescent hypertrophy
  ◊ Physiologic discoid subacute mass
  ◊ Resolves spontaneously
• Type II: Physiologic gynecomastia
  ◊ Generalized enlargement to greater degree
• Type III:
  ◊ Obesity simulates gynecomastia
• Type IV:
  ◊ Pectoral muscle hypertrophy
System(s) affected: Skin/Exocrine, Endocrine/Metabolic
Genetics: Some instance of familial gynecomastia may be inherited as a male-limited autosomal trait
Incidence/Prevalence in USA: 38-64% of pubertal males; rare except when drug-induced
Predominant age: Puberty; and over the age of 65 (especially with a weight gain)
Predominant sex: Male only

SIGNS AND SYMPTOMS
• Usually asymptomatic
• May be painful and tender if it has developed rapidly (drug-induced, refeeding gynecomastia)

CAUSES
• Physiologic - transient in neonatal boys and at puberty
• Exposure to a high level of estrogen compared to testosterone concentration
• Tumors - estrogen secreting, gonadotropin secreting and prolactin secreting pituitary adenomas
• Drug-induced (hormones, marijuana, digitalis, spironolactone, cimetidine, ketoconazole, cytotoxic drugs, antihypertensives, sedatives, antidepressants, amphetamine)
• Systemic disorders - cirrhosis, thyrotoxicosis, renal failure
• Androgen production deficiency
• Androgen resistant syndromes
• Trauma
• Idiopathic

RISK FACTORS
• Klinefelter's syndrome
• Obesity
• Testicular failure
• Recovery from prolonged severe illness associated with malnutrition and weight loss (refeeding gynecomastia)
• Family history
• Peutz-Jeghers syndrome
• Male pseudohermaphroditism

DIAGNOSIS

DIFFERENTIAL DIAGNOSIS
• Obesity with increase in adipose tissue
• Carcinoma of the male breast
• Lipomas
• Neurofibromas

LABORATORY
• Laboratory evaluation rarely indicated
• Human chorionic gonadotropin levels - high levels may lead to finding a choriocarcinoma or other hCG-secreting tumor
• Plasma testosterone and luteinizing hormone measurements - help diagnose hypogonadism
• Serum estradiol
• Serum prolactin
• Liver function
• Others if clinically indicated e.g., thyroid function, chromosomal analysis
Drugs that may alter lab results: N/A
Disorders that may alter lab results:
• Cirrhosis
• Thyrotoxicosis
• Renal failure

PATHOLOGICAL FINDINGS
• Dense, periductal hyaline, collagenous connective tissue
• Hyperplastic ductal lining
• Plasma cell infiltrate

SPECIAL TESTS Full endocrine investigations may be indicated

IMAGING CT, ultrasonography (rarely indicated)

DIAGNOSTIC PROCEDURES
• History and physical exam to determine possible etiology
• Biopsy, if suspicious

TREATMENT

APPROPRIATE HEALTH CARE
Outpatient

GENERAL MEASURES
• Correct underlying disorder
• Withdrawal of causative drug if feasible
• Observation with reassurance that problem is transient

SURGICAL MEASURES
• Biopsy if suspicious for cancer
• Subcutaneous mastectomy for severe, persistent cases or those with psychological concerns

ACTIVITY No restrictions

DIET
• No special diet
• If obesity a problem, weight loss diet

PATIENT EDUCATION N/A

MEDICATIONS

DRUG(S) OF CHOICE None
Contraindications: N/A
Precautions: N/A
Significant possible interactions: N/A

ALTERNATIVE DRUGS N/A

FOLLOWUP

PATIENT MONITORING
• Every 3-6 months for physiologic gynecomastia
• Until well for non-physiologic gynecomastia

PREVENTION/AVOIDANCE
In men taking estrogen for prostate cancer - low dose radiation prior to institution of diethylstilbestrol

POSSIBLE COMPLICATIONS
• Nipple inversion may occur following subcutaneous mastectomy
• Asymmetry of breasts

EXPECTED COURSE/PROGNOSIS
• Physiologic gynecomastia clears without treatment (may take up to 2 years)
• Drug withdrawal cures
• Other causes - outcome depends on etiology
• Little change in Type III without substantial weight loss
• Good results with subcutaneous mastectomy

MISCELLANEOUS

ASSOCIATED CONDITIONS Listed with Causes

AGE-RELATED FACTORS
Pediatric:
• Transient gynecomastia seen in neonatal boys
• At puberty, may be observed in 38-64% of boys
Geriatric: Drug induced form more common
Others: N/A

PREGNANCY N/A

SYNONYMS Male breast hypertrophy

ICD-9-CM
611.1 Hypertrophy of breast

SEE ALSO
• Klinefelter's syndrome

OTHER NOTES N/A

ABBREVIATIONS N/A

REFERENCES
• Becker KL, ed: Principles and Practice of Endocrinology and Metabolism. Philadelphia, J.B. Lippincott Co., 1990
• Holder TM, Ashcroft KW, eds: Pediatric Surgery. 2nd Ed. Philadelphia, W.B. Saunders Co., 1993
• Mahoney CP: Adolescent gynecomastia. Differential diagnosis and management. Pediatr Clin North Am 1990;37:1389
Illustrations: N/A
Internet references: http://www.5mcc.com

Author(s)
Timothy L. Black, MD, FACS, FAAP

Headache, cluster

BASICS

DESCRIPTION
Attacks of severe, unilateral headache typically localized in periorbital area and temple associated with ipsilateral lacrimation, rhinorrhea, ptosis, miosis, and nasal congestion. Individual attacks last 30-180 minutes and occur 1-6 times per day. Two forms exist: episodic with attack phases lasting 4-16 weeks, followed by a cluster-free interval of generally 6 months to years duration; and chronic, with a cluster-free interval of less than 1 week in a 12 month period of time.

System(s) affected: Nervous
Genetics: Unknown
Incidence/Prevalence in USA: 0.5-1% of adult population
Predominant age: Mean age of onset: 30 years in men, later in women
Predominant sex: Male > Female (6:1)

SIGNS AND SYMPTOMS
• Sudden onset of severe headache
• Headache reaches crescendo within 15 minutes, lasts < 3 hours
• Pain is unilateral, oculo-temporal or oculo-frontal; rare in other locations
• Severe, piercing, boring, exploding, penetrating (occasionally throbbing) pain
• Ipsilateral partial Horner's syndrome (ptosis and miosis)
• Lacrimation (84%)
• Injected conjunctiva (58%)
• Ptosis (57%)
• Nasal stuffiness (48%)
• Rhinorrhea (43%)
• Bradycardia (43%)
• Nausea (40%)
• Perspiration (26%)
• Restlessness and agitation during attacks
• Attacks may occur at same time for consecutive days; frequently an attack occurs within 90 minutes of falling to sleep (corresponding to first REM sleep)

CAUSES
Unknown, perhaps:
• Disruption of circadian rhythm based on hypothalamus
• Disturbed autoregulation of cerebral arteries
• Disorder of serotonin metabolism or transmission in CNS
• Disorder of histamine concentrations or receptors

RISK FACTORS
• Male gender
• Age > 30 years
• Small amounts of vasodilators, such as, alcohol or nitroglycerine
• Occasional relationship to previous head trauma or surgery

DIAGNOSIS

DIFFERENTIAL DIAGNOSIS
Diagnosis generally made through careful history. Differential includes other head and neck pathology, migraine, trigeminal and other facial neuralgias, chronic paroxysmal hemicrania (probably a cluster variant), temporal arteritis, pheochromocytoma.

LABORATORY
Not useful except to rule out differential diagnosis
Drugs that may alter lab results: N/A
Disorders that may alter lab results: N/A

PATHOLOGICAL FINDINGS   N/A

SPECIAL TESTS   N/A

IMAGING
Generally of little value except in atypical presentations or those unresponsive to therapy

DIAGNOSTIC PROCEDURES   N/A

TREATMENT

APPROPRIATE HEALTH CARE
Outpatient except in patient at suicidal risk

GENERAL MEASURES
• During cluster periods, avoid alcohol, bright lights and glare, excessive emotion and stress as these may precipitate attacks
• Avoid narcotic analgesics, especially oral preparations
• Tobacco (high predilection for tobacco abuse in this population) may make patients more refractory to therapy

SURGICAL MEASURES
Radiofrequency trigeminal gangliolysis in carefully selected refractory patients with strictly unilateral attacks

ACTIVITY
• Avoid self-injury during bouts of excruciating pain
• Vigorous physical activity at first symptom may abort attack in some
• Compression of ipsilateral carotid or temporal artery may reduce pain in some. Caution exercised in recommending carotid massage in patient at risk for occult carotid disease.

DIET
• During cluster phase, alcohol even in small amounts frequently precipitates attacks
• Rarely, specific foods may trigger attacks

PATIENT EDUCATION
• Focus on the validity, natural history, and pathology of the condition
• Advise patient to avoid known precipitants
• Assist patient with learning self-treatment methods
• Provide supportive relationship and follow-up
• Avoid high altitudes

MEDICATIONS

DRUG(S) OF CHOICE

• General information
◊ Prophylactic therapy is paramount
◊ Avoid pain therapy for acute attacks, especially narcotic analgesics
◊ Assess cardiovascular risk before instituting vasoactive drugs, such as, ergotamine or sumatriptan
• Acute attacks
◊ Oxygen 100% at 7-10 liters for 10-15 minutes administered through a tight-fitting face mask with patient in sitting position and breathing at normal respiratory rate
◊ Sumatriptan (Imitrex) 6 mg subcutaneous, maximum of 12 mg per 24 hours with at least 1 hour between injections
◊ Dihydroergotamine mesylate (DHE 45) 1 mg IM or IV. May teach self-administration with SC.
• Prophylaxis (to shorten cluster period or prevent expected attacks):
◊ Verapamil 80 mg PO qid spaced evenly through waking hours
◊ Lithium carbonate (Eskalith) 300 mg 2-4 times a day
◊ Methysergide (Sansert) 4-10 mg daily divided doses tid or qid. More useful in younger patient in early stage of disease.
◊ Ergotamine timed to be at peak serum level during anticipated attack, e.g., 2 mg rectal or 1-2 mg oral 2 hours before. This is especially useful to prevent nocturnal attacks.
◊ Prednisone, various schedules, e.g., 60-80 mg PO for 7 days followed by rapid tapering over 6 days or 40 mg/day for 5 days tapered over 3 weeks. This therapy is initiated while other long-term agent is being employed, such as, verapamil or lithium.

Contraindications: Refer to manufacturer's literature
Precautions: Refer to manufacturer's literature
Significant possible interactions: Refer to manufacturer's literature

ALTERNATIVE DRUGS

• Acute attack:
◊ Lidocaine intranasal instillation of 1 mL of 4% topical solution slowly on same side as symptoms. Position patient supine with head extended 45 degrees and rotated 40 degrees to the side of pain. May need to premedicate with 1-2 drops of intranasal 0.5% phenylephrine for nasal stuffiness.
• Prophylaxis
◊ Indomethacin up to 150 mg per day in divided doses. Absolute responsiveness in chronic paroxysmal hemicrania (CPH) and useful in female cluster patients.
◊ Nifedipine 40-120 mg/day
◊ Nimodipine up to 240 mg/day
◊ Combinations of verapamil and lithium with or without ergotamine may be useful when single drug therapy is ineffective
◊ Histamine desensitization done at certain major headache centers

FOLLOWUP

PATIENT MONITORING

• To anticipate cluster bouts and initiate early prophylaxis
• Monitor for adverse medication response and side-effects
• Monitor for unmasking of underlying cardiovascular disorder
• Education for patient and family

PREVENTION/AVOIDANCE

• Alcohol, nitroglycerine, and some foods can induce cluster attack
• Disturbances in sleep cycle can induce attacks (sleep cycle disruption common due to anticipation and occurrence of nocturnal attacks)
• Strong emotions, anger, excessive physical activity may induce attacks
• Tobacco may slow responsiveness to medication
• Narcotics may expedite transformation of episodic cluster to chronic cluster

POSSIBLE COMPLICATIONS

• Self-injury during attack
• Side-effects of medication including unmasking of coronary heart disease
• Potential for drug abuse

EXPECTED COURSE/PROGNOSIS

• Recurrent attacks
• Prolonged remissions
• Possibility of transformation of episodic cluster to chronic cluster and occasionally chronic cluster to episodic cluster

MISCELLANEOUS

ASSOCIATED CONDITIONS

• Significantly higher incidence of peptic ulcer and coronary heart disease (males)
• Prior history of migraine frequently in female patients
• Increased risk of suicide

AGE-RELATED FACTORS

Pediatric: Very rare cases reported
Geriatric: N/A
Others:
• With age - more likely to begin in women, often in peri- or post-menopausal years
• Characteristic appearance - "leonine" face, thickened skin, above average height, more likely to have hazel eye color, and be heavy smokers. No evidence of specific psychologic type.

PREGNANCY   Very rare in pregnancy

SYNONYMS

• Migrainous neuralgia
• Sphenopalatine neuralgia
• Histamine cephalalgia

ICD-9-CM

346.2 Variants of migraine (including cluster and histamine)
784.0 Headache

SEE ALSO

• Headache, tension
• Migraine

OTHER NOTES   N/A

ABBREVIATIONS   N/A

REFERENCES

• Cady RK, Fox AW, eds: Treating the Headache Patient. New York, Marcel Dekker, 1995
• Dechant KC, Clissol SP: Sumatriptan (review). Drugs 1992;43:776-98
• Dalessio DJ, Silberstein SD: Wolff's Headache and Other Head Pain. 6th Ed. New York, Oxford University Press, 1993
• Raskin NH: Headache. 2nd Ed. New York, Churchill Livingstone, 1988
Illustrations: N/A
Internet references: http://www.5mcc.com

Author(s)

Roger Cady, MD

Headache, tension

 BASICS

DESCRIPTION
Tension headache can be divided into two types:
- Episodic - usually associated with some stressful event, is of moderate intensity, self-limited, and usually responds to nonprescription preparations
- Chronic - often recurring daily, bilateral location, usually occipito-frontal and associated with contracted muscles of the neck and scalp

System(s) affected: Musculoskeletal
Genetics: 40% have a positive family history for headache
Incidence/Prevalence in USA: Common
Predominant age: 60% have onset after age 20 (unusual to begin after age 50)
Predominant sex: Female > Male

SIGNS AND SYMPTOMS
- Bilateral headache in 90%
- Located fronto-occipital or generalized
- Dull, pressing or band-like
- Intensity varies throughout the day
- Often present upon arising or shortly thereafter
- Chronic headaches have a duration greater than 5 years in 75% of patients
- Insomnia
- Teeth grinding
- Not aggravated by physical activity
- Difficulty concentrating
- Muscular tightness or stiffness in neck, occipital and frontal regions

CAUSES
- Poor posture
- Stress and/or anxiety
- Depression (found in 70% of those with daily headache)
- Low platelet serotonin
- Cervical osteoarthritis
- Intramuscular vasoconstriction

RISK FACTORS
- Obstructive sleep apnea
- Medications
- Excess caffeine

 DIAGNOSIS

DIFFERENTIAL DIAGNOSIS
- Cervical spondylosis
- TMJ syndrome
- Caffeine-dependency
- Non-prescription analgesic dependency
- Depression
- Head injury
- Severe anemia or polycythemia
- Uremia and hepatic disorders
- Toxic effects from drugs or fumes
- Dental disease
- Paget's disease of bone
- Chronic sinusitis
- Refractive error
- Hypertension
- Hypoxia
- Temporal arteritis
- Migraine
- Lesions of the eye or middle ear
- Lesions of the oral cavity

LABORATORY
- CBC
- SMAC-20
- Thyroid studies
- ESR in anyone over 50 years of age

Drugs that may alter lab results: N/A
Disorders that may alter lab results: Chronic hepatitis, renal and thyroid conditions

PATHOLOGICAL FINDINGS
Normal neurological examination, furrowed brow, tense masseter muscle, tight muscles in the scalp and neck

SPECIAL TESTS   N/A

IMAGING
- X-rays of cervical spine
- Head CT or MRI necessary only when headache pattern has recently changed or there is a positive finding on neurological exam

DIAGNOSTIC PROCEDURES   NA

TREATMENT

APPROPRIATE HEALTH CARE
Outpatient setting

GENERAL MEASURES
- Relief measures - use relaxation routines; rest in quiet, dark room with cold washcloth over eyes; hot bath or shower; massaging back of neck and temples
- Biofeedback training offers a nonpharmacologic alternative which is often beneficial

SURGICAL MEASURES   N/A

ACTIVITY
Encourage physical fitness, range of motion and strengthening exercises for the neck

DIET
No demonstrated link between diet and tension headache

PATIENT EDUCATION
- Life style changes to minimize stress. Suggest patient seek counseling, if appropriate.
- Encourage relaxation techniques, aerobic exercise, assertiveness training
- Patient information available from the National Headache Foundation, 5252 N. Western Ave., Chicago, IL 60625, (800)843-2256

MEDICATIONS

DRUG(S) OF CHOICE
• Acute attack - nonsteroidal anti-inflammatory drugs (NSAID's):
  ◊ Naproxen sodium (Naprosyn, Aleve) 500 mg/bid
  ◊ Fenoprofen calcium (Nalfon) 600 mg/day (200 mg q 4-6 hours)
  ◊ Ibuprofen (Motrin, Advil) 400 mg/tid
  ◊ Ketoprofen (Orudis) 50 mg/tid
• Prophylaxis for chronic tension headache - antidepressants
  ◊ Amitriptyline (Elavil) 50-100 mg/day
  ◊ Desipramine (Norpramin) 50-100 mg/day
  ◊ Imipramine (Tofranil) 50-100 mg/day
  ◊ Nortriptyline (Pamelor) 25-50 mg/day

Contraindications:
• NSAID's and antidepressants, in general, not suitable for use in children
• Antidepressants should not be used concomitantly with MAO inhibitors

Precautions:
• Do not use antidepressants in presence of acute myocardial infarction
• Avoid over dependence on nonprescription caffeine-containing preparations
• Use NSAID's with precaution in patients with history of previous peptic disease

Significant possible interactions:
Antidepressants and alcohol create accentuated depression

ALTERNATIVE DRUGS
• Beta blockers - prophylaxis (select one):
  ◊ Propranolol (Inderal LA) 80 mg/daily
  ◊ Nadolol (Corgard) 40 mg/daily
  ◊ Atenolol (Tenormin) 50-100 mg/daily
• Combination agent - prophylaxis
  ◊ Isometheptene - dichloralphenazone - acetaminophen (Midrin) one capsule tid
• Other NSAIDs

FOLLOWUP

PATIENT MONITORING
A warm, nonjudgmental, understanding relationship with the physician is the best predictor for a successful treatment program

PREVENTION/AVOIDANCE
• Physical therapy
• Biofeedback and relaxation therapy
• Cervical traction
• Injection of trigger points

POSSIBLE COMPLICATIONS
• Undue reliance on non-prescription caffeine-containing analgesics
• Dependence/addiction to narcotic analgesics
• GI bleed from NSAID use
• Risk of addiction to analgesics
• Risk of epilepsy is four times that of the general population

EXPECTED COURSE/PROGNOSIS
• Usually follows a chronic course when life stressors are not changed
• Most cases are intermittent and should not interfere with work or normal life span

MISCELLANEOUS

ASSOCIATED CONDITIONS
10% of patients with tension headache also have migraine headache

AGE-RELATED FACTORS
Pediatric: 15% will have onset at age less than 10 years
Geriatric: Onset of new headache in the elderly is always worrisome and cause for careful study
Others: Unusual for tension-type headaches to begin after age 50

PREGNANCY
No documented relationship

SYNONYMS
• Muscle contraction headache
• Cephalgia

ICD-9-CM
307.81 Tension headache

SEE ALSO
N/A

OTHER NOTES
N/A

ABBREVIATIONS
N/A

REFERENCES
• Maizels M: The clinician's approach to the management of headache. West J Med, March 1998;168:203-12
• DuBose D: Migraines and other headaches: An approach to diagnosis and classification. American Family Physician, May 1995;51:1498-1504
• Perchalsji JJ: Managing the Patient with Chronic Daily Headache. Family Practice Recertification 1994;16(11):34-42
• Smith R: Chronic Headaches in Family Practice. JABFP 15(6):589-599
Illustrations: N/A
Internet references: http://www.5mcc.com

Author(s)
Don McHard, MD

Hearing loss

BASICS

DESCRIPTION Complete or partial hearing loss that may involve the middle ear (mechanical, conductive) or the inner ear (nerve, sensorineural)
System(s) affected: Nervous
Genetics: Both types may be on a genetic basis
Incidence/Prevalence in USA:
• 140/100,000/year (134 adults, 6 school age children)
• 3,494 (cases/100,000), with 3,333 for adults and 161 for school age children
Predominant age: All ages, but more common in elderly
Predominant sex: Male = Female

SIGNS AND SYMPTOMS Obvious difficulty hearing, with possible association of other symptoms such as tinnitus, dizziness, pain, and fullness

CAUSES
• Conductive
  ◊ Cerumen impaction
  ◊ Perforation of tympanica membrane
  ◊ Middle ear fluid (serous otitis media)
  ◊ Acute otitis media
  ◊ Adhesive otitis media
  ◊ Damage to ossicles (trauma, infection, etc.)
  ◊ Tympanosclerosis (thickening of drum that may produce fixation)
  ◊ Otosclerosis (new bone growth that produces stapes fixation)
  ◊ Cholesteatoma (growth of skin into middle ear)
  ◊ Middle ear tumor (glomus, etc.)
  ◊ Congenital problems (atresia, ossicular fixation, etc.)
  ◊ Temporal bone fracture, injuries
• Sensorineural
  ◊ Acoustic tumor
  ◊ Meniere's disease
  ◊ Noise induced (industrial, recreational, occupational)
  ◊ Hereditary
  ◊ Congenital
  ◊ Viral (relatively common, esp. mumps)
  ◊ Ototoxicity (ASA, quinine, gentamicin, kanamycin, etc.)
  ◊ Syphilis - hearing loss, tinnitus, dizzy
  ◊ Presbycusis (hearing loss related to aging)
  ◊ Temporal bone injury, fracture
  ◊ Metabolic (hypothyroid, etc.)
  ◊ Perilymphatic (inner ear) fistula (usually secondary to pressure changes or trauma)
  ◊ Autoimmune disease

RISK FACTORS Nasal allergy and other causes of eustachian tube obstruction; exposure to loud noise levels; use of ototoxic antibiotics; prematurity; heredity (otosclerosis)

DIAGNOSIS

DIFFERENTIAL DIAGNOSIS
• In conductive loss, must rule out cholesteatoma
• In sensorineural loss, must rule out acoustic tumor

LABORATORY N/A
Drugs that may alter lab results: N/A
Disorders that may alter lab results: N/A

PATHOLOGICAL FINDINGS N/A

SPECIAL TESTS
• Audiometry including pure tone and speech testing, and impedance (middle ear pressure) testing. Both types of hearing loss may fluctuate, making audiometric results variable from test to test. Marked conductive loss in one ear may be difficult to exclude (mask) when testing opposite ear.
• Otoscopy with operating microscope (sometimes necessary to see small superior, attic perforation, indicating a cholesteatoma)

IMAGING
• CT scan (not routinely needed) is useful to demonstrate tumors and cholesteatoma of the temporal bone
• MRI scan is more useful to show acoustic and other cerebellopontine angle tumors (usually produce a sensorineural hearing loss)

DIAGNOSTIC PROCEDURES
• Exploratory tympanotomy sometimes necessary to confirm presence of middle ear fluid, tumor, etc.
• Underlying conditions are identified primarily on basis of history of hearing loss, otoscopy, and hearing test (audiometry)
• FTA or equivalent
• Sed rate for autoimmune disease

TREATMENT

APPROPRIATE HEALTH CARE
Outpatient

GENERAL MEASURES
• Conductive (mechanical)
  ◊ Cerumen: Remove with suction and irrigation (not if perforation is present). Don't direct water against drum but against canal wall. Manipulation with wire curette may help.
  ◊ Tympanic membrane perforation: Surgical correction
  ◊ Serous otitis (primarily in children). Treat underlying conditions. Use decongestants, antibiotics. Urge inflation of eustachian tube (hold nose and blow).
  ◊ Adhesive otitis: Looks like perforation. Treat eustachian tube problem. May need surgery.

  ◊ Damage to ossicles: Don't manipulate. Refer to otolaryngologist.
  ◊ Tympanosclerosis: Drum has white plaques. Treat only if hearing loss is present.
  ◊ Otosclerosis: Suspect on basis of history of onset, early in life, that is progressive, with positive family history of hearing loss. Consider surgery. Refer to otolaryngologist.
  ◊ Cholesteatoma: Identify by perforation that is located near margin of drum. Refer to otolaryngologist.
  ◊ Middle ear tumor: May see through drum. Most commonly will be glomus tumor, which has red color and may cause pulsation. Significant problem, needs prompt referral to otolaryngologist.
  ◊ Congenital deformity: Don't attribute all hearing loss in children to infections and middle ear fluid. Refer to otolaryngologist.
  ◊ Temporal bone injury: If limited, may only involve middle ear. Drum likely to appear blue. Refer to otolaryngologist.
• Sensorineural (nerve)
  ◊ Acoustic tumor: Most significant type of hearing loss. Very important to diagnose promptly. Suspect when unilateral hearing loss and tinnitus (with or without dizziness) are present. Needs much higher degree of suspicion on part of primary care physician. Refer to otolaryngologist.
  ◊ See topic on Meniere's disease
  ◊ Noise damage: The most common cause of hearing loss in this country. Very frequent on occupational basis, and has the attention of federal government (OSHA regulations). Also occurs secondary to sports and recreation (hunting, use of guns, loud music, chain saws, shop tools). Needs much greater level of recognition at primary care level. Refer to otolaryngologist.
  ◊ Hereditary/congenital: Needs immediate recognition early in life, so that if significant, hearing aids can be placed. Rarely, surgery may be effective.
  ◊ Viral: A relatively common cause of permanent hearing loss, frequently unilateral, e.g., mumps
  ◊ Ototoxic (medication): Needs much more recognition at primary care level. Suspect when hearing loss, and perhaps dizziness and tinnitus come on during course of treatment with certain antibiotics (and many other medications). See Medications.
  ◊ Syphilis: Treat with high dose penicillin given intravenously, as well as steroids
  ◊ Presbycusis: No specific treatment available, but important to provide hearing rehabilitation. This includes counseling patient to avoid factors that may cause further loss (noise exposure, ototoxic drugs). Emphasize development of lip reading skills, and counseling family to pronounce words clearly, face patient when speaking, etc. Offer hearing aid trial when patient is a suitable candidate.
  ◊ Temporal bone injury: No treatment available specifically for hearing loss unless middle ear is involved
  ◊ Metabolic: Treatment of specific problem (e.g. hyperlipidemia, hypothyroid)
  ◊ Perilymphatic fistula: Diagnosis based on history of injury to ear including barotrauma during diving. Treatment is early exploration to confirm fistula in round or oval window of middle ear, with repair of fistula. Refer to otolaryngologist.

◊ Total or near total sensorineural hearing loss: Cochlear implant (electronic device inserted into mastoid and inner ear)

◊ Autoimmune sensorineural hearing loss: Steroids and chemotherapy. Refer to otolaryngologist.

SURGICAL MEASURES
See General Measures

ACTIVITY
• Patients having perforation of the ear drum or ventilation tube in place should be advised not to swim or allow water to enter the ear
• Patients having hearing loss secondary to noise exposure should be advised to avoid loud noise, or to use suitable protection (ear plugs or ear muffs)

DIET
Patients whose hearing loss is due to Meniere's disease should avoid excessive use of salt

PATIENT EDUCATION
See information under other headings

MEDICATIONS

DRUG(S) OF CHOICE
• Cerumen impaction - it is frequently helpful to soften the wax prior to removing it. triethanolamine polypeptide oleate-condensate (Cerumenex) is popular, but should not be used in the presence of a perforation, and may produce a skin reaction. A good alternative is simply to place, or have the patient place mineral oil in the ear canal overnight prior to wax removal. Hexachlorophene (pHisoHex) and topical docusate sodium (Colace) are also useful to soften very hard wax.
• Acute otitis media - erythromycin or amoxicillin
• Chronic otitis media with purulent drainage - neomycin-polymyxin B-hydrocortisone (Cortisporin) otic drops (or an equivalent) placed into the ear canal (3-6 drops bid)
• Serous otitis media - decongestant, e.g., phenylephrine - phenylpropanolamine - guaifenesin (Entex) and erythromycin
• Sudden sensorineural hearing loss with no apparent cause - steroid therapy in high dosage form (80 mg/day of prednisone, or equivalent steroid) may be helpful

Contraindications: History of sensitivity to any of the antibiotics referred to above

Precautions: Avoid the temptation of over-diagnosing "red ear" and using antibiotics without a well thought out diagnosis

Significant possible interactions: Refer to manufacturer's literature

ALTERNATIVE DRUGS
• Acute otitis media - cefaclor
• Chronic ear infection with drainage - ear drops and powder containing ciprofloxacin. Gentamicin drops is another alternative.

FOLLOWUP

PATIENT MONITORING
Hearing testing (audiometry) is the primary means of monitoring patient progress

PREVENTION/AVOIDANCE
• Impaired eustachian tube function (serous otitis media, acute otitis media) - improve tubal function with treatment of allergic and sinus disease. Treat upper respiratory infections (URI) promptly and aggressively if ear problems are frequent.
• Sensorineural hearing loss due to noise exposure (or any type of nerve deafness) - advise against excessive noise exposure; recommend ear plugs/ear muffs
• Nerve deafness due to ototoxic medications may be prevented by the avoidance, or careful use of drugs known to be ototoxic (consider audiometric monitoring if used). The most frequently implicated antibiotics are gentamicin, kanamycin, neomycin, vancomycin, and streptomycin. Other implicated drugs include lidocaine, morphine, digitalis, quinidine, and furosemide. Use of these drugs cannot always be avoided. Be more suspicious of the possibility that a given medication might be ototoxic, and when hearing loss is a problem, to prescribe with care.
• Serious nerve deafness resulting from CNS disease (meningitis, lues) may be prevented by thorough treatment of the primary problem
• If URI present, avoid flying or diving

POSSIBLE COMPLICATIONS
• Middle ear problems may progress to chronic ear problems (perforations, cholesteatoma)
• Cholesteatoma is capable of producing major complications including permanent loss of hearing, balance problems, facial nerve paralysis, meningitis, lateral sinus thrombosis, and brain abscess. Glomus tumors and acoustic tumors must be identified, or major CNS complications may result.
• Meniere's disease may proceed to total and permanent hearing loss if not treated, and may occur in spite of treatment
• Severe nerve deafness, particularly associated with tinnitus may produce such an emotional impact on the patient that suicide may occur. Treat the patient with empathy and understanding, offer help even if it seems limited. Encouragement and followup care are extremely helpful in managing these patients.

EXPECTED COURSE/PROGNOSIS
Sensorineural hearing loss is usually permanent, but in a few instances, may be improved, cured or have progression halted

MISCELLANEOUS

ASSOCIATED CONDITIONS
Noise, allergy, sinus disease, trauma, heredity, ototoxicity, CNS infections (meningitis, lues), age, hyperlipidemia, hypothyroid, barotrauma and autoimmune disease

AGE-RELATED FACTORS
Pediatric: Eustachian tube problems and secondary middle ear problems are more common in infants and small children, usually becoming less frequent by approximately age 10
Geriatric: Presbycusis is common and is made worse by noise exposure and other factors
Others: N/A

PREGNANCY
Otosclerosis may become active during pregnancy

SYNONYMS
N/A

ICD-9-CM
380.4 Impacted cerumen
385.00 Tympanosclerosis, unspecified
387.9 Otosclerosis, unspecific
382.0 Acute suppurative otitis media

SEE ALSO
• Ménière's disease

OTHER NOTES
N/A

ABBREVIATIONS
SNHL = sensorineural hearing loss

REFERENCES
• Lucente FE, Gady HE: Essentials of Otolaryngology. 4th ed. Philadelphia, Lippincott Williams & Wilkins, 1999:116-125
Illustrations: N/A
Internet references: http://www.5mcc.com

Author(s)
Gale Gardner, MD, FACS

Heat exhaustion & heat stroke

BASICS

DESCRIPTION A continuum of increasingly severe heat illnesses caused by dehydration, electrolyte losses, and failure of the body's thermoregulatory mechanisms
• Heat exhaustion is an acute heat injury with hyperthermia due to dehydration
• Heat stroke is extreme hyperthermia with thermoregulatory failure and profound central nervous system dysfunction
System(s) affected: Endocrine/Metabolic, Nervous
Genetics: N/A
Incidence/Prevalence in USA: Dependent on predisposing conditions in combination with environmental factors
Predominant age: More likely in children or elderly
Predominant sex: Male = Female

SIGNS AND SYMPTOMS
• Heat Exhaustion
  ◊ Fatigue and lethargy
  ◊ Weakness
  ◊ Dizziness
  ◊ Nausea, vomiting
  ◊ Myalgias
  ◊ Headache
  ◊ Profuse sweating
  ◊ Tachycardia
  ◊ Hypotension
  ◊ Lack of coordination
  ◊ Agitation
  ◊ Intense thirst
  ◊ Hyperventilation
  ◊ Paresthesias
  ◊ Core temperature elevated but < 103°F (< 39.4°C)
• Heat Stroke
  ◊ Exhaustion
  ◊ Confusion, disorientation
  ◊ Coma
  ◊ Hot, flushed, dry skin
  ◊ Core temperature > 105°F (> 40.5°C)

CAUSES Failure of heat-dissipating mechanisms or an overwhelming heat stress leading to a rise in core temperature, dehydration and salt depletion

RISK FACTORS
• Poor acclimatization to heat or poor physical conditioning
• Salt or water depletion
• Obesity
• Acute febrile or gastrointestinal illnesses
• Chronic illnesses - uncontrolled diabetes or hypertension, cardiac disease
• Alcohol and other substance abuse
• High heat and humidity, poor air circulation in environment
• Heavy, restrictive clothing

DIAGNOSIS

DIFFERENTIAL DIAGNOSIS
• Other causes of elevated temperature, dehydration or circulatory collapse
  ◊ Febrile illnesses, sepsis
  ◊ Drug-induced fluid loss
  ◊ Cardiac arrhythmia or infarction
  ◊ Acute cocaine intoxication
  ◊ Malignant hyperthermia (an autosomally inherited disorder of skeletal and cardiac muscle in which patients have abnormal muscle metabolism on exposure to halothane or skeletal muscle reactants)

LABORATORY
• Used primarily to detect end-organ damage
• Electrolytes, urinalysis
• Creatinine, blood urea nitrogen
• Liver enzymes
• Complete blood count
• Increased urine specific gravity
• Results of above studies yield hypernatremia, hyperchloremia, hemoconcentration
Drugs that may alter lab results: Diuretics
Disorders that may alter lab results: N/A

PATHOLOGICAL FINDINGS Only those associated with major organ system failure

SPECIAL TESTS N/A

IMAGING N/A

DIAGNOSTIC PROCEDURES Rectal temperature monitoring

TREATMENT

APPROPRIATE HEALTH CARE
Emergency treatment - best in a hospital setting

GENERAL MEASURES
• Rapid cooling - remove clothing, wet patient down, ice packs
• Fluid and electrolyte replacement with hypotonic oral fluids or IV 0.5-1.0 liter normal saline
• Consider central venous pressure monitoring

SURGICAL MEASURES N/A

ACTIVITY Rest with legs elevated

DIET
• Cool or cold clear liquids only (non-carbonated)
• Avoid caffeine
• Unrestricted sodium

PATIENT EDUCATION
• Stress the importance of proper conditioning and acclimatization
• Instruct patients to recognize heat stress signs and symptoms
• Maintain as much skin exposure as possible in hot, humid conditions, while using proper sun block protection
• Avoid dehydration with proper fluids during activity or exercise - 8 oz fluid intake for every 15 minutes of moderate exercise

MEDICATIONS

DRUG(S) OF CHOICE No medications are required in the initial management. Use isotonic saline solution to rehydrate.
Contraindications: N/A
Precautions: N/A
Significant possible interactions: N/A

ALTERNATIVE DRUGS N/A

FOLLOWUP

PATIENT MONITORING
• Rectal temperature monitoring - cooling may be discontinued when the core temperature drops to 102°F (38.9°C) and stabilizes
• Heat stroke patients may require airway management, hemodynamic monitoring and careful fluid and electrolyte administration and monitoring
• Consider central venous pressure monitoring

PREVENTION/AVOIDANCE Most important factor in preventing heat stress is adequate fluid replacement. Allow acclimatization to hot weather through proper conditioning and activity modification. Dress appropriately with loose-fitting, open weave, light-colored clothing.

POSSIBLE COMPLICATIONS
• May involve failure of any major organ system
• Cardiac arrhythmias or infarction
• Pulmonary edema, adult respiratory distress syndrome
• Coma, seizures
• Acute renal failure
• Rhabdomyolysis
• Disseminated intravascular coagulation
• Hepatocellular necrosis

EXPECTED COURSE/PROGNOSIS
• Good when mental function is not altered and when serum enzymes are not elevated. Recovery is within 24-48 hours in most cases.
• The mortality rate for heat stroke (10-80%) is directly related to the duration and intensity of hyperthermia as well as to the speed and effectiveness of diagnosis and treatment

MISCELLANEOUS

ASSOCIATED CONDITIONS N/A

AGE-RELATED FACTORS
Pediatric: Children are more susceptible
Geriatric: Elderly are more susceptible
Others: N/A

PREGNANCY May be more prone to volume depletion with heat stress

SYNONYMS
• Heat illness
• Heat injury
• Hyperthermia
• Heat collapse
• Heat prostration

ICD-9-CM
992.5 Heat exhaustion
992.0 Heat stroke

SEE ALSO Hyperthermia, malignant

OTHER NOTES N/A

ABBREVIATIONS N/A

REFERENCES
• Mellion MB, Shelton GL: Safe exercise in the heat and heat injury. In: Mellion MB, Walsh AR, Shelton GL, eds. The Team Physician's Handbook. Philadelphia, Hanley & Belfus, 1990:59-69
• Knochel JP: Heatstroke and related heat stress disorders. Disease-A-Month 1989;35(5):301-377
• Brouchama A: Heat stroke: a new look at an ancient disease. Int Care Med 1995;21(8):623-625
• Lea-Chiong TL, Stith JT: Heat stroke and other heat related illnesses. The maladies of summer. Postgrad Med 1995;98(1):26-28
• Bross MH, Nash BT, Carlton F: Heat emergencies. Am Fam Phys 1994;50(2):389-396
Illustrations: N/A
Internet references: http://www.5mcc.com

Author(s)
Scott A. Fields, MD

Hemochromatosis

BASICS

DESCRIPTION A hereditary disorder in which the small intestine absorbs excessive iron. Since the body lacks any way to excrete iron, the excess is stored in glands and muscle, such as the liver, pancreas, and heart. Over the years, the involved organs begin to fail.

System(s) affected: Endocrine/Metabolic

Genetics: Autosomal recessive; acquired; mutation in HFE gene; associated with HLA-A3, HLA-B14, HLA-B7

Incidence/Prevalence in USA:
3 cases/1000 people (heterozygote frequency 1 in 10) - the most common abnormal gene in the US population

Predominant age: Present from birth, but symptoms usually present in the fifth and sixth decades

Predominant sex: Male = Female (clinical signs are more frequent in men (8:1 male to female ratio)

SIGNS AND SYMPTOMS
- Weakness (83%)
- Abdominal pain (58%)
- Arthralgia (43%)
- Loss of libido or potency (38%)
- Amenorrhea (22%)
- Dyspnea on exertion (15%)
- Neurologic symptoms (6%)
- Hepatomegaly (83%)
- Increased skin pigmentation (75%)
- Loss of body hair (20%)
- Splenomegaly (13%)
- Peripheral edema (12%)
- Jaundice (10%)
- Gynecomastia (8%)
- Ascites (6%)
- Testicular atrophy
- Hepatic tenderness
- Diabetes mellitus symptoms

CAUSES
- The mechanism for increased iron absorption in the face of excessive iron stores is unknown. Iron metabolism appears normal in this disease except for a higher level of circulating iron.
- Iron overload may be due to thalassemia, sideroblastic anemia, liver disease, excess iron intake, chronic transfusion

RISK FACTORS
- The disease is a genetic disorder. Some variables influence the age of onset and severity of symptoms
- Intake of iron, especially from vitamin supplements. These may contain large amounts of iron as well as vitamin C, which enhances iron absorption
- Alcohol increases the absorption of iron (as high as 41% of patients with symptomatic disease are alcoholic)
- Loss of blood delays the onset of symptoms, such as blood loss in women because of menstruation and pregnancy.

DIAGNOSIS

DIFFERENTIAL DIAGNOSIS
- Repeated transfusions
- Hereditary anemias with ineffective erythropoiesis
- Alcoholic cirrhosis
- Porphyria cutanea tarda
- Atransferrinemia
- Excessive ingestion of iron (rare)

LABORATORY
- Transferrin saturation (serum iron concentration divided by total iron-binding capacity x 100): greater than 70% is virtually diagnostic of iron overload; 45% or higher warrants further evaluation
- Serum ferritin: greater than 300 µg/L for men and post-menopausal women and 200 µg/L for pre-menopausal women
- Urinary iron
- Increased urine hemosiderin
- Hyperglycemia
- Decreased FSH
- Decreased LH
- Decreased testosterone
- Increased SGOT
- Hypoalbuminemia

Drugs that may alter lab results: Iron supplements, transfusions may elevate serum iron

Disorders that may alter lab results:
Inflammatory reactions, other forms of liver disease, certain tumors (e.g., acute granulocytic leukemia), rheumatoid arthritis may elevate serum ferritin

PATHOLOGICAL FINDINGS
- Increased hepatic parenchymal iron stores
- Hepatic fibrosis and cirrhosis with hepatomegaly
- Pancreatic enlargement
- Excess hemosiderin in liver, pancreas, myocardium, thyroid, parathyroid, joints, skin
- Cardiomegaly
- Joint deposition of iron

SPECIAL TESTS
After diagnosis established, consider oral glucose tolerance test to rule out diabetes and echocardiogram to rule out cardiomyopathy

IMAGING
CT scan, MRI, and magnetic susceptibility measurement (MSM) are being studied for measuring body iron, but have not yet reached validation and general availability

DIAGNOSTIC PROCEDURES
- Liver biopsy for stainable iron is the standard for diagnosis. Presence or absence of cirrhosis can also be ascertained.
- DNA PCR testing for HFE gene mutations C282Y and H63D - present in 85-90% of patients

TREATMENT

APPROPRIATE HEALTH CARE
Outpatient

GENERAL MEASURES
- Removal of excess iron by repeated phlebotomy once or twice weekly to establish and maintain a mild anemia (hematocrit of 37-39%)
- When the patient finally becomes iron deficient, a lifelong maintenance program of 4-6 phlebotomies a year to keep storage iron normal - maintain serum ferritin ≤ 50 µg/L

SURGICAL MEASURES N/A

ACTIVITY
Full activity unless significant heart disease

DIET
- An iron-poor diet is not of significant benefit
- Avoid alcohol, iron-fortified foods, iron-containing supplements, and uncooked shellfish
- Restrict vitamin C to small doses between meals
- Tea chelates iron and may be drunk with meals

PATIENT EDUCATION
- Iron Overload Diseases Association, Inc., 433 Westwind Dr., North Palm Beach, FL 33408
- American Hemochromatosis Society, Inc., 777 East Atlantic Ave, Z-363, Delray Beach, FL 33483-5352

Hemochromatosis

 MEDICATIONS

DRUG(S) OF CHOICE None. Only when phlebotomy is not feasible or in the presence of severe heart disease should the iron-chelating agent deferoxamine (Desferal) be considered.
Contraindications: N/A
Precautions: N/A
Significant possible interactions: N/A

ALTERNATIVE DRUGS None

 FOLLOWUP

PATIENT MONITORING
• Measure hematocrit before each phlebotomy - skip phlebotomy if hematocrit is less than 36%
• Schedule an additional phlebotomy when hematocrit is greater than 40%
• When anemia becomes refractory, repeat transferrin saturation and serum ferritin to confirm depletion of iron stores
• When iron stores are depleted, 4 to 6 phlebotomies a year should keep iron stores normal
• During maintenance therapy, measure transferrin saturation and serum ferritin yearly
• Liver biopsy to assess iron stores when serum iron transferrin and ferritin results have not normalized

PREVENTION/AVOIDANCE Family members should be screened

POSSIBLE COMPLICATIONS
• Cirrhosis
• Hepatoma (only in patients with cirrhosis)
• Diabetes mellitus
• Cardiomyopathy
• Arthritis
• Hypogonadism

EXPECTED COURSE/PROGNOSIS
• Patients diagnosed before cirrhosis develops and treated with phlebotomy have a normal life expectancy
• Life expectancy is reduced in patients with cirrhosis, diabetes mellitus, and patients that require longer than 18 months of phlebotomy therapy to return iron stores to normal

 MISCELLANEOUS

ASSOCIATED CONDITIONS See Possible complications

AGE-RELATED FACTORS
Pediatric: Although rare, iron overload can occur even as early as 2 years of age. The disorder can be diagnosed before iron overload is clinically apparent
Geriatric: N/A
Others: N/A

PREGNANCY Avoid iron supplements

SYNONYMS
• Bronze diabetes
• Troisier-Hanot-Chauffard syndrome

ICD-9-CM 275.0 Disorders of iron metabolism

SEE ALSO N/A

OTHER NOTES Most patients with hemochromatosis go undiagnosed. Since treatment with phlebotomy will prevent all complications when begun early, the diagnosis of hemochromatosis should be considered much more frequently by physicians

ABBREVIATIONS N/A

REFERENCES
• Bacon BR. Diagnosis and Management of Hemochromatosis. Gastroenterol 1997;113:995-9
• Powell LW, George DK, et al. Diagnosis of Hemochromatosis. Ann Intern Med 1998;129:925-31
• Barton JC, McDonnel SM, et al. Management of Hemochromatosis. Ann Intern Med 1998;129:932-9
Illustrations: 1 available on CD-ROM
Internet references: http://www.5mcc.com

Author(s)
Robert A. Marlow, MD, MA

Hemophilia

 BASICS

DESCRIPTION
• Hemophilia A and hemophilia B are clinically indistinguishable, inherited bleeding disorders due to a deficiency of coagulant factor VIII (hemophilia A) or factor IX (hemophilia B)
• Disease severity is determined by percent of coagulant factor present
◊ Severe; < 2%
◊ Moderate; 2-5%
◊ Mild; > 6%. Patients with greater than 25% factor activity rarely bleed, however bleeding after major surgery can occur in patients or carriers with factor VIII levels in the range of 25-35%.

System(s) affected:
Hemic/Lymphatic/Immunologic
Genetics: Both hemophilia A and hemophilia B are X-linked, recessive
Incidence/Prevalence in USA:
• Hemophilia A - 10 in 100,000 males
• Hemophilia B - 2 in 100,000 males
Predominant age:
• Both are congenital conditions
• Severe disease generally noted at birth or in first year
• Mild disease may not be diagnosed until young adulthood
Predominant sex: Females are generally asymptomatic carriers unless their factor level is < 40%. Rare exceptions occur from consanguinity within families, concomitant Turner's syndrome, or extremely disproportionate lyonization resulting in the preponderance of cells in the carrier female containing the X chromosome with the hemophilic gene.

SIGNS AND SYMPTOMS
• Bleeding into soft tissues, muscles, and weight-bearing joints
• Bleeding occurs hours to days after injury, can involve any organ, and can continue for hours to days
• Compartment syndromes and ischemic nerve damage from large hematomas
• Repeated bleeding into a joint causes osteoarthritis, articular fibrosis, and joint ankylosis
• Hematuria
• CNS bleeding, usually post-traumatic

CAUSES   Congenital

RISK FACTORS   Positive family history.
Can predict risk to offspring using simple Mendelian genetics for an X-linked recessive disorder.

 DIAGNOSIS

DIFFERENTIAL DIAGNOSIS
• Von Willebrand's disease
• Vitamin K deficiency (factor IX is vitamin K dependent)
• Other factor deficiencies, afibrinogenemia, dysfibrinogenemia, fibrinolytic defects, platelet disorders

LABORATORY
• Activated partial thromboplastin time (PTT) is prolonged while platelet count, and prothrombin time are normal
• Bleeding time is prolonged in 15-20% of patients with hemophilia A
• PTT is corrected when mixed with normal plasma
• Hemophilia A - diagnostic test is low factor VIII.
• Hemophilia B - diagnostic test is low factor IX
Drugs that may alter lab results: Recent aspirin use will increase bleeding time, leading to confusion with Von Willebrand's disease
Disorders that may alter lab results: N/A

PATHOLOGICAL FINDINGS
• Synovial hemosiderosis
• Articular cartilage degeneration
• Thickening of periarticular tissues
• Bony hypertrophy

SPECIAL TESTS   Hemophilia A - carrier
detection compares the ratio of factor VIII to von Willebrand's factor protein and is predictive in up to 95% of cases. Molecular diagnosis is preferred for carrier testing.

IMAGING   N/A

DIAGNOSTIC PROCEDURES   N/A

 TREATMENT

APPROPRIATE HEALTH CARE
• Outpatient
• Home infusion therapy
• Inpatient for infusions following significant bleeding episodes

GENERAL MEASURES
• Avoid aspirin or aspirin-containing drugs
• Treat early. Symptoms often precede obvious bleeding.
• An uncomplicated, soft tissue bleeding or an early hemarthrosis requires a single infusion to 20-30% activity
• More extensive hemarthrosis or retroperitoneal bleeding requires bid infusions for 72 or more hours to 25-50% activity
• Life-threatening bleeding into the CNS requires maintaining levels greater than 50% activity for 2 weeks
• Major surgery requires greater than 50% activity preoperatively, continued for 1-2 weeks postoperatively
• Orthopedic care and physical therapy to prevent contractures and maintain joint mobility
• Vaccinate against hepatitis B at time of diagnosis
• Maintain good dental care
• Annual evaluation in a comprehensive hemophilia center
• Consideration for three times weekly prophylaxis in severe factor VIII deficiency

SURGICAL MEASURES
• Surgical or radionucleotide synovectomy, in selected patients
• Joint replacement, in selected patients

ACTIVITY
• Attempt to lead as normal a life as possible
• Restrict activities in proportion to the degree of factor deficiency, but maintaining a trim physical condition is important

DIET   No special diet

PATIENT EDUCATION
• Teach patient and family about signs and symptoms to watch for
• Genetic counseling
• Home care with self administered replacement therapy is often used
• Printed patient information available from: National Hemophilia Foundation, 110 Green Street, Room 406, New York, NY, 10012, (212)219-8180

Hemophilia

MEDICATIONS

DRUG(S) OF CHOICE

• Hemophilia A: Recombinant or monoclonal factor VIII is treatment of choice for hemophilia A patients who are HIV negative and who have had minimal prior concentrate exposure. Less optimal are plasma products enriched in factor VIII [cryoprecipitate, factor VIII concentrate]

◊ 1 unit of factor VIII (the amount in 1 mL of plasma) per kg of body weight will raise the plasma level of the recipient by 2%

◊ Number units = [(desired percent activity - current percent activity) times (body weight in kilograms)] divided by 2

◊ For example: 70 kg patient with 5% activity needs to be taken to 25% activity. Units needed: [(25% - 5%) x (70 kg)] / 2 = [(25 - 5) x (70)] / 2 = 700 units of factor VIII needed

◊ Half-life of factor VIII is 8-12 hours, therefore need to infuse at least bid to maintain a chosen factor VIII level, and tid when tight control of the level is needed

• Hemophilia B: Recombinant factor IX became available in mid 1997 and is treatment of choice for hemophilia B patients who are HIV negative and who have had minimal prior concentrate exposure. Monoclonal antibody purified factor IX is an effective and apparently safe plasma derived product

◊ For mild patients: Desmopressin (DDAVP); 0.3 mcg/kg diluted in 10-20ml of saline IV over 20 minutes. An intranasal preparation is also available.

◊ Factor IX concentrate for moderate to severe hemorrhage and patients to undergo surgery. One unit/kg will raise levels 1%

◊ Number units = [(desired percent activity - current percent activity) times (body weight in kilograms)] divided by 1

◊ For example: 70 kg patient with 5% activity needs to be taken to 25% activity. Units needed: [(25% - 5%) x (70 kg)] / 2 = [(25 - 5) x (70)] / 1 = 1400 units of factor IX needed

Contraindications: None

Precautions: Hemophilia B - some factor IX concentrates contain trace amounts of activated vitamin K-dependent factors and therefore are thrombogenic and carry a risk for thromboembolism

Significant possible interactions: N/A

ALTERNATIVE DRUGS

• Aminocaproic acid (epsilon-aminocaproic acid, EACA) can be used for minor dental work following a single factor VIII infusion. Aminocaproic acid greatly enhances the risk of thromboembolism and should be used with caution with factor IX concentrates.

• Patients with inhibitors to factor VIII may require intensive plasmapheresis, large doses of concentrate, infusion of prothrombin complex concentrates (by-passing products), or porcine factor VIII

FOLLOWUP

PATIENT MONITORING
Regular evaluations every 6 to 12 months include a musculoskeletal evaluation, an inhibitor screen, liver tests, and tests for antibodies to hepatitis viruses and human immunodeficiency virus (HIV)

PREVENTION/AVOIDANCE
Genetic counseling

POSSIBLE COMPLICATIONS

• Factor VIII and IX preparations and transfusions may result in viral hepatitis, chronic liver disease, and acquired immunodeficiency syndrome (AIDS). However, recent advances in factor VIII concentrate preparation should prevent future HIV infection and hepatitis B and C.

• Hemophilia A - 10-20% of patients develop inhibitors to factor VIII, typically those with severe disease receiving multiple transfusions. Type I (high responders) inhibitors to factor VIII rapidly neutralize factor VIII and prevent effective transfusion therapy. Type II (low responders) inhibitors are low-titer and may respond to higher than normal doses of factor VIII.

EXPECTED COURSE/PROGNOSIS

• Repeated hemarthroses result in eventual deformity and crippling

• Survival is normal for those with mild disease, and mortality is increased 2 to 6 fold in those with moderate to severe disease, primarily due to complications of infection

• Median life expectancy with this condition peaked in late 1970's at 68 years, and is now declining due to the AIDS epidemic

• Up to 70% are HIV seropositive, especially those with severe disease, and 4% with severe disease develop AIDS. Younger patients whose treatment began since the mid-late 80's are largely HIV negative and are not expected to be exposed by modern replacement products. The proportion of HIV positive hemophiliacs is therefore declining.

MISCELLANEOUS

ASSOCIATED CONDITIONS
None

AGE-RELATED FACTORS

Pediatric: Mean age of onset of symptoms is 1.5 years for severe disease (often noted in first year), 3 years for moderate disease, and 5 years or later for mild disease

Geriatric: N/A

Others: N/A

PREGNANCY

• The vast majority of females are asymptomatic carriers, although an occasional carrier will bleed at time of surgery. They require no specific treatment during pregnancy or delivery.

• Prenatal diagnosis previously required sampling fetal blood for coagulant activity. Newer prenatal detection schemes detect an identifiable restriction fragment length polymorphism or a gene deletion or rearrangement in a sample of chorionic villus or from fluid obtained at amniocentesis.

SYNONYMS

• Hemophilia A
• Factor VIII deficiency
• Classic hemophilia
• Hemophilia B
• Factor IX deficiency
• Christmas disease

ICD-9-CM

286.0 Hemophilia A
286.1 Hemophilia B

SEE ALSO
N/A

OTHER NOTES
Recombinant factor VIII is available. It has biologic activity and clinical efficacy comparable to plasma factor VIII, while posing no risk of transmitting hepatitis viruses or HIV. There are factor VIII and factor IX concentrates prepared from human plasma using a monoclonal antibody method plus either heat or detergent treatment of the concentrate. These monoclonal-prepared concentrates have the lowest risk for hepatitis B and essentially no risk for HIV infection. (Recombinant factor IX became available in mid 1997, and has no risk of viral infection.)

ABBREVIATIONS
N/A

REFERENCES

• Jones PK, Ratnoff OD: The changing prognosis of classic hemophilia (factor VII "deficiency"). Ann Int Med 1991;114(8):641-8
• Schwartz RS, et al: Human Recombinant DNA-Derived Antihemophilic Factor (Factor VIII) in the Treatment of Hemophilia A. N Engl J Med 1990;323(26):1800-5

Illustrations: N/A

Internet references: http://www.5mcc.com

Author(s)

W. Paul Bowman, MD

Hemorrhoids

BASICS

DESCRIPTION Varicosities of the hemorrhoidal venous plexus. Usual course - acute; chronic; relapsing.
• External hemorrhoids are located below the dentate line and covered by squamous epithelium
• Internal hemorrhoids are located above the dentate line
System(s) affected: Gastrointestinal, Cardiovascular
Genetics: No known genetic pattern
Incidence/Prevalence in USA: Common
Predominant age: Adults, although may occur at any age
Predominant sex: Male = Female

SIGNS AND SYMPTOMS
• All cases:
  ◊ Constipation
  ◊ Straining with defecation
• Small or minimal
  ◊ Episodic bleeding on stool
• Extensive internal
  ◊ Feeling of incomplete evacuation
• Small or minimal external
  ◊ Pruritus
• Protruding but can be reduced
  ◊ Mass
  ◊ Prominent bleeding
  ◊ Pruritus
  ◊ Thrombosis with severe acute pain
• Protruding, not reducible
  ◊ Mass
  ◊ Inability to clean after stool
  ◊ Thrombosis common
  ◊ Strangulation possible
  ◊ Ulceration

CAUSES
• Dilated veins of hemorrhoidal plexus
• Tight internal anal sphincter

RISK FACTORS
• Pregnancy
• Colon malignancy
• Liver disease
• Portal hypertension
• Constipation
• Occupations that require prolonged sitting
• Loss of muscle tone in old age, rectal surgery, episiotomy, anal intercourse
• Obesity

DIAGNOSIS

DIFFERENTIAL DIAGNOSIS
• Rectal or anal neoplasia
• Condyloma

LABORATORY N/A
Drugs that may alter lab results: N/A
Disorders that may alter lab results: N/A

PATHOLOGICAL FINDINGS N/A

SPECIAL TESTS N/A

IMAGING N/A

DIAGNOSTIC PROCEDURES
• Ano-rectal examination including anoscopy
• Sigmoidoscopy
• Inspection following straining at stool

TREATMENT

APPROPRIATE HEALTH CARE
All of these treatments, except surgical, are outpatient with recovery and freedom from symptoms within 48 hours

GENERAL MEASURES
• Mild symptoms or prevention:
  ◊ Avoid prolonged sitting at stool
  ◊ Avoid straining
  ◊ Avoid constipation through stool softeners, and high fiber intake in diet or with supplements
  ◊ Use soap and water for cleanup after stool
• For pain, sitz baths with soapy water, or hypertonic epsom salts (cup per 2 quarts of water)
• Mild and minimal hemorrhoids respond to changed diet, relief of constipation, soap and water cleanup and brief stooling
• Pruritus or mild discomfort after stooling responds to hydrocortisone ointment, anesthetic ointments or sprays
• Mild bleeding with external hemorrhoids responds to sitz baths and ointments or suppositories

SURGICAL MEASURES
• Indications
  ◊ Persisting and soiling bleeding
  ◊ Prolapsed internal hemorrhoids
  ◊ Poor anal hygiene due to prolapsed hemorrhoids
  ◊ Persistent pain
• Treatments
  ◊ For severe pain:
    - Incision of thrombosed hemorrhoid
  ◊ Severe protruding hemorrhoids:
    - Rubber band ligation (internal hemorrhoids only)
    - Injection therapy (suitable for one or two)
    - Cryosurgery, infrared or laser surgery for external hemorrhoids
  ◊ Prolapsed rectum
    - Requires surgical correction
  ◊ Surgical resection - for major external or internal hemorrhoids

ACTIVITY
• No restrictions
• Encourage physical fitness
• Avoid prolonged sitting and straining on the toilet

DIET High fiber

PATIENT EDUCATION Explain recurrence benignity, need for good diet, exercise and stooling health

MEDICATIONS

DRUG(S) OF CHOICE
- Prevention:
  ◊ Fiber supplements
  ◊ Stool softeners
- Pain:
  ◊ Analgesic sprays or ointments - benzocaine (Hurricaine), dibucaine (Nupercainal)
- Pruritus:
  ◊ Hydrocortisone (Anusol-HC, Cortifoam) ointment
- Bleeding:
  ◊ Astringent suppositories (Preparation H)
  ◊ Hydrocortisone (Anusol; Cortifoam) ointment

Contraindications: Refer to manufacturer's literature

Precautions: Refer to manufacturer's literature

Significant possible interactions: Refer to manufacturer's literature

ALTERNATIVE DRUGS N/A

FOLLOWUP

PATIENT MONITORING As needed, depending on treatment

PREVENTION/AVOIDANCE
- Avoid constipation
- Lose weight, if overweight
- Avoid prolonged sitting on the toilet
- Avoid prolonged sitting at work. Get up and move around periodically.

POSSIBLE COMPLICATIONS
- Thrombosis
- Secondary infection
- Ulceration
- Anemia (rare)
- Incontinence

EXPECTED COURSE/PROGNOSIS
- Spontaneous resolution
- Recurrence

MISCELLANEOUS

ASSOCIATED CONDITIONS
- Liver disease
- Pregnancy
- Portal hypertension
- Constipation

AGE-RELATED FACTORS
Pediatric:
- Uncommon in infants and children. Look for underlying cause, e.g., venacaval or mesenteric obstruction, cirrhosis, portal hypertension.
- Occasionally, as in adults, hemorrhoids may result from chronic constipation, fecal impaction and straining at stool. Surgery is rarely required.

Geriatric: Common in elderly along with rectal prolapse

Others: N/A

PREGNANCY Common in pregnancy.
Usually resolves after pregnancy. No treatment required, unless extremely painful.

SYNONYMS Piles

ICD-9-CM
455.6 hemorrhoids, nos

SEE ALSO
- Colorectal malignancy
- Portal hypertension
- Portal vein thrombosis

OTHER NOTES N/A

ABBREVIATIONS N/A

REFERENCES
- Fazio VW: Anorectal Disorders. In Gastroenterology Clinics of North America, Philadelphia, W.B. Saunders Co., 1987
- Pfenninger JL: Modern treatments for internal hemorrhoids. Brit Med J 1997;314:1211-2
- Nagle D, Rolandelli RH: Primary care office management of perianal and anal disease. Primary Care; Clinics in Office Practice 1996;23:609-20
- Metcalf A: Anorectal disorders. Five common causes of pain, itching, and bleeding. Postgraduate Medicine 1995;98:81-94

Illustrations: N/A

Internet references: http://www.5mcc.com

Author(s)
Frank L. Iber, MD

Hepatic encephalopathy

BASICS

DESCRIPTION Altered mental and neuromotor functioning associated with acute or chronic liver disease and/or portal systemic shunting of blood. The prominent features are mild to marked forgetfulness, impaired arousability, and a "flapping tremor" (asterixis).
System(s) affected: Gastrointestinal, Nervous
Genetics: Unknown
Incidence/Prevalence in USA:
• Occurs in 1/3 cases of cirrhosis
• Occurs in all cases of fulminant hepatic failure
• Present in nearly half of patients who reach the stage of liver disease requiring transplantation
Predominant age: Parallels that of fulminant liver disease with peak in the 40's, and cirrhosis with peak in late 50's. May occur at any age.
Predominant sex: Male = Female (reflecting the underlying liver disease)

SIGNS AND SYMPTOMS
• Ages 10-60
◊ Prominent signs of underlying liver disease (50%), jaundice most common, ascites second most common
◊ Gastrointestinal hemorrhage with hematemesis or melena (20%)
◊ Systemic infection, urinary tract or pulmonary (20%)
◊ Four stages of confusion and obtundity described. (1) forgetfulness, disturbance in nocturnal sleep, daytime drowsiness, (2) mild confusion but arousability, (3) arousable, but markedly confused, limited orientation and thought content, (4) unarousable.
◊ Asterixis prominent in stages 2, 3
◊ Handwriting and hand coordination deteriorated in stages 1, 2
◊ Tremor prominent in stage 2
◊ Psychotic thoughts infrequent
◊ Reflexes symmetrically hyperactive
◊ Tremor and asterixis not observed in ocular muscles
◊ Mental and neurological signs change rapidly (over 6 to 12 hours)
• Age over 60
◊ Signs of underlying liver disease diminished (25%)
◊ Confusion more prominent
◊ Precipitating gastrointestinal hemorrhage or infection less often identified
◊ Remains in stage 1 or 2 for many days
◊ Progression slower
• Age under 10
◊ Signs of underlying liver disease prominent, usually fulminant hepatic failure or extremely advanced cirrhosis
◊ Progression through the stages very rapid, often 6 to 12 hours
◊ Precipitating cause frequently not identified

CAUSES
• Shunting of intestinal blood through the severely diseased liver without the intervention of viable liver cells. TIPS (transjugular intrahepatic portacaval shunt), a widely used radiologically inserted shunt to lower portal pressure, produces liver encephalopathy.
• Shunting of such blood through collateral circulation or surgically constructed portacaval shunts
• Thus hepatic coma may occur in extremely advanced acute liver disease (fulminant hepatic failure) or following portacaval shunting or transjugular intrahepatic portal shunt (TIPS). However, it is most common in long standing cirrhosis of the liver with spontaneous shunting of intestinal blood through collaterals.
• Failure of liver to detoxicate agents noxious to CNS, eg, ammonia, mercaptans, fatty acids
• Increased aromatic and reduced branched chain amino acids in blood
• Precipitation of acute event, search for:
◊ New overt or occult infection including spontaneous peritonitis
◊ Potassium, magnesium or other electrolyte depletion
◊ Use of opiate, sedative, tranquilizer, drugs
◊ Gastrointestinal bleeding

RISK FACTORS
• Infection
• Sedative or opiate drugs
• Electrolyte disturbance
• Anemia
• Gastrointestinal hemorrhage

DIAGNOSIS

DIFFERENTIAL DIAGNOSIS
• Head trauma, concussion, subdural hematoma
• Alcohol withdrawal syndrome
• Toxic confusion due to medication
• Toxic confusion due to illicit drug use
• Meningitis
• Metabolic encephalopathy related to anoxia, hypoglycemia, hypokalemia, hypo- or hypercalcemia, uremia

LABORATORY
• Screening blood, sputum and urine cultures to identify infection
• Hematology to identify anemia and signs of infection
• Standard biochemistry profile to identify hypokalemia, bilirubinemia, altered calcium status, hypomagnesemia, urea, hypoglycemia
• Arterial blood gases
• Liver tests to evaluate severity of underlying liver disease
• Prothrombin and partial thromboplastin time
• Venous ammonia (elevated in 70% of liver coma)
• Toxicology screen for illicit drugs

Drugs that may alter lab results:
• Infusion of amino acid solutions may affect ammonia level
• Opiate administration - producing severe constipation may affect ammonia level
Disorders that may alter lab results:
• Uremia may affect ammonia level
• Rapid and severe tissue breakdown, massive burns, trauma or infection may affect ammonia level

PATHOLOGICAL FINDINGS
• Brain edema in 100% of fatal cases
• Glial hypertrophy in chronic encephalopathy

SPECIAL TESTS
• Electroencephalogram shows symmetrical slowing of basic (alpha) rhythm in common with other forms of metabolic encephalopathy
• Visually-evoked potential specific in stages 2, 3 and 4

IMAGING
• Useful only to rule out other diagnoses
• CT scan of head most useful
• Brain MRI shows increased glutamine in basal ganglia

DIAGNOSTIC PROCEDURES
• Clinical setting and findings adequate in 80% of cases
• Venous ammonia of great aid in patients with chronic liver disease when the clinical findings are confusing
• EEG is useful to a limited extent, but findings are similar in other forms of metabolic encephalopathy
• Treatment response often confirms diagnosis

TREATMENT

APPROPRIATE HEALTH CARE
• Outpatient for stages 1 and 2 when diagnosis is clear and if recurrent can be managed satisfactorily
• Stage 3 or 4 requires inpatient management
• Stage 3 or 4 in fulminant hepatic failure is a strong indication for evaluation for liver transplantation. Transfer to a transplant center should be considered.

GENERAL MEASURES
• Identify and treat vigorously precipitating causes - gastrointestinal bleed, infection, sedative drugs, or electrolyte imbalance are most common
• Stage 2 or higher - attention to adequate fluid intake, and at least 1000 kcal (4.19 MJ) of food daily
• Give Fleet's enema to all patients without diarrhea
• Clumsiness and poor judgment prominent. Be sure patient has the care needed to avoid falls, cuts on broken glass, smoking burns, machinery or auto accidents.
• Avoid sedative or opiate medications. Benzodiazepine sedatives and opiate derivatives such as Lomotil have caused liver coma.

SURGICAL MEASURES N/A

ACTIVITY
• As tolerated
• Avoid driving and machinery

DIET
• Integrate with needs of underlying liver disease
• Lower total protein. Stage 1 - avoid protein gluttony. Stage 2 - limit red meat and consume small portions of all other protein foods, total protein for day 50-60 grams. Stage 3 - consume 40 gram protein or vegetable protein diet (about 20 grams). Stage 4 - consume 10 or fewer grams of protein. For all stages at least 1000 kcal (4.19 MJ) ingested daily.
• As coma improves, increase dietary protein as tolerated

PATIENT EDUCATION
• Include family in education
• Dietician instruction in eating lower protein diets, avoid protein bingeing
• Avoid unnecessary sedative or antianxiety medications and opiates
• Recognition of early signs and to get treatment promptly
• Pamphlets (quite good for family) - American Association for the Study of Liver Diseases, 6900 Grove Road, Thorofare, NJ 08086, (609)848-1000)

MEDICATIONS

DRUG(S) OF CHOICE
• Lactulose (Cephulac) syrup 30 mL of 50% solution four times daily. Diminish to bid when 3 or more bowel movements a day occur daily.
• If stage 4 is present, worsening occurs, or no improvement in 2 days, add antibiotics. Amoxicillin 4 gm/day is suitable. Neomycin 1-4 gm/day in 4 divided doses may be used if renal status is good.
• Antacids as needed
Contraindications:
• Total ileus
• Hypersensitivity reaction
Precautions:
• Potassium depletion
• Electrolyte imbalance
• Renal failure
Significant possible interactions: Refer to manufacturer's profile of each drug

ALTERNATIVE DRUGS
• Any antibiotic affecting intestinal flora such as:
  ◊ Metronidazole or vancomycin in refractory cases
  ◊ Dopamine agonists, e.g., bromocriptine have been tried
  ◊ Branched-chain amino acids IV
  ◊ Flumazenil

FOLLOWUP

PATIENT MONITORING
• To optimize treatment a trail-making test should be followed (provided by Cephulac makers). Apply to Stage 1 and 2 patients to determine how much maintenance treatment and diet needed. Should be run daily at first and then at each visit when changes in drugs and diet are made.
• Patients with changed findings should be seen twice weekly
• Stable patients should be seen monthly
• Trail-making test performed at each office visit

PREVENTION/AVOIDANCE
• Avoid unessential medications, particularly opiates, sedatives
• Avoid protein binges

POSSIBLE COMPLICATIONS
• Recurrence
• Stable, chronic, impaired status
• With many recurrences, permanent basal ganglion injury (non-Wilsonian hepatolenticular degeneration)
• Hepatorenal syndrome
• Acute tubular necrosis
• Bleeding
• Disseminated intravascular coagulation
• Bacteremia
• Shock

EXPECTED COURSE/PROGNOSIS
• In acute or fulminant
  ◊ With adequate aggressive treatment, disappears without residue or recurrence
• In chronic liver disease
  ◊ Coma returns
  ◊ With each recurrence it becomes more and more difficult to treat
  ◊ Plateau of maximum improvement shows a decrement over several years, such that the degree of improvement with treatment is less and less. Eventual 80% mortality.

MISCELLANEOUS

ASSOCIATED CONDITIONS
• Liver disease
• Rarely with portacaval shunt with normal liver function

AGE-RELATED FACTORS See under
Signs and symptoms
Pediatric: N/A
Geriatric: N/A
Others: N/A

PREGNANCY May occur as a complication
of pregnancy

SYNONYMS
• Hepatic coma
• Liver coma

ICD-9-CM 572.2 Hepatic encephalopathy

SEE ALSO N/A

OTHER NOTES N/A

ABBREVIATIONS N/A

REFERENCES
• Cordoba J, Blei AT: Treatment of hepatic encephalopathy. Am J Gastroenter 1997;92:1429-1439
Illustrations: N/A
Internet references: http://www.5mcc.com

Author(s)
Frank L. Iber, MD

Hepatitis, viral

BASICS

DESCRIPTION A group of systemic infections involving the liver with common clinical manifestations; caused by different viruses with typically distinctive epidemiological patterns
System(s) affected: Gastrointestinal
Genetics: Some predisposition to immunologic manifestations; DR4 - positive increase with concurrent immunologic disease
Incidence/Prevalence in USA:
• HAV - 33% of Americans have antibodies; 125,000-200,000 infections/yr; 70% symptomatic
• HBV - 140,000-320,000 infections/year; 1-1.25 million chronically infected; >500,000 carriers (10% of infected). Post-transfusion HBV<1% of blood recipients.
• HCV - 16% of sporadic hepatitis: 35,000-180,000 new infections year ; 3.9 million chronically infected (85% of infected)
• HDV - present in 1% of HBV
• HEV - unknown
• HGV - 0.3% of acute viral hepatitis; 900-2,000 infections/yr; found in 2% of nonA, nonB chronic hepatitis. Frequent co-infection with HCV. In cryptogenic cirrhosis, HGV present in 12%; clinical significance unclear.
Predominant age: HAV rare in infants; susceptibility increases with age. HBV, HCV, HEV occur in all ages.
Predominant sex: Fulminant HBV: Male > Female (2:1)

SIGNS AND SYMPTOMS
• Fever (60%); unusual with HBV and HCV
• Malaise (67%)
• Nausea (80%)
• Anorexia (54%)
• Jaundice (in adults, 62%); 66% of HCV anicteric
• Dark urine (84%)
• Abdominal pain (56%)
• Fatigue (major complaint in HCV)
• Headache
• Meningismus (occasional)
• Vomiting

CAUSES
• Multiple viruses possible
• HAV and HEV transmitted enterically (fecal-oral); parenteral route rare
• Maximum infectivity 2 weeks before jaundice
• May be endemic in institutions
• HBV transmitted sexually or by blood products including infection acquired perinatally; also enterically. HDV coinfection increases HBV severity.
• HCV transmitted through blood or its products; in 40%, mode unknown
• HDV identified only with HBV infection
• HGV has similar patterns to HCV

RISK FACTORS
• Health care workers/other occupational risks
• Hemodialysis
• Recipients of blood and/or blood products
• IV drug users (53% of new infections); individuals with tattoos
• Sexually active homosexual males
• Household exposure
• Intimate exposure
• Positive needlestick
• Transplanted organs

DIAGNOSIS

DIFFERENTIAL DIAGNOSIS Infectious mononucleosis, primary or secondary hepatic malignancy, ischemic hepatitis, drug-induced hepatitis, alcoholic hepatitis, autoimmune hepatitis, Wilson's disease

LABORATORY
• Marked elevation of AST/ALT (acute hepatitis, particularly ALT, 400-several thousand U/L); HCV may have normal ALT; AST/ALT ratio =>1 associated with cirrhosis in chronic HCV
• Mild elevation of alkaline phosphatase
• Bilirubin from normal to markedly elevated; with elevation, conjugated and unconjugated fractions usually increased
• Serological markers to identify viruses

```
Diagnosis  Biochemical markers
HAV:
  A, R      Anti-HAV IgM
  P         Anti-HAV IgG
HBV:
  A, E      HBsAg
  A         Anti-HBc IgM,
              HBsAg, HBeAg
  C         HBsAg, +/- HBeAg
HCV:
  A,C,Rcv   Anti-HCV (ELISA)
HDV:
  A         HDAg, Anti-HDV IgM
  P         Anti-HDV IgG
HEV:        Test not available
HGV:        PCR-RNA
```

A-acute infection, R-recent in fection, C-chronic infection P-previous infection, E-early/ carrier state, Rcv-Recovered

• For severe hepatitis, measure PT and PTT, albumin, electrolytes, glucose and CBC
• If HBV chronic, confirm by HBV-DNA titer
• Patients with severe HBV infection should be tested for coinfection with HDV
• HBeAg indicates high infectivity (horizontal and vertical transmission)
• Persistence > 10 weeks indicates probable chronic liver disease
• Acute, ongoing HCV, confirm by other markers, RIBA, esp. HCV-RNA (for chronic HCV); >viral titers in genotypes 1a, 1b than 2, 3
• In early acute HCV infection, anti-HCV may be negative; may need retest in 3-6 months
• HCV antibodies (ELISA, RIBA) are sensitive markers for patients with chronic HCV, but not sensitive enough for detection of asymptomatic carriers (blood donors)

• Chronic HCV, may find (+) ANA, ASMA, LKMA
• Subtyping HCV genotypes using RIBA may be useful
Drugs that may alter lab results: N/A
Disorders that may alter lab results: N/A

PATHOLOGICAL FINDINGS Liver biopsy in persistent or chronic disease shows wide range of histologic changes (variable inflammation and/or necrosis, cholestasis, steatosis, fibrosis, cirrhosis or chronic active hepatitis. Clinical course does not predict severity of histopathologic changes.

SPECIAL TESTS Liver biopsy usually needed for determining type and extent of liver injury in persistent disease and to exclude other diseases. Also, usually necessary prior to start of interferon alfa treatment.

IMAGING Usually not of diagnostic importance. Ultrasound may demonstrate ascites or exclude obstruction.

DIAGNOSTIC PROCEDURES
• History; exposure source; exclude drugs
• Tenderness on fist percussion over the liver; may be hepatomegaly
• Jaundice may or may not be present
• Serum "liver function tests" often elevated before bilirubin increases; measure aminotransferases in acute illnesses when there is no evident cause
• Serum biochemical markers for each virus, diagnosis in 90% of patients

TREATMENT

APPROPRIATE HEALTH CARE
• Outpatient care usual
• Segregation helpful for food handlers with HAV, or health care workers with HBV or HCV

GENERAL MEASURES
• Correct: coagulation defects, fluid and electrolytes, acid-base imbalance, hypoglycemia, impairment of renal function
• Report acute cases to public health dept

SURGICAL MEASURES Consider liver transplantation in fulminant acute hepatitis/end-stage liver disease (HCV)

ACTIVITY As tolerated

DIET Adequate calories; balanced nutrition

PATIENT EDUCATION
• Proper use and disposal of needles
• Proper hygiene, particularly food handlers
• HBV sexually transmitted; HCV sexual transmission low, but does occur
• HBV present in saliva also

MEDICATIONS

DRUG(S) OF CHOICE
• Interferon alfa-2b (IFN, Intron A) or Interferon alfa-2a (Roferon-A)(HCV), or with ribavirin (Virazole) 1 g/day. Induces remission (25-50% in HBV; 40% in HCV); decreases abnormal aminotransferase concentrations in chronic HBV/HCV. May be used safely post-transplant.
• Amantadine (Symmetrel) or rimantadine (Flumadine) may be useful in HCV non-responders (to IFN) - 100 mg bid for 6 mo. Famciclovir (Famvir) 500 mg tid has been used for HBV.
• Corticosteroids: In cholestatic HAV, a short course may shorten illness, but may be most effective in milder disease

Contraindications: Interferon: platelet count < 50,000. Mouse immunoglobulin, egg protein or neomycin allergy. Corticosteroids may add to morbidity/increased mortality.

Precautions:
• Other disorders of coagulation, myelosuppression, seizures, depression (esp. suicide ideation), pregnancy, fertile age group, lactation.
• Increased serum triglycerides may occur during IFN therapy; may cause abnormal ALT. Measure HCV-RNA to assess response in such patients.
• Psychiatric evaluation may be prudent prior to IFN treatment in chronic HCV

Significant possible interactions: Refer to manufacturer's profile of each drug

ALTERNATIVE DRUGS
Lamivudine 100 mg daily for chronic hepatitis B

FOLLOWUP

PATIENT MONITORING
• Serial measurement of serum AST/ALT
• Appropriate serum viral markers useful for evaluation of recovery or progression
• Liver biopsies in chronic disease
• Monitor for metabolic complications
• WBC, platelets with interferon alpha therapy
• Chronic HBV, HBV-DNA valuable for prediction of favorable response to IFN. High pretreatment ALT and low pretreatment HBV-DNA associated with favorable response.
• With HCV, quantitative serum HCV-RNA levels monitor response and post-treatment relapse (if negative after 3 months, sustained response likely)

PREVENTION/AVOIDANCE
• General
  ◊ Screen blood products
  ◊ Proper disposal of needles
  ◊ Good sanitation, hygiene

• HAV
  ◊ Immune globulin (passive immunization) - 0.02 mL/kg IM (given 1-2 weeks after exposure prevents illness in 80-90%). With prolonged exposure give q 5 months. Also use for close contacts, day care staff/children (if case occurs), institutions with multiple cases, travelers to areas of high prevalence (with 3 week lead time, use vaccine).
  ◊ Hepatitis A vaccine (Havrix, Vaqta) 0.5 mL dose IM in children > 2 yrs; 1.0 mL in adults IM; 2nd dose 6-12 mo later for >8 yrs. Separate syringe site from immune globulin. Use for travelers, day-care staff/children, custodial facility employees, sewage workers, military, homosexual men, food handlers, Native Americans/Alaskan natives.
• HBV
  ◊ Hepatitis B vaccine: 3 doses at 0, 1, and 6 months. Dose dependent on manufacturer. Merck Recombivax: 0.5ml (5 mcg)/dose age ≤ 19 and 1.0 ml (10 mcg)/dose age >19. SKB Engerix: 0.5ml (10 mcg)/dose age ≤19 & 1.0ml(20 mcg)/dose age >19.
  ◊ High risk groups, use hepatitis B human immune globulin within 24 hr of exposure (0.06 mL/kg IM)
  ◊ HBV screening in pregnant women; vaccinate all infants at birth. Schedule: 3 injections - birth, 2 mo, 6-18 mo. Children/adolescents may start series anytime, but complete by age 11-12 yrs.
• HCV: No specifics on prevention/avoidance
• HDV: Preventing HBV will prevent HDV
• HEV: No specifics on prevention/avoidance
• HGV: Recommendations same as for HCV

POSSIBLE COMPLICATIONS
Acute or subacute necrosis, chronic active or chronic hepatitis, cirrhosis, hepatic failure; hepatocellular carcinoma (HBV, HCV)

EXPECTED COURSE/PROGNOSIS
• Varies with causative virus
• Severity of hepatic encephalopathy best predictor of poor survival in hepatic failure
• HAV may cause mild disease at times, often no jaundice; no chronic liver disease; mortality < 1%; lifetime immunity usual with recovery. 3 rare variants: relapsing, cholestatic, fulminant.
• HBV (mortality 1%) and HDV (with icterus, mortality 2-20%) more severe symptoms; often leads to persistent/chronic liver disease, cirrhosis, liver failure, hepatocellular carcinoma (HCC); more severe problems if impaired immune function. Follow treatment with HBV-DNA levels.
• In HCV, regardless of severity, >80% progress to chronic hepatitis, 20-50% to cirrhosis, and some, liver failure. Typically slow progression 10-30 years. May progress to HCC, but IFN may decrease HCC risk. Association with type II AI. Chronic HCV unlikely to clear HCV-RNA spontaneously. HCV after needlestick, usually sustained IFN response. Final phase HCV rare cause of fulminant hepatic failure.
• Alcohol may be factor for HCC in chronic HCV
• Chronic HDV, 70% develop cirrhosis; low incidence of HCC
• HEV does not result in chronic disease

MISCELLANEOUS

ASSOCIATED CONDITIONS
• Arthritis, urticaria, immune complex nephritis (particularly membranous glomerulopathy), anemias (including aplastic anemia), dermatitis and cardiomyopathy (usually with HBV, rare with HCV). HCV implicated in sporadic form of idiopathic mixed cryoglobulinemia, porphyria cutanea tarda, polyarteritis nodosa.
• HIV-HCV: more severe course

AGE-RELATED FACTORS
Pediatric: HAV milder; usually anicteric; may be unrecognized. HBV more acute, less prolonged, less complications, but may become chronic.
Geriatric: N/A
Others: Alcohol abuse a major factor for chronic liver disease from HBV and HCV. Measure viral biochemical markers in patients with alcoholic liver disease (esp. anti-HCV).

PREGNANCY
• Test, in later gestation, for HBsAg
• HBV transmitted vertically (< 10%) as well as perinatally and produces carrier state in 30%. Give infant HBIg 0.5 mL and HBV vaccine (Recombivax HB; separate sites) within 12 hrs of birth followed by HBV vaccine, 0.5 mL IM at ages 1 and 6 months. Check HBsAg and HBsAb at age 1
• HCV vertical transmission increased in HIV

SYNONYMS N/A

ICD-9-CM
070 Viral hepatitis

SEE ALSO Immunizations

OTHER NOTES N/A

ABBREVIATIONS
PCR = polymerase chain reaction; HCC = hepatocellular carcinoma; AI = autoimmune hepatitis

REFERENCES
• Alter MJ, Mast EE: The epidemiology of viral hepatitis in the U.S. Gastroenterol Clin North Am 1994; 23:437-455
• Seeff LP: Natural history of hepatitis, type C. Semin Gastrointest Dis, 1995;6:20
1 additional references available at web site
Internet references: http://www.5mcc.com
Illustrations: N/A

Author(s)
Geoffrey R. Swain, MD

Hepatoma

BASICS

DESCRIPTION Primary malignant tumor of liver arising from hepatic parenchymal cells (hepatocytes), blood vessels or cholangioles within the liver, excluding gallbladder and biliary passages. With the exception of fibrolamellar type almost always associated with an underlying liver disease, usually cirrhosis.

System(s) affected: Gastrointestinal
Genetics: No known genetic pattern
Incidence/Prevalence in USA:
• 1-5 new cases per 100,000 of population per year
• Among known cirrhotics, 2-5 cases/100/year
Predominant age: 6th-8th decade (mean age 55-62 years) in USA and western countries. Among immigrants from Asia and Africa occurs 2-3 decades earlier.
Predominant sex: Male > Female (3-4:1)

SIGNS AND SYMPTOMS
• Early curable stage
  ◊ Paraneoplastic syndrome - feminization, precocious puberty
  ◊ Palpable nodule on liver
  ◊ Age 2 to 6 years - abdominal mass in liver, abdominal pain, irregular hepatomegaly
• Usual adult manifestations
  ◊ Known cirrhosis or prominent clinical signs of cirrhosis - 80%
  ◊ Abdominal pain - 80%, right upper quadrant, dull ache to severe, aggravated by jolting
  ◊ Hepatomegaly - 80-90%, irregular, nodular, firm to hard, tender
  ◊ Weight loss, 30%
  ◊ Hepatic arterial bruit, 20%
  ◊ Friction rub - rare, more common in metastatic liver disease
  ◊ Nausea, vomiting
  ◊ Fever - 10-50%, low grade, intermittent
  ◊ Paraneoplastic manifestations - hypertrophic osteoarthropathy, carcinoid syndrome, feminization, polycythemia
  ◊ Hemoperitoneum, most common tumor cause
  ◊ Unexplained deterioration of stable cirrhosis
  ◊ Budd-Chiari syndrome
  ◊ Blockage of portal vein, inferior vena cava, renal veins

CAUSES
• Cirrhosis - accounts for 60 to 80% of cases. Alcoholic cirrhosis most important in western world. Reported risk of hepatoma in alcoholic cirrhosis is 3-10% with micronodular pattern.
• Hepatitis B virus infection - associated with > 70% of cases worldwide. Most important factor in Africa and Asia but less important in western countries. In USA, HBsAg is positive in 20% cases of this tumor.
• Hepatitis C virus infection - 50-70% of HBsAg negative patients are positive for anti-HCV antibody, an important factor in hepatoma patients not due to HBV infection. Particular problem in Orientals.

• Mycotoxins (aflatoxins) - metabolite of fungus Aspergillus flavus that contaminates foods. Two series, B1 and derivatives and G1 and derivatives. B1 being the most potent carcinogen, important in Sub-Saharan Africa and Southeast Asia, no significant role in USA.
• Vinyl polymer, but not the finished product, produces angiosarcoma

RISK FACTORS
• Primary liver disease - cirrhosis, chronic active hepatitis
• HBsAg positivity, anti-HCV antibody
• Chronic use of oral contraceptives
• Hemochromatosis
• Alpha-1-antitrypsin deficiency
• Primary biliary cirrhosis
• Metabolic disorders (tyrosinemia, Niemann-Pick disease)
• Clonorchiasis, gallstones, choledochal cysts - cholangiocarcinoma

DIAGNOSIS

DIFFERENTIAL DIAGNOSIS
• Early asymptomatic tumor - underlying liver conditions, e.g., cirrhosis, chronic hepatitis; benign liver nodules, hamartoma, hemangioma, metastatic adenocarcinoma, gallstones, or gallbladder polyp
• Late symptomatic tumor with hepatomegaly - hepatic cyst, adenoma, hemangioma, abscess, metastatic malignancy of liver, cirrhosis with activity, infarction of liver, fatty infiltration, thrombosis of hepatic veins, portal vein, inferior vena cava, active viral hepatitis, alcoholic hepatitis
• Ruptured tumor - all causes of acute abdomen, traumatic hemoperitoneum

LABORATORY
• Erythrocytosis, elevated Ca, low glucose
• Liver function test abnormalities
• Tumor markers
  ◊ Alpha fetoprotein (AFP) - single most important lab test for screening and diagnosis of hepatoma - 70%. Negative in angiosarcoma, cholangiocarcinoma and fibrolamellar carcinoma. Level > 400 ng/mL (> 400 µg/L) is diagnostic, level does not correlate with prognosis.
  ◊ Other markers - des-gamma-carboxyprothrombin, gamma glutamyl transferase, carcinoembryonic antigen (CEA), variant alkaline phosphatase, isoferritins
Drugs that may alter lab results:
Hypoglycemic agents, calcitonin, vitamin D
Disorders that may alter lab results:
Acute or chronic hepatitis, germ cell tumors, pregnancy. All cause slight elevation of AFP.

PATHOLOGICAL FINDINGS
• Nodular - 75%, usually in cirrhotic liver
• Massive - common in children and non-cirrhotic livers, more prone to rupture
• Diffuse - rare, a large part of liver is involved
• Hepatocellular origin - most commonly multicentric, well differentiated, usually superimposed on underlying cirrhosis. Almost always produces bile. Anaplastic form often difficult to be certain of cell of origin or differentiate from metastatic malignancy.
• Fibrolamellar - single nodule, non-cirrhotic, extensive fibrous stroma
• Cholangiocarcinoma - multicentric, most often mixed with hepatocellular elements
• Angiosarcoma

SPECIAL TESTS   N/A

IMAGING
• Plain x-ray - useful to demonstrate metastatic involvement to lung and bone
• Ultrasound - best diagnostic imaging technique, capable of detecting tumor < 1 cm, and may be positive when AFP is normal. Has been useful in serially following cases of cirrhosis to identify hepatocellular cancer when under 2 cm and curable.
• CT scan - valuable in determining extrahepatic spread of the disease
• MRI - helpful in delineating the details of tumor, and invasion of vessels
• Hepatic arteriography - mostly done to see the anatomy of hepatic vessels and extent of tumor while considering resection, embolization, dearterialization or intra-arterial infusion of cytotoxic agents. Most useful in detecting angiosarcoma, separating benign vs. malignant.
• Lipiodal angiography and CT - lipiodal is readily taken up by tumor cells, this technique can detect even millimeter sized lesions. Lipiodal also serves as a vehicle to deliver chemotherapeutic or radioactive agents to the tumor.
• Gallium scans - 90% of hepatocellular carcinoma and 60% of other types of liver cell tumors take up and retain gallium for up to 48 hours

DIAGNOSTIC PROCEDURES
• Liver biopsy - recommended for all tumors and particularly small nodules detected on serial ultrasound
• Fine needle aspiration - under ultrasonography, may be difficult to determine cell origin when anaplastic, unable to diagnose fibrolamellar and angiosarcoma due to too small a sample of tissue
• Laparoscopy - to visualize the extent of tumor, to see whether non-tumorous liver is cirrhotic, peritoneal spread, and obtain diagnostic biopsy
• Exploratory laparotomy with operative biopsy, commonly used in children

TREATMENT

APPROPRIATE HEALTH CARE
Inpatient initially

GENERAL MEASURES
Precautions to avoid falls, attention to nutrition

SURGICAL MEASURES
• Surgery is lobectomy, liver segmentectomy or whatever required for complete removal
• Repeated alcohol injection of involved tumor sites under ultrasound guidance shrinks tumor mass and prolongs survival and improves quality of life
• Infarcting the tumor by radiological injection of its arterial supply does not prolong survival
• Liver transplantation curative in cancer with cirrhosis with 15% alive at 3 years
• Incidental hepatomas < 2 cm found at transplant do not influence survival.

ACTIVITY
As tolerated

DIET
High calorie, low protein diet

PATIENT EDUCATION
Important for prevention; abstinence from alcohol and IV drugs, vaccination against HBV

MEDICATIONS

DRUG(S) OF CHOICE
Only for unresectable hepatoma patients. Doxorubicin (Adriamycin) 60-75 mg/m2 every 3 weeks. Dose can be repeated depending on the response. Only partial response in 25% cases.
Contraindications:
• Cardiomyopathy
• Poor hepatic reserves (bilirubin > 2.0)
Precautions: Neutropenia with nadir at 10-14 days, septicemia, cardiotoxicity (25%) if cumulative dose > 550 mg/m2, hepatotoxicity
Significant possible interactions: N/A

ALTERNATIVE DRUGS
• Fluorouracil (5-FU), cyclophosphamide, methotrexate have been used but no promising results
• Immunotherapy: Radiolabeled antibodies like 131-I-antiferritin have been used. Can be used in conjunction with doxorubicin (Adriamycin), still experimental.
• Intra-arterial injection of 131-I Lipiodol or Lipiodol/Adriamycin, not in common use

FOLLOWUP

PATIENT MONITORING
• After successful resection there is high risk for recurrence
• Check AFP every 3 months
• Ultrasound every 4-6 months

PREVENTION/AVOIDANCE
• Prevention against HBV infection/cirrhosis
  ◊ General education regarding risks of exposure to HBV and precautions to avoid this
  ◊ Vaccination in high risk individuals - nurses, doctors, dialysis unit staff, lab technicians
  ◊ Vaccination of all children
  ◊ Abstinence from alcohol, IV drugs, homosexual behavior
  ◊ Persistent HBV and HCV infections eradicated with alpha interferon
• Screening and early diagnosis
  ◊ Early diagnosis to detect asymptomatic tumor (< 3 cm) at a potentially curable stage has been emphasized. The only screening test available so far is AFP testing which can detect 70-80% of tumors < 3 cm when used in conjunction with serial high resolution sonography.
  ◊ AFP should be done every 6 months in high risk individuals (cirrhosis, chronic active hepatitis) along with annual ultrasound. In moderate risk subjects (HBsAg positive but asymptomatic), AFP should be done yearly followed by ultrasound if it is abnormal.
  ◊ Patients exposed to 10 or more years of vinyl chloride polymerization should have q 6 months sonography. New nodules should be promptly biopsied.

POSSIBLE COMPLICATIONS
Rupture, hemoperitoneum, liver failure, cachexia, metastases to other organs

EXPECTED COURSE/PROGNOSIS
• Unresectable symptomatic tumors
  ◊ Grave prognosis, seldom live more than 6 months
  ◊ After liver transplantation - 2 year survival rate 15-20%
  ◊ After chemotherapy or chemoimmunotherapy, only partial remission in one quarter of cases
  ◊ Direct necrosis with alcohol injection
  ◊ Chemoembolization
• Resectable asymptomatic tumors
  ◊ Surgery is curative in > 70% of children without cirrhosis and in > 40% of adults without cirrhosis
  ◊ Surgery is curative in > 70% of cirrhosis when tumor nodules less than 2 cm; curative < 10% of the time if 3 cm or greater
  ◊ Liver transplantation curative in cancer with cirrhosis with 15% of patients alive at 3 years

MISCELLANEOUS

ASSOCIATED CONDITIONS
• Infections - chronic hepatitis B, hepatitis C, Delta hepatitis, clonorchiasis and schistosomiasis
• Primary liver diseases - alcoholic cirrhosis, primary biliary cirrhosis
• Metabolic diseases - Alpha1-antitrypsin deficiency, hemochromatosis, Wilson's disease, tyrosinemia

AGE-RELATED FACTORS
Can occur in all age groups
Pediatric: Second most common tumor in first year of life following Wilms' tumor. High cure rate.
Geriatric: N/A
Others: N/A

PREGNANCY
N/A

SYNONYMS
• Hepatocellular carcinoma
• Liver cancer
• Fibrolamellar carcinoma
• Cholangiocarcinoma

ICD-9-CM
155.0 Malignant neoplasm of liver, primary

SEE ALSO
N/A

OTHER NOTES
• In Africa and Southeast Asia:
  ◊ Incidence of hepatoma is high - 15-20 cases/100,000/year
  ◊ Age group is younger - 3rd and 4th decade
  ◊ Male to female ratio is high - 6:1 to 7:1
  ◊ Aflatoxin and HBV are the major factors and cirrhosis is less important
  ◊ Course is more progressive and fulminant
  ◊ Tumors are mostly at unresectable stage at first presentation

ABBREVIATIONS
• HBsAg = hepatitis B surface antigen
• HCV = hepatitis C virus
• HBV = hepatitis B virus
• AFP = alphafetoprotein

REFERENCES
• Hemming AW, Greig PD, Langer B: Current surgical management of primary hepatocellular carcinoma. Advances in Surg 1999;32:169-192
• Fried MW: Treatment of hepatocellular carcinoma: medical options. Liver Transplantation and Surg 1998;4(5 suppl1):s92-97
• Mor E, Kaspa RT, Sheiner P, Schwartz M: Treatment of hepatocellular carcinoma associated with cirrhosis in the era of liver transplantation. Ann of Int Med 1998;129:643-653
Illustrations: 1 available on CD-ROM
Internet references: http://www.5mcc.com

Author(s)
Frank L. Iber, MD

Hepatorenal syndrome

BASICS

DESCRIPTION An acute, functional and progressive reduction in renal blood flow and glomerular filtration rate (GFR) secondary to intense renal cortical vasoconstriction in the setting of decompensated cirrhosis. Other etiologies for renal failure in cirrhosis must be absent to diagnose hepatorenal syndrome (HRS). HRS may be classified as (1) type 1 HRS with a rapidly progressive decline in GFR (< 2 weeks); or (2) type II HRS which is not as rapidly progressive (> 2 weeks).
System(s) affected: Gastrointestinal, Nervous, Endocrine/Metabolic, Hemic/Lymphatic/Immunologic, Renal/Urologic
Genetics: Not important except as risk for liver disease (e.g., infantile or autosomal recessive polycystic kidney disease or alpha-1-antitrypsin deficiency, etc.)
Incidence/Prevalence in USA: Unknown (clear cut differentiation between hepatorenal syndrome and acute tubular necrosis [ATN] or pre-renal state not always made). Estimate: 32-41/100 admitted to the hospital for cirrhosis with ascites develop HRS at 2 and 5 years. One other study in patients with cirrhosis and ascites: 18% and 39% (of HRS) at 1 and 5 years.
Predominant Age: Usually > 4th decade (increased incidence of alcoholic cirrhosis) but may occur at any age
Predominant Sex: Male > Female (increased incidence and prevalence of alcoholic cirrhosis)

SIGNS AND SYMPTOMS
• Oliguria in the setting of cirrhosis
• Jaundice, ascites, encephalopathy
• GI bleeding
• Poor nutritional status
• Splenomegaly
• Spider angioma
• Peripheral vasodilatation
• Tachycardia and bounding pulse often present with HRS. Almost always develops during a hospitalization, not on admission.

CAUSES End stage liver disease from alcohol or toxins, viral hepatitis, fulminant hepatic failure, malignancy or any other injury which leads to cirrhosis (e.g., schistosoma) with accompanying risk factors

RISK FACTORS
• Any reduction of effective blood volume in cirrhosis including:
  ◊ Excessive diuresis and gastrointestinal blood loss (e.g., variceal bleeding)
  ◊ Excessive diarrhea (lactulose-induced)
  ◊ Bacteremia
  ◊ Reduction in venous return with tense ascites
  ◊ Vomiting; GI bleeding
  ◊ Protein-calorie malnutrition, especially with alcoholic cirrhosis

DIAGNOSIS

DIFFERENTIAL DIAGNOSIS
• For abrupt onset of oliguria in cirrhosis
  ◊ Volume contraction
  ◊ Cardiac failure (possibly alcoholic cardiomyopathy)
  ◊ Acute vasomotor nephropathy
  ◊ Obstruction
  ◊ Interstitial nephritis (drug-induced)

LABORATORY
• Azotemia in the setting of cirrhosis with appropriate spot urine values (consistent with tubular function): Na+ < 10 mEq/L, FeNa < 1%; urine/plasma creatinine > 30:1; osmolality mild to moderate reduction in concentrating ability (400-600 mOsm/kg/water). All reversible causes should be ruled out (e.g., pre-renal; obstruction).
• Urinalysis - absence of ATN casts; < 500 mg/dL protein
• Lack of improvement in renal function following diuretic withdrawal and expansion of plasma volume with 1.5 L of normal saline
• Minor criteria: urine volume < 500 cc/day; urine red cells < 50 hpf; serum sodium < 130 mcg/L
• Other: prolonged prothrombin time, decreased serum albumin concentration, elevated bilirubin
Drugs that may alter lab results: N/A
Disorders that may alter lab results: N/A

PATHOLOGICAL FINDINGS
• Liver: cirrhosis or acute fulminant failure
• Kidneys: would function if transplanted into hosts without liver disease, a functional renal derangement only

SPECIAL TESTS Xenon 133 washout curves show a profound reduction in renal cortical perfusion (historic interest)

IMAGING Renal ultrasound shows normal kidneys without obstruction

DIAGNOSTIC PROCEDURES Though experimental presently, renal duplex Doppler ultrasonography appears to have predictive value in separating cirrhotics who will develop HRS from those who won't based on resistive index

TREATMENT

APPROPRIATE HEALTH CARE
Maintenance of volume status in cirrhosis

GENERAL MEASURES
• Supportive
  ◊ Avoid iatrogenic events that precipitate HRS
  ◊ Diagnose and treat correctable causes of azotemia in cirrhosis: volume expanders (100 gm albumin in 500 cc normal saline) should always be tried if possible, left ventricular function maximized if possible, relief of urinary obstruction when present
• Other
  ◊ Large volume paracentesis
  ◊ Dialysis is only indicated as ancillary support for patients awaiting liver transplant or in patients with acute potentially reversible liver failure
  ◊ Head-out water immersion and LaVeen shunts of dubious value
  ◊ Acute liver failure with HRS may reverse if the liver regenerates

SURGICAL MEASURES Liver transplantation when feasible is the only curative treatment. The observed 3 month to estimated 6 months to 1 year survival in patients with transjugular intrahepatic portosystemic stent-shunts is improved. LeVeen shunt may provide similar benefit.

ACTIVITY Bedrest

DIET N/A

PATIENT EDUCATION In alcoholic cirrhosis, abstention from alcohol is essential and may prevent further deterioration of cirrhosis

MEDICATIONS

DRUG(S) OF CHOICE Low dose dopamine may provide temporary benefit. Not curative.
Contraindications: N/A
Precautions:
• Avoid NSAID's, demeclocycline, aminoglycosides or other nephrotoxins
• Judicious use of loop diuretics
• Avoid iatrogenic volume contraction in cirrhotic inpatients
Significant possible interactions: Refer to manufacturer's literature

ALTERNATIVE DRUGS Vasopressin analogues (terlipressin and ornipressin) combined with plasma volume expansion demonstrate some effect on the short-term reversibility of renal dysfunction. May act as a bridge to liver transplant. Questions of efficacy persist, however.

FOLLOWUP

PATIENT MONITORING N/A

PREVENTION/AVOIDANCE See Risk Factors

POSSIBLE COMPLICATIONS Death

EXPECTED COURSE/PROGNOSIS
• Grave without liver transplant in chronic cirrhosis or without regeneration of the liver in acute fulminant failure
• If a liver transplant is performed, actuarial patient survival after transplant is less in patients with preceding hepatorenal syndrome
• The patient may be supported with hemodialysis, continuous arterio-venous hemofiltration (CAVH) or continuous arterio venous hemodialysis (CAVHD) and transjugular portosystemic stent-shunt prior to organ availability for transplant

MISCELLANEOUS

ASSOCIATED CONDITIONS See Causes and Differential Diagnosis

AGE-RELATED FACTORS
Pediatric: See Genetics
Geriatric: N/A
Others: N/A

PREGNANCY May be associated with HRS if liver failure occurs during pregnancy

SYNONYMS
• Renal failure of cirrhosis
• Functional renal failure of cirrhosis
• Hepatic nephropathy
• Heyd's syndrome
• Oliguric renal failure of cirrhosis
• Hemodynamic renal failure of cirrhosis

ICD-9-CM
572.4 Hepatorenal syndrome
997.4 Hepatorenal syndrome, resulting from a procedure

SEE ALSO
• Acetaminophen poisoning
• Renal failure, acute (ARF)
• Cirrhosis of the liver
• Hepatitis, viral
• Schistosomiasis of the liver, chronic

OTHER NOTES N/A

ABBREVIATIONS
HRS = hepatorenal syndrome

REFERENCES
• Celeb H, Dondy E, Celikes H: Renal blood flow detection with Doppler ultrasonography in patients with hepatic cirrhosis. Arch Int Med 1997;157:564-566
• Arroyo V, Gines P, Gerbes AL et al: Definition and diagnostic criteria of refractory ascites and hepatorenal syndrome in cirrhosis. Hepatology 1996;23:164-176
• Roberts LR, Kamath PS: Ascites and hepatorenal syndrome; pathophysiology and management. Mayo Clin Proc 1996;71:874881
• Van Roey G, Moore K: The hepatorenal syndrome. Pediatr Nephrol 1996;10:100-107
• Brensing KA, Textor J, Strunk H, et al: Transjugular intrahepatic portosystemic stent-shunt for hepatorenal syndrome. Lancet 1997;349:697-698
• Sussman NL, Lake JR: Treatment of hepatic failure-1996: current concepts and progress toward liver dialysis. Am J Kid Dis 1996;27:605-621
• Gines P. Arroyo V, Rodes J: Ascites and hepatorenal syndrome: pathogenesis and treatment strategies. Advances In Internal Med 1998;43:99-143
• Bateller R, Sort P, Gines P, Arroyo V: Hepatorenal syndrome: definition, pathophysiology, clinical features and management. Kidney Intl `998;53(suppl 66):S47-S53
• Epstein M: Hepatorenal syndrome: emerging perspectives. Seminars in Nephrology 1997;17(6):563-575
Illustrations: N/A
Internet references: http://www.5mcc.com

Author(s)
Michael Youtsey, MD
Gregory W. Rutecki, MD

Herpangina

BASICS

DESCRIPTION Infectious disease caused by Coxsackievirus group A. Characteristics - fever of short duration, typical vesicular or ulcerated lesions in the post pharynx or on the soft palate. Usual course - acute.
System(s) affected: Endocrine/Metabolic, Gastrointestinal
Genetics: N/A
Incidence/Prevalence in USA: N/A
Predominant age: 3 months-16 years
Predominant sex: Male = Female

SIGNS AND SYMPTOMS
- Anorexia
- Drooling
- Sore throat
- Fever
- Malaise
- Irritability
- Listlessness
- Local pain
- Emesis
- Backache
- Headache
- Coryza
- Diarrhea
- Bilateral discrete vesicles, gray base
- Erythematous parchory
- Vesicles may rupture ulcers to form ulcers
- Posterior pharynx location - pharynx, tonsils, soft palate, little involvement of anterior 2/3 of mouth

CAUSES
- Coxsackievirus A
- Coxsackievirus B

RISK FACTORS Contact with infected person

DIAGNOSIS

DIFFERENTIAL DIAGNOSIS
- Herpes simplex - multiple ulcers on lips and anterior mouth. Diagnose with Herpes culture.
- Drug reactions - cutaneous lesions often present (urticaria, erythema multiforme)
- Recurrent aphthous stomatitis
  ◊ Buccal, labial, alveolar, mucosal ulcers
  ◊ Recurrent crops
  ◊ Few systemic symptoms
- Lichen planus - painful ulcer, white "lacey" pattern on mucosa or may have cutaneous lesions which are purple and pruritic

LABORATORY
- Slight leukocytosis (< 50%)
- Positive viral culture - mouth washings, stool
Drugs that may alter lab results: N/A
Disorders that may alter lab results: N/A

PATHOLOGICAL FINDINGS   N/A

SPECIAL TESTS
- Complement fixation
- Hemagglutinin inhibition tests

IMAGING   N/A

DIAGNOSTIC PROCEDURES   N/A

TREATMENT

APPROPRIATE HEALTH CARE
Outpatient

GENERAL MEASURES
- Self-limited
- Palliative and supportive
- Hydration

SURGICAL MEASURES   N/A

ACTIVITY   No restrictions

DIET   Clear liquids

PATIENT EDUCATION   N/A

MEDICATIONS

DRUG(S) OF CHOICE
- Analgesics - acetaminophen, NSAID's
- Topical anesthetics
- Mouthwash - aqueous solution of 1% dyclonine and 1% diphenhydramine (Benadryl) in 50% attapulgite (Kaopectate)
- 2% viscous lidocaine solution

Contraindications: N/A
Precautions: N/A
Significant possible interactions: N/A

ALTERNATIVE DRUGS   N/A

FOLLOWUP

PATIENT MONITORING   Hydration

PREVENTION/AVOIDANCE   Avoid contact with infected individual

POSSIBLE COMPLICATIONS
- Exanthem
- Meningitis
- Myocarditis
- Encephalitis

EXPECTED COURSE/PROGNOSIS
Complete recovery

MISCELLANEOUS

ASSOCIATED CONDITIONS   N/A

AGE-RELATED FACTORS
Pediatric: N/A
Geriatric: N/A
Others: N/A

PREGNANCY   N/A

SYNONYMS   N/A

ICD-9-CM
074.0 Herpangina

SEE ALSO
- Herpes simplex

OTHER NOTES   N/A

ABBREVIATIONS   N/A

REFERENCES   Bondi J, Jegasothy B, Lazarus G: Dermatology, Diagnosis and Therapy. Norwalk, CT, Appleton & Lange, 1991
Illustrations: N/A
Internet references: http://www.5mcc.com

Author(s)
Jeffrey A. Stearns, MD

Herpes eye infections

BASICS

DESCRIPTION Infections of the eye caused by one of the herpesviruses. Herpes simplex (HSV) types 1 and 2 or varicella-zoster virus. These infections may affect the eyelids and surrounding skin and may also cause conjunctivitis, keratitis, uveitis, as well as retinitis or optic neuritis. These viruses establish latent infections and eye involvement is most often from reactivation of latent viruses. Epstein-Barr virus may cause conjunctivitis or keratitis in infectious mononucleosis. Cytomegalovirus, which is also a herpesvirus, can cause a severe retinitis in immunocompromised patients with AIDS.

System(s) affected: Nervous, Skin/Exocrine

Genetics: No genetic pattern

Incidence/Prevalence in USA:
- HSV - 500,000 cases per year; 1/10,000 infants born with neonatal HSV
- Zoster - 300,000 new cases per year

Predominant age:
- HSV may affect any age
- Zoster usually affects older people

Predominant sex: Male = Female

SIGNS AND SYMPTOMS
Varies according to the virus and the ocular structures involved
- Eye pain
- Red eye (usually unilateral)
- Photophobia
- Tearing
- Decreased vision
- Skin/eyelid rash and pain
- Fever (varicella-zoster or infectious mononucleosis)
- Malaise (varicella-zoster or infectious mononucleosis)

CAUSES
- Primary infections:
  ◊ Neonatal HSV, usually HSV-2
  ◊ Primary ocular HSV, usually HSV-1
- Recurrent infections:
  ◊ Reactivation of HSV or herpes zoster virus (HZV) from trigeminal ganglion
- Reactivating factors:
  ◊ Fever
  ◊ Ultraviolet light
  ◊ Cold wind
  ◊ Systemic illness
  ◊ Menstruation
  ◊ Emotional stress
  ◊ Local trauma
  ◊ Immunosuppression

RISK FACTORS
- Family members/close contact with HSV
- History of varicella infection

DIAGNOSIS

DIFFERENTIAL DIAGNOSIS
- Viral conjunctivitis of other cause
- Bacterial keratoconjunctivitis
- Adult inclusion (chlamydial) conjunctivitis
- Allergic conjunctivitis
- Corneal abrasion
- Recurrent corneal erosion
- Toxic conjunctivitis
- Fungal keratitis
- Iritis/uveitis
- Scleritis

LABORATORY
- Laboratory tests are usually not required unless diagnosis in doubt
- Viral culture from cornea, conjunctiva, or skin; fluorescent antibody; polymerase chain reaction (PCR)
- Giemsa stain of corneal or skin lesion scrapings for multinucleated giant cells

Drugs that may alter lab results: N/A

Disorders that may alter lab results: N/A

PATHOLOGICAL FINDINGS
- Vesicular skin rash
- Zoster rash follows dermatome, does not cross midline and involves upper eyelid
- Dendritic keratitis
- HSV dendrites stain with fluorescein
- Large geographic corneal ulcers may occur
- Corneal stromal inflammation, opacity and neovascularization may occur
- Decreased corneal sensation
- Uveitis
- Secondary glaucoma

SPECIAL TESTS
- Fluorescein staining of the cornea - positive staining with HSV
- Rose bengal staining of cornea - positive with zoster and HSV
- Corneal sensation - usually decreased
- Slit-lamp exam
- Measure intraocular pressure
- Dilated funduscope exam
- Evaluate zoster patients under age 40 for immunodeficiency

IMAGING   N/A

DIAGNOSTIC PROCEDURES   As above

TREATMENT

APPROPRIATE HEALTH CARE
- Outpatient
- Hospitalize if severe systemic spread for IV therapy

GENERAL MEASURES
- Warm compresses to skin lesions
- Gentle debridement of corneal epithelial lesions

SURGICAL MEASURES   Occasionally, débridement of involved epithelium

ACTIVITY   As tolerated

DIET   Regular

PATIENT EDUCATION   American Academy of Ophthalmology

MEDICATIONS

DRUG(S) OF CHOICE
- Skin and eyelid lesions:
  ◊ Prophylactic topical antibiotic ointment, such as bacitracin or erythromycin bid for 1-2 weeks
  ◊ Trifluorothymidine (Viroptic) 1% drops or vidarabine 3% ointment 5 times per day if eyelid margin involved
  ◊ Zoster - acyclovir 800 mg po 5 times per day for 10 days or famciclovir 500 mg po tid for 7 days; useful if started within 7 days of onset and active lesions are present
  ◊ Severe or persistent zoster - hospitalize; acyclovir 5-10 mg/kg IV q 8 hours for 5-10 days
  ◊ For postherpetic neuralgia in herpes zoster:
   - Consider prednisone 60 mg po for 3-7 days and taper off over the next 1-2 weeks
   - Cimetidine 400 mg po bid during prednisone treatment
   - Consider antidepressant such as amitriptyline 25 mg po tid
- Corneal disease:
  ◊ HSV epithelial disease:
   - Trifluorothymidine 1% drops 9 times per day or vidarabine 3% ointment 5 times per day; taper over 10-21 days based on response
   - Cycloplegia with scopolamine 0.25% or cyclopentolate 1% drops tid
  ◊ Stromal keratitis or uveitis (without epithelial disease):
   - Cycloplegia with scopolamine 0.25% or cyclopentolate 1% drops tid
   - Topical steroid such as prednisolone acetate 1% drops qid
   - Trifluorothymidine 1% drops qid for prophylaxis while on topical steroids
- Optic neuritis, chorioretinitis, or cranial nerve involvement with zoster:
  ◊ Acyclovir 5-10 mg/kg IV q 8 hours for 1 week
  ◊ Prednisone 60 mg po for 3-7 days and taper over the next 1-2 weeks

- Secondary glaucoma
    ◊ Aqueous humor suppressant such as timolol 0.5% drops bid or methazolamide 50 mg po bid or tid
- Neurotrophic ulcer or persistent epithelial disease:
    ◊ Consider reducing or discontinuing topical antivirals to avoid toxicity
    ◊ Preservative-free lubricant ointment
    ◊ Erythromycin 3% ophthalmic ointment q hs or bid
    ◊ Consider patching or tarsorrhaphy

Contraindications:
- Topical steroids are contraindicated with active corneal epithelial disease
- Acyclovir is contraindicated in pregnancy
- Prednisone should not be used in immunocompromised patients

Precautions:
- Topical antiviral agents are toxic and may cause an allergic reaction; substitution with another agent may be tried
- Topical steroids can raise intraocular pressure
- Acyclovir dosage should be reduced in renal insufficiency
- See manufacturer's literature for additional precautions

Significant possible interactions: See manufacturer's literature

ALTERNATIVE DRUGS
- Idoxuridine 0.5% ointment or 0.1% drops 5 times per day is more toxic than the other antivirals, but may be substituted if allergic reaction develops to others
- Topical acyclovir ointment to skin lesions - effectiveness uncertain
- Medroxyprogesterone 1% drops in place of other steroids if corneal thinning
- Capsaicin 0.025% cream tid to 6 times per day for months to years for post-herpetic neuralgia
- Nonsteroidal anti-inflammatory agents po for scleritis associated with zoster
- Amitriptyline may also be helpful for postherpetic neuralgia
- Oral acyclovir 2 gm/day in divided doses x 10 days may be used in patients intolerant of topical antivirals

FOLLOWUP

PATIENT MONITORING
- Size of epithelial defect
- Vision
- Corneal opacity
- Anterior chamber inflammation
- Intraocular pressure

PREVENTION/AVOIDANCE
- Avoid close contact with patients with active lesions
- Herpes zoster virus can be spread to individuals who have not had chicken pox
- Avoid known precipitating factors for recurrent HSV
- Topical steroids alone do not reactivate the virus, but may exacerbate spontaneous recurrences
- Very slow taper of topical steroids over many months for corneal epithelial disease
- Antiviral prophylaxis while on topical steroids
- Varicella vaccination prior to infection
- Oral acyclovir 400mg bid reduces recurrence rate HSV keratitis by 50%

POSSIBLE COMPLICATIONS
- Corneal neovascularization and scarring resulting in poor vision
- Neurotrophic ulcer with perforation
- Secondary bacterial or fungal infection
- Secondary glaucoma from uveitis or steroid treatment
- Necrotizing interstitial keratitis
- Corneal transplant may be required
- Post-herpetic neuralgia with zoster
- Vision loss from optic neuritis or chorioretinitis
- Systemic involvement

EXPECTED COURSE/PROGNOSIS
- Neonatal primary HSV often disseminated with high mortality rate, 37% have vision worse than 20/200
- Primary HSV in children and adults often asymptomatic; overt disease usually self-limited
- Recurrent ocular HSV:
    ◊ Skin lesions in clusters last for 5-7 days
    ◊ HSV epithelial disease - without treatment, 40% resolve without sequelae; with treatment, 90-95% resolve without complication
    ◊ HSV stromal keratitis usually resolve in weeks to months with some scarring; neovascularization increases risk for severe scarring
- Ocular varicella - may produce a keratitis; usually self-limited, but with occasional complications
- Herpes zoster ophthalmicus
    ◊ Dermatitis 8-14 days acute phase with subsequent scarring possible
    ◊ Conjunctivitis, episcleritis and scleritis may occur
    ◊ Two-thirds of patients develop keratitis and decreased corneal sensation
    ◊ Uveitis occurs in about 40%
    ◊ Neurotrophic keratitis occurs in one-half; most recover sensation in 2-3 months
    ◊ Secondary glaucoma occurs in 10%
    ◊ Post-herpetic neuralgia in 20-40%; usually longer lasting in older patients
- Recurrence common for HSV and HZO

MISCELLANEOUS

ASSOCIATED CONDITIONS
- Immunosuppression
- AIDS
- Malignancy

AGE-RELATED FACTORS
Pediatric: Neonatal HSV often systemic and life-threatening
Geriatric: Zoster more common in older age groups
Others: Consider immunodeficiency in zoster patients under age 40

PREGNANCY
- May increase recurrence
- Avoid systemic steroids, acyclovir and other medications contraindicated in pregnancy
- Pregnant women who have not had chicken pox should especially avoid contact with patients with active zoster

SYNONYMS
- Herpes simplex keratitis
- Herpes zoster ophthalmicus
- Herpetic keratitis or keratouveitis

ICD-9-CM
054.40 herpes simplex (HSV) with ophthalmic complications
053.2 herpes zoster (HZV) with ophthalmic complications

SEE ALSO Conjunctivitis

OTHER NOTES N/A

ABBREVIATIONS
HSV = herpes simplex virus
HZV = herpes zoster virus
HZO = herpes zoster ophthalmicus
VSV = varicella-zoster virus (synonym for HZV)

REFERENCES
- Albert DM, Jakobiec FA, eds: Principles and Practice of Ophthalmology. Philadelphia, W.B. Saunders Co., 1994
- Cullom RD Jr, Chang B, eds: The Wills Eye Manual - Office and Emergency Room Diagnosis and Treatment of Eye Diseases. 2nd Ed. Philadelphia, J.B. Lippincott Co., 1994
- Pepose JS, Holland GN, Wilhelmus KR. Ocular Infection and Immunity. St. Louis, Mosby, 1996
Illustrations: N/A
Internet references: http://www.5mcc.com

Author(s)
Thomas W. Hejkal, MD, PhD

Herpes gestationis

BASICS

DESCRIPTION A rare dermatopathic, immune-mediated and self-limited eruption most often occurring during mid-pregnancy
• Onset is in second trimester of pregnancy with remission after delivery except for some postpartum flares. May recur in subsequent pregnancies.
• Characterized by pruritic polymorphous vesicles, papules, and/or bullae often located in peri-umbilical or other truncal areas. May affect the buttocks, forearms, palms, or soles; less frequently scalp and face may be involved. Clustered vesicles may coalesce to form bullae, rupture to form crusts, then heal with hyperpigmentation.
• Mucous membranes are spared but intestinal mucosa may have celiac-like lesions without significant clinical malabsorption
System(s) affected: Skin/Exocrine, Reproductive
Genetics: Genetic predisposition possible, suggested by increased HLA-A1, -B8, and -DR3 antigens in affected women
Incidence/Prevalence in USA: Rare; 1 per 4000-50,000 pregnancies
Predominant age: Child-bearing years
Predominant sex: Female only

SIGNS AND SYMPTOMS
Intensely pruritic papules and/or vesicles, occurring first in peri-umbilical area and spreading more generally

CAUSES
• Unknown but immune alterations suspected
• Not caused by herpes virus

RISK FACTORS
• Episode in prior pregnancy
• Herpes simplex does not increase risk

DIAGNOSIS

DIFFERENTIAL DIAGNOSIS
• Other pruritic conditions of pregnancy
◊ Besnier's prurigo gestationis with excoriated papules and no vesicles; usually limited to extensor surface of extremities
◊ Papular urticarial papules and plaques of pregnancy (PUPPP syndrome) which has urticarial plaques and small papules with a narrow, pale halo and no vesicles
◊ Impetigo herpetiformis has sterile pustules, not vesicles, and may involve mucous membranes, groin, and inner thighs
◊ Papular dermatitis of pregnancy
• Non-pregnancy conditions to consider
◊ Dermatitis herpetiformis (much more chronic and more often in middle-aged males)
◊ Bullous pemphigoid
◊ Toxic drug eruption including erythema multiforme

LABORATORY
• Tzanck smear negative
• Herpes simplex virus culture negative
• Peripheral eosinophilia may be present
Drugs that may alter lab results: N/A
Disorders that may alter lab results: N/A

PATHOLOGICAL FINDINGS
• Subepidermal vesicle often with eosinophils and edema of dermal papillae
• Acantholysis is rare
• Inflammation surrounds superficial and deep dermal vessels

SPECIAL TESTS
Biopsy with direct immunofluorescence shows intense deposition of C3 (100%) and IgG (30-40%) along basement membrane. Serum may have circulating IgG antibasement membrane autoantibodies (10-20%) by indirect immunofluorescence; if not, half have herpes gestationis (HG) factor (a protein that fixes complement to basement membrane in-vitro human skin preparations).

IMAGING N/A

DIAGNOSTIC PROCEDURES Biopsy

TREATMENT

APPROPRIATE HEALTH CARE
Outpatient

GENERAL MEASURES
• Differentiate from herpes virus infection
• Relieve pruritus
• Prevent secondary infection
• Soothing compresses such as Domeboro or Burrow's solution may help relieve itching

SURGICAL MEASURES N/A

ACTIVITY As tolerated

DIET No special diet

PATIENT EDUCATION
• Educate about difference between this and herpes virus infection
• Inform of possible fetal risks and possibility of limited disease in newborn

MEDICATIONS

DRUG(S) OF CHOICE
• Topical steroids and antihistamines for mild pruritus
• Most will require systemic corticosteroids in doses of 20-60 mg/day (at the minimum effective dose) through first month postpartum
Contraindications: Weigh risk of aggravating hyperglycemia, potential effects on maternal and fetal bone, increased susceptibility to infections versus benefit of relieving pruritus, and resolving the lesions
Precautions:
• Use prednisone cautiously in patients with immune impairment, diabetes, or thrombophlebitis
• If prednisone has been used over several weeks, taper when discontinuing to prevent cortisol deficiency
Significant possible interactions:
Methylprednisolone may enhance toxicity of erythromycin

ALTERNATIVE DRUGS   Pyridoxine

FOLLOWUP

PATIENT MONITORING   Watch for secondary bacterial infection

PREVENTION/AVOIDANCE
• Avoid other people with infections, since there is susceptibility of open skin lesions and decreased resistance secondary to corticosteroids
• Some authorities recommend cesarean section when mother is known to be infected
• Avoid scalp monitors if disease involves maternal genitalia
• Use of estrogens or progesterone may trigger flare-up

POSSIBLE COMPLICATIONS
• Secondary bacterial infection
• Excess systemic medication in pregnancy
• Fetal deaths
• Premature births
• Fetal growth retardation
• Conjunctivitis
• Keratitis
• Cataracts
• Shock
• Transient herpes gestationis in the neonate

EXPECTED COURSE/PROGNOSIS
• Spreads during 2nd-3rd trimester
• Remits after delivery
• Often flares in puerperium
• Tends to recur in subsequent pregnancies
• Systemic steroids may suppress new lesions, relieve pruritus, and dampen course; fetal outcome may be worsened

MISCELLANEOUS

ASSOCIATED CONDITIONS
• Pregnancy
• Hydatidiform mole
• Choriocarcinoma

AGE-RELATED FACTORS
Pediatric:
• Has been associated with preterm birth (22%) and still birth (< 10%)
• Rare cases of transient neonatal herpes gestationis are usually mild and resolve spontaneously; these are probably from passive transfer of antibasement membrane antibodies and HG factor
Geriatric: N/A
Others: N/A

PREGNANCY   By definition, a condition of pregnancy and puerperium

SYNONYMS
• Dermatitis gestationis
• Pemphigoid gestationis

ICD-9-CM
646.80 Other specified complications of pregnancy (unspecified relation to delivery)
646.83 Other specified complications of pregnancy (antepartum)

SEE ALSO   N/A

OTHER NOTES   Uncommon intrauterine infections are associated with microcephaly intracranial calcification and chorioretinitis

ABBREVIATIONS   N/A

REFERENCES
• Pritchard JA, MacDonald PC, Gant NF, eds: Williams Obstetrics. Norwalk, CT, Appleton-Century-Crofts, 1985
• Zone JJ, Provost T: Bullous Disease. In: Moschella SL, ed. Dermatology. Philadelphia, W.B. Saunders Co., 1985
• Roger D, et al: Specific pruritic diseases of pregnancy. Arch Dermatol 1994:130:734-739
• Borradori L, Saura J: Specific dermatoses of pregnancy. Arch Dermatol 1994;130:778-780
Illustrations: N/A
Internet references: http://www.5mcc.com

Author(s)
Arthur R. Slaughter, MD

Herpes simplex

BASICS

DESCRIPTION Viral disease with many manifestations, usually seen as painful vesicles that often occur in clusters on skin, cornea, or mucous membranes; may occur as encephalitis, pneumonia, or disseminated infection.
Usual course of primary disease is 2 weeks; duration of recurrences varies; viral shedding in recurrence is briefer than with primary disease. Newborns or individuals with immune compromise are at risk for major morbidity or mortality.
System(s) affected: Skin/Exocrine, Nervous
Genetics: N/A
Incidence/Prevalence in USA:
• 29.2/100,000 office visits/year
• Widespread; 0.65-20% of adults may be excreting HSV1 or HSV2 at any given time
• Prevalence of antibodies varies from 30% in higher socioeconomic strata to 100% in lower socioeconomic strata; 20,000-70,000/100,000
Predominant age: All ages
Predominant sex: Male = Female

SIGNS AND SYMPTOMS
• Vesicles - usually cluster and open as painful ulcerated lesions, often with erythematous base
• Primary disease classic variations include:
◊ Herpetic whitlow: localized primary infection on a finger with intense itching and pain, followed by vesicles that may coalesce with swelling, erythema, and may mimic pyogenic paronychia; neuralgia and axillary adenopathy sometimes; heals over 2-3 weeks without incision. Primary inoculation of other abraded skin can occur (e.g., herpes gladiatorum in wrestlers).
◊ Primary herpetic gingivostomatitis and pharyngitis: first infection with HSV1 usually in early childhood; incubation from 2-12 days, then fever, sore throat, pharyngeal edema and erythema; small vesicles develop on pharyngeal and oral mucosa, rapidly ulcerate and increase in number to involve soft palate, buccal mucosa, tongue, floor of mouth, and often lips and cheeks; tender gums may bleed; fetid breath, cervical adenopathy; fever, general toxicity, poor oral intake, and drooling contribute to dehydration; autoinoculation of other sites may occur; resolves in 10-14 days with slower resolution of adenopathy
◊ Primary genital herpes: see Herpes, genital topic
◊ Primary herpes keratoconjunctivitis: by HSV1 usually; can present as unilateral conjunctivitis with regional adenopathy, as blepharitis with vesicles on lid margin, as keratitis with dendritic lesions or with punctate opacities; lasts 2-3 weeks but systemic involvement prolongs process

◊ Eczema herpeticum: diffuse pox-like eruption complicating atopic dermatitis; one cause of Kaposi's varicelliform eruption; sudden appearance of lesions in typical atopic areas (upper trunk, neck, head); high fever, local edema, adenopathy, umbilicated vesicles develop hemorrhagic crust or become pustular; appear in crops for up to a week; significant fluid or blood loss and secondary bacterial infections can cause fatality; similar serious inoculations can occur with severe burn patients and go unrecognized under the eschar.
◊ Neonatal herpes simplex: perinatal primary infection is life-threatening and usually acquired by vaginal birth of infected mother; fetal risk and neonatal risk are greater in mothers with primary genital herpes infection since shedding is more prolonged and the inoculum is greater; incubation from 5-7 days usually (rarely 4 weeks); cutaneous, mucous membrane, or ocular signs in only 70%; congenital infection via prenatal transplacental virus transfer may present with jaundice, hepatosplenomegaly, DIC, encephalitis, seizures, temperature instability, chorioretinitis, and/or conjunctivitis with or without skin vesicles; neurologic morbidity worse with HSV2 than with HSV1 in neonates; fatal hepatic or adrenal necrosis may occur
• Recurrent diseases from endogenous reactivation include:
◊ Herpes labialis: recurrent lesions on lips with HSV1, usually less than one recurrence per six months, but 5-25% may have more than one attack per month; precipitating events may be sunlight, fever, trauma, menses, stress; prodrome of pain, burning, itching may last 6-48 hrs before vesicles appear, often at vermilion border with increased pain; will ulcerate and crust within 48 hrs; heals within 8-10 days generally; may have local adenopathy
◊ Ocular herpes: may recur as keratitis, blepharitis, or keratoconjunctivitis; may have dendritic ulcers, decreased corneal sensation, less visual acuity; uveitis may cause permanent visual loss
◊ Recurrent genital herpes (herpes progenitalis): see Herpes, genital topic

CAUSES Herpes simplex virus, a DNA virus of two major types: HSV1 and HSV2; most often HSV1 is associated with oral lesions and HSV2 with genital lesions but reverse occurs also

RISK FACTORS
• Immune compromise (brief as with occurrence of other illness or stress, or more chronic as with chemotherapy, malignancy, or AIDS)
• Newborns - if exposed to actively infected mother via birth canal or if exposed to case in nursery (insufficient maternal passive antibody transfer); risk greatest for neonate of mother with active primary H. simplex infection
• Prior HSV infection
• Sexual intercourse with infected person (condoms can help prevent but location of some lesions may permit spread even with condoms)
• Occupational exposure (medical/dental risk more for HSV1 whitlow and general community to HSV2 whitlow)

DIAGNOSIS

DIFFERENTIAL DIAGNOSIS
• Impetigo - straw-colored vesicles that crust
• Aphthous stomatitis - grayish, shallow erosions with ring of hyperemia, usually only anterior in mouth and lips
• Herpes zoster - unilateral dermatome distribution
• Syphilitic chancre - usually painless ulcer
• Herpangina - vesicles predominate on anterior tonsillar pillars, soft palate, uvula and oropharynx but not more anteriorly on lips or gums (usually caused by group A Coxsackievirus)
• Stevens-Johnson syndrome
• Other causes of Kaposi's varicelliform eruption are varicella and Coxsackievirus A16

LABORATORY
• Tzanck smear shows multinucleated giant cells often with intranuclear inclusions (scrape material from lesion onto slide, fix with ethanol or methanol, stain with Giemsa or Wright preparation; alternatively spray slide with cytological fixative and stain as for Pap smear)
• Herpes simplex virus culture - only half of true positives available in 2 days; rest may take 6 days or longer to be positive; not considered as reasonable means to follow activity of recurrent disease near labor and delivery
Drugs that may alter lab results: N/A
Disorders that may alter lab results:
Varicella (herpes zoster) has identical findings on Tzanck smear

PATHOLOGICAL FINDINGS
Multinucleated giant cells with 2-15 nuclei per cell with eosinophilic inclusion bodies within nuclei; intraepithelial edema (ballooning degeneration) and intracellular edema; brain biopsy (in encephalitis) has hemorrhagic necrosis of gray and white matter with acute and chronic inflammation, thrombosis and fibrinoid necrosis of parenchymal vessels, and intranuclear inclusions in astrocytes, oligodendroglia, and neurons

SPECIAL TESTS
• Clinically available antibody tests do not reliably distinguish between HSV-1 and HSV-2, but initially high titers or less than a fourfold rise of titers between acute and convalescent sera may help rule-out a primary infection
• IgM HSV antibodies may appear in first 4 weeks of life in infected infants

IMAGING N/A

DIAGNOSTIC PROCEDURES
• Occasionally biopsy is needed
• Screen for other sexually transmitted diseases with primary genital herpes

TREATMENT

APPROPRIATE HEALTH CARE
Outpatient

GENERAL MEASURES
- Limited skin lesions (as in recurrent herpes labialis) may benefit from early unroofing of vesicles and application of Campho-Phenique
- Intermittent cool moist dressings with Domeboro or Burow's solution
- Inability to void from severe periurethral lesions may be remedied by pouring a cup of warm water over genitals while urinating or sitting in a warm bath to urinate
- Children with gingivostomatitis may require IV hydration
- Extensive skin disease (as with neonates or with eczema herpeticum) may require vigorous volume replacement

SURGICAL MEASURES   N/A

ACTIVITY   No restrictions

DIET   Avoid acidic foods with gingivostomatitis

PATIENT EDUCATION
- Avoid contact with immunocompromised
- Wash hands often
- Genital herpes: avoid sexual contact while disease is active; discuss condom benefits and limits and reinforce benefits of mutually monogamous sexual relations.
- Reassure and reduce stigma

MEDICATIONS

DRUG(S) OF CHOICE
- Acyclovir (Zovirax)
  ◊ Primary genital herpes: 200 mg po q4h x 5 doses daily for 10 days
  ◊ Recurrent genital herpes: 200 mg po q4h x 5 doses daily for 5 days; for chronic suppression in persons with frequent recurrences - 400 mg bid
  ◊ Neonatal herpes simplex or encephalitis: 10 mg/kg IV over 1 hour q8h x 10-14 days
  ◊ Primary herpes gingivostomatitis, recurrent herpes labialis and other HSV skin infections: 200 mg po q4h x 5 doses daily for 10 days
- Penciclovir (Denavir)
  ◊ Oroherpes recurrence: 1% cream q2h while awake for 4 days
- Valacyclovir (Valtrex): better bioavailability orally than acyclovir, is converted to acyclovir; indicated for use only in immunocompetent
  ◊ Primary genital herpes: 1 gm po BID for 10 days
  ◊ Recurrent genital herpes: 500 mg po bid for 5 days; chronic suppression 1 g po qDay (10 or more recurrences per year) or 500 mg po qDay (9 or less recurrences per year)

- Famciclovir (Famvir): is converted to penciclovir, with longer intracellular half-life and higher levels than acyclovir
  ◊ Primary genital herpes: 250 mg po tid for 5-10 days
  ◊ Recurrent genital herpes: 125 mg po bid for 5 days; chronic suppression 250 mg po bid

Contraindications: Acyclovir, valacyclovir, or famciclovir: Hypersensitivity or intolerance

Precautions:
- Reduce dosage in renal insufficiency for acyclovir, valacyclovir and famciclovir
- Acyclovir may produce encephalopathic reactions, particularly in the elderly
- Valacyclovir: Thrombotic thrombocytopenia purpura/hemolytic uremic syndrome (TTP/HUS) reported in some immunocompromised persons in trials on high doses (8 grams daily) for CMV suppression
- Pregnancy - see Miscellaneous section

Significant possible interactions:
Probenecid with IV acyclovir, possibly probenecid with valacyclovir can reduce renal clearance and elevate antiviral drug levels

ALTERNATIVE DRUGS
- Foscarnet: Drug of choice for acyclovir-resistance in immunocompromised persons with systemic HSV; 40 mg/kg IV q8h (assume valacyclovir and famciclovir resistance also if acyclovir resistance occurs)
- Other topicals:
  ◊ Ophthalmic preparations for herpes keratoconjunctivitis: Acyclovir, vidarabine (Vira-A), idoxuridine and trifluorothymidine; refer to ophthalmologist

FOLLOWUP

PATIENT MONITORING   Observe for disappearance of lesions and resolution of systemic manifestations

PREVENTION/AVOIDANCE   See Patient Education

POSSIBLE COMPLICATIONS   Herpes encephalitis - brain biopsy may be needed for diagnosis; herpes pneumonia; aseptic meningitis; herpes viremia

EXPECTED COURSE/PROGNOSIS
Good for treatment of recurrent episodes. Expect frequent recurrences.

MISCELLANEOUS

ASSOCIATED CONDITIONS   Erythema multiforme

AGE-RELATED FACTORS
Pediatric: Previously described
Geriatric: Decreased immunological competence of old age may increase risk
Others: N/A

PREGNANCY
- Acyclovir for HSV in pregnancy is recommended for severe or complicated disease; contact manufacturer/CDC registry (1-800-722-9292- ext 58465 if acyclovir used in pregnancy.
- Risk of viral shedding at delivery from asymptomatic recurrent genital HSV low (~1.6%); not predicted by monitoring cultures
- Attack rate for neonatal HSV is 41% if primary maternal genital HSV present at time of delivery and about 4% for recurrent genital HSV at time of delivery. Avoid fetal scalp electrodes if maternal history of genital HSV.
- C-section indicated if any active genital lesions (or prodrome) present; consider if primary genital herpes occurred within 4 wks of expected delivery
- Obtain HSV cultures (urine, stool, CSF, eyes, throat) of neonates exposed to primary maternal genital HSV at delivery; treat with acyclovir if clinically ill, cultures positive, CSF abnormal
- Neonates with possible exposure to HSV with signs of infection: lethargy, poor feeding, fever, or lesions; admit, culture; treat immediately with IV acyclovir if HSV illness suspected

SYNONYMS   N/A

ICD-9-CM
054.0 Eczema herpeticum
054.9 Herpes simplex, any site
771.2 Neonatal herpes simplex
054.9 Herpes labialis

SEE ALSO   Herpes, genital

OTHER NOTES   N/A

ABBREVIATIONS   N/A

REFERENCES
- Dwyer DE, Cunningham AL: Herpes simplex virus infection in pregnancy. Ballieres Clin Obstet Gynaecol 1993;7:75-105
- Hirsch MS: Herpes simples virus. In: Mandell GL, et al, eds. Principles and Practice of Infectious Diseases. New York, Churchill Livingstone, 1990
- Easterbrook P, Wood MJ: Successors to acyclovir. J Antimicrob 1994;34:307-311
- Drugs for non-HIV viral infections. The Medical Letter 1997;39:69-76
1 additional references available at web site
Internet references: http://www.5mcc.com
Illustrations: 18 available on CD-ROM

Author(s)
Arthur R. Slaughter, MD

Herpes zoster

 BASICS

DESCRIPTION
A disease usually presenting as a painful unilateral dermatomal eruption. Zoster results from reactivation of varicella-zoster (chickenpox) virus that has been dormant in the dorsal root ganglia.

System(s) affected: Skin/Exocrine, Nervous

Genetics: N/A

Incidence/Prevalence in USA:
• 215/100,000/year; incidence is increasing as population ages
• Occurs in 10-20% of the population at some time
• Active herpes zoster 23.9/100,000
• Post herpetic neuralgia 86/100,000

Predominant age: Increasing incidence with aging. 80% of cases occur in persons over age 20 years (2-3 per 1000 age 20 to 50; 10 per 1000 > 80 years).

Predominant sex: Male = Female

SIGNS AND SYMPTOMS
• Prodromal phase (sensations over involved dermatome prior to rash)
  ◊ Tingling
  ◊ Itching
  ◊ Boring or knifelike pain
• Acute phase
  ◊ Constitutional symptoms
  ◊ Fatigue
  ◊ Malaise
  ◊ Headache
  ◊ Low-grade fever
  ◊ Dermatomal rash
  ◊ Weakness (1% may have weakness in distribution of rash - called herpes zoster motoricus)
  ◊ Initially erythematous and maculopapular that evolves rapidly to grouped vesicles
  ◊ Vesicles become pustular and/or hemorrhagic in 3 to 4 days
  ◊ Resolution of rash with crusts separating by 14 to 21 days
  ◊ Possible sine herpete (zoster without rash)
• Chronic phase
  ◊ Postherpetic neuralgia (15% overall; increases dramatically with age)
  ◊ A small percentage (1-5%) may affect the motor nerves causing weakness (herpes zoster motoricus), e.g., facial nerve (Ramsay Hunt syndrome), spinal motor radiculopathies

CAUSES
Reactivation of dormant varicella-zoster (chicken pox) virus in dorsal root ganglia or gasserian ganglia

RISK FACTORS
• Increasing age
• Compromised cell-mediated immunity in immunosuppressed patients or patients with malignancy (especially leukemia and lymphoma)
• Spinal surgery
• Spinal cord radiation

 DIAGNOSIS

DIFFERENTIAL DIAGNOSIS
• Rash - herpes simplex virus, Coxsackievirus, contact dermatitis, superficial pyoderma
• Pain - cholecystitis, pleuritis, myocardial infarction

LABORATORY
• Rarely necessary
• Viral culture
• Tzanck smear (does not distinguish from herpes simplex and false negatives occur)
• Monoclonal antibody tests
• Blood mononuclear cell testing for viral DNA (research tool)

Drugs that may alter lab results: N/A

Disorders that may alter lab results: N/A

PATHOLOGICAL FINDINGS
• Multinucleated giant cells with intralesional inclusion
• Lymphatic infiltration of sensory ganglia with focal hemorrhage and nerve cell destruction

SPECIAL TESTS
N/A

IMAGING
N/A

DIAGNOSTIC PROCEDURES
Biopsy for direct immunofluorescence testing (rarely done)

 TREATMENT

APPROPRIATE HEALTH CARE
Outpatient unless disseminated or occurring as complication of serious underlying disease requiring hospitalization

GENERAL MEASURES
• Wet dressings with tap water or 5% aluminum acetate (Burow's) applied 30 to 60 minutes 4-6 times per day
• Lotions such as calamine

SURGICAL MEASURES
N/A

ACTIVITY
No restrictions

DIET
No special diet

PATIENT EDUCATION
• Duration of rash is 2-3 weeks
• Potential for dissemination (worrisome signs, constitutional illness signs and/or spreading rash)
• Potential postherpetic neuralgia
• Potential risk of transmitting illness to susceptible persons

MEDICATIONS

DRUG(S) OF CHOICE
• Antiviral agents, if initiated early (within 48-72 hours of rash) are of benefit in relieving symptoms and speeding resolution of rash. Postherpetic neuralgia is probably reduced when antiviral agents prescribed in acute phase of zoster. Clearly indicated for zoster associated with serious underlying condition and in ophthalmic zoster.
• Antiviral agents
  ◊ Acyclovir (Zovirax) 800 mg every 4 hours (5 doses(daily) for 7-10 days
    ◊ Famciclovir 500 mg po tid for 7 days
    ◊ Valacyclovir 1000 mg po tid for 7 days
• Pain medications (acetaminophen, codeine, nonsteroidal anti-inflammatory drugs)
• Silver sulfadiazine (Silvadene) topically for secondarily infected rash
Contraindications: Refer to manufacturer's profile of each drug
Precautions:
• Assess renal function prior to using acyclovir
• Acyclovir - pregnancy category C
• Refer to manufacturer's profile of each drug
Significant possible interactions:
• Acyclovir-probenecid: may inhibit excretion of acyclovir

ALTERNATIVE DRUGS
• Sorivudine
• Vidarabine

FOLLOWUP

PATIENT MONITORING Symptom dependent

PREVENTION/AVOIDANCE
• Varicella vaccines currently available will theoretically reduce zoster incidence in the future
• Vaccines are being tested for prevention of herpes zoster in individuals previously infected with wild VZ virus
• Zoster patients may transmit virus causing varicella (chickenpox) to susceptible persons

POSSIBLE COMPLICATIONS
• Postherpetic neuralgia
• Ocular involvement with facial zoster
• Meningoencephalitis
• Cutaneous dissemination
• Superinfection of skin lesions
• Hepatitis
• Pneumonitis
• Peripheral motor weakness
• Segmental myelitis
• Cranial nerve syndromes especially ophthalmic and facial (Ramsay Hunt syndrome)
• Corneal ulceration
• Guillain-Barré syndrome

EXPECTED COURSE/PROGNOSIS
• Resolution of rash within 14 to 21 days
• Postherpetic neuralgia defined as pain persisting at least one month after rash has healed
• Postherpetic neuralgia incidence increases dramatically with age (4% age 30-50; 50% over age 80 years)

MISCELLANEOUS

ASSOCIATED CONDITIONS
Immunocompromise including HIV infection, transplant recipients, and malignancies

AGE-RELATED FACTORS
Pediatric:
• Occurs rarely in children (primarily immunosuppressed)
• Has been reported in infants primarily infected in utero
Geriatric:
• Increased incidence and prevalence
• Increased incidence of postherpetic neuralgia
Others: Consider HIV infection in young patients with zoster

PREGNANCY Can occur during pregnancy

SYNONYMS Shingles

ICD-9-CM
053.9 Herpes zoster, NOS

SEE ALSO
• Chickenpox
• Herpes simplex
• Herpes eye infections
• Bell's palsy

OTHER NOTES
• Corticosteroid efficacy to prevent postherpetic neuralgia remains controversial
• Some sources advocate symptomatic ganglionic block to prevent postherpetic neuralgia
• Tricyclic antidepressants are the only proven effective agents for postherpetic neuralgia
• Capsaicin cream and transcutaneous nerve stimulation are advocated by some clinicians for post herpeticneuralgia

ABBREVIATIONS N/A

REFERENCES
• Lancaster T, et al: Primary care management of acute herpes zoster: systematic review of evidence from randomized controlled trials. British Jour of General Practice 1995; 45(390): 39-45
• Donahue JG, et al: The Incidence of Herpes Zoster. Arch Intern Med 1995;155:1605
• Tyring S, et al: Famciclovir for the Treatment of Acute Herpes Zoster: Effects on Acute Disease and Postherpetic Neuralgia. Annals of Internal Medicine 1995;123:89
• Volmink J, Lancaster, T, Gray S, Silagy C: Treatments for postherpetic neuralgia: a systematic review of randomized controlled trials. Fam Prac 1996;13(1):84-91
• Ali NM: Does sympathetic ganglionic block prevent postherpetic neuralgia? Regional Anesthesia 1995;20(3):227-233
• Wood MJ: How to measure and reduce the burden of zoster-associated pain. Scandinavian J of Infectious Dis 1996;100:55-58
• Muradami S,et al. Rapid diagnosis of varicella zoster virus infection in acute facial palsy. Neurology. 1998 Oct;51(4):1202-5
Illustrations: 8 available on CD-ROM
Internet references: http://www.5mcc.com

Author(s)
Larry W. Halverson, MD

Herpes, genital

BASICS

DESCRIPTION Herpes (from Greek "to creep or crawl") simplex virus (usually HSV-2) infection involving the genitals
• Primary genital herpes: initial infection; no previous antibodies to HSV.
• First-episode (non-primary): prior infection with a herpes simplex serotype, first genital involvement
• Recurrent (secondary): reactivation of latent herpes virus infection, usually previous genital involvement
System(s) affected: Nervous, Skin/Exocrine, Reproductive
Genetics: N/A
Incidence/Prevalence in USA:
• 50-200/100,000 (300,000 - 700,000 cases/year)
• 10,000-30,000/100,000 people (45 million)
Predominant age: 18-40
Predominant sex: Female > Male

SIGNS AND SYMPTOMS
• 60-70% of patients infected with HSV-2 are asymptomatic or do not recognize clinical manifestations of disease
• Presence of multiple, shallow, tender ulcers has 94% specificity for diagnosis of genital HSV in males
• Primary genital herpes
  ◊ Fever; headache; malaise; myalgia
  ◊ Burning genital pain
  ◊ Dysuria (female)
  ◊ Dyspareunia
  ◊ Sacral paresthesia
  ◊ Inguinal adenopathy
  ◊ Aseptic meningitis in 30%
  ◊ Occasional urinary retention
  ◊ Vesicles, on an edematous erythematous base, which ulcerate, crust over, and resolve spontaneously within 21 days. Vesicles persist longer on dry skin.
  ◊ Bilateral lesions, primarily affecting the external genitalia: female - labia majora/minora, inner thighs, vaginal mucosa, cervix, perianal skin; male - penile glans, penile shaft, urethra
• Non-primary: first episode
  ◊ Burning genital pain
  ◊ Vesicles, on a non-edematous erythematous base, which ulcerate, crust over, and resolve spontaneously within 14-17 days
• Non-primary: recurrent
  ◊ Prodromal symptoms - burning, numbness, tingling, paresthesia of genitals at site of previous lesions which occur approximately 24 hours prior to the eruption of new vesicles
  ◊ Burning genital pain
  ◊ Vesicles, on a non-edematous erythematous base, which ulcerate, crust over, and resolve spontaneously within 7-10 days
  ◊ Unilateral lesions

CAUSES
• Herpes simplex virus; a double stranded DNA
  ◊ HSV-1: 10-30% (increasing incidence)
  ◊ HSV-2: 70-90% (99% with HSV-2 antibodies have genital lesions)

RISK FACTORS
• Primary inoculation
  ◊ Higher prevalence with increasing age, lower socioeconomic status, African-American race
  ◊ Sexual activity - number of lifetime partners, duration of sexual activity, and past history of STD's
  ◊ Fomites - wet towels (rare)
• Transmission:
  ◊ Incubation period: 1-45 days (mean 5.8)
  ◊ Male to female transmission greater than female to male
  ◊ Annual risk for susceptible female acquiring disease from an infected male partner is 10-30%; for susceptible male from infected female approximately 5%
  ◊ Patients without HSV-1 antibody are at greater risk for acquiring HSV-2 infection than those with HSV-1 antibody
  ◊ Over 50% of new cases result from transmission during asymptomatic shedding
  ◊ Risk of asymptomatic shedding is highest within 1 year of occurrence of first episode of genital herpes, occurs 2-3% of days, in HSV-2 infection, and in women with frequent symptomatic episodes
  ◊ Daily therapy with oral acyclovir suppresses shedding of HSV-2, but influence of acyclovir treatment on transmission is unknown
• Triggers (recurrent): genital trauma, menses, intercurrent infection, emotional stress, sunlight

DIAGNOSIS

DIFFERENTIAL DIAGNOSIS
• Primary syphilis
• Chancroid
• Lymphogranuloma venereum
• Atypical genital warts
• Scabies
• Molluscum contagiosum
• Allergic contact dermatitis
• Trauma
• Candidiasis
• Herpes zoster
• Behçet's syndrome
• Stevens-Johnson syndrome
• Inflammatory bowel disease
• Granuloma inguinale
• Folliculitis
• Ulcerative balanitis
• Neoplasia

LABORATORY
• Viral detection from lesion: swab vesicle fluid or ulcer; viral culture, EIA, DNA detection by PCR (2-3x more sensitive than viral culture)
• Tzanck prep: Sensitivity = 40-50% compared to culture; multinucleated giant cells.
• Pap smear
• Serology: ELISA, direct fluorescent assay (DFA), radioimmunoassay (RIA) and complement fixation. Do not reliably discriminate between HSV-1 and HSV-2. Sensitivity = 80% compared to culture. Primary herpes - 4 x increase acute/convalescent titer; recurrent herpes - no increase in acute/convalescent titer.

• Type specific serologic assays: Immunodot, Western Blot and monoclonal antibody blocking RIA - do discriminate between HSV-1 and HSV-2 infections (not generally available)
Drugs that may alter lab results: Calcium agglutinate swabs may be toxic to HSV and are not recommended for culture; use cotton or dacron tipped swabs instead
Disorders that may alter lab results: Varicella-zoster will give identical Tzanck prep results

PATHOLOGICAL FINDINGS
• Histopathologic-cytopathic changes
  ◊ Intracellular edema of epithelial cells
  ◊ Nuclear margination of chromatin
  ◊ Formation of Cowdry type A intranuclear inclusions
  ◊ Cell fusion into multinucleated giant cells
• Pathologic stages:
  ◊ Primary mucocutaneous infection
  ◊ Acute ganglionic infection
  ◊ Establishment of latency
  ◊ Ganglionic reactivation
  ◊ Recurrent infection

SPECIAL TESTS

Lesion†	Serology††	Stage†††
HSV1	Negative	P HSV1
HSV2	Negative	P HSV2
HSV1	HSV2	N HSV1
HSV2	HSV1	N HSV2
HSV1	HSV1 ± HSV2	R HSV1
HSV2	HSV2 ± HSV1	R HSV2

```
   † culture or EIA
  †† type-specific antibody
 ††† P=primary; N=non-primary;
     R=recurrent
```

IMAGING N/A

DIAGNOSTIC PROCEDURES N/A

TREATMENT

APPROPRIATE HEALTH CARE
Outpatient, self-care

GENERAL MEASURES
• Cool compresses (Burow's solution 4-6 times a day); ice packs to perineum; sitz baths
• Local perineal hygiene
• Analgesics (NSAID's); topical anesthetic

SURGICAL MEASURES N/A

ACTIVITY
• Avoid intercourse in the presence of symptomatic genital lesions
• Appropriate rest if systemic manifestations (primary) are present

DIET N/A

PATIENT EDUCATION Herpes Resource Center ASHA/HRC, P.O. Box 13827, Research Triangle Park, NC 27709-9940, HRC Hotline (919)361-8488

MEDICATIONS

DRUG(S) OF CHOICE
• Acyclovir (Zovirax)
◊ Primary episode: 400 mg tid x10 days or 200 mg po 5 qD x7-10 days
◊ Severe local or disseminated disease: 5 mg/kg IV q 8 hrs x7 days
◊ Encephalitis: 10 mg/kg IV, q 8 hrs x10 days
◊ Recurrent episodes: 200 mg po 5 qD x5 days (or 400 mg tid x5 days, or 800 mg bid x5 days)
◊ Chronic suppression: recommended for frequent (≥6/year) or disabling recurrences: 400 mg po bid (or 200 mg po 3-5 times/day) - appears safe and efficacious for at least 6 years duration of therapy
◊ HIV infection: 400 mg po 3-5 qD until clinical resolution attained
Contraindications: Allergy to acyclovir
Precautions:
• Acyclovir
◊ Not approved for routine use in pregnancy
◊ Drug is excreted in breast milk
◊ Modify dose in patients with significant renal insufficiency
◊ Acyclovir resistance (in conjunction with famciclovir and valacyclovir resistance) occurs mostly in HIV infected patients
Significant possible interactions:
• Acyclovir
◊ Methotrexate - use with caution in patients who have had a neurologic reaction to intrathecal methotrexate
◊ Interferon - acyclovir is synergistic in vitro with interferon. Clinical significance is unknown. Use with caution in patients with prior neurological reactions to interferon.
◊ Probenecid - will decrease renal excretion, increase serum concentration
◊ Use with caution in combination with nephrotoxic agents

ALTERNATIVE DRUGS
• Acyclovir topical ointment - less effective; use is discouraged
• Foscarnet: 40 mg/kg IV every 8 hours in severe disease with proven or suspected acyclovir resistant strains
• Vidarabine: 10 mg/kg/day infused over 10 hours; benefits HIV patients with HSV-1 infection failing acyclovir and foscarnet therapy
• Famciclovir (Famvir)
◊ Metabolized to penciclovir, inhibits viral replication
◊ Activity/side effects similar to acyclovir
◊ Pregnancy category B
◊ First episode: 250 mg po tid x 7-10 days (not FDA approved)
◊ Recurrent: 125 mg po bid x 5 days
◊ Chronic suppression: 250 mg po bid
• Valacyclovir (Valtrex)
◊ Metabolized to acyclovir and valine
◊ May cause thrombotic thrombocytopenia purpura/hemolytic uremic syndrome in immunocompromised patients
◊ Pregnancy category B
◊ First episode: 1 g po bid x 7-10 days
◊ Recurrent: 500 mg bid x 5 days
◊ Chronic suppression: 500-1000 mg po daily or 250 mg po bid

FOLLOWUP

PATIENT MONITORING
• Acute episode - followup if complications
• Latent infection - annual pap smear; careful exam of pregnant women during prenatal visits and at onset of labor
• Reassess need for chronic suppression therapy after1 year

PREVENTION/AVOIDANCE
• Condoms/spermicide in sexual activity
• Avoid multiple sexual partners
• Avoid stress when possible
• Abstain from sexual activity when lesions or prodromal symptoms are present
• Susceptible women (without evidence of HSV antibody) should avoid unprotected sexual contact during late pregnancy

POSSIBLE COMPLICATIONS
• Vaginal discharge
• Secondary bacterial infection
• Urinary retention
• Aseptic meningitis
• Transmission to neonate
• Spontaneous abortion, preterm birth, low birthweight infants
• Increased risk for HIV infection (relative risk of 2-3)

EXPECTED COURSE/PROGNOSIS
• Resolution of signs/symptoms: Primary in 14-21 days; first episode - non-primary 14-17 days; recurrent 7-10 days
• Latent infection - recurrences in 80% of patients within 1 year of initial HSV-2 infection; immunocompetent patients average 3-4/year

MISCELLANEOUS

ASSOCIATED CONDITIONS
• Herpes labialis
• Syphilis
• Gonorrhea
• Non-gonococcal urethritis/cervicitis
• Genital warts (HPV)
• AIDS (HIV)
• Trichomoniasis

AGE-RELATED FACTORS
Pediatric:
• Genital lesions in prepubertal child suggests sexual abuse
• Neonatal infection occurs in 10-20/100,000 live births (1500-2000 cases annually); results in death or significant neurologic impairment in 85% of individuals. Most neonatal infections result from maternal asymptomatic viral shedding
• High risk infant: acyclovir 30 mg/kg/day IV q8h for 10-14 days
• Low risk infant: if asymptomatic, culture eyes, nasopharynx, mouth at 24-36 hours old and observe
Geriatric: N/A
Others: N/A

PREGNANCY
• Primary/1st episode genital herpes infection associated with increased rate of spontaneous abortion (45%) and preterm labor (35%)
• Greatest risk for neonatal infection occurs with primary or non-primary first episode genital herpes infection of the mother at time of delivery (30% transmission rate) enhanced by prolonged rupture of membranes, use of fetal scalp electrode, presence of lesions on cervix, and premature infant
• Low risk - recurrent asymptomatic HSV shedding in mother (3%)
• Low risk of infection for infants of mothers with high titer of neutralizing antibodies
• Cesarean section is indicated if herpetic genital lesions are present during labor
• Culture any suspicious lesion for genital herpes during pregnancy
• Routine cultures indicated only at time of labor for women with genital herpes history
• Acyclovir therapy:
◊ Not approved for routine use in pregnancy
◊ It has been used by some clinicians during the last 1-2 weeks of pregnancy to avoid activation of lesions, and in the third trimester to treat life-threatening infections, both without apparent complications of therapy.
◊ In women with recurrent genital herpes, oral acyclovir prophylaxis from 37 weeks gestation may be more cost-effective than cesarean delivery in preventing neonatal infection
◊ Pregnant women on acyclovir: report to CDC/ Wellcome 800-722-9292, x38465

SYNONYMS Herpes genitalis

ICD-9-CM 054.10 Genital herpes, unspecified

SEE ALSO Herpes simplex

OTHER NOTES N/A

ABBREVIATIONS N/A

REFERENCES
• Centers for Disease Control and Prevention: 1998 Guidelines for treatment of STDs. MMWR 1998;47;RR-1:20-26
• Clark JL, et al: Management of genital herpes. Am Fam Phys 1995;51:175-182
• Patel R, Barton SE: Antiviral chemotherapy in genital herpes simplex virus infections. Internat J of STD & AIDS 1995;6:320-328
• Slomka MJ: Seroepidemiology and control of genital herpes. Communicable Disease Report. CDR Review 1996;6:R41-R45
• Randolph AG, Hartshorn RM: Acyclovir prophylaxis in late pregnancy to prevent neonatal herpes - a cost-effective analysis. Obstet-Gynecol 1996;88:603-610
• Schomogyi M, Weld A, Corey L: Herpes simplex virus-2 infection. Infectious Disease Clinics of North America 1998; 12: 47-61
• Riley LE: Herpes simplex virus. Seminars in Perinatology 1998; 22(4): 284-292
11 additional references available at web site
Internet references: http://www.5mcc.com
Illustrations: N/A

Author(s)
Gary Levine, MD

Hiccups

BASICS

DESCRIPTION Sudden, involuntary, contraction of the inspiratory muscles (predominantly the diaphragm) terminated by abrupt closure of the glottis stopping the inflow of air and producing the characteristic sound.
System(s) affected: Pulmonary, nervous
Genetics: N/A
Incidence/Prevalence in USA: Self limited hiccups are extremely common; intractable hiccups are rare
Predominant age: All ages (including fetus)
Predominant sex: Male > Female (4:1)

SIGNS AND SYMPTOMS Hiccup attacks usually occur at brief intervals and last only a few seconds or minutes. Bouts lasting more than 48 hours often imply an underlying physical or metabolic disorder. Intractable hiccups may occur continuously for months or years. Hiccups usually occur with a frequency of 4 to 60 per minute.

CAUSES
• Pathophysiologic significance is unknown; hiccups have been associated with more than 100 underlying disorders.
• Results from stimulation of one or more limbs of the hiccup reflux arc (vagus and phrenic nerves) with a "hiccup center" located in the upper spinal cord
• In men greater than 90% have an organic basis while in women a psychogenic cause is more likely
• Specific underlying causes include:
 ◊ Alcoholism
 ◊ CNS lesions (brainstem tumors, vascular lesions, Parkinson's disease)
 ◊ Diaphragmatic irritation (tumors, pericarditis, eventration, splenomegaly, hepatomegaly, peritonitis)
 ◊ Hair, insect or foreign body irritating tympanic membrane
 ◊ Pharyngitis, laryngitis
 ◊ Mediastinal and other thoracic lesions (pneumonia, aortic aneurysm, tuberculosis, myocardial infarction, lung cancer)
 ◊ Esophageal lesions (reflux esophagitis, achalasia, Candida esophagitis, carcinoma, obstruction)
 ◊ Gastric lesions (ulcer, distention, cancer)
 ◊ Hepatic lesions (hepatitis, hepatoma)
 ◊ Pancreatic lesions (pancreatitis, pseudocysts, cancer)
 ◊ Inflammatory bowel disease
 ◊ Cholelithiasis, cholecystitis
 ◊ Prostatic disorders
 ◊ Appendicitis
 ◊ Postoperative, abdominal procedures
 ◊ Toxic metabolic causes (uremia, hyponatremia, gout, diabetes)
 ◊ Drug induced (dexamethasone, methylprednisolone, benzodiazepines, alpha methyldopa)
 ◊ Psychogenic causes (hysterical neurosis, grief, malingering)
 ◊ Idiopathic

RISK FACTORS
• General anesthesia
• Post-operative state
• Irritation of the vagus nerve branches
• Structural, vascular, infectious or traumatic CNS lesions

DIAGNOSIS

DIFFERENTIAL DIAGNOSIS See Causes (burping [eructation] may be confused with hiccups)

LABORATORY N/A
Drugs that may alter lab results: N/A
Disorders that may alter lab results: N/A

PATHOLOGICAL FINDINGS N/A

SPECIAL TESTS N/A

IMAGING Fluoroscopy is useful to determine if one hemidiaphragm is dominant

DIAGNOSTIC PROCEDURES N/A

TREATMENT

APPROPRIATE HEALTH CARE
• Outpatient (usually)
• Inpatient (if elderly, debilitated or intractable hiccups)

GENERAL MEASURES
• Treat any specific underlying cause when identified.
 ◊ Dilate esophageal stricture or obstruction
 ◊ Remove hair or foreign body from ear canal
 ◊ Angostura bitters for alcohol induced hiccups
 ◊ Catheter stimulation of pharynx for operative and post-operative hiccups
 ◊ Anti-fungal treatment for Candida esophagitis
 ◊ Correct electrolyte imbalance
• Simple home remedies
 ◊ Swallowing a spoonful of sugar
 ◊ Sucking on a hard candy or swallowing peanut butter
 ◊ Holding breath and increasing pressure on diaphragm (Valsalva maneuver)
 ◊ Tongue traction
 ◊ Lifting the uvula with a cold spoon
 ◊ Drinking from the far side of a glass
 ◊ Inducing fright
 ◊ Smelling salts
 ◊ Rebreathing into a paper (not plastic) bag
 ◊ Sipping ice water
• Medical measures
 ◊ Relief of gastric distention (gastric lavage, nasogastric aspiration, induced vomiting)
 ◊ Counterirritation of the vagus nerve (supraorbital pressure, carotid sinus massage, digital rectal massage), to be used with caution
 ◊ Respiratory center stimulants (breathing 5% carbon dioxide)
 ◊ Phrenic nerve block of dominant hemidiaphragm; phrenic crush, transection
 ◊ Psychiatric (hypnosis, behavioral modification)
 ◊ Miscellaneous (cardioversion, acupuncture)

SURGICAL MEASURES N/A

ACTIVITY As tolerated

DIET Avoid gastric distension from overeating, carbonated beverages, aerophagia

PATIENT EDUCATION See General Measures

MEDICATIONS

DRUG(S) OF CHOICE
Possible drug remedies:
• Baclofen, a GABA analog, 5-10 mg tid (best choice)
• Chlorpromazine 25-50 mg IV
• Haloperidol 2-12 mg IM
• Phenytoin 200 mg IV then 100 mg qid
• Metoclopramide 5-10 mg qid
• Nifedipine 10-20 mg qd-tid
• Amitriptyline 10 mg tid
Contraindications: Refer to manufacturer's literature (baclofen is not recommended in patients with stroke or other cerebral lesions)
Precautions: Refer to manufacturer's literature (abrupt withdrawal of baclofen should be avoided)
Significant possible interactions: Refer to manufacturer's literature

ALTERNATIVE DRUGS
• Amantadine, carbidopa-levodopa in Parkinson's disease
• Steroid replacement in Addison's disease
• Antifungal agent in Candida esophagitis
• Ondansetron in carcinomatosis with vomiting

FOLLOWUP

PATIENT MONITORING   Until hiccups cease

PREVENTION/AVOIDANCE
• Correct underlying cause
• Maintenance drug therapy (e.g., baclofen 5-10 mg tid; phenytoin 100 mg qid; valproic acid 15 mg/kg undivided doses; nifedipine 10-20 mg qd-tid; metoclopramide 10 mg qid)

POSSIBLE COMPLICATIONS
• Inability to eat
• Weight loss
• Exhaustion, debility
• Insomnia
• Cardiac arrhythmias
• Wound dehiscence
• Death (rare)

EXPECTED COURSE/PROGNOSIS
• Hiccups often cease during sleep
• Most acute benign hiccups resolve with home remedies or spontaneously
• Intractable hiccups may last for years and decades
• Hiccups have persisted despite bilateral phrenic nerve transection

MISCELLANEOUS

ASSOCIATED CONDITIONS   See Causes

AGE-RELATED FACTORS
Pediatric: May persist from fetal state
Geriatric: Can be a serious problem among the elderly
Others: N/A

PREGNANCY   Fetal hiccups noted as rhythmic fetal movements (confirmed sonographically), fetal hiccups often recur in subsequent pregnancies

SYNONYMS
• Hiccoughs
• Singultus

ICD-9-CM
786.8 Hiccough

SEE ALSO   N/A

OTHER NOTES   N/A

ABBREVIATIONS   N/A

REFERENCES
• Lewis JH: Hiccups: Reasons and remedies. In: Lewis JH, ed. A Pharmacologic Approach to Gastrointestinal Disorders. Baltimore, Williams & Wilkins, 1994
• Lewis JH: Hiccups. In: Rakel RE, ed. Conn's Current therapy. Philadelphia, WB Saunders Co, 1996;11-16
Illustrations: N/A
Internet references: http://www.5mcc.com

Author(s)
James H. Lewis, MD, FACP, FACG

Hidradenitis suppurativa

 BASICS

DESCRIPTION Acute, tender, cyst-like abscesses in apocrine gland bearing skin (axillae, anogenital area, pubes, areolae, also apocrine glands scattered around umbilicus, scalp, trunk and face). In chronic cases, fibrotic sinus tracts develop with intermittent drainage and periodic acute abscesses.
System(s) affected: Skin/Exocrine
Genetics: Unknown, possibly single gene transmission (autosomal dominant)
Incidence/Prevalence in USA: 0.3-4%
Predominant age: Peak onset age 11-30, commonly 30-40; rare before puberty
Predominant sex: Female (perianal) > Male (axillary)

SIGNS AND SYMPTOMS
• Early signs of pruritus, erythema, and local hyperhydrosis
• Comedones may be present
• Distribution - area of apocrine glands with axillae and groin most common
• Papules (dome-shaped) 1-3 cm in size
• Nodules (dome-shaped) 1-3 cm in size
• Larger lesions fluctuant
• Multiple recurrences at the same site
• Healing sites accompanied by scarring and sinus tracts
• Associated arthritis (rare)

CAUSES
• Traditionally considered a disorder of apocrine glands but now felt to be due to occlusion of terminal follicular epithelium within apocrine gland-bearing skin. Bacteria involvement is not a primary pathogenic event, but secondary.
• Historically part of "follicular occlusive triad"; acne conglobata, dissecting cellulitis of scalp, hidradenitis suppurativa. Pilonidal sinus later added to form a tetrad.

RISK FACTORS
• Obesity
• African American
• Female
• Acne
• Diabetes Mellitus
• Hypercholesterolemia
• Low basal metabolic rate

 DIAGNOSIS

DIFFERENTIAL DIAGNOSIS
• Furunculosis. Differentiate by specific culture and also by the response to specific antibiotics.
• Carbuncles, granulomatous disease, infected epidermoid cysts, tuberculosis cutis, actinomycosis, tularemia and carcinoma. With inguinal involvement: granuloma inguinale and lymphogranuloma venereum.
• Inflammatory bowel disease with anogenital fistula (may also coexist with hidradenitis suppurativa or be mistaken for it)

LABORATORY
• Culture of exudate from lesion: Staphylococci, Streptococci, E. Coli, Proteus with chronic condition, usually not anaerobes. Increasing antibiotic resistance.
• Possibly increased ESR, leukocytosis, decreased serum iron, normocytic anemia, and changes in serum electrophoresis pattern - probably due to chronic inflammatory process
Drugs that may alter lab results: N/A
Disorders that may alter lab results: N/A

PATHOLOGICAL FINDINGS Acute and chronic inflammation, multiple comedones, sinus tracts when recurrent

SPECIAL TESTS Culture discharge from lesion(s)

IMAGING N/A

DIAGNOSTIC PROCEDURES
• Incision and drainage of lesion(s) with biopsy
• Clinical criteria for early diagnosis (proposed by Mortimer)
 ◊ Recurrent deep boils > 6 months in flexural sites
 ◊ Onset after puberty
 ◊ Poor response to conventional antibiotics
 ◊ Strong tendency toward relapse or recurrence
 ◊ Comedones in apocrine gland-bearing skin
 ◊ Routine culture of pus from boils - no pathogens
 ◊ Personal or family history of acne or pilonidal sinuses and exacerbation of boils premenstrually in women

 TREATMENT

APPROPRIATE HEALTH CARE
Generally outpatient

GENERAL MEASURES
• Symptomatic treatment acute lesions
• Prevent new lesions
• Local cleansing (germicidal soap)
• Improve environmental factors that cause follicular blockage

SURGICAL MEASURES
• Wide excision with healing by granulation (considered more efficacious then drug treatment); but medical treatment tried first because of extensive nature of surgery treatment
• Incision and drainage of lesions
 ◊ Remove sinus tracts
 ◊ Exteriorization with curettage and electrodesiccation
• Treatment for severe, intractable cases: excision and skin graft
• CO_2 laser stripping with healing by secondary intention

ACTIVITY Fully active

DIET No restrictions

PATIENT EDUCATION
• Minimize heat exposure and sweating
• Reduce weight if obese
• Avoid constrictive clothing
• Medication precautions

MEDICATIONS

DRUG(S) OF CHOICE
• Antibiotics (not curative, relapse almost always inevitable); treatment sometimes for 2 or more months:
  ◊ Tetracycline 250 mg qid or 500 mg tid
  ◊ Minocycline (Minocin) 100 mg bid po
  ◊ Clindamycin 2% lotion or neomycin cream topically to control odor. Topical clindamycin as effective as systemic tetracyclines for stage 1 or 2 disease. Oral clindamycin also effective.
  ◊ Erythromycin 1-1.5 gm qd po
  ◊ Doxycycline 100 mg bid 7-14 days
  ◊ Other antibiotics depending on culture
• Birth control pills (female only), if antibiotic therapy fails. Low-dose progesterone BCPs (e.g., Norinyl, Ortho-Novum, Enovid).
• Consider oral retinoids
  ◊ Isotretinoin (Accutane) 40-80 mg/day po for 4 months. No Accutane during pregnancy (highly teratogenic). Equivocal results, still frequent recurrences.
• Consider steroids
  ◊ Injection of lesions with depot-type steroids (e.g., triamcinolone)
  ◊ Consider brief course of systemic corticosteroids
  ◊ Anti-androgen therapy - controversial
Contraindications: Tetracycline - pregnancy, children < 8 years
Precautions:
• Tetracycline - use sunscreen (SPF 15 or better) to avoid phototoxicity.
• Review professional literature before prescribing birth control pills or Accutane
Significant possible interactions:
• Tetracycline - do not take dairy products, antacids, or iron preparations within 2 hours of tetracycline dose.

ALTERNATIVE DRUGS N/A

FOLLOWUP

PATIENT MONITORING Revisits monthly, or more often if needed

PREVENTION/AVOIDANCE
• Minimize heat exposure and sweating
• Lose weight if overweight
• Avoid constrictive clothing/frictional trauma
• Avoid underarm antiperspirants and deodorants

POSSIBLE COMPLICATIONS
• Contracture formation at the sites of lesions
• Restricted limb mobility
• Squamous cell carcinoma may develop in indolent sinus tracts (usually anogenital)
• Disseminated infection septicemia- unusual
• Lymphedema
• Urethral/rectal fistula
• Anemia
• Arthritis (asymmetrical pauciarticular to symmetrical polyarthritis/polyarthralgia. Typically larger joints of upper or lower extremities, particularly the knee)
• Amyloidosis
• Renal failure
• Interstitial keratitis

EXPECTED COURSE/PROGNOSIS
• Individual lesions (with or without drainage) heal slowly in 10-30 days
• Recurrences may last for several years
• Rare spontaneous resolution
• Relentlessly progressive scarring and sinus tracts

MISCELLANEOUS

ASSOCIATED CONDITIONS
• Acne
• Perifolliculitis capitis abscedens et suffodiens (dissecting cellulitis of scalp)
• Obesity with associated diabetes mellitus, atopy, acanthosis nigrans

AGE-RELATED FACTORS
Pediatric: Rarely occurs before puberty (1 case reported in a 2 year old)
Geriatric: Rare after menopause
Others: Common late puberty through age 40

PREGNANCY No Accutane treatment during pregnancy

SYNONYMS
• Apocrinitis
• Hidradenitis axillaris
• Acne inversa

ICD-9-CM
705.83 Hidradenitis

SEE ALSO
• Furunculosis
• Folliculitis

OTHER NOTES
• Some patients develop only two or three papules per year. Others develop new lesions and drain as rapidly as old ones resolve.
• Although 50% of patients receiving Accutane, in doses similar to those for acne, obtain appreciable improvement, relapse occurs quickly upon discontinuing

ABBREVIATIONS N/A

REFERENCES
• Brown TJ, Rosen T: Hidradenitis Suppurativa. Southern Med J 1998;91(12):1107-1114
• Moschella SL, Hurley HJ: Dermatology. 3rd Ed. Philadelphia, W.B. Saunders, 1992
• Lynch PJ: Dermatology for the House Officer. 3rd Ed. Baltimore, Williams & Wilkins, 1994
• Bell BA, Ellis H: Hidradenitis Suppurativa. Journal of the Royal Society of Medicine 1978;71:511-515
• Sauer GC: Manual of Skin Diseases. 6th Ed. Philadelphia, J.B. Lippincott, 1991
• Orkin M, ed: Dermatology. Los Altos, CA, Lange Medical Publishers, 1991
• Lapins J, Marcusson JA, Emtestam L: Surgical treatment of chronic hidradenitis suppurativa: CO2 laser stripping-secondary intention technique. British J of Dermatol 1994 131:551-556
Illustrations: N/A
Internet references: http://www.5mcc.com

Author(s)
Paul J. Jaster, MD

Hip fracture

BASICS

DESCRIPTION Fracture of the head or neck of the femur, usually as the result of a fall
- Types
  ◊ Neck, subcapital or transcervical
  ◊ Intertrochanteric
  ◊ Subtrochanteric; usually caused by more severe trauma and has higher incidence in males than the other types

System(s) affected: Musculoskeletal
Genetics: No known genetic factor
Incidence/Prevalence in USA:
- 200,000 patients per year over the age of 65 have fracture of hips
- In women over age 75, there is a 1% incidence per year

Predominant age: 80% occur in those over age 60
Predominant sex: Female > Male

SIGNS AND SYMPTOMS
- Pain in hip. If severe, it usually indicates a displaced fracture. Mild pain usually occurs in non-displaced fractures.
- Pain in knee. Pain is referred from hip and may occur in absence of hip pain.
- External rotation of leg
- Shortening of leg

CAUSES
- Falls
- Motor vehicle trauma
- Spontaneous in pathologic conditions

RISK FACTORS
- Osteoporosis, usually post menopausal
- Metastatic cancer
- Neurological disease
- Severe renal disease with secondary hyperparathyroidism
- Use of long-acting sedatives and hypnotics in the elderly

DIAGNOSIS

DIFFERENTIAL DIAGNOSIS Rule out primary or metastatic malignancy

LABORATORY Routine pre-operative laboratory including CBC, chemical profile, electrolytes
Drugs that may alter lab results: N/A
Disorders that may alter lab results: N/A

PATHOLOGICAL FINDINGS
Osteoporosis

SPECIAL TESTS N/A

IMAGING
- X-rays - AP and "frog leg" lateral of hip
- X-ray AP pelvis to rule out pelvis fracture as cause of pain. Also provides information regarding appearance of opposite side.
- X-ray remainder of femur to include knee
- X-ray any other tender or painful area as other fractures are common and symptoms may be ignored with severe pain of hip fracture
- CT or MRI scans are not routinely indicated as the diagnosis is usually obvious from plain radiographs

DIAGNOSTIC PROCEDURES N/A

TREATMENT

APPROPRIATE HEALTH CARE
- Treat as semi-emergency
- During transportation to hospital, gentle traction of the leg, especially Buck's traction 5# will help relieve discomfort. This can be maintained in bed, but requires close observation of circulation and skin changes.

GENERAL MEASURES
- Medical evaluation to have patient in best possible condition before surgery
- Surgery is almost always indicated. Older patients do not tolerate long periods of bed confinement.
- Protect pressure points to avoid decubitus ulcers, especially on the sacrum, heels and malleoli

SURGICAL MEASURES
- A hip prosthesis or pins are used in neck fractures. Nails or screws with side plates are used in intertrochanteric fractures. For subtrochanteric fractures, a nail with a long side plate, or intermedullary hip screws, or reconstructive rods may be used.

ACTIVITY
- Patients should be up (for toilet, and prevention of deep vein thrombosis and decubiti) as soon as possible after surgery, usually the next day
- Ambulate as soon as possible after surgery, e.g., with use of a walker. Close supervision by an experienced therapist necessary.

DIET No special diet

PATIENT EDUCATION Refer to physical therapy for walking instructions; usually non-weight bearing for several weeks at least

MEDICATIONS

DRUG(S) OF CHOICE Analgesics, as indicated. Drug of choice might be morphine sulfate 2-10 mg q3h prn with change to oral opioids as soon as possible.
Contraindications: Associated head injury or severe respiratory disease
Precautions: Dosage should be lower in older people to avoid respiratory problems
Significant possible interactions: Refer to manufacturer's literature

ALTERNATIVE DRUGS N/A

FOLLOWUP

PATIENT MONITORING
• X-rays of the hip taken prior to discharge from the hospital and every 8-12 weeks afterward until healed
• Monitor postoperative physical therapy for full recovery

PREVENTION/AVOIDANCE
• Prophylactic treatment for osteoporosis
• Avoid long-acting sedatives and hypnotics in the elderly
• Use walking canes or walkers if patient has unsteady gait
• Have older people use proper chair for sitting. Should not allow hip flexion greater than 90 degrees since rising from this position requires external rotation of the extremity with subsequent torsional forces which can cause fracture.
• Use sturdy rails in showers, bathrooms, stairs, or ramps

POSSIBLE COMPLICATIONS
• Mental deterioration. Present in 90% of older patients for varying periods of time after surgery. Usually subsides, but may persist due to pre-existing arteriosclerosis.
• Infection. More common in comminuted fractures and patients with diabetes. Surgical implants should be left in place and antibiotics given as indicated by culture and sensitivity. Some require the wound to be opened and drained.
• Aseptic necrosis of femoral head. Occurs in 25-30% of femoral neck fractures. Treatment requires a prosthetic replacement in older patients.
• Phlebitis. Prophylaxis with warfarin (Coumadin) to keep INR 2.0-2.5 or protime 15-18 scc - for at least 4 weeks; or enoxaparin (Lovenox) 30 mg SQ q12h beginning 12 hours after surgery and continuing until patient is mobile
• Nonunion
  ◊ In case of neck fractures, a prosthetic replacement is indicated
  ◊ In the intertrochanteric fracture, a bone graft, usually with replacement of the nail and plate, is indicated

EXPECTED COURSE/PROGNOSIS
• Hip fractures remain a serious injury in older people. There is a 15-20% three month mortality in trochanteric fractures and 10% in neck fractures.
• Sixty-five percent of patients can be expected to return to their former state of health

MISCELLANEOUS

ASSOCIATED CONDITIONS
• Osteoporosis
• Metastatic malignancy

AGE-RELATED FACTORS
Pediatric: N/A
Geriatric: Hip fractures common in geriatric age group
Others: N/A

PREGNANCY N/A

SYNONYMS
• Subcapital fracture
• Trochanteric fracture
• Femoral neck fracture

ICD-9-CM
820. Fracture of neck of femur (use appropriate modifier)

SEE ALSO
• Osteoporosis

OTHER NOTES None

ABBREVIATIONS N/A

REFERENCES
• Clinical Orthopedics #218, May, 1987; Symposium of hip fractures; pp. 2-104
• Bentley G: Impacted Fracture of the Neck of the Femur. Bone & Joint Surgery 1968, 50:B:551
• Sarmiento A, et al: Avoidance of Complications. Clinical Orthopedics 1967;53:47
Illustrations: N/A
Internet references: http://www.5mcc.com

Author(s)
Furnie W. Johnston, MD
R. Bruce Hall, MD

Hirsutism

BASICS

DESCRIPTION Excessive male-pattern hair growth due to increased androgenic hormones
• Often accompanied by menstrual irregularities
• Extreme androgenic effects (deep voice, clitorimegaly, balding) is known as virilization
System(s) affected: Endocrine/Metabolic, Reproductive
Genetics: Multifactorial
Incidence/Prevalence in USA: 8% of adult women
Predominant age: Postpubertal females
Predominant sex: Postpubertal females

SIGNS AND SYMPTOMS
• Hair thickens and darkens in "male" pattern - beard, moustache, chest hair
• Usually accompanied by irregular menses and anovulation
• Usually accompanied by acne
• May be accompanied by infertility
• Onset is usually gradual

CAUSES
• Excessive androgenic effects:
  ◊ Excess hormone production from the ovary or adrenal gland
  ◊ Increased peripheral sensitivity to androgens
  ◊ Decreased sex hormone binding globulin
• Causes with persistent anovulation:
  ◊ Polycystic ovary disease
  ◊ Hypothyroidism
  ◊ Hyperprolactinemia
• Ovarian causes:
  ◊ Polycystic ovaries
  ◊ Ovarian tumors
  ◊ Premature ovarian failure
• Adrenal causes:
  ◊ Tumor (rare)
  ◊ Cushing's (rare)
  ◊ Late onset congenital adrenal hyperplasia

RISK FACTORS
• Family history
• Anovulation

DIAGNOSIS

DIFFERENTIAL DIAGNOSIS All hirsutism is from relative excess of androgen. This can be produced by the ovaries, the adrenals, or caused indirectly by other hormone imbalances. A specific etiology is often not found.
• Excess ovarian androgen production (testosterone level)
• Excess adrenal androgen production (DHEAS [dehydroepiandrosterone sulfate])
• Late onset congenital adrenal hyperplasia (17 hydroxyprogesterone [17-OHP])
• Hypothyroidism (TSH)
• Hyperprolactinemia (prolactin level)
• Ovarian tumor (testosterone > 200)
• Adrenal tumor (DHEAS > 700)
• Idiopathic - possibly through peripheral conversion - no good test available
• Anabolic steroid use in performance athletes
• Cushing's disease - very rare

LABORATORY
• Basic workup - total testosterone, DHEAS, 17-OHP, TSH, prolactin
• If testosterone > 200, need ovarian tumor workup
• If DHEAS > 700, need adrenal tumor workup
• LH/FSH ratio is elevated in 75% of polycystic ovarian disease
• If testosterone, DHEAS or 17 OHP are elevated, but not in tumor range, treat
Drugs that may alter lab results: N/A
Disorders that may alter lab results: N/A

PATHOLOGICAL FINDINGS N/A

SPECIAL TESTS
• Fasting glucose to insulin ratio to rule out insulin resistance in polycystic ovary syndrome
• Some do endometrial biopsy if > 35 years old
• If strong suspicion of Cushing's disease, can do dexamethasone suppression test. Give 1 mg dexamethasone po at PM and draw plasma cortisol at 8:00 am. If cortisol > 5, borderline; if > 10, abnormal.
• If 17-OHP is 300-800, do ACTH (Cortrosyn) test (ACTH 0.25 mg IV and check 17-OHP at 0 and 1 hour)
• Some do 3 alpha-androstanediol glucuronide to check for peripheral conversion - but not a good test and doesn't change therapy
• If DHEAS is high, but not in tumor range, can do low dose dexamethasone test (0.5 mg dexamethasone qid x 5 days, then recheck DHEAS and testosterone - they will decrease if androgens are adrenal and won't if they are ovarian)

IMAGING
• If testosterone > 200 or DHEAS > 700, need CT of ovaries or adrenals
• Ultrasound can image polycystic ovaries as a supplement to clinical diagnosis

DIAGNOSTIC PROCEDURES N/A

TREATMENT

APPROPRIATE HEALTH CARE
Outpatient

GENERAL MEASURES
• Treatment is slow and often lifelong
• If patient desires pregnancy, ovulation induction may be necessary
• Provide contraception as needed
• Encourage patient to maintain ideal weight
• Treat accompanying acne

SURGICAL MEASURES N/A

ACTIVITY No special activity

DIET No special diet

PATIENT EDUCATION
• Hormonal treatment stops further hair growth but will not usually reverse present hair
• Treatment takes 6-24 months and may be life long
• Cosmetic measures include - plucking, bleaching, shaving, electrolysis, laser hair removal and cover up cosmetics
• Electrolysis should be by a licensed professional

MEDICATIONS

DRUG(S) OF CHOICE
After tumor has been ruled out:
- Hormonal therapy - the goal is to:
  ◊ Decrease androgens
  ◊ Increase sex steroid binding globulin (SBG)
  ◊ Increase testosterone clearance
  ◊ Decrease LH
- Oral contraceptives:
  ◊ Any brand is effective - monophasics, triphasics, estrogen dominant and progesterone dominant
  ◊ Estrogen and progesterone can be given separately
  ◊ Medroxyprogesterone (Depo-Provera) IM every 3 months
- Chronic dexamethasone therapy:
  ◊ Can be used in late onset congenital adrenal hyperplasia (0.5 mg qhs), but oral contraception also effective

Contraindications: Avoid giving medications in pregnancy
Precautions: N/A
Significant possible interactions: N/A

ALTERNATIVE DRUGS
- Metformin: experimentally decreases insulin secretion which decreases androgen production in polycystic ovaries
- Antiandrogenic drugs (often used when workup is negative and oral contraceptives not helping. They have low efficacy and many side effects):
  ◊ Spironolactone: up to 200 mg/day - onset of action is slow, side effects include menorrhagia, contraindicated in pregnancy
  ◊ Cyproterone: orphan drug not routinely available - usually combined with estrogen - contraindicated in pregnancy. Monitor LFTs.
  ◊ Flutamide: 250 mg tid - nonsteroidal antiandrogen. Monitor LFTs. Need concurrent oral contraceptives.
  ◊ Ketoconazole: 400 mg day - avoid with astemizole, triazolam, cisapride
  ◊ Leuprolide (Lupron): lowers LH. Side effects of menopause.
  ◊ Danazol: lowers LH. Side effects of menopause
  ◊ Serenoa repens (Saw Palmetto) - in small studies decreases hair growth via blocking 5-alpha-reductase activity

FOLLOWUP

PATIENT MONITORING
Monitor for known side effects of medications

PREVENTION/AVOIDANCE
- Tumor must be ruled out before beginning therapy
- As hormone balance improves, fertility may increase - provide contraception as needed
- Patients desiring pregnancy may need fertility intervention such as ovulation induction
- Women with late onset congenital adrenal hyperplasia may be carriers for the severe early onset childhood disease - counsel
- Avoid quackery and unlicensed electrolysis
- Prolonged amenorrhea may, over time, put the patient at risk for endometrial hyperplasia or carcinoma
- There is an increased incidence of diabetes and insulin resistance in polycystic ovarian disease which can increase risk of heart disease

POSSIBLE COMPLICATIONS
- Dysfunctional uterine bleeding and anemia
- Androgenic excess may adversely affect lipid status, cardiac risk and bone density
- Poor self image/shame

EXPECTED COURSE/PROGNOSIS
- Good (with long term therapy) for halting further hair growth
- Moderate to poor for reversing current hair growth

MISCELLANEOUS

ASSOCIATED CONDITIONS
- Acne
- Infertility
- Obesity
- Hyperinsulinemia

AGE-RELATED FACTORS
Pediatric: N/A
Geriatric: Can occur after menopause if peripheral conversion of estrogen is poor
Others: N/A

PREGNANCY
- May have related infertility
- If pregnancy occurs, must discontinue known contraindicated drugs
- Pregnancy outcome is related to underlying cause of hirsutism

SYNONYMS   N/A

ICD-9-CM   704.1 Hirsutism

SEE ALSO
- Fertility problems
- Acne vulgaris
- Obesity
- Polycystic ovarian disease
- Hyperprolactinemia
- Hypothyroidism, adult

OTHER NOTES   N/A

ABBREVIATIONS
LFTs = liver function tests

REFERENCES
- Speroff L, Glass R, Kase N: Clinical Gynecologic Endocrinology and Infertility. 5th Ed. Williams & Wilkins, Baltimore, 1994
- Franks S: Polycystic ovarian disease. NEJM 1995;333(13):853-868
- Kalve E, Klein JF: Evaluation of women with hirsutism. Am Fam Phys 1996;54)1):117-124
- Hirsutism amd polycystic ovarian syndrome. Society for Reproductive Medicine, 1995
Illustrations: 1 available on CD-ROM
Internet references: http://www.5mcc.com

Author(s)
Laura L. Novak, MD

Histoplasmosis

BASICS

DESCRIPTION Fungal infection with Histoplasma capsulatum, a dimorphic soil-dwelling saprophyte that has multiple clinical manifestations. Initial infection in the normal host is often asymptomatic. Other manifestations include a self-limited flu-like syndrome, mediastinal fibrosis, scar tissue residual, chronic cavitary disease in those with obstructive lung disease and disseminated histoplasmosis which is more frequent in the immunocompromised host and infants.
• H. capsulatum has worldwide distribution; the most endemic region in North America is the central U.S. The fungus exists in mycelial form in nature and in yeast phase when exposed to mammalian temperatures. Spores may remain active for up to ten years. Exposure to bird or bat excrement promotes growth of the fungus for unexplained reasons.
• Chronic pulmonary histoplasmosis - usually occurs in white males with obstructive lung disease and apical bullous lung pathology. These patients exhibit evidence of an indolent infectious process.
• Disseminated histoplasmosis infection in the immunocompromised is a rare opportunistic infection which may mimic sepsis syndrome and progress to multiple organ system failure
System(s) affected: Pulmonary, Gastrointestinal, Skin/Exocrine, Hemic/Lymphatic/Immunologic
Genetics: None known
Incidence/Prevalence in USA:
• Infection in endemic areas is virtually 100%; few patients develop active disease; approximately 500,000 new infections in the U.S./yr
• Occurrence in AIDS patients is 2%-5%
• Disseminated histoplasmosis occurs in < 0.05% of infections, one-third of these are infants < 1 year old, in adults there is an increased prevalence with age > 60 years
Predominant age:
• None in acute histoplasmosis
• Infants < 1 year old are at higher risk for disseminated histoplasmosis
Predominant sex:
• Acute histoplasmosis - Male = Female
• Disseminated histoplasmosis - Male > Female (5-10:1)

SIGNS AND SYMPTOMS
• Primary infection in the normal host is usually asymptomatic
• 1% immunocompetent individuals with low-level exposure develop symptoms
• 99% subclinical infection
• Arthralgia-erythema nodosum-erythema multiforme is associated with acute infection
• Low grade fever, anorexia, weight loss, night sweats, and productive cough are associated with chronic infections

CAUSES Dimorphic fungus Histoplasma capsulatum

RISK FACTORS
• Spelunking
• Cleaning chicken coops
• Excavation near bird roosts
• Demolition or remodeling of old buildings
• Exposure to decayed wood or dead trees
• Performing routine activities in areas with high accumulation of bird droppings
• Immunosuppression

DIAGNOSIS

DIFFERENTIAL DIAGNOSIS
• Atypical pneumonia and viral pneumonitis
• Other fungal diseases such as blastomycosis, coccidioidomycosis
• Other granulomatous diseases such as M. tuberculosis and sarcoidosis
• Pneumoconiosis
• Lymphoma
• Malignancies associated with hilar lymphadenopathy

LABORATORY
• For disseminated histoplasma antigen in AIDS patients, urinary and blood histoplasmosis
• Polysaccharide antigen detection is a rapid test for diagnosis and for monitoring relapse
• Complement fixation may be negative approximately 30% in acute histoplasmosis and 50% in disseminated histoplasmosis
• Immunodiffusion test may be negative in approximately 50% of patients with acute histoplasmosis. Maximum positivity of test occurs 4-6 weeks after exposure.
• Complement fixation antibodies at titers 1:8 or 1:16 are presumptive for diagnosis, > 1:32 is strongly supportive as is an acute 4-fold titer rise. Determining the presence of H and M bands may be helpful.
• For chronic histoplasmosis and disseminated disease, cultures of sputum, bronchoalveolar lavage, bone marrow, lymph nodes, blood, liver and cerebrospinal fluid may be positive. Demonstration of characteristic organisms by silver stain on biopsy and bronchoalveolar lavage and bronchial washing specimens is diagnostic.
Drugs that may alter lab results: N/A
Disorders that may alter lab results:
• Serologic tests may be falsely negative early in infection or in the immunocompromised
• False positive results may occur with tuberculosis and other fungal diseases
• Slow clearance of antibodies may identify patients with past Histoplasmosis infection who now present with a different disease
• False positive complement fixation titers may occur after histoplasmin skin antigen testing
• False positive H. capsulatum polysaccharide antigen test may occur with patients with disseminated blastomycosis and coccidiomycosis

PATHOLOGICAL FINDINGS Poorly formed caseating granulomas on biopsy or bronchoscopy specimens with identification of characteristic yeast forms by methenamine silver stain

SPECIAL TESTS
• Determine the presence of urinary H. capsulatum antigen
• Bronchoscopy
• Liver and bone marrow biopsies

IMAGING
• Routine chest roentgenogram may reveal focal mid-lung field infiltrates (27%), hilar or mediastinal adenopathy (25%) or both (30%). May see miliary or diffuse pattern with disseminated disease following large antigen load.
• If indicated, CAT scan of chest to differentiate mediastinal fibrosis from mediastinal granuloma

DIAGNOSTIC PROCEDURES
• Serologic blood work
• Bronchoscopy with bronchoalveolar lavage and transbronchial biopsy
• Liver and bone marrow biopsies for suspected disseminated disease
• Mediastinoscopy for lymph node biopsy

TREATMENT

APPROPRIATE HEALTH CARE
• Usually outpatient
• Disseminated histoplasmosis requires hospitalization for initial treatment

GENERAL MEASURES 99% of acute primary histoplasmosis resolve spontaneously; symptomatic treatment only

SURGICAL MEASURES N/A

ACTIVITY Avoid high risk exposures

DIET No restrictions

PATIENT EDUCATION Extended treatment needs in chronic cavitary histoplasmosis; maintenance therapy in AIDS

MEDICATIONS

DRUG(S) OF CHOICE
• Disseminated histoplasmosis
◊ Amphotericin B - test dose is 1 mg followed by 0.25 mg/kg/dose, which may be slowly increased to 0.5 mg/kg/dose. Cumulative dose to 1-2 gm (at least 35 mg/kg is indicated).
◊ Ketoconazole or itraconazole for mild disease
- Ketoconazole: Induction therapy with 400 mg/day for 3 days, then maintenance therapy 200 mg or 400 mg a day
- Itraconazole: Induction therapy with 200 mg twice a day for 3 days, then 200 mg once or twice daily

Histoplasmosis

- AIDS patients
  ◊ Itraconazole for mild disease: Induction therapy with 600 mg/day for 3 days, then 400 mg/day. Drug of choice for primary and maintenance therapy is itraconazole. Ketoconazole is not effective in AIDS-related histoplasmosis. Maintenance therapy with itraconazole 400 mg/day or amphotericin-B 50-100 mg weekly (1 mg/kg).
- Chronic cavitary histoplasmosis
  ◊ Amphotericin-B for severe or moderately severe disease, 2.0-2.5 g cumulative
  ◊ Ketoconazole or itraconazole for mild disease
    - Ketoconazole: Induction therapy with 400 mg/day for 3 days, then maintenance therapy 200 mg or 400 mg/day
    - Itraconazole: Induction therapy with 200 mg twice daily for 3 days, then 200 mg once or twice daily
- Acute pulmonary histoplasmosis
  ◊ Amphotericin B for severe or moderately severe disease; test dose is 1 mg followed by 0.25 mg/kg/dose which may be slowly increased to 0.5 mg/kg/dose. Cumulative dose at least 35 mg/kg
  ◊ Ketoconazole or itraconazole for mild disease
    - Ketoconazole: Induction therapy with 400 mg/day for 3 days, then maintenance therapy 200 mg or 400 mg/day
    - Itraconazole: Induction therapy with 200 mg twice daily for 3 days, then 200 mg once or twice daily
- Duration of treatment
  ◊ Optimal duration of treatment with antifungals has not been established
  ◊ Disseminated histoplasmosis - 6 months course
  ◊ Chronic cavitary histoplasmosis - at least 12 months course with stable chest roentgenogram findings over 3-6 months
  ◊ Acute pulmonary histoplasmosis - 2-3 month course
  ◊ AIDS-related or relapsed - chronic, lifelong, maintenance therapy
- Mediastinal granuloma
  ◊ Can mimic fibrosing mediastinitis, may respond to treatment with amphotericin B
- Fibrosing mediastinitis
  ◊ Has no active infection present and is not treatable

Contraindications: No contraindications to treatment in patients with progressive cavitary disease or disseminated histoplasmosis. The latter has a mortality rate of 80% if untreated.

Precautions:
- Amphotericin B
  ◊ Dosage probably does not need to be adjusted for creatinine clearance
  ◊ It is nephrotoxic. Renal function must be monitored closely. Monitor electrolytes, especially potassium and magnesium.
  ◊ Rigors can be prevented by pre-infusion meperidine. Fever and chills can be diminished by pre-infusion dose of acetaminophen plus diphenhydramine.
- Ketoconazole
  ◊ Is associated with gastrointestinal upset
  ◊ May inhibit testosterone synthesis and should be used with caution in patients with underlying hepatic dysfunction

Significant possible interactions:
- Expected benefits outweigh possible risks.
- Ketoconazole
  ◊ Requires an acid environment for dissolution. If the patient requires antacid or H2 blockade, administer at least 2 hours after dose of ketoconazole
  ◊ Co-administration of terfenadine may cause cardiac arrhythmias
  ◊ May increase cyclosporine levels
  ◊ May decrease Rifampin and INH levels as well as ketoconazole levels
  ◊ May increase phenytoin levels
- Itraconazole
  ◊ Rifampin levels may decrease itraconazole to undetectable levels
  ◊ May increase digoxin levels
  ◊ Questionable effect on cyclosporine levels
- Fluconazole
  ◊ May increase cyclosporine levels
  ◊ May increase warfarin effect
  ◊ Questionable effect of Rifampin on fluconazole

ALTERNATIVE DRUGS Fluconazole has not been approved for histoplasmosis therapy. Fluconazole is undergoing investigational studies in its use for chronic pulmonary and disseminated histoplasmosis. Preliminarily, fluconazole doses of 400 mg/day or higher may be necessary for therapeutic outcome.

FOLLOWUP

PATIENT MONITORING Renal function and liver chemistries every 1-2 months for chronic therapy patients; chest x-ray to evaluate therapy response at regular intervals

PREVENTION/AVOIDANCE
Maintenance therapy is required in AIDS

POSSIBLE COMPLICATIONS
- Bronchial, tracheal or esophageal obstruction secondary to adenopathy, broncholithiasis
- Pulmonary, splenic and hepatic calcifications, rarely pericarditis, pleurisy or effusion
- CNS histoplasmosis (rare): Chronic meningitis or intracranial histoplasmosis
- Endocarditis involving aortic or mitral valves
- Pericardial effusions (sterile exudates) not thought to be secondary to hematogenous spread
- Fibrosing mediastinitis can cause stenosis of vascular and bronchial structures within the mediastinum causing pulmonary hypertension, superior vena cava syndrome and bronchial obstruction
- Acute renal failure and hepatic dysfunction secondary to medications
- Amphotericin induced hypokalemia
- Relapse occurring in the immunocompromised or inadequately treated patient with disseminated histoplasmosis

EXPECTED COURSE/PROGNOSIS
- Primary histoplasmosis - 99% resolve spontaneously
- The prognosis for chronic cavitary pulmonary histoplasmosis is determined by the loss of lung parenchyma and pulmonary function
- Treatment of disseminated disease in AIDS/non-AIDS cases does improve outcome with ketoconazole having > 80% success rate and amphotericin B being 60-100% successful. Despite maintenance therapy, AIDS patients, have 10-50% relapse rate.

MISCELLANEOUS

ASSOCIATED CONDITIONS
- Disseminated histoplasmosis is an opportunistic infection in the immunocompromised host
- HIV infection

AGE-RELATED FACTORS
Pediatric: 1/3 of cases of disseminated histoplasmosis occur in infants < 1 year old
Geriatric: Increased incidence of disseminated histoplasmosis in males during 6th and 7th decades
Others: N/A

PREGNANCY No increased incidence

SYNONYMS N/A

ICD-9-CM 115.9 Histoplasmosis, unspecified

SEE ALSO N/A

OTHER NOTES N/A

ABBREVIATIONS N/A

REFERENCES
- Dismukes WE, Cloud G, Bowles C, et al: Treatment of blastomycosis and histoplasmosis with ketoconazole. Ann Intern Med 1985;103:861-872
- Como JA, Dismukes WE: Oral azole drugs as systemic antifungal therapy. N Engl J Med 1994;330:263-272
- Wheat JL, Connolly-Stringfield P, Kohler RB, et al: Histoplasma capsulatum polysaccharide antigen detection in diagnosis and management of disseminated histoplasmosis in patients with acquired immunodeficiency syndrome. Am J Med 1989;87:396-400
- Wheat JL, Connolly-Stringfield PA, Baker RL, et al: Histoplasmosis in the acquired immune deficiency syndrome: clinical findings diagnosis and treatment, and review of the literature. In Medicine 1990;69:361-374
- Wheat J: Histoplasmosis: recognition and treatment. Clin Infect Dis. (suppl) 1994;1:S19-27
Illustrations: 1 available on CD-ROM
Internet references: http://www.5mcc.com

Author(s)
Robert P. Baughman, MD

HIV infection & AIDS

BASICS

DESCRIPTION A chronic infection with variable course (requiring about 10 years from the time of infection for 50% of persons to develop AIDS). HIV infects cells with CD4 receptors, most notably the CD4 lymphocytes (also called T4 or T helper cells). Infection causes cell death and a decline in immune function resulting in opportunistic infections, malignancies, and neurologic problems. These opportunistic conditions define the acquired immunodeficiency syndrome (AIDS). As of 1/1/93 all HIV infected persons with < 200 CD4 cells are categorized as AIDS. HIV appears to have direct effects on the central nervous system, the GI tract and other systems.

System(s) affected:
Hemic/Lymphatic/Immunologic, Nervous, Pulmonary, Gastrointestinal
Genetics: Unclear
Incidence/Prevalence in USA: > 500,000 AIDS cases; > 300,000 deaths
Predominant age: Young adults - 25-44
Predominant sex: Male > Female

SIGNS AND SYMPTOMS

• Acute infection: Mononucleosis-like syndrome with fever, rash, myalgia, and malaise a self-limited syndrome occurring about 6-8 weeks postinfection, associated with the development of HIV antibody
• Asymptomatic infection: Follows initial infection; variable duration
• Persistent generalized lymphadenopathy: Characteristics - lymph node enlargement 1 cm or greater in two or more extra-inguinal sites. Adenopathy persists longer than 3 months.
• Other diseases:
  ◊ Constitutional: Fever lasting more than one month, involuntary weight loss of more than ten percent baseline weight, persistent diarrhea, skin rash, severe chronic fatigue
  ◊ Neurologic disease: Dementia, myelopathy or peripheral neuropathy not explained by other illness
  ◊ Secondary infectious disease:
    - AIDS-defining opportunistic infections: Pneumocystis carinii pneumonia; chronic cryptosporidial diarrhea; cerebral toxoplasmosis; extra -intestinal Strongyloides; isosporiasis; esophageal, bronchial/pulmonary candidiasis; cryptococcosis; histoplasmosis; coccidioidomycosis; disseminated mycobacterial disease; cytomegalovirus disease; chronic mucocutaneous or disseminated herpes simplex; progressive multifocal leukoencephalopathy.
    - Other specified infections: Oral hairy leukoplakia, dermatomal zoster, nocardiosis, tuberculosis (pulmonary), recurrent salmonella bacteremia, oral candidiasis.
  ◊ Secondary cancers: Kaposi's sarcoma, non-Hodgkin's lymphoma, and primary brain lymphoma, invasive cervical cancer.
• Other conditions not classified above that may be attributed to HIV infection: idiopathic thrombocytopenic purpura, seborrheic dermatitis, chronic lymphoid interstitial pneumonitis, alopecia, and renal disease.

• 1993 revised classification: For HIV infection and expanded surveillance case definition for AIDS among adolescents and adults (from MMWR)
• Categories:

A	B	C
Asymptomatic or persistent general lymph-adenopathy (includes acute [primary] infection)	Symptomatic; not category A or C conditions	AIDS indicator conditions

• CD4 cell categories:

1	2	3
≥ 500/μg	200-499/μg	< 200/μg
A1, B1, C1†	A2, B2, C2†	A3†, B3†, C3†

(† = expanded AIDS surveillance case definition)
• Conditions: Included in the AIDS surveillance case definition
  ◊ Candidiasis of bronchi, trachea, or lungs
  ◊ Candidiasis, esophageal
  ◊ Cervical cancer, invasive
  ◊ Coccidioidomycosis, disseminated or extrapulmonary
  ◊ Cryptococcosis, extrapulmonary
  ◊ Cryptosporidiosis, chronic intestinal (> 1 month duration)
  ◊ Cytomegalovirus disease (other than liver, spleen or nodes)
  ◊ HIV encephalopathy
  ◊ Herpes simplex: chronic ulcer(s) (> than 1 month duration) or bronchitis pneumonitis, or esophagitis
  ◊ Histoplasmosis, disseminated or extrapulmonary
  ◊ Isosporiasis, chronic intestinal (> 1 month duration)
  ◊ Kaposi's sarcoma
  ◊ Lymphoma, Burkitt's (or equivalent term)
  ◊ Lymphoma, immunoblastic (or equivalent term)
  ◊ Lymphoma, primary in brain
  ◊ Mycobacterium avium complex or M. kansasii, disseminated or extrapulmonary
  ◊ Mycobacterium tuberculosis, any site (pulmonary or extrapulmonary)
  ◊ Mycobacterium, other species or unidentified species, disseminated or extrapulmonary
  ◊ Pneumocystis carinii pneumonia
  ◊ Progressive multifocal leukoencephalopathy
  ◊ Salmonella septicemia, recurrent
  ◊ Toxoplasmosis of brain
  ◊ Wasting syndrome resulting from HIV infection

CAUSES
• Human immunodeficiency virus (HIV); a retrovirus

RISK FACTORS
• Sexual activity
• Injection drug use
• Recipients of blood products: Highest risk 1975 to 3/1985
• Hemophiliacs who received pooled plasma
• Children of HIV-infected women:
  ◊ 30% of the these children during pregnancy will be infected without treatment
  ◊ Breast feeding is a possible route of transmission
  ◊ Prenatal, intrapartum and postpartum zidovudine significantly decreases the risk of HIV transmission from mother to child (from 29% to 8%)

• Needle stick (estimate 1 in 250 for hollow needles)
  ◊ Postexposure treatment with zidovudine, lamivudine, and indinavir for significant exposures (MMWR 1998)

DIAGNOSIS

DIFFERENTIAL DIAGNOSIS Screen for HIV infection when there is prolonged illness without ready explanation.

LABORATORY
• ELISA
  ◊ Sensitivity and specificity > 98%
  ◊ Reported as reactive or non-reactive. Reactive tests should be repeated. Confirm repeatedly reactive tests by another test (most commonly the Western Blot).
• Western blot
  ◊ Test results are positive, negative, or indeterminate (indeterminate tests result from non-specific reactions of HIV-negative sera with some HIV proteins)
  ◊ The CDC recommends reaction with two of the following three bands as criteria for positivity: P24; gp41, and gp 120/160. If the test is indeterminate, repeat test in 3-6 months.
Drugs that may alter lab results: N/A
Disorders that may alter lab results: N/A

PATHOLOGICAL FINDINGS N/A

SPECIAL TESTS As indicated by suspicion of opportunistic infection or HIV-associated condition.

IMAGING N/A

DIAGNOSTIC PROCEDURES N/A

TREATMENT

APPROPRIATE HEALTH CARE
Outpatient setting. Consultation with infectious disease or HIV specialist prior to onset of acute situations.

GENERAL MEASURES
• The initial visit:
  ◊ Past medical history including STD's and TB with dates and treatment
  ◊ Review of systems to include fever, chills, diarrhea, weight loss, fatigue, adenopathy, oral sores, cough, shortness of breath, dyspnea on exertion, visual changes, headaches, skin rash, neurologic changes, sinusitis, odynophagia
  ◊ Social history
  ◊ Physical examination, with Pap smear
  ◊ Immunization review (pneumococcal, influenza, and Td recommended in adults. OPV contraindicated in children [use IPV]).

HIV infection & AIDS

◊ Studies: CBC with differential and platelets; SMAC; RPR; CD4 absolute count and %lymphocytes CD4; hepatitis B sAg and sAb; chest x-ray; PPD with control; HIV-1 RNA viral quantitation (viral load); toxoplasmosis IgG, CMV IgG, Pap smears in females
• Patients with CD4<500 or CD4 >500 and viral burden >10,000-30,000 copies/mL will benefit from antiretroviral treatment. Combination antiretroviral therapy has contributed to a 23% decline in AIDS deaths in 1996 as compared with 1995.
• Patients with CD4<200 or with oral candidiasis or other signs of significant immune suppression should receive Pneumocystis carinii prophylaxis
• Patients with CD4<100 and toxoplasmosis IgG should receive toxoplasmosis prophylaxis.
• Patients with CD4<50 should receive prophylaxis against Mycobacterium avium complex (MAC)

SURGICAL MEASURES N/A

ACTIVITY Encourage regular exercise.

DIET
• Encourage good nutrition
• Avoid raw eggs, unpasteurized milk and other potentially contaminated foods
• May require vitamin supplementation

PATIENT EDUCATION
• Provide frank, complete, non-judgmental information on the routes of transmission (primarily sexual and needle sharing). Teach HIV infected how to minimize risk to others.
• Pre-printed and additional information material is available from a wide variety of sources including: National AIDS Hotline - (800)342-2437 [Spanish (800)342-7432]
• National Institute of Health AIDS Clinical Trials Group (800)874-2572. Information on AIDS/HIV clinical trials.
• American Foundation for AIDS Research: (212)719-0033; new treatments and research

 MEDICATIONS

DRUG(S) OF CHOICE
• Nucleoside reverse transcriptase inhibitors:
  ◊ Abacavir (ABC, Ziagen)
  ◊ Didanosine (ddl, Videx)
  ◊ Lamivudine (3TC, Epivir)
  ◊ Stavudine (d4T, Zerit)
  ◊ Zalcitabine (ddC, Hivid)
  ◊ Zidovudine (AZT, Retrovir)
• Protease inhibitors:
  ◊ Amprenavir (Agenerase)
  ◊ Indinavir (Crixivan)
  ◊ Nelfinavir (Viracept)
  ◊ Ritonavir (Norvir)
  ◊ Saquinavir (Invirase)
• Non-nucleoside reverse transcriptase inhibitors:
  ◊ Delaviridine (Rescriptor)
  ◊ Efavirenz (Sustiva)
  ◊ Nevirapine (Viramune)

• Current standard of care requires the use of 3 drugs to attempt to prevent the emergence of resistance. Goal of therapy is to reduce viral load as much as possible and delay or reverse immunodeterioration.
Contraindications: Significant drug interactions
Precautions: Antiretroviral drugs have significant toxicities; refer to specific drug information
Significant possible interactions: Antiretroviral drugs, especially the protease inhibitors have potentially life-threatening interactions; refer to specific drug information

ALTERNATIVE DRUGS N/A

 FOLLOWUP

PATIENT MONITORING
• Frequency determined largely by the patient's clinical and psychological status and by the need to monitor drug toxicity and immune function
• Recheck CD4 counts and viral load at least every 3 months depending on stage of illness and medical regimen
• Check at subsequent visits:
  ◊ Complete, careful physical exam
  ◊ Complete review of systems especially focused on neurologic symptoms (CNS infection, malignancy, or dementia), visual changes (CMV retinitis), diarrhea, fever, night sweats, shortness of breath, dyspnea on exertion (early P. carinii pneumonia), and odynophagia (esophageal candidiasis)
• Genotypic and phenotypic tests for resistance to antiretrovirals are now available. Their clinical utility is not fully established.

PREVENTION/AVOIDANCE When possible: avoid unscreened blood products; avoid unprotected sexual intercourse; use condoms; avoid injection drug abuse; avoid contact with fluids of HIV infected

POSSIBLE COMPLICATIONS
• Immunodeficiency
• Opportunistic infections
• Neuropsychiatric symptoms
• HIV-associated malignancies

EXPECTED COURSE/PROGNOSIS
When untreated HIV infection leads to AIDS, life expectancy is two to three years. AIDS defining opportunistic infections usually do not develop until CD4<200. In HIV untreated infection, CD4 counts decline at a rate of 50-80/year with more rapid decline as counts drop below 200. The newer retroviral regimens may delay or reverse immune dysfunction.

 MISCELLANEOUS

ASSOCIATED CONDITIONS
• Syphilis: May be more aggressive in

HIV-infected persons. Definitive treatment for syphilis in HIV infected persons is controversial; consult with an STD specialist.
• Tuberculosis is co-epidemic with HIV. HIV infection changes the management of TB; should test all persons with TB for HIV, or if not tested, should treat with multiple drugs as if HIV-infected.

AGE-RELATED FACTORS
Pediatric: Progresses more rapidly in infants
Geriatric: Progresses more rapidly in age >50
Others: N/A

PREGNANCY Antiretroviral therapy has been demonstrated to decrease the risk of HIV transmission to infants. Pregnant women should be treated based on their HIV disease status. Current guidelines are cited below.

SYNONYMS
• Acquired immune deficiency syndrome

ICD-9-CM
042 Human immunodeficiency virus infection with specified conditions
043 Human immunodeficiency virus causing other specified conditions
044 Other HIV infection

SEE ALSO
• Pneumonia, Pneumocystis carinii (PCP)
• Kaposi's sarcoma
• Candidiasis
• Candidiasis, mucocutaneous
• Cytomegalovirus inclusion disease
• Tuberculosis
• Cryptococcosis
• Idiopathic thrombocytopenic purpura (ITP)
• Rhodococcus infections

OTHER NOTES Increased risk of cervical cancer in HIV-infected women. Perform PAP smears at least every 6 months.

ABBREVIATIONS N/A

REFERENCES
• CDC: Report of the NIH Panel to Define Principles of Therapy of HIV Infection and Guidelines for the use of Antiretroviral Agents in HIV-Infected Adults and Adolescents. MMWR 1998;47(NO. RR-5)
• Carpenter C, et al: Antiretroviral therapy for HIV infection in 1998. JAMA 1998;250:78-86
• CDC: 1997 USPHS/IDSA guidelines for the prevention of opportunistic infections in persons infected with human immuno deficiency virus. MMWR 1997;46(No. RR-12)
• U.S. Public Health Service Task Force Recommendations for Use of Antiretroviral Drugs During Pregnancy for Maternal Health and Reduction of Perinatal Transmission of HIV Type 1 in the US. Fed Reg, 12-97
• Sande M, Volberding P: The Medical Management of AIDS. 5th Ed. Philadelphia, WB. Saunders Co., 1997
Illustrations: 39 available on CD-ROM
Internet references: http://www.5mcc.com

Author(s)
Kevin Carmichael, MD

Hodgkin's disease

BASICS

DESCRIPTION A malignant disease of the lymphoid tissue, caused by the transformation of an uncertain progenitor cell to the pathognomonic Reed-Sternberg cell. Disease spreads to contiguous lymphoid tissue, and eventually to non-lymphoid tissue.
• Rye classification-based on pathologic findings (frequency by percent):
  ◊ Lymphocyte predominant (2-10)
  ◊ Mixed cellularity (20-40)
  ◊ Lymphocyte depleted (2-15)
  ◊ Nodular sclerosis (40-80)
System(s) affected:
Hemic/Lymphatic/Immunologic
Genetics:
• First degree relatives - 3 times risk
• Siblings of younger patients - 7 times risk
Incidence/Prevalence in USA:
• 3.1/100000
• About 7200 new cases expected in 1999
• Incidence is lower in underdeveloped countries
Predominant age:
• Bimodal age distribution
  ◊ Early peak in mid to late 20s
  ◊ Later peak around 60-70
• Rare under age 5
Predominant sex: Male > Female (1.4:1)

SIGNS AND SYMPTOMS
• Asymptomatic lymphadenopathy (usually cervical or supraclavicular)
• Fever (Pel-Ebstein pattern)
• Night sweats
• Weight loss
• Fatigue
• Anorexia
• Unexplained itching
• Alcohol-induced pain

CAUSES
• Unknown; EB virus may play a role

RISK FACTORS
• Immunodeficiency (inherited or acquired)
• Autoimmune disorders
• HIV infection

DIAGNOSIS

DIFFERENTIAL DIAGNOSIS
• Non-Hodgkin lymphoma
• Infectious lymphadenopathy
• Other solid tumor metastases
• Sarcoidosis
• Autoimmune disease
• AIDS/HIV infection
• Drug reaction

LABORATORY
• CBC
• Chemistry profile
• ESR
• Liver function tests
• Renal function tests
Drugs that may alter lab results:
Phenytoin may produce pseudolymphoma
Disorders that may alter lab results: N/A

PATHOLOGICAL FINDINGS
• Reed-Sternberg (RS) cell
  ◊ Abundant cytoplasm
  ◊ Two or more nuclei or nuclear lobes, each with a prominent nucleoli
• Background infiltrate of lymphocytes, histiocytes, granulocytes, plasma cells and fibroblasts

SPECIAL TESTS N/A

IMAGING
• Chest X-ray
• Thoracic CT scan
• Abdominal and pelvic CT scan (or possibly MR scan)
• Lymphangiogram
• Bone scan, gallium scan, abdominal ultrasound (used infrequently)

DIAGNOSTIC PROCEDURES
• Excisional lymph node biopsy (needle biopsy not sufficient)
• Exploratory laparotomy with splenectomy-only if treatment will be altered by results
• Bone marrow biopsy-especially with systemic symptoms
• Liver biopsy (in selected cases)

TREATMENT

APPROPRIATE HEALTH CARE
• Initial staging is critical to therapy
• Cotswold classification
  ◊ Stage I - single lymph node group
  ◊ Stage II - two or more node groups on same side of diaphragm
  ◊ Stage III - Node groups on both sides of diaphragm
  ◊ Stage IV - dissemination involving extra-nodal organs (not the spleen which is considered lymphoid tissue)
  ◊ Subclass designations: A = no symptoms; B = systemic symptoms (fever, night sweats, weight loss >10% body weight); X = bulky disease (widened mediastinum > 1/3 intrathoracic diameter or > 10 cm nodal mass); E = single extra-nodal site involvement in proximity with known nodal site

GENERAL MEASURES
• Treatment aimed for cure with minimum toxicity, including treatment-induce late mortality
• Treatment can be radiation therapy (RT), chemotherapy (Chemo), or combined radiation and chemotherapy (CMT), based on stage and tumor burden
  ◊ Stage IA, IIA, nonbulky - usually RT alone; chemo for selected high risk patients
  ◊ Stage IB, IIB, nonbulky - RT, if staging laparotomy is done: otherwise, CMT
  ◊ Stage IIAX, IIBX (bulky disease) - CMT
  ◊ Stage IIIA - possibly RT for carefully selected patients (minimal disease limited to upper abdomen); otherwise, CMT
  ◊ Stage IIIB, IV - CMT
• Autologous bone marrow transplant for selected patients who fail conventional therapy

SURGICAL MEASURES N/A

ACTIVITY As tolerated

DIET No restrictions

PATIENT EDUCATION
• Reproductive impact
  ◊ Spermatogenesis often impaired prior to therapy
  ◊ Gonadal side effects of therapy
  ◊ Sperm banking option for males
• Risks of secondary malignancy
• Careful oral and dental care during therapy
• Patient education material
  ◊ Leukemia Society of America, 733 3rd Avenue, New York, NY 10017

MEDICATIONS

DRUG(S) OF CHOICE
• Note: Must be monitored by experienced oncologist
• ABVD chemotherapy - 4 week cycles
  ◊ Doxorubicin (Adriamycin) - 25 mg/m2 IV days 1 and 15
  ◊ Bleomycin 10 mg/m2 IV days 1 and 15
  ◊ Vinblastine 6.0 mg/m2 IV days 1 and 15
  ◊ Dacarbazine 375 mg/m2 IV days 1 and 15
• Repeat cycles at least 6 times if blood counts permit
Contraindications: As in general for chemotherapy
Precautions: Chemotherapy toxicity, bone marrow suppression
Significant possible interactions: Refer to manufacturer's literature

ALTERNATIVE DRUGS
• MOPP chemotherapy - 4 week cycles
  ◊ Mechlorethamine (nitrogen mustard) 6.0 mg/m2 IV days 1 and 8
  ◊ Vincristine (Oncovin) 1.4 mg/m2 IV days 1 and 8
  ◊ Procarbazine 100 mg/m2 po days 1 through 14 (avoid vanilla, cheese and wine)
  ◊ Prednisone 40 mg/m2 po days 1 through 14 during cycles 1 and 4
• Alternate cycles with MOPP/ABVD to minimize toxicity

FOLLOWUP

PATIENT MONITORING   CBC, nutrition and hydration

PREVENTION/AVOIDANCE
• Pneumococcal vaccine, if splenectomy is planned for staging
• Consider vaccines for Haemophilus and Neisseria species as well

POSSIBLE COMPLICATIONS
• Secondary malignancies following therapy
• Sterility, gonadal dysfunction
• Hypothyroidism
• Bone marrow suppression
• Immunosuppressed infections, including herpes zoster
• Anemia
• ITP, TTP
• Coronary artery disease, cardiomyopathy
• Radiation pneumonitis, pulmonary fibrosis
• Transient radiation myelopathy (Lhermitte's sign)

EXPECTED COURSE/PROGNOSIS
• Overall 5 year survival 82%
• 75% long term survival
• 10 year survival rates correlate with stage at diagnosis
  ◊ Stage IA, IB, IIA nonbulky 85-95%
  ◊ Stage IIA bulky, IIB 80-85%
  ◊ Stage IIIA 75-90%
  ◊ Stage IIIB 60-65%
  ◊ Stage IV 55-60%

MISCELLANEOUS

ASSOCIATED CONDITIONS
• T lymphocyte defects, which persist after successful treatment
• Patients with HIV tend to present with more advanced disease

AGE-RELATED FACTORS
Pediatric: Increased risk for males
Geriatric: Usually presents in more advance stage and shows unfavorable histology
Others: N/A

PREGNANCY
• Pregnancy not known to affect course of disease
• Hodgkin's disease not known to affect pregnancy or fetus IF therapy can be postponed until delivery
• Normal pregnancy can occur after treatment, if fertility is maintained
• Risk of disease progression during pregnancy is variable. Management must be individualized

SYNONYMS   Malignant lymphoma

ICD-9-CM
201.90 Hodgkin's disease, unspecified

SEE ALSO
Lymphoma, non-Hodgkin's

OTHER NOTES   N/A

ABBREVIATIONS   N/A

REFERENCES
• Urba WJ, Longo DL: Hodgkin's disease. NEJM 1992;326(10):678-87
• Weinshel EL, Peterson BA: Hodgkin's disease. CA 1993;43:327-46
• Aisenberg AC: Problems in Hodgkin's disease management. Blood 1999;93(3):761-79
Illustrations: N/A
Internet references: http://www.5mcc.com

Author(s)
Rich Londo, MD

Hordeolum (stye)

BASICS

DESCRIPTION The common term "stye" refers to any inflammation or infection of the eyelid margin involving the hair follicles of the eyelashes (external hordeolum), meibomian glands (internal hordeolum), or granulomatous infection of the meibomian glands (chalazion)
System(s) affected: Skin/Exocrine
Genetics: No known genetic pattern
Incidence/Prevalence in USA: Extremely common
Predominant age: None
Predominant sex: Male = Female

SIGNS AND SYMPTOMS
• Redness of the margin of the eyelid with scaling, collection of discharge
• Localized inflammation of the eyelashes
• Patients may experience itching or scaling of the eyelids, chronic redness, eye irritation leading to localized tenderness and pain

CAUSES
• The most common causes of eyelid infections are staphylococcal, although other organisms may also be involved
• Seborrhea can predispose to infections of the eyelid

RISK FACTORS
• Predisposing blepharitis (low grade infections of the eyelid margin)
• Poor eyelid hygiene
• Contact lens wearers
• Application of make-up

DIAGNOSIS

DIFFERENTIAL DIAGNOSIS
• Blepharitis
• Eyelid neoplasms

LABORATORY Culture of the eyelid margins is usually not necessary
Drugs that may alter lab results: None
Disorders that may alter lab results: None

PATHOLOGICAL FINDINGS Bacterial contamination and white cells in eyelid discharge

SPECIAL TESTS None

IMAGING None

DIAGNOSTIC PROCEDURES History and eye examination

TREATMENT

APPROPRIATE HEALTH CARE
Outpatient

GENERAL MEASURES
• Warm compresses to the area of inflammation can help increase blood supply and potentiate spontaneous drainage
• Good personal hygiene with attention to cleansing the eyelids on a daily basis to prevent recurrent infections
• Application of an antibiotic ointment (such as erythromycin) to the margin of the eyelid after proper cleansing. (Except children under 12, where there is a risk of blurred vision and amblyopia.) Helps reduce bacterial proliferation.

SURGICAL MEASURES If the infection becomes localized to a single gland, incision, drainage, and curettage is sometimes necessary. This is an in-office procedure with a local anesthetic.

ACTIVITY No restrictions

DIET No special diet

PATIENT EDUCATION
• The patient should be instructed in proper cleansing of the eyelids using a solution of tap water and baby shampoo or a commercially prepared hypoallergenic cleanser
• The stye should not be squeezed

MEDICATIONS

DRUG(S) OF CHOICE
• Erythromycin ophthalmic ointment
• Occasionally use of an aminoglycoside ophthalmic ointment such as gentamicin may be necessary if refractory to simpler treatment
Contraindications: None
Precautions: None
Significant possible interactions: None

ALTERNATIVE DRUGS   None

 FOLLOWUP

PATIENT MONITORING   The patient should be seen within several weeks to assess the effectiveness of therapy

PREVENTION/AVOIDANCE   Eyelid hygiene

POSSIBLE COMPLICATIONS   None expected. An internal hordeolum, if untreated, may lead to generalized cellulitis of the lid.

EXPECTED COURSE/PROGNOSIS
Responds well to treatment, but tends to recur in some patients

 MISCELLANEOUS

ASSOCIATED CONDITIONS
• Acne
• Seborrhea

AGE-RELATED FACTORS
Pediatric: N/A
Geriatric: N/A
Others: N/A

PREGNANCY   N/A

SYNONYMS
• Internal hordeolum
• External hordeolum
• Chalazion hordeolum
• Zeisian sty
• Meibomian sty

ICD-9-CM
373.1 Hordeolum
373.2 Chalazion
373.0 Blepharitis

SEE ALSO   N/A

OTHER NOTES   N/A

ABBREVIATIONS   N/A

REFERENCES   None
Illustrations: N/A
Internet references: http://www.5mcc.com

Author(s)
Robert M. Kershner, MD, FACS

Horner's syndrome

BASICS

DESCRIPTION Horner's syndrome is caused by interruptions of the sympathetic nerve supply to the eye and results in miosis, ptosis, and absence of sweating of the ipsilateral face and neck
• Peripheral lesion - distal to superior cervical ganglion
• Central lesion - proximal to superior cervical ganglion
System(s) affected: Nervous, Skin/Exocrine
Genetics: Some autosomal dominant familial incidence
Incidence/Prevalence in USA: Unknown
Predominant age: May occur at any age
Predominant sex: Male = Female

SIGNS AND SYMPTOMS
• Ptosis (drooping of the eyelid)
• Miosis (narrowing of the pupil of the eye)
• Anhidrosis
• Enophthalmos is sometimes found
• Iris (in congenital Horner's) reduced - pigmentation, blue-gray, mottled of the affected eye
• Loss of ciliospinal reflex

CAUSES
• Interruption of the sympathetic nerve fibres that originate in the hypothalamus and travel down to the lateral part of the brain stem to exit in the thoracic area. These fibers synapse in the cervical sympathetic ganglia and the postganglionic fibers travel to the eye along the wall of the carotid and ophthalmic arteries.
• Idiopathic

RISK FACTORS
• Apical bronchogenic carcinoma
• Aneurysm of the carotid or subclavian artery
• Injuries to the carotid artery high in the neck
• Congenital Horner's syndrome
• Dissection of the carotid arteries
• Cluster headaches, approximately 20% of which have an accompanying ipsilateral Horner's syndrome. The syndrome may outlast the headaches.
• Carotid artery occlusion, approximately 15% of patients with carotid artery occlusion develop ipsilateral Horner's syndrome - may occur without evidence of cerebral ischemia, neck injuries or operative procedures
• Syringomyelia
• Inflammatory process

DIAGNOSIS

DIFFERENTIAL DIAGNOSIS
Neurological diseases

LABORATORY N/A
Drugs that may alter lab results: N/A
Disorders that may alter lab results: N/A

PATHOLOGICAL FINDINGS
• Brainstem lesion
• Massive hemisphere lesion
• Cervical cord lesion
• Root lesion
• Sympathetic chain lesion

SPECIAL TESTS
• Instillation of 4% solution of cocaine into conjunctival sac produces dilatation of the pupil in Horner's syndrome caused by a central sympathetic pathways lesion. (Response is absent in peripheral sympathetic lesion.)
• Instillation of 1:1000 solution of epinephrine into conjunctival sac produces dilatation of the pupil in Horner's syndrome caused by a peripheral sympathetic lesion

IMAGING CT/MRI of the brain, chest, spinal cord

DIAGNOSTIC PROCEDURES Spinal tap - occasionally indicated in addition to above.

TREATMENT

APPROPRIATE HEALTH CARE
Inpatient or outpatient, depending upon cause

GENERAL MEASURES
• Search for tumor or other compressive lesion is indicated for any patient who develops Horner's syndrome
• Horner's syndrome in itself does not produce any disability or require treatment
• Treatment is management of the underlying condition

SURGICAL MEASURES N/A

ACTIVITY Disease dependent

DIET Disease dependent

PATIENT EDUCATION N/A

MEDICATIONS

DRUG(S) OF CHOICE Therapy appropriate for the underlying disease
Contraindications: N/A
Precautions: N/A
Significant possible interactions: N/A

ALTERNATIVE DRUGS N/A

FOLLOWUP

PATIENT MONITORING Disease dependent

PREVENTION/AVOIDANCE None known

POSSIBLE COMPLICATIONS Chronic pupillary constriction

EXPECTED COURSE/PROGNOSIS Variable with cause

MISCELLANEOUS

ASSOCIATED CONDITIONS
• Wallenberg's syndrome
• Pancoast's tumor
• C8 radiculopathy

AGE-RELATED FACTORS
Pediatric: N/A
Geriatric: N/A
Others: N/A

PREGNANCY N/A

SYNONYMS
• Bernard-Horner syndrome
• Bernard's syndrome
• Cervical sympathetic syndrome
• Oculosympathetic syndrome

ICD-9-CM 337.9 Horner's syndrome

SEE ALSO N/A

OTHER NOTES N/A

ABBREVIATIONS N/A

REFERENCES Pryce-Phillips W, Murray TJ: Essential Neurology. New York, Scientific American Medicine, 1991
Illustrations: N/A
Internet references: http://www.5mcc.com

Author(s)
Stanley G. Smith, MA, MB, FCFPC

Huntington's disease

BASICS

DESCRIPTION An inherited disease characterized by dementia and chorea that has a gradual onset and slow progression. Symptoms usually don't develop until after 30 years of age. By the time of diagnosis the patient has usually reproduced and passed the disease to another generation.
System(s) affected: Nervous
Genetics: Autosomal dominant; genetic marker on chromosome 4
Incidence/Prevalence in USA: 4-8 cases/100,000 people in the U.S.
Predominant age: Young adult (16-40); middle age (40-75)
Predominant sex: Male = Female

SIGNS AND SYMPTOMS
• Chorea
• Dysphagia
• Dysarthria
• Impaired recent memory
• Impaired judgment
• Intellectual decline
• Emotional disturbances
• Depression
• Anxiety
• Delusions
• Aggressiveness
• Urinary incontinence
• Bowel incontinence
• Weight loss
• Hypotonia
• Gait disturbance
• Postural instability
• Hyperkinesia
• Abnormal eye movements
• Facial twitching
• Emotional lability
• Apathy
• Withdrawal
• Dementia
• Bradykinesia
• Rigidity
• Hypertonia
• Clonus
• Mania
• Hallucinations
• Delusions
• Paranoia
• Schizophrenia
• Impulsiveness
• Hostility
• Agitation
• Primitive reflexes

CAUSES HD is associated with a cytosine-adenine-guanine (CAG) trinucleotide repeat expansion in a large gene on the short arm of chromosome 4. The gene encodes the protein huntingtin, which selectively accumulates in clumps within brain cells. These cells appear sensitive to damage by the aggregated, toxic levels of huntingtin.

RISK FACTORS Family history is a definite risk factor. Although a small percent of patients with DNA-proven Huntington's disease will have a negative family history.

DIAGNOSIS

DIFFERENTIAL DIAGNOSIS
• Movement disorder - hereditary
◊ Huntington disease
◊ Hereditary nonprogressive chorea
◊ Neurocanthocytosis
◊ Wilson's disease
◊ Ataxia-telangiectasia
◊ Lesch-Nyhan syndrome
◊ Hallervorden-Spatz disease
◊ Fahr's disease
• Movement disorder - secondary
◊ Infections/immunologic
   - Sydenham chorea
   - Encephalitis
   - Systemic lupus erythematosus
   - Tertiary syphilis
◊ Drug induced
   - Levodopa
   - Anticonvulsants
   - Anticholinergics
   - Cimetidine
   - Isoniazid
◊ Metabolic and endocrine
   - Chorea gravidarum
   - Hyperthyroidism
   - Birth control pills
   - Hyperglycemic nonketoic encephalopathy
◊ Vascular
   - Hemichorea/hemiballism with subthalamic nucleus lesion
   - Periarteritis nodosa
• Movement disorder - unknown etiology
◊ Senile chorea
◊ Essential chorea
◊ Parkinson's disease
• Dementia
◊ Alzheimer's disease
◊ Creutzfeldt-Jacob
◊ Pick disease
• Emotional and perceptual disorders
◊ Bipolar disorder
◊ Schizophrenia
• Abnormal behavior
◊ Alcoholism
◊ Anti-social personality disorder

LABORATORY
• Decreased endogenous gamma-aminobutyric acid (GABA)
• Decreased glutamic acid decarboxylase
• Decreased choline-acetyltransferase
Drugs that may alter lab results: N/A
Disorders that may alter lab results: N/A

PATHOLOGICAL FINDINGS
• Gross - cerebral atrophy
• Gross - atrophic caudate nucleus
• Gross - atrophic putamen
• Gross - ventricular enlargement
• Gross - atrophic globus pallidus
• Gross - atrophic frontal lobes
• Gross - atrophic parietal lobes
• Gross - cortical atrophy
• Micro - loss of small neurons of striatum with fibrillary gliosis
• Micro - loss of small neurons with fibrillary gliosis in ventrolateral thalamic nucleus
• Micro - loss of small neurons with fibrillary gliosis in substantia nigra
• Electron microscopy - membranous whorls
• Electron microscopy - increased numbers of dense synaptic vesicles in presynaptic nerve terminals

SPECIAL TESTS Presymptomatic detection of the disease via genetic linkage analysis is possible; but widespread testing awaits the resolution of social and ethical considerations

IMAGING
• CT or MRI - cerebral atrophy and atrophy of caudate nucleus
• Positron emission tomography (PET) - reduced glucose utilization
• Head CT - enlarged lateral ventricle

DIAGNOSTIC PROCEDURES N/A

TREATMENT

APPROPRIATE HEALTH CARE
Outpatient

GENERAL MEASURES
• Genetic counseling
• Symptomatic treatment (dopamine receptor blocking drugs), such as phenothiazines or haloperidol
• Consider electroconvulsive therapy (ECT) for drug-resistant depression
• Speech and occupational therapy

SURGICAL MEASURES N/A

ACTIVITY Full activity as long as possible

DIET No special diet, but soft diet with liquid supplements may be needed. Coenzyme Q10 (Ubiquinone), a popular vitamin supplement, shows promise in reversing the generalized energy defect in HD.

PATIENT EDUCATION
• Counseling for offspring
• Newsletter and printed information available from: Huntington's Disease Society of America, 140 W. 22nd St, 6th Flr, New York, NY 10011-2420, phone (212)242-1968; fax (212)243-2443

MEDICATIONS

DRUG(S) OF CHOICE For dyskinesia and/or behavioral problems: Haloperidol (Haldol) 1 mg bid and increased every 3 or 4 days until satisfactory response. Suggested daily maximum 10 mg.
Contraindications: Refer to manufacturer's literature
Precautions: Extrapyramidal reactions, tardive dyskinesia may occur. Can be treated with anticholinergic medication.
Significant possible interactions: Do not administer with meperidine due to possibility of serotonin syndrome.

ALTERNATIVE DRUGS
• Presynaptic dopamine-depleting agents
• Reserpine
• Tetrabenazine
• Postsynaptic dopamine antagonists
• Tricyclic antidepressants
• Antipsychotics

FOLLOWUP

PATIENT MONITORING Periodically for behavioral changes

PREVENTION/AVOIDANCE Genetic counseling

POSSIBLE COMPLICATIONS
• Choking
• Subdural hematoma
• Chorea
• Personality changes
• Dementia
• Death
• Suicide

EXPECTED COURSE/PROGNOSIS
Poor, progressive impairment, fatal outcome within 20 years

MISCELLANEOUS

ASSOCIATED CONDITIONS N/A

AGE-RELATED FACTORS
Pediatric: Usually does not occur until after puberty
Geriatric: Usually fatal before geriatric age group; but onset is after age 50 in 20%
Others: About 20% of relatives at 1-in-2 risk of inheriting Huntington's disease from an affected parent now accept the offer of presymptomatic testing

PREGNANCY N/A

SYNONYMS
• Chronic progressive hereditary chorea
• Huntington's chorea

ICD-9-CM 333.4 Huntington's disease

SEE ALSO Wilson's disease

OTHER NOTES N/A

ABBREVIATIONS N/A

REFERENCES
• Adams RD, Victor M, Ropper AH: Principles of Neurology. 6th Ed. New York, Mcgraw-Hill, 1997
• Haddad MS, Cummings JL: Huntington's disease. Psychiatr Clin North Am 1997;20:791-807
• Koroshetz WJ, Jenkins BG, Rosen BR, Beal MF: Energy metabolism defects in Huntington's disease and effects of coenzyme Q10. Ann Neurol 1997;41:160-165
• Wahlin TB, Lundin A, Backman L, Almquist E, et al: Reactions to predictive testing in Huntington's disease: case reports of coping with a new genetic status. Am J Med Genet 1997;73:356-365
• Ranen NG, et al: ECT as a treatment for depression in Huntington's disease. J Neuropsychiatry Clin Neurosci 1994;6:154-159
• The American College of Medical Genetics/American Society of Human Genetics Hunting Disease Genetic Testing Working Group: Laboratory guidelines for Huntington disease genetic testing. Am J Hum Genet 1998;62:1243-1247
• Nance MA: Huntington disease: clinical, genetic, and social aspects. J Geriatr Psychiatry Neurol 1998 Summer;11(2):6170
• Quinn N, Schrag A: Huntington's disease and other choreas. J Neurol 1998 Nov;245(11):709-716
Illustrations: N/A
Internet references: http://www.5mcc.com

Author(s)
Richard Viken, MD

Hydrocele

BASICS

DESCRIPTION Hydrocele is a collection of fluid within the scrotum.
• Communicating hydrocele: Associated with a patent processus vaginalis, has associated indirect inguinal hernia
• Non-communicating hydrocele: Infantile type - no communication, frequent spontaneous resolution. Adult type - no communication, infrequent resolution.
• Hydrocele of the cord: Distal portion of processus vaginalis has closed, mid-portion patent and fluid filled, proximal portion may be open or closed
• Acute hydrocele: Acute fluid collection resulting from an acute process within the tunica vaginalis
System(s) affected: Reproductive
Genetics: Unknown
Incidence/Prevalence in USA: Estimated to be 1% of adult males; prevalence 1000/100,000
Predominant age: Childhood
Predominant sex: Male only

SIGNS AND SYMPTOMS
• Swelling in scrotum or inguinal canal
• Demonstrated fluctuation in size (communicating hydrocele)
• Usually not painful
• Sensation of heaviness in scrotum
• Pain radiating to back (occasionally)
• Fluid collection in scrotum that transilluminates

CAUSES
• Closure of processus vaginalis trapping peritoneal fluid (non-communicating)
• Closure of distal processus, trapping fluid in mid portion of processus vaginalis (hydrocele of cord)
• Failure of closure of processus vaginalis (communicating hydrocele)
• Infection
• Tumors
• Trauma
• Ipsilateral renal transplantation

RISK FACTORS
• Ventriculoperitoneal shunt
• Exstrophy of the bladder
• Ehlers-Danlos syndrome
• Peritoneal dialysis

DIAGNOSIS

DIFFERENTIAL DIAGNOSIS
• Indirect inguinal hernia
• Orchitis
• Epididymitis
• Traumatic injury to testicle
• Torsion of testicle or torsion of appendix testes

LABORATORY N/A
Drugs that may alter lab results: N/A
Disorders that may alter lab results: N/A

PATHOLOGICAL FINDINGS Patent processus vaginalis in communicating hydroceles

SPECIAL TESTS N/A

IMAGING
• Abdominal x-ray - may be useful to distinguish incarcerated hernias from hydrocele (rarely needed)
• Inguino-scrotal ultrasound - should be able to demonstrate presence of bowel, e.g., distinguish incarcerated hernia in child from a hydrocele of the cord
• Testicular nuclear scan or doppler ultrasound - to distinguish testicular torsion

DIAGNOSTIC PROCEDURES N/A

TREATMENT

APPROPRIATE HEALTH CARE
• Outpatient surgery
• Observation in early infancy until definite communication demonstrated or until 1-2 years of age

GENERAL MEASURES N/A

SURGICAL MEASURES
• Inguinal approach with ligation of processus vaginalis and drainage of hydrocele sac in children. (In hydrocele of cord, sac can be completely removed.)
• Scrotal approach with drainage of hydrocele and resection of tunica vaginalis in adults
• In adults no therapy is needed unless hydrocele causes discomfort or unless there is a significant underlying cause such as tumor
• Jaboulay-Winkelmann procedure (for thick hydrocele sac) - hydrocele sac wrapped posteriorly around cord structures
• Lord procedure (for thin hydrocele sac) - radial sutures used to gather hydrocele sac posterior to testis and epididymis
• Aspiration of hydrocele should not be done (with possible exception of postoperative hydrocele)

ACTIVITY Full activity after surgery

DIET For age

PATIENT EDUCATION N/A

TREATMENT

APPROPRIATE HEALTH CARE
Outpatient usually. Inpatient, if underlying disorder warrants.

GENERAL MEASURES
• A thorough search for correctable secondary causes and treating an underlying illness or removing an incriminated drug
• In case of primary hypertriglyceridemia, screening the other family members
• Treatment is indicated in distinct hypertriglyceridemia to prevent acute pancreatitis and in mild hypertriglyceridemia to prevent CAD in patients with high risk, strong family or personal history of atherosclerosis.
• Treatment of severe hypertriglyceridemia associated with pancreatitis - hospitalization, elimination of dietary fat; if diabetic, continuous IV infusion of insulin

SURGICAL MEASURES N/A

ACTIVITY Usually no restrictions. Exercise is important.

DIET Weight reduction to ideal body weight with AHA Step I Diet (50-55% carbohydrate, less than 30% fat)

PATIENT EDUCATION
• Smoking cessation
• Elimination of alcohol

MEDICATIONS

DRUG(S) OF CHOICE
• Fibrates: reduce triglycerides 20-70%, decrease hepatic VLDL synthesis and increase VLDL metabolism
  ◊ gemfibrozil (Lopid) 600 mg bid
  ◊ fenofibrate (Tricor) 67 mg 1-3 q day
• Niacin (Niaspan) 1-3 g/day
  ◊ Reduces triglycerides by 20-50%
  ◊ Inhibit hepatic VLDL synthesis
Contraindications: Refer to manufacturer's literature

Precautions:
• Gemfibrozil and fenofibrate
  ◊ Side effects - upper and lower GI side effects (usually mild and are the most frequent adverse effects), cholelithiasis, myalgia, hepatotoxicity
  ◊ May increase the incidence of myopathy/rhabdomyolysis if given with HMG-CoA reductase inhibitors
• Nicotinic acid
  ◊ Side effects - flushing and pruritus (prostaglandin mediated and alleviated by ASA)
  ◊ Upper GI discomfort and peptic ulcer disease (PUD)
  ◊ Hepatotoxicity (more with sustained release preparation)
  ◊ Hyperuricemia and gout, hyperglycemia, toxic amblyopia
  ◊ Flushing less with extended release forms
  ◊ Fulminant hepatic necrosis reported with extended release forms
Significant possible interactions:
Gemfibrozil with warfarin - enhanced anticoagulation effect; monitor PT closely following addition or withdrawal of gemfibrozil

ALTERNATIVE DRUGS
• HMG-CoA reductase inhibitors [lovastatin (Mevacor), pravastatin (Pravachol), simvastatin (Zocor), fluvastatin (Lescol), atorvastatin (Lipitor), cerivastatin (Baycol)] lower triglycerides 10-30%
• Fish oil
• Clofibrate (Atromid-S)

FOLLOWUP

PATIENT MONITORING
• Fasting lipid profile
• Liver function test, CPK, CBC diff
• Target goals
  ◊ For pancreatitis - TG < 500 mg/dL (< 5.65 mmol/L)
  ◊ For CHD - primary prevention: TG < 200 mg/dL (< 2.26 mmol/L); secondary intervention: TG < 150 mg/dL (< 1.70 mmol/L)

PREVENTION/AVOIDANCE Covered in other headings

POSSIBLE COMPLICATIONS
• Acute pancreatitis
• Atherosclerosis

EXPECTED COURSE/PROGNOSIS
• Good in secondary disorder if the underlying causes are eliminated
• In primary, may need life-long treatment

MISCELLANEOUS

ASSOCIATED CONDITIONS
• Mostly associated with low HDL cholesterol
• May be associated with hypercholesterolemia

AGE-RELATED FACTORS
Pediatric: In severe cases only, diet is recommended
Geriatric: N/A
Others: N/A

PREGNANCY All drugs are contraindicated during pregnancy

SYNONYMS
• Hyperlipidemia
• Chylomicronemia syndrome

ICD-9-CM
272.4 Hyperlipidemia
272.3 Type I or V hyperlipidemia (chylomicronemia syndrome)
272.1 Hypertriglyceridemia - type IV
272.2 Type III, Type II-B, hyperlipoproteinemia
272.0 Type II-A

SEE ALSO Hypercholesterolemia

OTHER NOTES N/A

ABBREVIATIONS
AHA = American Heart Association
CAD = coronary artery disease
HDL = high density lipoprotein
IDL = intermediate density lipoprotein
LDL = low density lipoprotein
LPL = lipoprotein lipase
PUD = peptic ulcer disease
TG = triglycerides
VLDL = very low density lipoprotein

REFERENCES
• NIH consensus conference, triglycerides, HDL and coronary heart disease. JAMA 1993;269:505-510
• Henkin Y, Kreisberg RA: Hypertriglyceridemia: Current concepts of a controversial issue. In: Mazzaferri EL, Kreisberg RA, eds. Advances in Endocrinology and Metabolism. St. Louis, C.V. Mosby, 1993
• Miller M (guest editor). Triglycerides as a Risk Factor in Cardiac heart disease. Clinical Cardiology, Supp II, June 1999
Illustrations: 5 available on CD-ROM
Internet references: http://www.5mcc.com

Author(s)
Reza Moattari, MD

Hypochondriasis

 BASICS

DESCRIPTION Hypochondriasis is a mental disorder associated with an excessive worry about one's health and a preoccupation with a variety of symptoms whereby the person is convinced he/she is suffering from some sort of disease. Patients suffering from this condition mostly seek medical attention searching for the physician that will diagnose them with a physical illness to explain their symptoms. This often leads to a variety of excessive work-ups, including many repetitive and expensive lab tests and diagnostic procedures. Even though these are necessary to rule out some serious physical disease, this diagnosis should not be made by exclusion alone, but should also be made by using inclusive criteria as mentioned below.

System(s) affected: Nervous

Genetics: Some studies show an increase prevalence of hypochondriasis in families, especially among identical twins and first degree relatives.

Incidence/Prevalence in USA:
• Some studies point out that hypochondriasis is present in 3-14% of patients seen by primary care physicians.
• Some surveys show that 10-20% of the general population worry about illness from time to time. About 45% of patients seen by mental health professional worry about illness from time to time.

Predominant age: The peak incidence is believed to happen during the fourth or fifth decade of life, although all age groups can be affected, including children, adolescents, and the elderly.

Predominant sex: It is found equally in men and women; however, women tend to seek help more often than men

SIGNS AND SYMPTOMS
• Preoccupation with fears of having, or the idea that one has, a serious disease based on the person's misinterpretation of bodily symptoms
• The preoccupation persists despite appropriate medical evaluation and reassurance
• The belief is not of delusional intensity (as in delusional disorder, somatic type) and is not restricted to a circumscribed concern about appearance (as in body dysmorphic disorder).
• The preoccupation causes clinically significant distress impairment in social, occupational, or other important areas of functioning.
• The duration of the disturbance is at least 6 months
• The preoccupation is not better accounted for by generalized anxiety disorder, obsessive-compulsive disorder, panic disorder, a major depressive episode, separation anxiety, or another somatoform disorder.

CAUSES
• Biological: There is some evidence suggesting that patients with hypochondriasis may be born with a tendency to amplify somatic sensations and that they have lower threshold and a lower tolerance of physical discomfort
• Life events: Medical diseases may predispose a patient to hypochondriasis, such as certain patients being highly sensitive to certain physical symptoms following an acute stroke, myocardial infarction, intensive treatment following malignant illness, organ transplantation, etc. These may be experienced by the patient or by a close family member or friend.
• Childhood events: The experience of numerous or serious actual medical illnesses during one's childhood may predispose the individual to hypochondriasis later on in life.
• Psychological: Many authors view hypochondriasis as the patient's psychodynamic defense against guilt, shame, low self-esteem, and a narcissistic over-indulgence with one's self. Other authors view it as the patient's way of seeking attention by overly identifying with the sick role which offers the patient a way to alleviate symptoms of anxiety and seek reassurance.
• Socio-cultural: Some societies and cultures view mental symptoms in a pejorative and stigmatized way, blaming the patient for his/her illness, however, if the patient has physical symptoms and a bona fide medical diagnosis, he/she are treated with greater empathy, dignity, and respect and are not blamed for causing their illness.

RISK FACTORS Exposure to life-threatening medical conditions and procedures in one's childhood, adolescence, or in adult life

 DIAGNOSIS

DIFFERENTIAL DIAGNOSIS
• Any patient suffering from hypochondriasis, as with any other psychiatric disorder is not immune from developing a medical/organic disease. Such organic diseases as those affecting many organ systems like connective tissue diseases, autoimmune diseases, as well as more focused single-organ type diseases must always be considered as a possibility in these patients.
• Underlying depressive disorders
• Schizophrenia
• Delusional disorders
• Conversion disorder
• Anxiety disorder
• Panic disorder
• Obsessive-compulsive disorder
• Factitious disorder with physical symptoms
• Somatization disorder
• Chronic pain disorder
• Body Dysmorphic disorder
• Malingering
• Munchausen syndrome

LABORATORY
• Lab tests are used to rule out organic diseases
Drugs that may alter lab results: N/A
Disorders that may alter lab results: N/A

PATHOLOGICAL FINDINGS N/A

SPECIAL TESTS N/A

IMAGING N/A

DIAGNOSTIC PROCEDURES
• Thorough mental status examination
• Psychological testing is used to rule out other psychiatric disorders and specifically confirm the diagnosis of hypochondriasis

 TREATMENT

APPROPRIATE HEALTH CARE
Outpatient

GENERAL MEASURES
• Treatment of choice is individual psychotherapy delivered on an outpatient basis
• Many patients do better with supportive psychotherapy and behavior modification focused on the alleviation of their symptoms
• Group therapy: Some patients do better in a group setting where they get social support and interaction with others
• Reassuring the patient by repeating lab tests is only short-lived and does not solve the underlying problem

SURGICAL MEASURES N/A

ACTIVITY Regular exercise in moderation

DIET Good nutrition

PATIENT EDUCATION Providing cognitive knowledge about the condition strengthens the patient's intellectual capacities and provides a structure for better response to somatic symptoms, cognitive behavioral and other psychotherapeutic interventions.

MEDICATIONS

DRUG(S) OF CHOICE
• No specific drug is known to cure hypochondriasis
• Anti-depressants and anti-anxiety medications are most successful in patients who have a preponderance of anxiety and depressive symptoms
• The SSRI group (selective serotonin reuptake inhibitors) are most helpful and have to be used selectively based on patient's tolerance to side effects
• Select patients with a preponderance of obsessive-compulsive symptoms have responded to such drugs as clomipramine 50-150 mg/day or fluoxetine 20-80 mg/day or fluvoxamine 100-300 mg/day
Contraindications:
• Avoid medications that patient is allergic to
• Avoid medications with many side effects
• Avoid medications with known drug interactions
Precautions: Avoid long term use of narcotics and other addictive medication
Significant possible interactions: N/A

ALTERNATIVE DRUGS
• Lithium carbonate: 300-900 mg/day with an optimal blood level of 0.5-0.9 mEq/L
• Valproic acid: 500-2000 mg/day or 15-60 mg/kg/day with an optimal plasma level of 50-100 µg/mL

FOLLOWUP

PATIENT MONITORING
• Patients should be seen on a regular basis in the primary care physician's office or with a psychotherapist
• Appointments should be scheduled regardless of whether the patient has new symptoms or not
• Avoid the use of long hospitalizations and unnecessary lab work-ups
• Avoid statements such as, "Call me if you have a problem" or "Make an appointment only if you have a problem"
• Provide reassurance by careful listening to the patient's concerns. Allow the patient to talk about psychosocial issues.
• Provide a safe environment for empathic listening and understanding

PREVENTION/AVOIDANCE   N/A

POSSIBLE COMPLICATIONS
• Risks of repeated and unnecessary lab and diagnostic procedures
• Narcotic and other drug addictions

EXPECTED COURSE/PROGNOSIS
• The natural history of this condition is usually chronic
• It has fluctuations in the intensity with periods of relative remission and exacerbation of acuity that may create destruction in the patient's life
• Prognosis varies depending on the patient's personality structure, education, social support system, intelligence, and motivation for change
• Many psychiatrists consider this condition to have a poor prognosis for psychoanalytic treatment

MISCELLANEOUS

ASSOCIATED CONDITIONS
Somatization disorder, conversion disorder, depressive disorder NOS, anxiety disorder NOS

AGE-RELATED FACTORS
Pediatric: Early childhood exposure to serious medical illness and diagnostic procedures predisposes these patients to develop hypochondriasis in adult life
Geriatric: Elderly patients usually have a higher frequency for chronic medical illness which may co-exist with hypochondriasis and complicates the treatment of hypochondriasis
Others: N/A

PREGNANCY   N/A

SYNONYMS
• Hypochondriacal neurosis
• Hypochondria

ICD-9-CM
300.7 Hypochondriasis

SEE ALSO   N/A

OTHER NOTES   N/A

ABBREVIATIONS   N/A

REFERENCES
• Noyes R Jr. The relationship of hypochondriasis to anxiety disorders. General Hosp Psychiatry 1999;21:8-17
• Clark DM, et al. Two psychological treatments for hypochondriasis. A randomized controlled trial. British J of psychiatry 1999;173:218-225
• Rief W, et al. Cognitive aspects of hypochondriasis and the somatization syndrome. J of Abnormal psychiatry 1998;107:587-595
• Bouman TK, Visser S. Cognitive and behaviorial treatment of hypochondriasis. Psychotherapy and Psychosomatics 1998;67:214-221
• Ferguson E. Hypochondriacal concerns symptoms reporting and secondary gain mechanism. British J of Medical Psychology 1998;71:281-295.
11 additional references available at web site
Internet references: http://www.5mcc.com
Illustrations: N/A

Author(s)
Moshe S. Torem, MD, FAPA

Hypoglycemia, diabetic

BASICS

DESCRIPTION An abnormally low concentration of glucose in the circulating blood of a diabetic. A side effect of insulin and/or sulfonylurea treatment in the course of normal treatment of diabetes mellitus. Hypoglycemia may also occur as a condition in itself or in association with other disorders. Often referred to as an "insulin reaction".
System(s) affected: Endocrine/Metabolic
Genetics: No known genetic pattern
Incidence/Prevalence in USA:
• Most type 1 diabetics experience hypoglycemia. Tightly controlled type 1 often experience hypoglycemia weekly.
• Type 2 diabetics experience hypoglycemia much less frequently than type 1 diabetics
• Most common in type 1 diabetics
• Common in type 2 diabetic patients treated with oral agents such as sulfonylureas, or meglitinides (repaglinide) agents and/or insulin
• Neither metformin, alpha-glucosidase inhibitors (acarbose and miglitol) or troglitazone cause hypoglycemia when used as monotherapy, but may enhance the risk of hypoglycemia when used in combination with insulin and/or sulfonylureas and/or meglitinides.
• Uncommon in diabetics treated with diet and exercise alone
• Studies comparing insulin lispro (human analog) with human regular insulin did not demonstrate a difference in frequency of hypoglycemia
Predominant age: All ages
Predominant sex: Male = Female

SIGNS AND SYMPTOMS
• Adrenergic hypoglycemia signs and symptoms include:
  ◊ Pallor
  ◊ Tremulousness
  ◊ Nervous anxiety
  ◊ Irritability
  ◊ Tachycardia
  ◊ Diaphoresis
  ◊ Weakness
• Neuroglycopenic hypoglycemia signs and symptoms include:
  ◊ Diplopia
  ◊ Lethargy
  ◊ Inability to concentrate or remember
  ◊ Confusion
  ◊ Behavior change
  ◊ Paresthesias
  ◊ Hunger
  ◊ Seizure
  ◊ Coma

CAUSES
• Loss of the hormonal counter-regulatory mechanism in glucose metabolism
• Diet - too little food (skipping a meal)
• Medication - too much insulin or oral hypoglycemic agent (improper dose or timing)
• Erratic absorption of insulin or oral hypoglycemics
• Adverse reaction from other medications
• Exercise - unplanned or excessive exercise
• Alcohol consumption
• Vomiting or diarrhea

RISK FACTORS
• Two or three times more common in the "tight control" patient (according to data from the Diabetes Control and Complications Trial).
• Most type 1 diabetics experience hypoglycemia. Type 2 diabetics experience hypoglycemia much less frequently unless insulin is used. Uncommon in those treated with diet and exercise alone.
• Nearly 3/4 of severe hypoglycemic episodes occur during sleep
• Autonomic neuropathy
• Illness, stress and unplanned life events
• Greater than 5 years duration of diabetes
• Elderly patient
• Renal disease
• Liver disease
• Congestive heart failure
• Hypothyroidism
• Hypoadrenalism
• Gastroenteritis
• Starvation
• Alcoholism

DIAGNOSIS

DIFFERENTIAL DIAGNOSIS
• Aspirin can induce hypoglycemia in some children
• Drinking alcohol can cause blood sugar to drop in sensitive individuals
• Hypoglycemia is well documented in chronic alcoholics and binge drinkers
• Eating unripe ackee fruit from Jamaica is a rare cause of low blood sugar
• Gastrointestinal dysfunction causing postprandial hypoglycemia or alimentary reactive hypoglycemia
• Hormonal deficiency states (hormonal reactive hypoglycemia)
• Idiopathic reactive hypoglycemia
• Hypoglycemia of sepsis
• Islet cell tumors
• Factitious hypoglycemia from surreptitious injection of insulin
• Hypoglycemia may be found in nondiabetics under certain conditions such as early pregnancy, prolonged fasting, and long periods of strenuous exercise
• Reactive hypoglycemia a popular diagnosis 20 years ago, is actually quite rare

LABORATORY
• Plasma glucose ≤ 45 mg/dL (≤ 2.5 mmol/L) or less
• "Suspect" low when plasma glucose is between 45 and 60 mg/dL (2.5 and 3.33 mmol/L)
• In children plasma glucose ≤ 40 mg/dL (≤ 2.22 mmol/L)
Drugs that may alter lab results: N/A
Disorders that may alter lab results: N/A

PATHOLOGICAL FINDINGS N/A

SPECIAL TESTS Chronic hypoglycemia is evidenced by a low glycohemoglobin level

IMAGING N/A

DIAGNOSTIC PROCEDURES
• History
• Physical exam
• Plasma, or whole blood glucose
• Severe hypoglycemia episodes are defined as those in which the patient has incapacity sufficient to require the assistance of another person

TREATMENT

APPROPRIATE HEALTH CARE
• Outpatient except for complicating emergencies (coma, unapparent cause, long acting oral hypoglycemic)
• Admit the patient if:
  ◊ There is any doubt of the cause
  ◊ Expectation of prolonged hypoglycemia
  ◊ Inability of the patient to drink

GENERAL MEASURES
• Education is the mainstay of prevention
• Blood glucose targets should be individualized
• Any sugar-containing food or beverage which can be rapidly absorbed, eg, juice (4-6 ounces), candy (5-6 pieces of hard candy) or non-diet soda
• OTC glucose tablets or gels
• Hypoglycemic unawareness (most commonly found in patients with long-standing type 1 DM) is a major risk factor for severe hypoglycemic reactions
• Intensive therapy for diabetes should be adjusted to minimize the occurrence of severe hypoglycemia
• Meticulous prevention of hypoglycemia can reverse hypoglycemia unawareness

SURGICAL MEASURES N/A

ACTIVITY Rest until glucose is normal

DIET Avoid extra calories without changing the source of the problem - excess insulin or oral hypoglycemic

PATIENT EDUCATION
• Most important measure is prevention
• Educate patients, their relatives and close friends, teachers and supervisors
• Teach home glucose monitoring and self-adjustment for insulin therapy, diet control, and exercise regimen
• Emergency medical assistance may be needed if the person does not recover within a few minutes
• Carry an ID tag
• Always keep some type of quick-acting carbohydrate close by

MEDICATIONS

DRUG(S) OF CHOICE
• General
◊ Oral administration of small molecule sugars (saccharose/glucose)
◊ Approximately 60-90 calories repeated every 15 minutes until blood sugar is 100 mg/dL (5.55 mmol/L) or more
◊ It takes about 15 minutes for the carbohydrates to be digested and to enter the blood stream as glucose
• In patients with loss of consciousness at home
◊ Administer glucagon IM or subcutaneous in the deltoid or anterior thigh:
◊ If under 5 years old, give 0.25 to 0.50 mg
◊ Older child (5-10 years old) give 0.50 to 1 mg
◊ Over 10 years old, give 1 mg
• If emergency medical personnel are present or patient hospitalized
◊ Give one-half amp 50% dextrose every 5-10 minutes until the patient awakens
◊ Then feed orally and/or administer 5% dextrose intravenously at a level that will maintain the blood glucose at a level above 100 mg/dL.
◊ Patients with hypoglycemia secondary to oral hypoglycemics should be monitored for 24-48 hours since hypoglycemia may recur after apparent clinical recovery

Contraindications: None

Precautions: Refer to manufacturer's literature

Significant possible interactions:
• Treatment may cause hyperglycemia (called Somogyi phenomenon)
• Clearance of certain oral hypoglycemics from plasma may be prolonged in persons with liver disease

ALTERNATIVE DRUGS
Acarbose, a potent alpha-glucosidase inhibitor slows the absorption kinetics of dietary carbohydrates by reversible competitive inhibition of alpha-glucosidase activity, and so reduces the post-prandial blood glucose increment and insulin response

FOLLOWUP

PATIENT MONITORING
Home glucose monitoring

PREVENTION/AVOIDANCE
• Educating patients, family and close friends
• Maintaining a routine schedule of diet, medication and exercise
• Regular blood-glucose testing
• Wearing a medical alert identification bracelet or necklace
• Those patients who experience recurrent hypoglycemic episodes should be individually evaluated and when appropriate, the employment position should be modified

POSSIBLE COMPLICATIONS
• Coma
• Seizure
• Prolonged or severe hypoglycemia may cause permanent neurological damage and/or cognitive impairment
• Evaluation of neuropsychological functioning of DCCT participants shows no evidence of significant cognitive deterioration associated with repeated episodes of severe hypoglycemia. Repeated episodes of severe hypoglycemia are not necessarily associated with cognitive dysfunction.
• Significant differences have been documented between adults and children in the incidence of hypoglycemia

EXPECTED COURSE/PROGNOSIS
Full recovery is usual depending on the rapidity of diagnosis and treatment

MISCELLANEOUS

ASSOCIATED CONDITIONS
• Autonomic dysfunction
• Neuropathies
• Cardiomyopathies

AGE-RELATED FACTORS
Pediatric: Significance of hypoglycemia in infants of diabetic mothers remains to be defined
Geriatric: Often not diagnosed in the elderly
Others: N/A

PREGNANCY
With hypoglycemic reactions during pregnancy the fetus is less likely to be hypoglycemic because of active transport of glucose across the placenta

SYNONYMS
• Low blood sugar
• Insulin reaction
• Insulin shock
• Reactive hypoglycemia

ICD-9-CM
250.8 Diabetic hypoglycemia
251.0 Hypoglycemia due to insulin
251.1 Hypoglycemia, other specified cause
251.2 Hypoglycemia, unspecified cause
300.19 Factious hypoglycemia
579.3 Post-op hypoglycemia
775.0 Perinatal hypoglycemia due to maternal DM
775.6 Neonatal hypoglycemia
962.3 Hypoglycemia due to therapeutic misadventure

SEE ALSO
• Diabetes mellitus, Type 1
• Diabetes mellitus, Type 2

OTHER NOTES
• The tighter the diabetic control the greater the importance of home glucose monitoring to avoid hypoglycemia
• In patients receiving beta blockers, the drug will mask tachycardia, but not the sweating

ABBREVIATIONS
N/A

REFERENCES
• Diabetes Control and Complications Trial (DCCT). Adverse events and their association with treatment regimens in the Diabetes Control and Complications Trial. Diabetes Care 1995;18(11):1415-27
• American Diabetes Association Clinical Practice recommendations. Diabetes Care 1999;22(s1):s1-119
• Service FJ: Hypoglycemia. Endocrinol Metab Clin NA 1997;26(4):411-414
• National Diabetes Information Clearinghouse (NDIC) a service of the National Institute of Diabetes and Digestive and Kidney Diseases (NIDDK)
• American Diabetes Association
Illustrations: N/A
Internet references: http://www.5mcc.com

Author(s)
Joseph A. Florence, MD

Hypoglycemia, nondiabetic

BASICS

DESCRIPTION Hypoglycemia is an abnormally low blood glucose level associated with some of the signs or symptoms listed below. Occurs often in diabetic patients (covered under a separate topic) and has a less common appearance in nondiabetic patients.
• Reactive hypoglycemia - in response to a meal, specific nutrients, or drugs. May occur within 2-3 hours after a meal, or later. Also seen after gastrointestinal surgery (in association with dumping syndrome in some patients).
• Spontaneous (fasting) hypoglycemia - may be associated with a primary condition, e.g., hypopituitarism, Addison's disease, myxedema, or in disorders related to liver malfunction, and renal failure. If hypoglycemia presents as a primary manifestation, other disorders to consider include hyperinsulinism and extrapancreatic tumors.
System(s) affected: Endocrine/Metabolic
Genetics: Some aspects may involve genetics (e.g., hereditary fructose intolerance)
Incidence/Prevalence in USA: Unknown
Predominant age: Older adult
Predominant sex: Female > Male

SIGNS AND SYMPTOMS
• Central nervous system (CNS); these symptoms predominate if glucose dropping gradually:
  ◊ Headache
  ◊ Confusion
  ◊ Visual disturbances
  ◊ Changes in personality
  ◊ Convulsions
  ◊ Coma
• Heart
  ◊ Palpitations
  ◊ Hypotension
• Gastrointestinal
  ◊ Hunger
  ◊ Nausea
  ◊ Belching
• Adrenergic; these symptoms are more prominent in acute drop in glucose (as in insulin reaction)
  ◊ Sweating
  ◊ Anxiety
  ◊ Tremulousness
  ◊ Dizziness
  ◊ Diaphoresis
  ◊ Nervousness

CAUSES
• Reactive: Post-prandial hypoglycemia
  ◊ Alimentary hyperinsulinism
  ◊ Meals (high in refined carbohydrates)
  ◊ Certain nutrients, e.g., fructose, galactose, leucine
  ◊ Glucose intolerance (prediabetic)
  ◊ Pseudohypoglycemia - patients with symptoms of hypoglycemia or self-diagnosis in whom low blood sugars may not be detectable and who may be impossible to convince that they do not suffer from hypoglycemia after all tests are found to be normal
  ◊ Gastrointestinal surgery
  ◊ Idiopathic (unknown)

• Spontaneous: Fasting hypoglycemia
  ◊ Drugs or alcohol (insulin or sulfonylureas, propranolol, salicylates, quinine, disopyramide, or pentamidine
  ◊ Surreptitious drug use (self-injection of insulin or taking oral hypoglycemic in nondiabetic patients
  ◊ Hepatic disease
  ◊ Islet cell hyperplasia or tumor
  ◊ Catecholamine deficiency
  ◊ Glucagon deficiency
  ◊ Extrapancreatic tumor
  ◊ Exercise
  ◊ Fever
  ◊ Pregnancy
  ◊ Renal glycosuria
  ◊ Large tumor
  ◊ Ketotic hypoglycemia of childhood
  ◊ Adrenal insufficiency
  ◊ Hypopituitarism
  ◊ Enzyme deficiencies or defects
  ◊ Severe malnutrition
  ◊ Sepsis

RISK FACTORS Listed with Causes

DIAGNOSIS

DIFFERENTIAL DIAGNOSIS
• CNS disorders
• Psychogenic

LABORATORY
• Lab studies best done when patient is symptomatic
• Measurement of blood and plasma glucose
• C-peptide measurement
• Check liver studies, serum insulin, cortisol
Drugs that may alter lab results: Many drugs can affect levels. Refer to a drug or laboratory reference.
Disorders that may alter lab results: N/A

PATHOLOGICAL FINDINGS N/A

SPECIAL TESTS
• Plasma glucose overnight fasting - < 60 mg/dL (< 3.33 mmol/L)
• Plasma glucose 72-hour fasting - < 45 mg/dL (< 2.5 mmol/L) for females and < 55 mg/dL (< 3.05 mmol/L) for males
• Oral glucose tolerance - < 50 mg/dL (< 2.78 mmol/L)
• IV tolbutamide test - normal
• Insulin radioimmunoassay - elevated insulin levels if islet cell tumor present

IMAGING Abdominal CT to rule out abdominal tumor

DIAGNOSTIC PROCEDURES
• Overinterpretation of glucose tolerance tests may lead to an overdiagnosis of hypoglycemia. More than 1/3 of normal patients have hypoglycemia with or without symptoms during a 4 hour glucose tolerance test. However, these individuals may be at risk for developing type II diabetes mellitus.

• For definitive diagnosis - patient should have
(1) documented occurrence of low blood glucose levels
(2) symptoms that occur when the blood glucose is low
(3) evidence that the symptoms are relieved specifically by the ingestion of sugar or other food
(4) identification of the particular type of hypoglycemia

TREATMENT

APPROPRIATE HEALTH CARE
Outpatient except for severe cases. May also be inpatient for testing.

GENERAL MEASURES
• Oral carbohydrate for alert patient without drug overdose (2-3 tablespoons of sugar in glass of water or fruit juice, 1-2 cups of milk, a piece of fruit, soda cracker)
• If patient unable to swallow, glucagon IM or subcutaneously
• In hypoglycemia caused by drugs or certain nutrients, avoid or control the causative agents
• In hypoglycemia following meals - try high protein diet with restricted carbohydrates
• Avoid stress
• "Nonhypoglycemic hypoglycemia" or "pseudohypoglycemia"
  ◊ Many patients (often females, ages 20-45) present with the diagnosis of reactive hypoglycemia (self-diagnosed or overinterpretation of tests)
  ◊ Symptoms usually pertain to chronic fatigue and somatic complaints (stress often has a role in these symptoms)
  ◊ Management is difficult. Listening is important. Dietary changes, e.g., 120 gm carbohydrate diet, low in simple sugars can be recommended.
  ◊ Counseling - for stress or other problems may be useful

SURGICAL MEASURES If islet cell tumor (insulinoma) - surgery is the treatment of choice. If it is inoperable, drug therapy may relieve symptoms.

ACTIVITY May need to revise exercise routine

DIET
• High protein, low carbohydrate
• Frequent small feedings (6) instead of 2-3 larger meals
• Avoid fasting

PATIENT EDUCATION
• Instructions about fasting tests and interpretations of results
• Dietary instruction
• Counseling for stress, if appropriate
• Recognition of early symptoms of hypoglycemia and how to take corrective action

MEDICATIONS

DRUG(S) OF CHOICE
• Once an established diagnosis is made, drug therapy appropriate to the underlying disorder
• In patient unable to swallow - glucagon IM or subcutaneously. If no response, give IV glucose. For serious hypoglycemia, give IV bolus of 25-50 g of 50% glucose solution followed by a constant infusion of glucose until the patient can take by mouth.
• Insulinoma - see separate topic in book
• Postsurgical gastrectomy patients unresponsive to diet changes may benefit from propantheline which delays gastric emptying
Contraindications: Refer to manufacturer's literature
Precautions: Refer to manufacturer's literature
Significant possible interactions: Refer to manufacturer's literature

ALTERNATIVE DRUGS N/A

FOLLOWUP

PATIENT MONITORING
• Dependent on type and severity of symptoms, and treatment of underlying cause
• Hypoglycemia from sulfonylurea can last for days

PREVENTION/AVOIDANCE
• Follow dietary and exercise guidelines
• Patient recognition of early symptoms and taking corrective action

POSSIBLE COMPLICATIONS   If tumor removed (insulinoma), some surgical risk involved

EXPECTED COURSE/PROGNOSIS
Favorable, with recognition and appropriate treatment

MISCELLANEOUS

ASSOCIATED CONDITIONS
• Insulinoma
• Severe liver disease
• Alcoholism
• Adrenocortical insufficiency
• Myxedema
• Malnutrition (patients with renal failure)
• Gastrointestinal surgery
• Panhypopituitarism
• Addison's disease

AGE-RELATED FACTORS
Pediatric: Usually divided into 2 syndromes (1) transient neonatal hypoglycemia and (2) hypoglycemia of infancy and childhood
Geriatric: More likely to have underlying disorders or be using causative drugs
Others: N/A

PREGNANCY N/A

SYNONYMS
• Postprandial hypoglycemia
• Functional hypoglycemia
• Idiopathic hypoglycemia
• Alimentary hypoglycemia
• Postgastrectomy hypoglycemia
• Alcohol-induced hypoglycemia
• Factitious hypoglycemia
• Iatrogenic hypoglycemia
• Exogenous hypoglycemia

ICD-9-CM 251.2 Hypoglycemia, unspecified

SEE ALSO
• Insulinoma
• Hypoglycemia, diabetic

OTHER NOTES N/A

ABBREVIATIONS N/A

REFERENCES
• Foster DW, Rubenstein AH: Hypoglycemia. In: Braunwald E, Isselbacher KJ, Petersdorf RG, et al, eds. Harrison's Principles of Internal Medicine. 14th Ed. New York, McGraw-Hill, 1997:2081-2087
• Flier JS: Hypoglycemia/pancreatic islet cell disorders. In: Bennett JC and Plum E, eds. Cecil: Texrbook of Medicine. 20th Ed. Philadelphia, WB Saunders Co, 1996:1278-1282
• Service FJ: Hypoglycemia. Endocrinology & Metabolism Clinics of NA 1997;26(4):936-955
Illustrations: N/A
Internet references: http://www.5mcc.com

Author(s)
F. David Schneider, MD, MSPH

Hypokalemia

BASICS

DESCRIPTION
Hypokalemia occurs when serum potassium (K) concentration is below the normal range, commonly 3.5-5.0 mEq/L (3.5-5.0 mmol/L).

System(s) affected: Endocrine/Metabolic, Nervous, Musculoskeletal, Renal/Urologic

Genetics:
• Some familial disorders are rare causes of hypokalemia
   ◊ Familial hypokalemic periodic paralysis
   ◊ Congenital adrenogenital syndromes
   ◊ Liddle's syndrome
   ◊ Familial interstitial nephritis

Incidence/Prevalence in USA: Common

Predominant age: N/A

Predominant sex: Male = Female

SIGNS AND SYMPTOMS
• Neuromuscular (most prominent manifestations) - skeletal muscle weakness (may range from mild weakness to total paralysis, including respiratory muscles); may lead to rhabdomyolysis in severe cases. Smooth muscle involvement may lead to gastrointestinal hypomotility producing ileus and constipation.
• Cardiovascular - ventricular arrhythmias, hypotension, cardiac arrest
• Renal - polyuria, nocturia due to impaired concentrating ability
• Metabolic - hyperglycemia

CAUSES
• General causes
   ◊ Decreased intake (uncommon): anorexia nervosa, deficient diet in alcoholics
   ◊ Gastrointestinal loss: vomiting, diarrhea, laxative abuse, fistulas, villous adenoma, ureterosigmoidostomy
   ◊ Intracellular shift of K: metabolic alkalosis, insulin excess, beta adrenergic catecholamine excess (acute stress, intake of B2 agonists), hypokalemic periodic paralysis, intoxications (theophylline, barium, toluene)
• Renal potassium loss
   ◊ Drugs: diuretics, penicillin antibiotics, aminoglycosides
   ◊ Mineralocorticoid excess states: primary hyperaldosteronism, secondary hyperaldosteronism (congestive heart failure, cirrhosis, nephrotic syndrome, malignant hypertension, renin-producing tumors), Bartter's syndrome, congenital adrenogenital syndromes, exogenous mineralocorticoids (glycyrrhizic acid in licorice, carbenoxolone, steroids in nasal sprays), Liddle's syndrome
   ◊ Glucocorticoid excess states: Cushing's syndrome, exogenous steroids, ectopic ACTH production, II ß mydroxysteroid dehydrogenase deficiency
   ◊ Renal tubular acidosis (RTA)
   ◊ Leukemia
   ◊ Magnesium depletion
   ◊ Thyrotoxic hypokalemic paralysis

RISK FACTORS
Any disorder or medication regimen requiring potassium supplementation

DIAGNOSIS

DIFFERENTIAL DIAGNOSIS
Spurious hypokalemia which occurs when blood with a high WBC count (> 100,000/mm3) is allowed to stand at room temperature (WBC's extract K from plasma), thyrotoxicosis

LABORATORY
Serum potassium < 3.5 mEq/L (< 3.5 mmol/L)

Drugs that may alter lab results: Diuretics

Disorders that may alter lab results: Leukemia and other conditions with high WBC

PATHOLOGICAL FINDINGS
• Vacuolization of proximal and distal renal tubular cells
• In severe hypokalemia, necrosis of cardiac and skeletal muscle

SPECIAL TESTS
• ECG - flattening or inversion of T waves, increased prominence of U waves, depression of ST segment, ventricular ectopia
• Work-up for etiology - excessive renal K loss is present when urinary K is in excess of 20 mEq/day in the presence of hypokalemia. In the patient with excessive renal K loss and hypertension (HTN), plasma renin and aldosterone levels should be determined to differentiate adrenal from non-adrenal causes of hyperaldosteronism. If HTN is absent and the patient is acidotic, RTA should be considered. If HTN is absent and serum pH is normal to alkalotic, a high urine chloride (> 10 mEq/day) (> 10 mmol/day) suggests hypokalemia secondary to diuretics or Bartter's syndrome and a low urine chloride (< 10 mEq/day) (< 10 mmol/day) suggests vomiting as the probable cause.

IMAGING
If there is evidence of mineralocorticoid excess (see Special tests), proceed with CT scan of adrenal glands

DIAGNOSTIC PROCEDURES
N/A

TREATMENT

APPROPRIATE HEALTH CARE
• Hypokalemia is usually not an emergency. For asymptomatic patients being treated with oral replacement, outpatient followup is sufficient.
• Patients with cardiac manifestations will require intravenous replacement with cardiac monitoring in an intensive care setting

GENERAL MEASURES
• Treatment of the underlying cause, if hypokalemia is mild
• When hypokalemia is severe, potassium replacement is necessary

SURGICAL MEASURES
N/A

ACTIVITY
No restrictions

DIET
In mild hypokalemia (K = 3.0-3.5 mEq/L) (K = 3.0-3.5 mmol/L) not caused by GI losses, dietary supplementation may be sufficient. Potassium-rich foods include oranges, bananas, cantaloupes, prunes, raisins, dried beans, dried apricots, and squash.

PATIENT EDUCATION
• Instructions for diet
• If potassium supplementation is necessary, stress need for compliance

Hypokalemia

MEDICATIONS

DRUG(S) OF CHOICE
• For non-emergent conditions (serum K > 2.5 mEq/L [K > 2.5 mmol/L], no cardiac manifestations), oral therapy is preferred and doses of 40-120 mEq/day (40-120 mmol/day) are usually adequate. Potassium chloride is suitable for all forms of hypokalemia. Other K salts may be indicated if there is a coexisting disorder: Potassium bicarbonate or bicarbonate precursor (gluconate, acetate, or citrate) in metabolic acidosis or phosphate in phosphate deficiency.
• For emergent situations (serum K < 2.5 mEq/L [< 2.5 mmol/L], arrhythmias), intravenous replacement is indicated. The rate of administration should not exceed 20 mEq/hour (20 mmol/hour) and maximum recommended concentration is 60 mEq/L (60 mmol/L) of saline for peripheral administration. Central may give higher concentration.
• In non-emergent situations, intravenous K should be given only when oral administration is not feasible (e.g., vomiting, postoperative state). In this setting, rate should not exceed 10 mEq/hour and concentration should not exceed 40 mEq/L.

Contraindications: None
Precautions:
• Any form of K replacement carries the risk of hyperkalemia
• Serum K should be checked more frequently in groups at higher risk: Elderly, diabetics, and patients with renal insufficiency
• Patients receiving digitalis and patients with diabetic ketoacidosis in whom intracellular shift in K is expected after insulin therapy is initiated must have more aggressive replacement

Significant possible interactions:
Concomitant administration of K sparing diuretics (spironolactone, triamterene, amiloride ACE inhibitors) magnify the risk of hyperkalemia

ALTERNATIVE DRUGS   None

FOLLOWUP

PATIENT MONITORING
• Patients receiving intravenous therapy should have their serum K level checked frequently (q4-6 h)
• Patients requiring potassium supplements should have serum potassium studied at intervals dictated by calculation of patient compliance

PREVENTION/AVOIDANCE   Patients being started on diuretics should be advised to increase their dietary K intake (see Diet)

POSSIBLE COMPLICATIONS
Hyperkalemia

EXPECTED COURSE/PROGNOSIS
The ease of correction of hypokalemia and the need for prolonged treatment rests on the primary cause. If this can be eliminated (e.g., resolution of diarrhea, discontinuation of diuretics, removal of adrenal tumor), hypokalemia is expected to resolve and no further treatment is indicated.

MISCELLANEOUS

ASSOCIATED CONDITIONS   N/A

AGE-RELATED FACTORS   N/A
Pediatric: Not common in this age group, but may occur in chronic gastrointestinal loss or secondary to hyperadrenalism
Geriatric:
• Diuretic therapy, diarrhea and chronic laxative abuse are most common causes for hypokalemia in this age group
• May need to correct magnesium depletion
Others: N/A

PREGNANCY   Treatment is same

SYNONYMS   N/A

ICD-9-CM   276.8 Hypokalemia

SEE ALSO
• Hyperkalemia
• Liddle's syndrome

OTHER NOTES   N/A

ABBREVIATIONS
RTA = renal tubular acidosis
K = potassium

REFERENCES
• Peterson LN, Moshe L: Disorders in potassium metabolism. In: Schreir RW, ed: Renal and Electrolyte Disorders. Philadelphia, Lippincott-raven, 1997:192-240
• Allon M: Disorders in potassium metabolism. In: Greenberg A, ed: Primer on Kidney Diseases. San Diego, Academic Press, 1998:98-106
• Mandal A: Hypokalemia and hyperkalemia. Med Clin of NA 1997;81(3):611-639
Illustrations: N/A
Internet references: http://www.5mcc.com

Author(s)
Mark D. Darrow, MD

Hypokalemic periodic paralysis

BASICS

DESCRIPTION Episodic weakness associated with low serum potassium (K+) levels.
• Two forms exist:
◊ Familial hypokalemic periodic paralysis; the more common form (HPP) is usually inherited as an autosomal dominant trait
◊ Hypokalemic periodic paralysis with thyrotoxicosis (TPP); rarer, usually affects Asian males.
System(s) affected: Endocrine/Metabolic, Nervous, Musculoskeletal
Genetics: Autosomal dominant (HPP)
Incidence/Prevalence in USA: 1:100,000 (estimated)
Predominant age: Onset of disease in late childhood or adolescence (HPP), early adulthood (TPP). Onset of disease after age 35 extremely rare.
Predominant sex:
• Male > Female (3:1) (HPP)
• Male > Female (20:1) (TPP)

SIGNS AND SYMPTOMS
• Episodic attacks of limb muscle weakness which last from a few hours to several days
• Typical attack comes on during sleep which was preceded by strenuous exercise
• Attacks also provoked by high carbohydrate or high sodium (Na+) meals
• Cold, stress, alcohol, diuretics, insulin, or epinephrine may also exacerbate attack
• Strength between attacks usually normal
• After years of prolonged, frequent attacks patient may develop persistent proximal weakness
• Myalgias
• Proximal weakness greater than distal weakness
• Muscles of the eyes, face, tongue, pharynx, larynx, diaphragm, and sphincters rarely involved
• Deep tendon reflexes hypoactive
• Sensation preserved

CAUSES
• Exact pathogenesis unknown
• Abnormality is in the muscle membrane
• Muscle fibers chronically depolarized by 10-15 mV, but membrane conductance normal between attacks
• Patients with HPP may have impairment of K-ATP channel leading to reduced sarcolemma K-ATP current
• Reduced K-ATP current may explain symptoms of paralysis
• A calcium channel mutation due to an abnormal gene (CACNL1A3) on chromosome 1q 31-32 has been identified (HPP only)
• Contractile apparatus normal
• Pathogenesis of HPP and TPP may be different since thyroid hormone doesn't worsen HPP

RISK FACTORS
• Male
• Age under 35
• Family history (HPP)
• Asian (TPP)

DIAGNOSIS

DIFFERENTIAL DIAGNOSIS
• Hyperkalemic periodic paralysis (adynamia episodica)
• Paramyotonia congenita
• Normokalemic periodic paralysis
• Barium poisoning
• Hyperventilation
• Secondary hypokalemia (laxative or diuretic use, diarrhea, vomiting, renal or adrenal disease, clay ingestion)
• Myasthenia gravis
• Guillain-Barré syndrome
• Tick paralysis
• Cataplexy
• Sleep paralysis
• Presyncope
• "Drop attacks"
• Akinetic epilepsy

LABORATORY
• Hallmark is low serum K+ (as low as 1.8 mEq/L [1.8 mmol/L])
• Urine K+ normal
• Elevated T3, T4, free thyroid index, and decreased TSH (TPP only)
Drugs that may alter lab results: N/A
Disorders that may alter lab results: N/A

PATHOLOGICAL FINDINGS
• Muscle biopsy may show atrophy, centrally placed vacuoles of sarcoplasm
• Electronmicroscopy studies show vacuoles are due to progressive dilatation of sarcoplasmic reticulum

SPECIAL TESTS
• With mild hypokalemia electrocardiogram (ECG) may show S-T depression, flattened T waves, presence of U waves
• With severe hypokalemia ECG may show peaked P waves, prolonged P-R interval, widened QRS
• Electromyography not helpful (usually normal between attacks)

IMAGING Thyroid scans using radioiodine (TPP only)

DIAGNOSTIC PROCEDURES
Provocative testing (50 to 100 g oral glucose with 2 to 4 g oral sodium followed by exercise, or 50 to 100 g oral glucose with 10-20 IU subcutaneous insulin) may be required. Patient should have cardiac monitoring during testing.

TREATMENT

APPROPRIATE HEALTH CARE
• Severe hypokalemia or weakness - inpatient with cardiac monitoring
• Mild hypokalemia or weakness - outpatient with close follow up

GENERAL MEASURES May rarely need respiratory support

SURGICAL MEASURES N/A

ACTIVITY As tolerated

DIET
• Avoid high carbohydrate, high sodium foods
• K+ rich fruit of dubious benefit

PATIENT EDUCATION N/A

MEDICATIONS

DRUG(S) OF CHOICE
• Acute attack
◊ Oral potassium chloride, 0.2 to 0.4 mEq/kg (0.2-0.4 mmol/kg), repeated every 15 to 30 min depending on response of ECG, serum K+, muscle strength (usual dose: 40 mEq [40 mmol])
◊ In life-threatening situation or if vomiting give intravenous (IV) KCl in mannitol [5% glucose or normal saline IV may worsen situation]. Bolus 0.1 mEq/kg (0.1 mmol/kg) every 5 to 10 min; monitor ECG, serum K+. (Usual dose: 15 mEq [15 mmol] over 15 minutes then 10 mEq/hr [10 mmol/hr] if peripheral IV, up to 60 mEq/hr [60 mmol/hr] if central IV and cardiac monitoring.)
• Prevention of attacks in HPP
◊ Oral KCl
◊ Acetazolamide (Diamox), 125 to 1000 mg/d divided qd to bid
• Prevention of attacks in TPP
◊ Treat underlying thyrotoxicosis with beta-adrenergic blocking agents (propranolol [Inderal] and others)
◊ Acetazolamide contraindicated

Contraindications:
• Acetazolamide - marked hepatic or renal dysfunction, hypersensitivity, adrenal failure, hyperchloremic acidosis, low serum Na+, K+
• Propranolol - cardiogenic shock, sinus bradycardia, 2nd or 3rd degree AV block, congestive heart failure, bronchial asthma

Precautions:
• Infusion of IV KCl must be monitored to avoid inadvertent infusion of large and potentially fatal doses
• Peripheral intravenous KCl infusion rates greater than 10 mEq/h (10 mmol/h) may be painful
• Acetazolamide - drowsiness or paresthesias at high doses
• Propranolol - impaired hepatic or renal function

Significant possible interactions:
• Acetazolamide - high dose aspirin
• Propranolol - reserpine, verapamil, aluminum hydroxide, phenytoin, rifampin, chlorpromazine, cimetidine, theophylline

ALTERNATIVE DRUGS
• Acute attack
◊ None
• Prevention of attacks in HPP
◊ Triamterene (Dyrenium) 25 to 100 mg/d
◊ Spironolactone (Aldactone) 25 to 100 200 mg/d
• Prevention of attacks in TPP
◊ Propylthiouracil, radioactive ablation of the thyroid

FOLLOWUP

PATIENT MONITORING
• Follow serum K+, electrolytes (if on acetazolamide)
• Follow thyroid function tests (if on propranolol or propylthiouracil)

PREVENTION/AVOIDANCE See
Medication (prevention of attacks) and Diet

POSSIBLE COMPLICATIONS Cardiac
arrhythmias, respiratory collapse

EXPECTED COURSE/PROGNOSIS
• Frequency of attacks usually lessens with age
• After years of prolonged, frequent attacks patient may develop persistent proximal weakness

MISCELLANEOUS

ASSOCIATED CONDITIONS
Hyperthyroidism with hypokalemic periodic paralysis with thyrotoxicosis, TPP

AGE-RELATED FACTORS
Pediatric: Onset of disease in late childhood or adolescence
Geriatric: Onset of disease after age 25-35 extremely rare; frequency of attacks usually lessens with age
Others: N/A

PREGNANCY N/A

SYNONYMS
• Paroxysmal myoplegia

ICD-9-CM 359.3 Hypokalemic familial
periodic paralysis

SEE ALSO
• Hypokalemia
• Hyperthyroidism
• Myasthenia gravis
• Guillain-Barré syndrome
• Tick paralysis

OTHER NOTES N/A

ABBREVIATIONS
• K+ = potassium
• Na+ = sodium
• ATPase = adenosine triphosphatase
• HPP = hypokalemic periodic paralysis (familial)
• TPP = thyrotoxic hypokalemic periodic

REFERENCES
• Antes LM, Kujuba DA, Fernandez PC: Hypokalemia and the pathology of ion transport molecules. Semin Nephrol 1998;18:31-45
• Barch R, Furman RE: Pathophysiology of myotonia and periodic paralysis. In: Asbury AK, McKhann GM, McDonald WI, eds. Diseases of the Nervous System, Clinical Neurobiology. 2nd Ed. Philadelphia, W.B. Saunders Co., 1992
• Hoffman EP: Voltage-gated ion channelopathies: inherited disorders caused by abnormal sodium, chloride, and calcium regulation in skeletal muscle. Annual Review of Medicine 1995;46:431-441
• Jurkat-Rott K, Lehmann-Horn F, et al: A calcium channel mutation causing hypokalemic periodic paralysis. Human Molecular Genetics 1994;3(8):1415-1419
• Ko GTC, Chow CC, Yeung HHL, et al: Thyrotoxic periodic paralysis in a Chinese population. QJ Med 1996;89:463-468
• Lapie P, Lory P, et al: Hypokalemic periodic paralysis: an autosomal dominant muscle disorder caused by mutation in a voltage-gated calciumchannel. Neuromuscular Disorders 1997;7:234-240
• Lehmann-Horn F, Rüdel A: Channelopathies: the nondystrophic myotonias and periodic paralyses. Seminars in Pediatric Neurology 1996;3(2):122-139
• Ober KP: Thyrotoxic periodic paralysis in the United States: Report of 7 cases and review of the literature. Medicine 1992;71(3):109-120
• Mendell JR, Griggs RC, Ptacek LJ: Diseases of muscle. In: Fauci AS, Braunwald E, Isselbacher KJ, et al (eds): Harrison's Principles of Internal Medicine. New York, Mcgraw Hill, 1998
• Stedwell R, Allen KM, Binder LS: Hypokalemic paralysis: A review of the etiologies, pathophysiology, presentation, and therapy. Am J Emerg Med 1992;10:143-148
• Sterns RH, Narins RG: Disorders of potassium balance. In: Stein JH, ed. Internal Medicine. 4th Ed. Boston, Little Brown & Co, 1994
• Ptacek L: The familial periodic paralyses and nondystrophic myotonias. Am J Med 1998;104:58-70
• Tricarico D, Servidei S, Tonali P, et al: Impairment of skeletal muscle adenosine triphosphate-sensitive K+ channels in patients with hypokalemic periodic paralysis. J Clin Invest 1999;104:675-682
Illustrations: N/A
Internet references: http://www.5mcc.com

Author(s)
Chris Vincent, MD

Hyponatremia

BASICS

DESCRIPTION
Defined as a plasma sodium concentration < 135 mEq/L (< 135 mmol/L)
- Hypovolemic hyponatremia - there is a decrease in total body water (TBW) and a greater decrease in total body sodium. The extracellular fluid (ECF) volume is decreased. Orthostatic hypotension and other changes consistent with hypovolemia are present.
- Euvolemic hyponatremia - there is an increase in TBW with a normal total body sodium. The ECF volume is minimally to moderately increased but there is no edema.
- Hypervolemic hyponatremia - there is an increase in total body sodium and a greater increase in TBW. The ECF is increased markedly and there is edema.
- Redistributive hyponatremia - there is a shift of water from the intracellular compartment to the extracellular compartment with a resultant dilution of sodium. TBW and total body sodium are unchanged. This occurs with hyperglycemia.
- Pseudohyponatremia - there is a dilution of the aqueous phase by excessive proteins or lipids. TBW and total body sodium are unchanged. This occurs in hypertriglyceridemia or multiple myeloma.

System(s) affected: Endocrine/Metabolic
Genetics: N/A
Incidence/Prevalence in USA: Described as the most common electrolyte disorder seen in a general hospital population. A recent study of hospitalized patients found an incidence of 1% and a prevalence of 2.5%.
Predominant age: All ages
Predominant sex: Male = Female

SIGNS AND SYMPTOMS
- Lethargy
- Disorientation
- Generalized weakness
- Muscle cramps
- Anorexia
- Hiccups
- Nausea and vomiting
- Agitation or delirium
- Stupor
- Coma
- Depressed deep tendon reflexes
- Hypothermia
- Positive Babinski responses
- Cheyne-Stokes respiration
- Pseudobulbar palsy
- Seizures
- Orthostatic hypotension
- Cranial nerve palsies

CAUSES
- Hypovolemic hyponatremia (extrarenal loss of sodium)
  ◊ Gastrointestinal loss - vomiting, diarrhea
  ◊ Third spacing - peritonitis, pancreatitis, burns, rhabdomyolysis
  ◊ Skin loss - burns, sweating, cystic fibrosis
  ◊ Lung loss - bronchorrhea
- Hypovolemic hyponatremia (renal loss of sodium)
  ◊ Salt losing nephritis
  ◊ Mineralocorticoid deficiency
  ◊ Diuretic

  ◊ Bicarbonaturia - renal tubular acidosis, metabolic alkalosis
  ◊ Ketonuria or anion gap acidosis
  ◊ Partial urinary tract obstruction
  ◊ Osmotic diuresis
- Euvolemic hyponatremia
  ◊ Hypothyroidism
  ◊ Pure glucocorticoid deficiency
  ◊ Drugs
  ◊ Stress
  ◊ Syndrome of inappropriate antidiuretic hormone release (SIADH). Causes include pulmonary and central nervous system disorders.
- Hypervolemic hyponatremia
  ◊ Nephrotic syndrome
  ◊ Cirrhosis
  ◊ Congestive heart failure
  ◊ Renal failure
- Redistributive hyponatremia
  ◊ Hyperglycemia
  ◊ Mannitol infusion
- Pseudohyponatremia
  ◊ Hypertriglyceridemia
  ◊ Multiple myeloma

RISK FACTORS
Excessive fluid intake

DIAGNOSIS

DIFFERENTIAL DIAGNOSIS
See Causes

LABORATORY
- Serum sodium less than 135 mEq/L (135 mmol/L)
- Plasma osmolality
- Urine sodium
- BUN
- Creatinine
- Hypovolemic hyponatremia
  ◊ Plasma osmolality low
  ◊ BUN/creatinine ratio greater than 20/1
  ◊ Urine sodium > 20 mEq/L (> 20 mmol/L) - renal loss
  ◊ Urine sodium < 10 mEq/L (< 10 mmol/L) - extrarenal loss
  ◊ Serum potassium > 5.0 mEq/L (> 5 mmol/L) - consider mineralocorticoid deficiency
- Euvolemic hyponatremia
  ◊ Plasma osmolality low
  ◊ BUN/creatinine ratio less than 20/1
  ◊ Urine sodium > 20 mEq/L (> 20 mmol/L)
- Hypervolemic hyponatremia
  ◊ Plasma osmolality low
  ◊ Urine sodium < 10 mEq/L (< 10 mmol/L) in nephrotic syndrome, CHF, cirrhosis
  ◊ Urine sodium > 20 mEq/L (> 20 mmol/L) in acute and chronic renal failure
- Redistributive hyponatremia
  ◊ Plasma osmolality normal or high
  ◊ Glucose or mannitol levels elevated
- Pseudohyponatremia
  ◊ Plasma osmolality normal
  ◊ Triglyceride or protein levels elevated

Drugs that may alter lab results: N/A
Disorders that may alter lab results: N/A

PATHOLOGICAL FINDINGS N/A

SPECIAL TESTS
For euvolemic hyponatremia a thyroid stimulating hormone (TSH) to rule out hypothyroidism and a one-hour cosyntropin stimulation test to rule out adrenal insufficiency

IMAGING
- CT of head if pituitary problem suspected or if SIADH from CNS problem suspected
- Chest x-ray to rule out pulmonary pathology if SIADH diagnosed

DIAGNOSTIC PROCEDURES N/A

TREATMENT

APPROPRIATE HEALTH CARE
- Inpatient treatment mandatory if acute hyponatremia or symptomatic
- Inpatient treatment advised if asymptomatic and serum sodium less than 125 mEq/dL

GENERAL MEASURES
- Assess all medications patient is taking
- Institute seizure precautions

SURGICAL MEASURES N/A

ACTIVITY
Varies according to patient mental status

DIET
- Euvolemic hyponatremia - water restriction to 1000 cc/day
- Hypervolemic hyponatremia - water and sodium restriction
- Hypovolemic hyponatremia - isotonic saline
- Redistributive or pseudohyponatremia - treat underlying cause

PATIENT EDUCATION N/A

MEDICATIONS

DRUG(S) OF CHOICE
• Severe symptomatic hyponatremia: The use of hypertonic saline (3%) is clearly indicated only in patients who are both severely symptomatic and have sodium concentrations less than 120 mEq/L (120 mmol/L). Three percent saline should be used at a rate of 1 cc/kg/hr. This will raise the serum sodium level by approximately 1 mEq/L/hr (1 mmol/L/hr). The hypertonic saline infusion should only continue until a serum sodium of 120 mEq/L (120 mmol/L) is reached or the patient becomes asymptomatic. Avoid correction by more than 12 mEq/L/day (12 mmol/day).
• Chronic hyponatremia: If hyponatremia does not improve with fluid restriction or other appropriate treatment, consider using demeclocycline. In doses of 600-1200 milligrams per day, the drug produces a nephrogenic diabetes insipidus.
• Maintenance: Clinical judgment

Contraindications: Demeclocycline can cause nephrotoxicity in patients with liver disease

Precautions:
• Demeclocycline - photosensitivity and nausea can occur
• Three percent saline-rapid correction of severe symptomatic hyponatremia has been associated with central pontine myelinolysis (CPM). This neurologic disorder induces loss of myelin and supportive structures in the pons and occasionally in other areas of the brain. CPM is seen one to several days after rapid correction of serum sodium and is characterized by gradual neurologic deterioration.

Significant possible interactions:
Demeclocycline - oral anticoagulants, oral contraceptives, penicillin

ALTERNATIVE DRUGS   N/A

FOLLOWUP

PATIENT MONITORING
• Serum sodium level should be monitored when clinically indicated. If three percent saline is used the sodium level should be checked hourly.
• Volume status should be monitored if 3% or 0.9% saline is used

PREVENTION/AVOIDANCE   Dependent on underlying condition

POSSIBLE COMPLICATIONS
• Occult tumor may present with SIADH
• Hypervolemia if saline used
• Central pontine myelinolysis

EXPECTED COURSE/PROGNOSIS
With recognition and proper treatment a return to normal serum sodium and resolution of neurologic symptoms is expected. Prognosis is dependent on underlying condition.

MISCELLANEOUS

ASSOCIATED CONDITIONS
• Hypothyroidism
• Hypopituitarism
• Adrenocortical hormone deficiency

AGE-RELATED FACTORS   N/A
Pediatric: N/A
Geriatric: N/A
Others: N/A

PREGNANCY   N/A

SYNONYMS   N/A

ICD-9-CM   276.1 Hyposmolality and/or hyponatremia

SEE ALSO   N/A

OTHER NOTES   N/A

ABBREVIATIONS
• TBW = total body water
• ECF = extracellular fluid
• SIADH = syndrome of inappropriate antidiuretic hormone

REFERENCES   Schrier RW: Renal and Electrolyte Disorders. 4th Ed. Boston, Little brown and Co., 1997
Illustrations: N/A
Internet references: http://www.5mcc.com

Author(s)
Peter Kozisek, MD

Hypoparathyroidism

BASICS

DESCRIPTION Deficiency of parathyroid hormone (PTH) from disease, injury or congenital malfunction of the parathyroid glands. Manifested as hypocalcemia producing neuromuscular symptoms ranging from paresthesia to tetany.
• Classifications:
◊ Hypoparathyroidism (follows accidental removal or damage to parathyroid glands during surgery; may be transient or permanent)
◊ Idiopathic (parathyroids absent or atrophied)
◊ Pseudohypoparathyroidism (no PTH deficiency, but target organs do not respond to its action)
System(s) affected: Endocrine/Metabolic, Nervous, Musculoskeletal
Genetics: Idiopathic hypoparathyroidism may have a genetic component
Incidence/Prevalence in USA: All forms are rare
Predominant age: All ages
Predominant sex: Male = Female

SIGNS AND SYMPTOMS
• Chronic hypocalcemia may be asymptomatic
• Neuromuscular excitability as carpopedal spasm
• Increased deep tendon reflexes
• Chvostek's sign: hyperirritability of the facial nerve when tapped
• Trousseau's sign: carpopedal spasm within 2 minutes of inflating a blood pressure cuff over systolic pressure
• Dysphagia
• Organic brain syndrome
• Psychosis
• Mental deficiency (children)
• Tetany (paresthesias, pain, difficulty walking, laryngospasm, stridor, cyanosis, seizures)
• Dry hair
• Brittle fingernails
• Dry, scaly skin
• Cataracts
• Cardiac arrhythmias

CAUSES
• Idiopathic
◊ DiGeorge syndrome
◊ Congenital absence
◊ Late onset, autoimmune
• Postsurgical (may be transient)
• Infiltrative - metastatic carcinoma and others
• Irradiation
• Hypomagnesemia
• Alcohol

RISK FACTORS
• Neck surgery
• Neck trauma
• Head and neck malignancies

DIAGNOSIS

DIFFERENTIAL DIAGNOSIS
• Rickets and osteomalacia
• Candidiasis
• Pseudohypoparathyroidism
• Addison's disease
• Pernicious anemia
• Hypocalcemia of severe illness

LABORATORY
• Serum total and ionized calcium - decreased
• Serum phosphorus - increased (> 5.4 mg/dL [> 1.74 mmol/L])
• RIA (radioimmunoassay) for parathyroid hormone - decreased
Drugs that may alter lab results:
Corticosteroids
Disorders that may alter lab results:
Other hormonal disorders; hypoalbuminuria

PATHOLOGICAL FINDINGS
• Complete or almost complete replacement of parathyroid gland parenchymal tissue by fat
• Brain blood vessels calcified

SPECIAL TESTS
• ECG - increased Q-T and S-T intervals (due to hypocalcemia)
• Serum beta-carotene (normal)
• D-xylose absorption
• 72 hour stool fat
• Slit-lamp - may show early posterior lenticular cataract formation

IMAGING
• X-ray:
◊ Increased bone density
◊ Tooth roots absent
◊ Calcification of cerebellum, choroid plexus, cerebral basal ganglia

DIAGNOSTIC PROCEDURES N/A

TREATMENT

APPROPRIATE HEALTH CARE
• Outpatient unless severe
• Inpatient for tetany
• Outpatient followup

GENERAL MEASURES
• Transient forms of hypoparathyroidism may not require treatment
• Acute attack hypoparathyroid tetany
◊ Is life-threatening and requires immediate IV treatment to raise calcium levels
◊ Verify adequate airway is present
◊ If patient is awake, breathing into paper bag can help raise serum ionized calcium levels also
◊ Seizure prevention
◊ May require tracheostomy
• Maintenance
◊ Lifelong calcitriol and calcium
◊ Maintain serum calcium in the low normal range 8.5-9 mg/dL (2.12-2.25 mmol/L)
◊ Skin softeners for scaly skin
◊ Adequate control requires careful attention to avoid overtreatment or undertreatment

SURGICAL MEASURES N/A

ACTIVITY As tolerated

DIET No special diet

PATIENT EDUCATION
• Careful and detailed instructions about maintenance therapy
• Importance of periodic blood chemical evaluations
• Signs and symptoms of overtreatment and undertreatment to watch for

MEDICATIONS

DRUG(S) OF CHOICE
• For tetany:
  ◊ Immediate IV calcium gluconate 10-20 mL of 10% solution given slowly until tetany ceases
  ◊ Calcium salts orally as soon as possible, 1-2 g daily
  ◊ Oral vitamin D (ergocalciferol) 500 IU/day or
  ◊ Calcitriol - pediatric dose: 0.04-0.08 µg/kg/24 hr. Adult dose: 0.25 µg/24 hr. Then 0.25 µg qod. Adjust based on calcium and phosphorus levels.
• Maintenance:
  ◊ Calcium - 1-2 g daily in divided doses
  ◊ Oral vitamin D or calcitrol
  ◊ If associated endocrinopathies - appropriate hormone replacement
  ◊ Thiazide diuretic - for some patients to increase phosphate excretion and decrease calcium excretion

Contraindications: Refer to manufacturer's literature

Precautions: Refer to manufacturer's literature

Significant possible interactions: Refer to manufacturer's literature

ALTERNATIVE DRUGS   N/A

FOLLOWUP

PATIENT MONITORING
• Outpatient after tetany corrected
• Periodic blood chemical evaluations

PREVENTION/AVOIDANCE   Care in surgical procedure that may cause damage to parathyroid glands

POSSIBLE COMPLICATIONS
• Neuromuscular symptoms (reversible)
• Cataracts
• Basal ganglia calcifications
• If condition starts early in childhood - stunting of growth, malformation of teeth, mental retardation
• Hypothyroidism
• Parkinsonian symptoms
• Ossification of the paravertebral ligaments
• Complications of overtreatment or undertreatment
• Institutionalized due to permanent mental damage

EXPECTED COURSE/PROGNOSIS
• Course - acute, chronic
• Transient hypoparathyroidism following surgery is reversible
• Fair outlook with diagnosis and treatment

MISCELLANEOUS

ASSOCIATED CONDITIONS
• DiGeorge's syndrome
• Addison's disease
• Mucocutaneous candidiasis

AGE-RELATED FACTORS
Pediatric:
• May occur in premature infants
• Congenital absence of parathyroids
• May appear later in childhood as idiopathic
Geriatric: Hypocalcemia fairly common in the elderly and may be due to multiple abnormalities
Others: N/A

PREGNANCY   N/A

SYNONYMS   Parathyroid tetany

ICD-9-CM   252.1 Hypoparathyroidism

SEE ALSO   N/A

OTHER NOTES   N/A

ABBREVIATIONS   N/A

REFERENCES
• Greenspan FS and Strewler GJ, 1997. Basic and Clinical Endocrinology, 5th ed. Stamford CT, Appleton & Lange pp 233-247
• Scriver CR, et al: The Metabolic Base of Inherited Disease. 7th Ed. New York, McGraw-Hill, 1995
• Guise TA, Mundy GR: Evaluation of hypocalcemia in children and adults. J Clin Endo & Metab 1995;80:1473-1478
• Obermayer-Straub P, et al: Autolmmune polyglandular syndromes. Baillieres Clin Gastroenterol 1998;12(2):293-315
• Mestman JH: Parathyrold disorders of pregnancy. Semin Perinatol 1998;22(6):485-96
Illustrations: N/A
Internet references: http://www.5mcc.com

Author(s)
Richard P. Levy, MD

Hypopituitarism

BASICS

DESCRIPTION Generalized condition caused by partial or total failure of the pituitary gland's vital hormones - ACTH, TSH, LH, FSH, GH, prolactin (PRL)
System(s) affected: Endocrine/Metabolic, Reproductive, Skin/Exocrine, Nervous, Gastrointestinal, Musculoskeletal
Genetics: Some pituitary defects are congenital
Incidence/Prevalence in USA: Relatively rare
Predominant age: Occurs in adults and children. In children it causes dwarfism and pubertal delay.
Predominant sex: Male = Female

SIGNS AND SYMPTOMS
• Usually starts with hypogonadism or gonadotropin failure (decreased FSH and LH)
• Signs of hypofunction of target glands
• Secondary amenorrhea
• Impotence
• Infertility
• Decreased libido
• Diabetes insipidus (rare)
• Lethargy
• Tiredness
• Sensitivity to cold
• Anorexia
• Nausea
• Abdominal pain
• Lactation failure
• Retarded growth
• Failure of secondary sexual characteristics to develop
• Mental aberrations
• Headache
• Visual field defects
• Blindness

CAUSES
• Lesions or tumors of the anterior pituitary gland (intrasellar or extrasellar)
• Congenital defects
• Pituitary apoplexy
• Hypophysectomy
• Infiltrative diseases (e.g., sarcoidosis, histiocytsosis X)
• Sometimes idiopathic
• Lymphocytic hypophysitis
• Irradiation
• Accidental or surgical trauma
• Hypothalamic disease

RISK FACTORS
• Trauma
• Pregnancy and delivery

DIAGNOSIS

DIFFERENTIAL DIAGNOSIS
• Primary hypothyroidism
• Anorexia nervosa
• Chronic liver disease
• Myotonia dystrophica
• Addison's disease
• Primary psychosis
• Primary hypogonadism

LABORATORY
• Confirms hormonal deficiencies
• Radioimmunoassay of pituitary and target gland hormones
• Provocative tests
Drugs that may alter lab results: Any hormone
Disorders that may alter lab results:
• Cushing's syndrome
• Addison's disease
• Hyperthyroidism
• Hypothyroidism

PATHOLOGICAL FINDINGS
• Destruction of anterior pituitary
• Atrophy of adrenal cortex, thyroid, gonads

SPECIAL TESTS
• Careful testing for smell
• Visual field examination by quantitative perimetry

IMAGING
• X-rays - chest, skull, hands, wrists (for bone age)
• Pituitary CT or MRI

DIAGNOSTIC PROCEDURES N/A

TREATMENT

APPROPRIATE HEALTH CARE
• Outpatient
• Inpatient for surgery when hypopituitarism is due to a pituitary tumor

GENERAL MEASURES
• Hormonal replacement
• Exercise program to rehabilitate
• Wear medical identification

SURGICAL MEASURES
• Surgery for pituitary tumor

ACTIVITY Encourage active physical exercise program

DIET High calorie, high protein

PATIENT EDUCATION
• Wear medical identification bracelet or necklace
• In patient with documented ACTH deficiency, stress need for additional cortisone at time of any major physical stress (e.g., fever above 101°F [38.3°C]; acute illness)

MEDICATIONS

DRUG(S) OF CHOICE
• Replacement of hormones secreted by the target glands:
  ◊ Hydrocortisone
  ◊ Thyroxine
  ◊ Androgen or cyclic estrogen
  ◊ Human growth hormone (for treating dwarfism and in selected adult patients)
  ◊ Dosages and administration schedule vary according to age and sex, refer to manufacturer's literature
Contraindications: Refer to manufacturer's literature
Precautions: Refer to manufacturer's literature
Significant possible interactions: Refer to manufacturer's literature

ALTERNATIVE DRUGS   N/A

FOLLOWUP

PATIENT MONITORING   3 and 12 month evaluations for post-treatment hormonal status. For patients with pituitary tumors include visual fields, thyroid and adrenal function, sellar computerized imaging.

PREVENTION/AVOIDANCE   None

POSSIBLE COMPLICATIONS
• Blindness
• Adrenal crisis
• Long-term medications

EXPECTED COURSE/PROGNOSIS
• Course - acute, chronic
• Variable, but guardedly favorable with replacement therapy
• If due to postpartum necrosis, may have complete or partial recovery

MISCELLANEOUS

ASSOCIATED CONDITIONS
• Childhood hypopituitarism
• Sheehan's syndrome
• Hypothyroidism
• Kallman's syndrome

AGE-RELATED FACTORS
Pediatric: Hypopituitarism in this age group leads to dwarfism due to lack of growth hormone
Geriatric: More difficult to diagnose
Others: N/A

PREGNANCY
• Severe postpartum hemorrhage can lead to hypopituitarism
• Lymphocytic hypophysitis may be triggered by pregnancy

SYNONYMS
• Pituitary cachexia
• Hypopituitarism syndrome
• Simmond's syndrome or disease
• Panhypopituitarism

ICD-9-CM
253.2 panhypopituitarism

SEE ALSO   N/A

OTHER NOTES   N/A

ABBREVIATIONS   N/A

REFERENCES
• Sheehan H, Summers VK: The syndrome of hypopituitarism. Q.J. Med 1949;42:319
• Vance M: Hypopituitarism. N Eng J Med 1994;330:1651
Illustrations: N/A
Internet references: http://www.5mcc.com

Author(s)
William F. Young, Jr., MD

Hypothermia

BASICS

DESCRIPTION
Hypothermia occurs when a core (rectal, tympanic or esophageal) temperature falls below 35°C (95°F). It may take several hours or several days to develop. As the body temperature falls, all organ system are affected; cerebral blood flow decreases and the metabolic rate declines rapidly. Patients who have been immersed for as long as 45 minutes in very cold water and appear to be dead have still been resuscitated.

System(s) affected: Endocrine/Metabolic, Cardiovascular, Nervous, Skin/Exocrine
Genetics: N/A
Incidence/Prevalence in USA: Estimates vary widely due to lack of pathological evidence, and that hypothermia is usually considered a secondary cause in diagnosing disorders
Predominant age: Very young and the elderly
Predominant sex: Male = Female

SIGNS AND SYMPTOMS
• Mild (34-35°C)
◊ Lethargy
◊ Mild confusion
◊ Shivering
◊ Loss of fine motor coordination
◊ Increased pulse and blood pressure
◊ Peripheral vasoconstriction
• Moderate (30-34°C)
◊ Delirium
◊ Bradycardia
◊ Hypotension
◊ Hypoventilation
◊ Cyanosis
◊ Arrhythmias
◊ Semicoma and coma
◊ Muscular rigidity
◊ Generalized edema
◊ Slowed reflexes
• Severe (< 30°C)
◊ Very cold skin
◊ Rigidity
◊ Apnea
◊ No pulse - ventricular fibrillation or asystole
◊ Areflexia
◊ Unresponsive
◊ Fixed pupils

CAUSES
• Decreased heat production
• Increased heat loss
• Impaired thermoregulation

RISK FACTORS
• Malnutrition
• Cold water immersion
• Homeless
• Outdoor workers
• Trauma victims (especially head)
• Alcohol consumption
• Mental illness
• Drug intoxication (barbiturates, phenothiazines, cyclic antidepressants, parasympatholytics, benzodiazepines, narcotics)

• Endocrinopathies (hypothyroidism, hypopituitarism, hypoadrenalism, hypoglycemia)
• Hypothalamic and CNS dysfunction
• Sepsis
• Cardiovascular disease
• Bronchopneumonia
• Hepatic failure
• Uremia
• Extensive skin disease
• Excessive fluid loss

DIAGNOSIS

DIFFERENTIAL DIAGNOSIS
• Cerebrovascular accidents
• Intoxication
• Drug overdose
• Complications of diabetes, hypothyroidism, hypopituitarism

LABORATORY
• Arterial blood gases (reported in the uncorrected form)
• Complete blood and platelet counts
• Toxicology screen
• Serum electrolytes
• Urinalysis
• Prothrombin time
• Partial thromboplastin time
• Fibrinogen levels
• Blood culture
• BUN/creatinine
• Glucose
• Amylase
• Liver function studies
• Thyroid function tests
• Serum cortisol
• Cardiac enzymes
Drugs that may alter lab results: Refer to laboratory test reference
Disorders that may alter lab results: Refer to laboratory test reference

PATHOLOGICAL FINDINGS
• Moderate dilation of right heart
• Pulmonary edema

SPECIAL TESTS
• Temperature measure - with special thermometers that can record low temperatures and measure core temperatures. Oral temperatures are of no value.
• Electrocardiogram - slowing of sinus rate with T-wave inversion, QT-interval prolongation, hypothermic J waves (Osburn waves) characterized by a notching of the QRS complex and ST segment
• Thyroid and pituitary function tests

IMAGING
X-rays of the cervical spine, chest, abdomen, if appropriate

DIAGNOSTIC PROCEDURES
History of prolonged exposure to cold may make the diagnosis obvious, but hypothermia may be overlooked, especially if patient is comatose

TREATMENT

APPROPRIATE HEALTH CARE
Inpatient (emergency room or intensive care)

GENERAL MEASURES
• Establish ABC's of basic life support; establish airway, intubate if necessary. Give warm humidified oxygen (42-46°C). Correct metabolic acidosis.
• Evaluate for frostbite and other trauma
• Rewarming
◊ Dependent on severity of hypothermia
◊ Rate of rewarming should be 0.5-2°C/hour. More rapid rewarming can cause ventricular fibrillation and hypovolemic shock.
• With all patients
◊ Remove wet garments
◊ Protect against heat loss and wind chill
◊ Maintain horizontal position
◊ Monitor core temperature and cardiac rhythm
• Mild hypothermia
◊ Passive rewarming (wrap in heated blanket or clothing)
◊ Administration of heated (43°C) IV solutions (D5NS)
◊ Warm fluids may be given if fully alert
• Moderate hypothermia
◊ Active external rewarming
◊ Heated blankets; heating pads
◊ Radiant heat sources
◊ Alcohol-circulating blankets
• Severe hypothermia
◊ Active internal (core) rewarming
◊ Peritoneal dialysis
◊ Gastrointestinal, colonic, or bladder lavage with warm fluids (43°)
◊ Heated intravenous fluids
◊ Heated humidified oxygen
◊ Thoracic cavity lavage (43°)
◊ Extracorporeal blood rewarming
• Cardiac arrhythmias
◊ Atrial fibrillation and sinus bradycardia are common, but patients usually convert to normal sinus rhythm with rewarming
◊ Transient type ventricular arrhythmias should not be treated. If treatment is required, bretylium is recommended.
◊ If cardiac pacing required, preferable to use external noninvasive pacemaker
• Sepsis bacterial infections
◊ In infants - signs may not be evident, initiate treatment with broad-spectrum antibiotic until culture results are available
◊ Older children and adults - if no signs, can usually wait for culture results
◊ Diabetic adults - consider prophylactic antibiotic coverage

SURGICAL MEASURES
N/A

ACTIVITY
Bedrest. Because of the cold, heart is irritable and susceptible to arrhythmias. Take special care in moving and transporting.

DIET
Warm fluids only, if alert and able to swallow

PATIENT EDUCATION
- Preventive measures to avoid recurrence
- If due to inadequate clothing or housing, refer patient to a social service agency
- Accidental hypothermia, NIH publication, No. 93-1464

MEDICATIONS

DRUG(S) OF CHOICE
- For sepsis or bacterial infection - antibiotics
- If ventricular fibrillation requires treatment, bretylium, 5 mg/kg, may be helpful. Magnesium sulfate, 100 mg/kg, is also effective.
- For hypoglycemia, D50W at a dose of 1 mg/kg IV
- Thiamine, 100 mg IV, should be given to any alcoholic or cachectic patient
- Naloxone, 2.0 mg IV, should be given to any patient with a depressed level of consciousness
- Levothyroxine 150-500 µg IV for hypothermic myxedema
- For severe acidosis - sodium bicarbonate

Contraindications:
- Medications, including epinephrine, lidocaine and procainamide can accumulate to toxic levels if used repeatedly in severely hypothermic patients
- Routine use of steroids, barbiturates or antibiotics have not been shown to increase survival or decrease postresuscitative damage

Precautions:
- If the patient fails to respond to the initial three defibrillation attempts or initial drug therapy, subsequent defibrillations or additional boluses of medication should be avoided until core temperature > 30°C. When temperature > 30°C, IV medications are indicated, but at longer than the standard intervals.
- Avoid vasopressors because of arrhythmogenic potential and delayed metabolism
- To prevent fluid overload, IV fluids should be slowly administered because of the decreased cardiac output
- Avoid lactated Ringer's solution because of decreased lactate metabolism

Significant possible interactions: Use all drugs cautiously because metabolism and renal elimination are impaired and once rewarming has occurred, there is mobilization of depot stores

ALTERNATIVE DRUGS   N/A

FOLLOWUP

PATIENT MONITORING
- During acute episode
  ◊ Lab work repeated frequently (with particular attention to electrolytes and glucose)
  ◊ Continuous cardiac monitoring
  ◊ Urinary output monitoring
  ◊ Temperature monitoring
  ◊ Follow blood gases, both corrected and uncorrected
- Following acute episode
  ◊ Continued therapy for any underlying disorder

PREVENTION/AVOIDANCE
- Appropriate clothing for cold weather, with particular attention to head, feet and hand coverings
- If walking or climbing in cold climate, carry survival bags lined with space blankets for use if stranded or injured
- Avoid alcohol, especially if anticipating exposure to cold weather
- Alertness to early symptoms and initiating preventive steps, e.g., drinking warm fluids
- Adequate heat in the home
- Review patient's medications that may predispose to hypothermia (e.g., neuroleptics, sedatives, hypnotics, tranquilizers) and decrease dosage or discontinue if appropriate and feasible
- Referral of patient to social service agency for help with adequate housing, heat or clothing

POSSIBLE COMPLICATIONS
- Cardiac arrhythmias
- Hypotension secondary to marked vasodilatation of rewarming
- Pneumonia (aspiration and broncho)
- Pulmonary edema
- Pancreatitis
- Peritonitis
- Gastrointestinal bleeding
- Acute tubular necrosis
- Intravascular thromboses
- Metabolic acidosis
- Gangrene of extremities
- Compartment syndromes

EXPECTED COURSE/PROGNOSIS
- Mortality rates are decreasing for hypothermia due to increased recognition and advanced therapy. Mortality usually dependent upon the severity of underlying cause of hypothermia.
- In previously healthy individuals, recovery is usually complete
- Mortality rate in healthy patients < 5%
- Mortality rate in patients with co-existing illness > 50%

MISCELLANEOUS

ASSOCIATED CONDITIONS
- Congestive heart failure
- Hypothyroidism
- Hypopituitarism
- Uremia
- Addison's disease
- Ketoacidosis
- Pulmonary infection
- Sepsis
- Brain injury, tumor
- Diabetes

AGE-RELATED FACTORS
Pediatric:
- All infants are at increased risk of hypothermia because of their limited ability to produce heat when placed in a cold environment. This is particularly true during the first 12 hours of life and in asphyxiated infants. Newborns should be placed under a radiant heat source and the amniotic fluid dried off.
- A child's body temperature drops faster than an adult's when immersed in cold water. This may increase tolerance of the heart's arrhythmias.

Geriatric:
- Mortality rates increase with increasing age
- Older adults have a lower metabolic rate and it is more difficult for them to maintain normal body temperature when environment drops below 18°C
- Aging also impairs the ability to detect temperature changes
- This population also has increased incidence of diseases that decrease heat production, increase or impair thermoregulation

Others: N/A

PREGNANCY
Controlled hypothermia in the operating suite is safe during pregnancy, especially with cerebrovascular surgery

SYNONYMS
Accidental hypothermia

ICD-9-CM
991.6 Accidental hypothermia
995.89 Anesthetic hypothermia
778.2-778.3 Newborn
780.9 Hypothermia not associated with low environmental temperature

SEE ALSO
- Frostbite
- Near drowning

OTHER NOTES   N/A

ABBREVIATIONS   N/A

REFERENCES
- Weinberg AD: Hypothermia. Annual of Emergency Medicine 1993; 22(part 2):370-377
- Danzl DT, Pozos R: Accidental hypothermia. New Engl J Med 1994;331:1756-1760

Illustrations: N/A

Internet references: http://www.5mcc.com

Author(s)
Scott T. Henderson, MD

Hypothyroidism, adult

BASICS

DESCRIPTION   A clinical state resulting from decreased circulating levels of free thyroid hormone or from resistance to hormone action. Myxedema connotes severe hypothyroidism.

System(s) affected: Endocrine/Metabolic

Genetics:
• No known genetic pattern for idiopathic primary hypothyroidism
• Hypothyroidism may be associated with Type II autoimmune polyglandular syndrome, which is associated with HLA-DR3, DR4
• Secondary hypothyroidism frequently results from treatment for Graves disease, which may be familial

Incidence/Prevalence in USA:
• 5-10/1000 in general population
• Over age 65, increases to 6-10% of women, 2-3% of men

Predominant age: Over 40

Predominant sex: Female > Male, 5-10:1

SIGNS AND SYMPTOMS
• Symptoms
  ◊ Onset may be insidious, subtle
  ◊ Weakness, fatigue, lethargy
  ◊ Cold intolerance
  ◊ Decreased memory
  ◊ Hearing impairment
  ◊ Constipation
  ◊ Muscle cramps
  ◊ Arthralgias
  ◊ Paresthesias
  ◊ Modest weight gain (10 pounds [4.5 kg])
  ◊ Decreased sweating
  ◊ Menorrhagia
  ◊ Depression
  ◊ Hoarseness
  ◊ Carpal tunnel syndrome
• Signs
  ◊ Dry, coarse skin
  ◊ Dull facial expression
  ◊ Coarsening or huskiness of voice
  ◊ Periorbital puffiness
  ◊ Swelling of hands and feet
  ◊ Bradycardia
  ◊ Hypothermia
  ◊ Reduced systolic blood pressure
  ◊ Increased diastolic blood pressure
  ◊ Reduced body and scalp hair
  ◊ Delayed relaxation of deep tendon reflexes
  ◊ Macroglossia
  ◊ Dilutional hyponatremia
  ◊ Anemia (usually normochromic, normocytic)
  ◊ Enlarged heart on chest x-ray (often due to pericardial effusion)

CAUSES
• Post-ablative follows radioactive iodine therapy or thyroid surgery. Delayed hypothyroidism may develop in patients treated with thioamide drugs (propylthiouracil, methimazole) 4 to 25 years later.
• Primary hypothyroidism may develop as a result of autoimmune thyroiditis, or be idiopathic
• With goiter, most commonly due to autoimmune disease, such as Hashimoto's thyroiditis; or heritable biosynthetic defects, iodine deficiency (rare in the US), or drug induced (iodides, lithium, phenylbutazone, aminosalicylic acid)
• Suprathyroid hypothyroidism, may be due to deficiency of thyrotropin-releasing hormone (TRH) from the hypothalamus or thyroid-stimulating hormone (TSH) from the pituitary
• Transient hypothyroidism may result from silent thyroiditis (most common in post partum period) and subacute granulomatous thyroiditis

RISK FACTORS
• Risk increases with increasing age
• Autoimmune diseases

DIAGNOSIS

DIFFERENTIAL DIAGNOSIS
• Nephrotic syndrome
• Chronic nephritis
• Neurasthenia
• Depression
• Euthyroid sick syndrome
• Congestive heart failure
• Primary amyloidosis
• Dementia from other causes

LABORATORY
• Total serum thyroxine (T4) - decreased
• T3 resin uptake - increased
• TSH (radioimmunoassay) - elevated
• Free T4 index (= T3 resin uptake x total serum T4) - low
• In severe hypothyroidism, anemia, elevated cholesterol, CPK, LDH, AST, hyponatremia

Drugs that may alter lab results:
• Thyroid supplement
• Cortisone
• Dopamine
• Phenytoin
• Estrogen or androgen therapy in excess of replacement
• Amiodarone
• Salicylates

Disorders that may alter lab results:
• Any severe illness
• Pregnancy
• Chronic protein malnutrition
• Hepatic failure
• Nephrotic syndrome

PATHOLOGICAL FINDINGS   Thyroid may be small, atrophic or enlarged

SPECIAL TESTS   Radioimmunoassay

IMAGING   None necessary

DIAGNOSTIC PROCEDURES   Elevated TSH (greater than 20 µU/mL [3-20 mIU/L]) is diagnostic of primary thyroid failure

TREATMENT

APPROPRIATE HEALTH CARE
Outpatient except for complicating emergencies (coma, hypothermia)

GENERAL MEASURES   Goals of treatment are to restore and maintain a euthyroid state

SURGICAL MEASURES   N/A

ACTIVITY   As tolerated

DIET
• High-bulk diet may be helpful to avoid constipation
• Low fat diet for obese patients

PATIENT EDUCATION
• Importance of compliance with thyroid replacement therapy
• Need for lifelong treatment
• Report to physician any signs of infection, heart problems
• Signs of thyrotoxicity

MEDICATIONS

DRUG(S) OF CHOICE
• Levothyroxine (Synthroid, Levothroid)
◊ 50-100 µg/day. Increase by 25 µg/day every 4-6 weeks until TSH is in normal range.
◊ Dosage requirements may vary with age, sex, residual secretory capacity of thyroid gland, other drugs being taken by patient, intestinal function
◊ Elderly patients may require lower dose because clearance is decreased
Contraindications:
• Thyrotoxic heart disease
• Uncorrected adrenocorticoid insufficiency
Precautions:
• Start with lower doses in the elderly and patients with heart disease
• Diabetic patients may need readjustment of hypoglycemic agents with institution of thyroxine
• Dosage of oral anticoagulants may need adjustment; monitor prothrombin time while initiating treatment
Significant possible interactions:
• Oral anticoagulants
• Insulin
• Oral hypoglycemics
• Estrogen
• Oral contraceptives
• Cholestyramine
• Ferrous sulfate may decrease absorption when taken concomitantly

ALTERNATIVE DRUGS   None currently recommended

FOLLOWUP

PATIENT MONITORING
• Every 6 weeks until stabilized, then every 6 months
• Follow cardiac status closely in older patients

PREVENTION/AVOIDANCE   N/A

POSSIBLE COMPLICATIONS
• Treatment induced congestive heart failure in people with coronary artery disease
• Myxedema coma - life threatening complication of hypothyroidism
• Increased susceptibility to infection
• Megacolon
• Organic psychosis with paranoia
• Adrenal crisis with vigorous treatment of hypothyroidism
• Infertility
• Hypersensitivity to opiates
• Overtreatment over long periods can lead to bone demineralization

EXPECTED COURSE/PROGNOSIS
• With early treatment, striking transformations in approved appearance and mental function. Return to normal state is the rule.
• Relapses will occur if treatment is interrupted
• If untreated, may progress to myxedema coma

MISCELLANEOUS

ASSOCIATED CONDITIONS
• Hyponatremia
• Anemia
• Idiopathic adrenocorticoid deficiency
• Diabetes mellitus
• Hypoparathyroidism
• Myasthenia gravis
• Vitiligo
• Hypercholesterolemia
• Mitral valve prolapse
• Depression
• Rapid cycling bipolar disorder

AGE-RELATED FACTORS
Pediatric: N/A
Geriatric:
• Characteristic signs and symptoms frequently changed or absent. Hypothyroidism is common in elderly. Diagnosis based on laboratory criteria.
• Replacement therapy is usually about two thirds of the dose used in young adults.
Others: N/A

PREGNANCY
• Replacement therapy may need adjustment. TSH levels should be monitored monthly during first trimester.
• Postpartum - check TSH levels at about 6 weeks
• Painless subacute thyroiditis may occur in the post partum period leading to transient hypothyroidism lasting about 3 months. Treatment with replacement therapy may be warranted. Up to 30% of these individuals develop permanent hypothyroidism.

SYNONYMS   Myxedema

ICD-9-CM
244 Acquired hypothyroidism
244.0 Postsurgical hypothyroidism
244.2 Iodine hypothyroidism

SEE ALSO
• Thyroiditis
• Hyperthyroidism

OTHER NOTES
• Surgical procedures
◊ Hypothyroid patients (mild to moderate) tolerate surgery with mortality and complications similar to euthyroid patients
◊ If surgery is elective, render patient euthyroid prior to procedure
◊ If surgery is urgent, proceed with the procedure with individualized replacement therapy preoperatively and postoperatively

ABBREVIATIONS   N/A

REFERENCES
• Barzel US: Hypothyroidism: diagnosis and management. Clin Geriatric Med 1995;11(2):239-249
• Ridgway EC: Modern concepts of primary thyroid gland failure. Clin Chemistry 1996;42(1)179-182
• Rudy DR, Tzagournis M: In: Rakel R, ed. Textbook of Family Medicine. 5th Ed. Philadelphia, WB Saunders Co, 1995:1099-1102
• Wallace K, Hofmann MT: Thyroid dysfunction: how to manage overt and subclinical disease in older patients. Geriatrics 1998;53(4):32-38
• Adlin V: Subclinical hypothyroidism deciding when to treat. Am Fam Phys 1998;57(4):776-780
Illustrations: N/A
Internet references: http://www.5mcc.com

Author(s)
Barbara A. Majeroni, MD

Id reaction

BASICS

DESCRIPTION A cutaneous eruption associated with, but distant to, the main lesion of the disease. Id is a word termination often combined with a root reflecting the causative factor. For example, bacterid, syphilid, and tuberculid. The dermatophytid is the most frequently referenced id reaction in dermatology. A dermatophytid is an autosensitization reaction where a secondary cutaneous reaction occurs at a site distant to a primary fungal infection. The distant eruption is due to circulating fungal antigen from the primary site reacting with antibodies at sensitized areas of the skin.
System(s) affected: Skin/Exocrine
Genetics: N/A
Incidence/Prevalence in USA: Not infrequent
Predominant age: All affect all ages
Predominant sex: Male = Female

SIGNS AND SYMPTOMS
USUAL
• Pruritic vesicles on the hands
• Tinea infection on the feet
• Generalized reactions can occur
LESS COMMON
• Papules
• Lichenoid eruption
• Eczematoid eruption

CAUSES Circulating antigens react with antibodies at sensitized areas of the skin

RISK FACTORS
• Fungal infection of the skin

DIAGNOSIS

DIFFERENTIAL DIAGNOSIS
• Pompholyx
• Contact dermatitis
• Drug eruptions
• Pustular psoriasis

LABORATORY
• Fungal infection at the primary site proven by potassium hydroxide (KOH) or fungal culture
• No fungal demonstrable at the site of the presumed id reaction
Drugs that may alter lab results: N/A
Disorders that may alter lab results: N/A

PATHOLOGICAL FINDINGS
• Vesicles in the upper dermis
• Moderate acanthosis
• Increased granular cell layer
• Lack of inflammation

SPECIAL TESTS Skin shows a positive trichophytin reaction

IMAGING N/A

DIAGNOSTIC PROCEDURES
• Potassium hydroxide (KOH) prep
• Fungal culture

TREATMENT

APPROPRIATE HEALTH CARE
Outpatient

GENERAL MEASURES
• treatment of the underlying fungal infection
• Symptomatic treatment of pruritus with antihistamines and/or topical steroids if needed
• Treatment for secondary bacterial infection

SURGICAL MEASURES N/A

ACTIVITY As tolerated

DIET No special diet

PATIENT EDUCATION
• Avoidance of hot humid conditions which promote fungal growth
• Aeration of susceptible body areas, eg, wear sandals or open foot wear
• If possible, wearing boxer shorts or loose fitting clothing, drying off wet skin after bathing, using powders and antiperspirants to make the environment less conducive to fungal growth

MEDICATIONS

DRUG(S) OF CHOICE Antifungals - topical and/or systemic
Contraindications: Refer to manufacturer's profile of each drug
Precautions: Refer to manufacturer's profile of each drug
Significant possible interactions: Refer to manufacturer's profile of each drug

ALTERNATIVE DRUGS
• Topical or systemic antibiotics for any secondary infection
• Antihistamines for any prutitus
• Topical steroids for pruritus
• Systemic steroids only if reaction is florid or generalized nature

FOLLOWUP

PATIENT MONITORING Followup in a few days or a week pending clinical course

PREVENTION/AVOIDANCE
• Minimize factors for developing fungal infections
• Prompt treatment of any developing fungal infection

POSSIBLE COMPLICATIONS
• Secondary bacterial infection (cellulitis)

EXPECTED COURSE/PROGNOSIS
After appropriate treatment, virtual resolution in a few days to two weeks

MISCELLANEOUS

ASSOCIATED CONDITIONS Primary fungal infection

AGE-RELATED FACTORS
Pediatric: N/A
Geriatric: N/A
Others: N/A

PREGNANCY N/A

SYNONYMS
• Dermatophytid
• Trichophytid

ICD-9-CM
692.89 Id reaction (due to bacteria)

SEE ALSO
• Tinea pedis
• Tinea corporis

OTHER NOTES N/A

ABBREVIATIONS N/A

REFERENCES Habif T: Clinical Dermatology. 3rd Ed. St. Louis, CV Mosby, 1996
Illustrations: 1 available on CD-ROM
Internet references: http://www.5mcc.com

Author(s)
Joseph Shrum, MD

Idiopathic hypertrophic subaortic stenosis (IHSS)

BASICS

DESCRIPTION This entity was the first known form of the hypertrophic cardiomyopathies (HCM) with the characteristic finding of inappropriate (disproportionate to the hemodynamic load) myocardial hypertrophy
• IHSS is characterized by a dynamic pressure gradient in the subaortic area leading clinically to both:
◊ Diastolic dysfunction with impaired ventricular filling and elevated atrial filling pressures producing dyspnea
◊ Systolic dysfunction with limitation of cardiac output response to exercise, exertional syncope, and secondary left ventricular hypertrophy
• Diagnosis usually is made by recognition of signs associated with outflow obstruction, but symptoms are predominantly characterized by diastolic dysfunction

System(s) affected: Cardiovascular
Genetics:
• Autosomal dominant with > 50% penetrance
• Evidence of disease (usually milder) is found in 25% of first degree relatives. Relatives usually do not have outflow obstruction, exhibit only localized hypertrophy, and are asymptomatic.
Incidence/Prevalence in USA: Uncommon
Predominant age: Most commonly presents in third decade (disease of young adulthood), but occurs from newborns to elderly
Predominant sex: Male = Female

SIGNS AND SYMPTOMS
• Dyspnea: mainly a result of diastolic dysfunction and initially exertional in onset (50-90%)
• Angina pectoris (50-90%)
• Syncope: exertional (50-90%)
• Presyncope: exertional (50-90%)
• Fatigue (50-90%)
• Palpitations (50-90%)
• Paroxysmal nocturnal dyspnea (50%)
• Double apical impulse due to prominent atrial system
• PMI displaced laterally
• Rapidly rising bifid carotid pulse
• Prominent S4
• S2 variable splitting (depending on degree of outflow obstruction)
• Harsh systolic crescendo-decrescendo murmur best heard between apex and left sternal border
• Murmur: increases and lengthens with Valsalva, standing, amyl nitrite; decreases with sudden squatting, lying down, passive leg raising, isometric handgrip

CAUSES Thickened septum impinging on the anterior mitral valve leaflet during systole causing outflow obstruction

RISK FACTORS Family history of HCM

DIAGNOSIS

DIFFERENTIAL DIAGNOSIS
• Fixed outflow obstruction such as aortic stenosis (AS). In AS the carotid pulse is slow-rising and reduced in volume versus the rapid-rising bifid pulse of IHSS. Bedside hemodynamic maneuvers (Valsalva, etc.) also help to differentiate.

LABORATORY N/A
Drugs that may alter lab results: N/A
Disorders that may alter lab results: N/A

PATHOLOGICAL FINDINGS
• Distinctive pattern of left ventricular (LV) hypertrophy - localized disproportionate hypertrophy of the LV septum with the ratio of septal to free wall thickness > 1.3:1 without anatomic evidence of pressure overload
• Dilated atria
• Increased LV mass and small chamber sizes
• Mural plaque of LV outflow tract
• Mitral valve thickening
• Anatomic variants:
◊ Apical form; not associated with intraventricular gradients
◊ Localized mid-ventricular obstructive form
• Disorganization and disarray septal muscle bundles
• Abnormal intramural coronary arteries

SPECIAL TESTS
• Electrocardiogram: Common findings (50-90%)
◊ Non-specific ST-T wave abnormalities
◊ Left ventricular hypertrophy
• Electrocardiogram: Less common findings (< 50%)
◊ Prominent and abnormal Q waves in anterior precordial and lateral limbs lead, simulating myocardial infarction
◊ P-wave abnormalities indicating left atrial enlargement
◊ Short PR interval with QRS morphology suggestive of pre-excitation without clear evidence of pre-excitation (rare in IHSS)
◊ Holter findings - frequent ventricular arrhythmias with up to 25% revealing ventricular tachycardia
◊ Atrial fibrillation - late finding and poor prognostic sign

IMAGING Chest x-ray - variable findings from normal cardiac size to cardiomegaly, none of which is pathognomonic

DIAGNOSTIC PROCEDURES
• Echocardiography
◊ Asymmetric septal hypertrophy with septal to free wall ratio > 1.3:1
◊ Abnormal systolic anterior leaflet motion of the mitral valve
◊ Left ventricular hypertrophy
◊ Left atrial enlargement
◊ Small ventricular chamber size with increased contractility
◊ Partial systolic closure of aortic valve in mid-systole
◊ Mitral valve prolapse
◊ Mitral regurgitation by Doppler
◊ Decreased mid-aortic flow coincident with systolic anterior leaflet motion of mitral valve by Doppler
• Radionuclide
◊ Thallium scintigraphy with stress at times reveals positive defects in setting of arteriographically normal coronary arteries
• Cardiac catheterization and angiocardiography
◊ Hemodynamic measurement documents degree and lability of outflow obstruction, and diastolic characteristics of left ventricle
◊ Angiocardiography documents left and right ventricular anatomy and coronary arterial anatomy

TREATMENT

APPROPRIATE HEALTH CARE
Outpatient usually. Inpatient for studies and/or surgery.

GENERAL MEASURES
• Therapy based on pathophysiology, namely interventions to reduce ventricular contractility or increase ventricular volume, ventricular compliance, and outflow tract dimensions
• Digitalis glycosides are contraindicated except for atrial fibrillation with uncontrolled response
• Nitrates and sympathomimetic amines (e.g., isoproterenol) are contraindicated except with concomitant coronary heart disease
• Diuretics are relatively contraindicated because of their effect on ventricular volume and left ventricular myotomy
• Pacemaker therapy - AV sequential pacing is frequently helpful in symptomatic patients with an outflow obstruction who do not respond to medical therapy

SURGICAL MEASURES Left ventricular myomectomy - done only in setting of severe symptoms refractory to medical therapy or sequential pacing in those patients with outflow gradient >50 mm Hg (<6.65 kPa), either at rest or with provocation. 95% successful in abolishing gradient with 70% of patients having a marked symptomatic improvement for at least 5 years.

ACTIVITY
• Strenuous exercise, especially competitive sports, should not be undertaken because of high risk of sudden death. Younger patients with little or no functional impairment have the greatest risk of sudden death.
• Sports participation by patients with IHSS is not permitted if any of the following are present: Marked left ventricle hypertrophy, significant outflow gradient, significant supraventricular and/or ventricular arrhythmias, or history of sudden death in relatives with hypertrophic cardiomyopathy

Idiopathic hypertrophic subaortic stenosis (IHSS)

DIET No special diet, but may need to reduce caloric intake, due to reduced activity

PATIENT EDUCATION
• Activity restrictions
• Refer for psychosocial counseling if appropriate (patient and family may suffer from restricted life-style and chronic disease problems)
• Recommend family learn cardiopulmonary resuscitation methods

MEDICATIONS

DRUG(S) OF CHOICE
• Beta blockers (propranolol, metoprolol, etc)
◊ May decrease outflow obstruction: Some evidence suggests that it may increase ventricular compliance. No clear evidence that it reduces incidence of sudden death.
◊ 1/3 to 2/3 of patients experience symptomatic improvement
◊ May titrate up to 320 mg/day of propranolol equivalent to obtain clinical effect provided patient tolerates dose
• Calcium channel blockers (primarily verapamil)
◊ Alternative to therapy with propranolol
◊ May have better effect on exercise performance
◊ Decrease in outflow gradient due to depression of cardiac contractility
◊ Improves diastolic filling by improved diastolic relaxation
• Amiodarone (Cordarone)
◊ Limited use in treating ventricular arrhythmias because of documented pro-arrhythmic effects in HCM
◊ Only to be used in patients with ventricular tachycardia associated with hemodynamic compromise. Use of drug is to be guided by initial and followup electrophysiological studies.
Contraindications:
• Verapamil:
◊ Major side effects include depression of impulse formation and A-V block, negative inotropism, and vasodilatation - all of which can result in hypotension, shock, pulmonary edema, and death
◊ Therefore, relatively contraindicated for use in patients with increased left ventricle end diastolic pressure (LVEDP), paroxysmal nocturnal dyspnea (PND), orthopnea, and/or in patients with sinus node disease and A-V block (unless there is an appropriate pacing device)
Precautions: See manufacturer's profile of each drug
Significant possible interactions: See manufacturer's profile of each drug

ALTERNATIVE DRUGS
• Diltiazem
• Disopyramide

FOLLOWUP

PATIENT MONITORING Yearly when symptoms and pharmacologic regimens become stable

PREVENTION/AVOIDANCE
• Avoid strenuous exercise, especially competitive sports
• Avoid rapid standing
• Avoid inotropic drugs and diuretics
• Use antitussives for infections that are accompanied by a cough

POSSIBLE COMPLICATIONS
• Sudden death
• Congestive heart failure
• Arrhythmia
• Atrial fibrillation with mural thrombosis formation
• Infective mitral endocarditis

EXPECTED COURSE/PROGNOSIS
• Annual mortality rate - 4% a year (sudden death most common reason)
• Chronic illness with restricted life-style

MISCELLANEOUS

ASSOCIATED CONDITIONS
• Mitral regurgitation
• Essential hypertension
• Mitral valve prolapse
• Angina pectoris

AGE-RELATED FACTORS
Pediatric:
• IHSS being recognized with increasing frequency
• Children may be asymptomatic. Evaluation of a heart murmur may disclose IHSS.
Geriatric: Occurrence is more frequent with increasing age. Female prevalence is greater in this age group.
Others: N/A

PREGNANCY N/A

SYNONYMS
• Hypertrophic obstructive cardiomyopathy (HOCM)
• Muscular subaortic stenosis

ICD-9-CM
425.1 Hypertrophic obstructive cardiomyopathy

SEE ALSO N/A

OTHER NOTES Genetic counseling may be appropriate

ABBREVIATIONS
• HCM = hypertrophic cardiomyopathy
• AS = aortic stenosis
• LV = left ventricle
• PMI = Point of maximal impulse

REFERENCES
• Braunwald E, ed: Heart Disease: A Textbook of Cardiovascular Medicine. 4th Ed. Philadelphia, W.B. Saunders Co., 1992
• Maron BJ, et al: Sudden death in hypertrophic cardiomyopathy. A profile of 78 patients. Circulation 1982;65:1388
• Goldman L, Braunwald E, eds: Primary Cardiology. 1st Ed. Philadelphia, WB Saunders Co, 1998
Illustrations: N/A
Internet references: http://www.5mcc.com

Author(s)
Peter Kozisek, MD

Idiopathic thrombocytopenic purpura (ITP)

 BASICS

DESCRIPTION A decrease in the circulating number of platelets (< 100,000 per microliter) in absence of toxic exposure or a disease associated with a low platelet count. It occurs as a secondary effect of peripheral platelet destruction as well as decreased platelet production. It is a diagnosis of exclusion.
• Acute ITP - a disease of childhood which often follows an acute infection and has spontaneous resolution within 2 months. Platelet counts < 20,000. This is a common disorder.
• Chronic ITP - a disease which persists after 6 months without a specific cause. Usually seen in adults and persists for months to years. Platelet count typically 30,000-80,000.
System(s) affected:
Hemic/Lymphatic/Immunologic
Genetics: No known genetic pattern
Incidence/Prevalence in USA: 1 in 10,000
Predominant age:
• Acute ITP - children ages 2-9 years old
• Chronic ITP - 20-50 years old
Predominant sex:
• Acute ITP - Male = Female
• Chronic ITP - Female > Male (3:1)

SIGNS AND SYMPTOMS
• Post traumatic bleeding at 40,000-60,000 platelet count
• Petechial hemorrhages
• Purpura
• Bruising tendency
• Gingival bleeding
• Gastrointestinal bleeding
• Mucocutaneous hemorrhages
• Menometrorrhagia
• Menorrhagia
• Recurrent epistaxis
• Neurological symptoms secondary to intracerebral bleeding
• Non-palpable spleen (absence of splenomegaly is an essential diagnostic criterion)
• Spontaneous bleeding < 20,000 platelet count

CAUSES IgG autoantibodies on platelet surface

RISK FACTORS
• Acute infection
• Age
• Cardiopulmonary bypass
• Hypersplenism
• Antiphospholipid antibody syndrome
• Preeclampsia
• HIV infection

 DIAGNOSIS

DIFFERENTIAL DIAGNOSIS
• Drug induced immune thrombocytopenia. Over 150 drugs have been implicated.
• Infections
• Acute leukemia
• Thrombotic thrombocytopenia purpura (TTP)
• Hemolytic uremic syndrome
• Factitious: "platelet clumping on the peripheral smear"
• Thrombocytopenia secondary to sepsis
• Myelodysplastic syndrome, particularly in the older patient
• Decreased production in marrow: malignancy, drugs, viruses, megaloblastic anemia
• Post transfusion
• Isoimmune neonatal purpura
• Disseminated intravascular coagulation (DIC)
• Alcohol induced

LABORATORY
• Decreased platelet count: 5,000-75,000
• Relative lymphocytosis and slight eosinophilia
• Prolonged bleeding time (not useful in the presence of thrombocytopenia)
• Anemia
• PT, PTT normal
Drugs that may alter lab results: N/A
Disorders that may alter lab results: N/A

PATHOLOGICAL FINDINGS
• Peripheral smear shows normal red and white cells with diminished but large platelets
• Marrow reveals abundant megakaryocytes with normal erythroid and myeloid precursors

SPECIAL TESTS
• Peripheral smear - routinely recommended
• Platelet associated antibody (PA-IgG) - optional

IMAGING CT of head to rule out intracranial bleeding if clinically indicated

DIAGNOSTIC PROCEDURES Bone marrow aspiration/biopsy (consider in refractory cases). Does not need to be done before giving gamma globulin.

 TREATMENT

APPROPRIATE HEALTH CARE
• Outpatient management unless patient at risk for bleeding (platelet count < 20,000)
• Admit patients with active bleeding

GENERAL MEASURES
• Children with platelet counts > 30,000 do not require treatment if they are asymptomatic or those with minor purpura do not need treatment
• Treatment for adults if platelet < 20,000, or platelets < 50,000 with symptoms or risks for bleeding such as HTN or peptic ulcers
• Specific treatment usually not necessary unless count is < 100,000; possibly < 30,000 with chronic ITP
• Platelet transfusions for significant bleeding

SURGICAL MEASURES Splenectomy in patients who fail medical therapy. Be sure to administer pneumococcal vaccine at least 2 weeks prior to splenectomy.

ACTIVITY Minimal activity to prevent injury or bruising. Avoid contact sports.

DIET No special diet

PATIENT EDUCATION Avoidance of ASA and other platelet inhibiting drugs

Idiopathic thrombocytopenic purpura (ITP)

MEDICATIONS

DRUG(S) OF CHOICE
• Acute ITP: prednisone 1-2 mg/kg/day for 4 weeks, then taper. If refractory, consider splenectomy.
• Chronic ITP: prednisone 60 mg/day for 4-6 weeks, then taper. May require repetition. If ineffective at non-toxic doses, consider splenectomy. Prednisone may then be effective. If still refractory, consider alternate drugs.
Contraindications: Do not administer gamma globulin if patient has IgA deficiency
Precautions: Refer to manufacturer's literature
Significant possible interactions: Anaphylaxis in patients with IgA deficiency who have IgA auto-antibodies

ALTERNATIVE DRUGS
• Acute ITP: IV immune globulin (IVIG, gamma globulin) 1-2 gm/kg single dose or 400 mg/kg/day for 5 days. Minor adverse reactions - chills, nausea, headache, joint pains in 2-7%. If this occurs, slow the rate of infusion. Gamma globulin may be effective alone or as a pretreatment to facilitate platelet transfusion. May delay need for splenectomy.
• Chronic ITP: high doses of intravenous gamma globulin in emergencies
• Anti-RHo(D) immune globulin 250 IU (50 µg/kg) as a single dose or in two divided doses given over 2 days; indications for use:
  ◊ Children with acute or chronic ITP
  ◊ Adults with chronic ITP
  ◊ ITP secondary to HIV infection
• Azathioprine or cyclophosphamide as single agents; either at doses of 2 mg/kg/day for 1-6 months
• Vincristine or vinblastine
• Danazol 200-400 mg bid
• Plasmapheresis
• Interferon

FOLLOWUP

PATIENT MONITORING
• Frequent platelet counts, daily to weekly, depending on severity and treatment
• Follow clinical status of hemostasis

PREVENTION/AVOIDANCE
Avoid medications (when feasible) that inhibit platelet function (such as aspirin), or those that suppress bone marrow

POSSIBLE COMPLICATIONS
• 1% mortality due to intracranial hemorrhage
• Severe blood loss
• Corticosteroid adverse effects
• Pneumococcal infections if patient must have splenectomy. Use pneumococcal vaccine.

EXPECTED COURSE/PROGNOSIS
• Acute ITP:
  ◊ 80-85% completely recover within 2 months
  ◊ 15% proceed to chronic ITP
• Chronic ITP:
  ◊ 10-20% recover spontaneously
  ◊ Remainder with diminished platelets for months to years
  ◊ May see spontaneous remissions (5%) and relapses

MISCELLANEOUS

ASSOCIATED CONDITIONS
• Acute ITP:
  ◊ Varicella
  ◊ Other viral infections
• Chronic ITP:
  ◊ HIV
  ◊ Graves' disease
  ◊ Hashimoto's thyroiditis
  ◊ Sarcoidosis
  ◊ Systemic lupus erythematosus
  ◊ Autoimmune hemolytic anemia (Evans' syndrome)

AGE-RELATED FACTORS
Pediatric:
• The acute form is primarily a childhood disease
• Better prognosis than adults
Geriatric: ITP is uncommon in this age group; look for other cause of low platelet count
Others: N/A

PREGNANCY
• Only if < 50,000 platelet count, may consider C-section
• Patient in labor should receive intravenous gamma globulin due to risk to the infant
• Platelet autoantibodies cross the placenta and may cause neonatal thrombocytopenia. Consider prednisone 10-20 mg/day for 10-14 days prior to delivery.
• Preeclampsia or gestational thrombocytopenia may cause thrombocytopenia unrelated to ITP

SYNONYMS
• Postinfectious thrombocytopenia
• Immune thrombocytopenic purpura
• Werlhof's disease

ICD-9-CM 287.3 Primary thrombocytopenia

SEE ALSO N/A

OTHER NOTES N/A

ABBREVIATIONS N/A

REFERENCES
• Diagnosis and treatment of idiopathic thrombocytopenia purpura. American Society of Hematology ITP practice guideline panel. Amer Fam Phys 1996;54:2437-2447
• George JN, El-harake MA, Raskob GE: Chronic idiopathic thrombocytopenic purpura. N Engl J Med 1994;331:1207-1210
• Blanchette V, et al: Management of chronic immune thrombocytopenia in adults and children. Semin Hematol 1998;35(suppl)36-51
• Lichtin A: Idiopathic thrombocytopenia purpura: guidance amid uncertainty. Clev Clin J Med 1998;65(10):510-514
Illustrations: N/A
Internet references: http://www.5mcc.com

Author(s)
Jeffery T. Kirchner, DO, FAAFP
Robert H. Scott, MD

Immunizations

BASICS

DESCRIPTION For the prevention of certain diseases. Specific indications include:
- Hepatitis B
  ◊ Infants
  ◊ Healthcare workers
  ◊ Laboratory personnel who might be exposed to the virus
  ◊ Intravenous drug users
  ◊ Male homosexuals
  ◊ Patients with a sexually transmitted disease
- Pneumococcal
  ◊ All persons over age 65
  ◊ All patients prior to splenectomy
  ◊ Patients with chronic liver, heart, lung or renal disease
  ◊ Patients with diabetes mellitus, HIV, asplenia
- Influenza
  ◊ All persons age 50 and older according to AAFP
  ◊ All persons age 65 and older according to ACIP
  ◊ Healthcare workers
  ◊ Patients with chronic heart, lung or renal disease (may begin at 6 months of age)
  ◊ Patients with diabetes mellitus, HIV
- Diphtheria, tetanus, acellular pertussis (DTaP)
  ◊ All children starting at age 2 months
  ◊ May be given up to the 7th birthday
  ◊ DTaP recommended
- Diphtheria and tetanus (pediatric)
  ◊ Children < 7 years who cannot take DTaP
- Tetanus and diphtheria (adult)
  ◊ Booster at ages 11-12 or 14-16 and either every 10 years thereafter or a single booster dose at age 50
- Measles, mumps and rubella (MMR)
  ◊ Children at age 12 to 15 months and again between 4 and 6 years
  ◊ Adults (especially medical personnel and daycare workers) without prior immunization or uncertain immunizations born after 1956
  ◊ International travelers
  ◊ College students - 2 doses total if not previously vaccinated
- Varicella
  ◊ Children at age 12 to 18 months (1 dose)
  ◊ Catch-up vaccination for children 18 months to 12 years (1 dose) without history of chickenpox
  ◊ Vaccination approved for persons ≥ 13 years without history of chickenpox (2 doses)
  ◊ Health care workers without a previous history of chickenpox
- Polio
  ◊ All children starting at 2 months of age
  ◊ Adults previously immunized who will travel to areas where polio is prevalent
  ◊ Unimmunized adults should receive the inactivated IPV vaccine
  ◊ 4 doses of IPV unless parents refuse or travel overseas

- Haemophilus influenzae type b
  ◊ All children starting at 2 months of age
- Hepatitis A
  ◊ Travelers to higher risk countries
  ◊ Patients with chronic liver disease
  ◊ Certain high-risk communities and ethnic groups, e.g., Native American/Alaskan
  ◊ Homosexual males
  ◊ Street drug users
  ◊ Laboratory personnel who might be exposed
- Rotavirus
  ◊ Infants at 2, 4 and 6 months
  ◊ Do not start series at age 7 months or older
  ◊ Decision on use of rotavirus pending intussusception studies

System(s) affected:
Hemic/Lymphatic/Immunologic
Genetics: N/A
Incidence/Prevalence in USA: N/A
Predominant age: N/A
Predominant sex: N/A

SIGNS AND SYMPTOMS N/A

CAUSES N/A

RISK FACTORS N/A

DIAGNOSIS

DIFFERENTIAL DIAGNOSIS N/A

LABORATORY N/A
Drugs that may alter lab results: N/A
Disorders that may alter lab results: N/A

PATHOLOGICAL FINDINGS N/A

SPECIAL TESTS N/A

IMAGING N/A

DIAGNOSTIC PROCEDURES N/A

TREATMENT

APPROPRIATE HEALTH CARE N/A

GENERAL MEASURES
- Informed patient consent should discuss consequences of specific diseases and risks of immunizations - Vaccine Information Statements should be given prior to vaccination
- Antipyretics (acetaminophen) are useful for the fever which may accompany immunizations

SURGICAL MEASURES N/A

ACTIVITY No restrictions after immunization

DIET No specific restrictions after immunization

PATIENT EDUCATION Report adverse events promptly. Minor redness, swelling, and or soreness at the site of injections can be expected; ice packs and acetaminophen may be helpful.

```
---IMMUNIZATION SCHEDULE------------------------------------
      <------- months --------> <------ years ----->
      0  1  2  4  6  12  15  18  4-6  11-12 14-16 65+
---------------------------------------------------------
Hep B†        1  2  3                  R
DTaP       1  2  3      4--->     5
Td                                     1-----> and q 10 yrs
Hib        1  2  3  4------->
IPV        1  2
OPV                1------->      2
Rotavirus  1  2  3
MMR                   1--->       2     R
Var                   1------->          R
INFL                                          1 yearly
PNEU                                          1 once
---------------------------------------------------------
Dash (-->) indicate range of acceptable ages for vaccination
R = Review immunizations/administer needed dose(s)
†Start hepB series at birth, if mother is HBsAg-positive
```

MEDICATIONS

DRUG(S) OF CHOICE

```
--IMMUNIZATION DOSES----------
Agent      Dose (mL)  Route
----------------------------------
DTaP         0.5       IM
MMR          0.5       SQ
Polio (OPV)  0.5       PO
Polio (IPV)  0.5       SQ
Rotavirus              PO
HBv†         ††        IM
Hib          0.5       IM
Influenza    0.5†††    IM
Td and DT    0.5       IM
Pneumococcal 0.5       IM or SQ
Varicella    0.5       SQ
----------------------------------
```

†Newborns of hepatitis B surface antigen positive mothers should also receive HBIG
††Variable
†††0.25mL for children 6-35 months old

```
--TETANUS WOUND PROPHYLAXIS---
    (for Td and TIG)
```

Type of wound	Prior tetanus immunizations		
	Uncertain or <3 doses		≥3 doses
	Td	TIG	Td‡
Clean†	Yes	No	10
Dirty††	Yes	Yes	5
Puncture	Yes	Yes	5
Major†††	Yes	Yes	5

For example, an adult with a puncture wound and 2 prior doses of tetanus toxoid should receive both Td and TIG.
‡TIG not needed; give Td if years indicated have passed since last immunization
†Clean: Minor wound
††Dirty: Contaminated with dirt, feces, or saliva
†††Major: Burn, frostbite, crush injury

Contraindications:
• Anaphylaxis to thimerosal: DTP, DT, TD, PRP-OMP, multi-dose vials of HbOC, influenza, and some brands of pneumococcal vaccine contraindicated. Thimerosal will be removed from most vaccines shortly.
• Anaphylaxis to neomycin: MMR, DTP, Hib, OPV, IPV, varicella contraindicated
• Anaphylaxis to streptomycin: OPV, IPV contraindicated
• Anaphylaxis to previous dose
• Encephalopathy within 7 days after DTP: Give DT for next dose(s)
• Pregnancy: MMR, varicella
• Known, active, untreated tuberculosis: varicella contraindicated
• Anaphylaxis to eggs: influenza
• Other
  ◊ Immunocompromised patients should, in general, not receive live viral vaccines (MMR, varicella and OPV), although patients with HIV may receive MMR if not severely immunocompromised
  ◊ Persons with unavoidable (e.g., household) contact with the immunocompromised should not receive OPV (give IPV)

Precautions:
• DTaP
  ◊ Suspected neurologic disease: Delay immunization until clarified
  ◊ Fever of ≥ 40.5°C (105°F) within 48 hours after previous DTP/DTaP
  ◊ Collapse or shock-like state (hypotonic-hyporesponsive episode) within 48 hours after DTP/DTaP
  ◊ Seizure within 3 days after DTP/DTaP
  ◊ Persistent, inconsolable crying lasting ≥ 3 hrs within 48 hours after DTP/DTaP
  ◊ The following are NOT contraindications and DTaP may be given if present:
    - Family history of convulsions: Pre-treat with acetaminophen and after DTaP q4h for 24 hrs
    - Family history of SIDS
    - Family history of adverse event following DTaP/DTP
    - Temperature < 40.5°C (105°F) following a prior DTaP/DTP
• Varicella
  ◊ Avoid salicylates for 6 weeks
Significant possible interactions: Avoid MMR and varicella vaccine within 3-11 months after gamma globulin (see ACIP)

ALTERNATIVE DRUGS None

FOLLOWUP

PATIENT MONITORING
• None routinely needed
• Hepatitis: Measure antibody (anti-HBs) response after HBv for healthcare workers, immunocompromised persons and offspring of hepatitis B carriers

PREVENTION/AVOIDANCE N/A

POSSIBLE COMPLICATIONS
Fever, malaise, local reactions (redness, pain) are most common. Rarely, allergic reactions, febrile seizures. Some believe DTP causes encephalopathy rarely. Rotavirus vaccine might cause intussusception.

EXPECTED COURSE/PROGNOSIS
Most patients develop antibodies

MISCELLANEOUS

ASSOCIATED CONDITIONS N/A

AGE-RELATED FACTORS
Pediatric: Most vaccines are given before entry into school. Do not delay DTaP immunization of the preterm infant unless specific contraindications exist.
Geriatric: Pneumococcal, influenza, and tetanus are needed in older age groups
Others: N/A

PREGNANCY MMR and varicella should not be routinely given to pregnant women or women who are planning pregnancy within 3 months (MMR) or next 1 month (varicella).

SYNONYMS
• Vaccinations
• Inoculations

ICD-9-CM
V05.9 Healthy person receiving prophylactic inoculation or vaccination

SEE ALSO
• Chickenpox
• Diphtheria
• Hepatitis, viral
• Influenza
• Measles, rubella
• Measles, rubeola
• Pertussis
• Pneumonia, bacterial
• Poliomyelitis
• Mumps
• Tetanus

OTHER NOTES
• PPD may be given at same time as MMR and/or OPV or wait 4 weeks after immunization to do skin test
• Culture-proven pertussis provides immunity; use DT instead of DTaP
• Haemophilus disease: Immunity not provided when child under 2 years; administer Hib as if no disease has occurred
• Combination vaccines are available

ABBREVIATIONS
DTaP = pediatric diphtheria and tetanus toxoids, and acellular pertussis vaccine
DT = pediatric diphtheria and tetanus toxoids
Td = adult diphtheria and tetanus toxoids
TIG = tetanus immune globulin
HBv = hepatitis B vaccine
HBIG = hepatitis B immune globulin
OPV = trivalent oral poliovirus vaccine
IPV = enhanced inactivated poliovirus vaccine
HbOC = Hib vaccine (hibTITER)
PRP-OMP = Hib vaccine (PedvaxHIB)
PRP-T = Hib vaccine (ActHIB, OmniHIB)
MMR = measles, mumps, and rubella vaccine
Hib = conjugated Haemophilus influenzae type b vaccine
INFL = influenza vaccine
PNEU = pneumococcal vaccine
PPD = purified protein derivative
VZIG = varicella-zoster immune globulin
Var = varicella zoster vaccine

REFERENCES
• Advisory Committee on Immunization Practices (ACIP)
• Red Book 1997 Report of the Committee on Infectious Diseases. American Academy of Pediatrics, 1997
• American Academy of Family Physicians
Illustrations: N/A
Internet references: http://www.5mcc.com

Author(s)
Richard Kent Zimmerman, MD, MPH
Richard D. Clover, MD

Immunodeficiency diseases

BASICS

DESCRIPTION
Disorders associated with disruption of the integrity of the immune system resulting in a wide spectrum of illnesses
• May be primary or secondary and involve any or all of the system's cells and their products (T cells, B cells, monocytes, macrophages, etc.) their receptors, metabolic pathways and products which are normally involved in health maintenance and protection
• Primary
  ◊ Combined immunodeficiencies, e.g., severe combined immunodeficiency (SCID), adenosine deaminase (ADA) deficiency, and reticular dysgenesis
  ◊ Antibody deficiencies, e.g., X-linked agammaglobulinemia, IgA deficiency, Ig deficiency with increased IgM (hyper-IgM syndrome), common variable immunodeficiency (CVID) and transient hypogammaglobulinemia of infancy
  ◊ Other well-defined syndromes, e.g., Wiskott-Aldrich syndrome (eczema, thrombocytopenia and repeated infections), ataxia telangiectasia (cerebellar ataxia, oculocutaneous telangiectasia and immunodeficiency) and DiGeorge's syndrome (isolated T cell deficiency)
  ◊ Associated syndromes e.g., Down syndrome, chronic mucocutaneous candidiasis, hyper-IgE syndrome, chronic granulomatous disease, partial albinism and WHIM syndrome (warts, hypogammaglobulinemia, infection, myelokathexis [retention of leukocytes in a hypercellular marrow]), phagocytic defects with early onset of periodontal disease.
  ◊ Complement deficiencies
• Secondary
  ◊ AIDS
  ◊ Other infections, malignancies, malnutrition, protein-losing enteropathy, drugs, and chronic stress

System(s) affected:
Hemic/Lymphatic/Immunologic
Genetics: Included in Description
Incidence/Prevalence in USA:
• 1 in every 500 (including IgA deficiency) born with an immune system defect
• Many more will acquire a defect which may be transient or permanent
Predominant age:
• All ages. Children most likely to present with primary or inherited deficiencies.
• Number of newborns with AIDS increasing. In part associated with: (1) increased premature infant survival, (2) improved treatment and care of other primary diseases, (3) use of immunosuppressive agents.
Predominant sex: Male > Female

SIGNS AND SYMPTOMS
• Common features
  ◊ Unusual susceptibility to infection. Frequency and severity vary with type of defect.
  ◊ Malignancies, especially lymphoreticular

  ◊ Increased tendency toward autoimmune disorders
  ◊ Weight loss
  ◊ Fever
• More specific features
  ◊ Combined T and B cell deficiencies associated with severe fungal, bacterial and viral infections. Enzyme deficiencies may be involved.
  ◊ T cell deficiencies may be acquired (as with the human immunodeficiency virus) or congenital with wide spectrum manifestations. Children with DiGeorge's syndrome show cardiac defects, micrognathia, hypertelorism and hypocalcemic tetany.
  ◊ B cell or immunoglobulin deficiency syndromes may be associated with chronic sinusitis, recurrent respiratory infection, chronic diarrheal disease, rheumatoid arthritis, systemic lupus erythematosus (SLE), atopy, splenomegaly, anemia, recurrent pneumococcal pneumonia and meningococcal meningitis
  ◊ Chronic giardiasis, fever of unknown origin and malabsorption should cause suspicion of immunodeficiency
  ◊ Miscellaneous syndromes include chronic mucocutaneous candidiasis, fatal Epstein-Barr virus infection, and complement component deficiencies

CAUSES
• Primary immunodeficiency diseases
  ◊ Faulty genes and gene products resulting in inherited defects of the immune system including: antibody, cellular, phagocytic cytokine production, and complement deficiencies
  ◊ Manifested by infections soon after birth but may not be expressed clinically until later in life
• Secondary immunodeficiency diseases
  ◊ Treatment with immunosuppressive agents
  ◊ Nutritional deficiencies
  ◊ Use of drugs and exposure to chemicals should be considered
  ◊ X-ray treatment
  ◊ IgA deficiency associated with phenytoin or penicillamine
  ◊ Thymoma associated with hypogammaglobulinemia
  ◊ Viruses e.g., HIV-1 and HIV-2

RISK FACTORS
• Family history
• Almost anything less than good health practices
• Drug abuse and parenteral blood exposure
• Sexual lifestyle
• Aging

DIAGNOSIS

DIFFERENTIAL DIAGNOSIS
• Must consider all immunodeficiency disorders
• Careful history and physical will direct proper search

LABORATORY
• High percentage of immunodeficiencies will be discovered by a CBC with a differential smear and immunoglobulin levels including: IgG, IgA, IgM and IgE. IgG subclasses should be included.
• Further assays include mononuclear cell populations which may be quantified
• Total lymphocyte a good screen
• Functional evaluation by skin testing (anergy battery) and antibody levels to common viruses and bacterial toxins
• Complement levels
• Phagocyte function
• Specific cytokine function
• Additional specific tests for suspected acquired causes for immunodeficiencies (AIDS, chronic diarrhea, malignancy, drugs, etc.)
Drugs that may alter lab results: N/A
Disorders that may alter lab results: N/A

PATHOLOGICAL FINDINGS
Vary with type of deficiency and resultant disease(s)

SPECIAL TESTS   N/A

IMAGING
• MRI helpful in evaluation of CNS lesions associated with toxoplasmosis
• Techniques and technology continue to improve dramatically

DIAGNOSTIC PROCEDURES
• Careful history and physical
• Try to deduce whether infections associated with T cell response inadequacies (fungal and other opportunistic infections) or lack of B cell (antibodies) response or both

TREATMENT

APPROPRIATE HEALTH CARE
• Outpatient or inpatient management appropriate to clinical problem

GENERAL MEASURES
• Depends mainly on complexity of the immune deficiency
• Bone marrow transplant with donor T cell engraftment in severe abnormalities of T cell function. Best done at referral research centers.
• Intravenous immunoglobulin - for patients deficient in IgG. Not appropriate for treatment for Ig deficiency other than IgG, but may be helpful in the hyper-IgM syndrome.

SURGICAL MEASURES   N/A

ACTIVITY   As appropriate

DIET   Severe immunodeficiencies require sterile conditions

PATIENT EDUCATION   Printed patient information available from: Immune Deficiency Foundation, 25 West Chesapeake Ave. Room 206, Rowson, MD 21204

MEDICATIONS

DRUG(S) OF CHOICE Surgeon's choice for prophylaxis
Contraindications: N/A
Precautions: N/A
Significant possible interactions: N/A

ALTERNATIVE DRUGS N/A

FOLLOWUP

PATIENT MONITORING Follow weekly postoperatively for 2-8 weeks

PREVENTION/AVOIDANCE N/A

POSSIBLE COMPLICATIONS
• Slow return of bowel function
• Higher risk of subsequent obstruction
• Sepsis

EXPECTED COURSE/PROGNOSIS
Usually excellent prognosis. In general, mortality from intestinal obstruction ranges from < 1% to > 20% depending upon etiology, bowel viability, co-morbidities, etc.

MISCELLANEOUS

ASSOCIATED CONDITIONS N/A

AGE-RELATED FACTORS
Pediatric:
• Different etiologies of obstruction in childhood
  ◊ Duodenal malformations
  ◊ Jejunoileal atresia
  ◊ Malrotation and midgut volvulus
  ◊ Meconium ileus
  ◊ Necrotizing enterocolitis
  ◊ Hirschsprung's disease
  ◊ Intussusception
  ◊ Duplications
  ◊ Meckel's diverticulum
  ◊ Imperforate anus
Geriatric:
• Colon neoplasms more common
• Chronic constipation/impactions more common
Others: N/A

PREGNANCY N/A

SYNONYMS N/A

ICD-9-CM
560.0 Intussusception
560.3 Impaction of intestine
560.9 Intestinal obstruction, unspecified

SEE ALSO N/A

OTHER NOTES Rectal examination showing occult blood may represent colon malignancy as etiology of the obstruction

ABBREVIATIONS N/A

REFERENCES Sleisenger MH, Fordtran JS, eds: Gastrointestinal Disease: Pathophysiology, Diagnosis, Management. 5th Ed. Philadelphia, W.B. Saunders Co., 1994
Illustrations: N/A
Internet references: http://www.5mcc.com

Author(s)
Leo C. Mercer, MD

Intestinal parasites

BASICS

DESCRIPTION

• The class of infectious agents called parasites is divided into two parts:
◊ Protozoa are single cell animals which characteristically divide and multiply within the host, are usually direct fecal-oral in transmission, and do not cause an eosinophilia
◊ Helminths (worms) are multi-cellular animals and with rare exceptions (i.e., Strongyloides stercoralis, Hymenolepis nana) do not multiply within the host and are often associated with some degree of eosinophilia. The level of eosinophilia is associated with the degree of mucosal invasiveness. The worms have a limited life span within the host and without reinfection would eventually die on their own.
• Not all of the parasites that start out by ingestion in the bowel will remain in the bowel. Some are invasive and some do not release their infective forms into the bowel. This later group, including Toxoplasma gondii, Echinococcus, Trichinella spiralis will not be covered in this topic.
• Most worms require either a prolonged incubation period outside the host before being infectious or need a specific vector for transmission. A notable exception to this rule is Enterobius vermicularis (pinworm), the eggs of which are infectious shortly after being passed, so auto-infection occurs readily.
• Direct person-to-person transmission of worms is uncommon
• The likelihood of acquiring an intestinal parasite depends on several factors - the presence of the specific infectious agent, an appropriate "vector" or mode of transmission, and a host who is susceptible to the infectious agent. The world-wide distribution of parasites is determined by geographic factors, socio-economics, age, and crowding with poor food preparation and a break in the standard of water and personal sanitation being the major factors.

System(s) affected: Gastrointestinal

Genetics: Genetic factors play a minor role in the acquisition, pathogenesis and clearance of these infections

Incidence/Prevalence in USA:

• From laboratory statistics: 5-30% general population
• From day care surveys: Asymptomatic 20-30%; symptomatic 50-80%
• Intestinal protozoa account for the majority of parasitological findings in North America (most considered to be non-pathogenic)
• In a random sampling, at least one parasite would be found in the stools of 5-10% of all people. If Blastocystis hominis were included in this accounting, 20-30% of specimens examined in parasitology will be positive.
• Helminths are considerably rarer and are highly dependent on population demographics and prior geographic exposure risk factors. In general, less than 10% of all parasitology reports include a helminth.

Predominant age: Pediatric
Predominant sex: Male = Female

SIGNS AND SYMPTOMS

• Diarrhea
• Abdominal pain/tenderness
• Excessive gas - bloating, eructation, flatulence, borborygmi
• Nausea or vomiting
• Weight loss and anorexia
• Dysentery, i.e., bleeding (rare, but associated with Entamoeba histolytica, Balantidium coli)
• Pruritus ani (E. vermicularis, Trichuris trichiura, S. stercoralis, tapeworms)
• Passing a worm or a worm segment
• Increased bowel sounds
• Peri-rectal or vulvar rash

CAUSES

• Protozoan pathogens:
◊ Giardia lamblia
◊ Entamoeba histolytica
◊ Cryptosporidium
◊ Isospora belli
◊ Balantidium coli
◊ Cyclospora cayetanensis
◊ Microsporida
• Possible protozoan pathogens:
◊ Dientamoeba fragilis
• Probable non-pathogenic protozoa
◊ All other Entamoeba species
◊ Endolimax nana
◊ All other intestinal flagellates
• Helminthic pathogens - nematodes (roundworms):
◊ Enterobius vermicularis
◊ Trichuris trichiura
◊ Ascaris lumbricoides
◊ Hookworm (Necator americanus, Ancylostoma duodenale)
◊ Strongyloides stercoralis
◊ Capillaria philippinensis
◊ Trichostrongylus sp
• Helminthic pathogens - trematodes (flukes)
◊ Fasciolopsis buski
◊ Clonorchis sinensis
◊ Opisthorchis viverrini
◊ Heterophyes heterophyes
◊ Fasciola hepatica
◊ Paragonimus westermani
◊ Schistosoma mansoni
◊ S. japonicum
◊ S. hematobium
◊ S. mekongi
• Helminthic pathogens - cestodes (tapeworms)
◊ Taenia saginata
◊ Taenia solium
◊ Diphyllobothrium latum
◊ Hymenolepis nana
◊ Hymenolepis diminuta
◊ Dipylidium caninum

RISK FACTORS

• Age (children)
• Low socioeconomic status
• Poor sanitation - personal, food, water
• International travel
• Crowding - day care centers, institutional care
• Intercurrent medical conditions, pregnancy, gastric hypoacidity, immunosuppression (AIDS)

DIAGNOSIS

DIFFERENTIAL DIAGNOSIS

• Other intestinal infections
• Food poisoning
• Malabsorption
• Inflammatory bowel disease
• Hemorrhoids
• Rectal fissures

LABORATORY

• Examination of a single stool specimen collected into a preservative (i.e., sodium acetate formalin [SAF]), well mixed to fix and preserve all elements, will provide an accurate diagnosis in 90% of patients. Additional specimens will need to be examined for greater diagnostic accuracy.
• Newer techniques of lab exam of stool specimens (such as monoclonal antibodies, other antigen detection techniques, DNA detection) are exciting developments but currently provide little advantage over routine techniques and represent additional costs. These techniques are needed to differentiate E. histolytica from E. dispar
• Serology - for specific infections, especially if they do not produce a patent infection in the bowel (i.e., no eggs or parasites released into the stool), or if low numbers of parasites. May be indicated rarely, but are usually available only through referral centers.

Drugs that may alter lab results: Use of antibiotics, oil based laxatives, and the presence of barium in the stool may make a parasitological diagnosis difficult or impossible

Disorders that may alter lab results: N/A

PATHOLOGICAL FINDINGS

• Majority of intestinal parasites are not invasive and produce no or non-specific changes in the histology of the bowel
• Invasive amebiasis of the bowel produces a classical endoscopic and histological picture of ulceration and inflammation in the colon
• Protozoa and helminths may be seen in bowel biopsies

SPECIAL TESTS

• Special techniques for the detection of Cryptosporidium, Isospora belli, Cyclospora, and microsporidia often require that the laboratory be informed of the "risk" profile of the patient before these tests will be done
• Pinworm paddles provide a greater diagnostic yield when Enterobius vermicularis is being considered. Multiple tests (5) may be needed to exclude the diagnosis of pinworms.
• Parasite culture is possible for a few organisms - Giardia lamblia, Entamoeba histolytica, Strongyloides stercoralis, but are rarely indicated and are usually available only in referral laboratories
• String tests and upper bowel intubations are rarely needed to diagnose the upper intestinal parasites

• Rarely, a biopsy will demonstrate the presence of an invasive helminth on tissue section. Worms can be extremely difficult to diagnose in this manner, usually needing the expertise of a tissue parasite pathologist. The other parasites may be visualized on the mucosa or in the mucous layer.

IMAGING Diagnostic radiology rarely needed. Exception is for invasive infections such as amebiasis where colitis, amebomas and liver abscesses may be demonstrated by the appropriate techniques.

DIAGNOSTIC PROCEDURES
• Invasive diagnostic procedures are rarely needed or indicated
• With hemorrhagic colitis and a possible diagnosis of invasive amebiasis, sigmoidoscopy will reveal a muco-purulent colitis with ulceration. A scraping from an ulcer, promptly examined by microscopy, will reveal the motile hematophagous trophozoites of E. histolytica.
• Upper intestinal endoscopy can yield fluid to be examined for Giardia lamblia and Strongyloides stercoralis. Impression smears and biopsies obtained with the endoscope can also be examined.

TREATMENT

APPROPRIATE HEALTH CARE
Outpatient except for rare surgery or inpatient medical treatment

GENERAL MEASURES
• Therapy must be assessed in the best interest of the patient. Not all patients need to be treated with drugs.
• Symptomatic treatment is indicated for patient comfort once specific therapy has been initiated
• Bowel paralyzing drugs, for diarrhea caused by invasive organisms, are relatively contraindicated

SURGICAL MEASURES
• Surgical procedures play little role in treatment except when amebic liver abscesses need to be drained, e.g., multiple or large abscesses not responding to medical management, or threatened rupture, especially left lobe abscesses. Drainage of such abscesses is often accomplished by directed catheter placement in radiology, with surgical back-up as required.
• Surgery may be required if bowel or other organ obstruction occurs, as can be seen with Ascaris lumbricoides migration

ACTIVITY As tolerated

DIET
• Nutritional support may be required
• Many patients during and following bowel infections, especially when infected with Giardia lamblia, will experience irritable bowel syndrome and/or lactose intolerance. The majority of these patients will respond to a lactose free diet, reduction of caffeine intake, and an increase in dietary fiber.

PATIENT EDUCATION
• Educating the patient is important to reduce the risk of reinfection or transmission
• Education will depend on the parasite, host characteristics and the environment that the two interact in

MEDICATIONS

DRUG(S) OF CHOICE
• Protozoa
  ◊ Entamoeba histolytica asymptomatic needs individual assessment
  ◊ Entamoeba histolytica symptomatic intestinal - iodoquinol or diloxanide furoate
  ◊ Entamoeba histolytica invasive disease - iodoquinol or diloxanide furoate. Plus metronidazole, alone or dehydroemetine or emetine plus chloroquine phosphate.
  ◊ Giardia lamblia - metronidazole or tinidazole or furazolidone or quinacrine. Note: albendazole, available in US only from manufacturer, may have activity against G. lamblia.
  ◊ Cryptosporidium - none proven effective
  ◊ Isospora belli protozoa - trimethoprim-sulfamethoxazole
  ◊ Balantidium coli - tetracycline or iodoquinol or metronidazole
  ◊ Cyclospora - sulfamethoxazole-trimethoprim
  ◊ Microsporidia - albendazole (some species)
• Helminths
  ◊ Nematodes (except Strongyloides and Trichostrongylus) - mebendazole or pyrantel pamoate or piperazine citrate or albendazole (available in US only from manufacturer)
  ◊ Strongyloides and Trichostrongylus - thiabendazole or albendazole (available in US only from manufacturer)
  ◊ Cestodes - praziquantel or niclosamide
  ◊ Trematodes - niclosamide or praziquantel
Contraindications: Refer to manufacturer's profile of each drug
Precautions: Refer to manufacturer's profile of each drug
Significant possible interactions: Refer to manufacturer's profile of each drug

ALTERNATIVE DRUGS N/A

FOLLOWUP

PATIENT MONITORING Repeat examination, to ensure clearance, should be timed taking into account: The life cycle of the parasite (how long would it take to regenerate and become patent) and the risk of reinfection, as well as the specific test likely to find the parasite (stool, pinworm paddle, culture, serology)

PREVENTION/AVOIDANCE The specific nature of the infection often dictates the specific methods needed to avoid reinfection. This usually involves matters of personal, food and/or water sanitation.

POSSIBLE COMPLICATIONS Chronic persistent diarrhea

EXPECTED COURSE/PROGNOSIS See specific text on individual parasite

MISCELLANEOUS

ASSOCIATED CONDITIONS N/A

AGE-RELATED FACTORS
Pediatric: Most common age group affected
Geriatric: Illness may cause more severe debilitation
Others: AIDS - susceptibility to infection, severity of disease

PREGNANCY Some of these infections can be particularly serious in pregnancy. Many of the drugs are contraindicated in pregnancy.

SYNONYMS N/A

ICD-9-CM 129 Intestinal parasitism, unspecified

SEE ALSO N/A

OTHER NOTES N/A

ABBREVIATIONS N/A

REFERENCES
• DuPont HL: Persistent diarrhea in travelers. Clin Infect Dis 1996;22:124-128
• Abramowicz M, ed: Drugs for parasitic infections. In The Medical Letter. New York, The Medical Letter Inc. 1998, Vol. 40:1-28
• Mandell GL, ed: Principles and Practice of Infectious Diseases. 4th Ed. New York, Churchill Livingstone, 1995
Illustrations: N/A
Internet references: http://www.5mcc.com

Author(s)
D. W. MacPherson, MD, MSc (CTM), FRCPC

Intussusception

 BASICS

 DIAGNOSIS

 TREATMENT

DESCRIPTION Invagination of a portion of intestine into itself (may involve any part of small intestine, ileocolic [95%], or colo-colic)
System(s) affected: Gastrointestinal
Genetics: N/A
Incidence/Prevalence in USA: 1.5-4/1000 live births
Predominant age: 5-10 months (65% are less than one year of age)
Predominant sex: Male > Female (3:2) - male preponderance is more notable in older infants

SIGNS AND SYMPTOMS
• Vomiting (80-100%)
• Blood per rectum - currant-jelly stools (65%-95%) highest percent in infants
• Intermittent, colicky abdominal pain (almost all children)
• Lethargy (22%) (more pronounced with longer duration of illness)
• Palpable mass (16-41%)
• Diarrhea (7%)
• Prolapse of intussusception through anus (3%)
• Fever
• Extreme pallor in some

CAUSES
• Children
  ◊ Marked hypertrophy of Peyer's patches (92-98%)
  ◊ Lead point in 2%-8% (polyp, Meckel's diverticulum, duplication cyst, ectopic pancreas, lymphoma, Henoch-Schönlein purpura, lipoma, carcinoma)
  ◊ Allergic reactions, diet changes, changes in intestinal activity may be other causes
  ◊ Possible adenovirus or rotavirus infection
• Adults
  ◊ Virtually always associated with lead point

RISK FACTORS
• Henoch-Schönlein purpura
• Leukemia
• Lymphoma
• Cystic fibrosis
• Recent upper respiratory infection (21%)
• Recent operation (1-24 days previously)

DIFFERENTIAL DIAGNOSIS
• Adhesive band small bowel obstruction
• Appendicitis
• Gastroenteritis

LABORATORY
• Electrolytes
• CBC
• Urinalysis
• Stool guaiac
Drugs that may alter lab results: N/A
Disorders that may alter lab results: N/A

PATHOLOGICAL FINDINGS
• Hyperplasia of Peyer's lymphatic patches of terminal ileum (92%) with or without mesenteric lymphadenopathy
• Recognizable lead point (see list in Causes) (2-8%)

SPECIAL TESTS N/A

IMAGING
• Ultrasound
• Plain film - flat and upright abdominal films may suggest the diagnosis

DIAGNOSTIC PROCEDURES
• Contrast enema (barium, water soluble contrast or air)
• Abdominal ultrasound

APPROPRIATE HEALTH CARE
Inpatient until resolved

GENERAL MEASURES
• IV fluid resuscitation
• Foley catheter (if child severely dehydrated)
• Nasogastric tube
• Antibiotics useful only if necrotic bowel present
• Non-operative care:
  ◊ Hydrostatic/pneumatic reduction of intussusception (50-80% success)
  ◊ Barium column should be 40-42 inches high
  ◊ Enema continued as long as progress is made. Bowel may be drained and the enema repeated.
  ◊ Pneumatic reduction pressure should not exceed 120-140 mm Hg (16-18.6 kPa)

SURGICAL MEASURES
• Right lower quadrant incision
• Gentle manipulation by pushing intussusception (not pulling)
• If unable to reduce or non-viable bowel, segmental resection with re-anastomosis
• Enterotomy if lead point suspected
• Incidental appendectomy commonly done

ACTIVITY As tolerated after reduction

DIET Liquids started after abdominal distension resolves and bowel function returns

PATIENT EDUCATION
• Instruct family on possibility of recurrence (5-13%)
• Most recurrences occur in first 24 hours postreduction

MEDICATIONS

DRUG(S) OF CHOICE N/A
Contraindications: N/A
Precautions: N/A
Significant possible interactions: N/A

ALTERNATIVE DRUGS N/A

FOLLOWUP

PATIENT MONITORING Office visit one week after discharge

PREVENTION/AVOIDANCE N/A

POSSIBLE COMPLICATIONS
• Bowel perforation during attempted reduction
• Prolonged ileus
• Adhesions with intestinal obstruction
• Incisional hernia
• Ischemic intestine requiring second operation
• Electrolyte abnormality
• Anemia
• Pleural effusion
• Sepsis
• Recurrence

EXPECTED COURSE/PROGNOSIS
• Mortality should not exceed 1-2%
• Possible recurrence (5-13%) after hydrostatic reduction
• Possible recurrence (3%) after operative reduction

MISCELLANEOUS

ASSOCIATED CONDITIONS
• Schönlein-Henoch purpura
• Cystic fibrosis

AGE-RELATED FACTORS
Pediatric:
• Usually no lead point
• Postoperative intussusception (1-24 days postoperatively) is virtually always in small bowel and only rarely can be reduced hydrostatically
Geriatric: 90% have lead point
Others: N/A

PREGNANCY N/A

SYNONYMS N/A

ICD-9-CM
560.0 Intussusception

SEE ALSO
• Intestinal obstruction
• Cystic fibrosis
• Schönlein-Henoch purpura

OTHER NOTES N/A

ABBREVIATIONS N/A

REFERENCES
• Pang .C: Intussusception revisited: Clinicopathologic analysis of 261 cases, with emphasis on pathogenesis. Southern Medical J 1989;82(2):215-228
• Skipper RP, Boeckman R, Klein R: Childhood intussusception. SGO 1990;171:151-153
• O'Neill JA, Rowe MI, Grosfeld JL, et al: Pediatric Surgery. 5th ed., St Louis, Mosby, 1998
• West KW, Stephens B, Rescorla FJ, et al: Postoperative intussusception: Experience with 36 cases in children. Surgery 1988;104:781-787
Illustrations: N/A
Internet references: http://www.5mcc.com

Author(s)
Timothy L. Black, MD, FACS, FAAP
James P. Miller, MD, FACS, FAAP

Iron deficiency anemia

BASICS

DESCRIPTION Anemia due to decreased iron stores. Poor iron utilization and poor iron re-utilization (e.g., anemia of chronic disease) are also due to iron deficiency, but iron stores are not depleted. Onset may be acute with rapid blood loss, or chronic with poor diet or slow blood loss. This is the most common cause of anemia in the U.S.
System(s) affected:
Hemic/Lymphatic/Immunologic
Genetics: No known genetic pattern
Incidence/Prevalence in USA: Affects 7-10% of the adult population, 10-20% of the infants and toddlers, and 15-45% of pregnant patients. Most likely the poor and in children who are under-immunized.
Predominant age: All ages but especially toddlers and menstruating women
Predominant sex: Female > Male

SIGNS AND SYMPTOMS
• Asymptomatic in most cases
• Cheilosis
• Dyspnea on exertion, fatigue, tachycardia, palpitation, vasomotor disturbances
• Effects of underlying GI ulceration, neoplasm, uterine disorders or bleeding varices
• Headache, inability to concentrate, irritability, listlessness
• Neuralgic pain, peripheral paresthesias
• Pica (dirt, paint, ice)
• Spoon-shaped, brittle nails
• Susceptibility to infection

CAUSES
• Blood loss (e.g., menses, GI bleed)
• Poor iron intake
• Poor iron absorption (e.g., postgastrectomy)
• Increased demand for iron (e.g., infancy, adolescence, pregnancy)
• Hookworm infestation
• Gastric carcinoma

RISK FACTORS See Causes

DIAGNOSIS

DIFFERENTIAL DIAGNOSIS
• Defective iron utilization (e.g., thalassemia, sideroblastosis, G6PD deficiency)
• Defective iron re-utilization (e.g., infection, inflammation, cancer, other chronic diseases)
• Hypoproliferation (e.g., decreased erythropoietin from hypothyroidism, renal failure, etc.)

LABORATORY
• Stainable iron in bone marrow aspiration is the gold standard
• Low serum ferritin is best non-invasive test in adults, but may miss some deficient patients since ferritin is an acute phase reactant. Fe/TIBC (transferrin ratio) is no longer recommended since it is less sensitive and less specific than ferritin.
• Peripheral smear usually shows hypochromia and microcytosis, but may be normal
• Hemoglobin is usually lower than 12 g/dL, but patients with higher premorbid hemoglobin (such as smokers and patients with chronic hypoxemia) may be anemic at higher Hgb levels. Abnormal values for infants and toddlers, and for pregnant persons, are less than 10.5-11.0 g/dL.
• Low RBC count helps to distinguish from thalassemia where count is normal or high
• Microcytosis with ovalocytosis and anemia unresponsive to iron suggest thalassemia trait
• Low MCV may be absent in mild anemia, or hidden by population of larger cells (e.g., reticulocytes or macrocytes)
• An empiric trial of iron at 3 mg/kg/day may be the best way to diagnose decreased iron stores in infants and children, if reticulocytes elevated in 7-10 days, or Hgb increased > 1.0 g/dL after 4 weeks
Drugs that may alter lab results: Iron supplements or multivitamin-mineral preparations that contain iron
Disorders that may alter lab results:
• Ferritin elevated by acute liver disease, cirrhosis, Hodgkin's disease, acute leukemia, solid tumors, fever, acute inflammation, renal dialysis
• Hemoglobin may be elevated by smoking or chronic hypoxemia, thereby hiding anemia if standard anemia limits are used

PATHOLOGICAL FINDINGS
• Absent marrow iron stores
• Marrow - hyperplastic, micronormoblastic

SPECIAL TESTS
• Cause of iron loss - stool guaiac testing, GI endoscopy, stool for O & P, clotting studies
• Rule-out thalassemia - review prior CBC's for persisting mild anemia and marked ovalomicrocytosis, elevated Hgb A2 or Hgb F, family history, and especially high or high normal RBC count
• Rule-out G6PD deficiency - assay at least 6 weeks after last drop in Hgb
• Rule-out poor re-utilization - trial of iron (oral or parenteral), bone marrow aspiration and iron stain
• Rule-out gastric carcinoma, especially in the elderly

IMAGING GI endoscopy to discover occult bleeding sites

DIAGNOSTIC PROCEDURES
• Bone marrow aspiration
• Sigmoidoscopy
• Gastroscopy
• Colonoscopy

TREATMENT

APPROPRIATE HEALTH CARE
Outpatient

GENERAL MEASURES
• Search for cause and correct it. There can be no excuse for not searching for a bleeding site.
• Avoid transfusions except in rare instances

SURGICAL MEASURES N/A

ACTIVITY Patients with hypoxemia, low cardiac output or angina may require reduced activity prescriptions

DIET
• Limit milk to 1 pint a day (adults)
• Emphasize protein- and iron-containing foods (meat, beans, leafy green vegetables)
• Increase dietary fiber to decrease likelihood of constipation during iron replacement therapy
• No milk, other dairy product, antacid, or tetracycline within two hours of drug dosage

PATIENT EDUCATION For patient education materials contact: National Heart, Lung & Blood Institute, Communications & Public Information Branch, National Institutes of Health, Building 31, Room 41-21, 9000 Rockville Pike, Bethesda, MD 20892, (301)251-1222

MEDICATIONS

DRUG(S) OF CHOICE
• Ferrous sulfate 300 mg tid on an empty stomach one hour before meals is an ideal dose that provides 180 mg of elemental iron a day. Dose can be reduced as needed for GI symptoms, which affect 15% of patients on standard iron therapy. Or the dose can be taken with meals, which may reduce the delivery of iron by 50%. People with a moderate anemia (Hgb = 10 g/dL) need only 1500-2000 mg of elemental iron replacement. Reducing the amount of iron per dose as much as necessary to abate symptoms will make parenteral iron therapy unnecessary in almost all cases. Special iron formulations and compounds are very expensive and reduce symptoms only to the degree that they reduce delivery of iron.
• Liquid iron preparations are useful for children with a recommended dose of 3 mg/kg/day given in a single dose.
• Consider parenteral iron for patients with malabsorption if higher doses and use of vitamin C fail
Contraindications:
• Antacids concomitantly
• Tetracycline concomitantly
Precautions:
• Iron preparations cause black bowel movements
• Iron overdose is highly toxic. Patients should be instructed to keep tablets and liquids out of the reach of small children.
Significant possible interactions:
• Allopurinol
• Antacids
• Penicillamine
• Tetracyclines
• Vitamin E

ALTERNATIVE DRUGS   N/A

FOLLOWUP

PATIENT MONITORING   Regularly after return to normal (in order to detect recurrences)

PREVENTION/AVOIDANCE
• Good nutrition with adequate iron intake
• Correction of gynecologic or other problems causing excess blood loss

POSSIBLE COMPLICATIONS
Neglecting to identify hidden bleeding points, particularly a bleeding malignancy

EXPECTED COURSE/PROGNOSIS
Curable with iron therapy if the underlying cause can be discovered and cured

MISCELLANEOUS

ASSOCIATED CONDITIONS   N/A

AGE-RELATED FACTORS
Pediatric: Frequent problem in infants whose major source of nutrition is cow's milk and juices
Geriatric: Accounts for 60% of anemias in people over 65
Others: N/A

PREGNANCY   Common during pregnancy unless iron supplements are included in the diet

SYNONYMS
• Anemia of chronic blood loss
• Hypochromic, microcytic anemia
• Chlorosis

ICD-9-CM   280.9 iron deficiency anemia, unspecified

SEE ALSO   N/A

OTHER NOTES   N/A

ABBREVIATIONS   N/A
• Hgb = hemoglobin
• TIBC = total iron binding capacity

REFERENCES
• Lee RG, Bithell TC, et al: Wintrobe's Clinical Hematology. 9th Ed. Philadelphia, Lea & Febiger, 1993
• Williams WJ, Beutler E, Erslev AJ, et al, eds: Hematology. 4th Ed. New York, McGraw-Hill, 1990
• Van den Broek et al: Iron status in pregnant women: which measurements are valid? Brit J Haem 1998;103(3):817-824
• Farrell R, LaMont JT: Rational approach to iron-deficiency anaemia in premenopausal women. Lancet 1998;352(9145):1953-1954
• Adams WG, et al: Anemia and elevated lead levels in underimmunized inner-city children. Pediatrics 1998;101(3)
• Fireman Z, Kopelman Y, Sternberg A: Endoscopic evaluation of iron deficiency anemia and follow-up in patients older than age 50. J Clin Gastroent 1998;26(1):7- 10
• Waterbury L. Anemia. In Barker LR, Burton JR, Zieve PD. (ed): Principles of Ambulatory Medicine 4th ed. Philadelphia, Lippincott Williams & Wilkins, 1995:593-607
Illustrations: N/A
Internet references: http://www.5mcc.com

Author(s)
Bruce Block, MD

Iron toxicity, acute

BASICS

DESCRIPTION Acute iron overload due to accidental or intentional ingestion. Accidental ingestion is not uncommon since iron-containing compounds are readily available, brightly colored, and are often sugar coated. Acute symptoms are characterized by vomiting, diarrhea, mild lethargy, upper abdominal pain, pallor, and hyperglycemia with more severe clinical findings including cyanosis, stupor, acidosis, hematemesis, shock, and coma.
System(s) affected: Gastrointestinal, Cardiovascular, Hemic/Lymphatic/Immunologic
Genetics: N/A
Incidence/Prevalence in USA: 3699 cases reported in 1988 along with 15,977 cases of intoxication with iron-fortified vitamins; leading cause of poisoning mortality of children in the US
Predominant age:
• Children most frequently involved (in 1984, 1337 out 1738 iron poisoning cases were reported in children < 6 years of age)
• From 1988-92, approximately 17% of children's deaths reported to poison control centers in the U.S. were iron poisonings
Predominant sex: N/A

SIGNS AND SYMPTOMS
• 0.5 to 2 hours - vomiting, hematemesis, abdominal pain, diarrhea, lethargy, shock, acidosis, and coagulopathy
• Apparent recovery may contribute to a false sense of security after initial ingestion, observe patient closely
• 2 to 12 hours - profound shock, severe acidosis, cyanosis and fever
• 12 to 48 hours - symptoms may recur and can include pulmonary edema, shock, acidosis, convulsions, anuria, hyperthermia, and death
• 2 to 6 weeks - if patient survives, pyloric or antral stenosis, hepatic cirrhosis and CNS damage can be seen
The phases listed above do not occur in all patients. For example, in massive overdose, patients may present in shock.

CAUSES
• Excessive iron ingestion - the average human lethal dose is 200 to 250 mg of elemental iron per kg of body weight (equivalent to about 230 ferrous sulfate based on 60 mg of elemental iron per tablet)
• Toxicity is likely following 60 mg/kg of elemental iron ingestion

RISK FACTORS Access to iron products by children resulting in accidental ingestion

DIAGNOSIS

DIFFERENTIAL DIAGNOSIS
If unknown iron ingestion
• Gastritis
• Small bowel obstruction
• Drug intolerance/overdose
• Alcohol toxicity
• Viral illness
• Diabetic ketoacidosis

LABORATORY
• CBC
• Electrolytes and glucose
• Serum iron; total iron binding capacity (TIBC) (may not be available in some hospitals)
• PT/INR (prothrombin time /International Normalized Ratio) and activated partial thromboplastin time (APTT)
• Serum bicarbonate
• Liver function tests in severe overdose
Drugs that may alter lab results:
Deferoxamine can falsely lower serum iron unless a reducing agent is added to the specimen. Should obtain a free iron concentration.
Disorders that may alter lab results:
TIBC rises factitiously in the presence of high iron levels

PATHOLOGICAL FINDINGS
• None (by definition)

SPECIAL TESTS   N/A

IMAGING   Abdominal and chest x-ray

DIAGNOSTIC PROCEDURES
Abdominal x-ray to evaluate for tablets in the gut

TREATMENT

APPROPRIATE HEALTH CARE
• Emergency room for acute ingestion
• Inpatient for severe ingestion
• Supportive treatment

GENERAL MEASURES
• Maintain proper airway, respiration and circulation
• Assess the amount of iron ingested
• Removal of iron from the gastrointestinal tract
• Hemodialysis, peritoneal dialysis, and exchange transfusion have also be used in lethal overdoses
• Maintain electrolyte balance, treat shock,hypotension, hyperglycemia
• Explore psychological issues if an intentional ingestion

SURGICAL MEASURES   N/A

ACTIVITY   N/A

DIET   N/A

PATIENT EDUCATION
• Prevention counseling on proper storage of iron products out of the reach of children
• Educational material from poison control centers may be available to use
• An informative poster is available, at no charge, from the Department of Health and Human Services, 5600 Fishers Lane (HFI-40), Rockville, MD 20857

MEDICATIONS

DRUG(S) OF CHOICE
• Decontamination with syrup of ipecac [1-12 years: 15 mL; adult: 30 mL] if a patient has recent iron ingestion and is a candidate for emesis. Contraindications are signs of oral pharyngeal/esophageal irritation, a depressed gag reflex, or CNS excitation/depression. Controversy exists as to whether to give ipecac to children < 6 mo of age.
• Criteria for emesis/lavage:
  ◊ > 20 mg/kg ingested
  ◊ Symptomatic
  ◊ Adults
• Gastric lavage, using tepid water, may be indicated in patients who are comatose or at risk for convulsing. Use if over 20 mg/kg or unknown amount of iron has been ingested.
• Whole bowel irrigation with a solution containing polyethylene glycol (Colyte, GoLYTELY) electrolyte lavage, gives rapid diarrhea with relatively little fluid and electrolyte imbalance; (children: 25 mL/kg/h; adults: 1.5-2 L/h); indicated when radiographic evidence of iron past the pylorus or if tablets persist in the GI tract after other attempts of decontamination. End point: clear rectal effluent, disappearance of radiopacities.
• If serum iron exceeds TIBC or peak serum iron is > 300 mcg/dL, administer IV deferoxamine, 15 mg/kg/hr, for not more than 24 hrs to chelate iron and prevent it from entering into chemical reactions. Serum iron levels drop usually within 12 to 48 hours.
Contraindications: Deferoxamine is relatively contraindicated in patients with severe renal disease or anuria, primary hemochromatosis
Precautions: Deferoxamine may cause flushing of skin, urticaria, hypotension and shock with rapid IV injections
Significant possible interactions: N/A

ALTERNATIVE DRUGS   N/A

FOLLOWUP

PATIENT MONITORING
• KUB until no pills are seen
• Serum iron concentration
• CBC, electrolytes, serum bicarbonate, blood glucose, serum iron, and TIBC
• Some patients' urine will turn a characteristic vin rose color after treatment (previously this was used as a diagnostic test of significant iron poisoning)

PREVENTION/AVOIDANCE
• Keep prescription and over-the-counter iron products/vitamins out of reach of children
• Keep syrup of ipecac on hand in case of accidental acute ingestion

POSSIBLE COMPLICATIONS   2-4 weeks
after severe ingestion has resulted in pyloric or antral stenosis, hepatic cirrhosis and CNS damage

EXPECTED COURSE/PROGNOSIS
Depends on amount ingested and length of time patient exposed

MISCELLANEOUS

ASSOCIATED CONDITIONS   N/A

AGE-RELATED FACTORS
Pediatric: For a 2 year old, the average lethal dose of elemental iron is 3 grams
Geriatric: N/A
Others: N/A

PREGNANCY   N/A

SYNONYMS   Iron poisoning

ICD-9-CM
964.0 poisoning by iron and its compounds

SEE ALSO   N/A

OTHER NOTES   N/A

ABBREVIATIONS   TIBC - total iron binding capacity

REFERENCES
• Aisen P, Cohen G, Kang JO: Iron Toxicosis. Int Rev Exp Pathol 1990;31:1-46
• Banner WJ, Tong TG: Iron poisoning. Ped Clin N Am, 1986;33:393-409
• Iron, Poisondex Toxicologic Management, 1974-1999 Micromedex Inc. Vol 00
• FDA Medical Bulletin 1995; 25.3. Washington, DC, Federal Food & Drug Administration, 1995
• Thompson DF: Reassessment of measuring total iron binding capacity in acute iron overdose. Ann Pharmacother 1994;28:63-66
• Chyka PA, Butler AY, Holley JE: Serum iron concentrations and symptoms of acute poisoning in children. Pharmacotherapy 1996;16:105301058
Illustrations: N/A
Internet references: http://www.5mcc.com

Author(s)
Julienne K. Kirk, PharmD

Irritable bowel syndrome

BASICS

DESCRIPTION   Altered bowel habits, abdominal pain, gaseousness, in the absence of organic pathology (divided into four types):
• Alternating diarrhea with constipation
• Diarrhea predominant
• Constipation predominant
• Upper abdominal bloating and discomfort
System(s) affected: Gastrointestinal
Genetics: Unknown, but more common in families of patients
Incidence/Prevalence in USA:
• Unknown, but 50% of gastrointestinal visits, and second to upper respiratory infection as cause for lost workdays
• At least 15% of population (uncommon in children and early teens)
Predominant age:
• Late 20's, rarely in late teens
• If over age 40, other disease more likely
Predominant sex:
• Female > Male (2:1) in the US
• In other parts of the world - Male > Female

SIGNS AND SYMPTOMS
• All present in most patients but not with every episode
• Abdominal pain, usually lower quadrant, relieved by defecation
• Mucus in stools
• Constipation
• Diarrhea
• Distention
• Upper abdominal discomfort after eating
• Straining for normal consistency stools
• Urgency of defecation
• Feelings of incomplete evacuation
• Scybalous stools
• Nausea, vomiting (rarely)

CAUSES   Unknown but patients show some gut motility abnormalities with increased response to stress and stimulants, and increase in the 3 cycles/minute smooth muscle contractions

RISK FACTORS
• Other members of the family with the same or similar gastrointestinal disorder
• History of childhood sexual abuse
• Sexual or domestic abuse in women

DIAGNOSIS

DIFFERENTIAL DIAGNOSIS
• Inflammatory bowel syndromes
• Lactose intolerance
• Infections (Giardia lamblia, Entamoeba histolytica, Salmonella, Campylobacter, Yersinia, Clostridium difficile)
• Diverticula
• Cathartic use
• Magnesium containing antacids
• Celiac sprue
• Pancreatic insufficiency
• Depression
• Somatization
• Adenocarcinoma of the colon
• Villous adenoma
• Endocrine tumors
• Hypo/hyperthyroidism
• Diabetes mellitus
• Radiation damage to colon or small bowel

LABORATORY
• As needed to rule out other pathology
  ◊ ESR
  ◊ CBC
  ◊ Stool for ova, parasites and culture
Drugs that may alter lab results: N/A
Disorders that may alter lab results: N/A

PATHOLOGICAL FINDINGS   All labs normal except for sigmoidoscopy

SPECIAL TESTS   Not needed for diagnosis

IMAGING
• Barium enema, if indicated is usually normal
• Small bowel series

DIAGNOSTIC PROCEDURES
Sigmoidoscopy (often normal), can show spasm that reproduces pain and increase mucosal folds

TREATMENT

APPROPRIATE HEALTH CARE
Outpatient

GENERAL MEASURES
• Heat to abdomen can help
• Biofeedback may help
• Reduce stress

SURGICAL MEASURES   N/A

ACTIVITY   As normal

DIET
• Increase fiber - may make some patients worse
• Avoid - large meals; spicy, fried, fatty foods; milk products, carbohydrates

PATIENT EDUCATION
• Many materials available nationally and locally
• Stress the organicity of the disease versus any psycho-social interpretation
• Teach patient to avoid problem stimulants

MEDICATIONS

DRUG(S) OF CHOICE
• Use from among this list according to need or response
  ◊ Bulk producing agents - psyllium containing products (Metamucil) 1 tbsp bid or tid
  ◊ Constipating agents (if diarrhea is significant) - loperamide (Imodium) 4 mg initial dose, then 2 mg after each unformed stool or Diphenoxylate-atropine (Lomotil) 2.5-5.0 mg (1-2 tablets) after each unformed stool
  ◊ Antispasmodics/anticholinergics - dicyclomine (Bentyl) 10-20 mg bid to qid or lactase (Lactaid) 1-3 caplets ac for lactose intolerance
  ◊ Anticholinergics/sedatives - chlordiazepoxide-clidinium (Librax) 1 or 2 ac and qhs; phenobarbital-hyoscyamine-atropine-hyoscine (Donnatal) 1 or 2 tablets ac and hs; amitriptyline HCL (Elavil) 25-50 mg qhs
  ◊ Antiflatulents - simethicone (Mylicon) 2 or 4 tablets pc and hs
  ◊ For milk intolerance - lactase capsules or tablets; 1-2 tablets prior to ingesting milk products
Contraindications: Refer to manufacturer's profile of each drug
Precautions: Refer to manufacturer's profile of each drug
Significant possible interactions: Refer to manufacturer's profile of each drug

ALTERNATIVE DRUGS   N/A

FOLLOWUP

PATIENT MONITORING   As needed for symptoms

PREVENTION/AVOIDANCE   See Diet

POSSIBLE COMPLICATIONS   N/A

EXPECTED COURSE/PROGNOSIS
• No progression to cancer or inflammatory disease
• Expect recurrences, when under stress, throughout life. Frequency lessens as age increases.

MISCELLANEOUS

ASSOCIATED CONDITIONS
• Migraine
• Bladder frequency
• Nocturia
• Urgency
• Fecal incontinence
• Fibromyalgia
• Dyspareunia
• Depression
• Stress incontinence

AGE-RELATED FACTORS   N/A
Pediatric: N/A
Geriatric: N/A
Others: N/A

PREGNANCY   Anecdotal information implies that irritable bowel syndrome gets worse in pregnancy. But there are no increased risks to fetus or mother.

SYNONYMS
• Mucous colitis
• Spastic colon
• Irritable colon

ICD-9-CM
564.1 Irritable colon

SEE ALSO   N/A

OTHER NOTES   Must not give patients the impression that this is a psychiatric illness

ABBREVIATIONS
IBS = irritable bowel sysdrome

REFERENCES
• Verne GN, Cerda JJ: Irritable bowel syndrome: streamlining the diagnosis. Post Grad Med 1997;102(3):197-208
• Dalton CB, Drossman DA: Diagnosis and treatment of irritable bowel syndrome. Am Fam Phys 1997;55(3):875-885
• Read NW, ed: Irritable Bowel Syndrome. London, Grune and Stratton, 1991
• Rakel R, ed: Textbook of Family Practice. 5th Ed. Philadelphia, W.B. Saunders Co., 1995
Illustrations: N/A
Internet references: http://www.5mcc.com

Author(s)
S. Shevaun Duiker, MD

Kaposi's sarcoma

 BASICS

DESCRIPTION
A neoplasm characterized by vascular tumors of skin and viscera in several different forms:
- Indolent (classic) Kaposi's sarcoma (KS)
- African (endemic) KS
- AIDS-related (epidemic) KS
- Form associated with immunosuppressive medications

System(s) affected: Skin/Exocrine, Hemic/Lymphatic/Immunologic
Genetics: Unknown
Incidence/Prevalence in USA:
- Indolent/lymphadenopathic - rare
- In AIDS patients - common
Predominant age: 16-75
Predominant sex: Male > Female

SIGNS AND SYMPTOMS
- Indolent Kaposi's
  ◊ Multicentric red-blue violaceous tumors on the skin
  ◊ Tender skin tumors
  ◊ Pruritic skin tumors
  ◊ In older men, lesions appear first on toes or legs
- African (endemic) Kaposi's
  ◊ Usually involves skin, viscera or lymph nodes
- In Kaposi's associated with HIV infection (epidemic)
  ◊ Skin lesions widely disseminated, on the face, arms, trunk
  ◊ Lesions on mucous membranes
  ◊ Lesions in lymph nodes
  ◊ Lesions in viscera

CAUSES
A herpes virus designated "Kaposi's sarcoma herpes virus" (KSHV) or human herpes virus type 8 (HHV8) has been strongly linked to KS. Samples from KS lesions have been found to contain DNA sequences identical with KSHV, and KSHV can be propagated from skin lesions of patients with KS.

RISK FACTORS
- HIV infection
- Living in endemic area (especially Zaire or Uganda)
- Immunosuppressant medications
- Transplantation and chemotherapy

 DIAGNOSIS

DIFFERENTIAL DIAGNOSIS
Bacillary angiomatosis, granuloma faciale, vascular proliferation and purpuric lesions

LABORATORY
Nothing specific
Drugs that may alter lab results: N/A
Disorders that may alter lab results: N/A

PATHOLOGICAL FINDINGS
- Micro - proliferation of atypical spindle cells
- Micro - proliferation of vascular channels
- Micro - large hyperchromic nuclei
- Micro - spindle-shaped perivascular cells
- Micro - hemosiderin laden macrophages

SPECIAL TESTS
Tissue examination

IMAGING
CT or MRI scan (chest, abdomen) may assess visceral involvement

DIAGNOSTIC PROCEDURES
- Biopsy of skin or lymph node
- Bronchoscopy with biopsy
- Liver biopsy

 TREATMENT

APPROPRIATE HEALTH CARE
- Outpatient
- Outpatient surgery

GENERAL MEASURES
- If KS due to immunosuppressant medications, eliminate or reduce medication dosage
- If KS is HIV-related, optimize anti-HIV therapy to reduce HIV viral load
- Treatment is otherwise determined by extent of the disease
- Observation
- Radiotherapy (electron beam) or x-ray therapy 1000 to 2000 rads
- Systemic chemotherapy, immunotherapy, or anti-viral therapy

SURGICAL MEASURES
- Cryotherapy
- Intralesional chemotherapy or immunotherapy
- Surgical excision

ACTIVITY
Remain active as long as possible

DIET
No special diet

PATIENT EDUCATION
N/A

MEDICATIONS

DRUG(S) OF CHOICE
• Chemotherapy
◊ Doxorubicin
or
◊ Bleomycin
or
◊ Vinblastine
or
◊ Vincristine
or
◊ Daunorubicin
or
◊ Interferon - parenteral or intralesional
Note: Both doxorubicin and danunorubicin are available and approved for use in liposomal forms
Contraindications: Refer to manufacturer's literature
Precautions: Refer to manufacturer's literature. Myelosuppression with chemotherapy.
Significant possible interactions: Refer to manufacturer's literature

ALTERNATIVE DRUGS
• Several studies have reported that some individuals have responded to anti-viral medications such as foscarnet (Foscavir), ganciclovir (Cytovene, Vitrasert), and cidofovir (Vistide)
• Several clinical studies are underway using newer agents including 9-cis-retinoic acid

FOLLOWUP

PATIENT MONITORING
In HIV patients with KS, other opportunistic infections must be aggressively treated

PREVENTION/AVOIDANCE
• Safe sex practices
• Possible prophylaxis with anti-viral medications

POSSIBLE COMPLICATIONS
Aggressive form affects at least 1/3 of HIV infected patients

EXPECTED COURSE/PROGNOSIS
• Improved HIV treatments may result in improved HIV-related KS survival
• Indolent form - 10 year survival

MISCELLANEOUS

ASSOCIATED CONDITIONS
• AIDS
• HIV infection

AGE-RELATED FACTORS
Pediatric: N/A
Geriatric: Indolent form most likely to occur in men in this age group
Others: N/A

PREGNANCY N/A

SYNONYMS
• Endotheliosarcoma
• Multiple, idiopathic hemorrhagic sarcoma

ICD-9-CM
173.9 Malignant neoplasm of the skin

SEE ALSO HIV infection & AIDS

OTHER NOTES N/A

ABBREVIATIONS
KS = Kaposi's sarcoma

REFERENCES
• Abrams D, Grieco M, McMeeking A: AIDS/HIV Treatment Directory. New York, American Foundation for AIDS Research (updated 4 times yearly)
• Cesarman E: Kaposi's sarcoma-associated herpes-like DNA sequences in AIDS-related body cavity-based lymphomas. NEJM 1995;332(18):1186-1191
• Moore PS, Chang Y: Detection of a herpesvirus-like DNA sequence in Kaposi's sarcoma in patients with and without HIV infection. NEJM 1995;331:1181-1185
• Martin JN, et al: Sexual transmission and the natural history of human herpesvirus 8 infection. NEJM 1997;338:948-954
• Kedes DH, Ganem D. Sensitivity of Kaposi's-associated herpesvirus replication to antiviral drugs: Implications for potential therapy. J Clin Invest 1997;99:2082-6.
Illustrations: 9 available on CD-ROM
Internet references: http://www.5mcc.com

Author(s)
R. Scott Gorman, MD

Kawasaki syndrome

BASICS

DESCRIPTION An acute, distinct, self-limited, febrile disease of children which is notable for vasculitis of coronary blood vessels with potential dilation, aneurysms, thrombosis, rupture, or myocardial ischemia. KS should be considered in febrile children with cervical adenitis (≥1.5 cm) unresponsive to antibiotics, without an obvious alternative diagnosis.
System(s) affected: Cardiovascular, Gastrointestinal, Hemic/Lymphatic/Immunologic, Musculoskeletal, Nervous, Pulmonary, Renal/Urologic, Skin/Exocrine
Genetics: Increased incidence of HLA-Bw 22 in Japanese patients; increased incidence of HLA-Bw 51 in US Caucasians and in Jewish, Israeli patients. Slight increase in siblings of cases. Worldwide, affects all races, but most prevalent in Japan.
Incidence/Prevalence in USA: Worldwide, affects all races but most prevalent in Japan. In the US, the annual incidence rate is 0.6 cases/100,000 children under 5 years old. Seasonal variation - increased in winter and spring. Increased outbreaks at 2-3 year intervals. In developed countries, more common than acute rheumatic fever as a cause of acquired heart disease in children
Predominant age: 1-5 years; 50% are < 2 years old, 80% are < 5 years old. Seldom seen after 8 years of age.
Predominant sex: N/A

SIGNS AND SYMPTOMS
• Fever for 5 days or more
  ◊ Fever is high (103-105°F [39.4-40.5°C]) and unresponsive to antibiotics
  ◊ May be prolonged (2-3 weeks with average duration of 11 days)
• Polymorphous rash
  ◊ May be maculopapular, scarlatiniform, morbilliform, erythema marginatum, or rarely vesiculopustular
  ◊ Frequently confluent in the perineum where it desquamates
• Bilateral conjunctival suffusion
  ◊ Nonpurulent
• Changes of lips and oral cavity
  ◊ Reddening of lips in the acute stage which crack, fissure and bleed in the subacute phase
  ◊ Strawberry or erythematous tongue
  ◊ Diffuse injection of oral and pharyngeal mucosa without exudate
• Acute, nonpurulent cervical lymphadenopathy (in 50-75% of patients)
  ◊ Lymph nodes 1 cm or greater in diameter
  ◊ Generalized lymphadenopathy usually absent
• Extremity changes
  ◊ Reddened palms and soles on days 3-5
  ◊ Indurative edema of hands and feet on days 4-7
  ◊ Membranous desquamation from fingertips in convalescent phase

• Other organ system involvement:
  ◊ Cardiovascular
    - Acutely may have tachycardia (disproportionate to fever), gallop rhythms, and ECG changes suggestive of myocarditis
    - Pericarditis, often subclinical
    - Coronary artery and other medium-sized arterial aneurysms
  ◊ Gastrointestinal
    - Anorexia
    - Vomiting or diarrhea
    - Acute, acalculous cholecystitis may present as a right upper quadrant mass and pain
    - Pancreatitis
  ◊ Renal
    - Nephritis
    - Urethritis
  ◊ Pulmonary
    - Pneumonitis, atelectasis, or pleural effusions
  ◊ Joints
    - Arthritis of wrists, knees, and ankles may appear in third week of illness
  ◊ Neurologic
    - Irritability
    - Aseptic meningitis
    - Peripheral neuropathies

CAUSES
• Unknown
• Microbial agent is favored because of acute, self-limited course and community-wide outbreaks
  ◊ Leading theory is that a staphylococcal or streptococcal superantigen, in the appropriate host, stimulates T cell populations which in turn cause activation of immune responses directed against endothelial cell antigens

RISK FACTORS Environmental - exposure to rug shampoo and residing in close proximity to bodies of water have been inconsistently associated risk factors in large epidemics

DIAGNOSIS

DIFFERENTIAL DIAGNOSIS
• Staphylococcal scalded skin syndrome
• Toxic shock syndrome
• Stevens-Johnson syndrome
• Reiter's syndrome
• Juvenile rheumatoid arthritis
• Scarlet fever
• Measles
• Rubella
• Roseola
• Epstein-Barr virus infections
• Mycoplasma infection
• Leptospirosis
• Lyme disease
• Rocky Mountain spotted fever
• Toxoplasmosis
• Acrodynia
• Drug reactions
• Other vasculitides

LABORATORY
• Anemia (normochromic, normocytic)
• Leukocytosis (12,000-40,000 cells/mm3) with immature forms
• Elevated CRP, ESR, and alpha1-antitrypsin concentrations
• Platelet counts rise in subacute phase and peak in convalescent at 750,000-1,500,000
• Thrombocytopenia associated with severe coronary disease and myocardial infarction
• Mildly elevated serum liver enzymes and bilirubin
• CSF pleocytosis may be seen
• Measles immunoglobulin (IgM) titer helpful in differentiating KS from measles
• Sterile urethral pyuria occurs in 30% of patients
Drugs that may alter lab results: N/A
Disorders that may alter lab results: N/A

PATHOLOGICAL FINDINGS
• During acute stage, neutrophilic infiltrates involving pericardium, myocardium, endocardium, and vascular endothelium may be present
• Necrosis may develop and result in aneurysmal dilatation of medium-sized arteries
• Mononuclear infiltration predominates in the second week of illness, gradually resolving with or without fibrosis
• In addition to cardiac involvement, arteritis may also develop in lungs, kidneys, gastrointestinal tract, and other organs

SPECIAL TESTS
• Quantitative serum immunoglobulins
• ANA, RF, VDRL, immune complexes, complement levels

IMAGING
• Electrocardiogram may show ischemia, arrhythmias
• Echocardiogram may show cardiomyopathy, pericardial effusion, coronary artery dilatation or aneurysms
• Radiography including angiography

DIAGNOSTIC PROCEDURES
• No laboratory study proves diagnosis; diagnosis rests on clinical features and exclusion of other illnesses in differential diagnosis
• Diagnosis of typical syndrome requires fever of at least 5 days' duration, plus 4 of the following 5 criteria:
  ◊ Mucous membrane changes
  ◊ Extremity changes
  ◊ Cervical lymphadenopathy of at least 1 cm in size
  ◊ Rash
  ◊ Conjunctival suffusion
• Atypical cases occur with incomplete clinical findings; frequency of coronary artery aneurysms may be higher in this subset of patients

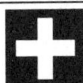

TREATMENT

APPROPRIATE HEALTH CARE When seen acutely, most children are hospitalized for diagnostic evaluation and supportive care. Older children with mild disease may be managed on an outpatient basis.

GENERAL MEASURES
• Antibiotics are given until bacterial etiologies are excluded
• Once KS is suspected, all patients need a cardiac evaluation, including electrocardiogram and echocardiogram
• Diuretics, inotropic agents, and pacemakers may be required for myocarditis

SURGICAL MEASURES
Aortocoronary artery bypass surgery for symptomatic patients with severe stenotic lesions (> 75% occluded)

ACTIVITY
May be limited if cardiac involvement

DIET
IV fluids may be needed if fever and irritability make feeding difficult

PATIENT EDUCATION N/A

MEDICATIONS

DRUG(S) OF CHOICE
• Aspirin: 80-100 mg/kg/day during the febrile phase. When child is afebrile, continue with low, single dose (5 mg/kg/day, to maximum of 80 mg) therapy for antithrombotic effects until active disease subsides.
• IV immune globulin (IVIG) 2 gm/kg at the time diagnosis is made (preferably within the first 10 days of illness) lowers the risk of coronary artery aneurysms and may shorten the duration of the acute phase. Retreatment is occasionally considered if clinical response is incomplete, although this has not been well studied.
Contraindications: Corticosteroids may increase the chance of aneurysm formation and should be avoided except in exceptional cases
Precautions: High dose salicylate therapy can cause tinnitus and hepatitis
Significant possible interactions: Aspirin therapy is associated with Reye's syndrome in children who develop viral infections, particularly influenza B and varicella. Influenza vaccination is recommended for children requiring aspirin therapy during influenza season, and aspirin should probably be discontinued if influenza or varicella infection occurs.

ALTERNATIVE DRUGS
• Dipyridamole, 4 mg/kg/d, is sometimes administered if coronary artery abnormalities develop
• Fibrinolytic agents (urokinase) for coronary artery thrombosis
• Alprostadil (prostaglandin E1) for peripheral artery ischemia
• Heparin followed by warfarin for large or multiple nonobstructive or obstructive aneurysms

FOLLOWUP

PATIENT MONITORING
• Monitor platelet count and acute phase reactant along with clinical course; when all return to normal, aspirin can be stopped
• Repeat ECG and echocardiogram at 3 and 8 weeks if initial studies are normal; may need further studies (e.g., angiography) if abnormal

PREVENTION/AVOIDANCE N/A

POSSIBLE COMPLICATIONS
• 20% of untreated patients develop coronary artery aneurysms in convalescent phase. Risk factors include:
  ◊ Male sex
  ◊ Age < 1 year old
  ◊ Fever > 2 weeks
  ◊ Elevated ESR for > 4 weeks
• Ischemic heart disease risk factors include:
  ◊ Aneurysms > 8 mm
  ◊ Diffuse or saccular aneurysm
  ◊ Fever > 21 days
  ◊ Steroid therapy
  ◊ Age > 2 years old
• Mortality 0.5%, related to cardiovascular disease

EXPECTED COURSE/PROGNOSIS
• Usually self-limited
• Only potentially permanent sequelae involve cardiovascular system
• Unknown but possible increased risk of atherosclerotic heart disease in adulthood
• Sudden death is possible

MISCELLANEOUS

ASSOCIATED CONDITIONS N/A

AGE-RELATED FACTORS
Pediatric: See Description
Geriatric: N/A
Others: N/A

PREGNANCY N/A

SYNONYMS
• Mucocutaneous lymph node syndrome
• Infantile periarteritis nodosa

ICD-9-CM 446.1 Kawasaki disease

SEE ALSO
• Polyarteritis nodosa
• Toxic shock syndrome

OTHER NOTES N/A

ABBREVIATIONS
KS = Kawasaki syndrome

REFERENCES
• Feigin RD, et al: Kawasaki disease. In: Oski FA, et al, eds. Principles and Practice of Pediatrics. 2nd Ed. Philadelphia, J.B. Lippincott Co.,1994
• American Academy of Pediatrics. Kawasaki disease. In: Peter G, ed. 1994 Red Book: Report of the Committee on Infectious Diseases. 23rd Ed. Elk Grove Village, IL, Academy of Pediatrics, 1994
• Wortmann DW, Nelson AM: Kawasaki syndrome. Rheum Dis Clin N Amer 1990;16:363
• Rowley AH. Kawasaki syndrome. Pediatr Clin North Am 1999 Apr;46(2):313-29
Illustrations: 2 available on CD-ROM
Internet references: http://www.5mcc.com

Author(s)
Mark R. Dambro, MD, FAAFP

Keloids

BASICS

DESCRIPTION Abnormally large overgrowth of fibrous tissue (scar) occurring as a result of trauma or irritation that does not subside with time
System(s) affected: Skin/Exocrine
Genetics:
• 5-15 times more common in blacks and Asians than Caucasians. In all races, more darkly pigmented individuals are at higher risk.
• Both autosomal dominant and autosomal recessive familial inheritance have been reported
Incidence/Prevalence in USA: Largely unknown, but does affect 4-16% of the black and Hispanic population
Predominant age: N/A
Predominant sex: Male = Female

SIGNS AND SYMPTOMS
• Pain
• Tenderness
• Hyperesthesia
• Pruritus
• Firm, smooth, elevated scar with sharply demarcated borders
• Initially may be pale or mildly erythematous
• Older lesion hypo- or hyperpigmented
• Scar extends beyond margins of the initial wound
• Over period of years, keloids continue to grow and may develop claw-like projections

CAUSES
• Wounds: traumatic, surgical, body piercing
• Burn injury
• Other injuries
  ◊ Insect bite
  ◊ Folliculitis barbae
  ◊ Acne

RISK FACTORS
• Family history of keloids
• Dark skin pigment
• Certain locations on the body, e.g., deltoids, chest, earlobes
• Pregnancy
• Adolescence

DIAGNOSIS

DIFFERENTIAL DIAGNOSIS
• Hypertrophic scar (usually spontaneously regress; do not cross wound margins)
• Dermatofibroma
• Infiltrating basal cell carcinoma

LABORATORY N/A
Drugs that may alter lab results: N/A
Disorders that may alter lab results: N/A

PATHOLOGICAL FINDINGS Histology
shows whorl-like arrangements of hyalinized collagen bundles with pressure thinning of papillary dermis and minimal elastic tissue

SPECIAL TESTS N/A

IMAGING N/A

DIAGNOSTIC PROCEDURES
• Biopsy, only if unable to differentiate from carcinoma, since a biopsy may increase the keloid's size. If possible, use a 2mm punch biopsy to minimize trauma.

TREATMENT

APPROPRIATE HEALTH CARE
Outpatient

GENERAL MEASURES
"Step care" is warranted, adding pressure and then radiation if steroid injections fail.
• Intralesional corticosteroid injections: cause atrophy and are most successful therapy
• Pressure bandages: must maintain 24 mm Hg, and should be worn for 6-12 months. Bandages should not be removed for more than 30 minutes/day. Pressure clips useful for earlobes.
• Radiation: no advantage over other methods, therefore use if other methods fail, and then use in conjunction with steroids and pressure
• Topical agents: No evidence to support efficacy; e.g., retinoic acid, vitamin E, antineoplastic agents, silicone gel

SURGICAL MEASURES
• Surgery - high recurrence rate (45-100%), therefore used only for debulking of large keloids or if a lesion is unresponsive to steroid injections alone
• Laser surgery - no definitive evidence of efficacy

ACTIVITY Full activity

DIET No special diet

PATIENT EDUCATION
• Stress possibility of recurrence despite appropriate treatment
• May require many months of treatment with combined modalities

MEDICATIONS

DRUG(S) OF CHOICE
• Triamcinolone suspension 10 mg/mL (Kenalog)
◊ Using 27-30 gauge needle and a TB syringe (total dose 20-30 mg of triamcinolone). May inject 3 lesions at a time, using 10 mg/lesion.
◊ Advance needle while injecting in order to evenly distribute medication
◊ Early keloids are more responsive to this therapy than older lesions
◊ Reinject every 4 weeks until keloid shrinks to near skin surface
◊ If no response to 10 mg/mL triamcinolone suspension, may try 40 mg/mL suspension
◊ May mix dilute triamcinolone (5-10 mg/mL) with local anesthetic for excision of keloids. Postoperative steroid injections at 2-4 weeks and then monthly for 6 months helps prevent recurrences.
Contraindications: None absolute
Precautions:
• Systemic absorption with adrenal suppression (reversible)
• Local affects - skin atrophy, ulceration, depigmentation, telangiectasias
• Both types of side effects more common with 40 mg/mL triamcinolone suspension
Significant possible interactions: Rare interactions (only with very large doses of corticosteroids and systemic absorption)

ALTERNATIVE DRUGS
• Verapamil locally may be helpful
• Interferon alpha 2b may be helpful after excision

FOLLOWUP

PATIENT MONITORING
Monthly visits, up to a year, for evaluation and possible steroid re-injections

PREVENTION/AVOIDANCE
• Primary prevention: avoid elective surgery or body piercing in high-risk patients
• Compressive pressure dressings may be useful in high risk (e.g., burn) patients. Local steroid injection postoperatively in high risk patients is also effective.

POSSIBLE COMPLICATIONS
Skin atrophy, ulceration, depigmentation, telangiectasias can occur as a result of local steroid injections

EXPECTED COURSE/PROGNOSIS
Lesions gradually diminish with therapy over a 6-18 month period, leaving a flat, shiny scar

MISCELLANEOUS

ASSOCIATED CONDITIONS
None

AGE-RELATED FACTORS
Keloid formation more common during adolescence
Pediatric: None
Geriatric: None
Others: N/A

PREGNANCY
Keloid formation more likely during pregnancy

SYNONYMS
• Razor bumps

ICD-9-CM
701.4 Keloid scar

SEE ALSO
N/A

OTHER NOTES
N/A

ABBREVIATIONS
N/A

REFERENCES
• Rook A, Wilkinson DS, Ebling FJG, et al: Textbook of Dermatology. 5th Ed. Oxford. Blackwell Scientific Publishing, 1992
• Berman B, Flores F. The treatment of hypertrophic scars and keloids. Eur J Derm 1998;8:591-5
• Lawrence WT. Treatment of earlobe keloids with surgery plus adjuvant intralesional verapamil and pressure earrings. Ann Plastic Surgery 1996;37:167-9
• Berman B, Bieley HC. Adjunct therapies to surgical management of keloids. Derm Surgery 1996;22:126-30
Illustrations: 4 available on CD-ROM
Internet references: http://www.5mcc.com

Author(s)
Ronald E Pust, MD

Keratosis, actinic

BASICS

DESCRIPTION Common, usually multiple premalignant skin lesions of sun-exposed areas. They are the most common indicator of excessive cumulative ultraviolet light exposure. The risk of transformation to squamous carcinoma is quite low: 1/4% risk of malignant transformation per lesion per year.

System(s) affected: Skin/Exocrine
Genetics: Relates to complexion
Incidence/Prevalence in USA: Common in blondes and redheads; rare in blacks
Predominant age: 40+; progressive with age (if child, look for freckling and other stigmata of xeroderma pigmentosum)
Predominant sex: Male > Female (from occupational sun exposure)

SIGNS AND SYMPTOMS
• Lesions usually fairly flat, red, and rough to palpitation
• Mild hyperesthesia common over lesions
• Hypertrophic verrucous lesions (called "cutaneous horns" if extreme) may be impossible to differentiate from squamous cell carcinoma clinically
• A pigmented variant also exists
• Actinic cheilitis usually involves lower lip
• Only photo-exposed areas involved, often with other stigmata of chronic actinic damage: lentigines, actinic elastosis, atrophy

CAUSES
• Short-wave ultraviolet light (UVB)
• Possibly ultraviolet (UVA)
• Bowen's disease can be caused by the carcinogenic types of human papilloma virus and arsenic exposure

RISK FACTORS
• Equatorial latitudes
• High elevations
• Outdoor occupation (farmers, sailors, ranchers)
• Outdoor athletics
• Sun worshippers
• Accompanying heat, wind, humidity augment carcinogenic effect
• Occupational exposure, i.e., petroleum products
• Immunosuppression, especially organ transplantation

DIAGNOSIS

DIFFERENTIAL DIAGNOSIS
• Squamous cell carcinoma (hypertrophic type)
• Verruca vulgaris (hypertrophic type)
• Seborrheic dermatitis or psoriasis (near hairline)
• Lentigo maligna (pigmented type)
• Lupus erythematosus

LABORATORY   N/A
Drugs that may alter lab results: N/A
Disorders that may alter lab results: N/A

PATHOLOGICAL FINDINGS
Diagnosis usually made clinically except where there is a suspicion of carcinoma
• Hyperkeratosis
• Hypertrophic, atrophic, Bowenoid, acantholytic, and pigmented varieties show the corresponding epidermal findings
• Malignant cells sparse except in Bowenoid variety
• Usually a sparse lymphocytic and plasma cell infiltrate

SPECIAL TESTS   N/A

IMAGING   N/A

DIAGNOSTIC PROCEDURES   Biopsy (shave)

TREATMENT

APPROPRIATE HEALTH CARE
Outpatient

GENERAL MEASURES   Sun-protective techniques (See Patient Education)

SURGICAL MEASURES
• Cryosurgery for smaller number of lesions
• For extensive lesions (but medical treatment usually preferred)
◊ Skin peels, i.e., 35% trichloracetic acid
◊ CO2 laser therapy
◊ Dermabrasion

ACTIVITY   No restrictions

DIET   No special diet

PATIENT EDUCATION
• Teach sun-protective techniques
• Transfer hobbies and other outdoor activities to early morning or late afternoon
• Wear protective clothing and hats
• Daily use of topically applied sunscreens with SPF greater than 15; preferably containing titanium dioxide or avobenzone (Parsol-1789) to afford protection in the UVA range also
• Teach self-examination for cutaneous carcinoma (melanoma, squamous cell, basal cell)

MEDICATIONS

DRUG(S) OF CHOICE
• Topical fluorouracil, destroys even subclinical lesions, also non-scarring; usually applied bid for 3-4 weeks (for larger number of lesions)
Contraindications: N/A
Precautions: Continue treatment to involved skin
Significant possible interactions: N/A

ALTERNATIVE DRUGS
• Topical tretinoin (Retin-A) may be used to enhance the efficacy of topical fluorouracil

FOLLOWUP

PATIENT MONITORING Dependent on associated malignancy and frequency with which new actinic keratoses appear

PREVENTION/AVOIDANCE Sun protective techniques (See Patient Education)

POSSIBLE COMPLICATIONS Actinic keratosis is a premalignant lesion and may undergo carcinomatous proliferation to become squamous cell carcinoma

EXPECTED COURSE/PROGNOSIS
Excellent, if prevention taken by patient

MISCELLANEOUS

ASSOCIATED CONDITIONS
• Squamous cell carcinoma

AGE-RELATED FACTORS
Pediatric: Rare
Geriatric: Frequent problem
Others: N/A

PREGNANCY   N/A

SYNONYMS   N/A

ICD-9-CM   701.1 Keratoderma, acquired

SEE ALSO
• Dermatitis, seborrheic

OTHER NOTES   N/A

ABBREVIATIONS   N/A

REFERENCES
• Dodson JM, et al: Malignant potential of actinic keratoses and controversy over treatment. Archives of Dermatology 1991;127:1029
• Lever WF, Schaumburg-Lever G: Histopathology of the Skin. 7th Ed. Philadelphia, J.B. Lippincott, 1990
Illustrations: 5 available on CD-ROM
Internet references: http://www.5mcc.com

Author(s)
John R. Person, MD

Labyrinthitis

BASICS

DESCRIPTION Inflammation of the vestibular labyrinth (a system of intercommunicating cavities and canals in the inner ear). There are many possible causes (see Differential Diagnosis). The most constant and pervasive symptom is vertigo.
System(s) affected: Nervous
Genetics: No known genetic pattern
Incidence/Prevalence in USA: Unknown
Predominant age: All ages beyond infancy
Predominant sex: Male = Female

SIGNS AND SYMPTOMS
• Vertigo
• Dizziness
• Hearing loss, fluctuating
• Nausea and vomiting
• Tinnitus
• Perspiration
• Increased salivation
• Generalized malaise
• Hypercapnia
• Nystagmus

CAUSES
• Physiological - mismatch of vestibular, visual and somatosensory systems triggered by an external stimulus, such as a stop after whirling turns, heights, motion sickness
• Pathological - imbalance in the vestibular system caused by a lesion within vestibular pathways (inner ear to cerebral cortex)
• Infections (especially viral)
• Tumors
• Vasculitis
• Infarction
• Ototoxic drugs, especially aminoglycosides
• Head injury
• Neuronitis

RISK FACTORS
• Trauma
• Stress
• Drug ingestion
• Predisposing virus infection
• Cardiovascular disease
• Cerebrovascular disease

DIAGNOSIS

DIFFERENTIAL DIAGNOSIS
• Acute viral labyrinthitis
• Benign positional vertigo
• Meniere's syndrome
• Postconcussion syndrome
• Chronic bacterial otomastoiditis
• Drug-induced damage to vestibular labyrinth
• Vascular insufficiency
• Cerebellopontine-angle tumors, such as acoustic neuroma
• Multiple sclerosis
• Para-infectious encephalomyelitis
• Para-infectious cranial polyneuritis
• Ramsay Hunt syndrome
• Cerebral or systemic vasculitis
• Temporal lobe epilepsy
• Benign positional vertigo

LABORATORY Routine laboratory studies not helpful
Drugs that may alter lab results: All drugs with potential ototoxicity
Disorders that may alter lab results: N/A

PATHOLOGICAL FINDINGS N/A

SPECIAL TESTS
• Electronystagmography
• Caloric test
• Doll's eye test
• Forced voluntary hyperventilation for 1 to 3 minutes to mimic symptoms if cause is physiologic or emotional

IMAGING CT or MRI for suspected lesions involving the eighth cranial nerve

DIAGNOSTIC PROCEDURES History and physical

TREATMENT

APPROPRIATE HEALTH CARE
Outpatient

GENERAL MEASURES
• Treat underlying disorder when possible
• Symptomatic treatment to accompany specific treatment

SURGICAL MEASURES N/A

ACTIVITY Lie still with eyes closed in darkened room during acute attacks. Otherwise, activity as tolerated.

DIET Reduced sodium

PATIENT EDUCATION Griffith, H.W.: Instructions for Patients, Philadelphia, W.B. Saunders Co.

MEDICATIONS

DRUG(S) OF CHOICE
• Meclizine (Antivert) 25 mg qid
• Diazepam (Valium) 5 mg qid
• Promethazine (Phenergan) 25 mg qid
• Prochlorperazine (Compazine) suppositories 25 mg, for vomiting
• Scopolamine transdermal where available
Contraindications: Refer to manufacturer's literature
Precautions: All the listed medications have significant adverse reactions. Use with caution. Avoid scopolamine in the elderly.
Significant possible interactions: Refer to manufacturer's literature

ALTERNATIVE DRUGS
• Diazepam 5 mg qid
• Prochlorperazine (Compazine) suppositories 25 mg

FOLLOWUP

PATIENT MONITORING As needed

PREVENTION/AVOIDANCE No preventive measures

POSSIBLE COMPLICATIONS
Permanent hearing loss

EXPECTED COURSE/PROGNOSIS
Depends on cause. Physiological labyrinthitis usually clears completely.

MISCELLANEOUS

ASSOCIATED CONDITIONS
• Ménière's disease
• Head injury

AGE-RELATED FACTORS
Pediatric: Unusual in this age group
Geriatric:
• Very common in this age group, especially benign positional vertigo
• Avoid scopolamine or use with extreme caution in this age group
Others: N/A

PREGNANCY Avoid medications

SYNONYMS
• Acute peripheral vestibulopathy
• Vestibular neuronitis

ICD-9-CM
386.30 Labyrinthitis, unspecified

SEE ALSO
• Ménière's disease
• Tinnitus

OTHER NOTES N/A

ABBREVIATIONS N/A

REFERENCES Baloh RW, Honrobia V: Clinical Neurology of the Vestibular System. 2nd Ed. Philadelphia, F.A. Davis Co, 1990
Illustrations: N/A
Internet references: http://www.5mcc.com

Author(s)
Marshall Godwin, MD

Lacrimal disorders

DESCRIPTION Lacrimal disorders refer to diseases and abnormalities of tear production and tear film. The most common lacrimal disorder is "dry eye." Lacrimal duct disorders, seen in the pediatric age group, often result in "overflow" tearing.
System(s) affected: Skin/Exocrine
Genetics: None
Incidence/Prevalence in USA: Very common and more often seen in arid climates of the desert Southwest
Predominant age: Dry eye symptoms increase with age. Most common in the elderly.
Predominant sex: Female > Male

SIGNS AND SYMPTOMS
• Gritty sensation to the eyes
• Visual blurring
• Redness
• Excessive tearing and mucus production
• Inadequate tears on the ocular surface

CAUSES Poor tear production and/or rapid evaporation of the tears

RISK FACTORS Individuals who live in arid regions, are on diuretics or have a history of collagen vascular diseases such as rheumatoid arthritis, Sjögren's syndrome, Bell's palsy, eyelid abnormalities and thyroid disease, are most at risk.

DIFFERENTIAL DIAGNOSIS Lacrimal disorders need to be differentiated from ocular infections and allergy. Another important consideration is the variety of anticholinergic affecting drugs that decrease tear production.

LABORATORY Tear production can be measured using a Schirmer's filter strip after instillation of topical anesthetic. Wetting of less than 10 mm of the slip after 5 minutes is indicative of insufficient tear production.
Drugs that may alter lab results: N/A
Disorders that may alter lab results: N/A

PATHOLOGICAL FINDINGS In Sjögren's syndrome infiltration of the lacrimal gland with inflammatory cells may be evident

SPECIAL TESTS N/A

IMAGING None

DIAGNOSTIC PROCEDURES Staining of the ocular surface with fluorescein will show areas of abnormal uptake and patches of drying. Rose bengal will be taken up by dead or dying epithelial cells and may be a more sensitive test.

APPROPRIATE HEALTH CARE
Outpatient

GENERAL MEASURES
• Those with systemic illnesses predisposed to dry eye should be informed and instructed in the appropriate use of artificial tear supplements
• Cool mist vaporizer and home humidification is helpful

SURGICAL MEASURES N/A

ACTIVITY No restrictions

DIET No special diet

PATIENT EDUCATION All individuals with systemic illnesses predisposed to dry eye, menopausal women, and those residing in arid climates or over the age of 60 should be instructed in the use of artificial tear supplements to combat dry eye symptoms

MEDICATIONS

DRUG(S) OF CHOICE
• Artificial tear drops excluding those that have preservatives. The dosage of the drop varies depending on the severity of the symptoms. Usually one drop in each eye several times throughout the day can prevent ocular discomfort.
• The use of a bland ophthalmic ointment at bedtime between the eyelid and the eye can help prevent drying of the eye at night
• Vitamin A supplements
Contraindications: N/A
Precautions: N/A
Significant possible interactions: N/A

ALTERNATIVE DRUGS   N/A

 FOLLOWUP

PATIENT MONITORING   Monitor early to determine the effectiveness of treatment. Occasionally the use of more viscous drops or increased frequency of tear supplements may be required.

PREVENTION/AVOIDANCE
• Prevent exposure to eye irritants from pollution, cigarette smoke, and sun exposure
• Ensure adequate vitamin A intake in the diet or as a supplement

POSSIBLE COMPLICATIONS   Severe dry eye can lead to corneal break-down, secondary invasion by bacteria and eye infections

EXPECTED COURSE/PROGNOSIS
Lacrimal disorders can be adequately managed with artificial tear supplements. Blocked tear ducts can be managed with probing and punctal dilation and/or dacryocysto-rhinostomy procedures in more severe cases.

 MISCELLANEOUS

ASSOCIATED CONDITIONS   Sjögren's syndrome and age-related factors more commonly seen in the elderly population

AGE-RELATED FACTORS
Pediatric: May find lacrimal duct blockage in infants
Geriatric: Most common in this age group
Others: N/A

PREGNANCY   Dry eyes can frequently be associated with pregnancy in an otherwise healthy individual. Vitamin A intake should not exceed 6000 IU a day.

SYNONYMS   Epiphoria (excessive tearing)

ICD-9-CM
375.11 Dacryops
375.15 Tear film insufficiency, unspecified

SEE ALSO
• Sjögren's syndrome

OTHER NOTES   Symptoms of dry eye are most often overlooked by practitioners when considering conjunctivitis (pink eye) and allergic disorders

ABBREVIATIONS   N/A

REFERENCES   Orbit Eyelids And Lacrimal System, Basic and Clinical Course. San Francisco, American Academy of Ophthalmology
Illustrations: N/A
Internet references: http://www.5mcc.com

Author(s)
Robert M. Kershner, MD, FACS

Lactose intolerance

BASICS

DESCRIPTION
Inability to digest lactose (the primary sugar in milk) into its constituents, glucose and galactose, due to low levels of lactase enzyme in the brush border of the duodenum
- Congenital lactose intolerance - very rare
- Primary lactose intolerance - common in adults in whom a low level of lactase has developed after childhood. Symptoms are experienced after consumption of milk. Intolerance varies with amount of lactose consumed.
- Secondary lactose intolerance - inability to digest lactose caused by any condition injuring the intestinal mucosa (e.g., diarrhea) or a reduction of available mucosal surface (e.g., resection). This is usually transient, with the duration of the intolerance determined by the nature and course of the primary condition.
- 50% or more of infants with acute or chronic diarrhea have lactose intolerance, especially with rotavirus disease. Also, fairly common with giardiasis and ascariasis, inflammatory bowel disease, and the AIDS malabsorption syndrome.
- Lactose malabsorption - inability to absorb lactose. This does not necessarily parallel lactose intolerance.

System(s) affected: Gastrointestinal, Endocrine/Metabolic

Genetics: Unknown

Incidence/Prevalence in USA:
- Primary lactose intolerance - varies according to race. 75-90% of American Indians, blacks, Asians, Mediterraneans and Jews, less than 5% of descendants of Northern and Central Europeans.
- Secondary lactose intolerance - 50% or more of infants with acute or chronic diarrheal disease have lactose intolerance, especially with rotavirus disease. Also fairly common with giardiasis and ascariasis, inflammatory bowel disease and the AIDS malabsorptive syndrome.

Predominant age:
- Primary - teenage and adult
- Secondary - depends on the underlying condition

Predominant sex: Male = Female. However, 44% of lactose intolerant women will regain the ability to digest lactose during pregnancy.

SIGNS AND SYMPTOMS
- Bloating
- Cramping
- Abdominal discomfort
- Diarrhea or loose stools
- Flatulence
- Rumbling (borborygmi)
- Only one-third to one-fifth of people with lactose malabsorption will develop symptoms. Degree of symptoms varies with lactose load and with other foods consumed at the same time.
- In children - vomiting is common; frothy, acid stools; malnutrition can occur

CAUSES
- Primary lactose intolerance - normal decline in the lactase activity in the intestinal mucosa after weaning which is genetically controlled and permanent
- Secondary lactose intolerance - associated with gastroenteritis in children
- Also nontropical and tropical sprue, regional enteritis, abetalipoproteinemia, cystic fibrosis, ulcerative colitis, immunoglobulin deficiencies in both adults and children

RISK FACTORS
- Race
- Age

DIAGNOSIS

DIFFERENTIAL DIAGNOSIS
Sucrase deficiency, diseases listed under secondary lactose intolerance

LABORATORY
Low fecal pH and reducing substances only valid when stools are collected fresh and assayed immediately. Fairly insensitive.
Drugs that may alter lab results: None
Disorders that may alter lab results: None

PATHOLOGICAL FINDINGS
Lactase deficiency in intestinal mucosa - may be patchy or focal. Rarely used in clinical practice.

SPECIAL TESTS
- Lactose breath hydrogen test - especially in children
- Lactose absorption test - alternative to lactose breath hydrogen test in adults

IMAGING
None

DIAGNOSTIC PROCEDURES
Small bowel biopsy for assay of lactase activity - may be normal if deficiency is focal or patchy (not readily available and usually not necessary)

TREATMENT

APPROPRIATE HEALTH CARE
Outpatient except severe cases of malnutrition

GENERAL MEASURES
No disease specific measures

SURGICAL MEASURES
N/A

ACTIVITY
Full activity

DIET
- Reduce or restrict dietary lactose to control symptoms
- Yogurt and fermented products such as hard cheeses are tolerated better than milk
- Supplement calcium in the form of calcium carbonate
- Commercially available "lactase" preparations (Lactaid or Lactrase) are effective in reducing symptoms in many people
- Prehydrolyzed milk (Lactaid) is available and effective

PATIENT EDUCATION
- Patients must read labels on commercial products since milk-sugar is used in many products and may cause symptoms
- Lactose intolerant patients may tolerate whole milk or chocolate milk better than skim
- Lactose consumed with other food products is better tolerated than when it is consumed alone
- Primary lactase deficiency is permanent; secondary lactose intolerance is usually temporary, though it may persist for several months after the inciting disease has been cured.

Lactose intolerance

MEDICATIONS

DRUG(S) OF CHOICE
• Lactase (Lactaid, Lactrase) tablets
  ◊ 1 to 2 capsules or tablets prior to ingesting milk products. These vary in effectiveness at preventing symptoms.
  ◊ Can add tablets or contents of capsules to milk before drinking
  ◊ Also available in milk in some areas
Contraindications: None
Precautions: Not effective for all people with lactose intolerance
Significant possible interactions: None

ALTERNATIVE DRUGS   None

FOLLOWUP

PATIENT MONITORING   N/A

PREVENTION/AVOIDANCE   Avoidance of lactose in large quantities will relieve symptoms. Patients can learn what level of lactose is tolerable in their diet.

POSSIBLE COMPLICATIONS   Calcium deficiency

EXPECTED COURSE/PROGNOSIS
• Normal life expectancy
• Symptoms can be controlled

MISCELLANEOUS:

ASSOCIATED CONDITIONS
• Tropical or nontropical sprue
• Giardiasis
• Immunoglobulin deficiencies
• Crohn's disease
• Cystic fibrosis

AGE-RELATED FACTORS
Pediatric:
• Primary lactose intolerance occurs after weaning - usually beginning in late childhood
• Breast milk contains a large quantity of lactose but does not seem to worsen diarrhea associated with viral or bacterial diseases
• Lactose free formulas are available
Geriatric: No increase in lactose intolerance in this age group
Others: Secondary lactose intolerance can begin at any age

PREGNANCY   44% of lactose intolerant women will be able to tolerate lactose while pregnant

SYNONYMS   Lactase deficiency

ICD-9-CM   271.3 intolerance or malabsorption (congenital) of lactose

SEE ALSO N/A

OTHER NOTES N/A

ABBREVIATIONS   N/A

REFERENCES
• Saavedra JM, Perman JA: Current Concepts in Lactose Malabsorption and Intolerance. Annu Rev Nutr 1989;9:475-502
• Hurst JW, ed: Medicine for the Practicing Physician. 2nd Ed. Boston, Butterworth, 1988
Illustrations: N/A
Internet references: http://www.5mcc.com

Author(s)
Kathryn Reilly, MD, MPH

Laryngeal cancer

BASICS

DESCRIPTION Most common cancer representing less than 1% of all malignant lesions. Squamous cell carcinomas comprise 5-98% of all malignant neoplasms of the larynx.
• Less than 2% of all carcinomas
• At the time of diagnosis, 62% will have local disease, 26% regional disease and 8% distant disease in the lungs, liver and/or bone
• No racial predilection
System(s) affected: Pulmonary
Genetics: Unknown
Incidence/Prevalence in USA: 5/100,00 (12,500 new cases per year)
Predominant age:
• Median age of occurrence in the 6th and 7th decades
• Less than 1% of laryngeal cancers arise in patients under 30 years of age
Predominant sex: Male > Female (5:1). However, increasing incidence in women who smoke.

SIGNS AND SYMPTOMS
• Persistent hoarseness in an elderly or middle aged cigarette smoker
• Dyspnea and stridor
• Ipsilateral otalgia
• Dysphagia
• Odynophagia
• Chronic cough
• Hemoptysis
• Weight loss due to poor nutrition
• Halitosis due to tumor necrosis
• Mass in the neck from metastatic lymph node
• Laryngeal tenderness due to tumor necrosis or suppuration
• Lump in the neck
• Broadening of the larynx on palpation with loss of crepitation
• Tenderness of the larynx
• Fullness of the cricothyroid membrane

CAUSES
• Smoking
• Alcohol abuse

RISK FACTORS Included in Causes

DIAGNOSIS

DIFFERENTIAL DIAGNOSIS
• Acute or chronic laryngitis
• Benign vocal cord lesions such as polyps, nodules, and papillomas
• Tuberculosis or fungal infection of the larynx

LABORATORY Liver function studies to rule out metastatic disease
Drugs that may alter lab results: N/A
Disorders that may alter lab results: N/A

PATHOLOGICAL FINDINGS N/A

SPECIAL TESTS
• Laryngoscopy - fungating, friable tumor with heaped up edges and granular appearance with multiple areas of central necrosis and exudate surrounding areas of hyperemia
• CT or MRI if chest and liver or brain metastasis suspected

IMAGING
• Bone scan if bone metastasis suspected
• Screening chest x-ray to rule out metastatic disease

DIAGNOSTIC PROCEDURES Indirect and/or direct laryngoscopy and biopsy to determine stage of disease as well as histologic confirmation

TREATMENT

APPROPRIATE HEALTH CARE
Outpatient primarily

GENERAL MEASURES Tracheotomy care, when applicable

SURGICAL MEASURES
• Tracheotomy may be necessary if tumor is large enough to cause upper airway obstruction
• Early disease may be treatable by either radiation therapy or laser cordectomy on an outpatient basis. 90% cure rates are the rule.
• More advanced disease needs inpatient care necessitating partial or total laryngectomy, and post-operative radiation therapy 4-5 weeks after surgery depending on the stage of disease

ACTIVITY Fully active unless the patient is debilitated from more advanced disease and/or greater degree of surgery

DIET
• Nasogastric or gastrostomy feeding may be necessary if tumor involves esophageal inlet
• No special diet otherwise

PATIENT EDUCATION Material is available from local cancer society

MEDICATIONS

DRUG(S) OF CHOICE
• Narcotics may be necessary for pain control during treatment for mucositis secondary to radiation therapy
• Nystatin mouth rinses for oral thrush
Contraindications: N/A
Precautions: N/A
Significant possible interactions: N/A

ALTERNATIVE DRUGS   N/A

FOLLOWUP

PATIENT MONITORING
• Repeat indirect laryngoscopy and complete head and neck examinations for at least five years after treatment to detect early recurrence or second primary
• Yearly chest x-ray and liver function tests
• Patients with dysphagia should undergo barium swallow and/or esophageal endoscopy to rule out second tumor in the esophagus
• Patients with unexplained pain should have appropriate radiological or nuclear medicine, bone scans
• Mental status change indicates CT scan of the brain to rule out brain metastases

PREVENTION/AVOIDANCE
• Indirect laryngoscopy for patients with persistent hoarseness lasting beyond one to two weeks
• Cessation of smoking and/or alcohol abuse

POSSIBLE COMPLICATIONS
• Temporary odynophagia or dysphagia secondary to mucositis and/or thrush during radiation therapy
• Persistent hoarseness despite adequate treatment necessitating further adjunctive procedures and/or speech therapy
• Tracheostomal stenosis requiring stenting with laryngectomy tubes or further surgery
• Dysphagia, secondary to upper esophageal stricture after total laryngectomy necessitating dilatation
• Aspiration, after partial laryngectomy necessitating completion laryngectomy or tracheotomy
• Inability to decannulate after partial laryngectomy due to laryngeal stenosis and/or aspiration
• Radiation induced chondronecrosis which mimics tumor recurrence
• Radiation edema necessitating emergent tracheotomy

EXPECTED COURSE/PROGNOSIS
• Early disease is expected to have greater than 90% cure

MISCELLANEOUS

ASSOCIATED CONDITIONS
• Less than 10% of patients may have a synchronous squamous cell carcinoma in the lower or upper aero-digestive tract; most notably in the esophagus or lungs

AGE-RELATED FACTORS
Pediatric: N/A
Geriatric: N/A
Others: N/A

PREGNANCY
• Very rare in young patients in general
• Natural history of disease and treatment side effects have to be weighed against the possibilities of continuing on to delivery

SYNONYMS   Cancer of larynx

ICD-9-CM   161.0 Malignant neoplasm of larynx

SEE ALSO   N/A

OTHER NOTES   N/A

ABBREVIATIONS   N/A

REFERENCES
• Suen JY, Myers EN: Cancer of the Head and Neck. 3rd Ed. Philadelphia, WB Saunders Co, 1996
• Ariyan S: Cancer of the Head and Neck. St. Louis, C.V. Mosby, 1987
Illustrations: N/A
Internet references: http://www.5mcc.com

Author(s)
Roy R. Casiano, MD

Laryngitis

 BASICS

DESCRIPTION
Inflammation of the mucosa of the larynx. Most common during peaks paralleling epidemics of individual viruses, late fall, winter, early spring. Course may be acute or chronic. Includes atrophic, hypertrophic, reflux, catarrhal, sicca, acute infectious, membranous, granulomatous.

System(s) affected: Pulmonary
Genetics: No known genetic pattern
Incidence/Prevalence in USA: Common
Predominant age: All ages
Predominant sex: Male = Female

SIGNS AND SYMPTOMS
- Hoarseness
- Abnormal sounding voice
- Aphonia or dysphasia
- Throat tickling
- Feeling of throat rawness
- Constant urge to clear the throat
- Fever
- Malaise
- Dysphagia
- Throat pain
- Cough
- Regional lymphadenopathy
- Stridor in children

CAUSES
- Virus infections - influenza A, B, parainfluenza, adenovirus, coronavirus, rhinovirus, HPV, CMV, HSV
- Bacterial infections - beta-hemolytic streptococcus, Streptococcus pneumoniae, H. influenza, tuberculosis, leprosy, Moraxella catarrhalis
- Excessive use of voice
- Inhaling irritating substances
- Aspiration of caustic chemical
- Aging changes - muscle atrophy, loss of moisture in larynx, bowing of vocal cords
- Esophageal reflux
- Fungal infections
- Parasites
- Spirochetes (syphilis)
- Allergic
- Autoimmune
- Idiopathic

RISK FACTORS
- Acute
  ◊ Upper respiratory tract infection
  ◊ Bronchitis
  ◊ Pneumonia
  ◊ Influenza
  ◊ Pertussis
  ◊ Measles
  ◊ Diphtheria
  ◊ Immunocompromised
- Chronic
  ◊ Allergy
  ◊ Chronic rhinitis
  ◊ Chronic sinusitis
  ◊ Voice abuse
  ◊ Reflux of gastric contents
  ◊ Smoking
  ◊ Alcohol abuse
  ◊ Constant exposure to dust or other irritants

 DIAGNOSIS

DIFFERENTIAL DIAGNOSIS
- Croup
- Measles
- Diphtheria
- Vocal nodules
- Laryngeal malignancy
- Thyroid malignancy

LABORATORY
WBC elevated in bacterial laryngitis
Drugs that may alter lab results: N/A
Disorders that may alter lab results: N/A

PATHOLOGICAL FINDINGS
N/A

SPECIAL TESTS
Virus culture (seldom necessary)

IMAGING
Only if needed for differential diagnosis

DIAGNOSTIC PROCEDURES
- Fiberoptic or indirect laryngoscopy - red, inflamed and occasionally hemorrhagic vocal cords, with rounded edges, and exudate
- Consider biopsy - chronic laryngitis in adults with history of smoking or alcohol abuse
- Consider 24° pH probe - chronic laryngitis in adults with gastroesophageal reflux

 TREATMENT

APPROPRIATE HEALTH CARE
Outpatient

GENERAL MEASURES
- Acute
  ◊ Usually a self-limited illness and not severe
  ◊ Voice rest
  ◊ Steam inhalations or cool-mist humidifier
  ◊ Increase fluid intake
  ◊ Analgesics
  ◊ Avoid smoking (or cigarette smoke from others) during acute phase
- Chronic
  ◊ Symptomatic treatment as above
  ◊ Voice therapy
  ◊ Stop smoking
  ◊ Reduce alcohol intake
  ◊ Occupational change or modification, if exposure
  ◊ For reflux laryngitis - elevate head of bed, other antireflux management

SURGICAL MEASURES
- Vocal cord stripping of hyperplastic mucosa and areas of leukoplakia (can be used for biopsy, may produce a more normal sounding voice)

ACTIVITY
Rest until fever subsides then, no restrictions

DIET
No special diet

PATIENT EDUCATION
- Provide assistance with smoking cessation
- Help patient with modification of other predisposing habits or occupational hazards

MEDICATIONS

DRUG(S) OF CHOICE
• Usually none
• Analgesics
• Antipyretics to reduce fever
• Cough suppressants
• Penicillin V 250 mg or erythromycin 250 mg - orally q6h for 10-12 days (for streptococcal or pneumococcal infections)
• Antacids or H2 blockers for GERD

Contraindications: Refer to manufacturer's literature

Precautions: Refer to manufacturer's literature

Significant possible interactions: Refer to manufacturer's literature

ALTERNATIVE DRUGS   N/A

FOLLOWUP

PATIENT MONITORING   None needed (usually)

PREVENTION/AVOIDANCE
• Avoid overuse of voice
• Prompt treatment of respiratory infections
• Influenza virus vaccine for high-risk individuals

POSSIBLE COMPLICATIONS   Chronic hoarseness

EXPECTED COURSE/PROGNOSIS
Complete clearing of the inflammation without sequelae

MISCELLANEOUS

ASSOCIATED CONDITIONS
• Viral pharyngitis
• Croup
• Bronchitis
• Pneumonitis

AGE-RELATED FACTORS
Pediatric: Common in this age group
Geriatric: May be sicker and slower to heal
Others: N/A

PREGNANCY   Use only safe antibiotics, if antibiotics are essential

SYNONYMS
• Acute laryngitis
• Chronic laryngitis

ICD-9-CM
464.0 Acute
476.0 Chronic

SEE ALSO   N/A

OTHER NOTES   N/A

ABBREVIATIONS   N/A

REFERENCES
• Avila MM, Carballal G, Rovaletti H, et al: Viral etiology in acute respiratory infections. Am Rev Respir Dis 1989;140:634
• Adams GL, et al: Fundamentals of Otolaryngology. 6th Ed. Philadelphia, W.B. Saunders Co., 1989
• Ballenger JI, Snow JB, eds: Otorhinolaryngology Head and Neck Surgery. 15 Ed. Philadelphia, Williams & Wlkins, 1996
Illustrations: N/A
Internet references: http://www.5mcc.com

Author(s)
Bruce T. Vanderhoff, MD
Anna N. Maxey, MD

Laryngotracheobronchitis

BASICS

DESCRIPTION Subacute viral illness, characterized by barking cough, stridor and fever, often causing upper airway obstruction in children. Most common cause of stridor in children.
System(s) affected: Pulmonary
Genetics: Unknown, though 15% have family history
Incidence/Prevalence in USA: 15,000-40,000/100,000
Predominant age: Childhood
Predominant sex: Male = Female

SIGNS AND SYMPTOMS
- Barking, spasmodic cough
- Biphasic stridor
- Low-grade to moderate fever
- Upper respiratory infection prodrome lasting 1-7 days
- Hypoxia/cyanosis
- Fatigue
- Non-toxic appearing child
- Normal voice, no drooling
- No change in stridor with positioning
- Non-tender larynx
- Inflamed subglottic region
- Normal appearing supraglottic region

CAUSES
- Parainfluenza 1
- Paramyxovirus
- Influenza virus type A
- Other parainfluenza and influenza viruses
- Respiratory syncytial virus
- Other viruses - adenovirus, rhinovirus, enterovirus, coxsackievirus, ECHO virus, reovirus, measles virus

RISK FACTORS
- Past history of croup
- Recurrent upper respiratory infections

DIAGNOSIS

DIFFERENTIAL DIAGNOSIS
- Epiglottitis
- Foreign body aspiration
- Subglottic stenosis (congenital or acquired)
- Bacterial tracheitis
- Simple upper respiratory infection
- Subglottic hemangioma
- Diphtheria

LABORATORY
- Leukopenia early
- Leukocytosis in severe later stage
Drugs that may alter lab results: N/A
Disorders that may alter lab results: N/A

PATHOLOGICAL FINDINGS
- Inflammatory reaction of respiratory mucosa
- Loss of epithelial cells
- Thick mucoid secretions

SPECIAL TESTS Rapid antigen tests are available in some centers

IMAGING
- PA and lateral neck films show funnel-shaped subglottic region with normal epiglottis - "steeple sign" or "pencil-point sign" (present in 40% of children with LTB)
- Patient should be monitored during imaging - progression of airway obstruction may be rapid

DIAGNOSTIC PROCEDURES
- Direct laryngoscopy - if child is not in acute distress
- Fiberoptic laryngoscopy - procedure of choice where available
- Bronchoscopy

TREATMENT

APPROPRIATE HEALTH CARE
- Outpatient in mild cases only
- Intensive care unit for patients with tachypnea, tachycardia, hypoxia, cyanosis, reactions, pneumonia, or congestive heart failure

GENERAL MEASURES
- Humidification - "croup tent"
- Intravenous fluids
- Electrocardiographic monitoring and pulse oximetry

SURGICAL MEASURES
- Intubation required in 6-10% for 3-5 days; use smallest tube possible
- Tracheotomy - rarely

ACTIVITY Must keep patient quiet; crying may exacerbate symptoms

DIET
- NPO with IV fluids for severe cases
- Frequent small feedings with increased fluids for mild cases

PATIENT EDUCATION
- Educate parents about when to seek emergency care if mild cases progress
- Emotional support and reassurance for the patient

MEDICATIONS

DRUG(S) OF CHOICE
• Dexamethasone: 1-1.5 mg/kg up to 20 mg every 8-12 hours for 8 doses
• Racemic epinephrine (Vaponefrin): 0.2-0.5 mL of 2.25 percent racemic epinephrine delivered in 2-3 mL of normal saline - one dose per 30 minutes, monitoring for side effects and rebound
• Antibiotics controversial in this viral illness
• Oxygen as needed
Contraindications: Refer to manufacturer's literature
Precautions: Avoid over sedation
Significant possible interactions: Refer to manufacturer's literature

ALTERNATIVE DRUGS
• Budesonide 2 mg nebulized; a topical glucocorticoid
• Ribavirin for respiratory syncytial virus
• Amantadine for influenza A

FOLLOWUP

PATIENT MONITORING
Severe cases require ICU care with respiratory monitoring for hypoxemia and hypercapnia

PREVENTION/AVOIDANCE   N/A

POSSIBLE COMPLICATIONS
• Subglottic stenosis in intubated patients
• Bacterial tracheitis
• Cardiopulmonary arrest
• Pneumonia

EXPECTED COURSE/PROGNOSIS
• Upper respiratory infection prodrome of 1-7 days
• If required, intubation is maintained for 3-5 days
• If required, tracheotomy is maintained for 3-7 days
• Recovery is usually full, without lasting effects

MISCELLANEOUS

ASSOCIATED CONDITIONS
If recurrent, search for underlying anatomic abnormality such as subglottic stenosis or consider foreign body

AGE-RELATED FACTORS
Pediatric: Common in children under the age of three
Geriatric: N/A
Others: N/A

PREGNANCY   N/A

SYNONYMS
• Croup
• Infectious croup
• Viral croup
• LTB

ICD-9-CM
464.20 Acute
464.21 With obstruction
476.1 Catarrhal, chronic, atrophic

SEE ALSO
• Bronchiolitis
• Common cold
• Epiglottitis
• Tracheitis, bacterial

OTHER NOTES
Less severe "variant" form, spasmodic croup, consists of croupy cough which becomes worse at night, but has no fever or x-ray changes. Usually resolves with mist therapy at home.

ABBREVIATIONS
LTB = laryngotracheobronchitis

REFERENCES
• Ballenger JJ: Diseases of the Nose, Throat and Ear. Philadelphia, Lea & Febiger, 1991
• Gates GA: Current Therapy in Otolaryngology - Head and Neck Surgery. 4th Ed. Philadelphia, B.C. Decker, Inc., 1990
Illustrations: N/A
Internet references: http://www.5mcc.com

Author(s)
Laurene L. Howell, MD
Gregg W. Suits, MD

Laxative abuse

BASICS

DESCRIPTION Diarrhea caused by self-medication or by a patient simulating diarrhea by the addition of fluid (e.g., urine) to the stool.
System(s) affected: Gastrointestinal, Nervous
Genetics: N/A
Incidence/Prevalence in USA: N/A
Predominant age:
• 18 to 40 years with bulimia nervosa
• 40 to 60 years without bulimia.
Predominant sex: Female > Male
Predominant race: N/A

SIGNS AND SYMPTOMS
• Diarrhea
• Additional symptoms - abdominal pain, rectal pain, nausea, vomiting, weight loss, muscle weakness, bone pain
• Additional signs - hypokalemia, skin pigmentation, finger clubbing, cyclic edema, kidney stones, melanosis coli
• The signs and symptoms will persist in spite of years of investigation and re-evaluation

CAUSES
• Ingestion of any laxative agent
• Psychological factors
  ◊ Bulimia nervosa
  ◊ Secondary gain of attention
  ◊ Hysterical behavior
  ◊ Multiple personality disorders
  ◊ Inappropriate perception of "normal" bowel habits
• Chronic constipation

RISK FACTORS See Causes

DIAGNOSIS

DIFFERENTIAL DIAGNOSIS Include any source of diarrhea of secretory or osmotic source

LABORATORY
• Serum test - hypokalemia, metabolic alkalosis
• Urinalysis may be abnormal
• Stool Na+, K+
• Stool pH (alkalinization suggests presence of phenolphthalein)
• Stool for laxative titers
• Urine volume and electrolytes
Drugs that may alter lab results: N/A
Disorders that may alter lab results: N/A

PATHOLOGICAL FINDINGS
• Melanosis coli
• "Cathartic colon" - refers to dilatation and ahaustral appearance on barium enema

SPECIAL TESTS Hospital room search

IMAGING Barium enema - cathartic colon

DIAGNOSTIC PROCEDURES
• Carefully selected when needed to rule out other diseases
• Try not to repeat prior evaluations
• Sigmoidoscopy
• High index of suspicion

TREATMENT

APPROPRIATE HEALTH CARE
Hospitalization may be needed (hypokalemia, malnutrition)

GENERAL MEASURES
• Psychological support is essential
• Confrontation of the patient, gently and with support and understanding
• Discontinue laxative use
• Long term laxative abuse requires weaning
• Treat constipation

SURGICAL MEASURES N/A

ACTIVITY Physical exercise program

DIET
• Ensure good nutritional habits
  ◊ Increase fiber intake
  ◊ Adequate calories, especially with bulimia

PATIENT EDUCATION See General Measures

MEDICATIONS

DRUG(S) OF CHOICE
• Based on psychological assessment
• Non-stimulant laxatives if needed
  ◊ Senna best during pregnancy and lactation
  ◊ Lactulose
  ◊ Fiber
Contraindications: Dantron - hepatotoxic
Precautions: Patients will be manipulative in attempts to hide problem, and often large quantities of laxatives
Significant possible interactions:
• Increased rate of intestinal flow may affect rate of absorption of medications: antibiotics, hormones, etc.
• Docusate sodium may potentiate hepatotoxicity of other drugs

ALTERNATIVE DRUGS N/A

FOLLOWUP

PATIENT MONITORING
• Careful psychological counseling
• Careful medical support. Show concern by frequent visits as needed.
• Assess serum electrolytes

PREVENTION/AVOIDANCE
• Suspicion in patients with unsolved chronic diarrhea
• Monitor "doctor hopping"
• Avoid exploratory surgery
• Avoid repeated testing for diagnosis

POSSIBLE COMPLICATIONS
• Risk of multiple tests and procedures and surgeries
• Malnutrition
• Electrolyte imbalances (hypokalemia)
• Renal failure
• Fatalities especially in children given laxatives by parents
• Renal calculi

EXPECTED COURSE/PROGNOSIS
• Protracted course
• Prognosis related to psychological response

MISCELLANEOUS

ASSOCIATED CONDITIONS N/A

AGE-RELATED FACTORS
Pediatric:
• Death
• Life long laxative dependence
Geriatric:
• Unusual to start beyond age of 60 years
• Rectal incontinence
Others: N/A

PREGNANCY N/A

SYNONYMS
• Factitious diarrhea
• Cathartic colon

ICD-9-CM 305.9 Other mixed, or unspecified drug abuse

SEE ALSO
• Bulimia nervosa
• Constipation
• Hypokalemia
• Renal failure, acute (ARF)
• Renal failure, chronic
• Renal calculi

OTHER NOTES N/A

ABBREVIATIONS N/A

REFERENCES
• Sleisenger MH, Fordtran JS., eds: Gastrointestinal Disease: Pathophysiology, Diagnosis, Management. 6th Ed. Philadelphia, WB Saunders Co, 1998
• Baker EH, Sandle GI: Complications of laxative abuse. Ann Rev of Med 1996;47:127
• Batal H, Johnson M, et al: Bulimia: a primary care approach. J Womens Health 1998;7(2):211
Illustrations: N/A
Internet references: http://www.5mcc.com

Author(s)
Duane C. Roe, MD

Lead poisoning

BASICS

DESCRIPTION Consequence of a high body burden of lead, an element with no known physiologic value
System(s) affected: Endocrine/Metabolic, Nervous, Gastrointestinal
Genetics: N/A
Incidence/Prevalence in USA:
• 17% of preschoolers in the US have a blood lead greater than 15 µg/dL (0.72 µmol/L). Sporadic cases in adults.
• Estimated (1990's) in children 6 months to age 5 years (≥ 15 µg/dL [0.72 µmol/L]): 17,000/100,000
Predominant age: 1-5 years old; adult worker
Predominant sex: Male = Female

SIGNS AND SYMPTOMS
• Often asymptomatic
• Mild to moderate toxicity
  ◊ May cause myalgia or paresthesia, fatigue, irritability, lethargy
  ◊ Abdominal discomfort, arthralgia, difficulty concentrating, headache, tremor, vomiting, weight loss, muscular exhaustibility
• Severe toxicity - leads to 3 major clinical syndromes
  ◊ Alimentary type - anorexia, metallic taste, constipation, severe abdominal cramps due to intestinal spasm and sometimes associated with rigidity of the abdominal wall
  ◊ Neuromuscular type (characteristic of adult plumbism) - peripheral neuritis usually painless and limited to extensor muscles
  ◊ Cerebral type or lead encephalopathy (more common in children) - seizures, coma, long-term sequelae including neurologic defects, retarded mental development, chronic hyperactivity
  ◊ Chronic exposure may cause renal failure

CAUSES Inhalation of lead dust or fumes, or ingestion of lead

RISK FACTORS
• Children with pica
• Children with iron deficiency anemia
• Residence or frequent visitor in deteriorating, pre-1960 housing with leaded-paint surfaces
• Children with seizures
• Children with hyperkinetic or autistic behavior
• Sibling or playmate with lead poisoning
• Dust from clothing of lead worker
• Lead dissolved in water from lead or lead-soldered plumbing
• Lead glazed ceramics, especially with acidic food or drink
• Food stored in inverted plastic bread bags printed with colored ink
• Colored comics
• Soil/dust near lead industries and roads
• Folk remedies (Mexican - azarcon, greta; Asian - chuifong tokuwan, pay-loo-ah, ghasard, bali goli, kandu; Middle Eastern - alkohl, surma, saoott, cebagin)

• Hobbies - glazed pottery making; target shooting at firing ranges; lead soldering; painting; preparing lead shot, fishing sinkers; stained-glass making; car or boat repair; home remodeling
• Occupational exposure - plumbers, pipe fitters, lead miners, auto repairers, glass manufacturers, shipbuilders, printers, plastic manufacturers, lead smelters and refiners, policemen, steel welders or cutters, construction workers, rubber product manufacturers, gas station attendants, battery manufacturers, bridge reconstruction workers
• Dietary - zinc or calcium deficiency

DIAGNOSIS

DIFFERENTIAL DIAGNOSIS
• Elevated erythrocyte protoporphyrin may be due to iron deficiency anemia, less commonly hemolytic anemia. Erythropoietic protoporphyria produces a very high erythrocyte protoporphyrin.
• Alimentary type may be confused with acute abdomen
• Neuromuscular type may be confused with other polyneuropathies
• Cerebral type may be confused with attention deficit disorder, mental retardation, autism, dementia, other causes of seizures

LABORATORY
• Blood lead (Pb) greater than 10 µg/dL (0.48 µmol/L), collected with lead-free container
CDC classification:

```
----------------------------
Class Lead (µg/dL)
I    < 10    (< 0.48 µmol/L)
II   10-19   (0.48-0.92 µmol/L)
III  20-44   (0.97-2.12 µmol/L)
IV   45-69   (2.17-3.33 µmol/L)
V    > 70    (> 3.38 µmol/L)
----------------------------
```

• Asymptomatic patient screening with erythrocyte protoporphyrin level (EP) greater than 35 µg/dL (0.62 µmol/L) indicates need for testing blood Pb
• Hgb and Hct slightly low. Eosinophilia or basophilic stippling on peripheral smear may be seen, but are not diagnostic of lead toxicity.
• Renal function decreased in late stages
Drugs that may alter lab results: N/A
Disorders that may alter lab results: N/A

PATHOLOGICAL FINDINGS N/A

SPECIAL TESTS Calcium ethylenediaminetetraacetic acid (Ca EDTA) mobilization test if blood Pb 25-44 µg/dL (1.21-2.12 µmol/L). This test is not widely used because it is technically difficult to perform and may delay diagnosis and treatment.

IMAGING Abdominal radiograph for lead particles in gut. X-ray of long bones for lines of increased density in the metaphyseal plate resulting from growth arrest.

DIAGNOSTIC PROCEDURES N/A

TREATMENT

APPROPRIATE HEALTH CARE
Outpatient unless parenteral chelation required

GENERAL MEASURES
• Case report to local health department for Class III-V. Complete inspection of home or work-place to determine source of lead. Screen all family members.
• Consider oral chelation for Class III or IV. Chelation (preferably parenteral) for Class V or symptomatic Class III or IV
• Remove from potential source of lead for Class IV or V, until complete inspection is performed

SURGICAL MEASURES N/A

ACTIVITY
• Avoid activity at any site of potential contamination

DIET
• If symptomatic, avoid excessive fluids
• Avoidance of pica
• Consume adequate calcium and iron
• Eat a low fat diet to reduce absorption and retention of lead

PATIENT EDUCATION
• Raising Children Toxic Free: How to keep your child safe from lead, asbestos, pesticides, and other environmental hazards. HL Needleman, PJ Landrigan. New York, Avon Books, 1994
• National Lead Information Center, 800-424-5323
• Alliance to End Childhood Lead Poisoning, 227 Massachusetts Ave, NE, Washington, DC 20002; 202-543-1147; http://www.aeclp.org

Lead poisoning

MEDICATIONS

DRUG(S) OF CHOICE
• Oral chelation:
◊ Succimer (Chemet, dimercaptosuccinic acid, DMSA) 10 mg/kg q8h x 5 days, then 10 mg/kg q12h x 2 weeks. May be repeated after 2 weeks off if lead levels are not stabilized below < 15 µg/dL (< 0.72 µmol/L).
• Parenteral chelation (begin after establishment of adequate urine output):
◊ Class V or symptomatic: dimercaprol (British anti-Lewisite, BAL) 75 mg/m2 given deep IM, then BAL 450 mg/m2/d divided q4h x 5 days + Ca EDTA (edetate calcium disodium) 1500 mg/m2/d continuous IV infusion x 5 days. If rebound lead level ≥ 45 µg/dL (≥ 2.17 µmol/L), chelation may be repeated after 2 day interval if symptomatic, after 5 day interval if symptomatic.
◊ Class IV asymptomatic: Ca EDTA 1000 mg/m2/d x 5 days. May be repeated after 5-7 days.
• Diazepam for initial control of seizures, further control maintained with paraldehyde

Contraindications:
• BAL should not be given to persons allergic to peanuts (the drug solution contains peanut oil)

Precautions:
• Succimer: Gastrointestinal upset, rash, nasal congestion, muscle pains, elevated liver function tests
• Ca EDTA: Renal failure, increased excretion of zinc, copper and iron
• BAL: Nausea, vomiting, fever, headache, transient hypertension, hepatocellular damage

Significant possible interactions:
• Vitamins should not be given concurrently with oral chelation
• BAL may precipitate hemolytic crisis in a patient with G6PD deficiency

ALTERNATIVE DRUGS
• Oral chelation with penicillamine (d-penicillamine, Depen, Cuprimine)
◊ Penicillin allergic patient should not receive D-penicillamine (cross-sensitivity is common)
◊ 10-20 mg/kg bid mixed in apple juice/sauce on empty stomach (not FDA approved)
◊ D-penicillamine may cause gastrointestinal upset, renal failure, granulocytopenia, liver dysfunction, iron deficiency, drug induced lupus-like syndrome

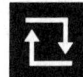

FOLLOWUP

PATIENT MONITORING
• After chelation, check for rebound Pb level in 7-10 days. Follow with regular monitoring, initially biweekly or monthly.
• Correct iron deficiency or any other nutritional deficiencies present
• For Class II or higher, repeat testing every 3 months until Class I level achieved

PREVENTION/AVOIDANCE
• Family should receive counseling on potential sources of lead and methods to decrease lead exposure. Wet mopping and dusting with a high phosphate solution (e.g., powdered automatic dishwasher detergent with 1/4 cup per gallon of water) will help control lead-bearing dust.
• If the source is in the home, the patient must reside elsewhere until the abatement process is completed

POSSIBLE COMPLICATIONS
• CNS toxicity may be long lasting or permanent
• Long-term lead exposure may cause chronic renal failure (Fanconi-like syndrome); gout; lead line (blue-black) on gingival tissue

EXPECTED COURSE/PROGNOSIS
• Symptomatic lead poisoning without encephalopathy generally improves with chelation, but subtle CNS toxicity may be long lasting or permanent
• If encephalopathy occurs, permanent sequelae (mental retardation, seizure disorder, blindness, hemiparesis) in 25-50%

MISCELLANEOUS

ASSOCIATED CONDITIONS
Iron deficiency anemia

AGE-RELATED FACTORS
Pediatric:
• Increasing evidence that low lead level exposure (as low as 10 µg/dL [0.48 µmol/L]) may produce neurotoxicity in children
• Children are at increased risk because of incomplete development of the blood-brain barrier before age 3 years allowing more lead into the central nervous system; ingested lead has 40% bioavailability in children compared with 10% in adults
• Common childhood behaviors such as frequent hand-to-mouth activity and pica (repeated ingestion of nonfood products) greatly increase the risk of ingesting lead
Geriatric: N/A
Others: N/A

PREGNANCY
• Lead exposure in pregnancy is associated with reduced birth weight and premature birth
• Lead is an animal teratogen

SYNONYMS
Lead poisoning, inorganic

ICD-9-CM
984.9 Toxic effect of unspecified lead compound

SEE ALSO
• Iron deficiency anemia
• Nephropathy, chronic lead

OTHER NOTES
Screening is recommended for asymptomatic children during their first 4 years of life living in high risk areas (> 12% elevated). Children in a low risk area should be screened by a questionnaire. Screening EP is not sensitive for blood Pb less than 25 µg/dL (1.20 µmol/L).

ABBREVIATIONS
Pb = lead
EP = erythrocyte protoporphyrin
BAL = British anti-Lewisite

REFERENCES
• Royce S: Case studies in environmental medicine: lead toxicity. US Dept. HHS, PHS, ATSDR, 1992
• Centers for Disease Control: Preventing lead poisoning in young children. US Dept. HHS, PHS, CDC, Atlanta, 1991
• Centers for Disease Control: Screening young children for lead poisoning: guidance for state and local public health officials. Atlanta, CDC, 1997
Illustrations: 1 available on CD-ROM
Internet references: http://www.5mcc.com

Author(s)
Jason Chao, MD, MS

Légg-Calvé-Pérthes disease

BASICS

DESCRIPTION Idiopathic necrosis of capital femoral epiphysis of the femoral head. 10-20% of cases are bilateral.
System(s) affected: Musculoskeletal
Genetics: No known genetic pattern identified
Incidence/Prevalence in USA: Incidence 15/100,000; prevalence 75/100,000
Predominant age: Susceptible age 2-12 years. However, approximately 80% occur between the ages of 4 and 9 years
Predominant sex: Males > Females (4:1). In bilateral cases males prodominate 7:1. However, females seem to have more severe involvement.

SIGNS AND SYMPTOMS
• Primarily hip or groin pain although with referred pain to the knee and thigh not uncommon
• Range of motion limited, especially in internal rotation and abduction
• Atrophy of thigh musculature due to disuse
• Leg length discrepancy secondary to collapse of the femoral head

CAUSES
• Etiology unclear
• Felt to be related to interruption of blood flow to femoral epiphysis
• Role of biochemical factors remains to be established

RISK FACTORS
• No genetic risk factors
• Increased incidence in children with low birth weight and delayed physical maturation

DIAGNOSIS

DIFFERENTIAL DIAGNOSIS
• Unilateral - septic arthritis, toxic synovitis, juvenile rheumatoid arthritis
• Bilateral - spondyloepiphyseal dysplasia, metaphyseal dysplasia

LABORATORY
• CBC
• Sedimentation rate (elevated in infection)
Drugs that may alter lab results: N/A
Disorders that may alter lab results: N/A

PATHOLOGICAL FINDINGS
• Early (necrosis, resorption) stage - necrosis of bone with subchondral bone fracture and subsequent collapse of subchondral bone
• Late (healing) stage - revascularization by creeping substitution of necrotic bone

SPECIAL TESTS

IMAGING
• Serial radiographs, AP and frog lateral, of the pelvis are crucial for determining of extent of involvement and progression of healing.
• Full extent of involvement may not be evident for several months as radiographic findings lag symptoms
• Technetium 99 bone scan - helpful in delineating the extent of avascular changes
• MRI - Most sensitive test; facilitates early diagnosis of necrosis and visualization of articular surface
• Dynamic arthrography - used to asses sphericity of femoral head

DIAGNOSTIC PROCEDURES Hip aspiration to rule out septic arthritis

TREATMENT

APPROPRIATE HEALTH CARE
• When necessary, a pediatric orthopaedic consultation
• Ambulatory treatment is usual, however, some patients may require inpatient traction or surgical procedures

GENERAL MEASURES
• Goals of treatment:
  ◊ Relieve weight bearing across affected hip, thus reducing irritability of the hip
  ◊ Obtain and maintain hip range of motion
  ◊ Maximize regeneration and spherical development of the femoral head by containing the femoral epiphysis within the acetabulum

SURGICAL MEASURES
• Adductor tonotomy to help restore range of motion secondary to adductor contracture
• Femoral and/or pelvic osteotomy to help contain femoral epiphysis within the confines of the acetabulum

ACTIVITY
• Ambulatory status depends on extent/stage of disease
• Limit weight bearing in cases of hip irritation

DIET No special diet

PATIENT EDUCATION
• Légg-Calvé-Pérthes disease is a self-limited disease with revascularization occurring within 3 years
• Treatment is directed at maintaining an appropriate range of motion and maximizing the containment of the femoral head

Légg-Calvé-Pérthes disease

 MEDICATIONS

DRUG(S) OF CHOICE
• Ibuprofen 10 mg/kg tid-qid
Contraindications: Allergy to ibuprofen
Precautions: GI irritation
Significant possible interactions: N/A

ALTERNATIVE DRUGS   N/A

 FOLLOWUP

PATIENT MONITORING
• Initially, close followup, with radiographic evaluation, is needed to determine extent of necrosis
• Once healing phase entered, followup can be every 6 months
• Long-term followup necessary to determine final outcome

PREVENTION/AVOIDANCE   Since etiology is not clearly understood, prevention is not possible

POSSIBLE COMPLICATIONS
• Permanent distortion of the femoral head
• Distorted joint susceptible to early degenerative joint disease

EXPECTED COURSE/PROGNOSIS
• Most patients have a favorable outcome
• Outcome is dependent on the patient's age at the time of the diagnosis (the younger the better)
• Prognosis is also related to the degree of involvement of the femoral head (as determined by radiography)

 MISCELLANEOUS

ASSOCIATED CONDITIONS   N/A

AGE-RELATED FACTORS
Pediatric:
• Physical maturation is delayed
• The younger the patient at the time of diagnosis, the greater the chance for remodeling
Geriatric: N/A
Others: N/A

PREGNANCY   N/A

SYNONYMS   N/A

ICD-9-CM   732.1 Juvenile osteochondrosis of hip and pelvis

SEE ALSO   N/A

OTHER NOTES   N/A

ABBREVIATIONS   N/A

REFERENCES
• Morrissy RT, Weinstein SL, ed. Pediatric Orthopaedics, 4th edition. Lovell and Winter, 1996
• Harring JA. Treatment of Légg-Calvé-Pérthes disease: Critical review of literature. J Bone Joint Surg 1998;73A(3):448-58
• Catterall, Chir M: Perthes Disease. In: Steinberg ME, ed. The Hip and its Disorders. Philadelphia, W.B. Saunders Co., 1991:419-439
• Tachdjian M: Pediatric Orthopedics. 2nd Ed. Philadelphia, W.B. Saunders Co., 1990:933-1003
• Wenger DR, Ward TW, Herring JA: Légg Pérthes Disease: Current Concepts Review. Journal of Bone and Joint Surgery 1991;73A:778-788
Illustrations: N/A
Internet references: http://www.5mcc.com

Author(s)
Francisco G. Valencia, MD

Legionnaires' disease

 BASICS

DESCRIPTION Legionnaires' disease was coined for an epidemic of lower respiratory tract disease occurring in Philadelphia in 1976 in war veterans. The causative bacterium was identified and named Legionella pneumophila and may cause pneumonia or flu-like illness.
System(s) affected: Pulmonary, Gastrointestinal
Genetics: None known
Incidence/Prevalence in USA:
2-4/100,000/year; 1-4% of community acquired pneumonias; up to 20% of nosocomial pneumonias; thought to be under reported
Predominant Age: 15 months-84 years, increased after age 50
Predominant sex: Male > Female

SIGNS AND SYMPTOMS
• Range of illness from asymptomatic seroconversion, mild febrile illness, to severe pneumonia
• Incubation 2-10 days
• Fever, chills
• Malaise, weakness, lethargy
• Anorexia
• Myalgia
• Headache
• Watery diarrhea in up to 50%
• Nausea and vomiting in 10-20%
• Dry cough which may become productive
• Pleuritic chest pain in up to 33%
• Relative bradycardia in up to 67% of patients
• Neuropsychiatric symptoms of confusion, disorientation, obtundation, depression, hallucinations, insomnia, seizures in up to 25%
• Blood streaked sputum; gross hemoptysis rare
• Hyponatremia
• Hypophosphatemia
• Elevated serum transaminases
• Hypotension (17%)

CAUSES Legionella pneumophila, a weakly gram negative organism widely distributed in soil and water, acquired by inhalation of infected aerosols

RISK FACTORS
• Smoking
• Alcohol abuse
• Immunosuppression/HIV
• Chronic cardiopulmonary disease
• Surgery
• Advanced age
• Renal failure

 DIAGNOSIS

DIFFERENTIAL DIAGNOSIS Other bacterial pneumonias, atypical pneumonias with mycoplasma and chlamydia, viral pneumonias

LABORATORY
• Sputum:
  ◊ Gram stain many neutrophils, few organisms
  ◊ Direct immunofluorescence 25-80% sensitive
  ◊ DNA probe 70% sensitive
  ◊ Cultures 50-90% sensitive
• Urine radioimmunoassay (RIA):
  ◊ > 90% sensitivity + specificity
  ◊ Intended for detection of L. pneumophilla serogroup 1 (which accounts for 70-80% of isolates)
• Blood:
  ◊ Indirect immunofluorescence 56% sensitive in three weeks and 90% sensitive after 6 weeks (acute and convalescent titers/seroconversion)
  ◊ Cultures 20% sensitive. Buffered charcoal yeast extract (BCYE) medium required.
• Polymerase chain reaction
  ◊ Experimental
Drugs that may alter lab results: N/A
Disorders that may alter lab results: Direct immunofluorescence can cross react with Pseudomonas and Bacteroides species, E. coli, Haemophilus

PATHOLOGICAL FINDINGS Multifocal pneumonia with alveolitis and bronchiolitis, with fibrinous pleuritis, and may have serous or serosanguinous pleural effusion. Abscess formation in up to 20%.

SPECIAL TESTS Silver and Gimenez stains for lung tissue/specimens

IMAGING
• Chest x-ray
  ◊ Not specific for Legionella
  ◊ Commonly with lower lobe patchy alveolar infiltrate with consolidation
  ◊ Cavitation or abscess, especially in immunocompromised
  ◊ Pleural effusion in up to 50%
  ◊ May take from 1-4 months for the x-ray to return to normal. Progression of infiltrate may be seen despite antibiotic therapy.

DIAGNOSTIC PROCEDURES
Transtracheal aspiration or bronchoscopy for sputum/lung samples

 TREATMENT

APPROPRIATE HEALTH CARE
Severity of illness and support available in the outpatient setting will dictate the appropriate site for care

GENERAL MEASURES
• Supportive care
• Maintaining oxygenation, hydration, and electrolyte balance while providing antibiotic therapy

SURGICAL MEASURES N/A

ACTIVITY As tolerated

DIET As tolerated

PATIENT EDUCATION Can educate patients regarding prevention/avoidance measures, lowering their risk status, and if infected already, about the expected course of the disease

MEDICATIONS

DRUG(S) OF CHOICE
• Erythromycin 30-60 mg/kg/day po or IV divided into four doses for 10-21 days
• Addition of rifampin 600 mg q 12 hours po or IV should be provided along with erythromycin in very ill patients
Contraindications: Hypersensitivity reactions
Precautions: Liver disease
Significant possible interactions:
• Erythromycin can increase theophylline, carbamazepine, and digoxin levels and can increase activity of oral anticoagulants
• Rifampin may decrease the effectiveness of oral anticoagulants, steroids, digoxin, quinidine, oral contraceptives and hypoglycemic agents

ALTERNATIVE DRUGS
• Tetracyclines may be used along with rifampin
  ◊ Doxycycline IV 200 mg every 12 hours x 2 doses, then 100 mg bid or po 200 mg x 1 dose, then 100 mg bid
• Trimethoprim-sulfamethoxazole, imipenem, and quinolones may also be effective
  ◊ Trimethoprim-sulfamethoxazole IV or po 5 mg/kg TMP every 8 hours
  ◊ Ofloxacin IV or po, 400 mg every 12 hours
  ◊ Ciprofloxacin IV 400 mg every 8 hours or po 750 mg every 12 hours
• Other macrolides (clarithromycin) or azalides (azithromycin)
  ◊ Clarithromycin 500 mg po bid
  ◊ Azithromycin 500 mg po qd

FOLLOWUP

PATIENT MONITORING
• Respiratory status, hydration and electrolyte status should be monitored closely
• Chest x-ray not useful to monitor clinical response

PREVENTION/AVOIDANCE
Heating water to 60-70 degrees centigrade may help prevent water contamination. UV light or copper-silver ionization are bactericidal.

POSSIBLE COMPLICATIONS
• Dehydration
• Hyponatremia
• Respiratory insufficiency requiring ventilator support
• Endocarditis
• Disseminated intravascular coagulation
• Renal failure
• Multiple organ dysfunction syndrome (MODS)
• Coma
• Death in 10% of treated non-immunocompromised patients, and in up to 80% of untreated immunocompromised patients
• Bacteremia or abscess formation in immunocompromised

EXPECTED COURSE/PROGNOSIS
• Recovery is variable, some patients experience rapid improvement with defervescence in 3-5 days and recovery in 6-10 days, while others may have a much more protracted course despite treatment
• Mortality rate can approach 50% with nosocomial infections

MISCELLANEOUS

ASSOCIATED CONDITIONS N/A

AGE-RELATED FACTORS
Pediatric: Less common
Geriatric: Increased incidence in those over age 50
Others: N/A

PREGNANCY N/A

SYNONYMS
• Legionella pneumonia
• Pontiac fever
• Legionellosis

ICD-9-CM
482.83 Pneumonia due to other gram negative bacteria

SEE ALSO
• Pneumonia, bacterial

OTHER NOTES
• Extrapulmonary disease can occur in the form of:
  ◊ Encephalitis
  ◊ Cellulitis
  ◊ Sinusitis
  ◊ Pancreatitis
  ◊ Pyelonephritis
  ◊ Endocarditis
  ◊ Pericarditis
  ◊ Perirectal abscess

ABBREVIATIONS N/A

REFERENCES
• Hoeprich P, Jordan MC: Infectious Diseases. 5th Ed. J.B. Lippincott, 1994
• Mandell GL, ed: Principles and Practice of Infectious Diseases. 4th Ed. New York, Churchill Livingstone, 1995
• Rubenstein E, Federman DD: Scientific American Medicine, 1999
• Edelstein PH: Legionnaire's disease. Clinical Infectious Diseases 1993;16:741-749
Illustrations: N/A
Internet references: http://www.5mcc.com

Author(s)
Mitchell S. King, MD

Leishmaniasis

BASICS

DESCRIPTION
An infective condition caused by several species of the protozoan Leishmania. Four major clinical syndromes are recognized.
• Visceral leishmaniasis (Kala-azar, Black fever) may be endemic, epidemic or sporadic. Different forms are:
◊ African Kala-azar: Found in the eastern half of Africa from the Sahara in the North to the Equator. Disease of older children and young adults (10-25 years) Males > females.
◊ Mediterranean or infantile Kala-azar: Seen primarily in the Mediterranean area, China and Latin America. Dogs, jackals, foxes and rats are potential reservoirs. The strains responsible for the Mediterranean and American disease are sometimes referred to as L. infantum and L. chagasi respectively.
◊ Indian Kala-azar: Age and sex distribution similar to African Kala-azar. Humans are the only known reservoir and transmission is by anthropophilic sandflies.
• Cutaneous leishmaniasis of the old and new worlds. Characterized by one or more localized lesions on exposed areas. These ulcerate centrally and spread centrifugally. Spontaneous healing less common in new world disease. Satellite lesions and lymphadenopathy may or may not occur.
• Mucocutaneous leishmaniasis (espundia). One or more lesions on the legs which may ulcerate. In 2-5% of patients, metastatic lesions appear in the nasopharynx after months or years, and may result in painful mutilating erosions of soft tissue. Lesions may occur rarely in perineum.
• Diffuse cutaneous leishmaniasis. Extensive skin lesions , but no visceral lesions. Clinical picture may be similar to lepromatous leprosy.
System(s) affected: Gastrointestinal, Pulmonary, Hemic/Lymphatic/Immunologic, Skin/Exocrine
Genetics: N/A
Incidence/Prevalence in USA: Rare, but reported in states bordering Mexico.
Predominant age: Children and young adults. (10-25 years). Mediterranean or infantile Kala-azar - usually < 4 years age.
Predominant sex: African Kala-azar, Indian Kala-azar: Male > female

SIGNS AND SYMPTOMS
• Incubation period - about 3 months for the visceral form and 2-24 months for others
• Onset - insidious/abrupt
• Malabsorption; failure to thrive in infants and children
• Fever - nocturnal, no signs of toxemia
• Cough
• Diarrhea, GI bleeding
• Lymphadenopathy
• Splenomegaly
• Moderate hepatomegaly
• Cirrhosis, portal hypertension (in 10% of patients)
• Anemia, pancytopenia
• Cutaneous lesions, may ulcerate and heal spontaneously
• Nasal stuffiness
• Epistaxis
• Edema, cachexia and hyperpigmentation in late stages
• Hypoalbuminuria
• Hypergammaglobulinemia

CAUSES
Several species of Leishmania including L. donovani (Kala-azar), L.infantum, L.chagasi (Mediterranean and American forms), L. tropica (cutaneous form), L. major (in Middle East, Afghanistan and India), L. mexicana, L. braziliensis and others. The organisms are transmitted by female sandflies of the genus phlebotomus in the old world and Lutzomyia in the new world.

RISK FACTORS
• Children > young adults in endemic areas
• Malnutrition
• AIDS
• Incomplete therapy of initial disease

DIAGNOSIS

DIFFERENTIAL DIAGNOSIS
• Malaria
• Brucellosis
• Tuberculosis
• Typhoid
• Hepatic abscess
• Lepromatous leprosy for diffuse leishmaniasis
Post Kala-azar dermal lesion (PKDL) must be differentiated from leprosy, syphilis and yaws

LABORATORY
• Demonstration of parasites in
◊ Bone marrow aspirate
◊ Splenic aspirate
◊ Lymph node aspirate or biopsy
◊ Biopsy material from suspicious skin lesions after cleaning with alcohol to reduce bacterial contamination
◊ The intracellular amastigote form in the macrophages, formerly known as the Leishman-Donovan (LD) body, has a characteristic pear-shaped body with a dark circular nucleus and short rod-shaped kinetoplasts
• Hypergammaglobulinemia
• Direct agglutination test detects IgM antibody which indicates acute disease
Drugs that may alter lab results: N/A
Disorders that may alter lab results: N/A

PATHOLOGICAL FINDINGS
• Marked lymphocytic infiltration
• Ulcerating lesions in the skin and mucosa of nasopharynx

SPECIAL TESTS
• Leishmanin skin test is positive 6-8 weeks after recovery in cutaneous forms, but not in diffuse leishmaniasis. It is negative in visceral leishmaniasis.
• Monoclonal antibodies or hybridization of tissue touch blots with labeled kinetoplast DNA probes used for identification of different strains of Leishmania
• ELISA highly sensitive and specific in visceral disease
• Montenegro skin test is nonstandardized and used only in epidemiological studies. It is negative in visceral leishmaniasis.
• An immune-chromato-graphic strip test for rapid detection of antibodies to leishmania antigen K39

IMAGING N/A

DIAGNOSTIC PROCEDURES
• Demonstration of the organism by smear or culture from aspirate or biopsy material. Novy-MacNeal-Nicolle medium or other liquid media used for cultures are maintained at 22-28°C for 21 days. Motile promastigotes can be observed microscopically.
• Speciation using monoclonal Ab or labeled DNA probes

TREATMENT

APPROPRIATE HEALTH CARE
Inpatient for blood transfusions and complicating superinfections. Outpatient care once the condition stabilizes.

GENERAL MEASURES
• Bed rest, oral hygiene, and good nutrition are important.
• Transfusions for anemia and antibacterial chemotherapy for bacterial complications must supplement specific therapy.
• Periodic ECG monitoring during prolonged therapy with pentavalent antimonials.

SURGICAL MEASURES
• Adjunctive splenectomy
• Reconstructive surgery for tissue damage

ACTIVITY
Bed rest during acute stages. Level of activity dependent on severity of disease and organ systems involved

DIET
Rich nutritious diet

PATIENT EDUCATION
Explain prevention measures

MEDICATIONS

DRUG(S) OF CHOICE
• Sodium antimony gluconate (Pentostam) 100 mg Sb5+/mL IV/IM: single daily dose of 20 mg/kg/day for 20-30 days
• Meglumine antimoniate (Glucantime) 85 mg Sb5+/mL, same dose and duration of treatment as above, can also be used
Note: In the U.S., these drugs are available only from the CDC, Atlanta, GA 30333; emergency telephone 404-639-2888 (http://www.cdc.gov)
• Relapses and incomplete responses should be treated with the same regimen for 40-60 days. Addition of oral allopurinol (Zyloprim) 20-30 mg/kg/day in three divided doses has been effective.
Contraindications: Refer to manufacturer's profile of each drug
Precautions: Refer to manufacturer's profile of each drug. Periodic ECG monitoring is recommended during prolonged therapy.
Significant possible interactions: Refer to manufacturer's profile of each drug

ALTERNATIVE DRUGS
Relapses with drug resistant organisms are usually treated with:
• Amphotericin B (Fungizone)IV: 0.5-1 mg/kg on alternate days
OR
• Pentamidine (Pentam): 3-4 mg/kg, 3 times a week for 5-25 weeks; investigational only
• Recombinant human interferon gamma: an adjunct to pentavalent antimony in treatment failures

FOLLOWUP

PATIENT MONITORING
• Follow-up at 3 and 12 months to detect relapses
• PKDL should be treated in the same fashion as the initial illness
• Periodic monitoring of ECG, liver function and renal function during prolonged therapy

PREVENTION/AVOIDANCE
• Use of pesticides (e.g., DDT) against sandflies
• Insect repellants - for travelers
• Permethrin - coated fine netting for travelers
• Early treatment of human cases
• Elimination of diseased dogs

POSSIBLE COMPLICATIONS
• Edema, cachexia, hyperpigmentation in late stages
• Superinfections and gastrointestinal bleeding may cause death in untreated patients with visceral disease (Kala-azar)
• 3-10% of the treated cases develop PKDL characterized by depigmented macules and wart-like nodules over the face and extensor surfaces of limbs
• Metastatic lesions in nasopharynx with tissue destruction in patients with mucocutaneous leishmaniasis

EXPECTED COURSE/PROGNOSIS
With early treatment, cure rate is over 90%, though in advanced cases, mortality remains at 15-25%. In untreated cases, death occurs in 3-20 months in up to 95% of adults and 85% of children.

MISCELLANEOUS

ASSOCIATED CONDITIONS
Fulminant Kala-azar has been described in association with AIDS and malnutrition

AGE-RELATED FACTORS
Pediatric:
• Pediatric Mediterranean or infantile Kala-azar usually a disease of children under 4 years
• African or Indian Kala-azar: usually a disease of children and young adults (10-25 years)
Geriatric: N/A
Others: N/A

PREGNANCY N/A

SYNONYMS
• Visceral leishmaniasis
• Kala-azar
• Black fever
• Dumdum fever

ICD-9-CM
085.0 Kala-azar

SEE ALSO N/A

OTHER NOTES N/A

ABBREVIATIONS
PKDL = Post Kala-azar Dermal Leishmaniasis
LD bodies = Leishman-Donovani bodies

REFERENCES
• Fauci AS, et al, eds: Harrison's Principles of Internal Medicine. 14th Ed. New York, McGraw Hill, 1998
• Dhanda V: Classics in Indian Medicine. The National Medical Journal of India 1994;7(4):201
• Tracy JW, Webster LT Jr: In: Hardman JG, Limbird LE, eds. The Pharmacological Basis of Therapeutics. 9th Ed. New York, Mcgraw-Hill, 1996:987-1008
• Sundar S, Reed SG, Singh VP, et al: Rapid accurate field diagnosis of Indian visceral leishmaniasis. Lancet 1998;351:563-565
Illustrations: N/A
Internet references: http://www.5mcc.com

Author(s)
V. Vasudeviah, BSc, MBBS

Leprosy

BASICS

DESCRIPTION
A chronic granulomatous infection caused by Mycobacterium leprae, an organism which has a high predilection for cooler regions - skin, mucous membrane and peripheral nerves. Leprosy is classified on a spectrum reflecting degrees of lost immunity (Ridley-Jopling classification).
• Indeterminate leprosy
Early cutaneous lesions; Findings are very subtle most commonly diagnosed in contacts of known leprosy cases. The lesions tend to heal spontaneously, but may progress to any of the other leprosy types.
• Tuberculoid leprosy (TT)
Characterized by early localized skin lesions and/or nerve lesions. Bacilli are few and difficult to find. Resistance to infection is high, and spontaneous recovery may occur; however peripheral nerves can be destroyed.
• Lepromatous leprosy (LL)
A generalized infection involving skin, oral, nasal, and upper respiratory mucous membrane, the anterior eye, cutaneous and peripheral nerve trunks, the RE system, adrenals, and testes. Numerous bacilli are easily found in tissue specimens. Patient's resistance to infection is low, and untreated disease is progressive
• Borderline (dimorphous) leprosy
This has features of both TT and LL poles in various combinations. Usually sub-divided into borderline tuberculoid (BT), mid-borderline (BB) and borderline lepromatous (BL). Borderline forms are unstable and may regress (reversal reaction) toward TT form or progress (Downgrading reaction) toward the LL form, depending on the effects of treatment and shifts in immune status
System(s) affected: Skin/Exocrine, Musculoskeletal, Nervous, Endocrine/Metabolic, Reproductive, Pulmonary, Hemic/Lymphatic/Immunologic
Genetics: Specific HLA-associated genes may be linked to different classes of disease, HLA-DR2 with TT and HLA-MT1 with LL
Incidence/Prevalence in USA: Extremely low; about 140 cases in 1992, mostly in immigrants from leprosy-endemic areas
Predominant age: Leprosy can present at any age, although cases in infants under 1 year are extremely rare
Predominant sex:
• Childhood: Male = Female
• Adults: Male > Female (2:1)

SIGNS AND SYMPTOMS
• Indeterminate leprosy
◊ One or more hypopigmented or hyperpigmented macules or plaques
◊ Anesthetic patches, though sensation is preserved in early stages
• TT
◊ Initial hypopigmented, hypesthetic macules with sharp demarcations
◊ Fully developed lesions are asymmetric and densely anesthetic with depressed atrophic central areas and elevated margins; loss of sweat glands and hair follicles near the lesion
◊ Nerve involvement occurs early
  - Ulnar, peroneal, and greater auricular nerves may be palpably and visibly enlarged
  - Neuritic pain
  - Muscle atrophy - small muscles of the hand
  - Facial nerve involvement leads to lagophthalmos, keratitis and corneal ulceration
◊ Hand and foot contracture
◊ Hand infection and plantar ulcers secondary to trauma
◊ Resorption and loss of phalanges may supervene
• LL
◊ Extensive cutaneous involvement, usually bilaterally symmetrical
◊ Highly variable cutaneous lesions macules, nodules, papules or plaques
◊ Sites of predilection are face, ears, wrists, elbows, buttocks and knees
◊ Loss of lateral eye brows
◊ Leonine facies
◊ Nasal stuffiness, epistaxis, septal perforation
◊ Nasal obstruction, laryngitis, hoarseness
◊ Saddle nose
◊ Keratitis, iridocyclitis
◊ Painless inguinal and axillary lymphadenopathy
◊ Testicular infiltrate and scarring - sterility
◊ Gynecomastia
• Borderline leprosy
Increasing variability in the appearance of skin lesions
◊ Papules and plaques may co-exist with macular lesions
◊ Anesthesia is less prominent than in TT
◊ Ear lobes slightly thickened, but eye brows and nasal region spared
◊ Skin lesions become even more numerous in BL type but without the symmetry typical of polar LL
◊ Skin lesions of BT generally resemble those of TT but are greater in number and have less well defined margins

CAUSES
Mycobacterium leprae: an acid fast rod is the causal agent. Incubation period is frequently 3-5 yrs although a range of 6 months to several decades has been seen

RISK FACTORS
• Close family contacts of untreated leprosy patients have 8 fold increased risk
• Compromised immunological status
• Poor socioeconomic status

DIAGNOSIS

DIFFERENTIAL DIAGNOSIS
• Lupus erythematosus
• Lupus vulgaris
• Sarcoidosis
• Yaws
• Dermal leishmaniasis
• Other skin conditions
• Peripheral neuropathy
• Syringomyelia

LABORATORY
• Demonstration of acid-fast bacilli in skin smears made by scraped-incision method is strong evidence of leprosy
• Skin biopsy
• Histologic involvement of peripheral nerves pathognomonic
• Mild anemia, elevated ESR and hyperglobulinemia
• Lepromin test: Usually positive in TT and negative in LL poles. It has no diagnostic value since it gives false positives in nearly all normal adults
• Sero-diagnostic assay: Based on the detection of antibody to phenolic glycolipid 1, this assay has a sensitivity of over 95% in LL and about 30% in TT
Drugs that may alter lab results: N/A
Disorders that may alter lab results: N/A

PATHOLOGICAL FINDINGS
• TT: Noncaseating granulomas containing lymphocytes, epithelioid cells, and perhaps giant cells; bacilli are difficult to demonstrate
• LL: granulomas comprising macrophages, large foam (virchow or lepra) cells, and many intracellular bacilli, frequently in spheroidal masses
• Borderline leprosy: granulomas change from an epithelioid cell predominance in BT to a macrophage predominance as the lepromatous pole is approached

SPECIAL TESTS
• Sero diagnostic assay
• Detection of M. Leprae in tissue by polymerase chain reaction

IMAGING N/A

DIAGNOSTIC PROCEDURES N/A

TREATMENT

APPROPRIATE HEALTH CARE
Outpatient usually, except in reactional states where inpatient care is called for

GENERAL MEASURES

• Manage with multi-disciplinary approach, including orthopedic surgery, ophthalmology and physical therapy in addition to specific drugs
• Rigid soled foot wear or walking plaster casts may prevent plantar ulcers
• Physical therapy and casts prevent hand contractures
• Utilize vocational retraining and rehabilitation along with psychological support
• Immediate recognition and treatment of eye problems essential
• Manage mild reactional states such as reversal reaction and erythema nodosum leprosum (ENL) with bed rest, analgesics and sedatives. Severe reactions require corticosteroids, thalidomide or clofazimine. Specific therapy must be continued without interruption.

SURGICAL MEASURES
Reconstructive surgery - nerve and tendon transplants, release of contractures and other cosmetic procedures can give more functional mobility and social acceptance

ACTIVITY
Dependent on severity of disease

DIET
Nutritious balanced diet

PATIENT EDUCATION
• Educate about the indolent course of the disease; importance of therapeutic completion
• Information pamphlets and awareness to ease psychological trauma and stigma
• Encourage case reporting

MEDICATIONS

DRUG(S) OF CHOICE
• Drugs and treatment duration are based on bacterial load (in skin smear) and clinical types. Multibacillary cases: bacterial load of 10 to the 11th power and clinical types BB, BL or LL. Paucibacillary cases: bacterial load of about 10 to the 6th power and clinical types TT, BT and indeterminate.
• Multibacillary standard regimen includes rifampin, clofazimine and dapsone:
  ◊ Adult outside USA >35 kg
  - Rifampin 600 mg once a month
  - Clofazimine 300 mg once a mo+ 50 mg/d
  - Dapsone 100 mg/d
  ◊ Adult outside USA < 35 kg
  - Rifampin 450 mg once a month
  - Clofazimine 300 mg once a mo+ 50 mg/d
  - Dapsone 50 mg/d
  ◊ Children ages 10-14
  - Rifampin 450 mg once a month
  - Clofazimine 200 mg once a mo+ 50 mg qod
  - Dapsone 50 mg/d
  ◊ Children underweight
  - Rifampin 12-15 mg/kg once a mo
  - Clofazimine 150 mg once a mo+ 50 mg qod
  - Dapsone 1-2 mg/kg/d

◊ Adults in the USA (recommended regimen)
  - Rifampin 600 mg/d for 3 years
  - Dapsone 100 mg/d for life
  - Clofazimine is given in dapsone-resistant cases: 50-100 mg/d for life
• Paucibacillary standard regimen
  ◊ Outside USA
  - Rifampin same doses as above
  - Dapsone 50-100 mg/d
  ◊ In USA
  - Rifampin 600 mg a day for 6 mos
  - Dapsone 100 mg/d for 3-7 years

Contraindications:
• Clofazimine and minocycline: pregnancy
• Ofloxacin: relative contraindication in children and adolescents

Precautions:
• Hemolysis and methemoglobinemia are common untoward reactions to dapsone
• Screen for G6-PD deficiency to prevent drug-induced hemolysis
• Reactionary states should be anticipated and treated aggressively
• Dapsone: GI upset, headaches, pruritus, agranulocytosis, fever, rash
• Clofazimine: GI upset and skin pigmentation
• Minocycline: reduce dose in renal damage

Significant possible interactions: Refer to manufacturer's literature for each drug

ALTERNATIVE DRUGS
• WHO recommended and widely used in countries where leprosy is endemic:
  ◊ Rifampin 600 mg monthly + ofloxacin 400 mg/d + minocycline 100 mg/d for up to 2 years
  ◊ Shorter duration of therapy in multi- and pauci-bacillary cases with rifampin 400 mg/d + ofloxacin 600 mg/d

FOLLOWUP

PATIENT MONITORING
• Frequent follow-up visits until therapy course is stabilized, then monthly supervision
• Periodic CBC, renal and hepatic function

PREVENTION/AVOIDANCE
• Early case finding and chemotherapy to suppress infectiousness and control spread
• Examine family and other close contacts regularly for leprosy
• Vaccination with BCG; 2 doses give good protection

POSSIBLE COMPLICATIONS
• Crippling of the hand and foot
• Trauma and secondary infection leading to loss of digits and extremities
• Blindness
• Lucio phenomenon - arteritis
• Secondary amyloidosis
• ENL: Rx with thalidomide 200 mg bid tapering to 50-100 mg/d in chronic patients
• Severe reversal reaction: prednisolone 40-60 mg/day, tapering slowly

EXPECTED COURSE/PROGNOSIS
Generally indolent, but may be interrupted by ENL and type I lepra reaction. Prognosis is good with early detection and therapy.

MISCELLANEOUS

ASSOCIATED CONDITIONS
HIV-positive patients with early or subclinical leprosy are more likely to develop overt disease. Concurrent leprosy may accelerate HIV-disease course.

AGE-RELATED FACTORS
Pediatric: Rare in infants under one year
Geriatric: N/A
Others: N/A

PREGNANCY
Clofazimine and minocycline contraindicated during pregnancy; dapsone may be used

SYNONYMS
• Hansen's disease

ICD-9-CM
030.9 Leprosy

SEE ALSO
N/A

OTHER NOTES
Indeterminate, TT and perhaps BT classified as paucibacillary. BB, BL or LL are classified as multibacillary. The National Hansen's Disease Center, Carville, LA 70721 (504-642-4722) provides consultation for physicians.

ABBREVIATIONS
TT = Tuberculoid type leprosy
LL = Lepromatous leprosy
BT = Borderline tuberculoid
BL = Borderline lepromatous
BB = Mid-borderline type
ENL = Erythema nodosum leprosum

REFERENCES
• Jacobson RR, Krahenbuhl JL: Leprosy. Lancet 1999;353:655-660
• Fauci AS, et al, eds: Harrison's Principles of Internal Medicine. 14th Ed. New York, McGraw Hill, 1998
• Mandell GL, Petri WA Jr: In: Goodman, Gilman, eds. The Pharmacological Basis of Therapeutics. 9th Ed. New York, McGraw-Hill, 1996:1169-1172
• WHO Tech Rep Ser 1998;No 874
• Reynolds EF, ed: The Extra Pharmacopoeia. 31st Ed. London 1996:146-147
Illustrations: N/A
Internet references: http://www.5mcc.com

Author(s)
V. Vasudeviah, BSc, MBBS

Leukemia

BASICS:

DESCRIPTION
Proliferation and accumulation of abnormal immature blood cell progenitors (blasts) in the bone marrow and other tissues. The outstanding characteristic is the development of marrow failure. Intracerebral leukostasis may develop if the blood blast count becomes greatly elevated. Leukemia is classified according to the type of blast and according to the course, if untreated:
• Acute lymphoblastic leukemia (ALL)
• Acute nonlymphoblastic leukemia (ANLL)
• Chronic myelocytic leukemia (CML)
• Chronic lymphocytic leukemia (CLL)

System(s) affected:
Hemic/Lymphatic/Immunologic

Genetics: Unknown, some are familial

Incidence/Prevalence in USA: The yearly incidence is 13.2:100,000 in males and 7.7:100,000 in females

Predominant age:
• 70% occurs in adults, mostly CLL and ANLL. 30% in children, mostly ALL.
• With the current cure rate especially good for childhood ALL, it is estimated that by the year 2010, one in 1,000 young adults (15-45 years of age) in the USA will be a childhood ALL survivor

Predominant sex: Males > Females

SIGNS AND SYMPTOMS
• Mostly nonspecific and related to marrow failure or infiltration
• Fever
• Bleeding (e.g., petechiae, purpura, easy bruising, or oozing)
• Bone pain, pallor, fatigue
• Splenomegaly
• Hepatosplenomegaly
• Lymphadenopathy
• If CNS is involved, symptoms of increased intracranial pressure can be present
• Gingival swelling

CAUSES   Precise causes unknown

RISK FACTORS
• Genetic and chromosomal abnormalities (e.g., trisomy 21, breakage and translocation)
• Radiation exposure
• Immunodeficiency states
• Chemical and drug exposure (nitrogen mustard and benzene)
• Preleukemia
• Cigarette smoking

DIAGNOSIS

DIFFERENTIAL DIAGNOSIS
• Viral induced cytopenia, lymphadenopathy and organomegaly
• Immune cytopenias
• Drug induced cytopenias
• Other marrow failure and infiltrative diseases: aplastic, hypoblastic and refractory anemias; paroxysmal nocturnal hemoglobinuria; myelodysplastic syndromes, Gaucher's disease, etc.

LABORATORY
• CBC, differential, platelets show subnormal RBC, neutrophils, and possibly subnormal platelets
• In some types, no circulating leukemic blasts are necessary to be present to establish the diagnosis. If 2 of the 3 above parameters are affected, or only one profoundly decreased, bone marrow failure should be ruled out.
• Reticulocyte count < 0.5
• Sedimentation rate usually elevated
• Chemistries LDH, and uric acid can be elevated
• Immunoglobulins IgG can be low or rarely elevated
• Coagulation profile can be normal or prolonged especially in promyelocytic leukemia (ANLL subtype)

Drugs that may alter lab results:
Chemotherapy agents, especially corticosteroids. Don't prescribe these before finalizing the bone marrow studies. Some leukemic blasts are very sensitive and can have massive cell kill from as little as one dose of corticosteroids.

Disorders that may alter lab results: N/A

PATHOLOGICAL FINDINGS
• The marrow will be hypercellular and the normal architecture effaced
• The percentage of leukemic cells compared to the remainder of the cell population is usually more than 30%
• Liver, spleen, and kidneys can be enlarged and infiltrated with leukemic cells

SPECIAL TESTS   Spinal tap may reveal fluid with leukemic cells

IMAGING
• Chest x-ray may reveal a large mediastinal mass
• Ultrasonography or CT scan of the abdomen may discover organomegaly

DIAGNOSTIC PROCEDURES
• Bone marrow studies are necessary to make the final diagnosis
• Aspirates are stained with a buffered Wright's stain and provide good resolution for cell morphology
• Biopsies are demineralized, sectioned and stained with hematoxylin-eosin (H&E) stain. They provide valuable information for cellularity, architecture, and megakaryocytic series.
• Marrow cell suspension used for:
  ◊ Cytochemistries (e.g., myeloperoxidase and Sudan black are positive in myeloblasts)
  ◊ Immunophenotyping especially useful for lymphoid leukemia and can indicate whether it is monoclonal or polyclonal, B lymphocytes or T lymphocytes, early or late, etc.
  ◊ Chromosome studies will show the ploidy and/or the presence of a translocation which is of prognostic value
  ◊ Immunofluorescent stain for terminal deoxyribonucleotidyl transferase (TdT), another marker that differentiates between myeloid and lymphoid blasts

TREATMENT

APPROPRIATE HEALTH CARE
• Consult with a chemotherapist
• Induction for acute leukemia treatment requires inpatient care

GENERAL MEASURES
• Assessment of liver, heart, and kidney functions and performance status
• In acute leukemia induction, establish good hydration and urine flow (especially in ALL patients)
• Give platelet transfusion if platelet count is < 20,000 or if patient is having bleeding symptoms
• Avoid aspirin products
• Give packed red blood cells transfusion if patient is symptomatic from the anemia (e.g., orthostatic hypotension, dizziness, fatigue, hyperactive precordium) or if a cerebral or a cardiopulmonary problem is present
• If the absolute neutrophil count (ANC) < 1000, exert close temperature monitoring. (ANC = WBC x (Percentage of Polys + Bands) ÷ 100). If patient becomes febrile (even low grade fever), appropriate cultures should be taken and patient placed on broad spectrum IV antibiotics covering pseudomonas and gram positive bacteria.
• Isolation (when the ANC is low) has no value because majority of the infecting agents in this situation are the patient's own normal flora of the skin, mouth, or gut
• In promyelocytic leukemia (ANLL subtype), patients are especially at risk for DIC when treatment is started. Heparinization is indicated with close followup of coagulation parameters.

SURGICAL MEASURES
• Bone marrow transplant
  ◊ Allogenic bone marrow transplantation in first remission for ANLL is advocated if a matched sibling is available. Autologous bone marrow transplant is also acceptable in first remission.
  ◊ Allogenic or autologous bone marrow transplant is acceptable in first remission in high risk ALL, especially in adults. They are acceptable in second remission for childhood ALL.
  ◊ Early studies using an allogenic non-related match donor seem to be promising and might replace the autologous route when a full sibling match is not available

ACTIVITY   Ambulatory as tolerated

DIET
• Special attention should be given to ensure adequately balanced calorie and vitamin intake
• Weight should be followed closely because patients usually have decreased appetite.

PATIENT EDUCATION

• Particularly regarding prognosis and treatment toxicity.
• Leukemia Society of America has pamphlets and coloring books for children. 33 Third Ave. New York, NY 10017, (212)573-8484
• NCI (Bethesda, Maryland) has pamphlets: "Chemotherapy and You," "Young People with Cancer" and about "ALL" and "ANLL." NCI has a telephone number for over-the-telephone education and recent updates of treatment options.
• "You and Leukemia, A Day At A Time" by Dr. Lynn S. Baker, W. B. Saunders Co., Philadelphia

MEDICATIONS

DRUG(S) OF CHOICE

Change frequently as result of research
• ALL
  ◊ Induction: vincristine plus prednisone plus asparaginase with or without doxorubicin or daunorubicin. CNS prophylaxis, intrathecal methotrexate with or without cranial irradiation.
  ◊ Maintenance: mercaptopurine (6-mercaptopurine) daily and methotrexate weekly for 2-3 years
• ANLL
  ◊ Induction: cytarabine plus daunorubicin or cytarabine plus idarubicin. Idarubicin seems to be superior to daunorubicin in the treatment of ANLL. Yeast derived granulocyte-macrophage colony stimulating factor (GM-CSF) and granulocyte colony stimulating factor(G-CSF) do not stimulate leukemia cell growth; but help in the resolution of marrow hypoplasia associated with chemotherapy.
  ◊ Maintenance: combined agents and high dose cytarabine
• Promyelocytic leukemia:
  ◊ All-trans-retinoic acid (ATRA) promotes maturation to normal granulocyte and provide remissions with lower toxicity
• CLL. An anti-CD33 monoclonal antibody has the potential for eradicating minimal residual disease in promyelocytic leukemia.
  ◊ Chlorambucil with or without prednisone used only if symptomatic or cytopenic. Fludarabine and cladribine (2-CDA), recently FDA approved, are showing great promise in refractory CLL. New agents such as somatostatin analog, cyclosporine, theophylline have significant activity in CLL.
• Hairy cell leukemia
  ◊ Interferon
• CML
  ◊ Chronic phase, allogenic bone marrow transplantation. If not possible, busulfan, hydroxyurea, or interferon alpha can prolong survival.
  ◊ Acute phase - daunorubicin plus cytarabine plus vincristine plus prednisone with or without thioguanine, or
• High dose cytarabine with or without daunorubicin

Contraindications:

No absolute contraindication is present due to the variety of protocol options

Precautions:

• Administration of chemotherapy agents should be by skilled and specifically trained individuals. IV vincristine, daunorubicin, and doxorubicin may lead to chemical burns in the event of extravasation.
• If liver injury is present, the toxicity of vincristine, anthracyclines and antimetabolites can be pronounced. If liver injury is advanced and hyperbilirubinemia is present, avoid those medications or reduce dosage.
• Anthracyclines can cause cardiomyopathy. Avoid them if patient has a pre-existing cardiac problem.
• Close monitoring of the WBC's, polys, RBC and platelets is required especially in CML (chronic phase or ALL maintenance in order not to induce profound myelotoxicity
• Patients will be immunosuppressed during treatment. Avoid live vaccines. Administer varicella-zoster, or measles immunoglobulin as soon as exposure of a patient at risk becomes known.

Significant possible interactions:

Allopurinol accentuates the toxicity of 6-mercaptopurine

ALTERNATIVE DRUGS   N/A

FOLLOWUP

PATIENT MONITORING

• Repeat bone marrow studies every week or every other week during induction of acute leukemia. Less frequently later. Also perform if a relapse is suspected.
• Follow uric acid level and urinary function closely
• Physical evaluation, including weight and blood pressure, should be done with every treatment and as frequently as once a week

PREVENTION/AVOIDANCE   No intense or contact sports and no aspirin due to low platelets and RBC

POSSIBLE COMPLICATIONS

• Side effects of chemotherapy
• Rarely in lymphoid leukemia, acute tumor lysis syndrome may develop leading to hyperuricemia, hyperkalemia, hyperphosphatemia, hypocalcemia, and/or uric acid nephropathy
• Late onset cardiomyopathy has been described in children treated with standard dose anthracyclines

EXPECTED COURSE/PROGNOSIS

• ALL remission rate is very good. In children, long term survival is the rule.
• AML remission rate is 60-80%, with only 20-40% long term survival
• CML invariably transforms into the acute phase within 2 years (median of 45 months). Afterward, survival rate is poor.

• CLL usually is asymptomatic for several years especially Rai, stages 0-II. In Rai's series the mean interval (in stages 0-II) is 5.3 years from diagnosis until therapy was needed. Median overall survival in CLL is thought to be 9 years.

MISCELLANEOUS

ASSOCIATED CONDITIONS   No specific condition is associated with leukemia. Leukemia can be the first manifestation of chromosomal abnormalities or an immunodeficiency.

AGE-RELATED FACTORS

Pediatric: Tolerate intense treatments better
Geriatric:
• Do not tolerate allogenic bone marrow transplant. Cut off age for transplant is usually 50 years.
• Autologous transplant may be tried in patients above 50 years, provided no organ failure is present and performance status is good
Others: N/A

PREGNANCY   Chemotherapy is a viable option in the 2nd and 3rd trimesters. Refer patient to an oncologist.

SYNONYMS   N/A

ICD-9-CM

204.0 ALL
202.4 Hairy cell leukemia
205.0 ANLL, AML or AGL
206.0 AMoL
204.1 CLL
205.1 CML or chronic granulocytic leukemia

SEE ALSO

• Leukemia, acute lymphoblastic in adults (ALL)

OTHER NOTES   N/A

ABBREVIATIONS

• ALL = acute lymphoblastic leukemia
• ANLL = acute nonlymphoblastic leukemia
• CML = chronic myelocytic leukemia
• CLL = chronic lymphocytic leukemia

REFERENCES

• Devita VT Jr, Helman S, Rosenberg SA, eds: Cancer: Principles & Practice of Oncology. 3rd Ed. Philadelphia, J.B. Lippincott, 1989
• The Medical Letter on Drugs and Therapeutics: Drugs of Choice for Cancer Chemotherapy. Vol. (33) (issue 840), March 22, 1991
• Yearbook of Hematology, 1997. St. Louis, C.V. Mosby and Co, 1997

Illustrations: 4 available on CD-ROM
Internet references: http://www.5mcc.com

Author(s)

Mustafa Barudi, MD

Leukemia, acute lymphoblastic in adults (ALL)

BASICS

DESCRIPTION A malignant proliferation and accumulation of immature lymphocytes
System(s) affected:
Hemic/Lymphatic/Immunologic
Genetics: Increased incidence in children with Down syndrome or in rare familial diseases such as ataxia-telangiectasia, Bloom's syndrome, Fanconi's anemia, Klinefelter's syndrome, and neurofibromatosis. Can rarely occur in adult identical twins.
Incidence/Prevalence in USA: 1000 adult cases/year
Predominant age: Median age is 35-40 years but incidence increases with age
Predominant sex: Male > Female (slightly)

SIGNS AND SYMPTOMS
• Anemia - fatigue, shortness of breath, lightheadedness, angina, headache
• Thrombocytopenia - petechiae, ecchymoses, epistaxis, retinal hemorrhages
• Granulocytopenia - fever, infection
• Lymphocytosis - lymphadenopathy, hepato/splenomegaly, bone pain
• Immunosuppression
• Metabolic abnormalities - hyperuricemia, renal failure, increased lactic acid dehydrogenase (LDH)
• Central nervous system - cranial nerve palsies, confusion

CAUSES Unknown. Epstein-Barr virus is implicated in Burkitt's leukemia/lymphoma.

RISK FACTORS
• Age over 60
• Incidence appears increased following exposure to chemical agents such as benzene or to radiation (but acute myeloid leukemia [AML] is more common)
• May follow aplastic anemia

DIAGNOSIS

DIFFERENTIAL DIAGNOSIS
• Malignant disorders - other leukemias, especially AML; prolymphocytic leukemia; malignant lymphomas; multiple myeloma; bone marrow metastases from solid tumors (breast, prostate, lung, renal); myelodysplastic syndromes
• Nonmalignant disorders - aplastic anemia; myelofibrosis; autoimmune diseases (Felty's syndrome, lupus); infectious mononucleosis; autoimmune thrombocytopenic purpura; leukemoid reaction to infection

LABORATORY
• Anemia - normochromic, normocytic
• Thrombocytopenia
• Peripheral blood lymphoblasts
• Elevated LDH
• Elevated uric acid
Drugs that may alter lab results: N/A
Disorders that may alter lab results: N/A

PATHOLOGICAL FINDINGS Diffuse replacement of marrow and lymph node architecture by sheets of malignant lymphoblasts

SPECIAL TESTS
• Immunophenotyping of marrow/blood lymphoblasts: B-lineage (CD19, CD20, CD24); T-lineage (CD2, CD5, CD7); CALLA ([common ALL antigen], CD10); human leukocyte antigen (HLA)-DR; terminal deoxynucleotidyl transferase (TdT); aberrant myeloid antigens (CG13); stem cell antigen (CD34)
• Cytochemical stains: Myeloperoxidase negative; Sudan black B usually negative; TdT positive; nonspecific esterase +/-; periodic acid Schiff (PAS) +/-
• Cytogenetics: Specific recurring chromosomal abnormalities have independent diagnostic and prognostic significance (hyperdiploidy > 50 chromosomes is favorable; the Philadelphia chromosome, t[9;22], the t[4;11], and the t[8;14] are unfavorable)
• Human leukocyte antigen (HLA) typing of patient and siblings for marrow transplantation

IMAGING
• Chest radiograph to evaluate for mediastinal mass or hilar adenopathy and for pulmonary infiltrates suggestive of infection
• Ultrasound exam to assess splenomegaly or renal enlargement suggestive of leukemic infiltration

DIAGNOSTIC PROCEDURES
• Bone marrow examination with aspiration, biopsy, immunophenotyping, cytochemistry, and cytogenetics
• Lymph node biopsy is rarely necessary but can be diagnostic
• Lumbar puncture should be done if neurological symptoms or signs are present. Repeat lumbar puncture after bone marrow remission is achieved to evaluate occult CNS involvement.

TREATMENT

APPROPRIATE HEALTH CARE
• Inpatient care during remission induction chemotherapy
• Post-remission therapy is usually outpatient
• Access to the resources and expertise of a major oncology center is important for appropriate support

GENERAL MEASURES Protective isolation from infection

SURGICAL MEASURES Surgical placement of a percutaneous silastic double-lumen central venous catheter

ACTIVITY Ambulatory as tolerated

DIET
• Nutritional support including intravenous hyperalimentation, if necessary
• Avoid alcohol

PATIENT EDUCATION
• Risks of infection, transfusion, chemotherapy
• Stop smoking

Leukemia, acute lymphoblastic in adults (ALL)

MEDICATIONS

DRUG(S) OF CHOICE
Optimal therapy is not yet known. All treatment regimens are still investigational, although clearly effective for some fraction of patients. CALGB protocol 9111 is an example of therapy (from Blood 1998; 92:1556-1564):
• Remission induction
  ◊ Cyclophosphamide 1200 mg/square meter on day 1 (800 mg/m2 if > 60 years old)
  ◊ Daunorubicin 45 mg/m2 on days 1, 2, and 3 (30 mg/m2 if > 60 years old)
  ◊ Vincristine 2 mg on days 1, 8, 15, and 22
  ◊ Asparaginase (L-asparaginase) 6000 units/m2 on days 5, 8, 11, 15, 18, and 22
  ◊ Prednisone 60 mg/m2 on days 1-21 (days 1-7 if > 60 years old)
  ◊ Filgrastim - G-CSF, 5 µg/kg/day SQ starting on day 4 has been shown to shorten the duration of neutropenia and improve the CR rate, especially in older patients
• Consolidation (repeat twice in 8 weeks
  ◊ Cyclophosphamide 1000 mg/m2 on day 1
  ◊ Intrathecal (IT) methotrexate 15 mg with hydrocortisone 50 mg on day 1
  ◊ Mercaptopurine (6-mercaptopurine) 60 mg/m2 on days 1-14
  ◊ Cytarabine 75 mg/m2 SC on days 1-4 and 8-11
  ◊ Vincristine 2 mg on days 15 and 22
  ◊ Asparaginase 6000 units/m2 on days 15, 18, 22, and 25
• CNS prophylaxis and interim maintenance - 2400 cGy cranial irradiation
  ◊ IT-methotrexate 15 mg with hydrocortisone 50 mg on days 1, 8, 15, 22, and 29
  ◊ Mercaptopurine (6-mercaptopurine) 60 mg/m2 on days 1-70
  ◊ Oral methotrexate 20 mg/m2 on days 36, 43, 50, 57, and 64
• Late intensification
  ◊ Doxorubicin 30 mg/m2 on days 1, 8, and 15
  ◊ Vincristine 2 mg on days 1, 8, and 15
  ◊ Dexamethasone 10 mg/m2 on days 1-14
  ◊ Cyclophosphamide 1000 mg/m2 on day 29
  ◊ Thioguanine (6-thioguanine) 60 mg/m2 on days 29-42
  ◊ Cytarabine 75 mg/m2 SC on days 29-32 and 36-39
• Prolonged maintenance
  ◊ Vincristine 2 mg/month for 16 months
  ◊ Prednisone 60 mg/m2 for 5 days with the vincristine
  ◊ Mercaptopurine (6-mercaptopurine) 60 mg/m2/day for 16 months
  ◊ Oral methotrexate 20 mg/m2/week for 16 months

Contraindications: Doses and schedule may need to be altered for older patients and for concurrent infection and organ toxicity

Precautions:
• Tumor lysis syndrome (elevated uric acid, potassium, and phosphate with decreased calcium leading to renal failure, disseminated intravascular coagulation, and cardiac arrhythmias) may be prevented by administering allopurinol 300 mg/day. Begin 2 days before chemotherapy begins. Reduce doses if used with mercaptopurine or azathioprine. Give increased fluids.
• Oral sulfamethoxazole-trimethoprim or aerosolized pentamidine is given for pneumocystis carinii prophylaxis
• Profound immunosuppression. Take appropriate precautions when patient is neutropenic
• High dose cyclophosphamide causes severe nausea and vomiting. Use appropriate antiemetic regimen to prevent.
• Neurotoxicity, ileus with vincristine
• Asparaginase may cause severe allergic reactions as well as impaired pancreatic and liver function. Monitor serum glucose concentrations frequently and carefully. Pancreatitis or thrombosis may occur.
Significant possible interactions: N/A

ALTERNATIVE DRUGS
Other anthracyclines, investigational chemotherapy agents

FOLLOWUP

PATIENT MONITORING
Daily during induction chemotherapy for metabolic and infectious complications. Weekly during remission consolidation chemotherapy. Monthly during maintenance therapy. Every 3 months thereafter.

PREVENTION/AVOIDANCE
N/A

POSSIBLE COMPLICATIONS
• Infections (pneumocystis carinii pneumonia, bacterial pneumonia or sepsis, fungal pneumonia)
• Bleeding
• Need for transfusions
• Sterility from treatment
• Arachnoiditis and CNS effects from intrathecal chemotherapy and irradiation
• Pancreatitis and liver dysfunction from chemotherapy
• Relapse of ALL in marrow or extramedullary sites (CNS, testis)

EXPECTED COURSE/PROGNOSIS
• 80-95% of patients < 60 years old will achieve a complete remission, and 35-60% will remain free of disease at 5 years
• Older patients (>60 years) do less well, but still 80% may achieve a complete remission
• Patients with unfavorable cytogenetic subtypes (especially t[9;22] and t[4:11]) should undergo allogeneic bone marrow transplantation in first remission if an HLA-identical donor were available

MISCELLANEOUS

ASSOCIATED CONDITIONS N/A

AGE-RELATED FACTORS
Pediatric: Bone growth and IQ development may be affected by treatment
Geriatric: N/A
Others: N/A

PREGNANCY
Many chemotherapy drugs are teratogenic

SYNONYMS Acute lymphocytic leukemia

ICD-9-CM 204.0 Lymphoid leukemia

SEE ALSO N/A

OTHER NOTES Burkitt's leukemia/lymphoma (ALL-L3) - the outcome is clearly better if high dose methotrexate and alkylating agents are used for initial therapy. Only 18 weeks of treatment is required.

ABBREVIATIONS HLA = human leukocyte antigen

REFERENCES
• Hoffman R, Benz EJ Jr, Shattil S, et al, eds: Hematology: Basic Principles and Practice. New York, Churchill Livingstone, 1995
• Laport GF, Larson RA: Treatment of adult acute lymphoblastic leukemia. Semin in Oncology 1997;24:70-82
• Finiewicz KJ, Larson RA: Dose-intensive therapy for adult acute lymphoblastic leukemia. Semin in Oncology 1999;26:6-20
• Larson RA, Dodge RK, Linker CA, et al: A randomized controlled trial of filgrastim during remission induction and consolidation chemotherapy for adults with acute lymphoblastic leukemia. Blood 1998;92:1556-1564
Illustrations: N/A
Internet references: http://www.5mcc.com

Author(s)
Richard A. Larson, MD

Leukoplakia, oral

BASICS

DESCRIPTION   A nonspecific clinical term used to describe a white patch in the oral mucosa which remains despite attempts to rub it off. It does not correlate with any specific microscopic findings and may be related to a variety of lesions, from benign hyperkeratosis to carcinoma.
System(s) affected: Gastrointestinal
Genetics: N/A
Incidence/Prevalence in USA:
• 3% of the adult population is affected, usually in men older than 40 years
Predominant age: 90% of lesions found in patients over 40 years of age
Predominant sex:
• Males > Female
• Some studies show no preference

SIGNS AND SYMPTOMS
• Location
  ◊ 50% on tongue, mandibular alveolar ridge, and buccal mucosa
  ◊ Also seen on maxillary alveolar ridge, palate and lower lip
  ◊ Infrequently - floor of the mouth and retromolar areas
• Appearance
  ◊ Varies from nonpalpable, faintly translucent white areas to thick, fissured, papillomatous, indurated lesions
  ◊ May feel rough or leathery
  ◊ Color may be white, gray, yellowish-white, or brownish-gray
  ◊ Cannot be wiped off
  ◊ Macular or plaque-like

CAUSES
• Tobacco use
• Alcohol consumption
• Oral sepsis
• Oral snuff (smokeless tobacco)
• Human papillomavirus, types 11 and 15
• Actinic radiation
• Vitamin deficiency
• Syphilis
• Dental restorations
• Prosthetic dental appliances
• Alcoholism
• Estrogen therapy

RISK FACTORS
• Age over 40
• Tobacco or alcohol use
• Repeated or chronic trauma to oral regions

DIAGNOSIS

DIFFERENTIAL DIAGNOSIS
• White oral lesions that can be wiped away:
  ◊ Candida
  ◊ Aspirin burn
• White oral lesions that cannot be rubbed off:
  ◊ Traumatic or frictional keratosis (e.g., linea alba)
  ◊ Leukoedema
  ◊ Galvanic keratosis
  ◊ Lichen planus
  ◊ Verrucous carcinoma
  ◊ Lupus
  ◊ Squamous cell carcinoma
  ◊ Oral hairy leukoplakia, commonly on the lateral border of the tongue with a bilateral distribution
  ◊ Leukokeratosis nicotina palati

LABORATORY   N/A
Drugs that may alter lab results: N/A
Disorders that may alter lab results: N/A

PATHOLOGICAL FINDINGS
• Biopsy specimens range from hyperkeratosis to invasive carcinoma
• 6% at initial biopsy are invasive carcinoma
• 4% subsequently undergo malignant transformation
• Location is important: 60% on floor of mouth are cancerous; rarely so on buccal mucosa

SPECIAL TESTS   N/A

IMAGING   N/A

DIAGNOSTIC PROCEDURES   Biopsy necessary to rule out carcinoma

TREATMENT

APPROPRIATE HEALTH CARE
Outpatient biopsy, only if lesion persists despite elimination of possible etiologic factors

GENERAL MEASURES
• Eliminate habitual lip biting
• Correct ill fitting dental appliances
• Stop smoking and alcohol
• If dysplasia evident, remove lesion. Consider otolaryngologist referral.
• Some small lesions may respond to cryosurgery
• Beta-carotene may cause partial regression (experimental)
• For hairy tongue: Tongue brushing

SURGICAL MEASURES
• Excision is the treatment of choice for lesions exhibiting dysplasia or malignant transformation

ACTIVITY   Full

DIET   Regular

PATIENT EDUCATION
• If biopsy negative, stress importance of periodic and careful followup
• Aid the patient in discontinuing tobacco and/or alcohol use. Referral to support groups, recommendations for stop smoking programs, etc.

Leukoplakia, oral

MEDICATIONS

DRUG(S) OF CHOICE
• Hairy leukoplakia
  ◊ Acyclovir 2-4 gm/day systemically is effective, but the lesions recur when the treatment is stopped
  ◊ Topical podophyllin 25% resin applied twice, one week apart, but the bad taste is poorly tolerated
• Leukoplakia
  ◊ isotretinoin (Accutan) 1-2 mg/kg/day may lead to temporary remission, but side effects are poorly tolerated
Contraindications: N/A
Precautions: N/A
Significant possible interactions: N/A

ALTERNATIVE DRUGS N/A

FOLLOWUP

PATIENT MONITORING Regular, close followup, even after successful treatment. Biopsy as needed.

PREVENTION/AVOIDANCE
• Avoid tobacco, alcohol, habitual biting
• Provide well-fitting dentures

POSSIBLE COMPLICATIONS
• Carcinoma
• New lesions may develop after treatment

EXPECTED COURSE/PROGNOSIS
• Curable if detected early
• 4-6% of initially benign lesions subsequently develop cancer
• More likely cancerous if on floor of mouth

MISCELLANEOUS

ASSOCIATED CONDITIONS
• Leukokeratosis nicotina palati is rarely malignant
• HIV infection

AGE-RELATED FACTORS
Pediatric: N/A
Geriatric: More common in elderly
Others: Rare before age 40

PREGNANCY N/A

SYNONYMS N/A

ICD-9-CM
528.6 Leukoplakia of oral mucosa or tongue

SEE ALSO
• HIV infection & AIDS
• Epstein-Barr virus infections

OTHER NOTES
• Uncommonly - other mucosal surfaces (vaginal, anal, etc.)
• Linea alba - a white line on the buccal mucosa, along the occlusal plane

ABBREVIATIONS N/A

REFERENCES
• Yeats D, Burn J: Common Oral Mucosal Lesions in Adults. Amer Fam Phys 1991;44:2043-50
• Fitzpatrick T, et al: Color Atlas and Synopsis of Clinical Dermatology. 2nd Ed. New York, McGraw-Hill, 1992
Illustrations: 1 available on CD-ROM
Internet references: http://www.5mcc.com

Author(s)
Mark R. Dambro, MD, FAAFP

Lichen planus

BASICS

DESCRIPTION A unique inflammatory disorder of the skin and mucous membranes. The disease is characterized by small flat, angular, violaceous, shiny, pruritic papules on the skin and white papules in the mouth. Onset abrupt or gradual. May be intermittent for years.
System(s) affected: Skin/Exocrine
Genetics: N/A
Incidence/Prevalence in USA: 450/100,000
Predominant age: 30-60 years, rare in children and the elderly
Predominant sex: Female > Male

SIGNS AND SYMPTOMS
• Skin
  ◊ Pruritus - often severe
  ◊ Papules - 1-10 mm, shiny, flat
  ◊ Color - violaceous, with white lace-like pattern (Wickham's striae) on papules. Wickham's striae best seen after topical application of mineral oil and if present, are almost pathognomonic for lichen planus.
  ◊ Shape - polygonal or oval shaped
  ◊ Arrangement - may be grouped, linear, annular, or scattered individual lesions.
  ◊ Koebner's phenomenon is often seen
  ◊ Distribution - ventral surface of wrists and forearms, glans penis, dorsa feet, groin, sacrum, shins and scalp. Hypertrophic (verrucous) lesions may occur on lower legs. An annular pattern may appear on trunk and mucous membranes. Linear arrangements of papules have been described.
• Mucous membranes
  ◊ Mucous membrane involvement is seen in 40-60% of patients with skin lesions. 20% of patients have mucous membrane lesions only.
  ◊ Milky-white papules with white lace-like pattern
  ◊ Usually seen on buccal mucosa, but may appear on tongue, gingiva, palate, and lips
  ◊ May be bullous or erosive
  ◊ Painful, especially if ulcers present
  ◊ Oral lesions may be precancerous (squamous cell carcinoma)
• Hair and nails
  ◊ Scalp - atrophic scalp skin and destruction of hair follicles. May result in permanent and total alopecia.
  ◊ Nails - (10%) may cause proximal to distal linear grooves and partial or complete destruction of nail bed with pterygium formation. Large toes most commonly affected.

CAUSES Etiology unknown. Possibly a disease of keratinization or an autoimmune disease. Emotional stress may antedate an attack.

RISK FACTORS Exposure to drugs or chemicals, graft versus host disease, or lupus erythematosus (LE-LP overlap syndrome)

DIAGNOSIS

DIFFERENTIAL DIAGNOSIS
• Chemical exposure (chemicals used in color developing)
• Drug eruption (chloroquine, quinacrine, gold salts, methyldopa, penicillamine, arsenic, bismuth, ACE inhibitors)
• Lichen nitidus
• Leukoplakia
• Psoriasis
• Candidiasis
• Squamous cell carcinoma; basal cell carcinoma
• Aphthous ulcers
• Herpetic stomatitis
• Secondary syphilis
• Scabies

LABORATORY N/A
Drugs that may alter lab results: N/A
Disorders that may alter lab results: N/A

PATHOLOGICAL FINDINGS
Inflammation with hyperkeratosis, increased granular layer, irregular acanthosis, basement-membrane thinning with "sawtoothing," hyaline bodies below the epidermis, band-like lymphocytic infiltrate of the upper dermis

SPECIAL TESTS N/A

IMAGING N/A

DIAGNOSTIC PROCEDURES Skin biopsy

TREATMENT

APPROPRIATE HEALTH CARE
Outpatient

GENERAL MEASURES
• Goal is to relieve itching with topical and systemic antibiotics
• Psoralens and ultraviolet A (PUVA) photochemotherapy may be helpful for generalized or resistant cases
• Behavior modification for stress reduction may prevent recurrence

SURGICAL MEASURES N/A

ACTIVITY Fully active

DIET No special diet

PATIENT EDUCATION Help with stress reduction if appropriate

MEDICATIONS

DRUG(S) OF CHOICE
• Skin
 ◊ Topical steroids (e.g., 0.1% triamcinolone acetonide) with occlusion
 ◊ Intralesional corticosteroids, e.g., triamcinolone (Kenalog) 5-10 mg/mL) for hypertrophic lesions
 ◊ Antihistamine (e.g., hydroxyzine, dosage - 25 mg q6h) if needed for itching
• Mucous membranes
 ◊ Topical oral retinoids, e.g., 0.05% tretinoin (retinoic acid) in Orabase or topical oral corticosteroids (0.1% triamcinolone (Kenalog in Orabase) bid
 ◊ Intralesional corticosteroids for erosive, painful lichen planus, e.g., 0.5-1.0 mL methylprednisolone (Depo-Medrol) 40 mg/mL
 ◊ Oral retinoids - isotretinoin (Accutane) or etretinate (Tegison)
Contraindications: Patients with history of hypersensitivity to corticosteroids or retinoids
Precautions:
• Systemic absorption of steroids may result in hypothalamic-pituitary-adrenal axis suppression, Cushing's syndrome, hyperglycemia, and glucosuria
• Increased risk with high potency - i.e., use over large surface area, prolonged use, occlusive dressings
• These medications are Category C teratogens. Avoid in pregnancy.
• Children may absorb a proportionally larger amount of topical steroid due to larger skin surface to weight ratio
Significant possible interactions: See manufacturer's profile of each drug

ALTERNATIVE DRUGS
• Oral prednisone - rarely used and only for a short course (e.g., prednisone 20 mg bid x 2-4 weeks)
• Cyclosporine may be used in severe cases, but cost and potential toxicity limits its use. Topical use for severe oral involvement refractory to other treatments.

FOLLOWUP

PATIENT MONITORING Serial skin exams

PREVENTION/AVOIDANCE Reduce stress

POSSIBLE COMPLICATIONS
• Alopecia
• Nail destruction
• Squamous cell carcinoma of the mouth

EXPECTED COURSE/PROGNOSIS
• Spontaneous resolution in weeks is possible, but disease may persist for years - especially in the mouth and on shins
• There is a tendency toward relapse, especially with emotional stress
• Recurrence 12-20% especially in those with generalized involvement

MISCELLANEOUS

ASSOCIATED CONDITIONS
• Hepatitis C
• Lichen nitidus
• Bullous pemphigoid
• Alopecia
• Myasthenia gravis
• Lupus erythematosus
• Biliary cirrhosis
• Vitiligo
• Ulcerative colitis
• Graft-versus-host reaction
• Morphea and lichen sclerosus et atrophicus

AGE-RELATED FACTORS
Pediatric: N/A
Geriatric: N/A
Others: N/A

PREGNANCY Avoid corticosteroids, retinoids

SYNONYMS N/A

ICD-9-CM 697.0 Lichen planus

SEE ALSO N/A

OTHER NOTES Remember the 5 p's of lichen planus - purple, planar, polygonal, pruritic papules

ABBREVIATIONS N/A

REFERENCES
• Habif T: Clinical Dermatology. 3rd Ed. St. Louis, CV Mosby, 1996
• Fitzpatrick TB, et al: Color Atlas and Synopsis of Clinical Dermatology. New York, McGraw-Hill, 1997
• Fitzpatrick TB, et al: Dermatology in General Medicine. 5th Ed. New York, McGraw-Hill, 1999
• Arnold HL Jr, Odom RB, James WD, eds: Andrews' Diseases of the Skin: Clinical pharmacology. 8th Ed. Philadelphia, W.B. Saunders Co., 1990
• Rakel RE (ed): Conn's Current therapy. 50th ed. Philadelphia, WB Saunders Co., 1998
• Howard R: Adult skin disease in the pediatric patient. Dermatologic Clin 1998:16(3):593-608
• Miles DA: Diagnosis and management of oral lichen planus. Dermatologic Clin 1996;14(2):281-290
Illustrations: 9 available on CD-ROM
Internet references: http://www.5mcc.com

Author(s)
Marc Darr, MD

Listeriosis

BASICS

DESCRIPTION Infection caused by the ubiquitous, weakly hemolytic, gram positive bacillus, Listeria monocytogenes, which is pathogenic to many animal species. Occurs most often in fetuses (disseminated infantile listeriosis), in neonates, and in immunosuppressed patients. Majority of adult patients have pre-existing disease (cirrhosis, lymphomas, solid tumors, AIDS, cancer therapy). Usual course - acute.
• In 1998-1999 at least 50 illnesses were reported from eleven states resulting from contaminated hot dogs and deli meats.
System(s) affected: Pulmonary, Endocrine/Metabolic, Gastrointestinal, Renal/Urologic, Hemic/Lymphatic/Immunologic, Nervous
Genetics: No known genetic pattern
Incidence/Prevalence in USA:
• 1,850 cases a year (425 deaths)
• Pregnant women are about 20 times more likely than healthy adults to get listeriosis
• Persons with AIDS are almost 300 times more likely to develop infection
Predominant age: Neonates, elderly
Predominant sex: Male > Female

SIGNS AND SYMPTOMS
• Asymptomatic
• Abdominal pain
• Adult respiratory distress syndrome
• Cervical lymphadenopathy
• Chills
• Conjunctivitis
• Decreased fetal movement
• Diarrhea
• Dysuria
• Fatigue
• Fever
• Hepatosplenomegaly
• Malaise
• Myalgia
• Nausea
• Pharyngitis
• Urinary frequency
• Vomiting
• Findings suggestive of meningitis - fever, headache, nausea and vomiting, stiff neck, delirium, coma
• Findings suggestive of sepsis - high fever and generalized severe illness without evidence of localized infection (in patients with alcoholism, malignancies, immunosuppression, AIDS)

CAUSES Listeria monocytogenes, a small gram-positive bacillus; infection with other species of Listeria are rare. Illnesses can begin 2-8 weeks after eating contaminated food.

RISK FACTORS
• Age - fetus, neonates, elderly
• Metastatic malignant disease
• HIV infection
• Alcoholism
• Renal hemodialysis
• Pregnancy
• Immunosuppressed
• Exposure to infected animals (veterinarians, butchers, etc.). Animal-to-human transmission is rare.
• Ingesting contaminated food or drink (e.g., soft Mexican style cheese or feta cheese)

DIAGNOSIS

DIFFERENTIAL DIAGNOSIS
• Other infections - Staphylococcal, gram negative Klebsiella, Candida, cryptococcosis, viral
• Infantile listeriosis, E. coli, Group B streptococci
• Infectious mononucleosis

LABORATORY
• CSF
  ◊ Gram stain - may reveal small, gram-positive rods or coccobacillary forms with "tumbling" motility. (Sometimes difficult to identify since organisms are not present in large numbers and may be confused with diphtheroids and other bacteria.)
  ◊ Cell count - in most cases, the predominant cell type is the neutrophil; however, mononuclear cells may predominate. Counts range from 0-1200/mm3. RBC's frequently seen.
  ◊ Protein concentration - within normal limits to 735 mg/dL
  ◊ Glucose - within normal limits to undetectable
  ◊ CSF cultures - demonstrates beta-hemolysis (L. monocytogenes grows well on 5% sheep's blood or chocolate agar)
  ◊ Counterimmunoelectrophor (CIE) latex agglutination (LA) - possibly useful for differential diagnosis
• Other tests
  ◊ Blood cultures should be done
  ◊ CBC - peripheral WBC may show an elevated neutrophil count and/or left shift
  ◊ Other cultures in newborn - cervical vaginal secretions and lochia from the mother; cord blood; grossly abnormal portions of the placenta, meconium, and exudate expressed from an incised skin papule of the neonate
Drugs that may alter lab results:
Antibiotics
Disorders that may alter lab results:
Cultures may be confusing in patients with mixed infections

PATHOLOGICAL FINDINGS
• Gross - multi-organ miliary granulomatosis
• Micro - nodular focal abscess
• Micro - necrotic amorphous basophilic debris
• Micro - increased tissue macrophages
• Micro - gram-positive bacilli
• Motile bacilli
• Chinese-letter aggregates

SPECIAL TESTS Specimens for serologic testing should be submitted to the local public health laboratory. In outbreaks, serotyping may be desirable.

IMAGING MRI with any patient having central nervous system symptoms

DIAGNOSTIC PROCEDURES Lumbar puncture

TREATMENT

APPROPRIATE HEALTH CARE
Inpatient during acute phase

GENERAL MEASURES
• Bedrest
• Isolation if immunosuppressed
• Secretion precautions
• Respiratory assistance (if apneic, or CNS depressed)

SURGICAL MEASURES N/A

ACTIVITY Bedrest

DIET
• Acute case, total parenteral nutrition, nasogastric tube, or softer diet if tolerated
• As a preventive, avoid eating raw or partially cooked foods and soft cheeses. Warm leftovers thoroughly and wash raw vegetables before cooking.

PATIENT EDUCATION
• Dietary guidelines for avoidance in high risk patients
• CDC - National Center for Infectious Diseases; www.cdc.gov/ncidod/ncid.htm/

Listeriosis

ICD-9-CM 027.0 Listeriosis

MEDICATIONS

DRUG(S) OF CHOICE
• Neonates - IV treatment 14-21 days:
◊ Meningitis - for infants older than one month: ampicillin 300-400 mg/kg/day IV
◊ Meningitis - neonate doses: < 2000 grams, less than 1 week old: ampicillin 50 mg/kg q12h. Older than 1 week: ampicillin 50 mg/kg every 8 hours. Plus gentamicin 7.5 mg/kg/day IV for 14 days. Discontinue gentamicin when cerebro-spinal fluid is sterile.
◊ Alternate therapy for neonates - penicillin G 100,000-200,000 units/kg/d IV x 14-21 days plus gentamicin as above
◊ Bacteremia or pneumonia - ampicillin 100-150 mg/kg/day (or penicillin G 200,000 units/kg/d IV) plus gentamicin 5.0 mg/kg/day. Discontinue gentamicin when blood cultures become negative.
• Pregnant women:
◊ Ampicillin 2 gm IV q4h for 14-21 days plus gentamicin 120 mg IV q8h. Adjust for peak 5-6 mcg/mL.
• Immunocompromised/elderly patients:
◊ Ampicillin 200 mg/kg IV x 3-4 weeks. Note: Some experts recommend addition of gentamicin 3-5 mg/kg/d IV plus intrathecal doses of 4 mg q12h or combination with TMX/sulfa.
• For endocarditis and typhoidal listeriosis:
◊ Penicillin G 75,000-100,000 units/kg IV q4h and continue for 14 days after defervescence. plus tobramycin 2 mg/kg load, then adjust based on levels. Aim for peak at 5-6. Continue for 4 weeks after defervescence.
• For oculoglandular:
◊ Erythromycin 30 mg/kg/day as 4 equal doses q6h and continue for 1 week after defervescence
Contraindications: Allergy to penicillins
Precautions: Cephalosporins are not adequate treatment. Refer to manufacturer's literature.
Significant possible interactions: Refer to manufacturer's literature

ALTERNATIVE DRUGS
• Trimethoprim-sulfamethoxazole may be the most effective treatment for adults because of its ability to penetrate cells. Total dose 10 mg/kg (based on trimethoprim component) in divided doses.
• Clarithromycin
• Ciprofloxacin

FOLLOWUP

PATIENT MONITORING
• Frequent arterial blood gases during acute phase
• Repeat lumbar puncture at 24-48 hours and at the end of treatment

PREVENTION/AVOIDANCE
• Avoid handling livestock during pregnancy
• Avoid contaminated silage
• Avoid contaminated sewage
• Avoid raw or contaminated milk products
• Avoid soft cheeses (Mexican and feta)
• Wash carefully all raw vegetables

POSSIBLE COMPLICATIONS
• Premature delivery
• Amnionitis
• Meningitis
• Septicemia
• Pulmonary abscess
• Hepatic abscess
• Placental abscess
• Splenic abscess
• Lymph node abscess
• Endocarditis
• Peritonitis
• Abortion
• Stillbirth
• Neonatal death

EXPECTED COURSE/PROGNOSIS
High mortality if symptomatic

MISCELLANEOUS

ASSOCIATED CONDITIONS
• Cirrhosis
• Lymphomas
• Solid tumors
• Immunodeficiencies
• Pregnancy

AGE-RELATED FACTORS
Pediatric:
• Infected fetuses are usually stillborn or premature. More than half are infected with lethal listeriosis.
• 50% mortality in treated neonates
Geriatric: Greater morbidity and mortality
Others: N/A

PREGNANCY
• Pregnant women are more susceptible to infection with Listeria monocytogenes; transmission to the fetus and neonates occurs with high mortality.
• Requires prompt and vigorous treatment to prevent transfer of disease to fetus (pregnant patient's symptoms may begin as a flu-like illness or be absent)

SYNONYMS
• Listeria monocytogenes
• Listerial disease

SEE ALSO N/A

OTHER NOTES
• Notify laboratory at time of sending any specimen that listeriosis is a possibility
• Laboratory specimens must be sent to laboratory promptly (few organisms more difficult to culture)
• Need at least 10 cc of spinal fluid for culture

ABBREVIATIONS N/A

REFERENCES
• Linnan MJ, Mascola L, Lou X, May S, Salimen C, et al: Epidemic listeriosis associated with Mexican-style cheese. N Engl J Med 1988;319, 823:828
• Von Lichtenberg F: Pathology of Infectious Diseases. New York, Raven Press, 1988
• Haft RF, Kasper D: Group B Streptococcus Infection in Mother and Child. Hospital Practice 1991;26
• Foodborne and Diarrhea Diseases Branch, CDC Personal Communication, 1997
• Southwick FS, Purich DL: Mechanisms of disease: Intracellular pathogenesis of listeriosis. NEJM 1996;334:770-776
• Update: Multistate outbreak of listeriosis-United States, 1998-1999: NMMWR. 1999;47:1117-1118
• Marron; Rosen B, Mascaro J, Carratala J: Listeria monocytogenes empyema in an HIV infected patient. Thorax;52:745-746
• Gilbert DN, Moellering RC, Sande MA: The Sanford Guide to Antimicrobial Therapy, 1998.
Illustrations: N/A
Internet references: http://www.5mcc.com

Author(s)
Susana May, MD, MPH

Low back pain

BASICS

DESCRIPTION
Mechanical low back pain is a diagnosis of exclusion. It is generally a self-limiting condition of the aging spine, responsive to conservative measures including rest and pain management. Patients typically present with pain at the posterior belt line with occasional referred pain to the buttocks and/or posterior thighs. These injuries often are the result of the mechanical stresses and functional demands placed on the low back area by everyday activities. The condition, for the vast majority of patients, is of short duration and complete recovery is the general rule. The primary goal of the clinician is to rule-out other more serious etiologies. It must be remembered that low back pain is a symptom, not a disease, and that the pathological basis of the pain frequently lies outside the spine.

System(s) affected: Musculoskeletal, Nervous

Genetics: N/A

Incidence/Prevalence in USA:
• 80% of Americans experience mechanical low back pain sometime in their lifetime
• One of the most common complaints for primary care visits
• Repetitive episodes are common

Predominant age: 25-45 years

Predominant sex: Male = Female

SIGNS AND SYMPTOMS
• History
  ◊ Onset of low back pain begins either suddenly after an injury or gradually over the next 24 hours
  ◊ Variable pain at posterior belt-line, typically bilateral
  ◊ Occasional radiation of pain to buttocks, and/or posterior thighs stopping at knees
  ◊ Pain pattern referred rather than radicular
  ◊ Back pain worse than leg pain
  ◊ Pain aggravated by back motion, sitting, standing, lifting, bending and twisting
  ◊ Pain relieved by rest (recumbency)
  ◊ Bowel and bladder function preserved
• Physical findings
  ◊ Normal motor, sensory, and reflex examinations
  ◊ Decreased lumbar range of motion, tenderness to palpation, paraspinous musculature spasm common
  ◊ Nerve root stretch tests are commonly negative
  ◊ Straight leg raise and other tests causing spinal motion may increase low back pain, but not leg pain

CAUSES
Normal aging process of musculoskeletal system aggravates an acute event

RISK FACTORS
• Age
• Activity
• Smoking
• Obesity
• Vibration, e.g., driving motor vehicles
• Sedentary lifestyle
• Psychosocial factors

DIAGNOSIS

DIFFERENTIAL DIAGNOSIS
• Structural
  ◊ Acute lumbar back pain
  ◊ Chronic lumbar back pain
  ◊ Low back strain/sprain
  ◊ Herniated lumbar intervertebral disc
  ◊ Degenerative disc disease
  ◊ Degenerative segmental instability
  ◊ Spinal stenosis
  ◊ Spondylolisthesis
  ◊ Fractures
• Inflammatory
  ◊ Ankylosing spondylitis and related inflammatory spondylopathies
  ◊ Infection: vertebral osteomyelitis, discitis
  ◊ Rheumatoid arthritis
• Neoplastic
  ◊ Primary tumors
  ◊ Metastases
• Referred pain
  ◊ Orthopaedic - osteoarthritis of hip
  ◊ Sacroiliac joint disease
  ◊ Gastrointestinal - duodenal ulcer, chronic pancreatitis, irritable bowel syndrome, diverticulitis
  ◊ Genitourinary - pyelonephritis, nephrolithiasis, prostatism
  ◊ Gynecological - pregnancy, endometriosis, ovarian cystic disease, pelvic inflammatory disease
  ◊ Cardiovascular - abdominal aortic aneurysm, vascular claudication

LABORATORY
• Generally negative and not typically indicated with initial presentation
• Indications
  ◊ Age > 50 years
  ◊ Nonmechanical nature of pain
  ◊ Atypical pain pattern or distribution
  ◊ Persistent symptomatology remittent to conservative treatment measures
• Screening laboratory studies
  ◊ CBC with differential
  ◊ Sedimentation rate
  ◊ Alkaline and acid phosphatase
  ◊ Serum calcium
  ◊ Serum protein electrophoresis

Drugs that may alter lab results: N/A

Disorders that may alter lab results: N/A

PATHOLOGICAL FINDINGS N/A

SPECIAL TESTS System directed investigation

IMAGING
• Plain radiographs
  ◊ Not indicated to initiate conservative management program
  ◊ Indicated for persistent symptoms > 1 week, patient age > 50 years, or suggestive history
  ◊ Radiographs utilized to rule-out tumor or identify other disease process
  ◊ Anteroposterior, lateral, spot lateral of L5-S1 and oblique x-rays are included in routine lumbo-sacral series
• Bone scan (scintigraphy)
  ◊ Technetium-99m labeled phosphorus indicates active mineralization of bone
  ◊ Rule-out tumor, trauma or infection

DIAGNOSTIC PROCEDURES MRI, CT/myelography only indicated with persistent symptoms, sciatica or the development of neurologic abnormalities

TREATMENT

APPROPRIATE HEALTH CARE
Outpatient for majority

GENERAL MEASURES
• Initial short-term bedrest 2-3 days
• Short-term analgesics
• NSAID's 10 day course initially, then prn
• Muscle relaxants 10 day course
• Physical therapy
• Manipulation

SURGICAL MEASURES N/A

ACTIVITY
• Restricted activities for 3-6 weeks
• Resume activities of daily living as tolerated

DIET Weight reduction - if appropriate

PATIENT EDUCATION
• Home based exercise program
• Posture and body mechanics training
• "Back school" for chronic mechanical low back pain

MEDICATIONS

DRUG(S) OF CHOICE   Nonsteroidal anti-inflammatory drugs - Ibuprofen, naproxen, salsalate. Less expensive, equally efficacious.
Contraindications: Refer to manufacturer's product information
Precautions:
• History of ulcer disease
• Elderly patients
• Renal disease
• Cardiac disease
Significant possible interactions: Refer to manufacturer's product information

ALTERNATIVE DRUGS   N/A

FOLLOWUP

PATIENT MONITORING   Estimated duration of care 1-6 weeks

PREVENTION/AVOIDANCE
• Smoking cessation
• Weight reduction
• General physical condition
• Avoid aggravating tasks, e.g., heavy lifting, bending, twisting, sudden unexpected movements or combination of above

POSSIBLE COMPLICATIONS
• Incorrect diagnosis
• Chronic low back pain
• Narcotic addiction
• Persistent psychosocial impairment

EXPECTED COURSE/PROGNOSIS
• Resumption of normal activity without residual symptoms in most cases
• May be hindered by secondary gain issues

MISCELLANEOUS

ASSOCIATED CONDITIONS
• Deconditioning
• Obesity
• Psychosocial disease

AGE-RELATED FACTORS
Pediatric: Thorough work-up imperative
Geriatric: Tumors, degenerative conditions, fractures and stenosis more common
Others: N/A

PREGNANCY   Commonly associated with low back pain and/or sciatica. Treatment is conservative.

SYNONYMS
• Low back syndrome
• Lumbar strain/sprain
• Lumbago

ICD-9-CM
722 Intervertebral disc disorders
724.2 Lumbago
724.5 Backache, unspecified

SEE ALSO   Lumbar (intervertebral) disk disorders

OTHER NOTES
• Adverse psychosocial factors to resolving back pain:
  ◊ Pending litigation or compensation
  ◊ Depressed or hostile patient
  ◊ Prolonged use of narcotics or alcohol

ABBREVIATIONS   N/A

REFERENCES
• American Academy of Orthopedic Surgeons: Clinical Policy; Low back musculoligamentous injury (sprain/strain). AAOS Bulletin 3638, April, 1991
• Macnab I, McCulloch J: Backache. 2nd Ed. Baltimore, Williams & Wilkins, 1986
Illustrations: N/A
Internet references: http://www.5mcc.com

Author(s)
Michael J. Smith, MD
Robert A. Cheney, MD

Lumbar (intervertebral) disk disorders

BASICS

DESCRIPTION Many patients with low back pain have lumbar disc disease and involvement of surrounding spinal ligaments, muscles and skeleton. Over time may progress to disc degeneration, disc herniation, spinal narrowing and arthritic proliferation of the facet joint. Management is based on symptoms and disability, because the distinction between the normal aging of the spine and pathological findings are hard to distinguish.
• Non-radicular low back pain (acute and chronic) - low back pain remaining near belt-line caused by soft tissue or disc injury
• Radicular low back pain (acute and chronic) - neuropathic pain is to a greater degree in the buttocks, hips or legs rather than the back. There may or may not be signs of weakness, numbness, or loss of reflex. In younger patients, the source of the pain is likely to be mechanical compression or chemical irritation of a nerve root.
• Spinal stenosis is more likely to be the etiology of radicular pain in patients over 55 years
System(s) affected: Musculoskeletal, Nervous
Genetics: N/A
Incidence/Prevalence in USA:
• One of the most frequent complaints for which adults seek medical attention and second to the common cold for most time off work
• Lifetime prevalence of low back pain is 60-90%. The annual incidence is 5%. Among patients with acute back pain, 1% have nerve root symptoms.
• 95% of diseased disks are localized to L4-5 and L5-S1
• Less than 2% of patients with low back pain have infections, neoplasms, or inflammatory spondyloarthropathies
Predominant age: 25-45 years, first episode in 20's and 30's, infrequent before 20 years or after age 65
Predominant sex: Male = Female

SIGNS AND SYMPTOMS
• Variable pain; usually dull, originating in back, extending below knee
• Pain may radiate (often unilaterally) in nerve root distribution
• Back pain decreases at night. Bedrest usually improves symptoms at least temporarily.
• Pain increases with walking
• Constitutional symptoms absent
• Sciatica can occur without back pain
• Often sensory aberrations in extremities, paresthesia and numbness
• Occasionally muscle group weakness
• Most disc ruptures are postero-lateral and press upon lumbar nerve root with radiating pain
• Lumbar scoliosis possible, trunk tilted toward or away from affected side, depending on location of extrusion
• Paraspinal muscle spasm

CAUSES
• Trauma, major or minor
• Frequent lifting of objects weighing 25 pounds (11.3 kg) or more, especially if lifted with arms extended and knees straight, and body twisted
• Vibration; e.g., driving motor vehicles

RISK FACTORS
• Normal aging process after age 20 years
• Cigarette smoking
• Narrow lumbar vertebral canal (for prolapsed disk)
• Stress, muscle tension
• Obesity
• Osteoporosis

DIAGNOSIS

DIFFERENTIAL DIAGNOSIS Acute lumbosacral strain, chronic lumbosacral strain, spondylosis, spondylolisthesis, spinal arthritis, fibrositis, cauda equina syndrome, compression fracture, poor posture, bursitis, metastatic and primary tumors, vertebral infection, pain referred from from hip, retroperitoneum, aneurysms, or pelvis, (geriatrics) neurogenic claudication

LABORATORY ESR - usually normal
Drugs that may alter lab results: N/A
Disorders that may alter lab results: N/A

PATHOLOGICAL FINDINGS Difficult to distinguish normal aging process of disc degeneration from specific lesions causing low back pain and sciatica

SPECIAL TESTS Electromyography - useful to exclude peripheral neuritis

IMAGING
• Lumbosacral plain films - rarely indicated just to initiate a conservative management program - indicated to rule out tumor or structural abnormality although presence of latter may not confirm source of pain
• Lumbosacral oblique views - controversial
• Myelography, CT scan, magnetic resonance have similar diagnostic accuracy for surgical candidate evaluation

DIAGNOSTIC PROCEDURES
• Sciatic stretch test - in supine position, elevation of affected leg (to 15-30% for severe, 30-60%, milder) elicits pain. Tip: can compare to sitting position to look for learned behavior.
• Laségue's sign - patient is supine, hip flexed, dorsiflexion of ankle accentuates sciatic pain or muscle spasm in posterior thigh
• Cross straight-leg-raising - elevating normal leg produces sciatica down other leg
• Doorbell sign - (insensitive) deep palpation of the spinous process over protruded disc reproduces sciatica
• Femoral stretch (for L2-3) in prone position, affected leg is extended from knee reproducing pain along femoral nerve

• Faber's test - (positive only for hip pain) in supine position, flexion, abduction and external rotation produces pain
• Neurologic defects of lower extremities and perineum will usually locate level of lesion. Test gait, reflexes, motor strength, muscle atrophy; pulses and abdominal bruits; rectal sphincter.

TREATMENT

APPROPRIATE HEALTH CARE
Outpatient for majority. Inpatient for severe disability and/or surgery.

GENERAL MEASURES
• Initial: ordinary activities as tolerated, local heat, pelvic traction, sedation, physical therapy (90% response)
• Following bedrest: up and about with midline support. Wean from support over next several weeks.
• For chronic non-radicular pain: improve physical fitness with low impact aerobic exercise. Manipulation and physical therapy have shown benefit.
• Transcutaneous electrical nerve stimulation (TENS): very short term benefit

SURGICAL MEASURES
• Procedures available
  ◊ Standard discectomy - discectomy techniques all have comparable results
  ◊ Microsurgical discectomy
  ◊ Percutaneous discectomy - relatively new, contraindicated in spinal stenosis and sequestered disc fragments
  ◊ Chemonucleolysis - lower rate of benefit and occasional severe complications
  ◊ Spinal fusion (arthrodesis) - indicated for spinal instability
• Absolute indications for discectomy
  ◊ Cauda equina syndrome
  ◊ Progressive neurological deficit despite conservative treatment
• Relative indications for discectomy
  ◊ Intolerable pain
  ◊ Multiple episodes of radiculopathy
  ◊ Severe postural tilt
  ◊ Persistent dysfunctional pain - these patients have been reported to improve more rapidly postoperatively but long term results show no difference from nonoperative treatment
  ◊ Static neurological deficit - no reported difference between operative or nonoperative treatment for improvement in weakness or sensory disturbance

ACTIVITY
• After pain is controlled (7-10 days), begin progressive walking program. Short walks initially 4 times a day and lengthen as tolerated.
• Return to work as soon as possible with avoidance of high risk activities, e.g., heavy lifting, vibration, smoking

DIET Weight reduction if appropriate

PATIENT EDUCATION Good posture, proper body mechanics, physical fitness, physical therapy if appropriate

MEDICATIONS

DRUG(S) OF CHOICE
• Analgesics
• Nonsteroidal anti-inflammatory medication
• Muscle relaxants (controversial)
• Mild sedatives
Contraindications: Refer to manufacturer's profile of each drug
Precautions: Elderly, hypertension, prior peptic ulcer disease or bleeding, renal disease, liver disease, cardiac dysfunction
Significant possible interactions: Refer to manufacturer's profile of each drug

ALTERNATIVE DRUGS N/A

FOLLOWUP

PATIENT MONITORING Outpatient - return visit about 10 days following initial visit, should be improved. Follow pain history and neurological status. Thereafter monitor every 2 weeks until fully functional. Monitor exercise program.

PREVENTION/AVOIDANCE
• Modification of jobs to reduce exposure to known risk factors
• Selection of workers by such means as strength testing for certain jobs
• Avoid smoking

POSSIBLE COMPLICATIONS
• Foot drop with weakness of anterior tibial, posterior tibial and peroneal muscles
• Loss of ankle jerk
• Bladder and rectal sphincter weakness with retention or incontinence
• Limitation of movement and restricted activity
• Narcotic addiction

EXPECTED COURSE/PROGNOSIS
• Acute low back pain (90%) and/or radiculopathy (60-80%) can be expected to recover spontaneously with conservative therapy
• Chronic nonradicular low back pain - most patients respond to conservative management such as manipulation, fitness, weight reduction, and education regarding back care
• Chronic radicular pain - good selection of surgical candidates have found satisfactory results (80% in long-term studies)

MISCELLANEOUS

ASSOCIATED CONDITIONS
• Poor physical conditioning/posture
• Obesity
• Osteoarthritis
• Osteoporosis
• Depression, other psychiatric disorders

AGE-RELATED FACTORS
Pediatric: Scoliosis, onset age 10 years, rarely symptomatic until adulthood. Detect difference in leg length.
Geriatric: Usually multifactorial lesions of spine. Degenerative spondylolisthesis (especially in women), spinal stenosis, and neurogenic claudication are more likely.
Others: N/A

PREGNANCY Commonly associated with low back pain and/or sciatica. Treatment is conservative.

SYNONYMS
• Degenerative disk disease
• Intervertebral disk dislocation

ICD-9-CM
722 Intervertebral disc disorders

SEE ALSO
• Low back pain

OTHER NOTES
• Features which predict best surgical outcome (90-95% improvement when all three exist)
  ◊ Definable neurological deficit
  ◊ Pathology in imaging which correlates with deficit
  ◊ Positive nerve root tension signs
• Adverse psychosocial factors to resolving back pain
  ◊ Sciatica with predominant back symptoms
  ◊ Pending litigation or compensation
  ◊ Depressed or hostile patient
  ◊ Low IQ or poorly educated may not be able to participate in assessment or decision
  ◊ Prolonged use of narcotics or alcohol

ABBREVIATIONS N/A

REFERENCES
• Beaty JH (ed): Orthopedic Knowledge Update, American Academy of Orthopedic Surgeons, 1997
• Kent OL, Haynor DR, Longstreth WT, Larson EB: The clinical efficacy of magnetic resonance imaging in neuroimaging. Ann Int Med 1994:120;856-871
• Frost H, Moffett JAK, Moser JS, Fairbank JCT: Randomized controlled trial for evaluation of fitness programme for patients with chronic low back pain. Brit Med Jour 1995;310:151-159
• Malmivaara A, Hakkinen U, Aro T, Heinrichs MJ, et al: The Treatment of Acute Low Back pain - bed rest, exercises, or ordinary activity?. NEJM 1995:332; 351-355
Illustrations: N/A
Internet references: http://www.5mcc.com

Author(s)
Claudia A. Peters, MD

Lung abscess

BASICS

DESCRIPTION A localized cavity in the lung with pus resulting from necrosis of lung tissue surrounded by lung infection. May be caused by aerobic or anaerobic infection. Usual course is sub-acute; progressive.
System(s) affected: Pulmonary
Genetics: No known genetic pattern
Incidence/Prevalence in USA: Unknown, relatively rare
Predominant age: Mainly 4th-6th decades
Predominant sex: Male > Female (4:1)

SIGNS AND SYMPTOMS
- Cough
- Sputum (purulent, foul-smelling)
- Fever
- Chest pain
- Dyspnea
- Chills, rigors
- Malaise
- Weight loss
- Anorexia
- Night sweats
- Hemoptysis
- Decreased breath sounds
- Crackles
- Wheezing
- Tachypnea
- Tachycardia
- Diaphoresis
- Dullness to percussion
- Consolidation by auscultation
- Cavernous breath sounds

CAUSES
- Lung infection
- Aspiration pneumonia
- Necrotizing pneumonia
- Cavitary infarction
- Septic embolism
- Bacteremia
- Bronchial stenosis or obstruction
- Tumors
- Dental abscess in loose tooth

RISK FACTORS
- Periodontal disease (gingivitis)
- Alcoholism
- Drug abuse
- Epilepsy
- Unconsciousness
- Lung neoplasia
- Immunosuppression/immunocompromised
- Diabetes mellitus
- Airway foreign body
- Gastroesophageal reflux with aspiration
- Sinusitis
- Gastric and esophageal surgery
- Dental and oropharyngeal surgery

DIAGNOSIS

DIFFERENTIAL DIAGNOSIS
- Bronchogenic carcinoma
- Bronchiectasis
- Empyema with bronchopulmonary fistula
- Tuberculosis
- Mycotic lung infections
- Actinomycosis
- Nocardiosis
- Infected pulmonary bulla
- Wegener's granulomatosis
- Pulmonary sequestration
- Subphrenic or hepatic abscess with perforation into a bronchus
- Bronchogenic or parenchymal cyst

LABORATORY
- Leukocytosis
- Anemia
- Hypoalbuminemia
- Sputum smear - mixed bacteria and neutrophils
- Sputum culture - mixed flora, anaerobes
- Gram-negative rods and cocci
- Pleural fluid - neutrophilia
- Bacteriology:
  ◊ Generally anaerobes
  ◊ Staphylococcus
  ◊ Klebsiella spp.
  ◊ Pseudomonas aeruginosa
  ◊ Other (uncommon)
Drugs that may alter lab results: Prior antibiotics
Disorders that may alter lab results: N/A

PATHOLOGICAL FINDINGS
- Gross - solitary abscess
- Multiple abscesses
- Micro - suppuration
- Cavitation

SPECIAL TESTS   N/A

IMAGING
- Chest x-ray: consolidation with radiolucency
- Air-fluid level
- Pleural effusion
- CT: define location and extent

DIAGNOSTIC PROCEDURES
- Bronchoscopy if obstruction suspected
- Bronchoscopic protected brushing
- Bronchoalveolar lavage
- Transthoracic needle aspiration

TREATMENT

APPROPRIATE HEALTH CARE
- Inpatient if ill, otherwise outpatient
- Inpatient surgery

GENERAL MEASURES
- Postural drainage
- Pulmonary physiotherapy
- Treat underlying etiology (e.g., with antibiotics)
- Bronchoscopy with selective therapeutic lavage - rarely

SURGICAL MEASURES   Rarely, surgery for complications (pulmonary resection)

ACTIVITY   Reduced activity until x-ray evidence of clearing

DIET   No restrictions

PATIENT EDUCATION   Pulmonary physiotherapy techniques

Lung abscess

MEDICATIONS

DRUG(S) OF CHOICE Antibiotics according to culture and sensitivity results. For presumed anaerobes, data from two prospective randomized trials have shown clindamycin 600 mg every 6-8 hours IV, followed by 300 mg every 6 hours orally for 4 weeks to result in fewer treatment failures than penicillin.
Contraindications: Refer to manufacturer's literature.
Precautions: Refer to manufacturer's literature
Significant possible interactions: Refer to manufacturer's literature

ALTERNATIVE DRUGS
• Anaerobes: standard therapy has been penicillin G 1-2 million units IV every 4 hours until improved, followed by 1.2 million units (750 mg) orally every 6 hours for 3-4 weeks. Metronidazole has not proven as effective as clindamycin.
• Bacteroides: cefoxitin, cefotetan, ticarcillin-clavulanate, chloramphenicol, imipenem
• Fusobacterium: first generation cephalosporin

FOLLOWUP

PATIENT MONITORING Continue treatment until cavity has resolved on serial x-rays (may take several months)

PREVENTION/AVOIDANCE Treat predisposing diseases

POSSIBLE COMPLICATIONS
• Extension
• Empyema
• Massive hemoptysis
• Pneumothorax
• Brain abscess

EXPECTED COURSE/PROGNOSIS
Without underlying disease, guardedly favorable. Increased sequelae and mortality with concomitant disease (up to 75% mortality).

MISCELLANEOUS

ASSOCIATED CONDITIONS
• Pneumonia
• Alcoholism
• Epilepsy
• Empyema
• Periodontal disease
• Unconsciousness
• Neoplasia
• Bronchogenic carcinoma
• Tuberculosis
• Fungal diseases

AGE-RELATED FACTORS
Pediatric: Occurs in children, Staphylococcus most common organism
Geriatric: Mortality higher in this age group
Others: N/A

PREGNANCY N/A

SYNONYMS Pulmonary abscess

ICD-9-CM
513.0 abscess of lung

SEE ALSO
• Pneumonia, bacterial

OTHER NOTES N/A

ABBREVIATIONS N/A

REFERENCES
• Bartlett JG: Anaerobic bacterial infections of the lung and pleural space. Clinical Infectious Diseases 1993;16;Suppl4:s248-255
• Murray JF, Nadel JA, eds: Textbook of Respiratory Medicine. 2nd Ed. Philadelphia, W.B. Saunders Co., 1994
• Guidiol F, Manresa F, Pallares R, et al: Clindamycin vs penicillin for anaerobic lung infections. Arch Int Med 1990;150:2525-2529
• Davis B, Systrom DM: Lung abscess: pathogenesis, doagnosis and treatment. Curr Clin Topics in Infect Dis 1998;18:252-273
Illustrations: N/A
Internet references: http://www.5mcc.com

Author(s)
J. P. W. Cunnington, MD, FRCPC

Lung, primary malignancies

 BASICS

DESCRIPTION
• The common lung cancers may be divided into two broad categories:
  ◊ Non-small cell cancer: includes squamous cell cancer, (most common); adenocarcinoma and large cell carcinoma
  ◊ Small cell cancer
• Other malignancies from the lung are numerous but uncommon (lymphoma, blastoma, sarcoma, etc.)
System(s) affected: Pulmonary
Genetics: N/A
Incidence/Prevalence in USA:
• 175,000 new cases per year
• 70/100,000 population
Predominant age: 50-70 years
Predominant sex: Male > Female

SIGNS AND SYMPTOMS
May be asymptomatic.
• Hypertrophic pulmonary osteoarthropathy
• Cough
• Shortness of breath
• Hemoptysis
• Exercise limitation
• Chest pain
• Hoarseness
• Wheezing
• Excess fatigue
• Dyspnea
• Shoulder/arm pain
• Dysphagia
• Bone pain
• Weight loss
• Superior vena cava syndrome
• Anemia

CAUSES
• Smoking (greater than 90%)
• Asbestos exposure
• Chronic interstitial pneumonitis
• Halogen ethers
• Inorganic arsenic
• Radioisotopes
• Atmospheric pollution
• Other metals

RISK FACTORS   Listed under Causes

 DIAGNOSIS

DIFFERENTIAL DIAGNOSIS
• Metastatic cancer
• Granuloma
• Hamartoma

LABORATORY
• CBC (look for anemia)
• SMA-18 (look for abnormalities of Na, K, Ca and liver enzymes)
• PT, PTT, platelet count
Drugs that may alter lab results: None likely
Disorders that may alter lab results: None likely

PATHOLOGICAL FINDINGS   Cancer cell type from positive histology or cytology (see Description)

SPECIAL TESTS
• Electrocardiogram
• Pulmonary function studies
• Exercise treadmill
• Stress thallium or Persantine scans when applicable

IMAGING
• Chest x-ray, CT scan of chest, split perfusion lung scan:
  ◊ Pulmonary nodule, mass, or infiltrate
  ◊ Mediastinal widening
  ◊ Atelectasis
  ◊ Hilar enlargement
  ◊ Pleural effusion
• Other CT scans:
  ◊ Of brain - when applicable
  ◊ Of abdomen (may not be necessary if CT of chest includes screen for hepatic or adrenal metastasis)
• Bone scan:
  ◊ When applicable

DIAGNOSTIC PROCEDURES
• Fiberoptic bronchoscopy
• Mediastinoscopy, when applicable
• Fine needle aspiration biopsy
• Scalene node biopsy, when applicable

 TREATMENT

APPROPRIATE HEALTH CARE
• Inpatient for surgery
• Outpatient chemotherapy or radiation therapy for small cell cancer

GENERAL MEASURES
• Radiotherapy
• Immunotherapy
• Pain relief when applicable

SURGICAL MEASURES   Surgical resection for non-small cell cancer, when possible - stage I and II and some stage III

ACTIVITY   Fully active

DIET   No special diet

PATIENT EDUCATION
• General verbal information on lung cancer
• American Cancer Society for support groups and other information

MEDICATIONS

DRUG(S) OF CHOICE Pain medication
Contraindications: Refer to manufacturer's instructions
Precautions: Refer to manufacturer's instructions
Significant possible interactions: Refer to manufacturer's instructions

ALTERNATIVE DRUGS N/A

FOLLOWUP

PATIENT MONITORING
• Surgically resectable
  ◊ First year each 3 months
  ◊ Second year each 6 months
  ◊ Third though fifth year once a year
• Surgically unresectable
  ◊ As necessary for palliation

PREVENTION/AVOIDANCE
• Stop smoking
• Avoid asbestos
• Avoid occupational exposure to metals
• Consider prophylaxis with retinoid, such as beta-carotene

POSSIBLE COMPLICATIONS
• Development of metastatic disease
• Local recurrence

EXPECTED COURSE/PROGNOSIS
• Stage I, post-surgical resection of squamous/adeno/large cell is 50% survival
• Stage II, post-surgical is 33% for squamous (stage IIIa, post-surgical survival is 15% for squamous), and 20% for adeno/large cell
• Note: Pre-surgical staging is less accurate so survival figures are lower
• If nonresectable, prognosis is poor with mean survival rate of 8 to 14 months

MISCELLANEOUS

ASSOCIATED CONDITIONS N/A

AGE-RELATED FACTORS
Pediatric: N/A
Geriatric: More common in elderly (> 75 years)
Others: N/A

PREGNANCY N/A

SYNONYMS
• Lung cancer

ICD-9-CM
162.9 Malignant neoplasm of bronchus and lung, unspecified

SEE ALSO N/A

OTHER NOTES N/A

ABBREVIATIONS N/A

REFERENCES
• Shields TW, ed: General Thoracic Surgery. 3rd Ed. Philadelphia, Lea and Febiger, 1989
• Baue AE, ed: Glenn's Thoracic and Cardiovascular Surgery. 5th Ed. East Norwich, Appleton and Lange, 1990
• Sabiston DC, ed: Surgery of the Chest. 4th Ed. Philadelphia, W.B. Saunders Co., 1983
Illustrations: N/A
Internet references: http://www.5mcc.com

Author(s)
John R. Burk, MD

Lupus erythematosus, discoid

BASICS

DESCRIPTION Discoid lupus erythematosus (DLE) is the most common form of chronic cutaneous lupus. It is a chronic skin disease characterized by sharply marginated dull, red macules with adherent scales extending into areas of atrophy, telangiectasias, or follicular plugging
• Localized DLE - more common form with lesions occurring on the face especially the malar areas, bridge of nose, lower lip, lower eyelids and ears
• Widespread DLE - lesions seen on upper extremities and thorax
System(s) affected: Skin/Exocrine
Genetics: N/A
Incidence/Prevalence in USA:
• 3/100,000 Caucasian females; 8/100,000 black females
• 100/100,000
Predominant age: 25 to 45
Predominant sex:
• Localized DLE - Female > Male (3:1)
• Widespread DLE - Female > Male (9:1)

SIGNS AND SYMPTOMS
• Red plaque-like lesions on face, thorax, or extensor aspect of upper extremities; rare below waist
• Older lesions atrophy and appear as smooth white or hyperpigmented scars with telangiectasias
• Scarring alopecia with scalp lesions
• "Carpet tack" appearance of skin when scale removed
• Lesions occasionally slightly pruritic or stinging
• Oral ulceration in 15 percent of patients
• Photosensitivity
• Koebner response (precipitation by cutaneous trauma)

CAUSES Unknown

RISK FACTORS Systemic lupus erythematosus (SLE)

DIAGNOSIS

DIFFERENTIAL DIAGNOSIS
• Actinic keratoses
• Polymorphous light eruption
• Drug eruptions
• Sarcoid
• Cutaneous leishmaniasis
• Lupus vulgaris
• Seborrheic dermatitis
• Lichen planus
• Plaque psoriasis
• Rosacea
• Pemphigus erythematosus
• Tinea faciei
• Jessner-Kanof disease
• Granuloma faciale

LABORATORY
• Localized DLE: positive ANA in low titer (30%)
• Widespread DLE, may occasionally find, increased sedimentation rate, positive ANA (30-40%), positive dsDNA (< 5%), leukopenia, hematuria and albuminuria if concomitant SLE
Drugs that may alter lab results: N/A
Disorders that may alter lab results: Concomitant SLE

PATHOLOGICAL FINDINGS
• Hyperkeratosis
• Epidermal atrophy
• Liquefactive degeneration of basal cell layer
• Edema, mucin, and inflammation of dermis
• Follicular plugging
• Basement zone thickened with strong periodic acid-Schiff reaction staining

SPECIAL TESTS Immunofluorescent staining of skin biopsies (lupus band test)

IMAGING N/A

DIAGNOSTIC PROCEDURES Skin biopsy

TREATMENT

APPROPRIATE HEALTH CARE
Outpatient

GENERAL MEASURES Avoid sun exposure, avoid excessive heat, cold, or trauma

SURGICAL MEASURES N/A

ACTIVITY Full activity

DIET Regular

PATIENT EDUCATION
• Teach patients proper use of sunscreens and other measures to prevent sun exposure (e.g., wide-brimmed hats, long sleeves, etc.)
• Advise patient about symptoms of systemic lupus erythematosus (SLE) that should be watched for
• Griffiths: Instructions for Patients, Philadelphia, W.B. Saunders Co.

MEDICATIONS

DRUG(S) OF CHOICE
• Localized DLE:
◊ Low to medium potency topical corticosteroid (eg, triamcinolone 0.1% bid to all active lesions
◊ If no response in 2-3 weeks, move to higher potency topical corticosteroid applied tid (eg, betamethasone)
◊ Intralesional corticosteroid (eg, triamcinolone 2.5-5 mg/mL for the face or 5-10 mg/mL elsewhere) for resistant lesions. Use 0.5 mL per 1 cm plaque.
• Widespread DLE:
◊ Hydroxychloroquine 200 mg or chloroquine 250 mg qd or bid and/or quinacrine 100 mg daily
◊ Short-term (1-2 weeks) of topical corticosteroids is helpful at the same time antimalarials are being started

Contraindications: Antimalarials such as hydroxychloroquine may have to be avoided in patients with preexisting retinal or hepatic disease. Do not give to individuals with G6PD deficiency. Quinacrine rarely causes hematologic cytopenia.

Precautions:
• Observe for skin atrophy with topical steroids especially with use on the face
• Patients on antimalarials should have an eye examination by an ophthalmologist at start of treatment and at 3-6 month intervals to monitor signs of retinal damage

Significant possible interactions: N/A

ALTERNATIVE DRUGS
• Localized DLE: Intralesional triamcinolone 2.5 mg/cc injected at monthly intervals. Prednisone 15 mg bid, then tapered after response.
• Widespread DLE: Quinacrine 100 mg qd, dapsone 100 mg qd, azathioprine 100 mg qd. Systemic retinoid, eg, etretinate 1 mg/kg; thalidomide is also effective

FOLLOWUP

PATIENT MONITORING
• Recheck patients once or twice per month
• Ophthalmology followup at 6 month intervals if patient on antimalarial
• If lesions subside, reduce dosage of antimalarials over 2-3 months, then discontinue

PREVENTION/AVOIDANCE   Avoid sun exposure or excessive heat, cold, or skin trauma

POSSIBLE COMPLICATIONS
Hypertrophic scarring, hypopigmentation (especially in blacks)

EXPECTED COURSE/PROGNOSIS
• 40% remit completely; 1-5% may develop systemic lupus (these patients usually have widespread DLE)
• Not life-threatening unless it turns into systemic type

MISCELLANEOUS

ASSOCIATED CONDITIONS
• Systemic lupus erythematosus
• Mixed connective tissue disease (MCTD)
• Antiphospholipid syndrome

AGE-RELATED FACTORS
Pediatric: Neonatal lupus erythematosus is a syndrome of cutaneous lupus and/or congenital heart block. It is caused by transplacental passage of one of several maternal antibodies.
Geriatric: N/A
Others: N/A

PREGNANCY   N/A

SYNONYMS
• Chronic cutaneous lupus erythematosus

ICD-9-CM
695.4 Lupus erythematosus (local, discoid)

SEE ALSO
• Systemic lupus erythematosus (SLE)

OTHER NOTES   N/A

ABBREVIATIONS   N/A

REFERENCES
• Habif T: Clinical Dermatology. 3rd Ed. St Louis, Mosby, 1996
• Goldstein A, Goldstein B: Practical Dermatology. 2nd Ed. St Louis, Mosby, 1997
• Freedberg IM, et al: Fitzpatrick's Dermatology in General Medicine, 5th ed. New York, McGraw Hill, 1999.
Illustrations: 8 available on CD-ROM
Internet references: http://www.5mcc.com

Author(s)
Gary J. Silko, MD

Lyme disease

BASICS

DESCRIPTION A multisystem infection caused by the spirochete Borrelia burgdorferi, which is transmitted primarily by Ixodid ticks
• Stage 1, early localized Lyme disease, includes a characteristic expanding skin rash (erythema migrans) and constitutional flu-like symptoms
• Stage 2, early disseminated Lyme disease, may present with involvement of one or more organ systems. Neurologic (15%) and cardiac (8%) disease are most common.
• Stage 3, chronic Lyme disease, involves arthritis (50%) and chronic neurological syndromes
System(s) affected: Skin/Exocrine, Musculoskeletal, Hemic/Lymphatic/Immunologic
Genetics: HLA - haplotype DR4 or DR2 may be more susceptible to prolonged arthritis
Incidence/Prevalence in USA: Overall incidence 4.4/100,000. Highest prevalence in Connecticut, Rhode Island, New York, New Jersey, Pennsylvania, Wisconsin, Maryland and Minnesota.
Predominant age: Can occur in all ages, but most common in children under 15 and in the 35-49 year age group
Predominant sex: Male = Female

SIGNS AND SYMPTOMS
• Stage 1:
  ◊ Erythema migrans (60-80%)
  ◊ Fever
  ◊ Headache
  ◊ Myalgias
  ◊ Arthralgias
  ◊ Some patients may be asymptomatic
• Stage 2: (involvement of one or more organ systems)
  ◊ Multiple erythema migrans
  ◊ Facial palsies, or other cranial neuropathies
  ◊ Aseptic meningitis
  ◊ Heart block
  ◊ Pericarditis
  ◊ Orchitis, hepatitis, or iritis
  ◊ Arthritis (usually large joint monarthritis)
• Stage 3:
  ◊ Recurrent synovitis
  ◊ Recurrent tendinitis and bursitis
  ◊ Neuropsychiatric symptoms, may include: Psychotic behavior, memory loss, dementia, depression, sleep disorders
  ◊ Encephalopathic symptoms: Headache, decreased memory, difficulty concentrating, confusion, fatigue
  ◊ Symptoms mimicking other CNS diseases: Multiple sclerosis-like syndromes, stroke-like symptoms, vestibular neuronitis, transverse myelitis, parkinsonian symptoms
  ◊ Peripheral neuropathic symptoms: Carpal tunnel syndrome, motor, sensory, or autonomic neuropathies
  ◊ Ophthalmic manifestations: Iritis, keratitis, retinal vasculitis, optic neuritis

CAUSES Infection with spirochete Borrelia burgdorferi, transmitted by the bite of Ixodid ticks

RISK FACTORS Exposure to tick infested area, most common from May to September

DIAGNOSIS

DIFFERENTIAL DIAGNOSIS
• Juvenile rheumatoid arthritis
• Viral syndromes
• Later stages may mimic many other diseases (see Signs and Symptoms)

LABORATORY
• ELISA for IgM and IgG B burgdorferi antibodies (frequently negative in stage 1 disease)
• Culture of CSF for B burgdorferi
Drugs that may alter lab results: Late stage disease with negative serology may be seen in patients who received early antibiotic treatment
Disorders that may alter lab results: False positive response has been seen with Rocky Mountain spotted fever, syphilis, systemic lupus erythematosus, and rheumatoid arthritis

PATHOLOGICAL FINDINGS Culture of B burgdorferi from blood or skin biopsy specimens has a very low yield

SPECIAL TESTS N/A

IMAGING N/A

DIAGNOSTIC PROCEDURES Lumbar puncture when neurologic findings are present, with ELISA of CSF for B burgdorferi antibodies

TREATMENT

APPROPRIATE HEALTH CARE
• Stage 1, clinical diagnosis, can be treated as an outpatient
• Stage 2 and 3 may require more intensive treatment, based on symptoms

GENERAL MEASURES Prevention of infection is possible by careful examination of skin for ticks after outdoor activities. Prompt removal of ticks may limit transmission. Clothing that covers the ankles should be worn in endemic areas, and the use of insect repellants is recommended.

SURGICAL MEASURES N/A

ACTIVITY No restriction

DIET No special diet

PATIENT EDUCATION
• In endemic areas, patients should be advised to protect themselves against tick exposure
• Information available from: American Lyme Disease Foundation, 293 Route 100, Suite 204, Somers NY 10589

MEDICATIONS

DRUG(S) OF CHOICE
• Stage 1:
 ◊ Doxycycline (Vibramycin) 100 mg po bid for 14-21 days (do not use in children under 12 or in pregnancy); or
 ◊ Amoxicillin 500 mg po tid for 14-21 days, (pediatric dose 25-100 mg/kg/day)
 ◊ Cefuroxime (Ceftin) axetil 500 mg bid for 14-21 days
• Stage 2:
 ◊ Normal CSF, treat for 28 days - doxycycline 100 mg po bid; or
 ◊ Amoxicillin 500 mg po tid
 ◊ Short course of corticosteroids (5-7 days) may be helpful
 ◊ With abnormal CSF, treat for 3-4 weeks - ceftriaxone (Rocephin) 2 g IV qd; or cefotaxime (Claforan) 2 g IV q 8 h; or penicillin G 20-24 million units/day IV
• Stage 3:
 ◊ Oral treatment for 28 days with doxycycline 100 mg bid; or
 ◊ Amoxicillin 500 mg tid
 ◊ If oral treatment fails, IV treatment for 2-3 weeks with ceftriaxone 2 g qd; or cefotaxime 2 g q 8 hr; or penicillin G 20-24 million units/day IV

Contraindications:
• Allergy to agent
• Doxycycline contraindicated in children and in women who are pregnant or breast feeding
Precautions: Refer to manufacturer's profile of each drug
Significant possible interactions:
• Oral anticoagulants may need reduced dose
• Oral contraceptives may be less effective

ALTERNATIVE DRUGS
• Cefuroxime (Ceftin) 500 mg bid for stage I disease, or tid for stage 2 or 3 disease

FOLLOWUP

PATIENT MONITORING
Stage 2 and 3 disease requires careful monitoring over a period of months to years, based on severity of symptoms

PREVENTION/AVOIDANCE
Awareness of the disease, protective clothing, and careful skin inspection with timely removal of ticks may reduce the incidence of disease. A 3 dose vaccine, LYMErix, is now available.

POSSIBLE COMPLICATIONS
• Recurrent synovitis, tendinitis, bursitis
• Chronic neurological symptoms
• Peripheral neuropathies
• See Signs and symptoms of Stage 3 disease

EXPECTED COURSE/PROGNOSIS
• Early treatment with antibiotics can shorten the duration of symptoms and prevent later disease
• Response of late stage disease is variable

MISCELLANEOUS

ASSOCIATED CONDITIONS N/A

AGE-RELATED FACTORS
Pediatric: Drug of choice in pediatrics is amoxicillin. Tetracyclines are contraindicated.
Geriatric: N/A
Others: Ixodid ticks are commonly found on deer. Hunters may be at increased risk.

PREGNANCY Because B burgdorferi can cross the placenta, pregnant patients with active disease should receive parenteral antibiotics. Doxycycline should not be used in pregnancy.

SYNONYMS Lyme arthritis

ICD-9-CM
088.81 Lyme disease

SEE ALSO N/A

OTHER NOTES Ixodid ticks require white footed mice to complete their life cycle. Investigators have had some success in eradicating the ticks by providing permethrin laced cotton in areas where the mice forage for bedding material.

ABBREVIATIONS N/A

REFERENCES
• The Medical Letter 1999;41(1049):29-30
• Nadelman RB, Wormser GP: Lyme borreliosis. Lancet 1998;352(9127):557-565
• The Medical Letter 1997; 39(1000);47-48
• MMWR 1996;45:481-484
• Rakel R, ed. Textbook of Family medicine. 5th Ed. Philadelphia, WB Saunders Co, 1995:337,1023
• Am J Med 1996;100;502-508
Illustrations: 3 available on CD-ROM
Internet references: http://www.5mcc.com

Author(s)
Barbara A. Majeroni, MD

Lymphogranuloma venereum

BASICS

DESCRIPTION
Lymphogranuloma venereum (LGV) is a rare, systemic, sexually transmitted disease caused by the three most virulent strains or serovars of *Chlamydia trachomatis*, the same organism responsible for chlamydial urethritis
• Tender inguinal lymphadenopathy, usually unilateral, is the most common clinical manifestation in heterosexual men. Women and homosexually active men might have proctocolitis or inflammatory involvement of perirectal or perianal lymphatic tissue. Painless vesicular or ulcerative lesions on the external genitalia may be seen in early disease and severe anogenital inflammation and scarring may result from untreated disease.
• Usually a disease of the tropics; especially Africa, but also seen in the Caribbean (Haiti and Jamaica), South America, East Asia and Indonesia. Chlamydial infections now require reporting in most states.

System(s) affected: Reproductive, Hemic/Lymphatic/Immunologic, Gastrointestinal
Genetics: N/A
Incidence/Prevalence in USA:
Approximately 300 cases reported to CDC each year. The prevalence of anorectal LGV is increasing in the USA in male homosexuals.
Predominant age: Third decade; corresponds with average age of peak sexual activity
Predominant sex: Male > Female (5:1)

SIGNS AND SYMPTOMS
Three stages:
• Primary:
◊ Superficial lesions such as papules, vesicles, ulcers or erosions appear on the external genitalia 3 days to 3 weeks after exposure. Lesions are painless and disappear in a few days leaving no scar. This stage often escapes notice.
• Secondary: the inguinal syndrome (bubonic stage) or hemorrhagic proctitis following rectal intercourse
◊ Predominantly in men (Male:Female > 10:1)
◊ Fever, chills
◊ Inguinal syndrome regional lymphadenopathy occurring a week to months after the primary stage
◊ Buboes begin as a mass of firm, tender, enlarged, matted lymph nodes, often unilateral and eventually involve the overlying skin with erythema and adhesions. They may have a groove through them formed by the inguinal ligament. As the buboes enlarge:
  - The patient experiences severe groin pain and often walks with a limp
  - Within one to two weeks, the buboes may become fluctuant and rupture relieving the pain and leaving fistulas to drain, heal and scar. Sometimes buboes simply involute and form firm inguinal masses.

• Proctitis:
◊ Anal pruritus and a mucous rectal discharge
◊ Multiple, discrete superficial ulcerations with irregular borders
◊ Rectal pain and tenesmus
◊ Rectal mucosa feels granular on digital exam
• Tertiary: the anogenital stage
◊ Lymphatic obstruction or scarring
◊ Genitalia or anorectal canal inflammation
◊ Predominantly women and homosexual men. The rectal or vaginal mucosa can become involved after direct inoculation by receptive intercourse or may become involved through posterior lymphatic spread.
◊ Lymphatic obstruction can produce either unusual perianal growths of lymphoid tissue resembling hemorrhoids or genital elephantiasis
◊ Perirectal abscesses, ischiorectal and rectovaginal fistulas, anal fistulas, and rectal strictures or stenosis can occur

CAUSES
Three of fifteen known strains of C. trachomatis described as serovars L1, L2, and L3 are responsible for LGV. While the strains of Chlamydia that cause urethritis appear to infect only squamocolumnar cells, LGV strains are more invasive and capable of replication in macrophages.

RISK FACTORS
• Unprotected intercourse, especially outside of a mutually monogamous and disease-free sexual relationship
• Anal intercourse
• Residing in or visiting tropical or developing countries
• With the increasing incidence of anorectal LGV in male homosexuals in the USA, LGV should be kept in mind when a patient presents with symptoms of proctocolitis
• Prostitutes

DIAGNOSIS

DIFFERENTIAL DIAGNOSIS
• Inguinal adenitis - chancroid, genital herpes or syphilis. In the USA, one or more of these is much more likely than LGV, especially if the adenitis is associated with a prominent genital ulceration. Other causes of inguinal adenitis include cat-scratch disease, HIV or reactive adenopathy due to skin lesions on the lower extremities. Less common: lymphoproliferative buboes.
• Buboes or suppurative adenitis - chancroid, donovanosis, plague, tularemia, sporotrichosis, actinomycosis and tuberculosis
• Retroperitoneal adenitis - may present as lower abdominal pain with subsequent extensive differential diagnosis
• Proctitis - gonococcal and non-LGV chlamydial proctitis as well as antibiotic-induced and infectious proctitis. Also inflammatory bowel disease.
• Lymphatic obstruction - consider schistosomiasis or malignancy

LABORATORY
• Mild leukocytosis with relative lymphocytosis or monocytosis
• Elevated erythrocyte sedimentation rate
• VDRL/RPR and HIV antibodies should be considered
Drugs that may alter lab results:
Antibiotics
Disorders that may alter lab results:
Chlamydial urethritis

PATHOLOGICAL FINDINGS N/A

SPECIAL TESTS
• Bubo pus, saline injected into a bubo and re-aspirated, infected tissue or primary lesion scrapings, preserved in proper transport media (ask your lab), can be studied with Giemsa stain or by immunofluorescence for inclusion bodies. They can also be cultured on McCoy cells. Yield is about 30% for all of these methods.
• Immunoglobulin M microimmuno-fluorescence (MIF) is a test used frequently to diagnose chlamydial pneumonia among infants, but can also be used for LVG
• Antibody levels to L1, L2, and L3 serovars of C. trachomatis can also be measured with complement fixation although cross-reactivity with other Chlamydial organisms is possible.
• A fourfold rise in MIF titer to LGV antigen or a complement fixation titer above 1:64, with the proper clinical scenario, is probably LGV. Complement levels above 1:128 confirm the LGV diagnosis. These levels are reached early in the disease. Acute and convalescent titers usually do not vary much at six weeks.
• MIF titers are more sensitive and specific than the complement fixation test, however they are only used in specialized research labs and are not routinely available
• Frei's intradermal test is obsolete
• Polymerase chain reaction (PCR) testing - recently developed to diagnose LGV

IMAGING
• Computerized tomography for retroperitoneal adenitis. Lymphography does not outline buboes, but may demonstrate the extent of lymph node involvement
• Barium enema may reveal the characteristic elongated stricture of rectal LGV

DIAGNOSTIC PROCEDURES Aspiration or incision and drainage of bubo for culture

TREATMENT

APPROPRIATE HEALTH CARE
Outpatient except for rare complications such as severe pain or for the surgical repair of complications. Surgery should only be attempted after antibiotic therapy.

GENERAL MEASURES Symptomatic treatment with nonsteroidal anti-inflammatories should be offered in those not contraindicated. Local heat may provide some analgesia.

SURGICAL MEASURES In the acute bubonic stage, fluctuant nodes should be aspirated before they burst and the occasional abscess should be incised and drained. Otherwise surgery should be avoided until antibiotics have been administered. Fever abates rapidly and bubo pain usually responds within a few days after starting antibiotics.

ACTIVITY Sexual abstention pending treatment, otherwise limited only by symptoms

DIET Avoid milk and milk products or any other agents that chelate tetracycline, such as iron supplements and antacids. Allow 2 hours for gastric emptying prior to medication administration if any of these agents are taken.

PATIENT EDUCATION
• LGV is a sexually transmitted disease. The patient should be counseled about other sexually transmitted diseases and safe sex practices
• Sexual partner(s) should be treated, especially those with contact in previous 30 days
• Offer HIV counseling and testing

MEDICATIONS

DRUG(S) OF CHOICE
• For acute cases: Doxycycline 100 mg po bid for 21 days
• For chronic or relapsing cases: Consider longer course of therapy
Contraindications: Tetracycline allergy or sensitivity
Precautions:
• For patients taking tetracyclines longer than 21 days, changes such as leukocytosis, atypical lymphocytes, toxic granulation of granulocytes, and thrombopenic purpura (rare) may be observed in the peripheral blood.
• Suprainfections such as antibiotic-induced diarrhea may ensue
• Tetracyclines may cause photosensitization. Advise patients to use sunscreen.
• Avoid tetracyclines in pregnancy and children under 8
Significant possible interactions:
• Avoid, when taking tetracyclines: milk and milk products, sodium bicarbonate, calcium and magnesium salts, silicate, iron preparations, and bismuth subsalicylate
• As opposed to the other tetracyclines, food does not otherwise interfere with absorption of doxycycline nor does doxycycline seem to have prolonged clearance in patients with impaired renal function
• Doxycycline's half-life is shortened from 20 to 7 hours in patients who are receiving chronic treatment with barbiturates or phenytoin and hence should be administered in the same dose three to four times a day in this group of patients

ALTERNATIVE DRUGS
• Erythromycin base 500 mg orally four times a day for 21 days, or
• Tetracycline 500 mg po qid for 21 days or
• Sulfisoxazole 500 mg po qid for 21 days or equivalent sulfonamide course

FOLLOWUP

PATIENT MONITORING
• Fever and bubo pain usually abate within 1 to 2 days after starting antibiotics. For persistent fever or malaise, monitor closely for complications such as abscesses or suprainfections.
• Treatment has no effect on preexisting scar tissue, therefore monitor for surgical complications
• Dual infections with other sexually transmitted diseases are common - appropriate monitoring should be performed, especially for syphilis and HIV

PREVENTION/AVOIDANCE
• Treat sexual contact(s)
• Abstinence or mutual monogamy in a proven disease-free sexual relationship is the only prevention. Condoms should be worn with sexual activity outside of such relationships.
• Condoms provide protection against genital-anogenital transmission but have no impact on transmission between other sites

POSSIBLE COMPLICATIONS
• Scarring - includes ureteral or bowel obstruction, persistent rectovaginal fistula or gross destruction of the anal canal, anal sphincter, or perineum. Repair of such complications as well as plastic repair of some of the complications of lymphatic obstruction such as genital elephantiasis are the more common surgical indications. Surgery should be performed only after antibiotic treatment.
• Mild rectal strictures can occasionally be dilated as an outpatient

EXPECTED COURSE/PROGNOSIS
• Early treatment improves the prognosis
• Complete resolution of symptoms is usual if treatment is undertaken before scarring
• Reinfection and/or inadequate treatment may result in relapse

MISCELLANEOUS

ASSOCIATED CONDITIONS Any of the sexually transmitted diseases. Screening should be done for syphilis and HIV.

AGE-RELATED FACTORS
Pediatric: N/A
Geriatric: N/A
Others: N/A

PREGNANCY
• Congenital transmission does not occur, but infection may be acquired during passage through an infected birth canal
• Pregnant and lactating women should be treated with erythromycin regimen

SYNONYMS
• Tropical bubo
• Climatic bubo
• Strumous bubo
• Poradenitis inguinalis
• Durand-Nicolas-Favre disease
• Lymphogranuloma inguinale
• Fourth and fifth or sixth venereal disease

ICD-9-CM
099.1 Lymphogranuloma venereum

SEE ALSO
• Chlamydial sexually transmitted diseases
• Chancroid
• Syphilis
• Herpes, genital

OTHER NOTES HIV infected patients with LGV should be treated with usual LGV regimen; may require long therapy

ABBREVIATIONS
• HIV = human immunodeficiency virus
• CDC = Centers for Disease Control
• LGV = lymphogranuloma venereum
• RPR = Rapid plasma reagin test for syphilis
• VDRL = Venereal Disease Research Laboratories test for syphilis

REFERENCES
• Centers for Disease Control: 1998 sexually transmitted diseases treatment guidelines. MMWR 47(RR-1), 1998
• Holmes KH, Mardh PA, Sparling PF, et al: Sexually Transmitted Diseases. 3rd ed. New York, McGraw Hill, 1999
Illustrations: 2 available on CD-ROM
Internet references: http://www.5mcc.com

Author(s)
Grant C. Fowler, MD

Lymphoma, Burkitt's

BASICS

DESCRIPTION Highly undifferentiated B cell lymphoma. It may involve sites other than lymph nodes or reticuloendothelial system, particularly bone marrow and central nervous system. Endemic areas - Central Africa; New Guinea. Rare in USA.
System(s) affected:
Hemic/Lymphatic/Immunologic
Genetics: Translocation of chromosome 8 onto chromosome 14 (70%); c–myc activation
Incidence/Prevalence in USA: Rare
Predominant age: 3 months to 16 years
Predominant sex: Male > female

SIGNS AND SYMPTOMS
- African:
  ◊ Mouth pain
  ◊ Loose teeth
  ◊ Loose deciduous molars
  ◊ Jaw mass
  ◊ Anemia
- North American:
  ◊ Abdominal mass
  ◊ Abdominal pain

CAUSES Unknown; high association with Epstein-Barr virus

RISK FACTORS Living in endemic areas

DIAGNOSIS

DIFFERENTIAL DIAGNOSIS N/A

LABORATORY
- Anemia
- Serum uric acid often elevated
Drugs that may alter lab results: N/A
Disorders that may alter lab results: N/A

PATHOLOGICAL FINDINGS
- Stage AR - completely resected intra-abdominal tumor
- Stages A and B - indicate single or multiple extra-abdominal sites
- Stage C - intra-abdominal disease, including kidneys and/or gonads
- Stage D - stage C findings plus extra-abdominal sites including bone marrow, pleura and/or central nervous system
- High mitotic rate
- Starry sky pattern
- A sea of monotonous cells
- Round to oval nuclei
- 2-5 prominent nucleoli
- Pyroninophilic cytoplasm

SPECIAL TESTS
- Cytogenic studies - translocation between chromosomes 8 and 14
- Immunologic studies - presence of B cell markers (usually IgM) on cell surface

IMAGING CT scan

DIAGNOSTIC PROCEDURES
- Bone marrow aspiration
- Lumbar puncture
- Lymph node biopsy

TREATMENT

APPROPRIATE HEALTH CARE
- Inpatient - for staging surgery and chemotherapy (may require ICU for stages C and D)
- Outpatient - after definitive treatment

GENERAL MEASURES
- Symptomatic treatment for respiratory, gastrointestinal, or psychosocial problems that may follow chemotherapy
- Be alert to increased risk for renal failure and life-threatening metabolic abnormalities due to tumor lysis

SURGICAL MEASURES
- Staging surgery
- Surgery to excise the abdominal mass if present

ACTIVITY As tolerated

DIET
- May have difficulty in swallowing or chewing (jaw involvement). Suggest small meals of a soft diet (protein milk shakes) to help prevent malnutrition.
- Adequate fluid intake

PATIENT EDUCATION
Leukemia Society of America
733 3rd Avenue
New York, NY 10017
(212)573-8424

MEDICATIONS

DRUG(S) OF CHOICE Combination chemotherapy according to most recent protocols. Type and extent of therapy depends on stage of disease.
Contraindications: Refer to manufacturer's literature
Precautions: Myelosuppression, alopecia, mucositis, neurotoxicity with chemotherapy
Significant possible interactions: Refer to manufacturer's literature

ALTERNATIVE DRUGS Intensive chemotherapy with or without bone marrow transplantation for advanced cass

FOLLOWUP

PATIENT MONITORING
• For effects of chemotherapy
• Follow for detection of recurrence

PREVENTION/AVOIDANCE Avoid endemic areas

POSSIBLE COMPLICATIONS
• Tumor lysis syndrome with renal failure:
  ◊ Hyperkalemia
  ◊ Hyperphosphatemia
  ◊ Hyperuricemia
  ◊ Hypocalcemia
  ◊ Tetany

EXPECTED COURSE/PROGNOSIS
• 90% of patients with stage A and over 70% of patients with stages B and C experience long-term remission and possible cure
• With recent protocols, some patients with stage D have also been cured
• Without treatment, prognosis is grave

MISCELLANEOUS

ASSOCIATED CONDITIONS N/A

AGE-RELATED FACTORS
Pediatric: Common age group for this disorder
Geriatric: Unusual in this age group
Others: N/A

PREGNANCY N/A

SYNONYMS
• Monomorphic undifferentiated lymphoma
• African lymphoma
• Maxillary lymphosarcoma

ICD-9-CM
200.2 Burkitt's tumor or lymphoma

SEE ALSO N/A

OTHER NOTES N/A

ABBREVIATIONS N/A

REFERENCES
• Vietti T, Fernbach D, eds: Clinical Pediatric Oncology. 4th Ed. St. Louis, C.V. Mosby, 1992
• Williams WJ, et al: Hematology. 4th Ed. New York, McGraw-Hill, 1990
• Bennett JC, Plum F, eds: Cecil Textbook of Medicine. 20th Ed. Philadelphia, W.B. Saunders Co., 1996
Illustrations: N/A
Internet references: http://www.5mcc.com

Author(s)
John J. Hutter, Jr., MD

Macular degeneration, age-related (ARMD)

BASICS

DESCRIPTION One definition of ARMD is pigmentary changes in the macula or typical drusen associated with visual loss to the 20/30 level or worse, not caused by cataract or other eye disease in individuals over 50 years of age. Other definitions do not include age or visual acuity criteria. ARMD is the leading cause of irreversible, severe visual loss in persons over 65 years of age.
• Stages:
◊ Atrophic/nonexudative: drusen and/or pigmentary changes in the macula
◊ Neovascular/exudative: growth of blood vessels underneath the retina
System(s) affected: Nervous
Genetics:
• The neovascular/exudative form is rare in blacks and more common in whites
• Genetic susceptibility may be a factor in senile macular degeneration, with approximately 1/4 of all senile cases being genetically determined
Incidence/Prevalence in USA:
• In the Framingham Eye Study (FES) drusen were noted in 25% of all participants who were ≥52 years of age. ARMD associated visual loss was noted in 5.7%.
• Prevalence increases with age. Over 75 years; one quarter of men and one third of women will have evidence of ARMD.
• The prevalence of severe visual loss from ARMD increases with age. 2.2% of patients over 65 years of age are blind in one or both eyes from ARMD.
• The atrophic/nonexudative stage accounts for 20% of cases of severe visual loss
• The neovascular/exudative stage accounts for 80% of cases of severe visual loss
Predominant age: FES prevalence rates:
• 1.6% of those individuals who were 52-64 years old
• 11% of those who were 65-74 years old
• 27.9% of those who were > 75 years
Predominant sex: Female > Male

SIGNS AND SYMPTOMS
• Atrophic/nonexudative stage
◊ Drusen
  - Small yellowish-white lesions
  - Can be subdivided into types such as hard drusen and soft drusen
◊ Atrophy of the retinal pigment epithelium (RPE), a pigment layer underneath the retina
• Neovascular/exudative stage
◊ Blood vessels growing underneath the retina from the choroid are called choroidal neovascular membranes (CNVMs) or subretinal neovascularization (SRN). The choroid is the vascular layer underneath the RPE.
  - Subretinal fluid
  - Exudates
  - Subretinal hemorrhage
  - Patients frequently notice distortion of central vision. On Amsler grid testing the horizontal or vertical lines may become broken, distorted or missing. Patients may notice straight lines appear crooked, e.g., telephone poles.
◊ Disciform scar: An advanced stage resulting in a fibrovascular scar

CAUSES
• Visible light can result in the formation and accumulation of metabolic byproducts in the RPE which normally helps remove metabolic byproducts from the retina. The excess accumulation of these metabolic byproducts interferes with the normal metabolic activity of the RPE and can lead to the formation of drusen.
• The neovascular stage generally arises from the atrophic stage
• Most patients do not progress beyond the atrophic/nonexudative stage; however, those that do are at a greater risk to develop severe visual loss

RISK FACTORS
• Excess sunlight exposure
• Blue or light iris color
• Hyperopia
• History of cardiovascular disease (hypertension, circulatory problems)
• Short height
• History of lung infection
• Cigarette smoking
• Low dietary intake of antioxidant nutrients
• Family history

DIAGNOSIS

DIFFERENTIAL DIAGNOSIS
Idiopathic subretinal neovascularization, presumed ocular histoplasmosis syndrome, diabetic retinopathy, and hypertensive retinopathy

LABORATORY N/A
Drugs that may alter lab results: N/A
Disorders that may alter lab results: N/A

PATHOLOGICAL FINDINGS
• Drusen: deposits of hyaline material between the retinal pigment epithelium (RPE) and Bruch's membrane (the limiting membrane between the RPE and the choroid)
• Breaks in Bruch's membrane allows CNVM's to invade the RPE and grow into the subretinal space

SPECIAL TESTS
• Fluorescein angiography: Can detect CNVM's. This test helps to differentiate between atrophic and neovascular ARMD.
• Indocyanine green videoangiography: May be useful in identifying occult or hidden CNVM's

IMAGING N/A

DIAGNOSTIC PROCEDURES
• Daily Amsler grid testing
• Eye examination with detailed fundus examination
• Fluorescein angiography

TREATMENT

APPROPRIATE HEALTH CARE
Outpatient for laser treatment. Inpatient or outpatient for vitrectomy surgery.

GENERAL MEASURES
• Atrophic/nonexudative macular degeneration
◊ No specific treatment alters the course
◊ Free radical formation in the retina, induced by visible light may play a role in cellular damage that results in ARMD.
◊ Vitamin A, E, C and beta-carotene may be useful in preventing cellular damage
◊ Oral zinc may retard visual loss
◊ Laser photocoagulation to treat drusen is unwarranted
• Neovascular/exudative macular degeneration
◊ The Macular Photocoagulation Study (MPS) demonstrated a treatment benefit for laser treatment of CNVM's which were 200 microns (200 microns = 0.2 mm) or greater from the center of the macula.
  - The MPS showed that the benefits of argon laser photocoagulation were greatest one year after treatment. At that time the proportion of eyes with severe visual loss was reduced 51% by treatment, from 43% in untreated eyes to 21% in treated eyes. The deterioration in treatment effect in the MPS is primarily due to recurrent CNVMs growing towards the center of the macula.
  - Fluorescein angiogram usually can determine whether a CNVM is present, if it is well defined, and if it is in a treatable position.
  - Recurrent CNVM's, after laser treatment, were seen in 59% of patients with ARMD. Recurrent CNVMs develop early after treatment; 73% of the recurrences occurred within the first year of treatment, usually within the first 6 months.
• Treatment of CNVMs from 1 to 199 microns from the center of the macula has been studied by the Age-Related Macular Degeneration Study-Krypton Laser (ARMDS-K). The benefit of laser treatment was greatest among patients without evidence of hypertension. No benefit was observed among patients who had highly elevated blood pressure and/or used antihypertensive medication.
◊ Because patients in the ARMDS-K treatment group had CNVM's closer to the center of vision, the magnitude of treatment benefit after laser photocoagulation is smaller in the ARMDS-K treatment group than in the argon laser trial for CNVM's further away from the center of the macula.
◊ Laser treatment can be applied to CNVM's directly underneath the center of vision; however, this can result in immediate worsening of vision. The long term benefits of laser treatment for these lesions makes this form of laser treatment an option.

Macular degeneration, age-related (ARMD)

• Vitrectomy has been used to remove CNVM's, but the benefits of this procedure are being studied

◊ CNVM's can bleed spontaneously leaving blood underneath the retina. Vitrectomy to remove subretinal blood may be of benefit and should be performed within 7 days of the bleed. Tissue plasminogen activator (tPA), instilled into the eye, may help remove a subretinal hemorrhage.

• Patients need to be monitored (usually with fluorescein angiography) after laser treatment, for recurrent CNVM's. After treatment, patients should report changes in the Amsler grid or their vision

• Low vision aids may be helpful

• Investigation/experimental treatments: transplanting of fetal RPE cells, photodynamic therapy using a light-activated drug and nonthermal light irradiation, laser treatment to drusen, low dose radiation therapy

SURGICAL MEASURES
See General Measures

ACTIVITY
Patients with the neovascular form of ARMD should avoid straining and anticoagulants if possible prior to laser treatment

DIET
• A diet high in vitamins A, E, C and beta-carotene along with zinc may be of benefit

• Eating dark green, leafy vegetables (spinach or collard greens) which are rich in carotinoids may decrease the risk of developing the neovascular/exudative stage

PATIENT EDUCATION
• American Academy of Ophthalmology, 655 Beach Street, San Francisco, CA 94109-1336

• Visually impaired patients should check with their local low vision center for aids

MEDICATIONS

DRUG(S) OF CHOICE Zinc and anti-oxidants may be of benefit. Zinc sulfate 100 mg bid with food has been recommended.
Contraindications: N/A
Precautions: Excess zinc ingestion can be associated with anemia and worsening of cardiovascular disease
Significant possible interactions: N/A

ALTERNATIVE DRUGS
• Interferon is currently undergoing investigation, but does not appear to be effective

• Thalidomide, investigational, is a potent inhibitor of angiogenesis and appears to be relatively safe in nonpregnant patients

FOLLOWUP

PATIENT MONITORING
• Laser treated patients should be re-examined promptly if new visual symptoms occur

• The Amsler grid can aid in discovering visual disturbances

• Patients with soft drusen or pigmentary changes in the macula are at an increased risk of visual loss. They should be instructed that it is important to monitor their vision, such as by Amsler grid testing and subjective measures of visual acuity, such as reading vision and image clarity. If there are no new symptoms, follow-up examination in 6-12 months.

• Follow-up examination for patients at increased risk of visual loss may permit early detection of treatable lesions

PREVENTION/AVOIDANCE
• Ultraviolet protection for eyes

• Well balanced diet which includes zinc, vitamins A, E, C, and beta-carotene

• Routine ophthalmologic visits; q2-4 years for patients 40-64 and q1-2 years after age 65

• Daily Amsler grid testing

POSSIBLE COMPLICATIONS   Blindness

EXPECTED COURSE/PROGNOSIS
• Patients with bilateral soft drusen, and pigmentary changes in the macula, but no evidences of exudation, have an increased likelihood of developing CNVM's and subsequent visual loss

• Patients with bilateral drusen carry a cumulative risk of 14.7% over five years of suffering significant visual loss in one eye from the neovascular stage of ARMD.

• Patient's with neovascular stage in one eye and drusen in the opposite eye are at a risk of 5-14% annually of developing the neovascular stage in opposite eye with drusen

• High incidence of recurrence after laser treatment for CNVM's

MISCELLANEOUS

ASSOCIATED CONDITIONS
• Presumed ocular histoplasmosis syndrome
• Exudative retinal detachment
• Vitreous hemorrhage
• Other causes of CNVM's

AGE-RELATED FACTORS
Pediatric: N/A
Geriatric: Prevalence will increase as population ages.
Others: N/A

PREGNANCY   N/A

SYNONYMS
• Senile macular degeneration
• Subretinal neovascularization

ICD-9-CM
362.51 Nonexudative senile macular degeneration
362.52 Exudative senile macular degeneration
362.57 Drusen (degenerative)

SEE ALSO   N/A

OTHER NOTES   N/A

ABBREVIATIONS
ARMD = age-related macular degeneration
SMD = senile macular degeneration
SRN = subretinal neovascularization
CNVM = choroidal neovascular membrane
RPE = retinal pigment epithelium
MPS = macular photocoagulation study
ARMDS-K = Age-related macular degeneration study-Krypton Laser

REFERENCES
• Leibowitz H, Krueger DE, Maunder LR, et al: The Framingham Eye Study Monograph; an ophthalmological and epidemiological study of cataract, glaucoma, diabetic retinopathy, macular degeneration, and visual acuity in a general population of 2631 adults, 1973-1975. Surv Ophthalmol 1980;24(Suppl):335-610
• The Macular Photocoagulation Study Group: Recurrent choroidal neovascularization after argon laser photocoagulation for neovascular maculopathy. Arch Ophthalmol 1986;104:503-512
• Macular Photocoagulation Study Group: Krypton laser photocoagulation for neovascular lesions of age-related macular degeneration. Results of a randomized clinical trial. Arch Ophthalmol 1990;108:816-824
• Macular Photocoagulation Study Group: Subfoveal neovascular lesions in age-related macular degeneration. Guidelines for evaluation and treatment in the macular photocoagulation study. Arch Ophthalmol 1991;109:1242-1257
• Sedden JM, Ajani UA, Sperduto RD, et al: Dietary carotenoids, vitamins A, C, and E, and advanced age-related macular degeneration. JAMA 1994;272:1413-1420
• Klaver CCW, Wolfs RCW, Assink JJM, et al: Genetic risk of age-related maculopathy: Population based familial aggregation study. Arch Ophthalmol 1998;115:1646-1651
4 additional references available at web site
Internet references: http://www.5mcc.com
Illustrations: 4 available on CD-ROM

Author(s)
Richard W. Allinson, MD

Malaria

BASICS

DESCRIPTION Malaria is an acute and chronic protozoan infection transmitted by Anopheles mosquitoes to humans. There are four species or Plasmodium that cause human infection.

System(s) affected:
Hemic/Lymphatic/Immunologic

Genetics: No known genetic pattern. Glucose-6-phosphate deficiency, sickle cell disease or trait, and hereditary ovalocytosis probably help protect against severe P. falciparum infection.

Incidence/Prevalence in USA: Rare primary outbreaks in US. Most cases are imported. In the US, in 1994, P. falciparum caused 44% of all reported cases, P. vivax 44%, P. malaria 4%, and P. ovale 3%.

Predominant age: All ages

Predominant sex: Male = Female

SIGNS AND SYMPTOMS
• Fever
• Malaise
• Chills
• Headache
• Nausea
• Splenomegaly (especially with chronic infection)
• Systolic hypotension
• P. falciparum (also known as malignant tertian malaria): Incubation period usually 12-14 days with subsequent high fevers every 48 hours within 2 months of infection. If large parasitemia, can lead to anemia, thrombocytopenia, and vascular collapse. Other complications include gastroenteritis, central nervous system impairment, renal failure, and pulmonary edema. Associated with fatal outcome if severe infection.
• P. vivax (benign tertian malaria) and P. ovale: Incubation period up to 12 months with high fever every 48 hours. Dormant parasites may remain in the liver causing relapse months after the initial infection.
• P. malariae (benign quartan malaria): Incubation period approximately 35 days with high fevers every 72 hours. May become chronic and lead to nephrotic syndrome.

CAUSES
• Plasmodium falciparum, P. malariae, P. vivax, P. ovale

RISK FACTORS
• Traveling and/or living in endemic area
• Bites from infected Anopheles mosquitoes, or transfusion of infected blood

DIAGNOSIS

DIFFERENTIAL DIAGNOSIS
• Infections such as localized (abscess), viral (mononucleosis), rickettsial, and mycobacterial infections. Collagen vascular diseases including systemic lupus erythematosis, primary vasculitides, and mixed connective tissue diseases. Neoplasms such as lymphoma and leukemia. Other causes of tropical splenomegaly and blood dyscrasias.
• Severe P. falciparum infection may mimic acute hepatitis, acute hemolytic anemia, pneumonia and stroke

LABORATORY
In uncomplicated infection:
• Elevated liver function tests and lactate dehydrogenase (>50% of cases)
• Thrombocytopenia (40%)
• Anemia (25%)
• Leukopenia (25%) vs leukocytosis (1-5%)

Drugs that may alter lab results:
Antimalarial agents may reduce parasitemia

Disorders that may alter lab results: N/A

PATHOLOGICAL FINDINGS
• Malaria causes hemolysis
• If infection is severe, hemolysis of parasitized red blood cells activate pro-inflammatory cytokines causing sludging within the microcirculation and localized necrosis
• Edema, localized hemorrhage, and the presence of malarial pigments are frequent findings

SPECIAL TESTS
• Malarial smear thick preparation obtained every 6-12 hours for 3 samplings. Best to obtain blood during or right after fever spike.
• Other very promising tests that are yet unapproved by the FDA include monoclonal antibody tests and a dipstick assay

IMAGING N/A

DIAGNOSTIC PROCEDURES Malarial peripheral blood smear showing intracellular parasite forms

TREATMENT

APPROPRIATE HEALTH CARE
Inpatient for most cases of falciparum malaria in nonimmune patients. Outpatient for others, except during acute phase if blood products or close observation is required.

GENERAL MEASURES In severe cases watch for complications, such as severe anemia, and renal failure, otherwise supportive care

SURGICAL MEASURES N/A

ACTIVITY May resume activity as soon as the fever is under control. Avoid strenuous exercise if splenomegaly.

DIET No restrictions; as tolerated

PATIENT EDUCATION Prevention of future exposures. These measures include prevention of mosquito bites and malarial chemoprophylaxis.

Malaria

MEDICATIONS

DRUG(S) OF CHOICE
• Oral therapy for chloroquine-resistant Plasmodium (resistant strains of P. falciparum and P. vivax)
  ◊ Quinine sulfate plus doxycycline or pyrimethamine-sulfadoxine (Fansidar) or clindamycin
    - Adults, quinine sulfate 650 mg tid for 3-7 days plus doxycycline 100 mg bid for 7 days or Fansidar 3 tablets on last day of quinine or clindamycin (P. falciparum only) 900 mg tid for 5 days
    - Children, quinine sulfate 7.5 mg base/kg (max 500 mg base) tid for 3-7 days plus doxycycline (not for < 8 years of age) 2 mg/kg daily for 7 days or Fansidar 1/2 pill/10 kg on last day of quinine or clindamycin (P. falciparum only) 10 mg/kg tid for 5 days
• Oral therapy for P. ovale, P. malariae, chloroquine-sensitive P. falciparum and chloroquine-sensitive P. vivax
  ◊ Chloroquine phosphate:
    - Adults, 600 mg base (1 gm salt) followed by 500 mg in 6 hours, then 500 mg at 24 and 48 hours
    - Children, 10 mg base/kg (maximum of 600 mg) then 5 mg/kg in 6 hours, then 5 mg/kg at 24 and 48 hours
  ◊ Primaquine phosphate (required for cure of dormant form of P. vivax and P. ovale only)
    - Adults, 30 mg base (52.6 mg) daily for 2 weeks or 45 mg base (79 mg) weekly for 8 weeks
    - Children, 0.3 mg base/kg daily for 2 weeks
• For severe infection requiring parenteral therapy
  ◊ Quinidine gluconate: adults and children, 10 mg/kg over 1-2 hours followed by 0.02 mg/kg/min continuous infusion or repeat initial dose every 8 hours until oral therapy can be started
Contraindications: Refer to manufacturer's literature
Precautions:
• Primaquine may cause hemolysis in patients with glucose-6-phosphate deficiency (G6PD)
Significant possible interactions: Refer to manufacturer's literature

ALTERNATIVE DRUGS
• Oral therapy for chloroquine-resistant Plasmodium (resistant strains of P. falciparum and P. vivax)
  ◊ Mefloquine: adults, 1250 mg once (may divide as 750 mg and 500 mg over 24 hours. Children, 25 mg/kg once.
  ◊ Atovaquone-proguanil (Malarone): adults, atovaquone 1000 mg and proguanil 400 mg daily for 3-7 days
• Oral therapy for P. ovale, P. malariae, chloroquine-sensitive P. falciparum and chloroquine-sensitive P. vivax
  ◊ Mefloquine: adults, 1250 mg once (may divide as 750 mg and 500 mg over 24 hours). Children, 50 mg/kg once

FOLLOWUP

PATIENT MONITORING Watch for relapse of clinical symptoms

PREVENTION/AVOIDANCE
• Use malarial chemoprophylaxis when in an endemic area
• Oral therapy for areas with chloroquine-resistant Plasmodium species (most areas)
  ◊ Mefloquine (begin 1 week before arrival and continue for 4 weeks after leaving area):
    - Adults: 250 mg (1 tablet) weekly
    - Children: 5-9 kg 1/8 tablet; 10-19 kg 1/4 tablet; 20-30 kg 1/2 tablet; 31-45 kg 3/4 tablet; > 45 kg 1 tablet
• Oral therapy for areas with chloroquine-sensitive Plasmodium species
  ◊ Chloroquine phosphate (begin 2 weeks before arrival and continue until 4-6 weeks after leaving area):
    - Adults: 300 mg base (500 mg) weekly
    - Children: 5 mg base/kg weekly (max 300 mg base)
• Oral therapy for areas with chloroquine and mefloquine resistance
  ◊ Doxycycline 100 mg daily. Not for pregnant women or children < 8 years. Begin 1-2 days before arrival and continue for 4 weeks after leaving area.

POSSIBLE COMPLICATIONS
• P. falciparum: if not treated early, may cause cerebral malaria, acute renal failure, acute gastroenteritis, pulmonary edema, massive hemolysis, and splenic rupture. Death from malaria is virtually limited to P. falciparum infection.
• P. malariae: nephrotic syndrome may develop in patients with chronic infection
• Other complications: seizures, anuria, delirium, coma, dysentery, algid malaria, blackwater fever, hyperpyrexia

EXPECTED COURSE/PROGNOSIS
Only falciparum infection carries a poor prognosis with high mortality if untreated. However, if diagnosed early and treated appropriately the prognosis is excellent.

MISCELLANEOUS

ASSOCIATED CONDITIONS N/A

AGE-RELATED FACTORS
Pediatric: N/A
Geriatric: More serious outcome in this age group
Others: N/A

PREGNANCY Chloroquine is safe. Mefloquine is not recommended unless there are no effective alternatives. Doxycycline, quinine and quinidine should not be used in pregnancy.

SYNONYMS N/A

ICD-9-CM
084.5 P. falciparum infection
084.8 Blackwater fever
771.2 Congenital malaria
573.2 Hepatitis
084.9 Cerebral malaria
084.5 Mixed malarial infection
084.1 Vivax malaria (benign tertian)
084.2 Quartan malaria
084.3 Ovale malaria
084.6 Recurrent malaria
084.6 Malaria, unspecified
084.0 Falciparum malaria (malignant tertian)

SEE ALSO N/A

OTHER NOTES
• Most areas of the world now have chloroquine-resistant P. falciparum (the form of malaria most prevalent world-wide). Some multi-drug resistant strains of P. falciparum and P. vivax are present in Southeast Asia.
• Current information regarding malaria treatment and prophylaxis is always available from Centers for Disease Control (CDC) in Atlanta, GA

ABBREVIATIONS N/A

REFERENCES
• Freedman DO (ed). Infectious Disease Clinics of North America. travel medicine 1998;12(2):267-284, 334-340, 364, 450-454
• Abramowicz A (ed). Drugs for Parasitic Infections. medical Letter 1998;40:5-7
• Centers for Disease Control and Prevention: Malaria Surveillance - United States, 1994. MMWR CDC Surveillance Summary 1997;46(suppl SS-5)
Illustrations: N/A
Internet references: http://www.5mcc.com

Author(s)
Beck Soderberg, MD

Malnutrition, protein-calorie

BASICS

DESCRIPTION
• Protein-calorie malnutrition (PCM) is present when sufficient energy and/or protein is not available to meet metabolic demands, leading to impairment in normal physiologic processes. PCM is classified according to degree of severity and by calculating the actual weight as a percentage of expected weight for height/length, using international standards (normal: 90-110%).
  ◊ 1st degree: mild form characterized by growth failure in children and wasting in adults. Weight as a percentage of expected weight: 85-90%
  ◊ 2nd degree: moderate form with additional biochemical changes, weight as a percentage of expected weight: 75-85%
  ◊ 3rd degree: severe PCM with the development of additional clinical signs, weight as a percentage of expected weight: < 75%
• Kwashiorkor is a condition which develops when there is gross protein deficiency though nonprotein calorie intake may be adequate.
• Marasmus occurs with deficiency of both protein and calories.
• Disease-related malnutrition is common, often not detected, and worsens during a hospital stay. In burns, trauma and infection: release of cytokines such as interleukins, tumor necrosis factor (TNF) and interferons worsens the nutritional status.
System(s) affected: Gastrointestinal, Endocrine/Metabolic, Musculoskeletal, Nervous, Hemic/Lymphatic/Immunologic
Genetics: N/A
Incidence/Prevalence in USA:
Institutionalized elderly, hospital patients and children of the poor have a significant prevalence
Predominant age: Infants and younger children (age 1-2) are more susceptible to PCM. However, PCM may occur at all ages.
Predominant sex: Male = Female

SIGNS AND SYMPTOMS
• Mild to moderate PCM
  ◊ Weight loss and reduction in subcutaneous fat in adults
  ◊ Stunted growth, wasted body habitus, delayed puberty and retarded cognitive and psychosocial development in children
  ◊ Decreased hand grip strength
  ◊ Impaired work capacity
  ◊ Risk of intrauterine growth retardation when pregnant women have PCM
  ◊ Reduced volume of breast milk with low fat content
• Severe PCM
  ◊ Severe alterations in the body habitus
  ◊ Muscle wasting in the extremities
  ◊ Associated micronutrient deficiency features
  ◊ Loss of subcutaneous fat
  ◊ Atrophy of interosseus hand muscles and temporalis
  ◊ Decreased skin elasticity
  ◊ Impaired immunity and susceptibility to infections
  ◊ Delayed wound healing and recovery
  ◊ Decubitus ulcers
  ◊ Dry, reddish-brown, sparse hair
  ◊ Lethargy, early satiety, vomiting and constipation
  ◊ Heart rate, BP and core body temperature may be subnormal
  ◊ Marasmic infants show gross weight loss, growth retardation and wasting of subcutaneous fat and muscle
  ◊ Kwashiorkor is characterized by generalized edema, flaky painful dermatoses, sparse and hair pigment changes, enlarged, fatty liver and petulant apathy

CAUSES
• Inadequate dietary intake
• Poor quality dietary protein
• Increased metabolic demands
• Increased nutrient losses

RISK FACTORS
• Nutritional
  ◊ Prolonged and severe reduction of intake
  ◊ Inadequate body reserves
  ◊ Concurrent deficiencies of the other nutrients
  ◊ Anorexia nervosa
• Underlying illnesses
  ◊ Fever, infection, trauma, burns and other hypercatabolic states
  ◊ Malabsorptive and maldigestive states
  ◊ Protein-losing enteropathy, nephrotic syndrome, enteric fistulas
  ◊ Metabolic disorders: Diabetes, hyperthyroidism
• Physiologic states in which requirements are increased
  ◊ Pregnancy and lactation
  ◊ Growth and development during infancy, childhood and adolescence

DIAGNOSIS

DIFFERENTIAL DIAGNOSIS
• Secondary growth failure due to malabsorption, congenital defects or deprivation
• Pellagra
• Nephritis or nephrosis
• Cardiac failure
• Disorders of glycogen metabolism
• Cystic fibrosis

LABORATORY
• Plasma albumin: Reduced
• Complete hemogram: Decreased lymphocyte count
• Serum chemistry
• Blood urea: Decreased
• Plasma transferrin: Decreased
• Plasma essential amino acids: Decreased
• Plasma betalipoprotein: Decreased
• Hypoglycemia with neuroglycopenia
• Plasma cortisol, GH: Increased, but insulin low
Drugs that may alter lab results: N/A
Disorders that may alter lab results: N/A

PATHOLOGICAL FINDINGS
• Marasmus
Muscle wasting and reduction in muscle mass due to gluconeogenesis. Mummified appearance. No edema. Fat depots reduced. Loss of subcutaneous fat.
• Kwashiorkor
Serum amino acid patterns distorted. Protein synthesis impaired. Hypoalbuminemia causes dependent edema. Impaired betalipoprotein synthesis causes fatty liver. Poor insulin response to glucose load. Growth, immune response, repair and production of enzymes and hormones are impaired in severe protein deficiency.

SPECIAL TESTS
• Triceps skin-fold thickness
• Mid-arm muscle area (MAMA)
• Protein index measurement
• Creatinine-height index
• Delayed-hypersensitivity index
• Prognostic-nutritional index (PNI)

IMAGING
Chest x-ray to rule out tuberculosis or other pulmonary infections

DIAGNOSTIC PROCEDURES
• History and physical examination
• MAMA = $[M - \pi(T)] \times [M - \pi(T)] \div 4\pi$
  M = mid-arm circumference (mm)
  T = triceps skin fold (mm)
  π = 3.1415
• Protein index = ratio of measured to predicted total body protein
• Creatinine-height index =
Actual 24 hr urinary creatinine excretion ÷ normative value for height and sex
• Delayed hypersensitivity index: This index quantitates the amount of induration elicited by skin testing with a common antigen such as Candida, Trichophyton or mumps.
Grading: 0 = < 0.5 cm; 1 = 0.5 cm; 2 = 1.0 cm
• Prognostic nutritional index is a weighted combination of 4 measures:
PNI% = 158 - [1.66 x A] - [0.78 x T] - [2.0 x F] - [5.8 x D]
where,
  A = serum albumin (g/L)
  T = triceps skin fold (mm)
  F = serum transferrin (g/L)
  D = delayed hypersensitivity index
All the above indices should be compared with the normative values in standard charts

TREATMENT

APPROPRIATE HEALTH CARE
Inpatient care for severe anemia, dehydration, electrolyte imbalance and superimposed infections. Outpatient care for stabilized cases.

GENERAL MEASURES
• Fluid and electrolyte balance should be restored and maintained
• In severe kwashiorkor, IV or SC infusion of amino acids
• Low-lactose formulas have been helpful in some cases with diarrhea due to disaccharidases deficiency
• Diarrhea due to other causes should be identified and treated
• Supplementary vitamins and micronutrients
• Mild anemia usually responds to oral protein, iron and folic acid supplements. Blood transfusion may be necessary in severe cases (Hb < 6 g/dL). Use oral iron with caution in kwashiorkor.

SURGICAL MEASURES   N/A

ACTIVITY   As tolerated

DIET
• Sufficient milk for infants and children to supply 2-5 g/kg/day protein. Lactic-acid fortified milk can be given.
• Adequate calories should be supplied by adding sugar and cereal to the milk diet (150-250 kcal/day)
• Gradual supplementation with high-energy foods such as candies, cake, puddings, meats, eggs and fruit juices
• Small, frequent feedings around the clock better tolerated in the early stages
• Prepared nutritional supplements available commercially are convenient

PATIENT EDUCATION
• Emphasis on nutrition education with the help of a dietician
• Need for a balanced food intake
• Educate about the composition of nutritional products to ensure balanced intake
• Awareness about risk factors and need for timely nutritional supplements

MEDICATIONS

DRUG(S) OF CHOICE
• Antibiotics may be indicated to treat infections
• Multivitamin-multimineral supplementation is required
Contraindications: N/A
Precautions: N/A
Significant possible interactions: N/A

ALTERNATIVE DRUGS   N/A

FOLLOWUP

PATIENT MONITORING
Initially periodic follow-up to ensure good nutritional status

PREVENTION/AVOIDANCE
• Emphasis on nutritional education and continuous nutritional care
• Routine record of height and weight
• Observe and record the patient's food intake
• Early recognition of increased nutritional needs during stress and infections
• Frequent interactions between physician, nurse and dietician to assess nutritional needs
• Avoidance of risk factors when possible

POSSIBLE COMPLICATIONS
Death in the first few days of treatment is usually due to electrolyte imbalance, infection, hypothermia or circulatory failure. Stupor, jaundice, petechiae and low serum sodium are ominous signs.

EXPECTED COURSE/PROGNOSIS
• Mortality varies between 15-40%
• Recovery is more rapid in kwashiorkor than in marasmus. Disappearance of apathy, edema and anorexia are favorable signs.
• In adequately treated cases, liver recovers fully without subsequent cirrhosis, but GI malabsorption and pancreatic deficiency may remain
• Compromised cell-mediated immunity returns to normalcy with recovery
• Behavioral and mental retardation is marked in the severely malnourished child. It is related to the duration of malnutrition and to the age of onset. Relatively mild degree of mental retardation persists into school age.

MISCELLANEOUS

ASSOCIATED CONDITIONS
• Malaria and other parasitic infections
• Multiple micronutrients deficiency
• Malabsorptive and maldigestive states

AGE-RELATED FACTORS
Pediatric:
Growth and development during infancy, childhood and adolescence increase nutritional requirements
Geriatric:
Institutionalized elderly are at special risk
Others: N/A

PREGNANCY
Pregnant women with mild to moderate PCM are at risk of delivering an infant with low weight/length for gestational age

SYNONYMS   N/A

ICD-9-CM
260 Kwashiorkor
261 Nutritional marasmus
263.9 Unspecified protein-calorie malnutrition

SEE ALSO   N/A

OTHER NOTES   N/A

ABBREVIATIONS
PCM = Protein - Calorie Malnutrition
PEM = Protein - Energy Malnutrition
MAMA = Mid - Arm Muscle Area
PNT = Protein Nutritional Index
TNF = tumor necrosis factor

REFERENCES
• Fauci AS, et al, eds: Harrison's Principles of Internal Medicine. 14th Ed. New York, McGraw Hill, 1998
• Golden GE: In: Garrow JS, James WPT, eds: Human Nutrition and Dietetics. 9th Ed. New York, Churchill Livingstone, 1996:440-455
• Dempster WS, Sive AA, et al: Eur J Clin Nut 1995; 49: 202-210.
Illustrations: N/A
Internet references: http://www.5mcc.com

Author(s)
V. Vasudeviah, BSc, MBBS

Marfan's syndrome

 BASICS

DESCRIPTION A dominantly inherited disorder of connective tissue affecting primarily the musculoskeletal system, the cardiovascular system and the eye
System(s) affected: Musculoskeletal, Endocrine/Metabolic
Genetics: Autosomal dominant with high penetrance; 15% spontaneous mutation
Incidence/Prevalence in USA: 1 in 10,000 - 20,000 (estimated 1 in 15,000)
Predominant age: Congenital, so disorder is present from birth. However clinical manifestations do not usually become apparent until adolescence or young adulthood.
Predominant sex: No gender, ethnic or racial predilection

SIGNS AND SYMPTOMS
• Musculoskeletal
  ◊ Tall stature
  ◊ Thin, gangly body habitus (limb length out of proportion to trunk)
  ◊ Arachnodactyly i.e. long, thin fingers
  ◊ Pectus deformity
  ◊ High arched palate
  ◊ Hyperextensible joints
  ◊ Kyphoscoliosis
  ◊ Joint laxity
• Cardiovascular
  ◊ Aortic root dilatation
  ◊ Aortic regurgitation
  ◊ Aortic dissection
  ◊ Mitral valve prolapse
  ◊ Mitral regurgitation
• Ocular
  ◊ Subluxation of lens, usually upward
  ◊ Myopia
  ◊ Retinal detachment (uncommon)
• Other
  ◊ Easy bruising (uncommon)
  ◊ Excessive bleeding (uncommon)

CAUSES Genetic; at least 5% are obviously familial, the remainder arise from apparent spontaneous mutations

RISK FACTORS Advanced paternal age gives rise to a slightly increased risk only in those cases which are not clearly familial

 DIAGNOSIS

DIFFERENTIAL DIAGNOSIS
Homocystinuria, contractural arachnodactyly, Ehlers-Danlos syndrome, trisomy, all of which are rare conditions and all of which have clear cut distinguishing clinical features from the Marfan's syndrome

LABORATORY
• There are no specific laboratory abnormalities in the Marfan syndrome
• It is recommended that suspected patients have urinary homocystine measured to rule out homocystinuria
Drugs that may alter lab results: N/A
Disorders that may alter lab results: N/A

PATHOLOGICAL FINDINGS
• Cystic medial necrosis of the aorta
• Myxomatous degeneration of the cardiac valves
• FBN1 gene on chromosome 15 codes for fibrillin, a large glycoprotein constituent of microfibrils. Mutations in this gene have been found in over 90% of patients with the Marfan's syndrome, when tested.

SPECIAL TESTS Slit lamp examination is necessary to detect lens subluxation

IMAGING
• Plain x-rays of spine are necessary during growth years to detect and quantify scoliosis
• Annual screening echocardiograms are recommended beginning in adolescence in order to detect presymptomatic aortic root dilatation or valvular degeneration

DIAGNOSTIC PROCEDURES N/A

 TREATMENT

APPROPRIATE HEALTH CARE
Outpatient

GENERAL MEASURES Multidisciplinary approach including primary care physician, cardiologist, ophthalmologist and possibly orthopedic surgeon. A clinical geneticist if available, would be ideal as primary care physician.

SURGICAL MEASURES Many, if not most, of these patients will ultimately require reconstructive cardiovascular surgery

ACTIVITY
• Fully active unless limited by symptoms
• Several highly-trained athletes with the Marfan syndrome have suffered sudden death during competition leading to some concern that people with Marfan syndrome should be discouraged from participating in aerobically demanding sports

DIET No special diet

PATIENT EDUCATION Information available from the National Marfan Foundation, 382 Main St., Port Washington, NY 11959; 800-8MARFAN

MEDICATIONS

DRUG(S) OF CHOICE
• No specific medical therapy is available, however drugs are used to try to prevent certain complications
• Propranolol or other beta-adrenergic blocking drugs are used to decrease the force of cardiac contraction, in the hope of delaying the development or progression of aortic root dilatation. The dosage of these drugs are adjusted to target heart rate, i.e., resting rate of 60 per minute, with a rise to no more than 80 per minute after moderate exertion.
• Estrogen combined with progestogen has been used to induce puberty in pre-adolescent girls in an attempt to shorten the growth spurt thereby ameliorating scoliosis and preventing excessively tall stature. Do this only under the supervision of an endocrinologist.
Contraindications:
• Congestive heart failure, asthma, diabetes for the beta-adrenergic blocking drugs
• Thromboembolic disease for the estrogen/progestogen
Precautions: Refer to manufacturer's profile of each drug.
Significant possible interactions:
Amphetamines, antihistamines, anti-diabetics, oral contraceptives

ALTERNATIVE DRUGS   N/A

FOLLOWUP

PATIENT MONITORING
• Frequent examinations (at least twice a year) while growing, with particular attention to cardiovascular system and scoliosis
• When cardiac symptoms develop or aortic root diameter becomes > 50 mm, surgical intervention must be considered
• When lens subluxation is detected, surgical correction is possible. However a high incidence of glaucoma results, so surgery should be offered only to those who cannot be treated with corrective lenses.

PREVENTION/AVOIDANCE
• No prenatal diagnosis yet available, but presymptomatic diagnosis may be possible at research centers using linkage analysis techniques
• Each child has a 50% chance of inheriting the disorder from an affected parent. Clinical manifestations are variable, however, so children may be more or less severely affected.
• Antibiotic prophylaxis for endocarditis should be prescribed for all Marfan syndrome patients with either a heart murmur or echocardiographic evidence of valvular or aortic root abnormalities

POSSIBLE COMPLICATIONS
• Bacterial endocarditis
• Aortic dissection
• Aortic or mitral valve insufficiency
• Dilated cardiomyopathy
• Retinal detachment

EXPECTED COURSE/PROGNOSIS
• Life-threatening complications are cardiovascular. Before routine corrective surgery was available most Marfan syndrome patients died before reaching the age of 35.
• With appropriate surgical intervention most patients can live a normal life span

MISCELLANEOUS

ASSOCIATED CONDITIONS   N/A

AGE-RELATED FACTORS
Pediatric: Early medical or surgical intervention may reduce the degree of scoliosis
Geriatric: N/A
Others: N/A

PREGNANCY   Pregnant women with the Marfan syndrome need to be managed as high-risk patients, preferably with involvement of a cardiologist. The outcome is usually excellent.

SYNONYMS   N/A

ICD-9-CM   759.82 Marfan syndrome

SEE ALSO   N/A

OTHER NOTES   N/A

ABBREVIATIONS   N/A

REFERENCES
• Pyeritz RE, McKusick VA: The Marfan Syndrome: Diagnosis and Management. New Engl J Med 1979;300:772-777
• Scriver RC, et al, eds: The Metabolic Basis of Inherited Disease. 7th Ed. New York, McGraw Hill, 1995
Illustrations: N/A
Internet references: http://www.5mcc.com

Author(s)
Robert J. Sliman, MD

Mastalgia

BASICS

DESCRIPTION Chronic breast pain often occurring prior to menses. Breast pain could also be acute and caused by other problems such as breast abscess.
System(s) affected: Skin/Exocrine
Genetics: Familial tendency
Incidence/Prevalence in USA: Mild form is common; severe form is uncommon
Predominant Age: > age 20
Predominant Sex: Female

SIGNS AND SYMPTOMS
• Breasts aching, heavy, or tender
• Enlarged breasts

CAUSES
• Associated with fibrocystic breast disease and premenstrual syndrome
• Hormonal influences; hormone replacement therapy

RISK FACTORS
• Caffeine consumption
• High fat diet

DIAGNOSIS

DIFFERENTIAL DIAGNOSIS
• The major alternate disease to consider is breast cancer
• Manipulation or trauma can also make symptoms worse
• Chest-wall pain must also be differentiated from mastalgia
• Often concurrent with premenstrual syndrome
• Ductal ectasia of the breast

LABORATORY No relevant findings
Drugs that may alter lab results: N/A
Disorders that may alter lab results: N/A

PATHOLOGICAL FINDINGS Fibrocystic changes

SPECIAL TESTS
• Possibly TSH
• Prolactin if galactorrhea
• Pap test of discharge, if present

IMAGING Mammography to differentiate from breast cancer

DIAGNOSTIC PROCEDURES
• Cysts may need to be aspirated for symptom relief and diagnostic verification
• Biopsies may be indicated based on exam or mammography

TREATMENT

APPROPRIATE HEALTH CARE
Outpatient

GENERAL MEASURES
• Stop or modify current hormonal therapy
• Repeat examination within 30 days will help establish any cyclic nodularity pattern
• Well-fitting support bra (maybe fitted by a professional).
• Reassurance (this is sufficient for most women)
• Weight reduction, if obese

SURGICAL MEASURES N/A

ACTIVITY No restrictions

DIET
• Decreased caffeine
• Decreased fat intake to 20% of total calories

PATIENT EDUCATION
• Explain that breast pain does not mean the patient has cancer
• Explain relationship to menses

Mastalgia

MEDICATIONS

DRUG(S) OF CHOICE
• No drugs are needed unless required by severity of symptoms. Reassurance, acetaminophen or ibuprofen may be all that is needed.
Contraindications: Refer to manufacturer's profile of each drug
Precautions: Refer to manufacturer's profile of each drug
Significant possible interactions: Refer to manufacturer's profile of each drug

ALTERNATIVE DRUGS
• Agents often used, whose value has been questioned:
◊ Diuretics (usually spironolactone) prior to menses
◊ Vitamin E 600 IU/day
◊ Evening primrose oil, includes high content of fatty acids, believed to decrease prostaglandin synthesis
◊ Oral contraceptives may help some patients
• Other possibilities for refractory patients, used infrequently because of potential side effects:
◊ Danazol 100 mg bid (possibly lower doses) - this may be the most effective. Major side effects - menstrual irregularities, weight gain, acne, hirsutism and voice change. May be used during luteal phase only.
◊ Bromocriptine 2.5-5.0 mg/day. Major side effects - nausea, dizziness, orthostatic hypotension.
◊ Tamoxifen 10 mg/day. Major side effects - cataracts, hepatocellular carcinoma, endometrial carcinoma. May be used during luteal phase only.
◊ Gonadotropin-releasing hormone agonists

FOLLOWUP

PATIENT MONITORING
• As needed for patients not on prescription medications
• Time of followup will vary by type of prescription medication and patient problems

PREVENTION/AVOIDANCE See Risk Factors

POSSIBLE COMPLICATIONS N/A

EXPECTED COURSE/PROGNOSIS
• Premenstrual mastalgia increases with age, then generally stops at menopause unless on hormone replacement therapy
• Most patients will have control of symptoms without hormonal treatment
• Several months of hormonal treatment may lead to several more months of relief, but the mastalgia usually recurs

MISCELLANEOUS

ASSOCIATED CONDITIONS
Premenstrual syndrome

AGE-RELATED FACTORS
Pediatric: N/A
Geriatric: N/A
Others: N/A

PREGNANCY N/A

SYNONYMS
• Mastodynia
• Breast pain

ICD-9-CM 611.71 mastalgia

SEE ALSO
• Premenstrual syndrome (PMS)

OTHER NOTES
• Cyclic mastalgia responds better than noncyclic mastalgia to treatment
• Effects of long-term hormonal treatment are unknown
• If other treatment fails, a final possibility is subcutaneous mastectomy (used rarely)
• Oophorectomy also provides relief and may be drastic treatment for some patients

ABBREVIATIONS N/A

REFERENCES
• Holland PA, Gately CA: Drug therapy of mastalgia. Practical Therapeutics 1994;48:709-716
• BeLieu RM: Mastodynia. Obstetrics and Gynecology Clin of No Amer 1994;21:461-477
• Ader DN, Shriver CD: Update on clinical and research issues in cyclical mastalgia. The Breast Jour 1998;4:25-32
Illustrations: N/A
Internet references: http://www.5mcc.com

Author(s)
Marjorie A. Bowman, MD, MPA

Mastoiditis

BASICS

DESCRIPTION   Inflammatory process in the mastoid air cells
• Acute mastoiditis - acute suppurative inflammatory process, typically after acute otitis media
• Chronic mastoiditis - usually associated with cholesteatoma and chronic ear disease
System(s) affected: Pulmonary
Genetics: No known genetic pattern
Incidence/Prevalence in USA: Unknown
Predominant age: Children, middle age
Predominant sex: Male = Female

SIGNS AND SYMPTOMS
• Otalgia
• Bulging erythematous tympanic membrane
• Post-auricular edema/mass
• Post-auricular erythema
• Post-auricular tenderness
• Protrusion of auricle
• Fever
• Increased WBC
• Clouding of mastoid air cells on plain films
• Fluid density in middle ear/mastoid air cells with or without loss of bony architecture
• Possible otorrhea if perforated tympanic membrane
• Subperiostial abscess

CAUSES
• Acute otitis media
• Inadequately treated suppurative otitis media
• Cholesteatoma
• Blockage of outflow tract of mastoid air cells (additus ad antrum)

RISK FACTORS
• Cholesteatoma
• Recurrent acute otitis media
• Immunocompromised host

DIAGNOSIS

DIFFERENTIAL DIAGNOSIS
• Post-auricular inflammatory adenopathy
• Severe external otitis
• Post auricular cellulitis
• Benign neoplasm - aneurysmal bone cyst, fibrous dysplasia
• Malignant neoplasm - rhabdomyosarcoma

LABORATORY   CBC with differential - increased WBC
Drugs that may alter lab results: N/A
Disorders that may alter lab results: N/A

PATHOLOGICAL FINDINGS
• Inflammatory tissue in air cell system
• Granulation tissue
• Osteitis

SPECIAL TESTS   Consider audiogram

IMAGING
• Plain mastoid films - clouding of mastoid air cells
• CT scan if complication suspected. Cloud air cells - loss of bony septation of the air cell system.

DIAGNOSTIC PROCEDURES   N/A

TREATMENT

APPROPRIATE HEALTH CARE
Hospitalized during acute phase

GENERAL MEASURES
• Keep ear dry

SURGICAL MEASURES
• Myringotomy; placement of pressure equalization (PE) tube
• Culture material obtained at myringotomy
• Frequent cleaning of ear canal under microscope to assure PE tube patency and adequate drainage of middle ear
• IV antibiotics to cover the most common organisms
• Topical antibiotic drops are also usually used after insertion of PE tube
• If subperiosteal abscess present, it should be aspirated. If aspiration is not sufficient, incision and drainage should be performed.
• Mastoidectomy is reserved for those patients failing to respond to above measures within 18-72 hours or those with meningeal or intracranial complications

ACTIVITY   Fully active, water precautions

DIET   No special diet

PATIENT EDUCATION   Griffith: Instructions for Patients; Philadelphia, W.B. Saunders Co., 1994

Mastoiditis

MEDICATIONS

DRUG(S) OF CHOICE
• IV antibiotics:
◊ Directed against most common organisms - group A beta-hemolytic strep, S. pneumonia, Hemophilus influenza
◊ In patients with cholesteatoma, consider Proteus, Bacteroides and occasional S. aureus and Pseudomonas organisms
◊ IV antibiotics for adult - ampicillin, 1-2 gm q6h or ampicillin-sulbactam (Unasyn) or cefuroxime, 750 mg q8h, to ensure coverage of beta-lactamase producing organisms
◊ IV antibiotics for children - ampicillin, 100-200 mg/kg/day divided q6h or cefuroxime, 750 mg q8h
• Topical/oral antibiotics:
◊ Topical drops - neomycin-polymyxin B-hydrocortisone (Cortisporin) otic drops or gentamicin ophthalmic solution
◊ Oral antibiotic - amoxicillin-clavulanate (Augmentin)
Contraindications: Refer to manufacturer's literature
Precautions: Refer to manufacturer's literature
Significant possible interactions: Refer to manufacturer's literature

ALTERNATIVE DRUGS Other antibiotics depending on pathogen sensitivity

FOLLOWUP

PATIENT MONITORING
• Postoperative - audiogram after acute process subsided
• Frequent cleansing of ear canal to keep PE tube patent

PREVENTION/AVOIDANCE
• Adequate antibiotic treatment for acute otitis media
• Treatment of chronic eustachian tube dysfunction (PE tubes)
• Early identification of cholesteatoma

POSSIBLE COMPLICATIONS
• Subperiosteal abscess
• Gradenigo's syndrome (sixth nerve palsy, draining ear and retro-orbital pain)
• Bezold's abscess
• Sigmoid sinus thrombosis
• Meningitis
• Intracranial abscess epidural/subdural/intraparenchymal

EXPECTED COURSE/PROGNOSIS
• Dependent on severity of disease
• Conductive hearing loss may require reconstructive surgery
• Expect to avoid complications with early treatment

MISCELLANEOUS

ASSOCIATED CONDITIONS N/A

AGE-RELATED FACTORS
Pediatric: N/A
Geriatric: N/A
Others: N/A

PREGNANCY N/A

SYNONYMS N/A

ICD-9-CM
383.9 Coalescent mastoiditis
383.00 Acute or subacute mastoiditis
383.02 Acute with Gradenigo's syndrome
383.02 Acute with petrositis
383.01 Acute with subperiosteal abscess

SEE ALSO N/A

OTHER NOTES N/A

ABBREVIATIONS PE = pressure equalization

REFERENCES Paparella MM, Shumrick DA, et al, eds: Otolaryngology. 4th Ed. Philadelphia, W.B. Saunders Co., 1991
Illustrations: N/A
Internet references: http://www.5mcc.com

Author(s)
Laurene L. Howell, MD
Sean O. McMenomey, MD

Measles, rubella

BASICS

DESCRIPTION
An endemic and epidemic viral exanthematous infection of children and adults, worldwide in distribution. Many infections are subclinical, but this virus can potentially cause fetal infection with resultant birth defects.

System(s) affected: Skin/Exocrine, Hemic/Lymphatic/Immunologic, Pulmonary, Nervous

Genetics: Children with congenital rubella syndrome and children with insulin dependent diabetes mellitus share a high frequency of HLA-DR3 histocompatibility antigen and a high prevalence of islet cell antibodies

Incidence/Prevalence in USA:
• Before rubella vaccine was introduced in 1969, epidemics occurred at 6-9 year intervals. Sporadic outbreaks continue to occur in hospitals, colleges, prisons, prenatal clinics and isolated religious communities.
• In 1998 the incidence of postnatal rubella was 0.12 cases per100,000 population, nearly a doubling of the 1997 rate. Presently, the source of the rubella outbreaks is from infected persons from countries where rubella is not included in routine immunization or just recently introduced schedules or administered in mass campaigns.

Predominant age: Children 5-9 years of age
Predominant sex: Male = Female

SIGNS AND SYMPTOMS
• Postnatal rubella
　◊ Adenopathy - posterior auricular, posterior cervical, suboccipital
　◊ Low-grade fever
　◊ Exanthem - descending, maculopapular, may desquamate
　◊ Enanthem - soft palate petechiae (Forschheimer's sign)
　◊ Conjunctivitis
　◊ Splenomegaly, rarely
　◊ Coryza
　◊ Malaise
　◊ Headache
　◊ Polyarthralgia/polyarthritis, especially in young women
　◊ Asymptomatic (25%-50%)
• Congenital rubella: (T = Transient, P = Permanent, D = Developmental)
　◊ Cataracts (P)
　◊ Microphthalmia (P)
　◊ Chorioretinitis (P)
　◊ Patent ductus arteriosus (P)
　◊ Pulmonic stenosis (P,D)
　◊ Atrial and ventricular septal defects (P)
　◊ Sensorineural deafness (P,D)
　◊ Microcephaly (P)
　◊ Meningoencephalitis (T)
　◊ Mental retardation (P,D)
　◊ Low birth weight (T)
　◊ Purpuric ("blueberry muffin") skin lesions (T)
　◊ Radiolucent bone disease (T)
　◊ Hepatosplenomegaly (T)
　◊ Large anterior fontanelle (T)
　◊ Language and behavior disorders (P,D)
　◊ Cryptorchidism (P)
　◊ Inguinal hernia (P)

CAUSES
Rubella virus is a single-stranded RNA virus in the togavirus family. Traveling via airborne droplets of nasopharyngeal secretions, the virus replicates in the nasopharynx and regional lymph nodes during a 16-18 day incubation period. After invading the bloodstream, it may spread to skin and other distal organs or, transplacentally, to the developing fetus. Fetal viremia may then produce disseminated fetal infection. Organogenesis occurs 2 to 6 weeks postconception, so that infection is a maximum hazard (40-80% risk) to heart and eyes at that time. During the second trimester, the fetus develops increasing immunologic competence, making it less susceptible (10% risk) to the effects of intrauterine infection.

RISK FACTORS
• Inadequate immunization
• Immunodeficiency states
• Immunosuppressive therapy
• Pregnancy
• Crowded living conditions
• School, day care
• Late winter, spring seasons
• International travel aboard commercial airplanes, cruise ships

DIAGNOSIS

DIFFERENTIAL DIAGNOSIS
• Postnatal rubella
　◊ Measles virus (rubeola)
　◊ Scarlet fever
　◊ Infectious mononucleosis
　◊ Toxoplasmosis
　◊ Roseola infantum (exanthem subitum)
　◊ Erythema infectiosum (fifth disease)
　◊ Drug eruptions
　◊ Other exanthematous enteroviral infections
• Congenital rubella
　◊ Cytomegalovirus
　◊ Varicella-zoster virus
　◊ Picornaviruses (coxsackievirus, echovirus)
　◊ Poliovirus
　◊ Herpes simplex virus
　◊ Western equine virus
　◊ Measles virus (rubeola)
　◊ Hepatitis B virus
　◊ Mumps virus
　◊ Influenza virus
　◊ Toxoplasmosis
　◊ Congenital syphilis
　◊ Malaria

LABORATORY
• Postnatal rubella
　◊ Mild leukopenia with relative lymphocytosis
　◊ Fourfold rise in serum levels of antibody to rubella virus
　◊ Pharynx, nose and blood culture positivity to rubella virus
• Congenital rubella
　◊ Presence of rubella-specific IgM antibody in serum up to one year of age, at which time, IgG becomes the dominant antibody
　◊ Isolation of rubella virus from pharynx, blood, urine, cerebrospinal fluid

Drugs that may alter lab results: N/A
Disorders that may alter lab results: After re-exposure to rubella, a person with a low level of antibody from past infection or vaccination may experience an acute rise in antibody. This is not associated with a high incidence of contagion to others nor of fetal risk.

PATHOLOGICAL FINDINGS
• Inhibition of cellular growth after infection
• Fetal vasculitis
• Placental angiopathy
• Tissue necrosis

SPECIAL TESTS
Cell-mediated immune responses (CMI) are impaired selectively in children with congenital rubella

IMAGING
N/A

DIAGNOSTIC PROCEDURES
Congenital rubella has been diagnosed by placental biopsy at 12 weeks

TREATMENT

APPROPRIATE HEALTH CARE
Outpatient usually

GENERAL MEASURES
• Postnatal rubella - mild and self-limited. Treat for symptomatic relief.
• Congenital rubella - supportive, unless neurologic or hemorrhagic complications develop

SURGICAL MEASURES
N/A

ACTIVITY
• For postnatal rubella - contact isolation for 7 days after onset of rash, bedrest is not necessary
• Contact isolation of congenitally infected infants for one year, unless nasopharyngeal and urine cultures after 3 months of age are negative for rubella virus

DIET
No special diet

PATIENT EDUCATION
Make every effort to avoid exposing infected patient to pregnant women

MEDICATIONS

DRUG(S) OF CHOICE Acetaminophen for fever every 4 hours if needed - 10-15 mg/kg/dose
Contraindications: N/A
Precautions: N/A
Significant possible interactions: N/A

ALTERNATIVE DRUGS None

FOLLOWUP

PATIENT MONITORING
• Persons immune to rubella via natural infection or vaccine may be reinfected when re-exposed. This infection is usually asymptomatic and detectable only by serologic means.
• In congenital rubella, it is extremely important to detect auditory and visual impairment early, so that adequate education and counseling can begin

PREVENTION/AVOIDANCE
• Rubella vaccine
 ◊ A 2-dose schedule in combination with measles and mumps (MMR) is recommended for those born after 1956. The first dose is recommended at age 12-15 months; the second dose is recommended either at 4-6 years of age or at 11-12 years of age. Children with HIV should receive MMR vaccine at 12 months of age if no contraindications exist.
 ◊ Recommended for susceptible individuals in the following groups: Prepubertal boys and girls, premarital or postpartum women, college students, day care personnel, health care workers, military personnel
 ◊ It is contraindicated in: Pregnancy, immunodeficiency or immunocompromised state (except HIV), receipt within the last 3 months of immunoglobulin (Ig) or blood, severe febrile illness, or hypersensitivity to vaccine components
 ◊ Persons who receive rubella vaccine do not transmit rubella to others, although the virus can be isolated from the pharynx
 ◊ During outbreaks of rubella, serologic screening before vaccination is not recommended, because rapid vaccination is necessary to stop the spread of the disease

POSSIBLE COMPLICATIONS
• Postnatal rubella
 ◊ Postinfectious encephalitis (1/5,000 cases)
 ◊ Thrombocytopenic purpura (1/3,000 cases)
 ◊ Testicular pain
 ◊ Mild hepatitis
• Congenital rubella
 ◊ Spontaneous abortion
 ◊ Stillbirth
 ◊ Premature delivery
 ◊ Progressive rubella panencephalitis
 ◊ Endocrine disturbances (diabetes, thyrotoxicosis, hypothyroidism)
• Rubella vaccine
 ◊ Lymphadenopathy
 ◊ Fever
 ◊ Rash
 ◊ Arthritis/arthralgia (older girls, women)
 ◊ Polyneuropathy

EXPECTED COURSE/PROGNOSIS
• Postnatal rubella
 ◊ Fever, 1-2 days
 ◊ Rash, 3 days
 ◊ Coryza, 5 days
 ◊ Lymphadenopathy, 1 week
 ◊ Arthralgia (when present), 2 weeks
 ◊ Complete and full recovery without sequelae is the rule
• Congenital rubella
 ◊ Varied and unpredictable spectrum of consequences, ranging from stillbirth to completely normal infancy and childhood
 ◊ Disease characterized by chronic infection; infants may remain contagious for months after birth
 ◊ Detectable levels of hemagglutination-inhibiting antibody (IgG) persist for years, then may decline. By age 5, 20% have no detectable antibody.
 ◊ Overall mortality 10%; greatest during first 6 months
 ◊ 70% of those with encephalitis develop residual neuromotor defects, including an autistic syndrome
 ◊ Prognosis is excellent when only minor defects are present

MISCELLANEOUS

ASSOCIATED CONDITIONS   N/A

AGE-RELATED FACTORS
Pediatric:
• Postnatal rubella is a milder disease in children than it is in adults
• Adolescents and young adults currently account for about 60% of all new cases
Geriatric: N/A
Others: N/A

PREGNANCY
• Women vaccinated against rubella are advised not to become pregnant for at least 3 months. The vaccine-type virus can cross the placenta. However, no case of congenital rubella has occurred after inadvertent vaccination

• If a pregnant woman is exposed to rubella (native disease, not vaccine associated), obtain an antibody titer. Presence of antibody implies immunity and no risk. If antibody is not detectable, obtain a second titer in 3 weeks. If antibody is present in the second specimen, infection has occurred. If antibody is again negative, obtain a third titer in 3 more weeks (6 weeks after exposure). At this time, a negative test means that infection has not occurred; a positive test means that infection did occur, and the fetus is at risk for congenital rubella.
• Human immunoglobulin (gamma globulin) in prophylaxis of rubella during pregnancy does not prevent rubella or the congenital rubella syndrome in a predictable or reliable fashion
• A reliable PCR-based method of detecting viral RNA may allow much more rapid prenatal diagnosis of rubella virus infection. Routine use is not yet available.

SYNONYMS
• German measles
• Three-day measles

ICD-9-CM
056.9 Uncomplicated postnatal rubella
771.0 Congenital rubella

SEE ALSO
• Measles, rubeola
• Immunizations

OTHER NOTES   Rubella vaccine is currently the only vaccine designed for the purpose of protecting someone other than the vaccine recipient

ABBREVIATIONS   N/A

REFERENCES
• Committee on Infectious Diseases, Elk Grove, Illinois, AAP Red Book, ed. 23, 1994
• Rudolph AM, ed: Rudolph's Pediatrics. 20th Ed. Norwalk, CT, Appleton & Lange, 1996
• Revello MG, et al: Prenatal diagnosis of rubella virus infection by direct detection and semiquantitation of viral RNA in clinical samples by reverse transcription-PCR. J Clin Microbiol 1997;35:708-713
• Watson JC, Hadler SC, Dykewicz CA, Reef S, et al: Measles, mumps, and rubella-vaccine use and strategies for elimination of measles, rubella, and congenital rubella syndrome and control of mumps: recommendations of the Advisory Committee on Immunization Practices (ACIP). MMWR Morb Mortal Wkly Rep 1998 May;22;47(RR-8):1-57
• Gorbach SL, Bartlett JG, Blacklow NR (eds): Infectious Diseases. 2nd Ed. Philadelphia, W.B. Saunders Company, 1998
• Rosa C: Rubella and rubeola. Semin Perinatol 1998 Aug; 22 (4):318-322
Illustrations: 1 available on CD-ROM
Internet references: http://www.5mcc.com

Author(s)
Richard Viken, MD

Measles, rubeola

BASICS

DESCRIPTION An acute epidemic viral exanthem which classically presents as a confluent erythematous maculopapular rash which begins over the head and spreads inferiorly to involve the trunk and extremities. The rash is preceded by the triad of cough, coryza, and conjunctivitis plus a pathognomonic enanthem (Koplik's spots).
System(s) affected: Skin/Exocrine, Hemic/Lymphatic/Immunologic, Pulmonary
Genetics: N/A
Incidence/Prevalence in USA: Number of cases peaked during 1990, 27,786; followed by marked decline, during 1997 the United States reported a provisional total of only 135 confirmed measles cases. Attack rate (# cases/100,000): 1991 - 3.82, 1992 - 0.87, 1993 - 0.12, 1994 - 0.37
Predominant Age: Between 1985 and 1994, children ≤ 2 years constituted largest proportion of cases (≥ 90% of these unvaccinated). During a 7 week period in 1997, no indigenous cases were reported, suggesting an interruption of measles transmission.
Predominant sex: Male = Female

SIGNS AND SYMPTOMS
- Incubation period:
  ◊ 10+/-2 days from exposure to symptoms
  ◊ 14 days average to onset of rash (range 7-18 days)
  ◊ Patients contagious from 1-2 days before symptoms (3-5 days before rash) to 4 days after onset of rash, immunocompromised patients contagious for the duration of the illness
- Prodromal period:
  ◊ Lasts 3+/-1 days
  ◊ Classic triad (brassy cough, coryza, and conjunctivitis)
  ◊ Fever
  ◊ Malaise
  ◊ Photophobia
  ◊ Enanthem (Koplik's spots) - minute, whitish spots over buccal/labial mucosa; number rapidly increases and these coalesce. Underlying mucosa bright red and granular; spots appear 2 days before rash and resolve within 3 days after rash onset.
- Exanthem period:
  ◊ Begins behind ears and at hairline
  ◊ Spreads centrifugally from head to feet
  ◊ Red, morbilliform, blanching rash
  ◊ Discrete lesions become confluent
  ◊ Confluence more prominent over upper body
  ◊ Clearing begins after 3-4 days
  ◊ Rash becomes coppery and nonblanching
  ◊ Fever resolves 2-3 days after onset of rash
  ◊ Pharyngitis
  ◊ Lymphadenopathy
  ◊ Croup, vomiting, and diarrhea (in young children)
  ◊ Patients contagious from 2 days before symptoms to 4 days after onset of rash

- Modified illness:
  ◊ Attenuated measles in partially immune patient
  ◊ Secondary prior immune globulin, transplacental measles antibody, live vaccine failure
- Atypical measles:
  ◊ Most cases secondary to natural infection following vaccination with killed vaccine (available in U.S. 1963-68; Canada until 1975)
  ◊ Maculopapular rash begins distally and spreads centrally
  ◊ Rash frequently is petechial, purpuric, or urticarial
  ◊ Pulmonary involvement in all cases
  ◊ Frequency decreasing

CAUSES Single antigenic type of a RNA morbillivirus in the paramyxovirus family

RISK FACTORS Not being vaccinated

DIAGNOSIS

DIFFERENTIAL DIAGNOSIS
- Typical measles:
  ◊ Any erythematous maculopapular rash
- Exanthems secondary to:
  ◊ Drug eruptions
  ◊ Infectious mononucleosis
  ◊ Mycoplasma pneumoniae
  ◊ Rubella
  ◊ Erythema infectiosum
  ◊ Roseola
  ◊ Enteroviruses
- Atypical measles:
  ◊ Rocky Mountain spotted fever
  ◊ Drug eruptions
  ◊ Anaphylactoid purpura
  ◊ Mycoplasma pneumoniae infection

LABORATORY
- Viral isolation in tissue culture
- Detection of measles antigen in exfoliative cells by immunofluorescence
- Demonstration of measles specific IgM or substantial rise in IgG tilers between acute and convalescent sera
Drugs that may alter lab results:
Immunosuppressive agents which may impair rise in specific antibody titers
Disorders that may alter lab results:
- Primary (severe combined immunodeficiency [SCID], etc.)
- Acquired immune deficiencies (HIV-1 infection, cancer chemotherapy)

PATHOLOGICAL FINDINGS
- Multinucleated giant cells
  ◊ Reticuloendothelial types (Warthin-Finkeldey) in lymphoid tissues
  ◊ Epithelial syncytial giant cells in skin, and respiratory mucosa
  ◊ Damaged respiratory ciliated epithelium

SPECIAL TESTS N/A

IMAGING N/A

DIAGNOSTIC PROCEDURES N/A

TREATMENT

APPROPRIATE HEALTH CARE
Outpatient except when complications develop (encephalitis, pneumonitis)

GENERAL MEASURES
- Symptomatic therapy (i.e., antipyretics, antitussives, humidification, encourage oral fluids)
- Control
  ◊ All cases should be placed in respiratory isolation until 4 days after the onset of the exanthem; immunocompromised patients should be isolated for the entire illness
  ◊ Notify public health officials of suspected cases
  ◊ Initiate preventive measures for all exposed susceptible persons or those at high risk for severe infection (i.e., symptomatic HIV infection, children less than 12 months)
  ◊ Live measles vaccine can provide protection to susceptible persons if given within 72 hours postexposure
  ◊ Immune globulin (Ig) given within 6 days postexposure can prevent or modify measles infection (0.25 mL/kg, maximum dose 15 mL; 0.5 mL/kg for immunocompromised patients)
  ◊ Patients with symptomatic HIV infection should receive Ig regardless of prior immunization
  ◊ Ig also indicated for susceptible household contacts of measles patient and pregnant women

SURGICAL MEASURES N/A

ACTIVITY Restricted during febrile phase

DIET As tolerated

PATIENT EDUCATION Avoid exposure to other children and potential secondary bacterial pathogens until respiratory symptoms resolve

MEDICATIONS

DRUG(S) OF CHOICE
• No proven specific antiviral agent is available
• Following the onset of infection, immune globulin has no significant effect on symptoms and duration of illness
• Antibiotics reserved for bacterial superinfection

Contraindications: Steroids contraindicated
Precautions: N/A
Significant possible interactions: N/A

ALTERNATIVE DRUGS
• Vitamin A
  ◊ 200,000 IU po per day for 2 days (100,000 IU between 6-12 months) has been shown to decrease the mortality and morbidity of severe measles in areas where vitamin A deficiency exists and mortality related to measles is ≥ 1%; efficacy in non-life-threatening infections not established
  ◊ Vitamin A currently recommended for the following patients:
    1. Children 6-24 months hospitalized with complications of measles
    2. Children over 6 months with immunodeficiency, malabsorption, moderate to severe malnutrition, ophthalmologic evidence of vitamin A deficiency, or recent immigration from areas with vitamin A deficiency
• Ribavirin
  ◊ Virus susceptible in vitro to ribavirin
  ◊ Immunosuppressed children with severe measles have been treated with IV or aerosolized ribavirin, but no controlled data and not approved by FDA

FOLLOWUP

PATIENT MONITORING   Not required unless complications develop

PREVENTION/AVOIDANCE
• Postexposure prophylaxis
  ◊ Vaccine use - protective if given within 72 hours postexposure
  ◊ Immune globulin (Ig) - prevents/modifies illness if given within 6 days postexposure. Dose - usually 0.25 mL/kg IM (for immunocompromised children 0.5 mL/kg IM) not to exceed 15 mL.
• Active immunization:
  ◊ Moraten strain vaccine - only currently licensed vaccine available as monovalent vaccine or in combination with mumps and rubella i.e., measles and rubella (MR); measles, mumps and rubella (MMR)
• Indications:
  ◊ Primary vaccination: Two doses of vaccine; 1st MMR at 12-15 months, 2nd dose of MMR at school age (4-6 years). Two dose vaccination schedule mandated by need to compensate for primary vaccine failures and global efforts to eradicate measles. During outbreaks, monovalent measles vaccine may be given to infants > 6 months. These children must be vaccinated with MMR as above. For a comprehensive discussion of the complete use and control of measles outbreaks, the reader is referred to the first listing in References.
  ◊ HIV infected children should be vaccinated while asymptomatic and before they develop profound immunosuppression. One case of a HIV infected young adult with advanced disease who developed measles vaccine virus associated pneumonitis post vaccination. The 2nd dose of vaccine may be given as early as 1 month after the 1st dose.
• Adverse events associated with vaccination (in 5-15% of susceptible vaccinees):
    ◊ Fever (7-12 days after)
    ◊ Transient rashes (in 5% of vaccinees)
    ◊ Convulsions (most likely febrile)

POSSIBLE COMPLICATIONS
• Otitis media (most common)
• Laryngotracheitis
• Bronchopneumonia - viral (Hecht's or giant cell pneumonitis) or bacterial in origin
• Encephalitis (incidence 1 per 1000)
• Hemorrhagic lesions ("black measles") of skin and bowel
• Thrombocytopenic purpura
• Myocarditis and pericarditis
• Subacute sclerosing panencephalitis - secondary to persistent infection following natural disease; disappearing as a result of mass vaccination

EXPECTED COURSE/PROGNOSIS
Self-limited; prognosis good

MISCELLANEOUS

ASSOCIATED CONDITIONS
• Primary measles in an immunosuppressed patient with leukemia or symptomatic HIV-1 infection may present with or without a rash and giant cell pneumonitis
• Giant cell pneumonitis
• Increased mortality with malnutrition
• Possible reactivation of latent tuberculosis secondary to measles

AGE-RELATED FACTORS
Pediatric: Infants have higher rate of complications than older children
Geriatric: N/A
Others: N/A

PREGNANCY   Increased fetal morbidity and mortality with infection during pregnancy

SYNONYMS   Rubeola

ICD-9-CM   055.9 Measles without mention of complication

SEE ALSO   Measles, rubella

OTHER NOTES   N/A

ABBREVIATIONS   N/A

REFERENCES
• Measles. In Report of the Committee on Infectious Diseases, 344-357, American Academy of Pediatrics, 1997
• Measles Prevention: Recommendations of the Immunization Practices Advisory Committee (ACIP). Morbidity and Mortality Weekly Report, Recommendations and Reports. 38 (S-9):1-13, 1989
• Cherry J: Measles. In: Feigin R, Cherry J, eds. Textbook of Pediatric Infectious Diseases. 4th Ed. Philadelphia, W.B. Saunders Co., 1998
Illustrations: N/A
Internet references: http://www.5mcc.com

Author(s)
Charles D. Mitchell, MD

Melanoma

BASICS

DESCRIPTION Malignant degeneration of cells from the melanocytic system. The overwhelming majority of melanoma arises in the skin, but it may also present as a primary lesion in any tissue pigmentation. Metastatic spread may be to any region in the body.
• Lentigo maligna - a cutaneous lesion that is the slowest growing malignant melanoma and has the least tendency to metastasize. Occurs most often on the face, beginning as a circumscribed macular patch of mottled pigmentation showing shades of dark brown, tan, or black.
• Ocular - a malignant progressive lesion of the eye
System(s) affected: Skin/Exocrine
Genetics:
• The only genetic predisposition is in the familial dysplastic nevus syndrome. If the family history of a person with dysplastic nevus syndrome includes one relative with melanoma, then the risk of developing melanoma is 100%.
• Skin pigmentation is the only other risk factor transmitted genetically
Incidence/Prevalence in USA:
• 4.5/100,000 people in the USA
• Estimated year 1995, 38,000 cases, 6,700 deaths
• Estimated year 2000, 1 in 75 persons then living will eventually die of malignant melanoma
Predominant age:
• A median age is 53 with the highest annual incidence rate of any cancer in whites between the ages of 25-29 and in white males between 35-39
• Greater than 50% of all individuals with melanoma are between ages 20-40
Predominant sex: Male = Female

SIGNS AND SYMPTOMS Any change in a pigmented lesion including hypo- or hyperpigmentation, bleeding, scaling, size change, texture change

CAUSES Under investigation. Probably radiation in the ultraviolet A+B range.

RISK FACTORS
• Adulthood
• Previous pigmented lesions (especially dysplastic nevi)
• Fair complexioned, freckling, blue eyes and blond hair
• Twice the risk in persons with adolescent blistering sunburn, family history of previous melanoma, congenital nevi
• Intermittent UV exposure (seasonal)
• Those with increased numbers of nevi
• Family history of melanoma

DIAGNOSIS

DIFFERENTIAL DIAGNOSIS
• Dysplastic nevi
• Vascular skin tumors
• Pigmented squamous cell and basal cell carcinomas, seborrheic keratoses, other changing nevi. It follows the ABCDE mnemonic which stands for (1) asymmetry, (2) border irregularity, (3) color variegation, and (4) diameter great than 6 millimeters with the location on whites being primarily back and lower leg, and on African Americans being hands, feet, and nails, (5) elevation above skin surface.

LABORATORY N/A
Drugs that may alter lab results: N/A
Disorders that may alter lab results: N/A

PATHOLOGICAL FINDINGS
• Gross pathologic features include four clinical types:
◊ Superficial spreading melanoma - 70% of all cases
◊ Nodular - 15% of all cases
◊ Acral lentiginous - 2-8% of all cases
◊ Lentigo-maligna - 4-10% of all cases
◊ Note: Nodular melanoma is primarily vertical growth while the other three types are horizontal

SPECIAL TESTS The only special tests that exist for melanoma are those designed to follow metastatic disease

IMAGING Imaging studies are of benefit only in detecting metastatic disease which is usually to the brain, lymph nodes and lungs

DIAGNOSTIC PROCEDURES Surgical biopsy is the only form of appropriate diagnostic procedure

TREATMENT

APPROPRIATE HEALTH CARE
Outpatient or inpatient surgery

GENERAL MEASURES The key to the cure of melanoma is prevention: Avoidance of blistering solar radiation and the use of a sunscreen when exposure is unavoidable

SURGICAL MEASURES The appropriate health care for melanoma is surgical excision. Much debate exists as to the extent of the margins of excision once diagnosis has been made. The tendency now is toward margins of 1 cm if the lesion is less than 2 mm thick. If thicker, then margins can be extended to 3 cm. Regional lymph node dissection is of some benefit in a few studies.

ACTIVITY Avoid sun exposure

DIET No restrictions

PATIENT EDUCATION
• It is critical that a patient with a history of melanoma or dysplastic nevi syndrome has frequent total body examinations for any abnormal appearing or changing nevi
• National Cancer Institute, Dept. of Health And Human Services, Public Inquiries Section, Office of Cancer Communications, Building 31, Room 101-18, 9000 Rockville Pike, Bethesda, MD 20892, (301)496-5583

MEDICATIONS

DRUG(S) OF CHOICE
• No one chemotherapeutic agent has shown unequivocal benefit in all cases
• Adjuvant chemotherapy has included bacillus Calmette-Guérin (BCG) and levamisole
• Standard chemotherapy includes dacarbazine
• Adoptive immunotherapy with leukapheresis and IL-2 with LAK's (under investigation)
• Some benefit with vaccines containing melanoma associated antigens (MAAs) has occurred. No treatment has shown unequivocal benefit.
Contraindications: Refer to manufacturer's literature
Precautions: Dacarbazine - myelosuppression, alopecia
Significant possible interactions: Refer to manufacturer's literature

ALTERNATIVE DRUGS
Many have been tried; recent trials show some promise

FOLLOWUP

PATIENT MONITORING
• Current recommendations after diagnosis of malignant melanoma are skin exams every 3-6 months
• Only chest x-rays on an annual basis have been shown to be of any benefit at all in that 6% of recurrences were detected. These findings did not appear to alter prognosis.
• The patient should conduct his/her own skin examinations on a weekly basis. They must be thorough.

PREVENTION/AVOIDANCE
Avoidance of burning solar exposures and the use of sunscreens is critical. Those at high risk should do all they can to avoid sunburn especially during the adolescent years.

POSSIBLE COMPLICATIONS
• Metastatic spread
• Unsatisfactory cosmetic results following the primary surgery

EXPECTED COURSE/PROGNOSIS
• Prognosis is entirely based on staging of the initial lesion
• Staging (falls into two categories)
◊ Breslow: This shows a 70% five-year survival of all patients who have no local or distant lymphatic spread.
◊ Clark's staging depends on depth of invasion by skin layer. The best prognosis is for those lesions which are less than .85 mm (especially if restricted to the stratum granulosum or higher) which carry 95-100% five-year survival. Spread to lymphatics or regional lymph nodes carries less than a 5% five-year survival.

MISCELLANEOUS

ASSOCIATED CONDITIONS As above

AGE-RELATED FACTORS
Pediatric: Rarely seen in pediatric age group
Geriatric: Lentigo maligna is most commonly seen in elderly patients who have had a slowly enlarging pigmented lesion, usually found on the face
Others: The most recent data on melanoma indicates that its highest incidence is between ages 30-50. However, it can occur at any age.

PREGNANCY
• Due to the facts that melanocyte-stimulating hormone (MSH) levels are markedly increased during pregnancy and that melanoma is one of the few carcinomas that can spread to the placenta, concern has been that pregnancy exacerbates melanoma. This has been neither proven nor disproven.
• If a person has had recent melanoma, many authors suggest waiting at least two years if further pregnancy is desired
• If invasion extends into the lymphatic structures, then further pregnancy is probably contraindicated
• If pregnancy occurs during metastatic melanoma, then there is clear risk to the fetus

SYNONYMS N/A

ICD-9-CM
172.9 Melanoma of skin, site unspecified

SEE ALSO N/A

OTHER NOTES
• It is imperative for the physician to realize that any nevus or pigmented lesion that is in any way suspect should be excised. A full thickness total excisional biopsy must be sent for pathologic specimen and never to be curetted, electrodesiccated, or shaved.
• Any irregularly pigmented lesion in a preadolescent individual > 2 cm should be considered for excision

ABBREVIATIONS N/A

REFERENCES
• Malignant melanoma-CA. American Cancer Society. July/Aug 1996;46:4
• Johnson TM, et al: Current therapy for cutaneous melanoma. J Am Acad Dermatol 1995;32:689-707
• Numerous authors: Symposium on Malignant Melanoma Parts II & IV. Mayo Clinic Prac 1997;72:356-371, 559-574
Illustrations: 16 available on CD-ROM
Internet references: http://www.5mcc.com

Author(s)
David P. Sealy, MD

Ménière's disease

BASICS

DESCRIPTION An inner ear (labyrinthine) disorder in which there is an increase in volume and pressure of the inner-most fluid of the inner ear (endolymph), resulting in recurrent attacks of hearing loss, tinnitus, vertigo, and fullness
• Usually unilateral, but in 10-50% may later involve the second ear
• Severity and frequency may diminish over the years, but with increasing loss of hearing. It is not a synonym for dizziness.
System(s) affected: Nervous
Genetics: N/A
Incidence/Prevalence in USA:
• No reliable figures are available to provide comprehensive numbers for incidence and prevalence by age and sex, but using incidence figures from a Swedish study conducted in 1973, it is estimated that the incidence of Ménière's disease in the US is 46 (new cases/100,000/year). No figures for sex and age are available, but the disease is relatively equal in males and females, and is extremely rare in children.
• Using extrapolation, the estimated prevalence is 1,150 (cases/100,000 population)
Predominant age: Usual age of onset 20-60
Predominant sex: Male = Female

SIGNS AND SYMPTOMS
• Hearing loss - low frequency, fluctuating
• Vertigo - spontaneous attacks, duration 20 minutes to several hours
• Ear fullness
• Occurs as attacks, with intervening remission
• During severe attacks
◊ Pallor
◊ Sweating
◊ Nausea and vomiting
◊ Falling
◊ Prostration
◊ All symptoms aggravated by motion
◊ Between attacks may experience motion-related imbalance without vertigo

CAUSES
• Unknown. Best theory is inner ear response to variety of injuries (reduced middle ear pressure, allergy, endocrine disease, lipid disorders, vascular, viral, luetic).
• Recent theory is intracranial compression of balance nerve by blood vessel

RISK FACTORS
• Caucasian
• Stress
• Allergy
• Increased salt intake
• Noise

DIAGNOSIS

DIFFERENTIAL DIAGNOSIS
• Acoustic tumor
• Syphilis
• Perilymph fistula
• Multiple sclerosis
• Viral labyrinthitis
• Vertebro-basilar disease
• Other labyrinthine disorders producing same symptoms (Cogan's syndrome, benign positional vertigo, temporal bone trauma)

LABORATORY
• Lab studies done to rule out other conditions
• Serologic tests specific for Treponema pallidum - microhemagglutination (MHA), fluorescent treponemal antibody (FTA), Treponema immobilization test (TPI)
• Thyroid studies
• Lipid studies
Drugs that may alter lab results: Any medication that produces a significant degree of sedation is likely to affect vestibular testing and invalidate it
Disorders that may alter lab results: Many conditions may produce auditory and vestibular findings identical to those associated with Ménière's disease, making it a diagnosis of exclusion. A low frequency sensorineural hearing loss (nerve loss as opposed to conductive loss) is seen on audiometry, and a reduced caloric response on caloric testing is usual.

PATHOLOGICAL FINDINGS
Autopsy only. Shows dilation of inner ear fluid system (endolymph).

SPECIAL TESTS
• Otoscopy with air pressure applied to the tympanic membrane
• Auditory
◊ Hearing test (audiometry using pure tone and speech) to show low frequency sensorineural [nerve] loss and impaired speech discrimination)
◊ Tuning fork test (Weber and Rinne) to confirm validity of audiometry
◊ Auditory Brainstem Response audiometry (ABR) to rule out acoustic neuroma
• Vestibular
◊ Spontaneous nystagmus (rapid rhythmic eye motion) seen visually. Must avoid eye fixation by having patient use 40 diopter glasses for test.
◊ Caloric testing - electronystagmography (ENG) may show reduced caloric response. Can obtain reasonably comparable information with use of 0.8 cc ice water instilled in ear canal, then noting duration and frequency of resulting nystagmus with 40 diopter lenses in place. Reduced activity on either side is consistent with Ménière's diagnosis, but is not diagnostic.

IMAGING
MRI to rule out acoustic tumor, which can produce identical symptoms and findings

DIAGNOSTIC PROCEDURES N/A

TREATMENT

APPROPRIATE HEALTH CARE Can usually be managed in outpatient setting. Inpatient for surgery.

GENERAL MEASURES
• Medications are given primarily for symptomatic relief of vertigo and nausea. There is no medication available that influences the disease process.
• For attacks, bedrest with eyes closed and protection from falling. Attacks rarely last longer than four hours.
• Streptomycin therapy for bilateral Ménière's disease, when conventional management has failed. Streptomycin may be administered over a period of several days or weeks intentionally to damage the neuro-epithelium of the balance centers and reduce their function. Hearing must be carefully monitored during this time so that the treatment does not proceed to the point of damaging the hearing structures. This form of treatment should be administered only by an otolaryngologist and after careful patient education.

SURGICAL MEASURES
• Hearing good: Endolymphatic sac surgery, either (1) decompression or (2) drainage of endolymph into mastoid or subarachnoid space. Alternative procedure is to cut the vestibular nerve (intracranial procedure). A newer procedure involves placement of gentamycin through the tympanic membrane into the middle ear space.
• Hearing poor, but usable: Can do sac procedure, nerve section, or gentamycin instillation depending on quality of hearing. For poor hearing, can decompress cochlea (cochleocentesis), or perfuse cochlea with streptomycin.
• Hearing not useful: Destruction of inner ear (labyrinthectomy)

ACTIVITY
• Limit activity during attacks
• Between attacks patient may be fully active, but this may be limited by (1) fear of impending attack, (2) unsteadiness following attacks, (3) ear fullness or tinnitus, or (4) hearing loss in involved ear that may severely limit the patient's ability to perform work duties or to participate in social life

DIET Limit total intake during attacks because of nausea. Otherwise diet is usually not a factor unless attacks are brought on by certain foods. A restricted salt diet may be useful in some cases.

PATIENT EDUCATION Many otolaryngologists keep booklets on Ménière's disease as handouts. Ask your otolaryngology consultant for a supply.

MEDICATIONS

DRUG(S) OF CHOICE
• Acute attack. For severe episode, one of the following may be used. Adult doses are indicated
◊ Atropine 0.2-0.4 mg IV
◊ Diazepam (Valium) 5-10 mg IV slowly
◊ Transdermal scopolamine, 1 patch, or smaller segment of patch, applied to skin surface and not replaced sooner than 3 days
• Maintenance. Adult doses are indicated (frequently must be reduced to avoid sedating effects)
◊ Meclizine (Antivert, Bonine) 25-100 mg orally, either at bedtime or in divided doses
◊ Ergotamine-belladonna-phenobarbital (Bellergal Spacetabs), one q 12 hr
◊ Diazepam (Valium), 2 mg (or less) tid
Contraindications:
• Atropine - cardiac disease, especially supraventricular tachycardia and other arrhythmias
• Scopolamine - children and elderly
Precautions:
• Sedating drugs should be used with caution, particularly in elderly people. The need to reduce the dosage is common. Patients should be cautioned not to operate motor vehicles when they are sedated.
• Atropine, scopolamine, and Bellergal should be used with particular caution. If not prescribed frequently, refer to manufacturer's literature.
Significant possible interactions:
• Bellergal - oral anticoagulants, tricyclic antidepressants, phenothiazines, narcotics, beta blockers, estrogens, and others
• Transdermal scopolamine - anticholinergics, belladonna products, antihistamines, tricyclic antidepressants, and others

ALTERNATIVE DRUGS
• Acute attack
◊ Droperidol, 1.5-2.5 mg IV slowly (in hospital setting)
◊ Promethazine (Phenergan) 12.5-25 mg IV slowly
◊ Diphenhydramine (Benadryl) 50 mg IV slowly
◊ Carbogen (5% carbon dioxide and 95% oxygen) by mask from tank
• Maintenance
◊ Dimenhydrinate (Dramamine) 50 mg q4-6h po
◊ Promethazine (Phenergan) 12.5-25 mg q4-6h po
◊ Diphenidol (Vontrol) 25-50 mg tid po
◊ Diphenhydramine (Benadryl), 25-50 mg q6-8h po. Maximum, 100 mg/24 hours
◊ Chlorothiazide (Diuril) 500 mg daily po with potassium supplement

FOLLOWUP

PATIENT MONITORING
The most common complaint by Ménière's patients regarding prior treatment is that the primary care physician did not take the condition seriously and that he or she didn't seem interested in providing ongoing care. Because of the emotional impact alone, these patients need close followup care. It is important to monitor the status of their hearing, since it is at risk, and to continue to consider the possibility of a more serious underlying problem such as an acoustic tumor.

PREVENTION/AVOIDANCE
• Reduce stress
• Reduce salt intake
• Don't smoke
• Avoid significant noise exposure, or use ear protectors
• Avoid use of ototoxic medications (aspirin, quinine, kanamycin, and many others)

POSSIBLE COMPLICATIONS
• Failure to diagnose acoustic neuroma
• Loss of hearing
• Injury during attack
• Inability to work

EXPECTED COURSE/PROGNOSIS
• Alternating attacks and remission
• Over time the balance problem tends to resolve, but the hearing worsens
• The great majority of patients can be managed successfully with medication. About 5-10% of patients require surgery for incapacitating vertigo.
• Very important not to overlook acoustic tumor, which produces an identical clinical picture

MISCELLANEOUS

ASSOCIATED CONDITIONS
• Cochlear hydrops (hearing problem only)
• Vestibular hydrops (balance problem only)
• Drop attacks

AGE-RELATED FACTORS
Pediatric: Unusual, but occasional. Dizziness in children likely to be on basis of significant central nervous system disease.
Geriatric: Less likely to occur in elderly. Patients exposed to loud noise levels over many years are more susceptible.
Others: Usual onset age 20-60

PREGNANCY
Not a common problem, but difficult to treat because of risk of producing fetal abnormalities with medication

SYNONYMS
• Ménière's syndrome
• Endolymphatic hydrops

ICD-9-CM
386.0 Meniere's disease

SEE ALSO
• Labyrinthitis
• Tinnitus

OTHER NOTES
• Hearing loss

ABBREVIATIONS
N/A

REFERENCES
• Lucente FE, Gady HE: Essentials of Otolaryngology. 4th ed. Philadelphia, Lippincott Williams & Wilkins, 1999:116-125
Illustrations: N/A
Internet references: http://www.5mcc.com

Author(s)
Gale Gardner, MD, FACS

Meningitis, bacterial

BASICS

DESCRIPTION Inflammation in response to bacterial infection of the pia-arachnoid and its fluid and the fluid of the ventricles. Meningitis is always cerebrospinal.
System(s) affected: Nervous
Genetics: Navajo Indian and American Eskimo may have genetic or acquired vulnerability to invasive disease
Incidence/Prevalence in USA: 3-10 cases per 100,000 population
Predominant age: Neonates, infants and geriatric aged
Predominant sex: Male = Female

SIGNS AND SYMPTOMS
• Antecedent URI
• Fever
• Headache
• Meningismus
• Signs of cerebral dysfunction
• Vomiting
• Photophobia
• Seizures
• Nausea
• Rigors
• Profuse sweats
• Weakness
• Altered mental status
• Focal neurologic deficits
• Elderly have subtle findings commonly including confusion
• Meningococcemia has rash - macular and erythematous at first, then petechial or purpuric

CAUSES
• Neonates: Group B or D Streptococcus, Escherichia coli, Listeria monocytogenes and non-group B Streptococcus
• Infants/children: H. influenzae (48%), Streptococcus pneumoniae (13%), and Neisseria meningitidis
• Adults: Streptococcus pneumoniae (30-50%), Haemophilus influenzae (1-3%), Neisseria meningitidis (10-35%), gram-negative bacilli (1-10%), Staphylococci (5-15%), Streptococci (5%) and Listeria species(5%)

RISK FACTORS
• Immunocompromised host
• Alcoholism
• Neurosurgical procedure or head injury
• Abdominal surgery for gram-negative

DIAGNOSIS

DIFFERENTIAL DIAGNOSIS
• Bacteremia
• Sepsis
• Brain abscess
• Seizures
• Other non-bacterial meningitides

LABORATORY
• Turbid CSF
• Neonates
  ◊ > 10 WBC's in CSF
  ◊ CSF: blood glucose ratio < 0.6
  ◊ CSF protein >150 mg/dL (> 1500 mg/L)
• Infants/children
  ◊ > 5 WBC's in CSF
  ◊ CSF: blood glucose ratio < 0.6
  ◊ CSF protein > 50 mg/dL (> 500 mg/L)
• Adults
  ◊ 1000-100,000 WBC's in CSF (average 5000-20,000)
  ◊ CSF: blood glucose ratio < 0.4
  ◊ CSF protein > 45 mg/dL (> 450 mg/L) (usually 150-400 mg/dL [1500-4000 mg/L])
  ◊ Suspect ruptured brain abscess when WBC count is unusually high (±100,000)
• In all age groups:
  ◊ CSF opening pressure > 180 mm H2O (1.77 kPa)
  ◊ CSF Gram stain + in 75% of untreated patients
  ◊ CSF culture + 70-80% of the time
  ◊ Blood culture + 40-60% of the time
  ◊ CSF bacterial antigen test (sensitivity varies)
Drugs that may alter lab results: N/A
Disorders that may alter lab results: N/A

PATHOLOGICAL FINDINGS N/A

SPECIAL TESTS N/A

IMAGING
• CT scan of head if concern for increased intracranial pressure (ICP)
• Chest x-ray may reveal silent area of pneumonitis or abscess
• Sinus/skull x-rays may reveal cranial osteomyelitis, paranasal sinusitis or skull fracture
• Later in course, head CT scan, if hydrocephalus, brain abscess, subdural effusions or subdural empyema are considered

DIAGNOSTIC PROCEDURES Lumbar puncture

TREATMENT

APPROPRIATE HEALTH CARE
Inpatient often with ICU. If diagnosis is suspected, lumbar puncture should be done in office with antimicrobial therapy begun before transfer to hospital.

GENERAL MEASURES
• Appropriate antibiotic therapy
• Vigorous supportive care with constant nursing to ensure prompt recognition of seizures and prevention of aspiration
• Therapy for any coexisting conditions
• Measures to prevent hypothermia and dehydration

SURGICAL MEASURES N/A

ACTIVITY As tolerated in hospital and on discharge

DIET Regular as tolerated, except when SIADH complicates course

PATIENT EDUCATION For patient education materials on this topic, contact: American Academy of Pediatrics, 141 Northwest Point Blvd., P.O. Box 927, Elk Grove Village, IL 60009-0927, (800)433-9016

MEDICATIONS

DRUG(S) OF CHOICE Empiric therapy until culture results available (need to consider local patterns of bacterial sensitivity)
• 0 to 4 weeks: ampicillin 300-400 mg/kg/d plus a third-generation cephalosporin (cefotaxime 200 mg/kg/d q4-6h OR ceftriaxone 100 mg/kg/d q12-24h); or ampicillin plus an aminoglycoside (tobramycin 7.5 mg/kg/d q6-8h prematures or infants < 1 week, 2.5 mg/kg q12h. 14-21 days treatment.
• Age 4 to 12 weeks: ampicillin plus a third-generation cephalosporin. 10 days treatment (same doses as above).
• Age 3 months to 18 years: third generation cephalosporin; or ampicillin plus chloramphenicol 75-100 mg/kg/d. 10 days treatment.
• For all ages > 1 month and < 50 years - evidence is convincing that corticosteroids decrease mortality and morbidity. Dexamethasone 0.15 mg/kg q6h, started 15-20 minutes before antibiotic x 4 days. (N Engl J Med 324:1525, 1991.)
• For all patients > 1 month with definite or probable meningitis - use vancomycin plus cefotaxime (2 gm q 4 hours) or ceftriaxone (2 gm/day)
Contraindications: Allergies to antibiotics
Precautions:
• Ototoxicity from aminoglycoside
• Hearing loss
• Developmental abnormalities related to meningitis
Significant Possible interactions: Refer to manufacturer's literature

ALTERNATIVE DRUGS
• Vancomycin
• Antipseudomonal penicillins
• Aztreonam
• Quinolones (e.g., ciprofloxacin)

FOLLOWUP

PATIENT MONITORING Brainstem auditory evoked response (BAER) test should be done with infants prior to hospital discharge. Further followup will depend on its results and course of meningitis while in hospital.

PREVENTION/AVOIDANCE
• Prompt medical treatment for infections
• Strict aseptic techniques when treating patients with head wounds or skull fractures
• Look for evidence of CSF fistula in patients with recurrent meningitis

POSSIBLE COMPLICATIONS
• Seizures (20-30% during course of illness)
• Focal neurologic deficit
• Cranial nerve palsies (III, VI, VII, VIII) 10-20% of cases, usually disappear within a few weeks
• Sensorineural hearing loss (10% in children)
• Neurodevelopmental sequelae (subtle learning deficits 30%)
• Obstructive hydrocephalus
• Subdural effusions

EXPECTED COURSE/PROGNOSIS
• Overall case fatality 14%
• H. influenza 6%
• Neisseria meningitidis 10.3%
• Streptococcus pneumoniae 26.3%

MISCELLANEOUS

ASSOCIATED CONDITIONS
Which worsen prognosis:
• Coma
• Seizures
• Alcoholism
• Old age
• Infancy
• Diabetes mellitus
• Multiple myeloma
• Head trauma

AGE-RELATED FACTORS
Pediatric: N/A
Geriatric: Several signs and symptoms may be less evident in elderly patients with other disorders (congestive heart failure, pneumonia)
Others: Different etiologic agents, antimicrobials and dosing, and CSF findings as listed above

PREGNANCY N/A

SYNONYMS N/A

ICD-9-CM
320 Bacterial meningitis

SEE ALSO
• Meningitis, viral
• Meningococcemia

OTHER NOTES N/A

ABBREVIATIONS N/A

REFERENCES
• Tunkel AR, Scheld WM: Issues in the management of bacterial meningitis. Am Fam Phys 1997;56(5):1355-62
• McIntyre PB, Berkey CS, King SM, et al: Dexamethasone as adjuvant therapy in bacterial meningitis. A meta-analysis od randomized clinical trials since 1988. JAMA 1997;278(11):925-31
• Anonymous: Therapy for children with invasive pneumococcal infections. American Academy of Pediatrics Committee on Infectious Diseases. Pediatrics;1997;99(2):289-99
Illustrations: N/A
Internet references: http://www.5mcc.com

Author(s)
Paul R. Gordon, MD

Meningitis, viral

BASICS

DESCRIPTION Viral infection of the meninges and spinal fluid. The usual cause is acute and may be relapsing. Peak incidence occurs in summertime.
System(s) affected: Nervous
Genetics: N/A
Incidence/Prevalence in USA: Average of 10,000 reported cases per year. Probably many more unreported.
Predominant age: May affect all ages, but most common in young adults
Predominant sex: Male = Female

SIGNS AND SYMPTOMS

- Fever
- Headache, often severe
- Stiff neck
- Nausea and vomiting
- Photophobia
- Generalized aches and pains
- Occasional rash

CAUSES

- Coxsackie A, B
- ECHO virus (enteroviruses 70-75% of all cases)
- Poliovirus
- Lymphocytic choriomeningitis (LCM)
- Mumps
- Herpes (simplex and zoster)
- Epstein-Barr virus (EBV)
- Arthropod borne viruses
- Cytomegalovirus (CMV)
- Adenovirus

RISK FACTORS

- No specifics known
- Immunocompromised hosts may be more susceptible to CMV and adenovirus

DIAGNOSIS

DIFFERENTIAL DIAGNOSIS

- Bacterial meningitis
- Encephalitis
- Acute encephalopathy
- Postinfectious encephalomyelitis
- Parameningeal infections (e.g., subdural empyema)
- Carcinomatous meningitis
- Meningeal leukemia
- Migraine headache
- Viral syndrome (e.g., influenza)
- Chemical meningitis
- Brain abscess
- Other infectious agents (TB, syphilis, ameba, leptospirosis)

LABORATORY

- CSF pleocytosis - usually predominantly mononuclear but may show more polys early on
- CSF cell count up to 3000-4000, but usually 50-200
- CSF - increased pressure
- CSF - serum antiviral antibody
- Elevated CSF protein, but usually < 150 mg/dL (< 1500 mg/L)
- CSF sugar usually normal (exceptions - herpes, mumps)
- Negative CSF Gram stain and culture for bacteria
- Negative CSF latex agglutination or CIEP for bacterial antigens
- Normal or mildly elevated WBC (blood)
- Viral cultures and/or antibody titers are seldom helpful

Drugs that may alter lab results:
Pretreatment with antibiotics may result in a "partially treated" bacterial meningitis, mimicking viral meningitis
Disorders that may alter lab results:
- Diabetes (alteration in spinal fluid sugar)
- Pre-existing neurologic diseases (e.g., brain tumor, demyelinating disease) could affect CSF findings

PATHOLOGICAL FINDINGS

Lymphocyte infiltration of meninges and ventricles

SPECIAL TESTS EEG in some cases, especially if encephalitis is a consideration

IMAGING

- CT scan or MRI scan of the brain
- Usually CT or MRI performed prior to lumbar puncture

DIAGNOSTIC PROCEDURES Lumbar puncture

TREATMENT

APPROPRIATE HEALTH CARE

- Usually inpatient, depending on severity of symptoms
- Private room indicated with moderate sterile precautions. Stress hand washing.

GENERAL MEASURES

- Fever control
- IV fluids if oral intake is poor or vomiting is present

SURGICAL MEASURES N/A

ACTIVITY Bedrest initially, then activity as tolerated

DIET Determined by symptoms; may need to NPO due to nausea or vomiting, advance to clear fluids and regular diet as tolerated

PATIENT EDUCATION

- Discuss possibility, but low probability, of transmission to contacts
- Expected duration of illness (2-7 days)
- For patient education materials favorably reviewed on this topic, contact: American Academy of Pediatrics, 141 Northwest Point Blvd., P.O. Box 927, Elk Grove Village, IL 60009-0927, (800)433-9016

MEDICATIONS

DRUG(S) OF CHOICE
• Analgesics (adult doses)
◊ Morphine 2-5mg IV q3h
◊ Nalbuphine (Nubain) 10mg IM
◊ acetaminophen-codeine or oxycodone-acetaminophen (Percocet), 1-2 q3h prn
• Anti-emetics
◊ Promethazine (Phenergan) 12.5-25 mg IV q4h
◊ Prochlorperazine (Compazine) 10 mg IM q4h, in adults
• Antipyretics
◊ Acetaminophen (Tylenol) 650 mg po or suppository q4h for adults. Approximately 60 mg per year of age in children or 10-15 mg/kg/dose.
• Antiviral agents are not indicated in the usual care of viral meningitis
• Antibiotics are not indicated for treatment of viral meningitis, but are often initiated until a diagnosis is firmly established. If all parameters suggest a viral etiology, it is usually prudent to treat symptomatically and follow the patient closely in the hospital setting. If in doubt, a broad spectrum antibiotic with good CSF penetration should be started intravenously. The choice may be dictated by local sensitivities, as well as a consideration of age related pathogens.
Contraindications: Refer to manufacturer's profile of each drug
Precautions:
• Aspirin should be avoided in children and adolescents due to a possible association with Reye's syndrome
• Phenothiazines may produce a dystonic reaction, especially in adolescents
Significant possible interactions: Refer to manufacturer's profile of each drug

ALTERNATIVE DRUGS
Symptomatic relief may be provided by a variety of anti-emetics and analgesics (e.g., nonsteroidal anti-inflammatory drugs)

FOLLOWUP

PATIENT MONITORING
• Once the acute illness begins resolving, follow at least once within 7-10 days
• Repeat of lumbar puncture is not necessary unless the clinical course is atypical

PREVENTION/AVOIDANCE   N/A

POSSIBLE COMPLICATIONS
• Deafness
• Fatigue
• Irritability
• Muscle weakness
• Seizures (rare)

EXPECTED COURSE/PROGNOSIS
Complete recovery in 2-7 days; headaches and other uncomfortable symptoms may sometimes persist intermittently for 1-2 weeks

MISCELLANEOUS

ASSOCIATED CONDITIONS
Encephalitis

AGE-RELATED FACTORS
Pediatric: N/A
Geriatric: Viral meningitis is rarely seen in the elderly, and suspicions should be raised about an alternative diagnosis, e.g., carcinomatous meningitis
Others: N/A

PREGNANCY   N/A

SYNONYMS
• Abacterial meningitis
• Aseptic meningitis

ICD-9-CM   047.9 Unspecified viral meningitis

SEE ALSO
• Meningitis, bacterial
• Encephalitis, viral

OTHER NOTES   Enteroviruses and arthropod-borne viruses predominate in warm months; mumps usually occurs in the winter and spring, often in epidemics

ABBREVIATIONS
• CIEP - counterimmunoelectrophoresis
• CSF - cerebrospinal fluid

REFERENCES
• Mandell G, Douglas RG Jr, Bennett JE: Principles and Practice of Infectious Diseases. 4th Ed. New York, Churchill Livingstone, 1995
• Krugman S, Katz S, Gershon A, Wilfert C: Infectious Diseases of Children. 9th ed. New York, C.V. Mosby, 1990
• Rotbart HA: Enteroviral infections in the central nervous system. Clin Infect Dis 1995;20(4):971-81
Illustrations: N/A
Internet references: http://www.5mcc.com

Author(s)
Gary M. Miller, MD

Meningococcemia

BASICS

DESCRIPTION The presence of Neisseria meningitidis in the blood. This encompasses a broad spectrum of clinical manifestations.
• Bacteremia without sepsis: the patient has upper respiratory symptoms only and recovers spontaneously without antibiotic
• Bacteremia without meningitis: the patient is acutely ill, may have skin manifestations (rashes, petechiae, ecchymosis) and hypotension
• Bacteremia with meningitis: this clinical picture of meningitis predominates (headache, decreased sensorium, neck rigidity). Patient may also have skin manifestations and hypotension.
• Bacteremia with acute arthritis dermatitis syndrome: the patient may have tenosynovitis typical of gonococcal etiology
System(s) affected: Cardiovascular, Nervous, Skin/Exocrine, Musculoskeletal, Endocrine/Metabolic, Hemic/Lymphatic/Immunologic, Renal/Urologic
Genetics: N/A
Incidence/Prevalence in USA: 1-3/100,000 population
Predominant age: Highest attack rate in infants ages 3 months to 1 year and then decreases with age; it may affect all ages
Predominant sex: Male = Female

SIGNS AND SYMPTOMS
• Malaise
• Fever
• Chills, rigor
• Sore throat
• Cough
• Headache
• Changes in mental status - restlessness, agitation, confusion, delirium, lethargy, stupor, coma
• Myalgia
• Vomiting
• Convulsions
• Stiff neck
• Focal neurologic signs
• Tachycardia
• Tachypnea
• Hypotension
• Cyanosis
• Maculo-papular rash
• Petechiae
• Ecchymosis, purpura
• Arthritis
• Tenosynovitis

CAUSES
• Neisseria meningitidis, a gram-negative diplococcus
  ◊ At least 13 serotypes
  ◊ Major serogroups: A, B, C, Y, W -135
  ◊ Serogroup A may cause epidemics in many parts of developing world
  ◊ Serogroup C caused recent outbreaks in the U.S.

RISK FACTORS
• Age 3 months to 1 year
• Late complement component deficiency (C5, C6, C7, C8 or C9)
• Household contacts
• Contacts in nurseries, day care centers, dormitories and other close institutions
• Campus bar patronage

DIAGNOSIS

DIFFERENTIAL DIAGNOSIS
• Septicemia due to other microorganism
• Meningitis due to other pyogenic bacteria
• Gonococcemia
• Acute bacterial endocarditis
• Rocky Mountain spotted fever
• Hemolytic uremic syndrome
• Gonococcal arthritis dermatitis syndrome
• Influenza

LABORATORY
• Leukocytosis or leukopenia
• Left shift of leukocytes, toxic granulation
• Thrombocytopenia
• Lactic acidosis
• Prolonged prothrombin time
• Prolonged partial thromboplastin time
• Low fibrinogen
• Elevated fibrin degradation products
• Blood culture growing N. meningitidis
• Cerebrospinal fluid (CSF):
  ◊ Cloudy
  ◊ Increased WBC's with PMN's predominant
  ◊ Gram stain showing gram-negative diplococci
  ◊ Glucose to blood glucose ratio < 0.4
  ◊ Protein > 45 mg/dL
  ◊ Positive for N. meningitidis antigen
  ◊ Culture grew N. meningitidis
Drugs that may alter lab results:
• Prior antibiotic administration may make blood and/or CSF culture negative
• Rifampin colors urine orange and may interfere with certain lab tests, e.g. urine dipstick
Disorders that may alter lab results: N/A

PATHOLOGICAL FINDINGS
• Disseminated intravascular coagulation
• Exudates on meninges
• PMN infiltration of meninges
• Hemorrhage of adrenal glands

SPECIAL TESTS N/A

IMAGING CT scan of head if concern for space-occupying lesions

DIAGNOSTIC PROCEDURES
• Blood culture
• Lumbar puncture, done immediately after a brief history and physical examination, if meningitis suspected

TREATMENT

APPROPRIATE HEALTH CARE
• If meningitis suspected, immediate lumbar puncture
• If lumbar puncture is delayed, administer antibiotic immediately
• Admit patient to ICU, if severe sepsis or meningitis suspected
• Respiratory isolation, for 24 hours from the beginning of antibiotic therapy, is appropriate

GENERAL MEASURES
• Appropriate antibiotic
• Supportive care including IV fluids, oxygen when needed
• Close monitoring of patient for seizure activity
• Treat complications, e.g., DIC, ARDS, renal failure

SURGICAL MEASURES N/A

ACTIVITY As tolerated depending on clinical condition

DIET As tolerated depending on clinical condition

PATIENT EDUCATION
• Educate family and close contacts regarding risk of contracting meningococcal infections
• Educate healthcare personnel who are not at risk of contracting meningococcal infections

MEDICATIONS

DRUG(S) OF CHOICE
• In patients with severe mental changes, consider administering dexamethasone 0.15 mg/kg q 6h x 16 doses, starting 15 minutes before first dose of antibiotic
• For meningitis - penicillin G 4 million units IV q 4h (children 0.25 mU/kg IV q 4-6h) or ampicillin 2 g IV q 4h (children 200-300 mg/kg IV q 6h)
• For other infections - use half the dose for meningitis
• Duration of treatment 7-10 days
• Chemoprophylaxis for close contacts (household members, personnel in nurseries, day care centers, nursing homes, dormitories and other closed institutions). Regimen: rifampin 600 mg (children 10 mg/kg) po q12h for 2 days or for adults only, one dose of ciprofloxacin 750 mg po. (No chemoprophylaxis is needed for casual contacts, health care personnel (except persons giving mouth-to-mouth resuscitation), schoolmates, office co-workers).
Contraindications: For patients with penicillin allergy, use alternate drugs
Precautions:
• Adjust dosage in patients with severe renal dysfunction
• Rifampin ingestion causes orange urine.
Significant possible interactions: Refer to manufacturer's literature

ALTERNATIVE DRUGS
• For meningitis - chloramphenicol 1 g IV q 6h (in children 75-100 mg/kg q 6h) or ceftriaxone 2 g IV q 12h (children 80-100 mg/kg q 12-24h)
◊ Ceftriaxone should not be used in patients with history of anaphylactic reactions to penicillin (hypotension, laryngeal edema, wheezing, hives, etc.)
◊ Chloramphenicol may cause aplastic anemia
• For other infections - ceftriaxone 1 g (children 40 mg/kg) IV q 24h

FOLLOWUP

PATIENT MONITORING In patients with neurologic deficits, follow-up with neurologist may be needed

PREVENTION/AVOIDANCE Before discharge, give patient rifampin 600 mg (children 10 mg/kg) po q 12h for 2 days to eradicate carriage or for adults only, one dose of ciprofloxacin 500-750 mg po

POSSIBLE COMPLICATIONS
• Disseminated intravascular coagulation
• Acute tubular necrosis
• Seizures
• Focal neurologic deficit
• Cranial nerve palsies
• Sensorineural hearing loss
• Obstructive hydrocephalus
• Subdural effusions

EXPECTED COURSE/PROGNOSIS
Overall mortality 10%

MISCELLANEOUS

ASSOCIATED CONDITIONS N/A

AGE-RELATED FACTORS
Pediatric: Age 3 months to 1 year - highest risk
Geriatric: Less common
Others: N/A

PREGNANCY N/A

SYNONYMS Spinal meningitis

ICD-9-CM
036.2 Meningococcemia
036.0 Meningococcal meningitis

SEE ALSO
• Sepsis
• Meningitis, bacterial

OTHER NOTES
• A vaccine containing polysaccharides of groups A, C, Y and W-135 is available for persons with late complement deficiency, anatomic or functional asplenia. Vaccination is also recommended for travelers to areas with epidemic meningococcal disease. It should also be considered for use in college students living in dormitories.

ABBREVIATIONS N/A

REFERENCES
• Apicella M: Neisseria meningitidis. In: Mandell GL, Bennett JR, Dolin R, eds. Principles and Practice of Infectious Diseases. 4th Ed. New York, Churchill Livingstone, 1995
• Marnejon T, Watanakunakorn C: Purpura fulminans and adrenal hemorrhage due to group Y meningococcemia in an elderly woman. South Med J 1991;84:527-529
• Rompalo AM, Hood EW, Roberts PL, et al: The acute arthritis dermatitis syndrome; The changing importance of Neisseria gonorrhea and Neisseria meningitidis. Arch Intern Med 1987;147:281-283
• Jackson LA, Schuchat A, Reeves MW, et al: Serogroup C meningococcal outbreaks in the United States. An emerging threat. JAMA 1995;273:383-389
• Imrey PB, Jackson LA, Ludwinski PH, et al: Outbreak of serogroup C meningococcal disease associated with campus bar patronage. Am J epidemiol 1996;143:624-630
Illustrations: N/A
Internet references: http://www.5mcc.com

Author(s)
Chatrchai Watanakunakorn, MD, FACP, FCCP

Meningomyelocele

BASICS

DESCRIPTION
• Incomplete closure of the vertebral column during embryogenesis, resulting in exposure of meninges and spinal cord
• Always associated with the constellation of findings known as the Chiari II malformation which include: small posterior fossa, hindbrain herniation into the upper cervical spinal canal, dysgenesis or agenesis of the corpus callosum, neuronal migration disorders of varying degree, and hydrocephalus
• Chiari II abnormality associated with myelomeningocele, anencephaly, and encephalocele all belong to a group of disorders known as neural tube defects. These serious congenital anomalies of the nervous system, which occur during the first 4 weeks of gestation, result from faulty formation of the neural tube.
• Post neurulation defects develop after 25 days of intrauterine life, when neurulation is complete
  ◊ Characterized by intact skin over the underlying lesion
  ◊ Lesions include simple meningocele, lipomyelomeningocele, diastematomyelia, myelocystocele, neurenteric cyst, intraspinal and pelvic meningoceles
System(s) affected: Nervous, Musculoskeletal, Renal/Urologic, Skin/Exocrine
Genetics:
• Myelomeningocele, as well as the neural tube defects (anencephaly and encephalocele) represent examples of multifactorial inheritance
• Parents of an affected infant have a 1:30 chance of producing a 2nd affected offspring. An affected patient, if able to have children, has a 3-4% chance of having an affected child. Parents with 2 affected children run the risk of 7-8% of having a third child so affected. 2nd degree relatives of an affected individual (nephews, nieces) have a 1:100 risk; the risk for 1st cousins is 1:200.
• Folic acid deficiency is an environmental factor strongly associated with neural tube defects
Incidence/Prevalence in USA:
• Neural tube defects (also referred to as spina bifida) incidence in caucasians is 1:700 live births
• Incidence among African-Americans is <1:3000
Predominant age: Congenital anomaly, apparent at birth
Predominant sex: Male = Female

SIGNS AND SYMPTOMS
• The myelomeningocele is usually single and involves the lumbosacral spine
• Hydrocephalus requiring CSF diversion, occurs in > 80% of infants with the Chiari II abnormality and myelomeningocele
• The Chiari II malformation (hindbrain herniation into the upper cervical spinal canal) requires surgical decompression in < 20% of affected children
  ◊ If symptomatic, can impair cranial nerve control of swallowing/respiration and, less frequently cause pyramidal signs

◊ Syringomyelia, cystic expansion of the central spinal canal, is often present
◊ Surgical hindbrain decompression, if done promptly after onset of symptoms of hindbrain compression, may reverse or arrest these symptoms (stridor, respiratory difficulties, laryngomalacia), but are often confused with respiratory infections, thus delaying treatment

CAUSES
• Ultimate cause of spinal dysraphism is unclear
• Dysraphic malformations probably occur when environmental agents impact an underlying hereditary risk factors

RISK FACTORS
• 1st trimester valproic acid and derivatives (valproate sodium) use
• High risk pregnancy – previous children with spina bifida
• Insufficient maternal levels of folic acid
• >90% of spina bifida infants are the product of low-risk pregnancies

DIAGNOSIS

DIFFERENTIAL DIAGNOSIS   N/A

LABORATORY
• Prenatal: maternal serum alpha-fetoprotein (AFP) levels – elevated AFP level at 16-18 weeks suggest fetal open neural tube defects, indicating further prenatal evaluation and genetic counseling
• Newborn: no specific lab studies indicated
Drugs that may alter lab results: N/A
Disorders that may alter lab results: N/A

PATHOLOGICAL FINDINGS   N/A

SPECIAL TESTS
• Prenatal diagnosis
  ◊ Amniocentesis: increased alpha-fetoprotein in amniotic fluid (by 14 weeks) suggests open neural tube defects
  ◊ Ultrasound: hydrocephalus usually diagnosed readily. Other signs associated with Chiari II anomaly may be discernable (Banana sign, callosal anomalies, mega choroid plexus).
• Neonate
  ◊ Neurological examination, including pinprick examination of trunk, legs, and perineum. Functional integrity present if stimulus causes purposeful limb movements, arousal, crying, anal wink, etc.

IMAGING
Neonate: cranial ultrasound most efficient way to assess ventricular size promptly; may demonstrate associated anomalies (callosal agenesis, etc)

DIAGNOSTIC PROCEDURES
• Neonate
  ◊ Myelomeningocele is usually apparent on physical examination
  ◊ Direct laryngoscopy is indicated for infants with stridor, an ominous sign suggesting the need for urgent CSF diversion and/or posterior fossa decompression

TREATMENT

APPROPRIATE HEALTH CARE
Inpatient

GENERAL MEASURES
• Multidisciplinary approach: Pediatric neurosurgery, orthopedics, urology, nursing, social services, pediatrics and physical therapy
• Most patients with myelomeningocele have neurogenic bladder necessitating intermittent catheterization to prevent severe secondary urologic disorders

SURGICAL MEASURES
• Myelomeningocele repair – ideally within 24-48 hours of birth
• CSF diversion (usually ventriculoperitoneal shunt) usually required at birth or shortly thereafter
• Orthopedic correction of extremity and spinal deformities is more elective but requires evaluation early
• Infants with clinical evidence of hindbrain compression despite adequate CSF diversion require prompt posterior fossa decompression

ACTIVITY
• Determined by level of the lesion
• Optimized by physical therapists and multidisciplinary team

DIET
• Obesity a major cause of morbidity in myelomeningocele patients
• Modified as needed to facilitate bowel and bladder training

PATIENT EDUCATION
• Genetic counseling
• Signs and symptoms of shunt malfunction
• Bowel/bladder care
• Patient resources: Spina Bifida Association of America, 4590 MacArthur Blvd, Suite 250, Washington, DC 20007-4226 (800) 621-3141

MEDICATIONS

DRUG(S) OF CHOICE   N/A
Contraindications: N/A
Precautions: Latex precautions
Significant possible interactions: Latex allergy

ALTERNATIVE DRUGS   N/A

FOLLOWUP

PATIENT MONITORING
• Regular followup in spina bifida clinic, with multidisciplinary assessment including pediatrics, neurosurgery, orthopedics, and urology

PREVENTION/AVOIDANCE
• Adequate folate (0.4 mg/day) intake before pregnancy and through first trimester. For women with prior NTD-affected pregnancy, give 4 mg/day of folate before conception and through first trimester.

POSSIBLE COMPLICATIONS
• Late deterioration due to tethering of spinal cord
• Shunt obstruction: headache, nausea and vomiting, visual disturbances, cognitive difficulty; the latter two problems may be chronic, unaccompanied by headache or vomiting
• Shunt obstruction may result in hydromyelia, which may manifest only with intrinsic muscle weakness of the hands
• Inadequate bladder hygeine can result in hydronephrosis progressing to renal failure
• Seizures may result from cortical migration disorders or herald shunt malfunction

EXPECTED COURSE/PROGNOSIS
• >80% of treated patients with open neural tube defects have normal IQ
• Since 1970's, management techniques have improved, a result of the creation of multidisciplinary spina bifida clinics
• Shunt infection and malfunction less common, but still a major cause of morbidity
• Generally, early prediction of motor and intellectual outcome in neonates with Chiari II and myelomeningocele is hazardous
• Infants with head circumference > 50 cm at birth have dismal cognitive prognosis

MISCELLANEOUS

ASSOCIATED CONDITIONS
• Infants with a "simple" meningocele may have associated intraspinal abnormalities requiring treatment

AGE-RELATED FACTORS
Pediatric: Congenital defect
Geriatric: N/A
Others: N/A

PREGNANCY
• Ultrasound key to the intrauterine diagnosis of this condition

SYNONYMS
• Myelomeningocele
• Spinal dysraphism
• Spina bifida
• Open neural tube defect

ICD-9-CM
741.0 Spina bifida with hydrocephalus (Chiari Type II)
741.9 Spina bifida without mention of hydrocephalus

SEE ALSO   N/A

OTHER NOTES
• Decisions about performing operative procedures or letting the disorder "take its natural course" in severely affected infants presents serious ethical problems, usually the more aggressive course is best.

ABBREVIATIONS
ACM = Arnold Chiari malformation
NTD = Neural tube defect

REFERENCES
• Czeizel AE, Dudas I. Prevention of the first occurrence of neural-tube defects by periconceptional vitamin supplementation. N Engl J Med 1992;327:1832-1835
• American Academy of Pediatrics. Folic acid for the prevention of neural tube defects. Committee on Genetics. Pediatrics 1999 Aug;104(2 Pt 1):325-7
• McLone DG, Knepper PA. The Cause of Chiari II malformation: a unified theory. Pediatr Neurosci 1989;15:1-12
• van Zalen-Sprock RM, van Vugt JM, van Geijn HP. First and early second trimester diagnosis of anomalies of the central nervous system. J Ultrasound Med 1995;14:603-610
Illustrations: N/A
Internet references: http://www.5mcc.com

Author(s)
David Donahue, MD

Menopause

BASICS

DESCRIPTION The cessation of spontaneous menstrual cycles
• Climacteric: That period of time during which there is a decline in ovarian function. Although a woman may continue to have periodic uterine bleeding, such cycles may be anovulatory. During this time estrogen production diminishes and a woman may experience early signs of estrogen deficiency, such as vasomotor symptoms, even though she still has periodic bleeding.
• Postmenopause: The period after menopause usually accounting for more than a third of a women's total life.
• Premature menopause: occurring before age 30 and may be associated with sex chromosome abnormalities
System(s) affected: Reproductive, Endocrine/Metabolic, Musculoskeletal, Cardiovascular
Genetics: N/A
Incidence/Prevalence in USA: Increasingly common as life span increases - currently affects over 30 million women
Predominant age:
• Average age is 51 (unrelated to the age of menarche) and virtually all women postmenopausal by age 58.
Predominant sex: Female only

SIGNS AND SYMPTOMS
• Cessation of menses - either abruptly or preceded by a period of irregular cycles and/or diminished bleeding
• Vasomotor symptoms - hot flashes, sweating (85%)
• Psychologic symptoms - depression, nervousness, insomnia
• Vaginal atrophy - dyspareunia
• Urinary tract atrophy - stress or urge urinary incontinence
• Skin atrophy - wrinkles
• Osteoporosis - fractures (20% by age 85)
• Arteriosclerosis - coronary artery disease

CAUSES
• Physiologic - when due to depletion of oocytes
• Surgical - when due to removal of functioning ovaries because of disease or incidental to hysterectomy
• Medical - as a result of treatment of endometriosis (danazol [Danocrine] or GnRH analogues) or of breast cancer (antiestrogens). This etiology is reversible. May occur after cancer chemotherapy and be permanent or reversible.

RISK FACTORS
• Increasing age
• Pelvic surgery
• Sex chromosome abnormalities

DIAGNOSIS

DIFFERENTIAL DIAGNOSIS
• Pregnancy
• Polycystic ovarian disease
• Microadenoma of pituitary
• Hypothalamic dysfunction
• Asherman's syndrome
• Obstruction of uterine outflow tract

LABORATORY
• Usually none is required because patient's age and symptoms readily establish the diagnosis
• If the diagnosis is questionable in a young patient, an elevated serum FSH indicates ovarian failure (FSH greater than 100 mIU/mL [100 IU/L]). Measurement of LH is not necessary. Estradiol (E2) levels will be less than 50 pg/mL.
• Peripheral blood karyotype if age < 30
Drugs that may alter lab results:
• Estrogens
• Androgens
Disorders that may alter lab results:
Temporary, reversible cessation of ovarian function, e.g., during chemotherapy

PATHOLOGICAL FINDINGS
• Atrophy of endometrium - virtually 100% if untreated. The uterus may seem smaller on bimanual examination.
• Atrophy of vagina - loss of rugae, appearance of petechiae - virtually 100% after several years if untreated
• Atrophy of urethra
• Osteoporosis - approximately 2% loss of bone mass/year. Most common in Caucasians and Orientals and least common in African-Americans.
• Arteriosclerosis
• Ovarian stroma only - or only a few inactive oocytes

SPECIAL TESTS
• Endometrial biopsy and/or D&C in patients who have intermenstrual or postmenopausal bleeding - may be accompanied by hysteroscopic examination of uterine cavity. Investigation for endometrial cancer is necessary even in the presence of an atrophic vagina (usually the cause of the bleeding).
• Bleeding may also be evaluated by vaginal sonography; if double wall thickness of endometrial stripe is less than 5 mm, endometrial carcinoma is highly unlikely

IMAGING
• None for physiologic menopause
• MRI scan of head if pituitary tumor suspected
• Some physicians monitor bone density with photon beam absorptiometry - abnormal only after bone loss has occurred

DIAGNOSTIC PROCEDURES
• Endometrial sampling if intermenstrual or post menopausal bleeding occurs
• Pap smear
• Bimanual pelvic examination
• Mammography annually

TREATMENT

APPROPRIATE HEALTH CARE
Periodic office visits

GENERAL MEASURES
• To retard development of osteoporosis: adequate calcium intake - at least 1500 mg elemental calcium/day (diet p;us supplemental calcium); exercise; avoid smoking, avoid excessive alcohol or caffeine intake
• ERT for prophylaxis against osteoporosis and coronary artery disease, relief of vasomotor symptoms and urogenital atrophy. Exceptions are women with contraindications to therapy and obese women (who usually have sufficient endogenous estrogens produced by peripheral conversion of androgens by adipose tissue).
• ERT has a favorable effect on lipoproteins; elevates HDL and may retard development of Alzheimer's disease.

SURGICAL MEASURES N/A

ACTIVITY Active, weight-bearing exercise.

DIET Increased calcium intake, adequate Vitamin D

PATIENT EDUCATION
• American College of Obstetricians and Gynecologists (ACOG), 409 12th St. S.W., Washington, D.C. 20024, (800)673-8444
• For a listing of sources for patient education materials favorably reviewed on this topic, physicians may contact: American Academy of Family Physicians Foundation, P.O. Box 8418, Kansas City, MO 64114, (800)274-2237, ext. 4400

MEDICATIONS

DRUG(S) OF CHOICE
• Estrogens: commonly oral estrogen, conjugated (Premarin) or estradiol
◊ For retarding osteoporosis 0.625 mg qd; lesser doses not effective
◊ If vasomotor symptoms persist at 0.625 mg, increase to 0.9 mg or 1.25 mg, however, optimal cardioprotective effect is 0.625mg
◊ Other forms of oral estrogen or the transdermal patch may be used and appear to be equally effective
• Progestogen: commonly medroxyprogesterone (Provera, Depo-Provera)
◊ Because estrogens are carcinogenic to the endometrium, a progestogen should be added for its protective effect against endometrial cancer. (If the uterus has been removed, a progestogen is not needed).
• Administration
◊ Estrogens and progestogens may be administered continuously (no withdrawal bleeding expected) or cyclically
◊ Common regimens: Premarin 0.625 mg + Provera 2.5 mg q day OR Premarin 0.625 mg for 25 days per month + Provera 5 mg during the last 14 days of estrogen therapy OR Premarin 0.625 mg daily + Provera 5 mg during 14 days of month. Fixed combinations (Prempro, Premphase) may be convenient. Another option is Premarin and micronized progesterone.
Contraindications:
• Estrogen dependent malignancies
• Unexplained abnormal uterine bleeding
• History of thrombophlebitis
• Active liver disease
Precautions:
• Continuous combination therapy should not result in uterine bleeding
• Women on cyclic therapy may bleed normally only during those days when no therapy is given. Any other bleeding must be evaluated (for the possibility of endometrial cancer).
Significant possible interactions: N/A

ALTERNATIVE DRUGS
• Oral: estropipate (Ogen) 0.625 mg, estradiol (Estrace) 1-2 mg
• Transdermal: estradiol (Estraderm, Vivelle, Alora, Climara) 0.05-0.1 mg/day applied twice weekly, or 0.05-0.1 mg/day applied weekly (Climara)
• Vaginal: conjugated estrogens (Premarin cream) - best for local therapy of atrophic vaginitis only; blood levels are unpredictable.
• Intramuscular: not recommended - may not be protective against coronary artery disease without first passing through the liver
• For women who cannot take estrogens - using progestogens (Depo-Provera) 150 mg IM every month is helpful in alleviating hot flashes. This may also retard the development of osteoporosis, but is not helpful in preventing coronary artery disease or urogenital atrophy.

• Clonidine (Catapres), oral or transdermal, may be used to treat vasomotor symptoms, but is not effective against other menopausal occurrences
• Vitamin D is not helpful as the sole treatment for preventing osteoporosis
• Calcitonin produces only a temporary increase in body calcium
• Sodium fluoride increases bone volume but has toxic side effects
• Alendronate (Fosamax) 10 mg/day (on empty stomach) to treat postmenopausal osteoporosis
• Raloxifene (Evista) 60 mg/day to prevent osteoporosis

FOLLOWUP

PATIENT MONITORING
• Annual Pap smear, pelvic and breast exams
• Monthly breast self-examination
• Annual mammography
• Endometrial sampling in patients with abnormal bleeding

PREVENTION/AVOIDANCE   Menopause is a physiological process. It cannot be avoided, but the untoward effects can be moderated or eliminated by ERT.

POSSIBLE COMPLICATIONS
• Vasomotor symptoms
• Uncomfortable psychologic symptoms
• Vaginal atrophy
• Skin wrinkles
• Osteoporosis
• Arteriosclerosis
• The estrogen dosage recommended is very low and is unlikely to cause some of the complications associated with higher doses of estrogen, including hypercoagulability, breast tenderness, gall bladder disease and hypertension. The possible relationship to breast cancer is controversial.

EXPECTED COURSE/PROGNOSIS
• If untreated
◊ Ultimate disappearance of vasomotor symptoms - usually takes several years
◊ Urogenital atrophy
◊ Osteoporosis - possible fractures especially of the hip, vertebrae and wrists. Mortality associated with hip fractures is 15%.
◊ Coronary artery disease
• If treated
◊ Minimal effects of estrogen deprivation
◊ Slower bone loss and reduced incidence of coronary artery disease. Delayed appearance of Alzheimer's disease
◊ Therapy may be continued indefinitely if no contraindications appear since osteoporosis will rapidly occur after stopping therapy
◊ If existent, increased risk for breast cancer from estrogen is minimal

MISCELLANEOUS

ASSOCIATED CONDITIONS   Any medical problems that may occur with increasing age, especially osteoporosis

AGE-RELATED FACTORS
Pediatric: N/A
Geriatric: N/A
Others: N/A

PREGNANCY   Mutually exclusive

SYNONYMS
• Climacteric
• Ovarian failure

ICD-9-CM
627.0 Premenopausal menorrhagia
627.2 Menopausal or female climacteric states
627.4 States associated with artificial menopause
716.3 Climacteric arthritis

SEE ALSO
• Osteoporosis
• Uterine bleeding postmenopausal

OTHER NOTES
• Estrogen replacement therapy is especially important in women having an early menopause, either spontaneous or surgical because of their long expected life without endogenous estrogens. Without such therapy, they may be at a significantly increased risk for osteoporosis and its life threatening or debilitating effects.
• Following surgical menopause, vasomotor symptoms often appear very rapidly. Estrogen replacement therapy may be started in the early postoperative period.
• In perimenopausal women bothered by severe vasomotor symptoms, cyclic estrogen and progestogen therapy may be started even though the patient is still having periodic uterine bleeding

ABBREVIATIONS
ERT = estrogen replacement therapy
HRT = hormone replacement therapy

REFERENCES
• Mishell DR Jr: Menopause. Physiology and Pharmacology. Chicago, Year Book Medical Publishers, 1987
• Achilles C, Leppert PC: The menopausal woman. In: Leppert PC, Howard FM (eds): Primary Care for Women. Philadelphia, Lippincott-raven, 1997::97-102
Illustrations: N/A
Internet references: http://www.5mcc.com

Author(s)
Alvin Langer, MD

Menorrhagia

BASICS

DESCRIPTION Excessive amount or duration of menstrual flow, at more or less regular intervals
• Distinguish from, but may overlap with:
  ◊ Metrorrhagia - irregular or frequent flow, noncyclic
  ◊ Menometrorrhagia - frequent, excessive, irregular flow (menorrhagia plus metrorrhagia)
  ◊ Polymenorrhea - frequent flow, cycles of 21 days or less
  ◊ Intermenstrual bleeding - bleeding between regular menses
  ◊ Dysfunctional uterine bleeding (DUB) - abnormal endometrial bleeding of hormonal cause and related to anovulation
System(s) affected: Reproductive
Genetics: N/A
Incidence/Prevalence in USA: Abnormal bleeding is common; prevalence varies with definition (endometrial carcinoma: about 40,000 new cases per year)
Predominant age:
• Menarche to menopause; about 50% of cases occur after 40 years of age
• Dysfunctional bleeding is fairly common in adolescence and near menopause
Predominant sex: Female only

SIGNS AND SYMPTOMS
• "Excessive" menstrual flow defined subjectively varies greatly from woman to woman (average normal menstrual flow is about 30 mL per cycle)
• Useful historical features include:
  ◊ Bleeding substantially heavier than the patient's usual flow
  ◊ Bleeding lasting more than 7 days
  ◊ Flow associated with passage of significant clots
  ◊ Anemia
• The following symptoms tend to suggest that cycles are ovulatory:
  ◊ Regular menstrual interval
  ◊ Mid-cycle pain (mittelschmerz)
  ◊ Dysmenorrhea
  ◊ Premenstrual symptoms - breast soreness, mood changes, etc.
• Abdominal pain or cramps at other times of the cycle may be associated with structural causes:
  ◊ Myomas
  ◊ Polyps
  ◊ Ovarian tumors
• Hirsutism or acne
  ◊ May accompany Stein-Leventhal syndrome

CAUSES
• Hypothyroidism
• Endometrial proliferation/excess/hyperplasia:
  ◊ Anovulation, oligo-ovulation
  ◊ Polycystic ovarian disease (PCOD), Stein-Leventhal syndrome
  ◊ Ovarian tumor
  ◊ Obesity
  ◊ Hormone (estrogen) therapy
• Endometrial atrophy:
  ◊ Postmenopause
  ◊ Prolonged progestin or oral contraceptive administration
• Local factors:
  ◊ Endometrial polyps
  ◊ Endometrial neoplasia
  ◊ Adenomyosis/endometriosis
  ◊ Uterine myomata (fibroids)
  ◊ Intrauterine device (IUD)
  ◊ Uterine sarcoma
• Coagulation disorders:
  ◊ Thrombocytopenia, platelet disorders
  ◊ von Willebrand's disease
  ◊ Leukemia
  ◊ Ingestion of aspirin or anticoagulants
  ◊ Renal failure/dialysis

RISK FACTORS
• Obesity
• Anovulation
• Estrogen administration (without progestin)
• Prior treatment with progestational agents or oral contraceptives increases the risk of endometrial atrophy, but decreases the risk of endometrial hyperplasia or neoplasia

DIAGNOSIS

DIFFERENTIAL DIAGNOSIS
• Pregnancy complications:
  ◊ Threatened abortion
  ◊ Incomplete abortion
  ◊ Ectopic pregnancy
• Nonuterine bleeding:
  ◊ Cervical ectropion/erosion
  ◊ Cervical neoplasia/polyp
  ◊ Cervical or vaginal trauma
  ◊ Condylomata
  ◊ Atrophic vaginitis
  ◊ Foreign bodies
• Pelvic inflammatory disease (PID):
  ◊ Endometritis
  ◊ Tuberculosis

LABORATORY
• Pregnancy test
• CBC to assess severity of blood loss, exclude thrombocytopenia and leukemia
• In selected cases:
  ◊ TSH - elevated in hypothyroidism
  ◊ Platelet count, bleeding time, prothrombin time (PT), partial thromboplastin time (PTT) for coagulation screen
  ◊ Creatinine, BUN
  ◊ Serum progesterone - 5-20 ng/mL (15.9-63.6 nmol/L) in luteal phase, < 1 ng/mL (< 3.18 nmol/L) in follicular phase or anovulatory cycle
Drugs that may alter lab results:
Progestins used prior to endometrial biopsy may cause decidualization and obscure true diagnosis
Disorders that may alter lab results: N/A

PATHOLOGICAL FINDINGS Vary with cause: see Causes

SPECIAL TESTS Endometrial biopsy detects hyperplasia, dysplasia, or atrophy. If done prior to expected menses, may also help make the diagnosis of anovulation or luteal phase defect.

IMAGING
• Ultrasonography to evaluate adnexal masses or fibroids suspected from pelvic exam
• Computerized tomography used in investigation of potentially malignant pelvic masses

DIAGNOSTIC PROCEDURES
• Pelvic and rectal examination
• Pap smear
• Endometrial biopsy
• Diagnostic dilatation and curettage
• Hysteroscopy

TREATMENT

APPROPRIATE HEALTH CARE
• Most cases can be managed as outpatients in office or emergency department
• Hospitalize for bleeding accompanied by orthostatic hypotension or hematocrit < 25%

GENERAL MEASURES
• Rule out pregnancy complications and non-uterine bleeding
• Treat severe or life-threatening bleeding acutely:
  ◊ Intravenous estrogen
  ◊ Curettage if necessary
  ◊ Hysterectomy in extreme case
• Proceed to identify underlying cause of bleeding and treat to prevent recurrence
  ◊ Hormonal therapy
  ◊ Dilatation and curettage for hormone-unresponsive cases
  ◊ Consider endometrial ablation or hysterectomy in persistent cases where fertility is not desired
  ◊ Specific treatment for neoplasia, polyps, systemic disease, etc.
  ◊ Patients who desire fertility may also need appropriate treatment for anovulation, endometriosis, myomata, etc.

SURGICAL MEASURES See general Measures

ACTIVITY As tolerated. Resting with feet elevated may be helpful.

DIET Iron supplementation may help correct for increased blood loss

PATIENT EDUCATION Information about side effects of medications

Menorrhagia

MEDICATIONS

DRUG(S) OF CHOICE
• For acute control of severe bleeding:
◊ Estrogen, conjugated (Premarin) 25 mg IV every 4 hours up to 6 doses until bleeding abates
• For less severe bleeding or after control of acute bleeding:
◊ Medroxyprogesterone acetate (Provera) 10-30 mg daily for 5-10 days
◊ Any combination oral contraceptive, (usually one of the "high dose" oral contraceptives) one tablet 4 times a day for 5-7 days
• To prevent heavy bleeding in subsequent cycles:
◊ Medroxyprogesterone acetate 10-20 mg daily for 10 days per month
◊ Usual cyclic dose of a combination oral contraceptive
• For endometrial atrophy in postmenopausal woman:
◊ Estrogen plus progesterone replacement therapy
Contraindications:
• To estrogen, oral contraceptives, or progestins:
◊ Pregnancy
◊ Breast or endometrial cancer
◊ Thromboembolic disease, past or present
◊ Impaired liver function
Precautions:
• Nausea and vomiting are common from IV estrogen; antiemetics are helpful
• Estrogen may precipitate acute intermittent porphyria or cholestatic jaundice in susceptible individuals
Significant possible interactions: Refer to manufacturer's profile of each drug

ALTERNATIVE DRUGS
• Norethindrone acetate (Norlutin, Norlutate) 2.5-10 mg daily for 10 days per month, during the assumed latter half of menstrual cycle
• Megestrol acetate (Megace) 40 mg daily for 10 days per month
• Megestrol acetate (Megace) 40 mg daily continuously to treat atypical hyperplasia
• Nonsteroidal prostaglandin-synthetase inhibitors (naproxen, mefenamic acid, ibuprofen, and others) can reduce blood loss with ovulatory cycles and reduce dysmenorrhea

FOLLOWUP

PATIENT MONITORING
• Varies with cause of bleeding
• Medical treatment of hyperplastic/dysplastic endometrium should be followed by repeat biopsy to confirm that histologic structure has returned to normal

PREVENTION/AVOIDANCE Pap smear and pelvic examination annually

POSSIBLE COMPLICATIONS Anemia

EXPECTED COURSE/PROGNOSIS
• Varies with cause of bleeding
• Most patients with hormonal causes will respond to hormonal manipulation

MISCELLANEOUS

ASSOCIATED CONDITIONS
Metrorrhagia; menometrorrhagia; androgenic disorders

AGE-RELATED FACTORS
Pediatric: Genital bleeding prior to puberty can result from trauma, foreign bodies, vaginal infection, or exogenous hormone administration
Geriatric: Genital atrophy may predispose to bleeding with minimal trauma. Neoplasm of ovary or endometrium must be ruled out.
Others:
• In adolescence, irregular bleeding due to anovulation and immaturity of the hypothalamic-pituitary-ovarian axis is common
• Beyond age 35-40, endometrial dysplasia and endometrial carcinoma are significant causes of bleeding. Obtain endometrial sampling before attempting hormonal treatment.

PREGNANCY Bleeding in pregnancy is not menorrhagia. Complications of pregnancy or cervical/vaginal lesions should be considered.

SYNONYMS N/A

ICD-9-CM
621.0 Endometrial polyp
621.3 Endometrial hyperplasia
621.8 Endometrial atrophy
626.2 Menorrhagia, menometrorrhagia, polymenorrhea
626.3 Pubertal menorrhagia
626.4 Irregular menses
626.6 Metrorrhagia
626.8 Dysfunctional uterine bleeding
627.0 Premenopausal (i.e., perimenopausal, climacteric) menorrhagia
627.1 Postmenopausal bleeding

SEE ALSO
• Amenorrhea
• Cervical dysplasia
• Cervical malignancy
• Cervical polyps
• Cervicitis
• Cervicitis, ectropion & true erosion
• Dysmenorrhea
• Uterine myomas
• Menopause
• Polycystic ovarian disease

OTHER NOTES N/A

ABBREVIATIONS N/A

REFERENCES
• Wentz AC: Abnormal Uterine Bleeding. In: Jones HW, ed. Novak's Textbook of Gynecology. 11th Ed. Baltimore, Williams & Wilkins, 1988
• Cowan BD, Morrison JC: Management of Abnormal Genital Bleeding in Girls and Women. N Engl J Med 1991;324(24):1710-1715
• Speroff L: Clinical Gynecologic Endocrinology and Infertility. 5th Ed. Baltimore, Williams & Wilkins, 1994
• Carlson JM: Menorrhagia and Metrorrhagia. In: Friedman EA, ed. Gynecologic Decision Making. 2nd Ed. Philadelphia, B.C. Decker, 1988
Illustrations: N/A
Internet references: http://www.5mcc.com

Author(s)
Donald A. F. Nelson, MD

Mental retardation

BASICS

DESCRIPTION Mental retardation (MR) is a symptom with multiple etiologies including chromosomal abnormalities, genetic defects, intrauterine, perinatal, neonatal, and postnatal causes. Mental retardation refers to substantial limitations in present functioning. It is characterized by significantly subaverage intellectual functioning, existing concurrently with related limitations in two or more of the following applicable adaptive skills areas: communication, self-care, home living, social skills, community use, self-direction, health and safety, functional academics, leisure and work. Cognitive and adaptive behavior deficits are manifested before age 18.
- Subgroups of mentally retarded:
  ◊ Mild: IQ 55-69 (85%)
  ◊ Moderate: IQ 40-54 (10%)
  ◊ Severe: IQ 25-39 (5%)
  ◊ Profound: IQ 0-24 (<1%)

System(s) affected: Nervous

Genetics:
- Autosomes: Trisomies and rearrangements - approximately 1500 variations are all associated with MR
- Sex chromosomes: 80 of 336 disorders cause MR
- Autosomal dominant: 180 of 3,000 disorders cause MR
- Autosomal recessive: 400 of 1,550 disorders cause MR

Incidence/Prevalence in USA: Incidence and prevalence are closely related to social, economic, and health conditions of the society. The general incidence of mental retardation in the United States has been estimated at 125,000 births per year by the American Association on Mental Retardation. This would correspond to approximately 3% of the population. The research on both incidence and prevalence of mental retardation in the US is exceedingly scant. A comprehensive Canadian study of the maritime Provinces found prevalences of 3.65 per 1000. Most professionals associated with the American Association on Mental Retardation accept a prevalence of 2.5% and they recognize that the prevalence varies with chronological age. Specifically, mildly retarded preschoolers are able to meet societies demands but are identified by the school system due to demands for cognitive processing. Conversely, once they leave the requirements of the educational system they may adapt to societies demands and the diagnosis need not apply.

Predominant age: By definition mental retardation occurs during the developmental period. Older adults who lose mental faculties are more accurately diagnosed as demented. Patients may present the MR after traumatic brain injury.

Predominant sex: Male > Female (1.5:1)

SIGNS AND SYMPTOMS
- Profoundly and severely retarded children are frequently diagnosed at the time of birth or during the newborn period. Children with profound or severe retardation are more likely to have dysmorphic features.
- Moderately retarded children may go undiagnosed until they fail to meet normal developmental milestones
- Mildly retarded children may go undiagnosed until well into the school years

CAUSES
- Chromosomal abnormalities
  ◊ Autosomal abnormalities
  ◊ Trisomy, e.g., Down syndrome
  ◊ Translocations
  ◊ Inversions
  ◊ Duplications
  ◊ Deletions, e.g., Prader-Willi
- Sex chromosome abnormalities
  ◊ Fragile X syndrome
  ◊ Turner syndrome
  ◊ Klinefelter syndrome
  ◊ Various multiple X and/or Y conditions
- Autosomal dominant conditions
  ◊ Neurocutaneous syndromes, e.g., neurofibromatosis, tuberous sclerosis
- Autosomal recessive conditions
  ◊ Amino acid metabolism, e.g., phenylketonuria, Maple syrup urine disease
  ◊ Carbohydrate metabolism, e.g., galactosemia, fructosuria
  ◊ Lipid metabolism
  ◊ Tay-Sachs
  ◊ Gaucher
  ◊ Niemann-Pick, e.g., mucopolysaccharidosis
  ◊ Purine metabolism, e.g., Lesch-Nyhan
  ◊ Other, e.g., Wilson
- Multifactorial and sporadic conditions
  ◊ Cornelia de Lange syndrome
  ◊ Spinal cord disorders (spina bifida, Arnold-Chiari malformation)
  ◊ Disorders of brain and skull
  ◊ Prenatal factors
  ◊ Rh incompatibility
  ◊ Maternal infections - all the TORCH viruses - rubella, toxoplasmosis, cytomegalic virus, and herpes simplex)
  ◊ Maternal diseases, e.g., diabetes mellitus, toxemia
  ◊ Maternal substance abuse, e.g., alcohol use/abuse. Fetal alcohol syndrome is a leading environmental cause of mental retardation.
  ◊ Prescription medications, such as Accutane or Dilantin
- Perinatal factors
  ◊ Prematurity
  ◊ Postmaturity
  ◊ Birth injuries
  ◊ High risk mothers
- Postnatal factors
  ◊ Childhood diseases, e.g., meningitis, encephalitis, general inflammatory disease with high fever, hypothyroidism
  ◊ Trauma, e.g., accidents, physical abuse, marked deprivation
  ◊ Poisoning, e.g., lead, carbon monoxide, household products

RISK FACTORS
Risk factors for future offspring of the parent couple must be calculated based upon the specific etiology of related retarded individuals

DIAGNOSIS

DIFFERENTIAL DIAGNOSIS
- Brain tumors
- Hearing and/or speech impairment
- Infantile autism
- Cerebral palsy
- Emotional disturbance
- Lack of environmental opportunities for appropriate development

LABORATORY
- Specific studies are available for those patients with identifiable genetic disease entities
- Chromosome studies
- Metabolic screens
- Amino acid
- Sugar substrates
- Molecular studies, e.g., DNA

Drugs that may alter lab results: N/A

Disorders that may alter lab results: N/A

PATHOLOGICAL FINDINGS N/A

SPECIAL TESTS
- Individually administered measure of intellectual abilities
  ◊ Measure utilized depends upon the age of the patient
  ◊ Birth through 42 months: Bayley's Scales of Infant Development
  ◊ 2 years of age through adulthood: Stanford Binet (form LM), Stanford Binet (4th edition), Wechsler Scales
  ◊ Preschool children: WIPPSI
  ◊ School age: WISC-III
  ◊ Adults: WAIS-III, and an adaptive behavior scale. All patients need a measure of adaptive behavior. The Vineland Adaptive Behavior Scales are widely utilized.
  ◊ Other measures are available; however, these are the most widely recognized and utilized measures of individual ability and adaptive behavior

IMAGING N/A

DIAGNOSTIC PROCEDURES See Special tests

Mental retardation

TREATMENT

APPROPRIATE HEALTH CARE
• Some specialized care may be necessary based upon the etiology of the retardation
• Care for the retarded is educational, not medical and should include early intervention

GENERAL MEASURES N/A

SURGICAL MEASURES N/A

ACTIVITY Full activity

DIET No research evidence supports the use of specific diets for mental retardation and/or Attention Deficit Hyperactivity Disorder (ADHD). Exception: Some metabolic and storage disorders, i.e., PKU.

PATIENT EDUCATION Parental education and consultation as to the development of appropriate behavioral and educational expectations are strongly advised. Families should be referred to the local Association for Retarded Citizens.

MEDICATIONS

DRUG(S) OF CHOICE None
Contraindications: N/A
Precautions: N/A
Significant possible interactions: N/A

ALTERNATIVE DRUGS N/A

FOLLOWUP

PATIENT MONITORING Regular pediatric care

PREVENTION/AVOIDANCE N/A

POSSIBLE COMPLICATIONS Learning inappropriate behaviors

EXPECTED COURSE/PROGNOSIS
• Mild retardation: Social and communication skills appropriate for community functioning, basic job skills, and functional literacy
• Moderate mental retardation: Speech deficits, social awareness, personal care skills, i.e., dressing, feeding, washing, sheltered employment, group home living
• Severe mental retardation: Limited speech and language, poor motor development, in need of supervision
• Profound mental retardation: Neurological defect, poor cognitive social ability, absent speech, possible self harm, extended care
• Specific etiologies, i.e., Down syndrome and fragile X patients show a decline in cognitive and adaptive behavior over time

MISCELLANEOUS

ASSOCIATED CONDITIONS
• Speech problems
• Seizures
• Maladaptive behaviors
• Attention deficit hyperactivity disorder (ADHD):
  ◊ Found with greater frequency among individuals with neuropsychological dysfunction
  ◊ Treatment for ADHD among the mentally retarded is not unlike that for the "normal" population
  ◊ Data indicates overuse of psychoactive substances to aid caretakers

AGE-RELATED FACTORS
Pediatric: N/A
Geriatric: N/A
Others: N/A

PREGNANCY Parents and first degree relatives could benefit from consultation with a genetic associate or counselor

SYNONYMS Mental deficiency

ICD-9-CM
317 Mild mental retardation
318.0 Moderate mental retardation
318.1 Severe mental retardation
318.2 Profound mental retardation
319 Unspecified mental retardation

SEE ALSO
• Cerebral palsy
• Down syndrome
• Fragile X syndrome
• Lead poisoning
• Attention deficit hyperactivity disorder

OTHER NOTES
• Extensive family history to aid in diagnosis is mandatory
• Genetic referral in cases without known etiology is appropriate

ABBREVIATIONS
MR = mental retardation

REFERENCES
• Jones KL: Smith's Recognizable Patterns of Human Malformations. 5th Ed. Philadelphia, W. B. Saunders, 1997
• Weiderman HR, Kunze J: Clinical syndromes. 3rd Ed. English translation. London, Mosby-Wolfe, 1997
• Baraitser M, Winter RM: Color Atlas of Congenital Malformation Syndromes. London, Mosby-Wolfe, 1996
Illustrations: N/A
Internet references: http://www.5mcc.com

Author(s)
Richard J. Simensen, PhD
Gene S. Fisch, PhD

Metatarsalgia

BASICS

DESCRIPTION A catch-all term for pain in the forefoot, usually in the plantar aspect
• Pain and inflammation along the medial and transverse arches of the mid - and forefoot, involving the muscles, tendons and ligaments
System(s) affected: Musculoskeletal
Genetics: N/A
Incidence/Prevalence in USA: Common
Predominant age: 30's-80's
Predominant sex: Female > Male

SIGNS AND SYMPTOMS
• Predominantly located in the dorsal and plantar forefoot, especially distal half of metatarsal shaft
• Pain
• Swelling
• Tenderness
• Occasionally erythema

CAUSES
• Excess strain (anatomical variations)
   ◊ Hallux valgus and rigidus
   ◊ Plantar flexed metatarsals
   ◊ Hammer toe
   ◊ Obesity
• Repetitive and/or excessive and/or unaccustomed walking and running
   ◊ Long distance
   ◊ Hard surfaces
   ◊ Poor shoe construction
   ◊ Skeletal abnormalities
• Systemic disorder
   ◊ Gout
   ◊ Rheumatoid arthritis

RISK FACTORS
• Pes planus (flat foot)
• Old or poorly constructed shoes
• Poor physical condition

DIAGNOSIS

DIFFERENTIAL DIAGNOSIS
• Stress fracture
• Cellulitis or infection
• Neuroma (plantar or Morton's)
• Inflammatory arthritis
• Traumatic arthritis
• Foreign body
• Tumor (rare)

LABORATORY
• WBC - normal (elevated in infection)
• Sedimentation rate - normal (elevated in infection and inflammatory arthritis)
• Tests for gout, rheumatoid arthritis, or other systemic disorders if strongly suspect
Drugs that may alter lab results: N/A
Disorders that may alter lab results: N/A

PATHOLOGICAL FINDINGS N/A

SPECIAL TESTS N/A

IMAGING
• Routine anteroposterior and lateral foot x-ray - normal
• Bone scan if high index of suspicion of stress fracture
• MRI if suspect mass lesion

DIAGNOSTIC PROCEDURES N/A

TREATMENT

APPROPRIATE HEALTH CARE
Outpatient

GENERAL MEASURES
• Ice initially
• Moist heat later
• Taping or Gelcast
• Walking cast - rarely
• Physical therapy - rarely
• Cane or crutch - temporary
• Arch support in a well-fitted, low-heel, air-soled shoe
• Energy-absorbing sole on shoe

SURGICAL MEASURES N/A

ACTIVITY
• Rest during active, symptomatic phase
• Weight bearing as tolerated
• Progressive return to previous level of activities and sports - bike riding to jogging to running (with an arch support in running shoes)

DIET No special diet

PATIENT EDUCATION Instruct about proper shoes for specific activity and gradual return to usual activities

MEDICATIONS

DRUG(S) OF CHOICE
- Nonsteroidal anti-inflammatories such as:
  ◊ Naproxen (Naprosyn) 500 mg bid 7-14 days
  ◊ Ibuprofen (Motrin) 800 mg tid 7-14 days
Contraindications:
- GI bleeding or ulcer history
- Liver diseases
Precautions:
- Renal disease
- Hepatic disease
- Fluid retention
- GI disorders, especially ulcers
- Coagulation disorders
- Anemia
Significant possible interactions:
- Anticoagulants
- Digoxin
- Lithium
- Methotrexate
- Cyclosporine

ALTERNATIVE DRUGS
New COX-2 - celecoxib (Celebrex) 100-200 mg 1d to bid for 7-10 days

FOLLOWUP

PATIENT MONITORING
Weekly for 2-4 weeks

PREVENTION/AVOIDANCE
- Appropriate shoes for appropriate activity
- Avoid overuse
- Treat systemic disorders

POSSIBLE COMPLICATIONS
Back and knee problems due to change in weight bearing dynamics

EXPECTED COURSE/PROGNOSIS
Expect complete healing with appropriate treatment

MISCELLANEOUS

ASSOCIATED CONDITIONS
See Causes

AGE-RELATED FACTORS
Pediatric: N/A
Geriatric:
- More frequent in older athletes and the aging
- Symptoms more pronounced
Others: N/A

PREGNANCY
N/A

SYNONYMS
N/A

ICD-9-CM
726.70 Metatarsalgia NOS

SEE ALSO
N/A

OTHER NOTES
N/A

ABBREVIATIONS
N/A

REFERENCES
Sullivan JA, Finberg L: The Pediatric Athlete. Park Ridge, Il, American Academy of Orthopedic Surgeons, 1990
Illustrations: N/A
Internet references: http://www.5mcc.com

Author(s)
Richard W. Cohen, MD

Migraine

BASICS

DESCRIPTION Paroxysmal headache lasting 4-72 hours. Episodes vary in frequency from more than once a week to less than one per year with symptoms abating completely between attacks. Prodromes consisting of non-specific symptoms occur frequently hours to days before headache. Most frequent sub-types are:
• Without aura - (common migraine) defining over 80% of attacks
• With aura - (classic migraine) characterized by focal disruption of neurological function begins and ends prior to headache onset
• Variants of migraine include:
◊ Transformed migraine - chronic headache pattern evolving from episodic migraine. Migraine-like attacks are superimposed on a daily or near-daily headache pattern, e.g., tension headache.
◊ Basilar migraine - occipital headache, with aura symptoms of dysarthria, vertigo, tinnitus, ataxia, and bilateral paresis or bilateral paresthesias
◊ Hemiplegic migraine - aura consisting of hemiplegia and/or hemiparesis
◊ Ophthalmoplegic - palsy of the ipsilateral third cranial nerve during the headache phase
◊ Retinal - symptoms of retinal vascular involvement during headache
◊ Childhood periodic syndromes - (migraine equivalents) recurrent often cyclic episodes of symptoms
◊ Status migrainous - persistent migraine which does not resolve spontaneously
◊ Migrainous stroke - persistent or permanent neurologic deficits persisting beyond migraine attack usually with neuro-imaging changes
System(s) affected: Nervous, Musculoskeletal, Cardiovascular, Gastrointestinal
Genetics: > 80% of patients have positive family history. Identification of a chromosomal abnormality has been confirmed in familial hemiplegic migraine.
Incidence/Prevalence in USA:
• Adults: 17.6% of females, 5.6% of males
• Childhood unknown; may be significant
Predominant age: Childhood; increase in early adolescence, through 30s and 40s; decreases with age, attacks may persist into mature adulthood
Predominant sex:
• Male ≥ Female in childhood
• Female > Male (3:1) after menarche to mid-adult life
• Female > Male (2:1) in postmenopausal female populations

SIGNS AND SYMPTOMS
Five phases of a migraine; symptoms vary from patient to patient or from attack to attack within the same individual
• Prodrome: A variety of "warnings" that precede migraine, frequently characterized by mood disruptions (e.g., euphoria, irritability, depression), fatigue, muscle tension, food craving, bloating, yawning, or subtle disruption of sensory processing

• Aura: Visual disruptions are most common, including scotoma, hemianopsia, fortification spectra, geometric visual patterns, and occasionally hallucinations. Somatosensory disruption in face or upper extremities is also common. Headache typically begins within 1 hour of aura resolution.
• Headache: Unilateral (30-40% bilateral), throbbing (40% non-throbbing) pain of 4-72 hours; intensified by movement; associated with systemic manifestations, e.g., nausea (87%), vomiting (56%), diarrhea (16%), photophobia (82%), phonophobia (78%), muscle tenderness (65%), lightheadedness (72%), vertigo (33%).
• Headache termination: Untreated, usually occurs with sleep; occasionally, vomiting or strong emotional experiences abort headache
• Postdrome: Headache pain resolved but another manifestation lingers on, such as, food intolerance, impaired concentration, fatigue, muscle soreness

CAUSES
• Exact etiology unknown; appears to be a genetically-linked, neuronal disease with vascular disruption as an epiphenomenon of underlying neurochemical disruption
• Serotonin and norepinephrine metabolism abnormalities may play a role
• Neurogenic inflammation and regional disruption of cerebral and/or extracranial blood flow may explain some clinical features

RISK FACTORS
• Specific foods, alcohol, missing meals, menstrual cycle, excessive sleep, fatigue, emotional stress, let down (relief of stress)
• Medications (estrogen replacement, BCP's, vasodilators)
• Family history of migraine
• Female gender
• Young age
• History of childhood cyclic vomiting, cyclic abdominal pain, motion sickness

DIAGNOSIS

DIFFERENTIAL DIAGNOSIS
• Other primary headache disorders
• Secondary headaches, such as tumor, infection, vascular pathology, or prescription or illicit drug, e.g., cocaine
• Drug seeking patients
• Psychiatric disease
• Rarely, migraine symptoms similar to certain forms of epilepsy

LABORATORY Only useful to rule out secondary causes of headache
Drugs that may alter lab results: N/A
Disorders that may alter lab results: N/A

PATHOLOGICAL FINDINGS
• Changes in blood serotonin levels and serotonin metabolites in the urine are reported
• Changes in regional blood flow
• Changes in sophisticated imaging studies

SPECIAL TESTS Only to rule out underlying pathology

IMAGING Occasionally required

DIAGNOSTIC PROCEDURES Based on careful history and physical findings

TREATMENT

APPROPRIATE HEALTH CARE
Outpatient. For status migrainous or cases complicated by concurrent medical problems or significant medication-withdrawal issues, hospitalization may be required.

GENERAL MEASURES
• Compression to ipsilateral temporal artery or tender areas of scalp or neck
• Cold compresses to area of pain
• Rest with pillows comfortably supporting head or neck in area devoid of sensory stimulation, including light, sound, and odors
• Withdrawal from stressful surroundings
• Sleep is desirable
• Biofeedback and early psychologic intervention in appropriate cases or when pain behaviors are first identified
• Most patients manage attacks with self-care

SURGICAL MEASURES N/A

ACTIVITY In bed in a dark quiet environment

DIET Maintain fluid intake. Avoid dietary precipitants of migraine.

PATIENT EDUCATION
• Emphasize migraine can not be cured, but symptoms can be managed
• Encourage use of diary and patient education
• Emphasize proper use of all medications
• Encourage lifestyle modifications

MEDICATIONS

DRUG(S) OF CHOICE
• 5-HT-1 agonists
◊ Sumatriptan (Imitrex), most effective during headache phase of migraine. 6 mg self-administered injection with efficacy of 70-85%; nasal spray of 20 mg, or 25 and 50 mg tablets with efficacy of 65%. 50 mg dose more effective than 25 mg. If initial injection fails to relieve migraine after 1 hour, don't repeat injection. If headache returns, repeat injection, nasal spray or oral tablets.
◊ Zolmitriptan (Zomig) 2.5 mg at onset of migraine. 5 mg tablet available. Efficacy approximately 65%.
◊ Naratriptan (Amerge) 2.5 mg initially; 1 mg tablet available. Slower to act than other "triptans", but well tolerated.

◊ Rizatriptan (Maxalt) initially 10 mg. 5 mg available and recommended for patients on propranolol. Efficacy similar to other "triptans".

◊ For all "triptans" - oral tablets slower in onset than injection or nasal spray; restore normal function for most; appropriate patient selection important

• Ergotamines

◊ Dihydroergotamine (DHE). Drug of choice in status migraines

- Most effective ergotamine; available as IV, IM, or SC injection. Also available as nasal spray (Migranol)

- 0.5-1 mg dose with up to 3 mg IM or 2 mg IV in 24 hours. Maximum weekly doses of 4-6 mg. Many protocols utilize antiemetic, such as, metoclopramide or prochlorperazine 5-10 mg IM or IV prior to DHE administration.

- DHE nasal spray (Migranol) 2 mg intranasal (0.5 mg in each nostril repeated in 15 minutes). Low recurrence rate of migraine reported in trials.

◊ Ergotamine tartrate

- Ergotamine-caffeine (Cafergot) suppositories 2 mg. Start with half and increase to 2 suppositories per attack. Avoid chronic use. Maximum 6 mg/attack; 10 mg/week.

- Oral preparations contain 1 mg of ergotamine and 100 mg of caffeine (Cafergot). Two tablets at onset of symptoms. Repeat after 30 minutes up to maximum dose of 6 mg per day. Cafergot PB contains 30 mg of pentobarbital and 0.25 mg of belladonna. Avoid chronic daily or near-daily use.

• Nonsteroidal anti-inflammatories: No clear efficacy established for any particular agent; early administration improves efficacy.

• Combination drugs

◊ Isometheptene - dichloralphenazone - acetaminophen (Midrin) 2 at onset then 1 q hr if needed up to 5 per 12 hour period

◊ Acetaminophen-butalbital (Phrenilin). 1 or 2 capsules at onset repeated q 4 hr prn up to 6/24 hours.

◊ Acetaminophen-butalbital (Fioricet) or acetaminophen-butalbital-codeine (Fiorinal #3, Fiorinal #4). 1 or 2 at onset q 4 hr prn up to 6/24 hours.

Contraindications:

• Avoid 5-HT-1 agonists in coronary heart disease, peripheral vascular disease, uncontrolled hypertension, and complex migraine, such as basilar or hemiplegic migraine. Avoid within 2 wks of MAO usage. Pregnancy category C.

• Selective 5-HT-1 agonists pregnancy category C. Ergotamines pregnancy category X.

• Avoid NSAIDs if danger of gastric erosion, renal, or hepatic disease

• Avoid acetaminophen in hepatic disease or with alcohol consumption

• Avoid drugs containing narcotics or butalbital in addiction prone patients

• Avoid vasoconstrictors in uncontrolled hypertension

Precautions:

• Administer ergotamines early

• Frequent use of acute treatment drugs may lead to changed migraine patterns

• Monitor use of aspirin and NSAID's for dyspepsia

• Monitor use of drugs with addictive potential

• Avoid concomitant sumatriptan and ergotamine

Significant possible interactions:

• Other sedatives, analgesics, alcohol, vasoconstrictors including decongestants

• Ergotamine and macrolide antibiotics

ALTERNATIVE DRUGS

• Any analgesic, antiemetic, or sedative

• Narcotics including butorphanol (Stadol) are reserved for rescue therapy

• In emergency department: sumatriptan, DHE, adequate analgesics, anti-emetic (chlorpromazine or prochlorperazine) and fluid replacement

• Other 5-HT-1 agonists

• A wide variety of vasoconstrictors, analgesics, anti-inflammatories, antiemetics, and sedatives used alone or in combination are prescribed based on symptoms and other factors. Except for parenteral 5-HT-1 agonists and antiemetics, drugs are most effective when taken early in migraine attacks.

FOLLOWUP

PATIENT MONITORING

• Early intervention assist management

• Monitor frequency of attacks, pain behaviors. medication usage

• Encourage lifestyle modifications

PREVENTION/AVOIDANCE

• Avoid precipitants of attacks

• Prescribe biofeedback and psychologic intervention early if pain behavior evident

• Prophylactic therapy: If attacks significantly interfere with lifestyle or are not adequately controlled by appropriate acute interventions, daily prophylactic therapy may be appropriate. Regularly scheduled follow-up is mandatory.

◊ Propranolol (Inderal) 80-320 mg daily
◊ Atenolol (Tenormin) 50-100 mg daily
◊ Nadolol (Corgard) 40-80 mg daily
◊ Timolol (Blocadren) 10-20 mg daily
◊ Metoprolol (Lopressor) 100-450 mg daily
◊ Amitriptyline (Elavil) 10-150 mg daily
◊ Nortriptyline (Pamelor) 10-150 mg daily
◊ Verapamil (Calan, Isoptin) 80-120 mg daily
◊ Isradipine (DynaCirc) 2.5-10 mg bid
◊ Methysergide (Sansert) 5-8 mg daily
◊ Cyproheptadine (Periactin) 4-16 mg daily
◊ Valproic acid (Depakene) or divalproex (Depakote) 250-1500 mg daily

• Consultation/referral

◊ Obscure diagnosis, concomitant medical conditions, significant psychopathology
◊ Unresponsive to usual treatment
◊ Analgesic dependent headache patterns

POSSIBLE COMPLICATIONS

• Rare status migrainosis

• Rare cerebral ischemic events

• Iatrogenic effects of treatment

EXPECTED COURSE/PROGNOSIS

• With age - reduction in severity, frequency, and disability of attacks

• Most attacks subside within 72 hours

MISCELLANEOUS

ASSOCIATED CONDITIONS Depression, panic disorders, sleep disturbance, cerebral vascular disease, myocardial disease, peripheral vascular disease and seizure

AGE-RELATED FACTORS

Pediatric: Recurrent abdominal pain and cyclic vomiting may predominate; attacks may be of shorter duration. Headache description by younger children may appear atypical.

Geriatric: Rare onset of acephalgic migraine (aura without subsequent headache) after the age of 40. Possible relationship to transient global amnesia. Late onset of migraine requires diagnostic evaluation.

Others: Migraine affects all races, social classes, intelligence levels

PREGNANCY Attacks frequently diminish, esp. in 2nd/3rd trimester. No treatment drug has FDA approval in pregnancy; ergotamines are contraindicated.

SYNONYMS

• Hemicrania
• Sick headache

ICD-9-CM

346.0 Classical migraine
346.2 Variants of migraine (including cluster)
346.9 Migraine, unspecified
784.0 Headache

SEE ALSO

• Headache, cluster
• Headache, tension

OTHER NOTES N/A

ABBREVIATIONS N/A

REFERENCES

• Cady RK, Fox AW, eds: Treating the Headache Patient. New York, Marcel Dekker, 1995
• Sandler M, Collins GM, eds: Migraine: A Spectrum of Ideas. New York, Oxford University Press, 1990
• Raskin NH: Headache. 2nd Ed. New York, Churchill Livingstone, 1986
• Dalessio DJ, ed: Wolff's Headache. 5th Ed. New York, Oxford University Press, 1987
Illustrations: N/A
Internet references: http://www.5mcc.com

Author(s)

Roger Cady, MD

Miliaria rubra

BASICS

DESCRIPTION Miliaria rubra or prickly heat is a papulovesicular eruption
System(s) affected: Skin/Exocrine
Genetics: N/A
Incidence/Prevalence in USA: N/A
Predominant age: Common in infants, less common in adults
Predominant sex: Male = Female

SIGNS AND SYMPTOMS
• Fine papules and vesicles on an erythematous base
• May become inflamed pustules (miliaria pustulosa)
• Prevalent in areas of friction caused by clothing and in areas of flexure
• In infants - trunk, diaper area, neck, groin, axilla, face
• Pilosebaceous follicles, palms, soles spared
• Lesions appear after individual has been in a hot humid environment, resulting in sweating
• Pruritus or prickly, mildly stinging sensation in affected areas

CAUSES
• Keratinous plugging of the sweat ducts as a result of toxins produced by resident bacteria
• This leads to rupture of sweat duct producing sweat retention vesicle

RISK FACTORS
• Hot humid environment
• Occlusive bandages
• Plastic undersheets
• High fever

DIAGNOSIS

DIFFERENTIAL DIAGNOSIS
• Acne
• Folliculitis
• Viral exanthems
• Drug eruptions
• Erythema toxicum
• Yeast infections
• Pyogenic infections

LABORATORY N/A
Drugs that may alter lab results: N/A
Disorders that may alter lab results: N/A

PATHOLOGICAL FINDINGS
• Keratinous plugging of sweat ducts
• Sweat retention vesicle

SPECIAL TESTS N/A

IMAGING N/A

DIAGNOSTIC PROCEDURES N/A

TREATMENT

APPROPRIATE HEALTH CARE
Outpatient

GENERAL MEASURES
• Avoid wearing heavy, tight clothing or garments causing friction
• Avoid plastic or occlusive dressings/garments in hot environments
• Avoid excessive use of soap and contact with irritants
• Frequent cool baths with Aveeno colloidal, oatmeal or cornstarch
• Provide cool, dry environment for 8-10 hours a day

SURGICAL MEASURES N/A

ACTIVITY Avoid vigorous activity leading to sweating

DIET No special diet

PATIENT EDUCATION
• Cause of eruption/avoidance
• General measures for home care

MEDICATIONS

DRUG(S) OF CHOICE
• Topical steroids to relieve pruritus - 0.1% betamethasone (Valisone) bid for 3 days
• Systemic antibiotics in cases of bacterial secondary infection - Staphylococcicidal antibiotic, e.g., dicloxacillin 250 mg qid for 10 days (unless resistance)
• If sweating due to fever, antipyretic drugs may be useful
Contraindications: N/A
Precautions: Care with fluorinated steroid application in children. They may cause systemic effects.
Significant possible interactions: N/A

ALTERNATIVE DRUGS
Over-the-counter preparations with menthol, camphor for pruritus, e.g., hydrocortisone (Sarna) or pramoxine (Prax)

FOLLOWUP

PATIENT MONITORING As needed for persistence of symptoms

PREVENTION/AVOIDANCE
• See General measures
• Acclimatize slowly to hot weather

POSSIBLE COMPLICATIONS
Secondary bacterial infections

EXPECTED COURSE/PROGNOSIS
• Benign - responds to cooling
• Avoidance of causative agents is key

MISCELLANEOUS

ASSOCIATED CONDITIONS N/A

AGE-RELATED FACTORS
Pediatric: More common
Geriatric:
• Less common
• Backs of hospitalized patients
Others: N/A

PREGNANCY N/A

SYNONYMS Prickly heat

ICD-9-CM
705.1 Prickly heat (disorders of sweat gland)

SEE ALSO N/A

OTHER NOTES N/A

ABBREVIATIONS N/A

REFERENCES Bondi E, Jegasothy B, Lazarus G: Dermatology, Diagnosis and Therapy, 1991
Illustrations: 4 available on CD-ROM
Internet references: http://www.5mcc.com

Author(s)
Jeffrey A. Stearns, MD

Milk-alkali syndrome

BASICS

DESCRIPTION A condition resulting from ingestion of excessive amounts of calcium and absorbable alkali (e.g., sodium bicarbonate and calcium carbonate) usually during self-treatment for peptic ulcer or gastro-esophageal reflux
System(s) affected: Gastrointestinal, Renal/Urologic, Endocrine/Metabolic
Genetics: Unknown
Incidence/Prevalence in USA: Infrequent
Predominant age: 40-75 years
Predominant sex: Male = Female

SIGNS AND SYMPTOMS
• Anorexia
• Band keratopathy
• Constipation
• Dehydration
• Depression
• Dizziness
• Food distaste
• Headache
• Irritability
• Mental status changes
• Myalgias
• Nausea
• Periarticular calcinosis
• Polydipsia
• Polyuria
• Vomiting
• Weakness

CAUSES Excess intake of milk and alkali as therapy for gastrointestinal problems accompanied with gastric hyperacidity (e.g., peptic ulcer, esophageal reflux)

RISK FACTORS
• Peptic ulcer
• Hiatal hernia
• Malignancies

DIAGNOSIS

DIFFERENTIAL DIAGNOSIS Other causes of hypercalcemia, such as excessive osteolysis with malignant disease, vitamin intoxication, thyroid disease, sarcoidosis, thiazide diuretic treatment, hyperparathyroidism

LABORATORY
• Mild alkalosis
• Hypercalcemia
• Normocalciuria
• Decreased urine phosphate
• Increased BUN and serum creatinine
• Normal alkaline phosphatase
Drugs that may alter lab results: N/A
Disorders that may alter lab results: N/A

PATHOLOGICAL FINDINGS
Nephrocalcinosis, ectopic calcification

SPECIAL TESTS   N/A

IMAGING   N/A

DIAGNOSTIC PROCEDURES   N/A

TREATMENT

APPROPRIATE HEALTH CARE
Inpatient

GENERAL MEASURES
• Withdraw milk and alkali
• Treat the hypercalcemia
• Intravenous treatment to cause calcinosis (usually with sodium chloride solution)
• Goal of treatment: Maintain urine volume of 3 liters per day
• With significant renal insufficiency, employ renal dialysis

SURGICAL MEASURES   N/A

ACTIVITY   Bedrest during active treatment

DIET   Increased fluid intake

PATIENT EDUCATION   N/A

MEDICATIONS

DRUG(S) OF CHOICE
• To treat hypercalcemia: Isotonic sodium chloride 0.9% intravenously when serum calcium exceeds 15 mg/dL (3.75 mmol/L) (see Hypercalcemia), plus
• Furosemide 80-100 mgm IV q2 for 24 hours after volume depletion has been corrected
Contraindications: Refer to manufacturer's literature
Precautions: Replace sodium and potassium losses associated with furosemide use
Significant possible interactions: Refer to manufacturer's literature

ALTERNATIVE DRUGS
Disodium phosphate and monopotassium phosphate. (HAZARDOUS - should be used only by experienced nephrologist and only if dialysis is unavailable.)

FOLLOWUP

PATIENT MONITORING
• Kidney function
• Fluid intake and output
• Urine electrolytes

PREVENTION/AVOIDANCE
Avoid excess milk and/or absorbable antacids

POSSIBLE COMPLICATIONS
• Renal failure
• Nephrocalcinosis

EXPECTED COURSE/PROGNOSIS
Favorable with appropriate therapy

MISCELLANEOUS

ASSOCIATED CONDITIONS
• Peptic ulcer disease
• Hiatal hernia
• Gastroesophageal reflux
• Hyperparathyroidism
• Hypercalcemia of malignancy

AGE-RELATED FACTORS
Pediatric: N/A
Geriatric: Occurs predominantly in this age group
Others: N/A

PREGNANCY N/A

SYNONYMS
• Burnett's syndrome
• Milk poisoning
• Milk drinker syndrome

ICD-9-CM
999.9 Complications of medical care, NEC

SEE ALSO N/A

OTHER NOTES N/A

ABBREVIATIONS N/A

REFERENCES
• Wilson JD, Foster DW, eds: Williams' Textbook of Endocrinology. 8th ed. Philadelphia, Saunders, 1992
• Labhart A: Clinical Endocrinology: Theory & Practice. 2nd Ed. Springhouse, PA, Springer-Verlag, 1987
Illustrations: N/A
Internet references: http://www.5mcc.com

Author(s)
Stanley G. Smith, MA, MB, FCFPC

Mitral stenosis

BASICS

DESCRIPTION
Resistance to diastolic filling of the left ventricle due to valvular narrowing. In the adult, the most common etiology is rheumatic heart disease.

System(s) affected: Cardiovascular

Genetics: Congenital mitral stenosis is a rare congenital malformation, manifested in only 0.42% of children with congenital heart disease

Incidence/Prevalence in USA: The overall incidence of rheumatic heart disease is decreasing. The mitral valve is the valve most commonly affected with rheumatic heart disease.

Predominant age: Symptoms primarily occur in middle age (40-70 years)

Predominant sex: Female > Male

SIGNS AND SYMPTOMS
- History:
  - ◊ History of murmur
  - ◊ History of rheumatic fever
  - ◊ History of pulmonary edema with pregnancy, exercise, infection or arrhythmia (commonly atrial fibrillation)
- Most common signs and symptoms:
  - ◊ Effort induced dyspnea
  - ◊ Palpitations
  - ◊ Effort fatigue
  - ◊ Hemoptysis (late)
  - ◊ Apical early diastolic low-pitched rumble often with presystolic accentuation (listen with bell of stethoscope in left lateral decubitus position)
  - ◊ Loud S1 (early in disease - as the valve becomes more stenotic and less mobile, this is less common)
  - ◊ Opening snap after S2 (may also diminish in intensity with increasing stenosis)
  - ◊ Right ventricle enlargement
- Other signs and symptoms:
  - ◊ Paroxysmal nocturnal dyspnea
  - ◊ Orthopnea
  - ◊ Recumbent cough
  - ◊ Hoarseness
  - ◊ Digital clubbing
  - ◊ Chest pain
  - ◊ Peripheral edema
  - ◊ Systemic embolization
  - ◊ Rales, atrial fibrillation, malar rash (rare)
  - ◊ Holosystolic murmur of mitral regurgitation may accompany the valvular deformity of mitral stenosis
  - ◊ If pulmonary hypertension is present: right ventricular lift, increased pulmonic second sound, a high pitched decrescendo diastolic murmur of pulmonic insufficiency (Graham Steell's murmur)
  - ◊ If right ventricular failure has developed: increased jugular venous distention, holosystolic murmur of tricuspid regurgitation at left sternal border, hepatomegaly and peripheral edema are often found
  - ◊ May also find associated aortic, or less commonly, tricuspid murmurs (due to aortic or tricuspid valve involvement with rheumatic heart disease)

CAUSES
In the adult, mitral stenosis is almost always secondary to rheumatic heart disease. Rarely, congenital in etiology.

RISK FACTORS
History of rheumatic fever

DIAGNOSIS

DIFFERENTIAL DIAGNOSIS
The major differential diagnosis to be considered in a patient with the relatively characteristic findings of mitral stenosis is the uncommon atrial myxoma or vegetation due to endocarditis obstructing left ventricle (LV) inflow. Diastolic flow murmurs can be also heard in the absence of true stenosis due to increased flow across a normal valve. These murmurs are generally limited to early diastole and may be associated with anemia, thyrotoxicosis, shunts as well as with significant mitral regurgitation.

LABORATORY
N/A

Drugs that may alter lab results: N/A

Disorders that may alter lab results: N/A

PATHOLOGICAL FINDINGS
- Scarring of the leaflets with fibrosis restricting valve mobility
- Retraction then leads to further valvular narrowing, often with a funnel shaped deformity
- Chordal involvement leads to fusion of the chords and obliteration of the interchordal spaces, further limiting LV inflow
- Left atrial dilatation
- Left atrial thrombi may be found
- Right ventricular hypertrophy
- Pulmonary arterial thickening

SPECIAL TESTS
- ECG:
  - ◊ Left atrial enlargement (manifested by broad, notched P waves in lead II with a negative terminal deflection of the P wave in lead V1)
  - ◊ Atrial fibrillation is commonly noted
  - ◊ With right ventricular hypertrophy, right axis deviation and a large R wave in V1 may be noted

IMAGING
- Chest x-ray:
  - ◊ Left atrial enlargement with straightening of the left heart border, a "double density", and elevation of the left main stem bronchus
  - ◊ Pulmonary venous patterns changes with redistribution of flow toward the apices
  - ◊ Prominent pulmonary arteries at the hilum with rapid tapering
  - ◊ Right ventricular enlargement
  - ◊ Kerley's B lines
  - ◊ Pulmonary edema pattern (late)

DIAGNOSTIC PROCEDURES
- Echocardiography: (2-D):
  - ◊ Mitral valve thickening with decreased diastolic excursion and "doming" of the anterior leaflet in diastole
  - ◊ Valvular calcification
  - ◊ Decreased mitral orifice as directly measured by planimetry
  - ◊ Enlarged left atrium
  - ◊ Right ventricular enlargement
  - ◊ Atrial thrombi
- Doppler:
  - ◊ Transvalvular pressure gradients
  - ◊ Calculated valve area
  - ◊ Concomitant mitral regurgitation (MR), pulmonary insufficiency (PI), tricuspid regurgitation (TR)
- Cardiac catheterization:
  - ◊ Increased left atrial or pulmonary capillary wedge pressure (PCWP)
  - ◊ Increased left atrial or PCWP to left ventricular pressure gradient
  - ◊ Calculated mitral valve orifice area
  - ◊ Calcified mitral valve
  - ◊ Concomitant mitral regurgitation
  - ◊ Presence of coronary artery disease

TREATMENT

APPROPRIATE HEALTH CARE
Outpatient except for complications or surgery

GENERAL MEASURES
- Mitral stenosis is generally a progressive disease. The asymptomatic patient with non-critical mitral stenosis can be followed with appropriate evaluation.
- The patient should avoid unusual stresses (emotional and physical)
- All patients should receive endocarditis prophylaxis, prior to dental work or invasive procedures, regardless of age, etiology or severity of the stenosis (as recommended by the American Heart Association in Circulation, 1997; 96: 358-366)
- Patients who have mitral stenosis on the basis of rheumatic fever should also receive rheumatic fever prophylaxis (in addition to endocarditis prophylaxis) if under 35 years of age or continues to be in contact with young children
- If atrial fibrillation develops, it is important to slow the heart rate to allow more time for diastolic filling through the stenotic valve
- The development of pulmonary edema is often associated with atrial fibrillation and a rapid ventricular response. It is important to slow the heart rate. Cardioversion could be considered, particularly if the patient is chronically anticoagulated.
- Consider anticoagulation with warfarin (Coumadin) in all patients with mitral stenosis, particularly if a history of systemic embolism, or have atrial fibrillation or a large left atrium

SURGICAL MEASURES Surgical intervention: If the patient is eligible for a commissurotomy or balloon valvuloplasty, the onset of symptoms clearly referable to the mitral stenosis is generally considered an indication for early surgical intervention. If, however, the patient requires placement of a mitral valve prosthesis, often the timing of the surgical intervention is delayed until the symptoms are more severe.

ACTIVITY Adequate rest and reasonable physical activity

DIET Low salt

PATIENT EDUCATION Educate the patient about symptoms of mitral stenosis and report them should they occur

MEDICATIONS

DRUG(S) OF CHOICE
• Judicious addition of diuretics if symptoms indicate
• Atrial fibrillation - consider digoxin plus anticoagulation with warfarin (Coumadin). Beta or calcium channel blockers have been used in place of digoxin. Digoxin is used for rate control, not to convert to normal sinus rhythm.
• Rheumatic fever prophylaxis - preferably penicillin G benzathine, 1.2 million units IM every four weeks or penicillin V 250 mg twice daily
• Bacterial endocarditis prophylaxis - depends on procedure. For dental procedures - amoxicillin 2.0 g given orally 1 hour before procedure for adults without contraindications.
Contraindications: Penicillin allergy
Precautions: Refer to manufacturer's profile of each drug
Significant possible interactions: There are many when using the combination of warfarin and digoxin. Use caution when adding new medications. Refer to manufacturer's profile of each drug.

ALTERNATIVE DRUGS
Erythromycin for rheumatic fever prophylaxis; Clindamycin for bacterial endocarditis prophylaxis

FOLLOWUP

PATIENT MONITORING
Close regular visits for assessment of the gradually progressive symptoms

PREVENTION/AVOIDANCE
• Bacterial endocarditis prophylaxis for dental and invasive procedures continued for life
• Strep throat - treat appropriately when it occurs
• Rheumatic fever prophylaxis when indicated (See General Measures)

POSSIBLE COMPLICATIONS
• Thromboembolism from mitral stenosis is a major potential complication (anticoagulation therapy has lessened this risk substantially)
• Recurrent rheumatic fever
• Bacterial endocarditis
• Pulmonary hypertension
• Pulmonary edema

EXPECTED COURSE/PROGNOSIS
• Although a milder course is now seen in North America, the classic mitral stenosis history is 10 years from the episode of rheumatic fever to the development of a murmur, another 10 years until symptomatic and another 10 years for the patient to develop serious disability
• Operative mortality 1-2% for mitral commissurotomy; 2-5% for mitral valve replacement

MISCELLANEOUS

ASSOCIATED CONDITIONS
Congestive heart failure

AGE-RELATED FACTORS
Pediatric: N/A
Geriatric:
• Atrial fibrillation and complicating arterial embolism more common
• Though there is an increased risk for bleeding, anticoagulation therapy recommended (unless specifically contraindicated) due to high risk of embolism and valve thrombosis (especially if atrial fibrillation present)
Others: N/A

PREGNANCY
• Can cause marked deterioration in cardiac function due to hemodynamic changes associated with increased intravascular volume and heart rate, with decreased diastolic filling time
• The associated pulmonary hypertension also poorly tolerated in pregnancy

SYNONYMS N/A

ICD-9-CM 394.0 Mitral stenosis

SEE ALSO N/A

OTHER NOTES N/A

ABBREVIATIONS N/A

REFERENCES
• Brandenburg RO, et al: Cardiology: Fundamentals and Practice, Chicago, Year Book Medical Publishers, 1987
• Dalen JE, Alpert JS: Valvular Heart Disease. 2nd Ed. New York, Little Brown, 1987
• Cotran RS, et al, eds: Robbins Pathological Basis of Disease. 4th Ed. Philadelphia, W.B. Saunders Co., 1989
• Hurst JW, et al: The Heart. 7th Ed. New York, McGraw-Hill, 1990
Illustrations: N/A
Internet references: http://www.5mcc.com

Author(s)
James M. Galloway, MD, FACP, FACC

Mitral valve prolapse

BASICS

DESCRIPTION Mitral valve prolapse (MVP) = a bulging of mitral valve leaflets into left atrium during systole. most often asymptomatic and nonprogressive. A subset of patients have MVP syndrome with signs and symptoms ranging from chest pain and fatigue to autonomic dysfunction (including syncope), cardiac dysrhythmias, strokes, and sudden death. Degeneration of prolapsing mitral valve with time also sometimes occurs.

System(s) affected: Cardiovascular, Endocrine/Metabolic, Nervous

Genetics: Autosomal dominant with variable expression. Part of inherited connective tissue disorders such as Marfan syndrome and Ehlers-Danlos syndrome.

Incidence/Prevalence in USA: Approximately 2.5-5% of the general population

Predominant age: Uncommon before adolescent growth spurt, usually detected in young adulthood

Predominant sex:
• Females > Males (under the age of 20)
• Females = Males (after age 20)
• Males more severely affected than females after age 50

SIGNS AND SYMPTOMS

• Usually asymptomatic, nonprogressive, and benign
• Subset of patients may have arrhythmias, emboli, endocarditis, severe mitral regurgitation, and sudden death.
• Characteristic systolic click (sound) and/or late systolic murmur, whose characteristics and timing change with body position and often fluctuate between exams.
• Chest pain: recurrent, located in left precordial and substernal areas, varies from instantaneous to hours in duration
• Fatigue
• Syncope/presyncope
• Dyspnea
• Body habitus: Thin, arm span greater than height, abnormal thoracic cage or spine including narrow AP chest and pectus excavatum, high arched palate
• "MVP" syndrome
 ◊ Low body weight
 ◊ Low blood pressure
 ◊ Minor skeletal abnormalities
 ◊ Orthostasis
 ◊ Palpitations
 ◊ Mitral regurgitation
 ◊ Autonomic dysfunction: chest pain, panic attacks, anxiety
 ◊ Neuroendocrine dysfunction
• Sudden death - new autopsy studies find evidence of small vessel disease (including AV nodal coronary arteries) and cardiomyopathic changes of ventricle (especially septum), suggesting some cases of sudden death due to VT/VF from ischemia or scarring

CAUSES

• Primary disorder: inherited; mitral valve and supportive structures disproportionately large for left ventricle
• Secondary disorder:
 ◊ Disorders of tissue structure: Marfan syndrome, Ehlers-Danlos, pseudoxanthoma elastica, osteogenesis imperfecta, myxomatous degeneration of connective tissue of the mitral valve
 ◊ Connective tissue diseases: rheumatic endocarditis, SLE
 ◊ Structural heart diseases: ruptured chordae tendineae, mitral stenosis
 ◊ Coronary artery disease
• Associated dysautonomia is cause of orthostasis and syncope, palpitations, anxiety, chest pain, fatigue, and dyspnea.

RISK FACTORS

• Positive family history
• Disorder of connective tissue/collagen
• Increased risk of complications
 ◊ Male sex and age over 50
 ◊ Posterior leaflet prolapse (associated with holo-systolic murmur)
 ◊ Mitral regurgitation (including exercise-induced MR)

DIAGNOSIS

DIFFERENTIAL DIAGNOSIS

• Click:
 ◊ Ejection clicks
 ◊ Opening snap (mitral/tricuspid stenosis)
 ◊ Split S2
 ◊ Ventricular aneurysm
 ◊ Constrictive pericarditis causing pericardial knock
• Late systolic murmur:
 ◊ Tricuspid valve prolapse
 ◊ Papillary muscle dysfunction
 ◊ Hypertrophic cardiomyopathy
 ◊ VSD

LABORATORY N/A

Drugs that may alter lab results: N/A
Disorders that may alter lab results: N/A

PATHOLOGICAL FINDINGS

• Myxomatous degeneration of the mitral valve
• Thickened, redundant mitral valve leaflets

SPECIAL TESTS

• ECG
 ◊ Usually normal
 ◊ Inferior ST-T wave changes
 ◊ Atrial arrhythmias, ventricular arrhythmias including complex arrhythmias, left atrial/ventricular enlargement secondary to mitral regurgitation
• Signal-averaged ECG helps predict ventricular and supraventricular arrhythmias

IMAGING Chest x-ray usually normal

DIAGNOSTIC PROCEDURES

• Echocardiogram (MVP may be an incidental discovery):
 ◊ The most useful test for confirming and defining mitral valve prolapse.
 ◊ Should not be used to screen for mitral valve prolapse. Clinically significant mitral valve prolapse usually obvious on physical exam. Silent mitral valve prolapse common and clinically insignificant.
 ◊ Other valves may have myxomatous degeneration and prolapse. Echocardiogram evaluates the other valves as well.
 ◊ Doppler echocardiogram detects and quantitates mitral regurgitation
 ◊ Serial echocardiograms useful in following mitral regurgitation
• Tilt table studies useful to diagnose autonomic dysfunction causing light-headedness and syncope
• Holter monitoring sometimes detects life-threatening arrhythmias. Atrial arrhythmias more common when mitral regurgitation present
• EKG stress test:
 ◊ Detects exercise-induced arrhythmias
 ◊ Detects exercise-induced mitral regurgitation which is associated with higher risk
 ◊ 50% false positive rate for ischemic changes
 ◊ Repeating the stress test after beta blockers improves specificity

TREATMENT

APPROPRIATE HEALTH CARE
Outpatient

GENERAL MEASURES
• 75% of cases have no increase in morbidity/mortality and no treatment required

SURGICAL MEASURES
• 25% of patients require valvular surgery after age 50, generally after long asymptomatic period
• Mitral valve and mitral annulus repair becoming preferred over mitral valve replacement

Mitral valve prolapse

ACTIVITY
• Generally unrestricted
• Certain patients have arrhythmias precipitated by exercise which often respond to beta blockers
• Associated decreased intravascular volume may cause orthostasis and syncope with vigorous sports and/or dehydration
• Competitive sports should be avoided in patients with aortic root enlargement, unexplained syncope, uncontrolled tachyarrhythmias, etc.

DIET
• Adequate salt intake important: low baseline intravascular volume, abnormal renin-aldosterone response to volume depletion, and autonomic dysregulation limit compensatory response.
• Caffeine, alcohol, and cigarettes should be avoided with palpitations

PATIENT EDUCATION
• Assurance of usually benign course
• Patient information can be obtained from: American Heart Association, 7320 Greenville Avenue, Dallas, TX 75231, (214)373-6300
• On Health; http://onhealth.com

MEDICATIONS

DRUG(S) OF CHOICE
• Usually none needed.
• Beta-blockers (e.g. atenolol) helpful if palpitations severe.
• Aspirin indicated for TIA
• When indicated (see Prevention/Avoidance):
  ◊ Antibiotics
  ◊ Warfarin (Coumadin)
Contraindications:
• Diuretics to be avoided (baseline low intravascular volume)
• Oral contraceptives to be avoided in patients with focal neurologic events
Precautions: Beta-blockers will increase fatigue and orthostasis/dizziness.
Significant possible interactions: Refer to manufacturer's literature

ALTERNATIVE DRUGS None

FOLLOWUP

PATIENT MONITORING
• Serial echocardiograms in patients with posterior leaflet prolapse, mitral regurgitation (including exercise-induced), thickened or redundant leaflets, increased left ventricular size.

PREVENTION/AVOIDANCE
• Endocarditis prophylaxis for auscultatory murmur or redundant, thickened leaflets by echocardiogram. Prophylaxis not needed in MVP without a murmur.
• Good dental hygiene
• Anticoagulation in patients with atrial fibrillation and atrial enlargement

POSSIBLE COMPLICATIONS
• Sudden death - rare. Some cases of MVP associated with proteoglycan deposition (valves as well as extravalvular) and with small vessel disease, causing ventricular arrhythmias and sudden death.
• Uncommon and related to advancing age, male sex, atrial/ventricular size rather than to presence/absence of valvular prolapse:
  ◊ Infective endocarditis
  ◊ TIA
  ◊ Stroke
  ◊ Congestive heart failure
  ◊ Heart block
  ◊ Severe mitral regurgitation
  ◊ Syncope

EXPECTED COURSE/PROGNOSIS
• 75% excellent with same morbidity/mortality over age-matched controls
• 25% progressive mitral regurgitation with a long (25 year) asymptomatic phase followed by rapid deterioration requiring valvular repair within a year once symptoms occur

MISCELLANEOUS

ASSOCIATED CONDITIONS
< 5% of all mitral valve prolapse:
• Marfan syndrome
• Osteogenesis imperfecta
• Ehlers-Danlos syndrome
• Adult polycystic kidney disease
• Stickler syndrome
• Pseudoxanthoma elasticum
• Turner's syndrome
• Rheumatologic diseases including SLE, PSS, MCTD
• Primary cardiac disorders including rheumatic endocarditis, mitral stenosis, hypertrophic cardiomyopathy, LV aneurysm, coronary artery disease, and congenital abnormalities
• Duchenne's muscular dystrophy
• Inherited disorders of metabolism (Hunter's, Hurler's, & Sanfilippo's syndromes)
• Autoimmune thyroid disease (including Grave's disease)

AGE-RELATED FACTORS
Pediatric: Rarely detected before adolescent growth spurt
Geriatric: Complications occur mostly in men over 50
Others: N/A

PREGNANCY
• Mitral valve prolapse itself is not a contraindication to pregnancy.
• Connective tissue diseases (e.g., Marfan syndrome), especially with an enlarged aortic root, may be a contraindication to pregnancy
• Increased blood volume of pregnancy may improve symptoms of mitral valve prolapse

SYNONYMS
• Systolic murmur-click syndrome
• Mitral click murmur syndrome

ICD-9-CM
424.0 Mitral valve disorders
394.0 Mitral stenosis
394.1 Rheumatic mitral insufficiency
394.2 Mitral stenosis with insufficiency
394.9 Other and unspecified mitral valve diseases

SEE ALSO
• Mitral stenosis
• Mitral regurgitation due to papillary muscle dysfunction
• Mitral regurgitation due to rheumatic fever
• Marfan's syndrome
• Systemic lupus erythematosus (SLE)
• Polycystic kidney disease
• Turner's syndrome
• Muscular dystrophy

OTHER NOTES N/A

ABBREVIATIONS
MVP = mitral valve prolapse

REFERENCES
• Hurst JW, et al: The Heart. 7th Ed. New York, McGraw-Hill, 1990
• Bennett JC, Plum F, eds: Cecil Textbook of Medicine. 20th Ed. Philadelphia, W.B. Saunders Co., 1996
• Devereux RB: Recent developments in the diagnosis and treatment of MVP. Current Opinion Cardiol 1995; 10(2): 107-16
• Kim S, et al: Relationship between severity of MR and prognosis of MVP. Am Heart J 1996; 132(2(pt1)): 348-55
• Burke AF. Farb, et al: Fibromuscular dysplasia of small coronary arteries and fibrosis in the basilar ventricular septum in mitral valve prolapse. Am Heart J 1997;134(2):282-291
• Corrado D: Sudden death in young people. G Ital Cardiol 1997;27(11):1097-1105
Illustrations: N/A
Internet references: http://www.5mcc.com

Author(s)
Hetty B. Hall, MD

Molluscum contagiosum

BASICS

DESCRIPTION Common, benign viral skin disorder consisting of small umbilicated papules which tend to occur on the face, trunk and extremities in children and on the groin and genitalia in adults. Incubation period is 2 weeks to 2 months. In immunocompromised individuals (e.g., HIV infection), the lesions can be extensive and atypical. They are occasionally giant (up to 3 cm), involve face, neck and trunk, and are recalcitrant to treatment.
System(s) affected: Skin/Exocrine
Genetics: No known genetic pattern
Incidence/Prevalence in USA: Common
Predominant age: Children and young adults
Predominant sex: Male = Female

SIGNS AND SYMPTOMS
• Discrete pearly to flesh colored firm papules
• Diameter 2 to 6 mm (rarely giant nodules up to 3 cm occur)
• Usually grouped in one or two areas
• Centrally umbilicated with erythematous base
• Lesions can be pruritic or tender
• Beneath umbilicated center is white curd-like core
• Distribution: Anywhere. Predilection for face, trunk and extremities in children and groin and genitalia in adults.

CAUSES DNA virus of the poxvirus group.
The virus cannot be grown in cell cultures. Incubation period is 2 weeks to 2 months after contact.

RISK FACTORS
• Close personal contact with infected persons
• In children, transmission can occur from swimming pools
• In adults, sexual transmission is common
• Immunocompromised individuals

DIAGNOSIS

DIFFERENTIAL DIAGNOSIS
• Basal cell carcinoma
• Furunculosis
• Keratoacanthomas
• Warts
• Pyodermas (folliculitis, furunculosis)
• Pyogenic granuloma
• Vesicular skin disorders
• Disseminated mycosis in AIDS patients

LABORATORY Virus particles cannot be cultured
Drugs that may alter lab results: N/A
Disorders that may alter lab results: N/A

PATHOLOGICAL FINDINGS
• Intracytoplasmic inclusion bodies in histological or cytological specimens
• Hypertrophied and hyperplastic epidermis

SPECIAL TESTS N/A

IMAGING N/A

DIAGNOSTIC PROCEDURES
• White, curd-like core easily expressed from beneath umbilication
• Biopsy

TREATMENT

APPROPRIATE HEALTH CARE
Outpatient

GENERAL MEASURES Spontaneous resolution common in 6-12 months. Individual lesions resolve in 2 months.

SURGICAL MEASURES
• Removal by curettage alone, or curettage followed by trichloracetic acid or light electrodesiccation
• Cryotherapy is also effective

ACTIVITY No restrictions

DIET No special diet

PATIENT EDUCATION Instructions for Patients, W.B. Saunders Co., Philadelphia

MEDICATIONS

DRUG(S) OF CHOICE Curettage or cryotherapy are treatments of choice. Use of topical trichloroacetic acid, silver nitrate, phenol, tincture of iodine, podophyllin and tretinoin have all been reported. No clinical trials comparing efficacy or risk exist. In HIV and immunocompromised patients, antiviral drugs such as cidofovir show promise in treating recalcitrant cases. However, large scale studies are lacking.
Contraindications: Refer to manufacturer's literature
Precautions: Refer to manufacturer's literature
Significant possible interactions: Refer to manufacturer's literature

ALTERNATIVE DRUGS N/A

FOLLOWUP

PATIENT MONITORING Recheck in 2 to 4 weeks after treatment for development of new lesions. Two to 4 visits are often required for complete course of treatment.

PREVENTION/AVOIDANCE In adults, avoid sexual contact with infected individuals

POSSIBLE COMPLICATIONS
• Autoinoculation is common
• Contagious to others
• Immunocompromised individuals may have extensive infections

EXPECTED COURSE/PROGNOSIS
• Untreated, the condition is usually self limited. Individual lesions spontaneously involute in 2 months. Total resolution usually takes 6 to 12 months.
• Recurrences are uncommon in immunocompetent individuals
• Lesions in HIV infected patients are more recalcitrant

MISCELLANEOUS

ASSOCIATED CONDITIONS Occurs in 5-18% of patients with HIV infection

AGE-RELATED FACTORS
Pediatric: Commonly seen on face, trunk and extremities. May be spread through swimming pools.
Geriatric: N/A
Others: In adults, is often a sexually transmitted disease.

PREGNANCY N/A

SYNONYMS N/A

ICD-9-CM
078.0 Molluscum contagiosum

SEE ALSO N/A

OTHER NOTES Spontaneous healing depends on triggering of a cell mediated immune response

ABBREVIATIONS N/A

REFERENCES
• Gottlieb SI, Myskowski PL: Molluscum contagiosum. Int'l J Dermatol 1994;33(7):453-461
• Janniger CK, Swartz RA: Molluscum contagiosum in children. Cutis 1993;52:194-196
• Lewis EJ, Lam M, Crutchfield CE 3rd: An update on Molluscum contagiosum. Cutis 1997;60:29-34
Illustrations: 2 available on CD-ROM
Internet references: http://www.5mcc.com

Author(s)
Nancy Elder, MD, MSPH

Mononucleosis

BASICS

DESCRIPTION
Mononucleosis is a viral illness caused by the Epstein-Barr virus (EBV) of the herpes family. It causes 90% of the mono-like syndromes. EBV infection causes general involvement of the lymphoreticular system. The "mono" syndrome is characterized by fatigue, fever, splenomegaly, adenopathy and pharyngitis. Transmission is fecal-oral, often attributed to kissing. Incubation period is 20-50 days.

System(s) affected:
Hemic/Lymphatic/Immunologic
Genetics: N/A
Incidence/Prevalence in USA:
• Lower socioeconomic status: 50-85% seropositive by age 4
• Middle-upper socioeconomic status: 14-50% seropositive by college age
• By young adult life, 90-95% of persons are antibody positive
• Incidence is about 50/100,000/year in general population to 5,000/100,000/year in susceptible college students
• No clear seasonal incidence
Predominant age: High school and college predominate
Predominant sex: Male = Female

SIGNS AND SYMPTOMS
• In most cases the clinical triad of sore throat (the most frequent complaint), fever, and lymphadenopathy are present
• Malaise (100%)
• Fatigue (100%)
• Headache (50%)
• Fever (85-90%)
• Adenopathy (85%)
• Tonsillitis (60%)
• Splenomegaly (45%)
• Hepatomegaly (35%)
• Petechiae (palate) (35%)
• Edema (periorbital) (35%)
• Rash (3-15%)
• Jaundice (9%)

CAUSES
Epstein-Barr virus a double-stranded DNA herpes virus

RISK FACTORS
• College and high school students
• Kissing
• 70-90% shed virus 2-6 months after initial infection
• 20-30% individuals shed virus at any one time after 6 months
• 10-20% culture rate from the oropharynx of normal adults and 50% from renal transplant and HIV positive patients
• Blood transfusion ("post pump perfusion syndrome")

DIAGNOSIS

DIFFERENTIAL DIAGNOSIS
• Cytomegalovirus (CMV)
• Toxoplasmosis
• Rubella
• Adenovirus
• Herpes simplex
• Drug side effects
• Streptococcal pharyngitis
• Viral tonsillitis
• Vincent's angina
• Diphtheria
• Viral hepatitis A and B
• Lymphoma or leukemia
• Human herpesvirus -6
• Roseola
• Mumps
• Drug reactions
• Primary HIV infection

LABORATORY
• Positive EBV titers (IgG or IgM) (100%)
• Lymphocytosis (95%)
• Atypical monocytosis (95%)
• Elevated liver function tests (80%)
• Hypergammaglobulinemia (80%)
• Positive heterophil antibodies (70%)
• Thrombocytopenia (50%)
• Elevated bilirubin (40%)
• Cold agglutinins (30-80%)
• Monospot test useful as screen
Drugs that may alter lab results: N/A
Disorders that may alter lab results:
• CMV most frequently confused with EBV-induced mononucleosis
• Group A beta streptococcus often present (30%); does not rule out mononucleosis

PATHOLOGICAL FINDINGS
• B-cell lymphocytes infected
• Polyclonal proliferation of B-cells
• Strong T-cell response

SPECIAL TESTS
Positive results most likely during 2nd to 3rd week of clinical illness
• Heterophil antibody tests (Monospot or differential absorption). Tends to be negative in young children.
• Specific EBV titers (use in heterophil negative or complications)
◊ Viral capsid antigen (VCA): IgG and IgM - peak at 3-4 weeks. IgG then declines, but persists for life. IgM declines rapidly and is undetectable by 3 months. High persisting IgG suggests remote infection, systemic lupus, chronic renal failure, Burkitt's lymphoma, nasopharyngeal cancer, leukemia, sarcoidosis, cancer, AIDS, Hodgkin's lymphoma, rheumatoid arthritis, and immunodeficiency state.
◊ Early antigen (EA): Occur in 70-90%, persist 2-3 months. May persist in up to 20% of remote infections. High persisting titers might suggest: Pregnancy, immunodeficiency states, Hodgkin's lymphoma, lymphoma, leukemia, AIDS, Burkitt's, nasopharyngeal carcinoma.

◊ Epstein-Barr nuclear antigen (EBNA): Develop after 2 months and persist indefinitely. E antigen in mononucleosis primarily. K antigen in nasopharyngeal carcinoma primarily. Absence suggests immunodeficiency.

IMAGING
Possible splenomegaly and/or hepatomegaly

DIAGNOSTIC PROCEDURES
• History and physical - fatigue, fever, splenomegaly, adenopathy, pharyngitis
• Heterophil antibodies - positive serology
• CBC/differential - abnormal white count
◊ Absolute lymphocytosis (> 4,000 cells/cc)
◊ Relative lymphocytosis (> 50%)
◊ Atypical lymphocytosis (10-20% or more)

TREATMENT

APPROPRIATE HEALTH CARE
Outpatient usually; 95% of patients recover uneventfully, without specific treatment

GENERAL MEASURES
• No specific treatment
• Quarantine not indicated
• General supportive measures
• Gargles
• Avoid vigorous splenic palpation

SURGICAL MEASURES
If splenic rupture, splenectomy (not always necessary) though probable mode of management for near future

ACTIVITY
• Rest (bedrest possibly during acute phase)
• Avoid contact sports, heavy lifting, strenuous athletics (during first 2-3 weeks or as long as splenomegaly persists)

DIET
• Healthy diet important
• To ease throat discomfort, patient may want to drink milk shakes, fruit juices and consume soft foods

PATIENT EDUCATION
• Convalescence may take several weeks
• Avoid stress
• Discuss feasibility of continuing with school or work
• Emphasize risk of splenic rupture from contact sports

Mononucleosis

MEDICATIONS

DRUG(S) OF CHOICE
- Antibiotics for secondary infections only
- Analgesics
  ◊ acetaminophen (Tylenol)
  ◊ codeine
- Steroids may be indicated in certain complications only - prednisone, 40-80 mg/d then less over 5-7 days. Consider in threatened airway obstruction, hemolytic anemia, and thrombocytopenic purpura.
- Specific antiviral therapy is of no benefit

Contraindications: Aspirin (associated with Reye's syndrome)

Precautions: Refer to manufacturer's profile of each drug

Significant possible interactions: Refer to manufacturer's profile of each drug

ALTERNATIVE DRUGS   N/A

FOLLOWUP

PATIENT MONITORING
- Re-evaluate as needed based on clinical findings
- Preferable documentation of resolution of splenomegaly before resuming contact sports

PREVENTION/AVOIDANCE
- Avoid saliva of infected persons
- DNA vaccine research in progress
- No blood donation for at least 6 months

POSSIBLE COMPLICATIONS
- Chronic EBV Infections (chronic fatigue syndrome- very controversial)
- Splenic rupture (rare, 0.1-0.5% of patients with proven mononucleosis)
- Hemolytic anemia (mild)
- Thrombocytopenic purpura
- Coagulopathy
- Aplastic anemia
- Hemolytic-uremic syndrome
- Seizures
- Cerebellar syndrome
- Nerve palsies
- Meningoencephalitis
- Optic neuritis
- Reye's syndrome
- Coma
- Transverse myelitis
- Guillain-Barré syndrome
- Psychosis
- Pericarditis
- Myocarditis
- ECG changes
- Airway obstruction
- Pneumonitis
- Pleural effusion
- Pulmonary hemorrhage
- Hepatitis/liver necrosis
- Malabsorption
- Dermatitis
- Urticaria
- Erythema multiforme
- Glomerulonephritis
- Nephrotic syndrome
- Mild hematuria/proteinuria
- Conjunctivitis
- Episcleritis
- Uveitis
- B-hemolytic streptococcal infections
- Staphylococcal infection
- Mycoplasma infection
- Bullous myringitis
- Orchitis
- Parotitis
- Monoarticular arthritis
- Jaundice

EXPECTED COURSE/PROGNOSIS
- Fever subsides in about 10 days
- Adenopathy and splenomegaly subside in about 4 weeks
- Children should be able to return to school when signs of infection have decreased, appetite returns, and alertness, strength, and sense of well-being allow.
- Death is uncommon (splenic rupture, blood dyscrasias, hypersplenism, or encephalitis)
- Potential role in some malignancies, especially in context of immune suppression

MISCELLANEOUS

ASSOCIATED CONDITIONS
Streptococcal pharyngitis

AGE-RELATED FACTORS
Pediatric:
- Children have subclinical or mild infections
- Most adolescents have clinically apparent infections

Geriatric: N/A

Others: N/A

PREGNANCY   No other specific recommendations

SYNONYMS
- Mono
- Infectious mononucleosis (IM)

ICD-9-CM   075 Infectious mononucleosis

SEE ALSO   Epstein-Barr virus infections

OTHER NOTES   N/A

ABBREVIATIONS   N/A

REFERENCES
- Neinstein L: Adolescent Health Care: A Practical Guide. 2nd Ed. Baltimore, Urban & Schwarzenberg, Inc., 1991
- Schroeder SA, Krupp MA, Tierney LM, McPhee SJ, eds: Current Medical Diagnosis and Treatment. Norwalk, CT, Appleton & Lange, 1989
- Isselbacher KJ, et al, eds: Harrison's Principles of Internal Medicine. 13th Ed. New York, McGraw-Hill, 1994
- Safran D, Bloom GP: Spontaneous Splenic Following Mononucleosis. American Surgeon 1990;56(10):601-605 (VI:91093752)
- Hanto DW: Clarification of EB virus associated posttransplant lymphoproliferative diseases. Ann Rev Med 1995:46:381-394
- Oren J, Sobel J: Human herpesvirus type 6. Review Clin Infectious Dis 1992;14:741-746
- Schuler J, Horst F: Spontaneous splenic rupture - the role of nonoperative management. Arch Surg 1995;130:662-665
- Goodman, Gilman: The Pharmacological Basis of Therapeutics. 9th Ed. New York, McGraw-Hill, 1996
- Mandell, et al: Principles and Practice of Infectious Disease, 4th ed. Churchill Livingstone, Inc. 1995.

Illustrations: 2 available on CD-ROM

Internet references: http://www.5mcc.com

Author(s)
Robert L. Weston, MD

Motion sickness

BASICS

DESCRIPTION Not a true sickness but a normal response to an abnormal situation in which there is a sensory conflict about body motion between the visual receptors, vestibular receptors and body proprioceptors. It can also be induced when patterns of motion differ from those previously experienced.
System(s) affected: Nervous
Genetics: N/A
Incidence/Prevalence in USA: N/A
Predominant age: N/A
Predominant sex: N/A

SIGNS AND SYMPTOMS
• Nausea
• Vomiting
• Diaphoresis
• Pallor
• Hypersalivation
• Yawning
• Hyperventilation
• Anxiety
• Panic
• Malaise
• Fatigue
• Weakness
• Confusion

CAUSES Motion (auto, plane, boat, amusement rides)

RISK FACTORS
• Travel
• Visual stimuli (i.e. moving horizon)
• Poor ventilation (fumes, smoke, carbon monoxide)
• Emotions (fear, anxiety)
• Zero gravity
• Other illness or poor health

DIAGNOSIS

DIFFERENTIAL DIAGNOSIS
• Mountain sickness
• Vestibular disease
• Gastroenteritis
• Metabolic disorders
• Toxin exposure

LABORATORY N/A
Drugs that may alter lab results: N/A
Disorders that may alter lab results: N/A

PATHOLOGICAL FINDINGS N/A

SPECIAL TESTS N/A

IMAGING N/A

DIAGNOSTIC PROCEDURES N/A

TREATMENT

APPROPRIATE HEALTH CARE
Remove triggers or noxious stimuli

GENERAL MEASURES
• Minimize exposure (seat in middle of plane or boat)
• Improve ventilation

SURGICAL MEASURES N/A

ACTIVITY
• Semi-recumbent seating
• Fix vision at 45 degree angle above horizon
• Avoid fixation of vision on moving objects (i.e., waves)
• Avoid reading

DIET
• Decrease oral intake or take frequent small feedings
• Avoid alcohol

PATIENT EDUCATION N/A

MEDICATIONS

DRUG(S) OF CHOICE
• Scopolamine transdermal where available; apply patch 6 hours before travel and replace every 3 days
or
• Dimenhydrinate (Dramamine) adults and adolescents 50-100 mg q4h, maximum 400 mg/day; children 6-12 years 25-50 mg q4h, maximum 150 mg/day
• Meclizine (Antivert) 25 mg qid

Contraindications: Glaucoma

Precautions:
• Young children
• Elderly
• Pregnancy
• Urinary obstruction
• Pyloric obstruction

Significant possible interactions:
• Sedatives (antihistamines, alcohol, antidepressants)
• Anticholinergics (belladonna alkaloids)

ALTERNATIVE DRUGS
• Antihistamines
  ◊ Meclizine (Antivert)
  ◊ Terfenadine (Seldane)

FOLLOWUP

PATIENT MONITORING N/A

PREVENTION/AVOIDANCE
• Minimize exposure (seat in middle of plane or boat)
• Improve ventilation
• Semi-recumbent seating
• Fix vision at 45 degree angle above horizon
• Avoid fixation of vision on moving objects (i.e., waves)
• Avoid reading
• Minimize food intake prior to travel

POSSIBLE COMPLICATIONS
• Hypotension
• Dehydration
• Depression
• Panic

EXPECTED COURSE/PROGNOSIS
• Symptoms should resolve when motion exposure ends
• Resistance to motion sickness seems to increase with age

MISCELLANEOUS

ASSOCIATED CONDITIONS N/A

AGE-RELATED FACTORS
Pediatric: Children more susceptible to motion sickness
Geriatric: Age confers some resistance to motion sickness
Others: N/A

PREGNANCY N/A

SYNONYMS
• Car sickness
• Sea sickness
• Air sickness
• Space sickness

ICD-9-CM
994.6 Motion sickness

SEE ALSO N/A

OTHER NOTES N/A

ABBREVIATIONS N/A

REFERENCES
• Dundee JW, McMillan C: Positive evidence for P6 acupuncture antiemesis. Postgrad Med 1991;67:417-422
• Bennett JC, Plum F, eds: Cecil Textbook of Medicine. 20th Ed. Philadelphia, W.B. Saunders Co., 1996
• Kohl RL, Calkins DS: Control of nausea & autonomic dysfunction with terfenadine, a peripherally acting antihistamine. Aviation, Space and Environmental Medicine 1991;62(5):392-396
Illustrations: N/A
Internet references: http://www.5mcc.com

Author(s)
Marshall Godwin, MD

Multiple myeloma

BASICS

DESCRIPTION Multiple myeloma (malignant tumor of plasma cells) is the most common primary malignancy of bone. It is the prototype of a monoclonal tumor cell proliferation that usually reveals monoclonal protein in the serum or urine of more than 90% of patients. The disease process encompasses a spectrum of localized and disseminated disease forms.

System(s) affected:
Hemic/Lymphatic/Immunologic, Nervous, Musculoskeletal

Genetics: Occasional familial occurrence, indicating recessive heredity

Incidence/Prevalence in USA: Multiple myeloma accounts for approximately 1% of all types of malignant disease and slightly more than 10% of hematologic malignancies

Predominant age: Ages 40 to 80 (with a peak incidence in the 70's)

Predominant sex: Male = Female

SIGNS AND SYMPTOMS
• The majority of patients (65%) present with bone pain
• Pathologic fracture occurs in approximately one-third of these patients
• Weakness and fatigue are common
• Bleeding (nose, gums), often evidenced by purpura or epistaxis, may occur in the presence of thrombocytopenia or secondary amyloidosis
• Recurrent infections may occur
• Patients may also present with renal insufficiency or renal failure
• Swelling on ribs, skull, sternum, vertebrae, clavicles, shoulder, pelvis
• Weight loss
• Hyperviscosity syndrome

CAUSES Unknown. There are tumor cells characteristic of plasma cells arising from bone marrow.

RISK FACTORS Family history of myeloma

DIAGNOSIS

DIFFERENTIAL DIAGNOSIS
Metastatic carcinoma, primary malignancy of bone (sarcoma, lymphoma), metabolic bone disease, monoclonal gammopathy of undetermined significance (MGUS)

LABORATORY
• Anemia is present in 70% of the patients at the time of diagnosis. Nearly all patients will develop anemia as the disease progresses.
• Peripheral blood smear - rouleaux formation
• Serum protein electrophoresis - usually shows a spike or a localized band (M spike in approximately 80% of patients). Of these, 50% are IgG protein, 20% IgA, and 17% free monoclonal light chains (Bence Jones protein).
• Urine electrophoresis - positive about 70% of the time for light chains, but inconsistencies hinder diagnosis
• Hypercalcemia
• Decreased platelets
• Elevated sedimentation rate
• Elevated creatinine and BUN

Drugs that may alter lab results: N/A
Disorders that may alter lab results: N/A

PATHOLOGICAL FINDINGS
• Secondary amyloidosis
• Myeloma kidney

SPECIAL TESTS N/A

IMAGING
• Skeletal x-rays often show a radiolucent or a lytic lesion when the long bones are involved. The skull often shows punched-out lytic lesions with no sclerotic or reactive border. Periosteal reaction is uncommon. Vertebral compression fractures, with occasional extraosseous or extradural cord compression, are commonly seen.
• Although technetium-99 bone scans have often been described as cold, they will actually show some slight uptake increase in involved skeletal regions, particularly in the presence of fracture; however, the amount of uptake is far less than that demonstrated in other malignancies of bone
• MRI scans can be extremely valuable in determining the extent of marrow involvement as well as the difference between benign compression fractures and multiple myeloma lesions

DIAGNOSTIC PROCEDURES The laboratory test most likely to yield a definitive diagnosis is a bone marrow biopsy. The bone marrow will contain increased numbers of plasma cells at various stages of maturation.

TREATMENT

APPROPRIATE HEALTH CARE
Outpatient, except during intensive chemotherapy periods

GENERAL MEASURES
• Radiation therapy is limited to patients with intractable bone pain (failing chemotherapy)
• Patients with impending or pathologic fractures should have those fractures rigidly stabilized along with removal of the tumor, if possible. Patients with impending paraplegia secondary to spinal cord involvement should undergo immediate radiation therapy and bracing and/or surgical decompression and stabilization.

SURGICAL MEASURES N/A

ACTIVITY As tolerated

DIET No special diet

PATIENT EDUCATION American Cancer Society has literature available

Multiple myeloma

MEDICATIONS

DRUG(S) OF CHOICE Chemotherapy is the primary treatment for symptomatic multiple myeloma, but the ideal chemotherapy is unknown. The most common initial protocol management includes the oral administration of melphalan (Alkeran) and prednisone. This protocol produces an objective response in 50-60% of the patients. This is usually given in oral doses of 0.25 mg/kg/day for four days, along with 50 mg of prednisone bid for the same period of time. The dosage should be repeated every six weeks with leukocyte and platelet counts evaluated at three-week intervals.
Contraindications: Refer to manufacturer's profile of each drug
Precautions:
• Melphalan - myelosuppression is the major dose-limiting toxicity of this drug (mainly leukopenia, thrombocytopenia). Monitor CBC, platelets every 3 weeks.
• Prednisone - usual hazards of long-term corticosteroid administration. Refer to manufacturer's literature.
Significant possible interactions: Refer to manufacturer's profile of each drug

ALTERNATIVE DRUGS In the event of failure of the above-mentioned regimen, alternate protocols include
◊ Cyclophosphamide, carmustine (BCNU), vincristine, and prednisone
◊ VAD - combination of vincristine, doxorubicin (Adriamycin), and dexamethasone

FOLLOWUP

PATIENT MONITORING CBC, platelets q 6 weeks

PREVENTION/AVOIDANCE N/A

POSSIBLE COMPLICATIONS
• Skeletal destruction
• Spontaneous fractures
• Secondary amyloidosis
• Renal insufficiency
• Recurrent infections (e.g., Streptococcus pneumoniae, Haemophilus influenzae)
• Hyperviscosity syndrome

EXPECTED COURSE/PROGNOSIS
• Average survival time varies considerably. The median survival of all patients is approximately 24 months. A significantly large number of patients survive for much longer periods of time with evidence of disease present.
• There are occasional temporary remissions with therapy
• Bone marrow transplantation should be considered in younger patients

MISCELLANEOUS

ASSOCIATED CONDITIONS Multiple myeloma has an association with systemic amyloidosis in which the amyloid is derived from immunoglobulin light chains. In one autopsy series, 15% of the patients had generalized amyloidosis with deposits in the kidneys, spleen, adrenal bodies, and liver. Kidney involvement often leads to azotemia and secondary renal failure.

AGE-RELATED FACTORS
Pediatric: N/A
Geriatric: More common in older adults
Others: N/A

PREGNANCY N/A

SYNONYMS Myeloma, plasma cell

ICD-9-CM 203.0 Multiple myeloma

SEE ALSO N/A

OTHER NOTES N/A

ABBREVIATIONS N/A

REFERENCES DeVita VT, Hellman S, Rosenberg SA: The Principles and Practices of Oncology. 4th Ed. Philadelphia, J.B. Lippincott, 1993
Illustrations: N/A
Internet references: http://www.5mcc.com

Author(s)
Mark C. Leeson, MD, FACS

Multiple sclerosis

BASICS

DESCRIPTION Multiple sclerosis (MS) is a recurrent (occasionally progressive) inflammatory progressive demyelinization of the white matter of the brain and spinal cord resulting in multiple and varied neurologic symptoms and signs. Usual course - intermittent, progressive and relapsing. It may pursue an acute course or slowly progressive. It is a major cause of disability in young adults.
System(s) affected: Nervous
Genetics: Appears to be a strong genetic component in determining susceptibility to the disease.
Incidence/prevalence in USA: 25,000 new cases each year
Predominant age: Young adult (16-40 years)
Predominant sex: Female > Male

SIGNS AND SYMPTOMS
• Ataxia
• Babinski sign
• Blurred, double or loss of vision in a single eye; often triggered by retro-bulbar neuritis and its visual sequelae
• Clonus
• Clumsiness
• Dysarthria
• Emotional lability
• Fatigue
• Genital anesthesia
• Hand paralysis
• Hemiparesis
• Hyperactive deep tendon reflexes
• Hyperesthesia
• Incoordination
• Loss of position sense
• Loss of vibration sense
• Monoparesis
• Ocular paralysis
• Paresthesias
• Sexual impotence in men
• Urinary frequency, hesitancy, incontinence
• Trigeminal neuralgia

CAUSES
• Unknown
• Autoimmune theory - supported by HLA linkage, hereditary pattern, immunocytes in plaques, changes in peripheral blood immunocytes
• Viral theory - supported by increasing incidence of disease at higher latitudes, clusters of cases with families, geographical clusters of cases, animal studies of infectious diseases of myelin
• Combined theory - autoimmune disorder triggered by environmental exposure to toxin or virus early in life

RISK FACTORS
• Living in temperate zone
• Northern European descent
• Family history of the disease

DIAGNOSIS

DIFFERENTIAL DIAGNOSIS
• Amyotrophic lateral sclerosis
• Behçet's disease
• Brain stem tumors
• Central nervous system infections
• Cerebellar tumors
• Friedreich's ataxia
• Hereditary ataxias
• Leukodystrophies
• Neurofibromatosis
• Pernicious anemia
• Progressive multifocal leukoencephalopathy
• Ruptured intervertebral disk
• Small cerebral infarcts
• Sarcoidosis
• Spinal cord tumors
• Syphilis
• Syringomyelia
• Systemic lupus erythematosus
• Vasculitides

LABORATORY
• Cerebrospinal fluid
  ◊ Abnormal colloidal gold curve
  ◊ Gamma globulin IgG elevated
  ◊ Mild mononuclear pleocytosis (less than 40 cells/mL)
  ◊ Myelin debris
  ◊ Negative serology for syphilis
  ◊ Protein normal or slightly elevated 50-100 mg/100 mL (50-100 mg/dL [500-1000 mg/L])
• Tests to exclude other disorders
  ◊ Fluorescent treponemal antibody absorption (FTA-ABS)
  ◊ Sedimentation rate
  ◊ Screens for clinically suspected vasculitic disorders
  ◊ Human T-lymphotropic virus-1 (HTLV-I) serology
Drugs that may alter lab results: N/A
Disorders that may alter lab results: N/A

PATHOLOGICAL FINDINGS
• Destruction of myelin sheaths of nerve fibers and axis cylinders, sparing axons, glia and other structures
• Atrophy of optic nerves and cerebral hemispheres
• T-cell lymphocytes about venules

SPECIAL TESTS
• Visual evoked response (VER) - abnormal in 75-97% of definite MS cases
• Somatosensory evoked potentials - abnormal in 72-96% of cases
• Brain stem auditory evoked responses - abnormal in 57-65% of cases
• CSF
  ◊ Oligoclonal bands
  ◊ Increased IgG

IMAGING N/A
• MRI (more sensitive than CT) - may show many plaques
• CT scan (double-dose, delayed) - plaques

DIAGNOSTIC PROCEDURES
• No test specific to diagnose MS
• History, physical, CSF analysis, MRI, evoked potential studies, repeated observations over a period of time

TREATMENT

APPROPRIATE HEALTH CARE
• Outpatient as long as possible
• Long-term care facility for physical therapy or complications such as pyelonephritis

GENERAL MEASURES
• No specific therapy. Remissions occur spontaneously and make treatment evaluations difficult.
• Emotional support, encouragement, and reassurances are necessary to help avoid a hopeless outlook
• Occupational therapy
• Urologic evaluation including any sexual dysfunction problems (impotence common in male patients)
• Self-catheterizations for inadequate bladder emptying (indwelling catheter may be necessary in a few patients)
• Custodial care, if patient cognitively impaired
• Physiotherapy to maintain range of movement and strength and to avoid contractures

SURGICAL MEASURES N/A

ACTIVITY
• Maintain activity, avoid overwork and fatigue
• Rest during periods of acute relapse

DIET If constipation a problem, high fluid intake, plus a high fiber diet

PATIENT EDUCATION For patient education materials favorably reviewed on this topic, contact: National Multiple Sclerosis Society, 205E 42nd Street, New York, NY 10017, (800)624-8236

Multiple sclerosis

MEDICATIONS

DRUG(S) OF CHOICE
Drug therapy directed toward relieving symptoms
• Methylprednisolone: IV 1000 mg for 5 days followed by tapered oral prednisone for acute attacks, especially retrobulbar neuritis (recommended by some clinicians)
• Spasticity: baclofen, low dosage to start, 5 mg 1-3 times a day, increase as needed, or diazepam 2-5 mg qhs
• Constipation: stool softeners, bulk producing agents, laxative suppositories
• Urinary problems: propantheline 7.5 mg every 3-4 hours to start, increase to 15 mg 3-4 times a day plus 15-30 mg at bedtime; or oxybutynin chloride 5 mg 3-4 times a day
• Prophylactic antibiotics: for urinary infections
• Incoordination or tremors: no ideal therapy; may try beta-blockers (if not contraindicated), primidone, or clonazepam.
• Depression and emotional lability: amitriptyline 10-25 mg at bedtime to start, increase as tolerated
• Paranoia or mania: haloperidol or lithium
• Musculoskeletal pain or discomfort: nonsteroidal anti-inflammatories
• Hemifacial and dysesthesias: carbamazepine 100-200 once or twice a day to start, increase to total daily dosage of 600-1600 mg 3-4 times a day. Must monitor serum levels.
• Immunosuppressive agents (e.g., azathioprine, ACTH (adrenocorticotropic hormone), methylprednisolone, cyclophosphamide, interferons, cyclosporine) still investigational
Contraindications: Refer to manufacturer's literature
Precautions: Refer to manufacturer's literature
Significant possible interactions: Refer to manufacturer's literature

ALTERNATIVE DRUGS
• Oral steroids: Poor evidence for use alone
• Chronic fatigue: amantadine 200-300 mg/day (no specific evidence that this works)
• Baclofen 40-80 mg/day in divided doses for reduction of spasticity
• Interferon beta approved for relapsing MS - 0.25 mg SC every other day
• Copolymer-1 and cladribine have shown promising results in clinical results

FOLLOWUP

PATIENT MONITORING Requires patient follow-up

PREVENTION/AVOIDANCE No known preventive measures. Avoid factors that may precipitate an attack, particularly stress from hot weather.

POSSIBLE COMPLICATIONS
• Coma
• Delirium
• Emotional lability
• Nystagmus
• Optic nerve atrophy
• Paraplegia
• Sexual impotence (men)
• Urinary tract infections

EXPECTED COURSE/PROGNOSIS
• Highly variable and unpredictable. Approximately 70% of patients lead active, productive lives with prolonged remissions.
• May disable the patient by early adulthood or cause death within months of onset
• Average duration exceeds 25 years
• 30% relapse in one year, 20% in 5-9 years, 10% in 10-30 years

MISCELLANEOUS

ASSOCIATED CONDITIONS N/A

AGE-RELATED FACTORS
Pediatric: Unlikely before puberty.
Geriatric: Remissions less frequent in this age group
Others: N/A

PREGNANCY A triggering factor for multiple sclerosis in some cases

SYNONYMS
• Disseminated sclerosis
• Insular sclerosis

ICD-9-CM 340 Multiple sclerosis

SEE ALSO N/A

OTHER NOTES
• Since the course is highly variable and unpredictable, avoid a hopeless outlook
• 30-40% of patients with optic neuritis alone eventually develop other signs

ABBREVIATIONS N/A

REFERENCES
• Sibley WA: Therapeutic claims in multiple sclerosis. 2nd Ed. New York, Demos, 1988
• Matthews WB, et al: McAlpine's Multiple Sclerosis. 2nd Ed. New York, Churchill Livingstone, 1991
• Adams RD, Victor M: Principles of Neurology. 5th Ed. New York, McGraw-Hill, 1993
• Rowlan LP, ed: Merritt's Textbook of Neurology. 9th Ed. Philadelphia, Williams & Wilkins, 1995
• Beck RW, et al: The effect of corticosteroids for acute optic neuritis on the subsequent development of multiple sclerosis. New Engl J Med 1994;329;24:1764-1769
Illustrations: 1 available on CD-ROM
Internet references: http://www.5mcc.com

Author(s)
Stanley G. Smith, MA, MB, FCFPC

Mumps

BASICS

DESCRIPTION Acute generalized paramyxovirus infection usually presenting with unilateral or bilateral parotitis. Epidemics late winter and spring with transmission by respiratory secretions. Incubation is approximately 14 to 24 days.
System(s) affected: Reproductive, Hemic/Lymphatic/Immunologic, Skin/Exocrine
Genetics: N/A
Incidence/Prevalence in USA:
• 0.29/100,000 (725 per year)
• 0 .0064/100,000
• 90% of adults are sero-positive even without history
Predominant age: 85% occur before age 15 years, but more severe in adults
Predominant sex: Male = Female

SIGNS AND SYMPTOMS
• Parotid pain and swelling in one or both glands
• Rare prodrome of fever, neck muscle ache, malaise
• Initial parotid swelling just behind jaw
• Swelling peaks in 1-3 days, lasts 3-7 days
• Obscures angle of mandible
• Elevates earlobe
• Redness at opening of Stensen's duct
• Sour foods cause pain in the parotid gland region
• Moderate fever, usually not above 104°F (40.0°C). High fever is frequently associated with complications.
• Meningeal signs in 15%, encephalitis in 0.5%
• Rarely arthritis, orchitis, thyroiditis, mastitis, pancreatitis
• Rare maculopapular erythematous rash
• Up to 50% of cases may be asymptomatic
• Swelling in the sternal area, rare, but pathognomonic of mumps

CAUSES
• Mumps paramyxovirus
• Other viruses, such as Coxsackie (rare)

RISK FACTORS
• Urban epidemics, non-vaccinated population
• Usual communicable period is 24 hours before to 72 hours after onset of parotitis
• Incubation period usually 18 days

DIAGNOSIS

DIFFERENTIAL DIAGNOSIS
• Parainfluenza parotitis, other viruses
• Suppurative parotitis - often associated with Staphylococcus aureus (presence of Wharton's duct pus nearly excludes diagnosis of mumps).
• Recurrent allergic parotitis
• Salivary calculus with intermittent swelling
• Lymphadenitis from any cause
• Cytomegalovirus parotitis in immunocompromised patients
• Mikulicz's syndrome (chronic, painless parotid and lacrimal gland swelling of unknown cause that occurs in tuberculosis, sarcoidosis, lupus, leukemia, and lymphosarcoma patients)
• Malignant or benign salivary gland tumors
• Drug-related parotid enlargement (iodides, guanethidine)
• Other causes of the complications of mumps (meningoencephalitis, orchitis, oophoritis, pancreatitis, polyarthritis, nephritis, myocarditis, prostatitis)
• Mumps orchitis must be differentiated from testicular torsion and from chlamydial or bacterial orchitis. (Testicular scan can be useful.)

LABORATORY
• Viral isolation from throat washings, urine, blood, or spinal fluid
• Serum amylase elevated
• Rise in paired antibodies: Anti-"S" antibodies peak early and may be seen at the time of presentation
• Cerebrospinal fluid (CSF) - leukocytosis
• Leukopenia
Drugs that may alter lab results: N/A
Disorders that may alter lab results: N/A

PATHOLOGICAL FINDINGS Periductal edema and lymphocytic infiltration

SPECIAL TESTS Rarely necessary, an easier salivary test for IgM is pending

IMAGING Useful to differentiate mumps orchitis from testicular torsion

DIAGNOSTIC PROCEDURES N/A

TREATMENT

APPROPRIATE HEALTH CARE
• Outpatient, if no complications
• High fever and testicular pain - may hospitalize for steroids or interferon

GENERAL MEASURES
• Supportive and symptomatic care
• For patients with orchitis, ice packs to scrotum can help relieve pain
• Scrotal support with adhesive bridge while recumbent and/or athletic supporter while ambulatory
• Use IV fluids if severe nausea or vomiting accompanies pancreatitis

SURGICAL MEASURES N/A

ACTIVITY Mumps orchitis - bedrest and local supportive clothing, such as wearing 2 pairs of briefs, or adhesive-tape bridge

DIET Liquids if cannot chew

PATIENT EDUCATION
• Must be out of school until no longer contagious - about 9 days after onset of pain
• Orchitis is common in older children but rarely results in sterility
• Immunization of family may protect against later exposures but not the present one

MEDICATIONS

DRUG(S) OF CHOICE Corticosteroids or a nonsteroidal anti-inflammatory may diminish pain and swelling in acute orchitis and arthritis mumps, but usually not necessary. May use acetaminophen for fever and/or pain.
Contraindications: Refer to manufacturer's profile of each drug
Precautions: Avoid aspirin for pain in children. There may be an association of aspirin, virus infection, and Reye's syndrome in children.
Significant possible interactions: Refer to manufacturer's profile of each drug

ALTERNATIVE DRUGS
• Mumps arthritis may improve with corticosteroids or a nonsteroidal anti-inflammatory
• Interferon alfa-2b for 7 days may be used in severe bilateral orchitis to prevent infertility

FOLLOWUP

PATIENT MONITORING Most cases will be mild. Monitor hydration status.

PREVENTION/AVOIDANCE
• 2 doses of live mumps vaccine recommended for active immunization: At 15 months and at entry to middle school. (Postexposure vaccination does not protect from recent exposure).
• Isolate hospitalized patients until 9 days past onset

POSSIBLE COMPLICATIONS
• May precede, accompany, or follow salivary gland involvement and may occur (rarely) without primary involvement of the parotid gland
• Meningitis or encephalitis may present 10 days after first symptoms of illness. Aseptic meningitis is typically mild, but meningo-encephalitis may lead to seizures, paralysis, hydrocephalus or, in 2% of cases, death.
• Cerebrospinal fluid (CSF) pleocytosis found in 65% of cases with parotitis
• Orchitis common (30%) in postpubertal boys, starts within 8 days after parotitis, fever, swollen testis of 4 day duration, fertility impaired in 13% but absolute sterility is rare
• Oophoritis in 7% of postpubertal females, no decreased fertility
• Pancreatitis, usually mild
• Nephritis, thyroiditis, or arthralgias are rare
• Myocarditis - usually mild, but may depress ST segment, may be linked to endocardial fibroelastosis
• Deafness - 1/15,000 unilateral nerve deafness, may not be permanent
• Inflammation about the eye (rare)
• Dacryoadenitis, optic neuritis

EXPECTED COURSE/PROGNOSIS
• Complete recovery is usual, immunity is permanent
• Sensorineural hearing loss in 4% of adults - transient
• Rare recurrence after 2 weeks may be recurrent nonepidemic parotitis

MISCELLANEOUS

ASSOCIATED CONDITIONS N/A

AGE-RELATED FACTORS
Pediatric:
• In adolescents - orchitis more common
• Most cases of acute epidemic mumps occur in children aged 5 to 15. Unusual in children less than 2 years. Most infants less than 1 year are immune.
• Less likely to develop complications
Geriatric: Most are immune
Others: Most complications occur in post-pubertal group

PREGNANCY
• No proven complications of vaccine, but theoretically should not vaccinate in pregnancy
• Disease may increase rate of spontaneous abortion in first trimester

SYNONYMS
• Epidemic parotitis
• Infectious parotitis

ICD-9-CM 072.9 Mumps without mention of complication

SEE ALSO N/A

OTHER NOTES A portion of people infected with mumps virus have no parotid swelling and a clinically inapparent infection

ABBREVIATIONS N/A

REFERENCES
• Behrman RE, ed: Nelson's Textbook of Pediatrics. Philadelphia, W.B. Saunders, 1996
• Report of the Committee on Infectious Diseases (Red Book). Elk Grove Village, Ill, American Academy of Pediatrics, 1997
• Casella R, Liebundgut B, Lehmann K, Gasser T: Mumps orchitis: report of a miniepidemic. J Urol 1997;158:2158-2161
• CDC: Measles, Mumps, and Rubella - Vaccine Use and Strategies for Elimination of Measles, Rubella, and Congenital Rubella Syndrome and Control of Mumps. MMWR 1998;47:No.RR-8:6-15
Illustrations: N/A
Internet references: http://www.5mcc.com

Author(s)
Frances Wu, MD

Muscular dystrophy

BASICS

DESCRIPTION Inherited, progressive diseases of muscle with wide ranges of clinical expression. Included:
- Congenital muscular dystrophy (CMD)
- Congenital myotonic dystrophy
- Duchenne's muscular dystrophy (DMD)
- Becker's muscular dystrophy (BMD)
- Myotonic dystrophy
- Fascioscapulohumeral dystrophy (FSH)
- Limb girdle dystrophy
- Emery-Dreifuss muscular dystrophy (ED)

System(s) affected: Musculoskeletal, Nervous
Genetics: See Causes and Risk factors
Incidence/Prevalence in USA:
- Duchenne's muscular dystrophy (DMD): 1 per 3000 male births
- Myotonic dystrophy: 1 per 10,000 births

Predominant age:
- Birth to infancy: Congenital muscular dystrophy with or without cerebral involvement, congenital myotonic dystrophy
- Infancy to early childhood: Duchenne's muscular dystrophy (DMD), Becker's muscular dystrophy (BMD), fascioscapulohumeral dystrophy (FHS)
- Late childhood to adolescence: BMD, FSH, myotonic dystrophy

Predominant sex: Male > Female (DMD and BMD caused by defect in same gene)

SIGNS AND SYMPTOMS
- DMD and BMD:
  ◊ Leg pain may be an early complaint
  ◊ Normal motor milestones until child begins to walk
  ◊ Clumsiness - frequent falls, toe-walking, waddling gait
  ◊ Weakness - inability to jump or climb stairs, weak neck flexors, Gower's sign, lumbar lordosis
  ◊ Pseudohypertrophy of calf muscles and contractures of heel cords
  ◊ Kyphosis and scoliosis
  ◊ Progressive decline in vital capacity
- Myotonic dystrophy:
  ◊ Facial weakness - open, triangular mouth and droopy eyelids
  ◊ Sustained muscle contraction with percussion of thenar eminence
  ◊ Weakness in distal limbs
  ◊ High forehead with receding hairline
  ◊ Neonatal form - hypotonia, respiratory distress, hip dislocations
  ◊ Cataracts, gonadal dysfunction, cardiac conduction defects/arrhythmias
  ◊ Difficulty in letting go (myotonia) after handshake
- FSH:
  ◊ Facial weakness - inability to completely close eyes or whistle, pouting expression with transverse smile
  ◊ Shoulder and proximal arm weakness: inability to do push-ups, horizontal clavicles, exaggerated bicep muscles size ("Popeye" arms), winging of the scapula
  ◊ Retinal vascular abnormalities in most patients
- ED:
  ◊ Toe walking and small biceps
  ◊ Contractures of neck, biceps, Achilles tendons - even without significant weakness
  ◊ Cardiac conduction abnormalities with risk of sudden death

CAUSES
- X-linked: DMD and milder allelic form BMD have gene deletion, in 2/3 of patients, at Xp21.2 for production of "dystrophin"; ED have abnormal gene at Xq 28
- Autosomal dominant: Myotonic dystrophy gene mapped to short arm of chromosome 19. FSH gene mapped to 4q35.

RISK FACTORS
- X-linked: affected male on maternal side of family (although female carriers may rarely be symptomatic)
- Autosomal dominant - affected parent: Myotonic dystrophy more severe if mother is affected parent.
- Autosomal recessive: CMD gene mapped to chromosome 6q2

DIAGNOSIS

DIFFERENTIAL DIAGNOSIS
- Onset from birth to early infancy: Encephalopathy, spinal muscular atrophy, infantile botulism, myasthenia gravis, congenital myopathies, metabolic myopathies, chromosomal disorders, paroxysmal disorders, neonatal spinal cord injury
- Onset from infancy to early childhood: Carnitine deficiency, acid maltase deficiency, spinal muscular atrophy, myotonia congenita
- Onset from childhood to adolescence: Other muscular dystrophies, spinal muscular atrophy, congenital myopathies, metabolic or inflammatory myopathies, myasthenia gravis, periodic paralysis

LABORATORY
- Creatine kinase:
  ◊ Marked elevation in DMD
  ◊ Moderate elevation in BMD, FSH
  ◊ Normal in congenital muscular dystrophy, late DMD

Drugs that may alter lab results:
- Opiates including codeine, heroin, meperidine, and morphine
- Dexamethasone
- Ethanol
- Digoxin
- Furosemide
- Aminocaproic acid
- Halothane
- Imipramine
- Phenobarbital
- Lithium
- Clofibrate

Disorders that may alter lab results:
- Polymyositis/dermatomyositis
- Muscle trauma - exercise, seizures, IM injections, needle EMG
- Hypothyroidism, hyperthyroidism
- Myocardial infarction, stroke, sepsis, shock

PATHOLOGICAL FINDINGS
- Muscle biopsy
  ◊ DMD: fiber splitting, necrosis, regeneration with interspersed fibrosis
  ◊ FSH: highest yield in supraspinatus muscle with occasional degenerating fibers and small angulated fibers with inflammatory cells
  ◊ ED: type I fiber atrophy

SPECIAL TESTS
EMG in myotonic dystrophy - high frequency repetitive, waxing and waning discharges ("dive-bomber" effect)

IMAGING
- Brain MRI in CMD shows diffuse white matter changes resembling leukodystrophy

DIAGNOSTIC PROCEDURES
- Muscle biopsy of moderately weak muscle (vastus lateralis, triceps) not studied by needle electromyography
- Dystrophin level from muscle biopsy. In DMD dystrophin content is <3% normal; in BMD dystrophin content is <20% normal.
- Prenatal diagnosis
  ◊ DMD and BMD: Dystrophin studies in chorionic villus sampling and amniocytes; analysis of fetal RBCs in maternal blood; Pre-implantation diagnosis
  ◊ CMD: Merosin-alpha-2 subunit in trophoblast

TREATMENT

APPROPRIATE HEALTH CARE
Outpatient with team approach - neurologist, orthopedic surgeon, physical and occupational therapists, social worker, and orthotist

GENERAL MEASURES
- Physical therapy to maintain neuromuscular function
- Orthoses to sustain walking and delay development of scoliosis
- Respiratory care, ventilation during sleep for nocturnal hypoventilation syndrome

SURGICAL MEASURES
Surgical release of contractures or fixation of joints

ACTIVITY
Exercise as desired, but stop short of muscle pain or exhaustion

DIET
Monitor nutrition and fat stores because of increased caloric requirements

PATIENT EDUCATION
- Family and individual counseling
- Genetic counseling
- Printed material and clinical services available through the Muscular Dystrophy Association, 3561 E. Sunrise Dr., Tucson, AZ 85718; (800)221-1142

Muscular dystrophy

MEDICATIONS

DRUG(S) OF CHOICE
• No drug treatment recommended at present
• Prednisone 0.15-0.75 mg/kg/day improves muscle strength in boys with DMD
Contraindications: N/A
Precautions: Careful monitoring for side effects of long-term steroid therapy is required; these include weight gain, hypertension, GI bleeding, immunosuppression
Significant possible interactions: N/A

ALTERNATIVE DRUGS   N/A

FOLLOWUP

PATIENT MONITORING
• Determined by interdisciplinary health care team
• In patients with ED, early detection of cardiac abnormalities may permit lifesaving pacemaker insertion

PREVENTION/AVOIDANCE
• Maternal carrier status evaluation in DMD (80% sensitive) and BMD (60% sensitive) by creatine kinase levels
• DNA probes for carrier status determination and antenatal diagnosis in DMD and BMD
• DNA linkage techniques in selected families for antenatal diagnosis of myotonic dystrophy

POSSIBLE COMPLICATIONS
• Cardiac arrhythmias or myopathy
  ◊ Especially in ED
  ◊ In DMD (< 80%)
  ◊ In BMD (< 40%)
• Hypertension - FSH
• Dysphagia or acute gastric dilation - DMD, myotonic dystrophy
• Malignant hyperthermia - DMD
• Respiratory failure and early death - congenital muscular dystrophy (15%), neonatal-onset myotonic dystrophy (> 50%)
• Endocrinopathies - myotonic dystrophy
• Cataracts - myotonic dystrophy
• Sensorineural hearing loss - FSH
• Seizures and cerebral dysplasia - congenital muscular dystrophy with cerebral involvement (> 50%)
• Increase in fetal breech presentation in female carriers of DMD

EXPECTED COURSE/PROGNOSIS
• DMD and BMD:
  ◊ Progressive weakness, contractures, inability to walk
  ◊ Kyphoscoliosis and respiratory compromise
  ◊ Early death (Duchenne's 16 +/- 4 years; Becker's 42 +/- 16 years)
• Myotonic dystrophy (neonatal onset) and congenital muscular dystrophy with cerebral involvement:
  ◊ Progressive hypotonia and weakness
  ◊ Respiratory failure and early death
• Other types
  ◊ Slow progression and near normal life span

MISCELLANEOUS

ASSOCIATED CONDITIONS
• Mental retardation - DMD (25%), myotonic dystrophy with early onset
• Malignant hypothermia may be seen in patients with DMD

AGE-RELATED FACTORS
Pediatric: N/A
Geriatric: N/A
Others: N/A

PREGNANCY   Refer mother with myotonic dystrophy to perinatologist

SYNONYMS
• Pseudohypertrophic muscular dystrophy
• Steinert's disease
• Landouzy-Déjèrine dystrophy
• Fukuyama syndrome

ICD-9-CM
359.0 Congenital muscular dystrophy
359.1 DMD, BMD, FSH, ED and others
359.2 Myotonic dystrophy

SEE ALSO   N/A

OTHER NOTES   N/A

ABBREVIATIONS
CMD = Congenital muscular dystrophy
DMD = Duchenne's muscular dystrophy
BMD = Becker's muscular dystrophy
FSH = fascioscapulohumeral dystrophy

REFERENCES
• Brooke MH: Clinician's View of Neuromuscular Diseases. 2nd Ed. Baltimore, Williams & Wilkins, 1986
• Abbs S: Prenatal diagnosis of Duchenne and Becker muscular dystrophy. Prenatal Diagnosis 16:1187-98, 1996
• Brown RH: Dystrophin-associated proteins and the muscular dystrophies. Ann Rev Med 1997;48:457-466
• Cwik VA: Disorders of muscle - dystrophies and myopathies. In: Berg BO, ed. Principles of Child Neurology. New York, McGraw-Hill, 1996:1665-1701
• Fassiti A, Murphy S, Dickson G: Gene therapy of Duchenne muscular dystrophy. Adv Genet 1997;35:117-153
• Leger P, Leger SS: Respiratory concerns in Duchenne muscular dystrophy. Pediatr Pulmon 1997;(suppl)16:137-139
• Tawil R, et al: Facioscapulohumeral dystrophy: a distinct regional myopathy with a novel molecular pathogenesis. Ann Neurol 1998;43:279-282
Illustrations: N/A
Internet references: http://www.5mcc.com

Author(s)
David A. Griesemer, MD
Nasir Waheed, MD

Myasthenia gravis

BASICS

DESCRIPTION
A disorder of the neuromuscular junction resulting in a pure motor syndrome characterized by weakness and fatigue particularly of the extraocular, pharyngeal, facial, cervical, proximal limb and respiratory musculature. Typical and neonatal forms are immunologically mediated. A number of congenital forms of obscure pathogenesis exist. Onset may be sudden and severe (myasthenic crisis) but, more typically, is mild and intermittent over many years.
System(s) affected: Musculoskeletal, Hemic/Lymphatic/Immunologic
Genetics:
• 15% of infants born to myasthenic mothers have neonatal myasthenia gravis, due to the transplacental passage of acetylcholine receptor antibodies. The condition completely resolves in weeks to months. Neonatal myasthenia gravis is not a genetic disorder.
• Infants with congenital myasthenia gravis syndromes are born to normal mothers. The onset is at birth or in early childhood. Inheritance is typically autosomal recessive. The condition is persistent.
• Typical adult and juvenile myasthenia gravis do have a familial predisposition (5% of cases) and an increased frequency of HLA-B8 and DR3.
Incidence/Prevalence in USA:
2-5/year/million; 3/100,000
Predominant age: Ages 20-40, but occurs at any age (1-80). Incidence in females peaks in the 3rd decade, in males in the 5th and 6th decades.
Predominant sex:
• Adults - Female > Male (3:2)
• Children - Female > Male (3:2)
• Children with myasthenia plus associated disease - Female > Male (5:1)

SIGNS AND SYMPTOMS
• Ptosis
• Diplopia
• Facial weakness
• Fatigue on chewing
• Dysphagia
• Dysarthria
• Dysphonia
• Neck weakness
• Proximal limb weakness
• Respiratory weakness
• Generalized weakness

CAUSES
Humoral and cellular immune-mediated injury of the post-synaptic neuromuscular junction acetylcholine receptors

RISK FACTORS
• Female
• Age 20-40
• Familial myasthenia gravis
• D-penicillamine ingestion
• Other autoimmune diseases

DIAGNOSIS

DIFFERENTIAL DIAGNOSIS
• Oculopharyngeal muscular dystrophy
• Thyrotoxic ophthalmopathy
• Other disorders of neuromuscular transmission (myasthenic syndrome, botulism)
• Polymyositis
• Other myopathies
• Guillain-Barre syndrome
• Intracranial focal lesions involving cranial nerves
• Multiple sclerosis
• Depression
• Chronic fatigue syndrome

LABORATORY
• Acetylcholine receptor antibody - generalized myasthenia 80% positive; ocular myasthenia 50% positive; myasthenia + thymoma 100% positive; congenital myasthenia 0% positive; no clear correlation between antibody titer and disease severity
• Check thyroid function tests
Drugs that may alter lab results: N/A
Disorders that may alter lab results: N/A

PATHOLOGICAL FINDINGS
• Muscle electron microscopy - receptor infolding and the tips of the folds are lost, synaptic clefts are widened
• Immunofluorescence - IgG antibodies and complement on receptor membranes

SPECIAL TESTS
• Motor nerve conduction velocity - normal
• Sensory nerve conduction velocity - normal
• Concentric needle (conventional) electromyography- normal in mild cases; low amplitude, short duration, polyphasic motor unit potentials with a varying morphology (may be called "myopathic")
• Repetitive nerve stimulation - shows a decremental response at 3Hz which is seen more frequently in the proximal, cervical or facial muscles. The decrement is less pronounced 30 seconds after a 30 second maximal voluntary contraction (post-tetanic facilitation) and most pronounced 120 seconds after the contraction (post-tetanic depression).
• Single fiber EMG (SFEMG) - highly sensitive but less specific, technically difficult to perform, limited availability. SFEMG assesses the temporal variability between two muscle fibers within the same motor unit (jitter). Myasthenia is one condition that increases jitter.
• Edrophonium (Tensilon) test - initial dose is 2 mg IV, followed in 30 seconds by 3 mg, followed in 30 seconds by 5 mg to a maximum dose of 10 mg. A positive test is characterized by improvement of strength (of striated muscle) within 30 seconds of administration. False positives make a saline placebo control desirable. Atropine 0.4 mg IV may rarely be required as an antidote for severe bradycardia, but should always be available.

IMAGING Chest CT scan - thymoma

DIAGNOSTIC PROCEDURES
• History and physical
• Electrodiagnostic studies; repetitive nerve stimulation (RNS)
• Edrophonium (Tensilon) test

TREATMENT

APPROPRIATE HEALTH CARE
• Typically outpatient
• Inpatient care for plasmapheresis, intravenous gamma globulin, management of pulmonary infections, myasthenic or cholinergic crises

GENERAL MEASURES
• Management of myasthenia gravis is difficult and should be carried out by a neurologist with experience in the field.
• Three basic approaches to treatment, 1) being symptomatic, 2) being immunosuppressive and 3) being supportive. No or few patients should receive single therapeutic modality.
• Symptomatic therapy consists of reversal of weakness with an acetylcholinesterase inhibitor (eg pyridostigmine bromide; also available as slow release oral preparation), or neostigmine methylsulfate which can be administered parenterally. Symptomatic therapy does nothing to stop the ongoing immunologically mediated damage to the muscle receptor. An overdose of these agents may induce severe weakness known as a cholinergic crisis. Suspect cholinergic crisis if there are other signs of cholinergic overactivity (excessive secretions, diarrhea, bradycardia).
• Immunosuppressive or immunomodulatory therapy in some form is necessary. This includes thymectomy, corticosteroids, plasmapheresis, immunosuppressive drugs (azathioprine, cyclophosphamide, cyclosporine) and/or intravenous human gamma globulin.
• Supportive therapy may be intermittently or occasionally eventually continually required; may include intubation, tracheostomy, artificial ventilation, respiratory therapy, administration of antibiotics, nasogastric tube and/or gastrostomy

SURGICAL MEASURES N/A

ACTIVITY As tolerated. Heat and exercise both temporarily exacerbate symptoms.

DIET As tolerated

PATIENT EDUCATION Printed materials, reference lists and other forms of patient and family support available from:
1. Myasthenia Gravis Foundation, 2225 Riverside Plaza, #1540, Chicago, IL 60606, (800)541-5454
2. Muscular Dystrophy Association, 3300 E. Sunrise Drive, Tucson, AZ 85718-3208, (800)572-1717, (520)529-2000

MEDICATIONS

DRUG(S) OF CHOICE
• Pyridostigmine bromide (Mestinon), 60 mg tablets and 180 mg sustained release tablets. Titrate dosage to clinical need. An average requirement would be 600 mg per day.
• Neostigmine methylsulfate (Prostigmin), 0.25, 0.5 and 1 mg/mL concentrations. Titrate dosage to clinical need. Starting dosages would be 0.5 mg SC or IM every 3 hours.
• Prednisone should be initiated with a daily, followed by a switch to an alternate day, regimen. Start with a 60-80 mg/day, taper the dosage every 3 days. Switch to an alternate day regimen within 2 weeks, continue to taper very slowly attempting to establish the minimum dosage necessary to maintain remission. A typical maintenance dosage would be 35 mg every other day.
• Azathioprine or cyclophosphamide 150-200 mg per day.
• Immune globulin

Contraindications: Refer to manufacturer's literature

Precautions: Numerous. Avoid aminoglycosides and other drugs with potential for neuromuscular blockade which may precipitate weakness. Refer to manufacturer's literature.

Significant possible interactions: Numerous. Refer to manufacturer's literature.

ALTERNATIVE DRUGS Cyclosporine

FOLLOWUP

PATIENT MONITORING Constant in an intensive care unit setting during myasthenic or cholinergic crises

PREVENTION/AVOIDANCE Not possible

POSSIBLE COMPLICATIONS
• Acute respiratory arrest
• Chronic respiratory insufficiency
• Atelectasis, aspiration, pneumonia

EXPECTED COURSE/PROGNOSIS
Highly variable, ranging from remission to death. Mortality is probably less than 10%.

MISCELLANEOUS

ASSOCIATED CONDITIONS
• Thymoma
• Thymic hyperplasia
• Thyrotoxicosis
• Other autoimmune diseases

AGE-RELATED FACTORS
Pediatric: N/A
Geriatric: N/A
Others: Occurs in patients of all ages

PREGNANCY N/A

SYNONYMS N/A

ICD-9-CM 358.0 Myasthenia gravis

SEE ALSO N/A

OTHER NOTES N/A

ABBREVIATIONS
MG = myasthenia gravis

REFERENCES
• Rowland LP, ed: Merritt's textbook of Neurology. 9th Ed. Philadelphia, Williams & Wilkins, 1995
• Kimura J: Electrodiagnosis in diseases of nerve and muscle: principles and practice. 2nd Ed. Philadelphia, F.A. Davis, 1989
• Snead OC, Benton JW, Dwyer D, et al: Juvenile myasthenia gravis. Neurology 1980;30:732-739
• Soliven BC, Lang DJ, Penn AS, et al: Seronegative myasthenia gravis. Neurology 1988;38:514-517

Illustrations: N/A
Internet references: http://www.5mcc.com

Author(s)
Colin R. Bamford, MD

Myelodysplastic syndromes (MDS)

BASICS

DESCRIPTION A heterogeneous group of acquired hematopoietic stem cell disorders, characterized by cytologic dysplasia in the bone marrow and blood and by various combinations of anemia, neutropenia, and thrombocytopenia
• There is a natural progression of disease between categories as cellular maturation becomes more arrested and blast cells accumulate. There is a great deal of overlap between arbitrary diagnostic subgroups.
• Refractory anemia (RA) - < 5% blasts in marrow; < 1% blasts in blood
• Refractory anemia with ringed sideroblasts (RARS) - < 5% blasts in marrow; > 15% ringed sideroblasts; < 1% blasts in blood. Also known as acquired idiopathic sideroblastic anemia (AISA).
• Refractory anemia with excess of blasts (RAEB) - 5-20% blasts in marrow; < 5% blasts in blood. This category is now generally considered to be acute myeloid leukemia (AML).
• Refractory anemia with excess of blasts in transformation (RAEBT) - 20-30% blasts in marrow; or > 5% blasts in blood; or Auer rods present
• Chronic myelomonocytic anemia (CMMOL) - 1-20% blasts in marrow; < 5% blasts in blood with > 1000 monocytes/µl
• Refractory cytopenia - same as RA but with leukopenia or thrombocytopenia without anemia
• Refractory cytopenia with multilineage dysplasia (RCMD) - marked trilineage dysplasia but without excess of blasts
• Acute MDS with sclerosis - RAEB with marked myelosclerosis
• Refractory anemia with 5q minus syndrome - RA or RAEB with erythroid hyperplasia, mono- or bilobulated megakaryocyte nuclei and normal or increased platelets. Incidence is 2:1 female > male. Characteristic interstitial deletion on the long arm of chromosome 5.
• Therapy-related (t-MDS) - seen 3-7 years after treatment with alkylating agents and/or radiation therapy. Evolves to acute myeloid leukemia (AML) over about 6 months.
System(s) affected:
Hemic/Lymphatic/Immunologic
Genetics: Most are clearly clonal neoplasms by cytogenetics, G6PD isoenzyme analysis, or RFLP analysis. Mutations in RAS oncogene have been reported.
Incidence/Prevalence in USA: Apparent increased incidence (1-2/100,000/year) in recent years may be due to more accurate diagnosis
Predominant age: Median age is > 65 years; uncommon in children and young adults
Predominant sex: Male = Female

SIGNS AND SYMPTOMS
• Anemia - fatigue, shortness of breath, lightheadedness, angina
• Leukopenia - fever, infection
• Thrombocytopenia - ecchymoses, petechiae, epistaxis, purpura
• Splenomegaly - uncommon; mild to moderate enlargement may be encountered, particularly in CMMOL
• Skin infiltrates

CAUSES   Unknown

RISK FACTORS
• Primary MDS is associated with occupational exposure to petroleum solvents (benzene, gasoline)
• Secondary (therapy-related) MDS is associated with prior treatment with alkylating agents or radiation therapy

DIAGNOSIS

DIFFERENTIAL DIAGNOSIS
• Other malignant disorders - evolving acute myeloid leukemia (AML) or erythroleukemia; chronic myeloproliferative disorders (chronic myelogenous leukemia (CML), polycythemia vera, myeloid metaplasia with myelofibrosis); malignant lymphoma; metastatic carcinoma
• Nonmalignant disorders - aplastic anemia; autoimmune disorders (Felty's syndrome, lupus); nutritional deficiencies (pyridoxine, vitamin B12, protein malnutrition); heavy metal intoxication; alcoholism; chronic liver disease; hypersplenism; chronic inflammation; recent cytotoxic therapy or irradiation; HIV infection; paroxysmal nocturnal hemoglobinuria (PNH).

LABORATORY
• Anemia - often macrocytic; occasional poikilocytosis, anisocytosis; variable reticulocytosis
• Granulocytopenia - hypogranular or agranular neutrophils with poorly condensed chromatin. Pelger-Huet anomaly with hyposegmented nuclei.
• Thrombocytopenia - occasionally giant platelets or hypogranular platelets
• Fetal hemoglobin - increased in 70%
• Sugar water (Ham's) test - increased RBC membrane sensitivity to complement lysis in some
• Direct antiglobulin (Coombs) test - positive in some
• Paraprotein - present in some
• Erythropoietin - usually normal or physiologically compensated levels unless renal failure is present
Drugs that may alter lab results: N/A
Disorders that may alter lab results: N/A

PATHOLOGICAL FINDINGS
• Ineffective hematopoiesis with dysplasia in one or more cell lineages dominates the bone marrow picture in MDS. Marrow cellularity is usually normal or increased for the patient's age but may be hypoplastic in about 10%.

• Reticulin fibrosis is usually minimal except in therapy-related MDS
• Myeloblasts may be clustered in the intertrabecular spaces, abnormal localization of immature precursors (ALIP)

SPECIAL TESTS
• Cytogenetics - at least half of patients with primary MDS and nearly all with therapy-related MDS have clonal chromosomal abnormalities (+8,-7,-5, del(5q), del(7q), del(20q), iso(17), and complex karyotypes). Detection of such a clonal abnormality establishes a diagnosis of neoplasm and rules out a nutritional, toxic, or autoimmune etiology.
• Granulocyte function tests - abnormal in half (decreased myeloperoxidase activity, phagocytosis, chemotaxis, and adhesion)
• Platelet function tests - impaired aggregation
• Marrow colony assays in vitro - results variable and correlate poorly with clinical course. Poor clonal growth may suggest more rapid evolution to AML.
• Immunophenotyping - nonspecific myeloid markers present. Occasionally evidence can be found for concomitant lymphoproliferative disorder. Loss of CD59 expression suggests PNH.

IMAGING   Liver/spleen scan or CT although rarely necessary may disclose occult splenomegaly or lymphadenopathy

DIAGNOSTIC PROCEDURES
• Bone marrow aspiration, biopsy, and cytogenetics
• Review peripheral blood smear

TREATMENT

APPROPRIATE HEALTH CARE   Usually outpatient except when necessary to hospitalize for treatment of infection, blood transfusions, or intensive chemotherapy

GENERAL MEASURES
• Immunize for pneumococcal pneumonia and influenza and hepatitis B
• RBC transfusions to alleviate symptoms
• Platelet transfusions only for bleeding or prior to surgery, in order to avoid alloimmunization
• Early use of antibiotics for fever, even while culture results are pending, due to quantitative and qualitative granulocyte disorder
• Iron chelation therapy to avoid iron overload from chronic transfusions

SURGICAL MEASURES   N/A

ACTIVITY   As tolerated

DIET   Reduce alcohol use. Reduce iron intake.

PATIENT EDUCATION
• Stop smoking
• Seek early medical attention for fever, bleeding, or symptoms of anemia
• Advise about the risks of chronic transfusion therapy

Myelodysplastic syndromes (MDS)

MEDICATIONS

DRUG(S) OF CHOICE
• No medication has been proven more effective for these heterogeneous disorders than supportive care with antibiotics and transfusions as needed. Vitamins, iron, corticosteroids, androgens, or thyroid hormone are rarely helpful unless evidence of a specific deficiency exists.
• Clinical trials with 5-azacitidine, 75 mg/m2 SC for 7 days; repeated every 28 days, decreases RBC transfusion requirements and yields longer times to AML or death and improvements in quality of life.
• Intensive chemotherapy: younger patients with MDS may benefit from AML chemotherapy, especially if Auer rods are present, but toxicity may be severe for older patients. Remission durations are variable (median, about 1 year).
• Allogeneic bone marrow transplantation: recommended for younger patients with HLA-matched donors to eradicate the malignant clone and re-supply normal hematopoietic stem cells
• Aminocaproic acid (epsilon-aminocaproic acid, EACA) or tranexamic acid may benefit patients with chronic, severe thrombocytopenia and bleeding.
Contraindications: Cytotoxicity of chemotherapy may increase the risk of bleeding and infection and the need for transfusion support
Precautions: Aspirin, salicylates, and NSAID's should be avoided
Significant possible interactions: N/A

ALTERNATIVE DRUGS
• Possible differentiating agents such as tretinoin (all-trans-retinoic acid, ATRA); or homoharringtonine and other hematopoietic growth factors are under investigation
• Danazol or prednisone may benefit concomitant autoimmune thrombocytopenia
• Investigational agents: low doses of cytarabine or 5-azacitidine, 13-cis retinoic acid, interferon, cyclosporine, granulocyte-macrophage colony stimulating factor (GM-CSF) or granulocyte colony stimulating factor (G-CSF), interleukin-3 (IL-3)
• Agents that inhibit production of tumor necrosis factor in the marrow are being investigated
• Amifostine may stimulate proliferation of normal hematopoiesis
• Topotecan has been reported to have cytotoxic benefit in CMMOL

FOLLOWUP

PATIENT MONITORING
At least monthly during supportive care. More frequently if receiving treatment.

PREVENTION/AVOIDANCE   N/A

POSSIBLE COMPLICATIONS
Infection, bleeding, complications of anemia and transfusions

EXPECTED COURSE/PROGNOSIS
• Median survival for RA and RARS is 5 years but may extend much longer. Refractory anemia with 5q minus syndrome is quite favorable.
• Median survival for RAEB, RAEBT, and CMMOL is about 1 year with half of patients evolving to AML and the other half dying of infection or bleeding

MISCELLANEOUS

ASSOCIATED CONDITIONS   N/A

AGE-RELATED FACTORS
Pediatric: Monosomy 7 syndrome; juvenile chronic myelogenous leukemia
Geriatric: N/A
Others: N/A

PREGNANCY   N/A

SYNONYMS
• Dysmyelopoietic syndrome
• Hemopoietic dysplasia
• Preleukemia
• Smoldering or subacute myeloid leukemia
• CMMOL; Chronic myelomonocytic anemia
• CMML; Chronic myelomonocytic anemia

ICD-9-CM
238.7 Myelodysplastic syndrome

SEE ALSO   N/A

OTHER NOTES   N/A

ABBREVIATIONS
PNH = paroxysmal nocturnal hemoglobinuria

REFERENCES
• Hoffman R, Benz EJ Jr, Shattil S, et al, eds: Hematology: Basic Principles and Practice. New York, Churchill Livingstone, 1995
• Greenberg P, Cox C, Le Beau MM, et al: International scoring system for evaluating prognosis in myelodysplastic syndromes. Blood 1997;89:2079-2088
• Thirman MJ, Larson RA: Therapy-related myeloid leukemia. Hematology/Oncology Clin of NA 1996;10:293-320
Illustrations: N/A
Internet references: http://www.5mcc.com

Author(s)
Richard A. Larson, MD

Myeloproliferative disorders

BASICS

DESCRIPTION The myeloproliferative disorders are neoplasms of the pluripotent hematopoietic stem cell. They include chronic myelogenous leukemia (CML), polycythemia vera (PV), agnogenic myeloid metaplasia with myelofibrosis (AMM/MF), and essential thrombocytosis (ET). PV is discussed in another chapter.
• With each disorder, the proliferation of one particular cell line tends to dominate. There is a variable tendency for reactive proliferation of the bone marrow fibroblast, which is not a part of the malignant clone, resulting in myelofibrosis, and for termination in an acute blastic leukemia.
• CML
◊ Characterized by marked splenomegaly and increased granulocytes, particularly neutrophils
◊ Runs a generally mild course until it transforms to a frankly leukemic (blastic) phase
• AMM/MF
◊ Characterized by the tendency of the neoplastic cells to lodge and grow in multiple sites outside the marrow
◊ Myelofibrosis appears to be a reaction to the presence of the abnormal, proliferating hematopoietic clone
• ET
◊ Dominated clinically by a markedly elevated platelet count
System(s) affected:
Hemic/Lymphatic/Immunologic
Genetics:
• CML - no genetic predisposition known
• AMM/MF - rare familial occurrence
• ET - may be familial
Incidence/Prevalence in USA:
• CML - annual incidence 1-2/100,000; 1/5 of all leukemia cases; incidence increases with age
• AMM/MF - annual incidence 0.5/100,000
• ET - annual incidence 0.1/100,000
Predominant age:
• CML - median age at diagnosis is 45-50
• AMM/MF; ET - median age at diagnosis is 60; distinct second peak incidence of ET occurs in younger patients
Predominant sex:
• CML - Male > Female 1.7:1
• AMM/MF - Male > Female (slightly)
• ET - Female > Male 1.3:1

SIGNS AND SYMPTOMS
• General
◊ Most are asymptomatic at the time of diagnosis
◊ Vague constitutional symptoms
◊ Hypermetabolic state (fever, sweating)
◊ Acute gouty arthritis
◊ Left-upper-quadrant abdominal pain or fullness from splenomegaly

• CML
◊ Marked splenomegaly (palpable in 90% of patients)
• AMM/MF
◊ Splenomegaly in virtually all patients, and can be massive
◊ Hepatomegaly in 50%
◊ Lymph node enlargement in 10%
◊ Jaundice, edema, and ascites in 10-20%
◊ Petechiae in up to 25%
• ET
◊ Easy bruiseability, unusual bleeding after minor dental procedures, large-vessel bleeding in the absence of trauma
◊ Transient ischemic attacks, or even frank strokes, may occur in patients with markedly elevated platelet counts

CAUSES Unknown. May be familial for some types.

RISK FACTORS
• Family history of myeloproliferative disorder (rare)
• CML - increased incidence in atomic bomb survivors and following radiation treatment of ankylosing spondylitis and cervical cancer

DIAGNOSIS

DIFFERENTIAL DIAGNOSIS
• CML
◊ Low or absent leukocyte alkaline phosphatase (LAP) also seen in paroxysmal nocturnal hemoglobinuria, and occasional cases of myelodysplasia and AMM/MF
◊ Leukemoid reaction
• AMM/MF
◊ Hepatomegaly in the absence of splenomegaly is extremely rare in AMM/MF, and suggests secondary myeloid metaplasia
◊ Spent PV (late stage of PV)
◊ Secondary myelofibrosis
• ET
◊ Secondary thrombocytosis (including inflammation, iron deficiency, and neoplasia)

LABORATORY
• Basophilia
• Elevated serum vitamin B12 level
• Hyperuricemia
• CML
◊ Marked leukocytosis consisting of mature polymorphonuclear neutrophils and myelocytes or metamyelocytes
◊ Chronic phase typically with less than 5% myeloblasts in peripheral blood
◊ Blast crisis is defined when 30% or more blast cells are present in the bone marrow and/or peripheral blood
◊ Markedly decreased leukocyte alkaline phosphatase (absent in 5-10% of patients)
• AMM/MF
◊ Mild anemia - in more than 50% of patients at time of diagnosis, eventually in almost all patients, and is progressive
◊ Leukocytosis in 50% of patients (up to 50,000 leukocytes per mL, up to 10% blasts)
◊ Leukoerythroblastic blood picture
◊ Occasional RBC autoantibodies

• ET - the Polycythemia Vera Study group diagnostic criteria are:
◊ Thrombocytosis persistently greater than 600,000 per mL in the absence of an identifiable cause
◊ Normal total RBC mass
◊ Presence of iron in the bone marrow
◊ Absence of fibrosis in bone marrow biopsy
◊ Absence of the Philadelphia chromosome
Drugs that may alter lab results: N/A
Disorders that may alter lab results: In CML, LAP rises during infection, glucocorticoid use, or successful therapy. False positive hyperkalemia can be seen in ET due to release of platelet potassium upon blood clotting

PATHOLOGICAL FINDINGS
• AMM/MF
◊ Foci of extramedullary hematopoiesis seen in kidneys, lymph nodes, adrenal glands, and lungs
◊ Special stains of the bone marrow reveal increased reticulin deposition, even in hypercellular areas

SPECIAL TESTS
CML > 95% of patients are Philadelphia chromosome positive (shortened chromosome 22 due to a reciprocal translocation between chromosomes 22 and 9)

IMAGING
AMM/MF - radiographic osteosclerosis in 50% of patients, particularly in the axial skeleton and proximal long bones

DIAGNOSTIC PROCEDURES
• Peripheral blood smear
• Bone marrow aspiration
• Cytogenetic studies

TREATMENT

APPROPRIATE HEALTH CARE
Outpatient therapy. Inpatient for surgery when required.

GENERAL MEASURES
• Treatment to relieve symptoms and prevent infections
• Splenectomy has no impact on mortality, but is occasionally done for symptomatic relief. Extreme thrombocytosis, progressive and massive liver enlargement may ensue.
• CML
◊ Bone marrow transplantation is the only curative option, with disease-free survival in 50-70%, and should be offered to young patients with HLA matched donors
◊ Interferon alpha may produce hematologic remissions, and is appropriate for older patients and those without HLA-matched donors
◊ Hydroxyurea or an alkylating agent is used for controlling the excessive myelopoiesis in chronic phase disease
◊ Accelerated phase and blast crisis usually treated with regimens designed for the treatment of acute leukemia

- AMM/MF
  ◊ No definitive therapy
  ◊ Rule out other treatable causes for anemia
  ◊ Anemia is treated with transfusions as required
  ◊ Radiotherapy for localized bone pain, or symptomatic extramedullary hematopoietic tumors
  ◊ Successful bone marrow transplantation leads to the reversal of established fibrosis
- ET
  ◊ Young, asymptomatic patients generally not treated
  ◊ Lower the platelet count in those > 60, history of thrombosis, or with other cardiovascular risk factors

SURGICAL MEASURES See General Measures

ACTIVITY Restrictions will be dependent on symptoms and progression of the disorder

DIET
- Maintain good nutrition
- Small frequent meals, high-protein drinks
- Antacids as needed

PATIENT EDUCATION
- Explanations about the disorder, treatment protocols, lab studies, and prognosis
- Symptoms of recurrence to watch for
- Importance of followup examinations

MEDICATIONS

DRUG(S) OF CHOICE
- Hydroxyurea 20-30 mg/kg/day as a single daily dose, generally favored over alkylating agents in the control of leukocytosis or thrombocytosis, as it has little to no known leukemogenic potential
- Allopurinol to control hyperuricemia - begin prior to hydroxyurea therapy
Contraindications: ET - because platelet function is often defective, drugs such as salicylates that impair platelet function are generally avoided
Precautions: ET - prolonged administration of platelet-antiaggregating agents may increase the risk of gastrointestinal hemorrhage
Significant possible interactions: Toxicity (bone marrow depression) of cyclophosphamide (Cytoxan) increased by allopurinol

ALTERNATIVE DRUGS
- Interferon controls leukocytosis and thrombocytosis
- AMM/MF
  ◊ Androgens and glucocorticoids may improve anemia
  ◊ Corticosteroids if autoimmune hemolysis present

- ET
  ◊ Aspirin, with or without dipyridamole, may prove useful in preventing thrombotic or ischemic symptoms in some patients
  ◊ Erythromelalgia (described below) responds to rapid reduction of the platelet count or to administration of nonsteroidal anti-inflammatory agents
  ◊ Ticlopidine (Ticlid) or anagrelide (Agrelin), to inhibit platelets

FOLLOWUP

PATIENT MONITORING Individualized and dependent on therapy, ongoing studies, and stage of the illness

PREVENTION/AVOIDANCE N/A

POSSIBLE COMPLICATIONS
- Transformation to acute leukemia
- Gout due to hyperuricemia
- Uric acid nephropathy
- AMM/MF
  ◊ Portal hypertension
  ◊ Splenic infarcts
  ◊ Budd-Chiari syndrome
- ET
  ◊ Thrombohemorrhagic complications in one third
  ◊ Erythromelalgia (a vaso-occlusive syndrome with localized pain, burning, warmth of distal extremities - may progress to gangrene)

EXPECTED COURSE/PROGNOSIS
- CML
  ◊ In the 2 years following diagnosis, 10% of patients per year will develop into the accelerated phase or blast crisis. This rate then increases to 15-20% per year.
  ◊ Median survival > 5 years from the time of diagnosis, approximately 12-18 months after development of the accelerated phase, and 3 months after developing blast crisis
  ◊ Adverse prognostic factors include advanced age, large liver size, degree of splenomegaly, elevated platelet count, degree of leukocytosis, presence of blasts or of large numbers of eosinophils or basophils, percent of immature cells in the marrow, and clonal evolution
  ◊ 85% will die in blast crisis
- AMM/MF
  ◊ Progressive splenomegaly, anemia and thrombocytopenia
  ◊ Median survival is 5 years from the time of diagnosis, and 10 years from disease onset
  ◊ Usually die of hemorrhagic or thrombotic complications, 10% terminate in a rapidly progressive form of acute leukemia
  ◊ Adverse prognostic factors include platelet count less than 100,000 per mL, hemoglobin of less than 10 gm/dL, complex cytogenic abnormalities, and hepatomegaly
- ET
  ◊ Overall life expectancy only slightly shortened

MISCELLANEOUS

ASSOCIATED CONDITIONS AMM/MF - associations have been reported with systemic lupus erythematosus, periarteritis nodosa, scleroderma, and vasculitis

AGE-RELATED FACTORS
Pediatric: Rare in the young
Geriatric: These disorders more often found in middle and later years
Others: N/A

PREGNANCY
- CML
  ◊ Pregnancy does not affect the course of the disease
  ◊ Greater than 95% of mothers survive to delivery, with greater than 80% fetal survival rate through gestation
  ◊ Severe congenital defects have been reported with busulfan
- ET
  ◊ Increased risk of 1st trimester abortion. No need to treat if asymptomatic.

SYNONYMS N/A

ICD-9-CM
205.1 CML
289.8 AMM/MF
238.7 Myeloproliferative disease, chronic
238.7 Essential thrombocythemia

SEE ALSO
- Leukemia
- Polycythemia vera

OTHER NOTES N/A

ABBREVIATIONS
CML = chronic myelogenous leukemia, chronic myelocytic leukemia, chronic granulocytic leukemia
PV = polycythemia vera
AMM/MF = agnogenic myeloid metaplasia with myelofibrosis, idiopathic myelofibrosis
ET = essential (primary) thrombocythemia, hemorrhagic thrombocythemia

REFERENCES Doll DC, et al, eds: Myeloproliferative disorders. Seminars in Oncology 1995;22(4):305-411
Illustrations: N/A
Internet references: http://www.5mcc.com

Author(s)
Robert Dolin, MD

Myocardial infarction

BASICS

DESCRIPTION Acute myocardial infarction (AMI) is the rapid development of myocardial necrosis resulting from a sustained and complete reduction of blood flow to a portion of the myocardium, produced by a superimposed thrombosis, generated by a ruptured atherosclerotic plaque
• Clinical consequences - dependent on the size and location of the infarction and the rapidity with which blood flow can be re-established by pharmacologic or mechanical modalities
• After total occlusion myocardial necrosis is complete in 4-6 hours. Flow to ischemic area must remain above 40% of pre-occlusion levels for that area to survive.
• Infarctions can be divided into Q-wave and non Q-wave, with the former being transmural and associated with totally obstructed infarct-related artery and the latter being non-transmural and associated with patent, but highly narrowed infarct-related artery
• Total occlusion of the left main coronary artery which usually supplies 70% of the LV mass is catastrophic and results in death in minutes

System(s) affected: Cardiovascular
Genetics: N/A
Incidence/Prevalence in USA: 600/100,000
Predominant age: Over 40
Predominant sex:
• Age 40-70: Male > Female
• Over age 70: Male = Female

SIGNS AND SYMPTOMS
• Pain - arm, back, jaw, epigastrium, neck, chest
• Anxiety
• Lightheadedness, pallor, weakness, syncope
• Nausea, vomiting, diaphoresis
• Chest heaviness, tightness
• Cough, diaphoresis, dyspnea, rales, wheezing
• S4 heart sound
• Arrhythmias
• Hypertension, hypotension
• Jugular venous distention
• Cannon jugular venous A waves (in presence of heart block or right ventricular failure)

CAUSES
• Coronary thrombosis - most common cause due to ruptured plaque inducing platelet aggregation and then thrombosis has been identified as the initiating factor in most cases
• Coronary artery spasm
• Arteritis
• Embolic infarction
• Congenital coronary anomalies
• Oxygen supply - demand imbalance; carbon monoxide poisoning
• In situ thrombosis - hematologic in origin (e.g., polycythemia rubra vera)
• Cocaine-induced vasospasm

RISK FACTORS
• Hypercholesterolemia (increased LDL; decreased HDL)
• Premature (<55) familial onset of coronary disease
• Smoking
• Diabetes mellitus
• Hypertension
• Sedentary life style
• Aging
• Hostile, frustrated personality
• Hypertriglyceridemia

DIAGNOSIS

DIFFERENTIAL DIAGNOSIS
• Unstable angina pectoris - serial ECG and enzymes to differentiate
• Aortic dissection
• Pulmonary embolism
• Pericarditis - differentiated by history of postural improvement of pain and pleuritic component, plus presence of a pericardial friction rub and upward concave diffuse ST segment elevation on ECG
• Esophageal spasm - no ECG or enzyme elevations
• Pancreatitis and biliary tract disease

LABORATORY
• Troponin I has been shown to be a specific indicator of myocardial infarction. It appears 3-6 hours after MI, peaks at 16 hours and decreases in 9-10 days.
• Creatine kinase (CK): rises following infarction; beginning in 4-8 hours; peaking in 18-24 hours and subsiding over 3-4 days. Is a specific indicator for myocardial necrosis, but has a 15% false positive rate.
• CK isoenzymes: MM, MB, and BB forms identified with skeletal muscle, BB in brain and kidney, and MB in cardiac. Elevation of CK-MB in serum is diagnostic of myocardial infarction.
• LDH: rises above normal values within 24 hours of an acute MI and reaches a peak within 3-6 days and returns to baseline within 8-12 days. Can be used to date recent episode of acute MI well past the acute episode.
• ESR: rises above normal level within 3 days and may remain elevated for several weeks
• Leukocytes: rise within several hours after an MI, peak in 2-4 days, and are normal within 1 week

Drugs that may alter lab results: Refer to standard cardiology texts
Disorders that may alter lab results: Refer to standard cardiology texts

PATHOLOGICAL FINDINGS
• Myocardial necrosis
• Atherosclerosis, if etiologic
• Thrombosis; usually not seen because spontaneous thrombolysis occurs within 24 hours in most patients

SPECIAL TESTS
• Electrocardiography
  ◊ ST segment elevation in a regional pattern - typical of acute transmural ischemia
  ◊ ST segment depression with T-wave inversions - typical of subendocardial ischemia
  ◊ ST segment elevation and depression are early findings of myocardial ischemia. A significant percent of patients will have non-specific findings on presentation, such as peaked T-waves and ST-segment elevation less than 0.1 mv. A small percentage of patients, with transmural infarction, present with normal ECG.
  ◊ Q-waves representing transmural myocardial necrosis appear with 24-48 hours
• Echocardiography
  ◊ 2D and M-mode echocardiography useful in evaluating wall motion abnormalities in MI and overall left ventricular function
  ◊ Useful in delineating and assessing mechanical complications

IMAGING
• Chest x-ray
  ◊ Findings dependent on severity of MI
• Radionuclide studies
  ◊ Thallium scanning. Accumulates in viable myocardium.
  ◊ Technetium-99 gated blood pool scanning-noninvasive means of measuring ventricular function. Accumulates in recently infarcted myocardium.

DIAGNOSTIC PROCEDURES
Angiography prior to procedures to re-establish coronary perfusion

TREATMENT

APPROPRIATE HEALTH CARE
Inpatient coronary care unit

GENERAL MEASURES
• General
  ◊ Analgesia, prevention and treatment of electrical and mechanical complications, limitation of infarct size, and salvage of myocardium
• Arrhythmias
  ◊ Ventricular tachycardia: DC countershock, lidocaine, procainamide (Pronestyl), or IV cordarone
  ◊ Ventricular fibrillation: DC countershock and CPR/IV cordarone
  ◊ Atrial flutter and fibrillation: digitalis or IV diltiazem (Cardizem) or verapamil. If hemodynamic compromise - DC countershock or rapid atrial pacing.
  ◊ Sinus bradycardia: no treatment unless accompanied by hypotension or hemodynamic compromise. Then treat with atropine and if ineffective, electrical pacing.
  ◊ Atrioventricular block: in inferior infarction requires transvenous pacing if patient hemodynamically compromised. In anterior infarction, pacing usually required as escape rhythm is unstable with ventricular asystole occurring quite suddenly.

SURGICAL MEASURES
- Coronary reperfusion
  ◊ Emergency percutaneous transluminal angioplasty (PTCA) or stenting - mechanical form of coronary reperfusion. Recent studies suggest this technique may be superior to intravenous thrombolysis if initiated within first hour.
  ◊ Emergency surgical reperfusion - can be accomplished with low mortality. Must be carried out within 4 hours of beginning of the event. Many consider this treatment to be rarely indicated.
- Pump failure
  ◊ Intra-aortic balloon counter pulsation
  ◊ PTCA/stenting

ACTIVITY
- Bedrest for first 24 hours; bedside commode
- Medically supervised rehabilitation plan

DIET
Nothing by mouth until stable; later, low fat, low salt diet

PATIENT EDUCATION
Printed patient information available from: American Heart Association, 7320 Greenville Avenue, Dallas, TX 75231, (214)373-6300

MEDICATIONS

DRUG(S) OF CHOICE
- Coronary reperfusion
  ◊ Alteplase (tissue plasminogen activator, TPA, Activase). 15 mg IV bolus, 50 mg over 30 minutes, then 35 mg over 60 minutes.
  ◊ Heparin by standard or weight-adjusted protocol
  ◊ Aspirin 325 mg po acutely
- Acute MI, general
  ◊ Nitrates 5 μg/min IV, increase slowly. Do not lower arterial blood pressure beyond 90 mm Hg. Change to oral or topical when patient stable.
  ◊ Lidocaine 1-2 mg/kg once, then 1-4 mg/min. Use for ventricular arrhythmias only. Do not expect arrhythmia prophylaxis.
  ◊ Oxygen (2-4 L/minute)
  ◊ Oxazepam 10 mg po or lorazepam 0.5 mg IV, if needed for sedation every 4-6 hours
  ◊ Morphine 2-6 mg IV q2-4h prn pain/sedation
  ◊ Metoprolol (Lopressor) 5 mg IV x 3, 2 minutes apart followed by 50 mg po q6h starting 15 minutes after past IV dose
  ◊ Stool softeners - milk of magnesia, docusate sodium (dioctyl sodium sulfosuccinate) 100 mg bid, etc. to avoid straining and constipation secondary to immobility and narcotic use
- Post MI
  ◊ Beta-blockers reduce mortality
  ◊ Nitrates may be needed for angina
  ◊ ACE inhibitors prevent adverse remodeling, may improve longevity

Contraindications:
- Beta-blockers relatively contraindicated in CHF or incipient heart failure and bronchospasm. May use IV esmolol (Brevibloc), a short acting beta blocker, if uncertain.
- IV thrombolysis (TPA/Streptokinase) contraindicated in patients with active internal hemorrhage; recent head trauma, intracranial neoplasm, hemorrhagic CVA; pregnancy; persistent hypertension (>200/120); prolonged (>10 minutes) or traumatic CPR; diabetic hemorrhagic retinopathy; severe trauma or major surgery within 2 weeks; calcium channel blockers, especially with LV dysfunction

Precautions:
- Use IV thrombolysis (TPA/Streptokinase) cautiously in patients with active peptic ulcer or heme positive stools; known bleeding disorders or current use of anticoagulants; uncontrolled hypertension; prior exposure to Streptokinase or Streptococcal infection in last 6 months; Trauma or major surgery within 2 months

Significant possible interactions: N/A

ALTERNATIVE DRUGS
- Thrombolytics
  ◊ Streptokinase: produces systemic lytic effect in addition to local thrombolysis. Less costly then TPA. 1.5 million units in 50 cc D5W given over 60 minutes.
- Beta-blockers for acute arrhythmia
  ◊ Atenolol 5 mg IV over 5 minutes. Follow with a second dose 10 minutes later. Follow with 50 mg po in 10 minutes after the 2nd IV dose. Then q12h for at least 7 days.

FOLLOWUP

PATIENT MONITORING
Determined by needs of patient

PREVENTION/AVOIDANCE
- Avoid risk factors
- Aspirin 81 mg/day may be helpful

POSSIBLE COMPLICATIONS
- Congestive heart failure
- Cardiogenic shock
- Myocardial rupture
- Left ventricular aneurysm
- Left ventricular thrombus and peripheral embolism
- Deep venous thrombosis and pulmonary embolism
- Pericarditis
- Dysrhythmias
- Mitral regurgitation
- Ventricular septal defect
- Dressler's syndrome
- Cardiac arrest
- Death

EXPECTED COURSE/PROGNOSIS
- Overall mortality rate is 10% during the hospital phase with an additional 10% mortality rate during the year after. More than 60% of the deaths occur within one hour of the onset of the event.
- Killip classification
  I - No CHF; mortality rate <5%
  II - Mild-Moderate CHF (bibasilar rales and/or S3 gallop); mortality rate 10%
  III - Severe CHF (rales over greater than 50% lung fields, S3 gallop, pulmonary edema); mortality rate 30%
  IV - Cardiogenic shock BP <90 mm Hg (<12 kPa) with hypoperfusion, e.g., oliguria, confusion, clammy skin; mortality rate >80%

MISCELLANEOUS

ASSOCIATED CONDITIONS
- Abdominal aortic aneurysm
- Extracranial cerebrovascular disease
- Atherosclerotic peripheral vascular disease

AGE-RELATED FACTORS
Pediatric: N/A
Geriatric: All incidences of complications are higher
Others: N/A

PREGNANCY
N/A

SYNONYMS
- Coronary thrombosis
- Coronary occlusion
- Heart attack

ICD-9-CM
410.0 Acute myocardial infarction of anterolateral wall
410.9 Acute myocardial infarction, unspecified site

SEE ALSO
- Ventricular tachycardia (VT)
- Ventricular standstill
- Congestive heart failure

OTHER NOTES
N/A

ABBREVIATIONS
CHF = congestive heart failure

REFERENCES
- Braunwald E: Heart Disease. 4th Ed. Philadelphia, W. B. Saunders Co., 1992
- Harvey AM: The Principles and Practice of Medicine. 22nd Ed. Norwalk, CT, Appleton & Lange, 1988
Illustrations: N/A
Internet references: http://www.5mcc.com

Author(s)
Phil Lobstein, MD

Narcolepsy

BASICS

DESCRIPTION A disorder of unknown etiology characterized by excessive sleepiness typically associated with cataplexy and other REM sleep phenomena, such as sleep paralysis and hypnogogic hallucinations. Commonly misconceived as representing low intelligence and/or poor motivation. The syndrome is frequently overlooked with an average of 15 years of symptoms prior to diagnosis. Onset is usually in teenage years.

System(s) affected: Nervous

Genetics:
• Inherited dominant with incomplete penetrance
• 60 fold increased incidence in families with positive history
• Incidence in first degree relative of index case is 30%
• Biologic marker HLA-DR2 allele on short arm of chromosome 6 in 100% of Caucasian patients; 1/3 normal subjects are also positive. 30% of black narcoleptic patients are non DR 2, but all with HLA-Dw1.

Incidence/Prevalence in USA: 1 in 3000 diagnosed

Predominant age: Mean age onset 18, 50% after age 40

Predominant sex: Male = Female

SIGNS AND SYMPTOMS
• Tetrad: 10-20% with all symptoms
• All with excessive daytime sleepiness (EDS)
• Sleep attacks - primary symptom, most severe form of EDS
  ◊ Instantaneous, irresistible REM sleep
  ◊ First and most disabling symptom
  ◊ Satisfied by naps lasting 5-10 minutes
  ◊ Lasts minutes to hours
  ◊ 1-8 naps per day, 24 hour duration of sleep normal
  ◊ Increased in monotonous environment, warm environment, after a large meal, or with strong emotions
  ◊ 20-25% of all patients with excessive somnolence
• Cataplexy (70%) auxiliary symptom
  ◊ Sudden bilateral weakness of skeletal muscles
  ◊ Provocation by sudden strong wave of emotion
  ◊ Lack of impairment of consciousness and memory
  ◊ Short duration (less than a few minutes)
  ◊ Responsiveness to treatment with clomipramine and imipramine
  ◊ Can be limited to a particular muscle group, e.g., jaw droop with inability to speak; arm, neck or leg weakness

• Sleep paralysis - auxiliary symptom (33%)
  ◊ When falling asleep or on awakening the patient wants to move but cannot
  ◊ The brain wakes from sleep while the body remains in REM sleep
  ◊ Lasts seconds to minutes
  ◊ Patients are aware of events around them, but cannot open eyes or move
  ◊ Can be preceded by hallucinatory phenomena
  ◊ 50% of normal population have at least one episode (nonspecific)
• Hypnagogic hallucinations - auxiliary symptom (33%)
  ◊ Vivid, frightening auditory or visual illusions or hallucinations at onset of sleep
  ◊ Dream-like experiences that occur during wakefulness or suddenly at sleep onset
  ◊ Characteristic hallucinations include seeing human or animal faces or feeling that someone else is in the room
• Disturbed nocturnal sleep (66%)
  ◊ Normal total sleep with decreased sleep efficiency
  ◊ More frequent transitions from wakefulness to sleep
  ◊ Retrograde amnesic and automatic behavior lasting minutes to hours
  ◊ Increased periodic leg movements (50%)

CAUSES
• Unknown
• Possible involvement of the immune system
• Widespread under-release of dopamine and a brainstem-specific proliferation of acetylcholine receptors and hypersensitivity to acetylcholine

RISK FACTORS
• Head trauma
• CNS infectious disease
• Anesthesia
• Family history

DIAGNOSIS

DIFFERENTIAL DIAGNOSIS
EDS present in 4% of population, most are not narcolepsy, causes include:
• Sleep apnea syndromes - 40-50% of those with excessive somnolence
• Epileptic seizures and syncope
• Idiopathic CNS hypersomnolence - 5-10% of those with excessive somnolence
• Nocturnal myoclonus
• Psychomotor seizures
• Abuse of sedative drugs
• Clinical diagnosis possible if cataplexy present

LABORATORY HLA-DR2
Drugs that may alter lab results: N/A
Disorders that may alter lab results: N/A

PATHOLOGICAL FINDINGS N/A

SPECIAL TESTS
• Nighttime polysomnography - monitoring of patients in a sleep laboratory will usually document fragmented sleep with a normal amount of REM sleep but a pattern of sleep onset REM. Polysomnography rules out other causes of excessive daytime sleepiness including sleep apnea syndromes and nocturnal myoclonus.
• Multiple sleep latency test (MSLT) - begins at least 90 minutes after nighttime test. Patient is monitored during 4-5 naps taken at two-hour intervals. The rapidity of sleep onset and type of sleep pattern are documented. A supportive test includes a mean sleep latency (time to fall asleep) of five minutes or less and at least two sleep-onset REM periods. Sensitivity 77%, specificity 97%, PPV 73%.
• HLA typing in ambiguous cases

IMAGING N/A

DIAGNOSTIC PROCEDURES
• REM periods during MSLT
• Diagnostic criteria - B and C, or A and D and E and G
A. Excessive sleepiness
B. Recurrent lapses into sleep daily for ≥ 3 months
C. Cataplexy
D. Associated features: sleep paralysis, hypnagogic hallucinations, disrupted sleep
E. Multiple sleep latency test abnormalities as described
F. Biologic markers (see Genetics)
G. Absence of medical or psychiatric disorder

TREATMENT

APPROPRIATE HEALTH CARE
Inpatient for sleep laboratory analysis, outpatient for followup

GENERAL MEASURES
• Usually managed with medication
• Regularly scheduled time for naps may help in mild cases

SURGICAL MEASURES N/A

ACTIVITY Exercise can sometimes decrease the number of sleep attacks. Seek to achieve optimal physical fitness.

DIET No special diet, avoid alcohol

PATIENT EDUCATION
• Symptoms can spontaneously improve or worsen
• The American Narcolepsy Association, P.O. Box 1187, San Carlos, CA 94070, (800)327-6085

MEDICATIONS

DRUG(S) OF CHOICE
• Recommended drugs either block norepinephrine uptake or cause central anticholinergic effects
• Excessive daytime sleepiness - stimulants that increase levels of daytime alertness:
 ◊ Methylphenidate (Ritalin) initial dose 30 mg/day divided 2-3/day; maximum dose 100 mg/day
 ◊ Pemoline (Cylert) - longer half life 8-10 hours; initial dose 37.5 mg/day divided AM and noon; maximum dose 150 mg/day. Monitor liver function studies 4 weeks after start and then once a year.
 ◊ Dextroamphetamine initial dose 15 mg/day divided 2-3/day; maximum dose 100 mg/day
 ◊ Combination of long and short acting - pemoline plus single or multiple doses of methylphenidate
 ◊ Modafinil (Provigil) 200 or 400 mg/day. structually distinct from amphetamines
• For auxiliary symptoms (cataplexy, hypnagogic hallucination, sleep paralysis) - tricyclic antidepressants suppress REM sleep. Imipramine 75-150 mg/day, protriptyline 10-40 mg/day, fluoxetine 20-60 mg/day, clomipramine 150-250 mg/day.
Contraindications: Stimulants in hypertensive patients
Precautions:
• If patient develops tolerance to stimulants, switch drugs rather than increasing the dose - there is little cross-tolerance
• Patient may develop tolerance to the anticataplectic effect of tricyclic antidepressants and can get a rebound in cataplexy when withdrawn
• Stimulants - headaches, irritability, hypertension, psychosis, anorexia, habituation
• Pemoline - less cardiovascular side effects, longer acting, liver toxicity, little abuse potential
• Imipramine - dry mouth, sedation, urinary retention, impotence
Significant possible interactions:
Combination of tricyclic antidepressants and stimulants can lead to significant hypertension

ALTERNATIVE DRUGS
• Selegiline - selective MAO-B inhibitor
 ◊ 20-40 mg/day divided AM and noon
 ◊ Anticatapletic and effective for excessive daytime sleepiness
 ◊ Doses > 20 mg must be on low tyramine diet since it begins to lose selectivity
• Excessive daytime sleepiness:
 ◊ Propranolol 280-480 mg/day, good for patients during withdrawal from stimulants or patients with hypertension
 ◊ Dextroamphetamines 5-60 mg/day
 ◊ L-Tyrosine 64-120 mg/day
• Ancillary symptoms
 ◊ Gamma-hydroxybutyrate 5.25-6.75 g during sleep, has little effect on sleep architecture of REM sleep but increases slow-wave sleep. Also has mild effect on excessive daytime sleepiness without tolerance development. Gamma-hydroxybutyrate can increase sleep walking by increasing slow-wave sleep.
 ◊ Codeine 150 mg/day
 ◊ Triazolam 0.25 mg improves nocturnal sleep quality

FOLLOWUP

PATIENT MONITORING
• Frequent blood pressure checks
• Followup every 6 months

PREVENTION/AVOIDANCE N/A

POSSIBLE COMPLICATIONS N/A

EXPECTED COURSE/PROGNOSIS
• Life-long disease
• Symptoms can worsen with aging
• In women, symptoms can improve after menopause

MISCELLANEOUS

ASSOCIATED CONDITIONS Obstructive sleep apnea

AGE-RELATED FACTORS
Pediatric: Uncommon syndrome of childhood
Geriatric: Symptoms worsen with aging
Others: N/A

PREGNANCY N/A

SYNONYMS N/A

ICD-9-CM
347 Cataplexy and narcolepsy

SEE ALSO
• Sleep apnea, obstructive

OTHER NOTES N/A

ABBREVIATIONS
• REM = rapid eye movement
• MSLT = multiple sleep latency test

REFERENCES
• Mitler M, Hajdukovic R, et al: Narcolepsy. Journal of Clinical Neurophysiology 1990;7(1):93-118
• Scharf M, Fletcher K, et al: Current Pharmacologic Management of Narcolepsy. AFP 1988;38(1):143-148
• Nahmias J, Karetzky M: Current Concepts in Narcolepsy. New Jersey Medicine 1989;86:617-622
• Chaudhary B, Husain I: Narcolepsy. Jour Fam Prac 1993;36(2);207-213
• Standards of Practice Committee of the American Sleep Disorders Association: Practice parameters for the use of stimulants in the treatment of narcolepsy. Sleep 1994;17(4):348-351
• Parkes JD, Clift SJ, Dahlitz MJ: The narcoleptic syndrome. J of Psychiatry 1995;59(3):221-224
• Green P, Stillman M: Signs, symptoms, differential diagnosis, and management of narcolepsy. Arch Fam Med 1998;7:472-478
Illustrations: N/A
Internet references: http://www.5mcc.com

Author(s)
Jeffrey F. Minteer, MD

Near drowning

BASICS

DESCRIPTION Multisystem, potentially fatal disease, resulting from near suffocation secondary to submersion of a person's face or head. Approximately 10% of drowned patients die without actually aspirating. Most near drowning victims do not aspirate large volumes of fluid.
System(s) affected: Pulmonary, Nervous, Cardiovascular
Genetics: N/A
Incidence/Prevalence in USA:
• 8500 deaths yearly; 90,000 near-drowning victims
• Drowning is the 4th leading cause of accidental death in the United States
Predominant age: Teenagers and toddlers
Predominant sex: Male > Female

SIGNS AND SYMPTOMS
• Altered level of consciousness or comatose
• Absent or thready pulse
• Tachypnea or agonal respirations
• Cyanosis
• Wheezing
• Hypothermia
• Poorly reactive, dilated and fixed pupils
• Poor peripheral perfusion

CAUSES
• Swimming accidents
• Hyperventilation before underwater swimming
• Boating mishaps
• Motor vehicle accidents (i.e., auto submerged in water)
• Suicide
• Drug overdose (including alcohol)

RISK FACTORS
• Low socioeconomic class
• Alcohol
• Seizure disorder
• Inability to swim
• Improper pool fencing
• Inadequate adult supervision of children
• Cardiac arrhythmias
• Living in sunbelt states

DIAGNOSIS

DIFFERENTIAL DIAGNOSIS The submersion may have resulted from loss of consciousness and accidentally falling into water because of another medical condition (i.e., head trauma, arrhythmia, seizure, etc.)

LABORATORY
• Salt water
  ◊ Hypoxemia
  ◊ Hypercarbia
  ◊ Hypokalemia
  ◊ Mixed acidosis
  ◊ Slight increase in serum sodium
  ◊ Normal or minimally increased Hb
  ◊ Rare albuminuria
  ◊ Rare oliguria
  ◊ Rare hemoglobinuria
  ◊ Hypovolemia possibly, or hypervolemia
• Fresh water
  ◊ Hypoxemia
  ◊ Hypercarbia
  ◊ Hypokalemia
  ◊ Mixed acidosis
  ◊ Slight decrease in serum sodium
  ◊ Normal or slightly decreased Hb
  ◊ Albuminuria rarely
  ◊ Oliguria rarely
  ◊ Rare hemoglobinuria
  ◊ Evidence of hemolysis
Drugs that may alter lab results: N/A
Disorders that may alter lab results: Any underlying condition that may alter normal fluid and electrolyte balance (i.e., congestive heart failure) or alter normal pulmonary function (i.e., emphysema)

PATHOLOGICAL FINDINGS
• "Dry lungs" 10% of time
• Loss of normal pulmonary architecture (fresh water). Alveolar consolidations, collapse, hyaline membrane formation.
• Increased lung weight and intra-alveolar hemorrhages (salt water)
• Lung hyperexpansion
• Pneumonia, abscess and adult respiratory distress (ARDS) in those who survive only a few hours or days
• Renal - acute tubular necrosis
• Neurologic - cerebral edema

SPECIAL TESTS
• Lung compliance (reduced)
• Central venous pressure monitoring
• ECG
• EEG
• Calculation of V/Q mismatch, shunt, $AaDO_2$

IMAGING Chest x-ray may show pulmonary edema, consolidation from aspiration, atelectasis or pneumothorax

DIAGNOSTIC PROCEDURES N/A

TREATMENT

APPROPRIATE HEALTH CARE
Hospitalize all patients initially. Monitor patients in an Intensive Care setting except for those few who present to the emergency room in an alert condition without evidence of respiratory compromise. The incidence of delayed drowning is 5%. Therefore all patients who have had a significant submersion accident should be hospitalized for 24-48 hours.

GENERAL MEASURES
• Begin resuscitation at the scene. Remove from water quickly and place in normal CPR position.
• Supplemental oxygen
• Positive airway pressure - positive end-expiratory pressure (PEEP) or continuous positive airway pressure (CPAP) for persistent hypoxia
• Avoid abdominal thrust unless airway obstruction is present
• Monitor pH and adjust bicarbonate administration accordingly
• Monitor arterial oxygenation
• Avoid steroids
• Avoid prophylactic antibiotics
• Hyperventilate patient (keep $PaCO_2$ 25-30 mm HG)

SURGICAL MEASURES N/A

ACTIVITY Bedrest for at least the initial 24 hours

DIET N/A

PATIENT EDUCATION Proper water safety techniques may help to avoid this problem

MEDICATIONS

DRUG(S) OF CHOICE
• All patients: Oxygen
• Unconscious patient without known pH: Sodium bicarbonate - 1.0 mEq/kg (1.0 mmol/kg)
• For bronchospasm: Aerosolized bronchodilator - albuterol (Proventil, Ventolin) 3cc of 0.083% solution OR 0.5mL of 0.5% solution diluted in 3cc saline
• Patients who develop pneumonia: Appropriate antibiotic based on sputum or endotracheal lavage culture
• Fresh water drowning patients with hemolysis: Transfusion may be necessary
• Prophylactic antibiotics and steroids are not helpful
Contraindications: Refer to manufacturer's profile of each drug
Precautions: Refer to manufacturer's profile of each drug
Significant possible interactions: Refer to manufacturer's profile of each drug

ALTERNATIVE DRUGS
• For bronchospasm
◊ Aerosolized bronchodilator - metaproterenol (Alupent) 0.3 mL in 3 mL normal saline
◊ Aminophylline

FOLLOWUP

PATIENT MONITORING
• Frequent check of vital signs
• Arterial blood gas monitoring
• Pulmonary artery catheter may be needed for hemodynamic monitoring
• Pulse oximeter for oxygen saturation trending
• Intracranial pressure monitoring in selected patients
• Serial chest x-rays
• Serum electrolyte determinations

PREVENTION/AVOIDANCE
• Proper adult supervision of children
• Knowledge of water safety guidelines
• Mandatory pool fencing
• Avoidance of alcohol or recreational drugs around water
• Swimming instruction at an early age
• Boating safety knowledge
• Personal flotation device (life preserver if necessary)

POSSIBLE COMPLICATIONS
• Prolonged neurologic sequelae
• Fear of water
• Pneumonitis/lung abscess
• Secondary drowning
• Adult respiratory distress syndrome

EXPECTED COURSE/PROGNOSIS
• Patients who are alert or mildly obtunded at the time they present to the hospital have an excellent chance for a full recovery
• Patients who are comatose or receiving CPR at the time of presentation or who have dilated and fixed pupils and no spontaneous respiratory activity have a more guarded and often poor prognosis

MISCELLANEOUS

ASSOCIATED CONDITIONS
• Cardiopulmonary arrest before the submersion
• Trauma, especially to the head causing altered mental status
• Seizure disorder
• Alcohol or drug overdose

AGE-RELATED FACTORS
Pediatric: Children frequently don't swim well
Geriatric: N/A
Others:
• Adolescents - may be intoxicated or using drugs
• Adults - most near-drownings are associated with boating accidents with or without alcohol

PREGNANCY N/A

SYNONYMS N/A

ICD-9-CM
994.1 Drowning and nonfatal submersion
518.5 Pulmonary insufficiency following trauma and surgery

SEE ALSO
• Respiratory distress syndrome, adult

OTHER NOTES Accomplished swimmers may drown by hyperventilation before prolonged underwater swimming or by becoming fatigued following a particularly strenuous or long swim. Approximately 10% of victims drown without aspiration.

ABBREVIATIONS N/A

REFERENCES
• Wintemute G: Childhood Drowning and Near-Drowning in the United States. AJDC 1990;144:663
• Modell J, Graves S, Ketover A: Clinical Course of 91 Consecutive Near-Drowning Victims. Chest 1976;70:231
Illustrations: N/A
Internet references: http://www.5mcc.com

Author(s)
Alan J. Cropp, MD, FCCP

Nephropathy, urate

BASICS

DESCRIPTION Renal parenchymal damage and dysfunction associated with disordered uric acid metabolism. Several syndromes can present.
• Gout: Acute urate crystal-induced arthritis related to chronic hyperuricemia due to uric acid renal underexcretion in 80-90% and uric acid overproduction in 10-20%.
• Hyperuricemic acute renal failure: Precipitated by distal tubular obstruction resulting from acute massive overproduction of uric acid due to cell lysis. Serum uric acid usually greater than 15-20 mg/dL (0.88-1.18 mmol/L).
• Uric acid nephrolithiasis: Most commonly seen in gouty patients who are uric acid overproducers and have hyperuricosuria. Frequency of stone formation increases with increasing serum uric acid levels and urinary uric acid excretion rates. About 22% of gouty patients will form uric acid stones.
• Hyperuricemia of chronic renal failure: Occurs when creatinine clearance less than 15. Serum uric acid usually greater than 10 mg/dL. Secondary gout rare. Acute deterioration of renal function can be precipitated by an abrupt rise in serum uric acid.
• Chronic urate nephropathy: Renal insufficiency attributed to parenchymal damage secondary to medullary urate deposition. Bulk of evidence supports conclusion that typical gout or asymptomatic hyperuricemia are unlikely to lead to serious renal insufficiency. In patients with gout, renal insufficiency can usually be attributed to a complicating medical condition, most often hypertension, diabetes, renal vascular disease, obstructive uropathy, urinary tract infection or lead intoxication.
System(s) affected: Renal/Urologic
Genetics: N/A
Incidence/Prevalence in USA: Gout 0.3%, Hyperuricemia 5-10%
Predominant age: Adults
Predominant sex: Male > Female

SIGNS AND SYMPTOMS
• Hyperuricemic acute renal failure
  ◊ Precipitated by chemotherapy for leukemia or lymphoma
  ◊ Precipitated by heat stress and exercise
  ◊ Oliguria
  ◊ Anuria
  ◊ Anorexia, nausea, vomiting, encephalopathy and other manifestations of uremia
  ◊ Hypertension
  ◊ Anemia
  ◊ Dehydration
• Uric acid nephrolithiasis
  ◊ Flank pain
  ◊ Groin pain
  ◊ Micro or gross hematuria
  ◊ Anorexia
  ◊ Nausea
  ◊ Vomiting
  ◊ Dehydration

• Hyperuricemia of chronic renal failure
  ◊ Established chronic renal failure with glomerular filtration rate (GFR) less than 15-20
  ◊ Serum uric acid greater than 10 mg/dL chronically
  ◊ Intercurrent cause of abrupt increase in serum uric acid
  ◊ Acute decrease in GFR
  ◊ Acute onset of uremic symptoms

CAUSES
• Primary
  ◊ Congenital gout, hypertension and hyperuricemia (autosomal dominant)
  ◊ Congenital HGPRT deficiency (X-linked recessive)
  ◊ Congenital PRPP overactivity (X-linked recessive)
  ◊ Congenital glycogen storage disease, type I
• Secondary
  ◊ Lead intoxication
  ◊ Diuretics
  ◊ Cytotoxic chemotherapy in leukemia or lymphoma
  ◊ Heat stress and exercise
  ◊ Diabetic ketoacidosis
  ◊ Starvation ketosis
  ◊ Chronic myeloproliferative disease
  ◊ Psoriasis

RISK FACTORS
• Sudden increase in uric acid load
• Dehydration
• Urine pH less than 5
• Hypertension
• Diabetes mellitus
• Renal insufficiency
• Renal vascular disease

DIAGNOSIS

DIFFERENTIAL DIAGNOSIS Other causes of acute renal failure, other causes of nephrolithiasis, other causes of chronic renal failure

LABORATORY
• Gout and hyperuricemia
  ◊ Hyperuricemia
  ◊ Hyperuricosuria in 10-20%
  ◊ Decreased urinary ammonia production
• Hyperuricemic acute renal failure
  ◊ Serum uric acid greater than 15-20 mg/dL (0.88-1.18 mmol/L)
  ◊ Rising BUN and creatinine
  ◊ Urinary uric acid to creatinine ratio > 1
  ◊ Uric acid crystals in urine
• Uric acid nephrolithiasis
  ◊ Uric acid crystals in urine
  ◊ Urinary uric acid greater than 600-700 mg (3.54-4.13 mmol) per 24 hours (hyperuricosuria) on purine-free diet
  ◊ Hyperuricemia
  ◊ Microhematuria
  ◊ Pyuria
  ◊ Positive urine culture
  ◊ Stone composition uric acid or mixed uric acid and calcium oxalate or calcium phosphate

• Hyperuricemia of chronic renal failure
  ◊ Acute exacerbation of hyperuricemia with serum uric acid greater than 10 mg/dL (0.59 mmol/L)
  ◊ Acute on chronic BUN and creatinine elevations
Drugs that may alter lab results: N/A
Disorders that may alter lab results: N/A

PATHOLOGICAL FINDINGS
• Renal tophi-medullary monosodium urate deposits with inflammatory reaction and interstitial fibrosis
• Poor correlation between severity of renal pathology and severity of gout
• Tubulointerstitial nephritis with obstruction, recurrent infection or lead intoxication

SPECIAL TESTS Stone analysis

IMAGING
• IVP
• Renal ultrasound

DIAGNOSTIC PROCEDURES
• Cystoscopy and retrograde pyelography
• Renal biopsy

TREATMENT

APPROPRIATE HEALTH CARE
Outpatient except for complicated nephrolithiasis and hyperuricemic acute renal failure

GENERAL MEASURES
• Hydration to increase urine output
• Normalize serum uric acid
• Normalize renal uric acid excretion
• Decrease uric acid production
• Maintain urine pH greater than 6
• Antibiotic treatment of urinary tract infection
• Hyperuricemic acute renal failure:
  ◊ IV hydration
  ◊ Hemodialysis

SURGICAL MEASURES Uric acid nephrolithiasis: Cystoscopic or surgical stone removal for persistent ureteral obstruction

ACTIVITY Limited during attacks of acute gouty arthritis

DIET
• Purine restriction
• Protein restriction
• For nephrolithiasis, fluid intake adequate to produce urine output at least 2 L per day unless urine output is limited by acute or chronic renal failure
• In acute renal failure restrict sodium for hypertension and potassium for hyperkalemia

PATIENT EDUCATION Griffith, H.W.: Instructions for Patients. Philadelphia, W.B. Saunders Co., 1994

MEDICATIONS

DRUG(S) OF CHOICE
• Gout and hyperuricemia
  ◊ Uricosuric agent - probenecid (Benemid) starting with 250 mg bid and doubling 7-10 day intervals up to 500-1000 mg bid (maximum 3 gm/day)
  ◊ Xanthine oxidase inhibitor preferred for hyperuricosuria - allopurinol (Zyloprim) 200-300 mg/day.
  ◊ Treatment of symptomatic or asymptomatic hyperuricemia with uric acid-lowering drugs has no apparent favorable or adverse effect with respect to development of renal insufficiency
• Hyperuricemic acute renal failure
  ◊ Prevent by pretreating with allopurinol and hydrating patient prior to administration of chemotherapeutic agents for leukemia or lymphoma
    ◊ Loop diuretic
    ◊ IV alkalinizing solution
• Uric acid nephrolithiasis
  ◊ Allopurinol 200-300 mg/day
  ◊ Alkali to maintain urine pH 6.0-6.5 - sodium bicarbonate or potassium citrate-citric acid 0.5-1.5 mEq/kg in 5 or 6 divided doses
• Hyperuricemia of chronic renal failure
  ◊ Allopurinol in patients with prior history of gout
Contraindications: Avoid uricosuric agents in patients with hyperuricosuria, uric acid nephrolithiasis or chronic renal failure
Precautions:
• Avoid abrupt decreases or increases in serum uric acid, which may precipitate acute gouty arthritis
• Administer colchicine 0.5-0.65 mg/day 1-4 times/week concomitantly with allopurinol first 2-3 months to prevent precipitation of acute gouty arthritis
Significant possible interactions:
Phenylbutazone, diflunisal, aspirin (1-2 gm/day), radio-contrast agents, glyceryl guaiacolate, pyrazinamide, ethambutol, ethanol, diuretics, ascorbic acid (high dose), nicotinic acid

ALTERNATIVE DRUGS
Sulfinpyrazone (Anturane)

FOLLOWUP

PATIENT MONITORING
• Serum uric acid, urinary uric acid excretion, BUN and/or serum creatinine at least twice a year
• Blood pressure screening at least once a year

PREVENTION/AVOIDANCE
• Appropriate pretreatment prior to chemotherapy of leukemia or lymphoma
• Avoid factors that can cause abrupt or persistent increases of serum uric acid or urinary uric acid excretion
• Prompt treatment of urinary obstruction or infection
• Control blood pressure in hypertensives

POSSIBLE COMPLICATIONS
• Gout and hyperuricemia
  ◊ No apparent renal complications
• Hyperuricemic acute renal failure
  ◊ Irreversible renal failure (end-stage renal disease)
  ◊ Residual renal insufficiency
  ◊ Persistent renal tubular functional defects
• Uric acid nephrolithiasis
  ◊ Urinary obstruction
  ◊ Urinary infection
  ◊ Renal insufficiency
• Hyperuricemia of chronic renal failure
  ◊ Progression to end-stage renal failure

EXPECTED COURSE/PROGNOSIS
• With effective drug therapy and general management prognosis is excellent in patients with gout, hyperuricemia, or nephrolithiasis
• Development or progression of renal insufficiency should not occur unless due to underlying renal disease or associated medical conditions with adverse renal effects

MISCELLANEOUS

ASSOCIATED CONDITIONS
• Hypertension
• Diabetes mellitus

AGE-RELATED FACTORS
Pediatric: Gout and uric acid nephrolithiasis may have onset in infancy or childhood with HGPRT deficiency or PRPP overactivity
Geriatric: Renal insufficiency more likely due to age and associated medical conditions
Others: N/A

PREGNANCY Women with nephrolithiasis have a slightly higher incidence of urinary tract infection, but no increase in stone formation rate

SYNONYMS N/A

ICD-9-CM
274.10 Gouty nephropathy
274.11 Uric acid nephrolithiasis

SEE ALSO N/A

OTHER NOTES N/A

ABBREVIATIONS N/A

REFERENCES
• Jacobson HR, Striker GE, Klahr S, eds: The Principles and Practice of Nephrology. Philadelphia, B.C. Decker, Inc., 1995
• Brenner B, Rector F: The Kidney.5th Ed. Philadelphia, W.B. Saunders Co., 1995
• Puig JG, et al: Hereditary nephropathy associated with hyperuricemia and gout. Arch Int Med 1993;153:357
Illustrations: N/A
Internet references: http://www.5mcc.com

Author(s)
Donald F. Eipper, MD

Nephrotic syndrome

BASICS

DESCRIPTION
A syndrome comprising glomerular proteinuria (3.5 g per 1.73m2 body-surface area/day), hypoalbuminemia, lipiduria, hypercholesterolemia and edema as a result of a primary renal disease or secondary to another disease process.
System(s) affected: Renal/Urologic, Endocrine/Metabolic
Genetics: N/A
Incidence/Prevalence in USA:
• Children - 2:100,000 new cases/year
• Adults - 3:100,000 new cases/year
Predominant age:
• Children - 1.5-6 years (MCD)
• Adults - all ages (FGS, MGN more common USA; IgG-IgA worldwide)
Predominant sex: Male = Female

SIGNS AND SYMPTOMS
• Fluid retention: abdominal distention, ascites, edema, puffy eyelids, scrotal swelling, weight gain, shortness of breath
• Anorexia
• Hypertension
• Oliguria
• Orthostatic hypotension
• Retinal sheen
• Skin striae

CAUSES
• Primary renal disease
  ◊ Fibrillary glomerulopathy (primary)
  ◊ Focal glomerulonephritis
  ◊ Focal glomerulosclerosis (FGS)
  ◊ IgA nephropathy
  ◊ Membranoproliferative glomerulonephritis (MPGN)
  ◊ Membranous glomerulonephritis (MGN)
  ◊ Mesangial proliferative glomerulonephritis
  ◊ Minimal change disease (MCD)
  ◊ Rapidly progressive glomerulonephritis (RPGN)
  ◊ Congenital nephrotic syndrome
• Secondary renal disease. Associated primary renal disease shown in brackets:
  ◊ Allergens (snake venoms, antitoxins, poison ivy, insect stings)
  ◊ Carcinoma (bronchogenic, breast, colon, stomach, kidney) [MGN, etc]
  ◊ Diabetes mellitus (most common)
  ◊ Erythema multiforme
  ◊ Fibrillary glomerulopathy (secondary: amyloid, cryoglobulins, multiple myeloma, chronic lymphocytic leukemia [CLL]
  ◊ Schönlein-Henoch purpura
  ◊ Heredofamilial (Alport's syndrome, Fabry's disease)
  ◊ HIV infection
  ◊ Hodgkin's lymphoma [MCD]
  ◊ Infections: ventriculo atrial shunt infection, bacterial endocarditis [MPGN], viral (hepatitis B [MPGN, mesangial, MGN]) other viral (hepatitis C), protozoal and helminthic

  ◊ Leukemias
  ◊ Lymphomas [MGN]
  ◊ Non-Hodgkin's lymphoma
  ◊ Focal glomerulosclerosis (reflux nephropathy, heroin abuse, nephron ablation, extensive glomerular scarring in acute glomerulonephritis, chronic renal allograft rejection, end stage kidney, morbid obesity, a thromboembolism)
  ◊ Malignant hypertension
  ◊ Melanoma
  ◊ Nephrotoxins and drugs (gold penicillamine, mercury [MGN])
  ◊ Nonsteroidal anti-inflammatory drug induced nephrotic syndrome [MCD] and interstitial nephritis.
  ◊ Polyarteritis nodosa
  ◊ Post streptococcal glomerulonephritis [PSGN] - 20% are nephrotic
  ◊ Sarcoid
  ◊ Serum sickness
  ◊ Sjögren's syndrome
  ◊ Systemic lupus erythematosus (SLE) [MGN, FGS, focal, mesangial, diffuse, proliferative]
  ◊ Toxemia of pregnancy

RISK FACTORS
• Drug addiction (e.g. heroin [FGS])
• Hepatitis B and C, HIV, other infections
• Immunosuppression
• Nephrotoxic drugs
• Vesicoureteral reflux (FGS)
• Cancer (usually MGN, may be nil disease (MCD)
• Chronic analgesic abuse

DIAGNOSIS

DIFFERENTIAL DIAGNOSIS See Causes.
Is the disease predominantly nephrotic (protein without hematuria) such as MCD or MGN; or predominantly nephritic (protein plus blood) such as MPGN or FGS?

LABORATORY
• Hypoalbuminemia
• Hyperlipidemia
• Lipiduria
• Low complement in some diseases
• Azotemia
• Hypercholesterolemia
• Increased serum beta-globulin
• Increased serum IgG
• Urine
  ◊ Proteinuria (> 3 gm/24 hr)
  ◊ Glycosuria
  ◊ Hematuria
  ◊ Aminoaciduria
  ◊ RBC casts
  ◊ Granular casts
  ◊ Proteinuria
  ◊ Hyaline casts
  ◊ Fatty casts
  ◊ Foamy appearance
Drugs that may alter lab results: See description
Disorders that may alter lab results: Many

PATHOLOGICAL FINDINGS
• Light microscopy
  ◊ May see nothing (e.g., MCD)
  ◊ Disease specific: sclerosis (e.g., FGS in diabetes)
• Immunofluorescence: Mesangial IgA (Schönlein-Henoch, IgG-IgA nephropathy). Other specific for disease.
• Electron microscopy (specific for disease as in sub-epithelial deposits of IgG in MGN)

SPECIAL TESTS
• Complement levels
• Antinuclear antibody
• Serum protein electrophoresis/quantitative immunoglobulins
• Urine immune electrophoresis
• Blood cultures
• Renal venogram for thrombosis

IMAGING
• X-ray
• Ultrasound
• CT
• MRI or venography for renal vein thrombosis

DIAGNOSTIC PROCEDURES   History, physical, basic laboratory including electrolytes, renal biopsy with light, immunofluorescence, electron microscopy for definitive diagnosis

TREATMENT

APPROPRIATE HEALTH CARE
Outpatient

GENERAL MEASURES
• Treat infections vigorously (especially bacteriuria, endocarditis, peritonitis)
• Anticoagulant (heparin and warfarin) if thromboses occur
• Vaccines: Pneumococcal, influenza and H. influenzae
• Avoid excess sunlight
• Avoid nephrotoxic drugs
• Judicious use of diuretics
• Severe anemia may be treated with erythropoietin
• Pneumococcal vaccine

SURGICAL MEASURES   N/A

ACTIVITY   Bedrest as tolerated

DIET
• Normal protein (1 g/kg/day)
• Low fat (cholesterol)
• Reduced sodium
• Liberal potassium (unless hyperkalemic)
• Supplemental multivitamins and minerals, especially D and iron
• Fluid restriction if hyponatremic
• Caloric restriction if obese or diabetic
• Hypercholesterolemia - low fat soy-protein diet, 7 g protein/kg/day

PATIENT EDUCATION
• Printed material for patients: National Kidney Foundation, 30 E. 33rd Street, Suite 1100, NY, NY 10016, (800)622-9010
◊ "Childhood Nephrotic Syndrome" (Order #02-23NN)
◊ "Diabetes and Kidney Disease" (Order #02-09CP) and "Focal Glomerulosclerosis" (Order #02-28NN)

MEDICATIONS

DRUG(S) OF CHOICE
• Treat underlying disorder (use decision analysis)
• For steroid-responsive disease: MCD and FGS
◊ Adults-MCD: prednisone 1.0-1.5 mg/kg/day for 4-6 weeks. After response, continue steroid for 2 additional weeks, then shift to maintenance dose of 2-3 mg/kg q od for 4 weeks. Taper to zero during the next 4-6 months, or 120 mg po qod same duration, same period of taper. FGS all adults should receive 3-4 months of glucocorticoids and a cumulative dose of 6 gm of prednisolone.
◊ Children: prednisone 60 mg/m2 or 2 mg/kg/day orally for 4 weeks. After response, continue steroid for 2 additional weeks, then shift to maintenance dose of 2-3 mg/kg q od for 4 weeks. Taper to zero during the next four months.
• MGN patients with a poor prognosis: persistent, heavy proteinuria > 8 gm/day for > 6 months; elevated serum creatinine; hypertension; male sex; over age 50 or have a biopsy with sclerosis. Probably benefit from cytotoxic therapy (chlorambucil or cyclophosphamide [Cytoxan]). For hepatitis B virus glomular disease - interferon.
• For edema
◊ Most importantly salt restriction; then judicious thiazide, loop diuretics
◊ If resistant, a combination of loop and distal diluting segment diuretics, e.g., metolazone (Zaroxolyn) are synergistic
◊ It is possible that furosemide (Lasix) and albumin mixed and given IV may potentiate diuresis (eg, 150 mg furosemide plus 25 gm human serum albumin). Be wary of possible thromboses (especially renal vein thrombosis).
• Other nephrotic renal diseases: frequently relapsing MCD, RPGN, ?MGN, SLE
◊ Bolus steroids and/or immune suppression (cyclophosphamide, chlorambucil, cyclosporine)
◊ Consultation often required
• Hypercholesterolemia
◊ Diet and cholesterol lowering drugs (cholestyramine and/or HMG-CoA reductase inhibitors)
◊ Anticoagulants (heparin, followed by warfarin) for thrombotic events. There is data to suggest prophylactic oral anticoagulation in all cases of membranous GN (Kid Int. 1994;45:578-585).

◊ Hypocalcemia from vitamin D loss should be treated with oral vitamin D (dihydrotachysterol) 0.2 mg q day
◊ ACE inhibitors to reduce proteinuria even in normotensive patients and to control hypertension if also present
Contraindications: See manufacturer's literature
Precautions: See manufacturer's literature
Significant possible interactions: See manufacturer's literature

ALTERNATIVE DRUGS   N/A

FOLLOWUP

PATIENT MONITORING   Frequent monitoring for azotemia, hypertension, edema, nephrotoxicity, serum cholesterol, weight

PREVENTION/AVOIDANCE
• Avoid causative factors whenever possible
• Detect and treat infections vigorously. Infections may involve the common (Pneumococcus) to the unusual (Strongyloides), especially with immunosuppression.

POSSIBLE COMPLICATIONS
• Low levels of: 25-hydroxycholecalciferol, serum calcium, adrenocortical hormones, thyroid hormones
• Hypercoagulability, thrombosis
• Pulmonary emboli
• Hyperlipidemia/accelerated cardiovascular disease
• Acute renal failure
• Progressive renal failure
• Renal vein thrombosis
• Protein malnutrition
• Infection
• Pleural effusion
• Ascites
• Iron deficiency (uncommon)

EXPECTED COURSE/PROGNOSIS
Varies with specific causes. Complete remission expected if basic disease is treatable (infection, malignancy, drug-induced). Otherwise may progress to dialysis dependence (e.g., diabetic glomerulosclerosis).

MISCELLANEOUS

ASSOCIATED CONDITIONS
• Cancer
• Diabetes mellitus
• Connective tissue disease (e.g., SLE)
• Multiple myeloma

AGE-RELATED FACTORS
Pediatric: Relatively common in children aged 1.5-4 years (MCD)
Geriatric: Occurs in this age group. Prognosis is worse.
Others: N/A

PREGNANCY   Toxemia of pregnancy may be nephrotic

SYNONYMS   N/A

ICD-9-CM
581.9 Nephrotic syndrome with unspecified lesion in kidney

SEE ALSO
• Renal failure, acute (ARF)
• Renal failure, chronic
• Diabetes mellitus, Type 1
• Diabetes mellitus, Type 2
• Multiple myeloma
• Systemic lupus erythematosus (SLE)
• Endocarditis, infective (part 1)
• Amyloidosis
• Breast cancer
• Colorectal malignancy
• HIV infection & AIDS
• Glomerulonephritis, acute
• Sjögren's syndrome

OTHER NOTES   N/A

ABBREVIATIONS
• FGS = focal segmental glomerulosclerosis
• MGN = membranous nephropathy
• MPGN = chronic hypocomplementemic glomerulonephritis, chronic mesangiocapillary glomerulonephritis
• MCD = lipid nephrosis, four process disease, nil disease
• RPGN = crescentic glomerulonephritis

REFERENCES
• Klein M, Radhakrishnan J, Appel G: Cyclosporine treatment of glomerular diseases. ANN Rev Med 1999;50:1-15
• Eddy AA, Schnaper HW: The nephrotic syndrome: from the simple to the complex. Semin in Nephrol 1998;18:304-326
• Cameron JS: Nephrotic syndrome in the elderly. Sem in Nephrol 1996;16:319-329
• Glassock RJ: Management of intractable edema in nephrotic syndrome. Kid Int Suppl 1997;58:S75-79
• Gansevoort RT, Vaziri NO, de Jong PE: Treatment of nephrotic syndrome with recombinant erythropoietin. Am J Kid Dis 1996;28:274-277
• Schnaper HW: Primary nephrotic syndrome of childhood. Curr Opin Pediatr 1996;8:141-147
• Orth SR, Ritz E: The nephrotic syndrome. NEJM 1998;338:1202-1211
Illustrations: N/A
Internet references: http://www.5mcc.com

Author(s)
Jonathan Maks, MD
Gregory W. Rutecki, MD

Neuroblastoma

BASICS

DESCRIPTION A neoplasm of neural crest origin which may arise anywhere along the sympathetic ganglion chain or in the adrenal medulla. The most common tumor in children less than 1 year of age in the USA.
System(s) affected: Nervous, Endocrine/Metabolic
Genetics:
• Familial cases reported
• Genetic abnormalities in 80%
• Deletions in short arm of chromosome 1p36
• Amplification of n-myc oncogene occurs on chromosome 2 (poor prognostic sign)
Incidence/Prevalence in USA: 27.8 cases/million children/year for 1st five years of life in USA; 8.7 cases/million in children/year for 1st 15 years of life in USA; Denmark: 1/12,000 - 14,000 live births; Japan: 1/15,000-18,749 infants
Predominant age:
• 90% occur in 1st 8 years of life
• 60% occur in < 2 years of age
• Most common intra-abdominal malignancy in the newborn
Predominant sex: Slightly more common in boys than girls(1.2:1)

SIGNS AND SYMPTOMS
• 50-60% present with metastatic disease
• Abdominal mass (50-75%)
• Weight loss
• Anemia
• Failure to thrive
• Abdominal pain and distension
• Bone pain
• Fever
• Diarrhea
• Hypertension (25%)
• Horner's syndrome (ptosis, miosis, enophthalmos, heterochromia of iris)
• Orbital ecchymosis (panda eyes)
• Respiratory distress
• Dysphagia
• Paraplegia
• Cauda equina syndrome
• Flushing, sweating, irritability
• Cerebellar ataxia (chaotic nystagmus): dancing eye syndrome

CAUSES
• Genetic abnormalities in 80% of cases

RISK FACTORS
• Beckwith-Wiedemann syndrome
• Pancreatic islet cell dysplasia
• Maternal phenytoin treatment
• Fetal alcohol syndrome
• Hirschsprung's disease

DIAGNOSIS

DIFFERENTIAL DIAGNOSIS
• Rhabdomyosarcoma
• Wilms' tumors
• Other tumors of neck, chest, abdomen and pelvis
• Hydronephrosis

LABORATORY
• CBC, platelet count
• Liver function studies
• Renal function studies
• Urinary catecholamines
• Uric acid
• Creatinine
• Magnesium, calcium
• LDH
• Electrolytes
• Bilirubin, SGOT, SGPT
• Gd2 monoclonal antibody levels
• Serum neuron-specific enolase
• Serum ferritin
• Bone marrow aspiration
• Assay for VIP
Drugs that may alter lab results: N/A
Disorders that may alter lab results: N/A

PATHOLOGICAL FINDINGS
• Small, dark, round cells
• Immature tumors tend to be large, red, lobular soft, friable
• Mature tumors are fibrous, contain calcification, hemorrhage, necrosis, cysts, rosettes, nerve filaments
• May be neuroblastoma, ganglioneuroblastoma, or benign neuroblastoma (depends on cell maturity)
• Favorable histology (Shimada): Stroma-rich, well-differentiated and intermixed tumors
• Unfavorable histology (Shimada): Stroma-rich nodular and stroma-poor, undifferentiated tumors
• Staging (Evans)
  ◊ I - confined to single organ, completely resected
  ◊ II - Extends beyond organ of origin but does not cross midline
  ◊ III - Extends across midline
  ◊ IV -Distant metastases
  ◊ IV-S - Infants under I year with metastases to liver, skin or bone marrow, sparing cortical bone
• Amplification of n-myc oncogene (poor prognosis)
• Normal DNA ploidy - worse prognosis than hyperploidy

SPECIAL TESTS N/A

IMAGING
• Chest x-ray
• Skeletal survey (including orbital views)
• Bone scan
• CT or MRI of neck, chest, abdomen or pelvis (depending on location of tumor)
• Myelogram for neurologic symptoms

DIAGNOSTIC PROCEDURES
• Myelogram if needed
• Bone marrow aspiration

TREATMENT

APPROPRIATE HEALTH CARE
Inpatient workup and treatment until stable and induction chemotherapy completed

GENERAL MEASURES
• Radiation therapy in Stage III over 1 year of age
• Chemotherapy for stage II and greater

SURGICAL MEASURES
• Surgical resection may be complete, incomplete or biopsy only (for Stage I, excision only)
• If resection incomplete or biopsy, chemotherapy followed by 2nd look operation
• Dumbbell extension through vertebral foramina, chemotherapy alone vs. laminectomy and decompression
• Stage IV-S: resection of primary tumor and chemotherapy
• Bone marrow transplantation considered in stages III & IV

ACTIVITY As tolerated

DIET No special diet

PATIENT EDUCATION
• Patient and family teaching regarding long term outlook
• Possibility of second malignancy
• Side effects of treatment

MEDICATIONS

DRUG(S) OF CHOICE
- Cyclophosphamide
- Melphalan
- Vincristine
- Dacarbazine
- Teniposide
- Etoposide
- Doxorubicin (Adriamycin)
- Cisplatin
- Peptichemio
- Carboplatin
- Ifosfamide [with mesna to protect against hemorrhagic cystitis]

Contraindications: See manufacturer's information

Precautions: See manufacturer's information

Significant possible interactions: See manufacturers information

ALTERNATIVE DRUGS
- By protocol
- Ondansetron (Zofran), dronabinol (Marinol), metoclopramide (Reglan), and others for nausea control

FOLLOWUP

PATIENT MONITORING
- Multi-agent chemotherapy every 3-4 weeks for 4 courses then re-evaluate with bone marrow or second look operation
- Follow every 3 months for 1st year, every 4 months for 2nd year, every 6 months for 3rd year, then at least yearly
- Follow with CT or MRI every 3-6 months initially, then yearly

PREVENTION/AVOIDANCE   N/A

POSSIBLE COMPLICATIONS
- Nausea, vomiting
- Alopecia
- Bone marrow depression
- Immunosuppression
- Hemorrhagic cystitis
- Azotemia
- Diarrhea
- ADH secretion
- Local tissue necrosis
- Myocardiopathy
- Renal toxicity
- Hearing loss
- Hypocalcemia, hypomagnesemia

EXPECTED COURSE/PROGNOSIS
- Overall survival 55%
- Stage I - expected survival approximates 100%
- Stage II - Survival 75%
- Stage III - Survival 43%
- Stage IV - Survival 15%
- Stage IV-S - Survival 70-80%
- Normal DNA ploidy, n-myc amplifications, unfavorable histology indicates worse than usual prognosis for same tumor
- Infants under 1 year of age have better outcome
- Patients with cervical, pelvic, and mediastinal tumors have better prognosis than those with retroperitoneal, paraspinal or adrenal tumors
- Survival for those presenting with opsoclonus and nystagmus is nearly 90% (seen especially in mediastinal tumors in infants under 1 year of age)

MISCELLANEOUS

ASSOCIATED CONDITIONS   See Risk factors

AGE-RELATED FACTORS
Pediatric: Occurs only in children
Geriatric: N/A
Others: N/A

PREGNANCY   N/A

SYNONYMS   N/A

ICD-9-CM
194.0 Malignant neoplasm of adrenal medulla
171.8 Malignant pelvo-abdominal neoplasm
195.1 Thoracic neoplasm
173.4 Cervical neoplasm

SEE ALSO   N/A

OTHER NOTES   N/A

ABBREVIATIONS   N/A

REFERENCES
- Ashcraft KW, Holder TM: Pediatric Surgery. 2nd Ed. Philadelphia, W.B. Saunders Co., 1993
- Grosfeld JL, Rscorla F, West KW, Goldman J: Neuroblastoma in the First Year of Life: Clinical and Biologic Factors Influencing Outcome. Seminars in Pediatric Surgery 1993;2(1):37-46
- O'Neill JA, Rowe MI, Grosfeld JL, et al: Pediatric Surgery. 5th ed., St Louis, Mosby, 1998
- Matthay KK: Neuroblastoma: A clinical challenge and biological puzzle. CA Cancer Jour Clin 1995;45:179-182
Illustrations: N/A
Internet references: http://www.5mcc.com

Author(s)
Timothy L. Black, MD, FACS, FAAP

Neurodermatitis

BASICS

DESCRIPTION   A chronic dermatitis resulting from continued, repeated rubbing or scratching part of the skin
System(s) affected: Skin/Exocrine
Genetics: None known
Incidence/Prevalence in USA: Common
Predominant Age: May occur in any age
Predominant sex: Female > Male

SIGNS AND SYMPTOMS
• Gradual onset
• Lichenified, pruritic, scaly patch on any part of the body
• Accentuation of normal skin lines
• Surface often excoriated
• Vesicles or weeping are rare
• Non-erythematous
• Postinflammatory hypopigmentation or hyperpigmentation may be present
• Scarring is rare except after serious secondary infections
• Most commonly involves nape of neck, lower legs, ankles, wrist, extensor surface of forearms, scalp, external ear or anogenital region
• Nuchal and suboccipital regions more commonly affected in women
• Perineal region more commonly affected in men

CAUSES
• Idiopathic in many instances
• Some causes of apparent idiopathic disease may be secondary to a previously unrecognized dermatosis
• Secondary forms may begin as another pruritic skin disease which evolves into neurodermatitis after resolution of the primary dermatitis
• Primary dermatoses from which neurodermatitis may develop include lichen planus, stasis dermatitis, atopic dermatitis, tinea corporis, seborrheic dermatitis, xerosis and eczema
• Social stress or obsessive-compulsive personality trait may play a role in development of this disease

RISK FACTORS
• Any pre-existing pruritic dermatosis as noted above
• Obsessive-compulsive personality/anxiety
• Exposure to irritants

DIAGNOSIS

DIFFERENTIAL DIAGNOSIS
• Atopic dermatitis
• Contact dermatitis
• Cutaneous T-cell lymphoma
• Drug reaction
• Lichen planus
• Lichenified psoriasis
• Photodermatitis
• Stasis dermatitis
• Cutaneous amyloidosis
• Fungal infections
• Seborrheic dermatitis

LABORATORY   None diagnostic
Drugs that may alter lab results: N/A
Disorders that may alter lab results: N/A

PATHOLOGICAL FINDINGS   Thickening of all skin layers with minimal cellular infiltration is noted on skin biopsy

SPECIAL TESTS   None

IMAGING   N/A

DIAGNOSTIC PROCEDURES   Skin biopsy

TREATMENT

APPROPRIATE HEALTH CARE
Outpatient management

GENERAL MEASURES
• Treat pruritis to interrupt the scratch-itch cycle
• Occlusive dressings to prevent rubbing/scratching may be beneficial
• Nail trimming

SURGICAL MEASURES   N/A

ACTIVITY   As tolerated. Encourage exercise in those cases where stress may play a role.

DIET   Regular

PATIENT EDUCATION
• Patients should understand the cause of this disease and their role in helping resolve the condition
• Various stress reduction techniques can also be used in those patients in whom stress plays a significant role

MEDICATIONS

DRUG(S) OF CHOICE
• Topical steroids
◊ High potency steroids alone, such as 0.05% betamethasone dipropionate cream or 0.05% clobetasol propionate cream can be used initially, but these should not be used on the face, anogenital region, or intertriginous areas. They should be used on small areas only , and for no longer than two weeks.
◊ An intermediate potency steroid such as 0.1% triamcinolone cream may be used initially under an occlusive dressing for one to two weeks instead
◊ Switch to intermediate or low potency steroids alone as response allows
◊ An intermediate potency steroid, such as 0.025% or 0.1% triamcinolone cream may be used for initial treatment of the face and intertriginous areas and for maintenance treatment of other areas. A low potency steroid, such as 1% hydrocortisone cream should be used for maintenance treatment of the face and intertriginous areas.
• Steroid tape (Cordran)
◊ Optimized penetration
◊ Provides some barrier to further trauma
Contraindications: High potency topical steroids are contraindicated for use on the face and intertriginous areas
Precautions: Topical and intralesional steroid therapy can cause epidermal and dermal atrophy as well as hypopigmentation
Significant possible interactions: N/A

ALTERNATIVE DRUGS
• Tar preparations are useful but cosmetically less appealing
• Menthol 0.25% solution can help relieve pruritis
• Oral antihistamines can be used for both their antipruritic and sedative effects
• In extreme cases, a short tapering course of oral prednisone could be considered
• Intralesional corticosteroids
• Capsaicin
• Anxiolytics or tricyclic antidepressants (e.g., lorazepam or amitriptyline)
• Topical doxepin cream
• Una boot as barrier protection
• Cold Burow's solution compresses

 FOLLOWUP

PATIENT MONITORING Patients should be followed closely and regularly for response to therapy and for development of complications from therapy

PREVENTION/AVOIDANCE Avoid known pruritic substances/exposure

POSSIBLE COMPLICATIONS
• Secondary infection
• Complications related to therapy, as mentioned

EXPECTED COURSE/PROGNOSIS
Often runs a chronic course, however, the prognosis is good for those patients in whom the scratch-itch cycle can be broken. After healing, the skin should have a normal appearance unless secondary infection has occurred.

 MISCELLANEOUS

ASSOCIATED CONDITIONS Prurigo nodularis is a nodular variety of the same disease process

AGE-RELATED FACTORS
Pediatric: Rare in pre-adolescents
Geriatric: N/A
Others: N/A

PREGNANCY N/A

SYNONYMS
• Lichen simplex chronicus

ICD-9-CM
698.3 Neurodermatitis (circumscripta) (local)

SEE ALSO
• Pruritus ani
• Pruritus vulvae
• Dermatitis, contact
• Dermatitis, stasis
• Dermatitis, seborrheic

OTHER NOTES N/A

ABBREVIATIONS N/A

REFERENCES
• Orkin M, Maibach HI: 1st Ed. Dermatology. San Mateo, CA, Appleton & Lange, 1991
• Moschella SL, Hurley HJ: Dermatology. 3rd Ed. Philadelphia, W.B. Saunders, 1992
• Arnold HL, Odom RB, James WD: Andrews' Diseases of the Skin. 8th Ed. Philadelphia, W.B. Saunders Co., 1990
• Sauer GC: Manual of Skin Disease. 7th Ed. Philadelphia, J.B. Lippincott, 1996
• Sams WM, Lynch, PJ: Principles and Practice of Dermatology. 2nd Ed. New York, Churchill Livingstone, 1996
• Muramatsu T, et al: Localized cutaneous amyloidosis simulating lichen simplex chronicus. J of Derm 1995;22:759-763
Illustrations: 6 available on CD-ROM
Internet references: http://www.5mcc.com

Author(s)
Mitchell S. King, MD
Amy Y. Wang, MD

Neurofibromatosis (Types 1 & 2)

BASICS

DESCRIPTION The most common of the neurocutaneous syndromes (phakomatosis), consisting of Neurofibromatosis Type 1 (1 in 4,000) and Neurofibromatosis Type 2 (1 in 50,000). Although named similarly, and both autosomal dominant disorders, they are two distinctly different conditions with genes now identified on two separate chromosomes.
• Type 1 (NF 1) is also known as von Recklinghausen disease
• Type 2 (NF 2) as bilateral acoustic neurofibromatosis
System(s) affected: Nervous, Skin/Exocrine, Musculoskeletal
Genetics:
• NF1: autosomal dominant inheritance. Nearly 50% of cases are attributed to new mutations. The NF 1 gene mapped to chromosome 17. Prenatal diagnosis possible.
• NF2: Autosomal dominant inheritance. The NF 2 gene mapped on chromosome 22.
Incidence/Prevalence in USA: NF 1 = 1/4,000; NF 2 = 1/50,000
Predominant age: N/A
Predominant sex: Male = Female

SIGNS AND SYMPTOMS
• NF1: Two or more of the following:
  ◊ Six or more café au lait spots measuring 5 mm or more in prepubertal individuals or 15 mm or more in adults (97%)
  ◊ Two or more neurofibromata or plexiform neurofibroma (15%)
  ◊ Axillary or inguinal freckling (91%)
  ◊ Two or more Lisch nodules (30%)
  ◊ Optic glioma (4%)
  ◊ Characteristic osseous lesions such as sphenoid dysplasia, long bone cortical thinning, ribbon ribs, angular scoliosis (6%)
  ◊ First degree relative with NF 1, according to above criteria
• NF2: When one or more present, diagnosis is likely:
  ◊ Bilateral vestibular schwannomas
  ◊ Family history of NF 2, plus unilateral 8th nerve mass or family history and any two of the following: neurofibroma, meningioma, glioma, schwannoma, and juvenile posterior subcapsular lenticular opacity.

CAUSES
• Congenital

RISK FACTORS
• Family history

DIAGNOSIS

DIFFERENTIAL DIAGNOSIS
• NF1:
  ◊ Familial café au lait spots (autosomal dominant) – no other NF1 features
• NF2:
  ◊ Solitary acoustic neuroma (develops later in life and is not hereditary)

LABORATORY N/A
Drugs that may alter lab results: N/A
Disorders that may alter lab results: N/A

PATHOLOGICAL FINDINGS
• NF1: Generalized disorder of cells of neural crest origin

SPECIAL TESTS N/A

IMAGING N/A

DIAGNOSTIC PROCEDURES
• NF1:
  ◊ Dictated by findings and clinical evaluation
  ◊ Slit lamp ocular exam
  ◊ Radiology of skull and spine
  ◊ Psychological testing
  ◊ Diagnostic criteria: two or more of the following:
    - Six or more cafe au lait spots measuring 5 mm or more in prepubertal individuals or 15 mm or more in adults (97%)
    - Two or more neurofibromata or plexiform neurofibroma (15%)
    - Axillary or Inguinal freckling (91%)
    - Two or more Lisch nodules (30%)
    - Optic glioma (4%)
    - Characteristic osseous lesions such as sphenoid dysplasia, long bone cortical thinning, ribbon ribs, angular scoliosis (6%)
    ◊ First degree relative with NF 1, according to above criteria
• NF2:
  ◊ Clinical examination: skin, eye, and hearing
  ◊ Audiologic evaluation: brain stem evoked response (BAER)
  ◊ Radiologic examination: MRI of head
  ◊ When one or more of the following are present, the diagnosis of NF 2 is likely:
    - Bilateral vestibular schwannomas
    - Family history of NF 2, plus unilateral 8th nerve mass or family history and any two of the following: neurofibroma, meningioma, glioma, schwannoma, and juvenile posterior subcapsular lenticular opacity

TREATMENT

APPROPRIATE HEALTH CARE
Outpatient

GENERAL MEASURES
• Access to patient support groups
• Referral of patient to National NF Organization
• NF1:
  ◊ General outpatient follow-up of symptomatic patients for early identification of complications
  ◊ Periodic exams with particular attention to CNS findings and close attention to any masses or focally arising "new" pain
  ◊ Referral for psychosocial issues of family and affected individuals
  ◊ Educational intervention for children with learning disabilities or ADHD (40%)
• NF2:
  ◊ Annual neurologic examination
  ◊ Annual ophthalmologic exam
  ◊ Annual hearing examination or more frequently as necessitated
  ◊ Hearing augmentation as needed
  ◊ Speech therapy as needed
  ◊ Counseling and education regarding insidious problems associated with hearing loss, balance, or sense of direction

SURGICAL MEASURES
• NF1: Surgical treatment if indicated for scoliosis, plexiform neurofibromata or malignancy
• NF2: excision of tumor as indicated

ACTIVITY
• NF2: Caution advised in swimming, diving, or climbing heights

DIET No restrictions

PATIENT EDUCATION
• Genetic counseling and patient education regarding future complications and decisions about family planning

MEDICATIONS

DRUG(S) OF CHOICE
- NF1:
  ◊ Anticonvulsants: for seizure control
  ◊ Stimulant medications: for attention deficit hyperactivity disorder (ADHD)

Contraindications: N/A

Precautions: N/A

Significant possible interactions: caution necessary with these classes of drugs. Refer to manufacturer's profiles.

ALTERNATIVE DRUGS   N/A

FOLLOWUP

PATIENT MONITORING
- Annual evaluation and periodic assessment for at risk individuals

PREVENTION/AVOIDANCE
- Genetic counseling

POSSIBLE COMPLICATIONS
- NF1:
  ◊ Disfigurement: skin neurofibromata develop primarily on exposed areas
  ◊ Scoliosis: common: most cases mild
  ◊ CNS: A large head is common but rarely associated with hydrocephalus. Optic glioma or other CNS tumors arise usually during childhood (5-10%).
  ◊ Learning disability: common; often diagnosed upon entering school. May be associated with attention deficit hyperactivity disorder (ADHD).
  ◊ Rare Complications:
  - Mental retardation
  - Epilepsy
  - Hypertension
  - Variable onset of puberty
  - Slightly higher risk for malignancy (e.g. Wilms, leukemia, rhabdosarcoma)

EXPECTED COURSE/PROGNOSIS
- NF1: Variable; most patients have a mild expression and lead normal lives
- NF2: Variable

MISCELLANEOUS

ASSOCIATED CONDITIONS   N/A

AGE-RELATED FACTORS
Pediatric: External stigmata subtle or absent in very young children
Geriatric: Cutaneous lesions and tumors increase in size and number with age
Others: N/A

PREGNANCY   Genetic counseling

SYNONYMS
Von Recklinghausen Disease (NF1)
Bilateral acoustic neurofibromatosis (NF2)

ICD-9-CM
237.3 neurofibromatosis

SEE ALSO
- Ataxia-telangiectasia
- Von Hippel-Lindau disease
- Tuberous sclerosis
- Sturge-Weber disease

OTHER NOTES   N/A

ABBREVIATIONS   N/A

REFERENCES
- Listernick R, Charrow J: Neurofibromatosis type 1 in childhood. J Ped 1990;116;6:845-853
- Gutmann DH, et al: The diagnostic evaluation and multidisciplinary management of NF 1 and NF 2 JAMA 1997;278;1:51-57
- Martuza RL, Eldridge R: Neurofibromatosis 2. NEJM 1988;318(11):684-688
- NIH Consensus Development Conf Statement: Neurofibromatosis, 6;12: July 13-15, 1987

Illustrations: N/A
Internet references: http://www.5mcc.com

Author(s)
Nuhad D. Dinno, MD

Nocardiosis

BASICS

DESCRIPTION Nocardiosis is an acute, subacute, or chronic infection occurring in cutaneous, pulmonary, and disseminated forms. Nocardiosis produces suppurative necrosis and abscess formation at sites of infection.
• Primary cutaneous nocardiosis presents as cutaneous infection (cellulitis or abscess), lymphocutaneous infection (similar to sporotrichosis), or subcutaneous infection (actinomycetoma)
• Pulmonary infection presents as an acute, subacute, or chronic pneumonitis
• Disseminated nocardiosis may involve any organ (lesions in the brain or meninges most frequent)
System(s) affected: Pulmonary, Renal/Urologic, Nervous, Skin/Exocrine
Genetics: N/A
Incidence/Prevalence in USA: 0.4/100,000 (it is estimated that 500-1000 new cases occur per year)
Predominant age: All ages are susceptible, mean age at diagnosis is the fourth decade of life
Predominant sex: Males > Female (3:1)

SIGNS AND SYMPTOMS
• Pulmonary nocardiosis:
  ◊ Fever (70%)
  ◊ Cough (52%)
  ◊ Pleuritic chest pain (32%)
  ◊ Dyspnea (16%)
  ◊ Anorexia
  ◊ Weight loss
  ◊ Hemoptysis
  ◊ Tachypnea
  ◊ Rales
  ◊ Central nervous system dysfunction in those with CNS involvement
  ◊ Other focal infections in those with disseminated infection
• Cutaneous nocardiosis
  ◊ Abscesses
  ◊ Lymphadenopathy
• Disseminated nocardiosis
  ◊ Confusion
  ◊ Disorientation
  ◊ Dizziness
  ◊ Headache
  ◊ Nausea and/or vomiting
  ◊ Seizures

CAUSES Nocardiosis is caused by traumatic or inhalation inoculation of Nocardia species bacteria (predominantly Nocardia asteroides, but also N. brasiliensis, N. caviae, N. farcinica, N. transvalensis, N. otitidiscavarium, and N. nova) from soil

RISK FACTORS
• Most cases occur as opportunistic infection of immunocompromised hosts or hosts with predisposing pulmonary abnormalities
• Solid organ transplantation, chronic granulomatous disease of childhood, dysgammaglobulinemias, pemphigus, Cushing's disease, hemochromatosis, cirrhosis, bronchiectasis, tuberculosis, sarcoidosis, anthrosilicosis, pulmonary alveolar proteinosis, lymphoma, leukemia, glucocorticoid and cytotoxic therapy, solid malignancies, and AIDS.

DIAGNOSIS

DIFFERENTIAL DIAGNOSIS Includes other causes of acute, subacute, or chronic pneumonitis, particularly those occurring principally in immunocompromised hosts; tuberculosis, histoplasmosis, mixed bacterial lung abscess, and carcinoma

LABORATORY The diagnosis is established by observing the characteristic microscopical appearance of the organism in Gram stained and modified acid-fast stained preparations of sputum or pus or histopathologic samples. Confirmation is by culture of these same specimens.
Drugs that may alter lab results: N/A
Disorders that may alter lab results: N/A

PATHOLOGICAL FINDINGS
Histopathology reveals a suppurative lesion with acute necrosis and abscess formation and the microorganism

SPECIAL TESTS N/A

IMAGING
• X-ray - confluent bronchopneumonia with or without cavitation. Pleural effusion is common (up to 50%). Other chest x-ray presentations include masses, nodules, cavities, interstitial infiltrates.
• Imaging of the brain (brain scan, CT, or MRI) may reveal single or multiple intracranial abscesses, and is indicated in all patients with pulmonary nocardiosis. Other sites of focal infection may be identified by imaging in disseminated disease.

DIAGNOSTIC PROCEDURES If evaluation of sputum is nondiagnostic, bronchoscopy for bronchoalveolar lavage and transbronchial lung biopsy may prove valuable for diagnosis. Percutaneous aspiration of lung lesion is often useful.

TREATMENT

APPROPRIATE HEALTH CARE
Patients with moderate or severe illness generally require hospitalization

GENERAL MEASURES Respiratory support is often necessary in such hospitalized patients

SURGICAL MEASURES Surgical drainage of abscesses other than intrapulmonary abscesses is generally indicated if technically feasible

ACTIVITY Acute phase usually requires bedrest. Increase activity as condition improves.

DIET No special diet

PATIENT EDUCATION
• Not a contagious disease
• Advise patients of the need for long-term antimicrobial therapy to reduce the likelihood of relapse

MEDICATIONS

DRUG(S) OF CHOICE
• Sulfonamides are the traditional mainstay of treatment for all forms of nocardiosis. Some prefer sulfadiazine because of possibly better CNS activity. Sulfadiazine should be given as 4-8 gm po per day in 4 divided doses. Dosage should be adjusted to maintain sulfonamide serum levels in the range of 8-16 mg/dL.
• Some prefer to use trimethoprim-sulfamethoxazole. This agent must be used if parenteral sulfonamide therapy is required. Initial dose based on trimethoprim component: 640 mg trimethoprim daily. Base subsequent doses on sulfamethoxazole level. Dosage should provide equivalent sulfonamide dosing and levels as when a sulfonamide is used alone.

Contraindications:
• Sulfonamides - in the last month of pregnancy (should only be used when the potential benefits outweigh the risks)
• All antimicrobial agents above are contraindicated in the presence of known hypersensitivity to the agent

Precautions: With the use of high dose sulfadiazine, high urine flow should be maintained to minimize risk of crystalluria. Generally, patient should be advised to drink 2-3 L/day.

Significant possible interactions:
• Sulfonamides can increase the therapeutic effects of oral anticoagulants, phenytoin, sulfonylurea hypoglycemic agents, methotrexate, and thiopental
• Decreased absorption of digoxin may be encountered

ALTERNATIVE DRUGS
Alternatives for sulfonamide allergic patients include doxycycline or minocycline, ampicillin plus erythromycin, amikacin, imipenem, ß-lactam/ß-lactamase inhibitor combinations, and cefotaxime or ceftriaxone. Clinical experience with these alternative regimens is limited.

FOLLOWUP

PATIENT MONITORING
Patients on high dose sulfonamide therapy should have a complete blood count and assessment of hepatic and renal function performed at least every other week

PREVENTION/AVOIDANCE
N/A

POSSIBLE COMPLICATIONS
• Central nervous system infection (brain abscess or meningitis) (16%)
• Secondary cutaneous nocardiosis (13%)
• Septic arthritis (2%)
• Hematogenous osteomyelitis (1%)
• Other focal manifestations of disseminated infection (13%)

EXPECTED COURSE/PROGNOSIS
Overall modern mortality is 7-44%. In renal transplant recipients: overall mortality 25%, 0% mortality with isolated cutaneous involvement, 29% mortality with localized pleuropulmonary disease, 42% mortality with central nervous system involvement. In patients with the acquired immunodeficiency syndrome, mortality is 30%.

MISCELLANEOUS

ASSOCIATED CONDITIONS
See Risk factors

AGE-RELATED FACTORS
Pediatric: Reported association between chronic granulomatous disease of childhood and nocardiosis
Geriatric: N/A
Others: N/A

PREGNANCY
Sulfonamides - in the last month of pregnancy should only be used when the potential benefits outweigh the risks

SYNONYMS
N/A

ICD-9-CM
039.9 Nocardiosis, NOS

SEE ALSO
N/A

OTHER NOTES
Unusual nocardial infections: keratoconjunctivitis associated with contact lenses, peritonitis in patients on continuous ambulatory peritoneal dialysis, upper respiratory and digestive tract infections, pericarditis, hematogenous endophthalmitis, prosthetic joint infections, natural or prosthetic valve endocarditis

ABBREVIATIONS
N/A

REFERENCES
• Kalb RE, Kaplan MH, Grossman ME: Cutaneous nocardiosis. J Am Acad Derm 198513:125-133
• Wilson JP, Turner HR, Kirchner KA, Chapman SW: Nocardial infection in renal transplant recipients. Medicine 1989;68:38-57
• Kim J, Minamoto GY, Grieco MH: Nocardial infection as a complication of AIDS: Report of six cases & review. Rev Infect Dis 1991;13:624-629
• Mamelak AN, Obano WG, Flaherty JF, Rosenblum ML: Nocardial brain abscess: Treatment strategies and factors influencing outcome. Neurosurgery 1994;35:622-631
• Marrie TJ: Pneumonia caused by Nocardia Species. Sem Resp Infect 1994; 9:207
Illustrations: 2 available on CD-ROM
Internet references: http://www.5mcc.com

Author(s)
Ronald A. Greenfield, MD
Douglas P. Fine, MD

Obesity

BASICS

DESCRIPTION
A condition of increased body weight (consisting of both lean and fat tissue) that leads to increased morbidity and mortality. Also defined as weight 20% greater than an individual's desirable weight as defined by the Metropolitan Life Insurance Company or BMI > 28.
• Android obesity (male pattern or abdominal obesity) is higher risk and gynecoid obesity (female pattern or gluteal obesity) is lower risk for long-term health problems.

```
Obesity threshold (BMI=28)
- - - - - - - - - - - - - - - - - - - - - - -
Height        Weight(lb)
 5' 0"          143
 5' 2"          153
 5' 4"          163
 5' 6"          173
 5' 8"          184
 5' 10"         195
 6' 0"          206
 6' 2"          218
 6' 4"          230
- - - - - - - - - - - - - - - - - - - - - - -
```

System(s) affected: Gastrointestinal, Endocrine/Metabolic
Genetics: 25-30% of the variance in body fat is genetically transmitted
Incidence/Prevalence in USA:
• Ages 35-44: 1600/100,000 males; 1400/100,000 females
• Ages 65-74: 500/100,000 males; 400/100,000 females
• 20-30% of adult men and 30-40% of adult women (according to an NIH panel)
Predominant age: All ages
Predominant sex: Female > Male

SIGNS AND SYMPTOMS
Increased body weight and adipose tissue

CAUSES
• Multifactorial
• Rare genetic syndromes have been described
• Idiopathic obesity is assumed to be due to an imbalance between food intake and energy expenditure (physical activity and metabolic rate)
• Insulinoma
• Hypothalamic disorders
• Cushing's syndrome
• Corticosteroid drugs

RISK FACTORS
• Parental obesity
• Pregnancy
• Sedentary lifestyle
• High fat diet
• Low socioeconomic status

DIAGNOSIS

DIFFERENTIAL DIAGNOSIS   N/A

LABORATORY
• Not needed for diagnosis
• Consider thyroid function tests
• Cardiac risk factors: serum cholesterol, triglycerides, glucose
Drugs that may alter lab results: N/A
Disorders that may alter lab results: Hypothyroidism

PATHOLOGICAL FINDINGS
• Hypertrophy and/or hyperplasia of adipocytes
• Cardiomegaly
• Hepatomegaly

SPECIAL TESTS
• Body mass index (BMI) = body weight (kg) divided by the square of body height (m). Obesity is BMI > 28 kg/m2.
• Determine fat distribution pattern by measuring waist and hips circumferences and calculating the waist to hips ratio (WHR)
• Android (male pattern, or abdominal obesity) has WHR greater than 0.85 for females; 0.95 for males
• Gynecoid (female pattern, or gluteal obesity) has WHR less than 0.85 for females; 0.95 for males

IMAGING   N/A

DIAGNOSTIC PROCEDURES   N/A

TREATMENT

APPROPRIATE HEALTH CARE
Outpatient

GENERAL MEASURES
• Appropriate functions for the primary care physician include: assessment of degree of health risk from BMI and WHR (see Diagnosis); assessment of motivation to lose weight; helping patients to set goals of therapy; office counseling or referral to a registered dietician or weight loss program for in depth counseling on diet, exercise, and behavior modification; and long term follow-up
• Many reputable commercial and community programs exist for obesity treatment. Desirable programs should include diets which meet the RDA for nutrients, exercise counseling, behavior modification, and provision for long term maintenance. Physicians can provide valuable additional monitoring and long term followup.

SURGICAL MEASURES
Occasionally, treat patients with severe obesity (BMI > 40 kg/m2) with a gastric bypass or stapling procedure. This involves complex pre-surgical evaluation, surgery and followup and should be done in a center skilled in this treatment. Surgical treatment is the most effective long term weight loss treatment available for morbid obesity.

ACTIVITY
• Exercise alone rarely causes significant weight loss, but may improve long term results of weight loss treatment and should be an integral part of any weight loss program.
• Exercise regimens involve 30 minutes 3-5 times/week. Increasing calories expended in activities throughout the day is also important.
• Many patients benefit from an "exercise prescription"

DIET
• Diet restriction is the cornerstone of obesity management (low-fat, high-complex carbohydrate and high-fiber)
• A 500 kcal (2.10 MJ) reduction in calorie per day intake will result in approximately 1 pound (.45 kg) weight loss per week
• Very low calorie diets (VLCD)
  ◊ 400-800 kcal (1.68-3.35 MJ) per day are usually based on liquid formulas and cause more rapid weight loss
  ◊ Complications of VLCD include: dehydration, orthostatic hypotension, fatigue, muscle cramps, constipation, headache, cold intolerance, and relapse after discontinuation
  ◊ Contraindications of VLCD include: recent myocardial infarction or cerebrovascular accident, renal or hepatic disease, cancer, pregnancy, insulin-dependent diabetes mellitus, some psychiatric disturbances
  ◊ Physician supervision is important for VLCD

PATIENT EDUCATION
• Educating the patient about the value of weight reduction is important
• Behavior modification can improve dietary adherence and long term results of weight loss and should be included in any weight loss program
• A self help brochure "On Your Way to Fitness" can be ordered for $1.00 per copy from Shape Up America, P.O. Box 9738, Bridgeport, CT 06699. It gives information for exercise self-assessment and increasing exercise for obese patients. Patients can also visit the web site www.shapeup.org.

MEDICATIONS

DRUG(S) OF CHOICE
Drug treatment is not usually recommended, although appetite suppressants may be indicated for short-term use (few weeks) in conjunction with a weight loss regimen
• Schedule IV drugs
  ◊ Diethylpropion
  ◊ Phentermine
  ◊ Mazindol
  ◊ Sibutramine 5-15 mg qd (starting dose 10 mg) is approved without restriction on length of use
• Schedule III drugs
  ◊ Phendimetrazine
  ◊ Benzphetamine
Contraindications: Advanced atherosclerosis, symptomatic cardiovascular disease, hypertension, hyperthyroidism, glaucoma, history of drug abuse, agitated states, use of MAO inhibitors
Precautions:
• Abuse potential, especially for Schedule III
• Relapse after discontinuation of drug
• Sibutramine can cause elevations in pulse and blood pressure
Significant possible interactions:
• Concurrent use with general anesthetics may cause arrhythmias
• Serotonergic agents may cause "serotonin syndrome" in combination with sibutramine

ALTERNATIVE DRUGS
• Phenylpropanolamine is used in over-the counter-weight loss preparations
• Orlistat (Xenical) is a lipase inhibitor which decreases absorption of dietary fat. 120 mg tid with meals. Separate taking fat soluble vitamin supplements by at least 2 hours.

FOLLOWUP

PATIENT MONITORING   Long term followup is crucial to prevent further weight gain or regain after weight loss

PREVENTION/AVOIDANCE   Counseling in regular exercise and prudent diet with regular follow-up, especially in children and young adults and those with family history of obesity or diabetes mellitus

POSSIBLE COMPLICATIONS
• Increased mortality due largely to cardiovascular disease
• Diabetes mellitus
• Hypertension
• Hyperlipidemia
• Gall bladder disease with cholelithiasis
• Osteoarthritis
• Gout
• Thromboembolism
• Hypoventilation and sleep apnea syndromes
• Poor self-esteem
• Occupational discrimination

EXPECTED COURSE/PROGNOSIS
• Long term maintenance of weight loss is extremely difficult
• If patient is not motivated, successful weight loss is unlikely

MISCELLANEOUS

ASSOCIATED CONDITIONS   See Possible complications

AGE-RELATED FACTORS
Pediatric: Prevalence of obesity is increasing. Among other factors, decreased physical activity and increased television viewing have been implicated.
Geriatric: Desirable weights (those associated with the lowest risk of mortality) increase with age
Others: Pre-puberty and young adulthood appear to be sensitive periods for development of obesity

PREGNANCY   Pregnancy is a common time for onset of, or increase in obesity

SYNONYMS
• Overweight
• Adiposis
• Adiposity

ICD-9-CM   278.0 Obesity

SEE ALSO   N/A

OTHER NOTES   N/A

ABBREVIATIONS
RDA = recommended daily allowance
BMI = body mass index

REFERENCES
• Danford D, Fletcher JW, eds: Methods for voluntary weight loss and control. National Institutes of Health Technology Assessment Conference. Ann Intern Med 1993;119 (7 Part 2) S6:41-763
• Bray GA, ed: Obesity. Endocrinology and Metabolism Clinics of N Am 1996;25(4)
• Jones TF, Eaton CB. Exercise prescription. Am Fam Phys 1995;52(2):543-550
Illustrations: N/A
Internet references: http://www.5mcc.com

Author(s)
David S. Gray, MD

Obsessive compulsive disorder

BASICS

DESCRIPTION Psychiatric condition classified as an anxiety disorder in Diagnostic and Statistical Manual of Mental Disorders (DSM-IV-R) and characterized by recurrent, intrusive thoughts (obsessions) and ritualistic behaviors (compulsions)
• Obsessions and compulsions consume more than an hour per day and cause occupational/social impairment
• Patients know thoughts (obsessions) come from their own minds and are not imposed from outside (as in thought insertion). Thoughts are not associated with another disorder (for example, thought of food if an eating disorder is present).
• Compulsions are ritualistic behaviors designed to relieve the anxiety of obsessions
• Common obsessive themes:
  ◊ Violence, such as harming a beloved child
  ◊ Doubt, such as whether doors or windows locked or iron turned off
  ◊ Blasphemous thoughts, such as in a devoutly religious person
  ◊ Contamination, dirt or disease
  ◊ Symmetry or orderliness
• Common rituals or compulsions:
  ◊ Hand washing
  ◊ Checking
  ◊ Counting
  ◊ Hoarding
  ◊ Repeaters - such as dressing rituals
System(s) affected: Nervous
Genetics: Positive family history in about 20% of cases, no mode of transmission identified
Incidence/Prevalence in USA: 2.5% lifetime prevalence, 1.5-2.1% one year prevalence
Predominant age: Mean age 20. 1/3 cases present by age 15, new cases after age 50 rare, 80% of cases before age 35
Predominant sex: Male = Female (males tend to present at a younger age)

SIGNS AND SYMPTOMS
• Obsessions and/or compulsions that consume more than an hour a day and cause significant distress or impairment
• Obsessions (thoughts) are recurrent; patient attempts to ignore or neutralize thoughts with another thought or action
• Neither obsessions nor compulsions are related to another mental disorder
• Compulsions (actions) are repetitive, purposeful behaviors in response to thoughts in attempt to neutralize the thought - such as checking in response to doubt (locks, doors, windows or driving back over route to check for any possible damage inadvertently done while driving one's car)
• Repeated handwashing or ritualistic handwashing in response to fear of contamination
• 80-90% of patients have obsessions and compulsions
• 10-19% are pure obsessional
• 5% perform rituals until they "feel right" and may not have an identifiable obsession
• Hoarding and obsessional slowness comprise two other categories

CAUSES Dysregulation of neurotransmitter, serotonin

RISK FACTORS Greater concordance in monozygotic twins family history as above

DIAGNOSIS

DIFFERENTIAL DIAGNOSIS
• Impulse control disorders: Compulsive gambling, sex or substance abuse - the "compulsive" behavior is not in response to obsessive thought and patient derives pleasure from the activity, unlike OCD where obsessions and compulsions are ego dystonic
• Depression: Can see brooding, but ideas not perceived as senseless as in OCD
• Schizophrenia: Patient perceives thought to be true and from an external source
• Obsessive compulsive personality disorder: Not to be confused with OCD. In personality disorder, traits are ego-syntonic. Traits include perfectionism, preoccupation with detail, trivia or procedure and regulation. Patient tends to be rigid, moralistic and stingy. Often traits are rewarded in patient's job as desirable traits.
• Generalized anxiety, phobic disorders, separation anxiety: Similar response of heightened anxiety, but presence of obsessions or rituals clarifies OCD diagnosis

LABORATORY N/A
Drugs that may alter lab results: N/A
Disorders that may alter lab results: N/A

PATHOLOGICAL FINDINGS N/A

SPECIAL TESTS
• Yale Brown obsessive-compulsive scale (Y-BOCS)
• Maudsley obsessive-compulsive inventory (MOCI)

IMAGING PET scan - abnormal metabolism in frontal cortex and caudate nuclei (not generally available other than in research centers)

DIAGNOSTIC PROCEDURES
Psychiatric interview

TREATMENT

APPROPRIATE HEALTH CARE
Outpatient

GENERAL MEASURES
• Combine medications and cognitive behavior therapy
• Psychiatric referral for therapy (in vivo exposure and response prevention)
• Family psycho-education
• Parent behavior mangement training if OCD patient child/adolescent

SURGICAL MEASURES Psychosurgery (last resort)

ACTIVITY No restriction

DIET With use of phenelzine must have tyramine-free diet to prevent precipitation of hypertensive crisis

PATIENT EDUCATION
• Obsessive-Compulsive Foundation, P. O. Box 70, Milford, CT 06460-0070 (203) 878-5669 or (203) 874-3843 for recorded information
• Printed patient information available from: Obsessive-Compulsive Anonymous, P.O. Box 215, New Hyde Park, NY 11040, (516)741-4901

MEDICATIONS

DRUG(S) OF CHOICE
• Serotonin reuptake inhibitor, fluoxetine (Prozac)
   ◊ Adults: begin with 20 mg/day q morning and increase every 4-6 weeks to obtain maximal clinical response. Dose range: 20-60 mg/day. Doses >20 mg/day should be divided.
   ◊ Children: safety and efficacy has not been established
• Sertraline (Zoloft)
   ◊ Adults: begin with 50 mg per day and increase every week until clinical response. Dose range: 50-200 mg per day. Doses > 100 mg/day should be divided.
   ◊ Children: safety and efficacy have not been established
• Paroxetine (Paxil)
   ◊ Adults: begin with 20 mg/day, increase weekly in 10 mg increments until maximal clinical response
   ◊ Children: begin with 20 mg/day, increase weekly in 10 mg increments until maximal clinical response
• Fluvoxamine (Luvox)
   ◊ Adult - begin with 100 mg/day and increase every week until clinical response (dosage range 200-300 mg)
   ◊ Children (8-17) - begin with 25 mg/day, increase in small increments (25-50 mg) until clinical response

Contraindications:
• Absolute fluoxetine, paroxetine, and sertraline contraindications
   ◊ Hypersensitivity to the selective serotonin re-uptake inhibitors
   ◊ Within 14 days of MAO inhibitor
• Relative fluoxetine and sertraline contraindications
   ◊ Severe liver impairment
   ◊ Seizure disorders (lowers seizure threshold)
• Clomipramine is of the tricyclic antidepressant class, so carries same contraindications as drugs in that class
• Absolute clomipramine contraindications:
   ◊ Within 6 months of myocardial infarction
   ◊ Narrow angle glaucoma
   ◊ 3rd degree AV block
   ◊ Within 14 days of MAO inhibitor
• Relative clomipramine contraindications:
   ◊ Prostatic hypertrophy (urinary retention)
   ◊ Seizure disorder (lower seizure threshold)
   ◊ 1st, 2nd degree AV block, bundle branch block and CHF (pro-arrhythmic effect)

Precautions:
• Drug should to be taken for a minimum of 10 weeks before considering it a treatment failure
• Because patients with OCD may have concomitant depression, suicide potential must be assessed
• Long half-life may be troublesome if patient has an adverse reaction
• May cause drowsiness and dizziness when therapy is initiated - warn patients about driving and heavy equipment hazards
• May alter glucose control by lowering blood glucose levels while on the medication and increase blood glucose after stopping the medication
• Tricyclic class of antidepressants dangerous in overdose

Significant possible interactions:
• Clomipramine
   ◊ Not yet fully elucidated
   ◊ May interfere with guanethidine, clonidine
   ◊ Serum level increased if used concomitantly with haloperidol
   ◊ Probable plasma increase if used with cimetidine, fluoxetine, methylphenidate
   ◊ Increases serum level of phenobarbital
• Fluoxetine and sertraline
   ◊ Causes increased concentrations of the following medications: warfarin, phenytoin, carbamazepine, diazepam, tricyclic antidepressants, and neuroleptics

ALTERNATIVE DRUGS
• Clomipramine
   ◊ Adults - beginning at 25 mg/day and increased gradually to 100 mg over first 2 weeks. Then to 250 mg over next several weeks, as tolerated.
   ◊ Children - beginning at 25 mg /day over first two weeks as in adults. Then titrated up to 3 mg/kg or 200 mg/day (which ever is smaller) over the next several weeks.

FOLLOWUP

PATIENT MONITORING
• Y-BOCS
• MOCI

PREVENTION/AVOIDANCE N/A

POSSIBLE COMPLICATIONS
• Depression in 1/3 of OCD patients
• Avoidant behavior (phobic avoidance)
• Anxiety and panic-like episodes associated with obsessions

EXPECTED COURSE/PROGNOSIS
• Chronic waxing and waning course in majority
• 24-33% fluctuating course
• 11-14% phasic with periods of remission
• 54-61% chronic progressive course

MISCELLANEOUS

ASSOCIATED CONDITIONS
• Depression
• Panic disorder
• Social phobia
• Phobia
• Tourette's
• Alcoholism
• Substance abuse

AGE-RELATED FACTORS
Pediatric: Child/adolescent onset in 33%. At this age males outnumber females 3:1.
Geriatric: Diagnosis not generally made after age 50
Others: N/A

PREGNANCY
• Onset of OCD has been noted after delivery
• Safety of fluoxetine and clomipramine has not been established in pregnancy nor lactation

SYNONYMS
Obsessive compulsive neurosis

ICD-9-CM
300.3 Obsessive-compulsive disorders

SEE ALSO
• Anxiety
• Depression

OTHER NOTES Not to be confused with obsessive compulsive personality disorder (see Differential Diagnosis)

ABBREVIATIONS
Y-BOCS = Yale Brown obsessive compulsive scale
OCD = obsessive compulsive disorder
MOCI = Maudsley obsessive-compulsive inventory

REFERENCES
• Diagnostic and Statistical Manual of Mental Disorders (DSM-IV-R). 4th Ed. American Psychiatric Association, Washington, D.C., 1994
• Kaplan HI, Sadock BJ (eds). Comprehensive Textbook of Psychiatry, 6th ed. Williams & Wilkins, Baltimore, MD, 1995.
• Hohagen F. New perspectives in research and treatment of obsessive-compulsive disorder. Br J Psychiatry Suppl1998; (3 5):1-96
• Eddy MF, Walbroehl GS. Recognition and treatment of obsessive-compulsive disorder. Am Fam Phys 1998;57(7):1623-8, 1632-4.
• AACAP. Practice parameters for the assessment and treatment of children and adolescents with obsessive-compulsive disorder. J Am Acad Child Adolesc Psychiatry 1998;37(10 Suppl):27S-45S
Illustrations: N/A
Internet references: http://www.5mcc.com

Author(s)
Doug Post, PhD

Ocular chemical burns

BASICS

DESCRIPTION Chemical exposure to the eye can result in rapid, devastating, and permanent damage and is one of the true emergencies in ophthalmology
• Separate alkaline from acid chemical exposure:
◊ Alkaline burns - more severe, alkali penetrates and saponifies tissues easily, may produce injury to lids, conjunctiva, cornea, sclera, iris, lens, and retina
◊ Acid burns - usually acid does not damage internal structures since protein coagulation limits acid penetration. Injury often limited to lids, conjunctiva, and cornea.
System(s) affected: Nervous, Skin/Exocrine
Genetics: N/A
Incidence/Prevalence in USA: Estimated 300/100,000/year
Predominant age: 18-65
Predominant sex: Male > Female

SIGNS AND SYMPTOMS
• Mild burns:
◊ Pain and blurred vision
◊ Eyelid skin erythema and edema
◊ Corneal epithelial defects or superficial punctate keratitis
◊ Conjunctival chemosis, hyperemia, and hemorrhages without perilimbal ischemia
◊ Mild anterior chamber reaction
• Moderate to severe burns:
◊ Severe pain and markedly reduced vision
◊ Second and third degree burns of eyelid skin
◊ Corneal edema and opacification
◊ Corneal epithelial defects
◊ Marked conjunctival chemosis and perilimbal blanching
◊ Moderate anterior chamber reaction
◊ Increased intraocular pressure
◊ Local necrotic retinopathy
◊ In alkaline burns, can have initial pain which later diminishes

CAUSES
• Alkali:
◊ Ammonia (NH3)
◊ Lye (NaOH)
◊ Magnesium hydroxide [Mg(OH)2]
◊ Potassium hydroxide (KOH)
◊ Lime [Ca(OH)2]
• Acids:
◊ Hydrochloric (HCl)
◊ Hydrofluoric (HF)
◊ Acetic (CH3COOH)
◊ Nitrous (HNO2)
◊ Sulfuric (H2SO4)

RISK FACTORS
• Construction work (plaster, cement, whitewash)
• Use of cleaning agents (drain cleaners, ammonia)
• Automobile battery explosions (sulfuric acid)
• Industrial work (many possible agents)
• Alcoholism

DIAGNOSIS

DIFFERENTIAL DIAGNOSIS
• Thermal burns
• Ocular cicatricial pemphigoid
• Other causes of corneal opacification
• Ultraviolet radiation keratitis

LABORATORY None
Drugs that may alter lab results: N/A
Disorders that may alter lab results: None

PATHOLOGICAL FINDINGS
• Precipitation of glycosaminoglycans causes corneal opacification
• Saponification of cell membranes causes cell death
• Cation binding to collagen results in hydration, thickening, and shortening of collagen fibrils. This can mechanically elevate intraocular pressure.

SPECIAL TESTS Measure pH of tear film with litmus paper or electronic probe (irrigating fluid with non-neutral pH [e.g., normal saline has pH of 4.5] may alter results)

IMAGING Not necessary unless suspicion of intraocular or orbital foreign body is present

DIAGNOSTIC PROCEDURES
• Careful slit lamp examination, fundus ophthalmoscopy, tonometry, and measurement of visual acuity
• Full extent of damage from alkaline burns may not be apparent until 48-72 hours after exposure

TREATMENT

APPROPRIATE HEALTH CARE
Emergency room with inpatient admission and ophthalmology consultation, depending on severity

GENERAL MEASURES Copious irrigation and removal of corneal or conjunctival foreign bodies are always the initial treatment. Continue irrigation until the tear film is of neutral pH and pH is stable. Sweep the conjunctival fornices every 12-24 hours to prevent adhesions.

SURGICAL MEASURES
• Punctal occlusion for tear film preservation and corneal epitheliopathy
• Tarsorrhaphy for persistent epithelial defects
• Tissue adhesive (e.g., isobutyl cyanoacrylate) for impending or actual corneal perforation
• Conjunctival or limbal autograft transplantation for epithelial stem cell restoration
• Lamellar or penetrating keratoplasty for tectonic stabilization or visual rehabilitation

ACTIVITY Ambulatory

DIET Usual for patient

PATIENT EDUCATION
• Safety glasses
• Need for immediate ocular irrigation with any available water following chemical exposure to the eyes

MEDICATIONS

DRUG(S) OF CHOICE
• Immediate treatment (any non-toxic irrigant):
◊ In hospital setting, sterile water, normal saline, lactated Ringer's solution are effective
◊ In the field, use what is available (tap water). Rapidity of irrigation is critical.
◊ Irrigation is continued until pH of superior/inferior cul-de-sac is neutral
◊ It is impossible to over-irrigate
• Further treatment: (depending on severity and associated conditions)
◊ Topical prophylactic antibiotics: Any broad spectrum agent, e.g., bacitracin-polymyxin B (Polysporin) ointment q2-4h, ciprofloxacin (Ciloxan) drops q 2-4h, chloramphenicol (Chloroptic) ointment q2-4h
◊ Tear substitutes: hydroxypropyl methylcellulose (Hypotears PF, Refresh Plus) drops q4h, carboxymethylcellulose (Refresh P.M.) ointment qhs
◊ Cycloplegics for photophobia and/or uveitis: Cyclopentolate 1% tid, or scopolamine 1/4% bid
◊ Anti-glaucoma for elevated intraocular pressure (IOP): latanoprost (Xalatan) 0.005% q24h or timolol (Timoptic) 0.5% bid or levobunolol (Betagan) 0.5% bid and/or acetazolamide (Diamox) 125-250 mg po q6h or methazolamide (Neptazane) 25-50 mg po bid and/or mannitol 20% 1-2 g/kg IV prn
◊ Corticosteroids for intraocular inflammation: Prednisolone (Pred-Forte) 1% or equivalent q1-4h for 10-14 days; if severe, prednisone 20-60 mg po qd for 5-7 days. Taper rapidly if epithelium intact by this time.
◊ Consider vitamin C (ascorbic acid) 500 mg po qid and/or acetylcysteine (Mucomyst) 10-20% top q4 h if corneal melting occurs
Contraindications: None
Precautions:
• For timolol and levobunolol - history of congestive heart failure or chronic obstructive pulmonary disease
• For acetazolamide and methazolamide - history of nephrolithiasis or metabolic acidosis
• For mannitol - history of congestive heart failure or renal failure
• For scopolamine - history of urinary retention
• Topical corticosteroids must be used with caution in the presence of damaged corneal epithelium as iatrogenic infection can occur. Daily follow-up or consultation with an ophthalmologist is recommended.
Significant possible interactions: Refer to manufacturer's literature

ALTERNATIVE DRUGS
Where available - topical fibronectin, epidermal growth factor, prokinase inhibitors

FOLLOWUP

PATIENT MONITORING
• Depending on severity of ocular injury, from daily to weekly visits initially
• May be inpatient
• If on mannitol or prednisone, consider frequent serum electrolytes

PREVENTION/AVOIDANCE
Safety glasses to safeguard uninvolved eye

POSSIBLE COMPLICATIONS
• Persistent epitheliopathy
• Fibrovascular pannus
• Corneal ulcer/perforation
• Progressive symblepharon and entropion
• Neurotrophic keratitis
• Glaucoma
• Cataract
• Hypotony
• Phthisis bulbi

EXPECTED COURSE/PROGNOSIS
• Depends on severity of initial injury
• Increasing amounts of limbal ischemia and corneal opacification correlate with poorer prognosis
• For severely injured eyes, permanent loss of vision is not uncommon
• Autologous cultivated corneal epithelium has been used for long term restoration of vision.
• Autologous nasal mucosal transplantation has also been successfully employed

MISCELLANEOUS

ASSOCIATED CONDITIONS Facial cutaneous chemical or thermal burns

AGE-RELATED FACTORS
Pediatric: N/A
Geriatric:
• Compromised ocular surface from keratitis sicca or other disease associated with poorer prognosis
• Compromised corneal endothelium or pre-existing glaucoma may also complicate clinical management
Others: N/A

PREGNANCY N/A

SYNONYMS Chemical ocular injuries

ICD-9-CM
940.2 Alkali burn of cornea and conjunctival sac
940.3 Acid burn of cornea and conjunctival sac

SEE ALSO
• Burns
• Keratitis, superficial punctate

OTHER NOTES N/A

ABBREVIATIONS N/A

REFERENCES
• Fraunfelder FT, Roy FH: Current Ocular Therapy. 3rd Ed. Philadelphia, W.B. Saunders Co., 1990
• McCulley JP: Chemical Injuries. In: Smolin G, Thoft RA, eds. The Cornea: Scientific Foundations and Clinical Practice. New York, Little, Brown, 1987
• Shingleton BJ, Hersh PS, Kenyon KR: Eye Trauma. St. Louis, Mosby Year Book, 1991
• Ralph RA: Chemical Burns of the Eye. In: Tasman W, ed. Clinical Ophthalmology. Philadelphia, J.B. Lippincott, 1994
Illustrations: N/A
Internet references: http://www.5mcc.com

Author(s)
Robert G. Fante, MD

Onychomycosis

BASICS

DESCRIPTION Infection of nail by fungi (dermatophytes, Candida, molds).
System(s) affected: Skin/Exocrine
Genetics: N/A
Incidence/Prevalence in USA: 22-130 cases/1000 population
Predominant age:
• Dermatophytes common in adults; even molds in older adults
Predominant sex:
• Candidal: adult women

SIGNS AND SYMPTOMS
• Dermatophytes: Commonly preceded by dermatophyte infection at another site; 80% involve toenails - especially hallux; simultaneous infection of finger and toe nails rare. Four clinical forms occur:
  ◊ Distal subungual onychomycosis
   - Spreads from hyponychium to nailbed to nailplate
   - Subungual hyperkeratosis
   - Subungual paronychia
   - Onycholysis
   - Nail dystrophy
   - Discoloration: yellow-brown
   - Bois vermoulu ("worm-eaten wood")
   - Onychomadesis
  ◊ Lateral onychomycosis (common)
   - Yellowish discoloration lateral nail groove
   - Onycholysis, proximal or distal
  ◊ Proximal onychomycosis (rare)
   - Hands or feet
   - Leukonychia: begins under posterior nail groove, spreading to nail plate and lunula
  ◊ White superficial onychomycosis (rare)
   - Hallux preferentially affected
   - Infection of upper part of nailplate
   - Opaque white spots on nail plate eventually merge to involve entire surface of the nail
• Candidal:
  ◊ Hands 70% - especially dominant hand
  ◊ Middle finger most common
  ◊ Pain mild, unless secondarily infected
  ◊ Pain increases on prolonged contact with water
  ◊ Primarily affects tissue surrounding nail
  ◊ Begins with cuticle detachment
  ◊ Dark yellowish to blackish-brown zone along lateral border of nail
  ◊ Secondary ungual changes - convex, irregular, striated nailplate with dull rough surface
  ◊ Onycholysis, especially on hands
  ◊ Distal subungual onychomycosis may occur
  ◊ Primary involvement of the nailplate uncommon (thin, crumbly, opaque, brownish nailplate deformed by transverse grooves)
  ◊ Periungual edema/erythema may occur (club-shaped, bulbous fingertips)
  ◊ Superficial white onychomycosis - young children
• Molds
  ◊ More common over 60 years old
  ◊ More common in nails of hallux
  ◊ Resembles distal and lateral onychomycosis

CAUSES
• Dermatophytes (invade normal keratin)
  ◊ *Trichophyton rubrum* - most common
  ◊ *Trichophyton mentagrophytes* var. interdigitale - 25% as common as *T. rubrum* (most common pathogen for white superficial onychomycosis)
  ◊ *Epidermophyton floccosum, T. violaceum, Microsporum* less common
• Candida
  ◊ 70% *Candida albicans*
  ◊ *C. parapsilosis, C. tropicalis, C. krusei* (less common)
• Molds (invade altered keratin)
  ◊ *Scopulariopsis brevicaulis, Hendersonula toruloidea, Aspergillus species, Alternaria tenuis, Cephalosporium, Scytalidium hyalinium*

RISK FACTORS
• Dermatophytes
  ◊ Warmth, moisture, hyperhidrosis
  ◊ Tight fitting shoes, rubber shoes
  ◊ Peripheral vascular disease
  ◊ Depressed cell-mediated immunity
  ◊ Indirect contamination
• Candidal
  ◊ Direct contamination - ano-vulvar, perirectal pruritus
  ◊ Chemical or mechanical damage to cuticle
  ◊ Maceration or occlusion
  ◊ Contact with substances containing sugar
  ◊ Hyperhidrosis
  ◊ Chilblain
  ◊ Cold hands (Raynaud's phenomenon)
  ◊ Psoriatic onycholysis
  ◊ Diabetes mellitus
  ◊ Hyperparathyroidism
  ◊ Addison's disease
  ◊ Malnutrition
  ◊ Malabsorption
  ◊ Dyscrasias
  ◊ Malignancies
  ◊ Postoperative conditions
  ◊ Altered immune function
• Molds
  ◊ Soil contamination
  ◊ Peripheral vascular disease
  ◊ Overlapping toes
  ◊ Onychogryposis (deforming overgrowth of nails resulting in hooked or curved state)

DIAGNOSIS

DIFFERENTIAL DIAGNOSIS
• Black nail paronychia
• Herpetic whitlow
• Eczema
• Pustular psoriasis
• Tumor
• Darier's disease
• Pityriasis rubra pilaris
• Trophic changes, peripheral vascular disease
• Endocrine disease
• Drugs; chemicals
• Trauma

• Alopecia areata
• Lichen planus
• Yellow-nail syndrome (icterus, carotenemia, amyloidosis)
• White acquired nail disease (trauma, acute infection, chronic disease, thallium or arsenic poisoning, hepatic cirrhosis, chronic albuminemia)
• Brown-black pigment (melanotic, hematoma)
• Green dyschromia (*Pseudomonas aeruginosa*)
• Connective tissue disorders: dermatomyositis, scleroderma, Reiter's

LABORATORY
• KOH preparation: clip or file away some of nailplate as needed, collect scales from stratum corneum of most proximal area (beneath nail or crumbling nail itself with 1 mm currette), 5% KOH + gentle heat, 100% sensitive if > 2 preps examined
• Cultures - negative in 30% (secondary to loss of dermatophyte viability; improved by immediate culture on Sabouraud's and CC media)
• Histologic examination of keratin, punch or scalpel biopsy - proximal lesions with PAS stain
• All are influenced by quality of sampling
• CD4 < 450
Drugs that may alter lab results:
Discontinue all topical medication several days before obtaining sample
Disorders that may alter lab results: N/A

PATHOLOGICAL FINDINGS Pathogens within the nail keratin

SPECIAL TESTS N/A

IMAGING N/A

DIAGNOSTIC PROCEDURES N/A

TREATMENT

APPROPRIATE HEALTH CARE
• Outpatient - unless secondary cellulitis/osteomyelitis

GENERAL MEASURES
• Avoid factors that promote fungal growth (heat, moisture)
• Treat underlying disease risk factors
• Treat other fungal infections
• Treat secondary infections

SURGICAL MEASURES
• Nail removal to remove infected keratin
  ◊ Mechanical: soften with occlusive dressing, detach from nailbed with tweezers or file with abrasive paper/grinding stone
  ◊ Chemical: protect peripheral tissue with adhesive strips, apply ointment of 30% salicylic acid, 40% urea or 50% potassium iodide under occlusive dressing
  ◊ Surgical avulsion: for involvement of a few nails

ACTIVITY
Restrictions based on promoting factors, underlying disease or secondary infection

DIET
No special diet

PATIENT EDUCATION
N/A

MEDICATIONS

DRUG(S) OF CHOICE
• Dermatophytes - local: Less effective than systemic, apply under occlusive dressing, may mix with keratinolytic chemicals
  ◊ Imidazoles: Clotrimazole (Lotrimin, Mycelex), miconazole (Monistat), butoconazole, tioconazole, econazole (Spectazole), ketoconazole (Nizoral), sulconazole (Exelderm), oxiconazole (Oxistat), terbinafine (Lamisil)
  ◊ Unsaturated fatty acid derivatives: Propionic acid, undecylenic acid; haloprogin (Halotex), tolnaftate (Tinactin)
  ◊ Amorolfine (Loceryl) 5% topical lacquer
• Dermatophytes - systemic:
  ◊ Fluconazole (Diflucan) 400 mg po weekly for 6 months (pulse therapy), overall better tolerated than ketoconazole; expensive; reserve for extreme cases (disseminated disease, immunocompromised)
  ◊ Itraconazole (Sporanox): 400 mg po qd for a week per month for 2 months for fingernails and 3-4 months for toenails (pulse therapy)
  ◊ Terbinafine (Lamisil) 250 mg po qd for 3 months
• Candida:
  ◊ Imidazole derivative
  ◊ If bacterial infection present, use antibacterial plus anti-Candidal, e.g., nystatin (Mycostatin), topical amphotericin B (Fungizone), itraconazole (Sporanox) 200 mg po qd for 3 months, or fluconazole 400 mg po weekly for 6 months (pulse therapy)
• Mold:
  ◊ 1% iodinated alcohol, Whitfield's ointment, silver nitrate, glutaraldehyde, imidazole derivatives, itraconazole

Contraindications:
• Griseofulvin: porphyria, hepatocellular failure, serious side effects (leukopenia, persistent anemia), pregnancy
• Ketoconazole: hepatocellular disease, pregnancy
• Fluconazole: hepatocellular failure, pregnancy

Precautions:
• Topical agents: use with caution on broken skin, vascular compromise, decreased sensation
• Griseofulvin: monitor for hepatic, renal, hematopoietic side effects; photo-sensitivity; lupus-like symptoms or exacerbation. Take with meals to enhance absorption.
• Ketoconazole: hepatotoxicity (may be severe or fatal), anaphylaxis may (rarely) occur with first dose, decreased testosterone levels
• Fluconazole: decrease dose in renal failure, hepatotoxicity

Significant possible interactions:
• Griseofulvin: warfarin, barbiturates, alcohol, oral contraceptives
• Ketoconazole: warfarin, rifampin, cyclosporine, phenytoin, terfenadine
• Fluconazole: phenytoin (Dilantin), cyclosporine, oral hypoglycemics, oral anticoagulants, rifampin, hydrochlorothiazide
• Itraconazole and ketoconazole require gastric acid for absorption - effectiveness reduced with antacids, H2 blockers, omeprazole, etc.

ALTERNATIVE DRUGS
• Dermatophytes - local: ciclopirox (Loprox), naftifine (Naftin), cationic surfactants, e.g., benzalkonium chloride (Cetylcide), cetrimide, cetylpyridinium chloride (Ony-Clear, Fungoid)], halogenated / chlorinated derivatives [chloramine, tincture of iodine], dyes [malachite green, crystal violet], mercury derivatives [thimerosal], phenols, glutaraldehyde
• Dermatophytes - systemic: griseofulvin (Fulvicin, Gris-PEG, Grisactin) ultramicrosize, usual adult dose 250-500 mg bid with meals for 6-12 months

FOLLOWUP

PATIENT MONITORING
• Topical agents: slow response expected; visits q 6-12 weeks
• Griseofulvin: CBC and liver function tests initially, then q 3 months
• Ketoconazole: liver function tests q 3 weeks for the first 3 months, then monthly
• Itraconazole and fluconazole - liver function tests at start and at 4 weeks
• Terbinafine - liver function and hematologic tests at start and at 4 weeks
• Treatment duration (months): fingernails 6-9s, toenails 9-12, great toenail 12-24

PREVENTION/AVOIDANCE
• Keep affected area clean and dry
• Avoid rubber or other occlusive footwear
• Avoid tight or ill-fitting footwear
• Wear absorbent cotton socks - avoid wool or synthetic fibers
• Change clothing and towels frequently and launder in hot water

POSSIBLE COMPLICATIONS
• Secondary infections with progression to cellulitis/osteomyelitis

EXPECTED COURSE/PROGNOSIS
• Relapse common; prognosis especially poor if one hand, 2 feet or multiple nails involved
• 20-40% of nails fail to respond
• 40-70% of patients show long term relapse

MISCELLANEOUS

ASSOCIATED CONDITIONS
• Immunodeficiency or chronic metabolic disease

AGE-RELATED FACTORS
Pediatric:
• Rare before puberty
• Candidal infection presents more commonly as superficial white onychomycosis
Geriatric:
• Mold onychomycosis more common
• Predisposing diseases more common
• Hepatic/renal reserve limited
• Decreased ability for topical self-treatment
Others: N/A

PREGNANCY
Drug choices limited

SYNONYMS
• Tinea unguium
• Ringworm of the nail

ICD-9-CM
110.1 Dermatophytosis of nail
112.3 Candidiasis of skin and nails

SEE ALSO
• HIV infection & AIDS

OTHER NOTES
• Onycholysis = detachment of nailplate from nailbed
• Dystrophy = thickening, deformation, crumbling
• Onychomadesis = shedding of nail
• Leukonychia = yellowish-white spots

ABBREVIATIONS
N/A

REFERENCES
• Pariser DM: Superficial fungal infections. Postgraduate medicine 1990;87(5):205-214
• Baden HP: Diseases of the Hair and Nails. Chicago, Year Book Medical Publishers, 1987
• Doncker PDe, Gupta AK, Marynissen G, et al. Itraconazole pulse therapy for onychomycosis and dermatomycoses: an overview. J Am Acad Dermatol 1997;37:969-74
Illustrations: 4 available on CD-ROM
Internet references: http://www.5mcc.com

Author(s)
Samuel L. Moschella, MD, FACP

Optic atrophy

BASICS

DESCRIPTION End result of loss of ganglion cells or axons of the optic nerve
System(s) affected: Nervous
Genetics: Inherited forms may be autosomally recessive, autosomally dominant or X-linked recessive
Incidence/Prevalence in USA: Unknown
Predominant age:
• Inherited forms occur shortly after birth to the third decade
• Acquired forms tend to occur later
Predominant sex: Male > Female (inherited forms)

SIGNS AND SYMPTOMS
• Loss of visual acuity
• Pallor of the optic disk
• Loss of pupillary reactions
• Visual field defects

CAUSES
• Glaucoma
• Post central retinal artery or vein occlusion
• Ischemic optic neuropathy
• Chronic optic neuritis
• Chronic papilledema
• Compression of the optic nerve or chiasm or tract by tumor or by aneurysm
• Trauma
• Syphilis
• Retinal degeneration (e.g., retinitis pigmentosa)
• Congenital optic atrophy
• Radiation neuropathy
• Drugs (amiodarone, chloroquine, ethambutol, oral contraceptives, streptomycin, vincristine)
• Thiamine deficiency

RISK FACTORS
• Hereditary
  ◊ Family history
• Acquired
  ◊ Diabetes mellitus
  ◊ Hypertension
  ◊ Radiation exposure
  ◊ Alcoholism
  ◊ Renal failure
  ◊ Arteriosclerosis

DIAGNOSIS

DIFFERENTIAL DIAGNOSIS
• Myopia
• S/p cataract extraction (no natural yellow color from the human lens)

LABORATORY
• CBC
• Antinuclear antibody (ANA)
• ESR
• Rapid plasma reagin (RPR)
• Fluorescent treponemal antibody absorption (FTA-ABS)
• Serological test for syphilis
• Heavy metal screen
Drugs that may alter lab results: N/A
Disorders that may alter lab results: N/A

PATHOLOGICAL FINDINGS N/A

SPECIAL TESTS
• Automated visual field test (i.e., Humphrey)
• Color vision testing

IMAGING CT or MRI of head

DIAGNOSTIC PROCEDURES
• Carotid Doppler (adult acquired optic atrophy)
• Complete ophthalmologic exam including dilated evaluation of retina

TREATMENT

APPROPRIATE HEALTH CARE
Outpatient

GENERAL MEASURES
• Treat underlying cause (rarely possible)
• Discontinue causative drug if possible
• If pressure against optic nerve is cause, neurosurgery to relieve it may help if done early

SURGICAL MEASURES N/A

ACTIVITY Fully active

DIET No special diet

PATIENT EDUCATION
• Low vision counseling if bilateral
• Genetic counseling if inherited
• For patient education materials favorably reviewed on this topic, contact: National Eye Institute, Information Officer, Dept. of Health and Human Services, 9000 Rockville Pike, Bethesda, MD 20892, (301)496-5248

MEDICATIONS

DRUG(S) OF CHOICE None
Contraindications: N/A
Precautions: N/A
Significant possible interactions: N/A

ALTERNATIVE DRUGS N/A

FOLLOWUP

PATIENT MONITORING Annual evaluations if stable

PREVENTION/AVOIDANCE N/A

POSSIBLE COMPLICATIONS N/A

EXPECTED COURSE/PROGNOSIS
• Rarely possible to treat the underlying cause effectively
• Visual loss occurs over weeks to months
• Optic atrophy secondary to vascular, trauma, degenerative changes and some toxic causes has a very bad prognosis

MISCELLANEOUS

ASSOCIATED CONDITIONS
• Inherited neurodegenerative conditions
◊ Hereditary ataxia
◊ Charcot-Marie-Tooth disease
◊ Storage diseases
◊ Leukodystrophies

AGE-RELATED FACTORS
Pediatric: Optic atrophy in small children is difficult to recognize because disks normally have a pale appearance
Geriatric: None
Others: None

PREGNANCY None

SYNONYMS N/A

ICD-9-CM 377.10 optic atrophy, unspecified

SEE ALSO N/A

OTHER NOTES American Council of the Blind (800)424-8666

ABBREVIATIONS N/A

REFERENCES
• Miller NR: Walsh and Hoyt's Clinical Neuro-Ophthalmology. 4th Ed. Baltimore, Williams & Wilkins, 1982
• Fraunfelder FT, Roy FH: Current Ocular Therapy. 3rd Ed. Philadelphia, W.B. Saunders Co., 1990
Illustrations: 1 available on CD-ROM
Internet references: http://www.5mcc.com

Author(s)
Robert Noecker, MD

Optic neuritis

BASICS

DESCRIPTION Inflammation of the optic nerve
System(s) affected: Nervous
Genetics: N/A
Incidence/Prevalence in USA: N/A
Predominant age: Typically 18-50 years
Predominant sex: Female > Male

SIGNS AND SYMPTOMS
• Loss of vision, deteriorating from hours to days, usually reaching lowest level in one week
• Usually unilateral in adults, bilateral disease more common in children
• Tenderness of the globe, deep orbital pain or brow ache, especially with eye movement
• Central, cecocentral or arcuate visual field deficits
• Decreased color vision
• Apparent dimness of light intensities
• Impairment of depth perception
• Increase in visual symptoms with increased body temperature (Uhthoff's sign)
• May be either swollen optic disk (most commonly seen in children) or normal optic disc
• Relative afferent pupillary defect (Marcus Gunn pupil)

CAUSES
• Idiopathic
• Multiple sclerosis
• Viral infections of childhood (measles, mumps, chickenpox)
• Other viral infections (mononucleosis, herpes zoster, encephalitis)
• Contiguous inflammation of the meninges, orbit, or sinuses
• Granulomatous inflammations (syphilis, tuberculosis, cryptococcus, sarcoidosis)
• Intraocular inflammations
• Lead toxicity
• Chronic high doses chloramphenicol
• Posterior uveitis
• Vascular lesions of optic nerve
• Tumors
• Fungal infections

RISK FACTORS N/A

DIAGNOSIS

DIFFERENTIAL DIAGNOSIS
• Acute papilledema
• Anterior ischemic optic neuropathy
• Severe systemic hypertension
• Toxic/nutritional optic neuropathy
• Orbital tumor compressing the optic nerve
• Intracranial tumor pressing on the afferent visual pathway
• Leber's congenital optic neuropathy

LABORATORY
• CBC
• Antinuclear antibody (ANA)
• ESR
• Rapid plasma reagin (RPR)
• Fluorescent treponemal antibody absorption (FTA-ABS)
• Serological test for syphilis
Drugs that may alter lab results: N/A
Disorders that may alter lab results: N/A

PATHOLOGICAL FINDINGS N/A

SPECIAL TESTS
• Visual field test (preferably automated Humphrey or Octopus)
• Color vision testing

IMAGING
• Chest x-ray
• MRI head or CT head/orbits in atypical cases or when patient is not improving after 10-14 days and other tests are negative

DIAGNOSTIC PROCEDURES
• Check blood pressure
• Complete ophthalmologic exam including pupillary assessment, color vision evaluation with color plates, dilated retinal examination with optic nerve assessment
• Neurologic work-up

TREATMENT

APPROPRIATE HEALTH CARE
Outpatient observation

GENERAL MEASURES No disease specific measures

SURGICAL MEASURES N/A

ACTIVITY Fully active

DIET No special diet

PATIENT EDUCATION
• Reassurance about recovery of vision
• If felt to be secondary to demyelinating disease, patient should be informed of the risk of developing multiple sclerosis
• For patient education materials favorably reviewed on this topic, contact: National Eye Institute, Information Officer, Dept. of Health and Human Services, 9000 Rockville Pike, Bethesda, MD 20892, (301)496-5248

MEDICATIONS

DRUG(S) OF CHOICE None
Contraindications: N/A
Precautions: N/A
Significant possible interactions: N/A

ALTERNATIVE DRUGS
• Pulse steroids: methylprednisolone 250 mg IV q6h x 12 doses in the hospital followed by prednisone 1 mg/kg/day po for 11 days, taper over 1-2 weeks
• Anti-ulcer medication is given with steroids

FOLLOWUP

PATIENT MONITORING Monthly followup to monitor visual changes

PREVENTION/AVOIDANCE N/A

POSSIBLE COMPLICATIONS
Permanent loss of vision

EXPECTED COURSE/PROGNOSIS
• Visual acuity begins to improve 2-3 weeks after onset
• Improvement continues over several months and vision often returns to normal or near normal levels
• Those patients with poor vision and who receive IV steroids often recover faster
• When baseline vision is good, IV steroids have no beneficial effect

MISCELLANEOUS

ASSOCIATED CONDITIONS Over 50% of adult optic neuritis patients will develop multiple sclerosis

AGE-RELATED FACTORS
Pediatric: N/A
Geriatric: N/A
Others: N/A

PREGNANCY N/A

SYNONYMS
• Papillitis
• Retrobulbar neuritis

ICD-9-CM 377.30 Optic neuritis

SEE ALSO Multiple sclerosis

OTHER NOTES N/A

ABBREVIATIONS N/A

REFERENCES
• Sergott R, Brown M: Current concepts of the pathogenesis of optic neuritis associated with multiple sclerosis. Surv Ophthalmol 1988;33:108-116
• Miller N: Walsh and Hoyt's Clinical Neuro-Ophthalmology. 4th Ed. Baltimore, Williams & Wilkins, 1982
• Fraunfelder FT, Roy FH: Current Ocular Therapy. 3rd Ed. Philadelphia, W.B. Saunders Co., 1990
Illustrations: 1 available on CD-ROM
Internet references: http://www.5mcc.com

Author(s)
Robert Noecker, MD

Oral cavity neoplasms

BASICS

DESCRIPTION Malignant tumors affecting the lip, tongue, floor of the mouth, salivary glands, inside of cheeks, gums, and palate. 90% of the neoplasms are squamous cell carcinomas and the remainder are lymphomas, melanomas, adenocarcinomas from minor salivary gland origin and sarcomas.
System(s) affected: Gastrointestinal
Genetics: N/A
Incidence/Prevalence in USA:
• 12/100,000 (30,300 new cases a year). 5000 persons die of this disease annually.
• Oral cavity neoplasms account for 4% of all cancers occurring in men and 2% in women
• High incidence in Asia, related to the habit of chewing betelnut, fresh betel leaf, and habitual reverse smoking in which the lighted end of the cigarette is held within the oral cavity
Predominant age: 50 and over. However, increasingly being seen in younger age group with the use of smokeless tobacco.
Predominant sex: Male > Female

SIGNS AND SYMPTOMS
• Dysphagia
• Odynophagia
• Problems articulating
• Regurgitation of liquids secondary to nasopharyngeal incompetence from the tumor
• Ipsilateral otalgia from referred pain
• Friable granular exophytic and/or infiltrative mass or ulcer which frequently is tender and confused with infection. Usually has hard indurated margins by palpation which extend beyond the confines of the ulcer itself.
• Hard neck mass suggesting metastatic disease in the nodal chain along the internal jugular vein

CAUSES
• Tobacco use (smokeless or smoked)
• Use of snuff
• Excess alcohol consumption
• Exposure to ultraviolet light in the instances of lip carcinoma
• Riboflavin or iron deficiency anemia, and Plummer-Vinson syndrome associated with oral cancers
• Betel nut or leaf chewing

RISK FACTORS N/A

DIAGNOSIS

DIFFERENTIAL DIAGNOSIS
• Exudative tonsillitis (usually bilateral involvement)
• Stomatitis or glossitis secondary to infectious etiology, most commonly candidiasis
• Benign tumors of the oral cavity (slow growing and usually not erosive or ulcerative)
• Kaposi's sarcoma
• Mycosis fungoides
• Premalignant lesions such as leukoplakia or erythroplasia
• Lichen planus

LABORATORY Liver function test to rule out metastasis to the liver
Drugs that may alter lab results: N/A
Disorders that may alter lab results:
• Alcoholism
• Hepatitis

PATHOLOGICAL FINDINGS Malignant changes characteristic of cell types

SPECIAL TESTS N/A

IMAGING
• Chest x-ray to rule out metastasis to the lungs
• Imaging bone scans if there is pain in the bones suggesting bone metastasis
• CT or MRI scan if clinical suggestion of intracranial or liver metastasis

DIAGNOSTIC PROCEDURES Transoral biopsy as an outpatient makes the definitive diagnosis

TREATMENT

APPROPRIATE HEALTH CARE
• Inpatient for surgery
• The treatment varies depending on location, i.e., tongue, buccal wall, pharynx, palate, lip

GENERAL MEASURES
• Unresectable lesions usually are treated with radiation therapy and/or chemotherapy for palliation
• Nutrition is of prime importance for normal wound healing should patient require surgery. Patients may need naso-gastric and/or gastrostomy feedings if orally disabled.

SURGICAL MEASURES
• Wide resection with or without radiation therapy and/or chemotherapy is the treatment of choice
• Tracheotomy may be necessary if the patient has problems handling secretions or difficulty breathing

ACTIVITY As tolerated by patient's nutritional and physical status

DIET
• Depends on the extent of disease and whether the patient is able to chew or swallow
• Usually early lesions can be managed with a regular diet. As disease progresses, a soft diet is necessary.

PATIENT EDUCATION Literature is available from American Cancer Society

MEDICATIONS

DRUG(S) OF CHOICE Narcotics for pain relief
Contraindications: N/A
Precautions: N/A
Significant possible interactions: N/A

ALTERNATIVE DRUGS N/A

FOLLOWUP

PATIENT MONITORING Routine periodic head and neck exams to detect possible second primary or recurrence in the upper respiratory and digestive tract

PREVENTION/AVOIDANCE
• Avoidance of smoking or the use of smokeless tobacco
• Avoid alcohol use

POSSIBLE COMPLICATIONS
• Functional and/or cosmetic disabilities proportional to the degree of surgery and stage of tumor
• Stomatitis with or without candidiasis secondary to radiation therapy or chemotherapy
• Persistent dysphagia secondary to surgery or radiation therapy
• Persistent problems with articulation or deglutition depending on the amount of tongue resection

EXPECTED COURSE/PROGNOSIS
Early lesions with adequate treatment leads to a greater than 80% cure

MISCELLANEOUS

ASSOCIATED CONDITIONS
Leukoplakia or erythroplasia should be biopsied, since they are considered premalignant and associated with carcinoma at least 10% of the time

AGE-RELATED FACTORS None
Pediatric: N/A
Geriatric: Greater incidence after 50
Others: N/A

PREGNANCY N/A

SYNONYMS N/A

ICD-9-CM
145.9 Malignant neoplasm of mouth, unspecified
198.89 Secondary malignant neoplasm, other specified sites, other
230.0 Carcinoma in situ lip, oral cavity and pharynx
210.4 Benign neoplasm other and unspecified parts of mouth
235.1 Neoplasm of uncertain behavior of lip, oral cavity and pharynx

SEE ALSO N/A

OTHER NOTES
• High incidence in Asia related to the habit of chewing the betel nut, fresh betel leaf, and habitual reverse smoking (lighted end is held within the oral cavity).

ABBREVIATIONS N/A

REFERENCES Cummings CW, Fredrickson JM, Harker LA, Crause CJ, Schuller DE: Otolaryngology: Head and Neck Surgery. Volume 2. New York, C.V. Mosby Company, 1986
Illustrations: 1 available on CD-ROM
Internet references: http://www.5mcc.com

Author(s)
Roy R. Casiano, MD

Oral rehydration

BASICS

DESCRIPTION
• Dehydration and ongoing fluid losses from infectious gastroenteritis (GE) can be effectively treated with oral rehydration solutions (ORS), except in the most severe cases where initial parenteral fluid resuscitation is required. This therapy takes advantage of the coupled transport of sodium and glucose in the small intestine even during course of GE. Water follows osmotically after sodium entry. Potassium is passively absorbed via solvent drag. A glucose concentration of 2% allows maximal sodium absorption.
• ORS for rehydration should have a sodium content of about 75 mEq/L (75 mmol/L). Maintenance ORS, with sodium content of 40-50 mEq/L (40-50 mmol/L), are useful for mild dehydration and treatment of ongoing losses with a relatively low sodium content (e.g., rotavirus). High sodium diarrheal losses as from cholera require higher sodium content ORS (WHO solution = 90 mEq/L Na).

System(s) affected: Gastrointestinal, Endocrine/Metabolic
Genetics: N/A
Incidence/Prevalence in USA: N/A
Predominant age: Primarily infants and children; effective for all ages
Predominant sex: Male = Female

SIGNS AND SYMPTOMS See
Dehydration

CAUSES N/A

RISK FACTORS N/A

DIAGNOSIS

DIFFERENTIAL DIAGNOSIS N/A

LABORATORY N/A
Drugs that may alter lab results: N/A
Disorders that may alter lab results: N/A

PATHOLOGICAL FINDINGS N/A

SPECIAL TESTS N/A

IMAGING N/A

DIAGNOSTIC PROCEDURES N/A

TREATMENT

APPROPRIATE HEALTH CARE
Primarily outpatient. Designed to be administered by family members.

GENERAL MEASURES
• Estimate replacement at 60 mL/kg for mild- and 80-100 mL/kg for moderate dehydration over the first 4-8 hours. Very important to replace any ongoing losses and add maintenance fluids.
• Replace ongoing stool losses with ORS. In infant, estimate 5-10 mL/kg per stool or weigh diapers.
• Add maintenance requirements to replacement:
 ◊ Estimate:
  0-10 kg - 4 mL/kg/hr
  Plus 10-20 kg - 2 mL/kg/hr
  Plus > 20 kg - 1mL/kg/hr
 ◊ Use maintenance ORS. Traditional clear fluids (e.g., fruit juice, soda) are inappropriate for oral rehydration therapy.
• If the patient has hypertonic dehydration, oral rehydration should be planned for 12-24 hours
• If vomiting occurs, small amounts of ORS given frequently is usually effective
• If patient is not vomiting and is alert, patient's thirst is excellent indicator of fluid needs
• ORS is not to be diluted
• Maintenance oral rehydration therapy begins when the deficit is replaced and provides for ongoing losses. Maintenance ORS or a combination of ORS and water or other clear liquids can be used.
• Effective at all ages. If child refuses because of taste, flavor with a commercial artificially sweetened flavoring, such as, Nutrasweet-flavored Kool-Aid; use approximately 1/4 teaspoon to 4 oz ORS.
• Effective at all ages: prepackaged ORS flavored freeze pops (often well accepted)
• Begin feeding as soon as rehydration achieved

SURGICAL MEASURES N/A

ACTIVITY As tolerated

DIET
• For breast feeding infants - mother should continue nursing
• For bottle fed babies - early institution of lactose-free formulas. Delay using milk-based formula for several days.
• Age appropriate - complex carbohydrate rich (eg, rice, bread, potato, cereal), low fat foods should be offered as soon as the dehydration deficit is replaced. Cow's milk can be added to diet after several days.

PATIENT EDUCATION
• Awareness and availability of ORS markedly diminishes morbidity from gastroenteritis
• Travelers concerned with severe diarrhea should carry ORS packets on trips

Oral rehydration

MEDICATIONS

DRUG(S) OF CHOICE
• The prototype ORS is the World Health Organization solution. In developed countries, when GE is unlikely to be caused by cholera, a lower sodium solution is advisable.
WHO ORS:
  ◊ 1 liter of clean water
  ◊ 1/2 tsp sodium chloride (salt)
  ◊ 1/2 tsp trisodium citrate
  ◊ 1/4 tsp potassium chloride (salt substitute)
  ◊ 2 tbsp glucose
Notes:
  ◊ Glucose can be replaced by either sucrose (table sugar) or rice powder which are less expensive.
  ◊ Trisodium citrate can be replaced by sodium bicarbonate (baking soda). (Sodium bicarbonate was used in previous formulation.)

Comparison of ORS's

Solution	Type†	Na+	Storage form
WHO ORS	R	90	Powder
Rehydralyte	R	75	Liquid
Pedialyte	M	45	Liquid
Kaolectro	M	50	Powder
Beech-nut-Ped. Electrolyte	M	50	Liquid

† R = rehydration
  M = maintenance
Na+ = Sodium (mEq/L or mmol/L)

Contraindications:
• Conditions predisposing to risk of aspiration: Altered consciousness, seizure activity, severe hypotension, shock
• Persistent vomiting (as in pyloric stenosis)
• Absent bowel sounds
Precautions:
• The ingredients should be provided in pre-mixed packets in order to avoid iatrogenic errors in mixing
• If water safety is questionable, it should be boiled or treated for purification
• Discard the solution after 12 hours if held at room temperature, or 24 hours if refrigerated
• After rehydration is complete, ORS's should not be used as the only fluid intake because the high sodium content may lead to hypernatremia
Significant possible interactions: N/A

ALTERNATIVE DRUGS   N/A

FOLLOWUP

PATIENT MONITORING   The patient needs to be frequently evaluated to ensure establishment of an improving clinical status and an adequate urine output

PREVENTION/AVOIDANCE   N/A

POSSIBLE COMPLICATIONS   Change to IV hydration if the patient has increasing weight loss (fluid deficit), clinical deterioration, or intractable vomiting.

EXPECTED COURSE/PROGNOSIS
• Rapid clinical improvement despite continuing diarrhea is the usual course
• The overall complication rate for oral rehydration is the same as that for parenteral rehydration in cases of mild and moderate dehydration.

MISCELLANEOUS

ASSOCIATED CONDITIONS   N/A

AGE-RELATED FACTORS   N/A
Pediatric: See Diet
Geriatric: N/A
Others: N/A

PREGNANCY   N/A

SYNONYMS   N/A

ICD-9-CM   N/A

SEE ALSO
• Dehydration
• Cholera
• Diarrhea, acute
• Gastroenteritis, viral
• Hypernatremia

OTHER NOTES   Advantages of oral rehydration include a much lower cost, minimal storage requirements (for powder forms) and no need for sterile conditions

ABBREVIATIONS
• GE = gastroenteritis
• ORS = oral rehydration solutions

REFERENCES
• Provisional Committee on Quality Improvement, Subcommittee on Acute Gastroenteritis Practice Parameter: The management of acute gastroenteritis in young children. Pediatrics 1996;97:424-436
• Duggen C, Nurko S: Feeding the gut: the scientific basis for continued enteral nutrition during acute diarrhea. J Pediatr 1997;131:801-808
• Meyers A: Modern management of acute diarrhea and dehydration in children. Am Fam Phys 1995;51:1103-18
• Santosham M, et al: A double-blind clinical trial comparing WHO ORS with a reduced osmolarity solution containing amounts of sodium and glucose. J Pediatr 1996;128:45-51
Illustrations: N/A
Internet references: http://www.5mcc.com

Author(s)
William A. Primack, MD
Charles N. Jacobs, MD

Osgood-Schlatter disease

BASICS

DESCRIPTION The syndrome associated with traction apophysitis in adolescent boys and girls consisting of pain of the tibial tubercle with swelling
System(s) affected: Musculoskeletal
Genetics: Unknown
Incidence/Prevalence in USA: Not known, but common (13% of athletes in one Finnish study)
Predominant age:
• Females 10-16
• Males 11-18
Predominant sex: Male > Female

SIGNS AND SYMPTOMS
• Unilateral or bilateral (30%) tibial tuberosity pain
• Pain exacerbated by exercise, especially jumping and landing after jumping
• Tibial tuberosity swelling
• Pain increased with knee extension against resistance or kneeling
• Knee pain with squatting or crouching
• Absence of effusion or condyle tenderness
• Erythema of tibial tuberosity

CAUSES Basic etiology unknown, but clearly exacerbated by exercise - jumping and pivoting sports are the worst

RISK FACTORS
• Age between 11 and 18
• Male sex
• Rapid skeletal growth
• Involvement in repetitive jumping sports

DIAGNOSIS

DIFFERENTIAL DIAGNOSIS
• Stress fracture of the proximal tibia
• Pes anserinus bursitis
• Quadriceps tendon avulsion
• Patellofemoral stress syndrome
• Chondromalacia patellae
• Proximal tibial neoplasm
• Osteomyelitis of the proximal tibia
• Tibial plateau fracture
• Patellar tendonitis
• Sinding-Larson-Johansson syndrome

LABORATORY No blood tests indicated unless other diagnostic considerations are entertained
Drugs that may alter lab results: N/A
Disorders that may alter lab results: N/A

PATHOLOGICAL FINDINGS
• Osteochondritis of the tibial tubercle
• Heterotopic bone formation at insertion of the patellar tendon
• Bony fusion of the tibial metaphysis
• Inflammatory infiltrate of the epiphysis in severe cases
• Complete avulsion of the tibial tubercle with nonunion of the tubercle with the tibia - possible complication (extremely rare)

SPECIAL TESTS N/A

IMAGING
• X-ray imaging of the proximal tibia and knee may show heterotopic calcification in the patellar tendon. X-rays are rarely diagnostic.
• Calcified thickening of the tibial tuberosity with irregular ossification at insertion of tendon to tibial tubercle
• Bone scan may show increased uptake in the area of the tibial tuberosity; will have increased uptake in apophysis in any child, but may be more than opposite side

DIAGNOSTIC PROCEDURES N/A

TREATMENT

APPROPRIATE HEALTH CARE
Outpatient

GENERAL MEASURES
• Frequent ice applications post exercise with pain
• Rest
• Knee immobilization in extension
• In more severe cases, avoidance of activities that increase pain or swelling
• Quadriceps isometric strengthening, hip extensions, adductor strengthening, hamstring and quadriceps stretching exercises

SURGICAL MEASURES Débridement of a thickened cosmetically unsatisfactory tibial tubercle (rare)

ACTIVITY Activity to be restricted to those activities not causing pain

DIET N/A

PATIENT EDUCATION
• Consider avoidance of jumping sports. Assure family that symptoms and findings will diminish with time and rest.
• OK to play sport with mild pain

MEDICATIONS

DRUG(S) OF CHOICE None in particular, but all analgesics may be considered. NSAID's are of minimal benefit.
Contraindications: N/A
Precautions: N/A
Significant possible interactions: N/A

ALTERNATIVE DRUGS More potent analgesics such as narcotics may be considered for short term use or in extreme situations

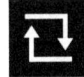

FOLLOWUP

PATIENT MONITORING Follow up on a prn basis for management of pain and disability

PREVENTION/AVOIDANCE
• Avoidance of those sports involving heavy quadriceps loading
• Patients may compete if the pain is minimal
• Increase hamstring and quadriceps flexibility

POSSIBLE COMPLICATIONS
• Nonunion of the tubercle to the tibia
• Upriding of the patella
• Patellar tendon avulsion
• Genu recurvatum
• Patellofemoral degenerative arthritis
• Patella alta
• Chondromalacia

EXPECTED COURSE/PROGNOSIS
Except in rare complicated cases, this is a self-limiting illness resolved within two years after full skeletal maturation. However, up to 50% of adults with prior Osgood-Schlatter disease will still report occasional symptoms.

MISCELLANEOUS

ASSOCIATED CONDITIONS N/A

AGE-RELATED FACTORS
Pediatric: In skeletally mature boys and girls, with boys more frequent than girls
Geriatric: N/A
Others: Participants in sports involving heavy quadriceps activity

PREGNANCY N/A

SYNONYMS Osteochondritis of the tibial tubercle

ICD-9-CM 732.4 Juvenile osteochondrosis of lower extremity, excluding foot

SEE ALSO Tendinitis

OTHER NOTES N/A

ABBREVIATIONS N/A

REFERENCES
• Outerbridge AR, Micheli LJ: Overuse injuries in the young athlete. Sports Med 1995;14(3):503-516
• Peck DM: Apophyseal injuries in the young athlete. Am Fam Phys 1995;51(8):1891-1895
• Reider B: Sports Medicine: The School Age Athlete. 2nd Ed. Philadelphia, WB Saunders Co, 1996
Illustrations: N/A
Internet references: http://www.5mcc.com

Author(s)
David P. Sealy, MD

Osteitis deformans

BASICS

DESCRIPTION Inflammatory focal or generalized condition of the skeleton characterized by rapid, chaotic bone resorption followed by equally chaotic and excessive bone formation. Leads to enlarged but weakened and highly vascularized bone which is painful, easily deformed and subject to fractures with minimal trauma. Cranial and vertebral involvement can also cause neurologic deficits.
System(s) affected: Musculoskeletal
Genetics: 15-50% of patients have one or more involved first order relatives with osteitis deformans. Recent data suggest an 18q locus is involved, but other chromosomal sites may also confer susceptibility.
Incidence/Prevalence in USA: 3% of Caucasian individuals above age 50 have at least one focus. Rare in African Americans and Asians.
Predominant age: Above age 50, occasional cases ages 20-50
Predominant sex: Male = Female

SIGNS AND SYMPTOMS
• Asymptomatic frequently
• Bone pain
• Skeletal deformities
• Bowing of extremities
• Acetabular protrusion
• Headaches
• Head enlargement
• Frequent fractures
• Secondary osteoarthritis
• Vertebral compression
• Neurologic deficits
• High output congestive heart failure (rare)
• Hypercalcemia (rare)
• Renal calculi (calcium, uric acid)
• Peyronie's syndrome
• Angioid streaks (rare)
• Mottled retinal degeneration (rare)
• Increased skin temperature over affected areas
• Bone sarcomas (rare)
• Peripheral neuropathies
• Carpal/tarsal tunnel syndromes
• Valvular/endocardial calcification
• Accelerated atherosclerosis
• Gouty diathesis
• Hyperparathyroidism
• Sensorineural hearing loss
• Conductive hearing loss

CAUSES Unknown; best evidence to date is for slow virus infection in genetically susceptible individuals

RISK FACTORS None known

DIAGNOSIS

DIFFERENTIAL DIAGNOSIS
• Polyostotic fibrous dysplasia
• Osteitis fibrosis cystica (skeletal hyperparathyroidism)
• Primary bone neoplasms
• Osteolytic, osteoblastic metastases

LABORATORY
• Serum calcium - usually normal, rarely increased
• Serum alkaline phosphatase (total or bone specific) - usually increased
• Serum GGT - normal
• Serum osteocalcin (BGP) - usually increased
• Urinary pyridinoline collagen crosslinks - usually increased
• N- and C-telopeptide (collagen crosslinks) - usually increased
Drugs that may alter lab results:
• Vitamin D and its metabolites
• Hepatotoxic drugs
Disorders that may alter lab results:
• See Differential diagnosis
• Osteomalacia
• Liver disorders
• Traumatic fractures

PATHOLOGICAL FINDINGS
• Chaotic bone resorption at advancing edge of disease. Osteoclasts are large, contain 10-100 nuclei and have abnormal configuration.
• Electronphotomicroscopically, the nuclei and cytoplasm contain myriad of inclusion bodies resembling viral nucleocapsids
• Later, excessive osteoblastic bone formation predominates with sclerotic bone containing cement lines forming mosaic pattern

SPECIAL TESTS
• Neurologic examination
• Audiogram, if skull involvement
• Visual field study, if skull involvement

IMAGING
• X-rays show irregular pattern of alternating bone formation and resorption in enlarged deformed bones. Resorptive fronts at advancing edge.
• Bone scans show intense uptake in focal pattern
• CT/MRI show extra-bony extension if sarcomatous degeneration occurs

DIAGNOSTIC PROCEDURES Bone biopsy needed only in confusing cases (rare)

TREATMENT

APPROPRIATE HEALTH CARE
Outpatient, except when intravenous treatment is used

GENERAL MEASURES
• Rarely, splints for severely resorbed areas with high risk of fracture
• Hearing aids for severe deafness; of some (but not great) value in sensorineural deafness

SURGICAL MEASURES
• Joint replacement (hip, knee) sometimes needed
• Osteotomy procedures for extreme deformity
• Decompression procedures (skull, spinal column) for acute neurologic deficits (rarely needed)
• Bone biopsy (rarely needed)
• Extirpative surgery for sarcomatous complications
• Open reduction of fractures

ACTIVITY
• Full activity to maintain function
• Avoid excessive mechanical stress on involved bones

DIET No special diet

PATIENT EDUCATION Paget Foundation, 120 Wall St., Suite 1602, New York, NY 10005 (212)509-5335; fax (212)509-8492; Email: pagetfdn@aol.com

MEDICATIONS

DRUG(S) OF CHOICE
• Synthetic injectable salmon calcitonin (Miacalcin): 50 IU three times weekly to 100 IU qd, courses 1.5 to 3 years
or
• Etidronate (Didronel), 5 mg/kg/day (approximately 400 mg) x 6 mos (taken on an empty stomach). Rarely, 20 mg/kg/day x 1 month. Courses may be repeated after a 3-6 month rest period
or
• Alendronate (Fosamax) 40 mg/day (taken on an empty stomach) for 6 mos
or
• Tiludronate (Skelid) 400 mg/day (taken on an empty stomach) for 3 months
or
• Risedronate (Actonel) 30 mg/day (taken on an empty stomach) for 2 months
or
• Pamidronate (Aredia) 60 mg/day by 4-6 hour infusions for 2-3 days. Alternately, 30 mg/day by 4-6 hour infusions once a week for 6 weeks. May be repeated several months later if effect wears off.
or
• Plicamycin (Mithracin), 25 mcg/kg/day or qod by 4-6 hr infusions x 9-10 infusions
• Add nonsteroidal anti-inflammatories (NSAID's) to above drugs for secondary osteoarthritis. COX-2 inhibitors may be substituted.
Contraindications:
• Prior history of allergy or hypersensitivity
• For alendronate, tiludronate, and risedronate, esophageal dysfunction, severe upper GI symptoms, GERD, etc.
• For plicamycin, manifest hepatic or renal impairment or bone marrow depression
Precautions:
• Adverse side effects may require ameliorative measures or temporary dose reduction
• Salmon calcitonin - nausea, vomiting, anorexia, flushing, rash, including urticaria (rare)
• Etidronate disodium - nausea, vomiting, diarrhea, increased bone pain
• Alendronate, tiludronate and risedronate - heartburn, epigastric pain, musculoskeletal pain. Take on an empty stomach with copious water. No food, beverages or other medications for 30-60 minutes hour. Remain upright for 1 hour.
• Pamidronate disodium - transient fever, leukopenia, hypocalcemia, headache, malaise, loss of appetite
• Plicamycin - vomiting, anorexia, malaise, abnormal liver/renal function, thrombocytopenia with bleeding
Significant possible interactions: None

ALTERNATIVE DRUGS
NSAID's or COX-2 inhibitors for mildly symptomatic disease in nonstrategic areas

FOLLOWUP

PATIENT MONITORING
• Followup visits every 2-4 months during drug therapy; yearly if drugs not being used. Alkaline phosphatase (total or bone specific) before each visit.
• Repeat x-rays and bone scan every 3-5 years or as needed

PREVENTION/AVOIDANCE
Avoid excessive mechanical stress on afflicted bones to reduce chance of fractures and other complications

POSSIBLE COMPLICATIONS
Fractures, severe deformities, head enlargement, acetabular protrusion, carpal/tarsal tunnel syndromes, neurologic deficits, deafness, visual impairment, congestive heart failure (high output), renal calculi, Peyronie's syndrome, sarcomatous degeneration

EXPECTED COURSE/PROGNOSIS
• Depends on severity, often asymptomatic
• Slow progression if untreated
• Significant amelioration with treatment (85% or greater)
• Poor prognosis if bone sarcoma develops

MISCELLANEOUS

ASSOCIATED CONDITIONS
• Hyperparathyroidism
• Gouty diathesis
• Secondary osteoarthritis
• Angioid streaks
• Mottled retinal degeneration
• Bone sarcoma (rare)
• Peyronie's disease

AGE-RELATED FACTORS
Pediatric: N/A
Geriatric: Common
Others: More prevalent if ancestry Caucasian, especially United Kingdom, Northern Europe (excluding Scandinavia), Italy, Australia and New Zealand. Rare in African Americans and Asians.

PREGNANCY N/A

SYNONYMS Paget's disease of bone

ICD-9-CM
731.0 Osteitis deformans without mention of bone tumor

SEE ALSO
• Hyperparathyroidism
• Arthritis, osteo
• Bone tumor, primary malignant

OTHER NOTES N/A

ABBREVIATIONS N/A

REFERENCES
• Hadjipavlou A, Lander P, Srolovitz H, Enker IP. Malignant transformation in Paget's disease of bone. Cancer. 1992;70:2802-2808
• Morales-Piga AA, Rey-Rey JS, Corres-Gonzalez J, Garcia-Sagredo JM, Loopez-Abente G. Frequency and characteristics of familial aggregation of Paget's disease of bone. J Bone Miner Res. 1995;10:663-670
• Singer FR, Minoofer PN. Biphosphonates in the treatment of disorders of mineral metabolism. Adv Endocrinol Metab, 1995;6:259-288
• Delmas PD, Meunier PJ: The management of Paget's disease of bone. NEJM 1997;336:558-566
• Wallach S. Identifying and controlling Paget's disease. J Musculoskel Med 1997;14(6):66-82
• Papapoulos SE: Paget's disease of bone: clinical, pathogenetic and therapeutic aspects. Bailliere's Clin Endocrinol Metab 1997;2:117-143
• Siris ES: Paget's disease of bone. Journal of Bone and Mineral Research 1998;13(7):1061-1065
• Ankrom MA, Shapiro JR: Paget's disease of bone (osteitis deformans). J Am Geriatr Soc 1998;46(8):1025-1033
Illustrations: N/A
Internet references: http://www.5mcc.com

Author(s)
Stanley Wallach, MD

Osteochondritis dissecans

BASICS

DESCRIPTION Condition in which segment of articular and underlying subchondral bone becomes separated from surrounding bone.
System(s) affected: Musculoskeletal
Genetics: No distinct genetic pattern known
Incidence/Prevalence in USA: Unknown
Predominant Age: 2 main age groups; children under 12 years old and young adults
Predominant Sex: Male > Female (3:1)

SIGNS AND SYMPTOMS
• Intermittent joint pain, clicking, swelling, locking and stiffness
• May be asymptomatic until the fragment detaches, then experience locking of the joint or giving way in the knee
• Focal tenderness over involved part of joint
• May have effusion, atrophy of supporting musculature, crepitus, decreased range of motion

CAUSES
Most widely accepted theories are:
• Trauma (direct or indirect)
versus
• Ischemic theory due to focal insufficiency in end-arterial blood supply leading to necrosis
• Accessory growth centers that may have arterial supply disrupted leading to typical osteochondritis dissecans lesion (unlikely)

RISK FACTORS No apparent genetic predisposition

DIAGNOSIS

DIFFERENTIAL DIAGNOSIS
• Meniscal tear
• Osteochondral fractures
• Patellalgia
• Anomalous ossification center especially in lat condyle

LABORATORY No specific tests
Drugs that may alter lab results: N/A
Disorders that may alter lab results: N/A

PATHOLOGICAL FINDINGS
• Primary change in the bone
• Avascular necrosis occurs in a focal area
• Overlying cartilage changes are secondary to the bony changes
• Loss of subchondral bone support leads to degenerative cartilage changes - softening, fibromatous, fissuring
• Fragment may detach and become loose body with traumatic event
• Healing occurs by revascularization and "creeping substitution"

SPECIAL TESTS N/A

IMAGING
• Plain radiographs - AP, lateral and "tunnel" view, first study to confirm diagnosis. Appears as a well demarcated fragment of bone surrounded by a radiolucent zone. If separated, the fragment may be seen elsewhere in the joint and a defect is present in the articular surface.
• Technetium 99 bone scan - now of historic value; was used to evaluate healing potential.
• CT scan - provides architectural description of lesion. Essentially replaced by MRI.
• MRI
  ◊ Very useful to delineate bony lesion
  ◊ Difficult to assess and identify the status of overlying articular cartilage. Healing progression difficult to follow.

DIAGNOSTIC PROCEDURES
• Arthroscopy - definitive procedure to assess the underlying cartilage and for definitive treatment

TREATMENT

APPROPRIATE HEALTH CARE
Outpatient usually; inpatient for surgery

GENERAL MEASURES
• Goals of treatment - maintain smooth congruous joint surface. Alleviate pain. Prevent degenerative joint disease. Promote revascularization of necrotic fragment.
• Splinting, crutches, non-weight bearing with active range of motion is the norm

SURGICAL MEASURES On occasion, early surgical intervention is needed. Orthopedic consultation recommended.

ACTIVITY
• Non-weight bearing, immobilization with intermittent maintenance of range of motion
• Follow closely for 12 weeks for healing; fragment displacement may occur, in which case arthroscopy is indicated.

DIET No specific diet recommended

PATIENT EDUCATION
• Compliance with immobilization and possibility of further trauma should be emphasized.
• Most lesions heal without surgical intervention.

MEDICATIONS

DRUG(S) OF CHOICE
• NSAIDs (e.g., ibuprofen 20-30 mg/kg/day)
Contraindications: N/A
Precautions: N/A
Significant possible interactions: N/A

ALTERNATIVE DRUGS   N/A

FOLLOWUP

PATIENT MONITORING
Initially should be followed every 6-8 weeks with serial radiographs to check for healing and possible displacement. Expect healing in 3 months. In one year radiographs usually show no residual abnormality.

PREVENTION/AVOIDANCE   No clear way to avoid its development.

POSSIBLE COMPLICATIONS
• Failure to revascularize and heal
• Displacement of fragment becoming loose body within a joint

EXPECTED COURSE/PROGNOSIS
• Most will heal without morbidity
• An incongruous joint surface may lead to degenerative changes if not managed adequately

MISCELLANEOUS

ASSOCIATED CONDITIONS   N/A

AGE-RELATED FACTORS
Pediatric: N/A
Geriatric: N/A
Others: N/A

PREGNANCY   N/A

SYNONYMS   N/A

ICD-9-CM   732.7 Osteochondritis dissecans

SEE ALSO   N/A

OTHER NOTES   N/A

ABBREVIATIONS   N/A

REFERENCES
• Federico DJ, et al: Osteochondritis Dissecans of the Knee: A historical review of etiology and treatment. Arthroscopy 1990;6(3):190-197
• Garrett JC: Clinics in Sports Med 1991;10(3):569-593
• Green WT, Banks HH: CORR; Osteochondritis Dissecans in Children 1990;(255):3-12
• Tachdjian MO: Pediatric Orthopedics 1990;2:1515-1534
Illustrations: N/A
Internet references: http://www.5mcc.com

Author(s)
Russell G. Cohen, MD
Francisco G. Valencia, MD

Osteomalacia & rickets

BASICS

DESCRIPTION Osteomalacia (referred to as rickets in children) is defined as an excess organic bone matrix secondary to defective or inadequate bone mineralization
System(s) affected: Musculoskeletal
Genetics: N/A
Incidence/Prevalence in USA: N/A
Predominant age: All ages. In adults, osteomalacia is usually a disease of the older population (50-80).
Predominant sex: Female > Male (slightly)

SIGNS AND SYMPTOMS
• Bone pain, tenderness, muscle weakness
• Bone pain is dull and tends to be poorly localized, usually affecting the ribs and upper thighs
• Muscle weakness is usually proximal
• Other symptoms of malnutrition or an underlying problem such as chronic renal disease may also be clinically evident
• Weight loss
• Anorexia
• Tetany
• In young children - restlessness, poor sleep patterns, craniotabes, costochondral beading, bowlegs, kyphoscoliosis

CAUSES
• Can be caused by a wide variety of pathogenic processes, including, but not limited to, vitamin D deficiency (reduced exposure to sunlight, poor nutrition, malabsorption syndromes)
• Defective metabolism of parent vitamin D to active metabolites (drug-induced, i.e., anticonvulsants - phenytoin (Dilantin), chronic renal failure), hypophosphatemia (renal tubular acidosis, hypophosphatemic syndrome), miscellaneous (long-term hemodialysis, malnutrition, vitamin D-dependent rickets)

RISK FACTORS
• Poverty
• Inadequate nutrition and sunlight exposure

DIAGNOSIS

DIFFERENTIAL DIAGNOSIS
• Osteoporosis
• Metastatic bone disease
• Primary bone malignancies (lymphoma, myeloma)

LABORATORY
• Alkaline phosphatase - increased
• Serum calcium is low or normal (never high)
• Hypophosphatemia
• Aminoaciduria
• Acidosis
• Glucosuria
• Hypouricemia
Drugs that may alter lab results: N/A
Disorders that may alter lab results: N/A

PATHOLOGICAL FINDINGS
• Defective calcification of growing bone
• Hypertrophy of epiphyseal cartilages

SPECIAL TESTS   N/A

IMAGING   Radiographic changes are non-specific. Earliest manifestations are thinning of cortical bone. In long-term osteomalacia: bone softening (protrusio acetabuli), looser lines, stress fractures, and pathologic fractures.

DIAGNOSTIC PROCEDURES   Bone biopsy and subsequent histopathologic evaluation deliver the most accurate diagnosis of osteomalacia. The biopsy is usually taken from the iliac crest, and both calcified, and non-calcified studies, as well as special stains (including von Kossa's stain) are helpful.

TREATMENT

APPROPRIATE HEALTH CARE   Can be managed on an outpatient basis, except for complicating emergencies/fractures

GENERAL MEASURES
• Treatment of osteomalacia depends upon the cause, i.e., gastrointestinal, renal, or nutritional.
• For nutritional osteomalacia, calcium and vitamin D have been shown to correct the disease process
• Treatment can be monitored by observing simple bone biochemistry
• Treatment results depend on identifying and correcting the cause

SURGICAL MEASURES   N/A

ACTIVITY   Full activity is encouraged, including a neuroconditioning program

DIET
• Ensure adequate vitamin D intake
• Provide instructions for a high calcium diet and information on calcium supplements, if appropriate

PATIENT EDUCATION   Educate family and patient on nutrition

MEDICATIONS

DRUG(S) OF CHOICE For adults and uncomplicated rickets: vitamin D (ergocalciferol) 2000-4800 IU once a day for one month. Then reduce dose gradually.
Contraindications: N/A
Precautions: N/A
Significant possible interactions: N/A

ALTERNATIVE DRUGS
• IV calcium salts if tetany complicates. Single IM dose of 100,000 IU in adolescents each Fall.
• Alfacalcidol
• Calcitriol

FOLLOWUP

PATIENT MONITORING Office visits every 6 months

PREVENTION/AVOIDANCE
• Adequate dietary intake of vitamin D
• Adequate sunlight exposure
• Fortified cow's milk

POSSIBLE COMPLICATIONS
• Fractures
• Osteomyelitis
• Renal failure
• Renal tubular acidosis
• Seizures
• Growth deformity; bowing long bones in children

EXPECTED COURSE/PROGNOSIS
Variable

MISCELLANEOUS

ASSOCIATED CONDITIONS
• Chronic renal disease
• Epilepsy
• Malnutrition
• Previous gastric surgery
• Pregnancy-nutritional factors

AGE-RELATED FACTORS
Pediatric: N/A
Geriatric: Studies have suggested that vitamin D deficiency osteomalacia is a relatively common condition in the acutely ill elderly population, with an estimated prevalence of about 3-5%; however, it often goes undiagnosed
Others: N/A

PREGNANCY N/A

SYNONYMS Rickets

ICD-9-CM 268.2 Osteomalacia, unspecified

SEE ALSO N/A

OTHER NOTES N/A

ABBREVIATIONS N/A

REFERENCES Mare GM, McKenna MJ, Frame B: Osteomalacia. Bone Mineral Res 1986;4:335
Illustrations: N/A
Internet references: http://www.5mcc.com

Author(s)
Mark C. Leeson, MD, FACS

Osteomyelitis

BASICS

DESCRIPTION Osteomyelitis is an acute or chronic infection of the bone and its structures caused most commonly by bacteria and rarely by other microorganisms. This infection may be acquired either by hematogenous, contiguous, or direct inoculation such as trauma or surgery.
System(s) affected: Musculoskeletal
Genetics: There is no genetic predisposition known in this disease
Incidence/Prevalence in USA: Uncommon
Predominant age: This infection is commonly seen in older adults; hematogenous is bimodal, also seen in infants and children
Predominant sex: Males > Females

SIGNS AND SYMPTOMS

• Hematogenous long bone infection
(in children with hematogenous osteomyelitis)
 ◊ Abrupt onset of high fever
 ◊ Irritability
 ◊ Malaise
 ◊ Restriction of movement of the involved extremity
 ◊ Signs of localized inflammation
• Hematogenous vertebral infection
(in adults with vertebral osteomyelitis)
 ◊ Illness is insidious and behaves more like a chronic infection
 ◊ History of an acute bacteremic episode associated with infection of a specific organ may be found in some patients
• Contiguous and vascular insufficiency associated infection
 ◊ Acute constitutional manifestations are seldom seen
 ◊ Localized signs and symptoms of inflammation with or without drainage frequently found
• Chronic osteomyelitis
 ◊ Non-healing ulcer or draining sinus
 ◊ Constitutional symptoms, when present, indicate acute suppurative condition in the bone or surrounding tissues
• Prosthetic device associated infection
 ◊ Infection may be acquired either by hematogenous route, or by contiguous foci such as local infection, operative contamination, or postoperative infection
 ◊ Acute postoperative infection may present as fever, localized swelling, tenderness, and drainage
 ◊ Chronic infection is characterized by joint discomfort, swelling, erythema, and joint dysfunction

CAUSES

• Acute hematogenous osteomyelitis
 ◊ Staphylococcus aureus (most common)
 ◊ Streptococcus, coagulase negative Staphylococcus, Haemophilus influenzae, and gram negative organisms (less common)
• Vertebral osteomyelitis
 ◊ Staphylococcus aureus and gram negative enteric organisms (common)
 ◊ Other microorganisms to consider include Mycobacterium tuberculosis, and fungi
• Contiguous focus osteomyelitis and vascular insufficiency osteomyelitis
 ◊ Mixed aerobic/anaerobic microorganisms are frequently found
• Prosthetic device infection
 ◊ Coagulase negative Staphylococcus, and S. aureus (most common)
 ◊ Diphtheroids, and gram negative bacteria (less common)

RISK FACTORS

• Sickle cell disease
• Other conditions which predispose to bone infarcts
• IV drug use
• Hemodialysis
• Local trauma
• Open fractures
• Presence of prosthetic orthopedic implant
• Vascular insufficiency
• Neuropathy
• Diabetes mellitus

DIAGNOSIS

DIFFERENTIAL DIAGNOSIS

• Systemic infection from other source
• Aseptic bone infarction
• Localized inflammation or infection of overlying skin and soft tissues
• Neuropathic joint disease
• Fractures
• Gout

LABORATORY

• Definitive diagnosis is made by needle aspiration or bone biopsy and demonstration of the microorganism by culture or histology
• Blood culture may be positive in about 50% of younger patients with acute hematogenous disease
• Leukocyte count is usually elevated in the acute cases, but not in the chronic cases
• Sedimentation rate or c-reactive protein is usually elevated, but non-specific
Drugs that may alter lab results:
Antimicrobial agents given before bone culture
Disorders that may alter lab results:
• Cultures from the sinus tract are unreliable because of frequent contamination
• Superficial cultures only helpful in identifying methicillin-resistant S. aureus

PATHOLOGICAL FINDINGS
Inflammatory process of the bone with pyogenic bacteria

SPECIAL TESTS   N/A

IMAGING

• No technique can absolutely confirm or exclude osteomyelitis
• Radiographic - routine x-ray (findings on plain x-ray often delayed for 10-14 days in acute infection)
• Radionuclide (technetium, indium, or gallium) are also useful, but limited by low specificity
• CT with good resolution, artifact may decrease specificity
• MRI excellent, but limited by costs

DIAGNOSTIC PROCEDURES   Needle biopsy or open bone biopsy for bacterial culture (which is the "gold standard")

TREATMENT

APPROPRIATE HEALTH CARE
Hospitalize the patient with suspected acute osteomyelitis for diagnostic work-up and initial treatment

GENERAL MEASURES   Symptomatic treatment of pain

SURGICAL MEASURES
• Surgical drainage and removal of necrotic tissues are of utmost importance to effect cure
• In patients with vascular insufficiency or severe gangrenous infection, amputation may be the only effective treatment

ACTIVITY   Bedrest and immobilization of the involved bone and joint

DIET   No restriction

PATIENT EDUCATION   Stress need for long-term treatment and follow up

MEDICATIONS

DRUG(S) OF CHOICE
These are essentially empiric choices; recommendations based on data from a very small number of studies. Antimicrobial agent/agents based on susceptibility testing and known clinical efficacy. The duration of therapy for acute osteomyelitis should be at least 4-6 weeks. In chronic osteomyelitis, longer duration of therapy may be needed.
• Staphylococcus aureus and coagulase negative staphylococcus: nafcillin 2 g IV q4-6h. Vancomycin 1 g q12h for methicillin resistant Staph.
• Streptococcus spp.: penicillin G 2-4 million units q4h IV
• Enteric gram negative bacilli and Pseudomonas aeruginosa: piperacillin 4 g q4-6h IV, plus aminoglycoside
• Mixed aerobic/anaerobic infection (diabetic foot, bite wound): beta-lactamase inhibitor combination (ticarcillin-clavulanate 3.1 g q6h IV; ampicillin-sulbactam 3 g q6h IV); piperacillin-tazobactam 3.375 g q6h IV
Contraindications: Allergy
Precautions: In patients with renal or hepatic insufficiency, antimicrobial dose may need adjustment
Significant possible interactions: Refer to manufacturer's literature

ALTERNATIVE DRUGS
• Staphylococcus aureus and coagulase negative staphylococcus: clindamycin 600 mg IV q6h, nafcillin 2 g q4h, or cefazolin 1 g q8h IV, or vancomycin 1 g q12h
• Streptococcus spp.: penicillin G 2 million units q4h, cefazolin 1 g q8h IV, or clindamycin 600 mg q6h IV
• Enteric gram negative bacilli and Pseudomonas aeruginosa: ceftazidime 1 g q8h IV or ciprofloxacin [or other quinolone] 750 mg q12h orally.
• Mixed aerobic/anaerobic infection (diabetic foot, bite wound): clindamycin plus third generation cephalosporin or quinolone
• Home therapy often used - consider a simplified antibiotic regimen for outpatient use or oral therapy
• Some published studies recommend use of hyperbaric oxygen (HBO), but none are randomized, controlled trials

FOLLOWUP

PATIENT MONITORING
Blood level of antimicrobial agents, serum antibacterial titers, sedimentation rate, repeat plain x-ray to confirm healing

PREVENTION/AVOIDANCE
Avoid further stress and weight bearing until healing

POSSIBLE COMPLICATIONS
• Abscess formation
• Bacteremia
• Fracture
• Loosening of the prosthetic implant
• Postoperative infection

EXPECTED COURSE/PROGNOSIS
• Cure of osteomyelitis with medical treatment is notoriously unpredictable especially when not accompanied by surgical debridement
• In patients with acute hematogenous osteomyelitis, the prognosis is usually good even without surgery. Cure takes about 6 weeks.
• The prognosis is improved if all infected bone has been removed

MISCELLANEOUS

ASSOCIATED CONDITIONS
Listed with Causes

AGE-RELATED FACTORS
Pediatric: Occurs most often in 5-14 age group and more frequently in boys
Geriatric:
• Vertebral osteomyelitis more common
• Contiguous focus of infection more common
• Vascular insufficiency is most common cause of osteomyelitis in 50-70 age group (usually due to presence of associated conditions)
Others: N/A

PREGNANCY N/A

SYNONYMS N/A

ICD-9-CM
730.0 Acute osteomyelitis
730.1 Chronic osteomyelitis
526.4 Jaw osteomyelitis
376.03 Orbital osteomyelitis

SEE ALSO N/A

OTHER NOTES N/A

ABBREVIATIONS N/A

REFERENCES
• Haas DW, McAndrew MP. Bacterial osteomyelitis in adults. Am J Medicine 1996;101:550-561
• Lipsky BA. Osteomyelitis of the foot in diabetic patients. Clin Infect Dis 1997;26:1318-1326
• Lew DP, Waldvogel FA: Osteomyelitis. NEJM 1997;336
Illustrations: 1 available on CD-ROM
Internet references: http://www.5mcc.com

Author(s)
Jeffery T. Kirchner, DO, FAAFP

Osteonecrosis

 BASICS

DESCRIPTION
Death of the cellular components of bony tissue

System(s) affected: Musculoskeletal

Genetics: The underlying condition of hemoglobinopathies, especially sickle cell disease, diabetes, and type II or IV hyperlipemia are inheritable and associated with a high incidence of osteonecrosis. Other forms have no proven genetic relationship.

Incidence/Prevalence in USA: Dependent upon the underlying condition

Predominant age: 3rd to 6th decade

Predominant sex: Male > Female

SIGNS AND SYMPTOMS
• The symptoms may be acute as in osteonecrosis of sickle cell disease or renal transplant. Usually insidious in other forms. Diagnosis may not be made for two years after onset of symptoms.
• Pain, the prominent symptom, is made worse with activity
• Loss of motion of the affected joint
• Stiffness (especially early morning)
• Swelling if the involved joint is superficial
• Locking may occur if a loose body has developed
• Proximal femur is the most common site and more prevalent in males in the 3rd-6th decade
• The distal femur, especially the medial femoral condyle, is the second most frequent site. This area is unique in that night pain is a prominent early symptom. Most common in females in the 6th-7th decade.
• Other sites in decreasing frequency are the proximal humerus, talus, carpal lunate (Kienböck's disease) and the humeral capitulum

CAUSES
• Idiopathic
• Fractures, especially the femoral neck
• Traumatic (fractures, dislocation)
• Dislocations
• Legg-Calvé-Perthes (seen in 6-12 year age group)
• Hemoglobinopathies (especially sickle cell disease)
• Metabolic (hemoglobinopathies, alcohol, steroids, renal failure/transplantation)

RISK FACTORS
• Gaucher's disease - especially likely as a postoperative infection
• Diabetes mellitus
• Alcoholism - the most frequent cause
• Type II or IV hyperlipemia
• Cortisone therapy (may be seen with Cushing's disease)
• Obesity
• Oral contraceptives
• Organ transplant, especially kidney
• Pregnancy
• Decompression sickness ("bends")

 DIAGNOSIS

DIFFERENTIAL DIAGNOSIS
Rheumatoid arthritis, septic necrosis and severe secondary parathyroidism. A crescent sign (a linear subchondral lucency indicates collapse of subchondral bone. Patchy lucencies reflect resorption; patchy sclerosis indicates growth of new bone over the scaffolding of dead trabeculae) in these conditions may occur because the bone may be so soft that it collapses producing a crescent sign.

LABORATORY N/A
Drugs that may alter lab results: N/A
Disorders that may alter lab results: N/A

PATHOLOGICAL FINDINGS
The subchondral fracture occurs during bone repair as necrotic bone is resorbed. Later, a collapse of the bone occurs with subsequent irregularities at the joint surface. This will eventually produce osteoarthritic changes.

SPECIAL TESTS
Bone scan shows decreased bone uptake (sometimes increased uptake depending on the stage). Later, the uptake increases as reparative processes begin within the bone.

IMAGING
MRI will show a decreased signal intensity of the involved bone and is the most sensitive diagnostic exam.

DIAGNOSTIC PROCEDURES
The presence of a crescent sign is practically diagnostic (see Differential Diagnosis of osteonecrosis). It is caused by a subchondral fracture.

 TREATMENT

APPROPRIATE HEALTH CARE
Outpatient normally; inpatient if surgery indicated

GENERAL MEASURES
• Only four conditions can be treated to decrease the incidence of osteonecrosis
  ◊ Alcoholism - abstinence is obvious, but quite difficult to attain
  ◊ Dysbarism - new tables of decompression, if followed, will lower osteonecrosis incidence of divers
  ◊ Transplant patients - decreased doses of cortisone and regulation of calcium and phosphorous metabolism
  ◊ Sickle cell disease - treat a crisis vigorously with hydration, possible exchange transfusion and oxygenation, especially hyperbaric oxygen

SURGICAL MEASURES
Bone grafts, arthroplasty, allografts and arthrodesis may be used, dependent upon the joint involved

ACTIVITY As tolerated

DIET No special diet

PATIENT EDUCATION
The patient should be instructed in the use of crutches and/or canes when the lower extremity is involved. Proper use of a walking cane can decrease the pressure on the femoral head 20-30% when walking.

MEDICATIONS

DRUG(S) OF CHOICE
• NSAID's - consistent with the underlying disease may be used for painful episodes
• Acetaminophen - 500 mg qid can be quite helpful in alleviating symptoms
Contraindications: See manufacturer's profile of each drug
Precautions: NSAIDs - if history of peptic ulcer is present, the use of ranitidine (Zantac) 150 mg bid or 300 mg hs can be given. Misoprostol (Cytotec) 100 μg bid will usually prevent gastritis (not needed with acetaminophen).
Significant possible interactions: See manufacturer's profile of each drug

ALTERNATIVE DRUGS Other
H2-receptor antagonists in patients with a history of peptic ulcer disease

FOLLOWUP

PATIENT MONITORING X-rays should be made every 12-18 months, more frequently if symptoms become more severe

PREVENTION/AVOIDANCE Early diagnosis and treatment of underlying disease

POSSIBLE COMPLICATIONS
• Progression of disease
• The progression of osteonecrosis leads to osteoarthritis of the involved joint to a varying degree. Arthroplasty of the hip carries a much poorer prognosis than osteoarthritis alone. It should be postponed as long as possible.

EXPECTED COURSE/PROGNOSIS
Gaucher's disease is associated with a high risk of infection following surgery

MISCELLANEOUS

ASSOCIATED CONDITIONS N/A

AGE-RELATED FACTORS
Pediatric: Legg-Calvé-Perthes occurs in the 6-12 year age group. Prognosis is better in younger patients.
Geriatric: N/A
Others: N/A

PREGNANCY Is a risk factor

SYNONYMS
• Idiopathic osteonecrosis
• Avascular necrosis
• lunatomalacia, Kienböck's disease
• Subchondral fracture

ICD-9-CM 730.1 Osteonecrosis

SEE ALSO
• Arthritis, osteo
• Legg-Calvé-Perthes disease

OTHER NOTES N/A

ABBREVIATIONS N/A

REFERENCES
• Harris WH: Total Hip Replacement. American Academy of Orthopedic Surgeons, Institutional Course Lectures, Vol 23. St. Louis, C.V. Mosby Company, 1974
• Eftekhaur Khaur NS, Keirwam H: Systemic and Local Complications following low friction. Arthroplasty. In Archives of Surgery 1976;111:150
• Nicholson OR: Total Hip Replacement. In Clinical Orthopedics 1973;95:217
Illustrations: N/A
Internet references: http://www.5mcc.com

Author(s)
Furnie W. Johnston, MD
R. Bruce Hall, MD

Osteoporosis

BASICS

DESCRIPTION
A multifactorial skeletal disease characterized by severe bone loss and disruption of skeletal micro-architecture sufficient to predispose to atraumatic fractures of the vertebral column, upper femur, distal radius, proximal humerus, pubic rami and ribs. Five types recognized:
• Postmenopausal (Type I): The most common form in Caucasian and Asian women. Due to excessive and prolonged acceleration of bone resorption following menopausal loss of estrogen secretion.
• Involutional (Type II): Occurs in both sexes above age 75. Due to a subtle, prolonged imbalance between rates of bone resorption and formation. A mixture of Types I and II is common.
• Idiopathic: A rare form of primary osteoporosis occurring in premenopausal women and in men below age 75. Not related to secondary causes or risk factors predisposing to bone loss.
• Juvenile: A rare form of variable severity in prepubertal children. Self-limited with cessation of fractures at puberty.
• Secondary: Due to extrinsic factors
System(s) affected: Musculoskeletal, Endocrine/Metabolic
Genetics: Familial predisposition. More common in Caucasians and Orientals than in Black and Latino ethnic groups.
Incidence/Prevalence in USA:
• 30-40% cumulatively in women, 5-15% in men
• Prevalence of idiopathic and juvenile types unknown
• Secondary osteoporosis cumulatively 5-10%, both sexes
Predominant age: Elderly
Predominant sex: Female > Male

SIGNS AND SYMPTOMS
• Back ache/pain; acute/chronic
• Loss of height
• Kyphosis/scoliosis
• Atraumatic fractures
• No peripheral bone deformities
• Sclerae not blue/green/grey
• Restrictive lung disease
• Gastrointestinal symptoms
• Depression, loss of self esteem
• Excess mortality, 5-20% during 1-5 years post acute fracture

CAUSES
• Postmenopausal (Type I): Hypoestrogenemia
• Involutional (Type II): Unknown
• Idiopathic: Unknown
• Juvenile: Unknown
• Secondary: Eating disorders, corticosteroid excess, rheumatoid arthritis, chronic liver/kidney disease, malabsorption syndromes, systemic mastocytosis, hyperparathyroidism, hyperthyroidism, a variety of hypogonadal states, idiopathic hypercalciuria, and others

• Aging: Bone loss is a consequence of aging, however, osteoporosis occurs in individuals who fail to achieve optimal skeletal mass or lose bone rapidly thereafter (e.g., excessive postmenopausal and/or involutional bone loss, or conditions/risk factors that increase bone loss).

RISK FACTORS
• Dietary - inadequate calcium or vitamin D; excessive phosphate/protein
• Physical - immobilization, sedentary lifestyle
• Social - alcohol, cigarettes, caffeine
• Medical - chronic diseases, malabsorption, endocrinopathies, (see also secondary osteoporosis in Description)
• Iatrogenic - corticosteroids, excess thyroid hormone replacement, chronic heparin, chemotherapy, loop diuretics, anticonvulsants, radiation therapy
• Genetic/familial - suboptimal bone mass at maturity, "familial fast bone losers"

DIAGNOSIS

DIFFERENTIAL DIAGNOSIS
• Multiple myeloma
• Other neoplasia
• Osteomalacia
• Osteogenesis imperfecta tarda (Type I)
• Skeletal hyperparathyroidism (primary and secondary)
• Hyperthyroidism
• Mastocytosis (rare)

LABORATORY
• CBC, multipanel tests usually normal
• Alkaline phosphatase (bone specific and total) may be transiently increased following fractures
• Serum and/or urine protein electrophoresis normal
• Thyroid function tests and urinary free cortisol normal in primary types
• Serum osteocalcin, if high, indicates high turnover type
• Urine calcium normal (except if idiopathic hypercalciuria)
• Serum and urinary pyridinoline and N- and C-telopeptide collagen crosslinks, if high, indicate high turnover type
Drugs that may alter lab results:
• Hepatotoxins: changes in total alkaline phosphatase
• Estrogens: changes in thyroid function tests
Disorders that may alter lab results:
• Multiple myeloma or other neoplasia
• Osteomalacia
• Hyperparathyroidism
• Hyperthyroidism

PATHOLOGICAL FINDINGS
• Reduced skeletal mass, trabecular bone more so than cortical bone. Loss of trabecular connections.
• Osteoclast and osteoblast number variable
• No evidence of other metabolic bone diseases and no increase in unmineralized osteoid
• Marrow normal or atrophic

SPECIAL TESTS   N/A

IMAGING
• Plain film "early" changes: increased width of intervertebral spaces, relative accentuation of cortical plates, vertical striations of vertebral bodies
• Plain film "late" changes: cortical plate fractures, vertebral compression, wedge and crush fractures, peripheral fractures at ends of long bones, rib fractures
• Bone scan: increased uptake at previous fracture sites
• Bone mineral density (BMD). Data Analysis: Normative data for DXA, QUS, and QCT are incorporated into each instrument, allowing calculation of T and Z scores. T scores represent the number of standard deviations (SD) a measurement deviates from the mean for young normal (age 25-40) controls of same sex and in some cases, ethnic group. T scores indicate severity of bone loss as follows: T scores of ±1 SD are normal; a T score between -1 and -2 indicates an osteopenic state; T scores below -2 indicate established osteoporosis with high risk of fracture. Z scores indicate number of standard deviations compared to age matched controls and are not generally used to determine severity or need for treatment.
◊ Whole body DXA: BMD of whole body, lumbar spine, forearm, and upper femur
◊ Peripheral (p) DXA: BMD of the calcaneus, distal tibia, and distal radius. Reasonable correlation with whole body DXA but does not reflect changes from baseline during treatment.
◊ Quantitative CT (QCT): Quantitates either trabecular or cortical bone mass (or both) of lumbar spine.
◊ Quantitative ultrasound (QUS): Uses US attenuation at calcaneus. Correlates with whole body and peripheral DXA, but does not reflect changes during treatment. May be influenced by microarchitecture as well as BMD.

DIAGNOSTIC PROCEDURES
Bone biopsy needed rarely, to rule out other metabolic bone diseases. Sometimes used to quantitate bone loss, utilizing quantitative histomorphometric technique.

TREATMENT

APPROPRIATE HEALTH CARE
• Usually outpatient
• Inpatient care for acute back pain, especially for new vertebral fractures and for acute treatment of upper femoral and pelvic fractures
• Nursing home or home care may be needed following peripheral fractures

GENERAL MEASURES
As required by pain and disability, e.g., heat, analgesics, physical therapy. Decrease falls.

SURGICAL MEASURES   N/A

ACTIVITY
• Maintain ambulation, walking 1 mile twice a day, if possible, swimming, tricycling
• Avoid exercises and maneuvers that increase compressive forces and mechanical stress on spine and peripheral bone sites
• Rehabilitation procedures for back muscle spasm, to increase agility (e.g., decrease falls), and encourage ambulation

DIET
• Reducing diet if overweight
• Calcium intake 1500 mg/day from all sources, if not hypercalciuric or with past medical history of calcium stones
• Avoid excess phosphate or protein intake, i.e., avoid phosphoric-acid-containing beverages and excess meat intake
• 600-1000 IU vitamin D daily from all sources

PATIENT EDUCATION Teaching resources and patient literature available from National Osteoporosis Foundation, 2100 M St., Suite 602, Washington, DC 20037

MEDICATIONS

DRUG(S) OF CHOICE
• Hormone replacement therapy (HRT)
 ◊ Estrogen-medroxyprogesterone (PremPro) q day
 ◊ Estrogen, conjugated (Premarin) 0.625 mg q day, if post-hysterectomy. 0.3 mg q day is advocated as effective, but is not approved at this dose.
 ◊ Estradiol (Estraderm) 0.05 mg q/day; patch applied biweekly; other estrogen patches may require only one weekly application
• Calcitonin (Miacalcin Nasal Spray) 200 IU intranasally; 1 puff per day, alternating nostrils or injectable calcitonin (Miacalcin) 100 IU SC qd or qod preferred, 50 IU qd or 3 times a week may be effective in high turnover types. Should be used in conjunction with adequate calcium and vitamin D.
• Alendronate (Fosamax) 10 mg q AM on an empty stomach

Contraindications:
• Calcitonins - none except allergy
• For alendronate, esophageal dysfunction, severe upper GI symptoms, GERD
• HRT absolute - past medical history of endometrial or breast cancer (with estrogen receptors) or premalignant breast conditions
• HRT relative - medical history uncontrolled hypertension, thromboembolic conditions, edematous conditions, endometriosis, migraine, severe hepatic dysfunction; family history of breast or uterine cancer, breast cancer (without estrogen receptors)

Precautions:
• Calcitonins: none
• HRT: annual gynecology exam with Pap smear or endometrial biopsy, breast exam and mammography. Check BP twice a week during initiation of HRT.
• Alendronate: take on empty stomach in the morning with 1-2 glasses of water. Nothing by mouth and remain seated or standing for 30 minutes to 1 hour.

Significant possible interactions: None

ALTERNATIVE DRUGS
• Other bisphosphonates: etidronate (Didronel), pamidronate (Aredia), tiludronate (Skelid), risedronate (Actonel) - inhibitors of bone resorption (not FDA approved)
• Sodium fluoride: stimulates bone formation, but effects on cortical bone uncertain. Sustained release preparations may be better tolerated.
• Tamoxifen: has some estrogen effects on bone without potential for breast stimulation. May stimulate uterus and cause other side effects.
• Under study: droloxifene, androgens/anabolics, parathyroid hormone analogues

FOLLOWUP

PATIENT MONITORING
• Bimonthly initially, then q 6 months
• Periodic multiphasic screening, annual gynecological exam, breast exam, and mammography
• Annual BMD using same technique
• Repeat x-rays for acute pain, suspected fractures
• Serial serum or urinary pyridinoline or N- or C-telopeptide collagen cross-links, in selected patients

PREVENTION/AVOIDANCE
• General guidelines: Diet, exercise, calcium, vitamin D
• Prevention during the osteopenic phase (prolonged, usually asymptomatic phase prior to fracturing)
 ◊ Identification of osteopenia
 ◊ Correction of treatable medical conditions and other risk factors; will also help achieve optimal skeletal mass during development
 ◊ HRT if postmenopausal and no absolute contraindications
 ◊ Low dose alendronate (Fosamax) 5 mg qd, if no contraindications
 ◊ Raloxifene (Evista) 60 mg q day, a selective estrogen receptor modulator (SERM) with positive effects on BMD and fracture risk, but no stimulatory action on breast or uterus. Relative contraindications include hot flashes, history of thromboembolic conditions.

POSSIBLE COMPLICATIONS
• Severe disabling pain
• Dorsal/lumbar neurologic deficits secondary to vertebral fracture (rare)
• Respiratory and GI symptoms
• Invalidism/death secondary to complications of upper femoral fractures

EXPECTED COURSE/PROGNOSIS
• With treatment, 70% of patients stabilize skeletal manifestations; increase bone mass, increase mobility, and have reduced pain
• 20-40% of upper femoral fractures lead to chronic care and/or premature death

MISCELLANEOUS

ASSOCIATED CONDITIONS
• Corticosteroid excess
• Rheumatoid arthritis
• Chronic liver/kidney disease
• Malabsorption syndromes
• Systemic mastocytosis
• Hyperparathyroidism; Hyperthyroidism including iatrogenic
• Various hypogonadal states
• Eating disorders

AGE-RELATED FACTORS
Pediatric: Juvenile osteoporosis not discussed herein
Geriatric:
Postmenopausal/involutional/mixed types
Others: Primary types uncommon in African Americans. Patients with British, North European, Scandinavian, and Oriental ancestry most susceptible.

PREGNANCY Rare acute osteoporosis of pregnancy, not discussed here

SYNONYMS N/A

ICD-9-CM 733.0 Osteoporosis

SEE ALSO N/A

OTHER NOTES N/A

ABBREVIATIONS
BMD = bone mineral density
HRT = hormone replacement therapy

REFERENCES
• Eastell R: Treatment of post menopausal osteoporosis. NEJM 1998;338(11):736-746
• Brunelli MP, Einhorn TA: Medical management of osteoporosis. Fracture prevention. Clinical Orthopaedics & Related Research 1998;348:15-21
• Heaney RP: Pathophysiology of osteoporosis. Endocrinology & Metabolism Clin of NA 1998;27(2):255-265
• Termine JD, Wong M: Post-menopausal women and osteoporosis: available choices for maintenance of skeletal health. Maturitas 1998;30(3):241-245
• Miller PD: Management of osteoporosis. Advances in Internal Med 1999;44:175-207
• Lyles KW. Management of patients with vertebral compression fractures. Pharmacotherapy 1999;19(1pt2):21s-24s)
Illustrations: N/A
Internet references: http://www.5mcc.com

Author(s)
Stanley Wallach, MD

Otitis externa

BASICS

DESCRIPTION Inflammation of the external auditory canal
• Acute diffuse otitis externa - the most common form, an infectious process usually bacterial, occasionally fungal
• Acute circumscribed otitis externa - synonymous with furuncle. Associated with infection of the hair follicle.
• Chronic otitis externa - same as acute diffuse, but of longer duration (greater than 6 weeks)
• Eczematous otitis externa - may accompany typical atopic eczema or other primary skin conditions
• Necrotizing "malignant" otitis externa - an infection which extends into the deeper tissues adjacent to the canal. May include osteomyelitis and cellulitis. Rare in children.
System(s) affected: Skin/Exocrine
Genetics: N/A
Incidence/Prevalence in USA:
• Unknown; incidence is higher in the summer months
• Acute, chronic and eczematous - common
• Necrotizing - uncommon
Predominant age: All ages
Predominant sex: Male = Female

SIGNS AND SYMPTOMS
• Itching
• Plugging of the ear
• Otalgia
• Periauricular adenitis
• Erythematous canal
• Purulent discharge
• Eczema of pinna
• Cranial nerve involvement (VII, IX-XII)

CAUSES
• Acute diffuse otitis externa
  ◊ Traumatized external canal
  ◊ Bacterial infection - pseudomonas (67% cases); staphylococcus; streptococcus; gram negative rods
  ◊ Fungal infection - aspergillus (90% cases); Phycomycetes; Rhizopus; actinomyces; Penicillium; yeast
• Chronic otitis externa
  ◊ Bacterial infection - pseudomonas
• Eczematous otitis externa (associated with primary skin disorder):
  ◊ Eczema
  ◊ Seborrhea
  ◊ Neurodermatitis
  ◊ Contact dermatitis
  ◊ Purulent otitis media
  ◊ Sensitivity to topical medications
• Necrotizing otitis externa
  ◊ Invasive bacterial infection - pseudomonas

RISK FACTORS
• Acute and chronic otitis externa
  ◊ Traumatization of external canal
  ◊ Swimming
  ◊ Hot humid weather
  ◊ Use of a hearing aid
• Eczematous
  ◊ Primary skin disorder
• Necrotizing otitis externa in adults
  ◊ Elderly
  ◊ Diabetes
  ◊ Debilitating disease
• Necrotizing otitis externa in children (rare)
  ◊ Leukopenia
  ◊ Malnutrition
  ◊ Diabetes mellitus
  ◊ Diabetes insipidus

DIAGNOSIS

DIFFERENTIAL DIAGNOSIS
• Ear pain
• Purulent ear discharge
• Hearing loss
• Cranial nerve palsy (VII, IX-XII) with necrotizing otitis externa
• Wisdom teeth eruption

LABORATORY Gram stain and culture of canal discharge (occasionally helpful)
Drugs that may alter lab results:
Antibiotic pretreatment
Disorders that may alter lab results: N/A

PATHOLOGICAL FINDINGS
• Acute and chronic otitis externa - desquamation of superficial epithelium of external canal with infection
• Eczematous otitis externa - pathologic findings consistent with primary skin disorder, secondary infection on occasion
• Necrotizing otitis externa - vasculitis, thrombosis and necrosis of involved tissues; osteomyelitis

SPECIAL TESTS N/A

IMAGING Radiologic evaluation of deep tissues in necrotizing otitis externa

DIAGNOSTIC PROCEDURES N/A

TREATMENT

APPROPRIATE HEALTH CARE
Outpatient, except for resistant cases and necrotizing otitis externa

GENERAL MEASURES
• Thorough cleansing of external canal
• Pain medications
• Antipruritic and antihistamines (eczematous form)

SURGICAL MEASURES N/A

ACTIVITY No restrictions

DIET No restrictions

PATIENT EDUCATION Methods for prevention

MEDICATIONS

DRUG(S) OF CHOICE
- Acute bacterial and chronic otitis externa
  ◊ Topical therapy for approximately 10 days
  ◊ 2% acetic acid
  ◊ Antibiotics
  ◊ Corticosteroids
- Fungal otitis externa
  ◊ Topical therapy anti-yeast for candida or yeast - nystatin
  ◊ Parenteral antifungal therapy - amphotericin B
- Eczematous otitis externa - topical therapy
  ◊ Aluminum acetate 8%
  ◊ Acetic acid 2% in aluminum acetate
  ◊ 5% aluminum acetate (Burrow's) solution
  ◊ Steroid cream, lotion, ointment
  ◊ Antibacterial, if superinfected
- Necrotizing otitis externa
  ◊ Parenteral antibiotics - antistaphylococcus and antipseudomonal
  ◊ 4-6 weeks of therapy

Contraindications:
- Hypersensitivity to topical or parenteral therapy
- Renal or hepatic failure when using amphotericin B

Precautions: Dosage adjustment for amphotericin B in patients with renal or hepatic dysfunction

Significant possible interactions:
- Hypokalemia associated with amphotericin B may lead to digitalis toxicity
- Concurrent administration of nonabsorbable anions, such as carbenicillin, may exacerbate hypokalemia

ALTERNATIVE DRUGS Azole antifungals for fungal otitis externa

FOLLOWUP

PATIENT MONITORING
- Acute otitis externa
  ◊ 48 hours after therapy instituted to assess improvement
    ◊ At the end of treatment
- Chronic otitis externa
  ◊ Every 2-3 weeks for repeated cleansing of canal
  ◊ May require alterations in topical medication, including antibiotics and steroids
- Necrotizing otitis externa
  ◊ Daily monitoring in hospital for extension of infection
  ◊ Baseline auditory and vestibular testing at beginning and end of therapy

PREVENTION/AVOIDANCE
- Avoid prolonged exposure to moisture
- Utilize preventive antiseptics
- Treat predisposing skin conditions
- Eliminate self-inflicted trauma to canal
- Diagnose and treat underlying systemic conditions

POSSIBLE COMPLICATIONS
- Mainly a problem with necrotizing otitis externa. May spread to infect contiguous bone and CNS structures.
- Acute otitis externa may spread to pinna causing a chondritis

EXPECTED COURSE/PROGNOSIS
- Acute otitis externa - rapid response to therapy with total resolution
- Chronic otitis externa - with repeated cleansing and antibiotic therapy the majority of cases will resolve. Occasionally, surgical intervention is required for resistant cases.
- Eczematous otitis externa - resolution will occur with control of the primary skin condition
- Necrotizing otitis externa - can usually be managed with debridement and prolonged parenteral antibiotics. Recurrence rate is 100% when treatment is inadequate. Surgical intervention may be necessary in resistant cases or if there is cranial nerve involvement. Mortality rate is significant, probably secondary to the underlying disease.

MISCELLANEOUS

ASSOCIATED CONDITIONS See Risk Factors

AGE-RELATED FACTORS N/A
Pediatric: N/A
Geriatric: N/A
Others: N/A

PREGNANCY N/A

SYNONYMS
- Swimmer's ear

ICD-9-CM
380.10 infective otitis externa, unspecified

SEE ALSO N/A

OTHER NOTES N/A

ABBREVIATIONS N/A

REFERENCES
- Marcy SM: Swimmer's Ear. Contemporary Pediatrics 1986;3:20
- Bluestone C, Stool S, eds: Pediatric Otolaryngology. 3rd Ed. Philadelphia, W.B. Saunders Co., 1996

Illustrations: N/A
Internet references: http://www.5mcc.com

Author(s)
James A. Nard, MD

Otitis media

BASICS

DESCRIPTION Inflammation of the middle ear
• Acute otitis media (AOM): Usually a bacterial infection accompanied by viral upper respiratory infection; rapid onset of signs and symptoms
• Recurrent AOM: 3 or more AOM in 6 months, or 4 or more AOM in 1 year
• Otitis media with effusion (OME): Persistent inflammation manifested as asymptomatic middle ear fluid that follows AOM or arises without prior AOM

System(s) affected: Nervous

Genetics: May be influenced by skull configuration or immunological defects

Incidence/Prevalence in USA: (Incidence) By age 7 years 93% of children have 1 or more AOM; 39% have 6 or more AOM; after AOM 10 to 20% still have OME 3 months later

Predominant age: Peak incidence age 6-18 months; declines after age 7 years; rare in adults

Predominant sex: Male > Female (for AOM and recurrent AOM)

SIGNS AND SYMPTOMS
• AOM:
  ◊ Earache
  ◊ Fever, although more often afebrile
  ◊ Accompanying URI symptoms
  ◊ Decreased hearing
  ◊ Otorrhea if eardrum perforated
  ◊ Eardrum mobility decreased (as observed by pneumatic otoscopy)
  ◊ Eardrum bulging, opaque, often yellowish or inflamed. Redness alone is not a reliable sign.
• AOM in infants:
  ◊ May cause no symptoms in the first few months of life
  ◊ Irritability is sometimes the only indication of earache
  ◊ Eardrum bulging, opaque, often yellowish or inflamed. Redness alone not a reliable sign.
• OME:
  ◊ Usually asymptomatic
  ◊ Decreased hearing probably universal, but not always measurable, and rarely appreciated by parents
  ◊ Eardrum often dull, but not bulging
  ◊ Eardrum mobility decreased (as observed by pneumatic otoscopy)

CAUSES
• AOM: A preceding viral upper respiratory infection produces eustachian tube dysfunction that is thought to promote bacterial infection via eustachian tube. Bacteriology:
  ◊ Pneumococci: 30-35%
  ◊ Haemophilus influenzae: 20-25%; 40% of these produce beta-lactamases that hydrolyze amoxicillin and some cephalosporins
  ◊ Moraxella (Branhamella) catarrhalis: 10-15%; 90% of these produce beta-lactamases that hydrolyze amoxicillin and some cephalosporins
  ◊ Group A streptococci: 3%
  ◊ Staphylococcus aureus: 1-2%
  ◊ Sterile/non-pathogens: 25-30%
• OME:
  ◊ 20-40% silent bacterial infection
  ◊ Eustachian tube dysfunction thought important
  ◊ Allergic causes rarely substantiated

RISK FACTORS
• Day care
• Formula feeding
• Smoking in household
• Male gender
• Family history of middle ear disease
• AOM in 1st year of life is a risk factor for recurrent AOM
• Sibling history of otitis media

DIAGNOSIS

DIFFERENTIAL DIAGNOSIS
• Tympanosclerosis
• Redness due to crying
• Earache with a normal ear exam may be caused by referred pain from the jaw or teeth

LABORATORY WBC higher in bacterial AOM than in sterile AOM
Drugs that may alter lab results: N/A
Disorders that may alter lab results: N/A

PATHOLOGICAL FINDINGS N/A

SPECIAL TESTS
• To document the presence of middle ear fluid - tympanometry, acoustic reflex measurement or acoustic reflectometry
• Hearing testing helpful to assess the need for early surgical intervention in OME
• Nasopharyngoscopy

IMAGING N/A

DIAGNOSTIC PROCEDURES
Tympanocentesis for microbiologic diagnosis recommended for treatment failures, may be followed by myringotomy

TREATMENT

APPROPRIATE HEALTH CARE
Outpatient except when surgery is indicated

GENERAL MEASURES
• AOM: Outpatient except for febrile infants < 2 months
• May use watchful waiting approach, treating symptoms without antibiotics for first 2-3 days. If symptoms persist, then amocicillin is first line treatment.

SURGICAL MEASURES
• OME: Referral for surgery if: > 4-6 months bilateral OME, and/or > 6 months unilateral OME, and/or hearing loss > 25 decibels
• Recurrent AOM: Referral for surgery if > 2 or 3 AOM while on chemoprophylaxis. Tympanostomy tubes and adenoidectomy effective surgical procedures for OME and recurrent AOM, but not in all cases.

ACTIVITY No restrictions

DIET No special diet

PATIENT EDUCATION N/A

MEDICATIONS

DRUG(S) OF CHOICE
• AOM: Amoxicillin 40-45 mg/kg bid >age 2 years, 5-7 day course with no complications; probably the most effective of penicillins/cephalosporins against relatively resistant (but not highly resistant) pneumococci
• Recurrent AOM: Amoxicillin 20 mg/kg daily for 3-6 months or until summer
• OME: Antihistamines and decongestants ineffective, indications for steroids not defined, amoxicillin promotes resolution in 10-15% but effect is usually transitory - not recommended.
• Note: if patient not toxic appearing, may choose to treat with antipyrine-benzocaine (Auralgan) drops and acetaminophen (Tylenol) as long as close follow up available - see evidence based web site. Spontaneous clinical resolution is 81%.
Contraindications: Allergy to penicillins
Precautions: Refer to manufacturer's profile of each drug
Significant possible interactions: Refer to manufacturer's profile of each drug

ALTERNATIVE DRUGS
• Alternative drugs are indicated for the following AOM patients:
  ◊ Patients with penicillin allergy
  ◊ Persistent symptoms after 48-72 hrs of amoxicillin
  ◊ AOM within 1 month of amoxicillin therapy
  ◊ AOM with severe earache
  ◊ Infants less than 6 months with high fever
  ◊ Immunocompromised hosts
  ◊ AOM due to Chlamydia trachomatis will respond to macrolides and sulfonamides
  ◊ AOM due to Mycoplasma pneumoniae will respond to macrolides
• AOM: Alternative drugs (treat for 10 days):
  ◊ Amoxicillin-clavulanate (Augmentin) 40 mg/kg/day of amoxicillin component tid - effective against resistant H. influenzae and M. catarrhalis, amoxicillin component effective against relatively resistant pneumococci
  ◊ Cefaclor (Ceclor) 40 mg/kg/day bid or tid is less effective than other alternatives
  ◊ Cefixime (Suprax) 8 mg/kg/day bid or single daily dose - effective against resistant H. influenzae and M. catarrhalis less effective than amoxicillin for pneumococci
  ◊ Cefpodoxime (Vantin) 10 mg/kg/day bid - less effective in vivo against H. influenzae than other drugs
  ◊ Ceftriaxone (Rocephin) 50 mg/kg IM single dose - effective against major pathogens, but expensive and painful so reserved for sick infants
  ◊ Clarithromycin (Biaxin) 15 mg/kg/day divided bid - not effective in vivo against H. influenzae
  ◊ Trimethoprim-sulfamethoxazole (Septra, Bactrim) 8 mg TMP/kg/day divided bid: up to 30% of pneumococci are resistant
  ◊ Erythromycin-sulfisoxazole (Pediazole) 40 mg erythromycin component/kg/day divided qid - some strains of pneumococci are resistant

• Recurrent AOM:
  ◊ Sulfisoxazole 75 mg/kg single daily dose for penicillin allergic patients
• Analgesics and antipyretics as needed

FOLLOWUP

PATIENT MONITORING
• AOM: Otoscopic examination 4 weeks after diagnosis
• OME: Monthly otoscopic or tympanometric exams as long as OME persists

PREVENTION/AVOIDANCE
• Breast-feeding decreases incidence of AOM
• Eliminate cigarette smoking in the household

POSSIBLE COMPLICATIONS
• AOM: Perforation/otorrhea, acute mastoiditis, facial nerve paralysis, otitic hydrocephalus, meningitis
• OME: Hearing loss. Extent and significance of impaired speech and language is controversial.
• Recurrent AOM and OME: Atrophy and scarring of eardrum, chronic perforation and otorrhea, cholesteatoma, permanent hearing loss, chronic mastoiditis, brain abscess and other intracranial suppurative complications

EXPECTED COURSE/PROGNOSIS
• AOM: Symptoms usually improve in 48-72 hrs; OME following AOM resolved in 90% by 3 months
• OME: Approximately 50% resolve after 8 weeks of observation
• Recurrent AOM and OME: Usually subside in school age children; only a small percentage have complications

MISCELLANEOUS

ASSOCIATED CONDITIONS
• Upper respiratory infection
• Bacteremia
• Meningitis
• Allergies

AGE-RELATED FACTORS
Pediatric: Primarily a pediatric disease
Geriatric: N/A
Others: N/A

PREGNANCY N/A

SYNONYMS
• Secretory otitis media
• Serous otitis media

ICD-9-CM
382.0 Acute otitis media
381.0 Acute suppurative otitis media

SEE ALSO N/A

OTHER NOTES In first few months of infancy, the eardrum is normally at an angle and less mobile in older adults

ABBREVIATIONS
AOM = acute otitis media
OM = otitis media
OME = otitis media with effusion

REFERENCES
• Rosenfield RM, Vertrees JE, Carr J, et al: Clinical efficacy of antimicrobial drugs for acute otitis media: meta analysis of 5400 children from 33 randomized trials. J Pediatr 1994;124:355-67
• Stool SE, Berg AO, Bernan S, et al: Otitis media with effusion in young children. Clinical practice guideline. AHCPR Publication no 94-0622, 1994
• Kozyrsky AL, Hildes-Ripstein GE, et al: Treatment of acute otitis media with a shortened course of antibiotics. JAMA 1998;279(21):1736-41
Illustrations: N/A
Internet references: http://www.5mcc.com

Author(s)
John Kilbourne, MD

Otosclerosis (otospongiosis)

BASICS

DESCRIPTION A primary bone dyscrasia involving the otic capsule. It is the leading cause of conductive hearing loss in adults.
• Histologic otosclerosis: Asymptomatic form in which abnormal bone spares vital structures of the ear
• Clinical otosclerosis: Abnormal spongy bone involves ossicular chain or other structures leading to altered physiology
System(s) affected: Nervous
Genetics:
• 60% of those affected give positive family history
• Appears to be transmitted by autosomal dominant gene with variable penetrance
Incidence/Prevalence in USA:
• 4-8% among Caucasians; 1% among African-Americans (histologic form)
• Caucasians 5000/100,000; Blacks 1000/100,000 (histologic form)
Predominant age: Clinical onset usually in early 20's. Peak incidence fourth and fifth decades.
Predominant sex: Female > Male (2:1)

SIGNS AND SYMPTOMS
• Progressive conductive hearing loss, usually with well preserved speech discrimination. May have sensorineural hearing loss with cochlear involvement.
• Carhart's notch: A dip in bone conductive threshold at 2000 Hz. on audiometric testing
• Schwartze's sign: Reddish hue on promontory upon otoscopic examination
• Patients often soft spoken and aware they seem to hear better in noisy environments

CAUSES Unknown; fluoride metabolism felt by some authorities to play a role in etiology

RISK FACTORS Unknown

DIAGNOSIS

DIFFERENTIAL DIAGNOSIS
• Chronic suppurative otitis media
• Serous otitis media
• External auditory canal occlusion
• Ossicular chain disruption
• Congenital fixation of stapes
• Presbycusis

LABORATORY N/A
Drugs that may alter lab results: N/A
Disorders that may alter lab results: N/A

PATHOLOGICAL FINDINGS
• Gross: Off-white to reddish bone formation, most often located anterior to the oval window and extending to involve the stapedial footplate. Sometimes covers entire oval window (obliterative). May be found anywhere in otic capsule. Bilateral in 75% of cases.
• Micro: "Spongy" appearing bone with increased vascular spaces. Osteoblasts and osteoclasts are plentiful.

SPECIAL TESTS Tuning fork and audiometric testing for conductive and/or sensorineural hearing loss. Will lateralize to more impaired ear with Weber's test.

IMAGING Coaxial or computerized tomography sometimes helpful

DIAGNOSTIC PROCEDURES N/A

TREATMENT

APPROPRIATE HEALTH CARE
Inpatient for surgery. Outpatient if surgery not feasible.

GENERAL MEASURES Hearing aids

SURGICAL MEASURES
• Surgical correction (stapedectomy): Usually involves mobilization or removal of the stapedial foot plate with placement of a stapes prosthesis. Recent procedural innovations have involved use of lasers.
• Relative indications for surgery include: Negative Rinne's test (air-bone audiometric gap at least 20 dB); bilateral involvement

ACTIVITY No restrictions

DIET No special diet

PATIENT EDUCATION
• Because speech discrimination is usually preserved, patients should be advised of the possible benefit from hearing aids (as an alternative or adjunct to surgery)
• Mayo Foundation for Medical Education and Research, Section of Patient and Health Education, Sieber Subway, Rochester, MN 55905, (507)284-8140

MEDICATIONS

DRUG(S) OF CHOICE No specific drug therapy but sodium fluoride, vitamin D and calcium gluconate have been tried, especially in cases of predominantly sensorineural hearing loss
Contraindications: Refer to manufacturer's literature
Precautions: Refer to manufacturer's literature
Significant possible interactions: Refer to manufacturer's literature

ALTERNATIVE DRUGS N/A

FOLLOWUP

PATIENT MONITORING Interval audiometric testing

PREVENTION/AVOIDANCE N/A

POSSIBLE COMPLICATIONS Surgical risks include chorda tympani nerve injury, tympanic membrane laceration, ossicular chain disruption, otitis media and externa, labyrinthitis, granuloma formation, perilymph fistulae, and total deafness ("dead ear")

EXPECTED COURSE/PROGNOSIS
Progressive hearing loss if not treated. Surgery improves hearing by at least 15 dB in 90% of cases.

MISCELLANEOUS

ASSOCIATED CONDITIONS
• Van der Hoeve's syndrome (rare triad of osteogenesis imperfecta, blue sclera, and otospongiosis)
• Tinnitus
• Vertigo

AGE-RELATED FACTORS
Pediatric: N/A
Geriatric: Important differential diagnosis for presbycusis
Others: N/A

PREGNANCY Progression may accelerate during pregnancy. Some women first notice hearing loss at this time.

SYNONYMS N/A

ICD-9-CM
387.9 Otosclerosis, unspecified

SEE ALSO Hearing loss

OTHER NOTES N/A

ABBREVIATIONS N/A

REFERENCES
• English GM: Otolaryngology: A Textbook. New York, Harper & Rowe, 1976
• Lee KJ: Essential Otolaryngology: Head & Neck Surgery. 4th Ed. New Hyde Park, NY, Medical Examination Pub. Co., 1987
Illustrations: N/A
Internet references: http://www.5mcc.com

Author(s)
Jeffrey D. Wolfrey, MD

Ovarian cancer

BASICS

DESCRIPTION   A variety of malignancies that arise from the epithelium (85-90%), stromal cells, or germ cells, or are metastatic to the ovary. These include:
- Epithelial:
  ◊ Serous (Fallopian tube-like epithelium)
  ◊ Mucinous (Cervical and GI mucinous epithelium)
  ◊ Endometrioid (Endometrial epithelium)
  ◊ Clear cell (Mesonephroid)
  ◊ Brenner (Transitional cell epithelium)
  ◊ Carcinosarcoma and mixed mesodermal
- Stromal:
  ◊ Granulosa cell tumor
  ◊ Theca cell tumor
  ◊ Sertoli-Leydig cell tumors
  ◊ Gynandroblastoma
  ◊ Lipid cell tumor
- Germ cell:
  ◊ Teratoma (mature [e.g., dermoid cyst] and immature)
  ◊ Dysgerminoma
  ◊ Embryonal carcinoma
  ◊ Gonadoblastoma
  ◊ Endodermal sinus tumor
  ◊ Embryonal carcinoma
  ◊ Choriocarcinoma
- Metastatic disease from:
  ◊ Breast
  ◊ Endometrium
  ◊ Lymphoma
  ◊ Gastrointestinal tract (Krukenberg tumor)

System(s) affected: Reproductive, endocrine/metabolic, gastrointestinal

Genetics: For a woman who has a first-degree relative with a history of ovarian cancer, her risk for disease increases from 1.4% to 5%. With 2 or more such relatives lifetime risk is 7%. In families with hereditary ovarian cancer syndrome (site-specific familial ovarian cancer syndrome, breast-ovarian cancer syndrome, and Lynch syndrome II) risk rises to 40-50%. Transmission is autosomal dominant. These syndromes are associated with a variety of mutations in BRCA-1 and BRCA-2, and commercial screens for these genes are available. The clinical utility of such screening is under study. Patients with germ-line mutations of BRCA-1 appear to have better survival rates compared to patients who do not. The overexpression of certain oncogenes (her-2/neu, K-ras, c-myc) and of a mutant form of the tumor suppression factor p53 are associated with poor outcome.

Incidence/Prevalence in USA:
- 1/56 women develop disease
- 26,500 new cases/yr, 14,500 deaths/year
- Leading cause of gynecologic cancer death in women. Despite the development of novel technologies, surgical procedures, and chemotherapeutic/radiotherapeutic protocols, the mortality of ovarian cancer has not decreased significantly during the last six decades.

Predominant age:
- Epithelial: 40-75 years
- Germ cell malignancies: usually observed in patients < 20 yrs.

Predominant sex: Females only

SIGNS AND SYMPTOMS   (Often secondary to pressure on surrounding abdominopelvic organs)
- Vague gastrointestinal symptoms
- Bloating and dyspepsia
- Sense of abdominal fullness
- Increased abdominal girth
- Abdominopelvic cramping
- Occasional vaginal discharge
- Irregular vaginal bleeding
- Urinary frequency in absence of infection
- Fatigue
- Ascites
- Cul-de-sac and/or pelvic nodularity
- Pelvic mass
- Dyspareunia
- Weight loss/loss of appetite
- Severe pain secondary to ovarian rupture (with hemoperitoneum) or torsion. Most commonly seen with germ cell tumors.
- Precocious puberty (choriocarcinoma, embryonal carcinoma)
- Hirsutism in androgen secreting germ cell tumors

CAUSES   Multiple genetic factors as above. Epidemiologic data suggest a role for environmental factors as yet undefined. Professional occupations and jobs requiring administrative roles are associated with an increased incidence of ovarian cancer; possibly because of delayed child-bearing, but race and socioeconomic factors also likely play parts.

RISK FACTORS   Family history

DIAGNOSIS

DIFFERENTIAL DIAGNOSIS
- Gastrointestinal or other gynecologic malignancies
- Irritable bowel syndrome
- Colitis
- Hepatic failure with ascites
- Diverticulitis
- Tubo-ovarian abscess
- Uterine fibroids
- Pelvic kidney

LABORATORY
- Cancer antigen (CA) 125 (normal < 35 u/mL)
- Liver function tests (LFTs) to rule out hepatic involvement
- CBC
- Urinalysis
- Carcinoembryonic antigen (CEA) if gastrointestinal primary suspected
- Chorionic gonadotropin (beta-hCG [dysgerminoma, choriocarcinoma, embryonal carcinoma]), alpha-fetoprotein (endodermal sinus tumor, embryonal carcinoma), or LDH (dysgerminoma)

Drugs that may alter lab results: N/A
Disorders that may alter lab results: CA 125 may be elevated with benign gynecologic disease (endometriosis, peritonitis, myomas, PID, Meig's syndrome) and with nongynecologic disease (CHF, pancreatitis, SLE, liver diseases)

PATHOLOGICAL FINDINGS   At surgery, most common type will be epithelial ovarian cancer and most common subtype will be serous cystadenocarcinoma

SPECIAL TESTS   N/A

IMAGING   Pelvic ultrasound to evaluate structural features of adnexal mass. If malignancy is suggested, then expeditious laparotomy is indicated. CXR, mammogram. Abdominopelvic CT scan with contrast, IVP, and barium enema only as warranted.

DIAGNOSTIC PROCEDURES
- Surgery is definitive
- Paracentesis for cytology is no longer advised

TREATMENT

APPROPRIATE HEALTH CARE
Inpatient

GENERAL MEASURES   N/A

SURGICAL MEASURES
- Surgical staging and optimal debulking are critical. New emphasis has been placed on maximal cytoreduction of tumor burden (enhances effectiveness of adjuvant therapy and associated with longer survival). Chemotherapy and/or radiotherapy as recommended.
- For epithelial malignancies staging, tumor excision/debulking includes:
  ◊ Peritoneal fluid (or washings from peritoneal lavage) is aspirated and cytology evaluated
  ◊ Omentum is biopsied or completely excised in the presence of tumor implants
  ◊ Peritoneal surfaces, the inferior aspect of the diaphragm, liver surface, and the small intestine and bowel are inspected and palpated for tumor.
  ◊ Cytologic smear of right hemidiaphragmatic undersurface
  ◊ Biopsy of adhesions
  ◊ Biopsy of paracolic recesses, pelvic sidewalls, and bladder cul-de-sac
  ◊ Pelvic and para-aortic lymph node biopsy
  ◊ TAH-BSO and extirpation of all associated masses as feasible
- For germ cell cancers (which are less likely to be bilateral)
  ◊ Salpingo-oophorectomy (unilateral if only one ovary involved) in young patient
  ◊ Careful staging, including lymph node dissection, may be adequate. Adjuvant therapy for higher stage or grade or with recurrence, depending on tumor type.

ACTIVITY   As tolerated

DIET
- High protein diet
- Follow serum protein closely with significant ascites

Ovarian cancer

PATIENT EDUCATION
• "What you need to know about ovarian cancer" and "Chemotherapy and you: A guide to self-help during treatment" - National Institutes of Health pamphlets

MEDICATIONS

DRUG(S) OF CHOICE
Chemotherapy: Women with stage 1a grade 1 and most 1b grade 1 tumors do not require adjuvant therapy. Patients with clear cell carcinomas, grade 3 tumors, or tumors staged at 1c or worse that are not of low malignant potential require adjuvant therapy. Patients should be encouraged to participate in ongoing clinical trials whenever possible.
• Platinum-based regimen (cisplatin or carboplatin)
• Paclitaxel (Taxol)
• Cyclophosphamide (Cytoxan)
• These and other drugs are currently being used in combination according to current GOG protocols (e.g., Protocol 111, which compares treatment with cisplatin and Taxol or Cytoxan) In addition to causing tumor regression, chemotherapy also limits the formation of ascites and pleural effusions.
Contraindications: Patient too ill to receive chemotherapy, excessive toxicity
Precautions: All regimens cause bone marrow suppression. Cisplatin associated with ototoxicity, renal toxicity, and peripheral neuropathy. Taxol can cause neutropenia and, less commonly, neuropathy.
Significant possible interactions: Refer to manufacturer's literature

ALTERNATIVE DRUGS
• Etoposide
• 5-fluorouracil
• Doxorubicin (Adriamycin)
• Other members of the alkylating agent family (melphalan, hexamethylmelamine, ifosfamide [with mesna to protect against hemorrhagic cystitis], thiotepa)
• Ondansetron (Zofran), dronabinol (marinol), metoclopramide (Reglan), prochlorperazine (Compazine), and promethazine (Phenergan) and others for nausea control

FOLLOWUP

PATIENT MONITORING
• A logarithmic or sevenfold fall in CA-125 suggests a good response, but normal values correlate poorly (<50%) with absence of disease. Persistent elevations reflect a poor response to therapy.
• A rise in CA-125 usually requires a change in therapy, while an inadequate drop after 3 courses of chemotherapy may require a change.
• In germ cell cancers, serum markers should fall to normal range. Normal levels correlate closely with absence of disease.

PREVENTION/AVOIDANCE
For epithelial cancer, frequency of ovulation appears to be important. Ovulation causes the surface epithelium to be in a state of flux and this may promote the genetic changes necessary for uncontrolled growth and malignant transformation. Consistent with this, the following factors are protective:
• Use of oral contraceptives
• Multiparity
• Late menarche
• Early menopause
◊ Women without contraindications should be encouraged to use OCPs. The progestin component of OCPs may protect against ovarian cancer by regulating apoptosis of the ovarian epithelium.
◊ Clomiphene use in infertile women may increase the incidence of ovarian neoplasia, but newer studies are refuting this
◊ Acetaminophen use may be protective by lowering leutinizing hormone levels
◊ Women with strong family histories of ovarian cancer (2 or more first-degree relatives) should be counselled by a gynecologic oncologist concerning cancer risk
◊ Patients with hereditary ovarian cancer syndromes should be counseled about prophylactic oophorectomy after child-bearing is completed or by age 35. Even after oophorectomy, there is a small risk of developing intra-abdominal carcinomatosis histologically identical to ovarian carcinoma.
• Screening - there are no adequate screening measures for the early detection of ovarian cancer in asymptomatic women. The routine use of serum CA-125 and transvaginal ultrasound for screening is discouraged. Annual pelvic examinations are recommended. An adnexal mass in a premenarchal female or a palpable adnexa in a postmenopausal female warrants further immediate evaluation because of increased risk of malignancy. Women with a hereditary ovarian cancer syndrome should have annual pelvic examinations, serum CA-125 quantitation, and transvaginal ultrasound.

POSSIBLE COMPLICATIONS
• Pleural effusion
• Pseudomyxoma peritonei
• Ascites
• Radiotherapy and chemotherapy adverse reactions
• Bowel obstruction
• Malnutrition
• Electrolyte disturbances
• Fistula formation

EXPECTED COURSE/PROGNOSIS
Expected 5 yr survival rates, based on FIGO data are:

Stage	Survival rate
I	a 84%, b 79%, c 73%
II	a 65%, b 54%, c 51%
III	a 52%, b 29%, c 18%
IV	14%

• In germ cell and stromal tumors, outcome related to histologic cell type in addition to clinical stage and histologic grade.
• In epithelial cell cancers, prognosis is determined by stage, histologic grade, and the amount of residual disease rather than the histologic cell type.

MISCELLANEOUS

ASSOCIATED CONDITIONS
• Ascites
• Pleural effusion
• Decrease of serum albumin
• Breast carcinoma

AGE-RELATED FACTORS
Pediatric: N/A
Geriatric: Generally, poorer prognosis compared to younger patients
Others: Patients under 65 have a better prognosis, possibly because they present in earlier stages of disease

PREGNANCY Dermoid cyst and serous cystadenoma most common.

SYNONYMS N/A

ICD-9-CM 183.0 Malignant neoplasm of ovary and other uterine adnexa

SEE ALSO N/A

OTHER NOTES N/A

ABBREVIATIONS N/A

REFERENCES
• Bell DA, Scully RE. Early de novo ovarian carcinoma. Cancer. In: DiSaia PJ, Creasman, WT, eds: Clinical Gynecologic Oncology. 5Th ed. St Louis, Mosby, 1997
• NIH Consensus Development Panel on Ovarian Cancer. Ovarian cancer: screening, treatment, and follow-up. JAMA 1995;273:491-497.
• Rubin SC, et al: Clinical and pathological features of ovarian cancer in women with germ-line mutations of BRCA-1. NEJM 1996;335:1413-1416
• Sala M, et al: A death certificate-based study of occupation and mortality from reproductive cancers among women in 24 states. J Occup Environ Med 1998;40:632-639
5 additional references available at web site
Internet references: http://www.5mcc.com
Illustrations: N/A

Author(s)
Peter P. Toth, MD, PhD

Ovarian tumor, benign

BASICS

DESCRIPTION   The ovaries are a source of many tumor types (benign and malignant) because of the histologic variety of their constituent cells. Benign ovarian tumors create difficulties in differential diagnosis because of the need to identify malignancy and discriminate a tumor from cysts, infectious lesions, ectopic pregnancy, and endometriomas. The tumors are often clinically silent until well developed; they may be solid, cystic, or mixed; and they may be functional (producing sex steroids as with arrhenoblastomas and gynandroblastomas) or nonfunctional.

System(s) affected: reproductive, endocrine/metabolic
Genetics: N/A
Incidence/Prevalence in USA: N/A
Predominant age:
• All ages
• Concern for malignancy greater in premenarchal girls and postmenopausal women
Predominant sex: Female only

SIGNS AND SYMPTOMS
• Usually asymptomatic
• Pain related to torsion, endometriosis, or rupture
• Increased abdominal girth
• Bowel pressure or bladder pressure sensations
• Menstrual irregularities
• Hirsutism or sexual precocity
• Early satiety
• Dyspepsia/bloating

CAUSES
• Endometriosis with localized, repeated ovarian hemorrhage
• Physiologic cysts
• Tumorigenesis with genetics as yet poorly defined

RISK FACTORS   Not yet characterized

DIAGNOSIS

DIFFERENTIAL DIAGNOSIS
• Ovarian malignancies
• Uterine myomas
• Appendicular cysts
• Diverticulitis or bowel abscess
• Pelvic inflammatory disease with tubo-ovarian abscess
• Distended urinary bladder
• Ectopic pregnancy
• Hydrosalpinx
• Functional cysts (follicular and corpus luteum cysts)
• Polycystic ovaries

LABORATORY
• CBC
• Serum tumor markers as indicated
 ◊ Cancer antigen (CA) 125
 ◊ Alpha fetoprotein
 ◊ Chorionic gonadotropin (beta-hCG)
 ◊ Serum LDH
 ◊ Serum estrogens and androgens
Drugs that may alter lab results: N/A
Disorders that may alter lab results:
• CA 125
 ◊ Endometriosis
 ◊ Peritonitis
 ◊ Pelvic inflammatory disease (PID)
 ◊ Meig's syndrome
 ◊ Uterine fibroids
 ◊ Hepatitis
 ◊ Pancreatitis
 ◊ Systemic lupus erythematosis
 ◊ Diverticulitis
• Beta-hCG
 ◊ Pregnancy
 ◊ Hydatidiform mole
• LDH
 ◊ Liver disease, drug-induced hepatotoxicity
• AFP
 ◊ Hepatocellular carcinoma
 ◊ Hepatic cirrhosis
 ◊ Acute or chronic hepatitis

PATHOLOGICAL FINDINGS
• Follicular (fluid distention of atretic follicle) and corpus luteum cysts (corpus luteum hematoma)
• Endometrioma
• Pregnancy luteoma (comprised of hyperplastic stromal theca-lutein cells)
• Serous and mucinous cystadenomas and mixed serous/mucinous cystadenomas
• Granulosa cell tumors
• Benign connective tissue tumors (thecomas, fibromas, Brenner tumors)
• Cystic teratoma (dermoid cyst)
• Germinal inclusion cyst (regarded by some as the precursor for epithelial ovarian cancer)

SPECIAL TESTS
• Pelvic exam is the most important
• Careful history and physical exam

IMAGING
• Transabdominal or transvaginal ultrasonography may differentiate tumors from other pelvic lesions and identify features that place the patient at greater risk for malignancy (solid component, papillations, multiple septations, ascites, bilaterality, fixed and irregular, rapidly enlarging, accompanied by cul-de-sac nodules). Color flow Doppler evaluation may also be helpful.
• Abdominopelvic CT scan with contrast
• Barium enema, colonoscopy, or IVP as indicated

DIAGNOSTIC PROCEDURES
• Exploratory laparoscopy or laparotomy

TREATMENT

APPROPRIATE HEALTH CARE
Inpatient if surgery necessary

GENERAL MEASURES   N/A

SURGICAL MEASURES
• Cystectomy or wedge resection for cyst with benign features
• Surgical removal of tumor to establish diagnosis when:
 ◊ Premenopausal cysts greater than 5 cm that persist more than 6-8 wks
 ◊ Mass that is solid
 ◊ Mass greater than 10 cm
 ◊ Mass in a premenarchal or postmenopausal female
 ◊ Suspicion of torsion or rupture
 ◊ Postmenopausal cysts
 ◊ Cysts with worrisome ultrasound features (e.g., papillations)

ACTIVITY   As tolerated

DIET   No special diet

PATIENT EDUCATION   A variety of excellent patient education materials (e.g., "Ovarian Cyst") can be downloaded from the AAFP (http://www.aafp.org/afp) and ACOG (http://www.acog.com) internet sites.

MEDICATIONS

DRUG(S) OF CHOICE In premenopausal patients with cystic masses less than 10 cm in diameter, therapy with a monophasic oral contraceptive pill for 4-6 wks may stimulate regression. Such cysts may also regress through simple resorption. If the cyst remains unchanged after 4-6 wks of observation, then surgical exploration is warranted.
Contraindications: Those established for OCPs (e.g., hypercoagulable state or history of DVT, ischemic heart disease, history of CVA, hypertension, hepatic adenoma).
Precautions: Refer to manufacturer's profile of each drug
Significant possible interactions: Refer to manufacturer's profile of each drug

ALTERNATIVE DRUGS N/A

FOLLOWUP

PATIENT MONITORING
• Most require only yearly exams
• Varies by diagnosis

PREVENTION/AVOIDANCE Use of oral contraceptives may decrease risk

POSSIBLE COMPLICATIONS
Complications of untreated dermoid and mucinous cysts may include pseudomyxoma peritonei

EXPECTED COURSE/PROGNOSIS
Complete cure

MISCELLANEOUS

ASSOCIATED CONDITIONS N/A

AGE-RELATED FACTORS
Pediatric: Malignancy must be ruled out in premenarchal patients
Geriatric: Because incidence of malignancy increases with age, postmenopausal patients warrant comprehensive evaluation and follow-up.
Others: N/A

PREGNANCY The majority of cysts discovered during pregnancy are corpus luteum or follicular cysts. The two most commonly encountered tumors during pregnancy are cystadenomas (serous or mucinous) and dermoid cysts.

SYNONYMS N/A

ICD-9-CM 220 Benign neoplasm of the ovary

SEE ALSO N/A

OTHER NOTES N/A

ABBREVIATIONS N/A

REFERENCES
• Benacerrif BR, Finkler NJ, et al: Sonographic accuracy in the diagnosis of ovarian masses. J Reprod Med 1990;35:491-495.
• Bird C, et al: Benign neoplasms of the ovary. In Sciarra J, Droegmuller W, eds. Clinical Gynecology. Philadelphia, JB Lippincott, 1990
• DiSaia PJ, Creasman, WT: Clinical Gynecologic Oncology. 5Th ed. Mosby, St Louis, 1997
• Drake J: Diagnosis and management of the adnexal mass. Amer Fam Phys 1998;57: 2471-2476
• Jones, HW: Ovarian cysts and tumors. In: Jones HW, Wentz, AC, Burnett, LS, eds: Novak's Textbook of Gynecology. 11th ed. Baltimore, Williams and Wilkins, 1988
• Mishell DR: Noncontraceptive benefits of oral contraceptives. J Reprod Med 1993;38: 1021-1029.
Illustrations: N/A
Internet references: http://www.5mcc.com

AUTHOR(S)
Peter P. Toth, MD, PhD

Paget's disease of the breast

BASICS

DESCRIPTION Rare type of carcinoma that appears unilaterally as dermatitis of the nipple, representing an extension to the epidermis of an underlying carcinoma of a mammary duct.

System(s) affected: Skin/Exocrine

Genetics: No known genetic pattern

Incidence/Prevalence in USA:
• 1000-4000 new cases each year
• Approximately 1-2% of all cases of breast cancer

Predominant age: 40-75

Predominant sex: Female

SIGNS AND SYMPTOMS
• Nipple skin changes that do not respond to conservative treatment
• Nipple itching
• Nipple burning
• Nipple oozing
• Nipple bleeding
• Eczematoid nipple changes
• Breast mass
• Nipple fissures
• Nipple ulceration
• Local hyperemia
• Local edema

CAUSES   Unknown

RISK FACTORS
• Same as for non-heritable breast carcinoma
  ◊ Early menarche
  ◊ Late menopause
  ◊ Nulliparity
  ◊ First birth after age 30
  ◊ Family history of breast cancer
  ◊ History of radiation exposure
  ◊ History of alcohol use
  ◊ Proliferative benign breast disease

DIAGNOSIS

DIFFERENTIAL DIAGNOSIS
• Eczema
• Psoriasis
• Skin tumors (e.g., Bowen's disease)
• Squamous cell carcinoma
• Basal cell carcinoma

LABORATORY   N/A

Drugs that may alter lab results: N/A

Disorders that may alter lab results: N/A

PATHOLOGICAL FINDINGS
• Micro - malignant cell invasion of the epidermis with large pale staining cells
• Underlying ductal adenocarcinoma

SPECIAL TESTS   N/A

IMAGING   Mammography - useful, but cannot exclude malignancy without clinicopathological correlation

DIAGNOSTIC PROCEDURES   Any chronic or non-healing nipple lesion should be biopsied

TREATMENT

APPROPRIATE HEALTH CARE
Treatment of the underlying breast cancer with surgery. Additional adjuvant chemotherapy and/or radiation therapy dependent on cancer histology, size and stage.

GENERAL MEASURES
• Radiotherapy
• Chemotherapy
• Hormonal manipulation

SURGICAL MEASURES   To be determined by surgeon

ACTIVITY   Full activity

DIET   No special diet

PATIENT EDUCATION   National Cancer Institute, Dept. of Health And Human Services, Public Inquiries Section, Office of Cancer Communications, Building 31, Room 101-18, 9000 Rockville Pike, Bethesda, MD 20892, (301)496-5583

Paget's disease of the breast

MEDICATIONS

DRUG(S) OF CHOICE
- Chemotherapy per oncology study protocols
  ◊ Doxorubicin (Adriamycin) based regimen
  ◊ CMF - cyclophosphamide, methotrexate, 5-fluorouracil
  ◊ Tamoxifen
  ◊ Paclitaxel (Taxol)

Contraindications: Refer to manufacturer's literature
Precautions: Refer to manufacturer's literature
Significant possible interactions: Refer to manufacturer's literature

ALTERNATIVE DRUGS   N/A

FOLLOWUP

PATIENT MONITORING
- Routine screening for women over age 40
  ◊ Annual mammogram
  ◊ Monthly self-exams
  ◊ Annual physician exams

PREVENTION/AVOIDANCE   None known

POSSIBLE COMPLICATIONS
Metastases

EXPECTED COURSE/PROGNOSIS
- Dependent on stage of underlying breast carcinoma

```
Stage                          10YR†
---------------------------------------
1    ≤ 2 cm tumor;          70-95%
       - nodes
2    > 2 cm tumor or        40-45%
       + nodes
3    > 5 cm tumor;
       + nodes or
       fixed nodes          10-15%
4    metastatic disease     <5%
---------------------------------------
†10 year disease-free survival
```

MISCELLANEOUS

ASSOCIATED CONDITIONS   Underlying carcinoma

AGE-RELATED FACTORS
Pediatric: N/A
Geriatric: N/A
Others: N/A

PREGNANCY   N/A

SYNONYMS   N/A

ICD-9-CM
174.0 malignant neoplasm of breast and areola

SEE ALSO   Breast cancer

OTHER NOTES   Extramammary Paget's disease can also occur

ABBREVIATIONS   N/A

REFERENCES
- Bland KI, Copeland EM, eds: The Breast. Philadelphia, W.B. Saunders Co., 1998
- Fitzpatrick TB, et al, eds: Dermatology In General Medicine. 5th Ed. New York, McGraw-Hill, 1999
- DeVita VT Jr, Hellman S, Rosenberg A, eds: Cancer: Principles and Practices of Oncology. 5th Ed. Philadelphia, J.B. Lippincott, 1997
Illustrations: N/A
Internet references: http://www.5mcc.com

Author(s)
Mark Horattas, MD, FACS

Pancreatic cancer, exocrine

BASICS

DESCRIPTION
Pancreatic exocrine malignancies (including adenocarcinoma, 90%; cystadenocarcinoma; and acinar cell carcinoma) represent 3% of all cancers but the fifth most common cause of cancer deaths in the United States.

These malignancies are divided into two broad categories:
• Periampullary lesions - most commonly adenocarcinoma of the head of the pancreas. Of lesser frequency are malignant lesions of the ampulla, duodenum and common bile duct. Lesions in these areas are characterized by jaundice, weight loss and abdominal pain.
• Lesions of body and tail - account for thirty percent of adenocarcinomas of the pancreas. Due to retroperitoneal location and distance from common bile duct, lesions tend to be much larger at diagnosis. Common symptoms are those of weight loss and pain.

System(s) affected: Gastrointestinal
Genetics: More common in blacks, diabetic patients
Incidence/Prevalence in USA:
• Approximately 28,000 new cases diagnosed per year
• Varies among ethnic groups, highest in Blacks and Hawaiians
Predominant age: Mean age in males = 63 years, females = 67 years
Predominant sex: Male > Female (1.5-2:1)

SIGNS AND SYMPTOMS
• Weight loss (90%)
• Pain (75%)
• Jaundice (65%)
• Anorexia (60%)
• Pruritus (40%)
• Diabetes mellitus (15%)
• Malnutrition (75%)
• Hepatomegaly (65%)
• Jaundice (70%)
• Palpable gallbladder (25%)
• Abdominal tenderness (20%)
• Mass (10%)
• Ascites (5%)

CAUSES
• No known etiology, though many associations
• Associations include race, diabetes mellitus, tobacco, environmental and occupational exposures, and dietary lipids
• Of interest, seemingly no association between pancreatitis, alcohol and coffee consumption when data adjusted for effect of tobacco use

RISK FACTORS
• Probable: Race, diabetes mellitus, tobacco
• Possible: Environmental/occupational exposures, dietary lipids

DIAGNOSIS

DIFFERENTIAL DIAGNOSIS
• Choledocholithiasis
• Pancreatitis
• Pancreatic pseudocyst
• Cholangiocarcinoma
• Carcinoma of the ampulla of Vater
• Duodenal neoplasms
• Endocrine tumors of pancreas
• Miscellaneous malignancies with extrinsic bile duct compression
• Biliary tract stricture
• Choledochal cyst

LABORATORY
• Bilirubin level mean of 15 mg/dL (256.5 μmol/L) in patients with jaundice due to pancreatic cancer; considerably higher than that in patients with benign diseases (choledocholithiasis, strictures)
• Patients with recent onset of jaundice with bilirubin greater than 10 mg/dL (171.0 μmol/L) should be considered to have neoplastic obstruction of common bile duct until proven otherwise
• Alkaline phosphatase elevated in most patients. Mean of 550 U/L not significantly different from level in patients with bile duct obstruction from benign disease
• Anemia present in approximately 60% of patients
• Stool occult blood present in approximately 90% of patients with periampullary tumors
• Elevated amylase found in less than 5% of patients
• Tumor markers:
  ◊ In general, useful for screening and assessment of extent of disease. Likely to have good specificity when multiple marker assays combined. Represent a dynamic area of research and discovery of new markers and development of sensitive and specific assays likely in the future.
  ◊ CA 19-9: Elevated in serum and pancreatic juice of patients with pancreatic cancer. Sensitivity/specificity in differentiating pancreatitis is undetermined.
  ◊ Carcinoembryonic antigen (CEA): Serum and pancreatic juice levels elevated beyond 10 ng/ml (10 μg/L) and 30 ng/mL (30 μg/L) respectively in patients with pancreatic cancer
  ◊ Pancreatic-oncofetal antigen: Sensitivity of 68% when used as screening test. Combining test with CEA and alpha-fetoprotein increases specificity.
Drugs that may alter lab results: N/A
Disorders that may alter lab results: N/A

PATHOLOGICAL FINDINGS
• Adenocarcinoma (90%)
• Acinar cell carcinoma (1.2%)
• Other (0.8%)
• Uncertain (9.2%)

SPECIAL TESTS
Pancreatic juice - for cytology and CEA, CA 19-9 assays

IMAGING
• Upper GI series - widening of duodenal sweep in large tumors
• CT scan - most useful imaging modality
• Ultrasound - limited by overlying bowel, less accuracy in staging
• MRI
• Endoscopic retrograde cholangiopancreatography (ERCP) - particularly useful in ampullary or duodenal lesions where biopsy may be performed, pancreatic juice sampled and pancreatic duct cytology
• PTC - delineates proximal biliary tree, important data in planning reconstruction following surgical procedure
• Angiography - role in preoperative staging, not in tumor localization

DIAGNOSTIC PROCEDURES
• Biopsy:
  ◊ CT-guided percutaneous needle aspiration has sensitivity of 85% with specificity of approximately 100% in pancreatic adenocarcinoma. Few complications and extremely low risk of tract seeding.
  ◊ Pseudocyst aspiration can differentiate benign pseudocysts from cystadenocarcinoma. Fluid in cystadenocarcinoma has low amylase, high CEA and lactate dehydrogenase (LDH) levels, and malignant cells are usually present.
  ◊ Liver biopsy may be useful in patients with hepatic metastases
  ◊ Laparoscopy with biopsy is becoming a popular technique and is likely to be more frequently used in the future for staging
• Esophagogastroduodenoscopy:
  ◊ Useful for evaluation of ampulla and duodenal regions in patients with periampullary and duodenal tumors

TREATMENT

APPROPRIATE HEALTH CARE
Inpatient for testing, preliminary therapy, surgery or other protocols

GENERAL MEASURES
• Management highly variable and influenced by the overall health of the patient, presence of metastases, and location and size of tumor
• Analgesia
• Management of pruritus
• Control of diabetes (usually "brittle") if total pancreatectomy performed
• Non-operative procedures
  ◊ Biliary decompression by use of endoprostheses, transhepatic drainage catheters
  ◊ Celiac blockade and epidural catheter placement for analgesia
  ◊ Chemotherapy - multiple protocols
  ◊ Radiation therapy - external beam (intraoperative - largely investigational)

SURGICAL MEASURES
• Pancreaticoduodenectomy (Whipple's procedure)
• Total pancreatectomy
• Regional pancreatectomy - resection pancreas, portal vein, regional nodes, subtotal gastrectomy
• Biliary decompression for unresectable disease - T-tube, bilio-enteric anastomoses
• Gastrojejunostomy for gastric outlet obstruction in unresectable disease

ACTIVITY   Ad lib

DIET   As tolerated. Serve small frequent meals.

PATIENT EDUCATION   Printed patient information available from: National Cancer Institute, Dept. of Health And Human Services, Public Inquiries Section, Office of Cancer Communications, Building 31, Room 101-18, 9000 Rockville Pike, Bethesda, MD 20892, (301)496-5583

MEDICATIONS

DRUG(S) OF CHOICE
• Analgesics
• Management of pruritus, e.g., phenothiazines or cholestyramine
• Chemotherapy - multiple protocols
• Antacids
• Pancreatic enzymes
• Diabetes control
Contraindications: N/A
Precautions: N/A
Significant possible interactions: N/A

ALTERNATIVE DRUGS   N/A

FOLLOWUP

PATIENT MONITORING   Variable

PREVENTION/AVOIDANCE   Avoid tobacco

POSSIBLE COMPLICATIONS
• Pain
• Jaundice
• Malnutrition
• Diabetes - especially in patients undergoing total pancreatectomy
• Operative mortality - varies from 10-40%

EXPECTED COURSE/PROGNOSIS
• Three year survival - 2.5%
• Five year survival - 1%
• Following surgery for potentially curable disease, five year survival is about 4%. Reflects high likelihood of metastases at the time of diagnosis.

MISCELLANEOUS

ASSOCIATED CONDITIONS
• Diabetes
• Other findings associated with metastases, e.g., superior vena cava syndrome, Horner's syndrome

AGE-RELATED FACTORS
Pediatric: N/A
Geriatric: More common in this age group, particularly males
Others: N/A

PREGNANCY   N/A

SYNONYMS   N/A

ICD-9-CM
157.0 Malignant neoplasm of pancreas (site specified 157.x)

SEE ALSO   N/A

OTHER NOTES   N/A

ABBREVIATIONS
CEA = carcinoembryonic antigen
CA = cancer antigen

REFERENCES   Howard JM, Jordan GL, Reber HA, eds: Surgical Diseases of the Pancreas. Philadelphia, Lea and Febiger, 1987
Illustrations: N/A
Internet references: http://www.5mcc.com

Author(s)
Leo C. Mercer, MD

Pancreatitis

BASICS

DESCRIPTION An inflammatory, auto-digestive process of the pancreas
- Acute pancreatitis
  ◊ Inflammatory episode with symptoms related to intrapancreatic activation of enzymes with pain, nausea and vomiting, and associated intestinal ileus
  ◊ It varies widely in severity, complications and prognosis
- Chronic pancreatitis
  ◊ Progressive functional destruction of the pancreas that may exist in the absence of an etiology
  ◊ Results in both exocrine and endocrine deficiencies
  ◊ Pain, maldigestion and diabetes mellitus are the major features

System(s) affected: Gastrointestinal
Genetics: Hereditary pancreatitis is a very rare condition with an autosomally dominant inheritance pattern
Incidence/Prevalence in USA: Urban - 22/100,00; rural - 10/100,000
Predominant age:
- Acute pancreatitis - none
- Chronic pancreatitis - 35-45 years (usually related to alcohol)
Predominant sex: Male = Female

SIGNS AND SYMPTOMS
- Abdominal pain - epigastric, may radiate straight through to back
- Nausea and/or vomiting
- Mild abdominal distention
- Fever (100-101°F [37.7-38.3°C])
- Hypotension/shock (40%)
- Mild jaundice
- Diminished or absent bowel sounds
- Flank discoloration (Grey Turner's sign)
- Umbilical discoloration (Cullen's sign)
- Pleural effusion

CAUSES
- Gallstones
- Alcohol
- Trauma/surgery
- Post endoscopic retrograde cholangiopancreatography (ERCP)
- Medications
- Metabolic
  ◊ Hypertriglyceridemia
  ◊ Hypercalcemia
  ◊ Renal failure
- Hereditary
- Systemic lupus erythematosus
- Infections
  ◊ Mumps
  ◊ Coxsackie B
  ◊ Hepatitis A and B
  ◊ Ascariasis
  ◊ Salmonella
- Penetrating peptic ulcer (rare)
- Cystic fibrosis
- Tumor
- Idiopathic
- Pancreas divisum
- Scorpion venom

RISK FACTORS   See Causes

DIAGNOSIS

DIFFERENTIAL DIAGNOSIS
- Acute pancreatitis
  ◊ Penetrating or perforated peptic ulcer
  ◊ Acute cholecystitis
  ◊ Choledocholithiasis
  ◊ Macroamylasemia, macrolipasemia
  ◊ Mesenteric vascular obstruction and/or infarction
  ◊ Perforation of a viscus
  ◊ Intestinal obstruction
  ◊ Aortic aneurysm
- Chronic pancreatitis
  ◊ Pancreatic cancer
  ◊ Other malabsorptive processes
  ◊ Other cause of biliary obstruction

LABORATORY
- Acute pancreatitis
  ◊ Elevated serum amylase
  ◊ Elevated serum lipase
  ◊ Elevated (mild) alanine aminotransferase (ALT) and/or aspartate aminotransferase (AST) - when associated with alcoholic hepatitis or choledocholithiasis
  ◊ Elevated alkaline phosphatase (mild) - when associated with alcoholic hepatitis or choledocholithiasis
  ◊ Hyperbilirubinemia - when associated with alcoholic hepatitis or choledocholithiasis
  ◊ Glucose increased - in severe disease
  ◊ Calcium decreased - in severe disease
  ◊ WBC 10,000 - 25,000
- Chronic pancreatitis
  ◊ Sometimes none
  ◊ Hyperglycemia
  ◊ Steatorrhea
  ◊ Flare-ups may mimic acute pancreatitis
  ◊ Elevated alkaline phosphatase, bilirubin
Drugs that may alter lab results: Insulin and corticosteroids
Disorders that may alter lab results:
- Biliary tract disease
- Penetrating peptic ulcer
- Intestinal obstruction
- Intestinal ischemia/infarction
- Ruptured ectopic pregnancy
- Renal insufficiency
- Burns
- Macroamylasemia, macrolipasemia

PATHOLOGICAL FINDINGS
- Acute pancreatitis: autodigestion of the pancreas, interstitial edema, hemorrhage, cell and fat necrosis
- Chronic pancreatitis: calcification, fibrosis

SPECIAL TESTS   N/A

IMAGING
- Acute pancreatitis
  ◊ Plain film of abdomen - signs of ileus
  ◊ Chest x-ray - pleural effusion
  ◊ Ultrasound/CT scan of abdomen
  ◊ Endoscopic retrograde cholangiopancreatography (ERCP)
  ◊ Dynamic CT scan

- Chronic pancreatitis
  ◊ X-ray of abdomen - pancreatic calcification
  ◊ Ultrasound and/or CT scan of abdomen - pseudocyst formation/calcification
  ◊ Endoscopic retrograde cholangiopancreatography (ERCP) - ductal deformity, retained common bile duct (CBD) stone, pancreatic duct stones and strictures
  ◊ Endoscopic sphincterotomy - early CBD stone removal improves outcome in severe cases
  ◊ Endoscopic ultrasound

DIAGNOSTIC PROCEDURES
- Acute pancreatitis
  ◊ CT guided aspiration of necrotic areas
  ◊ ERCP for common duct stone removal
- Chronic pancreatitis
  ◊ Secretin stimulation test
  ◊ Para-aminobenzoic acid test (bentiromide [Chymex] test)
  ◊ Lunch test meal

TREATMENT

APPROPRIATE HEALTH CARE
- Acute pancreatitis - hospitalization, unless very mild and able to maintain oral intake
- Chronic pancreatitis - outpatient except for complications

GENERAL MEASURES
- Acute pancreatitis
  ◊ P - pain control: meperidine
  ◊ A - arrest shock: IV fluids
  ◊ N - nasogastric tube for vomiting
  ◊ C - calcium monitoring
  ◊ R - renal evaluation
  ◊ E - ensure pulmonary function
  ◊ A - antibiotics
  ◊ S - surgery or special procedures in selected cases
- Chronic pancreatitis
  ◊ Pain - alcohol abstinence, analgesia (avoid narcotics if possible), celiac ganglion block, surgery, pancreatic enzyme preparations
  ◊ Maldigestion - pancreatic enzyme supplements, H2-blockers
  ◊ Diabetes mellitus - insulin

SURGICAL MEASURES
- Acute pancreatitis
  ◊ Infected necrosis
  ◊ Peritoneal lavage
- Chronic pancreatitis
  ◊ Pain
  ◊ Pseudocyst drainage

ACTIVITY
- Acute pancreatitis - usually bedrest although sitting in a chair may be more comfortable. Advance as able.
- Chronic pancreatitis - not restricted

DIET
• Acute pancreatitis: begin diet after pain, tenderness and ileus have resolved; small amounts of high carbohydrate, low fat and low protein foods. Advance as tolerated. NPO or nasogastric tube, if vomiting
• Chronic pancreatitis: small meals high in protein. Adjust if diabetes mellitus is present.

PATIENT EDUCATION
For patient education materials favorably reviewed on this topic, contact: National Digestive Diseases Information Clearinghouse, Box NDDIC, Bethesda, MD 20892, (301)468-6344

MEDICATIONS

DRUG(S) OF CHOICE
• Acute pancreatitis
◊ Meperidine (Demerol) 50-100 mg IM/IV every 3-4 hours
• Antibiotics
• Somatostatin
• Chronic pancreatitis
◊ Analgesics: acetaminophen (Tylenol), oxycodone-acetaminophen (Tylox), hydrocodone-acetaminophen (Vicodin), propoxyphene napsylate
◊ Pancreatic enzyme (Pancrease MT, Creon) supplements
◊ H2-blockers (reducing gastric acid increases availability of pancreatic enzymes)
Contraindications:
• Nor-meperidine, a metabolite of meperidine, may accumulate following several days of round-the-clock dosing. May cause mental status changes or seizures.
• Antibiotic allergy
Precautions: Narcotic addiction
Significant possible interactions: Refer to manufacturer's profile of each drug

ALTERNATIVE DRUGS   N/A

FOLLOWUP

PATIENT MONITORING
• Assure alcohol abstinence
• Follow and correct any etiologic cause - hypertriglycerides, choledocholithiasis
• Persistent elevation of amylase weeks after acute pancreatitis suggests possibility of pseudocyst - should perform imaging study

PREVENTION/AVOIDANCE
• Avoid alcohol
• Correct underlying causes, i.e., lipids, drug use, ARDS

POSSIBLE COMPLICATIONS
• Acute pancreatitis - pseudocyst
• Chronic pancreatitis - pseudocyst, abscess, biliary/duodenal obstruction, portal/splenic vein thrombosis, diabetes mellitus

EXPECTED COURSE/PROGNOSIS
• Acute pancreatitis: 85-90% resolve spontaneously, 3-5% mortality
◊ Poor prognosis indicated by:
- On admission: age > 55 years, WBC > 16,000/mm, blood glucose > 200 mg/dL (11.1 mmol/L), serum LDH > 2 x normal, serum SGOT > 6 x normal
- Within 48 hours: hematocrit decrease > 10%, serum calcium < 8 mg/dL, BUN increase > 5 mg/dL, arterial pO2 < 60 mm Hg, base deficit > 4 mEq/L, fluid retention > 6L
• Chronic pancreatitis: may have recurrent episodes of "acute pancreatitis", slow progression, may "burn out" with resolution of symptoms. Narcotic addiction frequent.

MISCELLANEOUS

ASSOCIATED CONDITIONS   N/A

AGE-RELATED FACTORS
Pediatric: Mumps, sometimes complicated by pancreatitis
Geriatric: Vascular disease
Others: N/A

PREGNANCY   Acute fatty liver of pregnancy

SYNONYMS   N/A

ICD-9-CM
577.0 Acute pancreatitis
577.1 Chronic pancreatitis

SEE ALSO
• Alcoholism
• Choledocholithiasis
• Peptic ulcer disease
• Systemic lupus erythematosus (SLE)
• Pseudocyst pancreas

OTHER NOTES   N/A

ABBREVIATIONS   N/A

REFERENCES
• Sleisenger MH, Fordtran JS, eds: Gastrointestinal Disease: Pathophysiology, Diagnosis, Management. 6th Ed. Philadelphia, WB Saunders Co, 1998
• Frank B, Gottlieb K: Amylose normal, lipase elevated: is it pancreatitis? Am J Gastrol 1999;94(2):463
• Pitchumoni CS: Chronic pancreatitis: pathogenesis and management of pain. J Clin Gastrol 1998;279(2):101
• Powell JJ, Miles R, Siriwardena AK: Antibiotic prophylaxis in the initial management of severe acute pancreatitis. Br J Surg 1998;85(5)582
• Linnemoe KD, Yeo CJ: Management of complications of pancreatitis. Curr Prob in Surg 1998;35(1):1
• Naruse S, Kitagawa M, et al: Chronic pancreatitis: overview of medical aspects. Pancreas 1998;16(3):323
• Watanabe S: Acute pancreatitis: overview of medical aspects. Pancreas 1998;16(3):307
• Greenfeld JI, Harmon, CM: Acute pancreatitis. Curr Opin In Pediatr 1997;9(3):260
Illustrations: N/A
Internet references: http://www.5mcc.com

Author(s)
Duane C. Roe, MD

Parkinson's disease

BASICS

DESCRIPTION An adult-onset neurodegenerative disorder of the extrapyramidal system characterized by a combination of tremor at rest, rigidity and bradykinesia. The diagnosis requires therapeutic response to levodopa which implies normal striatal neurons. This is the only neurodegenerative disease which is treatable long-term.
System(s) affected: Nervous, Musculoskeletal
Genetics: Genetic factors do not play a major role in causing typical PD, especially when onset after age 50
Incidence/Prevalence in USA: 50,000 per year; .3% 55-64, 1% 65-74, 3.1% 75-84; 4.3% 85-94
Predominant age: Age 60 with 5% between the ages of 21 and 39
Predominant sex: Male > Female (1.4:1)

SIGNS AND SYMPTOMS
• Cardinal signs
  ◊ Tremor (48 Hz) in repose: Diagnostic, but not required; relieved with activity, concentration, and sleep; increases with stress; 10% of patients present with only tremor, 30% present without; most begin with unilateral tremor.
  ◊ Bradykinesia: required for diagnosis; most disabling symptom; movement initiation difficult, can be overcome with will; causes the gait and postural abnormalities
  ◊ Rigidity: lead pipe type; cogwheeling with tremor
• Other associated signs and symptoms
  ◊ Speech is poorly enunciated, low volume, clipped
  ◊ Ocular abnormalities: Decreased blinking, blepharospasm, impaired upward gaze
  ◊ Seborrhea
  ◊ Dysautonomia with constipation, incontinence, sexual dysfunction
  ◊ Depression in 2/3 of patients
  ◊ Dementia in 20% of patients; more common in patients whose disease onset was bilateral - mild to moderate, 90% with Folstein MMSE >15
  ◊ Gait disturbances including no arm swing, en mass turning, problems getting up from chair, festination, freezing
  ◊ Leaning posture
  ◊ Propulsion or retropulsion
  ◊ Micrographia
  ◊ Mask faces
  ◊ Neglect of swallowing with drooling
• Hoehn and Yahr scale of disability in Parkinson's disease
  ◊ Stage 1 unilateral, minimal functional impairment
  ◊ Stage 2 bilateral without impairment of balance
  ◊ Stage 3 bilateral, positive instability, physically independent
  ◊ Stage 4 severe disability, can walk or stand without assist, but markedly incapacitated
  ◊ Stage 5 wheelchair bound or bedridden unless aided

CAUSES
• Unknown
• Loss of dopaminergic neurons in the substantia nigra with rate of loss 1% per year in patients with Parkinson's versus 0.5% in normal aging.
• Probably not genetic rather toxic or infectious
• Known toxins: MPTP, pesticides. Other non-dopaminergic neurons can be affected.

RISK FACTORS Unknown in the idiopathic disease

DIAGNOSIS

DIFFERENTIAL DIAGNOSIS
• Parkinsonism: bradykinesia and occasionally tremor with little or no response to levodopa indicating that the striatal neurons are also degenerated
  ◊ Progressive supranuclear palsy
  ◊ Multisystem atrophy
  ◊ Alzheimer's with extrapyramidal features
  ◊ Side effects of neuroleptic medications
  ◊ Infectious - postencephalitic
  ◊ Vascular - lacunar state
  ◊ Toxins
  ◊ Metabolic - Wilson's disease: onset <40
• Benign essential tremor: positive family history and relief with alcohol

LABORATORY N/A
Drugs that may alter lab results: N/A
Disorders that may alter lab results: N/A

PATHOLOGICAL FINDINGS Typical changes that allow precise pathological diagnosis. Lewy bodies.

SPECIAL TESTS N/A

IMAGING
• CT or MRI help rule out other disorders
• PET scanning

DIAGNOSTIC PROCEDURES
Diagnostic criteria:
• Clinically possible - any one of:
  ◊ Rest tremor
  ◊ Rigidity
  ◊ Bradykinesia
• Clinically probable - any 2 of:
  ◊ Rest tremor
  ◊ Rigidity
  ◊ Bradykinesia
  ◊ Impaired postural reflexes, or
One of first three displaying asymmetry
• Clinically definite - any 3 of:
  ◊ Rest tremor
  ◊ Rigidity
  ◊ Bradykinesia
  ◊ Impaired postural reflexes, or
  ◊ Any 2 of above with one of first 3 displaying asymmetry

TREATMENT

APPROPRIATE HEALTH CARE
Outpatient

GENERAL MEASURES
• Drugs have therapeutic and toxic effects
• Acute worsening may indicate depression, non-compliance or supervening illness
• Course is progressive with or without drugs. Life-long therapy directed toward symptom control - treat disability
• Investigate for drug-induced cause; if found, discontinue drug. Symptom resolution may take weeks to months.
• Physical, occupational and speech therapy
• Physical limitations require adjustments in the home, e.g., special chairs, elevated toilet seat, eating utensils, dressing oneself

SURGICAL MEASURES
• Adrenal medullary transplants, fetal midbrain with substantia nigra neurons
• Thalamotomy - akinesia
• Stereotactic pallidotomy - akinesia
• Deep brain stimulation - dyskinesia, tremor response 88%

ACTIVITY Maintain activity to whatever degree possible; use cane for walking

DIET
• Small frequent meals if difficulty in eating
• High liquid intake important; high bulk foods
• Reduced protein diet is unnecessary

PATIENT EDUCATION
• Local support groups
• United Parkinson Foundation, 360 W. Superior St., Chicago, IL 60610, 312-664-2344
• American Parkinson's Disease Foundation, 1250 Hyland Blvd., Staten Island, NY 10305, 800-223-2732

MEDICATIONS

DRUG(S) OF CHOICE
• Selegiline 5 mg in AM and noon: for patients with no limiting disability (neuroprotection unproven)
• Levodopa-carbidopa (Sinemet): for patients with manifested disability; although neuro-vegetative symptoms such as speech disorders and falls are resistant to levodopa
  ◊ Sinemet SR 50-200 (start with 1/2 tab) qid after food. Increase by 100 mg levodopa per day until desired effect or side effects occur. If early morning symptoms, add Sinemet 25-100 immediate release one half hour before arising.
  ◊ If switching to the SR, increase daily dose by 25%
  ◊ Add agonist if "wear off" or dyskinesia appears or when 800-1000 mg levodopa SR per day being taken

Parkinson's disease

• Dopamine agonists. Low potency; long half-life; reduces wearing-off effects of levodopa. Add when levodopa > 600 mg/day. early monotherapy may reduce levodopa use and long-term effects.
  ◊ Bromocriptine - start with 1.25 mg qd or bid
  ◊ Pergolide - 0.05 mg/d for 2 days and increase by 0.1 mg/d q 3 days x 12 days. If higher doses needed, then increase by 0.25 mg q 3 days. Mean dose is 3 mg.
  ◊ Pramipexole non-ergoline 0.125 mg tid, max 4.5 mg/day.
  ◊ Ropinirole non-ergoline. 0.25 mg tid, max 24 mg/day
  ◊ Cabergoline - ergoline with long half life - 0.5 mg/day to max 6 mg/day
  ◊ Titrate the levodopa-carbidopa combination downward as these agents are added such that 1 mg of bromocriptine equals 10 mg of levodopa and 1 mg of pergolide equals 10 mg of bromocriptine
• MAO inhibitors. May prolong time prior to need for levodopa/carbidopa. Blocks metabolism of dopamine. May be neuro-protective.
  ◊ Selegiline 5 mg - start with 1/2 tab qAM and 1/2 q noon; increase to 5mg bid. If add to levodopa-carbidopa, lower dosage 20%.
• Anticholinergics. For tremor in early stages or as an adjunct (30% improvement in 50% of patients).
  ◊ Trihexyphenidyl (Artane): 1 mg/day, increase by 2 mg every 3 days until 6-10 mg/day
  ◊ Benztropine (Cogentin): 1-2 mg/day. Start with 0.5 mg/day and increase slowly by 0.5 mg every 6 days. Maximum 6 mg/day.
• Amantadine, mode of action unknown
  ◊ Similar to anticholinergics; improves bradykinesia and rigidity; rapid onset 48-72h
  ◊ Synergistic with L-dopa
  ◊ 100-200 mg/day
• COMT inhibitor use as adjunct to L-dopa as in dopamine agonists, may decrease motor fluctuation in late stage disease
  ◊ Tolcapone - 100 mg tid, max 1200 mg/day
  ◊ Entacapone - 100 mg tid, max 1200 mg/day
Contraindications: Refer to manufacturer's literature
Precautions:
• L-dopa/carbidopa - late effects
  ◊ Time related dosage problems occur in 50% of patients in 4-5 years
  ◊ Dyskinesias probably secondary to receptor hypersensitivity.
  - Inter dose dyskinesia: occurs at peak level of drug 2 hours after immediate release form, limb choreoathetosis and grimacing; change to sustained release, reduce levodopa dose plus add agonist or clozapine 100-200 mg.
  - Diphasic dyskinesia: mobile dystonia of limbs occurs as the dose is rising and falling; increase individual dose or subcutaneous apomorphine pulses.
  - "Off" period dyskinesia: may begin as early morning dystonia (foot); reduce inter-dose interval or switch to sustained release or agonist

◊ Wear-off phenomena: usually occurs 3-4 hours after last dose. Usually first sign of drug-response problems caused by increased severity of nigral degeneration. Use sustained release form with an agonist or selegiline.
◊ On/off phenomena: 15-20% of patients develop severe fluctuation of response. Long-term high dose levodopa may be cause. Try low protein diet, slow release preparations, continuous subcutaneous infusions, or enteral infusion into duodenum. Also can decrease dose until on-off phenomena disappears and then restart drug.
◊ Hourly liquid preparation - 10 tablets 25-100 plus 2g abscorbic acid crystals in 1l of tap water; 75 mL in AM, then 35-50 mL/h
◊ Freezing: find a visual clue to "step over" or counting numbers in head
◊ Psychiatric side effects: confusion, hallucinations (well-formed visual or auditory) paranoia, nightmares. If mainly at night, reduce last evening dose or try clozapine.
• Agonists
  ◊ Nausea, nightmares, agitation, orthostatic hypertension, hallucinations
  ◊ Raynaud's phenomena in doses > 30 mg/day, edema, hypertension, worsening CHF
• MAO inhibitor: Anxiety/sleep disturbance
• Anticholinergics: Confusion, constipation, urinary retention, dry mouth and glaucoma
• Dopamine release stimulator: Confusion, hallucinations, edema, livedo reticularis, and worsening CHF
Significant possible interactions: Most have additive therapeutic and side effects

ALTERNATIVE DRUGS
• Tricyclic antidepressants for night time sedation and associated depression (50% of patients with Parkinson's)
• Antioxidants or vitamin E have shown no definite benefit
• Selective COMT inhibitors
• Apomorphine as agonist or for "freezing" (use limited by adverse effects [vomiting] and need for parenteral administration)
• Clozapine: 70-200 mg/day can suppress frequency of dyskinesia and increase "on" time; also useful for hallucinations. Side effects include sedation and sialorrhea, and most serious, agranulocytosis. Use 50 mg or less per day for drug-induced psychosis.

FOLLOWUP

PATIENT MONITORING Life-long for medication adjustment and physical therapy

PREVENTION/AVOIDANCE Avoid drugs known to cause tardive dyskinesia, such as: Fluphenazine, perphenazine, prochlorperazine, thiopropazate, trifluoperazine, promazine, thioridazine, haloperidol, droperidol, benperidol, fluspirilene, pimozide, trifluperidol, chlorprothixene, clopenthixol, thiothixene

POSSIBLE COMPLICATIONS Dementia, depression, aspiration pneumonia, falls, freezing, dyskinesias; also associated with a twofold increase risk of death

EXPECTED COURSE/PROGNOSIS
• More rapid progression: Older at disease onset; dementia
• Milder disease, the predominant feature is tremor

 MISCELLANEOUS

ASSOCIATED CONDITIONS Psychosis; depression

AGE-RELATED FACTORS
Pediatric: May occur as secondary parkinsonism in this age group
Geriatric: Common among elderly
Others: N/A

PREGNANCY N/A

SYNONYMS
• Paralysis agitans
• Shaking palsy

ICD-9-CM
332.0 paralysis agitans

SEE ALSO
• Depression
• Dementia
• Benign essential tremor syndrome

OTHER NOTES New approaches in treatment undergoing study

ABBREVIATIONS
COMT = catechol-O-methyltransferase

REFERENCES
• Sweeny PJ: Considerations in the diagnosis and management of Parkinson's disease. Fam Prac Recertification 1996;18(4)
• Poewe WH, Wenning GK: The natural history of Parkinson's disease. Neurology 1996;47(3):s146-s151
• Krauss JK, Jankovic J: Surgical treatment of Parkinson's disease. Am Fam Phys 1996;54(5):1621-1628
• Gottwald MD, et al: New pharmacotherapy for Parkinson's disease. Ann of Pharmacother 1997;31:1205-1217
4 additional references available at web site
Internet references: http://www.5mcc.com
Illustrations: N/A

Author(s)
Jeffrey F. Minteer, MD

Paronychia

BASICS

DESCRIPTION Infectious inflammation of the folds of skin surrounding the fingernail or toenail. May be acute or chronic.
System(s) affected: Skin/Exocrine
Genetics: No known genetic pattern
Incidence/Prevalence in USA: Common
Predominant age: All ages
Predominant sex: Female > Male (3:1)

SIGNS AND SYMPTOMS
• Separation of nail fold from nail plate
• Red, painful swelling of skin around nail plate
• Purulent
• Secondary changes of nail plate
• Green changes in nail (pseudomonas)

CAUSES
• Acute - Staphylococcus aureus. Less frequently by Streptococci and Pseudomonas
• Chronic - Candida albicans. Less frequently by fungi - dermatophytes and occasionally, by molds (Scytalidium fusarium)

RISK FACTORS
• Acute - trauma to skin surrounding nail, ingrown nails
• Chronic - frequent immersion of hands in water, diabetes mellitus

DIAGNOSIS

DIFFERENTIAL DIAGNOSIS
• Herpetic whitlow
• Felon
• Reiter's disease
• Psoriasis

LABORATORY
• Gram stain
• Culture and sensitivity
• KOH preparation plus fungal culture
Drugs that may alter lab results: Use of over-the-counter antimicrobials or antifungals
Disorders that may alter lab results: N/A

PATHOLOGICAL FINDINGS N/A

SPECIAL TESTS None

IMAGING N/A

DIAGNOSTIC PROCEDURES N/A

TREATMENT

APPROPRIATE HEALTH CARE
Outpatient

GENERAL MEASURES
• Acute - warm compresses or vinegar soaks, elevation
• Chronic - keep fingers dry

SURGICAL MEASURES Incision and drainage (I&D) of abscess, if present. If there is a subungual abscess or ingrown nail present, will need partial or complete removal of nail.

ACTIVITY Full activity

DIET No special diet

PATIENT EDUCATION Chronic - keep fingers dry

Paronychia

MEDICATIONS

DRUG(S) OF CHOICE
• Acute (if diabetic, suppurative or more severe cases):
  ◊ Dicloxacillin 125-500 mg q6h
  ◊ Cloxacillin 250-500 mg q6h
  ◊ Erythromycin 500 mg q6h
  ◊ Cephalexin (Keflex) 250 mg q6h
• Chronic:
  ◊ Bacterial - mupirocin (Bactroban)
  ◊ Yeast or dermatophyte - topical imidazoles (econazole, ketoconazole, terbinafine
• Systemic:
  ◊ Itraconazole (Sporanox) 200 mg/day for 90 days (may have longer action because incorporated in nail plate). Pulse therapy may be useful: 200 mg BID for 7 days, repeated monthly for 2 months
  ◊ Terbinafine (Lamisil) 250 mg q/d for 90 days
  ◊ Fluconazole (Diflucan) 150 mg/week for 4-6 months
Contraindications: Allergy to antibiotic
Precautions: Erythromycin may cause significant gastrointestinal upset
Significant possible interactions:
• Erythromycin affects levels of theophylline and effects of carbamazepine, digoxin and corticosteroids. Cardiac toxicity with terfenadine or astemizole.
• Ketoconazole, astemazole, itraconazole, fluconazole - terfenadine,

ALTERNATIVE DRUGS
Antipseudomonal drugs, e.g., third generation cephalosporin, aminoglycosides

FOLLOWUP

PATIENT MONITORING   Routine followup until healed

PREVENTION/AVOIDANCE
• Chronic - avoid frequent wetting of hands, wear rubber gloves with cloth liner
• Good diabetic control

POSSIBLE COMPLICATIONS
• Acute - subungual abscess
• Chronic - secondary ridging, thickening and discoloration of nail, nail loss

EXPECTED COURSE/PROGNOSIS
With adequate treatment and prevention, healing can be expected

MISCELLANEOUS

ASSOCIATED CONDITIONS   Diabetes mellitus

AGE-RELATED FACTORS
Pediatric: Anaerobes may be involved in cases with thumb/finger sucking
Geriatric: N/A
Others: N/A

PREGNANCY   N/A

SYNONYMS
• Eponychia
• Perionychia

ICD-9-CM
681.02 Onychia and paronychia of finger
112.3 Candidiasis of skin and nails

SEE ALSO
• Onychomycosis

OTHER NOTES   May be considered work-related in bartenders, waitresses, nurses and others who often wet their hands

ABBREVIATIONS   N/A

REFERENCES
• Fitzpatrick TB, et al, eds: Dermatology In General Medicine. 3rd Ed. New York, McGraw-Hill, 1987
• Moschella SC, Hurley HJ, eds: Dermatology. 3rd Ed. Philadelphia, W.B. Saunders Co., 1992
• Baran R, Dawber RPR, eds: Diseases of the Nail and Their Management. 2nd Ed. Boston, Blackwell Scientific, 1994
Illustrations: 2 available on CD-ROM
Internet references: http://www.5mcc.com

Author(s)
Larry Millikan, MD

Parvovirus B19 infection

BASICS

DESCRIPTION Human parvovirus B19 is the primary cause of erythema infectiosum (EI, or fifth disease). It also causes aplastic anemia in patients with increased RBC turnover (e.g., sickle cell anemia), chronic anemia in immunodeficient individuals, and arthritis and arthralgias in normal hosts. There is also the potential for intrauterine infection after maternal parvovirus B19 infection.

System(s) affected: Skin/Exocrine, Musculoskeletal, Hemic/Lymphatic/Immunologic

Genetics: Erythrocyte P antigen-negative individuals are resistant to infection

Incidence/Prevalence in USA: Extremely common; 50% of adults have evidence of prior infection. Most common as community epidemics in winter and spring in non-tropical regions.

Predominant age:
• Infection is common in childhood; approximately 2-11% of children under 11 years of age are parvovirus B19 seropositive
• Peak age for EI is 4-12 years

Predominant sex: Male = Female

SIGNS AND SYMPTOMS
• Erythema infectiosum (EI)
  ◊ Incubation period 4-14 days
  ◊ No preclinical symptoms most commonly. Fever is absent or low grade.
  ◊ Onset of rash noted first on the face ("slapped cheek appearance") with diffuse erythema of the face followed 1-4 days later by a second stage of a lacy reticular rash on the trunk and limbs
  ◊ A third stage of the rash is characterized by marked evanescence and recrudescence, sometimes associated with bathing, exercise, or sun exposure
  ◊ Pruritus and mild arthralgia may occur
  ◊ Headache, pharyngitis, coryza, myalgia, arthralgias, arthritis, and GI disturbances are more frequent and severe in adults
• Joint disease
  ◊ In adults, 80% of patients may manifest arthritis and/or arthralgia
  ◊ In children, joint symptoms are less common
  ◊ Knees, hands, and ankles (frequently symmetrical) are most commonly involved
  ◊ Joint symptoms usually subside in weeks but may persist for months. Joint destruction generally not seen.
• Transient aplastic crisis
  ◊ Seen in patients with chronic hemolysis, such as sickle cell anemia, spherocytosis, thalassemia, and pyruvate kinase deficiency
  ◊ Aplastic event is self-limited with reticulocytes reappearing in 7-10 days and full recovery in 2-3 weeks
• Chronic anemia
  ◊ Seen in immunodeficient individuals
  ◊ No manifestations of fever, rash, or joint symptoms usually

• Fetal/neonatal infection
  ◊ Risk of transplacental spread of virus approximately 33% in infected mothers
  ◊ Clinical manifestations range from asymptomatic seroconversion (most commonly), no seroconversion, second trimester fetal death, or stillbirth secondary to severe anemia and the development of fetal hydrops
  ◊ The principal organ involved in the fetus is the bone marrow: RBC survival is shortened and profound anemia can result from B19 induced erythroid bone marrow aplasia
  ◊ Risk of fetal loss in pregnancy is highest in first trimester B19 infection (9%)
  ◊ Anemia is the most common manifestation of later infection
  ◊ In one study, 84% of B19 infected pregnant women who carried to term delivered normal infants
  ◊ No known long-term developmental problems in infant survivors

CAUSES
• Small (20-25 mm), nonenveloped, single stranded DNA virus
• In EI, the period of viral shedding precedes the development of the rash, suggesting the pathogenesis of the rash is immune related
• In fetal infection, maternal viremia with transplacental passage is the source of infection. Respiratory secretions and rarely blood products are sources of human spread of virus.

RISK FACTORS
• Aplastic crisis - increased RBC turnover (e.g., sickle cell anemia)
• Chronic anemia - immunodeficient individuals
• Intrauterine infection - pregnant, non-immune woman

DIAGNOSIS

DIFFERENTIAL DIAGNOSIS
• Rubella
• Enteroviral disease
• Systemic lupus erythematosus
• Drug reaction
• Lyme disease
• Rheumatoid arthritis

LABORATORY
• Anemia with reticulocytopenia
• Serum IgM antibody to B19 is usual method of confirming diagnosis. During acute infection B19 IgM persists for 1-2 months (less in neonates).
• To exclude congenital B19 in infants with negative B19 IgM, one must follow an infant's B19 IgG serology in the first year of life
• Maternal serum alpha-fetoprotein may be increased in fetuses with hydrops fetalis
Drugs that may alter lab results: N/A
Disorders that may alter lab results: N/A

PATHOLOGICAL FINDINGS
• Skin biopsy usually normal or mild inflammation, usually consisting of perivascular infiltrations of mononuclear cells
• In hydrops fetalis, may see intranuclear inclusions in nucleated red blood cells
• In stillbirths, virus can be detected in all tissues

SPECIAL TESTS
• Antigen detection in tissue or fluids by nucleic acid hybridization or polymerase chain reaction is available on an investigational basis in many academic centers
• B19 cannot be grown in traditional tissue culture systems, but can be isolated in special cell lines in research laboratories

IMAGING Maternal infection - fetal ultrasound

DIAGNOSTIC PROCEDURES Amniotic fluid and chorionic villus sampling may be useful diagnostically in investigation of some maternal infections

TREATMENT

APPROPRIATE HEALTH CARE
• Outpatient management for EI
• Inpatient for aplastic crisis, other severe manifestations

GENERAL MEASURES None

SURGICAL MEASURES N/A

ACTIVITY
• Unrestricted for EI
• Arthritis patients may require physical therapy/exercise program

DIET No special diet

PATIENT EDUCATION
• Patients with chronic hemolytic diseases should be aware of risks for aplastic crisis if exposed to EI
• Pregnant women should avoid exposure to patients with active or chronic infections. However, most adults have already had inapparent infection are therefore not at risk. Exclusion of pregnant women from the workplace where EI is occurring is not recommended.
• Children with symptoms are not infectious and may attend child care or school (e.g., transmission of virus occurs in the asymptomatic interval between infection and symptom expression)

MEDICATIONS

DRUG(S) OF CHOICE
• No therapy needed usually
• IV immune globulin (IVIG) has been used for refractory anemias
• Red blood cell transfusions may be required for aplastic crisis
• Anti-inflammatory agents may alleviate arthritic symptoms
Contraindications: None
Precautions:
• Contact and respiratory isolation for patients hospitalized with aplastic crisis
• EI not contagious once rash has appeared
Significant possible interactions: None

ALTERNATIVE DRUGS None

FOLLOWUP

PATIENT MONITORING Periodic blood counts for anemic patients

PREVENTION/AVOIDANCE
• Standard hygienic practices can minimize spread
• Because EI is so common, it is not possible to avoid exposure completely. Also, period of contagion is before clinical illness (rash) appears.
• Pregnant health care workers should avoid caring for patients with aplastic crises
• Pregnant child care workers are at some increased risk; however, exclusion from the work place will not eliminate this risk, and therefore is not recommended

POSSIBLE COMPLICATIONS
Rare, but more commonly seen in adults than children
• Arthritis
• Persistent anemia
• Hemophagocytic syndrome
• Pneumonitis
• Encephalopathy
• Reports of congenital anomalies but no clear-cut association

EXPECTED COURSE/PROGNOSIS
• Usually self-limited
• Joint symptoms subside in weeks
• Full recovery from aplastic crisis in 2-3 weeks

MISCELLANEOUS

ASSOCIATED CONDITIONS None

AGE-RELATED FACTORS
Pediatric: N/A
Geriatric: None known
Others:
• School-related epidemic and non-immune household contacts have a secondary attack rate of 50%
• Health care workers have a secondary attack rate of 35% with the highest rate being among nurses exposed to children with aplastic crises

PREGNANCY See above

SYNONYMS
• Fifth disease
• Erythema infectiosum

ICD-9-CM
057.0 Erythema infectiosum (fifth disease)

SEE ALSO
• Abortion, spontaneous
• Anemia, sickle cell
• Schönlein-Henoch purpura
• Systemic lupus erythematosus (SLE)
• Arthritis, rheumatoid (RA)

OTHER NOTES N/A

ABBREVIATIONS
EI = erythema Infectiosum

REFERENCES
• Kumar ML: Human parvovirus B19 and its associated diseases. Clin Perinatol 1991;18:209
• Adler SP: Risk of human parvovirus B19 infections among school and hospital employees during endemic periods. J Infect Dis 1993;168:361
• Harris JW: Parvovirus B19 for the hematologist. Am J Hematol 1992;39:119
Illustrations: 4 available on CD-ROM
Internet references: http://www.5mcc.com

Author(s)
Mark R. Dambro, MD, FAAFP

Patent ductus arteriosus

 BASICS

 DIAGNOSIS

 TREATMENT

BASICS

DESCRIPTION Patent ductus arteriosus (PDA) is the failure of the ductus arteriosus to close after birth. 75% of time occurs as isolated defect.
System(s) affected: Cardiovascular
Genetics: No Mendelian inheritance. 1% chance of PDA in infant if one parent affected.
Incidence/Prevalence in USA: 8/1000 live births
Predominant age: Infancy
Predominant sex: Female > Male (2-3:1)

SIGNS AND SYMPTOMS
- Children
  ◊ Failure to grow
  ◊ Recurrent respiratory infections
  ◊ Easy fatigability
  ◊ Dyspnea on exertion
- Adult
  ◊ Leg fatigue
  ◊ Fatigue
  ◊ Shortness of breath
  ◊ Angina
  ◊ Syncope
- Signs (left-to-right shunt)
  ◊ Rough systolic murmur
  ◊ Continuous "machinery" murmur
  ◊ Thrill at left upper sternal border
  ◊ Bounding pulse with wide pulse pressure
  ◊ Prominent, displaced apical impulse
  ◊ Systolic ejection click
  ◊ Diastolic flow murmur (across mitral valve)
  ◊ Excessive sweating
  ◊ Tachypnea, tachycardia, rales if failure ensues
- Signs (right-to-left shunt)
  ◊ Cyanosis, especially lower extremities
  ◊ Clubbing
  ◊ Diastolic Graham-Steele murmur (pulmonic insufficiency)
  ◊ Right ventricular heave
  ◊ Polycythemia

CAUSES
- Prematurity
- Congenital
- Hypoxia
- Prostaglandins

RISK FACTORS
- Premature birth
- High altitudes
- Maternal rubella
- Coexisting cardiac anomalies
- Any condition resulting in hypoxia (pulmonary, hematologic, etc.)

DIAGNOSIS

DIFFERENTIAL DIAGNOSIS
- Venous hum
- Total anomalous pulmonary venous return
- Ruptured sinus of Valsalva
- Arteriovenous communications
- Anomalous origin of left coronary artery from pulmonary artery
- Absence or atresia of pulmonary valve
- Aortic insufficiency with ventricular septal defect
- Peripheral pulmonary stenosis (maternal rubella)
- Truncus arteriosus
- Aortopulmonary fenestration
- Coronary artery fistula

LABORATORY Arterial blood gas
Drugs that may alter lab results: None
Disorders that may alter lab results: None

PATHOLOGICAL FINDINGS
- Left ventricular and atrial enlargement
- Patent ductus may have abnormal intima (maternal rubella)

SPECIAL TESTS
- ECG in children and adults may show left ventricle and left atrial hypertrophy
- ECG in infants usually normal

IMAGING
- Echocardiography/Doppler
- Contrast echocardiography
- Radionuclide angiography
- Magnetic resonance imaging (MRI)
- Chest x-ray usually normal in infants
- Chest x-ray in children and adults (shunt vascularity, calcifications, left ventricle and left atrial enlargement, dilated ascending aorta, dilated pulmonary arteries)

DIAGNOSTIC PROCEDURES
- Cardiac catheterization and angiography - will demonstrate the shunt and determine the amount of shunt, pulmonary pressures, and other coexisting cardiac abnormalities
- Echocardiography - left atrial enlargement
- Doppler - displays direction of shunt and size of the patent ductus

TREATMENT

APPROPRIATE HEALTH CARE
Inpatient surgery

GENERAL MEASURES
- Small, asymptomatic shunts may not need closure
- Pulmonary support
- Oxygen to correct hypoxia
- Sodium and fluid restriction
- Correction of anemia (hematocrit > 45)

SURGICAL MEASURES
- Surgical transection and ligation for moderate/large shunts
- Transfemoral catheter technique to occlude PDA with foam plastic plug or double umbrella

ACTIVITY As tolerated

DIET No special diet

PATIENT EDUCATION Discuss prematurity and explain different treatments of premature infants and full-term infants

MEDICATIONS

DRUG(S) OF CHOICE
• Indomethacin 0.2-0.25 mg/kg/dose IV preferred. Repeat every 12-24 hours x 3 doses. (Decreased efficacy in term infants; not effective in children or adults.)
• Oxygen
• Diuretics
• Antibiotic prophylaxis if not surgically repaired

Contraindications:
• To treatment with indomethacin
  ◊ Renal dysfunction
  ◊ Overt bleeding
  ◊ Shock
  ◊ Necrotizing enterocolitis
  ◊ Myocardial ischemia

Precautions: With indomethacin treatment - oliguria, hyponatremia

Significant possible interactions: Refer to manufacturer's profile of each drug

ALTERNATIVE DRUGS   Alprostadil

FOLLOWUP

PATIENT MONITORING
• Annual, routine followup after closure
• Shunts that have not been closed should be followed more closely

PREVENTION/AVOIDANCE   N/A

POSSIBLE COMPLICATIONS
• Left heart failure
• Pulmonary hypertension
• Right heart hypertrophy and failure
• Eisenmenger's physiology
• Bacterial endocarditis
• Myocardial ischemia
• Necrotizing enterocolitis

EXPECTED COURSE/PROGNOSIS
• Spontaneous closure after 3 months is rare
• Before 3 months, closure in premature infants is 75%
• Before 3 months, closure in term infants is 40%
• Best postoperative results if closed before age 3 years
• Increased pulmonary vascular resistance and pulmonary hypertension more common if closed after age 3 years
• No firm statistics but decreased survival for large shunts

MISCELLANEOUS

ASSOCIATED CONDITIONS
• Coarctation of the aorta
• Pulmonary valve stenosis or atresia
• Peripheral pulmonary stenosis (maternal rubella)
• Aortic stenosis
• Ventricular septal defect
• Necrotizing enterocolitis
• Club feet, cataracts, blindness, systemic arterial stenosis (associated with maternal rubella)

AGE-RELATED FACTORS   Moderate to large shunts usually diagnosed in infancy or childhood. Small shunts occasionally diagnosed in adults.
Pediatric:
• Symptoms and signs depend largely on size of shunt
• Some infants with coexisting cardiac anomalies benefit temporarily from a patent ductus to provide shunting to the lungs (right heart obstructions) or periphery (coarctation of the aorta). This benefit is short lived, so definitive treatment should proceed as soon as feasible
Geriatric: Good results expected with repair age 50-70 years
Others: N/A

PREGNANCY
• Women with small to moderate sized ductus and left-to-right shunt can expect an uncomplicated pregnancy
• High risk in those with high pulmonary resistance and right-to-left shunt

SYNONYMS
• Aorticopulmonary shunt
• Aorticopulmonary communication

ICD-9-CM
747.0 Patent ductus arteriosus

SEE ALSO   N/A

OTHER NOTES   No need for antibiotic prophylaxis after surgical repair

ABBREVIATIONS   N/A

REFERENCES
• Adams FH, Emmanouilides GC, Riemenschneider TA: Moss' Heart Disease in Infants, Children and Adolescents. 5th Ed. Baltimore, Williams & Wilkins, 1995
• Braunwald E: Heart Disease. 4th Ed. Philadelphia, W.B. Saunders Co., 1992
• Makowitz JS, et al: Transcatheter versus surgical closure of patent ductus arteriosus. New Engl J Med 1994;330(14);1014
Illustrations: N/A
Internet references: http://www.5mcc.com

Author(s)
Karil Bellah, MD

Pediculosis

BASICS

DESCRIPTION Pediculosis is an infestation by lice
• Characteristics of lice:
  ◊ Lice are ectoparasites that when removed from their human host die of starvation within ten days
  ◊ Lice feed solely on human blood by piercing the skin, injecting saliva, and then sucking blood
  ◊ Lice are mobile and can move quickly
  ◊ A mature adult female lays 3-6 eggs, or nits, a day. Nits are 0.8 mm long, white, and appear cemented to the base of the hair. They hatch in 8-10 days and reach maturity in 8-18 days.
  ◊ Nits may survive three weeks when removed from host
• Two species of lice infest humans:
  ◊ Pediculus humanus has two subspecies, the head louse (Pediculus humanus capitis), and the body louse (Pediculus humanus corporis). The head and body lice are anatomically identical, although the head louse is smaller. Both species are smaller than 2 mm, are flat, wingless, and have three pairs of legs that attach closely behind the head.
  ◊ Phthirus pubis (pubic or crab louse). The pubic louse resembles a sea crab and is shorter than the Pediculosis species with large, widespread claws on the 2nd and 3rd legs.
System(s) affected: Skin/Exocrine
Genetics: No genetic pattern
Incidence/Prevalence in USA: 10-40% in schools where accurate surveys have been conducted
Predominant age:
• Most common in adults - pubic lice
• Most common in children - Pediculosis capitis
Predominant sex: Female > Male

SIGNS AND SYMPTOMS
• Pediculosis capitis (head louse)
  ◊ Found most often on the back of the head and neck and behind the ears (warmer areas of the hair)
  ◊ Nits are white spheres found on the hair shaft. They cannot be moved.
  ◊ Itching common, mostly at night
  ◊ Scratching can cause inflammation and secondary bacterial infection, with pyoderma and posterior cervical lymphadenopathy
  ◊ Eyelashes may be involved
• Pediculosis corporis (body louse)
  ◊ Poor hygiene
  ◊ Adult lice and nits in the seams of clothing
  ◊ Pruritus
  ◊ Secondary infection

  ◊ Uninfected bites present as red papules, 2-4 mm in diameter, with an erythematous base
• Phthirus pubis (pubic louse)
  ◊ Anogenital pruritus
  ◊ May have no symptoms during 30-day incubation period
  ◊ Nits are present at the base of hair shafts
  ◊ Delay in treatment may lead to development of widespread groin inflammation, infection, and regional adenopathy
  ◊ Pubic hair most common site
  ◊ Lice may spread to hair around anus, abdomen, axillae, chest, beard, eyebrows, and eyelashes
  ◊ Infested adult patients may spread lice to eyelashes of children. This may induce blepharitis with localized pruritus and/or infection.

CAUSES
• Lice are transmitted by close personal contact and contact with objects such as combs, hats, clothing, and bed linen
• Infected sexual contacts

RISK FACTORS
• Pediculosis corporis - inability to change and launder clothing, overcrowded sleeping quarters
• Phthirus pubis - sexual contact with an infected person
• Immunosuppression
• Sharing combs, hats, etc.

DIAGNOSIS

DIFFERENTIAL DIAGNOSIS
• Scabies and other mite species that can cause cutaneous reactions in humans
• Dandruff for head lice

LABORATORY N/A
Drugs that may alter lab results: N/A
Disorders that may alter lab results: N/A

PATHOLOGICAL FINDINGS N/A

SPECIAL TESTS
• Scalp and pubic lice are apparent with careful examination of individual hairs
• Lice and nits can easily be seen under a microscope
• On Wood's lamp exam, live nits fluoresce white, empty nits fluoresce gray
• Examination of the seams of clothing reveals body lice and their eggs

IMAGING N/A

DIAGNOSTIC PROCEDURES History and physical exam

TREATMENT

APPROPRIATE HEALTH CARE
Outpatient

GENERAL MEASURES
• Nit removal:
  ◊ After treatment with shampoo or lotion, nits remain in scalp or pubic hair
  ◊ Nits are best removed with a very fine comb (nit comb). Removal may be made easier by soaking the hair in a solution of equal parts water and white vinegar and wrapping wet scalp in a towel for at least 15 minutes.
  ◊ Repeat treatment periodically as needed for stubborn nits
  ◊ All family contacts possibly infested with head lice should be treated concomitantly
  ◊ Discarding the clothes or washing them in hot water
  ◊ Evaluate for other sexually transmitted diseases (for pubic lice)

SURGICAL MEASURES N/A

ACTIVITY No restrictions

DIET No special diet

PATIENT EDUCATION
• Poor hygiene is not a risk factor in acquiring pediculosis capitis
• Printed patient information available from: Mayo Foundation for Medical Education and Research, Section of Patient and Health Education, Sieber Subway, Rochester, MN 55905, (507)284-8140

Pediculosis

MEDICATIONS

DRUG(S) OF CHOICE
• Head lice - many topical preparations are effective. 1% lindane (Kwell) can be used but may have to be repeated in one week. 1% permethrin (Nix, Elimite) or pyrethrin (Rid) are also effective. They should be applied and washed off after 10 minutes.
• Pubic lice - treatments available include lindane, synergized pyrethrins, or permethrin. These can be used either as the shampoo left on for 10 minutes or the lotion which can be left on for several hours for best results.
• Body lice - best treated with lindane or synergized pyrethrins lotion applied once and left on for several hours
• Eyelash infestation - treated by careful manual removal of lice and nits, or by application of petroleum jelly (Vaseline) three or four times a day for 5 days

Contraindications: Avoid lindane in infants and pregnant women

Precautions:
• Pediculicides should never be used to treat eyelash infections
• Accidental ingestion and gross overuse of lindane may be associated with CNS toxicity

Significant possible interactions: N/A

ALTERNATIVE DRUGS
For resistant head lice, shaving the head or oral antibiotics may be indicated

FOLLOWUP

PATIENT MONITORING As needed

PREVENTION/AVOIDANCE
• Ability to change and launder clothing eliminates risk of acquiring Pediculosis corporis
• Careful followup in schools by public health nurses may help prevent recurrence and spread of head lice
• Washing combs, brushes, hats, coats, collars, sheets, pillow cases, etc., will help to prevent reinfestation by head lice
• Safe sex (pubic lice)

POSSIBLE COMPLICATIONS
• Persistent itching may be caused by too-frequent use of the pediculicide
• Secondary bacterial infections

EXPECTED COURSE/PROGNOSIS
• With appropriate treatment over 90% cure rate
• Recurrence common, mainly from reinfection, failure to comply with treatment

MISCELLANEOUS

ASSOCIATED CONDITIONS
• Pubic lice are readily transmitted by sexual contact, with a 90% transmission rate. Up to 1/3 of patients have at least one concomitant sexually transmitted disease.
• Eyelash infestation on a child may be a sign of sexual abuse

AGE-RELATED FACTORS N/A
Pediatric: N/A
Geriatric: N/A
Others: Typhus, relapsing fever, and trench fever are spread by body lice during wartime and in underdeveloped countries

PREGNANCY N/A

SYNONYMS
• Lice
• Crabs

ICD-9-CM
132.9 Pediculosis, unspecified

SEE ALSO
• HIV infection & AIDS
• Typhus fevers

OTHER NOTES N/A

ABBREVIATIONS N/A

REFERENCES
• Rakel RE (ed): Conn's Current Therapy. Philadelphia, WB Saunders Co, 1997
• Habif T: Clinical Dermatology. 3rd Ed. St. Louis, CV Mosby, 1996
Illustrations: N/A
Internet references: http://www.5mcc.com

Author(s)
George E. Kikano, MD

Pelvic inflammatory disease (PID)

BASICS

DESCRIPTION PID is a clinical syndrome caused by the ascent of microorganisms from the vagina and endocervix to the endometrium, fallopian tubes, ovaries, and contiguous structures. PID is a broad term that includes a variety of upper genital tract infections, unrelated to pregnancy or surgical procedures, such as salpingitis, salpingo-oophoritis, endometritis, tubo-ovarian inflammatory masses, and pelvic or diffuse peritonitis.
• Pathogenesis: The precise mechanism by which microorganisms ascend from the lower genital tract is not known. One possibility is that chlamydial or gonococcal endocervicitis alters the defense mechanisms of the cervix allowing ascent of the vaginal flora with or without the original pathogen. Other possibilities suggest that polymicrobial infection can occur without N. gonorrhoeae or C. trachomatis. Factors that predispose to the ascent of bacteria include the use of an intrauterine device (IUD) and the hormonal and physical changes associated with menstruation.
System(s) affected: Reproductive
Genetics: N/A
Incidence/Prevalence in USA: Estimated 1 million women are treated each year; 100-200/100,000
Predominant age: 16-40 years
Predominant sex: Female only

SIGNS AND SYMPTOMS
• May be asymptomatic
• Lower abdominal pain
• Fever and malaise
• Vaginal discharge
• Irregular bleeding
• Urinary discomfort, proctitis
• Nausea and vomiting
• Abdominal tenderness
• Tenderness with cervical motion
• Adnexal tenderness
• Unilateral or bilateral tender adnexal mass

CAUSES
Bacteriology - multiple organisms act as etiologic agents in PID and most cases are polymicrobial. Chlamydia trachomatis, Neisseria gonorrhoeae, and a wide variety of aerobic and anaerobic bacteria are recognized as etiologic agents. Mycoplasmas have also been implicated but their role is less clear. The proportion of cases infected with chlamydia or gonorrhea varies widely depending on the population studied. The most common anaerobes include Bacteroides, Peptostreptococcus, and Peptococcus species. The organisms involved in bacterial vaginosis are similar to the nongonococcal, nonchlamydial bacteria often found in the upper genital tract of women with PID, however, the relationship between these conditions is unclear.

RISK FACTORS
• Sexually active, reproductive age
• Most common in adolescents
• Multiple sexual partners
• Use of an IUD, greatest risk in first few months after insertion
• Previous history of PID; 20-25% will have a recurrence
• Chlamydial or gonococcal cervicitis; 8-10% will develop PID
• Gonococcal salpingitis occurs commonly within 7 days of onset of menses
• Condoms and vaginal spermicides lessen the risks of PID
• Oral contraceptives may reduce the risk of PID

DIAGNOSIS

DIFFERENTIAL DIAGNOSIS
• Appendicitis
• Ectopic pregnancy
• Ovarian torsion
• Hemorrhagic or ruptured ovarian cyst
• Endometriosis
• Irritable bowel syndrome
• Somatization disorder

LABORATORY
• Pregnancy test
• Leukocyte count greater than 10,000 cells per mm3
• Endocervical gram stain for gram-negative intracellular diplococci
• ESR of 15 mm/hour or higher
• Endocervical culture for gonorrhea
• Endocervical culture or antigen test for chlamydia
• Plasma cell endometritis on endometrial biopsy
Drugs that may alter lab results: N/A
Disorders that may alter lab results: N/A

PATHOLOGICAL FINDINGS N/A

SPECIAL TESTS
• Culdocentesis with culture of aspirated material
• Diagnostic laparoscopy with culture of fallopian tubes

IMAGING Pelvic ultrasound

DIAGNOSTIC PROCEDURES
• PID diagnosis is elusive and even asymptomatic patients are at risk for sequelae. Diagnosis incorrect in up to a third of women diagnosed. Laparoscopic diagnosis best but impractical as routine and generally reserved for problem situations. In general, wiser to over-treat lower tract genital infection than to miss an upper tract infection.
• Suggested criteria for diagnosis (sufficient for empiric treatment):
  ◊ Lower abdominal tenderness
  ◊ Cervical motion tenderness
  ◊ Adnexal tenderness

• Additional criteria:
  ◊ Temperature greater than or equal to 38°C
  ◊ WBC greater than or equal to 10,500/mm3
  ◊ Purulent material by culdocentesis
  ◊ Adnexal mass
  ◊ ESR > 15 mm/hour
  ◊ Laboratory evidence of gonorrhea or chlamydia
  ◊ Elevated C-reactive protein
• Definitive criteria:
  ◊ Histopathologic endometritis on biopsy
  ◊ Adnexal abscess on sonography
  ◊ Laparoscopic evidence of PID

TREATMENT

APPROPRIATE HEALTH CARE
• Outpatient, normally
• Hospitalization recommended in the following situations:
  ◊ Uncertain diagnosis
  ◊ Surgical emergencies cannot be excluded, e.g., appendicitis
  ◊ Suspected pelvic abscess
  ◊ Pregnancy
  ◊ Adolescent patient with uncertain compliance with therapy
  ◊ Severe illness
  ◊ Cannot tolerate outpatient regimen
  ◊ Failed to respond to outpatient therapy
  ◊ Clinical follow-up within 72 hours of starting antibiotics cannot be arranged
  ◊ HIV-infected

GENERAL MEASURES
• Avoidance of sex until treatment is completed
• Insure that sex partners are referred for appropriate evaluation and treatment. Partners should be treated, irrespective of evaluation, with regimens effective against chlamydia and gonorrhea.

SURGICAL MEASURES
• Reserved for failures of medical treatment and for suspected ruptured adnexal abscess with resulting acute surgical abdomen
• Conservative surgery preferred. This allows a 10-15% postoperative fertility rate.
• Hysterectomy and adnexectomy for older patients with completed childbirth
• Failure of medical therapy generally associated with adnexal abscess which may be amenable to transabdominal or transvaginal drainage under guidance by ultrasonography, computed tomography, or laparoscopy

ACTIVITY According to severity of illness

DIET According to severity of illness

PATIENT EDUCATION Information on written materials for patient distribution can be obtained from local and state health departments or from Information Services, CDC, E06, Atlanta, GA 30333, (404)639-1819

Pelvic inflammatory disease (PID)

MEDICATIONS

DRUG(S) OF CHOICE
Several antibiotic regimens are highly effective with no single regimen of choice, however, coverage should include chlamydia, gonorrhea, anaerobes, gram-negative rods, and streptococci. The CDC regimens that follow are recommendations and the specific antibiotics named are examples.
• Inpatient treatment; regimen A
◊ Cefoxitin 2 g IV every 6 hours or cefotetan IV 2 g every 12 hours (or other cephalosporins such as ceftizoxime, cefotaxime, and ceftriaxone) plus doxycycline 100 mg orally or IV every 12 hours
◊ Therapy for 24 hours after clinical improvement and doxycycline continued after discharge for a total of 10-14 days
• Inpatient treatment; regimen B
◊ Clindamycin 900 mg IV every 8 hours plus gentamicin loading dose IV or IM (2 mg/kg of body weight) followed by a maintenance dose (1.5 mg/kg) every 8 hours
◊ Therapy for 24 hours after clinical improvement with doxycycline after discharge as above, or clindamycin 450 mg orally qid for a total of 14 days
• Outpatient treatment; regimen A
◊ Cefoxitin 2 g IM plus probenecid, 1 g orally, concurrently or ceftriaxone 250 mg IM or equivalent cephalosporin plus doxycycline 100 mg orally bid for 10-14 days or tetracycline 500 mg orally qid for 10-14 days or erythromycin 500 mg orally qid for 10-14 days in patients who do not tolerate tetracyclines
• Outpatient treatment; regimen B
◊ Ofloxacin 400 mg orally bid for 14 days plus either clindamycin 450 mg orally qid, or metronidazole 500 mg orally bid for 14 days
Contraindications: Refer to manufacturer's profile of each drug
Precautions: Refer to manufacturer's profile of each drug
Significant possible interactions: Refer to manufacturer's profile of each drug

ALTERNATIVE DRUGS
Many other antibiotic regimens have been proposed and used with success. For example, tobramycin in place of gentamicin, tetracycline in place of doxycycline.

FOLLOWUP

PATIENT MONITORING
• Close observation of clinical status, in particular for fever, symptoms, level of peritonism, white cell count
• Follow adnexal abscess size and position with ultrasonography

PREVENTION/AVOIDANCE
• Educational programs about safe sex practices
• Education, particularly for those who have had an episode of PID
• IUD contraindicated in women with history of PID or lifestyle associated with STD
• Oral contraceptive appears to decrease risk of PID in cases with cervicitis and the PID cases which do occur are generally less severe
• Barrier contraceptives, especially condoms, and spermicidal creams or sponges provide protection, the extent of which is not well documented
• Insure evaluation and treatment of sex partners
• Comply with management instructions
• Seek medical care early when genital lesions or discharge appear
• Seek routine check-ups for STD if in non-mutually monogamous relationship(s)

POSSIBLE COMPLICATIONS
• A tubo-ovarian abscess will develop in approximately 7-16% of patients
• Recurrent infection occurs in 20-25% of patients
• Risk of ectopic pregnancy increased by 7-10-fold to about 8% of women who have had PID
• Tubal infertility in 15, 35, and 55% of women after one, two, and three episodes of PID, respectively
• Chronic pelvic pain in 20% related to adhesion formation, chronic salpingitis, or recurrent infections

EXPECTED COURSE/PROGNOSIS
• Wide variation with good prognosis if early, effective therapy instituted and further infection avoided
• Poor prognosis related to late therapy and continued unsafe lifestyle

MISCELLANEOUS

ASSOCIATED CONDITIONS
• In PID patients with an IUD in situ, especially if an adnexal abscess is present, the possibility of actinomyces infection requiring penicillin treatment must be kept in mind
• The IUD is contraindicated in women with a previous episode of PID
• Rupture of an adnexal abscess is rare but life-threatening. Early surgical exploration is mandatory.
• Chlamydia or gonococcal perihepatitis may occur with PID. This combination is termed the Curtis-Fitz-Hugh Syndrome.

AGE-RELATED FACTORS
Pediatric:
• PID is rare before puberty
• Adolescents are highly vulnerable to sexually transmitted diseases (STD) including PID. Early vigorous therapy to prevent infertility is especially important in this age group.
Geriatric: PID is rare after menopause, although postmenopausal adnexal abscess is a well-documented entity
Others: N/A

PREGNANCY PID is rare during pregnancy but occurs occasionally and the possibility must be kept in mind

SYNONYMS
• Salpingitis
• Salpingo-oophoritis
• Adnexitis
• Pyosalpinx
• Tubo-ovarian abscess
• Pelvic peritonitis

ICD-9-CM
614.9 Unspecified inflammatory disease of female pelvic organs and tissue

SEE ALSO
• Chlamydial sexually transmitted diseases
• Gonococcal infections
• Syphilis

OTHER NOTES N/A

ABBREVIATIONS N/A

REFERENCES
• Pelvic inflammatory disease: Guidelines for prevention and management. MMWR. 40:1-25, 1991
• 1998 Guidelines for treatment of sexually transmitted diseases MMWR. 47-RR-1
Illustrations: N/A
Internet references: http://www.5mcc.com

Author(s)
Michel E. Rivlin, MD

Pemphigoid, bullous

BASICS

DESCRIPTION Chronic benign bullous eruption considered to be an autoimmune disease. Most frequently affects people over 60.
System(s) affected: Skin/Exocrine, Hemic/Lymphatic/Immunologic
Genetics: HLA typing does not reveal any typical pattern
Incidence/Prevalence in USA: Uncommon
Predominant age: Greater than 60 years
Predominant sex: Female > Male

SIGNS AND SYMPTOMS
• Large bullae 2 to 5 cm in diameter. Occasional tiny peripheral vesicles.
• Bullae that arise from normal-appearing skin (sometimes) or erythematous skin (usually)
• Bullae stay intact for many days
• Located on extremities at first, trunk later
• Occasionally located on the scalp, palms, and soles; mucous membranes (infrequently)
• Intact blisters outnumber erosions (reverse is true with pemphigus)
• Clear fluid fills bullae (usually)
• Blood tinged fluid in bullae (sometimes)
• Itching (sometimes severe)
• Some patients are asymptomatic
• 10-20% of skin surface is continuously involved
• Pruritus may antedate onset of blisters (weeks to months)

CAUSES Autoimmune disorder

RISK FACTORS
• Female, age over 60
• Drug associated: furosomide, phenacetin, various penicillins

DIAGNOSIS

DIFFERENTIAL DIAGNOSIS
• Pemphigus
• Bullous erythema multiforme
• Dermatitis herpetiformis
• Drug eruptions
• Epidermolysis bullosa acquisita

LABORATORY Circulating autoantibodies in 70% directed at the basement membrane (by immunofluorescence). These can be demonstrated in serum or skin.
Drugs that may alter lab results: N/A
Disorders that may alter lab results: N/A

PATHOLOGICAL FINDINGS
• Bullae located in a subepidermal location
• Light microscopy reveals subepidermal blister with perilesional inflammation containing many eosinophils and mononuclear cells
• Immunofluorescent studies - deposition of C3 (100%) and IgG (65-90%) in lamina lucida

SPECIAL TESTS N/A

IMAGING N/A

DIAGNOSTIC PROCEDURES
• History and physical
• Biopsy and immunofluorescence studies - essential for precise diagnosis

TREATMENT

APPROPRIATE HEALTH CARE
Outpatient, unless significant complications

GENERAL MEASURES
• Soak active lesions to debride and remove crusts
• Analgesic mouth washes (see Medications)

SURGICAL MEASURES N/A

ACTIVITY Depends on severity of disease and/or complications

DIET Liquid. Regular diet when tolerated.

PATIENT EDUCATION
• Use of oral analgesics
• Teach side effects and adverse reactions of steroids

MEDICATIONS

DRUG(S) OF CHOICE
• Prednisone 60 to 80 mg in single morning dose. Gradually taper in several weeks to maintenance level of 20 to 40 mg per day. Attempt switch to alternate day treatment.
• Consider adjunctive drugs:
  ◊ azathioprine 100-150 mg to reduce prednisone maintenance therapy dosage or even as only drug to maintain control of the disease
  ◊ Methotrexate 10-25 mg per week as another adjunctive drug
  ◊ Mycophenolate mofetil (CellCept) 250 mg bid po
  ◊ Cyclosporine for resistant disease.
• Topical intralesional corticosteroids may be sufficient for patients with localized disease
• Oral analgesics prn:
  ◊ Elixir of diphenhydramine (Benadryl) for oral ulcers
  ◊ lidocaine (Xylocaine) viscous
  ◊ Dyclonine solution
Contraindications: Refer to manufacturer's literature
Precautions: Some patients (who have only occasional lesions) can be managed without the need for internal medication
Significant possible interactions: Refer to manufacturer's literature

ALTERNATIVE DRUGS Dapsone

FOLLOWUP

PATIENT MONITORING Blood levels mandatory if prescribing cyclosporine

PREVENTION/AVOIDANCE N/A

POSSIBLE COMPLICATIONS
• Superimposed infection (may result in death in elderly debilitated patient)
• Complications of steroid therapy
• Associated malignancy
• Untreated severe disease can be fatal

EXPECTED COURSE/PROGNOSIS
• A chronic disease that lasts indefinitely
• Old lesions heal rapidly as new lesions appear
• Accompanying debilitation not as great as with pemphigus

MISCELLANEOUS

ASSOCIATED CONDITIONS May have an associated malignancy

AGE-RELATED FACTORS
Pediatric: Not a problem in pediatric age group
Geriatric: Older people with pemphigoid may have higher than expected rate of malignancy
Others: N/A

PREGNANCY N/A

SYNONYMS Pemphigoid

ICD-9-CM 694.5 pemphigoid

SEE ALSO N/A

OTHER NOTES N/A

ABBREVIATIONS N/A

REFERENCES
• Fitzpatrick TB, et al, eds: Dermatology in General Medicine. 3rd Ed. New York, McGraw-Hill, 1987
• Habif T: Clinical Dermatology. 3rd Ed. St. Louis, CV Mosby, 1996
Illustrations: 6 available on CD-ROM
Internet references: http://www.5mcc.com

Author(s)
Samuel L. Moschella, MD, FACP

Pemphigus vulgaris

BASICS

DESCRIPTION Uncommon, debilitating, potentially fatal skin disorder characterized by painful intraepidermal bullae that appear on normal appearing skin without surrounding inflammation, often starting in the mouth
System(s) affected: Skin/Exocrine, Gastrointestinal
Genetics: HLA-A10 and HLA-DR4 and HLA-DRW6 antigens; higher incidence among persons of Jewish or Mediterranean descent
Incidence/Prevalence in USA: Rare
Predominant age: 30-60 years of age
Predominant sex: Male = Female

SIGNS AND SYMPTOMS
• Oral mucous membrane lesions (particularly in the posterior mouth) often precede the cutaneous lesions (sometimes by several weeks or months)
• Lesion distribution - upper trunk or back initially. Gradual extension to face, groin, and axillae.
• Bullae arise from normal appearing skin
• Multiple shallow erosions which heal slowly
• Blisters are fragile
• Intact bullae are found only on the first day or two of their existence
• After blister roof breaks, a bright red or crusted shallow erosion follows which requires weeks or months to heal
• Outer layer of skin can easily be rubbed off (Nikolsky's sign)

CAUSES An autoimmune disorder with specific IgG antibodies and sometimes complement arising from bone marrow plasma cells which are deposited at sites of epidermal cell damage; a few cases from captopril, penicillamine, piroxicam, penicillin, phenobarbital, pyritimol, heroin

RISK FACTORS
• Genetic factors (more common in persons of Jewish or Mediterranean descent)
• Medications (particularly penicillamine)

DIAGNOSIS

DIFFERENTIAL DIAGNOSIS
• Eczematous disorders
• Herpes
• Tinea
• Varicella-zoster
• Erythema multiforme
• Bullous impetigo
• Pemphigoid
• Dermatitis herpetiformis
• Drug eruptions
• Transient acantholytic dermatosis

LABORATORY
• Autoantibody titers (by immunofluorescent studies) 80-90%
• Titer corresponds to severity of the disease. Increasing titer found prior to relapse.
Drugs that may alter lab results: N/A
Disorders that may alter lab results: N/A

PATHOLOGICAL FINDINGS
• Causative antigens are located on the exterior surface of the cytoplasmic membrane of epithelial cells
• Biopsy shows acantholytic intraepidermal bullae
• IgG deposition in the epidermal intercellular space is found 100% of time in perilesional skin

SPECIAL TESTS N/A

IMAGING N/A

DIAGNOSTIC PROCEDURES
• Biopsy of lesions
• Light microscopy - suprabasal cleft formation and acantholysis

TREATMENT

APPROPRIATE HEALTH CARE
Depends on severity of the disease and medical status of patient

GENERAL MEASURES
• May require reverse isolation procedures
• Topical treatment to prevent oozing skin from adhering to bed sheets
• Soak active lesions to debride and remove crusts
• Analgesic mouth washes (see Medications)
• Plasmapheresis, or cyclosporine, if patient fails to respond to an adequate trial of recommended regimens

SURGICAL MEASURES N/A

ACTIVITY As severity of disease and medical status of patient dictates

DIET Liquid or soft for patient with mouth lesions. Regular diet when tolerated.

PATIENT EDUCATION
• Use of oral analgesics
• Teach side effects and adverse reactions of steroids

MEDICATIONS

DRUG(S) OF CHOICE
• Prednisone: high doses 60-100 mg, higher if necessary. Start at 80 mg, increase by 50% every 7 days until no new blisters. Reduce to every other day dosage when possible. Taper over 6-8 months to every other day maintenance therapy, continued for life.
• Consider concomitant immunosuppressants, such as azathioprine 2-3 mg/kg/day, less effective than cyclophosphamide, but less toxic. Use with steroid, or cyclophosphamide 1-3 mg/kg/day - second best therapy, more toxic
• Severe cases require combination plasmapheresis, cyclophosphamide and prednisone
• Oral analgesics prn, choose one:
  ◊ Diphenhydramine (Benadryl) elixir
  ◊ Lidocaine (Xylocaine) viscous
  ◊ Dyclonine solution or lozenges
Contraindications: Refer to manufacturer's literature
Precautions: Refer to manufacturer's literature
Significant possible interactions: Refer to manufacturer's literature

ALTERNATIVE DRUGS
• Gold therapy (with or without concomitant corticosteroids)
• Dapsone controls some cases
• Methotrexate often helpful, but too toxic due to need for high doses
• Chlorambucil
• Cyclosporine
• Gold

FOLLOWUP

PATIENT MONITORING
• Frequent visits during acute phases
• If immunosuppressants prescribed, monitor blood levels frequently
• In elderly patients, chest x-ray to rule out reactivation of old tuberculosis, test urine daily for glycosuria

PREVENTION/AVOIDANCE   N/A

POSSIBLE COMPLICATIONS
• Steroid complications that can lead to morbidity and mortality
• Inadequate nutrition and debilitation due to pain of oral lesions
• Sepsis/death for untreated or poorly controlled cases

EXPECTED COURSE/PROGNOSIS
• Chronic. Inevitably fatal if not treated.
• 10% fatality with vigorous treatment
• Ruptured bullae require weeks to heal

MISCELLANEOUS

ASSOCIATED CONDITIONS
• Thymomas
• Other internal malignancies
• Other autoimmune diseases

AGE-RELATED FACTORS
Pediatric: Unusual in this age group
Geriatric:
• This is the age group in which pemphigus is most likely to occur
• Close followup is needed for elderly patients on high doses of steroids
Others: N/A

PREGNANCY   N/A

SYNONYMS   Pemphigus

ICD-9-CM   694.4 Pemphigus

SEE ALSO   N/A

OTHER NOTES
• Atypical presentation - pemphigus foliaceus has infrequent oral lesions and is not as debilitating
• In mild disease, gold salts alone can sometimes produce remission. This has the obvious advantage of avoiding immunosuppression, However, not uniformly beneficial and no controlled trials.

ABBREVIATIONS   N/A

REFERENCES
• Fitzpatrick TB, et al, eds: Dermatology In General Medicine. 3rd Ed. New York, McGraw-Hill, 1987
• Habif T: Clinical Dermatology. 3rd Ed. St. Louis, CV Mosby, 1996
• Olson GL: Blistering disorders: which ones can be deadly? Postgrad Med 1994;46(1):53-64
• Thevolet J: Pemphigus: past, present and future. Dermatology 1994;189(sup2):26-29
• Huilgol SC, Black MM: Management of the immunobullous disorders. II pemphigus. Clinical & Experimental Dermatology 1995;20:283-293
Illustrations: 8 available on CD-ROM
Internet references: http://www.5mcc.com

Author(s)
Douglas M. Hoy, MD

Peptic ulcer disease

BASICS

DESCRIPTION A chronic ulcer in the lining of the gastrointestinal tract.
- Duodenal ulcer (DU): Most located in the duodenal bulb. Multiple ulcers, and if distal to the bulb raise the possibility of Zollinger-Ellison syndrome.
- Gastric ulcer (GU): Much less common than DU (in the absence NSAID's). Most commonly located along the lesser curvature of the antrum near the incisura and in the pre-pyloric area.
- Esophageal ulcers: A peptic ulcer in the distal esophagus may be part of Barrett's epithelial change due to chronic reflux of gastroduodenal contents
- Ectopic gastric mucosal ulceration: May develop in patients with Meckel's diverticula or other sites of ectopic gastric mucosa

System(s) affected: Gastrointestinal

Genetics: Higher incidence with HLA-B12, B5, Bw35 phenotypes, identical twins

Incidence/Prevalence in USA:
- DU: 4 times more common than GU. Lifetime prevalence = 10% for men; 5% for women (gender gap is closing). 200,000-400,000 new DU cases/annually.
- GU: 87,500 new cases annually. Incidence of new GU in adults; 50/100,000

Predominant age:
- DU 25-75 years (rare before age 15)
- GU peak incidence age 55-65; rare < age 40

Predominant sex:
- DU: Male > Female (slightly)
- GU: Male = Female (female predominance among NSAID users)

SIGNS AND SYMPTOMS
- In adults (DU)
  ◊ Gnawing or burning epigastric pain 1-3 hours after meals, relieved by food, antacids, or antisecretory agents
  ◊ Nocturnal pain causing early morning awakening
  ◊ Epigastric pain in 60-90% (often vague discomfort, cramping, hunger pangs). Non-specific dyspeptic complaints (belching, bloating, abdominal distention, food intolerance) in 40-70%.
  ◊ Symptomatic periods occur in clusters lasting a few weeks followed by symptom-free periods for weeks to months. Some seasonal occurrence (spring and fall).
  ◊ Early satiety, anorexia, weight loss, abnormal saline load test, succussion splash, gastric retention of barium, nausea, vomiting suggest pyloric obstruction
  ◊ Heartburn (suggesting reflux disease)
  ◊ Sudden, severe mid-epigastric pain radiating to right shoulder, peritoneal signs and free peritoneal air may indicate perforation
  ◊ Dizziness, syncope, hematemesis or melena suggest hemorrhage
- In adults (GU)
  ◊ Symptom complex similar to DU
  ◊ NSAID-induced ulcers often silent; perforation or bleeding may be initial presentation
  ◊ Epigastric pain following a meal an uncommon finding; early satiety, nausea, vomiting suggest gastric outlet obstruction
  ◊ Weight loss can occur with either benign or malignant gastric ulcers
- in children (DU)
  ◊ Positive family history in 50% of early onset DU patients (under age 20)
  ◊ May account for chronic abdominal pain syndrome in young children
  ◊ Gastric outlet obstruction from ulcer must be distinguished from congenital infantile hypertrophic pyloric stenosis (seen within the first month after birth along with visible peristalses and a palpable pyloric mass)

CAUSES
Etiology of DU and GU is multifactorial. H. pylori gastritis is present in >80% of DU and > 60% of GU.
- Imbalance between aggressive factors (e.g., gastric acid, pepsin, bile salts, pancreatic enzymes) and defensive factors maintaining mucosal integrity (e.g., mucus, bicarbonate, blood flow, prostaglandins, growth factors, cell turnover) which may relate to H. pylori infection
- Ulcerogenic drugs (e.g., NSAID's)
- Zollinger-Ellison syndrome
- Other hypersecretory syndromes

RISK FACTORS
- Strongly associated: Drugs (e.g., NSAID use), family history of ulcer, Zollinger-Ellison syndrome (gastrinoma), cigarettes (>1/2 pack/day)
- Possibly associated: Corticosteroids (high dose and/or prolonged therapy); blood group O; HLA-B12, B5, Bw35 phenotypes; stress; lower socioeconomic status; manual labor
- Poorly or not associated: Dietary spices, alcohol, caffeine, acetaminophen
- Annual risk of DU developing in H. pylori - positive individual ≤1%

DIAGNOSIS

DIFFERENTIAL DIAGNOSIS
- Non-ulcer dyspepsia
- Gastric carcinoma
- H. pylori-associated gastritis (without ulcer)
- Gastroesophageal reflux (with or without esophagitis)
- Crohn's disease (gastroduodenal)
- Pancreatitis
- Variant angina pectoris
- Cholelithiasis syndrome
- Atrophic gastritis

LABORATORY
- Anemia uncommon in absence of hemorrhage. Fecal occult blood requires colonic evaluation before attributing positive test to ulcer alone (esp. in patients > 40 years).
- Elevated serum gastrin (to rule out Zollinger-Ellison syndrome)
- Gastric analysis (to rule out achlorhydria, acid hypersecretion)
- Secretin stimulation test (paradoxical rise seen in ZE)
- Serum pepsinogen

Drugs that may alter lab results:
Antisecretory medications may give falsely low gastric analysis or elevated gastrin

Disorders that may alter lab results: N/A

PATHOLOGICAL FINDINGS
- Helicobacter pylori gastritis
- Ulcer crater usually > 5 mm diameter; extends through the mucosa (in contrast to stress-related ulceration)

SPECIAL TESTS Serology or urea breath test for H. pylori

IMAGING
- Endoscopy more accurate than radiography
- Radiographic features of benign GU include ulcer projecting beyond the lumen, radiolucent band (Hampton line) paralleling ulcer base, radiating folds

DIAGNOSTIC PROCEDURES
- Endoscopy (accuracy > 95%)
- Barium meal (accuracy 70-90%)
- Mucosal biopsy, cytology (excludes malignancy in > 99%)
- Exploratory laparotomy
- Histology or urea breath test for H. pylori

TREATMENT

APPROPRIATE HEALTH CARE
- Empiric treatment for young healthy patients with dyspepsia, otherwise endoscopy or barium meal for suspected complications, weight loss, persistent vomiting, etc., or symptom onset after age 50 years
- Emergency endoscopy and hospitalization for suspected ulcer bleeding
- ICU care for severe hemorrhage
- Surgical consult: suspected perforation/obstruction, uncontrolled bleeding

GENERAL MEASURES
- Reduce use of NSAID's and psychic stress
- Avoid or eliminate cigarette smoking

SURGICAL MEASURES For bleeding complication, obstruction or perforation

ACTIVITY Fully active for uncomplicated disease

DIET 3 regular meals daily with avoidance of dietary irritants

PATIENT EDUCATION National Digestive Diseases Information, Box NDDIC, Bethesda, MD 20892, (301)468-6344

MEDICATIONS

DRUG(S) OF CHOICE
Acute healing of DU and GU
• Acid suppression
  ◊ H2 blocker: ranitidine or nizatidine 150 bid or 300 mg hs; cimetidine 400 mg bid or 800 mg hs; famotidine 150 mg bid or 300 mg hs for 8-12 weeks
  ◊ Proton pump inhibitor, e.g., omeprazole 20 mg or lansoprazole 15 mg qd for 4 weeks
• Eradication of Helicobacter pylori (HP), single antibiotic regimens discouraged
  ◊ Classic "triple therapy": bismuth subsalicylate (Pepto-Bismol) 600 mg qid plus tetracycline 500 mg qid plus metronidazole 250 mg qid for 2 weeks; (amoxicillin 500 mg qid has been used in place of tetracycline)
• Currently optimal HP eradication regimens
  ◊ Omeprazole 20 mg or lansoprazole 30 mg bid plus 2 antibiotics (e.g., clarithromycin 500 mg bid and amoxicillin 1 gm bid for 2 weeks)
  ◊ Ranitidine-bismuth-citrate 400 mg bid plus clarithromycin 500 mg bid and amoxicillin 1 gm bid for 2 weeks
  ◊ Alternative antibiotics: Tetracycline and metronidazole
• Other:
  ◊ Treatment of H. pylori-negative ulcers: Most are due to NSAID's; treat acutely with H2-receptor antagonists or proton pump inhibitor for 4-12 weeks. Optimally, the NSAID should be discontinued.
  ◊ Unhealed refractory ulcers: higher doses of H2 blockers or proton pump inhibitors or surgery

Contraindications: Known hypersensitivity to the drug or another member of the class

Precautions:
• Renal insufficiency (GFR < 30 mL/min): reduce H2 blocker dose by 50%. Avoid magnesium-containing antacids
• Give sucralfate distant from meals to avoid binding with food proteins
• Bacterial resistance to metronidazole (50-60%) and clarithromycin (5-10%)
• Antibiotic-related side effects:
  ◊ Diarrhea (10%): change amoxicillin to tetracycline
  ◊ Nausea/vomiting (20%): avoid alcohol with metronidazole
  ◊ Unpleasant taste with metronidazole and clarithromycin
  ◊ Rash (5%): stop antimicrobial
  ◊ Pseudomembranous colitis (< 1%): treat with vancomycin
  ◊ Anaphylaxis, Stevens-Johnson syndrome (rare)

Significant possible interactions:
• Cimetidine interacts with many drugs (e.g., theophylline, warfarin, phenytoin, lidocaine) via inhibition of cytochrome P-450 isozymes, leading to reduced drug clearance; avoid cimetidine with interacting drugs.
• Ranitidine and famotidine have rarely been associated with increased theophylline levels
• Nizatidine has not been associated with drug interactions
• Omeprazole may prolong the elimination of diazepam, warfarin and phenytoin

• Sucralfate reduces absorption of tetracycline, norfloxacin, ciprofloxacin, and theophylline leading to subtherapeutic levels

ALTERNATIVE DRUGS
• Alternative ulcer healing drugs
  ◊ Sucralfate 1 gm qid or 2 gm bid for 4-8 wks
  ◊ Antacids, e.g., magnesium hydroxide, aluminum hydroxide 1 and 3 hours after meals (4-7 doses daily)

FOLLOWUP

PATIENT MONITORING
• Eradication of H. pylori: Expected in >90% (with 2 antibiotic regimen)
  ◊ Confirm eradication by CLOtest biopsy, urea breath test or serology in patients who remain symptomatic or relapse
  ◊ Treatment failure: use different antimicrobial regimen or test for sensitivity
• Acute DU: monitor clinical response. No need to repeat endoscopy or x-ray exam to document healing unless recurrence or complication suspected.
• Acute GU: confirm healing (endoscopy after 6-12 weeks for cytology and biopsy of poorly or unhealed ulcer to rule out malignancy)
• Symptomatic response to therapy does not preclude malignancy

PREVENTION/AVOIDANCE
• Eradication of HP: recurrence < 10% in the first year, off of all therapies
• Maintenance therapy (e.g., H2 blocker in 1/2 the acute healing dose at bedtime) suppresses ulcer relapse indefinitely while treatment is continued - however, relapses occur in most patients who remain HP positive
• Bleeding ulcers require continued maintenance therapy (e.g., H2 blocker or PPI if H. pylori not eradicated
• NSAID-related ulcers are best managed by avoiding salicylates and NSAID's. If NSAID's needed, add misoprostol (Cytotec), an H2 blocker or proton pump inhibitor.
• Selective COX-2 NSAID's (eg celecoxib, rofecoxib) produce significantly fewer GI ulcers; consider for use in patients at risk for ulceration

POSSIBLE COMPLICATIONS
• Hemorrhage in up to 25% of cases (initial presentation in 10%)
• Perforation occurs in < 5%, usually related to NSAID use
• Gastric outlet obstruction occurs in up to 5% of patients with duodenal or pyloric channel ulcers. Men predominate.

EXPECTED COURSE/PROGNOSIS
• Ulcer relapse rates after H. pylori eradication low; suspect surreptitious NSAID use
• Reinfection rates < 1% per year
• The risk of rebleeding after H. pylori therapy alone remains less well defined
• NSAID-related ulcers may occur independently of H. pylori status
• Intractability now rare; cost effectiveness proven for H. pylori eradication

MISCELLANEOUS

ASSOCIATED CONDITIONS
• Zollinger-Ellison syndrome (gastrinoma)
• Systemic mastocytosis
• MEN Type 1
• COPD, chronic renal failure, cirrhosis, hyperparathyroidism, carcinoid syndrome, polycythemia rubra vera, basophilic leukemia, porphyria cutanea tarda

AGE-RELATED FACTORS
Pediatric: Uncommon before puberty; hemorrhage and perforation more common
Geriatric: N/A
Others: N/A

PREGNANCY Unusual in gestation; safety of H2 blockers not established in first 16 wks, but considered reasonably safe later; sucralfate and antacids preferred as initial therapy

SYNONYMS
• Duodenal ulcer
• Gastric ulcer
• Helicobacter ulcer

ICD-9-CM DU 532.9, GU 531.9

SEE ALSO
• Zollinger-Ellison syndrome
• Pyloric stenosis

OTHER NOTES N/A

ABBREVIATIONS HP = Helicobacter pylori

REFERENCES
• Soll AH: Medical treatment of ulcer disease: Practice guidelines. JAMA 1996;275:622-629
• Peura DA: Proceedings of the ADHF International Update Conference on Helicobacter Pylori, Gastroenterol 1997;113(6):s1-169
• Silverstein MD, Petterson T, Talley NJ: Initial endoscopy or empirical therapy with or without testing for Helicobacter pylori for dyspepsia: A decision analysis. Gastroen 1996;110:72-83
• Ofman JJ, Etchason J, Fullerton s, et al: Management strategies for Helicobacter pylori-seropositive patients with dyspepsia: Clinical and economic consequences. Ann Int Med 1997;126:280-291
• Vakil N, Fennerty MB: Cost-effectiveness of treatment regimens for the eradication of Helicobacter pylori in duodenal ulcer. Am J Gastroenterology 1996;91:239-246
• Hawkey CJ: COX-2 inhibitors. Lancet 1999:353:307-314
5 additional references available at web site
Internet references: http://www.5mcc.com
Illustrations: N/A

Author(s)
James H. Lewis, MD, FACP, FACG

Pericarditis

BASICS

DESCRIPTION The clinical manifestations of disease processes involving the pericardial sac surrounding the heart
• Acute pericarditis: an inflammatory process from a wide spectrum of etiologies of the pericardium with or without associated effusion. The most common etiology is idiopathic or nonspecific pericarditis.
• Pericardial tamponade: cardiac compression from pericardial effusion causing hemodynamic compromise and disruption of compensatory mechanisms
• Constrictive pericarditis: thickening and adherence of the pericardium to the heart after chronic inflammation
System(s) affected: Cardiovascular
Genetics: Unknown
Incidence/Prevalence in USA: 2% penetration trauma develop tamponade
Predominant age: Adolescents and young adults
Predominant sex: Male > Female

SIGNS AND SYMPTOMS
• Acute pericarditis
◊ Chest pain, typically sharp, retrosternal with radiation to the trapezial ridge
◊ Pain frequently sudden in onset, with inspiration or movement
◊ Pain reduced by leaning forward and sitting up
◊ Splinted breathing
◊ Odynophagia
◊ Fever
◊ Myalgia
◊ Anorexia
◊ Anxiety
◊ Pericardial friction rub
◊ Cardiac arrhythmias often intermittent, supraventricular tachycardia (SVT)
◊ Tachypnea
◊ Localized rales
• Pericardial tamponade
◊ Dyspnea
◊ Tachycardia
◊ Distended jugular neck veins
◊ Cyanosis
◊ Relative or absolute hypotension
◊ Quiet precordium with little palpable cardiac activity
◊ Pericardial friction rub
◊ Lungs clear
◊ Ewart's sign - dullness and bronchial breathing between the tip of the left scapula and vertebral column
◊ Rapid thready pulse
◊ Varying degrees of consciousness
◊ Pulsus paradoxus: > 10 mm Hg (1.33 kPa) decrease in systolic pressure with inspiration
◊ Beck's triad - distended neck veins, hypotension and muffled heart sounds

• Constrictive pericarditis
◊ Asymptomatic, early
◊ Dyspnea, pulmonary congestion
◊ Fatigue very common
◊ Peripheral edema
◊ Hepatomegaly
◊ Ascites
◊ Jugular venous distention - elevated, deep Y trough (not seen in tamponade)
◊ Kussmaul's sign - inspiratory increase in jugular venous pressure
◊ Pericardial "knock" - follows S2 by 0.06-0.12 sec, increases with squatting
◊ Hypovolemia may mask the signs of constriction

CAUSES
• Idiopathic
• Viral: Coxsackie, echo, adenovirus, Epstein-Barr, mumps
• Bacterial: Haemophilus (especially children), Staphylococcus, Pneumococcus, Salmonella, Meningococcus, Lyme disease, Legionella, Mycoplasma
• Fungal: Candida, Histoplasmosis, Aspergillus, Nocardia
• Mycobacterial: Mycobacterium tuberculosis
• Parasites, protozoa
• Neoplastic: Breast, lung, lymphoma, mesothelioma
• Drug-induced: Procainamide, hydralazine, bleomycin, phenytoin, minoxidil, mesalamine, azathioprine and perhaps others
• Connective tissue disease: Systemic lupus erythematosis, rheumatoid arthritis, scleroderma, acute rheumatic fever
• Radiation
• Myocardial infarction, Dressler's
• Postpericardiotomy
• Uremia
• Myxedema
• Cholesterol pericarditis
• Aortic dissection
• Sarcoidosis
• Pancreatitis
• Inflammatory bowel disease
• AIDS
• Chylopericardium
• Familial - autosomal recessive (Mulibrey nanism)

RISK FACTORS
• Chest trauma

DIAGNOSIS

DIFFERENTIAL DIAGNOSIS
• Acute myocardial infarction
• Pneumonia with pleurisy
• Pulmonary emboli
• Aortic dissection
• Pneumothorax
• Mediastinal emphysema
• Cholecystitis
• Pancreatitis
• Esophageal perforation, rupture, inflammation or tear

LABORATORY
• Leukocytosis and increased ESR
• May see elevated creatine kinase (CK), lactate dehydrogenase (LDH), serum glutamic-oxaloacetic (SGOT)
Drugs that may alter lab results: N/A
Disorders that may alter lab results: N/A

PATHOLOGICAL FINDINGS
Micro: acute inflammation

SPECIAL TESTS
4 stages in pericarditis
• Electrocardiogram - electrical alternans in tamponade
• Echocardiogram - determines fluid, RA or RV collapse
• Right heart catheterization - eaualization of mean and diastolic pressure in all wave forms

IMAGING
• Chest x-ray - small pleural effusion, transient infiltrates; "water bottle" silhouette in large associated pericardial effusion
• Chest CT or MRI in suspected constrictive pericarditis may reveal calcified or thickened pericardium; delineate effusions

DIAGNOSTIC PROCEDURES
• Pericardiocentesis
• Pericardial biopsy

TREATMENT

APPROPRIATE HEALTH CARE
• Outpatient unless signs of complications
• Inpatient with complications (hemodynamic compromise or effusion present)

GENERAL MEASURES N/A

SURGICAL MEASURES Pericardiectomy may be required if drugs are not effective

ACTIVITY No restrictions; limited by patients symptoms only

DIET No restriction. If patient overweight, suggest a weight loss program.

PATIENT EDUCATION Since 15% of patients have a recurrence, must educate for return of symptoms and followup

MEDICATIONS

DRUG(S) OF CHOICE
Uncomplicated: aspirin 650 mg q4h. If effective, continue for 2 weeks.
Contraindications: Hypersensitivity to aspirin, known coagulopathy
Precautions: Use with caution in patients with asthma, nasal polyps, severe carditis, pregnancy in the third trimester, history of GI disturbances or bleeding, bleeding disorders or diathesis, telangiectasis, anticoagulation, renal or hepatic dysfunction
Significant possible interactions:
Acetaminophen, acetazolamide, ammonium chloride, antacids, aurothioglucose, chlorpropamide, cimetidine, corticosteroids, diclofenac, dicumarol, diltiazem, dipyridamole, etodolac, flurbiprofen, ibuprofen, indomethacin, insulin, ketorolac, meclofenamate, mefenamic acid, methotrexate, metoclopramide, naproxen, nitroglycerin, nizatidine, penicillin G, phenprocoumon, phenylbutazone, phenytoin, piroxicam, probenicid, protirelin, quinidine, spironolactone, sulfinpyrazone, sulfonylureas, sulindac, suprofen, tolmetin, valproic acid, warfarin

ALTERNATIVE DRUGS
• Ibuprofen 400-600 mg q6h for 2 weeks
• Indomethacin 25-75 mg q6-8h for 2 weeks
• Colchicine 1 mg q day
• Azathioprine, phenylbutazone, prednisone 60 mg q day x 2-3 days and quickly taper (last resort) over 2-4 weeks. Risk of recurrence with withdrawal.

FOLLOWUP

PATIENT MONITORING
• Followup patients in office in 2 weeks and re-evaluate cardiac status and symptomatology
• Repeat chest x-ray and electrocardiogram should be considered at 4 weeks

PREVENTION/AVOIDANCE N/A

POSSIBLE COMPLICATIONS
• Pericardial tamponade
• Recurrence of pericarditis
• Non-compressive effusion
• Chronic, constrictive pericarditis

EXPECTED COURSE/PROGNOSIS
• The majority of patients have complete resolution of pain and symptoms during the 2 weeks of therapy
• Fifteen per cent will have at least one recurrence in the first few months
• A rare patient may become refractory and require corticosteroids or pericardiectomy
• The hemodynamic effects of effusions depends on the volume and rapidity of development
• A very small percentage of patients can develop signs of right sided heart failure secondary to constriction. These patients are best treated with pericardiectomy.

MISCELLANEOUS

ASSOCIATED CONDITIONS Dependent on etiology

AGE-RELATED FACTORS
Pediatric: N/A
Geriatric: N/A
Others: N/A

PREGNANCY N/A

SYNONYMS Acute nonsuppurative pericarditis

ICD-9-CM
420.91 Acute idiopathic pericarditis
420.99 Other acute pericarditis

SEE ALSO N/A

OTHER NOTES N/A

ABBREVIATIONS N/A

REFERENCES
• Bennett JC, Plum F, eds: Cecil Textbook of Medicine. 20th Ed. Philadelphia, W.B. Saunders Co., 1996
• Shabetai R: Diseases of the Pericardium. Cardio Clinics Nov;1990
• Estok DE, et al: Cardiac tamponade in patients with AIDS: a review of pericardial disease in patients with HIV infection. Mt Sinai J Med 1998;65:33-39
• Pawsat DE, et al: Inflammatory disorders of the heart. pericarditis, myocarditis, and endocarditis. Emerg Med Clin of NA 1998;16:665-681
Illustrations: N/A
Internet references: http://www.5mcc.com

Author(s)
Darell E. Heiselman, DO, FCCM, FACP, FACC, FCCP

Peritonitis, acute

BASICS

DESCRIPTION Acute inflammation of the visceral and parietal peritoneum
System(s) affected: Gastrointestinal, Endocrine/Metabolic, Cardiovascular
Genetics: No known genetic pattern
Incidence/Prevalence in USA: Common
Predominant age: None
Predominant sex: Male > Female

SIGNS AND SYMPTOMS
- Acute abdominal pain
- Fever
- Nausea
- Vomiting
- Constipation
- Abdominal pain exacerbated by motion
- Abdominal distention
- Dyspnea
- Diffuse abdominal rebound
- Generalized abdominal rigidity
- Decreased bowel sounds
- Abdominal hyper-resonance to percussion
- Hypotension
- Tachycardia
- Hippocratic facies
- Tachypnea
- Dehydration
- Ascites

CAUSES
- Primary - spontaneous bacterial peritonitis
  ◊ Ascites associated with cirrhosis, nephrotic syndrome
- Secondary
  ◊ Following abdominal trauma
  ◊ Penetrating wounds
  ◊ Continuous ambulatory peritoneal dialysis
  ◊ Perforation
  ◊ Appendicitis
  ◊ Colitis - infectious, inflammatory
  ◊ Peptic ulcer perforation
  ◊ Gangrene of the bowel
  ◊ Diverticulitis
  ◊ Pancreatitis
  ◊ Postoperative
  ◊ Acute cholecystitis

RISK FACTORS
- Recent surgery
- Advanced liver disease
- Corticosteroid medication
- Nephrotic syndrome
- Continuous ambulatory peritoneal dialysis

DIAGNOSIS

DIFFERENTIAL DIAGNOSIS
- Abscess formation (subdiaphragmatic, subhepatic, peritoneal, pelvic)
- Other causes of ileus (volvulus, intussusception)
- Mesenteric adenitis
- Appendicitis
- Pancreatitis

LABORATORY
- Positive culture of peritoneal aspirate
- Leukocytosis
- Increased BUN
- Hemoconcentration
- Positive blood culture
- Metabolic acidosis
- Respiratory acidosis
- elevated amylase
- Ascitic fluid analysis

Drugs that may alter lab results:
Antibiotics prior to blood studies
Disorders that may alter lab results: N/A

PATHOLOGICAL FINDINGS
- Peritoneum - generalized fibrinopurulent exudate
- Peritoneum - polymorphonuclear infiltration

SPECIAL TESTS   N/A

IMAGING
- Abdominal film: free air in peritoneal cavity, large bowel dilatation, small bowel dilatation, intestinal wall edema
- Chest x-ray: elevated diaphragm
- CT: intra-abdominal mass, ascites
- Sonograph: intra-abdominal mass, ascites

DIAGNOSTIC PROCEDURES   N/A

TREATMENT

APPROPRIATE HEALTH CARE
Inpatient with intensive care as indicated

GENERAL MEASURES
- Treat paralytic ileus (nasogastric decompression)
- Treat dehydration
- Antibiotics are started empirically to cover a broad spectrum of organisms. The choice of antibiotic may be altered after culture results are obtained.
- Respiratory support if needed
- IV fluids
- Blood transfusions (sometimes)

SURGICAL MEASURES   Treat underlying condition(s) and infection (by surgery if necessary)

ACTIVITY   Bedrest until infection is under control

DIET
- IV fluids and electrolytes
- Oral feedings only after return of bowel sounds, and passage of flatus and/or feces
- Total parenteral nutrition may be necessary

PATIENT EDUCATION   N/A

Peritonitis, acute

 MEDICATIONS

DRUG(S) OF CHOICE
• Monotherapy:
◊ Cefotaxime 2 g IV q8h
or
◊ Ceftriaxone 2 g IV q24h
• Combination therapies:
◊ Ampicillin 1-2 g q6h plus gentamicin 1.5 mg/kg/dose plus clindamycin 600-900 mg q8h
or
◊ Ampicillin plus gentamicin plus metronidazole 500 mg q6-8h
or
◊ Gentamicin plus clindamycin
or
◊ Imipenem 0.5-1.0 g q6-8h
• Continuous abdominal peritoneal dialysis:
◊ Intraperitoneal vancomycin 20 mg/L dialysate + 1 gm IV "load" plus gentamicin (6-8 mg/L dialysate)
or
◊ Intraperitoneal ceftazidime
• Other:
◊ Morphine 2-10 mg IV q3-4h, as needed, for pain
Contraindications: Refer to manufacturer's literature
Precautions: Refer to manufacturer's literature
Significant possible interactions: Refer to manufacturer's literature

ALTERNATIVE DRUGS
• Initial therapy with a third-generation cephalosporin (e.g., cefotaxime or ceftriaxone)
• Antibiotics, other than those mentioned, if indicated by culture of blood or peritoneal fluid
• Meperidine 50-100 mg IM

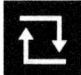 **FOLLOWUP**

PATIENT MONITORING
Frequent monitoring acutely

PREVENTION/AVOIDANCE
Prophylactic antibiotics during abdominal surgery

POSSIBLE COMPLICATIONS
• Hypovolemic consequences
• Septicemia
• Septic shock
• Acute renal failure
• Acute respiratory insufficiency
• Liver failure
• Abscess formation

EXPECTED COURSE/PROGNOSIS
• Fully developed paralytic ileus requires 48 hours for recovery
• Mortality dependent on - age, duration, cause, and on pre-existing conditions

 MISCELLANEOUS

ASSOCIATED CONDITIONS
• Abscesses: Subdiaphragmatic, subhepatic, peritoneal, pelvic
• Ileus

AGE-RELATED FACTORS
Pediatric: Get pediatric and surgical consultation, if available
Geriatric: Mortality greater in this age group. Symptoms may be muted.
Others: N/A

PREGNANCY
Ruptured ectopic pregnancy may lead to peritonitis

SYNONYMS
N/A

ICD-9-CM
567.2 acute generalized peritonitis

SEE ALSO
• Appendicitis, acute
• Crohn's disease
• Diverticular disease
• Ectopic pregnancy
• Pancreatitis

OTHER NOTES
N/A

ABBREVIATIONS
N/A

REFERENCES
• Shands JW Jr: Empiric antibiotic therapy of abdominal sepsis and serious perioperative infections. Surg Clinics of North Amer 1993;73(2):291-306
• Isselbacher KJ, et al, eds: Harrison's Principles of Internal Medicine. 13th Ed. New York, McGraw-Hill, 1994
• Sleisenger MH, Fordtran JS, eds: Gastrointestinal Disease: Pathophysiology, Diagnosis, Management.5th Ed. Philadelphia, W.B. Saunders Co., 1994
• Bennett JC, Plum F, eds: Cecil Textbook of Medicine. 20th Ed. Philadelphia, W.B. Saunders Co., 1996
• Sabiston DC Jr, ed: Textbook of Surgery: The Biological Basis of Modern Surgical Practice. 14th Ed. Philadelphia, W.B. Saunders Co., 1991
• Ewald GA, McKenziem CR, eds: Manual of Medical Therapeutics. 28th Ed. Boston, Little-Brown & Co., 1995
• Sanford JP, Gilbert DN, Moellering RC, Sande MA. The Sanford Guide to Antimicrobial Therapy - 1997. Antimicrobial Therapy, Inc: Vienna, VA, 1997
Illustrations: N/A
Internet references: http://www.5mcc.com

Author(s)
Alan Adelman, MD, MS

Pertussis

BASICS

DESCRIPTION Pertussis or whooping cough is a highly communicable, respiratory bacterial infection. Characteristically, it produces a paroxysmal spasmodic cough, ending in prolonged high-pitched inspiratory whoop or crow. Transmission is by direct contact and patients are contagious for 3 weeks. Incubation period averages 7 to 14 days (maximum 3 weeks). Usual course - acute, but protracted (lasts 4-12 weeks after catarrhal period).
System(s) affected: Pulmonary
Genetics: N/A
Incidence/Prevalence in USA:
• 1.740 cases/100,000 people
• Annual average cases - 3,500, with 10 deaths
• Increasing as immunization rates decline.
Predominant age: 3 months-6 years (infants comprise about half of the cases)
Predominant sex: Female > Male

SIGNS AND SYMPTOMS
• Cough paroxysms
• Staccato cough
• Mild fever
• Rhinorrhea
• Anorexia
• "Whoop" cough
• Apnea, episodic
• Posttussive inspiratory gasp
• Posttussive emesis

CAUSES Bordetella pertussis. Bordetella parapertussis and Bordetella bronchiseptica produce a similar, but milder clinical illness.

RISK FACTORS
• Unimmunized children
• Contact with an infected person
• Epidemic exposure
• Pregnancy

DIAGNOSIS

DIFFERENTIAL DIAGNOSIS
• Common cold
• Adenoviral syndromes
• Bronchiolitis
• Influenza
• Bacterial pneumonias
• Cystic fibrosis
• Tuberculosis
• Interstitial pneumonitis
• Foreign body

LABORATORY
• ELISA: IgA against Bordetella pertussis
• WBC: elevated (15,000-60,000) with marked lymphocytosis
• Bordetella pertussis on Bordet-Gengou culture medium
Drugs that may alter lab results: N/A
Disorders that may alter lab results: N/A

PATHOLOGICAL FINDINGS
• Focal emphysema
• Mucopurulent exudate
• Patchy ulceration of respiratory epithelium

SPECIAL TESTS N/A

IMAGING Chest x-ray - focal atelectasis, peribronchial cuffing, emphysema

DIAGNOSTIC PROCEDURES N/A

TREATMENT

APPROPRIATE HEALTH CARE
Hospitalization for seriously ill infants. Outpatient for milder cases.

GENERAL MEASURES
• General supportive, skilled nursing care
• Isolation and quarantine for 4 weeks; 1 week after erythromycin started
• Parenteral fluid therapy if needed
• Oxygen
• Careful observation for apnea in young infants, and, to avoid stimuli that trigger paroxysms
• Mechanical ventilation
• Nutritional support - may require tube feedings in infants

SURGICAL MEASURES N/A

ACTIVITY Rest during active phase in quiet environment

DIET Encourage extra fluids. May need to provide small frequent meals to assure adequate nutrition.

PATIENT EDUCATION For patient education materials favorably reviewed on this topic, contact: American Academy of Pediatrics, 141 Northwest Point Blvd., P.O. Box 927, Elk Grove Village, IL 60009-0927, (800)433-9016

Pertussis

MEDICATIONS

DRUG(S) OF CHOICE
• Erythromycin, 30-40 mg/kg/day divided doses every 6 hours for 14 days
• Other antibiotics for bacterial complications such as bronchopneumonia or otitis media
• Antibiotics do not alter course of illness unless given very early. They prevent transmission.
Contraindications: Do not use cough suppressants
Precautions: N/A
Significant possible interactions: N/A

ALTERNATIVE DRUGS
• Steroids and/or theophylline have been suggested for treatment of severely ill patients (their effectiveness and potential hazards require further controlled studies)
• Beta-2 agonists may help with cough paroxysms.

FOLLOWUP

PATIENT MONITORING
• Intensive care unit may be necessary for severely ill infants
• Older children and adults with mild cases do not need to be confined to bed

PREVENTION/AVOIDANCE
• Isolate infected persons until treated with erythromycin 5 days
• Active immunization for all infants, usually combined with diphtheria and tetanus toxoids (DPT). Immunization or booster not recommended after age 6 years.
• Erythromycin - for susceptible children (under 2 months or unvaccinated) if they are exposed to an infected person during the contagious period

POSSIBLE COMPLICATIONS
• Can infect up to 90% of household members who are not immune
• Death in infants
• Pneumonia
• Hypoxic encephalopathy
• Coma
• Otitis media
• Tuberculosis activation
• Epistaxis
• Hernia
• Re-induction of paroxysmal coughing (for several months) especially with upper respiratory infections
• Convulsions
• Cerebral hemorrhage
• Neurologic disorders
• Weight loss
• Hemoptysis
• Atelectasis

EXPECTED COURSE/PROGNOSIS
Complete recovery

MISCELLANEOUS

ASSOCIATED CONDITIONS
• Otitis media
• Bronchopneumonia
• Failure to thrive

AGE-RELATED FACTORS
Pediatric: Most serious and highest mortality in infants less than 6 months of age (death usually due to complications)
Geriatric: May be more serious in this age group
Others: N/A

PREGNANCY N/A

SYNONYMS
Whooping cough

ICD-9-CM
033 Whooping cough

SEE ALSO
• Immunizations
• Otitis media
• Failure to thrive (FTT)
• Common cold
• Adenovirus infections
• Bronchiolitis
• Influenza
• Pneumonia, bacterial
• Cystic fibrosis
• Tuberculosis

OTHER NOTES
• Do not use cough suppressants
• Reporting of selected adverse reactions with certain vaccines is now required by the National Childhood Vaccine Injury Act of 1986. Toll-free information number - (800)822-7967.

ABBREVIATIONS N/A

REFERENCES
• Mandell GL, ed: Principles and Practice of Infectious Diseases. 4th Ed. New York, Churchill Livingstone, 1995
• Centers for Disease Control: National Childhood Vaccine Injury Act: Requirements for permanent vaccination records and for reporting of selected events after vaccination. MMWR 1988;37:197-200
Illustrations: N/A
Internet references: http://www.5mcc.com

Author(s)
Nancy N. Dambro, MD

Pharyngitis

BASICS

DESCRIPTION Inflammation of the pharynx most commonly caused by acute infection. Group A streptococcus is a focus of diagnosis due to its potential for preventable rheumatic sequelae.

System(s) affected: Gastrointestinal

Genetics: Individuals with a positive family history of rheumatic fever have a higher risk of rheumatic sequelae following an untreated group A beta hemolytic streptococcal infection

Incidence/Prevalence in USA:
• Estimated 30 million cases diagnosed yearly
• 11% of all school age children visit a physician annually with pharyngitis
• 12-25% of sore throats seen by physicians
• Incidence of rheumatic fever is decreasing with estimate of 64 cases per 100,000

Predominant age:
• Pharyngitis occurs in all age groups
• Streptococcal infection has greatest incidence 5 to 18 years of age

Predominant sex: Male = Female

SIGNS AND SYMPTOMS
• Sore throat
• Enlarged tonsils
• Pharyngeal erythema
• Tonsillar exudates
• Soft palate petechiae
• Cervical adenopathy
• Absence of cough, hoarseness, or lower respiratory symptoms
• Fever (> 102.5°F [39.1°C] suggests Streptococcus)
• Scarlet fever rash: punctate erythematous macules with reddened flexor creases and circumoral pallor (Streptococcal pharyngitis)
• Gray pseudomembrane found in diphtheria and occasionally, mononucleosis
• Characteristic erythematous based clear vesicles in herpes stomatitis
• Anorexia
• Chills
• Malaise
• Headache
• Conjunctivitis, more commonly with adenovirus infections

CAUSES
• Acute - bacterial:
  ◊ Group A beta-hemolytic streptococci
  ◊ Neisseria gonorrhoeae
  ◊ Corynebacterium diphtheriae (diphtheria)
  ◊ Haemophilus influenzae
  ◊ Moraxella (Branhamella) catarrhalis
  ◊ Group C and G streptococcus, rarely
• Acute - virus:
  ◊ Rhinovirus
  ◊ Adenovirus
  ◊ Parainfluenza virus
  ◊ Coxsackievirus
  ◊ Coronavirus
  ◊ Echovirus
  ◊ Herpes simplex virus
  ◊ Epstein-Barr virus (mononucleosis)
  ◊ Cytomegalovirus
• Chronic
  ◊ More likely non-infectious
  ◊ Irritation from post-nasal discharge of chronic allergic rhinitis
  ◊ Chemical irritation
  ◊ Neoplasms and vasculitides

RISK FACTORS
• Group A beta hemolytic streptococcal epidemics occur
• Age (young are more susceptible)
• Family history
• Close quarters, such as in new military recruits
• Immunosuppression
• Fatigue
• Smoking
• Excess alcohol consumption
• Oral sex
• Diabetes mellitus
• Recent illness

DIAGNOSIS

DIFFERENTIAL DIAGNOSIS
• See causative factors
• Sore throat can be seen with leukopenia

LABORATORY
• Blood agar throat culture from swab. Bacitracin disc sensitivity of hemolytic colonies suggest group A streptococci.
• Rapid screening for streptococci can be done from throat swab with antigen agglutination kits. 5-10% false negatives lead some to suggest routine backup of all negatives with blood agar culture.
• Leukocytosis (if bacterial)

Drugs that may alter lab results: N/A
Disorders that may alter lab results: N/A

PATHOLOGICAL FINDINGS Culture of pathogens to identify causes

SPECIAL TESTS
• Special tests usually done only if history is suggestive
• Screening for gonococcal infection requires warm Thayer-Martin plate
• Viruses can be cultured in special media
• Mono spot test for Epstein-Barr virus
• Gram stain can be suggestive
• Streptococcal isolates can be immunologically typed

IMAGING N/A

DIAGNOSTIC PROCEDURES History and physical probably only 50% accurate. Laboratory required unless in epidemic setting.

TREATMENT

APPROPRIATE HEALTH CARE
Outpatient

GENERAL MEASURES
• Salt water gargles
• Acetaminophen
• Dyclonine lozenges
• Cool-mist humidifier

SURGICAL MEASURES N/A

ACTIVITY As tolerated

DIET No restrictions. Encourage extra fluids.

PATIENT EDUCATION
• Important to complete 10 day course of antibiotics regardless of symptom response
• Patients presumed to be non-infectious after 24 hours of antibiotic coverage

MEDICATIONS

DRUG(S) OF CHOICE
For streptococcal pharyngitis, penicillin is the standard. All choices should have complete 10 day course.
• Penicillin V 250 mg tid (25-50 mg/kg/day), or
• For penicillin allergic patients, erythromycin ethylsuccinate 300 to 400 mg tid (30 mg/kg/day), or
• Cephalexin 250 mg tid (30 mg/kg/day)
Contraindications: Allergy to specific antibiotic
Precautions: Refer to manufacturer's profile of each drug
Significant possible interactions: Refer to manufacturer's profile of each drug

ALTERNATIVE DRUGS
• Treatment of carrier state is difficult, usually requiring addition of rifampin to penicillin regimen
• Penicillin is the treatment most documented to prevent rheumatic sequelae but cephalosporins have lower rate of bacteriologic failure
• Bacterial eradication rates ≥ 10 days therapy with penicillin have been achieved with 6 days of amoxicillin and 5 days with various cephalosporins
• The newer macrolides, azithromycin and clarithromycin, are also effective against streptococcal pharyngitis, but more expensive. The chief advantage of azithromycin is its 5 day course with 10 day effective duration.
• Other cephalosporins are generally effective for streptococcal pharyngitis, but more expensive than cephalexin

FOLLOWUP

PATIENT MONITORING
• Routine followup cultures not necessary
• Telephone consult for duration of symptoms

PREVENTION/AVOIDANCE   Avoid contact with infected people

POSSIBLE COMPLICATIONS
• Rheumatic fever
• Post-streptococcal glomerulonephritis
• Peritonsillar abscess
• Systemic infection
• Otitis media
• Mastoiditis
• Septicemia
• Rhinitis
• Sinusitis
• Pneumonia

EXPECTED COURSE/PROGNOSIS
• Streptococcal pharyngeal infection runs a 5-7 day course with peak of fever at 2-3 days
• Symptoms will resolve spontaneously without treatment, but rheumatic complications are still possible
• Suppurative complications such as peritonsillar abscess require surgical intervention

MISCELLANEOUS

ASSOCIATED CONDITIONS   N/A

AGE-RELATED FACTORS
Pediatric: N/A
Geriatric: N/A
Others: N/A

PREGNANCY   N/A

SYNONYMS
• Sore throat
• Tonsillitis
• Streptococcal throat

ICD-9-CM
462 Acute pharyngitis
463 Acute tonsillitis
472.1 Chronic pharyngitis
474.0 Chronic tonsillitis
034.0 Streptococcal sore throat
034.1 Scarlet fever

SEE ALSO
• Rheumatic fever
• Herpes simplex
• Mononucleosis

OTHER NOTES   Unless clinical presentation is unusual, treatment is based on presence or absence of group A streptococci

ABBREVIATIONS   N/A

REFERENCES
• Pichichero ME: Controversies in the treatment of streptococcal pharyngitis. Amer Fam Phys 1990;42(6):1558-1560
• Bennett JC, Plum F, eds: Cecil Textbook of Medicine. 20th Ed. Philadelphia, WB Saunders Co, 1996
• Bisno AL, et al: Diagnosis and management of group A streptococcal pharyngitis: a practice guideline. Clin Infect Dis 1997;25(3):574-583
• Pichichero ME, Cohen R: Shortened course of antibiotic therapy for acute otitis media, sinusitis and tonsillopharyngitis. Pediatr infect Dis 1997;16(7):680-695
Illustrations: N/A
Internet references: http://www.5mcc.com

Author(s)
David E. Burtner, MD

Pheochromocytoma

BASICS

DESCRIPTION Catecholamine-producing tumor. In 90% of cases, the tumors are found in the adrenal medulla, but may also be found in other tissues derived from neural crest cells.
System(s) affected: Endocrine/Metabolic
Genetics: N/A
Incidence/Prevalence in USA:
• 0.01% to 0.1% of the hypertensive population
Predominant age: Any age, peak incidence ages 30 to 60 years
Predominant sex: Male = Female

SIGNS AND SYMPTOMS
• Paroxysmal spells (the "5 P's")
  ◊ Pressure - sudden increase in blood pressure
  ◊ Pain - headache, chest and abdominal pain
    ◊ Perspiration
    ◊ Palpitation
    ◊ Pallor
• Additional symptoms
    ◊ Constipation
    ◊ Tremor
    ◊ Weight loss
    ◊ Anxiety
• Signs
  ◊ Hypertension - paroxysmal in half of the patients
    ◊ Orthostatic hypotension
    ◊ Grade II to IV retinopathy
    ◊ Fever
    ◊ Hyperglycemia
    ◊ Hypercalcemia
    ◊ Erythrocytosis
    ◊ 10% of patients are asymptomatic

CAUSES
• Catecholamine-producing tumor - "Rule of 10:"
    ◊ 10% are extra-adrenal
    ◊ 10% are multiple or bilateral
    ◊ 10% are malignant
    ◊ 10% recur after surgical removal
    ◊ 10% occur in children
    ◊ 10% are familial
    ◊ 10% present as adrenal incidentalomas

RISK FACTORS
• Familial pheochromocytoma
• Multiple endocrine neoplasia types II A and B
• Neurofibromatosis
• Von Hippel-Lindau syndrome

DIAGNOSIS

DIFFERENTIAL DIAGNOSIS
• Labile essential hypertension
• Anxiety and panic attacks
• Paroxysmal cardiac arrhythmia
• Thyrotoxicosis
• Menopausal syndrome
• Hypoglycemia
• Mastocytosis
• Withdrawal of adrenergic-inhibiting medications
• Angina
• Hyperventilation
• Migraine headache
• Amphetamine or cocaine use
• Sympathomimetic ingestion

LABORATORY
• Elevated 24-h urine metanephrine
• Elevated 24-h urine or plasma catecholamines measured by high performance liquid chromatography (HPLC)
• If results equivocal or normal, repeat 24-h urine collection with a spell
Drugs that may alter lab results:
• Increased by:
    ◊ Amphetamines
    ◊ Tricyclic antidepressants
    ◊ Clonidine or other drug withdrawal
    ◊ Labetalol
    ◊ Ethanol
    ◊ Methyldopa
    ◊ Sotalol
    ◊ Levodopa
• Decreased by:
    ◊ Central alpha-2 agonists
    ◊ Reserpine
Disorders that may alter lab results:
Major physical stress (e.g., surgery, stroke)

PATHOLOGICAL FINDINGS
Catecholamine-producing tumor in the adrenal medulla, para-aortic sympathetic chain, wall of the urinary bladder, sympathetic chain in the neck or mediastinum

SPECIAL TESTS Clonidine suppression test, suppression/provocative tests

IMAGING
• Computerized abdominal imaging (MRI preferred over CT)
• I-123: I-metaiodobenzylguanidine scan
• In-111: pentetreotide scan

DIAGNOSTIC PROCEDURES N/A

TREATMENT

APPROPRIATE HEALTH CARE
Inpatient surgery

GENERAL MEASURES
• Combined alpha- and beta-adrenergic blockade
• Cardiovascular and hemodynamic variables must be monitored closely

SURGICAL MEASURES
• High risk surgical procedure
• Experienced surgeon/anesthesiologist team required

ACTIVITY No limitations

DIET High in salt content preoperatively

PATIENT EDUCATION National Adrenal Disease Foundation (NADF), 505 Northern Blvd, Great Neck, NY 11021; 516-407-4992; e-mail: nadf@aol.com

Pheochromocytoma

MEDICATIONS

DRUG(S) OF CHOICE
- Combined alpha- and beta-adrenergic blockade required preoperatively
- Initiate alpha-blockade first - phenoxybenzamine (Dibenzyline) 10 mg daily and increase by 10-20 mg every 2 days as needed to control blood pressure and paroxysmal spells (average dose is 0.5-1.0 mg/kg daily)
- Beta-blockade after alpha-blockade is established - propranolol (Inderal) 10 mg q 6 hrs initially and increase as necessary to control tachycardia
- Acute hypertensive crises should be treated with phentolamine (Regitine) or nitroprusside administered intravenously

Contraindications: Beta-adrenergic blockade in patients with asthma, sinus bradycardia and greater than first degree block, or congestive heart failure. Avoid beta-blockers with intrinsic sympathomimetic activity

Precautions:
- Beta-adrenergic blockade alone may result in more severe hypertension due to the unopposed alpha-adrenergic stimulation; patients should be cautioned about postural hypotension
- Beta-adrenergic blockade is initiated at low doses of a short acting agent due to the possible side effect of pulmonary edema in the patient with catecholamine myocardiopathy

Significant possible interactions: For beta-adrenergic blockade - verapamil, phenytoin, phenobarbitone, rifampin, chlorpromazine, cimetidine

ALTERNATIVE DRUGS
- Alpha-adrenergic blocking agents - prazosin (Minipress), terazosin (Hytrin), doxazosin (Cardura)
- Beta-adrenergic blocking agents - nadolol (Corgard), atenolol (Tenormin), metoprolol (Lopressor)
- Combined beta- and alpha-adrenergic blocker - labetalol (Normodyne, TranDate)
- Catecholamine synthesis inhibitor - metyrosine (Demser)

FOLLOWUP

PATIENT MONITORING
- Daily blood pressure monitoring prior to surgery
- Intra-operative hemodynamic monitoring
- Two weeks postoperatively - 24-h urine for measurement of catecholamines and metanephrines; if normal, re-check annually for five years

PREVENTION/AVOIDANCE   N/A

POSSIBLE COMPLICATIONS
- Postural hypotension with alpha-adrenergic blockade
- Pulmonary edema with beta-adrenergic blockade
- Intra-operative hypertensive crisis

EXPECTED COURSE/PROGNOSIS
- The survival rate after removal of a benign pheochromocytoma is nearly that of age- and sex-matched controls
- For malignant pheochromocytoma, the 5-year survival rate is less than 50%

MISCELLANEOUS

ASSOCIATED CONDITIONS
- Multiple endocrine neoplasia type IIA (medullary thyroid carcinoma and primary hyperparathyroidism)
- Multiple endocrine neoplasia type IIB (medullary thyroid carcinoma and mucosal neuromas)
- Neurofibromatosis
- Von Hippel-Lindau syndrome (retinal angiomatosis and cerebellar hemangioblastoma)
- Ataxia-telangiectasia
- Tuberous sclerosis
- Sturge-Weber syndrome
- Cholelithiasis
- Renal artery stenosis

AGE-RELATED FACTORS
Pediatric: N/A
Geriatric: N/A
Others: N/A

PREGNANCY
- First and second trimester - surgical resection
- Third trimester - cesarean section and removal of the pheochromocytoma in the same operation

SYNONYMS   Paraganglioma

ICD-9-CM
194.0 Malignant neoplasm of adrenal gland

SEE ALSO
- Hypertension, essential

OTHER NOTES   All patients with paroxysmal spells and hypertension or with difficult to control hypertension should be screened

ABBREVIATIONS   HPLC = high performance liquid chromatography

REFERENCES
- Young WF Jr: Pheochromocytoma: 1926-1993: Trends in Endocrinology and Metabolism 1993;4:122
- Bravo EL, Gifford RW: Pheochromocytoma: Diagnosis, localization, and management. N Engl J Med 1984;311:1298
- Young WF Jr: Spells: In search of a cause. Mayo Clin Proc 1995;70:757-765
Illustrations: 2 available on CD-ROM
Internet references: http://www.5mcc.com

Author(s)
William F. Young, Jr., MD

Phimosis & paraphimosis

BASICS

DESCRIPTION
• Phimosis: tightness of the penile foreskin which prevents it from being drawn back from over the glans
• Paraphimosis: constriction of glans penis by proximally placed phimotic foreskin
System(s) affected: Renal/Urologic, Reproductive, Skin/Exocrine
Genetics: N/A
Incidence/Prevalence in USA: 1% of males over 16 years of age
Predominant age: Infancy and adolescence
Predominant sex: Male only

SIGNS AND SYMPTOMS
• Phimosis
  ◊ Unretractable foreskin
  ◊ Pain on erection
  ◊ Superimposed balanitis
• Paraphimosis
  ◊ Penile pain
  ◊ Drainage
  ◊ Ulceration
  ◊ Swelling

CAUSES
• Phimosis
  ◊ "Physiologic" - present at birth and resolves spontaneously during the first 2-3 years of life by nocturnal erections which slowly dilate the phimotic ring
  ◊ Congenital - unresolved physiologic phimosis
  ◊ Acquired - recurrent infection or irritation
• Paraphimosis
  ◊ Foreskin not pulled back over the glans after cleaning, cystoscopy or catheter insertion

RISK FACTORS
• Phimosis
  ◊ Poor hygiene
  ◊ Diabetes
  ◊ Frequent diaper rash in infant
• Paraphimosis
  ◊ Presence of foreskin
  ◊ "Inexperienced" health care provider, i.e., leaving foreskin retracted after catheter placement

DIAGNOSIS

DIFFERENTIAL DIAGNOSIS
Penile lymphedema which can be related to insect bites, trauma or allergic reactions

LABORATORY   N/A
Drugs that may alter lab results: N/A
Disorders that may alter lab results: N/A

PATHOLOGICAL FINDINGS   N/A

SPECIAL TESTS   N/A

IMAGING   N/A

DIAGNOSTIC PROCEDURES   N/A

TREATMENT

APPROPRIATE HEALTH CARE
Outpatient except for complications

GENERAL MEASURES
Paraphimosis: Reduction if possible (should be done with the patient sedated). Place the middle and index fingers of both hands on the engorged skin proximal to the glans. Place both thumbs on glans and with gentle pressure pushing on the glans and pulling on foreskin, attempt reduction. If unsuccessful, a dorsal slit will be necessary with eventual circumcision after the edema resolves.

SURGICAL MEASURES
• Phimosis: Circumcision
• Paraphimosis: Dorsal slit with subsequent circumcision

ACTIVITY   No sexual activity following circumcision until healing is complete

DIET   No limitations

PATIENT EDUCATION   If the patient is uncircumcised, appropriate hygiene and care of the foreskin is necessary to prevent phimosis and paraphimosis

MEDICATIONS

DRUG(S) OF CHOICE N/A
Contraindications: N/A
Precautions: N/A
Significant possible interactions: N/A

ALTERNATIVE DRUGS N/A

FOLLOWUP

PATIENT MONITORING 1 week after reduction of paraphimosis and 1 to 2 weeks after a circumcision

PREVENTION/AVOIDANCE Good patient and parental education

POSSIBLE COMPLICATIONS
• Unreduced paraphimosis can lead to gangrene of the glans
• Posthitis (inflammation of the prepuce)

EXPECTED COURSE/PROGNOSIS
Complete resolution if treatment is carried out effectively

MISCELLANEOUS

ASSOCIATED CONDITIONS N/A

AGE-RELATED FACTORS
Pediatric:
• Recurrent balanitis, either chemical or infectious, can lead to an acquired phimosis
• Forced reduction of a physiologic foreskin can lead to chronic scarring and acquired phimosis
Geriatric: Recurrent infection and irritations (condom catheters) can lead to phimosis
Others: N/A

PREGNANCY N/A

SYNONYMS N/A

ICD-9-CM
605 Phimosis
605 Paraphimosis

SEE ALSO N/A

OTHER NOTES N/A

ABBREVIATIONS N/A

REFERENCES
• Kelalis PP, King LR, Belman AB: Clinical Pediatric Urology. 3rd Ed. Philadelphia, W.B. Saunders Co., 1991
• Stringer MD, Oldham KT, Mouriquand PD, Howard ER: Pediatric Surgery and Urology: Long Term Outcomes. Philadelphia, WB Saunders Co., 1998
Illustrations: N/A
Internet references: http://www.5mcc.com

Author(s)
James P. Miller, MD, FACS, FAAP
Timothy L. Black, MD, FACS, FAAP

Phobias

BASICS

DESCRIPTION A persistent irrational fear of a specific object, activity or situation that results in a compelling desire to avoid the perceived fear. Psychiatric conditions classified in Diagnostic and Statistical Manual of Mental Disorders (DSM-IV-R) as anxiety disorders. When confronted with the phobic stimulus, patient reacts with intense anxiety, usually realizes the fear is excessive or exaggerated. When a fear causes significant distress and interferes with normal functions of life, then it is considered a psychiatric disorder.
• Agoraphobia: Fear of being trapped in a situation where escape is impossible or difficult. Fear centers on (1) fear of being alone, (2) fear of being away from home and (3) fear of being in a place from where escape is difficult - seen most often in association with panic disorder.
• Simple phobia: Fear of a discrete stimulus such as animals, insects, heights, flying, closed spaces (claustrophobia), blood-injury phobia
• Social phobia: Fear of humiliation or embarrassment in social situations where person may be under scrutiny by others, e.g., performance anxiety, speaking in public, or fear of using public toilets
System(s) affected: Nervous
Genetics: No consistent genetic pattern
Incidence/Prevalence in USA: 1 month prevalence of all phobic conditions: 6.2%; lifetime prevalence: 12.5%
Predominant age:
• Agoraphobia - onset 18-35 (mean 24)
• Simple phobia fear of animals - onset usually in childhood (mean 4.4 years)
• Simple phobia fear of heights, claustrophobia - 4th decade
• Other simple phobias - mean 22.7 years
• Social phobia - late childhood, adolescence (mean 19 years)
Predominant sex:
• Female > Male, overall phobias
• Male = Female, social phobia

SIGNS AND SYMPTOMS
• Extreme anxiety when exposed to phobic stimulus
• Tremors
• Palpitations
• Sweating
• Blushing
• Dyspnea
• Dizziness
• Associated nausea

CAUSES
• Persistence or exaggeration of learned response, learned initially as a protective mechanism (such as avoidance of large dogs by small children)
• Social - learned maladaptive anxiety response to social situation

RISK FACTORS
• For all phobias - presence of another psychiatric disorder
• Separation anxiety in childhood
• Introverted or dependent personality

DIAGNOSIS

DIFFERENTIAL DIAGNOSIS
• For agoraphobia:
  ◊ Paranoid and psychotic states
  ◊ PTSD (posttraumatic stress disorder)
  ◊ Depression - but do not see the other aspects of depression (anhedonia, loss of appetite and libido, sleep disturbance-early morning awakening, frequent night awakening, difficulty falling asleep)
• For simple phobia:
  ◊ Schizophrenia - avoidance can be seen but usually in response to a delusion and patient does not realize that fear is excessive. Schizophrenia is intimately intertwined with delusion.
  ◊ PTSD - phobic avoidance seen and is associated with the original trauma
  ◊ Obsessive compulsive disorder (OCD) - avoidance associated with obsessions (such as dirt avoidance)
• For social phobia:
  ◊ Avoidant personality disorder - central fear in avoidant personality disorder is that of rejection, not of humiliation or embarrassment as in social phobia
  ◊ Paranoid personality disorder
  ◊ Schizophrenia

LABORATORY None
Drugs that may alter lab results: N/A
Disorders that may alter lab results: N/A

PATHOLOGICAL FINDINGS N/A

SPECIAL TESTS None

IMAGING N/A

DIAGNOSTIC PROCEDURES
• Careful history and observation of the patient
• Description of the behavior by patient, family or friends
• Psychiatric examination

TREATMENT

APPROPRIATE HEALTH CARE
Outpatient

GENERAL MEASURES
• Agoraphobia:
  ◊ Behavioral treatment
  ◊ Graduated exposure
  ◊ Different treatment required when agoraphobia is associated with panic disorder
• Simple phobia:
  ◊ In vivo or graduated exposure
  ◊ Fear of flying specifically - benzodiazepine
• Social phobia:
  ◊ Social skills training
  ◊ Graduated exposure
  ◊ Performance anxiety or situations where patient in a circumscribed setting - beta blocker

SURGICAL MEASURES N/A

ACTIVITY No restriction

DIET Consider restriction of stimulants - such as caffeine, nicotine, xanthines, sympathomimetics, which can overdrive anxiety. Phenelzine - requires tyramine free diet.

PATIENT EDUCATION
• Cognitive therapy
• Phobia clinic or group therapy, if available

MEDICATIONS

DRUG(S) OF CHOICE
• Agoraphobia - none recommended
• Simple phobia - none recommended, except for fear of flying. A benzodiazepine, such as alprazolam, may help. Initial dose as low as 0.25 mg titrated upward as needed.
• Social phobia (acute) - beta-blocker, e.g., propranolol (Inderal) 20-40 mg, 45-60 minutes before anticipated performance, atenolol 50-100 mg/day for more generalized social phobia
• Social phobia (chronic) - phenelzine , a MAO inhibitor, up to 60 mg/day, if social phobia more generalized and requires more constant medication (as opposed to the sporadic treatment for performance anxiety)

Contraindications:
• Beta-blocker - asthma or bronchospasm, congestive heart failure, bradycardia
• Phenelzine - not with other antidepressants, tyramine in diet, decongestants, diet pills, meperidine (Demerol), dextromethorphan, levodopa, and sympathomimetics

Precautions:
• Do not abruptly discontinue alprazolam due to potential for withdrawal seizures
• Monitor blood pressure in patients taking beta-blockers
• Consult drug information before using phenelzine

Significant possible interactions:
• Phenelzine - significant dietary restrictions due to potential for hypertensive crisis.
• Drugs to avoid include: Sympathomimetics, TCA's, fluoxetine, CNS depressants.
• Consult drug information sources before adding new medications in patients.

ALTERNATIVE DRUGS   N/A

FOLLOWUP

PATIENT MONITORING   Outpatient as needed

PREVENTION/AVOIDANCE   N/A

POSSIBLE COMPLICATIONS
• Avoidance behavior
• Episodic alcohol, barbiturate and anxiolytic abuse/overuse and dependence as patients try to self-medicate to ameliorate symptoms
• Development of mild depression

EXPECTED COURSE/PROGNOSIS
• Agoraphobia - usually associated with panic disorder, chronic. Often patient becomes more and more home-bound as condition continues.
• Simple phobia - some spontaneously remit as person ages (as in some simple phobias of childhood), alternatively some become chronic. Impairment can be minimal if object can be avoided (such as snakes). Although improvement occurs with in vivo exposure, phobia can recur after successful treatment.
• Social phobia - chronic course

MISCELLANEOUS

ASSOCIATED CONDITIONS
• For all phobias - depression, substance abuse
• Social and agoraphobia - panic attacks or panic disorder

AGE-RELATED FACTORS
Pediatric: Animal phobia mean age of onset 4.4 years
Geriatric: N/A
Others: N/A

PREGNANCY   No data

SYNONYMS   N/A

ICD-9-CM
300.22 Agoraphobia
300.29 Simple phobia
300. 23 Social phobia

SEE ALSO
• Obsessive compulsive disorder
• Post-traumatic stress disorder (PTSD)
• Anxiety
• Depression
• Schizophrenia
• Dissociative disorders

OTHER NOTES   N/A

ABBREVIATIONS
PTSD = posttraumatic stress disorder

REFERENCES
• Diagnostic and Statistical Manual of Mental Disorders (DSM-IV-R). 4th Ed. American Psychiatric Association, Washington, DC, 1994
• Cutis GC, et al: Specific fears and phobias. Epidemiology and classification. Brit J Psych 1998;173:212-217
Illustrations: N/A
Internet references: http://www.5mcc.com

Author(s)
Brian J. Murray, MD

Photodermatitis

BASICS

DESCRIPTION Light-induced eruptions seen in a pattern of photo-distribution
• Phototoxic reactions - result of the acute toxic effect on skin of ultraviolet light alone (sunburn) or together with a photosensitizing substance (non-allergic)
• Photoallergic eruptions - a form of allergic dermatitis resulting from combined effects of a photosensitizing substance (drugs or chemical) plus ultraviolet light (immunologic/delayed hypersensitivity)
• Polymorphous light eruption (PLE) - chronic, intermittent light-induced eruption with erythematous papules, urticaria, or vesicles on areas exposed to sunlight
System(s) affected: Skin/Exocrine
Genetics: Predisposition occurs in inbred populations (e.g., Pima Indians)
Incidence/Prevalence in USA: Unknown
Predominant age: All ages
Predominant sex: Male = Female

SIGNS AND SYMPTOMS
• Phototoxic
  ◊ Erythema
  ◊ With increasing severity - vesicles and bullae
  ◊ Classic example - sunburn
  ◊ Nails may exhibit onycholysis
  ◊ Chronic - epidermal thickening, elastosis, telangiectasia and pigmentary changes
  ◊ Sharp lines of demarcation between involved and uninvolved skin (sunlight exposure)
  ◊ Phototoxic eruption due to topicals - area of application
  ◊ Usually develops shortly after sun exposure
  ◊ Hyperpigmentation may follow resolution
  ◊ Pain
• Photoallergic
  ◊ Papules with erythema and occasionally vesicles
  ◊ Area exposed to light with less distinct borders
  ◊ Usually delayed - 24 hours or more after exposure
  ◊ May spread to unexposed areas
  ◊ Pruritus
• Polymorphous light eruption (PLE)
  ◊ Erythematous papules
  ◊ Occasionally urticaria or vesicles
  ◊ Scattered over sun exposed areas with normal skin in between
  ◊ Can spread to non-exposed areas
  ◊ Often flares in spring or early summer
  ◊ Desensitization affect (less over the course of the summer)
  ◊ Burning or pruritus may precede lesions

CAUSES
• Sunlight
• Phenothiazines
• Diuretics
• Tetracyclines
• Sulfonamides
• Oral contraceptives
• Topicals - psoralens, coal tars, photo-active dyes (eosin, acridine orange)

RISK FACTORS   N/A

DIAGNOSIS

DIFFERENTIAL DIAGNOSIS Systemic lupus erythematosus

LABORATORY Antinuclear antibody (ANA) to rule out systemic lupus erythematosus
Drugs that may alter lab results: N/A
Disorders that may alter lab results: N/A

PATHOLOGICAL FINDINGS
Nonspecific

SPECIAL TESTS
• Photo-testing
• Photopatch testing
• Skin biopsy - to rule out other disorders

IMAGING   N/A

DIAGNOSTIC PROCEDURES Physical examination and medical history

TREATMENT

APPROPRIATE HEALTH CARE
Outpatient

GENERAL MEASURES
• Avoid sunlight/limit exposure
• Protective clothing/sunscreens
• Ice packs/cold water compresses

SURGICAL MEASURES   N/A

ACTIVITY   Avoid sunlight

DIET   No special diet

PATIENT EDUCATION
• Avoidance of sunlight
• Avoidance of photosensitizing drugs
• Protective clothing
• Sunscreens

MEDICATIONS

DRUG(S) OF CHOICE
• Topical corticosteroids (betamethasone valerate 0.1% cream)
• NSAIDs (indomethacin 25 mg tid; aspirin; others)
• Prednisone for severe reactions (0.5-1 mg/kg/d) for 3-10 days
• Antihistamines for pruritus (hydroxyzine 25-50 mg qid)
• Sunscreens for prevention. Use broad-spectrum sunscreen to block both UVA and UVB. PABA may aggravate photodermatitis in sensitized patients (due to the sulfa moiety).
Contraindications: Refer to manufacturer's profile of each drug
Precautions: Refer to manufacturer's profile of each drug
Significant possible interactions: Refer to manufacturer's profile of each drug

ALTERNATIVE DRUGS   N/A

FOLLOWUP

PATIENT MONITORING   As necessary for persistence or recurrence

PREVENTION/AVOIDANCE
• Sunlight avoidance/protective clothing
• Identification and avoidance of causative drugs (see under Causes)
• Sunscreens - apply before exposure
  ◊ Zinc oxide - opaque, cosmetically less acceptable
  ◊ Chemical - use sun-protective factor > 15 for maximum protection; substantively resistant to sweat and swimming; cosmetically more acceptable

POSSIBLE COMPLICATIONS   N/A

EXPECTED COURSE/PROGNOSIS
Good with avoidance/protection measures

MISCELLANEOUS

ASSOCIATED CONDITIONS
• Sunlight aggravation of systemic lupus
• Persistent light reactivity
• Actinic reticuloid

AGE-RELATED FACTORS   N/A
Pediatric: N/A
Geriatric: More likely to experience adverse reactions to causative drugs
Others: N/A

PREGNANCY   N/A

SYNONYMS
• Sun poisoning

ICD-9-CM
692.79 due to solar radiation, other
692.89 due to other specified agents, other

SEE ALSO   N/A

OTHER NOTES   N/A

ABBREVIATIONS
NSAID = nonsteroidal anti-inflammatory drugs

REFERENCES   Bondi J, Jegasothy B, Lazarus G: Dermatology, Diagnosis and Therapy. Norwalk, CT, Appleton & Lange, 1991
Illustrations: N/A
Internet references: http://www.5mcc.com

Author(s)
Jeffrey A. Stearns, MD

Pinworms

BASICS

DESCRIPTION   Intestinal infection with Enterobius vermicularis. Characterized by perianal itching, usually worse at night.
System(s) affected: Gastrointestinal, Skin/Exocrine
Genetics: N/A
Incidence/Prevalence in USA:
Approximately 20% of young children (ages 5-10)
Predominant age: 5 to 14
Predominant sex: Female > Male

SIGNS AND SYMPTOMS
• Perianal itching
• Perineal itching
• Vulvovaginitis
• Enuresis
• Abdominal pain
• Insomnia

CAUSES   The intestinal nematode Enterobius (Oxyuris) vermicularis

RISK FACTORS
• Institutionalization (50-90% of institutionalized children have pinworms)
• Crowded living conditions
• Poor hygiene
• Warm climate

DIAGNOSIS

DIFFERENTIAL DIAGNOSIS
• Idiopathic pruritus ani
• Atopic dermatitis
• Contact dermatitis
• Psoriasis
• Lichen planus
• Infection with human papilloma virus
• Herpes simplex
• Fungal infections
• Erythrasma
• Scabies
• Vaginitis

LABORATORY N/A
Drugs that may alter lab results: N/A
Disorders that may alter lab results: N/A

PATHOLOGICAL FINDINGS
Identification of ova on low power microscopy or direct visualization of the female worm (10 mm in length). Ova are asymmetric, flattened on one side, and measure 30 by 60 µm.

SPECIAL TESTS
• Transparent tape test - a piece of transparent cellophane tape is adhered to the perianal skin in the early morning and then affixed to a microscope slide. This procedure must be performed at least 3 times to achieve 90% sensitivity.
• Flashlight to perianal region at night for direct observation
• Digital rectal examination with saline slide preparation of stool on gloved finger

IMAGING N/A

DIAGNOSTIC PROCEDURES N/A

TREATMENT

APPROPRIATE HEALTH CARE
Outpatient

GENERAL MEASURES
• All symptomatic family members should be treated simultaneously
• Bedclothes and underwear of infected individuals should be washed in hot water at the time of treatment (ova can remain viable for 2-3 weeks in a moist environment)
• Strict hand washing can help prevent fecal-oral transmission
• Practice good hygiene (showers, nail cleaning)
• Topical use of antipruritic creams or ointments may help relive itching in the perianal region

SURGICAL MEASURES N/A

ACTIVITY   No restrictions

DIET   No restrictions

PATIENT EDUCATION   For patient education materials on this topic: Centers for Disease Control, Dept. of Health and Human Services, Office of Public Affairs, Atlanta, GA 30333, (404)329-3534

Pinworms

MEDICATIONS

DRUG(S) OF CHOICE
Some clinicians recommend repeat treatment after 2 weeks.
• Mebendazole (Vermox) chewable tablet 100 mg as a single dose. Use with caution in children < age 2
or
• Pyrantel pamoate (Antiminth) oral suspension 11 mg/kg as a single dose. Maximum dose 1 gram. Use with caution in children < age 2
or
• Albendazole 400 mg orally as a single dose
Contraindications: Refer to manufacturer's profile of each drug
Precautions:
• All family members should be treated
• Take medicine on empty stomach
• May cause diarrhea and/or nausea
Significant possible interactions: Refer to manufacturer's profile of each drug

ALTERNATIVE DRUGS   N/A

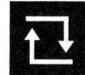

FOLLOWUP

PATIENT MONITORING   Unnecessary unless symptoms do not abate following drug therapy

PREVENTION/AVOIDANCE
• Careful hand washing, keep nails short and clean
• Wash anus and genitals at least once a day, preferably in a shower
• Don't scratch anus or put fingers near nose or mouth

POSSIBLE COMPLICATIONS
• Perianal scratching may cause impetigo or excoriation
• Young girls - vulvovaginitis, urethritis, endometritis, salpingitis
• Urinary tract infections

EXPECTED COURSE/PROGNOSIS
• Asymptomatic carriers are common
• Symptomatic infections are cured > 90% of the time with drug therapy
• Reinfection is common

MISCELLANEOUS

ASSOCIATED CONDITIONS   Pruritis ani

AGE-RELATED FACTORS
Pediatric: More common in children and more likely to get reinfected
Geriatric: N/A
Others: N/A

PREGNANCY   Drug therapy is contraindicated in pregnancy

SYNONYMS   Enterobiasis

ICD-9-CM   127.4 Enterobiasis

SEE ALSO   N/A

OTHER NOTES   N/A

ABBREVIATIONS   N/A

REFERENCES
• Bennett JC, Plum F, eds: Cecil Textbook of Medicine. 20th Ed. Philadelphia, WB Saunders Co., 1996
• Berman RE, et al, eds: Nelson Textbook of Pediatrics. 15th Ed. Philadelphia, WB Saunders Co., 1996
• Sanford JP, et al: Guide to Antimicrobial Therapy. New York, Pfizer, 1998
• Feigin RD, Cherry JD, eds: Textbook of Pediatric Infectious Diseases. 4th Ed. Philadelphia, WB Saunders Co., 1998
Illustrations: N/A
Internet references: http://www.5mcc.com

Author(s)
Steven Eisenstein, MD

Pityriasis alba

BASICS

DESCRIPTION A chronic skin disorder characterized by one or more groups of poorly marginated, white patches and plaques that appear on the cheeks, neck and lateral arms of children and young adults
System(s) affected: Skin/Exocrine
Genetics: Unknown, but is primarily seen in children with a genetic predisposition to atopic disease
Incidence/Prevalence in USA: Common, exact incidence unknown. Common, especially in dark-skin individuals in sunnier climates (90% for ages 6-12).
Predominant age: 3-10 years. Rare after 25.
Predominant sex: Male = Female

SIGNS AND SYMPTOMS
• Description - small, ill-defined white patches
• Location - cheeks and lateral arms
• Number - 1-12 or more patches
• Palpation - smooth or slightly rough, and dry
• Appearance - pinpoint white papules (representing accentuation and keratinization of follicular orifices)
• Scale is either invisible or fine and light
• More common in dark skinned individuals
• Usually asymptomatic
• Pruritic (rare)
• More apparent in summertime in light skinned individuals
• Lesions do not tan in summer
• Even a small amount of sunlight exposure causes lesions to redden

CAUSES
• Unknown. Maybe part of an atopic diathesis.
• Possibly defects in melanin production or transfer

RISK FACTORS Children with a genetic predisposition to atopic disease

DIAGNOSIS

DIFFERENTIAL DIAGNOSIS
• Pityriasis versicolor
• Vitiligo
• Milia
• Keratosis pilaris
• Indeterminate or uncharacteristic leprosy

LABORATORY N/A
Drugs that may alter lab results: N/A
Disorders that may alter lab results: N/A

PATHOLOGICAL FINDINGS Irregular melanin pigmentation of basal layer, follicular plugging, follicular spongiosis, and atrophic sebaceous glands

SPECIAL TESTS N/A

IMAGING N/A

DIAGNOSTIC PROCEDURES History and physical exam. Atopic diathesis is of diagnostic significance.

TREATMENT

APPROPRIATE HEALTH CARE
Outpatient

GENERAL MEASURES No truly effective therapy available. Lubricating cream application may improve roughness and/or dryness.

SURGICAL MEASURES N/A

ACTIVITY No restrictions

DIET No special diet

PATIENT EDUCATION Stress long-term chronicity and permanent resolution in second or third decade of life

Pityriasis alba

 ## MEDICATIONS

DRUG(S) OF CHOICE
• Coal tar preparations - Alphosyl, Estar, Balnetar, applied topically once or twice a day. Treatment is not mandatory.
• Topical steroids if needed to reduce redness due to sunburn or spontaneous inflammation
• Note: Neither will change the pigmentation, but may improve pruritus, roughness and/or dryness, if the lubricating cream is not sufficient
• Phototherapy (e.g., UVB)
• Anecdotal evidence supports use of Lacticare HC 1% (Lac-Hydrin + 1% hydrocortisone lotion)
Contraindications: N/A
Precautions: Refer to manufacturer's literature
Significant possible interactions: N/A

ALTERNATIVE DRUGS   N/A

 ## FOLLOWUP

PATIENT MONITORING   As needed only if lesions become symptomatic

PREVENTION/AVOIDANCE   No known preventive measures

POSSIBLE COMPLICATIONS   None expected

EXPECTED COURSE/PROGNOSIS
Permanent resolution during second or third decade of life

 ## MISCELLANEOUS

ASSOCIATED CONDITIONS   Atopic dermatitis

AGE-RELATED FACTORS
Pediatric: More common in children 3 to 10 years
Geriatric: Rare in this age group
Others: N/A

PREGNANCY   N/A

SYNONYMS
• Pityriasis streptogenes
• Pityriasis simplex
• Pityriasis sicca faciei
• Erythema streptogenes
• Furfuraceous impetigo

ICD-9-CM
696.5 Other and unspecified pityriasis

SEE ALSO
• Tinea versicolor
• Vitiligo
• Keratosis, actinic

OTHER NOTES   N/A

ABBREVIATIONS   N/A

REFERENCES
• Habif T: Clinical Dermatology. 3rd Ed. St. Louis, CV Mosby, 1996
• Sams WM, Lynch PJ, eds: Principles and Practices of Dermatology. 2nd Ed. New York, Churchill Livingstone, 1996
• Fitzpatrick TB, et al, eds: Dermatology in General Medicine. 4th Ed. New York, McGraw-Hill, 1993
• Arnold KL, Odom RB, James WD: Andrews' Diseases of the Skin. 8th Ed. Philadelphia, W.B. Saunders Co., 1990
• Vargas-Ocampo F: Pityriasis alba: a histologic study. Int J Dermatol 1993;32(12):870-3
Illustrations: 2 available on CD-ROM
Internet references: http://www.5mcc.com

Author(s)
Mitchell S. King, MD
Anne C. Reitz, MD

Pityriasis rosea

 BASICS

DESCRIPTION An idiopathic self-limited skin eruption characterized by widespread papulosquamous lesions
System(s) affected: Skin/Exocrine
Genetics: Less than 5 percent of those affected give a positive family history
Incidence/Prevalence in USA: Relatively common but exact frequency unknown
Predominant age: 10-35, but occurs in all age groups
Predominant sex: Male = Female

SIGNS AND SYMPTOMS
• Salmon to light brown oval plaques with fine scales centrally and "collarette" of loose scales along borders
• Lesions average 1-2 cm in diameter and usually spare face, hands and feet in adults
• Lesions frequently oriented along skin cleavage lines in "Christmas tree" pattern
• Eruption often preceded by 2-6 cm "herald patch" of similar appearance days to weeks before generalized rash
• Mild pruritus, rarely severe
• Fever and malaise rare
• Variant forms include purpuric, urticarial, and vesicular lesions

CAUSES Unknown, may be a viral agent or an autoimmune disorder

RISK FACTORS Unknown

 DIAGNOSIS

DIFFERENTIAL DIAGNOSIS
• Secondary syphilis
• Viral exanthems
• Drug rashes
• Psoriasis
• Parapsoriasis
• Eczema
• Lichen planus
• Tinea corporis

LABORATORY WBC normal. No specific lab markers. Serology to rule out syphilis.
Drugs that may alter lab results: N/A
Disorders that may alter lab results: N/A

PATHOLOGICAL FINDINGS Chronic inflammation with cytolytic degeneration of keratinocytes adjacent to Langerhans cells

SPECIAL TESTS KOH preparation to distinguish from tinea corporis

IMAGING N/A

DIAGNOSTIC PROCEDURES N/A

 TREATMENT

APPROPRIATE HEALTH CARE
Outpatient

GENERAL MEASURES
• Symptomatic treatment
• Topical antipruritics as needed
• Ultraviolet therapy has been used but efficacy not proven
• Lukewarm oatmeal baths (not hot as it can intensify itching)

SURGICAL MEASURES N/A

ACTIVITY Full activity with good skin hygiene to prevent secondary infection

DIET N/A

PATIENT EDUCATION
• Reassurance as to self-limited nature of condition
• Printed patient information available from: American Academy of Dermatology (708) 330-0230.

MEDICATIONS

DRUG(S) OF CHOICE
- Topical steroids to reduce itching, if needed
  ◊ Triamcinolone 0.1% cream
- Oral antihistamines
  ◊ Diphenhydramine (Benadryl) 25 mg tid
  ◊ chlorpheniramine 8 mg tid

Contraindications: N/A
Precautions: N/A
Significant possible interactions: N/A

ALTERNATIVE DRUGS   N/A

FOLLOWUP

PATIENT MONITORING
- Check syphilis serology
- Return visit for reevaluation, if lesions persist longer than 8-10 weeks

PREVENTION/AVOIDANCE   N/A

POSSIBLE COMPLICATIONS
Secondary infection (e.g., impetigo)

EXPECTED COURSE/PROGNOSIS
Gradual resolution in 1-14 weeks (usually 2-6)

MISCELLANEOUS

ASSOCIATED CONDITIONS   N/A

AGE-RELATED FACTORS
Pediatric: Face, distal extremities more often involved in children and lesions may be more papular
Geriatric: N/A
Others: N/A

PREGNANCY   N/A

SYNONYMS   N/A

ICD-9-CM
696.3 Pityriasis rosea

SEE ALSO
- Pityriasis alba
- Dermatitis, exfoliative
- Tinea versicolor

OTHER NOTES   N/A

ABBREVIATIONS   N/A

REFERENCES
- Fitzpatrick TB, et al, eds: Dermatology In General Medicine. 3rd Ed. New York, McGraw-Hill, 1987
- Cheong WK, Wong KS: Pityriasis Rosea. Singapore Medical Jour 1989
Illustrations: 10 available on CD-ROM
Internet references: http://www.5mcc.com

Author(s)
Jeffrey D. Wolfrey, MD

Placenta previa

BASICS

DESCRIPTION Placental implantation in the lower uterine segment in advance of the presenting fetal part.
• Total previa: placenta covers entire cervical os
• Partial previa: placenta covers part of the cervical os
• Marginal previa: placental edge just reaches cervical os
• Low lying placenta: placental edge is in the lower uterine segment but does not encroach on the internal cervical os
System(s) affected: Reproductive, Cardiovascular
Genetics: N/A
Incidence/Prevalence in USA: 0.5% to 0.8% of all pregnancies, approximately 1/200 deliveries; low lying placenta 4-8% in early pregnancy with < 10% persisting to term
Predominant age: Childbearing ages
Predominant sex: Female only

SIGNS AND SYMPTOMS
• Typically painless bright red bleeding 2nd or 3rd trimester
• Average time of first bleed, 27-32 weeks
• Contractions variably present
• First bleed usually self limited
• Maternal hemodynamic status consistent with clinical blood loss estimate
• Complete previas may bleed earlier and not "migrate"

CAUSES Prior uterine insult or injury or other uterine factors

RISK FACTORS
• Prior previa (4%-8%)
• First subsequent pregnancy following a cesarean section delivery
• Multiparity (5% in grand multiparous patient)
• Advanced maternal age
• Multiple gestation
• Prior spontaneous or induced abortions
• Smoking
• Cocaine use

DIAGNOSIS

DIFFERENTIAL DIAGNOSIS Abruptio placentae, vasa previa, vaginal and cervical causes including marked "bloody show" and infections

LABORATORY
• Maternal blood type and Rh
• Hemoglobin and hematocrit
• Platelet count
• PT, PTT, fibrinogen
• Type and cross match packed RBC (at least three units)
• Apt test: To determine fetal origin of blood (as in vasa previa). Mix vaginal blood with small amount tap water to cause hemolysis, centrifuge for several minutes, mix 1 cc of 1% NaOH with each 5 cc of the pink-hemoglobin-containing supernatant, observing pink fluid if fetal hemoglobin, and yellow-brown if adult origin.
• Wright's stain applied to a slide smear of vaginal blood looking for nucleated RBC's which are usually from cord blood and not adult blood
• L/S ratio for fetal maturity if needed
Drugs that may alter lab results: Drugs altering cell counts or clotting studies
Disorders that may alter lab results:
• Coagulopathies from other causes
• Red cell and hemoglobin disorders from other causes

PATHOLOGICAL FINDINGS
• Normocytic, normochromic anemia with acute bleed
• Coagulopathy rare, but may occur
• Positive Kleihauer-Betke if fetal/maternal transfusion

SPECIAL TESTS
• Kleihauer-Betke if concerned about fetal-maternal transfusion
• Bedside clot test: Draw red top tube from mother and observe for clot quality at 7-10 minutes. If there is no clot or if clot is friable may indicate disseminated intravascular coagulation (DIC).

IMAGING
• External sector sonography with moderately full and empty bladder
• Vaginal probe sonography may be done if not actively bleeding. Place the probe just inside vaginal os and use 5 or 6.5-mHz transducers.
• Magnetic resonance imaging (MRI) accurate, but more expensive, less available, and time consuming

DIAGNOSTIC PROCEDURES
• If placental location unknown and sonography not available, a double setup bimanual vaginal exam may be done in operating room with complete cesarean section readiness

• Careful vaginal speculum exam is not contraindicated and allows checking for cervical or vaginal source of bleeding, fern and nitrazine testing, cultures, and fluid for determining bleeding source
• Since fibrin degradation products rise in pregnancy, these levels are less helpful

TREATMENT

APPROPRIATE HEALTH CARE
• Inpatient observation at bedrest initially; once stable, and preterm, may be followed as outpatient
• May consider transfer to high risk center based on condition and local services

GENERAL MEASURES
• Optimizing maternal stability while delaying delivery, if possible, or if preterm to improve perinatal outcome
• Cesarean section indicated for partial or complete previa if fetus is mature or if the situation is urgent and the fetus is immature
• A trial of labor may be considered with anterior marginal previa, including oxytocin (Pitocin) augmentation IV
• Amniocentesis for L/S ratio for maturity as needed
• IV fluid support, oxygen, transfusions of packed RBC's, platelets and fresh frozen plasma if needed
• External fetal and labor monitoring
• Other intervention or observation based on maternal condition
• DIC risk low unless massive bleed. Follow coagulation studies and give fresh frozen plasma (FFP), platelets as needed, or cryoprecipitate if fibrinogen < 100-150 mg/dL (< 1.0-1.5 g/L).
• Transfuse platelets at < 20,000 or < 50,000 if surgery needed
• Low lying posterior marginal previa associated with dystocia and greater need for cesarean section
• Blood volume increased in pregnancy; can lose > 30% maternal blood volume before shock findings
• Central line placement only after checking coagulation studies
• May use sector probe with condom at introitus if vaginal probe unavailable
• With significant hemorrhage, Rh negative women should receive Rho(D) immune globulin (Rhogam) with each bleed

SURGICAL MEASURES Cervical cerclage does not significantly improve maternal or neonatal outcome

ACTIVITY
• Bedrest
• Pelvic rest; intercourse abstinence, avoid douching

DIET NPO initially, then based on delivery decisions

PATIENT EDUCATION
- First bleed rarely fatal
- Rebleed risk with activity or cervical stimulation
- Greatest cause of perinatal mortality is prematurity
- Risks and conditions associated with previa

MEDICATIONS

DRUG(S) OF CHOICE
- For IV fluids: Lactated Ringer's or saline
- Oxygen for all, since O2 consumption up 20% in pregnancy and fetus is more prone to hypoxia
- Fresh frozen plasma and platelets as needed
- Cryoprecipitate and fibrinogen if above unsuccessful
- Tocolytics may have role in certain preterm patients, but tachycardia of B-agonists (terbutaline) and risk of placental hypoperfusion with calcium channel blockers may make MgSO4 the drug of choice. For MgSO4, use 4 grams IV load and 1-4 grams/hour as indicated.

Contraindications:
Avoid tocolytics with term infant or unstable mother

Precautions:
- Beta-agonists and calcium channel blockers may complicate clinical picture
- Cryoprecipitate and fibrinogen may increase infection transmission risk

Significant possible interactions: Refer to manufacturer's profile of each drug

ALTERNATIVE DRUGS
- Ritodrine (Yutopar) IV may be an alternate beta-agonist, but carries same concerns as terbutaline

FOLLOWUP

PATIENT MONITORING
- Inpatient followup
- Outpatient care with frequent visits

PREVENTION/AVOIDANCE
- Decrease activity to avoid rebleeding
- All vaginal exams, sexual intercourse, douching, or other vaginal manipulation may cause rebleeding

POSSIBLE COMPLICATIONS
- Maternal mortality is rare with cesarean section available. Greatest fetal risk is preterm delivery.
- Attempted tocolysis may compromise maternal status
- Rebleeding risk may be more risky than delivery and management
- If previa present after 30 weeks, there is greater risk of persisting previa
- Placental accreta strongly associated with placenta previa (up to 15% of patients). Higher incidence in women with placenta previa and multiple prior cesarean sections
- Vasa previa
- IUGR - 16% incidence
- Congenital anomalies: Most common major anomalies of the central nervous system, cardiovascular system, respiratory and gastrointestinal tracts.
- Fetal anemia and Rh isoimmunization

EXPECTED COURSE/PROGNOSIS
- If term and complete or partial: Cesarean delivery
- If term and anterior marginal: Trial of labor may be okay
- If preterm and maternal and fetal status stable: May observe and delay delivery

MISCELLANEOUS

ASSOCIATED CONDITIONS
- Abnormal presentations such as oblique and/or transverse lie
- Persistent high fetal station
- Postpartum hemorrhage
- Increased incidence of small for gestational age (SGA) babies with previas

AGE-RELATED FACTORS
Pediatric: N/A
Geriatric: N/A
Others: Advanced maternal age increases risk

PREGNANCY   As above

SYNONYMS   N/A

ICD-9-CM
641.0 Placenta previa without hemorrhage
641.1 Hemorrhage from placenta previa
641.2 Premature separation of placenta
762.1 Premature separation of placenta (when causing newborn complications)

SEE ALSO
- Abruptio placentae

OTHER NOTES   N/A

ABBREVIATIONS
DIC = disseminated intravascular coagulation
L/S ratio = lecithin/sphingomyelin ratio
PT = prothrombin time
PTT = partial thromboplastin time

REFERENCES
- Cunninghma FG, et al: Williams Obstetrics. Norwalk, CT, Appleton-Century-Crofts, 1993:836-841
- Lavery JP: Placenta Previa. Obstetrics and Gyn 1990;33(3)
- Creasy RD, Resnik R: Maternal - Fetal Medicine, 3rd ed. WB Saunders Company 1994;602-609
- Anath CV, et al: The association of placenta previa with history of cesarean delivery and abortion: A meta-analysis. Am J Obstect Gynecol Nov 1997;1071-1078
- Baron F, et al: Placenta previa, placenta abruptio. Clin Ob Gyn, Vol 41, No3, 1998;527-532
Illustrations: N/A
Internet references: http://www.5mcc.com

Author(s)
Sandra M. Sulik, MD

Plague

BASICS

DESCRIPTION
- Acute infection
- Sporadic limited geographic distribution, especially Third World nations and Southwestern USA
- Epidemics associated with war, famine, and disaster
- Disease of rats and other small vertebrates
- Transmitted to humans by rat flea or human flea
- Occasional transmission to humans handling infected tissues
- Occasional human to human transmission by pulmonary secretions
- Recently shown that infected cats may transmit disease to humans by bite, licking or scratch

System(s) affected:
Hemic/Lymphatic/Immunologic, Skin/Exocrine, Pulmonary
Genetics: N/A
Incidence/Prevalence in USA: Few cases annually in Southwestern states, usually Spring, Summer, Fall
Predominant age: N/A
Predominant sex: Male = Female

SIGNS AND SYMPTOMS
- Bubonic plague
  ◊ Acute onset after 2-8 days incubation
  ◊ Fever
  ◊ Chills
  ◊ Weakness
  ◊ Headache
  ◊ Bubo - painful, very tender enlargement of regional lymph node(s) draining inoculation site. Overlying edema. Typically, absence of overlying skin lesion, ascending lymphangitis.
  ◊ Skin lesions - pustules, vesicles, eschars in area of flea bite(s), purpura
- Septicemic plague
  ◊ Features of bubonic plague
  ◊ Occasional occurrence without bubo
  ◊ Hypotension
  ◊ Hepatosplenomegaly
  ◊ Delirium
  ◊ Seizures in children
  ◊ Shock
- Secondary pneumonic plague
  ◊ Features of bubonic and septicemic plague
  ◊ Cough
  ◊ Chest pain
  ◊ Hemoptysis
- Primary pneumonic plague
  ◊ Acute onset within hours to one day after inhalation of bacteria
  ◊ Fever
  ◊ Chills
  ◊ Cough
  ◊ Chest pain
  ◊ Dyspnea
  ◊ Hemoptysis
  ◊ Lethargy
  ◊ Hypotension
  ◊ Shock

CAUSES
- Yersinia pestis, transmitted by bite of a flea from an infected rodent; secondary - other infected animal or human contact
- Untreated bubonic plague may progress to secondary pneumonic type which can be transmitted by contaminated respiratory droplets

RISK FACTORS
- Exposure to rats and fleas
- Close contact with infected cat
- Close contact with pneumonic plague patient
- Plague bacillus in laboratory
- Hunters who skin wild animals

DIAGNOSIS

DIFFERENTIAL DIAGNOSIS
Other causes of fulminant bacteremia, pneumococcal sepsis, meningococcemia; other causes of acute suppurative lymphadenitis (bubo), or rapidly pregoressive pneumonitis

LABORATORY
- Elevated white cell count, predominantly mature and immature neutrophils. Leukemoid reaction sometimes.
- Stained smears of aspirate of bubo, sputum, peripheral blood reveal gram-negative coccobacilli with bipolar staining, "safety pin" appearance
- Aspirate, blood, sputum cultures (infusion broth, blood and MacConkey agar) grow typical bacteria. Public health authorities arrange definitive identification and serological followup.

Drugs that may alter lab results:
Antibiotics - prior use of antibiotics
Disorders that may alter lab results: N/A

PATHOLOGICAL FINDINGS
Acute lymphadenitis with inflammation dominated by neutrophils, necrosis, masses of plague bacilli, seropurulent pericarditis

SPECIAL TESTS
Low platelet number; evidence of disseminated intravascular coagulation may be seen

IMAGING
Chest x-ray - patchy or confluent pulmonary consolidation in pneumonic plague

DIAGNOSTIC PROCEDURES
N/A

TREATMENT

APPROPRIATE HEALTH CARE
Hospitalization. For suspected pneumonic plague, respiratory isolation until 48 hours after initial effective therapy or after sputum negative.

GENERAL MEASURES
- Do not create aerosol
- Handle blood and bubo aspirate with gloves
- Notify laboratory to take precautions
- Intravenous fluids as required
- Hot, moist compresses for buboes

SURGICAL MEASURES
N/A

ACTIVITY
Bedrest until convalescent

DIET
As tolerated during recovery

PATIENT EDUCATION
- Avoid contact with wild animals
- Reduce rat and flea population in environment

Plague

MEDICATIONS

DRUG(S) OF CHOICE
• Aminoglycoside (gentamicin 5.1 mg/kg/day or streptomycin 15 mg/kg)
• If condition allows oral medication: tetracycline 25-50 mg/kg/day, equally divided, every 6 hours for 10 days
• For meningitis: chloramphenicol 25 mg/kg followed by 60 mg/kg in 4 equally divided doses, daily for 10 days
• Fluoroquinolones (levofloxacin, ofloxacin) and third generation cephalosporins (cefotaxime) may also be effective
Contraindications: Tetracyclines - contraindicated in pregnancy and ages under 8
Precautions:
• Reduce dose of aminoglycoside for renal impairment
• Pregnant women and those with hearing disorders (aminoglycosides)
• Chloramphenicol associated with hematologic toxicity
Significant possible interactions: N/A

ALTERNATIVE DRUGS   None
demonstrated to be as effective or less toxic

FOLLOWUP

PATIENT MONITORING
• CBC for hematologic toxicity of chloramphenicol
• Aminoglycoside blood levels if indicated
• Clinical testing for antibiotic toxicity if indicated

PREVENTION/AVOIDANCE
• Avoid contact with vectors, infected tissue or aerosol, e.g., pneumonic plague case
• Killed vaccine for people at high risk to reduce risk and/or severity; tetracycline prophylaxis. Vaccine available from C.D.C., Atlanta.

POSSIBLE COMPLICATIONS
• Progression of bubonic form to septicemic and pneumonic forms
• Necrosis of bubo may require aspiration or incision and drainage
• Pericarditis
• Adult respiratory distress syndrome
• Meningitis
• Death

EXPECTED COURSE/PROGNOSIS
• Untreated plague mortality > 50%; 100% in primary pneumonic plague
• Plague may be fulminant, e.g., exposure, first symptoms and death in one day in primary pneumonic plague. Must not delay treatment of suspected cases until laboratory-confirmed diagnosis. Delay of initial therapy beyond 24 hours after onset of primary pneumonic plague regularly followed by death.

MISCELLANEOUS

ASSOCIATED CONDITIONS N/A

AGE-RELATED FACTORS N/A
Pediatric: N/A
Geriatric: N/A
Others: N/A

PREGNANCY N/A

SYNONYMS Black death

ICD-9-CM
020.0 Bubonic plague
020.2 Septicemic plague
020.5 Unspecified pneumonic plague
020.3 Primary pneumonic plague
020.4 Secondary pneumonic plague

SEE ALSO N/A

OTHER NOTES N/A

ABBREVIATIONS N/A

REFERENCES
• Mandell GL, Douglas RG, Bennett JE, eds: Principles and Practice of Infectious Diseases. 4th Ed. New York, Churchill Livingstone, 1995
• Freem JA, et al. Invitro activities of 14 antibiotics against 100 human isolates of Yersinia pestis from a southern African plague focus. Antimicrobial Agents & Chemotherapy 1996;40:2646-2647
• Anonymous. Human plague in 1995. Weekly Epidemiological Record 1997;S72:344-347
Illustrations: N/A
Internet references: http://www.5mcc.com
•
Author(s)
D. W. MacPherson, MD, MSc (CTM), FRCPC

Pleural effusion

BASICS

DESCRIPTION A pleural effusion occurs when there is excessive fluid released into the pleural space or if there is lymphatic obstruction precluding normal drainage. Under normal conditions there is a small volume of pleural fluid in the pleural space which functions as a lubricant. Under pathological conditions, effusions develop and are classified as either transudates or exudates. Transudates are due to an imbalance between hydrostatic and oncotic pressures (as in hepatic cirrhosis, congestive heart failure, nephrotic syndrome, and obstruction of the superior vena cava). Exudates are secondary to a disturbance of the systems regulating pleural fluid formation and absorption/drainage (as in bacterial, viral, or fungal infection, rheumatologic disease, or malignancy). Distinguishing between these types of effusions, when etiology is uncertain or if there is inadequate response to therapy, can be helpful.
System(s) affected: Pulmonary, Cardiovascular
Genetics: N/A
Incidence/Prevalence in USA: Not known
Predominant age: Can occur at any age
Predominant sex: Male = Female

SIGNS AND SYMPTOMS
• None in small volume effusion
• Pleuritic chest pain and referred abdominal or shoulder pain
• Cough, may be productive or nonproductive, depending on etiology
• Chest wall splinting
• Dyspnea
• Tachypnea, particularly with lung compression or more severe infections
• Diminished chest wall excursion
• Decreased tactile fremitus
• Dullness to percussion over effusion
• Diminished or absent breath sounds
• Friction rub
• Chills
• Mediastinal shift (on chest radiograph)
• Weight loss
• Night sweats
• Hemoptysis
• Anorexia
• General malaise

CAUSES
• Congestive heart failure, effusion usually bilateral, but if unilateral R > L.
• Hypoalbuminemic states (cirrhosis, nephrotic syndrome)
• Constrictive pericarditis
• Dressler's syndrome with pericardial effusion
• Infection: parapneumonic effusion or empyema. Etiologic agents include bacteria, viruses, fungi, Mycoplasma, parasites, and tuberculosis. Empyema usually caused by polymicrobial anaerobic infection, Pseudomonas, Staphylococcus aureus, Escherichia coli, and occasionally Streptococcus pneumoniae.
• Pulmonary embolism/infarction

• Neoplastic processes: mesothelioma from asbestos exposure, bronchogenic carcinoma, breast carcinoma, lymphoma, leukemia, metastatic disease
• Rheumatologic disease (systemic lupus erythematosus, rheumatoid arthritis)
• Pancreatitis (left-sided exudate with high amylase concentration)
• Esophageal rupture
• Drug reaction, possibly accompanied by eosinophilia
• Uremia
• Atelectasis
• Meig's syndrome
• Subdiaphragmatic abscess
• Cirrhosis with ascites
• Chylous or pseudochylous effusion (thoracic duct injury)
• Trauma leading to intrapleural hemorrhage
• Idiopathic

RISK FACTORS N/A

DIAGNOSIS

DIFFERENTIAL DIAGNOSIS See causes

LABORATORY
• Leukocytosis with bandemia
• Anemia
• Hypoalbuminemia
• ANA titer
• Rheumatoid factor
• Pancreatic enzymes
• CA-125
• CA-19-9
• Creatinine/BUN
• Aerobic/anaerobic blood cultures
• Microbial cultures of pleural effusion fluid
Drugs that may alter lab results: N/A
Disorders that may alter lab results: N/A

PATHOLOGICAL FINDINGS See causes

SPECIAL TESTS
• Evaluation of pleural fluid withdrawn by thoracentesis. Transudates and exudates must be distinguished. A transudate has none of the following characteristics; however, an exudate must meet one:
  ◊ Pleural fluid protein/serum protein
  ◊ Pleural fluid LDH/serum LDH > 0.6
  ◊ Pleural fluid LDH > 2/3 upper limit of that in serum
• All exudates must be evaluated for:
  ◊ Differential cell count
  ◊ Amylase level
  ◊ Glucose level
  ◊ Comprehensive microbiologic culturing and Gram staining
  ◊ Cytology for tumor cells
• Additional studies: pH, RBC count (hemorrhagic effusion if > 100,000/cc, consider trauma as etiology for effusion).

IMAGING
• Chest radiography: AP and lateral decubitus views
• Thoracic ultrasound
• CT scan

DIAGNOSTIC PROCEDURES
• Pleural biopsy if suspicion of tuberculosis or neoplasm
• Thoracentesis
• Thoracoscopy (provides direct view of both parietal and visceral aspects of pleura)

TREATMENT

APPROPRIATE HEALTH CARE
Inpatient

GENERAL MEASURES
• Supportive care
  ◊ Supplemental oxygen
  ◊ IV fluid hydration
  ◊ Chest physiotherapy
  ◊ Therapeutic/diagnostic thoracentesis
• Antibiotics
  ◊ Empirically by age/social circumstances and modified by blood and pleural effusion fluid culture results
• Empyema
  ◊ Consider antibiotics alone with close monitoring in children
  ◊ Antibiotics with chest tube drainage in adults
  ◊ Pleurectomy in cases of trapped lung
• Pleural fluid loculation
  ◊ May inject 250,000 units of streptokinase or 100,000 units of urokinase intrapleurally to dissolve fibrin meshes creating loculation. If unsuccessful, then either thoracoscopic adhesiolysis or decortication via thoracotomy are indicated.
• Malignancy
  ◊ Consider treatment of primary source. However, most malignancies accompanied by malignant pleural effusions are advanced and cure is unlikely with chemotherapeutic intervention.
  ◊ If effusion is causing dyspnea, perform therapeutic thoracentesis and, if fluid reaccumulates rapidly, then place chest tube for continuous drainage.
  ◊ Other therapeutic interventions include placement of a pleuroperitoneal shunt and chemical pleurodesis
• Chylothorax - radiation therapy if from malignant cause or surgical repair of thoracic duct trauma.
• Hemothorax - diagnosed if hematocrit of pleural fluid > 50% that seen in blood. Usually caused by trauma or rupture of a tumor. Drainage via tube thoracostomy indicated. If bleeding persists or is of high volume then emergent thoracotomy is indicated

SURGICAL MEASURES See General Measures

ACTIVITY As tolerated

DIET Depends on clinical circumstances

PATIENT EDUCATION American Lung Association, 1740 Broadway, New York, New York 10038

MEDICATIONS

DRUG(S) OF CHOICE
• Antimicrobial therapy according to pathogens and associated sensitivities
• Chemical pleurodesis with doxycycline 500 mg, bleomycin 60 units, or talc in a slurry, as indicated
• Chemotherapy according to current oncologic protocols
• Steroids and nonsteroidal anti-inflammatory drugs for rheumatologic and inflammatory etiologies
• Diuresis as appropriate for effusions secondary to congestive heart failure and ascites
Contraindications: Refer to manufacturer's drug profiles
Precautions: Refer to manufacturer's drug profiles
Significant possible interactions: Refer to manufacturer's drug profiles

ALTERNATIVE DRUGS   N/A

FOLLOWUP

PATIENT MONITORING
• Serial chest radiographs, with frequency/interval determined by patient status/diagnosis
• Pulmonary function testing as indicated
• Serum studies, echocardiography, renal/hepatic function tests as indicated to monitor for stability/progression of nonmalignant/noninfectious factors precipitating effusions

PREVENTION/AVOIDANCE   N/A

POSSIBLE COMPLICATIONS
• Chronic empyema
• Drainage through chest wall - pleurocutaneous fistula
• Bronchopleural fistula
• Toxic shock syndrome

EXPECTED COURSE/PROGNOSIS
Mortality rate around 20% for exudative effusions; worse for elderly patients or those with serious underlying conditions

MISCELLANEOUS

ASSOCIATED CONDITIONS   N/A

AGE-RELATED FACTORS   N/A
Pediatric: N/A
Geriatric: N/A
Others: N/A

PREGNANCY   N/A

SYNONYMS   N/A

ICD-9-CM
511.9 Unspecified pleural effusion
511.1 Pleurisy with effusion, with mention of a bacterial cause other than tuberculosis
197.2 Secondary malignant neoplasm of respiratory and digestive system, pleura

SEE ALSO   N/A

OTHER NOTES   N/A

ABBREVIATIONS   N/A

REFERENCES
• Dowdeswell I. Pleural Diseases. In Internal Medicine (Stein J et al., eds). 5th Ed. St. Louis, Mosby, 1998
• Kendig R, Chernick V. Disorders of the Respiratory Tract in Children 5th Ed. Philadelphia, WB Saunders Co., 1990
• Light RW: Disorders of the pleura, mediastinum and diaphragm. In: Fauci AS, et al, eds: Harrison's Textbook of Internal Medicine. New York, McGraw Hill, 1998
Illustrations: N/A
Internet references: http://www.5mcc.com

Author(s)
Peter P. Toth, MD, PhD

Pneumonia, bacterial

BASICS

DESCRIPTION An acute, bacterial infection of the lung parenchyma. Infection may be community-acquired or nosocomial (hospital acquired by an inpatient for at least 48 hours or inpatient in the previous 1-3 weeks). Most commonly, community-acquired disease is caused by Streptococcus pneumoniae or Mycoplasma pneumoniae. Hospital-acquired pneumonia is usually due to gram negative rods (60%) such as Pseudomonas; 14.5% from Staphylococcus.

System(s) affected: Pulmonary
Genetics: No known genetic pattern
Incidence/Prevalence in USA:
• Incidence - community-acquired: 1200 cases/100,000 population per year
• Incidence - nosocomial: 800 cases/100,000 admissions per year
Predominant age: Age extremes
Predominant sex: Male > Female

SIGNS AND SYMPTOMS
• Cardinal signs and symptoms
  ◊ Cough and fever
  ◊ Chest pain (pleuritic)
  ◊ Chill, with sudden onset
  ◊ Dark, thick or bloody (rusty) sputum
• Respiratory
  ◊ Signs of consolidation
    - Rales
    - Egophony
  ◊ Signs of pleural involvement
    - Decreased breath sounds
    - Dullness to percussion
    - Friction rub
• Signs of respiratory distress
  ◊ Tachypnea/tachycardia (or bradycardia)
  ◊ Cyanosis
• Central nervous system
  ◊ Mentation changes to include anxiety, confusion and restlessness
• Gastrointestinal
  ◊ Abdominal pain
  ◊ Anorexia

CAUSES
• Sources
  ◊ Aspiration from the oropharynx
  ◊ Inhalation
  ◊ Hematogenous spread
• Bacterial pathogens
  ◊ Streptococcus pneumoniae (pneumococcus)
  ◊ Haemophilus influenzae
  ◊ Mycoplasma pneumoniae
  ◊ Staphylococcus aureus
  ◊ Legionella pneumophila
  ◊ Chlamydia pneumoniae, C. psittaci
  ◊ *Moraxella catarrhalis* (Branhamella catarrhalis)
  ◊ *Pseudomonas aeruginosa*
  ◊ *Klebsiella pneumoniae* (and other gram-negative rods)
  ◊ Anaerobes

RISK FACTORS
• Recent/concurrent viral infections
• Hospitalization to include mechanical ventilation, antecedent antibiotics, NG tubes
• Age extremes
• Alcoholism
• AIDS or other immunosuppression
• Tobacco smoking
• Renal failure
• Cardiovascular disease
• Functional asplenia
• Chronic obstructive pulmonary disease
• Diabetes mellitus
• Malnutrition
• Malignancy
• Altered level of consciousness or gag (e.g., seizures, stroke, neuromuscular disease, etc.)
• Occupational exposure
• Poorly implemented infection control practices

DIAGNOSIS

DIFFERENTIAL DIAGNOSIS Other causes of infectious pneumonitis: Viruses (respiratory syncytial, adenovirus, CMV, parainfluenza, influenzae A and B, varicella, measles, rubella, hantavirus); Nocardia; Fungi (Blastomyces, Cryptococcus, Aspergillus, Histoplasma, Coccidioides, Pneumocystis carinii); Protozoans (Toxoplasma); Rickettsia (Coxiella burnetii - Q fever). Also tuberculosis, pulmonary embolism with infarction, bronchiolitis obliterans with organizing pneumonia (BOOP), pulmonary contusion, pulmonary vasculitis, acute sarcoid, hypersensitivity pneumonitis, ARDS, pneumothorax, and other causes.

LABORATORY
• Leukocytosis with an immature shift on differential
• Hyponatremia (SIADH)
• Hypoxemia
• Hypocapnia initially, then hypercapnia
• Blood culture - positive in 10-20% of patients with community-acquired pneumonia, 8-20% nosocomial pneumonia
Drugs that may alter lab results:
Antecedent antibiotics
Disorders that may alter lab results:
Refer to lab test reference

PATHOLOGICAL FINDINGS
• Lung:
  ◊ Segmental, lobar, or multifocal peribronchial consolidation
  ◊ Positive gram stain for bacteria

SPECIAL TESTS
• Decubitus chest roentgenograms to investigate for empyema or parapneumonic effusion
• Gram stain and culture of pleural fluid
• pH of pleural fluid (iced, airless sample sent to blood gas laboratory)

IMAGING
• Chest roentgenogram (with lateral decubitus views if pleural effusion present)
  ◊ Lobar or segmental consolidation (air bronchogram)
    ◊ Bronchopneumonia
    ◊ Interstitial infiltrate
    ◊ Pleural effusion (free-flowing or loculated)

DIAGNOSTIC PROCEDURES
• Gram stain and culture of sputum (induced, if necessary)
• Nasotracheal suctioning for culture
• Transtracheal aspirate for culture
• Bronchoscopy with bronchoalveolar lavage or protected telescoping catheter brushing for culture
• Thoracentesis for pleural fluid studies
• Blood culture, especially if hospitalized - prior to antibiotics

TREATMENT

APPROPRIATE HEALTH CARE
• Community-acquired - outpatient for mild case, inpatient for moderate to severe case such as hypoxemia, altered mental status, hypotension, significant co-morbid illness, and age extremes.
• Nosocomial - patients already hospitalized

GENERAL MEASURES
• Empiric antimicrobial therapy for most likely pathogen(s)
• Consider oxygen for patients with cyanosis, hypoxia, dyspnea, circulatory disturbances or delirium
• Mechanical ventilation for respiratory failure
• Chest physiotherapy
• Hydration
• Nasotracheal suction
• Analgesia for pain
• Electrolyte correction
• Respiratory isolation if TB is a possibility

SURGICAL MEASURES   N/A

ACTIVITY   Bedrest and/or reduced activity during acute phase

DIET
• Nothing by mouth if there is incipient respiratory failure
• Consider soft, easy-to-eat foods

PATIENT EDUCATION   Printed patient information available from: American Lung Association, 1740 Broadway, New York, NY 100019 (212)315-8700; web site http://www.lungusa.org

MEDICATIONS

DRUG(S) OF CHOICE

• Initial therapy
◊ Usually empiric for most likely pathogens given clinical scenario (if specific etiology is identified, adjust antimicrobial therapy)
◊ Otherwise healthy young adult with mild community-acquired pneumonia: erythromycin 500 po q6h (the new macrolides should be considered in those intolerant of erythromycin or doxycycline and in smokers [to treat H. influenzae])
◊ Older patients or patients with preexistent illnesses, with mild community-acquired pneumonia: pneumococcal-active fluoroquinolone or 2nd generation cephalosporin or amoxicillin-clavulanate with or without erythromycin or other macrolide
◊ Patients with community-acquired pneumonia requiring hospitalization: second or third generation cephalosporin or beta-lactam/beta-lactamase inhibitor plus macrolide or a pneumococcal-active fluoroquinolone
◊ For nosocomial pneumonia: either ceftazidime or an antipseudomonal penicillin (piperacillin, mezlocillin, or ticarcillin) plus an aminoglycoside. Vancomycin should be considered if strong suspicion of Staphylococcus aureus.
• Therapy for specific organisms
◊ S. pneumoniae: penicillin G or oral amoxicillin/penicillin V. If high incidence of penicillin resistant S. pneumoniae in the area, consider either vancomycin or pneumococcal-active fluoroquinolone
◊ H. influenzae: trimethoprim-sulfamethoxazole. For severe infections - cefotaxime, ceftriaxone, or carbapenems
◊ S. aureus: nafcillin; vancomycin (if high incidence of methicillin resistant S. aureus)
◊ Klebsiella species: carbapenems, 3rd generation cephalosporin
◊ Pseudomonas: aminoglycoside plus antipseudomonal penicillin or ceftazidime
◊ Moraxella catarrhalis: 2nd generation cephalosporin (cefuroxime axetil), ß-lactam/ß-lactamase inhibitors
◊ Chlamydia pneumoniae: doxycycline, fluoroquinolone
◊ Mycoplasma pneumoniae: erythromycin, fluoroquinolone
◊ Legionella pneumophila: erythromycin (add rifampin for documented disease), fluoroquinolone
◊ Anaerobes: clindamycin, ß-lactam/ß-lactamase inhibitors
Contraindications: Allergy or likely cross-allergy to the prescribed antibiotic

Precautions: Possible significant sodium overload with antipseudomonal penicillins
Significant possible interactions: Refer to manufacturer's literature

ALTERNATIVE DRUGS

• S. pneumoniae: erythromycin; cephalosporin
• H. influenzae: cefuroxime; fluoroquinolones; extended macrolides; beta-lactam/beta-lactamase inhibitor
• S. aureus: a first generation cephalosporin; clindamycin
• Klebsiella: fluoroquinolone
• Pseudomonas: carbapenems, aztreonam
• Moraxella catarrhalis: trimethoprim-sulfamethoxazole; fluoroquinolone; cefixime, extended macrolide
• Chlamydia pneumoniae: clarithromycin; azithromycin
• Mycoplasma pneumoniae: clarithromycin; doxycycline; azithromycin
• Legionella pneumophila: clarithromycin; azithromycin; doxycycline

FOLLOWUP

PATIENT MONITORING

• If outpatient therapy, daily assessment of the patient's progress, and reassessment of therapy if clinical worsening or no improvement in 48-72 hours
• Chest roentgenograms take time to clear and may not show clearing, even though patient is improving. Repeat study about 9 weeks after recovery to verify the pneumonia was not caused by an obstructing endobronchial lesion in selected patients.
• Repeating the cultures after treatment has been started is unnecessary unless there has been treatment failure or if treating TB

PREVENTION/AVOIDANCE

• Reduce risk factors where possible
• Bedridden and postoperative patients - deep breathing and coughing exercises; prevent aspiration during nasogastric tube feedings
• Avoid indiscriminate use of antibiotics during minor viral infections
• Annual influenza vaccine for high risk individuals
• Polyvalent pneumococcal vaccine

POSSIBLE COMPLICATIONS

• Empyema
• Pulmonary abscess
• Superinfections
• Multiple organ dysfunction syndrome (MODS)
• Adult respiratory distress syndrome (ARDS)

EXPECTED COURSE/PROGNOSIS

• Usual course - acute. In otherwise healthy individual, improvement seen and fever resolved in 1-3 days; sometimes up to 1 week
• Overall mortality is about 5% in community acquired; (~15% if hospitalized and < 1% if not hospitalized) 30-50% in nosocomial
• Poorest prognosis - age extremes, positive blood cultures, low WBC, presence of associated disease, immunosuppression respiratory failure, inappropriate antecedent antibiotics, delayed treatment >8 hours

MISCELLANEOUS

ASSOCIATED CONDITIONS

• Alcoholism
• Tobacco smoking
• Upper respiratory infection

AGE-RELATED FACTORS

Pediatric: Morbidity and mortality high in children under age 1
Geriatric: Morbidity and mortality high if > 70, especially if associated disease or risk factor
Others: N/A

PREGNANCY   N/A

SYNONYMS

• Lobar pneumonia
• Classic pneumococcal pneumonia

ICD-9-CM   481 Pneumococcal pneumonia

SEE ALSO

• Pneumonia, viral
• Pneumonia, mycoplasma
• Rhodococcus infections

OTHER NOTES   Pneumococcal vaccine for all adults over age 65 and children over 2 years (and adults) with risk (cardio, pulmonary or metabolic disorders)

ABBREVIATIONS   N/A

REFERENCES

• Bartlett JD, Mundy LM: Community-acquired pneumonia. N Engl J Med 1995;333:1618-1624
• Laforce FM: Antibacterial therapy for lower respiratory tract infections in adults - A review. Clin Infect Dis 1992;14(S2):S233-237
• American Thoracic Society: Guidelines for the initial management of adults with community-acquired pneumonia. Am Rev Respir Dis 1993;148:1418-1426
• American Thoracic Society: Hospital acquired pneumonia in adults: diagnosis, assessment of severity, initial antimicrobial therapy, and preventive strategies. Am J Res Crit Care 1996;153:1711-1725
• Bartlett JD, et al: Community acquired pneumonia in adults: guidelines for management. Clin Infect Dis 1998;26:811-838
Illustrations: N/A
Internet references: http://www.5mcc.com

Author(s)
James K. Radike, MD
Ronald A. Greenfield, MD

Pneumonia, mycoplasma

BASICS

DESCRIPTION Interstitial pneumonia caused by extensive infection of the lungs and bronchi, particularly the lower lobes of the lungs, by Mycoplasma pneumoniae. Usual course - acute. Incubation period is about 18-21 days and includes prodromal symptoms.
• Little seasonal variation of incidence, therefore a greater percentage of pneumonia in summer and fall are from Mycoplasma. Epidemics in communities tend to be prolonged (over many months) and occur every 4-5 years.
System(s) affected: Pulmonary
Genetics: None
Incidence/Prevalence in USA:
• 130 cases/100,000 people
• Estimated to be most common cause of pneumonia in school children and young adults (without chronic underlying condition). The incidence varies considerably each year. Major outbreaks are repeated every 3-5 years.
Predominant age: Ages 5-15, but occurs at any age
Predominant sex: Male > Female

SIGNS AND SYMPTOMS
• Gradual onset with upper respiratory infection symptoms that progress
• Most will develop fever, cough, headache, sore throat, rales, and wheeze
• Many will develop myalgias, nasal congestion, chest pain
• Some will develop pleural effusion, pleural friction rub, cervical adenopathy, bullous myringitis, skin rash

CAUSES Mycoplasma pneumoniae infection

RISK FACTORS
• Close community living (e.g., hospitals, prisons, military bases, fraternity houses). Some of largest outbreaks have been in army recruits.
• Family exposure
• Immunocompromised patients

DIAGNOSIS

DIFFERENTIAL DIAGNOSIS
• Viral pneumonia
• Bacterial pneumonia (including plague and tularemia in severe cases)
• Fungal pneumonias
• *Pneumocystis carinii* pneumonia
• Chlamydia pneumonia, TWAR or psittaci
• Legionella pneumonia

LABORATORY
• Increased sedimentation rate
• Positive cold agglutinins (titer of 1:258 or greater; or rising fourfold) in 50% of infections
• False-positive VDRL
• M. pneumoniae culture (requires 7-10 days)
• Peripheral white blood cell count - normal
• Complement fixation serologic assay shows fourfold rise in titer at 2-4 weeks after symptom onset
• IgM antibody to M. pneumoniae in 80% of patients after 1-2 weeks of illness (enzyme immunoassay)
Drugs that may alter lab results: N/A
Disorders that may alter lab results: N/A

PATHOLOGICAL FINDINGS Absence of bacterial pathogens on Gram stain and culture of sputum or transtracheal aspirate. Mycoplasma is a fastidious and slow-growing organism.

SPECIAL TESTS Radiolabeled DNA probe which detects M. pneumoniae ribosomal RNA in respiratory secretions, 90% sensitive

IMAGING Chest x-ray - diffuse interstitial infiltrates; small bilateral pleural effusion present in 25% of cases

DIAGNOSTIC PROCEDURES N/A

TREATMENT

APPROPRIATE HEALTH CARE
Outpatient usually; inpatient if symptoms severe

GENERAL MEASURES N/A

SURGICAL MEASURES N/A

ACTIVITY Rest during acute phase

DIET Drink plenty of fluids

PATIENT EDUCATION Printed patient information available from American Lung Association, 1740 Broadway, New York, NY 10019, (212)315-8700

MEDICATIONS

DRUG(S) OF CHOICE
• Erythromycin - children 30-50 mg/kg/day for 10-14 days; adults 500 mg every 6 hours for 10-14 days
• Clarithromycin - children 15 mg/kg/d for 10-14 days; adults 500 mg bid for 10-14 days or azithromycin - children 10 mg/kg po first day, 5 mg/kg po for days 2-5; adults 500 mg first day, then 250 mg every day for 5 days. These newer macrolides might be used first if H. influenza is also suspected.
• Antibiotics such as penicillins are ineffective against M. pneumoniae

Contraindications: Refer to manufacturer's literature

Precautions: Refer to manufacturer's literature

Significant possible interactions:
Erythromycin and other macrolides inhibit the cytochrome P-450 microsomal enzyme system and can reduce elimination of other drugs such as carbamazepine, phenytoin, lovastatin, and theophylline. Prolongation of the QT interval and ventricular tachycardia has occurred in some patients receiving astemizide or terfenadine concomitantly with erythromycin.

ALTERNATIVE DRUGS
• Quinolones (Levofloxacin, Sparfloxacin) show good activity against Mycoplasma
• Adjunctive drugs - albuterol inhaler, 2 puffs qid for wheezing
• Children 9 yr and older - doxycycline 100 mg po bid

FOLLOWUP

PATIENT MONITORING
• Phone or in person followup
• Clearing of chest x-ray should be documented if the patient is older than 50. In smokers, document a clear x-ray in 6-8 weeks.

PREVENTION/AVOIDANCE   Isolation of
active cases. M. pneumoniae is carried in respiratory droplets. Antibiotic prophylaxis of contacts is not indicated.

POSSIBLE COMPLICATIONS
Note: All complications are rare except reactive airway disease, hemolytic anemia, and erythema multiforme.
• Reactive airway disease
• Hemolytic anemia
• Erythema multiforme
• Meningoencephalitis
• Polyneuritis
• Polyarthritis
• Stevens-Johnson syndrome
• Pericarditis
• Myocarditis
• Respiratory distress syndrome
• Cerebral ataxia
• Thromboembolic phenomena
• Pleural effusion

EXPECTED COURSE/PROGNOSIS
• Mycoplasma infection symptoms usually resolve in about 2 weeks
• Some constitutional symptoms may persist for several weeks
• With correct therapy, even most severe cases can expect complete recovery

MISCELLANEOUS

ASSOCIATED CONDITIONS   N/A

AGE-RELATED FACTORS
Pediatric:
• Unusual in infants
• M. pneumoniae is associated with an increased incidence of asthma attacks in older children
Geriatric: Unusual in this age group
Others: N/A

PREGNANCY   Tetracycline contraindicated
in pregnancy

SYNONYMS
• Primary atypical pneumonia (PAP)
• Eaton agent pneumonia
• Cold agglutinin-positive pneumonia

ICD-9-CM   483 Mycoplasma pneumonia

SEE ALSO
• Pneumonia, bacterial
• Pneumonia, viral
• Pneumonia, pneumocystis carinii (PCP)

OTHER NOTES   N/A

ABBREVIATIONS   N/A

REFERENCES
• Mandell GL, ed: Principles and Practice of Infectious Diseases. 4th Ed. New York, Churchill Livingstone, 1995
• Luby JP: Pneumonia caused by Mycoplasma pneumonia infection. Clinics in Chest Medicine 1991;12:237-99
• Luthan-Sadler BA, Morell VW: Viral and atypical pneumonias. Primary Care 1996;23:837-848
• Block S, Hedrick J, et al: Mycoplasma pneumonia and chlamydia pneumonia in pediatric community acquired pneumonia. Ped Infect Dis 1995;14:471-477
• O'handley JG, Gray LD: The incidence of Mycoplasma pneumoniae. J Am Board Fam Pract 1997;10:425-9
Illustrations: N/A
Internet references: http://www.5mcc.com

Author(s)
George R. Bergus, MD
Steven J. Havener, MD

Pneumonia, Pneumocystis carinii (PCP)

BASICS

DESCRIPTION A pneumonia arising in immunosuppressed persons caused by Pneumocystis carinii (PCP). This is one of the most common opportunistic infections occurring in patients with human immunodeficiency virus (HIV) infections. Pneumocystis infection can cause organ involvement and disseminated disease as well as pneumonia.
System(s) affected: Pulmonary
Genetics: N/A
Incidence/Prevalence in USA: PCP is the AIDS indicator disease in 43% of patients; with effective prophylaxis and antiretroviral therapy - incidence is decreasing
Predominant age:
• In HIV infected children, not taking prophylaxis, median age of onset is 5 months of age
• In HIV infected adults, PCP may occur at any age
Predominant sex: Male > Female (reflecting prevalence of HIV infection)

SIGNS AND SYMPTOMS
• Usually insidious but occasionally abrupt in onset
• Dyspnea on exertion progressing to continuous dyspnea
• Weakness, fatigue, malaise
• Fever, chills
• Cough - non-productive or productive of scant white or clear sputum
• Tachypnea
• Extrapulmonary Pneumocystis may occur (visceral, cutaneous, eyes) particularly in patients on aerosolized pentamidine for prophylaxis

CAUSES The ubiquitous Pneumocystis carinii may cause infection in normal hosts (65-100% of young children have positive serology) but will rarely cause symptoms in immunocompetent individuals

RISK FACTORS
• Immunodeficiency (premature infants, neoplasia, congenital, acquired or drug-induced immunodeficiency states, CD4 counts < 200 in adults)
• Patients with a history of previous PCP

DIAGNOSIS

DIFFERENTIAL DIAGNOSIS
• Tuberculosis
• Mycobacterium avium intracellulare
• Viral pneumonias
• Fungal pneumonias
• Lymphoid interstitial pneumonitis (in children)
• Bacterial pneumonia
• CMV pneumonia (cytomegalovirus)

LABORATORY
• Serum LDH frequently elevated (mean elevation of 362 IU)
• Arterial blood gases reveal hypoxemia and increased alveolar-arterial gradient (varies with severity of disease)
• Sputum induced with inhaled 3-5% hypertonic saline may reveal pneumocystis on cytologic evaluation using various stains. An IF (immunofluorescence) technique is also available. (Sensitivity may be as high as 78% in labs with experienced personnel.)
• CD4 cell count generally below 200 in HIV infected patients with PCP.
Drugs that may alter lab results: Inhaled pentamidine used to prevent PCP may change radiographic picture to infiltrates in predominantly upper-lobe distribution
Disorders that may alter lab results: N/A

PATHOLOGICAL FINDINGS
Pneumonitis caused by presence of organism and inflammatory response

SPECIAL TESTS Gallium scanning of the lungs is highly sensitive for PCP but is not very specific. May be useful when sputum studies are inconclusive and bronchoscopy is not available.

IMAGING
• Chest x-ray
  ◊ Shows bilateral diffuse interstitial or perihilar infiltrate in 75% of cases
  ◊ May also show a normal chest x-ray, unilateral disease, pleural effusions, abscesses or cavitations, pneumothorax, and lobar consolidations
  ◊ Upper lobe infiltrates may be present in patients on pentamidine prophylaxis

DIAGNOSTIC PROCEDURES
• Fiberoptic bronchoscopy with bronchoalveolar lavage or transbronchial biopsy is the preferred method of diagnosis when sputums are negative
• Open lung biopsy is rarely required
• A PCR test for pneumocystis may be useful in the future (on sputum, bronchoalveola fluid)

TREATMENT

APPROPRIATE HEALTH CARE
Outpatient in mild cases, otherwise inpatient

GENERAL MEASURES Oxygen therapy often necessary

SURGICAL MEASURES N/A

ACTIVITY As tolerated

DIET No special diet

PATIENT EDUCATION For patient education materials on this topic, contact: American Lung Association, 1740 Broadway, New York, NY 10019, (212)315-8700 or Project Inform - http://www.projinf.org

Pneumonia, Pneumocystis carinii (PCP)

MEDICATIONS

DRUG(S) OF CHOICE
• Trimethoprim-sulfamethoxazole (Bactrim, Septra) 15 mg/kg/day of trimethoprim component po in 3 divided doses or IV for 14-21 days. Reduce dose of trimethoprim-sulfamethoxazole in patients with renal failure.
• Adjunctive corticosteroid (prednisone or methyl prednisolone) therapy begun within 72 hours of diagnosis decreases mortality in AIDS patients (adults and children) with moderate to severe PCP (those with pO2<70 mmHg)
Contraindications: Use with care in pregnant patient and infants less than 2 months
Precautions:
• History of sulfa allergy
• A high percentage of patients with AIDS will develop intolerance to trimethoprim/ sulfamethoxazole. Especially common are dermatologic reactions, hematologic toxicity, or fever.
• Avoid sunlight
Significant possible interactions:
Phenytoin, oral anti-coagulants, oral sulfonylureas, digitalis

ALTERNATIVE DRUGS
• Pentamidine 3 mg/kg/day IV for 14-21 days
• Dapsone 100 mg po daily plus trimethoprim 15 mg/kg/day po in 3-4 divided doses. Check G6PD level before beginning dapsone as hemolysis may result.
• Clindamycin 300-400 mg po tid for 21 days plus primaquine 30 mg po daily for 21 days
• Trimetrexate glucuronate 45 mg/m2 IV qd over 60-90 minutes with leucovorin 20 mg/m2 IV or po q6h - continue for 72 hours after last dose of trimetrexate. Recommended course of therapy is 21 days of trimetrexate and 24 days of leucovorin. Doses may need to be adjusted for hematologic toxicity - monitor CBC/differential and platelets.
• Atovaquone 750 mg po tid or atovaquone suspension 750 mg bid for 21 days

FOLLOWUP

PATIENT MONITORING Serum LDH, pulmonary function tests and arterial blood gases generally normalize with treatment

PREVENTION/AVOIDANCE
• All AIDS patients with a history of PCP (or CD4 cells < 200 or evidence of immunodeficiency) require life-long prophylaxis with daily or thrice-weekly trimethoprim-sulfamethoxazole (double-strength), daily dapsone (100 mg/day biw or twice weekly) or monthly aerosolized pentamidine (300 mg). In patients intolerant of TMP-SMX, consider a rechallenge or desensitization with TMP-SMX - various protocols exist.
• All babies born to HIV infected mothers need to be on prophylaxis after the first month of life. Drug of choice is TMP-SMX; 150 mg/m2/day (TMP component) 3 times weekly. This should be continued until the baby is proven HIV negative or for the first year of life, after which CD4 cell count may be used to guide prophylaxis.

POSSIBLE COMPLICATIONS
• Respiratory failure
• Pneumothorax (even after successful treatment)
• Extrapulmonary pneumocystis (especially in patients on inhaled pentamidine prophylaxis)

EXPECTED COURSE/PROGNOSIS
• Mortality from first episode PCP is 10-15%. With prophylactic therapy, mean survival has increased.
• 40% of patients with PCP will have a recurrence without prophylaxis

MISCELLANEOUS

ASSOCIATED CONDITIONS
• AIDS
• HIV infection

AGE-RELATED FACTORS
Pediatric:
• Early onset (5 months of age) and high mortality (median survival 1 month)
• Important to distinguish from lymphoid interstitial pneumonitis (LIP) as treatment and prognosis differ
• PCP prophylaxis with TMP-SMX, dapsone or pentamidine for all HIV positive children less than 1 year old is recommended. For older HIV positive children, prophylaxis individualized based on CD4 counts (see Prevention/Avoidance section).
Geriatric: N/A
Others: N/A

PREGNANCY
Trimethoprim-sulfamethoxazole has been used for treatment and prophylaxis. Avoid pentamidine.

SYNONYMS
• Pneumocystosis
• Pulmonary pneumocystosis
• Interstitial plasma cell pneumonia

ICD-9-CM 136.3 Pneumocystosis

SEE ALSO
• HIV infection & AIDS

OTHER NOTES N/A

ABBREVIATIONS
• LDH = lactic acid dehydrogenase
• G6PD = glucose 6-phosphate dehydrogenase

REFERENCES
• Miller RF, Mitchell DM. Pneumocystis carinii pneumonia. Thorax 1995;50:191-200
• Sistek CJ, et al: Adjuvant corticosteroid therapy for Pneumocystis carinii pneumonia in AIDS patients. Ann Pharmacother 1992;9:1127-1133
• Simonds RJ, Hughes WT, Feinberg J, et al. Preventing Pneumocystis carinii pneumoni in persons infected with human immunodeficiency virus. Clin Infect Dis 1995;21(suppl 1):544-548
• Gluckstein D, Ruskin J: Rapid oral desensitization to trimethoprim-sulfamethoxazole: use in prophylaxis for pneumocystis carinii pneumonia in patients with AIDS who were previously intolerant of TMP/SMX. Clin Infect Dis 1995;20:849-53
Illustrations: N/A
Internet references: http://www.5mcc.com

Author(s)
Cynthia Gail Carmichael, MD

Pneumonia, viral

BASICS

DESCRIPTION Inflammatory disease of the lungs. Most viral pneumonia results from exposure of a non-immune individual to infected aerosolized secretions.
System(s) affected: Pulmonary
Genetics: No known genetic pattern
Incidence/Prevalence in USA:
• Approximately 90% of childhood pneumonia is viral
• 4-39% of pneumonia in adults has been attributed to viral etiologies in different series
• Prevalence is unknown and variable due to seasonal variation, though more common in winter months
• Mixed infections with bacterial pathogens common
Predominant age:
• More common in children than in adults
Predominant sex: Male = Female

SIGNS AND SYMPTOMS
• Fever
• Chills
• Cough (with or without purulent sputum production)
• Dyspnea
• Pulmonary rales and rhonchi
• Altered breath sounds
• Pleurisy
• Friction rub
• Headache
• Myalgias
• Malaise
• Gastrointestinal symptoms

CAUSES
• Influenza A, B and C
• Parainfluenza 1, 2, 3, and 4
• Respiratory syncytial virus (RSV, especially in young children)
• Adenovirus
• Cytomegalovirus (CMV), particularly in immunocompromised patients)
• Varicella (chickenpox)
• Herpes simplex
• Enterovirus
• Coronavirus
• Rubeola (measles)
• Epstein-Barr virus
• Hanta virus

RISK FACTORS
• Immunocompromised
• Living in close quarters
• Seasonal - epidemic upper respiratory illness
• Elderly
• Cardiac disease
• Chronic pulmonary disease
• Recent upper respiratory infection

DIAGNOSIS

DIFFERENTIAL DIAGNOSIS
• Bacterial pneumonia (especially atypical etiologies - *Chlamydia pneumoniae* and psittaci, *Mycoplasma pneumoniae*, *Legionella pneumophila*)
• Pulmonary edema
• *Pneumocystis carinii* pneumonia (PCP)
• Aspiration pneumonia
• Hypersensitivity pneumonitis
• Bronchial carcinoma with lymphangitic spread
• Bronchiolitis obliterans with organizing pneumonia (BOOP)
• Pulmonary embolus/infarction
• Cystic fibrosis (in infants)

LABORATORY
• Sputum gram stain and culture to identify bacterial co-pathogens if present
• Appropriate direct fluorescent antibody from throat swab, tracheal aspirate, or bronchoalveolar lavage specimens (HSV, VZV, Influenza A and B, RSV, adenovirus)
• Viral culture
• Cytopathology (CMV, HSV, Rubeola)
• Normal or near normal granulocyte count, occasionally leukopenic with increased lymphocyte percentage
• Hypoxemia with severe disease
• Hemoconcentration (Hanta virus)
• Serology (4-fold rise in acute vs convalescent titers)
• Polymerase chain reaction (PCR) detection if available
Drugs that may alter lab results: N/A
Disorders that may alter lab results: N/A

PATHOLOGICAL FINDINGS
• Heavy lungs
• Enlarged regional lymph nodes
• Cytoplasmic inclusion bodies (CMV)
• Intranuclear inclusion bodies (adenovirus, CMV, herpes virus, varicella)
• Intense inflammatory reaction with mononuclear cells
• Multinucleated giant cells (parainfluenza virus, Rubeola, HSV, varicella)

SPECIAL TESTS   N/A

IMAGING
• Chest roentgenogram - interstitial or alveolar infiltrates, peribronchial thickening, pleural effusion

DIAGNOSTIC PROCEDURES
• Nasopharyngeal throat swab
• Tracheal aspiration (seldom needed)
• Bronchoscopy with bronchoalveolar lavage (BAL)

TREATMENT

APPROPRIATE HEALTH CARE
Outpatient for most cases. Inpatient for infants under 4 months of age or elderly, or for any patient with diffuse, severe infection (hypoxemia, hypercarbia, hypotension or shock, adult respiratory distress syndrome) or significant comorbidity (CHF, CAD, COPD, etc.)

GENERAL MEASURES
• Encourage coughing and deep breathing exercises to clear secretions
• Careful disposal of secretions/universal precautions
• Hydration
• Respiratory isolation for varicella which is highly contagious (i.e., negative pressure)

SURGICAL MEASURES   N/A

ACTIVITY
• Rest

DIET
• Increase fluids, high calorie, high protein, soft diet

PATIENT EDUCATION
For patient education materials on this topic, contact: American Lung Association, 1740 Broadway, New York, NY 100919, (212)315-8700

MEDICATIONS

DRUG(S) OF CHOICE
• Amantadine (Symmetrel): Influenza A (not effective for influenza B)
◊ Age < 10: 4-8 mg/kg/day in 2 divided doses. Not to exceed 150 mg/day.
◊ Age 10-65: 100 mg orally q12 h (adults may be given a loading dose of 200 mg initially)
◊ Age > 65: 100 mg orally once a day
• Acyclovir (Zovirax): Pulmonary infections involving herpes simplex, herpes zoster or varicella
◊ Adults 5 mg/kg IV q8h for HSV pneumonia and 10 mg/kg IV q8h for varicella pneumonia
◊ Children 250 mg/square meter body surface area IV q8h
• Ganciclovir (Cytovene): CMV infection, HSV infection
◊ 5 mg/kg IV 12h
• Ribavirin (Virazole): RSV, possibly Hanta and Influenza B virus (20 mg/mL via continuous aerosol administration for 12-18 hours/day for 3-7 days). Indicated only in severe RSV infections, given via small particle aerosol generator (SPAG).
Contraindications: Refer to manufacturer's literature
Precautions:
• Amantadine should be used cautiously in patients with liver disease, epilepsy, renal disease, eczematoid rash, and those with a history of psychotic illness
• Ribavirin is teratogenic and should not be administered by pregnant health-care personnel
Significant possible interactions: Refer to manufacturer's literature

ALTERNATIVE DRUGS
• Rimantadine (Flumadine), an amantadine analog, is equally effective as amantadine and has fewer CNS adverse effects. Useful for Influenza A.
• Antibiotics for superimposed bacterial infections.
• Foscarnet (Foscavir) for CMV, HSV, varicella infections, 60 mg/kg IV q8h
• IV immune globulin (IVIG) may increase response in non-AIDS, immunosuppressed patients with CMV pneumonia. Dose and dosage regimen not well established, but 500 mg/kg IV qod x 10 doses may be beneficial.

FOLLOWUP

PATIENT MONITORING
• Physical examinations and/or chest roentgenograms
• Oxygenation if illness severe enough for hospitalization

PREVENTION/AVOIDANCE
• Influenza A and B vaccine: Use for patients with chronic cardiovascular lung disease, residents of chronic care facilities, medical personnel with extensive contact with high risk patients, people over 65 years of age or those with chronic diseases, immunosuppressed patients
• For those patients unable to receive influenza vaccine (egg allergy or other) and are at high risk because of age, co-morbid illness, or other risk factor, amantadine or rimantadine can be given throughout the infectious season if tolerated
• For those who did not receive the vaccine and have been exposed to influenza, or there is an influenza A outbreak, amantadine or rimantadine may also be taken for 2 weeks until vaccination has produced immunity
• Health care workers who are pregnant need to take proper precautions to avoid infectious patients
• Measles vaccine
• Varicella vaccine

POSSIBLE COMPLICATIONS
• Superimposed bacterial infections such as S. pneumoniae, S. aureus, H. influenzae and others
• Respiratory failure requiring mechanical ventilation
• Adult respiratory distress syndrome (ARDS)
• Reye's syndrome after influenza in children

EXPECTED COURSE/PROGNOSIS
Usually favorable prognosis with illness lasting several days to a week. Post-viral fatigue is common. However, death can occur, especially in pediatric or bone-marrow transplant adenovirus infections or in elderly influenza infections.

MISCELLANEOUS

ASSOCIATED CONDITIONS
• Bacterial pneumonias
• Fungi, Pneumocystis carinii in immunosuppressed patients

AGE-RELATED FACTORS
Pediatric: Adenovirus infections in children are serious. More serious RSV infections are almost always seen in infants and immunocompromised patients.
Geriatric: Greatest morbidity and mortality
Others: N/A

PREGNANCY Should avoid contact with persons who may have viral infections

SYNONYMS N/A

ICD-9-CM
480.9 Viral pneumonia, unspecified

SEE ALSO N/A

OTHER NOTES N/A

ABBREVIATIONS
• RSV = respiratory syncytial virus
• PCP = Pneumocystis carinii pneumonia
• ARDS = adult respiratory distress syndrome
• BOOP = bronchiolitis obliterans with organizing pneumonia
• CMV = cytomegalovirus
• PCR = Polymerase chain reaction

REFERENCES
• Mandell GL, ed: Principles and Practice of Infectious Diseases. 4th Ed. New York, Churchill Livingstone, 1995
• Fields BN, ed: Virology. 2nd Ed. New York, Raven Press, 1990
• Greenburg SB: Viral Pneumonia. Infectious Disease Clinics of North America. vol. 5 (3), September 1991
• Gorbach SL, ed: Infectious Diseases. Philadelphia, W.B. Saunders Company, 1992
Illustrations: N/A
Internet references: http://www.5mcc.com

Author(s)
Gene W. Voskuhl, MD
Ronald A. Greenfield, MD

Pneumothorax

BASICS

DESCRIPTION Accumulation of air or gas between the parietal and visceral pleurae.
- Spontaneous pneumothorax - may be primary or secondary
  ◊ Primary in young and otherwise healthy patients
  ◊ Secondary - as a complication of an underlying lung disease
- Traumatic pneumothorax - may coexist with hemothorax
- Tension pneumothorax - the air in the pleural space is under higher pressure than air in adjacent lung and vascular structures

System(s) affected: Pulmonary, Cardiovascular
Genetics: No known genetic pattern, possible congenital predisposition in thin, tall young men
Incidence/Prevalence in USA: 9/100,000
Predominant age: Adults 20-40 years
Predominant sex: Male > Female

SIGNS AND SYMPTOMS
- Chest pain, sudden, sharp, made worse by breathing, coughing or moving the chest
- Chest movements - asymmetrical
- Dyspnea
- Cyanosis (sometimes)
- Moderate to severe - profound respiratory distress
- Tension pneumothorax - weak, rapid pulse, pallor, neck vein distension, anxiety, tracheal deviation
- Shock
- Circulatory collapse
- Diminished breath sounds and voice sounds

CAUSES
- Perforation of the visceral pleura and entry of gas from the lung
- Gas generated by microorganisms in an empyema
- Penetration of the chest wall, diaphragm, mediastinum, or esophagus
- Blunt trauma to thorax

RISK FACTORS
- Trauma (broken rib, ruptured bronchus, perforated esophagus)
- Rupture of superficial lung bulla following cough or blowing a musical instrument
- Vigorous or stretching exercises
- Flying (high altitude) after loss of pressurization
- Diving (at ascension or rapid decompression)
- Pneumoconioses
- Tuberculosis
- Pneumonia due to TB, Klebsiella, Staph aureus
- Subpleural Pneumocystis carinii pneumonia (PCP) (in AIDS patients on PCP prophylaxis via pentamidine aerosol)
- Bronchial obstruction
- COPD (particularly emphysema)
- Asthma
- Neoplasms

- Endometriosis (during menstruation)
- Rare diseases (Marfan's, Ehlers-Danlos)
- Rupture of an infected abscess
- Lymphangioleiomyomatosis
- Cystic fibrosis
- Cigarette smoking
- Intubation ventilation

DIAGNOSIS

DIFFERENTIAL DIAGNOSIS
- Pleurisy
- Pericarditis
- Myocardial infarction
- Pulmonary embolism
- Diaphragmatic hernia
- Stomach herniation through diaphragm
- Dissecting aneurysm

LABORATORY
- Arterial blood gases in significant pneumothorax
  ◊ pH < 7.35
  ◊ pO_2 < 80 mm Hg (10.6 kPa)
  ◊ pCO_2 > 45 mm Hg (6.0 kPa)
Drugs that may alter lab results: N/A
Disorders that may alter lab results: N/A

PATHOLOGICAL FINDINGS N/A

SPECIAL TESTS N/A

IMAGING
- Chest x-ray:
  ◊ Air without lung markings peripherally, mediastinal shift to contralateral side
  ◊ Small pneumothorax may be evident only with expiratory or lateral decubitus film

DIAGNOSTIC PROCEDURES Careful history and physical. The physical findings depend on size of pneumothorax.

TREATMENT

APPROPRIATE HEALTH CARE
- Outpatient - lung collapse less than 30%, no dyspnea, no signs of tension pneumothorax, no underlying lung disease
- Inpatient - if more than 30% collapse, tension or underlying lung disease

GENERAL MEASURES
- Outpatient
  ◊ Bed rest
  ◊ Monitoring blood pressure, pulse rate, respirations
  ◊ Oxygen at high concentration will accelerate rate of absorption by 4 times
  ◊ Treatment of any underlying condition

SURGICAL MEASURES
- Inpatient
  ◊ Simple aspiration - insert 16 gauge cannula into 2nd anterior intercostal space at midclavicular line and attach a 3-way stopcock and 60 mL syringe. Withdraw air manually until no more can be aspirated.
  ◊ Thoracotomy tube - inserted in 4th, 5th or 6th intercostal space at midaxillary line and connect underwater seal
  ◊ Tension pneumothorax - insert 19 gauge or larger needle into the chest and attach a 3-way stopcock. Use a large syringe to withdraw air. Follow with tube insertion
  ◊ Pulmonary edema can be a complication of re-expansion
- Recurrent pneumothorax (more often occurs with larger pneumothoraces)
  ◊ Can cause severe disability
  ◊ Consider thoracoscopy or thoracotomy following 2 or more spontaneous pneumothoraces, if lungs not expanded after 7 days therapy or persistent bronchopleural fistula
  ◊ Consider pleurodesis with talc or other agents

ACTIVITY
- Bed rest until re-expanded
- No air travel until x-ray normal

DIET No special diet

PATIENT EDUCATION Stop smoking

MEDICATIONS

DRUG(S) OF CHOICE
• Pleurodesis for recurrent pneumothorax:
  ◊ Intrapleural doxycycline, 5 mg/kg in a total volume of 50 mL. Intrapleural doxycycline is painful so premedicate with short-acting benzodiazepine and give 4 mg/kg lidocaine in a total volume of 50 mL intrapleurally before doxycycline is injected.
  ◊ Intrapleural talc, 5g in 250 mL isotonic saline
Contraindications: If patient a possible candidate for future lung transplant, do not do sclerosing pleurodesis (sclerosing agents increase risk of bleeding at surgery so patients are not eligible for transplant)
Precautions:
• Talc procedure precipitated respiratory distress syndrome in 2 reports
• Pain at time of intrapleural instillation and postprocedure are most common side effects
Significant possible interactions: Refer to manufacturer's literature

ALTERNATIVE DRUGS   None

FOLLOWUP

PATIENT MONITORING
• Blood pressure, respiratory rate, arterial blood gases, for hospitalized patients
• After simple aspiration - clamp chest tube for 24 hours, then remove if no recurrence on x-ray. If lung not fully re-expanded after 7 days, consider persistent air leak/bronchopleural fistula.

PREVENTION/AVOIDANCE   No
preventive measures known, but patients may avoid some risk factors, e.g., exposure to high altitudes, flying in unpressurized aircraft, scuba diving, smoking

POSSIBLE COMPLICATIONS
• Re-expansion pulmonary edema following suction
• Bronchopleural fistulae requiring surgical repair
• Surgery indicated following 2 spontaneous pneumothoraces on the same side

EXPECTED COURSE/PROGNOSIS
• Air reabsorbed from small spontaneous pneumothorax in a few days
• Air reabsorbed from larger air space in 2-4 weeks
• Risk of recurrence is 30-50%

MISCELLANEOUS

ASSOCIATED CONDITIONS   Listed with Causes

AGE-RELATED FACTORS
Pediatric: Unusual in this age group except following trauma
Geriatric: Higher morbidity and mortality
Others: N/A

PREGNANCY   A known, but unusual complication of labor and delivery. It should be suspected in the pregnant patient with dyspnea and chest pain.

SYNONYMS   N/A

ICD-9-CM
512.0 Spontaneous tension pneumothorax
512.1 Iatrogenic pneumothorax
512.8 Other spontaneous pneumothorax

SEE ALSO   N/A

OTHER NOTES   Chest pain may simulate an acute MI or acute abdomen

ABBREVIATIONS
MI = myocardial infarction

REFERENCES
• Massad G, Thomas P, Wihlm JM: Minimally invasive management for first and recurrent pnemothorax. Ann Thorac Surg 1998;6:592-9
• Tschopp JM, Brutsche M, Frey JG: Treatment of complicated spontaneous pneumothorax by simple talc pleurodesis. Thorax 1997;52:329-32
• Sadikot RT, Greene T, Meadows K, Arnold AG: Recurrence of primary spontaneous pneumothorax. Thorax 1997;52:805-9
• Light RW: Management of spontaneous pneumothorax. Ann rev Respir Dis 1993;148:245
• Miller AC, Harvey JE: Guidelines for the management of spontaneous pneumothorax. Br Med J 1993;307:114
• Baumann MH: The clinician's perspective on pneumothorax management. Chest 1997;112:822-28
Illustrations: N/A
Internet references: http://www.5mcc.com

Author(s)
Barbara J. Moront, MD
Benito B. Perez, MD

Poliomyelitis

BASICS

DESCRIPTION Acute illness, symptomatic cases present as aseptic meningitis. Only a small number of cases with residual neurologic disease. Most symptomatic cases have nonspecific manifestations of infection. Illness is biphasic, paralysis occurs in second phase. Paralytic disease occurs with rapid onset. Spread by direst contact - fecal/oral. More common in warm months. Virus secreted for weeks in stool.
- Three types
  ◊ Encephalitic - coma
  ◊ Bulbar - cranial nerve paralysis
  ◊ Spinal - arm(s) and leg(s) weakness
System(s) affected: Nervous, Musculoskeletal
Genetics: N/A
Incidence/Prevalence in USA: Two new cases per year
Predominant age: 3 months-16 years; rarely adults
Predominant sex: Male = Female

SIGNS AND SYMPTOMS
- Nonspecific
- Meningitis
- Neurologic symptoms

CAUSES
Poliovirus - most common types are Brunhilde, Lansing and Leon

RISK FACTORS
- Living in areas where sanitation and hygiene are poor
- Low socioeconomic status
- Increasing age, if not immunized
- Pregnancy
- Recent tonsillectomy
- Inoculation (e.g., DPT injection)

DIAGNOSIS

DIFFERENTIAL DIAGNOSIS
- Guillain-Barré syndrome
- Mumps, herpes, coxsackievirus infection
- Aseptic meningitis
- Tick paralysis

LABORATORY
- Pleocytosis
- Increased protein
- Normal glucose
- Serology
- Virus culture - should be done when suspected
Drugs that may alter lab results: N/A
Disorders that may alter lab results: N/A

PATHOLOGICAL FINDINGS
- Spinal cord - perivascular cuffing, abnormal motor nuclei, chromatolysis of motor neurons, intermediate column inflammation, posterior column inflammation
- Diffuse mononuclear infiltrate
- Abnormal anterior horn cells
- Hypothalamic lesion
- Thalamic lesion
- Brainstem lesion
- Vestibular nuclei lesions
- Cerebellar deep nuclei lesions
- Reticular formation lesions
- Cortical motor area lesions
- Cerebral edema
- Edematous cord

SPECIAL TESTS
Spinal fluid virus isolation from throat (early in disease) and/or feces (early and late in the disease)

IMAGING N/A

DIAGNOSTIC PROCEDURES
Viral culture of CSF, stool and throat

TREATMENT

APPROPRIATE HEALTH CARE
Inpatient for acute phase. Outpatient or rehabilitation facility for therapy.

GENERAL MEASURES
- Provide bed that has firm mattress, footboard, foam rubber pads or sandbags. Change positions frequently. Give good skin care.
- Mechanical ventilation, if required
- Management of fecal impaction and urinary retention. Catheterization may be necessary.
- Non-narcotic analgesics
- Hot, moist packs
- Physical therapy
- Public health - all suspected cases, report immediately to public health department

SURGICAL MEASURES
Tracheostomy is frequently required in respiratory paralysis

ACTIVITY
- Bedrest during active phase. With paralysis, may require an extended period.
- Long-term rehabilitation plan - using physical therapy, braces, special shoes, possibly orthopedic surgery. Team effort with doctors, physical and occupational therapists, and social worker or psychiatrist, if necessary.

DIET
Be sure patient has adequate well-balanced diet. May require tube feedings.

PATIENT EDUCATION
For patient education materials favorably reviewed on this topic, contact: International Polio Network, 4502 Maryland Avenue, St. Louis, MO 63108, (314)361-0475

MEDICATIONS

DRUG(S) OF CHOICE
• Aspirin or other non-narcotic analgesics
• Antibiotics, if other infection develops
• Parasympathomimetic (bethanechol) may help patient with urinary retention, 10-50 mg po bid-qid. Up to 100 mg qid may be required.
Contraindications: Refer to manufacturer's literature
Precautions: Bethanechol - adverse affects are rare, but may occur if dose increased. Includes colicky feeling, urinary urgency, skin flushing.
Significant possible interactions: Refer to manufacturer's literature

ALTERNATIVE DRUGS   N/A

FOLLOWUP

PATIENT MONITORING   Individualized depending on severity and long-term physical therapy requirements

PREVENTION/AVOIDANCE
• Poliovirus vaccines; live oral and inactive. Vaccine recommendations shifting toward using inactive vaccine in order to prevent vaccine-associated paralytic poliomyelitis (VAPP)
(Note: Use of these vaccines has effectively eliminated the disease in the industrialized world.)

POSSIBLE COMPLICATIONS
• Urinary tract infection
• Atelectasis
• Pneumonia
• Myocarditis
• Postpoliomyelitis progressive muscular atrophy (PPMA) - characterized by progressive weakness beginning 30 years or more after an attack of poliomyelitis
• Postpoliomyelitis motor neuron disease - occurs many years after acute poliomyelitis, less common than PPMA

EXPECTED COURSE/PROGNOSIS
• Often irreversible paralysis; less than 5% mortality during acute disease
• Increased mortality over age 40
• Poor recovery for totally paralyzed muscle groups
• Good recovery for partially paralyzed muscle groups

MISCELLANEOUS

ASSOCIATED CONDITIONS   N/A

AGE-RELATED FACTORS
Pediatric: Most common in this age group. Polio is an extremely rare infection in U.S. since introduction of effective vaccines. (See Immunizations topic).
Geriatric: Extremely rare. Primary vaccination not recommended (except when traveling to endemic areas).
Others: N/A

PREGNANCY   A risk factor for developing polio

SYNONYMS
• Infantile paralysis
• Acute anterior poliomyelitis
• Acute lateral poliomyelitis

ICD-9-CM   045.1 Acute poliomyelitis with other paralysis

SEE ALSO
• Immunizations
• Tick paralysis

OTHER NOTES
WHO goal: eliminate polio in Americas by 2001

ABBREVIATIONS
WHO = World Health Organization

REFERENCES
• Bennett JC, Plum F, eds: Cecil Textbook of Medicine. 20th Ed. Philadelphia, W.B. Saunders Co., 1996
• Mandell GL, ed: Principles and Practice of Infectious Diseases. 4th Ed. New York, Churchill Livingstone, 1995
Illustrations: N/A
Internet references: http://www.5mcc.com

Author(s)
Mark M. Shelton, MD

Polyarteritis nodosa

BASICS

DESCRIPTION Polyarteritis nodosa (PAN) presents pathologically as an ongoing segmental inflammatory response within the media of small and medium sized muscular arteries
• Organ involvement - kidney, GI tract, skin, muscles, joints, genitourinary tract, peripheral and central nervous system, heart, testes, epididymis and ovaries
• One of the vasculitic syndromes which vary in involvement from mild, self-limited skin lesions to severe systemic isolated and combined, multi-organ dysfunction and death
• Although heterogeneity and "overlap" manifestations abound, PAN is classified as a systemic necrotizing vasculitis
System(s) affected: Cardiovascular, Nervous, Skin/Exocrine, Renal/Urologic, Gastrointestinal, Musculoskeletal
Genetics: Unknown
Incidence/Prevalence in USA: No definite figures because of inclusive grouping of different types of vasculitic syndromes
Predominant age: Childhood to geriatric age groups. Mean is 45 years.
Predominant sex: Male > Female (2.5:1)

SIGNS AND SYMPTOMS
• General (often nonspecific)
  ◊ Fever
  ◊ Weakness
  ◊ Weight loss
  ◊ Malaise
  ◊ Myalgia
  ◊ Livido reticularis
  ◊ Headache
  ◊ Abdominal pain and vague discomfort
• Related to organ system involved (may dominate clinical picture and course)
  ◊ Renal - hypertension, hematuria (usually microscopic), proteinuria, progressive renal failure
  ◊ Musculoskeletal - myalgia, migratory arthralgia and arthritis
  ◊ Skin - purpura, urticaria, subcutaneous hemorrhages, polymorphic rashes, subcutaneous nodules (uncommon but characteristic), persistent livedo reticularis and Raynaud's phenomenon (rare)
  ◊ Gastrointestinal - recurrent and severe pain, hepatomegaly, nausea, vomiting and bleeding
  ◊ Lung - Hilar adenopathy, patchy infiltrates, reticular or nodular lesions, often fleeting
  ◊ CNS - seizures, CVA's, headache, papillitis, altered mental states
  ◊ Peripheral nervous system - mononeuritis multiplex
  ◊ Cardiac - pericarditis, CHF associated with hypertension and/or myocardial infarction
  ◊ Genitourinary - usually asymptomatic but may have testicular, epididymal, ovarian pain. Neurogenic bladder reported.

CAUSES
• Unclear. Suggestive evidence for immunological involvement.
  ◊ Tissue deposition of immune complexes
  ◊ Hepatitis B antigenemia in 30% of cases
  ◊ Hepatitis B antigen in circulating immune complexes
  ◊ Hepatitis B antigen, complement and IgM demonstrated in vascular walls

RISK FACTORS N/A

DIAGNOSIS

DIFFERENTIAL DIAGNOSIS
• Systemic lupus erythematosis
• Cryoglobulinemia
• Subacute endocarditis
• Trichinosis
• Some rickettsial diseases
• Microscopic polyangiitis
• The key differences from other necrotizing vasculitides are lack of granuloma formation, sparing of veins and pulmonary arteries

LABORATORY
• Non specific:
  ◊ Abnormal urine sediment
  ◊ High neutrophil count
  ◊ Eosinophilia rare. Suggests granulomatous involvement when present
  ◊ Anemia of chronic disease
  ◊ Elevated sedimentation rate
  ◊ Hypergammaglobulinemia
  ◊ Hepatitis B surface antigen positive in 30% of cases (strong circumstantial evidence)
• Specific
  ◊ Mainly based on pathological findings of biopsy material from involved organs
  ◊ Careful examinations of biopsies from "acute abdomens", especially in males between the second and fourth decade
  ◊ Negative anti-neutrophil cytoplasm antibodies
Drugs that may alter lab results:
• Corticosteroids
Disorders that may alter lab results:
Allergic reactions and other immunologic disorders

PATHOLOGICAL FINDINGS
• Necrotizing inflammation, in various stages, of small and medium muscular arteries. Segmental in distribution, often seen at bifurcations and branchings. Involvement of venules not seen in classic PAN.
• Acute lesions show infiltration of polymorphonuclear cells through vessel wall and perivascular area
• Subsequent proliferation, degeneration, appearance of monocytes, necrosis with thrombosis and infarction of the involved tissue. Aneurysmal dilatations characteristic.
• Aortic dissection reported attributed to necrotizing vasculitis of the vasa vasorum

SPECIAL TESTS Angiographic demonstration of aneurysmal changes of small and medium sized arteries involving renal hepatic and mesenteric arteries represents strong evidence supporting the diagnosis

IMAGING Angiography: Mesenteric artery aneurysm, renal aneurysm, hepatic aneurysm, intestinal aneurysm

DIAGNOSTIC PROCEDURES N/A

TREATMENT

APPROPRIATE HEALTH CARE
Depends on extent and involvement of specific organs

GENERAL MEASURES The same as those needed for patients under treatment with steroids (high risk of infections), cytotoxic agents and plasmapheresis

SURGICAL MEASURES N/A

ACTIVITY As tolerated

DIET Low salt if hypertensive

PATIENT EDUCATION Arthritis Foundation, 1314 Spring Street N.W., Atlanta, GA 30309, (800)283-7800

MEDICATIONS

DRUG(S) OF CHOICE
• Favorable results reported with prednisone and cyclophosphamide. Reports differ as to the benefits of adding plasmaphoresis.
• Hepatitis B vaccine may be considered for the amelioration of any subsequent development of life-threatening complications of hepatitis B virus-associated polyarteritis nodosa
Contraindications: Refer to manufacturer's profile of each drug
Precautions: Refer to manufacturer's profile of each drug
Significant possible interactions: Refer to manufacturer's profile of each drug

ALTERNATIVE DRUGS   N/A

FOLLOWUP

PATIENT MONITORING
• Careful monitoring for infection
• Delayed appearance of neoplasms
• Angiographic changes may improve rapidly with combination steroid/cyclophosphamide therapy
• Acute phase reactants such as Interleukin-6 and C-reactive protein may be useful in diagnosis and monitoring activity level during treatment and followup

PREVENTION/AVOIDANCE   N/A

POSSIBLE COMPLICATIONS
• Glomerulonephritis
• Thrombosis
• Infarction
• Tissue/organ necrosis

EXPECTED COURSE/PROGNOSIS
• Expected course of untreated polyarteritis nodosa is poor
• 5 year survival rate 13%
• Steroid treatment may increase percentage survival rate to 50-60% (prospective studies in progress)
• Renal and GI signs most serious prognostic factors

MISCELLANEOUS

ASSOCIATED CONDITIONS
• Churg-Strauss syndrome
• Benign cutaneous periarteritis nodosa (bears watching and investigating because not necessarily benign)

AGE-RELATED FACTORS
Pediatric: N/A
Geriatric: N/A
Others: N/A

PREGNANCY   One case report suggests that if a patient attains remission before becoming pregnant, the chance of a successful delivery is reasonable

SYNONYMS
• Periarteritis
• Panarteritis
• Necrotizing arteritis

ICD-9-CM   446.0 Polyarteritis nodosa

SEE ALSO   N/A

OTHER NOTES
• Recommended reading: Jennette JC, Falk RJ. Small vessel vasculitis in N Engl J Med 1997: 337(21) 1512-1523

ABBREVIATIONS   N/A

REFERENCES
• Isselbacher KJ, et al, eds: Harrison's Principles of Internal Medicine. 13th Ed. New York, McGraw-Hill, 1994
• Bennett JC, Plum F, eds: Cecil Textbook of Medicine. 20th Ed. Philadelphia, W.B. Saunders Co., 1996
• Iino T, et al: Polyarteritis nodosa. J Rheumatol 1992;19(10):1632-36
• Nakayama H: Distinct response interleukin-6 and other laboratory parameters to treatment in a patient with polyarteritis nodosa. Angiology 1992;43(6):512-6
• Garanger TA, et al: Anti-neutrophil cytoplasmic antibodies in patient's with the Americal College of Rheumatology criteria for pain. Autoimmunity 1995;20(1):33-7
Illustrations: N/A
Internet references: http://www.5mcc.com

Author(s)
J. Harlan Dix, MD, FACP

Polycystic kidney disease

BASICS

DESCRIPTION Inherited disorders characterized by the development and growth of cysts in the kidneys; lined by epithelium, filled with fluid or semi-solid debris; accounts for 5-10% of patients with end stage renal disease
System(s) affected: Renal/Urologic
Genetics: See Causes
Incidence/Prevalence in USA: 1/200-1/1000
Predominant age: Usually diagnosed by age 45
Predominant sex: Male = Female

SIGNS AND SYMPTOMS
• Hypertension
• Hematuria; microscopic or macroscopic
• Palpable kidneys
• Hepatomegaly
• Abdominal pain
• Flank pain (60%)
• Headache
• Nocturia
• Dysuria
• Urinary frequency
• Polyuria

CAUSES
• Inherited autosomal dominant abnormality linked to chromosome 16. 90% penetrance by age 90 in gene carriers. A second gene on chromosome 4 recently identified. Rare autosomal recessive form exists in neonates. Offspring of affected individuals with 50% chance of acquiring disease. Can be detected in amniocentesis.
• Acquired polycystic kidney disease – found in 50% of patients on dialysis > 3 years

RISK FACTORS Dialysis

DIAGNOSIS

DIFFERENTIAL DIAGNOSIS
• Simple cysts
• Nephronophthisis-medullary cystic disease
• Medullary sponge kidney

LABORATORY
• Hematocrit - elevated in 5% of cases
• Urinalysis - may have hematuria and mild proteinuria
• Serum creatinine - may be elevated
• Kidney stones - usually calcium oxalate
Drugs that may alter lab results: N/A
Disorders that may alter lab results: N/A

PATHOLOGICAL FINDINGS N/A

SPECIAL TESTS
• Gene linkage analysis
  ◊ Helpful for suspected cases with nondiagnostic imaging
  ◊ Expensive
  ◊ Requires other family members

IMAGING
• Ultrasonography: > 5 cysts in the renal cortex or medulla of each kidney, in children, 2 or more cysts in either kidney
• CT scan more sensitive
• 85% of patients can be detected by age 25

DIAGNOSTIC PROCEDURES N/A

TREATMENT

APPROPRIATE HEALTH CARE
Outpatient except for complicating emergencies (infected cysts require 2 weeks IV antibiotics then long-term oral antibiotics)

GENERAL MEASURES
• Pain – bed rest and analgesics
• Hematuria (due to ruptured cyst) – bed rest, sedation, IV hydration

SURGICAL MEASURES
Renal transplant, by age 6-8 years, for autosomal recessive form

ACTIVITY Avoid contact activities that may damage enlarged organs.

DIET Low protein diet may retard progression of renal disease.

PATIENT EDUCATION
• Genetic counseling is critical
• Avoidance of nephrotoxic drugs

MEDICATIONS

DRUG(S) OF CHOICE
• No drug therapy available for polycystic kidney disease
• Hypertension – ACE inhibitors; avoid diuretics (possible adverse effects with cyst formation)
Contraindications: N/A
Precautions: N/A
Significant possible interactions: N/A

ALTERNATIVE DRUGS N/A

FOLLOWUP

PATIENT MONITORING Serum creatinine and blood pressure monitoring twice a year; more frequently as disease progresses

PREVENTION/AVOIDANCE Genetic counseling

POSSIBLE COMPLICATIONS
• Progression to renal failure
• Renal calculi in up to 30%
• Cyst infection
• Cyst rupture

EXPECTED COURSE/PROGNOSIS
• The disease is slowly progressive and has a variable outcome
• End stage renal disease occurs in 70% of patients by age 65
• Acquired disease with 5% adenocarcinoma, cysts regress after renal transplant, once nonazotemic

MISCELLANEOUS

ASSOCIATED CONDITIONS
• Cerebral aneurysms present in 10-40% of patients
• Colonic diverticuli in 80%
• Liver cysts in approximately 50%
• Pancreatic and ovarian cysts
• Mitral valve prolapse in 26%

AGE-RELATED FACTORS
Pediatric: N/A
Geriatric: Renal insufficiency in 50% of patients by age 70, accounts for 5-10% of dialysis patients.
Others: Hypertension is secondary to high renin. Responds to angiotensin converting enzyme (ACE) inhibitors.

PREGNANCY Higher frequency of new onset hypertension than in women without polycystic kidney disease. No adverse effect on the course of the polycystic kidney disease in asymptomatic patients. Patients with hypertension, proteinuria or renal insufficiency are at increased risk of complications. Also an increase in hepatic cysts with pregnancy (rarely a problem).

SYNONYMS N/A

ICD-9-CM
753.12 Polycystic kidney, unspecified type
753.13 Polycystic kidney, autosomal dominant
753.14 Polycystic kidney, autosomal recessive

SEE ALSO
• Renal failure, chronic
• Renal calculi

OTHER NOTES N/A

ABBREVIATIONS N/A

REFERENCES
• Welling LW, Granthem JJ: Cystic and developmental diseases of the kidney. In: Brenner BM, Rector FC, eds. The Kidney. Philadelphia, W.B. Saunders, 1991
• Chapman AB, Johnson A, Gabow PA, Schrier RW: The renin-angiotensin-aldosterone system and autosomal dominant polycystic kidney disease. N Engl J Med 1990;323:1091-1096
• Beebe DK: Autosomal dominant polycystic kidney disease. Amer Fam Phys 1996;53(3):925-931
Illustrations: N/A
Internet references: http://www.5mcc.com

Author(s)
Douglas M. Hoy, MD

Polycystic ovarian disease

BASICS

DESCRIPTION Polycystic ovarian disease (PCOD) is characterized by a state of chronic oligo-ovulation and/or anovulation culminating in oligomenorrhea and/or amenorrhea

System(s) affected: Reproductive, Endocrine/Metabolic, Skin/Exocrine

Genetics: N/A

Incidence/Prevalence in USA: Unknown, but is a common cause of oligomenorrhea and/or amenorrhea

Predominant age: Women of reproductive age

Predominant sex: Female only

SIGNS AND SYMPTOMS
• Amenorrhea
• Oligomenorrhea
• Obesity
• Hirsutism
• Acne
• Dysfunctional uterine bleeding
• Infertility
• Acanthosis nigricans
• Hypertension
• Virilism
• Enlarged ovaries
• Enlarged clitoris
• Deep voice

CAUSES
Disruption of hypothalamic-pituitary-ovarian axis (high normal luteinizing hormone and low normal follicle stimulating hormone leading to ovarian hyperandrogenism and follicular atresia and anovulation)

RISK FACTORS
• Endometrial hyperplasia
• Endometrial carcinoma
• Obesity
• Hypertension
• Diabetes mellitus
• Breast cancer
• Infertility

DIAGNOSIS

DIFFERENTIAL DIAGNOSIS
• Cushing's syndrome
• Hairan syndrome (hyperandrogenism, insulin resistance, acanthosis nigricans)
• Testosterone-producing ovarian or adrenal tumor
• Prolactin-producing pituitary adenoma
• Hyperthecosis
• Adult-onset adrenal hyperplasia
• Partial congenital adrenal hyperplasia (21-hydroxylase deficiency)
• Other adrenal enzyme deficiencies
• Endometrial hyperplasia
• Endometrial carcinoma

LABORATORY
• Luteinizing hormone/follicle stimulating hormone (LH/FSH) ≥ 2.5-3.0/1
• Testosterone increased, but less than 200 ng/dL (6.94 nmol/L)
• Dehydroepiandrosterone sulfate (DHEA-S) increased, but less than 800 µg/dL (20.8 µmol/L)
• Dehydroepiandrosterone (DHEA) increased
• 17-OH progesterone increased
• Estrone increased
• Androstenedione increased
• Sex hormone binding globulin decreased
• Prolactin

Drugs that may alter lab results:
• Oral contraceptives
• Steroids
• Antidepressants

Disorders that may alter lab results: N/A

PATHOLOGICAL FINDINGS
• Ovary usually enlarged with a smooth white glistening capsule
• Ovarian cortex lined with follicles in all stages of development but most are atretic
• Theca cell proliferation with an increase in the stromal compartment

SPECIAL TESTS
• Fasting serum glucose and insulin level to rule out insulin resistance and glucose intolerance
• Overnight dexamethasone suppression test (Decadron 1 mg po at 11:00PM and fasting serum cortisol at 8:00AM the next morning) to rule out Cushing's syndrome

IMAGING
Pelvis ultrasound revealing enlarged ovaries with multiple small follicular cysts

DIAGNOSTIC PROCEDURES
• History and physical examination
• Endometrial biopsy to rule out hyperplasia and or carcinoma

TREATMENT

APPROPRIATE HEALTH CARE
• Outpatient
• Inpatient, if surgery for wedge resection recommended

GENERAL MEASURES
No ideal treatment exists. Treatment must be individualized according to the needs and desires of the patient.

SURGICAL MEASURES N/A

ACTIVITY Full activity

DIET
Regular (weight loss recommended, if overweight)

PATIENT EDUCATION
Counsel the patient regarding the risk of endometrial and breast carcinoma, insulin resistance and diabetes mellitus, obesity and infertility

MEDICATIONS

DRUG(S) OF CHOICE
• If pregnancy not desired:
  ◊ Cyclic withdrawal bleeding with medroxyprogesterone acetate (Provera) 10 mg po x 12-14 days/month
or
  ◊ Low dose oral contraceptives
• If pregnancy desired:
  ◊ Ovulation induction with clomiphene citrate (Clomid, Serophene)
or
  ◊ Human menopausal gonadotropins - menotropins (Pergonal, Humegon)
or
  ◊ Pure follicle-stimulating hormone (Follistim, Fertinex, Gonal-F) with or without the addition of gonadotropin releasing hormone (GnRH) agonist [leuprolide acetate (Lupron) or nafarelin acetate (Synarel)]
  ◊ Troglitazone (Rezulin) - one 200 mg tablet twice daily; or metformin (Glucophage) 500 mg po daily or bid have been shown to improve hyperandrogenism and restore ovulation

Contraindications: None, but if using oral contraceptive agents to prevent sequelae of anovulation, be aware of contraindications

Precautions:
• Risks of multiple fetuses with clomiphene citrate is 8%
• Risks of multiple fetuses with HMG, FSH is 25%
• Risk of severe ovarian hyperstimulation syndrome (OHS) is less than 1%
• Diarrhea and GI symptoms with metformin
• Check liver function monthly with troglitazone

Significant possible interactions: Refer to manufacturer's profile of each drug

ALTERNATIVE DRUGS
Bromocriptine if prolactin is elevated

FOLLOWUP

PATIENT MONITORING
Monitor patient frequently throughout the menstrual cycle depending upon which drug combination is utilized for ovulation induction

PREVENTION/AVOIDANCE
Prevent endometrial and breast carcinoma

POSSIBLE COMPLICATIONS
• Multiple pregnancies
• Ovarian hyperstimulation syndrome (OHS)
• Oral contraceptives are not without risk

EXPECTED COURSE/PROGNOSIS
• Prognosis for fertility is excellent depending upon other fertility factors
• Proper treatment and followup of chronic anovulation, can prevent endometrial hyperplasia and/or carcinoma

MISCELLANEOUS

ASSOCIATED CONDITIONS
• Obesity
• Hypertension
• Endometrial hyperplasia and/or carcinoma
• Breast carcinoma
• Diabetes mellitus
• Hairan syndrome
• Infertility
• Hyperthecosis

AGE-RELATED FACTORS
Pediatric: May begin at puberty
Geriatric: N/A
Others: N/A

PREGNANCY
Does not cure the syndrome

SYNONYMS
• Stein-Leventhal syndrome
• Polycystic ovary syndrome

ICD-9-CM
256.4 Polycystic ovaries
628.0 Female infertility associated with anovulation

SEE ALSO
• Amenorrhea
• Forbes-Albright syndrome

OTHER NOTES
• Drug costs high
• Monitoring (ultrasounds, estradiols) costs high

ABBREVIATIONS
OHS = ovarian hyperstimulation syndrome
HMG = human menopausal gonadotropins
FSH = follicle stimulating hormone

REFERENCES
Danforth DM, Scott JR, et al, eds: Obstetric and Gynecology. 6th Ed. Philadelphia, J.B. Lippincott, 1990
Illustrations: N/A
Internet references: http://www.5mcc.com

Author(s)
Nicholas J. Spirtos, DO

Polycythemia vera

BASICS

DESCRIPTION   A clonal cell hematologic malignant disorder with excessive erythroid, myeloid and megakaryocytic elements in the bone marrow. It is one of a group of myeloproliferative disorders.
System(s) affected:
Hemic/Lymphatic/Immunologic
Genetics: Unknown genetic pattern (some suggestion that a chromosomal abnormality may be involved)
Incidence/Prevalence in USA: 0.5 per 100,000
Predominant age: Middle to late years, mean is 60 years (range 15-90)
Predominant sex: Male > Female (slightly)

SIGNS AND SYMPTOMS
- Early stages may produce no symptoms
- Headaches
- Tinnitus
- Vertigo
- Blurred vision
- Epistaxis
- Increased blood viscosity
- Spontaneous bruising
- Upper GI bleeding
- Peptic ulcer disease
- Arterial and venous occlusive events
- Pruritus
- Sweating
- Weight loss
- Plethora (face, hands, feet)
- Splenomegaly
- Hepatomegaly
- Hyperhistaminemia
- Bone pain (ribs and sternum)
- Bone tenderness (ribs and sternum)

CAUSES   Unknown, all three hematopoietic cell lines originate in a single clone

RISK FACTORS
- Jewish ancestry (may have increased frequency)
- Familial history (rare)

DIAGNOSIS

DIFFERENTIAL DIAGNOSIS
- Secondary polycythemias
- Hemoglobinopathy
- Spurious polycythemia

LABORATORY
- Tests used for diagnosis of polycythemia vera
  ◊ A1: Increased RBC mass - female ≥ 32 mL/kg, male ≥ 36 mL/kg
  ◊ A2: Normal arterial oxygen saturation (≥ 92%)
  ◊ A3: Splenomegaly
  ◊ B1: Thrombocytosis platelet count > 400,000/μL
  ◊ B2: Leukocytosis > 12,000/μL
  ◊ B3: Leukocyte alkaline phosphatase increased
  ◊ B4: Increased serum B12 or increased unsaturated vitamin B12 binding capacity (UB12CB)
- Diagnosis acceptable with following combinations:
  ◊ A1 + A2 + A3
  ◊ A1 + A2 + any 2 from B category (splenomegaly absent in about 25% of patients)
- Other lab findings
  ◊ Hyperuricemia
  ◊ Hypercholesterolemia
  ◊ Elevated blood histamine level
Drugs that may alter lab results: Diuretics may cause a spurious polycythemia
Disorders that may alter lab results: Excessive use of alcohol or tobacco

PATHOLOGICAL FINDINGS
- Plethoric congestion in all organs and tissues
- Major vessels contain thick, viscous blood
- Sinuses of spleen packed with red blood cells

SPECIAL TESTS   Bone marrow aspiration (red cell hyperplasia, absent iron stores) and biopsy (fibrosis during spent phase of the disease)

IMAGING   CT - splenomegaly

DIAGNOSTIC PROCEDURES   Bone marrow aspiration - hyperplastic and panmyelosis

TREATMENT

APPROPRIATE HEALTH CARE
Outpatient

GENERAL MEASURES
Individualized management necessary. Dependent on many factors - age, disease duration, disease phenotype, complications, disease activity.
Currently, phlebotomy is mainstay of therapy. Beyond that, differences exist among authorities about use and effectiveness of myelosuppressives.
- Phlebotomy
  ◊ To reduce hematocrit to approximately 45%
  ◊ Performed as often as every 2 or 3 days until normal hematocrit reached. Phlebotomies of 250-500 m/L. Reduce to 250-350 m/L in elderly patients or patients with cardiovascular disease.
  ◊ Concomitant therapy possibilities, e.g., some form of myelosuppression, radioactive phosphorus (in elderly patients)
  ◊ Phlebotomy repeated as necessary for maintenance
  ◊ If patient cannot tolerate phlebotomy - chemotherapy (hydroxyurea is the least mutagenic agent) or radiation therapy
- Other therapy
  ◊ Maintain hydration
  ◊ Pruritus therapy
  ◊ Manage thrombotic or hemorrhagic complications the same as with nonpolycythemic patient
  ◊ Uric acid reduction therapy

SURGICAL MEASURES   N/A

ACTIVITY   No restrictions

DIET
- No special diet (iron replacement not necessary)
- Phlebotomy regimen will produce pica, resulting in craving for crisp green vegetables (lettuce, celery) and ice

PATIENT EDUCATION
- Lifelong maintenance
- Complications to watch for

MEDICATIONS

DRUG(S) OF CHOICE
• Adjunctive
  ◊ Allopurinol 300 mg/day for uric acid reduction
  ◊ Cyproheptadine for pruritus, 4-16 mg as needed
  ◊ H2-receptor blockers or antacids for GI hyperacidity
• Myelosuppression
  ◊ Radioactive phosphorous in selected cases
  ◊ Busulfan or alkylating agents (e.g., hydroxyurea)
  ◊ The use of low-dose aspirin is controversial in view of bleeding risk, but small doses may be given if required
  ◊ Note: Refer to hematologist/oncologist for dosages and instructions
Contraindications: Refer to manufacturer's literature
Precautions: Refer to manufacturer's literature
Significant possible interactions: Refer to manufacturer's literature

ALTERNATIVE DRUGS
• Myelosuppression: chlorambucil, some authors believe contraindicated
• Interferon is an emerging treatment

FOLLOWUP

PATIENT MONITORING
• Frequent during early treatment until satisfactory hematocrit is reached
• Monitor hematocrit often and phlebotomize when needed

PREVENTION/AVOIDANCE
No known preventive measures

POSSIBLE COMPLICATIONS
• Uric acid stones
• Secondary gout
• Vascular thromboses (major cause of death)
• Transformation to leukemia
• Hemorrhage
• Peptic ulcer
• Increased risk for complications and mortality from surgery procedures. Assess risk-benefits and assure optimal control of disorder before any elective surgery.

EXPECTED COURSE/PROGNOSIS
• Median survival without treatment - 6 to 18 months following diagnosis
• Survival up to 10 years with treatment
• Some patients live, symptom-free, for 20 or more years

MISCELLANEOUS

ASSOCIATED CONDITIONS
• Budd-Chiari syndrome
• Mesenteric artery thrombosis

AGE-RELATED FACTORS
Pediatric: Rare in this age group
Geriatric: Phlebotomies and other therapies need to be adjusted for patients over 70
Others: N/A

PREGNANCY
Treat with phlebotomy alone

SYNONYMS
• Primary polycythemia
• Vaquez disease
• Polycythemia, splenomegalic
• Vaquez-Osler disease

ICD-9-CM
238.4 polycythemia vera

SEE ALSO
Myeloproliferative disorders

OTHER NOTES
N/A

ABBREVIATIONS
N/A

REFERENCES
• Williams WJ, Beutler E, Erslev AJ, et al, eds: Hematology. 4th Ed. New York, McGraw-Hill, 1990
• Conley CL: Polycythemia vera, diagnosis and treatment. Hosp Practice 1987;22:107
Illustrations: N/A
Internet references: http://www.5mcc.com

Author(s)
Stanley G. Smith, MA, MB, FCFPC

Polymyalgia rheumatica

BASICS

DESCRIPTION A clinical syndrome characterized by aching and stiffness of the shoulder and hip girdle muscles affecting older patients, associated with an elevated ESR, lasting over 1 month and responsive to low dose steroids
System(s) affected: Musculoskeletal, Hemic/Lymphatic/Immunologic
Genetics: Associated with HLA determinants
Incidence/Prevalence in USA:
Approximately 50/100,000 patients over age 50/year
Predominant age: 60 or older. Incidence increases with age (rare under 50 years old).
Predominant sex: Females > Male (2:1)

SIGNS AND SYMPTOMS
• Onset - abrupt or insidious
• Pain and stiffness shoulder and hip girdle
• Usually symmetrical
• Symptoms more common in the morning
• Gel phenomena (stiffness after prolonged inactivity)
• Constitutional symptoms - fatigue, malaise, depression, weight loss, low grade fever
• Arthralgias/arthritis (non inflammatory)
• No weakness (pain may limit strength)
• Muscle tenderness mild to moderate
• No muscle atrophy
• Decreased range-of-motion of joints on active motion usually due to pain
• May have signs and symptoms of giant cell arteritis (seen in approximately 15% of patients)

CAUSES Unknown

RISK FACTORS
• Age greater than 50
• Presence of giant cell arteritis

DIAGNOSIS

DIFFERENTIAL DIAGNOSIS
• Rheumatoid arthritis
• Other connective tissue disease
• Fibromyalgia
• Depression
• Polymyositis/dermatomyositis (check CPK, aldolase)
• Thyroid disease
• Viral myalgia
• Osteoarthritis
• Occult infection
• Occult malignancy (extensive search usually not necessary)
• Myopathy (steroid, alcohol, electrolyte depletion)

LABORATORY
• ESR (Westergren) elevation greater than 50
• Anemia - normochromic/normocytic
• Creatine phosphokinase (CPK)- normal
• Rheumatoid factor (RF) - negative (5-10% patients over 60 will have positive RF without disease)
• Mild elevations in liver function tests
Drugs that may alter lab results:
Prednisone
Disorders that may alter lab results:
Disorders causing acute phase reactants can elevate ESR (e.g., infection, neoplasm, renal failure)

PATHOLOGICAL FINDINGS
• None in muscle biopsy
• Mild non-specific synovitis

SPECIAL TESTS N/A

IMAGING N/A

DIAGNOSTIC PROCEDURES
• None, although in patients with symptoms suggesting giant cell arteritis, a temporal artery biopsy may be indicated. (Although the temporal artery biopsy may be positive, if there are no symptoms of giant cell arteritis, there is no reason to treat with high dose steroids. Increased morbidity has not been shown.)

TREATMENT

APPROPRIATE HEALTH CARE
Outpatient unless needs temporal artery biopsy

GENERAL MEASURES Physical therapy
for range-of-motion exercises if necessary

SURGICAL MEASURES N/A

ACTIVITY Do not overexercise to cause exertion

DIET
• Adequate calcium and electrolyte intake (1500 mg/day)
• Regular diet

PATIENT EDUCATION
• Precautions regarding steroid use
• Instruct the patient about symptoms of giant cell arteritis and to report them immediately
• For a listing of sources for patient education materials favorably reviewed on this topic, physicians may contact: American Academy of Family Physicians Foundation, P.O. Box 8418, Kansas City, MO 64114, (800)274-2237, ext. 4400
• Excellent materials also available from Arthritis Foundation, 1330 W. Peachtree St, NW, Atlanta, GA 30309, (800)475-4700

MEDICATIONS

DRUG(S) OF CHOICE
• Prednisone
◊ 10 mg/day initially (average initial effective dose 10-15 mg/d)
◊ Usually dramatic (diagnostic) response.
◊ May increase gradually to 20 mg if no response
◊ Begin slow taper at 4-6 weeks by only 1 mg every 1-4 weeks to a dose of 5-7.5 mg. Continue at this dose for approximately 18 months to 2 years, if no recurrence of symptoms.
◊ Then attempt to taper by 1 mg every 2-4 weeks until drug discontinued. Patient may, however, require steroids for 3 or more years.
◊ Increase prednisone for recurrence of symptoms (relapse common).
Contraindications: Use steroids with caution in patients with chronic heart failure, diabetes mellitus, systemic fungal or bacterial infection. Must treat infections concurrently if steroids are absolutely necessary.
Precautions: Long term steroid use associated with several significant adverse effects including sodium and water retention, exacerbation of chronic heart failure, hypokalemia, increased susceptibility to infection, osteoporosis, cataracts, avascular necrosis.
Significant possible interactions: Refer to manufacturer's literature

ALTERNATIVE DRUGS
NSAID's have been used, rarely successful

FOLLOWUP

PATIENT MONITORING
• Follow monthly initially and during taper of medication, every 3 months otherwise
• Follow ESR as steroids tapered
• Followup with patient for symptoms of giant cell arteritis. Educate patient to report such symptoms immediately (headache, visual and neurologic symptoms).

PREVENTION/AVOIDANCE N/A

POSSIBLE COMPLICATIONS
• Medication - complications related to steroid use
• Disease - exacerbation of disease with taper of steroids; development of giant cell arteritis (may occur when PMR is being adequately treated)

EXPECTED COURSE/PROGNOSIS
• Average length disease is 3 years (range 1-5 years)
• Exacerbation if steroids tapered too fast
• Prognosis very good if treated (may gradually remit even if no treatment)
• Relapse common

MISCELLANEOUS

ASSOCIATED CONDITIONS
• Giant cell arteritis
• Temporal arteritis

AGE-RELATED FACTORS
Pediatric: Does not occur in this age group
Geriatric: Incidence increases with age
Others: N/A

PREGNANCY N/A

SYNONYMS
• Senile rheumatic gout
• Anarthritic syndrome
• Forestier-Certonciny syndrome
• Polymyalgia rheumatica syndrome
• Rhizomelic pseudoarthrosis

ICD-9-CM
725 polymyalgia rheumatica

SEE ALSO
• Giant cell arteritis
• Arthritis, rheumatoid (RA)
• Fibromyalgia
• Arthritis, osteo
• Polymyositis/dermatomyositis
• Depression

OTHER NOTES
Westergren ESR is the preferred laboratory technique. If other types of ESR studies are used (e.g., Wintrobe, or zeta sedimentation rate [ZSR]), the guidelines listed in this chapter cannot be used for abnormal levels.

ABBREVIATIONS
PMR = polymyalgia rheumatica

REFERENCES
• Hunder GG: Giant Cell Arteritis and Polymyalgia Rheumatica. In: Kelly WN, Harris ED, Ruddy S, Sledge CB, eds. Textbook of Rheumatology. 3rd Ed. Philadelphia, W.B. Saunders Co., 1989
• Healey LA: Polymyalgia Rheumatica and Giant Cell Arteritis. In: McCarty DJ, ed. Arthritis and Allied Conditions: A Textbook of Rheumatology. Philadelphia, Lea and Febiger, 1989
• Wayland CM, Goronzy JJ: Polymyalgia rheumatica and giant cell arteritis. In:Koopman WJ, ed: Arthritis and Allied Disorders. 12th Ed. Philadelphia, Lea & Febiger, 1997
Illustrations: N/A
Internet references: http://www.5mcc.com

Author(s)
Bridget T. Walsh, DO
Eric P. Gall, MD

Polymyositis/dermatomyositis

BASICS

DESCRIPTION Systemic connective tissue disease characterized by inflammatory and degenerative changes in proximal muscles sometimes accompanied by characteristic skin rash.
• If skin manifestations are associated, it is designated as dermatomyositis
• Different types of myositis include:
◊ Idiopathic PM
◊ Idiopathic DM
◊ Childhood PM/DM
◊ PM/DM with malignancy
◊ PM/DM as an overlap
◊ Inclusion body myositis
◊ HIV associated myopathy
System(s) affected: Musculoskeletal, Pulmonary, Skin/Exocrine, Cardiovascular
Genetics: Mild association with HLA-DR3, HLA-DRw52
Incidence/Prevalence in USA: Estimated at 0.5-0.8 new cases/100,000; 1-2 patients/100,000
Predominant age: 5-15 years, 40-60 years
Predominant sex: Female > Male (2:1)

SIGNS AND SYMPTOMS
• Symmetrical proximal muscle weakness causing:
◊ Difficulty when arising from sitting or lying positions
◊ Difficulty kneeling
◊ Difficulty climbing stairs
◊ Difficulty descending stairs
◊ Difficulty raising arms
• Joint pain/swelling
• Dysphagia
• Respiratory impairment
• Decreased deep tendon reflexes of proximal muscle groups
• Muscle swelling, stiffness, induration
• Rash over face (eyelids, nasolabial folds), upper chest, dorsal hands, (especially knuckle pads)
• Periorbital edema
• Calcinosis cutis (childhood cases)
• Mesenteric arterial insufficiency/infarction (childhood cases)
• Cardiac impairment; arrhythmia, failure

CAUSES
• Unknown; potential factors:
◊ Inciting viral infection
◊ T cell activation
◊ Cytokine release
◊ Immune-mediate muscle destruction
◊ Genetic predisposition
◊ HTLV I

RISK FACTORS Family history of
autoimmune disease or vasculitis

DIAGNOSIS

DIFFERENTIAL DIAGNOSIS
• Vasculitis
• Progressive systemic sclerosis
• Systemic lupus erythematosus
• Rheumatoid arthritis
• Muscular dystrophy
• Eaton-Lambert syndrome
• Sarcoidosis
• Amyotrophic lateral sclerosis
• Endocrine disorders
◊ Thyroid disease
◊ Cushing's syndrome
• Infectious myositis (viral, bacterial, parasitic)
• Drug-induced myopathies
◊ Cholesterol lowering agents
◊ Colchicine
◊ Corticosteroids
◊ Ethanol
◊ Chloroquine
◊ Zidovudine (AZT)
• Electrolyte disorders (magnesium, calcium, potassium)
• Heritable metabolic myopathies

LABORATORY
• Increased creatine kinase (CK)
• Increased aldolase
• Increased SGOT
• Increased LDH
• Myoglobinuria
• Increased ESR
• Positive rheumatoid factor (less than 50% of patients)
• Positive ANA (more than 50% of patients)
• Leukocytosis (less than 50% of patients)
• Anemia (less than 50% of patients)
• Hyperglobulinemia (less than 50% of patients)
• Increased creatinine (less than 50% of patients)
• Myositis specific antibodies have been described in a minority of patients - most are anti-synthetase antibodies, anti-Jo-1 is the most common and has been found in about 20% of patients; associated with an increased incidence of interstitial lung disease
Drugs that may alter lab results: N/A
Disorders that may alter lab results: N/A

PATHOLOGICAL FINDINGS
• Micro - muscle fiber degeneration
• Micro - phagocytosis of muscle debris
• Micro - perifascicular muscle fiber atrophy
• Micro - inflammatory cell infiltrates in adult form
• Micro (electron microscopy) - inclusion bodies (inclusion body myositis only)
• Sarcoplasmic basophilia
• Muscle fiber increased in size
• Vasculopathy (childhood PM/DM)

SPECIAL TESTS
• ECG - arrhythmias, conduction disturbances
• Electromyography (EMG) - muscle irritability, low amplitude potentials, polyphasic action potentials, fibrillations
• Muscle biopsy (deltoid or quadriceps femoris)

IMAGING Chest x-ray: pulmonary interstitial
disease

DIAGNOSTIC PROCEDURES Diagnosis
usually relies on 4 findings - weakness, CPK elevation, abnormal EMG, findings on muscle biopsy. Presence of skin rash of dermatomyositis also helpful.

TREATMENT

APPROPRIATE HEALTH CARE
Outpatient

GENERAL MEASURES
• Search for malignancy in all adults
• Follow serum muscle enzymes carefully

SURGICAL MEASURES N/A

ACTIVITY
• Curtailed until after inflammation subsides
• Range-of-motion exercises to prevent contractures

DIET No special diet

PATIENT EDUCATION Muscular
Dystrophy Association, 3561 E. Sunrise Dr., Tucson, AZ 85718. Telephone (800)221-1142.

MEDICATIONS

DRUG(S) OF CHOICE
• Prednisone 40-60 mg/day initially in divided doses. Consolidate doses and reduce prednisone slowly when enzyme levels are normal. Probably need to continue 5-10 mg/day for maintenance.
• For steroid refractory cases:
 ◊ Azathioprine 1.0 mg/kg (arthritis dose) once or twice a day. Maintain at lowest possible dose.
 ◊ Methotrexate 10-25 mg weekly useful in some steroid-resistant cases
Contraindications: Refer to manufacturer's literature. Methotrexate contraindicated in patients with previous liver disease or current alcohol use.
Precautions:
• Prednisone - adverse effects associated with long-term steroid use include adrenal suppression, sodium, water retention, hypokalemia, osteoporosis, cataracts, increased susceptibility to infection
• Azathioprine - adverse effects include bone marrow suppression, increased LFT's, increased susceptibility to infection
• Methotrexate - adverse effects include stomatitis. bone marrow suppression, pneumonitis, and risk of liver fibrosis and cirrhosis with prolonged use
Significant possible interactions: Refer to manufacturer's literature

ALTERNATIVE DRUGS Other immunosuppressant drugs such as cyclophosphamide, chlorambucil, cyclosporine can be added to steroids. IV immune globulin (IVIG) added to steroids being evaluated in resistant cases, also tacrolimus. Combination methotrexate and azathioprine may also be useful in refractory cases.

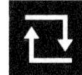
FOLLOWUP

PATIENT MONITORING
• Serial serum muscle enzyme testing
• Any adult should be studied for malignancy
• Monitor for steroid-induced metabolic complications (hypokalemia, hypertension, hyperglycemia, etc.)
• Bone densitometry and consideration of calcium, vitamin D, and Alendronate (Fosamax) therapy
• If azathioprine, methotrexate or other immunosuppressant used, then appropriate laboratory monitoring should be done periodically.

PREVENTION/AVOIDANCE N/A

POSSIBLE COMPLICATIONS
• Pneumonia
• Infection
• Myocardial infarction
• Carcinoma (especially breast, lung)
• Severe dysphagia
• Respiratory impairment due to muscle weakness, interstitial lung disease
• Aspiration pneumonitis
• Steroid myopathy
• Steroid induced diabetes, hypertension, hypokalemia, osteoporosis

EXPECTED COURSE/PROGNOSIS
• 30% residual weakness
• 20% persistent active disease
• 75% 5-year survival
• Survival worse for women and African-Americans
• Most patients improve with therapy
• 50% have full recovery
• Possibly relapsing
• Inclusion body myositis tends to be more steroid-refractory and includes more distal weakness

MISCELLANEOUS

ASSOCIATED CONDITIONS
• Malignancy
• Progressive systemic sclerosis
• Vasculitis
• Systemic lupus erythematosus
• Other connective tissue disorders

AGE-RELATED FACTORS
Pediatric:
• Childhood dermatomyositis occurs
• May be possible to discontinue prednisone gradually after a year or so
Geriatric:
• Rare after age 60
• Elderly male patient with polymyositis more likely to have underlying neoplasm
Others: N/A

PREGNANCY N/A

SYNONYMS
• Neuromyositis
• Wagner-Unverricht syndrome

ICD-9-CM
710.3 Dermatomyositis
710.4 Polymyositis

SEE ALSO
• Osteoporosis

OTHER NOTES Classification of types of myositis: Childhood dermatomyositis, primary idiopathic dermatomyositis, dermatomyositis or polymyositis associated with malignancy, primary polymyositis, myositis associated with overlap syndrome. Inclusion-body myositis represents a variant with atypical presentation and variable response to therapy.

ABBREVIATIONS N/A

REFERENCES
• Kelley W, et al: Textbook of Rheumatology. 5th Ed. Philadelphia, W.B. Saunders Co., 1997
• Villalba L, et al: Treatment of refractory myositis. A randomized crossover trial of two new cytotoxic regimens. Arthritis Rheum 1998;41:392-399
• Kagen LJ, ed: Inflammatory disorders of muscle. Rheum Dis Clin of No Amer 1994;20:811-1057
• Plotz PH, et al: Myositis: Immunologic contributions to understanding cause, pathogenesis, and therapy. Ann Int Med 1995;122:715-724
Illustrations: 4 available on CD-ROM
Internet references: http://www.5mcc.com

Author(s)
Christopher M. Wise, MD

Porphyria

BASICS

DESCRIPTION Several heme synthesis pathway enzyme deficiencies with overproduction and accumulation of intermediate metabolic products and resultant neuropsychiatric-abdominal or dermatologic symptoms and syndromes. All more common in Caucasians than Blacks or Asians.
• Porphyria cutanea tarda (PCT) - dermatologic
• Acute intermittent porphyria (AIP) - pyrroloporphyria; neuropsychiatric-abdominal
• Protoporphyria (PP) - erythropoietic or hepatoerythropoietic; mild dermatologic
• Variegate porphyria (VP) - South African porphyria, prevalence in S. Africa is 1/400
• Hereditary coproporphyria (HCP) - neuropsychic, occasionally dermatologic
• Porphobilinogen synthetase deficiency (PBD) - delta-aminolevulinic aciduria; neuropsychiatric-abdominal
• Congenital erythropoietic porphyria (CEP) - Günther's disease; severe dermatologic
• Other rare genetic variants reported
System(s) affected: Gastrointestinal, Skin/Exocrine, Hemic/Lymphatic/Immunologic
Genetics:
• Autosomal dominant - PCT, AIP, PP, VP, HCP
• Autosomal recessive - PBD, CEP
• Latency common with variable expression, many asymptomatic or minimally symptomatic carriers
• PCT also sporadic and acquired
Incidence/Prevalence in USA:
• PCT - 1/10,000
• AIP, PP, VP - 1/10,000 to 1/100,000
• HCP - less than 1/100,000
• PBD, CEP - very rare
Predominant age:
• CEP - early childhood
• PP - older childhood
• AIP, VP, HCP, PBD - young adult
• PCT - middle age
Predominant sex:
• PP, CEP - male=female
• PCT - seen more commonly in male
• AIP, VP, HCP, PBD - seen more commonly in female

SIGNS AND SYMPTOMS
• All usually reversible, lasting days to weeks
• May be permanent
• Urine may turn dark red or brown on standing (word porphyria from Greek porphyra = purple)
• Abdominal:
  ◊ Rather severe abdominal pain, occasionally in back and extremities
  ◊ Generalized more often than localized
  ◊ Often colicky
  ◊ Can mimic acute abdomen
  ◊ No fever should be present
  ◊ Chronic constipation common
  ◊ Severity of symptoms often out of proportion to physical findings
• Neurologic:
  ◊ Essentially anything
  ◊ Includes sensory and motor systems
  ◊ Includes autonomic nervous system
  ◊ May include seizures
  ◊ May lead to quadriplegia and/or respiratory paralysis with death
• Psychiatric:
  ◊ Essentially anything
  ◊ Psychosis most common
  ◊ Visual hallucinations common
  ◊ Disorientation frequent
  ◊ Chronic depression frequent
• Dermatologic:
  ◊ Photosensitivity
  ◊ Scrapes, ulcerations, blisters with minimal trauma
  ◊ Hyperpigmentation, especially hands and face
  ◊ Scarring frequent
  ◊ CEP - mutilating, with hemolysis, erythrodontia, splenomegaly
  ◊ PP - occasional hepatic disease, including hepatic failure

CAUSES
• Genetic enzyme deficiencies
• PCT - uroporphyrinogen decarboxylase
• AIP - porphobilinogen deaminase
• PP - ferrochelatase
• VP - protoporphyrinogen oxidase
• HCP - coproporphyrinogen oxidase
• PBD - porphobilinogen synthetase
• CEP - uroporphyrinogen III synthetase (cosynthetase)
• Acquired PCT causes:
  ◊ Decreased enzyme associated with alcohol, steroids, hormones
  ◊ Specific exposure to polyhalogenated hydrocarbons (e.g., hexachlorobenzene)
  ◊ Lead poisoning may alter pathways
  ◊ HIV
  ◊ Hepatitis C virus
  ◊ Ascorbic acid deficiency?

RISK FACTORS
• Multiple precipitating factors, especially AIP, VP, HCP
• Drugs (e.g., barbiturates and sulfas in AIP)
• Estrogens, especially oral contraceptives
• Steroids
• Liver disease
• Menstrual cycles
• Infection
• Fasting
• Heavy alcohol use

DIAGNOSIS

DIFFERENTIAL DIAGNOSIS Vast and protean

LABORATORY
• Urine for porphyrins during acute attack. Urine may be normal at other times.
• Individual enzyme activity in erythrocytes or other body cells/tissues
• Stool for porphyrins in PP, VP, HCP, CEP
• Bile for porphyrin in VP
• Plasma for fluorescence emission spectroscopy in VP
• Saliva for porphyria in PCT
• Erythrocyte uroporphyrin in CEP
• PP exception - urine unremarkable. Test erythrocyte protoporphyrin.
• Ferritin typically elevated in PCT
Drugs that may alter lab results: Unknown
Disorders that may alter lab results:
• Numerous conditions may cause slight increase in porphyrinuria, but patients asymptomatic
• Acute liver disease
• Hepatoma
• Hodgkin's lymphoma
• Multiple neurologic diseases

PATHOLOGICAL FINDINGS N/A

SPECIAL TESTS Genetic studies when applicable

IMAGING N/A

DIAGNOSTIC PROCEDURES N/A

TREATMENT

APPROPRIATE HEALTH CARE Outpatient, except for crises

GENERAL MEASURES
• Neuropsychiatric-abdominal - avoid drugs, alcohol, known toxins
• Dermatologic - shade, protective clothing; avoid skin trauma; PCT - phlebotomy weekly to monthly may help prevent
• CEP - consider bone marrow transplantation

SURGICAL MEASURES N/A

ACTIVITY Normal, except dermatologic avoid sun

DIET Neuropsychiatric - large quantities of carbohydrates have been reported to help

PATIENT EDUCATION American Porphyria Foundation, P.O. Box 22712, Houston, TX 77227, (713)266-9617

MEDICATIONS

DRUG(S) OF CHOICE
- Neuropsychiatric-abdominal
  ◊ Intravenous glucose 400 grams daily for one to two days
  ◊ Hematin (ferriprotoporphyrin IX, hemin [Panhematin]) IV 1-4 mg/kg/d over 10-15 minutes x 3-14 days
  ◊ Epilepsy - consider clonazepam or gabapentin
  ◊ Depression - consider selective serotonin re-uptake inhibitors
- Dermatologic:
  ◊ Oral carotenoids, e.g., beta-carotene (Solatene), 30 mg, 1-10 capsules per day

Contraindications: Known sensitivity to drug

Precautions: Hematin - phlebitis at IV site, reduced clotting ability

Significant possible interactions: None

ALTERNATIVE DRUGS
- PCT - chloroquine 125 mg twice weekly, or hydroxychloroquine 250 mg tid, in conjunction with phlebotomy
- PCT with hepatitis C virus - interferon beneficial for both
- Menstruating women - hematin premenstrual; cycle suppressors, e.g., luteinizing hormone releasing hormone (LHRH) analogues
- Autonomic manifestations - beta blockers
- Other symptoms - treat symptomatically
Note: AIP - antioxidants ineffective

FOLLOWUP

PATIENT MONITORING   Individualized

PREVENTION/AVOIDANCE
- Avoid precipitating drugs
  ◊ Alcohol
  ◊ Barbiturates
  ◊ Carbamazepine
  ◊ Chlorpropamide
  ◊ Danazol
  ◊ Ergots
  ◊ Estrogens and progestins
  ◊ Ethchlorvynol
  ◊ Glutethimide
  ◊ Griseofulvin
  ◊ Mephenytoin
  ◊ Meprobamate
  ◊ Methotrexate
  ◊ Methyprylon
  ◊ Metoclopramide
  ◊ Phenytoin
  ◊ Pyrazolones
  ◊ Succinimides
  ◊ Sulfonamide antibiotics
  ◊ Valproic acid
- Eat an adequate diet with high carbohydrate intake

POSSIBLE COMPLICATIONS   See list in Signs and Symptoms

EXPECTED COURSE/PROGNOSIS
- In all porphyrias:
  ◊ Patients who are asymptomatic or minimally symptomatic - unaffected longevity
  ◊ Patients who are more symptomatic - treatable and do well
  ◊ Neurologic complications (e.g., peripheral neuropathy, neurosis or hemiplegia), at times permanent
- In AIP
  ◊ Acute attacks have 25% mortality
  ◊ Increased risk of hepatocellular carcinoma
- Acquired PCT
  ◊ HIV
  ◊ Hepatitis C virus
  ◊ Hepatic malignancies

MISCELLANEOUS

ASSOCIATED CONDITIONS   N/A

AGE-RELATED FACTORS
Pediatric: N/A
Geriatric: N/A
Others: N/A

PREGNANCY   Unpredictable disease activity

SYNONYMS
- Delta-aminolevulinic aciduria
- Erythropoietic porphyria
- Günther's disease
- Hepatoerythropoietic porphyria
- Pyrroloporphyria
- South African porphyria

ICD-9-CM   277.1 disorders of porphyrin metabolism

SEE ALSO   N/A

OTHER NOTES   Some drugs considered safe - acetaminophen, aspirin, atropine, bromides, diazepam (in small doses), dicumarol, digoxin, diphenhydramine, ether, glucocorticoids, guanethidine, heparin, insulin, neostigmine, nitrous oxide, penicillin and derivatives, phenothiazines, narcotic analgesics, propranolol, streptomycin, succinylcholine, thiazides

ABBREVIATIONS
PCT = Porphyria cutanea tarda
AIP = Acute intermittent porphyria
PP = Protoporphyria
VP = Variegate porphyria
HCP = Hereditary coproporphyria
PBD = Porphobilinogen synthetase deficiency
CEP = Congenital erythropoietic porphyria

REFERENCES
- Fauci, et al, eds: Harrison's Principles of Internal Medicine. 14th Ed. New York, McGraw-Hill, 1998:2152-2158
- Bennett JC, Plum F, eds: Cecil Textbook of Medicine. 20th Ed. Philadelphia, W.B. Saunders Co., 1996
- Kelly WN, et al (eds): Textbook of Internal Medicine. 3rd ed. New York, Lippincott-Raven, 1997:880-882
Illustrations: 5 available on CD-ROM
Internet references: http://www.5mcc.com

Author(s)
Emil S Dickstein, MD, FACP

Portal hypertension

BASICS

DESCRIPTION Increased portal venous pressure (> 10 mm Hg.) that occurs in association with splanchnic vasodilatation, portosystemic collateral formation and a hyperdynamic circulation. Course is generally progressive and may produce one or more devastating clinical disorders.
System(s) affected: Gastrointestinal, Cardiovascular, Nervous
Genetics: No known genetic patterns except those associated with specific hepatic diseases that cause portal hypertension
Incidence/Prevalence in USA: Unknown. (Incidence of bleeding from gastroesophageal varices is approximately 120 episodes per 100,000 population per year.)
Predominant age: Adult
Predominant sex: Male > Female

SIGNS AND SYMPTOMS
May be general or related to specific complications
• General
  ◊ Splenomegaly
  ◊ Caput medusa
  ◊ Umbilical bruit
  ◊ Hemorrhoids
  ◊ Spider angiomata
  ◊ Gynecomastia
  ◊ Testicular atrophy
  ◊ Digital clubbing
  ◊ Palmar erythema
• Gastroesophageal varices
  ◊ Hematemesis
  ◊ Melena
  ◊ Anemia
  ◊ Hypotension
  ◊ Tachycardia
• Ascites
  ◊ Distended abdomen
  ◊ Fluid wave
  ◊ Shifting percussion dullness
• Hepatic encephalopathy
  ◊ Confusion
  ◊ Asterixis
  ◊ Hyperreflexia
• Hepatorenal syndrome
  ◊ Oliguria

CAUSES
May be intrahepatic or extrahepatic
• Cirrhosis present. Accounts for > 90% of cases.
  ◊ Alcoholic
  ◊ Viral (HBV, HCV, HGV)
  ◊ Wilson's disease
  ◊ Hemochromatosis
  ◊ Primary biliary cirrhosis
  ◊ Schistosomiasis
• Cirrhosis not present.
  ◊ Portal vein thrombosis
  ◊ Hepatic vein obstruction (Budd-Chiari syndrome)
  ◊ Right ventricular failure
  ◊ Myeloproliferative disorders

RISK FACTORS Many different chronic liver diseases and hepatotoxins

DIAGNOSIS

DIFFERENTIAL DIAGNOSIS
Usually related to specific complications/presentations.
• Gastroesophageal varices with hemorrhage vs:
  ◊ Portal hypertensive gastropathy
  ◊ Hemorrhagic gastritis
  ◊ Peptic ulcer disease
  ◊ Mallory-Weiss tear
• Ascites vs:
  ◊ Spontaneous bacterial peritonitis
  ◊ Pancreatic ascites
  ◊ Peritoneal carcinomatosis
  ◊ Tuberculous peritonitis
  ◊ Nephrotic syndrome
  ◊ Cardiac ascites
• Hepatic encephalopathy vs:
  ◊ Delirium tremens
  ◊ Intracranial hemorrhage
  ◊ Sedative abuse
  ◊ Uremia
• Hepatorenal syndrome vs
  ◊ Drug nephrotoxicity
  ◊ Renal tubular necrosis

LABORATORY
Non-specific changes associated with underlying disease.
• Hypersplenism
  ◊ Anemia
  ◊ Leukopenia
  ◊ Thrombocytopenia
• Hepatic dysfunction
  ◊ Hypoalbuminemia
  ◊ Hyperbilirubinemia
  ◊ Elevated alkaline phosphatase
  ◊ Elevated liver enzymes
  ◊ Abnormal clotting factors (PT, PTT.)
• Gastrointestinal bleeding
  ◊ Iron deficiency anemia
  ◊ Elevated serum ammonia
• Hepatorenal syndrome
  ◊ Elevated serum creatinine, BUN
  ◊ Urine Na < 20 mEq/L.
Drugs that may alter lab results: N/A
Disorders that may alter lab results: N/A

PATHOLOGICAL FINDINGS Specific for underlying disease

SPECIAL TESTS Specific for underlying disease

IMAGING
• UGI series. May outline varices in esophagus and stomach.
• CT scan and ultrasound. May detect cirrhosis, splenomegaly, ascites and varices.
• Duplex-Doppler (ultrasound.) Can determine presence and direction of flow in portal and hepatic veins. Useful in diagnosing portal vein and/or shunt thrombosis.
• Angiography. Demonstrates cork-screwing of intrahepatic vessels (cirrhosis); can identify varices and vascular anomalies.

DIAGNOSTIC PROCEDURES
• Endoscopy. Can diagnose esophageal and gastric varices and portal hypertensive gastropathy or can directly visualize other bleeding sites (peptic ulcers, gastritis, Mallory-Weiss tears.)
• Hepatic venous wedge pressure. Correlates with portal pressure; risk of variceal bleeding is increased if HVWP > 12 mm./Hg.

TREATMENT

APPROPRIATE HEALTH CARE
Inpatient

GENERAL MEASURES
• Treat underlying disease and support metabolic/nutritional needs.
• Avoid sedatives; may precipitate encephalopathy
• Transfuse packed RBCs as needed. Use caution; circulation is already hyperdynamic.
• Correct coagulopathy. Administer vitamin K and/or fresh-frozen plasma.
• Limit sodium administration; cirrhotic patients avidly retain sodium

SURGICAL MEASURES
• Liver transplantation may be recommended for selected patients with far-advanced hepatic disease. Other less aggressive approaches are available for specific complications of portal hypertension.
• Gastroesophageal varices with hemorrhage
  ◊ Endoscopic variceal sclerosis
  ◊ Endoscopic variceal banding
  ◊ Portacaval shunting
  ◊ Transjugular portosystemic shunt (TIPS)
• Ascites refractory to medical management
  ◊ Large volume paracentesis
  ◊ Peritoneovenous shunt

ACTIVITY Bed rest for acute complications (bleeding, encephalopathy or hepatorenal syndrome)

DIET Restrict sodium and protein

PATIENT EDUCATION N/A

MEDICATIONS

DRUG(S) OF CHOICE
• Therapy for variceal hemorrhage:
  ◊ For acute control: intravenous somatostatin or octreotide - synthetic analogue
  ◊ Alternative: vasopressin; but, has more complications (decreased by addition of nitroglycerin)
  ◊ For prevention of recurrence: propranolol
• Therapy for encephalopathy:
  ◊ Lactulose. Induces diarrhea and traps intracolonic ammonia.
  ◊ Neomycin. Reduces bacterial production of nitrogenous substances in colon.
• Therapy for ascites:
  ◊ Furosemide (Lasix)
  ◊ Spironolactone.
Contraindications: Vasopressin is a systemic vasodilator and may cause hypotension, bradycardia and cardiac and peripheral ischemia. Cardiac monitoring is advisable.
Precautions: Vasopressin may cause hypertension, bradycardia, arrhythmias. Patient must be on a cardiac monitor while receiving this drug. Co-administration of nitroprusside may reduce cardiotoxicity.
Significant possible interactions: Refer to manufacturer's literature

ALTERNATIVE DRUGS
Glypressin and terlipressin are more selective splanchnic vasoconstrictors and may be associated with fewer complications. Studies are continuing.

FOLLOWUP

PATIENT MONITORING
Acute complications of portal hypertension require intensive monitoring of vital signs and organ function. Long-term management includes regular follow-up of all affected organ systems.

PREVENTION/AVOIDANCE
Abstinence from alcohol. Adequate and appropriate nutrition.

POSSIBLE COMPLICATIONS
As described above

EXPECTED COURSE/PROGNOSIS
• Variceal bleeding: 50% re-bleed, usually within 2 years unless portal pressure is reduced by shunt or TIPS procedure
• Ascites: Generally recurs. Frequency and severity can be reduced if salt restriction is observed.
• Hepatic encephalopathy. Often recurs especially if re-bleeding develops. Low protein diet advised.

MISCELLANEOUS

ASSOCIATED CONDITIONS
As described above

AGE-RELATED FACTORS
Pediatric: Uncommon. Generally different etiology than in adults.
• Intrahepatic
  ◊ Biliary atresia
  ◊ Viral hepatitis
  ◊ Metabolic liver disease.
• Extrahepatic
  ◊ Congenital anomalies of portal vein
  ◊ Neonatal omphalitis (umbilical vein catheterization, sepsis, abdominal trauma)
Geriatric: Mortality and complication rate are increased
Others: N/A

PREGNANCY N/A

SYNONYMS N/A

ICD-9-CM 572.3 Portal hypertension

SEE ALSO
• Cirrhosis of the liver
• Hepatitis, viral

OTHER NOTES
• Other treatment approaches (inadequately studied with non-control protocols)
  ◊ Transhepatic obliteration of varices
  ◊ Concomitant treatment with non-selective beta-adrenergic blockers

ABBREVIATIONS N/A

REFERENCES
• Sleisenger MH, Fortran JS, eds: Gastrointestinal Disease: Pathophysiology, Diagnosis, Management. 5th Ed. Philadelphia, WB Saunders Co., 1994
• Jaffe DL, Chung RT, Friedman LS: Management of portal hypertension and its complications. Med Clin N Am 1996;80:1021-1034
• Pagliaro L, D'Amico G, Luca A, et al: Portal hypertension: diagnosis and treatment. J. Hepatol. 1995: 23 (Suppl 1):36-44
• Teran JC, Imperiale TF, Mullen KD, et al: Primary prophylaxis of variceal bleeding in cirrhosis: a cost-effectiveness analysis. Gastroent 1997;112:473-482
Illustrations: N/A
Internet references: http://www.5mcc.com

Author(s)
Wayne H. Schwesinger, MD

Post-concussive syndrome

BASICS

DESCRIPTION
• CNS dysfunction occurring after minor head injury with or without initial loss of consciousness. The primary cause is diffuse axonal injury and small vessel injury. Diffuse axonal injury is a result of shearing forces caused by rapid deceleration, flexion-extension injury, and rotatory injury. Neuronal injury continues for 6-12 hours secondary to free radical formation and other factors.
• Occurs in up to 50% of patients with mild traumatic brain injury (TBI)
• Most patients recover within 12 weeks but 15% with minor TBI will be symptomatic at 1 year and some never become asymptomatic
• By definition, these patients have an initial GCS of 13-15
• Concussion Grades:
  ◊ 1: transient confusion, no LOC, duration of mental status changes < 15 minutes
  ◊ 2: transient confusion, no LOC, duration of mental status change > 15 minutes
  ◊ 3: any LOC (including seizures), either brief or prolonged
System(s) affected: Nervous
Genetics: N/A
Incidence/Prevalence in USA: 180/100,000 with 27/100,000 being persistent
Predominant age: 15-24 years. Patients over 55 are more likely to have persistent deficits
Predominant sex: Male > Female

SIGNS AND SYMPTOMS
• Chronic headache; some may be severe
• Chronic neck pain
• Dizziness or vertigo
• Poor concentration
• Memory deficits
• Personality changes
• Irritability, depression, anxiety
• Decrease in ability to smell or taste (5%)
• Sleep-wake disturbances
• Other cognitive disturbances

CAUSES
Falls, motor vehicle accidents (MVA), assault, etc

RISK FACTORS
Those that predispose to falls, MVA, etc. including drugs and alcohol. Additionally, there is some association with litigation, female gender, preexisting headaches, and low socioeconomic status. However, these factors account for only a minority of the cases (eg, men are almost as likely as women to have symptoms, patients without pending litigation are almost as likely as those with pending litigation to have symptoms, etc.)

DIAGNOSIS

DIFFERENTIAL DIAGNOSIS N/A

LABORATORY N/A
Drugs that may alter lab results: N/A
Disorders that may alter lab results: N/A

PATHOLOGICAL FINDINGS Diffuse axonal injury has been demonstrated on post mortem specimens

SPECIAL TESTS Neuropsychometric testing will demonstrate subtle abnormalities not demonstrable on instruments such as mini mental status exam

IMAGING
• CT scan is usually normal
• MRI may show small petechial hemorrhages or focal cortical contusions. SPECT scanning may show small areas of focal edema. MRI and SPECT scanning should be considered research tools at this time since the diagnosis is primarily clinical.

DIAGNOSTIC PROCEDURES
Neuropsychometric testing

TREATMENT

APPROPRIATE HEALTH CARE An outpatient setting with involvement of a primary care physician, neurologist, and psychologist as appropriate. Many cases can be handled solely by the patient's primary care physician.

GENERAL MEASURES
• Address the patient's symptoms such as neck pain, headaches, depression, etc. using the usual medications
• Involvement of vocational rehabilitation may be necessary
• Behavioral therapy, etc. can be tried, but there is no good evidence that this is effective

SURGICAL MEASURES N/A

ACTIVITY As tolerated. Sports activity, etc., should be limited based on degree of injury. Parents and coaches will often try to return an athlete to sports competition prematurely. The American Academy of Neurology has published these guidelines (226 MMWR March 14, 1997). A second impact syndrome phenomenon occurs. The second injury, while in and of itself may be mild, is cumulative with the first and may be fatal. Recommendations are verbatim from MMWR.
• Grade 1 concussion:
  ◊ Management: the athlete should be removed from sports activity, examined immediately and at 5-minute intervals, and allowed to return that day to the sports activity only if postconcussive symptoms (headache, vomiting, etc.) resolve within 15 minutes. Any athlete who incurs a second Grade 1 concussion on the same day should be removed from sports activity until asymptomatic for 1 week.
• Grade 2 concussion:
  ◊ Management: The athlete should be removed from sports activity and examined frequently to assess the evolution of symptoms, with more extensive diagnostic evaluation if the symptoms worsen or persist for > 1 week. The athlete should return to sports activity only after asymptomatic for 1 full week. Any athlete who incurs a Grade 2 concussion subsequent to a Grade 1 concussion on the same day should be removed from sports activity until asymptomatic for 2 weeks.
• Grade 3 concussion:
  ◊ Management: the athlete should be removed from sports activity for 1 full week without symptoms if the loss of consciousness is brief or 2 full weeks without symptoms if the loss of consciousness is prolonged. If still unconscious or if abnormal neurologic signs are present at the time of initial evaluation, the athlete should be transported by ambulance to the nearest hospital emergency department. An athlete who suffers a second Grade 3 concussion should be removed from sports activity until asymptomatic for 1 month. Any athlete with an abnormality on computed tomography or magnetic resonance imaging brain scan consistent with brain swelling, contusion, or other intracranial pathology should be removed from sports activities for the season and discouraged from future return to participation in contact sports.

DIET N/A

PATIENT EDUCATION Discussion with patient and family about long term prospects, etc.

MEDICATIONS

DRUG(S) OF CHOICE
• Sleep disorders/depression/headache:
◊ Amitriptyline in age appropriate doses or other tricyclic drug
◊ SSRIs are less well studied in PCS, but can be used for depression
◊ Benzodiazepines should be avoided if possible
• Neck pain/headache:
◊ NSAIDs
◊ Avoid narcotics if possible
Contraindications: N/A
Precautions:
• NSAIDs may cause ulcer disease, elevated blood pressure, renal dysfunction and bleeding among other side effects
• Tricyclics can cause arrhythmias and should not be used in the suicidal patient; tricyclics can also cause urinary retention, constipation and other anticholinergic side effects
Significant possible interactions:
• NSAIDs: warfarin, ACE inhibitors, and lithium.
• Ibuprofen-oral hypoglycemics: hypoglycemia
• Tricyclics: multiple drug interactions including cimetidine and MAOIs. Check a drug reference.
• SSRIs-MAOI: should never be given together; risk of serotonin syndrome. These may also cause tricyclic toxicity when used together.

ALTERNATIVE DRUGS N/A

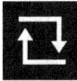

FOLLOWUP

PATIENT MONITORING As needed. Each case is individualized.

PREVENTION/AVOIDANCE Discussing the avoidance of drugs and alcohol with teens at the time of a sports physical. Discussion of seat-belt use.

POSSIBLE COMPLICATIONS Loss of source of income and resulting problems such as loss of house, strain on the family, etc.

EXPECTED COURSE/PROGNOSIS
Those not better by 1 year will probably not get better. It is of note that the resolution of litigation does not generally result in improvement of this disorder.

MISCELLANEOUS

ASSOCIATED CONDITIONS See Risk factors

AGE-RELATED FACTORS
Pediatric: Tend to improve more quickly
Geriatric: Tend not to improve
Others: Those over age 55 are more likely to have permanent deficits

PREGNANCY N/A

SYNONYMS N/A

ICD-9-CM
310.2 Postconcussion syndrome

SEE ALSO
• Brain injury, traumatic
• Cervical spine injury
• Depression
• Migraine
• Headache, tension

OTHER NOTES Consider a repeat head CT within the first couple of weeks if symptoms persist. The symptoms of PCS can also be due to subdural hemorrhages.

ABBREVIATIONS
TBI = traumatic brain injury
MVA = motor vehicle accident
PCS = post concussive syndrome
GCS = Glascow Coma Score
SPECT = single photon emission computed tomography

REFERENCES
• Alexander MP: Mild traumatic brain injury: pathophysiology, natural history, and clinical management. Neurology 1995;45:1253-1260
• Borczuk P. Neurologic emergencies: Mild head trauma. Emergency Clinics of NA 1997;15(3):653-679
Illustrations: N/A
Internet references: http://www.5mcc.com

Author(s)
Mark A. Graber, MD

Post-traumatic stress disorder (PTSD)

BASICS

DESCRIPTION A condition seen in people who experienced an event that would be extremely distressing to most human beings, e.g., serious threat to one's life, physical or psychological integrity; serious threat or harm to one's children, spouse, siblings, parents or other close relatives or friends; sudden destruction of one's home or community; seeing another person who has recently been (or is being) injured or killed as a result of a man-made violent act or natural disaster.
• The person's response involved intense fear, helplessness, or horror. Note: In children, this may be expressed instead by disorganized or agitated behavior.
• Symptoms of this condition did not exist prior to the trauma, and symptoms persist for at least one month following the trauma
• There is a subtype of post-traumatic stress disorder (PTSD) with a delayed onset of the symptoms which starts at least six months after the trauma
• The acute form of PTSD is defined as the duration being less than 3 months
• Chronic form is defined when the duration of symptoms is more than 3 months
System(s) affected: Nervous
Genetics: N/A
Incidence/Prevalence in USA: Up to 30% of victims of disasters develop PTSD. Lifelong prevalence in general population ranges from 1-14%.
Predominant age: The elderly and the very young are more vulnerable
Predominant sex: Adult women are more inclined to ask for help. Young boys may be more vulnerable to trauma than girls. Most men with PTSD have experienced combat or exposure to trauma on the job. Most women with PTSD have a history of rape or being physically assaulted.

SIGNS AND SYMPTOMS
• The traumatic event is persistently re-experienced in one or more of the following ways:
◊ Recurrent and intrusive distressing recollections of the event, including images, thoughts or perceptions. Note: In young children repetitive play may occur in which themes or aspects of the trauma are expressed.
◊ Recurrent distressing dreams of the event. Note: In children, there may be frightening dreams without recognizable content.
◊ Acting or feeling as if the traumatic event were recurring (includes a sense of reliving the experience, illusions, hallucinations, and dissociative flashback episodes, including those that occur on awakening or when intoxicated). Note: In young children, trauma-specific reenactment may occur.
◊ Intense psychological distress at exposure to internal or external cues that symbolize or resemble an aspect of the traumatic event

◊ Physiological reactivity on exposure to internal or external cues that symbolize or resemble an aspect of the traumatic event, such as increased heart rate, changes in blood pressure, discoloration of the skin, blurred vision, hyperperistalsis in smooth muscle, nausea, vomiting, diarrhea, urinary urgency, etc.
• Persistent avoidance of the stimuli associated with the trauma, or numbing of general responsiveness (not present before the trauma) as indicated by three (or more) of the following:
◊ Efforts to avoid thoughts, feelings or conversations associated with the trauma
◊ Efforts to avoid activities, places or people that arouse recollections of the trauma
◊ Inability to recall an important aspect of the trauma (psychogenic amnesia)
◊ Markedly diminished interest or participation in significant activities (in young children, loss of recently acquired developmental skills such as toilet training or language skills)
◊ Feelings of detachment or estrangement from others
◊ Restricted range of affect (e.g., unable to have loving feelings)
◊ Sense of a foreshortened future (e.g., does not expect to have a career, marriage, or a normal life span)
• Persistent symptoms of increased arousal (not present before the trauma), as indicated by two or more of the following:
◊ Difficulty falling or staying asleep (insomnia)
◊ Irritability or outbursts of anger
◊ Difficulty in concentrating
◊ Hypervigilance
◊ Exaggerated startle response
• Others:
◊ Duration of the disturbance is more than 1 month
◊ The disturbance causes clinically significant distress or impairment in social, occupational, or other important areas of functioning

CAUSES Events which are insults to one's personal integrity, self-esteem and security are psychologically traumatic and may lead to PTSD

RISK FACTORS Individuals with a history of childhood neglect or dysfunctional families, children of alcoholic parents, or childhood abuse, are predisposed and more susceptible to developing PTSD in response to trauma

DIAGNOSIS

DIFFERENTIAL DIAGNOSIS
• Organic mental disorders
• Generalized anxiety disorder
• Phobic disorders
• Depressive disorder
• Panic disorder
• Conversion disorder
• Somatization disorder
• Personality disorders
• Substance and chemical dependency

LABORATORY N/A
Drugs that may alter lab results: N/A
Disorders that may alter lab results: N/A

PATHOLOGICAL FINDINGS Character pathology as shown on the Minnesota multiple personality inventory (MMPI)

SPECIAL TESTS
• Neuropsychological testing is helpful in cases of dementia and more subtle cognitive dysfunction
• EEG to rule out any brain damage (results may be altered by any drug affecting EEG patterns such as - sleeping pills, antidepressants, neuroleptics and other psychotropic medications)
• Psychological testing and a thorough mental status examination are valuable in a complete, thorough assessment of the patient
• Sleep lab studies of 8 hour EEG help in diagnosis of sleep disorders
• Through an examination and interview, assisted by sodium amytal (given intravenously) or similar substances, one may uncover traumatic material in patients with amnesia. Similarly, an examination assisted by hypnosis may help in the diagnosis.
• Tests may be affected by withdrawal or intoxication from drugs and alcohol; any organic brain syndromes such as multiple infarct dementia, other forms of dementia, and forms of epilepsy

IMAGING CT scan of the head and MRI of the brain are valuable to rule out any brain damage

DIAGNOSTIC PROCEDURES
• Psychiatric examination
• Psychological testing
• Note: The American Psychiatry Association has implemented in 1994, a new diagnostic and classification manual for psychiatric disorders. This includes a new diagnostic category entitled Acute Stress Disorder. The signs and symptoms are essentially the same as those described for PTSD, except for the fact that in acute stress disorder, the disturbance lasts for a minimum of 2 days and the maximum of 4 weeks and occurs within 4 weeks of the traumatic event. If the symptoms last more than 4 weeks, or begin more than 30 days after the original trauma, the condition is diagnosed as PTSD.

TREATMENT

APPROPRIATE HEALTH CARE
• Most treatment is done on an outpatient basis
• In case of crisis such as a patient being suicidal or dysfunctional with activities of daily living, inpatient intensive treatment on a psychiatry unit is indicated

Post-traumatic stress disorder (PTSD)

GENERAL MEASURES
- As indicated by the patient's general condition, treatment includes individual psychotherapy, group therapy, hypnotherapy, narcoanalysis and narcosynthesis, and behavior therapy
- Crisis intervention shortly after the traumatic event is very valuable for the immediate distress and may prevent the development of a chronic or delayed form of post-traumatic stress disorder
- Relaxation exercises to help reduce anxiety and improve sleep have been found helpful

SURGICAL MEASURES N/A

ACTIVITY
- As indicated by patient's physical condition
- Restoration of regular sleep at night is essential in cases of insomnia

DIET A healthy diet of complex carbohydrates, proteins, and multi-vitamins and minerals. Avoid fatty foods.

PATIENT EDUCATION Lenore Terr: Too Scared to Cry. Harper & Row, NY, 1990

MEDICATIONS

DRUG(S) OF CHOICE
- Selective serotonin reuptake inhibitors (SSRI): (this group has recently been proven to be safe and effective for the control of many symptoms of PTSD)
    ◊ Fluoxetine 20-80 mg/day
    ◊ Sertraline 50-200 mg/day
    ◊ Paroxetine 20-60 mg/day
    ◊ Citalopram 20-60 mg/day
    ◊ Venlafaxine 75-325 mg/day
- Tricyclic antidepressants:
    ◊ Doxepin 50-150 mg/day
    ◊ Nortriptyline 30-100 mg/day
    ◊ Imipramine 50-300 mg/day
    ◊ Desipramine 50-300 mg/day
    ◊ Amitriptyline 50-300 mg/day
    ◊ Trimipramine 50-300 mg/day
    ◊ Protriptyline 15-60 mg/ day
    ◊ Amoxapine 50-300 mg/day
    ◊ Maprotiline 50-225 mg/day (increased risk of seizures with higher doses)
- Monoamine oxidase inhibitors:
    ◊ Phenelzine 45-75 mg/day is useful especially in PTSD patients with panic attacks
- Others:
    ◊ Trazodone 100-400 mg/day, given mostly at bedtime is helpful in patients with insomnia
    ◊ Nefazodone 200-600 mg/day in patients with insomnia improves REM sleep
    ◊ Small doses of neuroleptics are helpful in selective patients
    ◊ Bupropion 100-450 mg/day
    ◊ Neuroleptics - small doses are helpful in selective patients
    ◊ Benzodiazepines should be used selectively and with caution

Contraindications:
- Allergic reactions to specific drugs
- Use with caution in alcoholic patients with poor liver functions

Precautions:
- Do not mix tricyclic antidepressants with monoamine oxidase inhibitors
- Long-term use of benzodiazepines may lead to increased tolerance and drug dependency

Significant possible interactions:
Monoamine oxidase inhibitors may interact with other antidepressants, sympathomimetics such as pseudoephedrine and any foods with tyramine or its precursors

ALTERNATIVE DRUGS
- Clomipramine 75-250 mg/day or fluvoxamine 100-300 mg/day or fluoxetine 20-80 mg/day in patients with obsessive compulsive symptoms has been helpful in some cases
- Buspirone 30-80 mg/day has been found helpful in cases with severe anxiety
- Propranolol and clonidine have been used with limited results to control the psychophysiological hyperactivity during intense flashbacks

FOLLOWUP

PATIENT MONITORING Psychotherapy for at least one hour per week is necessary in the first phase of treatment

PREVENTION/AVOIDANCE Crisis intervention immediately after the traumatic event involving intensive support and treatment may prevent the development of chronic PTSD later

POSSIBLE COMPLICATIONS Suicide; self-inflicted violence in reenactment of trauma

EXPECTED COURSE/PROGNOSIS
- The lack of crisis intervention immediately following the trauma may lead to the persistence of symptoms. If symptoms last less than 3 months, the patient is still in the acute form of PTSD. If symptoms persist over 3 months, patients may develop chronic PTSD which may lead to loss of job, marital conflicts, total disability and repeated and/or lengthy hospitalizations with severe morbidity.
- If the onset of symptoms is at least 6 months or more after the original traumatic event, the patient suffers from a delayed onset type
- The more chronic and delayed the onset, the worse the prognosis. Early treatment in acute phase associated with better prognosis.

MISCELLANEOUS

ASSOCIATED CONDITIONS Personality disorders such as borderline personality disorder, depression, panic disorder, anxiety disorder, and dissociative disorders

AGE-RELATED FACTORS
Pediatric: Young children are susceptible to abuse and neglect; can develop chronic PTSD with failure to progress and grow in healthy way
Geriatric: Have fewer social support resources; adjustment to trauma less flexible; more sensitive to medication and need dose adjustment.
Others: N/A

PREGNANCY Avoid psychotropics in the first trimester. Focus on non-pharmacologic treatment techniques such as psychotherapy, hypnotherapy, relaxation therapy, etc.

SYNONYMS
- Trauma syndrome
- Battle fatigue
- Shell shock
- Post-disaster syndrome
- Trauma survivor's syndrome
- Traumatic neurosis

ICD-9-CM
293.9 Unspecified transient organic mental disorder

SEE ALSO N/A

OTHER NOTES N/A

ABBREVIATIONS
PTSD = post-traumatic stress disorder

REFERENCES
- Van derKolk, et al. Traumatic stress: the effects of overwhelming experiences on mind, body, and society. New York, Guilford Press 1996
- Field LH. Post-traumatic stress disorder; a reappraisal. J of the Royal Soc of Med. 1999;92:35-37
- Rauch SL, et al. A symptom provocation study of PTSD using PET and script driven imagery. Arch Gen Psychiatry. 1996;53:380-387
- Burton JK, Marshall RD. Categorizing fear and the role of trauma in a clinical formulation. Am J of Psychiatry 1999;156:761-766
- Yul W. Post-traumatic stress disorder. Archives of Disease in Childhood. 1999;80:107-109
- Yehuda R. Biological factors associated with susceptibility to post traumatic stress disorder. Canadian J of Psychiat 1999;44:34-39
16 additional references available at web site
Internet references: http://www.5mcc.com
Illustrations: N/A

Author(s)
Moshe S. Torem, MD, FAPA

Preeclampsia

 BASICS

DESCRIPTION Hypertension associated with proteinuria, edema, and acute excessive weight gain developing during pregnancy after 20 weeks gestation
System(s) affected: Reproductive, Cardiovascular, Nervous
Genetics: N/A
Incidence/Prevalence in USA: 5-10% of all pregnancies
Predominant age:
• Young, primigravid women
• Women over 35 years of age
Predominant sex: Female only

SIGNS AND SYMPTOMS
• Elevated BP (> 140/90 [18.6/12 kPa] or increased 30 [4 kPa] systolic or increased 15 [2 kPa] diastolic) recorded on 2 BP readings 6 hours apart
• Proteinuria (> 300 mg/24 hours or > 1 gram/L)
• Edema
• Rapid excessive weight gain (> 5 lb/week) (2.3 kg/week)
• Epigastric pain
• Headache
• Hyperreflexia
• Visual disturbances
• Apprehension
• Retinal arteriolar spasm
• Papilledema
• Retinal cotton-wool exudate
• Amnesia
• Oliguria
• Anuria

CAUSES
• Altered cardiovascular reactivity
• Increased capillary permeability
• Widespread vasospasm
• Microthrombi
• Hypertension
• Improper implantation of placenta to uterine wall limiting blood and nutrients to fetus

RISK FACTORS
• Familial incidence
• Lower socio-economic
• Multiple fetuses
• Teenage
• Collagen disorders
• Females > 35 years old
• Primigravida
• First subsequent pregnancy with a different father
• Diabetes mellitus of pregnancy
• Chronic hypertension
• Hydatid mole
• Fetal hydrops
• History of renal disease

 DIAGNOSIS

DIFFERENTIAL DIAGNOSIS
• Chronic hypertension
• Pregnancy worsened hypertension
• Pregnancy induced hypertension

LABORATORY
• Proteinuria (> 300 mg/24 hrs or > 1 gram/L)
• Uric acid increased (mild increase > 5.5 mg/dL [0.32 mmol/L]);
(severe increase > 9.5 mg/dL [0.56 mmol/L])
• Thrombocytopenia
• CrCl < 90 mL/min/1.73m2 (0.87 mL/s/m2)
• Increased BUN (> 16 mg/dL [5.7 mmol/L])
• Increased creatinine (> 1.0 mg/dL [88 μmol/L])
• Abnormal increased liver function tests
• Increased fibrin degradation products
• Increased PT
• Decreased fibrinogen
• Granular casts in urine
• Red blood cell casts in urine
• Renal tubular cell casts in urine
• White blood cell casts in urine
• Increased urine specific gravity
• Increased T4
• Thrombocytopenia
• Decreased fibrinogen
• Disseminated intravascular coagulation
• Hyperbilirubinemia
Drugs that may alter lab results: N/A
Disorders that may alter lab results: Chronic renal disease

PATHOLOGICAL FINDINGS
• Fibrin deposits in kidneys
• Fibrin deposits in liver with necrosis and periportal hemorrhages
• Placental vascular abnormalities

SPECIAL TESTS N/A

IMAGING N/A

DIAGNOSTIC PROCEDURES 24 hour urine for protein

 TREATMENT

APPROPRIATE HEALTH CARE
• Outpatient care if mild
• Inpatient care if deterioration
• Delivery of fetus as soon as possible if severe
• Admit to hospital if blood pressure > 160/110 (21.3/14.6 kPa), proteinuria > 5 gm/24 hr, oliguria, cerebral or visual disturbances (scotoma, blurred vision), severe headache, altered consciousness, pulmonary edema, thrombocytopenia, impaired liver function tests, epigastric pain

GENERAL MEASURES
• If outpatient, keep a daily weight record; use a home test to check for proteinuria
• If outpatient, twice a week blood pressure tests

SURGICAL MEASURES N/A

ACTIVITY
• Bedrest on left side
• Ambulatory only to void

DIET
• Salt restriction is not good because the patient is in an intravascular contracted state
• Protein 80-100 gm/day

PATIENT EDUCATION Avoid excessive weight gain during pregnancy (> 25-30 lb [11.4-13.6 kg])

MEDICATIONS

DRUG(S) OF CHOICE For seizure prophylaxis - magnesium sulfate (MgSO4) loading dose 4 grams IV in 200 mL normal saline over 20-30 min. Maintenance dose - 1-2 grams/hr IV.

Contraindications: Refer to manufacturer's profile of each drug

Precautions:
• Therapeutic magnesium levels are 4-7 mEq/L (2-3.5 mmol/L)
• Toxicity (flushing, sweating, hyporeflexia, flaccid paralysis, CNS depression, oliguria, decreased cardiac function)
• Spinal/epidural anesthesia contraindicated
• Continue 24 hour postpartum
• Toxicity therapy with 10% calcium gluconate, 1 gram over 2-3 minutes plus oxygen
• Give oxytocin (Pitocin) postpartum to prevent bleeding (60 unit/L at 50 cc/hr)
• Keep urine flow > 25 cc/hr
• Recheck reflexes often. They may be hypoactive, but should be present.

Significant possible interactions: Refer to manufacturer's profile of each drug

ALTERNATIVE DRUGS
• Hypertension:
  ◊ Hydralazine (Apresoline) 5-10 mg IV q 20-30 minutes, or
  ◊ Diazoxide 30 mg minidose if refractory to hydralazine
  ◊ Avoid nitroprusside (decreased uterine blood flow plus possible lethal fetal cyanide levels)
• Seizures:
  ◊ MgSO4 - not as effective for treatment of seizures as it is for prophylaxis
  ◊ Diazepam (Valium) 10 mg IV followed by 10 mg IM q4h if MgSO4 unavailable or ineffective

FOLLOWUP

PATIENT MONITORING
• Keep urine output > 25 cc/hr
• Continue MgSO4 for 24 hr postpartum
• Give oxytocin (Pitocin) postpartum to prevent bleeding (60 unit/L at 50 cc/hr)

PREVENTION/AVOIDANCE
• Weight control
• Large scale studies do not support low dose aspirin for prevention

POSSIBLE COMPLICATIONS
• Eclampsia (seizures)
• Hypertensive crisis
• Acute pyelonephritis
• Acute fatty liver
• Acute pulmonary edema

EXPECTED COURSE/PROGNOSIS
• Prevention of seizures
• Delivery of viable fetus

MISCELLANEOUS

ASSOCIATED CONDITIONS Abruptio placenta

AGE-RELATED FACTORS
Pediatric: Increased incidence in teenagers
Geriatric: N/A
Others: Older pregnant females (> 35 years old) have increased incidence

PREGNANCY N/A

SYNONYMS
• Pregnancy-induced hypertension
• Toxemia of pregnancy

ICD-9-CM
642.4 Preeclampsia, mild
642.5 Preeclampsia, severe

SEE ALSO
• Eclampsia (toxemia of pregnancy)

OTHER NOTES N/A

ABBREVIATIONS
MgSO4 = magnesium sulfate
CrCl = creatinine clearance

REFERENCES
• Burrow GN, Ferris TF, eds: Medical complications during pregnancy. 4th Ed. Philadelphia, WB Saunders, 1995:1-28
• Cunningham FG, MacDonald PC, Gant NF, eds: Williams' Obstetrics. 19th Ed. Norwalk, CT, Appleton and Lange, 1993
• Fisher S: J of Clin Investigation 1997;5
• Caritis S: N Engl J Med 1998; 338: 701-705
Illustrations: N/A
Internet references: http://www.5mcc.com

Author(s)
Stoney A. Abercrombie, MD

Premature labor

BASICS

DESCRIPTION Labor occurring prior to the completion of 36 weeks' gestation
System(s) affected: Reproductive
Genetics: N/A
Incidence/Prevalence in USA: 8-12% of all births in the USA
Predominant age: Childbearing
Predominant sex: Female only

SIGNS AND SYMPTOMS
• Regular uterine contractions, with or without pain, continuing for 1 hour
• Dull, low backache, pressure, or pain
• Intermittent lower abdominal or thigh pain
• Intestinal cramping, with or without diarrhea or indigestion
• Change in vaginal discharge
• Contractions every 5-10 minutes
• Dilatation of the cervix greater than 1 cm
• Effacement of the cervix more than 50%
• Signs of ruptured membranes (pH paper turns blue; fern positive)

CAUSES
• Infections (UTI, pyelonephritis, pneumonia)
• Subclinical chorioamnionitis (intra-amniotic infections from aerobes, anaerobes, mycoplasma, and ureaplasma)
• Uterine abnormalities (incompetent cervix, leiomyomata; septa, diethylstilbestrol DES exposure)
• Over-distention (by multiple gestation or hydramnios)
• Premature rupture of membranes
• Trauma
• Iatrogenic
• Abruption of placenta
• Immunopathology (eg, antiphospholipid antibodies)

RISK FACTORS
• Prior preterm delivery
• Multiple gestation
• Bacterial vaginosis
• Three or more first-trimester abortions
• Previous second-trimester abortion
• Cervical incompetence
• Abdominal surgery during pregnancy
• Uterine or cervical anomalies
• Placenta previa
• Premature placental separation (trauma or drug abuse - especially cocaine)
• Fetal abnormalities
• Hydramnios
• Serious maternal infection
• Vaginal bleeding in pregnancy
• Prepregnancy weight less than 45 kg (100 lb)
• Single parent
• No prenatal care
• Lower socioeconomic status
• Substance abuse (e.g., cocaine, tobacco)
• IUGR

DIAGNOSIS

DIFFERENTIAL DIAGNOSIS
Dehydration, urinary tract infections, round ligament pain, viral gastroenteritis, lumbosacral muscular back pain, vaginal infections, Braxton-Hicks contractions, adnexal torsion

LABORATORY
• Urinalysis and urine culture for evaluation of urinary tract infection
• Gonorrhea, and chlamydial cultures
• Vaginal-rectal-perineal culture for group B strep
• Drug screen when appropriate
• CBC with differential
• Electrolytes, creatinine and BUN for dehydration
Drugs that may alter lab results: N/A
Disorders that may alter lab results: N/A

PATHOLOGICAL FINDINGS
Placental inflammation. Acute inflammation usually caused by infection. Chronic inflammation caused by immunopathology.

SPECIAL TESTS
Consider amniocentesis if ≥32 weeks' gestation for evaluation of lecithin/sphingomyelin (L/S) ratio and desaturated phosphatidylcholine (DSPC). If L/S ratio is greater than 2:1, and DSPC greater than 1000, hyaline membrane disease is unlikely. Also consider amniocentesis to evaluate for intra-amniotic infection (cell count with differential; glucose; gram stain; aerobic, anaerobic, mycoplasma and ureaplasma cultures.

IMAGING
• Consider uterine ultrasound to quantitate gestational age, estimated fetal weight, multiple gestations, amount of amniotic fluid, and fetal growth
• Transvaginal ultrasound to evaluate cervical length and dilatation

DIAGNOSTIC PROCEDURES
• Uterine monitoring for at least two hours or until contractions stop
• Speculum vaginal examination for signs of infection (purulent discharge, opaque membranes) and cultures
• pH and fern testing for ruptured membranes
• Digital cervical examination for effacement and dilatation (if membranes intact)

TREATMENT

APPROPRIATE HEALTH CARE
Outpatient or inpatient depending on circumstances

GENERAL MEASURES
• Treat underlying risk factors with appropriate measures (antibiotics for infections, hydration for dehydration)
• If delivery is inevitable, but not immediate, consider transport to a tertiary care center or hospital equipped with a neonatal intensive care unit
• If mother is at 24-34 weeks' gestation and has no evidence of infection, consider administering glucocorticoids to reduce incidence of neonatal respiratory distress, intraventricular hemorrhage and necrotizing enterocolitis

SURGICAL MEASURES
For malpresentation or fetal compromise, consider cesarean delivery

ACTIVITY
• Pelvic rest (no douching or sexual intercourse)
• Bedrest. Discontinue work or other physical activities.
• Hospitalization may be necessary if on intravenous tocolysis or if bedrest is impossible at home

DIET
Liquids only or npo, if delivery becomes imminent

PATIENT EDUCATION
Call physician or proceed to hospital whenever contractions last over an hour, low back pain that comes and goes, change in vaginal discharge, "menstrual cramping." or intestinal cramping. In the presence of risk factors, patient should be counselled early in pregnancy.

Premature labor

MEDICATIONS

DRUG(S) OF CHOICE
• Hydrate with 500 mL D5NS or D5LR for first half hour
• For tocolysis, protocols include:
◊ Terbutaline 0.25 mg subcutaneously every 30 minutes up to 3 doses until contractions stop. Then 0.25 SQ every 6 hours for 4 doses (optional). Consider oral terbutaline 2.5-5 mg every 4-6 hours. If contractions persist or pulse is greater than 120, change to another tocolytic.
◊ Magnesium sulfate solution of 40 g per 1000 mL of D5NS. Bolus 4-6 g over 20 min, then begin infusion at 2 g/hr, increasing by 0.5 g/hr every 15-30 min to a maximum of 4 g/hr; check reflexes and serum magnesium levels (therapeutic is 6-8 mg/dL [2.47-3.29 mmol/L]). Stop for significant side effects. When tocolysis occurs, decrease dose by 0.5 g/hr each hour to a minimum of 2 g/hr and then consider switch to oral therapy after 12 -24 hours.
• Antibiotics for group B strep prophylaxis pending cultures
• Glucocorticoids to reduce incidence of neonatal respiratory distress, protocols include:
◊ Betamethasone 12 mg IM two doses 24h apart
or
◊ Dexamethasone 6 mg IM bid x 4 doses
or
◊ Betamethasone 12 mg IM single dose can be repeated every 7 days as long as preterm delivery is likely; discontinue at 34 weeks gestation

Contraindications:
• Severe preeclampsia, hemorrhage, chorioamnionitis, advanced labor, intrauterine growth retardation, fetal heart decelerations or lethal fetal abnormalities
• Relative contraindications to terbutaline include maternal cardiac rhythm disturbance or poorly controlled diabetes or thyrotoxicosis
• Relative contraindications to magnesium sulfate are myasthenia gravis, hypocalcemia, renal failure, or concurrent use of calcium channel blockers

Precautions:
• Palpitations, nausea, intractable vomiting, pulse greater than 140, decreased urine output
• Long-term terbutaline may adversely affect glucose tolerance. Consider repeating glucose screen if using terbutaline for more than 1 week.

Significant possible interactions:
Pulmonary edema from rehydration fluids and tocolytic agents, nifedipine and magnesium sulfate

ALTERNATIVE DRUGS
Nifedipine for tocolysis or indomethacin; caution due to significant fetal risk

FOLLOWUP

PATIENT MONITORING
• Weekly office visits and cervical checks for those at high risk for preterm labor
• Ambulatory external tocodynamometry has not yet been proven efficacious for prevention of preterm labor
• Treating bacterial vaginosis in second trimester with metronidazole 250 mg tid for 7 days, erythromycin base 333 mg tid for 14 days; alternatively, using clindamycin 300 mg bid for 7 days may reduce risk of premature delivery
• Controversy exists on whether maintenance tocolysis is useful
• The role of cervico-vaginal fetal fibronectin testing to assist risk assessment is controversial

PREVENTION/AVOIDANCE
• Patient education at each visit in 2nd and 3rd trimester for those at risk; for general population, periodically during the 2nd and 3rd trimester
• Consider cerclage placement before 20 week's gestation for those at high risk because of an incompetent cervix

POSSIBLE COMPLICATIONS
Labor resistant to tocolysis; pulmonary edema

EXPECTED COURSE/PROGNOSIS
If membranes are ruptured and no infection, manage expectantly, but delivery generally occurs within 3-7 days. If membranes are intact, treat until 36-37 weeks, gestational age.

MISCELLANEOUS

ASSOCIATED CONDITIONS
See Risk Factors

AGE-RELATED FACTORS
N/A
Pediatric: N/A
Geriatric: N/A
Others: N/A

PREGNANCY
By definition, a problem of pregnancy

SYNONYMS
Preterm labor

ICD-9-CM
644.2 Premature labor

SEE ALSO
N/A

OTHER NOTES
N/A

ABBREVIATIONS
IUGR = intrauterine growth retardation

REFERENCES
• ACOG Technical Bulletin, No. 206, June, 1995
• Anon: Effect of corticosteroids for fetal maturation on perinatal outcomes. NIH Consensus Development Panel on the Effect of Corticosteroids for Fetal Maturation on Perinatal Outcomes. JAMA 1995;273(5):413-418
• Hauth JC, Goldenberg RY, Andrews WW, et al: Reduced incidence of preterm delivery with metronidazole and erythromycin in women with bacterial vaginosis. NEJM 1995;333(26):1732-1736
Illustrations: N/A
Internet references: http://www.5mcc.com

Author(s)
Cathryn Heath, MD
John C. Smulian, MD, MPH

Premenstrual syndrome (PMS)

BASICS

DESCRIPTION Premenstrual syndrome is a constellation of symptoms that occurs prior to menstruation and is severe enough to interfere significantly with the patient's life. DSM-IV diagnosis is premenstrual dysmorphic disorder.
System(s) affected: Endocrine/Metabolic, Reproductive, Nervous
Genetics: Unknown, probably familial incidence
Incidence/Prevalence in USA: Almost all women have some symptoms prior to menses (this is not PMS). A low percentage have actual PMS.
Predominant age: Childbearing years, worse during late 20's and 30's
Predominant sex: Females only

SIGNS AND SYMPTOMS
Symptoms can involve any organ system but the following are more common:
• Depressed mood
• Mood swings
• Irritability
• Difficulty concentrating
• Fatigue
• Edema
• Breast tenderness
• Headaches
• Sleep disturbances

CAUSES Unknown, presumed hormonal; perhaps interacting with neurotransmitters

RISK FACTORS
• Premenstrual exacerbations can occur with other diseases (i.e., depression)
• Caffeine and high fluid intake exacerbate PMS symptoms
• Stress may precipitate
• PMS increases with age

DIAGNOSIS

DIFFERENTIAL DIAGNOSIS The major differentials are psychiatric syndromes, particularly depressive disorders and/or dysthymia. Other entities may be suggested by history or physical.

LABORATORY There are no laboratory tests which confirm or refute PMS. History and physical may disclose a need for specific laboratory tests.
Drugs that may alter lab results: N/A
Disorders that may alter lab results: N/A

PATHOLOGICAL FINDINGS N/A

SPECIAL TESTS N/A

IMAGING N/A

DIAGNOSTIC PROCEDURES Patients complete questionnaires over a minimum of two months to confirm premenstrual exacerbation of symptoms and lack of substantial symptoms in the follicular phase

TREATMENT

APPROPRIATE HEALTH CARE
Outpatient

GENERAL MEASURES
• Increase daily exercise
• Eat regular, balanced meals
• Stop smoking
• Get regular sleep
• Stress reduction techniques
• Individual or couples counseling
• Support groups
• Light therapy

SURGICAL MEASURES N/A

ACTIVITY
• No restrictions
• Exercise is recommended

DIET Low-salt; low-caffeine; low-fat; frequent, small meals; high complex carbohydrates

PATIENT EDUCATION Explain PMS and treatment

MEDICATIONS

DRUG(S) OF CHOICE

No single drug works for all women. Drugs that are used with varying degrees of success are listed.
- Anti-depressants (fluoxetine, sertraline, clomipramine, citalopram or nortriptyline), particularly for patients with depressive symptoms. Antidepressants may work when used only during the luteal phase of the menstrual cycle.
- Diuretics (usually spironolactone) during luteal phase
- Symptomatic treatment of pain (ibuprofen or acetaminophen)
- Magnesium 300-500 mg/day
- Elemental calcium 1000 mg/day
- Vitamin B6 in modest doses (50 mg bid, may be toxic in higher doses)
- Vitamin E - up to 600 IU/day
- Evening primrose oil, high content of fatty acids, 500 mg qd to 1000 mg tid for breast tenderness, believed to decrease prostaglandin synthesis
- Oral contraceptives may help
- Bromocriptine 2.5 mg tid at time of symptoms and danazol 100 mg bid may also work for breast tenderness, but have more side effects
- Danazol for the total PMS symptom complex
- Gonadotropin-releasing hormone agonists with or without concurrent estrogens/progestins

Contraindications: Refer to manufacturer's profile of each drug

Precautions: Refer to manufacturer's profile of each drug

Significant possible interactions: Refer to manufacturer's profile of each drug

ALTERNATIVE DRUGS   N/A

FOLLOWUP

PATIENT MONITORING   See patient to provide general support and further patient education

PREVENTION/AVOIDANCE   N/A

POSSIBLE COMPLICATIONS   N/A

EXPECTED COURSE/PROGNOSIS

Many patients can have their symptoms adequately controlled. Disappears at menopause.

MISCELLANEOUS

ASSOCIATED CONDITIONS   N/A

AGE-RELATED FACTORS
Pediatric: N/A
Geriatric: N/A
Others: N/A

PREGNANCY   N/A

SYNONYMS   N/A

ICD-9-CM   625.4 Premenstrual tension syndromes

SEE ALSO   Mastalgia

OTHER NOTES   Treatment may need to be continued for a long time. PMS sometimes continues after hysterectomy. Effects of long-term hormonal treatment unknown.

ABBREVIATIONS   N/A

REFERENCES
- Demonico SO, Brown CS, Ling F: Premenstrual syndrome. Current Opinion in Obstetrics and Gynecology 1994;6:499-502
- Carter T, Verhoef MJ: Efficacy of self-help and alternative treatments of premenstrual syndrome. Womens Health Issues 1994;4:130-137
- Barnhart KT, Freeman EW, Sandheimer SJ: A clinician's guide to premenstrual syndrome. Med Clin of NA 1995:70:1457-1472
- Korzekwa MI, Steiner M: Premenstrual syndromes. Clinical OB & Gyn 1997;40:564-576
- Freeman EW: Premenstrual syndrome: current perspectives on treatment and etiology. Curr Opin in OB & Gyn 1997;9:147-153
Illustrations: N/A
Internet references: http://www.5mcc.com

Author(s)
Marjorie A. Bowman, MD, MPA

Pressure ulcer

BASICS

DESCRIPTION Skin breakdown is a common and serious complication affecting usually frail, disabled, acutely ill or immobile elderly patients, especially within long-term care settings. Most common sites are over bony prominences, such as elbows, hips, heels, outer ankles, and base of spine. Over 95% of ulcers develop on lower part of body. Median length of hospital stay to treat pressure sore is 46 days. Risk of death in elderly patient increases fourfold when sores heal and sixfold when sores do not heal.

System(s) affected: Skin/Exocrine
Genetics: N/A
Incidence/Prevalence in USA:
• 9% of all hospitalized and 23% of all nursing home patients
• 2 million patients develop these pressure sores each year
• Incidence is 43/100,000 population every year; 65% of elderly with femoral fractures; 33% of critical care patients, and a 60% prevalence among quadriplegic patients
• Estimated prevalence in nursing home residents ranges from 2.6-24%

Predominant age: 60-70% are elderly patients; age >85 at greatest risk
Predominant sex: Female > Male (due to survival differential); cost to heal pressure ulcer ranges from $5,000-$40,000

SIGNS AND SYMPTOMS
• Stage I - non-blanching erythema, warmth, tenderness
• Stage II - skin breakdown limited to dermis, excoriation, blistering, drainage, more sharply defined erythema, variable skin temperature, local swelling or edema
• Stage III - ulcer formation into subcutaneous tissues, crater formation, slough, eschar, and/or drainage
• Stage IV - ulcers extend beyond deep fascia into muscle or bone, decayed area may be larger than visibly apparent wound, osteomyelitis or sepsis may be present, granulation tissue and epithelialization may be present at wound margins

CAUSES
• Uneven application of pressure over a bony hard site; high pressure applied for two hours produces irreversible tissue ischemia and necrosis
• Shearing forces which develop when a seated person slides toward floor or toward foot of bed if supine
• Frictional forces which develop when pulling a patient across a bed sheet
• Moisture from incontinence or perspiration can increase the friction between two surfaces

RISK FACTORS
• Immobility (e.g., quadriplegia)
• Malnutrition and low body weight
• Hypoalbuminemia
• Fecal incontinence
• Urinary incontinence
• Bone fracture (especially femoral)
• Vitamin C deficiency
• Low diastolic blood pressure

• Age-related skin changes, such as diminished pain perception, thinning of epidermis, loss of dermal vessels, altered barrier properties, reduced immunity, and slowed wound healing
• Anemia
• Infections
• Peripheral vascular disease
• Dementia
• Malignancies
• Diabetes mellitus
• Cerebral vascular accidents
• Dry skin (low humidity, < 40%, and cold)
• Fractures
• Edema
• Assessment scale for evaluating risk factors include: Norton, Braden (Braden Q version for children), Waterlow and Walsall

DIAGNOSIS

DIFFERENTIAL DIAGNOSIS
• Stasis or ischemia ulcers
• Vasculitides
• Cancers
• Radiation injury
• Pyoderma gangrenosum and other dermatologic conditions

LABORATORY
• Culture of wound if there is evidence of infection (surrounding erythema, purulent drainage, foul odor)
• White blood cell count and differential if fever is present (greater than 37°C)
• Erythrocyte sedimentation rate
• If leucocytosis present, urinalysis to identify causative agents
• If above tests positive, blood and urine cultures

Drugs that may alter lab results: N/A
Disorders that may alter lab results: N/A

PATHOLOGICAL FINDINGS Extensive necrosis of affected part

SPECIAL TESTS N/A

IMAGING
• If leukocytosis present, chest radiograph
• Plain radiographs involved bone

DIAGNOSTIC PROCEDURES N/A

TREATMENT

APPROPRIATE HEALTH CARE
• An interdisciplinary approach usually indicated in nursing home, inpatient or home care settings if trained supervision available
• Complications will require inpatient setting to treat systemic infection, extensive debridement or skin grafting

GENERAL MEASURES
• Improve overall nutritional status (adequate protein intake)
• Clean wound each time dressing is changed to remove dead tissue, excess fluid and other debris
• Healing enhanced with body temperature maintained at 37°C (97.7°F) and an acidic pH
• Never use antiseptics and skin cleansers which harm the tissue
• Surgery for wounds not responding to treatment within 2-4 weeks
• Débridement of necrotic pressure ulcers using occlusive dressings, hydrotherapy, proteolytic enzymes, and surgical or laser débridement
• Pressure reduction products such as, specialized beds and repositioning every two hours to relieve pressure at site of ulceration (air-fluidized or low-air-loss beds); static-pressure and foam mattresses are less expensive. Water mattresses, sheepskins, and egg-crate mattresses are other less expensive devices.
• Avoid agents that delay wound healing, such as topical corticosteroids, hydrogen peroxide, povidone iodine solution, and hypochlorite solutions
• Control of fecal and/or urine incontinence Specific measures by stage as follows:
• Stage I: Nonblanchable erythema of intact skin
  ◊ Relieve pressure (floatation or airflow mattress/bed)
  ◊ Use moisture barrier lubricant, transparent bio-occlusive dressings (Opsite) or Granulex Spray on reddened areas
  ◊ Keep all skin areas clean and dry
  ◊ Assess skin every 8-12 hours
• Stage II: Partial thickness skin loss of epidermal and/or dermal layers
  ◊ Use saline soaked 4 x 4's to cleanse pressure sore followed by topical antibiotic
  ◊ Rinse with saline soaked 4 x 4's
  ◊ Pat dry with 4 x 4's
  ◊ Apply protective barrier film to unbroken skin surrounding pressure sore
  ◊ Apply occlusive hydrocolloid dressing (Duoderm)
  ◊ Repeat every three days
  ◊ Loosely pack wound
  ◊ Whirlpools useful for necrotic wounds
• Stage III: Full thickness skin loss through subcutaneous tissue to fascia
  ◊ Irrigate wound with saline solution
  ◊ Scrub and debride with dry gauze and gels for autolytic débridement
  ◊ Re-rinse wound
  ◊ Blot excess moisture with dry 4 x 4 gauze
  ◊ Apply protective barrier film
  ◊ Apply skin care product (occlusive hydrocolloid dressing, granules, or paste)
  ◊ If wound highly exudating, use absorption dressing (exudate absorbers) and change daily; consider wound culture

• Stage IV: Exposure or destruction of muscle, bone and other supportive structure
◊ If eschar present, need to be debrided or sloughed
◊ Irrigate wound with saline solution x 2
◊ Blot excess moisture with 4 x 4 dry gauze
◊ Apply protective barrier film to unbroken skin surrounding sore
◊ Moisten packing gauze (Kerlix) in saline and pack wound
◊ Apply outer dressing
◊ Surgical intervention for definitive treatment of deep and complicated pressure ulcers, such as myocutaneous flaps, split-thickness skin grafts and primary closure

SURGICAL MEASURES See under various stages in General Measures

ACTIVITY
• Any activity consistent with patient's ambulatory status and relief of pressure on wound
• Perform passive range-of-motion exercises for patient or encourage patient to do active exercises if possible

DIET
• Oral high-calorie and high-protein supplements
• Oral zinc sulfate, vitamin A and C, and iron

PATIENT EDUCATION
• Patient Care 1993; 27(7):65-66
• National Action Group for the Prevention and Treatment of Decubitus Ulcers, P.O. Box 1098, Union City, CT 06770
• AHCPR publication No. 92-0048, Preventing Pressure Ulcers: A Patient's Guide, May 1992.
• Patient information handout from: Findley D: Practical management of pressure ulcers. Amer Fam Phys 1996;54(3):1519-1536

MEDICATIONS

DRUG(S) OF CHOICE
• Clindamycin or gentamicin for complications such as cellulitis, osteomyelitis, or sepsis
• Supplements - vitamin C 500 mg twice a day, zinc sulfate
• Antibiotic prophylaxis for bacterial endocarditis if valvular lesions present
• Two week trial of topical antimicrobials (e.g., silver sulfadiazine or triple antibiotics) should be used only for a clean superficial ulcer not healing or producing moderate amount of exudate; cultures are necessary to determine whether antifungal (miconazole, clotrimazole, or haloprogin) or specific antibacterial agents (silver sulfadiazine, neomycin-polymyxin B-bacitracin, gentamicin, mupirocin 2%) are indicated
• Enzymatic debriding agents such as collagenase (Santyl), trypsin (Granulex), fibrinolysin-deoxyribonuclease (Elase), papain (Panafil) or sutilains (Travase) used with a moisture barrier to protect surrounding normal tissue

• Recommended dressings include polyurethane films (Op-site, Tegaderm), absorbent hydrocolloid dressings (Duoderm, Comfeel Ulcus)
Contraindications: Refer to manufacturer's literature
Precautions: Refer to manufacturer's literature
Significant possible interactions: Refer to manufacturer's literature

ALTERNATIVE DRUGS
• Calendula ointment or a 5% flower extract with allantoin stimulates new epithelial growth in surgical wounds
• Two drops of tea tree oil in 8 ounces of water - used as a rinse to decrease risk of infection
• Marshmellow root ointment over wound daily

FOLLOWUP

PATIENT MONITORING
• Frequent evaluation of all patients with history of pressure sores, especially if limited mobility. Include nutritional status and dietary intervention.
• Early identification of areas of skin redness to prevent subsequent breakdown
• Skin cleansing as soon as soiled and at routine intervals

PREVENTION/AVOIDANCE
• Up to 95% of all pressure ulcers are preventable
• Pressure relief
• Early identification of at risk individuals and elimination of risk factors (risk assessment tools: Brader Scale for Predicting Pressure Sore Risk for nursing home patients and The Norton Scale for hospitalized patients)
• Underpads (non-cloth) to absorb moisture
• Quality nursing care
• Early interdisciplinary supportive care - include staff, patient, family/caregiver
• Nutritional assessment of patient, especially if cannot take food by mouth or has experienced involuntary change in weight. Additional protein and calories should be provided (vitamin C and zinc).
• Frequent patient repositioning if immobile - every hour if wheelchair bound and every 2 hours if bedridden
• Functional assessment of patient and treatment of incontinence
• Frequent physical examination of skin areas affected by pressure, moisture, shearing or friction sources
• Use mattress overlays, seat cushions or special mattresses and beds to reduce pressure on pressure points

POSSIBLE COMPLICATIONS
• Growth of resistant organisms if antibiotics used for local or systemic infection
• Gangrene

EXPECTED COURSE/PROGNOSIS
• Though pressure ulcers are associated with an increased rate of mortality, with good medical care, most can be expected to heal
• In a recent study among long-term care hospital patients, 79% of pressure sores improved and 40% completely healed during a six-week followup period using ordinary therapies

MISCELLANEOUS

ASSOCIATED CONDITIONS
• Malnutrition
• Fecal and/or urinary incontinence
• Immobility
• Impaired mental status
• Skin atrophy
• Low body weight
• Compromised immune states

AGE-RELATED FACTORS
Pediatric: N/A
Geriatric: Over 60% occur in elderly
Others: N/A

PREGNANCY N/A

SYNONYMS
• Decubitus ulcer
• Bedsore
• Trophic ulcer
• Pressure sore

ICD-9-CM 707.0 Decubitus ulcer

SEE ALSO N/A

OTHER NOTES N/A

ABBREVIATIONS N/A

REFERENCES
• Findley D: Practical management of pressure ulcers. Amer Fam Phys 1996;54(3):1519-1536
• Levine JM, Totolus E: Pressure ulcers; A strategic plan to prevent and heal them. Geriatrics 1995;50(1): 32-37
• Pressure Ulcer Guideline Panel: Pressure ulcer treatment. Amer Fam Phys 1995;51(5):1202-1222
• Panel for the Prediction and Prevention of Pressure Ulcers in Adults. Pressure Ulcers in Adults: Predicting and Prevention. Clinical Practice Guidelines, No. 3. AHCPR Publication No. 92-0047, May, 1992
Illustrations: N/A
Internet references: http://www.5mcc.com

Author(s)
Evan W. Kligman, MD

Priapism

BASICS

DESCRIPTION   Painful and/or abnormally prolonged penile erection
System(s) affected: Reproductive
Genetics: N/A
Incidence/Prevalence in USA: Unknown
Predominant age: Young adult
Predominant sex: Male only

SIGNS AND SYMPTOMS
• Penile erection that is persistent, prolonged, painful, and tender
• Urination difficult during erection
• Loss of sexual function if treatment is not prompt and effective
• Low flow or ischemic priapism - glans penis flaccid
• High flow or arterial priapism - glans penis rigid

CAUSES
• Intracavernosal injections of vasoactive drugs for erectile dysfunction; most common cause
• Pelvic vascular thrombosis
• Prolonged sexual activity
• Sickle cell anemia
• Leukemia
• Other blood dyscrasias
• Pelvic hematoma or neoplasia
• Cerebrospinal tumors
• Tertiary syphilis
• Bladder calculus
• Injury to penis
• Urinary tract infections, especially prostatitis, urethritis, cystitis
• Several drugs suspected as causing priapism, such as chlorpromazine, prazosin, trazodone, and certain corticosteroids, anticoagulants, antihypertensives
• Intracavernous fat emulsion

RISK FACTORS
• Dehydration

DIAGNOSIS

DIFFERENTIAL DIAGNOSIS   List with Causes

LABORATORY
• CBC
• Sickle prep and hgb electrophoresis
• Coagulation profile
• Platelet count
• Urinalysis
Drugs that may alter lab results: N/A
Disorders that may alter lab results: N/A

PATHOLOGICAL FINDINGS
• Pelvic vascular thrombosis
• Partial thrombosis of corpora cavernosa
• Corpus spongiosum, glans penis: No involvement
• Arterial priapism will show arteriocavernosus fistula

SPECIAL TESTS   N/A

IMAGING
• Penile doppler testing may be necessary to differentiate high-flow from low-flow priapism

DIAGNOSTIC PROCEDURES   Physical examination

TREATMENT

APPROPRIATE HEALTH CARE
Inpatient

GENERAL MEASURES
• Reassurance about outcome if warranted
• Continuous caudal or spinal anesthesia if etiology is neurogenic
• Treat any underlying cause
• In sickle cell anemia: Intravenous hydration; partial exchange or repeated transfusions to reduce percent of sickle cells below 50%
• Pain relief

SURGICAL MEASURES
• Introduction of 12 or 16 gauge needles into corpora cavernosa (best done by urologist if available)
  ◊ First: aspiration of 20-30 cc of blood from corpora cavernosum with 12-16 gauge needle
  ◊ Then: if caused by injected vasodilator, use intracavernous injection of 10-25 mg ephedrine sulfate or 5-10 µg epinephrine or 125-250 µg phenylephrine
  ◊ May repeat one time in 20-30 minutes if no response
• Create fistula between glans and corpus cavernosum (with biopsy needle by urologist)
• Semipermanent diversion by saphenous shunt from one or both corpora
• Cavernoso-spongiosum shunt to permit reestablishment of pelvic circulation

ACTIVITY   Bedrest until relieved

DIET   N/A

PATIENT EDUCATION
• Information about long-term outlook, referral for counseling
• Reduction of vasoactive drug therapy, if responsible for priapism and elimination of offending drugs if causal

MEDICATIONS

DRUG(S) OF CHOICE
• Narcotics for pain if needed
• Vasoconstrictors may be injected after dilution, e.g., metaraminol 1 mg into the penis
Contraindications: Refer to manufacturer's literature
Precautions: Refer to manufacturer's literature
Significant possible interactions: Refer to manufacturer's literature

ALTERNATIVE DRUGS N/A

FOLLOWUP

PATIENT MONITORING Close followup after surgery

PREVENTION/AVOIDANCE
• Avoid dehydration
• Avoid excessive sexual stimulation
• Avoid causative drugs (see Causes) when possible

POSSIBLE COMPLICATIONS
• Erectile dysfunction (impotence)

EXPECTED COURSE/PROGNOSIS
• Even with excellent treatment, detumescence may require several weeks
• Impotence is likely

MISCELLANEOUS

ASSOCIATED CONDITIONS Sickle cell anemia

AGE-RELATED FACTORS
Pediatric: > 85% likelihood of sickle cell in African American children
Geriatric: Treatment more difficult and less likely successful
Others: N/A

PREGNANCY N/A

SYNONYMS N/A

ICD-9-CM
607.3 Priapism

SEE ALSO
• Anemia, sickle cell
• Erectile dysfunction

OTHER NOTES N/A

ABBREVIATIONS N/A

REFERENCES
• Smith DR: General Urology. 14th Ed. Los Altos, CA, Lange Medical Publications, 1995
• Tanagho EA, McAninch JW, eds: Smith's General Urology. 12th Ed. Norwalk, CT, Appleton & Lange, 1988
• Harmon WJ and Nehra A: "Priapism: Diagnosis and Management," Mayo Clinic Proceedings. Vol 12 (4) April 1997: 350-355.
Illustrations: N/A
Internet references: http://www.5mcc.com

Author(s)
Bruce Block, MD

Primary pulmonary hypertension

BASICS

DESCRIPTION Pulmonary arterial hypertension of unknown cause, where secondary causes have been ruled out. Three pathologic subtypes have been identified: (1) thrombotic (56%), (2) plexogenic (28%), (3) veno-occlusive (16%).

System(s) affected: Pulmonary, Cardiovascular

Genetics: 7% familial; autosomal dominant with variable expression and "genetic anticipation"

Incidence/Prevalence in USA: 1-2 cases/million. 1% of all causes of cor pulmonale at autopsy. 0.5-2% of patients with portal hypertension or HIV

Predominant age: Mean age 34-36 years; second incidence peak in males 50-59 years

Predominant sex: Female > Male (3:1)

SIGNS AND SYMPTOMS

- Loud P2 (> 80%)
- Right ventricular lift (> 80%)
- Dyspnea (> 75%)
- Murmur of tricuspid insufficiency (50-80%)
- Increased jugular venous pressure (50-80%)
- Right ventricular S4 (50-80%)
- Chest pain (> 50%)
- Fatigue (> 50%)
- Palpitations (< 50%)
- Syncope; dizziness (< 50%)
- Cough (< 50%)
- Raynaud's phenomenon (< 10%)
- Hepatomegaly (< 50%)
- Pulmonic ejection click (< 50%)
- Right ventricular S3 (< 50%)
- Murmur of pulmonic insufficiency (< 50%)
- Lower extremity edema (< 50%)
- Superficial thrombophlebitis (5%)

CAUSES

- Unknown; possible pulmonary arteriolar hyperactivity and vasoconstriction; occult thromboembolism; possible autoimmune (high frequency antinuclear antibodies)
- In Europe, reports of PPH associated with anorectic agent aminorex fumarate in late 1960's; tainted rapeseed oil
- HIV positive patients may have an increased incidence of primary pulmonary hypertension
- Anorectic agents (fenfluramine and dexfenfluramine)
- Amphetamines

RISK FACTORS Female sex

DIAGNOSIS

DIFFERENTIAL DIAGNOSIS

- Pulmonary parenchymal disease (COPD, asthma, pulmonary fibrosis, granulomatous disease, malignancy)
- Pulmonary vascular disease (pulmonary thromboembolism, collagen vascular disease, pulmonary arteritis, schistosomiasis, sickle cell disease)
- Cardiac disease (cardiomyopathy, valvular heart disease, congenital heart disease, persistent fetal circulation, pulmonary venous hypertension)
- Other disorders of respiratory function (sleep apnea syndromes, neuromuscular diseases, pleural diseases, thoracic cage abnormalities)
- IV drug abuse

LABORATORY

- ANA positive (1/3 of patients)

Drugs that may alter lab results:
Hydralazine, procainamide, isoniazid, etc.

Disorders that may alter lab results:
Many other diseases, e.g., lupus, scleroderma

PATHOLOGICAL FINDINGS

- Medial hypertrophy and arterial thrombosis are common in all subtypes
- Plexogenic pulmonary arteriopathy (30-70%): laminar "onion skin" intimal proliferation, focal medial disruption, aneurysmal dilatation
- Microthromboemboli (20-50%)
- Veno-occlusive disease (10-15%)

SPECIAL TESTS

- ECG - right ventricular hypertrophy and right axis deviation
- Pulmonary function testing - arterial hypoxemia, reduced diffusion capacity, hypocapnea
- V/Q scan - must rule out proximal pulmonary artery emboli
- Exercise test: reduced maximal O2 consumption, high minute ventilation, low anaerobic threshold, reduced maximal oxygen pulse, increased DO2A-a. Correlation to severity of disease with 6 minute walk test.

IMAGING

- Chest x-ray: enlarged central pulmonary arteries with pulmonary arterial branches attenuated. Right ventricular enlargement a late finding. If increased interstitial markings, consider lung parenchymal disease or veno-occlusive disease.
- Echo-Doppler: right ventricular enlargement and overload; important to rule out underlying cardiac disease such as atrial septal defect with secondary pulmonary hypertension or mitral stenosis
- Ultra fast CT -sensitivity probably equal to pulmonary angiogram with lower contrast dose

DIAGNOSTIC PROCEDURES

- Chest x-ray, pulmonary function tests, arterial blood gases, and V/Q scan should be done
- Cardiac catheterization - right heart catheterization is necessary to measure pulmonary artery pressures and hemodynamics; rule out underlying cardiac disease and response to vasodilator therapy
- Pulmonary angiography - should be done if segmental or larger defect on V/Q scan. Caution in pulmonary hypertension as can lead to hemodynamic collapse; use low osmolar agents, subselective angiograms.
- Lung biopsy not recommended

TREATMENT

APPROPRIATE HEALTH CARE

- Medical therapy is first line and primarily palliative; health care is guided by clinical status
- Hospitalization with invasive monitoring is needed to screen vasodilator responsiveness and initiate vasodilator therapy
- There is a national registry established by the National Heart, Lung, and Blood Institute

GENERAL MEASURES

- Primary modalities are oxygen supplementation, vasodilators, anticoagulants, and treatment of heart failure (e.g., diuretics)
- Oxygen supplementation is indicated for rest, exercise, or nocturnal hypoxemia
- The acute response to vasodilators may improve survival; hydralazine, calcium channel blockers and prostacyclin

SURGICAL MEASURES

- Surgical procedures - patients with documented large vessel thromboembolic disease should be considered for pulmonary thrombectomy
- Heart-lung or lung transplantation is an option for appropriate patients when medical therapy has failed
- Blade-balloon atrial septostomy

ACTIVITY Restricted; exercise worsens pulmonary vascular resistance

DIET Low salt with heart failure

PATIENT EDUCATION

- Need to discuss prognosis; options such as transplantation
- Avoidance of pregnancy

MEDICATIONS

DRUG(S) OF CHOICE
• Medical therapy may be guided by suspected subtype:
◊ Plexogenic (clear lung fields, normal perfusion scan) - vasodilators potentially useful. Vasodilators - calcium channel blockers, first line, may be more effective in high doses. Other agents: ACE-inhibitors, alpha-antagonists, hydralazine - none shown to improve survival.
◊ Thrombotic (clear lung fields, patchy perfusion scan) - anticoagulants potentially useful. Anticoagulants - warfarin, heparin, antiplatelet agents.
◊ Veno-occlusive (pulmonary venous congestion, patchy perfusion scan) - vasodilators probably useless
All types: Heart failure may be treated with diuretics. Digoxin use controversial - not shown to be beneficial or detrimental. Digoxin may adversely affect exercise capacity due to increase in pulmonary vascular resistance.
• Chronic vasodilator therapy
◊ Nifedipine, diltiazem
◊ Prostacyclin
◊ Hydralazine
◊ Isoproterenol
◊ Terbutaline
◊ Prazosin
◊ Phentolamine
◊ Phenoxybenzamine
• Screening for responsiveness
◊ Prostacyclin
◊ Iloprost
◊ Acetylcholine
◊ Adenosine
◊ Nitrous oxide
◊ Nitroprusside
◊ Isoproterenol
◊ Hydralazine
◊ Phentolamine
• Anticoagulation: 2 small studies suggest prolonged survival. Warfarin with INR ~2.0.
Contraindications: Avoid warfarin in patients with syncope or hemoptysis
Precautions: Vasodilator therapy and response should be evaluated with invasive monitoring. Short acting agents such as prostacyclin, adenosine, or acetylcholine are useful for screening.
Significant possible interactions: Refer to manufacturer's literature

ALTERNATIVE DRUGS   N/A

FOLLOWUP

PATIENT MONITORING   Frequent

PREVENTION/AVOIDANCE   None

POSSIBLE COMPLICATIONS
Thromboembolism, heart failure, sudden death

EXPECTED COURSE/PROGNOSIS
• Mean survival 2-3 years from time of diagnosis, 75% mortality at 5 years, although survival is quite variable as learned from the NIH registry.
• Mean age at diagnosis 34 years
• Mode of death:
◊ Right heart failure 63%
◊ Indeterminate 15%
◊ Pneumonia 7%
◊ Sudden death 7%
◊ Cardiac death 5%
• Poor prognostic factors:
◊ PaO2 < 63%
◊ RA pressure > 20 mm Hg
◊ Cardiac index < 2 L/min/m2
◊ Mean pulmonary arterial (PA) pressure > 85 mm Hg
◊ New York Heart Association (NYHA) class 3 or 4
◊ Raynaud's phenomenon

MISCELLANEOUS

ASSOCIATED CONDITIONS
• Portal hypertension
• Systemic lupus erythematosus
• HIV
• Raynauds

AGE-RELATED FACTORS
Pediatric: N/A
Geriatric: N/A
Others: N/A

PREGNANCY   Must be avoided; high mother and fetal wastage

SYNONYMS   Primary pulmonary vascular disease

ICD-9-CM
416.0 Primary pulmonary hypertension

SEE ALSO
• Cor pulmonale
• Pulmonary embolism

OTHER NOTES   N/A

ABBREVIATIONS
V/Q = ventilation/perfusion

REFERENCES
• Palevsky HE, Fishman AP: The management of primary pulmonary hypertension. JAMA 1991;265:1014-1020
• Hawkins JW, Dunn MI: Primary pulmonary hypertension in adults. Clinical Cardiology 1990;13:382-387
• Rich S: Primary pulmonary hypertension. In: Isselbacher KJ, et al, eds. Harrison's Principles of Internal Medicine. 13th Ed. McGraw-Hill, New York, 1994
• Cremona G, Higenbottom T: Role of prostacycline in the treatment of pulmonary hypertension. AF Cardio 1995;75(3):67A-71A
Illustrations: N/A
Internet references: http://www.5mcc.com

Author(s)
Darell E. Heiselman, DO, FCCM, FACP, FACC, FCCP

Proctitis

BASICS

DESCRIPTION An acute or chronic inflammation of the rectal mucosa
System(s) affected: Gastrointestinal
Genetics: Higher incidence in Jews
Incidence/Prevalence in USA:
0.5-3/100,000 (ulcerative proctitis)/10-30/100,000 (ulcerative proctitis)
Predominant age: Adult
Predominant sex: Male > Female

SIGNS AND SYMPTOMS
• Rectal and/or perianal discomfort
• Rectal bleeding and/or mucous discharge
• Diarrhea
• Tenesmus
• Urgency
• Constipation
• Fever
• Weight loss

CAUSES
• Idiopathic
• Rectal gonorrhea
• Crohn's disease
• Syphilis (usually secondary)
• Nonspecific sexually transmitted infection
• *Herpes simplex*
• Chlamydia
• Papillomavirus
• Amebiasis
• *Lymphogranuloma venereum*
• Ischemia
• Radiation therapy
• Toxins (e.g., hydrogen peroxide enemas)
• Vasculitis

RISK FACTORS
• Rectal intercourse
• Radiation
• Rectal injury
• Rectal medications
• Jewish heritage

DIAGNOSIS

DIFFERENTIAL DIAGNOSIS
• Traumatic proctitis
• Radiation proctitis
• Ulcerative colitis
• Crohn's disease
• Infections such as shigellosis or amebiasis

LABORATORY
• Serological tests for syphilis, ameba
• Smear, culture from rectal wall
• Stool cultures
Drugs that may alter lab results: N/A
Disorders that may alter lab results: N/A

PATHOLOGICAL FINDINGS
• Inflammation of rectal mucosa
• Ulceration
• Disruption of crypts

SPECIAL TESTS   N/A

IMAGING   N/A

DIAGNOSTIC PROCEDURES
• Flexible sigmoidoscopy
• Biopsy for histology, culture, viral studies, chlamydia culture
• Colonoscopy to exclude more proximal involvement

TREATMENT

APPROPRIATE HEALTH CARE
Outpatient, unless severe and refractory to usual measures

GENERAL MEASURES
• Treatment depends upon the cause
• Rectal gram stains have significant false-negative rate and if clinician has strong suspicion of gonorrheal proctitis, empiric treatment warranted while culture results pending
• Avoidance of causative factors
• Sitz baths may provide some relief

SURGICAL MEASURES   N/A

ACTIVITY   No restrictions

DIET   No special diet

PATIENT EDUCATION   Counseling regarding HIV infection risk

Proctitis

MEDICATIONS

DRUG(S) OF CHOICE
- Ulcerative proctitis - topical steroids (enemas or foam), mesalamine (Rowasa, 5-ASA, 5-aminosalicylic acid) enemas or suppositories; oral mesalamine (Asacol, Pentasa), olsalazine (Dipentum), sulfasalazine; systemic steroids when refractory to above drugs
- Gonorrheal - IM ceftriaxone 250 mg in a single dose plus doxycycline 100 mg orally bid for 7 days
- Herpetic - oral acyclovir 200-400 mg 5 times a day for 10 days
- Chlamydial - oral tetracycline 500 mg tid or doxycycline 100 mg bid

Contraindications: Refer to manufacturer's literature

Precautions: Refer to manufacturer's literature

Significant possible interactions: Refer to manufacturer's literature

ALTERNATIVE DRUGS
For gonorrheal - in patients unable to take ceftriaxone - IM spectinomycin 2 g in a single dose or ciprofloxacin 500 mg orally in a single dose. Perform culture 4-7 days after treatment to verify efficacy of treatment.

FOLLOWUP

PATIENT MONITORING
Follow until completely healed and monthly thereafter for 6 months

PREVENTION/AVOIDANCE
Safe sex, if sexually transmitted

POSSIBLE COMPLICATIONS
- Chronic ulcerative colitis
- Fistulae/abscess formation
- Treatment failure (may be as much as 35% in gonorrhea proctitis)
- Perforation

EXPECTED COURSE/PROGNOSIS
Satisfactory cure or control with appropriate treatment

MISCELLANEOUS

ASSOCIATED CONDITIONS
- Syphilis
- Gonorrhea
- Other sexually transmitted disease
- Prostate cancer (radiation therapy)

AGE-RELATED FACTORS
Pediatric:
- Not common, but if found, is more apt to spread to full-blown disease in more proximal areas of the colon
- Consider sexual abuse, if gonorrheal infection

Geriatric: Slower to heal, consider ischemia

Others: N/A

PREGNANCY N/A

SYNONYMS N/A

ICD-9-CM 569.49 Proctitis nos

SEE ALSO
- Ulcerative colitis
- Crohn's disease
- Syphilis
- Gonococcal infections
- Lymphogranuloma venereum
- Herpes simplex

OTHER NOTES N/A

ABBREVIATIONS N/A

REFERENCES
- Wexner SD: Sexually transmitted diseases of the colon, rectum, and anus. The challenge of the nineties. Dis Colon Rectum 1990;33:1048-62
- Kirsner JB, Shorter G, eds: Diseases of the Colon, Rectum and Anal Canal. Baltimore, Williams & Wilkins, 1989

Illustrations: N/A

Internet references: http://www.5mcc.com

Author(s)
Philip E. Jaffe, MD

Prostatic cancer

BASICS

DESCRIPTION The prostate is composed of acinar glands and their ducts arranged in a radial fashion with the stroma containing blood vessels, lymphatics and nerves. 95% of prostate cancers are acinar adenocarcinomas.
• Tumor grading:
  ◊ A1, A2 & B1, B2 - confined within capsule
  ◊ C1 - extension beyond the capsule
  ◊ C2 - involving the seminal vesicles
  ◊ D1 - metastatic disease in regional lymph nodes
  ◊ D2 - metastatic disease in bone or other organs

System(s) affected: Reproductive
Genetics: Unknown
Incidence/Prevalence in USA: 69 per 100,000
Predominant Age: Sixth or seventh decade
Predominant sex: Male only

SIGNS AND SYMPTOMS
• May be asymptomatic early or late in the course of disease
• Induration of the prostate on digital rectal exam
• Hard prostate, localized or diffuse
• Bladder outlet symptoms
• Acute urinary retention
• Hematuria (rare)
• Urinary tract infection (usually unrelated)
• Bone pain
• Weight loss
• Anemia
• Shortness of breath
• Lymphedema
• Neurologic symptoms
• Lymphadenopathy

CAUSES Unknown

RISK FACTORS
• Genetic predisposition (risk of prostatic cancer increases if a malignancy has occurred in a first degree relative)
• Endogenous hormonal influences
• Exposure to chemical carcinogens
• Sexually transmitted diseases
• Male over 60 years of age
• Increased risk with vasectomy has been newly proposed but is unsupported

DIAGNOSIS

DIFFERENTIAL DIAGNOSIS
• Benign nodule prostate growth
• Prostate stones
• Nodular whorls of adenoma
• Seminal vesicle enlargement

LABORATORY
• Prostate specific antigen (PSA), elevated
• Free PSA - low in cancer (Catalana, et al: JAMA 1995;274:1213-1220)
• Alkaline phosphatase, elevated with metastasis
• Urine cytology, rarely helpful
Drugs that may alter lab results: None
Disorders that may alter lab results:
• Rectal manipulation will not significantly increase PSA
• Prior liver or bone disease

PATHOLOGICAL FINDINGS
• Size and shape of prostatic acini almost always altered
• Small closely packed interposed stroma
• Eosinophilic crystalloids present
• Architecture disrupted
• Cells invade perineural space

SPECIAL TESTS
• Prostate specific antigen (PSA)
• Free PSA

IMAGING
• Bone scan, positive with metastasis
• Skeletal survey, positive with metastasis
• Lymph node aspiration, positive with metastasis
• Computerized tomography of pelvic lymph nodes, positive with metastasis
• Prostatic ultrasound
• Lymphoscintigraphy
• Magnetic resonance imaging of little value

DIAGNOSTIC PROCEDURES
• Biopsy, fine needle aspiration or core
• Ultrasound
• Bone marrow aspiration
• Bone biopsy
• Lymph node aspiration
• Lymph node biopsy
• Lymphoscopic lymph node dissection

TREATMENT

APPROPRIATE HEALTH CARE
Inpatient for surgery, outpatient for other treatment

GENERAL MEASURES
• Therapy by tumor grade
  ◊ A1, A2 or age > 70: Observation may be appropriate or palliative as needed
  ◊ B1, B2: Prostatectomy, radiotherapy (external beam or brachytherapy with implants)
  ◊ C1: Prostatectomy for selected patients, radiotherapy
  ◊ C2, D1, D2: Hormonal (androgen) ablation, chemotherapy, radiotherapy, palliative therapy

SURGICAL MEASURES
• Under age 70, aggressive surgery for cure
• Surgical for stages A-B and selected C under age 70
• Orchiectomy

ACTIVITY Full activity

DIET No special diet

PATIENT EDUCATION Printed material available from:
• American Cancer Society
• National Kidney & Urologic Diseases Information Clearinghouse, Box NKUDIC, Bethesda, MD 20893, (301)468-6345

Prostatic cancer

MEDICATIONS

DRUG(S) OF CHOICE
• None specific
• For androgen ablation:
◊ Flutamide (Eulexin) 250 mg tid
◊ Leuprolide (Lupron) 1 mg subcutaneously daily or 7.5 mg IM depot monthly or 30mg IM depot-4 months sustained q 4 months
• Goserelin (Zoladex) 3.6 mg q month
Contraindications: None
Precautions:
• Flare phenomenon with metastatic disease
• Fluid retention
• Nausea
• Vomiting
• Hot flashes
• Liver enzyme changes
Significant possible interactions: Refer to manufacturer's profile of each drug.

ALTERNATIVE DRUGS None

FOLLOWUP

PATIENT MONITORING
• Routine clinical examination q 3 months for 1 year, the q 6 months for a year
• Annual examinations indefinitely
• PSA q 3 months for 1 year, q 6 months 1 year, then yearly
• Chest x-ray, bone scan, q 6 months for 1 year, then as suggested by rising PSA

PREVENTION/AVOIDANCE None

POSSIBLE COMPLICATIONS
• Cardiac failure
• Phlebitis
• Pathologic fracture

EXPECTED COURSE/PROGNOSIS
• Early diagnosis and treatment of lesions should be curable
• Advanced disease favorable prognosis if endocrine sensitive
• Advanced unresponsive disease progresses in 18 months average

MISCELLANEOUS

ASSOCIATED CONDITIONS N/A

AGE-RELATED FACTORS
Pediatric: N/A
Geriatric: N/A
Others: N/A

PREGNANCY N/A

SYNONYMS
Cancer of the prostate

ICD-9-CM
185 Malignant neoplasm of prostate

SEE ALSO N/A

OTHER NOTES N/A

ABBREVIATIONS
PSA = Prostate specific antigen

REFERENCES
• Walsh PC, Gittes RF, Perlmutter AD: Campbell's Urology. 6th Ed. Philadelphia, W.B. Saunders Co., 1992
Illustrations: N/A
Internet references: http://www.5mcc.com

Author(s)
Jack L. Summers, MD, PhD

Prostatic hyperplasia, benign (BPH)

BASICS

DESCRIPTION Benign adenomatous growth of prostate which may result in bladder outlet obstruction
System(s) affected: Reproductive, Renal/Urologic
Genetics: Genetic factors may be involved. Risk higher if father had clinical BPH in his 50's.
Incidence/Prevalence in USA:
• Universal pathologic phenomenon seen in older men
• No hard evidence suggesting racial predisposition
Predominant age:
• Rarely seen in men < 40
• Seen in 50% of men > 50; 80% of men > 70
Predominant sex: Male only

SIGNS AND SYMPTOMS
Prostate size correlates poorly with symptoms
• Obstructive symptoms: Due to mechanical obstruction and/or detrusor muscle decompensation
   ◊ Decrease force or caliber of stream
   ◊ Hesitancy
   ◊ Post-void dribbling
   ◊ Sensation of incomplete bladder emptying
   ◊ Overflow incontinence
   ◊ Inability to voluntarily stop stream
   ◊ Urinary retention
• Irritative symptoms: Due to incomplete bladder emptying and/or detrusor muscle instability
   ◊ Frequency
   ◊ Nocturia
   ◊ Urgency
   ◊ Urge incontinence
• Other symptoms and signs:
   ◊ Gross hematuria
   ◊ Observation of weak stream
   ◊ Distended bladder (> 150 cc in order to detect by percussion)
   ◊ Increased post-void residual (> 100 cc)
   ◊ Prostate enlarged (normal 20 gram prostate - size of horse chestnut)
   ◊ Clinical clues suggesting renal failure due to obstructive uropathy (edema, pallor, pruritus, ecchymoses, nutritional deficiencies, etc.)
   ◊ American Urological Association (AUA) symptom index score > 7

CAUSES Exact etiology unknown, but evidence suggests BPH arises from a systemic hormonal alteration which may or may not act in combination with growth factors stimulating stromal or glandular hyperplasia

RISK FACTORS
• Intact testes (BPH rare in eunuchs)
• Aging (thus, rare in men < 40 years old)
• Dietary and environmental may be implicated

DIAGNOSIS

DIFFERENTIAL DIAGNOSIS
• Obstructive conditions:
   ◊ Prostate cancer
   ◊ Urethral stricture
   ◊ Bladder neck contracture (acquired or congenital)
   ◊ Anterior or posterior urethral valves
   ◊ Mullerian duct cysts
   ◊ Inability of bladder neck or external sphincter to relax appropriately during voiding
• Non-obstructive conditions:
   ◊ Neurogenic bladder (detrusor denervation)
   ◊ Myogenic cause (detrusor muscle failure)
   ◊ Medications (parasympatholytics, sympathomimetics, etc.)
   ◊ Psychogenic
• Irritative conditions:
   ◊ Neurogenic bladder
   ◊ Inflammatory disorders (prostatitis, urethritis, radiation cystitis, interstitial cystitis, etc.)
   ◊ Neoplasm (bladder carcinoma, especially carcinoma in situ)

LABORATORY
• BPH is a pathologic diagnosis - lab data is only suggestive
• Urinalysis: pyuria, pH changes due to chronic residual urine
• Elevated serum creatinine (if obstructive uropathy present)
• Urine culture positive (sometimes due to chronic residual urine)
• Prostate specific antigen (PSA) may be elevated but usually < 10 ng/mL (10 µg/L)
• Increased post-void residual (> 100 mL)
• Acute urinary retention, transurethral instrumentation may elevate the PSA
Drugs that may alter lab results:
• Finasteride (Proscar) may lower the PSA
Disorders that may alter lab results:
• Acute urinary retention, prostatitis, urinary tract instrumentation or prostatic infarction may elevate the PSA

PATHOLOGICAL FINDINGS
Confirmation obtained by biopsy, resection or extirpation surgery. 5 types: Stromal (fibrous), fibromuscular, muscular ("leiomyoma"), fibroadenoma, fibromyoadenoma.

SPECIAL TESTS
• Transrectal prostate ultrasound gives volumetric estimate of gland
• Needle biopsy (to rule out cancer)
• Have patient complete IPSS (see below)
   ◊ Mild Symptoms (score 0-7): Offer watchful waiting only
   ◊ Moderate symptoms (score 8-19) to severe symptoms (score 20-35): Offer treatment options

IMAGING
• IVP - increased post-void residual, large prostatic impression on bladder, trabeculated bladder, bladder diverticula, upper tract dilation, bladder stones

• CT scan or MRI of pelvis - enlarged prostate
• Ultrasound - increase postvoid residual, prostate or hydronephrosis

DIAGNOSTIC PROCEDURES
• Uroflow - volume voided per unit time. Peak flow < 10 mL/sec suggests obstruction (accurate when voided volume is > 200 mL).
• Pressure-flow curve (urine flow versus voiding pressures) - decreased urine flow and increased pressure indicates obstruction
• Cystoscopy shows occlusive prostatic lobes, bladder trabeculation. Indicated if diagnosis is in doubt or helps guide the surgical approach (if surgery is an option)
• Post-void residual by catheterization or bladder ultrasound

TREATMENT

APPROPRIATE HEALTH CARE
Inpatient or outpatient treatment required, either for surgery or medical treatment. Inpatient emergent treatment required to manage fluid and electrolyte abnormalities of obstructive uropathy.

GENERAL MEASURES
• Avoid large boluses of oral or IV fluids
• Avoid prolonged periods of not voiding
• Avoid sympathomimetic or anticholinergic medications (e.g., cold/flu preparations)
• Urethral catheterization if in retention

SURGICAL MEASURES
• Surgery (indicators to determine necessity) One of the following:
   ◊ Urinary retention due to prostatic obstruction
   ◊ Intractable symptoms due to prostatic obstruction (gauged by AUA symptom index; score at least > 8)
   ◊ Obstructive uropathy
   ◊ Recurrent or persistent urinary tract infections due to prostatic obstruction
   ◊ Recurrent gross hematuria due to enlarged prostate
   ◊ Medical therapy indicated when surgery indicators not met.
• Surgical procedures - minimally invasive
   ◊ Interstitial laser coagulation (ILC)
   ◊ High frequency focused ultrasound (HIFU)
   ◊ Transurethral needle ablation (TUNA)
   ◊ Transurethral microwave thermotherapy (TUMT)
   ◊ Water-induced thermotherapy (WIT)
   ◊ Prostate stenting
   ◊ Transurethral balloon dilation (TUDP)
   ◊ Transurethral ethanol ablation of prostate
• Surgical procedures - more invasive
   ◊ TURP
   ◊ Open prostatectomy
   ◊ Transurethral laser ablation, laser-indeced prostatectomy or laser enucleation of prostate
   ◊ Transurethral vaporization of prostate

ACTIVITY No restriction

DIET Avoid caffeinated or alcoholic beverages, excessively spiced foods

PATIENT EDUCATION
• The Prostate Book, published by Krames Communications, 312 90th St, Daly City, CA 94015-1898
• National Kidney & Urologic Diseases Information Clearinghouse, Box NKUDIC, Bethesda, MD 20893, (301)468-6345

 MEDICATIONS

DRUG(S) OF CHOICE
Indicated when no strong indication for surgery exists or patient declines surgery
• Alpha adrenergic antagonist: terazosin (Hytrin) 1-10 mg/day, doxazosin (Cardura) 1-8 mg/day, tamsulosin (Flomax) 0.4-0.8 mg/day
• Hormonal (anti-androgens) agents: finasteride (Proscar) 5 mg/day works best for larger prostates; turosteride, flutamide (Eulexin) and leuprolide (Lupron) are rarely used; phytotherapy (e.g., serenoa repens (Saw Palmetto), similar to finasteride in efficacy)
Contraindications:
• Use alpha adrenergic antagonists with caution in patients with cardiac or cerebrovascular disease or those who operate machinery. Give the first dose at bedtime to avoid orthostatic hypotension
• Hormones may cause impotence (less with flutamide) and lower the PSA
• The semen of men taking finasteride may cause effects on the fetus of pregnant sex partners
Precautions: Refer to manufacturer's profile of each drug
Significant possible interactions:
• Tamsulosin-cimetidine: do not administer together

ALTERNATIVE DRUGS N/A

 FOLLOWUP

PATIENT MONITORING
• Symptom index (IPSS) monitored every 1-6 months
• Urodynamics every 3-12 months
• Digital rectal exam yearly
• PSA yearly

PREVENTION/AVOIDANCE Appears to be part of the aging process

POSSIBLE COMPLICATIONS
• Bladder stones
• Prostatitis
• Renal failure
• Hematuria

EXPECTED COURSE/PROGNOSIS
• Symptoms improve or stabilize in 70-80% of patients; 20-30% require treatment because of worsening symptoms
• 11-33% men with BPH have occult prostate cancer

 MISCELLANEOUS

ASSOCIATED CONDITIONS N/A

AGE-RELATED FACTORS
Pediatric: N/A
Geriatric: Much more prevalent in elderly men
Others: N/A

PREGNANCY N/A

SYNONYMS
• Prostatic hyperplasia
• Prostatic hypertrophy

ICD-9-CM 600 hyperplasia of prostate

SEE ALSO N/A

OTHER NOTES N/A

ABBREVIATIONS
IPSS = International Prostate Symptom Score
IVP = intravenous pyelogram
AUA = American Urological Association

REFERENCES
• Proceedings of 94th annual American Urological Association Meeting, Dallas, 1999
• McConnel JD: Benign prostatic hypertrophy. In: Walsh PC, et al, eds. Campbell's Urology. Philadelphia, W.B. Saunders Co., 1998
• Kirby RS, McConnel JD: Benign prostatis hypertrophy, Fast Facts. Oxford, Health Press, 1997
• Kapoor DA, Reddy PK: Surgical alternatives to TURP in the management of BPH. AUA Update Series 1993;3(12)
Illustrations: N/A
Internet references: http://www.5mcc.com

Author(s)
Charles Jennings, MD, FACS

IPSS
Circle the numerical score for each question below.
OVER THE LAST MONTH OR SO:

1. How many times did you most typically get up to urinate from the time you went to bed at night until the time you got up in the morning?
• None--------0
• 1 time------1
• 2 times-----2
• 3 times-----3
• 4 times-----4
• 5 or more---5
2. How often have you had a sensation of not emptying your bladder completely after you finished urinating?
• Not at all--------------0
• Less than 1 time in 5----1
• Less than half the time--2
• About half the time------3
• More than half the time--4
• Almost always-----------5
3. How often have you had to urinate again less than two hours after you finished urinating?
• Not at all--------------0
• Less than 1 time in 5----1
• Less than half the time--2
• About half the time------3
• More than half the time--4
• Almost always-----------5
4. How often have you found that you stopped and started again several times when you urinate?
• Not at all--------------0
• Less than 1 time in 5----1
• Less than half the time--2
• About half the time------3
• More than half the time--4
• Almost always-----------5
5. How often have you found it difficult to postpone urination?
• Not at all--------------0
• Less than 1 time in 5----1
• Less than half the time--2
• About half the time------3
• More than half the time--4
• Almost always-----------5
6. How often have you had a weak urinary stream?
• Not at all--------------0
• Less than 1 time in 5----1
• Less than half the time--2
• About half the time------3
• More than half the time--4
• Almost always-----------5
7. How often have you had to push or strain to begin urination?
• Not at all--------------0
• Less than 1 time in 5----1
• Less than half the time--2
• About half the time------3
• More than half the time--4
• Almost always-----------5

Total score:_____
(sum of questions 1-7)

Prostatitis

BASICS

DESCRIPTION One of several inflammatory and/or painful conditions affecting the prostate gland
• Acute bacterial prostatitis – generally associated with urinary tract infection, has characteristically abrupt onset
• Chronic bacterial prostatitis –major cause of recurrent bacteriuria, less fulminant
• Nonbacterial prostatitis –findings similar to chronic bacterial, but bacterial cultures negative
System(s) affected: Reproductive, Renal/Urologic
Genetics: No known genetic pattern
Incidence/Prevalence in USA: Common
Predominant age:
• Mostly ages 30-50, sexually active
• Chronic more common in ages over 50
Predominant sex: Male only

SIGNS AND SYMPTOMS
• Acute bacterial
  ◊ Fever; chills
  ◊ Tense, boggy, very tender and warm prostate
  ◊ Low back pain
  ◊ Perineal pain
  ◊ Frequency
  ◊ Urgency
  ◊ Dysuria
  ◊ Nocturia
  ◊ Bladder outlet obstruction
• Chronic bacterial
  ◊ Symptoms often absent
  ◊ Perineal pain
  ◊ Dysuria
  ◊ Irritative voiding
  ◊ Lower abdominal pain
  ◊ Low back pain
  ◊ Scrotal pain
  ◊ Penile pain
  ◊ Pain on ejaculation
  ◊ Hematospermia
• Nonbacterial
  ◊ Similar to chronic prostatitis

CAUSES
• Acute and chronic bacterial
  ◊ Ascending infection through urethra
  ◊ Refluxing urine into prostate ducts
  ◊ Direct extension or lymphatic spread from rectum
  ◊ Hematogenous spread
  ◊ Calculi serving as nidus for infection
  ◊ Aerobic gram negative bacteria (*Escherichia coli, Pseudomonas, Klebsiella, Proteus*), *N. gonorrhea, Enterobacteriaceae*
  ◊ Miscellaneous – *Chlamydia trachomatis*
  ◊ Gram positive bacteria (*Streptococcus faecalis, Staphylococcus. aureus*)
  ◊ Organisms suspected, but unproven (*Staphylococcus epidermidis*, Micrococci, non-group D streptococcus, Diphtheroids)
• Nonbacterial
  ◊ Currently unknown
  ◊ Ureaplasma, trichomonas vaginalis, and Chlamydia postulated, but not proven

RISK FACTORS
• Male sex
• Age over 50
• Prostatic calculi
• Urinary tract infection

DIAGNOSIS

DIFFERENTIAL DIAGNOSIS
• Cystitis
• Urethritis
• Pyelonephritis
• Malignancy
• Obstructive calculus
• Foreign body
• Acute urinary retention

LABORATORY
• Fractional urine examination (initial 10 mL from urethra for voided bladder 1 (VB1) test, next 200 mL discarded, then midstream from bladder for VB2 test, then expressed prostate secretion (EPS), lastly urine after prostate massage for VB3 test. Some feel vigorous massage may lead to bacteremia.
• Urinalysis, culture, sensitivities on all samples
• Over 10-15 white cells per high powered field or positive culture in EPS or VB3 but not VB1 or VB2 diagnostic of bacterial prostatitis
• Bacteria count generally less in chronic than acute
• Nonbacterial will show white blood cells with a negative culture
• No abnormal findings with prostatodynia
Drugs that may alter lab results:
Antibiotics
Disorders that may alter lab results: N/A

PATHOLOGICAL FINDINGS
Inflammatory changes (except prostatodynia)

SPECIAL TESTS   N/A

IMAGING
• CT or ultrasound, if malignancy or abscess suspected
• Transrectal ultrasound (if prostatic calculi or abscess suspected)

DIAGNOSTIC PROCEDURES
• Needle biopsy or aspiration for culture
• Urodynamic testing (prostatodynia)
• Cystoscopy (in persistent nonbacterial prostatitis to rule out bladder cancer, interstitial cystitis)

TREATMENT

APPROPRIATE HEALTH CARE
• Inpatient (proven or suspected abscess, urosepsis, immunocompromised)
• Outpatient, if nontoxic

GENERAL MEASURES
• Analgesics
• Antipyretics
• Stool softeners
• Hydration
• Sitz baths to relieve pain and spasm
• Suprapubic catheter for severe urinary retention

SURGICAL MEASURES   Surgical resection for intractable chronic disease, or to drain an abscess; transurethral microwave thermotherapy for chronic nonbacterial prostatitis

ACTIVITY   Bedrest in severe cases

DIET
• Nonbacterial and prostatodynia – avoid spicy foods, excess caffeine and alcohol
• Acute and chronic bacterial – no special diet

PATIENT EDUCATION
• Printed patient information available from: National Kidney & Urologic Diseases Information Clearinghouse, Box NKUDIC, Bethesda, MD 20893, (301)468-6345

Prostatitis

MEDICATIONS

DRUG(S) OF CHOICE
• Acute bacterial (outpatient): Trimethoprim-sulfamethoxazole (Septra), double strength, two tablets, twice daily for 30 days
• Acute bacterial (inpatient): Ampicillin 150-200 mg/kg/d IV divided q6h plus aminoglycoside – gentamicin 2.0 mg/kg loading dose; 1.7 mg/kg q8h maintenance
• Chronic bacterial: A fluoroquinolone (norfloxacin 400 mg bid, ciprofloxacin 500 mg bid) at standard dose for ≥ 3 months
• Nonbacterial: May benefit from erythromycin, doxycycline, trimethoprim-sulfamethoxazole
• Prostatodynia: Alpha-adrenergic blocking agents may be useful
• Analgesics
• Antipyretics
• Stool softeners

Contraindications: Drug allergies

Precautions:
• Renal disease
• Hepatic disease
• Elderly
• G6PD deficiency

Significant possible interactions:
Fluoroquinolones with magnesium/aluminum antacids, theophylline, probenecid, NSAID's, warfarin

ALTERNATIVE DRUGS Carbenicillin
with aminoglycoside, erythromycin, tetracycline, cephalexin, fluoroquinolones

FOLLOWUP

PATIENT MONITORING
• Acute bacterial - urinalysis and culture 30 days after initiating treatment
• Chronic bacterial - urinalysis and culture every 30 days (may take several months)

PREVENTION/AVOIDANCE
Suppression therapy may benefit patient with chronic bacterial prostatitis

POSSIBLE COMPLICATIONS
• Abscess
• Sepsis
• Urinary retention

EXPECTED COURSE/PROGNOSIS
Often prolonged and difficult to cure. Studies with 55-97% cure rate depending on population and drug used.

MISCELLANEOUS

ASSOCIATED CONDITIONS
• Prostatic hypertrophy
• Cystitis
• Urethritis

AGE-RELATED FACTORS
Pediatric: None
Geriatric: Consider prostatic hypertrophy and urinary retention more seriously
Others: N/A

PREGNANCY N/A

SYNONYMS N/A

ICD-9-CM
601.0 Prostatitis, acute
601.1 Prostatitis, chronic

SEE ALSO
• Prostatic cancer
• Prostatic hyperplasia, benign (BPH)

OTHER NOTES
• Prostatodynia: pain in the area of prostate. Sometimes inaccurately designated as a diagnosis.

ABBREVIATIONS
VB = voided bladder
EPS = expressed prostate secretion

REFERENCES
• Isselbacher KJ, et al, eds: Harrison's Principles of Internal Medicine. 13th Ed. New York, McGraw-Hill, 1994
• Moul JN: Prostatitis: Sorting out the different courses. Postgrad Med 1993;94-5:191-194
• Daneshgari F, Crawford ED: Benign prostatic disease: A growing challenge in the 1990's. Postgrad Med 1993;93(7):84-92
• Sable CA, Scheld WM: Fluoroquinolones: How to use (but not overuse) these antibiotica. Geriatrics 1993;48(6):41-51
• Nickel JC, Sorensen R: Transurethral microwave thermotherapy for nonbacterial prostatitis: a randomized double blind controlled study using new prostatitis specific assessment questionnaires. J Urol 1996;155(6):1950:1954
Illustrations: N/A
Internet references: http://www.5mcc.com

Author(s)
Gary A. Goforth, MD, MTMH

Pruritus ani

BASICS

DESCRIPTION Intense chronic itching in the anal and perianal skin. Usual course - acute. Chronic pruritus ani is a symptom, not a diagnosis or disease.
System(s) affected: Skin/Exocrine
Genetics: No known genetic pattern
Incidence/Prevalence in USA: Common
Predominant age: All ages
Predominant sex: Male > Female (4:1)

SIGNS AND SYMPTOMS
- Primary
  ◊ Rectal itching
  ◊ Anal erythema
- Secondary
Secondary infections with yeast, fungus, and/or bacteria are possible after prolonged scratching
  ◊ Anal itching
  ◊ Anal fissures
  ◊ Maceration
  ◊ Lichenification
  ◊ Excoriations

CAUSES
- Dermatologic disorders
  ◊ Allergies (soap, topical anesthetics, oral antibiotics)
  ◊ Fistulas
  ◊ Fissures
  ◊ Neoplasms
  ◊ Psoriasis
  ◊ Eczema
  ◊ Seborrheic dermatitis
  ◊ Contact dermatitis
- Infections
  ◊ Pinworms and other worms
  ◊ Scabies
  ◊ Pediculosis
  ◊ Candidiasis
  ◊ Tinea
- Other
  ◊ Poor hygiene (fecal material allowed to dry on the skin)
  ◊ Diabetes mellitus
  ◊ Chronic liver disease
  ◊ Diarrheic alkalotic irritation
  ◊ Trauma from scented toilet paper

RISK FACTORS
- Overweight
- Hairy, tendency to perspire a great deal
- Anxiety-itch-anxiety cycle

DIAGNOSIS

DIFFERENTIAL DIAGNOSIS
- Allergies
- Psoriasis
- Atopic dermatitis
- Fungus infection
- Bacterial infection
- Parasites
- Hyperhidrosis
- Diabetes mellitus
- Liver disease
- Neoplasia
- Anxiety

LABORATORY
- Glycosuria
- Hyperglycemia
- Skin scraping, yeast
- Fungi
- Parasites
- Stool - ova plus parasites
Drugs that may alter lab results: N/A
Disorders that may alter lab results: N/A

PATHOLOGICAL FINDINGS Excoriation of epithelial layer of skin

SPECIAL TESTS Blood sugar levels

IMAGING N/A

DIAGNOSTIC PROCEDURES
- Inspection
- Anoscopy biopsy (to exclude neoplasia)

TREATMENT

APPROPRIATE HEALTH CARE
Outpatient

GENERAL MEASURES
- Treat predisposing factors, such as parasites, diabetes, liver disease, cryptitis, scabies, pediculosis
- Resist overmeticulous use of soap and rubbing
- Avoid tight clothing and under clothing
- Cleanse anal area after bowel movements with moistened absorbent cotton and plain water; baby wipes may be a convenient alternative
- Dust anal area with non-medicated talcum powder
- If unable to completely empty rectum with defecation, use small plain water enema (infant bulb syringe) after each bowel movement. This may prevent postevacuation soilage and irritation.

SURGICAL MEASURES N/A

ACTIVITY Avoid getting overheated

DIET If suspicious of food allergy, eliminate as a trial: Coffee, beer, cola, vitamin C tablets in excessive doses, spices, citrus fruits

PATIENT EDUCATION See information in General Measures

MEDICATIONS

DRUG(S) OF CHOICE
• Specific treatment for allergies, micro-organisms, bacteria and worm infestation
• For symptomatic treatment - hydrocortisone cream 0.5-1% applied sparingly, usually at night. If severe, may need to apply several times a day. Discontinue once itching stops.
Contraindications: Refer to manufacturer's literature
Precautions: Refer to manufacturer's literature
Significant possible interactions: Refer to manufacturer's literature

ALTERNATIVE DRUGS
Albendazole for pinworms: 200 mg orally once for children <2 yrs, 400 mg for children over 2 and adults

FOLLOWUP

PATIENT MONITORING   As needed

PREVENTION/AVOIDANCE
• Avoid topical agents
• Avoid laxatives
• Avoid tight underclothing made from synthetic material
• Practice good hygiene
• Use talcum powder
• Possibly lactobacillus acidophilus (tablets or in milk); possibly malt soup extract
• Eat yogurt when taking broad-spectrum antibiotics

POSSIBLE COMPLICATIONS
• Secondary bacterial infection
• Chronicity
• Excoriation
• Lichenification

EXPECTED COURSE/PROGNOSIS
• Depends upon etiology; usually good
• May be persistent and recurrent

MISCELLANEOUS

ASSOCIATED CONDITIONS
• Diabetes mellitus
• Psoriasis
• Hyperhidrosis
• Parasite infestations
• Hemorrhoids

AGE-RELATED FACTORS
Pediatric:
• Usually secondary to enterobiasis, anal fissures, other local inflammatory lesions, or coarse or moist undergarments. Nocturnal itching may be due to pinworms.
• Exposure to sunlight or dry heat may be helpful for infants with inflamed anal area
Geriatric: Common in this age group
Others: N/A

PREGNANCY   N/A

SYNONYMS   N/A

ICD-9-CM
698.0 Pruritus ani

SEE ALSO
• Pruritus vulvae
• Pinworms

OTHER NOTES   N/A

ABBREVIATIONS   N/A

REFERENCES
• Sleisenger MH, Fordtran JS, eds: Gastrointestinal Disease: Pathophysiology, Diagnosis, Management. 5th Ed. Philadelphia, W.B. Saunders Co., 1994
• Kirsner JB, Shortet G, eds: Diseases of the Colon, Rectum and Canal. Baltimore, Williams & Wilkins, 1988
Illustrations: N/A
Internet references: http://www.5mcc.com

Author(s)
Stanley G. Smith, MA, MB, FCFPC

Pruritus vulvae

BASICS

DESCRIPTION Pruritus vulvae is both a symptom and a pathologic process affecting the vulva. It is a symptom of underlying disease in the vast majority of the patients. As a primary diagnosis, it consists of irritation and vulvar itching without an underlying pathologic etiology.
System(s) affected: Skin/Exocrine
Genetics: Unknown
Incidence/Prevalence in USA: The exact incidence is unknown, although most women will complain of vulvar pruritus at some time during their life
Predominant age:
• Any age can be affected
• In young girls, it is usually caused by an infection
• Frequent in postmenopausal women
Predominant sex: Female only

SIGNS AND SYMPTOMS
• Constant itching of the vulva
• Constant burning of the vulva

CAUSES
• Infectious causes - vaginal yeast infections, Gardnerella, other vaginal infections, and yeast dermatitis of the vulva itself
• Urinary tract infections will produce vulvar burning on occasion
• Vulvar vestibulitis (inflammation of the vestibular glands) produces a constant burning with pruritus and dyspareunia
• Human papillomavirus (HPV) has been associated with burning and itching of the vulva
• Vulvar tissues are estrogen sensitive. Estrogen deprivation can produce burning and itching.
• A search for underlying malignancy should be paramount. Carcinoma in situ (Bowen's disease) and invasive malignancy will often be associated with pruritus.
• Changes in the epidermis, such as lichen sclerosis et atrophicus (LSA) (thinning of the vulvar tissues and homogenization at the basement membrane) or hyperkeratosis of the vulva produce pruritus
• Anal incontinence with fecal soilage produces pruritus
• Excessive heat produces symptoms from sweat and irritation
• Environmental and dietary irritants such as nylon, soaps, perfumes, and over-zealous cleansing can produce symptoms
• Dietary irritants include methylxanthines (coffee, cola), tomatoes, peanuts

RISK FACTORS N/A

DIAGNOSIS

DIFFERENTIAL DIAGNOSIS
• The diagnosis of primary idiopathic vulvar pruritus must be made by exclusion
• A search for infectious causes should be undertaken with treatment of yeast and other vaginitis
• Biopsy of any abnormal-appearing epithelium on the vulva to insure that malignant changes are not present
• Only when all other factors have been ruled out can the diagnosis primary idiopathic vulvar pruritus be established

LABORATORY
• Vaginal secretions can be evaluated by wet mount (NaCl for trichomonas or Gardnerella, and KOH for yeast). Cultures seldom required.
• Gram stain of the vagina is non-diagnostic as multiple organisms are present in the normal flora
Drugs that may alter lab results: N/A
Disorders that may alter lab results: N/A

PATHOLOGICAL FINDINGS These are related to the underlying etiology. In primary vulvar pruritus, no changes will be noted. If HPV is present, these changes will be seen in the cornified layer of the squamous epithelium.

SPECIAL TESTS Whenever necessary, biopsy of the vulva should be used to establish the primary diagnosis

IMAGING N/A

DIAGNOSTIC PROCEDURES Biopsy when needed

TREATMENT

APPROPRIATE HEALTH CARE
Outpatient

GENERAL MEASURES
• Treatment of any underlying cause must be undertaken
• In cases of idiopathic primary vulvar pruritus, conservative measures include sitz baths, topical steroid creams, avoidance of chemical irritants and dietary changes
• When conservative measures fail, advanced cases can be treated with alcohol block or laser

SURGICAL MEASURES Bowen's disease and premalignant changes are treated with excision or laser vaporization

ACTIVITY Unlimited

DIET A trial of dietary alteration should be attempted for idiopathic pruritus. Coffee and caffeine-containing beverages should be avoided. Other foods to avoid include tomatoes, peanuts.

PATIENT EDUCATION See Prevention/Avoidance

MEDICATIONS

DRUG(S) OF CHOICE
• Infectious sources should be treated with appropriate antimicrobials or antifungals
• Lichen sclerosis is treated with 2% testosterone in petrolatum
• Hyperkeratotic lesions are treated with topical steroid
• Idiopathic primary vulvar pruritus can be treated with topical steroids such as triamcinolone (Kenalog) or desoximetasone (Topicort) cream
Contraindications: N/A
Precautions: N/A
Significant possible interactions: N/A

ALTERNATIVE DRUGS   N/A

FOLLOWUP

PATIENT MONITORING   These women should be followed closely for the development of premalignant or malignant changes within the area of pruritus

PREVENTION/AVOIDANCE
• Irritants to the vulva such as perfumes, soaps (use non-allergenic) or perfume douches must be avoided
• Only cotton underwear should be worn
• No tight fitting clothes or nylon pantyhose

POSSIBLE COMPLICATIONS   Chronic course

EXPECTED COURSE/PROGNOSIS
• Vulvar pruritus can be kept under control with conservative measures and topical steroids
• When it advances to uncontrollable symptoms, alcohol block or laser may be necessary

MISCELLANEOUS

ASSOCIATED CONDITIONS   N/A

AGE-RELATED FACTORS
Pediatric: N/A
Geriatric: More frequent
Others: N/A

PREGNANCY   N/A

SYNONYMS
• Vulvar pruritus
• Vulvodynia
• Burning vulva syndrome

ICD-9-CM   698.1 Pruritus of genital organs

SEE ALSO   N/A

OTHER NOTES   N/A

ABBREVIATIONS   N/A

REFERENCES
• McKay M: Vulvodynia vs. Pruritus vulvae. Clin Obstet Gynecol 1985;28:123-133
• Smith L, Henricks D, McCullah R: Prospective studies on the etiology and treatment of pruritus ani. Dis Colon Rectum 1982;25:258-363
• Hopkins MP: Anatomy and pathology of the vulva and vagina. In: Rebar R, Baker V, eds. Gynecology & Obstetrics, An Integrated Approach. New York, Churchill Livingstone, 1993
Illustrations: N/A
Internet references: http://www.5mcc.com

Author(s)
Michael P. Hopkins, MD

Pseudofolliculitis barbae

BASICS

DESCRIPTION   Foreign body inflammatory reaction surrounding an ingrown hair (usually in beard area, especially submandibular region, but can occur on scalp, axilla, or pubic area if these sites are shaved or plucked). Characterized by red papule/pustule at point of entry. A mechanical problem.
System(s) affected: Skin/Exocrine
Genetics: Curly haired people, especially Blacks
Incidence/Prevalence in USA: Widespread. Incidence of 45% in black soldiers who shave. Adult male blacks - 50,000/100,000; adult male Caucasians - 3000-5000/100,000.
Predominant age: Postpubertal, middle age (40-75)
Predominant sex: Male > Female

SIGNS AND SYMPTOMS
• Tender exudative, erythematous follicular papules or pustules in beard area (less commonly in scalp, axilla, pubic areas)
• Range from 2-4 mm in size
• Painful upon shaving
• Alopecia
• Lusterless brittle hair

CAUSES
• Reentry penetration of skin by external pointed tip of growing curved whisker, or sharp tipped whisker can grow into follicular wall if shaved too close
• Plucking of hair can cause abnormal hair growth in injured follicles

RISK FACTORS
• Curly hair
• Shaving too close with multiple razor strokes
• Plucking hairs
• Black race

DIAGNOSIS

DIFFERENTIAL DIAGNOSIS
• Bacterial folliculitis
• Impetigo

LABORATORY   N/A
Drugs that may alter lab results: N/A
Disorders that may alter lab results: N/A

PATHOLOGICAL FINDINGS
• Clinical pathology - follicular papules and pustules
• Histopathology - because of its curvature, the advancing hair's sharp-tipped free end causes an epidermal invagination as it approaches the skin. This is accompanied by inflammation and often an intra-epidermal abscess. As hair enters dermis, more severe inflammation occurs with downgrowth of epidermis in an attempt to ensheath hair. An abscess forms within the pseudofollicle and a foreign body reaction forms at the tip of invading hair.

SPECIAL TESTS   Culture of pustules - usually sterile. May show coagulase-negative micrococcus (normal skin flora).

IMAGING   N/A

DIAGNOSTIC PROCEDURES   Clinical diagnosis

TREATMENT

APPROPRIATE HEALTH CARE
Outpatient

GENERAL MEASURES
• Acute treatment
  ◊ Dislodge embedded hair with sterile needle
  ◊ Discontinue shaving until red papules have resolved (minimum 3-4 weeks)
  ◊ Massage beard area with washcloths, coarse sponge or brush several times daily
  ◊ Systemic antibiotics if secondary infections present

SURGICAL MEASURES   N/A

ACTIVITY   Unlimited

DIET   No restrictions

PATIENT EDUCATION
• Dunn 88, Pseudofolliculitis Barbae, pages 170-172
• American Family Physician (see References)

Pseudofolliculitis barbae

MEDICATIONS

DRUG(S) OF CHOICE
• Topical or systemic antibiotic for secondary infection
  ◊ Application of clindamycin (Cleocin-T) solution bid
  ◊ Low doses erythromycin or tetracycline 250 mg bid
  ◊ Administer until papule/pustule resolution
• Mild cases
  ◊ 5% benzoyl peroxide - apply after shaving
  ◊ 1% hydrocortisone cream - apply at bedtime
• Moderate disease - chemical depilatories
  ◊ Disrupt cross-linking of disulfide bonds of hair causing blunt hair tip
  ◊ Apply no more frequently than every 3rd day - 2% barium sulfide (Magic Shave) or calcium thioglycolate (Surgex)
• Moderate disease - adjunct treatment
  ◊ Tretinoin (Retin-A) liquid/cream, applied daily or every other day
Contraindications:
• Clindamycin - history of regional enteritis or ulcerative colitis; history of antibiotic associated colitis
• Erythromycin, tetracycline, tretinoin hypersensitivity only
Precautions:
• Clindamycin - colitis, eye burning and irritation, skin dryness, pregnancy category B
• Erythromycin - cautious use in patients with impaired hepatic function, GI side effects especially abdominal cramping, pregnancy category B
• Tetracycline - permanent discoloration of teeth if given during last half of pregnancy
• Tretinoin - severe skin irritation, pregnancy category C
• Benzoyl peroxide - skin irritation and dryness, allergic contact dermatitis
• Hydrocortisone cream - local skin irritation, skin atrophy with prolonged use
Significant possible interactions:
• Erythromycin - increases theophylline and carbamazepine levels, decreases clearance of warfarin; cardiac toxicity with terfenadine and astemizole
• Tetracycline - depresses plasma prothrombin activity (therefore need to decrease warfarin dosages)

ALTERNATIVE DRUGS Topical application of glycolic acid lotion (8% buffered glycolic acid in a suitable carrier, either oil-in-water lotion or a non-lipid soap) twice daily. This treatment may allow shaving comfortably every day.

FOLLOWUP

PATIENT MONITORING As needed.
Educate patient on curative and preventive treatment.

PREVENTION/AVOIDANCE
• Mild cases
  ◊ Use tiny plastic hook for removing ingrown hairs before shaving
  ◊ Shave either with a manual adjustable razor at coarsest settings (avoids close shaves), a twin blade razor (Trac-II, The Bump-Fighter), a foil guarded razor (PFB razor), electric triple "O" head razor, or electric hair clipper with polyester skin cleansing pad (Buf-Puf by Riker Labs)
  ◊ Shave beard in direction of hair growth
  ◊ Do not stretch skin when shaving
  ◊ Use correct shaving cream/gel (Ef-Kay Shaving Gel, Edge Shaving Gel, Easy Shave Medicated Shaving Cream)
  ◊ Consider 5% benzoyl peroxide after shaving and application of 1% hydrocortisone cream at bedtime
• Moderate cases
  ◊ Chemical depilatories (barium sulfide)
  ◊ Consider 0.05% tretinoin (Retin-A) liquid or cream
• Severe cases
  ◊ Avoidance of shaving completely
  ◊ Electrolysis to destroy remaining hair follicles - controversial

POSSIBLE COMPLICATIONS
• Scarring (occasionally keloidal)
• Foreign body granuloma formation
• Disfiguring postinflammatory hyperpigmentation
• Impetiginization of inflamed skin

EXPECTED COURSE/PROGNOSIS
• Course is recurrent if preventative measures not followed
• Prognosis is poor in presence of progressive scarring and foreign body granuloma formation

MISCELLANEOUS

ASSOCIATED CONDITIONS Keloidal folliculitis

AGE-RELATED FACTORS
Pediatric: N/A
Geriatric: N/A
Others: N/A

PREGNANCY Do not use tretinoin (Retin-A), tetracycline, benzoyl peroxide

SYNONYMS
• Chronic sycosis barbae
• Pili incarnati
• Folliculitis barbae traumatica
• Razor bumps

ICD-9-CM
704.8 Other specified diseases of hair and follicles

SEE ALSO
• Folliculitis
• Impetigo
• Tinea barbae

OTHER NOTES N/A

ABBREVIATIONS N/A

REFERENCES
• Lever WF, Schaumburg-Lever G: Histopathology of the Skin. Philadelphia, J.B. Lippincott, 1990
• Dunn JF Jr: Pseudofolliculitis Barbae. Amer Fam Phys 1988;9
• Habif TP: Clinical Dermatology. St Louis, CV Mosby, 1995
• Sams W Jr, Lynch P: Principles and Practice of Dermatology. New York, Churchill Livingstone, 1990
• Perricone NV: Treatment of pseudofolliculitis barbae with topical glycolic acid: A report of two studies. Cutis 1993;52(4):232-235
• Lewis CW, Coquilla BH: Management of pseudofolliculitis barbae. Military Medicine, Vol 160, May 1995
Illustrations: N/A
Internet references: http://www.5mcc.com

Author(s)
W. Paul Slomiany, MD

Pseudogout (CPPD)

BASICS

DESCRIPTION An acute inflammatory arthritic disease usually involving large joints which primarily affects the elderly and is caused by calcium pyrophosphate dihydrate (CPPD) crystal deposition in joints. Associated with chondrocalcinosis.
• CPPD crystal deposition may cause a progressive degenerative arthritis in numerous joints
• CPPD crystal deposition may cause a more insidious, smoldering, symmetrical, polyarthritis which is similar to rheumatoid arthritis

System(s) affected: Musculoskeletal
Genetics:
• Uncommonly seen in familial pattern with autosomal dominant inheritance (< 1% of cases)
• Most cases sporadic
Incidence/Prevalence in USA: Unknown, primarily a disease of the elderly; chondrocalcinosis is present 1 in 10 in ages 60-75, over age 80 in 1 in 3. Only a small percentage develop pseudogout.
Predominant age: 80% of patients > than 60
Predominant sex: Male = Female

SIGNS AND SYMPTOMS
• Acute pain and swelling of one or more joints. Knee is involved in one-half of all attacks, ankle, wrist and shoulder also common.
  ◊ Inflammation, joint effusion, limitation of motion
  ◊ 50% associated with fever
  ◊ Any other synovial joint may be involved including first metatarsophalangeal
• Can present with a chronic progressive arthritis upon which acute inflammation attacks are superimposed
• Progressive degenerative arthritis in numerous joints including: wrists, metacarpophalangeal, hips, shoulders, elbows, and ankles without inflammatory attacks also seen
• Low grade inflammatory arthritis with multiple symmetrical joint involvement (mimics rheumatoid arthritis) < 5% of cases

CAUSES
• Acute inflammatory reaction to CPPD crystals shed into synovial cavity
• Physical and chemical changes in aging cartilage that favor crystal growth

RISK FACTORS
• Aging
• Trauma
• Pseudogout will often occur as a complication in patients hospitalized for other medical and surgical illnesses
• Metabolic diseases (10% or less of the cases)
  ◊ Hyperparathyroidism
  ◊ Hemochromatosis
  ◊ Gout
  ◊ Hypophosphatasia
  ◊ Hypothyroidism
  ◊ Ochronosis
  ◊ Wilson's disease
  ◊ Amyloidosis
  ◊ Hypomagnesemia

DIAGNOSIS

DIFFERENTIAL DIAGNOSIS
• Illness that may cause an acute inflammatory arthritis in a single or multiple joint(s): Gout, septic arthritis or trauma
• Other illnesses that may present with an acute inflammatory arthritis: Reiter's syndrome, Lyme disease, acute rheumatoid arthritis

LABORATORY
• Elevated sedimentation rate
• Leukocytosis with mild left shift
Drugs that may alter lab results: N/A
Disorders that may alter lab results: N/A

PATHOLOGICAL FINDINGS
CPPD crystal deposition in articular cartilage, synovium, ligaments and tendons

SPECIAL TESTS
• Synovial fluid analysis consistent with an inflammatory effusion:
  ◊ Cell count from 2000 to 100,000 WBC/mL
  ◊ Differential predominantly neutrophils (80-90%)
  ◊ Wet prep with polarized microscopy demonstrates small numbers of weakly positively birefringent crystals in the fluid and within neutrophils
• Metabolic studies
  ◊ To exclude an underlying cause should always be obtained in patients under age 50 and considered in the elderly
  ◊ Serum calcium
  ◊ Serum phosphorus
  ◊ Serum alkaline phosphatase
  ◊ Serum parathormone
  ◊ Serum iron, total iron binding capacity, and serum ferritin
  ◊ Serum magnesium
  ◊ Serum thyroxine and thyroid stimulating hormone (TSH) level

IMAGING
• X-rays of joints
  ◊ May demonstrate punctate and linear calcification in articular hyaline or fibrocartilage: Knees, hips, symphysis pubis, and wrists most often affected, may also be found in asymptomatic individuals
  ◊ In the chronic destructive indolent form of the disease: Subchondral cyst formation, fragmentation with formation of intra-articular radiodense bodies in joints not typically affected by degenerative joint disease.

DIAGNOSTIC PROCEDURES
• Aspiration of joint fluid with synovial fluid analysis required for proper confirmation of pseudogout; aspiration may relieve symptoms and speed resolution of inflammatory process

TREATMENT

APPROPRIATE HEALTH CARE
• If septic arthritis is considered possible, inpatient care may be required for empiric antibiotic therapy pending culture results
• If patient does not have adequate support system inpatient care may be required until patient is able to walk

GENERAL MEASURES
• Rest and elevate affected joint(s)
• Apply moist warm compresses to affected joints

SURGICAL MEASURES   N/A

ACTIVITY
• Non-weight bearing on affected joint while painful. Use crutches or walker.
• Perform isometric exercises to maintain muscle strength during the acute stage, i.e., quadriceps isometric contractions and leg lifts, if knee affected
• Begin range of motion of joint as inflammation and pain subside
• Resume weight bearing when pain subsides

DIET   No special diet

PATIENT EDUCATION   Specific instructions on exercise and activity

MEDICATIONS

DRUG(S) OF CHOICE
• Nonsteroidal anti-inflammatory drugs (choose one of the following):
◊ Indomethacin (Indocin) 50 mg tid with food
◊ Naproxen (Naprosyn) 500 mg bid with food
◊ Sulindac (Clinoril) 150-200 mg bid with food
◊ Ibuprofen (Motrin) 600-800 mg tid-qid with food. Maximum of 3.2 gm daily.
◊ Other NSAID's at anti-inflammatory doses are effective

Contraindications:
• History of hypersensitivity to NSAID's or aspirin
• Active peptic ulcer disease or history of recurrent upper gastrointestinal lesions
• Use with extreme caution when impaired renal function exists. Monitor serum creatinine.

Precautions:
• May interfere with platelet aggregation and prolong bleeding time. This effect is much shorter lived than with aspirin.
• May cause fluid retention and worsen congestive heart failure
• Abnormal liver function tests may develop in approximately 15% of patients. Discontinue if findings worsen or systemic manifestations occur.
• Serious gastrointestinal bleeding can occur without warning. Follow patient carefully for internal bleeding. Administer misoprostol 200 µg qid in patients with a history of peptic ulcer disease.

Significant possible interactions:
• May blunt the antihypertensive effects of angiotensin converting enzyme inhibitors
• May prolong the prothrombin time in patients taking oral anticoagulants
• Avoid concomitant usage of aspirin
• May blunt the diuretic effect of furosemide and hydrochlorothiazide
• May increase plasma lithium level in patients taking lithium carbonate
• May increase methotrexate levels

ALTERNATIVE DRUGS
• Intra-articular instillation of methylprednisolone acetate, 20-80 mg for large joints; 10-40 mg for medium joints. Available in 20, 40 and 80 mg/mL ampules.
• Intravenous colchicine 2 mg IV; may repeat 0.5 mg IV q6h; not to exceed 4 mg in 24 hours (oral colchicine ineffective). Contraindication: significant bone marrow dysfunction, renal insufficiency (creatinine clearance < 10 mL/min), biliary obstruction, sepsis.

FOLLOWUP

PATIENT MONITORING Reevaluate patient for response to therapy 48-72 hours after treatment instituted. Reexamine 1 week later, then as needed.

PREVENTION/AVOIDANCE None known

POSSIBLE COMPLICATIONS
• Erosive destructive arthritis in pattern of joints not usually affected by degenerative joint disease
• Recurrences may occur and a destructive arthritis may complicate CPPD

EXPECTED COURSE/PROGNOSIS
• Acute attack usually resolves in 10 days. Prognosis for resolution of acute attack is excellent.
• Some patients experience progressive joint damage with functional limitation

MISCELLANEOUS

ASSOCIATED CONDITIONS Consider in patients with pseudogout - hyperparathyroidism, hemochromatosis, gout, hypophosphatasia, hypothyroidism, ochronosis, Wilson's disease, amyloidosis, hypomagnesemia

AGE-RELATED FACTORS
Pediatric: Not seen in children
Geriatric: Most cases are in patients over 60
Others: N/A

PREGNANCY N/A

SYNONYMS
• Calcium pyrophosphate deposition disease

ICD-9-CM 712.2 Chondrocalcinosis due to calcium phosphate crystals

SEE ALSO N/A

OTHER NOTES N/A

ABBREVIATIONS CPPD = calcium pyrophosphate deposition disease

REFERENCES
• Schumacher H: Crystal induced arthritis: an overview. Am J of Med 1996;100(2A):465-525
• Jasmine J, McGrath H: Gout or 'pseudogout'? How to differentiate crystal induced arthropathies. Rheumatic Clin of NA 1995;21:151-161
• Rosenthal A, Ryan L: Treatment of refractory crystal-associated arthritis. Rheumatic Dis Clin of NA 1995;21:151-161
Illustrations: N/A
Internet references: http://www.5mcc.com

Author(s)
Paul T. Cullen, MD

Pseudomembranous colitis

BASICS

DESCRIPTION Inflammatory bowel disorder associated with antibiotic use. May be mild diarrhea, or move through several stages to a severe colitis. Usual course - acute, relapsing.
System(s) affected: Gastrointestinal
Genetics: No known genetic factors
Incidence/Prevalence in USA:
• Epidemic or endemic in hospitals and nursing homes
  ◊ Nursing homes: 2-8%
  ◊ Hospitals: 7-15%
• Community: 6.7/100,000 patients treated with antibiotics
• Healthy adults: 5% colonized with C. difficile
• Hospitalized patients: 10-20% are colonized
• Neonates: 40% are colonized
Predominant age: 40-75 years
Predominant sex: Male = Female

SIGNS AND SYMPTOMS
• Diarrhea (classically watery, green, foul-smelling, bloody)
• Abdominal tenderness, pain, cramps
• Fever (up to 8% report fever only)
• Hypovolemia/dehydration
• Hypoalbuminemia

CAUSES Pathogenic Clostridium difficile toxins (A & B)

RISK FACTORS
• Antibiotic exposure (prior 6 weeks) particularly: clindamycin, lincomycin, ampicillin, cephalosporins. However, may also rarely occur with penicillins, erythromycin, sulfa-trimethoprim, chloramphenicol, tetracycline. In fact, nearly all antibiotics have been implicated.
• Cancer chemotherapy: fluorouracil, methotrexate, combination regimens.
• Recent surgery, especially bowel surgery
• Uremia or hemolytic-uremic syndrome
• Intestinal ischemia
• Shock
• Tube feedings
• Enemas
• GI stimulants
• Stool softener
• H2 blockers and antacids
• Immunocompromise (e.g., low CD4)
• Prolonged hospitalization
• Advancing age
• Hirschsprung's
• Inflammatory bowel disease

DIAGNOSIS

DIFFERENTIAL DIAGNOSIS
• Other enteric pathogens
• Nonspecific inflammatory bowel diseases

LABORATORY
• Fecal leukocytosis
• Leukocytosis
• ELISA for C. difficile toxin, positive
• Culture
Drugs that may alter lab results: N/A
Disorders that may alter lab results: A high percentage of infants are normal carriers of C. difficile and are positive for toxin B

PATHOLOGICAL FINDINGS
• Mild, nonspecific colitis without plaques
• Gross - yellow-white plaques on colonic and small intestinal mucosa
• Micro - pseudomembrane arising from point of superficial ulceration
• Micro - fibrin
• Micro - thick confluent pseudomembrane
• Polymorphonuclear cells

SPECIAL TESTS
• Sigmoidoscopy - may be normal in 10-33%
• Colonoscopy may show involvement of the rectum and sigmoid colon and occasionally only right colon and/or distal ileum. Some patients do not have pseudomembrane.

IMAGING
• Abdominal film - distorted haustral markings, colonic distention
• CT - thickened or edematous colonic wall with pericolonic inflammation
• Note: Avoid barium enemas

DIAGNOSTIC PROCEDURES
Endoscopic visualization and sample collection

TREATMENT

APPROPRIATE HEALTH CARE
• Outpatient for most patients
• Inpatient for severe or patients with co-morbidities

GENERAL MEASURES
• Fluid replacement
• Fluid plus electrolyte therapy
• Discontinue antimicrobial agent
• Successful in 25%

SURGICAL MEASURES Colectomy, not diversion, may be required

ACTIVITY Bedrest during acute phase

DIET Nothing by mouth during fulminant phase

PATIENT EDUCATION N/A

MEDICATIONS

DRUG(S) OF CHOICE
If drugs are not able to be taken orally, give via NG, enema, or direct instillation by colostomy/ileostomy or IV.
• Metronidazole (Flagyl) 250 mg po qid for 10 days
• Vancomycin 125 mg po qid (only for severe or resistant cases) for 10 days
• Teicoplanin 50 mg po qid for 3 days then 100 mg bid for 4 days
Contraindications: Refer to manufacturer's literature
Precautions: Avoid antiperistaltic drugs such as diphenoxylate, atropine, loperamide to reduce risk of toxic megacolon
Significant possible interactions: Alcohol and metronidazole. Refer to manufacturer's literature.

ALTERNATIVE DRUGS
• Bacitracin 500 mg qid
• For flora repletion: Lactobacilli capsules or saccharomyces bouldardii enema of mixed colonies
• For chronic recurrences, adjunct therapy with full colon irrigation with Golytely

FOLLOWUP

PATIENT MONITORING
Careful monitoring through fulminant phase

PREVENTION/AVOIDANCE
• Judicious use of antimicrobial agents
• Keep courses of antibiotics as brief as possible
• Avoidance of recurrences
  ◊ Prolonged therapy
  ◊ Lactobacillus
  ◊ Repletion of other organisms which compete with C. Difficile
  ◊ In children, some success with IV gamma globulin

POSSIBLE COMPLICATIONS
• Reactive arthritis; Reiter's syndrome
• Hypoalbuminemia
• Ascites
• Dehydration, hypovolemia, shock
• Bowel perforation
• Toxic megacolon
• Death

EXPECTED COURSE/PROGNOSIS
• If treated, usual improvement in 3 days and virtually all patients recover
• Relapses do occur
• Untreated, 10-30% mortality
• In severely ill, colectomy sometimes required
• Significant morbidity and mortality in critical ill patients
• Poor prognostic factors: hypoalbuminemia, rapid fall in albumin, over 3 antibiotics, persistent C. difficile toxin after 7 days of treatment

MISCELLANEOUS

ASSOCIATED CONDITIONS
• Surgery
• Spinal fracture
• Intestinal obstruction
• Colon cancer

AGE-RELATED FACTORS
Pediatric:
• Unusual in children, but does occur
• Most infants are carriers; may become invasive in children with malignancy or Hirschsprung's disease
Geriatric: The elderly have a higher mortality rate from pseudomembranous colitis
Others: N/A

PREGNANCY
Serious complication if it occurs during pregnancy

SYNONYMS
• Antibiotic associated colitis
• Pseudomembranous enterocolitis

ICD-9-CM
008.45 Intestinal infection, Clostridium difficile

SEE ALSO N/A

OTHER NOTES N/A

ABBREVIATIONS N/A

REFERENCES
• Fekety R, Akshay S: Diagnosis and treatment of Clostridium difficile. JAMA 1993;269:71-75
• Leung D, et al: Treatment with intravenously administered gamma globulin of chronic relapsing colitis induced by Clostridium difficile toxin. Jour of Pediatr 1991;118:633-7
• Bartlett JG: Antibiotic-associated diarrhea. Clinical Infect Dis 1992;15:573-81
• Fualman S, et al: Clostridial difficile invasion & toxin circulation in fatal pediatric pseudomembranous colitis. Amer J Clin Pathol 1990;94:410-6
• McFarland L, Surawicz C, Stamm W: Risk factors for C. difficile carriage and C. difficile associated diarrhea in a cohort of hospitalized patients. J of Infect Dis 1990;162:678-84
• Ramaswamy R, et al: Prognostic criteria in Clostridium difficile colitis. Amer J Gastro 1996;91(3):460-4
• Hirschorn LR, et al: Epidemiology of community-acquired Clostridium difficile-associated diarrhea. J Infec Dis 1994;169:127-33
• Chatila W, Constantine M: Clostridium difficle causing sepsis and an acute abdomen in critically ill patients. Crit Care Med 1995;23(6):1146-1150
• Walker KJ, et al: Clostridium difficile colonization in residents in long-term care facilities: prevalence and risk factors. J Amer Geriatric Soc 41(9):940-6
• Simor AE, et al: Infection due to Clostridium difficile among elderly residents of a long term care facility. Clin Infec Dis 1993;17(4):672-8
• Reinke C, Messik CR: Update on Clostridium-difficile-induced colitis, Part 2. Amer J Hosp Pharm 1994;51(15):1892-901
• Tumbarello M, et al: Clostridium difficile-associated diarrhoea in patients with human immunodeficiency virus infection: a case control study. European J Gastro & Hepatol 1995;7(3):259-63
• Wenisch C, et al: Comparison of vancomycin, teicoplanin, metronidazole and fusidic acid for the treatment of Clostridium difficle associated diarrhea. Clin Infec Dis 1996;5:813-818
• Grundfest, et al: Clostridium difficile colitis in the critically ill. Dis of Colon Rectum 1996;6:619-623
• Liacouras CA, Piecol DA: Whole bowel irrigation as an adjunct to the treatment of chronic relapsing Clostridium difficle colitis. J Clin Gastroenterology 1996;22(3):186-189
Illustrations: N/A
Internet references: http://www.5mcc.com

Author(s)
Elizabeth I McCord, MD, MS

Psittacosis

BASICS

DESCRIPTION Psittacosis is the clinical manifestation of a respiratory infection with the bacteria *Chlamydia psittaci*. The infection is virtually always contracted from an infected bird. Human to human transmission is rare.
• Pneumonia, bronchitis and fever of unknown origin (FUO) are most common diagnoses
• Can range from sub-clinical respiratory infection to severe systemic infection. Severity of illness may vary with strain of C. psittaci.
System(s) affected: Pulmonary
Genetics: No known genetic predisposition
Incidence/Prevalence in USA:
• .04-.08/100,000. 100-200 cases/year reported to Centers for Disease Control. True incidence probably greater.
• Outbreaks may occur, usually associated with occupational exposure to infected turkeys or ducks
Predominant age: Adults
Predominant sex: Male = Female

SIGNS AND SYMPTOMS
• Onset usually acute but may be insidious
• Fever (often > 39°C)
• Chills
• Cough (may develop later, usually non-productive)
• Headache (may be severe)
• Malaise
• Anorexia
• Myalgias
• Confusion
• Vomiting and/or diarrhea
• Abdominal pain
• Pleuritic chest pain
• Hemoptysis
• Dyspnea without wheezing
• Arthralgias
• Sore throat
• Hoarseness
• Epistaxis
• Photophobia
• Tachycardia
• Retractions
• Flaring
• Cyanosis
• Crepitations more common than signs of consolidation
• Auscultation may be normal even with pneumonia
• Relative bradycardia
• Tender hepatomegaly and splenomegaly
• Horder's spots (faint, reddish brown, blanching rash)
• Petechiae

CAUSES Infection with Chlamydia psittaci

RISK FACTORS Exposure to infected bird(s), usually a pet pigeon or parakeet, or occupational exposure at a turkey or duck processing plant. Infected birds may appear healthy. Incubation period is 5-15 days. Human-to-human transmission possible, but rare.

DIAGNOSIS

DIFFERENTIAL DIAGNOSIS
• Consider other common bacterial respiratory pathogens including
  ◊ Streptococcus pneumoniae
  ◊ Hemophilus influenzae
  ◊ Klebsiella pneumoniae
  ◊ Chlamydia pneumoniae
  ◊ Mycoplasma pneumoniae
  ◊ Legionella species
• Typhoid fever, Q fever, Brucellosis

LABORATORY
• Leukocyte count often normal or low
• Erythrocyte sedimentation rate (ESR) usually elevated
• Sputum usually negative by gram stain and routine culture
• Proteinuria possible during febrile period
• Liver enzymes may be elevated
• Increased IgG, IgM, IgA
• Leukocytes with left shift
• Hypoxemia
• Hypocapnia
• Eosinophilia
Drugs that may alter lab results:
Serologic response may be blunted by early treatment with tetracycline
Disorders that may alter lab results: N/A

PATHOLOGICAL FINDINGS
• Alveolar phagocyte and lymphocyte infiltrate
• Granuloma formation
• Bronchial wall thickening
• Type III and IV immune complex deposition
• Diffuse miliary nodules

SPECIAL TESTS
• Culture requires special facilities and is rarely done
• Sera for serology should be collected 2 to 3 weeks apart (3-4 weeks for micro-immunofluorescence, and a second convalescent sera at 6-8 weeks if the pattern is uninterpretable)
• Complement fixation (CF) test most common serologic test for psittacosis, but is also positive with C. pneumoniae (a much more common respiratory pathogen) and C. trachomatis infections
• A fourfold rise in CF titer is diagnostic of an acute infection with Chlamydia
• A single or stable CF titer of > 1:64 suggests a recent infection
• The species specific micro-immunofluorescence test for C. psittaci is preferred, but not as widely available as the CF test

IMAGING
• Chest radiograph often shows patchy alveolar infiltrates of interstitial pneumonitis and small nodular densities
• Lobar consolidation also common
• Hilar adenopathy
• Pleural effusion possible but usually scanty
• Radiographic abnormalities may persist for several months after successful treatment

DIAGNOSTIC PROCEDURES N/A

TREATMENT

APPROPRIATE HEALTH CARE
• Outpatient
• Patients with dyspnea, hypoxia, confusion or other signs or severe disease should be hospitalized

GENERAL MEASURES
• History of avian exposure (particularly to a sick bird) is key to making early diagnosis
• Treatment depends primarily on severity of respiratory symptoms. Severely ill patients may require oxygen, intravenous fluids and antibiotics.
• While human to human transmission is rare, sputum and respiratory secretion precautions should be observed

SURGICAL MEASURES N/A

ACTIVITY Based on disease severity. No disease-specific restrictions.

DIET No special diet

PATIENT EDUCATION American Lung Association, 1740 Broadway, New York, NY 10019, (800)586-4872

MEDICATIONS

DRUG(S) OF CHOICE
• Doxycycline (Vibramycin) 100 mg po bid for 14-21 days or 100 mg IV q12h
• Tetracycline 500 mg po qid for 14-21 days. If severely ill, tetracycline 5-7.5 mg/kg q12h IV.
• Clarithromycin (Biaxin) 500 mg q12h (length of treatment not established for psittacosis)
Contraindications: History of allergic reaction to the medication
Precautions: Tetracycline and doxycycline - avoid dairy products and sun exposure. Reduce dosage in renal failure. Avoid using in pregnancy or in children less than 8 years old (causes permanent discoloration of teeth).
Significant possible interactions: Refer to manufacturer's profile of each drug

ALTERNATIVE DRUGS
• Erythromycin also has in vitro activity and can be used at doses of 500 mg po qid for 14 to 21 days
• Azithromycin (Zithromax) 500 mg on first day; then 250 mg qd (length of treatment not established for psittacosis)
• Rifampin (Rifadin, Rimactane) has in vitro activity and has been used in doses of 600 to 1200 mg po per day with erythromycin to treat endocarditis due to C. psittaci
• Beta-lactam (penicillin based) antibiotics not effective

FOLLOWUP

PATIENT MONITORING
Determined by severity of illness in the acute period. No disease-specific monitoring.

PREVENTION/AVOIDANCE
• Report to local health department
• Identify source of the infection if possible
• Public health surveillance of poultry flocks and pet shops
• Prophylactic antibiotic treatment with doxycycline (100 mg po qd for 10 days) has been advocated for people with known exposure

POSSIBLE COMPLICATIONS
• Meningitis and encephalitis
• Endocarditis, pericarditis and myocarditis
• Renal failure
• Erythema nodosum
• Sinusitis
• Respiratory failure
• Hepatitis
• Reactive arthritis (rare)
• Disseminated intravascular coagulation (rare)
• Valvular heart disease (rare)
• Spontaneous abortion (rare)
• Thyroiditis (rare)
• Pancreatitis (rare)
• Transverse myelitis (rare)

EXPECTED COURSE/PROGNOSIS
• Mortality rate less than 1% with appropriate treatment
• Patients usually respond within 24 to 48 hours following initiation of appropriate antibiotic therapy
• Full recovery may take weeks to months
• Relapse may occur necessitating second course of antibiotics
• Chest radiograph may not return to normal for up to 4 months

MISCELLANEOUS

ASSOCIATED CONDITIONS
None known

AGE-RELATED FACTORS
Pediatric: Uncommon in pediatric age group
Geriatric: Mortality rate may be higher in elderly or debilitated patients
Others: None

PREGNANCY
Spontaneous abortion has been reported with infection with some C. psittaci strains, primarily acquired from contact with sheep

SYNONYMS
• Ornithosis
• Bird breeder's disease
• Bird fancier's lung

ICD-9-CM
073.0-073.9 Ornithosis
495.8 Other specified allergic alveolitis and pneumonitis

SEE ALSO
• Chlamydia pneumoniae
• Q fever

OTHER NOTES
• Incubation period ranges from 5 to 40 days; usually 7 to 15 days
• No persistent immunity to reinfection

ABBREVIATIONS
N/A

REFERENCES
• Crosse BA: Psittacosis: a clinical review. J Infect 1990l;21:251-259
• Gregory DW, Schaffner W: Psittacosis. Sem Resp Infect 1997;12:7-11
• Schlossberg D: Chlamydia psittaci (psittacosis). In: Mandel Gl, Bennett JE, Dolin R (eds): Principles and Practices of Infectious Disease. 4th ed. New York, Churchill Livingstone, 1995:1693-1696
Illustrations: N/A
Internet references: http://www.5mcc.com

Author(s)
David H. Thom, MD, PhD

Psoriasis

BASICS

DESCRIPTION Genetically determined (sporadic) common, chronic, epidermal proliferative disease. Clinically characterized by erythematous, dry scaling patches, recurring remissions and exacerbations. Flares may be related to systemic and environmental factors. Usual course - acute, chronic; unpredictable.
• Clinical forms:
◊ Discoid or plaque psoriasis - most common, patches appear on scalp, trunk and limbs, nails may be pitted and/or thickened
◊ Guttate psoriasis - occurs most frequently in children, numerous small papules over wide area of skin, but greatest on the trunk
◊ Pustular psoriasis - small pustules over the body or confined to one area (i.e., palms and soles) or arranged in annular patterns (especially children)
◊ Inverse, flexural psoriasis - affects the flexural areas, lesions are moist and without scales (common in older people)
◊ Erythroderma (exfoliative psoriasis or red man syndrome) - patients skin turns red, may result from a flare of pre-existing dermatosis
◊ Ostraceous - grossly hyperkeratotic
System(s) affected: Skin/Exocrine
Genetics:
• Genetic predisposition (probably polygenic)
• Type I psoriasis - young, strong family history = more aggressive disease
• Type 2 psoriasis - older, no family history = more stable disease
• Higher incidence in Caucasians and atopic families
• Increased incidence of human leukocyte antigens (HLA antigens)
Incidence/Prevalence in USA: 1000-2000 cases/100,000 people in the U.S.
Predominant age: Two peaks of onset, age 16-22 and age 57-60; can develop in infants
Predominant sex: Male = Female

SIGNS AND SYMPTOMS
• Arthritis
• Pruritus
• Silvery scales on red plaques
• Knee-elbow-scalp distribution
• Stippled nails and pitting
• Positive Auspitz sign (underlying pinpoints of bleeding following scraping)
• Koebner's phenomenon (psoriatic response in previously unaffected area 1-2 weeks after skin injury)

CAUSES Possible genetic error in mitotic control. Activation of lymphocytes (antigen? autoimmune?). Epidermal cell cycle 10 times shorter than normal, leading to epidermal hyperproliferation.

RISK FACTORS
• Local trauma; local irritation
• Infection (streptococcal pharyngitis can stimulate acute guttate psoriasis, HIV)
• Endocrine changes
• Stress (physical and emotional)
• Sudden withdrawal of systemic and/or potent topical steroids
• Alcohol use
• Obesity

DIAGNOSIS

DIFFERENTIAL DIAGNOSIS
• Scalp - seborrheic dermatitis
• Body folds - intertrigo or candidiasis
• Diaper dermatitis
• Nails - onychomycosis
• Trunk - pityriasis rosea, pityriasis rubra pilaris, tinea corporis
• Squamous cell carcinoma
• Secondary and tertiary syphilis
• Cutaneous lupus erythematosus
• Eczema (nummular)
• Lichen planus
• Localized scratch dermatitis (lichen simplex chronicus)
• Mycosis fungoides
• Reiter's disease
• Subcorneal pustulosis
• Pustular eruptions

LABORATORY
• Negative rheumatoid factor
• Latex fixation test
• Leukocytosis and increased sedimentation rate often seen, especially in pustular psoriasis
• Fungal studies - may show a superimposed infection
• Uric acid increases in 10-20%
• In severe cases, anemia, B12, folate and iron deficiency can be present
Drugs that may alter lab results: N/A
Disorders that may alter lab results: N/A

PATHOLOGICAL FINDINGS
• Parakeratosis (focal), especially with neutrophils
• Hyperkeratosis
• Hypogranulosis
• Epidermal hyperplasia
• Elongation and thickening of rete ridges
• Thin epidermis above dermal papillae
• Spongiform pustule of Kogoj
• Munro's microabscess
• Abnormal mitoses
• Dilated tortuous capillary loops
• "Squirting" papillae

SPECIAL TESTS Biopsy

IMAGING N/A

DIAGNOSTIC PROCEDURES Usually diagnosis accomplished by inspection, occasionally biopsy required

TREATMENT

APPROPRIATE HEALTH CARE
• Outpatient usually
• May require inpatient for severe or resistant cases. Emergency: Severe and unstable forms like acute pustular psoriasis (Von Zumbusch's) or acute erythroderma.

GENERAL MEASURES
• Solar radiation
• Mild disease - ultraviolet radiation (UVA, UVB)
• Medication to soften scale, followed by soft brush while bathing
• Oatmeal baths for itching
• Tar shampoos
• Avoid excessive sun exposure
• Desert climates provide a favorable effect for some patients
• Wet dressings may help relieve pruritus
• For extensive, recalcitrant psoriasis, a referral to a specialist in psoriatic therapy is suggested

SURGICAL MEASURES N/A

ACTIVITY No restrictions

DIET No special diet

PATIENT EDUCATION
• Provide patient reassurance and anxiety relief to the extent possible
• Assurance to patient and family the condition is non-contagious
• For a listing of sources for patient education materials favorably reviewed on this topic, physicians may contact: American Academy of Family Physicians Foundation, 11400 Tomahawk Creek Parkway, Leawood, KS, 66211, (800)274-2237, ext. 4406
• National Psoriasis Foundation, Suite 300, 6600 S.W. 92nd Avenue, Portland, OR 97223, (503)244-7404; toll free (800)723-9166; fax (503)245-0626; E-mail 76135.2746@comserve.com

MEDICATIONS

DRUG(S) OF CHOICE
• Mild to moderate disease:
◊ Emollients: to start treatment; bid soft yellow paraffin or aqueous cream; petrolatum or aquaphor cream greasier and more effective
◊ Topical, **low potency** corticosteroids on delicate skin (eg, face, genitals or flexures) to prevent cutaneous atrophy. Alclometasone dipropionate, triamcinolone acetonide 0.25%, hydrocortisone 2.5%
◊ Topical, **medium potency** corticosteroids (fluticasone propionate, triamcinolone acetonide 0.1%, hydrocortisone valerate, mometasone furoate usually for lesions on the torso) tid-qid (overnight occlusion with plastic wrap will hasten resolution). Switching products prevents tachyphylaxis. Non-fluorinated is less atrophigenic.
◊ Topical, **strong potency** corticosteroids - betamethasone dipropionate halcinonide, fluocinonide, desoximetasone
◊ Topical, **super potency** corticosteroids - augmented betamethasone dipropionate, diflorasone diacetate, clobetasol propionate, halobetasol propionate. Limit use to 2 weels if possible, avoid occlusive dressings. Taper to prevent rebound. Usually reserved for recalcitrant plaques or lesions on palms or soles of feet.

◊ Intralesional corticosteroid: 2-5 mg/mL triamcinolone acetonide

◊ Coal tar (Estar, PsoriGel) may be beneficial when alternated with topical steroids. Apply and air dry for 15 minutes before going to bed or apply in AM for 15 minutes, then shower. Tar bath preparations for widespread involvement.

◊ Keratolytic agents: salicylic acid 6% gel (or 2-10% salicylate acid ointment) bid several weeks. Even 20% for 2 weeks, except in children. alpha hydroxy acid, glycolic acid or lactic acid. Decreased scale allows greater effectiveness of other topical medications. Alternate keratolytics with other topicals.

◊ Corticosteroid solutions and tar shampoos - scalp lesions

◊ Ultraviolet lamps and sun light effective. May be best treatment option during pregnancy or in young children.

◊ UVB + emollients in erythremogenic dose in fair-skinned patients - less toxic than PUVA

◊ Anthralin ointment 1% applied for 10 minutes, then washed off, useful adjunctive treatment. Use prior to ultraviolet light (UVA, UVB). Indicated for quiescent or chronic psoriasis, contraindicated in acute or actively inflamed psoriatic eruptions. Start with 0.1% and gradually increase to 3.5%. Irritates unaffected skin, protect areas with zinc oxide or petrolatum. Avoid face, eyes, mucous membranes.

• Severe disease:

◊ Triamcinolone, intralesional - mix with procaine or normal saline for concentrate of 4 mg/mL. Administer with syringe or dermajet. Effective in treating solitary resistant plaques and psoriasis involving the nails.

◊ Vitamin D analogs (calcipotriene ointment 0.005% for moderate plaque psoriasis). Results may not be maximal for 2 months. Too irritating for facial lesions. Watch for hypercalcemia. Weekly cumulative dose < 100-120 gram. Associated with little or no tachyphylaxis.

◊ Etretinate (Tegison) - especially pustular and erythrodermic psoriasis disease not responsive to standard treatments. Remains in body up to 2 years after treatment. Extremely fetotoxic. Do not use if pregnant or could become pregnant within 2 years of treatment. Safe for use on face.

◊ Tazarotene (Tazorac) - for psoriasis involving up to 20% body surface area. Avoid face and groin due to irritation. Daily or every other day treatment. Retinoid induced dermatitis major side effect.

◊ Oral corticosteroids only for severe or life-threatening disease (risk of rebound)

◊ Isotretinoin: may work on some patients

◊ PUVA (psoralen plus ultraviolet light) - very effective, but causes skin-aging, cataracts and increases risk of skin cancers

◊ Goeckerman's regimen - tar/UV light

◊ Methotrexate - single weekly dose (up to 25 mg) or 2.5-5 mg q12h for 3-4 days per week, but precautions necessary. Hydroxyurea for methotrexate failure. Azathioprine and intralesional cyclosporine, not common.

◊ Cyclosporine or tacrolimus: only for recalcitrant psoriasis (possible nephrotoxicity)

Contraindications: Refer to manufacturer's literature

Precautions: Refer to manufacturer's literature

Significant possible interactions: Refer to manufacturer's literature

ALTERNATIVE DRUGS

• Cyclosporin: In recalcitrant disease for short-term use only, perhaps alternating with other agents

FOLLOWUP

PATIENT MONITORING

• Continuous supportive care
• Medications used in treatment require close followup. Certain lab studies may be necessary. Long-term use of topicals is not recommended.
• With methotrexate therapy check CBC, SGOT, albumin every month. Some recommend liver biopsy before treating or 3 months after treatment started and then regularly (usually every 2 years) based on a cumulative methotrexate dose of 1.5 grams.

PREVENTION/AVOIDANCE

• Avoid alcoholic beverages
• Avoid irritating drugs
• Avoid stimulating drugs (lithium, ACE inhibitors, beta-adrenergic blockers, tetracycline, NSAID's, amiodarone, morphine, procaine, potassium iodide, salicylates, sulfapyridine, sulfonamides and penicillin. Pustular flares may occur with steroids).
• Avoid antimalarial medications (aminoquinolone compounds)

POSSIBLE COMPLICATIONS

• Pustular psoriasis
• Exfoliative erythrodermatitis
• Rebound of the psoriatic process after corticosteroids are discontinued
• Topical corticosteroids may cause thinning of skin, striae, masking local infection, hypopigmentation and tachyphylaxis (reduce tachyphylaxis by a corticosteroid-free interval or lower potency once improved)
• Hypercalcemia with excessive calcipotriene
• Salicylism possible in children with high dose topical salicylic acid.

EXPECTED COURSE/PROGNOSIS

• Usually benign
• Life-threatening forms do occur
• May be refractory to treatment

MISCELLANEOUS

ASSOCIATED CONDITIONS

• Extensive erythrodermic psoriasis may accompany AIDS
• Arthritis
• Psoriatic arthritis
• Myopathy
• Enteropathy
• Spondylitic heart disease
• Acute anterior uveitis

AGE-RELATED FACTORS

Pediatric:
• Onset common <10, rarely <3
• Disease may be atypical in its course

Geriatric:
• About 3% of psoriasis patients acquire the disease after age 65
• Detailed drug history important, since many drugs (e.g., beta-blockers) can exacerbate psoriasis
• If using cytotoxic medications for treatment of psoriasis, closely follow hepatic and renal functions, and creatinine clearance
• Elderly patients may have difficulty with application of topicals over all affected body parts

Others: N/A

PREGNANCY Unpredictable effect on disease. Avoid tars, topical corticosteroids, calcipotriene, and systemic therapies. Etretinate is fetotoxic.

SYNONYMS N/A

ICD-9-CM

696.1 Other psoriasis
696.2 Parapsoriasis

SEE ALSO N/A

OTHER NOTES N/A

ABBREVIATIONS N/A

REFERENCES

• Burrall B, Dijkstra J, Lowe N, Maibach H: Psoriasis therapies: Old, new and borrowed. Patient Care 1995;10:38-65
• Greaves MW, Weinstein GD: Treatment of psoriasis. NEJM 1995;332(9):581-588
• Habif T: Clinical Dermatology. 3rd Ed. St. Louis, CV Mosby, 1996
• Abel E: Diagnosis of drug induced psoriasis. Seminars in Dermatology 1992;11(4)
• Jegsothy B, et al: Tacrolimus (FK 506): A new therapeutic agent for severe recalcitrant psoriasis. Arc Dermatol 1992;128
• Ho C, Zioty D: Immunosuppressive Agents in Dermatology. Dermatology Clinics 1993;11(1)
• Moschella S, et al, eds: Dermatology. 3rd Ed. Philadelphia, W.B. Saunders Co., 1992
• Federman DG, Froelich CW: Topical psoriasis therapy. Am Fam Phys 1999;59(4):957-962
Illustrations: 15 available on CD-ROM
Internet references: http://www.5mcc.com

Author(s)
Paul J. Jaster, MD

Puerperal infection

BASICS

DESCRIPTION
Bacterial infection of the genital tract following delivery. Endometritis (infection of the endometrium, myometrium and parametrial tissues) is the most common infection. Less common are vaginal and cervical infections, perineal cellulitis, pelvic cellulitis, septic pelvic vein thrombophlebitis and parametrial phlegmon.

System(s) affected: Reproductive

Genetics: N/A

Incidence/Prevalence in USA:
- Vaginal deliveries - <3%
- Cesarean sections - 15 - 95%
- Accounts for 7% of maternal death
- Fourth leading cause of maternal mortality

Predominant age: N/A

Predominant sex: Female only

SIGNS AND SYMPTOMS
- Oral temperature >38.7°C (101.6°F) in first 24 hours post-partum or
- Oral temperature >38°C (100.4°F) in two of first 10 days post-partum (excluding first 24 hours)
- Uterine tenderness on exam
- Other localized tenderness on exam
- Ileus
- Tachycardia
- Chills, malaise, headache, anorexia
- Abdominal or localized pain
- Purulent or malodorous lochia
- Note: Group A or Group B strep bacteremia may have no localizing signs

CAUSES
- The risk of endometritis increases 5-30 fold following Cesarean delivery
- Endometritis commonly follows chorioamnionitis
- Other infections follow trauma to the perineum, vagina, cervix and uterus
- Infection is nearly always polymicrobial and involves organisms that have ascended from the lower genital tract:
  ◊ Aerobic isolates in 70% - *S. faecalis, S. agalatiae, S. viridans, Staphylococcus aureus, E. coli, Klebsiella sp., Proteus sp., Gardnerella vaginalis*
  ◊ Anaerobic isolates in 80% - *Peptococcus sp., Peptostreptococcus sp., Clostridium sp., Bacteroides bivius, B. fragilis, Fusobacterium sp.*
  ◊ Other - genital mycoplasmas - role in endometritis is unclear
  ◊ *Chlamydia trachomatis* - responsible for some late (7-10 days) post-partum endometritis
  ◊ Range of number of isolates is 1-8

RISK FACTORS
- Cesarean section
- Pre-existing chorioamnionitis
- Multiple vaginal examinations
- Indigent status
- Bacterial vaginosis or group B strep colonization of genital tract
- Prolonged rupture of membranes, prolonged labor and the use of internal fetal monitoring have been shown to be significant factors in univariate but not multivariate analysis

DIAGNOSIS

DIFFERENTIAL DIAGNOSIS
- Fever from other sources
  ◊ Urinary tract infection
  ◊ Viral syndrome
  ◊ Dehydration
  ◊ Pneumonia
  ◊ Wound infection
  ◊ Thrombophlebitis
  ◊ Thyroid storm

LABORATORY
- CBC - interpret with care as physiologic leukocytosis may be as high as 20,000
- Blood cultures - if sepsis is suspected
- Amniotic fluid gram stain - usually polymicrobial
- Uterine tissue cultures - difficult to obtain without contamination
- Genital tract cultures and rapid test for group B strep - usually done when patient is in labor
- Note: Diagnosis is usually made clinically

Drugs that may alter lab results: N/A

Disorders that may alter lab results: N/A

PATHOLOGICAL FINDINGS
- Microscopic sections of uterine lining show superficial layer of infected necrotic tissue
- Thrombosis of any of the pelvic veins including the vena cava
- Phlegmon on leaves of the broad ligament
- Abscess

SPECIAL TESTS
N/A

IMAGING
- If patient is not responsive to antibiotics
  ◊ CT or MRI for pelvic thrombophlebitis
  ◊ U/S, CT or MRI for abscess, pelvic masses or deep-seated wound infections

DIAGNOSTIC PROCEDURES
Paracentesis or culdocentesis with culture - rarely necessary

TREATMENT

APPROPRIATE HEALTH CARE
- Inpatient for severe infection
- Low grade endometritis may respond to outpatient treatment with oral antibiotics

GENERAL MEASURES
- IV antibiotics and close observation for severe infections
- Open and drain infected wounds
- Normalize fluid status
- Note: Amnioinfusion during labor may decrease infections when membranes have been ruptured for more than 6 hours.

SURGICAL MEASURES
- Curettage of retained products of conception
- Surgery to establish drainage of abscess
- Surgery to decompress the bowel
- Surgical drainage of a phlegmon is not advised unless suppurative

ACTIVITY
As tolerated

DIET
As tolerated although may be limited by ileus.

PATIENT EDUCATION
Call doctor if fever >38°C (100.4°F) post-partum or other symptoms of infection (see Signs and Symptoms)

MEDICATIONS

DRUG(S) OF CHOICE
• Cefoxitin 2 gms IV q6hrs. Add ampicillin if clinical failure after 48 hours.
• Cefotetan 2 IV q8hrs. Add ampicillin if clinical failure after 48 hours.
• Piperacillin 4 gms IV q6hrs
• Ampicillin-sulbactam (Unasyn) 2/1 gm IV q6hr
• Note: Base therapy on cultures, sensitivities, and clinical response

Contraindications:
• Drug allergy
• Renal failure (aminoglycosides)
• Avoid chloramphenicol, sulfa, tetracyclines, fluoroquinolones before delivery and if breast-feeding.

Precautions:
• Chloramphenicol rarely causes bone marrow suppression
• Clindamycin and other antibiotics occasionally cause pseudomembranous colitis

Significant possible interactions: Refer to manufacturer's literature

ALTERNATIVE DRUGS
• Clindamycin 600-900 mg IV q8hr plus gentamicin 2 mg/kg IV qd (traditional 'gold standard' but may cause nephrotoxicity, ototoxicity, pseudomembranous colitis, diarrhea (in up to 6%) and may require gentamicin peak and trough levels)
• Metronidazole 7.5 mg/kg IV q6hr plus gentamicin 2 mg/kg IV qd (see above)
• Amoxicillin-clavulanate (Augmentin) 500 mg po tid for mild infections as outpatient
• Note: Heparin may be indicated for septic pelvic vein thrombophlebitis - requires 10 days at full anticoagulation

FOLLOWUP

PATIENT MONITORING
• Individualize according to severity
• IV antibiotics can be stopped when afebrile for 24 - 48 hours
• Oral antibiotics on discharge are not necessary except in cases of bacteremia

PREVENTION/AVOIDANCE
• Treat chorioamnionitis during labor
• Treat prophylactically with cephazolin for high risk C/S deliveries after the cord is clamped
• Avoid unnecessary vaginal exams
• Avoid retained placental fragments or membranes

POSSIBLE COMPLICATIONS
• Resistant organisms
• Pelvic abscess
• Septic pelvic vein thrombosis
• Septic shock
• Death

EXPECTED COURSE/PROGNOSIS
• With supportive therapy and appropriate antibiotics most patients improve within a few days
• If no improvement on antibiotics, consider retained placental fragments or membranes, abscess, would infection, hematoma, abscess, cellulitis, phlegmon or septic pelvic vein thrombosis.

MISCELLANEOUS

ASSOCIATED CONDITIONS
• Chorioamnionitis

AGE-RELATED FACTORS
Pediatric: N/A
Geriatric: N/A
Others: N/A

PREGNANCY   A complication of pregnancy

SYNONYMS
• Endometritis
• Endoparametritis
• Endomyometritis
• Myometritis
• Endomyoparametritis
• Metritis
• Metritis with pelvic cellulitis

ICD-9-CM
670 Major puerperal infection

SEE ALSO   N/A

OTHER NOTES   N/A

ABBREVIATIONS   N/A

REFERENCES
• Hamadeh G, et al: Postpartum Fever. Amer Fam Phys 1995; 52(2):531-538
• Casey BM, Cox SM: Chorioamnionitis and Endometritis. Infect Dis Clin of NA 1997;11(1):203-222
• Creasy RK, Resnick R: Maternal-Fetal Medicine. 4th Ed. Philadelphia, WB Saunders Co., 1999
Illustrations: N/A
Internet references: http://www.5mcc.com

Author(s)
Carol Cordy, MD
Robert H. Scott, MD

Pulmonary edema

BASICS

DESCRIPTION Pulmonary interstitial and/or alveolar fluid accumulation that results when the forces moving fluid out of the pulmonary capillary exceed the forces restraining that fluid
System(s) affected: Cardiovascular, Pulmonary
Genetics: Multifactorial
Incidence/Prevalence in USA:
Approximately 150,000 persons per year in U.S. affected with non-cardiogenic pulmonary edema
Predominant age: Middle age and elderly
Predominant sex: Male = Female

SIGNS AND SYMPTOMS
• Respiratory
  ◊ Shortness of breath
  ◊ Dyspnea with exertion
  ◊ Orthopnea, paroxysmal nocturnal dyspnea
  ◊ Cough, often accompanied by pink or blood-tinged and frothy sputum
  ◊ Wheezing, rhonchi, gurgles
  ◊ Moist, crepitant rales noted initially at bases and progressing to apices
  ◊ Breathlessness, air hunger
  ◊ Noisy respirations
  ◊ Tachypnea
  ◊ Dilated alae nasi
  ◊ Inspiratory retraction of the intercostal spaces and/or supraventricular fossae
  ◊ Cheyne-Stokes respirations
• Cardiovascular
  ◊ Tachycardia
  ◊ Elevated jugular venous pulse
  ◊ Increased P2
  ◊ S3
  ◊ S4
  ◊ Nocturnal angina
  ◊ Pulsus alternans or presence of valvular heart disease
• General
  ◊ Weakness, fatigue
  ◊ Other symptoms depending on etiology
  ◊ Anxiety
  ◊ Diaphoretic, cold, ashen, or cyanotic skin
  ◊ Lower extremity edema

CAUSES
• Cardiogenic
  ◊ Left heart failure
  ◊ Ischemic heart disease
  ◊ Acute myocardial infarction
  ◊ Aortic and mitral valvular disease
  ◊ Hypertensive heart disease
  ◊ Cardiomyopathy
  ◊ Volume overload
  ◊ Arrhythmias
  ◊ Endocarditis
  ◊ Myocarditis
  ◊ Congenital heart disease
  ◊ Acute rheumatic fever and rheumatic heart disease
  ◊ Septal defects
  ◊ Cardiac tamponade
  ◊ High cardiac output states (e.g., thyrotoxicosis, beriberi)

• Noncardiogenic
  ◊ Shock
  ◊ Multiple trauma
  ◊ Infection/sepsis (especially pneumonia)
  ◊ Liquid aspiration (e.g., drowning, gastric contents)
  ◊ Inhaled toxic gases
  ◊ Pulmonary lymphatic obstruction
  ◊ Drug overdose (especially narcotics)
  ◊ High-altitude illness
  ◊ Pancreatitis
  ◊ Embolism (thrombus, fat, air, amniotic fluid)
  ◊ Neurogenic
  ◊ Hematologic and immunologic disorders
  ◊ Disorders associated with high negative pleural pressure
  ◊ Radiation pneumonitis
  ◊ Disseminated intravascular coagulation
  ◊ Eclampsia
  ◊ Decreased plasma oncotic pressure (e.g., hypoalbuminemia)
  ◊ Postcardioversion, postanesthesia, postcardiopulmonary bypass
  ◊ Oxygen toxicity
  ◊ ARDS
  ◊ Renal failure

RISK FACTORS Dependent on etiology

DIAGNOSIS

DIFFERENTIAL DIAGNOSIS
Important to distinguish between cardiogenic and non-cardiogenic pulmonary edema
• Pneumonia
• Asthma
• COPD exacerbation
• Pulmonary embolism
• Hyperventilation syndrome

LABORATORY
• None specific for pulmonary edema; laboratory abnormalities (e.g., creatine kinase [CK], amylase, etc.) may point to underlying etiology
• Hypoxemia
• Hypocarbia
• Respiratory alkalosis
• Increased A-a gradient
• Leukocytosis
Drugs that may alter lab results:
Administered oxygen may complicate arterial blood gas interpretation
Disorders that may alter lab results:
Underlying pulmonary disease from an unrelated etiology may complicate arterial blood gas interpretation

PATHOLOGICAL FINDINGS
• Cardiogenic
  ◊ Heavy, wet, subcrepitant lungs
  ◊ Intra-alveolar granular pink precipitate
  ◊ Alveolar microhemorrhages and hemosiderin-laden macrophages
  ◊ "Brown induration," chronic passive congestion
  ◊ Hypostatic bronchopneumonia

• Noncardiogenic
  ◊ Heavy, firm, red, and boggy lungs
  ◊ Interstitial and intra-alveolar edema, inflammation, fibrin deposition, hemorrhage, and patchy atelectasis
  ◊ Hyaline membrane formation
  ◊ Interstitial and intra-alveolar fibrosis

SPECIAL TESTS
• Arterial blood gas
• Electrocardiogram
• Pulmonary function tests
• Mixed venous oxygen saturation

IMAGING
• Two-dimensional echocardiography with Doppler may be useful in some cases of cardiogenic pulmonary edema (e.g., valvular heart disease, systolic vs. diastolic dysfunction)
• Chest x-ray (may be difficult or impossible to differentiate cardiogenic from non-cardiogenic pulmonary edema)
  ◊ Cardiogenic chest x-ray; Interstitial edema, cardiomegaly, pulmonary venous redistribution, Kerley's B lines, alveolar edema (initially perihilar), pleural effusions (more common)
  ◊ Non-cardiogenic chest x-ray; alveolar edema, cardiomegaly absent, pulmonary venous redistribution absent, pleural effusions less common

DIAGNOSTIC PROCEDURES
• Swan-Ganz catheter may help differentiate cardiogenic from non-cardiogenic pulmonary edema
• Cardiac catheterization - occasionally beneficial

TREATMENT

APPROPRIATE HEALTH CARE
Generally inpatient or intensive care; outpatient for mildest forms

GENERAL MEASURES
• Treat underlying condition
• Patient sitting, with legs dangling
• Oxygen
• Rotating tourniquets or phlebotomy selectively
• Mechanical ventilation, often requiring positive end-expiratory pressure support
• Rapid reduction in altitude in cases of high altitude pulmonary edema

SURGICAL MEASURES N/A

ACTIVITY Bedrest in most cases

DIET Low sodium diet

PATIENT EDUCATION
• Low sodium, fluid restriction
• Symptoms and signs of pulmonary edema
• Importance of medical compliance

Pulmonary edema

MEDICATIONS

DRUG(S) OF CHOICE
- Acute cardiogenic pulmonary edema
  ◊ Morphine sulfate 2-5 mg IV
  ◊ Furosemide 20-80 mg IV
  ◊ Nitroglycerin paste 1-2 inches
  ◊ In selected cases: Nitroglycerin drip beginning at 5 µg/min and increasing by 5-10 µg/min every few minutes, titrating to blood pressure, etc. Nitroprusside IV drip beginning at 10 µg/min and increasing by 5-10 µg/min every few minutes, titrating to blood pressure, etc. Dobutamine 2 µg/kg/min IV titrating to blood pressure, cardiac output, pulmonary capillary wedge pressure, etc.
- Chronic management of cardiogenic pulmonary edema
  ◊ Furosemide 20-400 mg daily
  ◊ Angiotensin converting enzyme inhibitors (e.g., captopril 6.25-25 mg po tid, lisinopril 2.5-20 mg po qd, enalapril 2.5-15 mg po qd-bid)
  ◊ Digoxin 0.125-0.25 mg po qd
  ◊ Carvedilol 3.125-25 mg po bid
  ◊ Isosorbide dinitrate 10-60 mg po tid-qid
  ◊ Thiazide diuretics (e.g., hydrochlorothiazide [HCTZ] 25-50 mg po qd)
- Noncardiogenic pulmonary edema
  ◊ Oxygen
  ◊ Selected cardiovascular drugs to optimize tissue oxygen delivery

Contraindications: Refer to manufacturer's profile of each drug

Precautions:
- Avoid liberal intravenous fluids, especially normal saline or lactated Ringer's
- Avoid use of carvedilol and other beta blockers in decompensated cardiac failure, bronchospastic disease, second or third degree AV block, sick sinus syndrome and severe bradycardia
- Avoid calcium channel blockers and other negative inotropic agents in the setting of cardiogenic pulmonary edema
- Avoid high forced inspiratory O2 (FiO2) > 50% for prolonged periods of time if possible
- Avoid prolonged administration of nitroprusside due to risk of cyanide toxicity. If nitroprusside administered for > 72 hrs, obtain a thiocyanate level.

Significant possible interactions: Additive hypotensive effects of nitrates, afterload reducers, diuretics, etc.

ALTERNATIVE DRUGS
- Chlorothiazide
- Metolazone
- Acetazolamide
- Bumetanide
- Potassium-sparing diuretics
- Other ACE inhibitors

FOLLOWUP

PATIENT MONITORING
- Inpatient
  ◊ Serial arterial blood gases or pulse oximetry, often in the intensive care unit with one-on-one nursing
  ◊ Strict measurement of intake and output
  ◊ Attention to optimal fluid management
  ◊ Attention to optimal ventilator settings
  ◊ Serial chest x-rays
- Outpatient
  ◊ Attention to clinical status
  ◊ Serial weights to assess fluid accumulation

PREVENTION/AVOIDANCE
Compliance with medications and diet

POSSIBLE COMPLICATIONS
- Death
- Reversible or irreversible organ ischemia
- Pulmonary fibrosis, particularly with noncardiogenic pulmonary edema

EXPECTED COURSE/PROGNOSIS
- Dependent on underlying etiology
- Mortality approximately 50-60% for noncardiogenic pulmonary edema and up to 80% for cardiogenic shock

MISCELLANEOUS:

ASSOCIATED CONDITIONS (see Causes)

AGE-RELATED FACTORS
Pediatric: Usually secondary to lung immaturity, congenital heart disease, or associated with trauma
Geriatric: Higher mortality
Others: N/A

PREGNANCY
Pulmonary edema may occur as a complication of tocolytic therapy with magnesium sulfate, terbutaline or ritodrine

SYNONYMS N/A

ICD-9-CM
428.1 Acute pulmonary edema with heart disease
518.4 Acute edema of lung, NOS

SEE ALSO
- Congestive heart failure
- Respiratory distress syndrome, adult
- Altitude illness

OTHER NOTES N/A

ABBREVIATIONS
ARDS = adult respiratory distress syndrome

REFERENCES
- Ingram RH, Braunwald E: Pulmonary edema. In: Braunwald E, ed. Heart disease - A Textbook of Cardiovascular Medicine. 4th Ed. Philadelphia, WB Saunders, Co, 1992
- Fauci A, et al: Harrison's Textbook of Internal Medicine. 14th Ed. New York, McGraw-Hill Inc, 1998

Illustrations: N/A
Internet references: http://www.5mcc.com

Author(s)
Peter Kozisek, MD

Pulmonary embolism

BASICS

DESCRIPTION Pulmonary embolism occurs when venous thrombi in the deep venous system of the legs dislodge and enter the pulmonary arterial circulation
• Pulmonary embolism presents as three different syndromes
◊ Acute cor pulmonale - due to massive pulmonary embolism, obstructing > 60-75% of the pulmonary circulation
◊ Pulmonary Infarction - occurs in patients with submassive pulmonary embolism with complete obstruction of a distal branch of the pulmonary circulation
◊ Acute unexplained dyspnea - occurs in patients who do not develop acute cor pulmonale or pulmonary infarction
System(s) affected: Pulmonary, Cardiovascular
Genetics: Hypercoagulability
Incidence/Prevalence in USA:
• 600,000-700,000 cases/year
• 100,000-200,000 deaths/year
Predominant age: Very rare in children, incidence increases with advancing age
Predominant sex: Male = Female

SIGNS AND SYMPTOMS
• Acute cor pulmonale
◊ Syncope
◊ Hypotension or cardiac arrest
◊ Dyspnea
◊ Anxiety
◊ Tachypnea
◊ Tachycardia
◊ Distended neck veins
◊ S3 gallop
◊ Clear lungs on auscultation
◊ ± Signs of deep venous thrombosis
◊ ECG - S1Q3T3 pattern or incomplete right bundle branch block
◊ Chest x-ray - usually normal
◊ Arterial blood gases (room air) decreased PO2, decreased PCO2
• Pulmonary infarction
◊ Pleuritic chest pain
◊ Dyspnea
◊ ± Hemoptysis
◊ Tachypnea
◊ Lungs - rales, wheezes and/or signs of pleural effusion
◊ ± Signs of deep venous thrombosis
◊ ECG - normal
◊ Chest x-ray - elevated hemidiaphragm, infiltrate or small pleural effusion
◊ Arterial blood gases (room air) - normal or decreased PO2, decreased PCO2, alkalosis
• Acute unexplained dyspnea
◊ Dyspnea
◊ ± Anxiety
◊ ± Tachycardia
◊ Tachypnea
◊ Clear lungs
◊ ± Signs of deep venous thrombosis
◊ ECG - usually normal
◊ Chest x-ray - normal

CAUSES
• Hypercoagulability
• Deep vein thrombosis responsible for 95% of pulmonary embolism

RISK FACTORS
• Prolonged bed rest
• Advanced age
• Congestive heart failure
• Malignancy
• Stroke
• Pregnancy
• Oral contraceptives
• Postoperative
• Trauma to legs
• Obesity

DIAGNOSIS

DIFFERENTIAL DIAGNOSIS
• Pneumonia
• Myocardial infarction
• Congestive heart failure
• Viral pleuritis
• Pericarditis

LABORATORY N/A
Drugs that may alter lab results: N/A
Disorders that may alter lab results: N/A

PATHOLOGICAL FINDINGS Pulmonary infarction

SPECIAL TESTS N/A

IMAGING
• The diagnosis is confirmed by V/Q lung scan (multiple segmental or lobar perfusion defects with normal ventilation), or pulmonary angiogram (intraluminal filling defects and/or arterial cutoffs)
• Chest x-ray may reveal parenchymal infiltrate, pleural effusion

DIAGNOSTIC PROCEDURES
• Lung scan
• Pulmonary angiogram
• Echocardiogram
• Spiral CT scan
• Diagnosis suspected on basis of signs and symptoms consistent with one of the three syndromes in a patient with deep venous thrombosis (DVT) or with risk factors for DVT

TREATMENT

APPROPRIATE HEALTH CARE
Hospitalization, ICU if hemodynamically unstable

GENERAL MEASURES
• Designed to maintain adequate cardiovascular and pulmonary functions and to prevent recurrence of emboli
• Oxygen therapy as needed

SURGICAL MEASURES
• Interruption of inferior vena cava may be indicated in patients who can not take anticoagulants or those who have recurrent emboli despite anticoagulant therapy
• In patients with massive embolism who have persistent hypotension, pulmonary embolectomy may be life saving despite a mortality of approximately 30%. An alternative to embolectomy is thrombolytic therapy in patients without a contraindication.

ACTIVITY
• Bed rest, move legs frequently
• Ambulation when patient stable

DIET No special diet, need to maintain adequate nutrition and fluids

PATIENT EDUCATION N/A

MEDICATIONS

DRUG(S) OF CHOICE
• Intravenous heparin by continuous infusion, at dose to prolong partial thromboplastin time to 1.5-2.0 times control for five to seven days. Usual regimen requires beginning with 80 units/kg load followed by 18 unit/kg/hr. Check PTT 6 hours after beginning infusion, then daily.
• Warfarin beginning day one or day two of hospitalization for at least three months. Warfarin dose adjusted to prolong prothrombin time to an INR of 2.5 (range 2.0 to 3.0).
• In event of hypotension requiring vasopressors in a patient with angiographically documented pulmonary embolism, pulmonary embolectomy or intravenous thrombolytic agents may be required
Contraindications: Refer to manufacturer's profile of each drug
Precautions:
• Refer to manufacturer's profile of each drug
• The major complication of heparin is the possibility of hemorrhage. If PTT is appropriately adjusted, the major hemorrhage rate should be low.
Significant possible interactions: Refer to manufacturer's profile of each drug

ALTERNATIVE DRUGS
• Thrombolytics (streptokinase, urokinase, tissue plasminogen activator [TPA])

FOLLOWUP

PATIENT MONITORING
After hospital discharge, prothrombin time should be prolonged to an INR of 2.5 (range 2.0 to 3.0). Warfarin should be continued for at least three months. In patients with continuous predisposition to DVT, it should be continued indefinitely.

PREVENTION/AVOIDANCE
Recognition of hospitalized patients with multiple risk factors for deep venous thrombosis and implementation of prophylactic therapy including low dose heparin, warfarin or leg compression devices

POSSIBLE COMPLICATIONS
• Pulmonary infarction
• Acute cor pulmonale
• Recurrent deep venous thrombosis or pulmonary embolism, post phlebitic syndrome
• Treatment failure requiring surgical venous interruption

EXPECTED COURSE/PROGNOSIS
With appropriate therapy hospital mortality is less than 5%. Long-term prognosis determined by coexisting disease(s).

MISCELLANEOUS

ASSOCIATED CONDITIONS
• Deep vein thrombosis
• Occult cancer (lung, GI tract, breast, uterus, prostate)

AGE-RELATED FACTORS
Pediatric: Quite rare
Geriatric: More common, more often fatal.
Others: N/A

PREGNANCY
Risk of occurrence during pregnancy and puerperium

SYNONYMS
N/A

ICD-9-CM
415.1 Pulmonary embolism and infarction

SEE ALSO
• Thrombosis, deep vein (DVT)

OTHER NOTES
N/A

ABBREVIATIONS
N/A

REFERENCES
• Isselbacher KJ, et al, eds: Harrison's Principles of Internal Medicine. 13th Ed. New York, McGraw-Hill, 1994
• Rippe JM, et al, eds: Intensive Care Medicine. 2nd Ed. New York, Little, Brown, 1991:308-316
Illustrations: N/A
Internet references: http://www.5mcc.com

Author(s)
James E. Dalen, MD, MPH

Pulmonic valvular stenosis

BASICS

DESCRIPTION A congenital deformity consisting of obstruction to right ventricular outflow at the pulmonic valve level
System(s) affected: Cardiovascular
Genetics: N/A
Incidence/Prevalence in USA: 10% of congenital heart disease
Predominant age: Newborn, but often asymptomatic for years
Predominant sex: Male = Female

SIGNS AND SYMPTOMS
• History of heart murmur since birth
• Acyanotic
• Dyspnea and fatigue are the most frequent symptoms
• Occasionally dizziness or syncope occurs, particularly exertional, due to the low fixed cardiac output
• Chest pain can occur
• Myocardial infarction of the hypertrophied right ventricle has been noted
• Prominent A wave of the jugular venous pulse
• Right ventricular impulse
• Midsystolic murmur (increased duration and later peaking with increased severity)
• Pulmonic ejection sound
• Soft, delay in P2
• Occasional tricuspid regurgitation

CAUSES
• Congenital
• Rubella embryopathy

RISK FACTORS   Family history

DIAGNOSIS

DIFFERENTIAL DIAGNOSIS
• Dysplastic pulmonic valve stenosis
• Discrete infundibular stenosis
• Subinfundibular obstruction
• Isolated pulmonary artery stenosis
• Supravalvar pulmonary stenosis
• Tetralogy of Fallot (Pink)

LABORATORY   N/A
Drugs that may alter lab results: N/A
Disorders that may alter lab results: N/A

PATHOLOGICAL FINDINGS   N/A

SPECIAL TESTS   ECG - generally sinus rhythm, occasional supraventricular arrhythmias, tall peaked P waves, rightward axis, severity correlates with R/S ratio in leads V1 and V6, right ventricular hypertrophy

IMAGING
• X-ray - post stenotic dilatation of the pulmonary trunk, prominence of right atrium and ventricle
• Echocardiogram - mobile dome, thickened pulmonic valve, post stenotic dilatation of the pulmonary trunk, small valve annulus; continuous wave Doppler provides an estimate of the transvalvular gradient
• Color-flow Doppler - delineates area of obstruction

DIAGNOSTIC PROCEDURES
• Cardiac catheterization
   ◊ Not indicated in mild pulmonic stenosis
   ◊ Essential in severe pulmonic stenosis
   ◊ Used to assess morphology of the right ventricle, pulmonary outflow tract and the pulmonary arteries
   ◊ Also used to rule out associated lesions e.g., atrial septal defect (ASD), though echocardiography may suffice.

TREATMENT

APPROPRIATE HEALTH CARE Usually outpatient. Inpatient, if surgery indicated.

GENERAL MEASURES
• Though infective endocarditis is rare, SBE prophylaxis is advisable
• Diagnostic treatment for critical pulmonary stenosis in newborns
• Intervention
   ◊ None required for mild pulmonic stenosis
   ◊ Intervention of asymptomatic patients with moderate PS is controversial. At minimum, regular assessment is advisable.

SURGICAL MEASURES Percutaneous balloon valvotomy (preferred) or surgical pulmonic valvotomy required for patient with severe obstruction

ACTIVITY No specific prescription. The lesion, if significant, will limit activity.

DIET No specific regimen

PATIENT EDUCATION American Heart Association, 7320 Greenville Avenue, Dallas, TX 75231, (214)373-6300

Pulmonic valvular stenosis

MEDICATIONS

DRUG(S) OF CHOICE
• No specific regimen in the absence of congestive heart failure
• Endocarditis prophylaxis
Contraindications: Refer to manufacturer's literature
Precautions: Refer to manufacturer's literature
Significant possible interactions: Refer to manufacturer's literature

ALTERNATIVE DRUGS   N/A

FOLLOWUP

PATIENT MONITORING
• Postoperative (or post-balloon valvotomy) Doppler ultrasound suggested at approximately 1 year after procedure
• Post valvotomy SBE prophylaxis still required
• Regular followup assessment for patients not undergoing surgical correction

PREVENTION/AVOIDANCE   N/A

POSSIBLE COMPLICATIONS
• Up to 10% late mortality following valvotomy in critical pulmonary stenosis in neonates
• Slower recovery in those with chronic severe right ventricular hypertrophy
• Post valvotomy pulmonic regurgitation reported in up to 50% (variable severity)
• Residual ASD or patent foramen ovale
• Persistent repolarization abnormalities on ECG associated with severe postoperative pulmonic regurgitation
• Late atrial arrhythmias

EXPECTED COURSE/PROGNOSIS
Outcome following either balloon or surgical valvotomy is excellent in general

MISCELLANEOUS

ASSOCIATED CONDITIONS   Other cardiac abnormalities, e.g., ventricular and atrial septal defects

AGE-RELATED FACTORS
Pediatric: Congenital disorder
Geriatric: N/A
Others: N/A

PREGNANCY   In asymptomatic young women with mild to moderate PS, pregnancy is generally well tolerated

SYNONYMS   Pulmonic stenosis

ICD-9-CM
424.3 Pulmonary valve disorders
746.02 Stenosis, congenital

SEE ALSO   Tetralogy of Fallot

OTHER NOTES   N/A

ABBREVIATIONS
• SBE = subacute bacterial endocarditis
• PS = pulmonic stenosis

REFERENCES
• Braunwald E, ed: Heart Disease: A Textbook of Cardiovascular Medicine. 4th Ed. Philadelphia, W.B. Saunders Co., 1992
• Liberthson R: Congenital Heart Disease: Diagnosis & Management in Children and Adults. Boston, Little Brown & Co., 1989
• Perloff J: Clinical Recognition of Congenital Heart Disease. 4th Ed. Philadelphia, WB Saunders Co, 1994
Illustrations: N/A
Internet references: http://www.5mcc.com

Author(s)
Sylvia A. Mamby, MD

Pyelonephritis

BASICS

DESCRIPTION
• Acute pyelonephritis is a syndrome caused by an infection of the pyelo-caliceal system, producing localized flank or back pain combined with systemic symptoms such as fever, chills and prostration. It is accompanied by bacteriuria, and often by bacteremia, which can progress to "septic shock" and death.
• Chronic pyelonephritis is the pathological result of progressive inflammation on the renal interstitium and tubules, and the radiologic diagnosis of the renal scarring and destructive changes in the caliceal system that are presumed to be caused by bacterial infection, vesicoureteral reflux, or both.
System(s) affected: Renal/Urologic
Genetics: N/A
Incidence/Prevalence in USA:
• Community acquired acute pyelonephritis - 15.7 per 100,000/per year
• Hospital acquired acute pyelonephritis - 7.3 per 10,000 hospital persons
Predominant age: All ages, especially > 50
Predominant sex: Female > Male

SIGNS AND SYMPTOMS
• In adults
  ◊ Fever; above 38.5°C
  ◊ Chills
  ◊ Unilateral vs. bilateral pain in the lumbar flank area
  ◊ Malaise
  ◊ Myalgia
  ◊ Anorexia
  ◊ Nausea
  ◊ Vomiting
  ◊ Diarrhea
  ◊ Headache
  ◊ Dysuria
  ◊ Frequency
  ◊ Urgency
  ◊ Suprapubic discomfort
  ◊ Flank pain on palpation
  ◊ From no physical findings to septic shock
• In infants and children
  ◊ Sepsis
  ◊ Fever
  ◊ Irritability
  ◊ Poor skin perfusion
  ◊ Inadequate weight gain or weight loss
  ◊ Gastrointestinal symptoms
  ◊ Jaundice to gray skin color
  ◊ Flank mass
  ◊ Enuresis
  ◊ Vaginal discharge, vulval soreness or pruritus in girls

CAUSES
• E. coli (75%)
• Other gram-negative rods, Proteus mirabilis, Klebsiella and Enterobacter account for 10-15%
• Enterococcus
• Staphylococcus - epidermis, saprophyticus (number two cause in young women) and aureus
• Leptospira
• Salmonella typhi
• Mycoplasma
• Anaerobes

RISK FACTORS
• Underlying urinary tract abnormalities
• Indwelling catheter
• Nephrolithiasis
• Diabetes mellitus
• Immunocompromised conditions
• Elderly, institutionalized women
• Acute pyelonephritis within the prior year
• Prostatic enlargement
• Recent urinary tract instrumentation
• Childhood UTI
• Symptoms longer than 7 days at presentation

DIAGNOSIS

DIFFERENTIAL DIAGNOSIS
• Renal infarction
• Acute renal vein thrombosis
• Acute renal artery dissection
• Obstructive uropathy
• Acute glomerulonephritis
• Acute bacterial pneumonia
• Myocardial infarction
• Acute hepatitis
• Cholecystitis
• Acute pancreatitis
• Appendicitis
• A perforated viscus
• Splenic infarct
• Aortic dissection
• Acute pelvic inflammatory disease
• Kidney stone
• Ectopic pregnancy

LABORATORY
• Urine culture (> 100,000 colony-forming units [CFU/mL]) and sensitivities
• Urine gram stain
• Pyuria
• The leukocyte esterase test in the urine
• Leukocyte casts
• Hematuria and mild proteinuria
• Leukocytosis
• Blood culture(s)
Drugs that may alter lab results:
Antibiotics
Disorders that may alter lab results: N/A

PATHOLOGICAL FINDINGS
• Acute:
  ◊ Abscess formation with neutrophils
  ◊ Glomeruli spared
  ◊ The area of the infection is wedge-shaped toward the medulla
• Chronic:
  ◊ Fibrosis
  ◊ Reduction in renal tissue
  ◊ Scarring
  ◊ Calyceal clubbing, dilatation and distortion

SPECIAL TESTS
• Bladder washout
• Antibody coated bacteria or ACB test

IMAGING
67gallium or 131I-Hippuran scanning

DIAGNOSTIC PROCEDURES
• If febrile for longer than 72 hours or if obstruction/anatomic abnormality suspected
  ◊ Cystoscopy with ureteral catheterization
  ◊ Contrast-enhanced computed tomography (CT) - spiral more sensitive than conventional
  ◊ Ultrasound
  ◊ Intravenous pyelogram (IVP)

TREATMENT

APPROPRIATE HEALTH CARE
• Outpatient therapy if mild to moderate illness (not pregnant, no nausea or vomiting; fever and pain not severe)
• Inpatient therapy for severe illness (pregnant, high fevers, severe pain, marked debility, intractable vomiting, possible urosepsis)

GENERAL MEASURES
• Intravenous fluids when needed
• Broad-spectrum antibiotics initially, tailoring therapy to culture and sensitivity results
• Analgesics and antipyrectics
• Urinary analgesics (e.g., phenazopyridine 200 mg tid) for severe dysuria

SURGICAL MEASURES
Percutaneous drainage of abscess if necessary

ACTIVITY
As tolerated

DIET
Encourage fluid

PATIENT EDUCATION
• Griffith, H. W.: Instructions for Patients; Philadelphia, W.B. Saunders Co. 1994:211

Pyelonephritis

MEDICATIONS

DRUG(S) OF CHOICE
Severe Illness: IV therapy until afebrile 48 hours and tolerating oral hydration and medications, then oral agents to complete 2 weeks
• IV agents (assuming normal creatinine clearance):
◊ Cefotaxime I g q 12 hours up to 2 g q 4 hours
◊ Ceftriaxone 1-2 g q day
◊ Cefoxitin 2 g q 8 hours
◊ Ciprofloxacin 400 mg q 12 hours
◊ Levofloxacin 250 mg q day
◊ Ofloxacin 400 mg q 12 hours
◊ Gentamicin 3-5 mg/kg of body weight q day or I mg/kg body weight q 8 hours (with or without ampicillin I g q 6 hours)
◊ Trimethoprim-sulfamethoxazole 160-800 mg q 12 hours (Note: Up to 30% E. coli resistant to ampicillin and trimethoprim/sulfamethoxazole in community acquired infections. If enterococcus suspected based on gram stain, ampicillin plus gentamicin is reasonable empiric choice, unless penicillin allergic, then use vancomycin.
• Oral agents:
◊ Ciprofloxacin 500 mg q 12 hours
◊ Levofloxacin 250 mg q day
◊ Norfloxacin 400 mg q 12 hours
◊ Cephalexin 500 mg qid
◊ Amoxicillin-clavulanate 875/125 mg q 12 hours or 500/125 mg tid
Contraindications:
• Allergies to penicillin, sulfa, or other agents listed
• Fluoroquinalones contraindicated in adolescents, children and pregnant women
• Nitrofarantoin does not achieve reliable tissue levels for pyelonephritis treatment
Precautions:
• Most antibiotics require adjustments in dosage with renal insufficiency • Follow aminoglycoside levels and renal function
Significant possible interactions: N/A

ALTERNATIVE DRUGS   N/A

FOLLOWUP

PATIENT MONITORING
• Response within 48 hours (95% of patients): discharge on oral agent (see above) after patient is afebrile for 48 hours to complete 2 weeks
• No response within 48 hours (5% of patients): reevaluate, review cultures; CT (spiral CT most sensitive), IVP or ultrasound; adjust therapy as needed; may need urological consult
• Mild/moderate Illness - oral therapy for 2 weeks as outpatient: ciprofloxacin, levofloxacin, norfloxacin, cephalexin, amoxicillin/clavulanate. (Up to 30% E. coli resistance to ampicillin and trimethoprim/sulfamethoxazole in community acquired UTI's). If enterococcus suspected based on urine gram stain, add amoxicillin to fluoroquinolone pending culture and sensitivity.
• All patients: follow-up urine analysis I to 2 weeks after completing therapy; if persistent hematuria despite eradication of infection, refer for urologic evaluation
• Women: routine follow-up cultures not recommended unless symptoms resolve but recur within 2 weeks; obtain urine culture, sensitivity, gram stain and CT or renal ultrasound. If symptoms resolve but recur after 2 weeks, treat as sporadic episode of pyelonephritis, unless 2 or more recurrences, then urologic evaluation necessary.
• Men, children, adolescents, patients with recurrent infections, patients with risk factors: repeat cultures I to 2 weeks after completing therapy; urologic evaluation after first episode of pyelonephritis and with recurrences.

PREVENTION/AVOIDANCE   N/A

POSSIBLE COMPLICATIONS
• Kidney abscess
• Metastatic infection: skeletal system, endocardium, eye, meningitis with subsequent seizures
• Septic shock and death
• Chronic renal insufficiency
• Complications of antibiotics

EXPECTED COURSE/PROGNOSIS
95% respond in 48 hours

MISCELLANEOUS:

ASSOCIATED CONDITIONS   N/A

AGE-RELATED FACTORS
Pediatric: Nonspecific systems, jaundice, enuresis, sepsis
Geriatric:
• May present as confusion
• Characteristics may change
Others: N/A

PREGNANCY
• The most common medical complications requiring hospitalization
• May complicate the pregnancy course and produce low weight babies

SYNONYMS
• Acute upper urinary tract infection

ICD-9-CM
590.1 Acute pyelonephritis
590.10 Acute pyelonephritis without lesion of medullary necrosis
590.0 Chronic pyelonephritis

SEE ALSO
• Urinary tract infection in males
• Urinary tract infection in females

OTHER NOTES   N/A

ABBREVIATIONS   N/A

REFERENCES
• Schrier RW, Gottschalk CW: Diseases of the Kidney. 6th Ed. Boston, Little, Brown, 1996
• Hooton TM, Stamm WE: Diagnosis and treatment of uncomplicated urinary tract infections. Infect Dis Clin NA 1997;11(3):551-581
• Bacheller CD, Bernstein JM: Urinary tract infections. Med Clin NA 1997;81(3):719-730
Illustrations: N/A
Internet references: http://www.5mcc.com

Author(s)
John Spangler, MD, MPH
Julienne K. Kirk, PharmD

Pyloric stenosis

 BASICS

DESCRIPTION   A progressive stenosis of the pyloric canal occurring in infancy
System(s) affected: Gastrointestinal
Genetics: Multifactorial inheritance risk; recurrence risk 3-9% if first degree relative affected
Incidence/Prevalence in USA: 1/300-1/1000 live births (male 1/150 live births; female 1/750 live births)
Predominant age: Infancy; onset usually at 3-4 weeks of age, rarely in the newborn period or as late as 5 months of age
Predominant sex: Male > Female (5:1)

SIGNS AND SYMPTOMS
• Intermittent, non-bilious, projectile vomiting of increasing frequency and severity
• Initially hunger, later weakness
• Epigastric distention
• Visible gastric peristalsis, sometimes retrograde
• Palpable tumor (olive) in right upper quadrant
• Jaundice, occasional
• Late signs: dehydration, weight loss
• Diminished stools

CAUSES
• Obscure, sometimes familial; 6% risk of recurrence if either parent had pyloric stenosis, much higher if the mother was affected

RISK FACTORS   2.5 times more common in Caucasians than in blacks

 DIAGNOSIS

DIFFERENTIAL DIAGNOSIS
• Inexperienced or inappropriate feeding
• Gastroesophageal reflux
• Gastritis
• Congenital adrenal hyperplasia, salt-losing
• Pyloric diaphragm
• Pylorospasm

LABORATORY
• Early - evidence hypochloremic alkalosis, with low serum chloride and high bicarbonate
• Later - may have acidosis with low bicarbonate and low potassium
• Elevated unconjugated bilirubin level
Drugs that may alter lab results: N/A
Disorders that may alter lab results: N/A

PATHOLOGICAL FINDINGS   Concentric hypertrophy of pyloric muscle

SPECIAL TESTS   Abdominal ultrasound by experienced radiologist will usually outline the pyloric tumor

IMAGING
• Upright plain film of abdomen may reveal dilated stomach (filled with fluid and/or air) and relative lack of air in intestines
• Ultrasound (first choice if available)
• Barium swallow (performed only when diagnosis is not clinically clear) reveals strong gastric contractions and elongated, narrow pyloric canal (string sign); now rarely performed if ultrasound available

DIAGNOSTIC PROCEDURES   None

 TREATMENT

APPROPRIATE HEALTH CARE
• Inpatient
• Surgery: Fredet-Ramstedt pyloromyotomy

GENERAL MEASURES   N/A

SURGICAL MEASURES   Surgery must be preceded by preoperative preparation, including: Empty stomach with nasogastric tube, fluid replacement, correction of electrolyte imbalance

ACTIVITY   N/A

DIET
• No preoperative feeding
• No feeding for 8-16 hours postoperative
• Gradual increase in feedings thereafter
• Should reach full feedings 48-72 hours after surgery

PATIENT EDUCATION   Instructions about preoperative and postoperative care

MEDICATIONS

DRUG(S) OF CHOICE N/A
Contraindications: N/A
Precautions: N/A
Significant possible interactions: N/A

ALTERNATIVE DRUGS N/A

FOLLOWUP

PATIENT MONITORING Routine pediatric health maintenance

PREVENTION/AVOIDANCE N/A

POSSIBLE COMPLICATIONS
• No long term morbidity
• Occasional postoperative wound infection with staph aureus

EXPECTED COURSE/PROGNOSIS
Complete recovery with catch-up growth and weight gain

MISCELLANEOUS

ASSOCIATED CONDITIONS
• Usually none
• Rarely
◊ Hiatal hernia
◊ Esophageal atresia
◊ Malrotation
◊ Gastro-esophageal reflux

AGE-RELATED FACTORS
Pediatric: N/A
Geriatric: N/A
Others: N/A

PREGNANCY N/A

SYNONYMS
• Infantile hypertrophic pyloric stenosis

ICD-9-CM
537.0 Acquired hypertrophic pyloric stenosis
750.5 Congenital hypertrophic pyloric stenosis

SEE ALSO N/A

OTHER NOTES N/A

ABBREVIATIONS N/A

REFERENCES
• Walker, Durie, Hamilton, Walker-Smith, Watkins. Pediatric Gastrointestinal Disease, 2nd ed. CV Mosby, 1996.
• Garcia VF, Randolph TG: Pyloric Stenosis: Diagnosis and Management. Pediatrics in Review 1990;11:292-296
• Dolgin SE: Pyloric stenosis. In: FD Burg (ed): Gellis and Kagan's Current Pediatric Therapy. Philadelphia, WB Saunders, 1999
Illustrations: N/A
Internet references: http://www.5mcc.com

Author(s)
Kurt J. Wegner, MD

Rabies

BASICS

DESCRIPTION A rapidly progressive infection of the central nervous system caused by an RNA virus and affecting mammals, including humans
• The disease is essentially 100% fatal once symptoms develop
• Infection can be prevented by prompt, postexposure treatment of persons bitten by, or otherwise exposed to, animals known, or suspected to be, carrying the disease
System(s) affected: Nervous
Genetics: N/A
Incidence/Prevalence in USA: 0-5 cases per year in humans; about 7000 cases per year in animals; about 30,000 postexposure treatments. In US citizens - rate of rabies < 0.001/100,000/year.
Predominant age: Any
Predominant sex: Male = Female

SIGNS AND SYMPTOMS
Usually proceed through four stages, although they may overlap
• Incubation
  ◊ The incubation period is the time between bite and first symptoms of disease. This time is between one and three months in 2/3 of the cases. Sometimes can be as short as 6 days or longer than 6 years. It is shortest in patients with extensive bites about the head and trunk.
  ◊ No symptoms except bite trauma
• Prodrome
  ◊ Lasts 2 to 10 days
  ◊ Pain or paresthesia at the bite site is the most specific symptom at this stage
  ◊ Symptoms are often extremely variable and nonspecific, including fever, headache
  ◊ May be referable to any of a number of organ systems
  ◊ May suggest any of a number of common infections
• Acute neurologic period
  ◊ Lasts 2 to 10 days
  ◊ Symptoms referable to central nervous system dominate clinical picture
  ◊ Generally takes one of two forms
  ◊ Furious rabies: Episodes of hyperactivity last about 5 minutes and include hydrophobia, aerophobia, hyperventilation, hypersalivation and autonomic instability interspersed with periods of normalcy
  ◊ Paralytic rabies: Paralysis dominates clinical picture, may be ascending (like Guillain-Barré syndrome) or affect one or more limbs differentially
• Coma
  ◊ Last hours to days; with intensive care, may rarely last months
  ◊ May evolve over a few days following acute neurologic period
  ◊ May be sudden, with respiratory arrest
• Death
  ◊ Usually occurs within three weeks of onset as result of complications
  ◊ Only 4 survivors reported in the world's literature

CAUSES
Rabies virus, a neurotropic virus present in saliva of infected animals

RISK FACTORS
For exposure to rabies:
• Professions or activities that may expose a person to wild or domestic animals, e.g., animal handlers, some lab workers, veterinarians, spelunkers (cave explorers)
• International travel to countries where canine rabies is endemic (most common risk factor)
• In the United States, most cases appear due to exposure to bats

DIAGNOSIS

DIFFERENTIAL DIAGNOSIS
• Any rapidly progressive encephalitis; important to exclude treatable causes of encephalitis, especially herpes
• Diagnosis should be considered if there is a bite by an animal capable of transmitting the disease; however, most patients in the U.S. do not recall exposure

LABORATORY
• WBC count in cerebrospinal fluid (CSF) exam may be normal or show moderate pleocytosis
• CSF protein may be normal or moderately elevated
• Viral isolation from saliva or CSF
• Serum CSF for rabies antibody
• Corneal smear stains positive by immunofluorscence in 50% of patients
Drugs that may alter lab results:
Immunosuppressive agents
Disorders that may alter lab results:
None

PATHOLOGICAL FINDINGS
Encephalitis may be found in brain biopsy, but abnormal findings may be confined to parts (brainstem, midbrain, cerebellum) only examined postmortem

SPECIAL TESTS
• Only available in state and federal reference laboratories
• Rabies antibody titer should be obtained on serum and CSF
• Skin biopsy from nape of neck should be obtained for direct fluorescent antibody examination
• Saliva culture for rabies virus

IMAGING Normal, or nonspecific findings consistent with encephalitis

DIAGNOSTIC PROCEDURES
• Spinal tap
• Skin biopsy to detect rabies antigen in hair follicles

TREATMENT

APPROPRIATE HEALTH CARE
• Suspect rabies encephalitis - inpatient with isolation
• Exposure to rabies - inpatient if wounds serious; outpatient for prophylactic treatment

GENERAL MEASURES
• Since there is no treatment for clinical rabies, this section is directed at prevention of disease following exposure to potentially rabid animals
• Physicians should evaluate each possible exposure to rabies and consult with local or state public health officials about the need for rabies prophylaxis
  ◊ In the United States, raccoons, skunks, bats, foxes, coyotes are the animals most likely to be infected, but any carnivore can carry the disease
  ◊ Postexposure prophylaxis should be considered for any person who reports direct contact with bats, unless it is known that an exposure did not occur.
• Outside the United States, dogs are a main reservoir especially in developing countries
• Before specific antirabies treatment is initiated, consider: Types of exposure (bite or nonbite), epidemiology of rabies in involved species, circumstances of biting incident and vaccination status of exposing animal

SURGICAL MEASURES N/A

ACTIVITY As tolerated

DIET No restrictions

PATIENT EDUCATION
• Avoid wild and unknown domestic animals
• Seek treatment promptly if bitten
• Careful wound cleansing is first line of treatment

MEDICATIONS

DRUG(S) OF CHOICE
• Postexposure prophylaxis regimen (do all 3)
◊ Local wound treatment: Immediate and thorough washing of all bite wounds and scratches with soap and water
◊ Passive vaccination: rabies immune globulin (RIG, Hyperab) administered once - 20 IU/kg body weight (formula is applicable for all ages). If anatomically feasible, all of the RIG should be thoroughly infiltrated in the area around the wound. Any remaining RIG should be administered IM. RIG should never be administered in the same syringe or into the same anatomical site as vaccine.
◊ Active vaccination: rabies vaccine, human diploid cell (HDCV) or Rabies vaccine adsorbed (RVA) IM in the deltoid or purified chick embryo cell vaccine (PCEC). For children, the anterolateral aspect of the thigh is acceptable. Gluteal area should never be used for vaccine injections. Give the first dose, 1 mL, as soon as possible after exposure; one additional dose should be given on days 3, 7, 14, and 28.
For previously vaccinated patients, two IM doses (1 mL each) of vaccine should be administered, one immediately and one 3 days later. RIG not necessary in these patients.
• Preexposure vaccination: For persons in high risk groups, such as veterinarians, animal handlers, certain laboratory workers, and persons spending time (e.g., one month or more) in foreign countries where rabies is enzootic
◊ Primary preexposure: IM vaccination regimen consists of three 1.0 mL injections of HDCV or RVA given in deltoid area, one each on days 0, 7, and 28. HDCV may also be given in intradermal (ID) doses, administered with a special syringe developed for that purpose (Imovax Rabies I.D. Vaccine); the 0.1 mL ID dose is administered in the deltoid area, follow the same schedule as for IM doses.
◊ For persons at frequent risk of exposure to rabies, serum should be tested every 2 years. A preexposure booster should be administered if this is less than acceptable level. If titer cannot be obtained, a booster can be administered instead.

Contraindications: None for postexposure treatment
Precautions: About 6% of persons develop mild serum sickness reaction following HDCV boosters. Mild local and systemic reactions are very common following vaccination. Mild reactions should not be a cause for interruption of immunization.
Significant possible interactions: Antibody response may be suppressed by diseases that suppress immune system

ALTERNATIVE DRUGS None

FOLLOWUP

PATIENT MONITORING After primary vaccination, serologic testing only necessary if patient has disease or takes medications that may suppress immune system

PREVENTION/AVOIDANCE See Treatment

POSSIBLE COMPLICATIONS None

EXPECTED COURSE/PROGNOSIS No postexposure failures reported in the United States since the 1970's

MISCELLANEOUS

ASSOCIATED CONDITIONS N/A

AGE-RELATED FACTORS
Pediatric: N/A
Geriatric: N/A
Others: N/A

PREGNANCY N/A

SYNONYMS Hydrophobia

ICD-9-CM 071 (clinical rabies) or V01.5 (rabies exposure) or V04.5 (inoculation or prophylactic vaccination)

SEE ALSO Animal bites

OTHER NOTES N/A

ABBREVIATIONS
• RIG = rabies immune globulin
• HDCV = human diploid cell rabies vaccine
• RVA = rabies vaccine adsorbed
• PCDC = purified chick embryo cell vaccine

REFERENCES
• Fishbein DB: Rabies in humans. In: Baer G, ed. Natural History of Rabies. 2nd Ed. Boca Raton, CRC Press, 1991:519-549
• Fishbein DB, Bernard KW: Rabies virus. In: Mandell GI, et al. Principles and Practice of Infectious Disease. 4th Ed. New York, Churchill Livingstone, 1995
• Rabies Prevention - United States, 1999. Morbidity and Mortality Weekly Reports 1999;48(RR-1):1-20
• Noah DL, Drenzek CL, Smith JS, et al: Epidemiology of human rabies in the United States, 1980-1996. Ann Intern Med 1998;128:922-30
Illustrations: N/A
Internet references: http://www.5mcc.com

Author(s)
Daniel B. Fishbein, MD

Radiation sickness

BASICS

DESCRIPTION Any somatic or genetic disruption of function or form caused by electromagnetic waves or accelerated atomic particles
• Acute radiation sickness: Symptoms occurring within 24 hours of exposure
• Chronic radiation syndrome: Symptoms occurring greater than 24 hours after exposure, and generally over an extended time
• Radiation measures
  ◊ 1 rad is the absorption of 100 ergs of energy by 1 gram of tissue
  ◊ 100 rads = 1 gray (Gy)
  ◊ The REM (Radiation Equivalent Man) unit was developed because different tissues have different sensitivities to radiation. 1 REM (Radiation Equivalent Man) is radiation dose in rads multiplied by a relative biologic effectiveness factor for the tissue involved. 100 REM = 1 sievert (Sv).
• Radiation includes:
  ◊ Electromagnetic emissions. Energy (and hence penetration) is inversely proportional to wave length, eg x-rays, gamma rays
  ◊ Particles. Alpha particles are the nuclei of helium atoms and beta particles are electrons. Both have low penetrance externally but are dangerous if ingested. Neutrons are damaging and penetrate well. Includes electrons, protons, alpha particles, neutron, negative pi-mesons, and heavy charged ions.
System(s) affected: Reproductive, Renal/Urologic, Cardiovascular, Nervous, Gastrointestinal, Skin/Exocrine, Hemic/Lymphatic/Immunologic, Pulmonary, Musculoskeletal
Genetics: Females tolerate better than males. The exception is pregnant females with risk of fetal injury at low dose.
Incidence/Prevalence in USA:
• Most acute radiation injury is related to accidents or radiation therapy
• 400,000 patients receive radiation therapy yearly for malignancies
• Accidents are sporadic and usually involve small numbers of individuals
• Historically:
  ◊ 120,000 individuals developed acute radiation syndrome in Japan as a result of nuclear explosions
  ◊ 7,266 natives of the Marshall Islands were exposed to radiation due to errors in judging winds after a nuclear test in the South Pacific
  ◊ Chernobyl accident in Russia in 1986 where an estimated 50,000 individuals received at least 0.5 Sv of exposure.
Predominant age: N/A
Predominant sex: N/A

SIGNS AND SYMPTOMS
• Acute radiation exposure is divided into several syndromes:
  ◊ Less than 200 rads = no disease. There may be some nausea more than 3 hours after the event. Nausea is not a reliable sign of exposure since most people involved in an accident of this type will complain of some nausea when questioned.
  ◊ 200-1000 rads = hematopoietic syndrome. Acute nausea and vomiting within 3 hours. Acute granulocyte elevation, then lymphopenia, then thrombocytopenia and neutropenia, then anemia. Peak lowering of platelets and granulocytes at 3 weeks (resolving in 12 weeks). Lymphopenia may last years. Survivors may get lung or kidney changes months after. Death rate 0-80% depending on dose received and treatment. Ld 50 for humans is 650 rads.
  ◊ 1000-5000 rads = gastrointestinal syndrome. Nausea and vomiting 30-60 minutes postexposure. Loss of the villus structure of small bowel. Severe GI bleeding, diarrhea and abdominal pain develop in 3 days and precede the hematopoietic syndrome. Death due to blood loss or gram negative sepsis. Survivors usually die late of bone marrow suppression. Death rate 80-100%.
  ◊ Over 5000 rads = neurovascular syndrome or "Spock syndrome". After a 15-30 minute asymptotic period; tremors, ataxia, vomiting, hypotension, seizures and death. Death rate 100%.

CAUSES
• Nuclear weapons
• Industrial accidents
• Nuclear power accidents
• Radiation therapy

RISK FACTORS
• Young patients more susceptible than old
• Men more sensitive than women
• Debilitated more susceptible than healthy

DIAGNOSIS

DIFFERENTIAL DIAGNOSIS
Was the patient exposed to radiation?
• Acute viral illness or anxiety cause nausea and vomiting
• Blast or heat cause skin redness
• Chemical exposure causes blistering, pain

LABORATORY
• Lymphocyte count at 48 hours post event
  ◊ Over 1500 = trivial or no exposure
  ◊ Over 1000 = survival without treatment
  ◊ 500-1000 = survival with treatment
  ◊ 100-400 = death without bone marrow transplant
  ◊ Under 100 = certain death
Drugs that may alter lab results:
Chemotherapeutic agents cause bone marrow suppression identical to radiation exposure
Disorders that may alter lab results: N/A

PATHOLOGICAL FINDINGS
• Hypocellular marrow with the hematopoietic syndrome
• The GI syndrome with loss of villus margin and sloughing of villus structure
• Late cases with fibrosis of lung, liver and kidney tissues
• Loss of hair indicates exposure of 350 rads and is complete at 700 rads

SPECIAL TESTS   Total body dosimetry may suggest dose of compound ingested. Most radioisotopes are not excreted well.

IMAGING N/A

DIAGNOSTIC PROCEDURES   N/A

TREATMENT

APPROPRIATE HEALTH CARE
Inpatient

GENERAL MEASURES
• Step 1 is decontamination to reduce external radiation and collateral exposure
• IV fluids, antinauseants and bedrest
• Platelet, RBC and WBC transfusion if needed
• Antibiotics for sepsis and neutropenia
• Treatment of collateral injuries such as burns and lacerations only after decontamination

SURGICAL MEASURES
• All wounds débrided to decontaminate
• All surgery within two days before loss of white cell and platelet function
• Bone marrow transplant for severe exposure

ACTIVITY   Isolation techniques for immune system injury

DIET   As tolerated. Hyperalimentation for severe GI syndromes.

PATIENT EDUCATION   Recommend genetic counseling and screening to persons who have been exposed to significant amounts of radiation

MEDICATIONS

DRUG(S) OF CHOICE
• Supportive therapy
◊ Antibiotics for enteric organisms for GI syndrome, e.g., trimethoprim-sulfamethoxazole, ciprofloxacin
◊ Broad spectrum antibiotics for infections common with bone marrow suppression, e.g., neutropenia
◊ If radioactive iodine - potassium iodide (SSKI) in doses proportional to the exposure
◊ If radioactive phosphorus - use parenteral magnesium sulfate
◊ Nonspecific ingestions - use laxatives to increase GI transit rate
Contraindications: Refer to manufacturer's literature
Precautions: Refer to manufacturer's literature
Significant possible interactions: Refer to manufacturer's literature

ALTERNATIVE DRUGS   N/A

FOLLOWUP

PATIENT MONITORING
• Daily CBC, platelet, granulocyte, lymphocyte counts
• Stools for blood
• Vital signs q4h looking for sepsis

PREVENTION/AVOIDANCE   Follow safety procedures

POSSIBLE COMPLICATIONS
• Long-term fibrosis of kidneys, liver and lung. Occur within 6 months of acute exposure and with as little as 300 rads of exposure.
• Radiation exposure can induce malignancies
• Increased long-term risk of leukemia (acute lymphocytic or chronic myelogenous)
• Multiple myeloma and cancers of the breast, esophagus, stomach, colon, lung, ovary, bladder, thyroid
• Sterility

EXPECTED COURSE/PROGNOSIS
• Patients surviving 12 weeks have excellent prognosis but should be monitored for long-term complications
• Hair lost usually returns within 2 months

MISCELLANEOUS

ASSOCIATED CONDITIONS   N/A

AGE-RELATED FACTORS
Pediatric: More sensitive to injury
Geriatric: Less sensitive to injury
Others: N/A

PREGNANCY   Injury to fetus likely

SYNONYMS   N/A

ICD-9-CM
990 Radiation effects, unspecified

SEE ALSO   N/A

OTHER NOTES   N/A

ABBREVIATIONS   N/A

REFERENCES
• Bennett JC, Plum F, eds: Cecil Textbook of Medicine. 20th Ed. Philadelphia, W.B. Saunders Co., 1996
• Kissane JM, ed: Anderson's pathology. 9th Ed. St. Louis, Mosby, 1990
• Cotran RS, Ramzi S, et al, eds: Robbins Pathological Basis of Disease. 5th Ed. Philadelphia, Saunders 1994
• Fauci AS, ed: Harrison's Principles of Internal medicine. 14th ed. New York, McGraw-Hill, 1998
Illustrations: 2 available on CD-ROM
Internet references: http://www.5mcc.com

Author(s)
Vicente J. Arano, MD

Rape crisis syndrome

 BASICS

DESCRIPTION
• Definitions (legal definitions may vary slightly from state to state)
◊ Sexual contact - intentional touching of a person's intimate parts (including thighs) or the clothing covering such areas, if it is construed as being for the purpose of sexual gratification
◊ Sexual conduct - vaginal intercourse between a male and female, or anal intercourse, fellatio, or cunnilingus between persons regardless of sex
◊ Rape - any sexual penetration, however slight, using force or coercion against the person's will
◊ Sexual imposition - similar to rape but without penetration or the use of force (i.e., non-consenting sexual contact)
◊ Gross sexual imposition - non-consenting sexual contact with the use of force
◊ Corruption of a minor - sexual conduct by an individual 18 years old or greater with an individual less than 15 years of age
System(s) affected: Nervous, Reproductive
Genetics: N/A
Incidence/Prevalence in USA:
• Over 100,000 cases of alleged rape reported in US every year
• Estimated that only 1 in 5 to 1 in 10 adult cases reported
• Estimated only 1 in 15 to 1 in 20 pediatric cases reported
• Estimated incidence of reported rape is 80/100,000 females (7% of violent crime)
Predominant age:
• Majority of adult victims are female in teens and 20's, (reported as high as 97 years)
• Pediatric victims may be either gender with predominance of females. Reported as young as 2 months.
• Increasing numbers of adult male victims presenting for treatment
Predominant sex: Female > Male

SIGNS AND SYMPTOMS
• In adults
◊ History of sexual penetration
◊ Sexual contact, or sexual conduct without consent and/or with the use of force
• In pediatrics
◊ Actual observation of, or suspicion of, sexual penetration, sexual contact, or sexual conduct
◊ Signs include evidence of the use of force and/or evidence of sexual contact (e.g., presence of semen and/or sperm)

CAUSES   Listed with Description

RISK FACTORS
• Numerous
• About 50% of rapes occur in the home, with 1/3 of these involving a male intruder

 DIAGNOSIS

DIFFERENTIAL DIAGNOSIS   Consenting sex among adults

LABORATORY
• Record results of wet mount noting the presence or absence of sperm and, if present, whether or not it is motile or immotile
• If indicated, a serum or urine pregnancy test should be obtained and the results recorded
Drugs that may alter lab results: N/A
Disorders that may alter lab results: N/A

PATHOLOGICAL FINDINGS   N/A

SPECIAL TESTS   N/A

IMAGING   N/A

DIAGNOSTIC PROCEDURES
• History:
◊ Record in patient's own words in so far as possible. Include date, approximate time, and general location as best possible. Document physical abuse other than sexual. Describe all types of sexual contact whether actual/or attempted. History of alcohol and/or drugs before or after alleged incident.
◊ Document time of last activity which could possibly alter specimens (e.g., bath, shower, or douche). Thorough gynecologic history is mandatory including last menstrual period (LMP), last consenting sexual contact, contraceptive practice, and prior gynecologic surgery.
• Physical examination:
◊ Use of drawings and/or photographs is encouraged. Use of UV light (Wood's lamp) to detect seminal stains on clothing or skin. Document all signs of trauma or unusual marks. Documentation of mental status/emotional state.
◊ Complete genital-rectal examination including evidence of trauma, secretions, or discharge. Use of a non-lubricated, water moistened speculum is mandatory since commonly used lubricants may destroy evidence.

 TREATMENT

APPROPRIATE HEALTH CARE
• Contact appropriate social services agency
• Majority of adult victims can be treated as outpatients unless associated trauma (physical or mental) requires admission
• Majority of pediatric sexual assault/abuse victims will require admission or outside placement until appropriate social agency can evaluate home environment

GENERAL MEASURES
• Providing health care to victims of sexual assault/abuse requires special sensitivity and privacy
• All such cases MUST be reported immediately to the appropriate law enforcement agency
• With the victim's permission, utilize personnel from local support agency(ies) (e.g., Rape Crisis Center). When available, use of in-house Social Services is extremely helpful to victim/family.
• Sedation and tetanus prophylaxis should be utilized when indicated
• Venereal disease prevention for gonorrhea/Chlamydia should be administered
• A discussion of possible pregnancy and pregnancy termination should be held with the victim. If hospital policy precludes such a discussion, then information about this option should be offered the victim via the followup mechanisms.
• Suspected HIV and hepatitis B exposure and testing should be discussed with the victim and be in keeping with hospital policies/protocols. The initial HIV test should be completed within seven days of the suspected exposure.

SURGICAL MEASURES   N/A

ACTIVITY   No restrictions

DIET   No restrictions

PATIENT EDUCATION
• Information and help available from local rape crisis support organizations
• National Institute of Mental Health, Public Inquiries Branch, Office of Scientific Information, Dept. of Health and Human Services, Parklawn Bldg., Room 15C-05, 5600 Fishers Lane, Rockville, MD 20857, (301)443-4513

MEDICATIONS

DRUG(S) OF CHOICE
• Gonorrhea: ceftriaxone 250 mg IM once or cefixime 400 mg po.
• Chlamydia: azithromycin (Zithromax) 1.0 g po single dose; or doxycycline 100 mg po bid or tetracycline 250 mg qid for 10 days. If the patient is pregnant, erythromycin should be used, 500 mg every 6 hours.
• Specific treatment for vulvovaginitis if present
• Note - gonorrhea and chlamydia medications may be given concomitantly
Contraindications: Refer to manufacturer's literature
Precautions: Refer to manufacturer's literature
Significant possible interactions: Refer to manufacturer's literature

ALTERNATIVE DRUGS
• Gonorrhea: spectinomycin, ciprofloxacin, norfloxacin, ampicillin/probenecid, or amoxicillin/probenecid. Note: Be aware of drug resistance in your region. In NE Ohio, for example, a 20% resistance of gonorrhea to ciprofloxacin has been reported.

FOLLOWUP

PATIENT MONITORING
• The patient should be seen in seven to ten days for followup care, including pregnancy testing, and counseling by a gynecologist or appropriate gynecologic clinic
• Close examination for vaginitis and treatment if necessary
• Followup test for syphilis and gonorrhea should occur in five to six weeks
• Followup testing for AIDS and hepatitis B should occur in six months
• Telephone numbers of counseling agency(ies) which can provide counslling/legal services to the patient should be provided
• Consider Sexual Assault Nurse Examiner (SANE) if available in area

PREVENTION/AVOIDANCE
• Scope of rape prevention is too complex and too broad to be discussed in these pages. True prevention will require many changes.
• Women may benefit from assertiveness training and self-defense training

POSSIBLE COMPLICATIONS
• Sexually transmitted disease and subsequent treatment
• Pregnancy (with the possibility of abortion)
• Trauma (physical and mental)

EXPECTED COURSE/PROGNOSIS
• Acute phase (usually 1-3 weeks following rape) - shaking, pain, wound healing, mood swings, appetite loss, crying. Also feelings of grief, shame, anger, fear, revenge or guilt.
• Late or chronic phase female victim may develop fear of intercourse, fear of men, nightmares , sleep disorders, daytime flashbacks, fear of being alone, loss of self-esteem, anxiety, depression, post-traumatic stress syndrome
• Recovery may be prolonged. Patients who are able to talk about their feelings seem to have a faster recovery.

MISCELLANEOUS

ASSOCIATED CONDITIONS N/A

AGE-RELATED FACTORS
Pediatric: Assurance to the child that he or she is a good person and was not the cause of the incident
Geriatric: N/A
Others: N/A

PREGNANCY Baseline pregnancy test conducted. Pregnancy prevention discussed with patient.

SYNONYMS
• Sexual assault
• Rape trauma

ICD-9-CM
V71.5 Alleged rape examination

SEE ALSO
• Chlamydial sexually transmitted diseases
• Gonococcal infections
• Hepatitis, viral
• HIV infection & AIDS
• Syphilis

OTHER NOTES
• Rape is a legal term and the examining physician is encouraged to use terminology such as "alleged rape" or "alleged sexual conduct".
• In majority of states, wife may now accuse husband of rape if they are estranged and living apart
• Since "consent defense" is common, documentation of evidence supporting the use of force or the administration of drugs/alcohol is imperative
• The use of a protocol is encouraged to assure every victim a uniform, comprehensive evaluation regardless of the expertise of the examining physician. The protocol must ensure that all evidence is properly collected and labeled, chain-of-custody is maintained, and the evidence is sent to the most appropriate forensic laboratory.
• All medical records must be well documented and legible
• All medical personnel must be willing and able to testify on behalf of the patient

ABBREVIATIONS N/A

REFERENCES
• Harwood-Nuss A, ed: The Clinical Practice of Emergency Medicine 2nd ed. Philadelphia, J.B. Lippincott-Raven, 1996
• Tintinalli JE, ed: Emergency Medicine: A Comprehensive Study Guide 4th ed. New York, McGraw-Hill, 1996
• Rosen P, ed: Emergency Medicine Concepts and Clinical Practice, 4th ed. St. Louis, Mosby, 1998
Illustrations: N/A
Internet references: http://www.5mcc.com

Author(s)
Daniel T. Schelble, MD, FACEP

Raynaud's phenomenon

BASICS

DESCRIPTION Bilaterally occurring vasospastic disorder manifested by intermittent attacks of extreme pallor, then cyanosis of the fingers (rarely, of the toes) brought on by cold exposure. With warming, vasodilatation and intense redness develops, followed by swelling, throbbing, paresthesias. Resolves with warming. May accompany emotional upset. Thumbs rarely involved. 13% may progress to atrophy of digital fat pads, ischemic ulcers of fingertips. 50% idiopathic or primary Raynaud's disease, 50% secondary (Raynaud's phenomenon).
• Disease: progressive, symmetrical. Involves fingers; rarely toes. Ages 15 to 45. Spasm is more frequent, more severe with time. No gangrene; rarely ulcerates. Diagnose only after 2 years if no underlying associated disease. May be associated with coronary vasospasm or primary pulmonary hypertension. No histologic abnormality found in digital arteries.
• Phenomenon: may be unilateral, asymmetric; may affect only one or two fingers. Underlying condition usually identifiable with time. Usually has a worse morbidity and prognosis than primary disease.
System(s) affected: Skin/Exocrine, Musculoskeletal, Hemic/Lymphatic/Immunologic
Genetics: Little information available, but some suggest a dominant inheritance pattern. One study suggests there is a 5-fold increase in Raynaud's in family members of a Raynaud's patient. (Arthritis Rheum 1996; 39:1189-91)
Incidence/Prevalence in USA: 4 to 10% of population (based on reporting of characteristic color changes, cold intolerance)
Predominant age: After 40
Predominant sex:
• Female > Male (4:1 in primary form)
• Male = Female (secondary form)

SIGNS AND SYMPTOMS
• Pallor/whiteness of fingertips with cold exposure, followed by cyanosis, then redness and pain with warming
• Ulceration of finger pads, progressing to autoamputation in severe, prolonged cases (10-13% of cases)
• Normal physical exam in primary; may show signs of underlying vasospastic or autoimmune disease in secondary form

CAUSES Unknown. May involve increased sensitivity of alpha-2-adrenergic receptors in digital vessels in primary type. Serotonin receptors (5-HT2 type) may be involved in secondary Raynaud's. Platelet and blood viscosity abnormalities also implicated.

RISK FACTORS
• Smoking (men only)
• Existing autoimmune or connective tissue disorder
• Alcohol use (women only)

• Unopposed estrogen therapy was associated with higher incidence of Raynaud's phenomenon in postmenopausal women. Not seen in women receiving combined hormone therapy.
• Helicobacter pylori may play a role in vascular diseases including Raynaud's phenomenon. Some patients showed significant improvement following eradication of H. pylori.

DIAGNOSIS

DIFFERENTIAL DIAGNOSIS
• Thromboangiitis obliterans (Buerger's disease) - primarily affects men; involves legs and feet; less than 5% have hand involvement, 90% have Raynaud's; smoking related
• Rheumatoid arthritis
• Progressive systemic sclerosis (scleroderma) - 90% have Raynaud's; Raynaud's may precede other symptoms by years
• Systemic lupus
• Carpal tunnel syndrome
• Thoracic outlet syndrome
• CREST syndrome (calcinosis cutis, Raynaud's phenomenon, esophageal dysmotility, sclerodactyly and telangiectasia)
• Cryoglobulinemias
• Waldenström's macroglobulinemia
• Acrocyanosis
• Polycythemia
• Occupational injury (especially from vibrating tools, masonry work, etc.)
• Drugs (beta-blockers, clonidine, ergotamine, methysergide, amphetamines, bromocriptine, bleomycin, vinblastine, cisplatin, cyclosporine).

LABORATORY
Tests for underlying secondary causes (CBC, ESR, RA, ANA, immunoelectrophoresis, esophageal motility studies)
Drugs that may alter lab results: N/A
Disorders that may alter lab results: N/A

PATHOLOGICAL FINDINGS
Histology of skin biopsy correlates poorly with clinical presentation. May show edema, necrotizing or non-necrotizing vasculitis, and/or perivasculitis.

SPECIAL TESTS
• Cold challenge test to elicit characteristic color changes in hands
• Nailfold capillaroscopy to detect enlarged, irregular capillary loops of other connective tissue diseases (primary Raynaud's should show normal vasculature)

IMAGING
Rarely, cases may demonstrate osteolysis of distal metaphyseal portions of phalanges, tapering and calcification of soft tissues

DIAGNOSTIC PROCEDURES
Diagnosis largely determined by history, provocative exposure to cold

TREATMENT

APPROPRIATE HEALTH CARE
Outpatient management usually sufficient

GENERAL MEASURES
• Dress warmly, wear gloves, avoid cold
• No smoking
• Avoid beta-blockers, amphetamines, ergot alkaloids, sumatriptan
• Biofeedback techniques to teach patients to increase hand temperature
• Finger guards over ulcerated fingertips

SURGICAL MEASURES
Cervical sympathectomy effect is transient - symptoms return in 1 to 2 years

ACTIVITY
Avoidance of situations in which exposure to cold is likely; avoid vibrating tools

DIET
No special diet

PATIENT EDUCATION
Emphasis on smoking cessation. Avoidance of aggravating factors (trauma, vibration, cold, etc.).

Raynaud's phenomenon

MEDICATIONS

DRUG(S) OF CHOICE
• Nifedipine 30-90 mg daily (sustained release form). (May only be needed during winter). Up to 75% experience improvement.
• Symptomatic responses do not correlate with objective evidence of improvement
Contraindications: Allergy to drug, pregnancy, congestive heart failure
Precautions: May cause headache, dizziness, lightheadedness, hypotension
Significant possible interactions:
• Increases serum level of digoxin - monitor digoxin levels closely after nifedipine added
• Cimetidine increases nifedipine level - may require dosage adjustment
• May increase prothrombin time in patients taking warfarin

ALTERNATIVE DRUGS
• Amlodipine, isradipine, nicardipine, and felodipine also appear to be effective and may be associated with fewer adverse effects
• Use of diltiazem, verapamil, reserpine, methyldopa, prazosin have equivocal support in literature
• Captopril studies suggest benefit, but need further evaluation (not FDA approved)
• Parenteral and oral prostacyclin have offered subjective improvement, but the effect is short-lived and not statistically significant
• Nitroglycerin patches may also be helpful, but limited by the incidence of severe headache

FOLLOWUP

PATIENT MONITORING
• Management of fingertip ulcers, including rapid treatment of infection
• Continue to observe for signs of associated illnesses, since Raynaud's may precede overt development of these conditions by an average of 11 years

PREVENTION/AVOIDANCE
• Avoid trauma to fingertips
• Avoid exposure to cold
• Smoking cessation

POSSIBLE COMPLICATIONS
Gangrene, autoamputation of fingertips

EXPECTED COURSE/PROGNOSIS
• Prolonged course with recurrent ischemia, ulceration
• In case of secondary phenomenon, many eventually develop hallmarks of underlying disease
• Between 12-50% of Raynaud's patients developed a secondary disorder, many of which were connective-tissue diseases

MISCELLANEOUS

ASSOCIATED CONDITIONS
• Lupus
• Rheumatoid arthritis
• Scleroderma
• Polymyositis
• Sjögren's
• Occlusive vascular disease
• Cryoglobulinemia
• Use of vibrating tools

AGE-RELATED FACTORS
Pediatric: Associated with systemic lupus erythematosus and scleroderma in children
Geriatric: Appearance of Raynaud's after 40 almost always indicates an underlying disease
Others: N/A

PREGNANCY N/A

SYNONYMS N/A

ICD-9-CM
443.0 Raynaud's syndrome

SEE ALSO
• Sjögren's syndrome

OTHER NOTES N/A

ABBREVIATIONS N/A

REFERENCES
• Isselbacher KJ, et al, eds: Harrison's Principles of Internal Medicine. 13th Ed. New York, McGraw-Hill, 1994
• Maricq HR, et al: Prevalence of Raynaud phenomenon in the general population. A preliminary study by questionnaire. J Chronic Dis 1986;39:423
• Coffman JD: Raynaud's phenomenon: an update. Hypertension 1991;17:593
• Gasbarrini A, et al: Helicobacter pylori eradication ameliorates primary Raynaud!s phenomenon. Dig Dis Sci 1998;43(8):1641-5
• Palesch YY, et al: Association between cigarette and alcohol consumption and Raynaud'sphenomenon. J Clin Epidemiol 1999;52(4):321-8
• Williams HJ, et al: Early undifferentiated connective tissue disease (C7D). VI. An inception cohort after 10 years: disease remissions and changes in diagnoses in well established and undifferentiated CTD. J Rheumatol 1999;26(4)-816-25
• Fraenkel L, et al: Different factors influencing the expression of Raynaud's phenomenon in men and women. Arthritis Rheum 1999;42(2):306-10
• Sturgill MG, Seibold JR: Rational use of calcium-channel antagonists in Raynaud's phenomenon. Curr Opin Rheumatol 1998; 10(6):584-8
• Lekakis J, et al: Short-term estrogen administration improves abnormal endothelial function in women with systemic sclerosis and Raynaud's phenomenon. Am Heart J 1998; 136(5):905-12
• Fraenkel L, et al: The association of estrogen replacement therapy and the Raynaud phenomenon in postmenopausal women. Ann Intern Med 1998; 129(3):208-11
• Spencer-Green G: Outcomes in primary Raynaud phenomenon: a meta-analysis of the frequency, rates, and predictors of transition to secondary diseases. Arch Intern Med 1998;158(6):595-600
Illustrations: 2 available on CD-ROM
Internet references: http://www.5mcc.com

Author(s)
John E. Perchalski, MD, FAAFP

Rectal prolapse

BASICS

DESCRIPTION Protrusion of the rectum through the anus
• Partial prolapse - involves only mucosa. This frequently follows anal operative procedures. (Radial rectal folds prolapsed through anus).
• Complete prolapse - involves the entire rectal wall (procidentia). This type occurs most commonly as a spontaneous event in children and complication of other disorders in the elderly. (Concentric rectal folds prolapsed through anus).
System(s) affected: Gastrointestinal
Genetics: Unknown
Incidence/Prevalence in USA: 4.2:1000 overall; 10:1000 after age 65 years
Predominant age: 2 years in children, 60-70 years in adults
Predominant sex: Male > Female (5:1 in adults, and a slight predominance in children)

SIGNS AND SYMPTOMS
• Children
  ◊ Sensation of anal mass
  ◊ Pain
  ◊ Rectal bleeding
  ◊ Protruding mass
• Adults
  ◊ Anorectal pain or discomfort during defecation
  ◊ Feeling of incomplete evacuation
  ◊ Rectal and urinary incontinence
  ◊ Rectal bleeding or discharge

CAUSES
• Children
  ◊ Idiopathic (most common)
  ◊ Abnormal innervation of levator ani muscle complex, puborectalis or anal sphincters or abnormal anatomic relationships of these muscle groups
• Adults
  ◊ Diastasis of levator ani
  ◊ Loose endopelvic fascia
  ◊ Loss of normal horizontal position of rectum
  ◊ Weak anal sphincter

RISK FACTORS
• Myelomeningocele
• Exstrophy of the bladder
• Cystic fibrosis
• Chronic constipation or diarrhea
• Imperforate anus
• Multiple sclerosis
• Stroke/paralysis
• Dementia

DIAGNOSIS

DIFFERENTIAL DIAGNOSIS
• Intussusception
• Rectal polyps
• Hemorrhoids

LABORATORY   N/A
Drugs that may alter lab results: N/A
Disorders that may alter lab results: N/A

PATHOLOGICAL FINDINGS   N/A

SPECIAL TESTS   N/A

IMAGING   Barium enema is useful in selected cases of recurrent rectal prolapse

DIAGNOSTIC PROCEDURES
Sigmoidoscopy is useful in recurrent prolapse to rule out rectal lesions

TREATMENT

APPROPRIATE HEALTH CARE
Outpatient, unless complications occur or surgical intervention required

GENERAL MEASURES
• Acute
  ◊ Prompt manual reduction of prolapse
  ◊ Treatment of diarrhea or constipation

SURGICAL MEASURES
• Recurrent
  ◊ Sub-mucosal injection of 5% phenol in glycerine in four quadrants under general anesthesia (outpatient)
  ◊ Linear electrocauterization (inpatient)
  ◊ Transabdominal Ripstein's procedure (suspension of rectum from sacrum by means of artificial material)
  ◊ Posterior sagittal rectal suspension and levator repair
  ◊ Ivalon sponge wrap procedure
  ◊ Anterior resection of rectum
  ◊ Transabdominal proctopexy (no artificial material used)
  ◊ Perineal rectosigmoidectomy
  ◊ Thiersch's wire (outpatient procedure; may be modified by using Marlex or Silastic strip instead of wire); used more commonly in children and elderly, poor-risk adults
  ◊ Gracilis Sling procedure

ACTIVITY   Full activity, when able

DIET   High fiber

PATIENT EDUCATION
• Particular reassurance to parents of infants with prolapse regarding benign nature of problem and high rate of spontaneous resolution
• Diet instructions
• Teach measures to avoid constipation
• Teach family/patient to reduce prolapse

MEDICATIONS

DRUG(S) OF CHOICE
• Mineral oil
• Stool softeners
• Lactulose
Contraindications: N/A
Precautions: N/A
Significant possible interactions: N/A

ALTERNATIVE DRUGS N/A

FOLLOWUP

PATIENT MONITORING Monthly visits until possible need for surgery has been determined or until prolapse has resolved

PREVENTION/AVOIDANCE Avoid constipation and diarrhea

POSSIBLE COMPLICATIONS
• Mucosal ulcerations
• Necrosis of rectal wall

EXPECTED COURSE/PROGNOSIS
• Spontaneous resolution expected in most children
• 5-10% recurrence rate for most procedures
• Good prognosis with treatment

MISCELLANEOUS

ASSOCIATED CONDITIONS
• Cystic fibrosis
• Myelomeningocele
• Exstrophy of the bladder
• Chronic constipation or diarrhea
• Imperforate anus
• Paraplegia
• Stroke
• Incontinence

AGE-RELATED FACTORS
Pediatric: Idiopathic most common type of rectal prolapse in children
Geriatric: Common problem in the elderly
Others: N/A

PREGNANCY N/A

SYNONYMS N/A

ICD-9-CM
569.1 Rectal prolapse

SEE ALSO
• Intussusception
• Hemorrhoids

OTHER NOTES N/A

ABBREVIATIONS N/A

REFERENCES
• Ashcraft KW, Garred JL, Holder TM, et al: Rectal prolapse: 17 year experience with the posterior repair and suspension. J Ped Surg 1990; 25(9): 992-995
• Holder TM, Ashcraft KW, eds: Pediatric Surgery. 2nd Ed. Philadelphia, W.B. Saunders Co., 1993
• Schwartz SI, Shires GT, Spencer FC, et al, eds: Principles of Surgery. 6th Ed. New York, McGraw-Hill Book Co., 1994
• O'Neill JA, Rowe MI, Grosfeld JL, et al: Pediatric Surgery. 5th ed., St Louis, Mosby, 1998
Illustrations: N/A
Internet references: http://www.5mcc.com

Author(s)
Timothy L. Black, MD, FACS, FAAP
James P. Miller, MD, FACS, FAAP

Refractive errors

BASICS

DESCRIPTION An inability of the eye to produce a focused image on the fovea or central part of the retina
• Emmetropia: When light rays are in perfect focus, the image being viewed is seen clearly
• Ametropia: Any refractive error of the eye which prevents normal focusing of the image
• Hyperopia: When the cornea of the eye is too flat or the eye is too short, light rays fall in focus behind the retina, and an individual is "farsighted"
• Myopia: When the cornea is too steep or the length of the eyeball is too long, light rays fall short of the retina, and the human eye is "nearsighted"
• Presbyopia: The natural tendency of the human crystalline lens to harden or become sclerotic, limiting the focusing of the eye on near objects (accommodation). The human crystalline lens thickens with age. By the age of 40, most people do not have enough room within the eye to allow normal excursion of the lens and accomodation: viewing of near objects are blurred and reading glasses are required.
• Astigmatism: When the cornea is steeper in one meridian more than the other or the globe is not round (oval or almond-shaped), visual blurriness occurs
System(s) affected: Nervous
Genetics: Refractive errors are inherited
Incidence/Prevalence in USA: 70% of the general population have some form of ametropia
Predominant age: Refractive errors are present at birth, but not usually detected until puberty
Predominant sex: Male = Female

SIGNS AND SYMPTOMS
• Difficulty seeing objects at a distance
• Difficulty focusing on near objects
• Difficulty reading
• Squinting
• Headaches (from squinting)

CAUSES
• Developmental (most common)
• Ocular trauma
• Iatrogenic (e.g. post cataract removal)

RISK FACTORS N/A

DIAGNOSIS

DIFFERENTIAL DIAGNOSIS
• Corneal disease
• Cataract
• Retinal abnormalities
• Diseases of the optic nerve

LABORATORY N/A
Drugs that may alter lab results: N/A
Disorders that may alter lab results: N/A

PATHOLOGICAL FINDINGS N/A

SPECIAL TESTS
• Pinhole vision test: To distinguish a refractive error from an organic cause of visual blurring, have the patient look through a pinhole in a card without a corrective lens. Patient's with a pure refractive error improve their vision since the pinhole blocks nonparallel and unfocusable rays of light.

IMAGING N/A

DIAGNOSTIC PROCEDURES
• Methods:
  ◊ Objective streak retinoscopy can be used to measure the degree of refractive error in spherocylinder correction for the proper spectacle or contact lens
  ◊ Antimuscarinic agents, e.g., clopentolate (Cyclogyl), tropicamide (Mydriacyl) applied topically paralyze the ciliary body, preventing accommodation. Cycloplegic refraction can then be performed.
• Age-related testing:
  ◊ Newborns should be examined for general eye health; ophthalmologic evaluation indicated for any discovered problems
  ◊ Vision screening should occur at each well child visit
  ◊ Visual acuity testing should be performed at approximately 3 1/2 years
  ◊ Visual acuity and motility testing should be performed at age 5
  ◊ Visual acuity should be retested prior to obtaining a driver's license, at age 40, and every 2-4 years until age 65, when evaluations are recommended every 1-2 years

TREATMENT

APPROPRIATE HEALTH CARE
Outpatient

GENERAL MEASURES
• Spectacle lenses (glasses)
• Soft and hard contact lenses

SURGICAL MEASURES
• Radial keratotomy (RK). With topical anesthesia, using a surgical keratome, multiple (4-8) radial incisions are placed onto the surface of the peripheral cornea to flatten the central, optical zone. The length, depth and proximity of the incision to the central optical zone determines its effect, and degree of correction obtained. Radial keratotomy is safe and effective and corrects nearsightedness, astigmatism or a combination of both, after the age of 18 when the prescription has stabilized.
• Photorefractive keratectomy (PRK). Surface corneal tissue is removed, with the excimer laser, to re-shape the cornea thus correcting nearsightedness, farsightedness, or astigmatism. Risks and disadvantages include pain, keratitis, and potential scarring. Healing requires 3 months with topical antibiotics and steroids with associated risks of glaucoma, cataract, and chronic inflammation.
• Automated lamellar keratoplasty (ALK). A microsurgical dermatome removes a layer of the superficial cornea to induce flattening. Investigational.
• Excimer laser. The laser photoablates corneal tissue from the central visual axis, thus flattening it. Following the procedure, the cornea must re-epithelialize. Healing takes several months, during which there is a mild haze and blurring of vision. FDA approved Oct, 1995. Investigational.
• Laser-assisted in-situ keratomileusis (LASIK). A superficial corneal flap is created with the keratome and the excimer laser removes a small amount of tissue thus reshaping the cornea. Corrects all refractive errors. Healing is rapid since re-epithelialization is not needed. Considered an adjunctive procedure for use with the excimer laser.
• Implantable contact lens (ICL). A thin, plastic lens is permanently implanted in the posterior chamber between the iris and the human crystalline lens. All refractive errors can be corrected. Risks include damage to the natural lens during surgery, cataract formation, and intraocular inflammation or infection.
• Several expansion procedures - presently under investigation - are methods to increase the space within the ciliary by surgical means to restore lens movement and accomodation

ACTIVITY N/A

DIET N/A

PATIENT EDUCATION
• All patients should have their eyes examined when starting school, and periodically thereafter
• The options of eyeglasses, contact lenses and permanent surgical correction of refractive errors should be considered
• Aggressive control of diabetes mellitus should be encouraged

MEDICATIONS

DRUG(S) OF CHOICE N/A
Contraindications: N/A
Precautions: Antimuscarinic agents may induce acute glaucoma, via acute angle closure
Significant possible interactions: N/A

ALTERNATIVE DRUGS N/A

FOLLOWUP

PATIENT MONITORING
• Routine annual adult eye exams in individuals < age 40 are not indicated
• Individuals with risks will need ocular exams as indicated by their conditions

PREVENTION/AVOIDANCE N/A

POSSIBLE COMPLICATIONS
• Amblyopia
• Poor school performance

EXPECTED COURSE/PROGNOSIS
Good if discovered early and corrected appropriately.

MISCELLANEOUS

ASSOCIATED CONDITIONS Patients with diabetes mellitus have fluctuating myopia as a result of poorly controlled blood glucose and concomitant swelling of the crystalline lens

AGE-RELATED FACTORS
Pediatric: Refractive errors can be detected early in life
Geriatric: Presbyopia occurs in later life
Others: Individuals over the age of 40 are more likely to experience presbyopia or normal loss of accommodation which occurs with age, necessitating the use of reading glasses for close work

PREGNANCY It is not unusual for refractive errors to be temporarily worsened during pregnancy due to hormonal changes in tear function and corneal swelling

SYNONYMS N/A

ICD-9-CM
367.0 Hyperopia
367.1 Myopia
367.4 Presbyopia
367.21 Astigmatism, regular

SEE ALSO
• Amblyopia

OTHER NOTES Fax-On-Demand service of American Academy of Ophthalmology for policy statement and patient education materials (908)935-2761

ABBREVIATIONS N/A

REFERENCES
• Kershner RM: Lessons from the Practice: The Gift of Sight – A Guide to Understanding Your Eyes. Thorofare, NJ, Slack, Inc., 1994
• Infant and Children's Vision Screening. American Academy of Ophthalmology - Policy Statement (#812), June, 1991
• Frequency of Ocular exams. American Academy of Ophthalmology - Policy Statement (#808), Sept, 1990
Illustrations: N/A
Internet references: http://www.5mcc.com

Author(s)
Robert M. Kershner, MD, FACS

Reiter's syndrome

BASICS

DESCRIPTION A triad of features including arthritis, conjunctivitis, and urethritis or cervicitis. Epidemiologically similar to other reactive arthritis syndromes characterized by sterile inflammation of joints from infections originating at non-articular sites. A fourth feature may be buccal ulceration or balanitis. (It is possible for only two features to be present.)
• Two forms:
 ◊ Sexually transmitted; symptoms usually begin 7-14 days after exposure
 ◊ Post-dysentery
System(s) affected: Musculoskeletal, Skin/Exocrine, Renal/Urologic
Genetics: HLA-B27 tissue antigen present in 60-80% of patients
Incidence/Prevalence in USA: 0.24-1.5% incidence after epidemics of bacterial dysentery; complicates 1-2% cases of non-gonococcal urethritis
Predominant age: 20-40 years
Predominant sex: Male > Female

SIGNS AND SYMPTOMS
• Musculoskeletal:
 ◊ Asymmetric arthritis (especially knees, ankles, MTP joints)
 ◊ Enthesopathy (inflammation at tendinous insertion into bone) such as plantar fasciitis, digital periostitis, Achilles tendinitis
 ◊ Spondyloarthropathy (spine and sacroiliac joint involvement)
• Urogenital tract:
 ◊ Urethritis
 ◊ Prostatitis
 ◊ Occasionally cystitis
 ◊ Balanitis
 ◊ Cervicitis - usually asymptomatic
• Eye:
 ◊ Conjunctivitis of one or both eyes
 ◊ Occasionally scleritis, keratitis, corneal ulceration
 ◊ Rarely uveitis and iritis
• Skin:
 ◊ Mucocutaneous lesions (small, painless, superficial ulcers on oral mucosa, tongue, glans penis)
 ◊ Keratoderma blennorrhagica (hyperkeratotic skin lesions of palms and soles and around nails)
• Cardiovascular:
 ◊ Occasionally pericarditis, murmur, conduction defects, aortic incompetence
• Nervous system:
 ◊ Rarely peripheral neuropathy, cranial neuropathy, meningoencephalitis, neuropsychiatric changes
• Constitutional:
 ◊ Fever, malaise, anorexia, weight loss
 ◊ Can appear seriously ill (fever, rigors, tachycardia, exquisitely tender joints)

CAUSES
• *Chlamydia trachomatis* the usual causative organism of postvenereal variety
• Dysenteric form following enteric bacterial infection due to Shigella, Salmonella, Yersinia, and Campylobacter organisms. This form more likely in women, children and the elderly.

RISK FACTORS
• Sexual intercourse 7-14 days prior to illness
• Food poisoning or bacterial dysenteric outbreak

DIAGNOSIS

DIFFERENTIAL DIAGNOSIS
• For specific diagnosis, arthritis associated with urethritis for longer than one month
• Rheumatoid arthritis
• Ankylosing spondylitis
• Arthritis associated with inflammatory bowel disease
• Psoriatic arthritis
• Juvenile rheumatoid arthritis
• Bacterial arthritis including gonococcal

LABORATORY
• Blood
 ◊ WBC 10,000-20,000
 ◊ Neutrophilic leukocytosis
 ◊ Elevated erythrocyte sedimentation rate
 ◊ Moderate normochromic anemia
 ◊ Hypergammaglobulinemia
• Synovial fluid
 ◊ WBC 1000-8000 cells/mm3
 ◊ Bacterial culture negative
• Collaborative tests
 ◊ Cultures or serology positive for Chlamydia trachomatis, or stools positive for Salmonella, Shigella, Yersinia or Campylobacter support the diagnosis
Drugs that may alter lab results: Antibiotics may affect isolation of the bacterial pathogens
Disorders that may alter lab results: N/A

PATHOLOGICAL FINDINGS
• A seronegative spondyloarthropathy (similar to ankylosing spondylitis, enteric arthritis and psoriatic arthritis)
• Villous formation in joints
• Joint hyperemia
• Joint inflammation
• Prostatitis
• Seminal vesiculitis
• Skin biopsy similar to psoriasis
• Non-specific conjunctivitis

SPECIAL TESTS Histocompatibility antigen HLA-B27 positive in 60-80% of cases in non-HIV related Reiter's

IMAGING
• X-ray
 ◊ Periosteal proliferation, thickening
 ◊ Spurs
 ◊ Erosions at articular margins
 ◊ Residual joint destruction
 ◊ Syndesmophytes (spine)
 ◊ Sacroiliitis

DIAGNOSTIC PROCEDURES N/A

TREATMENT

APPROPRIATE HEALTH CARE
Inpatient possibly, during acute phase

GENERAL MEASURES
• Treatment is symptomatic
• No treatment necessary for conjunctivitis. Iritis may require treatment.
• Treatment unnecessary for mucocutaneous lesions
• Physical therapy during recovery phase
• Arthritis may be prominent and disabling during the acute phase

SURGICAL MEASURES N/A

ACTIVITY Bedrest until joint inflammation subsides

DIET No special diet

PATIENT EDUCATION
• Teach home physical therapy techniques
• For a listing of sources for patient education materials favorably reviewed on this topic, physicians may contact: American Academy of Family Physicians Foundation, P.O. Box 8418, Kansas City, MO 64114, (800)274-2237, ext. 4400
• Arthritis Foundation, 1314 Spring Street N.W., Atlanta, GA 30309, (404)872-7100

MEDICATIONS

DRUG(S) OF CHOICE
• Symptomatic management - NSAID's including indomethacin, naproxen; intraarticular or systemic corticosteroids for refractory arthritis and enthesitis
• Specific treatment of pathogenic microorganism should be attempted:
  ◊ C. trachomatis - doxycycline 100 mg po bid for 7-14 days
  ◊ Salmonella, Shigella, Yersinia Campylobacter infections - ciprofloxacin 500 mg po bid for 5 days (course may be extended to 14-28 days to eradicate chronic carrier state)
• For gastrointestinal upset - antacids
• For iritis - intraocular steroids
• For keratitis - topical steroids

Contraindications:
• Gastrointestinal bleeding
• Patients with peptic ulcer, gastritis, ulcerative colitis
• Renal insufficiency

Precautions: Refer to manufacturer's literature

Significant possible interactions: Refer to manufacturer's literature

ALTERNATIVE DRUGS
• Aspirin or other NSAID's
• Sulfasalazine is promising, but not yet approved
• Methotrexate or azathioprine in severe cases (still experimental and not approved or agreed to be effective. Contraindicated, if HIV related Reiter's).
• Consultation with specialist recommended when considering immunomodulatory agents such as sulfasalazine, methotrexate or azathioprine
• Role of antibiotics under investigation, maybe helpful in some cases

FOLLOWUP

PATIENT MONITORING
Monitor clinical response to medications. Surveillance for complications of therapy, sulfasalazine, immunosuppressives.

PREVENTION/AVOIDANCE N/A

POSSIBLE COMPLICATIONS
• Chronic or recurrent disease in 5-50%
• Ankylosing spondylitis develops in 30-50% of HLA-B27 positive patients
• Urethral strictures
• Cataracts and blindness
• Aortic root necrosis

EXPECTED COURSE/PROGNOSIS
• Urethritis within 1-15 days after sexual exposure
• Onset of Reiter's syndrome within 10-30 days of infection
• Mean duration 19 weeks
• Poor prognosis associated with local disease involving heel, eye or heart

MISCELLANEOUS

ASSOCIATED CONDITIONS
• Prior shigellosis
• Salmonellosis
• Yersinia infection
• Mycoplasma or ureaplasma infection
• Chlamydia urethritis
• HIV infection

AGE-RELATED FACTORS
Pediatric: Enteric etiology more likely than chlamydia
Geriatric: Enteric etiology more likely than sexually transmitted
Others: N/A

PREGNANCY
No special considerations other than usual precautions regarding drugs

SYNONYMS
• Idiopathic blennorrheal arthritis
• Arthritis urethritica
• Urethro-oculo-articular syndrome
• Fiessinger-Leroy-Reiter disease

ICD-9-CM 099.3 Reiter's disease

SEE ALSO
• Behçet's syndrome
• Ankylosing spondylitis
• Arthritis, psoriatic

OTHER NOTES
Effects of antibiotics on the development and long-term outcome of Reiter's syndrome not known

ABBREVIATIONS N/A

REFERENCES
• Kean WF, MacPherson DW: Reiter's syndrome. In: Bellamy N, ed. Prognosis in the Rheumatic Diseases. London, Kluwer Academic Publishers, 1991
• McCormack WM, Rein MF: Urethritis. In: Mandell GL, Douglas RG, Bennett JE, eds. Principles and Practice of Infectious Diseases. 4rd Ed. New York, Churchill Livingstone, 1995
• Hughes RA, Keat AC: Reiter's syndrome and reactive arthritis: A current view. Sem in Arthritis and Rheumatism 1994;24(3):190-210
Illustrations: 3 available on CD-ROM
Internet references: http://www.5mcc.com

Author(s)
D. W. MacPherson, MD, MSc (CTM), FRCPC

Renal calculi

BASICS

DESCRIPTION Condition related to the presence of stones in the urinary tract. Stones form in the proximal tract and migrate distally, commonly lodging at three points along the ureter:
• Ureteropelvic junction
• Pelvic brim, as ureter crosses the iliac vessels
• Ureterovesical junction
System(s) affected: Renal/Urologic
Genetics:
• Familial tendency
• Some cases of hypercalciuria-autosomal dominant metabolic defect
• Cystinuria-autosomal recessive metabolic defect of amino acid transport
Incidence/Prevalence in USA:
• 1-4/1000 annual incidence
• 5-12% lifetime incidence
• Higher incidence in the "stone belt" (southeastern USA)
• Recurrence rate - 50% in five years
Predominant age: 20-40
Predominant sex: Male > Female (3-4:1), except for struvite (infection) stones which are more common in females

SIGNS AND SYMPTOMS
• Renal colic
  ◊ Sudden onset
  ◊ Agonizing flank pain, waxing and waning
  ◊ Radiation to lower abdomen, groin, testicles, or labia
    ◊ Causes patient to be restless
• Tachycardia
• Diaphoresis
• Nausea, with or without vomiting
• Abdominal tenderness, on deep palpation
• Ileus
• Costovertebral angle tenderness
• Hematuria
• Urinary frequency
• Chills, fever, pyuria (if infection present)
• Asymptomatic stones may be found on abdominal radiograph done for other reasons

CAUSES
• Metabolic abnormalities (a patient may show more than one)
  ◊ Supersaturation of urine with stone-forming salts
    - Hypercalciuria (>300 mg/24hr): 40-60% of cases
    - Hyperuricosuria (>750 mg/24hr): 20-35% of cases
    - Hyperoxaluria (>40 mg/24hr): 10-20% of cases
    - Cystinuria (>250 mg/L): 1-2% of cases
  ◊ Reduced inhibitors of stone formation
    - Hypocitraturia (<320 mg/day): 10-40% of cases
    - Hypomagnesiuria
    - Abnormal nephrocalcin, or other glycoprotein defects (Tamm-Horsfall protein, glycosaminoglycan, uropontin, crystal matrix protein)
• Infection with urease-producing organisms (mostly Proteus): 10-20% of cases
• Alterations in urinary pH
  ◊ pH<5.5 leads to uric acid stones
  ◊ pH>7.5 seen with struvite stones

RISK FACTORS
• Low urine output (<1100 ml/24hr)
• Strenuous work
• Dehydration
• Diet high in protein, oxalate, salt
• Medications
  ◊ Antacids
  ◊ Vitamins A, C, D
  ◊ Triamterene
  ◊ Ritonavir
  ◊ Some sulfa drugs
  ◊ Carbonic anhydrase inhibitors
  ◊ Some anti-epileptic drugs
  ◊ Corticosteroids
  ◊ Acetazolamide
• Immobility
• Weightlessness (as in space travel)

DIAGNOSIS

DIFFERENTIAL DIAGNOSIS
• Acute abdomen
• Acute lumbosacral strain, ruptured lumbar disc
• Aortic aneurysm
• Endometriosis
• Gastroenteritis
• Malingering or drug seeking behavior
• Pancreatitis
• Peptic ulcer disease
• Pyelonephritis or perinephric abscess
• Salpingitis
• Ureteral clot or sloughed papilla (secondary to diabetes, infection, analgesic abuse)

LABORATORY
• CBC
• Urinalysis
  ◊ Hematuria
  ◊ Crystals
  ◊ pH
  ◊ Pyuria, bacteruria
• Urine culture, if indicated
• Chemistry profile
• Parathyroid hormone, if calcium elevated
• For patients with recurrent episode (4 to 8 weeks after acute episode):
  ◊ 24 hour urine collection for volume, calcium, creatinine, uric acid, oxalate, citrate, sodium, magnesium
  ◊ If abnormal, consider repeating same tests on 24 hour urine after one week of dietary restrictions
Drugs that may alter lab results:
Allopurinol, diuretics, pyridium
Disorders that may alter lab results:
Other underlying infections, renal abnormalities

PATHOLOGIC FINDINGS
• Stone analysis:
  ◊ Calcium oxalate: 36-70%
  ◊ Calcium phosphate: 6-20%
  ◊ Mixed calcium stones: 11-31%
  ◊ Uric acid: 6-17%
  ◊ Struvite ("triple phosphate" or "infection") stone: 6-20%
  ◊ Cystine: 0.5-3%

SPECIAL TESTS Nitroprusside test on urine if cystinuria suspected

IMAGING
• Plain film of abdomen (KUB): 80-90% of stones are at least partially radiopaque
• IVP
• Ultrasound, especially if allergic to contrast dye
• CT scan

DIAGNOSTIC PROCEDURES Antegrade or retrograde pyelogram-rarely needed except in possible case of allergy to contrast dye

TREATMENT

APPROPRIATE HEALTH CARE
• Outpatient management possible for 80-90%
• Inpatient management and urology consult if:
  ◊ Intractable pain, nausea, or vomiting
  ◊ Signs of infection
  ◊ Imaging studies show non-functioning kidney, solitary or horseshoe kidney, or urine extravasation
  ◊ Stone larger than 6 mm

GENERAL MEASURES
• Pain control
• Hydration (2-3 L/day)
• Strain urine to recover the stone

SURGICAL MEASURES
• Cystoscopy with basket extraction or laser lithotripsy
• Extracorporeal shock wave lithotripsy
• Percutaneous lithotripsy or nephrolithotomy
• Open removal-required in less than 5% of patients

ACTIVITY As tolerated

DIET
• During acute episode-push fluids
• To reduce likelihood of recurrence:
  ◊ Fluid intake of 2 L/day (eight 8 ounce glasses/day besides meals)
  ◊ Moderate protein intake (60 gm/day)
  ◊ Moderate salt intake (3-4 gm/day)
  ◊ Avoid foods high in oxalate (spinach, rhubarb, beans, peanuts, tea, chocolate, cola)
  ◊ Avoid excess vitamin C (intake should be <1000mg/day total)
  ◊ Significant restriction of calcium intake is not recommended (1000-1500 mg/day probably reasonable)
  ◊ For cystine stones, reduce methionine in diet

PATIENT EDUCATION
• Instruction in straining urine
• Fluid and dietary instruction

MEDICATIONS

DRUG(S) OF CHOICE
• Acute therapy:
◊ Oral NSAID's (ibuprofen 600-800 mg tid)
◊ Oral narcotics (acetaminophen-codeine, acetaminophen-hydrocodone, acetaminophen-oxycodone)
◊ Oral indomethacin 50 mg qid (also available as a suppository)
◊ Injectable meperidine 50-100 mg or morphine 10-15 mg q3-4h
• Maintenance therapy:
◊ Calcium stones: hydrochlorothiazide (HCTZ) 25-50 mg/day or bid (consider potassium citrate 20 mEq bid or amiloride 5-10 mg/day to avoid low potassium); indapamide 2.5 mg/day; neutral phosphate 500 mg tid or qid with meals
◊ Uric acid stones: potassium citrate 20 mEq bid to maintain urine pH 6-7; allopurinol 300 mg/day
◊ Cystine stones: potassium citrate titrated to achieve urine pH>7.5; tiopronin 200-500 mg bid; penicillamine (d-penicillamine) 1-2 gm/day
◊ Struvite stones: antibiotics for 3 to 4 months after removal of stone; acetohydroxamic acid 250 mg tid or qid
Contraindications: Renal failure - neutral phosphate, d-penicillamine; pregnancy, lactation- tiopronin, d-penicillamine, acetohydydroxamic acid; medication allergy
Precautions: Monitor CBC, liver and renal function with tiopronin, d-penicillamine; monitor CBC, renal function with acetohydroxamic acid
Significant possible interactions: See manufacturer's profile of each drug

ALTERNATIVE DRUGS
Ketorolac po, IM or IV for pain (short term use only)

FOLLOWUP

PATIENT MONITORING
• Acute episode:
◊ Signs of infection
◊ Repeat KUB radiograph or ultrasound every 1-2 weeks
◊ Consider urologic referral if not resolved in 2-4 weeks
◊ Strain urine until stone passed

PREVENTION/AVOIDANCE
• Recurrent stones:
◊ Fluid intake to maintain urine output >2L/day
◊ Dietary compliance
◊ Struvite stones: periodic culture to confirm sterile urine

POSSIBLE COMPLICATIONS
• Hydronephrosis
• Infection/sepsis
• Renal impairment, especially in struvite stones (most "malignant" of the stones)
• Related to ESWL:
◊ Skin bruising
◊ Perinephric hematoma
◊ Hematuria
◊ Hypertension (possibly)

EXPECTED COURSE/PROGNOSIS
• Overall, 80-90% of stones pass spontaneously
◊ 50% of 6-10 mm stones pass
◊ Most stones >10 mm require surgical removal
• Recurrence - 50% in 5 years

MISCELLANEOUS

ASSOCIATED CONDITIONS
• Crohn's disease
• Gout
• Jejunoileal bypass, ileostomy, ileal conduit
• Laxative abuse
• Medullary sponge kidney
• Milk-alkali syndrome
• Myeloproliferative disorder
• Paraplegia/neurogenic bladder
• Primary hyperparathyroidism
• Renal tubular acidosis (type I)
• Sarcoidosis

AGE-RELATED FACTORS
Pediatric: Rare; consider inborn error of metabolism
Geriatric: N/A
Other: N/A

PREGNANCY
Consider urologic referral

SYNONYMS
• Nephrolithiasis
• Kidney stone

ICD-9-CM
592.0 Calculus of kidney

SEE ALSO
• Urolithiasis

OTHER NOTES
Black males have fewer stones than white males (approximately 1:3)

ABBREVIATIONS
CBC = complete blood count
KUB = kidney, ureter, bladder
IVP = intravenous pyelogram
CT = computerized tomography
NSAID = nonsteroidal anti-inflammatory drug
HCTZ = hydrochlorthiazide
ESWL = extra-corporeal shock wave lithotripsy

REFERENCES
• Pak CYC. Kidney stones. Lancet 1998;351:1797-1800
• Saklayen MG. Medical management of nephrolithiasis. Med Clin N Am 1997;81(3):785-99
• Trivedi BK. Nephrolithiasis. Post Grad Med 1996;100(6):63-78
• Wasserstein AG. Nephrolithiasis: acute management and prevention. Dis Mon 1998;44(5):196-213
Illustrations: N/A
Internet references: http://www.5mcc.com

Author(s)
Rich Londo, MD

Renal cell adenocarcinoma

BASICS

DESCRIPTION The most common solid renal neoplasm, renal cell adenocarcinoma, represents 2-3% of all adult malignancies; 9th most common male malignant tumor, 13th most common female malignant tumor. Characterized by obscure and varied presentations including paraneoplastic syndromes, vascular findings, and uncommon metastatic sites. Paraneoplastic and vascular syndromes do not indicate incurability or unresectability. Early, aggressive surgical management provides the best opportunity for cure.

System(s) affected: Renal/Urologic

Genetics:
- Oncogenes localized to the short arm of chromosome 3 may have etiologic implications. Chromosome 3p12-p26 are specific for clear cell RCC; 4% of RCC is familial.
- People with HLA antigen types Bw44 and DR8 are prone to develop renal cancer. These are rare familial renal carcinomas.

Incidence/Prevalence in USA:
- 30,000 new cases per year (1996); 12,000 deaths per year
- Men: 9.6/100,000
- Women: 4.2/100,000

Predominant age: 5th and 6th decades

Predominant sex: Male > Female (2:1)

SIGNS AND SYMPTOMS
- Solid renal masses, most 6-7 cm (incidentally discovered in asymptomatic patient due to increased use of CT and MRI)
- Hematuria 50-60%
- Elevated erythrocyte sedimentation rate 50-60%
- Abdominal mass 24-45%
- Anemia 21-41%
- Flank pain 35-40%
- Hypertension 22-38%
- Weight loss 28-36%
- Pyrexia 7-17%
- Hepatic dysfunction 10-15%
- Classic triad (hematuria, abdominal mass, flank pain) 7-10%
- Hypercalcemia 3-6%
- Erythrocytosis 3-4%
- Varicocele 2-3%
- Patients with vena caval thrombus present with lower extremity edema, new varicocele, dilated superficial abdominal veins, albuminuria, pulmonary emboli, right atrial mass or non-function of the involved kidney

CAUSES Unknown

RISK FACTORS
- Smoking
- Obesity
- Urban environment
- Cadmium
- Asbestos
- Petroleum by-products
- Herpes simplex virus exposure
- Phenacetin or analgesic abuse for transitional cell of the renal pelvis

DIAGNOSIS

DIFFERENTIAL DIAGNOSIS
- Hydronephrosis
- Polycystic kidneys
- Renal tuberculosis
- Renal calculi
- Renal infarction
- Benign renal cyst
- Transitional cell carcinoma (rare)

LABORATORY
- Anemia (21-41% of patients)
- Polycythemia
- Hematuria
- Alkaline phosphate may be elevated
- Increased erythrocyte sedimentation rate
- Urine - neoplastic cells
- Hypercalcemia
- Increased renin
- Transitional cell cancer (rare)

Drugs that may alter lab results: N/A

Disorders that may alter lab results: N/A

PATHOLOGICAL FINDINGS
- Renal cell tends to bulge out from the cortex producing a mass effect
- 48% of renal cell carcinomas measure < 5 cm and is grossly yellow to yellow/orange due to its high lipid content in the clear cell variety. Average renal cell size has been decreasing due to incidental discovery.
- The granuloma cell type more likely gray to white
- Small tumors are homogenous
- Large tumors may have areas of necrosis and hemorrhage
- A pseudocapsule covers some tumors
- Tumor thrombi into the vena cava generally do not invade the vena caval wall
- Microscopically there is a mixture of clear granular and occasionally sarcomatoid cells

SPECIAL TESTS
- Arteriography (rarely needed) - for tumors larger than 10 cm, it may identify parasitic capsular vessels for early control
- Cystoscopy - to rule out bladder cancer
- ECG as needed

IMAGING
- Intravenous pyelography with infusion nephrotomography remains the primary screening test for renal malignancy
- Ultrasonography - if there appears to be a mass on IVP, confirms the presence of a lesion and determines whether it is solid or cystic. Cystic lesions may either be observed or subjected to percutaneous cyst puncture.
- CT scan and, occasionally, arteriography - if solid or complex masses upon ultrasonography require further evaluation. 3% of RCC are bilateral by CT scan. The most common alteration with RCC is deletion of chromosome 3p. Recent evidence implicates gene p53 on chromosome 17p13.1 to be critical in renal cell carcinogenesis.

- Rapid sequence CT can demonstrate tumor enhancement
- MRI has not been shown to be superior to CT for tumors smaller than 8 cm, for larger tumors it may have advantage in delineating the vena cava
- Bone scans are indicated if the alkaline phosphatase is elevated or the patient has bone pain
- Brain CT is indicated if the patient has neurologic symptoms

DIAGNOSTIC PROCEDURES
- Simple cyst need not be aspirated unless painful
- Calcified cysts may contain renal cell cancer and therefore require open renal biopsy of the wall of the cyst or partial nephrectomy
- Hemorrhagic cyst - aspiration cytology may be helpful but needle biopsy of solid masses is to be discouraged, particularly if the patient has a normal contralateral kidney
- In solitary kidneys, open renal biopsy with wedge resection (not enucleation) can be performed if mass is ≤ 4 cm
- Doppler flow ultrasound of the renal veins or CT (thin cuts) that shows the renal vein entering the vena cava can be used to rule out tumor thrombus
- Venogram - when tumor thrombus is identified. The venogram can demonstrate when the thrombus goes above the hepatic veins or diaphragm (i.e., rarely cardiopulmonary bypass needed to remove the thrombus above the diaphragm at the time of nephrectomy).

TREATMENT

APPROPRIATE HEALTH CARE
Inpatient

GENERAL MEASURES N/A

SURGICAL MEASURES
- Surgery is indicated. Cytotoxic drug therapy has been only erratically effective. Lesions are fairly radiation resistant.
- Maintain hydration during iodine injection diagnostic studies to prevent acute tubular necrosis
- Consider a mechanical bowel preparation to ease the nephrectomy
- Consider antibiotic bowel preparation for larger tumors (> 10 cm) where possible bowel injury or resection may be more likely
- Exploration wedge resection for solitary kidney or tumors less than 4 cm, otherwise radical nephrectomy in the face of a normal contralateral kidney is preferred
- Usual preoperative pulmonary toilet, pulmonary function tests if indicated
- Renal cell carcinoma (85% of renal parenchymal malignant tumors) - CT solid mass larger than 3 cm, radical nephrectomy if there is a normal contralateral kidney; smaller than 3 cm, wedge resection. Intraoperative Doppler ultrasound is undergoing study to determine the optimum partial nephrectomy approach to small tumors. Laparoscopy nephrectomy is still investigational.

• Angiomyolipoma (80% of tuberous sclerosis patients have these benign tumors) - classic CT findings, may be followed with CT
• Hemorrhage into a cyst - aspiration cytology
• Complex cyst (calcified cyst wall or irregular wall) - open cyst wall biopsy if cytology is inconclusive
• Transitional cell carcinoma of the renal pelvis or calyces - nephroureterectomy
• Oncocytoma - larger than 3 cm, radical nephrectomy
• Sarcoma - wide excision
• Adult Wilms' tumor - radical nephrectomy for unilateral disease
• Metastasis (lymphoma > lung > breast > stomach) - depends on prognosis of primary tumor; nephrectomy for uncontrolled bleeding
• Cortical adenoma smaller than 3 cm (7-22% at autopsy) - wedge resection

ACTIVITY
• No special preoperative activity
• Postoperatively - as tolerated; full activity in 8 weeks

DIET Low protein diet for patients with proteinuria

PATIENT EDUCATION
• Preoperative nursing education is indicated for pulmonary toilet
• Pre-anesthesia education is needed if the patient is to have a patient controlled analgesia pump or epidural catheter for postoperative pain relief
• Printed patient information available from: National Kidney & Urologic Diseases Information Clearinghouse, Box NKUDIC, Bethesda, MD 20893, (301)468-6345

MEDICATIONS

DRUG(S) OF CHOICE
• For advanced renal cell carcinoma - interleukin-2 (IL-2) plus lymphokine-activated killer (LAK), or IL-2 alone, includes 4% complete responders and 11% partial responders. Dose schedules are under study.
Contraindications: N/A
Precautions: IUL monitoring for IL-2
Significant possible interactions: IL-2 associated with capillary leak syndrome (CLS)

ALTERNATIVE DRUGS
• Hormones - progesterone agents yield a 5-10% response rate
• Chemotherapy - vinblastine alone or with lomustine (CCNU) yields a 10-15% response rate

FOLLOWUP

PATIENT MONITORING
• One CT scan of the abdomen and renal fossa can be done 3-6 months later, particularly if the capsule or lymph nodes are positive, to monitor recurrences and repeat resection if needed for flank pain or mass
• For partial nephrectomy - renal ultrasound every 6 months for 3 years, then annually
• Chest x-rays to rule out pulmonary metastasis are performed quarterly for 2 years, then less often
• Skeletal x-rays and bone scan can be useful in detecting skeletal metastasis but should only be obtained if patient complains of bone pain or an alkaline phosphatase elevation
• Postoperative followup may be possible with plasma transcobalamin II or serum haptoglobin level to detect or monitor recurrences

PREVENTION/AVOIDANCE
• Do not smoke
• Eat a sensible diet
• Avoid stress, asbestos, cadmium, and petroleum distillates

POSSIBLE COMPLICATIONS
• Paraplegia can result with little warning from spinal vertebral metastasis
• CNS metastasis are not uncommon
• Approximately 30% of patients with RCC have metastatic disease when the diagnosis is established. The most common sites of metastasis are the lung (50-60%), bone (30-40%), regional nodes (15-30%), brain (10%) and adjacent organs (10%).

EXPECTED COURSE/PROGNOSIS
---STAGING---

		Robson's staging	5 year survival
Small tumor		I	60-70%
Large tumor		I	60-70%
Perinephric fat		II	50-65%
Renal vein		IIIa	50-60%
IVC involvement†		IIIa	5-35%
Adjacent structure		IVa	0-5%
Single node		IIIb	35%
Multiple node		III	5-35%
Fixed nodes		IIIb	5%
Distant metastases		IVb	0-5%

		TNM staging	5 year survival
Small tumor		T1	60-70%
Large tumor		T2	60-70%
Perinephric fat		T3	50-65%
Renal vein		T3b	50-60%
IVC involvement†		T3c	5-35%
Adjacent structure		T4a	0-5%
Single node		N1	35%
Multiple node		N2	5-35%
Fixed nodes		N3	5%
Distant metastases		M1	0-5%

†Infradiaphragmatic vena caval

MISCELLANEOUS

ASSOCIATED CONDITIONS
• Von Hippel-Lindau disease (30-45% of these patients develop renal cell)
• Adult polycystic kidney disease
• Horseshoe kidney
• Acquired renal cystic disease from chronic renal failure

AGE-RELATED FACTORS
Pediatric: Extremely rare in children
Geriatric: Most commonly presents in the 5th and 6th decade
Others: N/A

PREGNANCY N/A

SYNONYMS
• Kidney cancer
• Hypernephroma
• Grawitz's tumor
• Hypernephroid cancer

ICD-9-CM 189.0 Malignant neoplasm of the kidney

SEE ALSO N/A

OTHER NOTES N/A

ABBREVIATIONS
• RCC = renal cell carcinoma
• IVC = inferior vena cava

REFERENCES
• Resnick MY: Current Therapy in Genitourinary Surgery. 2nd Ed. St. Louis, Mosby-Year Book Publishers, 1992
• Novick AC, Streem SB, et al: Conservative surgery for renal cell carcinoma; A single center experience with 100 patients. J Urol 1989;141:835
• Issac W: Molecular diagnosis of RCC. AUA Today, Dec, 1994
• Novick AC: Partial nephrectomy gaining wider acceptance as alternative treatment in surgery for RCC. The Kidney Cancer Jour 1994;1(2)
• Seminars in Urologic Oncology 1996;14(4):208-215/230-243
• Riglin RA. Renal cell carcinoma: management of advanced disease. J Urol 1999 Feb;161(2):381-6; discussion 386-7
4 additional references available at web site
Internet references: http://www.5mcc.com
Illustrations: N/A

Author(s)
Mark R. Dambro, MD, FAAFP

Renal failure, acute (ARF)

BASICS

DESCRIPTION A syndrome of rapidly deteriorating kidney function with the accumulation of nitrogenous wastes
System(s) affected: Renal/Urologic, Cardiovascular
Genetics: No known genetic pattern
Incidence/Prevalence in USA: 5% of patients admitted to the hospital develop ARF; 10-15% of ICU patients develop ARF; 2-7% post open heart patients develop ARF; 50% of hospital ARF is iatrogenic.
Predominant age: All ages (average age increasing)
Predominant sex: Male = Female

SIGNS AND SYMPTOMS
- Anorexia
- Asterixis
- Back pain
- Coma
- Delirium
- Diarrhea
- Dyspnea
- Ecchymosis
- Edema
- Encephalopathy
- Epistaxis
- Fasciculation
- Fatigue
- GI hemorrhage
- Headache
- Hiccups
- Hyperpnea
- Hypertension
- Left ventricular failure
- Lethargy
- Muscle cramps
- Myoclonus
- Nausea
- Oliguria
- Pericarditis
- Petechiae
- Purpura (vasculitis)
- Rales
- Rash (acute interstitial nephritis)
- Retinopathy
- Seizure
- Somnolence
- Tachycardia
- Tachypnea
- Uriniferous odor
- Vomiting
- Weakness
- Xerostomia

CAUSES
- Pre-renal (30-60% of all cases)
  ◊ Hypovolemia
  ◊ Ineffective circulating volume: Congestive heart failure, cirrhosis, nephrotic syndrome and early sepsis
- Renal
  ◊ Tubular, interstitial: Acute interstitial nephritis (AIN) (drugs, infection); nephrotoxins; acute tubular necrosis; reflex anuria; contrast media (40-70% of all cases)
  ◊ Glomerular: Rapidly progressive (crescentic) glomerulonephritis (RPGN) (Immunofluorescence biopsy staining: linear, immune complex or pauci-immune); pregnancy (2%); systemic lupus erythematosus
- Vascular
  ◊ Ischemic nephropathy (renal artery stenosis)
    ◊ Dissecting aortic aneurysm
    ◊ Ruptured abdominal aortic aneurysm
- Post-renal
  ◊ Obstruction (See topic for Hydronephrosis) (1-10% of all cases)

RISK FACTORS
- Surgery (especially with increased age, elevated creatinine, simultaneous cardiac valve and bypass surgery)
- Volume depletion (especially in diabetes)
- Aminoglycoside therapy, congestive heart failure, contrast exposure, septic shock
- Nephrotoxic drugs (e.g., ACE inhibitors in renal artery stenosis)
- Rhabdomyolysis
- Administration of contrast (parenteral) in susceptible individuals
- Dopamine and mannitol appear to increase the risk of acute renal failure in some groups; particularly patients with diabetes mellitus.

DIAGNOSIS

DIFFERENTIAL DIAGNOSIS See causes

LABORATORY
- Urinalysis
  ◊ Proteinuria
  ◊ Hematuria
  ◊ Brown granular urinary casts
  ◊ Urinary renal tubular epithelial cells
- Urine sediment
  ◊ Coarse granular casts
  ◊ Renal tubular epithelial cells
  ◊ Eosinophils (AIN?)
  ◊ Red cell or hemoglobin casts (RPGN)
  ◊ Crystals (lithiasis, obstruction)
- Urine electrolytes/osmolality
  ◊ Increased urine sodium (> 20 mEq/L [>20 mmol/L]), increased fractional excretion of sodium (> 3%) (e.g., renal).
  Calculation: Fractional excretion of sodium = [(urine Na+/serum Na+) / (urine creatinine/serum creatinine)] X 100
  ◊ Urine isotonic to plasma
  ◊ Low urine sodium (< 10 mEq/L), low fractional excretion of sodium (≤ 1%), concentrate urine osmolality (≥ 500 mOsm/liter) (e.g., pre-renal)
- Other
  ◊ Azotemia
  ◊ Decreased creatinine clearance
  ◊ Hyperosmolarity
  ◊ Hyperphosphatemia
  ◊ Hyperkalemia
  ◊ Decreased serum bicarbonate
  ◊ Increased plasma volume
  ◊ Decreased hemoglobin
  ◊ Decreased hematocrit
  ◊ Hypocapnia
  ◊ Increased serum magnesium
  ◊ Acidemia (increased anion gap)
  ◊ Increased serum amylase/lipase
  ◊ Hyponatremia
  ◊ Hypocalcemia
  ◊ Increased serum uric acid
  ◊ Increased bleeding time
  ◊ Impaired phagocytic function
Drugs that may alter lab results: Too many to list
Disorders that may alter lab results: Too many to list

PATHOLOGICAL FINDINGS
- Kidney biopsy:
  ◊ Not particularly helpful in acute tubular necrosis (ATN)
  ◊ Diagnostic in AIN and RPGN
  ◊ In acute ischemic or toxic injury, necrosis or apoptosis of renal tubular cells

SPECIAL TESTS
- Angiogram (renal vascular disease)
- Cystoscopy - retrograde
- Bleeding time

IMAGING
- Obstruction - renal scan, CT scan
- Kidney ultrasound
  ◊ Renal cause: "Medical" renal disease (renal echogenicity = liver), normal size kidneys, kidney size disparity: ischemia
  ◊ Post renal cause - hydronephrosis

DIAGNOSTIC PROCEDURES Renal biopsy (ARF, unknown cause), diagnostic for AIN, RPGN

TREATMENT

APPROPRIATE HEALTH CARE
Inpatient and intensive care

GENERAL MEASURES
- Correction of underlying hemodynamic abnormalities, especially volume
- Hemodialysis as soon as diagnosis of uremia is established (or continuous renal replacement therapy). The use of biocompatible membranes (e.g., polymethyl methylacrylate) as opposed to cuprophane results in a higher rate of recovery of renal function, more rapid recovery and better patient survival.
- Decrease catabolism
- Convert oliguria to nonoliguria
- Daily weight
- Correct reversible causes (volume and mannitol)
- Modify dosages of renal excreted drugs (see under Medications - Precautions)
- If drug induced, discontinue offending agent
- Meticulous aseptic technique
- Continuous arteriovenous hemofiltration
- Intravenous human immunoglobulin G
- Correct easy bleeding with DDAVP, estrogen and cryoprecipitate
- Question prednisone in AIN
- Hyperkalemia - severe (1 amp Ca gluconate IV); other IV insulin + glucose, if acidosis also present (1 amp NaHCO3) Kayexalate po 15-60 gm/day if gastrointestinal tract functions
- Mannitol - alkaline diuresis in rhabdomyolysis

Renal failure, acute (ARF)

SURGICAL MEASURES N/A

ACTIVITY As tolerated

DIET
• Restrict fluids to volume of urine output plus 500 mL/day
• Eliminate potassium if serum level increased
• Oral and IV amino acids
• Increase carbohydrates to decrease catabolism
• Alimentation to decrease catabolism

PATIENT EDUCATION
National Kidney & Urologic Diseases Information Clearinghouse, Box NKUDIC, Bethesda, MD 20893, (301)468-6345 and The National Kidney Foundation, Inc., 30 East 33rd Street, NY, NY 10016. "What Everyone Should Know About Kidneys and Kidney Disease" (Order #01-01BP - English), (Order #01-02BP -Spanish).

MEDICATIONS

DRUG(S) OF CHOICE Prior to fixed renal failure: IV volume expansion with normal saline followed by mannitol, furosemide (Lasix), and calcium channel blockers. Low dose dopamine has not been shown to have a beneficial effect on survival. Volume expansion alone is beneficial in contrast injury. Dopamine-1 selective agonists may have promise for future treatment.
Contraindications: N/A
Precautions:
• Pharmacokinetics of all drugs used during renal failure should be reviewed for appropriate adjustment. For example, antiarrhythmic drugs:
◊ Quinidine: decrease dose, closely monitor drug level
◊ Procainamide: avoid in renal failure
◊ Disopyramide: reduction in maintenance dose
◊ Mexiletine: no dose adjustment-liver metabolized, etc.
Significant possible interactions:
Nonsteroidals plus other nephrotoxic drugs, male gender, increasing age, cardiovascular comorbidity and recent hospitalization are synergistic in causing ARF

ALTERNATIVE DRUGS N/A

FOLLOWUP

PATIENT MONITORING As needed

PREVENTION/AVOIDANCE
• See risk factors
• Allopurinol prior to chemotherapy for hematologic malignancy
• Hydration most important, especially prior to contrast and chemotherapy
• Non biocompatible membranes
• Hypotension

POSSIBLE COMPLICATIONS
• Sepsis - infection (leading cause of mortality)
• Convulsions
• Edema
• Pulmonary edema
• Congestive heart failure
• Hyperkalemia
• Paralysis
• Arrhythmias
• Death (50%)
• Pericarditis/tamponade
• Uremia
• Bleeding
• Hypotension

EXPECTED COURSE/PROGNOSIS
Recover usually in days to 6 weeks. High mortality rate (5-80%) depending on cause/multi-organ involvement, and age.

MISCELLANEOUS

ASSOCIATED CONDITIONS
• Hyperphosphatemia
• Hydronephrosis
• Muscle injury
• Congestive heart failure
• Cirrhosis
• Malignant hypertension
• Vasculitis
• Bacterial infections
• Drug reactions
• Hypercalcemia
• Hyperuricemia
• Sepsis
• Severe trauma
• Burns
• Transfusion reactions
• Internal bleeding

AGE-RELATED FACTORS
Pediatric: Congenital
Geriatric: Greater occurrence in this age group especially after surgery
Others: N/A

PREGNANCY
• Infected uterus (e.g., C. welchii [C. perfringens])
• Toxemia and a related obstetric complication
• Cortical necrosis
• Postpartum renal failure

SYNONYMS N/A

ICD-9-CM
584.9 acute renal failure unspecified

SEE ALSO
• Multiple myeloma
• Hepatorenal syndrome
• Reye's syndrome
• Rocky Mountain spotted fever
• Hydronephrosis
• Renal failure, chronic
• Rhabdomyolysis
• Glomerulonephritis, rapidly progressive

OTHER NOTES N/A

ABBREVIATIONS
• ATN = acute tubular necrosis
• AIN = acute interstitial nephritis
• RPGN = rapidly progressive glomerulonephritis
• ACE = angiotensin converting enzyme

REFERENCES
• Humes HD: Acute renal failure - the promise of new therapies. N Engl J Med 1997;336:870871
• Klahr S, Miller SB: Acute oliguria. NEJM 1998;338:671-675
• Alkhunaizi AM, Schrier RW: Management of acute renal failure: new perspectives. Am J Kid Dis 1996;28:315-328
• Thadoni R, Pascual M, Bonventre JV: Acute renal failure. N Engl J Med 1996;334:1448-1460
• Gutthann SP, Rodriguez LAG, Raiford DS, et al: Nonsteroidal drugs and the risk of hospitalization. Arch Int Med 1996;156:2433-2439
• Nolon CR, Anderson RJ: Hospital-acquired acute renal failure. J Am Soc Nephrol 1998;9:710-718
• Rao TK: Acute rnal failure syndromes in human immunodeficiency virus infection. Semin in Nephrol 1998;18(4):378-395
• Nissenson AR: Acute renal failure: definition and pathogenesis. Kid Intl 1998;53(suppl66):s7-s10
• Andreussi VE, Fuiano G, Stanziale P, et al: Role of renal biopsy in the diagnosis and prognosis of acute renal failure. Kid Intl 1998;53(suppl66):s91-s95
Illustrations: N/A
Internet references: http://www.5mcc.com

Author(s)
Michael Youtsey, MD
Gregory W. Rutecki, MD

Renal failure, chronic

BASICS

DESCRIPTION The result of any renal injury that decreases renal excretory and regulatory function chronically. Characteristic findings: nitrogen retention, acidosis, and anemia.

System(s) affected: Renal/Urologic, Hemic/Lymphatic/Immunologic, Endocrine/Metabolic

Genetics:
• Compared to the general population, African Americans are 3.9 x more likely to have ESRD (irreversible, dialysis dependent renal failure) and 6.7 x more likely to have hypertensive ESRD
• Hereditary renal diseases can lead to chronic renal failure in children and some adults (Alport's syndrome, autosomal recessive polycystic kidney disease)
• Autosomal dominant polycystic kidney disease is a relatively common cause of chronic renal failure in adults affecting approximately 10% of dialysis population. Inherited in an autosomal dominant pattern with mutation on short arm chromosome 16.

Incidence/Prevalence in USA:
• Common (estimated that 160,000 persons per year are treated for end stage renal disease). Prevalence in the USA: 2.8/100,000 people in USA (estimate) with a chronic elevation of creatinine greater than 2.0 mg/dL (176.8 µmol/L). ESRD (end stage renal disease) experienced an annual growth rate of 8.8% from 1982 to 1991.
• By the end of the decade, HIV-associated nephropathy will be the 3rd leading cause of ESRD in African Americans ages 20-64

Predominant age: All ages - much more common in adults. In children, chronic renal failure affects between 2 and 6 per 1 million population. The elderly represent 33,8% of new patients with ESRD from 1988-1991.

Predominant sex: Male = Female

SIGNS AND SYMPTOMS
• Anemia (normochromic, normocytic)
• Anorexia
• Confusion (late sign)
• Emotional lability
• Encephalopathy
• Endocrine dysfunction (thyroid, pituitary)
• Fatigue on slight exertion
• Hypertension
• Insomnia
• Intractable hiccups
• Lassitude
• Mental depression
• Metallic taste in mouth
• Muscle cramps
• Muscle twitching
• Nausea
• Neuropathy
• Nocturia
• Pallor
• Polyuria
• Pruritus
• Seizures (late sign)
• Serositis
• Skin dry
• Stomatitis
• Slight breathlessness
• Vomiting

CAUSES
• Renal parenchymal: Glomerular: membranous nephropathy, membrano-proliferative glomerulonephritis, systemic lupus erythematosus, focal glomerulosclerosis, diabetes mellitus, proliferative glomerulonephritis, amyloidosis, Alport's syndrome, connective tissue disease.
• Interstitial-tubular: Heavy metals, drugs, nephrotoxins, multiple myeloma, hypertension, gout(?), thrombotic microangiopathies, oxalate deposition, infection, renal artery stenosis or ischemic stenosis, connective tissue disease, autosomal dominant polycystic kidney disease, congenital.
• Post-renal: See hydronephrosis causes
• Pre-renal: Cirrhosis, cardiac, volume, nephrotic, drugs (e.g., NSAID's)

RISK FACTORS
• Contrast (diabetes, myeloma)
• Circulatory failure
• Urinary tract obstruction
• Analgesic abuse
• Untreated hypertension
• Diabetes mellitus
• The greater the proteinuria, the quicker the progression of CRF
• Cigarette smoking

DIAGNOSIS

DIFFERENTIAL DIAGNOSIS See causes

LABORATORY
• Blood:
  ◊ Smear - normochromic, normocytic anemia
  ◊ Decreased immune responsiveness
  ◊ Thrombocytopenia
  ◊ Decreased hematocrit
  ◊ Increased capillary fragility
  ◊ Increased bleeding time
• Chemistry:
  ◊ Azotemia
  ◊ Elevated ammonia
  ◊ Type IV hyperlipidemia
  ◊ Decreased active Vitamin D
  ◊ Increased parathyroid hormone
  ◊ Elevated glucose, insulin resistance
  ◊ Elevated phosphate
  ◊ Elevated potassium
  ◊ Elevated sulfate
  ◊ Elevated uric acid
  ◊ Reduced calcium
  ◊ Serum CO2 content - 15-20 mEq/L (15-20 mmol/L)
• Urine
  ◊ Proteinuria
  ◊ Casts

Drugs that may alter lab results:
• Cimetidine
• Trimethoprim
• Cefazolin: increase creatinine

Disorders that may alter lab results:
Ketosis may artificially raise creatinine

PATHOLOGICAL FINDINGS
• Kidney biopsy
• Glomerulonephritis
• Interstitial nephritis

SPECIAL TESTS
• 24 hour urine studies (protein, clearance)
• Glofil clearance
• Complement studies
• Antinuclear antibody
• Serum protein electrophoresis
• Urine immune electrophoresis
• Hepatitis B surface antigen

IMAGING
• Ultrasound - shows decreased kidney size, may show obstructed ureter and bladder outlet (diabetic kidneys and ADPKD kidneys are not small)
• CT scan

DIAGNOSTIC PROCEDURES Kidney biopsy

TREATMENT

APPROPRIATE HEALTH CARE
Inpatient or outpatient depending on severity

GENERAL MEASURES
• Treat any aggravating cause aggressively (salt and water depletion, nephrotoxins, congestive heart failure, infection, hypercalcemia, urinary obstruction)
• Drugs may exacerbate chronic renal failure
• Pay careful attention to dosing, and avoid use of nephrotoxic agents. When possible, treat anemia with erythropoietin (HCT ≤ 30%).
• Dialysis: hemo, peritoneal, transplant
• Vitamin D (active) and calcium supplements (dihydrotachysterol 0.2-0.4 mg q day); calcium acetate tablets with meals tid
• Strict control of blood pressure. For patients with proteinuria > 1 gm/d ≤ 125/75; < 1 gm/d 130/80. ACE inhibitors in diabetes mellitus.
• Earlier referral to a nephrologist decreases mortality on dialysis
• Control glucose in diabetic patients
• Vaccines: Pneumococcal, influenza and H. influenzae

SURGICAL MEASURES Transplantation

ACTIVITY Restricted only by patient's condition

DIET
• Adequate caloric intake
• Restricted protein intake (.8 gm/kg/day for GFR between 25-55 cc/min per 1.73m2 and .6 gm for GFR between 13-25 cc/min)
• Restricted intake of phosphate
• Water intake limited to maintain serum sodium concentration of 135 to 145 mEq/L
• Sodium restriction if volume expanded
• Potassium restriction if hyperkalemic
• Vitamin supplementation (avoid extra-dietary intake of magnesium)
• Strict dietary restrictions in the elderly may not be necessary, since they often have a low protein and salt intake

PATIENT EDUCATION
• For patient education materials favorably reviewed on this topic, contact: National Kidney and Urologic Diseases Information Clearinghouse, Box NKUDIC, Bethesda MD 20893. (301)468-6345
• The National Kidney Foundation, Inc. 30 East 33rd Street, New York, New York 10016. "Bone Disease in Chronic Renal Failure" (Order #02-27CP), "Diabetes and Kidney Disease" (Order #02-09CP). "Drug Abuse Can Hurt Your Kidneys" (Order #02-22N) or "Nutrition and Changing Kidney Function" (Order #0401).

MEDICATIONS

DRUG(S) OF CHOICE
• Multivitamin
• Lipid lowering agents appropriate for disorder (cholesterol lowering specifically for nephrotic syndrome); may use cholestyramine or HMG-CoA reductase inhibitor
• Erythropoietin for anemia, approximately 100-150 units/kg thrice weekly IV or subcutaneous
• Salt restriction and diuretics for edema. Thiazides do not work at glomerular filtration rate (GFR) < 30 cc/min (creatinine > 2.5 mg/dL).
• Calcium acetate and oral vitamin D for renal failure osteodystrophy (see information under General Measures)
• Hypertension: drugs to lower blood pressure. For diabetic CRF, angiotensin converting enzyme inhibitors slow progression to dialysis dependence (captopril 25-50 bid to decrease diastolic < 90).
• Muscle cramps: Vitamin E
• Pruritus: Skin moisturizers, diphenhydramine, activated charcoal
• Bleeding: DDAVP, cryoprecipitate, dialysis in uremia
Contraindications: Refer to manufacturer's literature
Precautions:
• Monitor serum electrolytes carefully
• Monitor loop diuretic use to avoid volume depletion
• Adjust the dose of all medications with a renal route of excretion
Significant possible interactions: Refer to manufacturer's literature

ALTERNATIVE DRUGS
• Multivitamin preparation excluding fat-soluble vitamins and magnesium containing products
• Angiotensin converting enzyme inhibitors may prevent or slow progression to end stage renal failure (non renal vascular) in some diseases; definitely in diabetic CRF

FOLLOWUP

PATIENT MONITORING
• Blood, urine, chemistries and clinical status
• Blood pressure, volume monitored frequently
• Diagnose uremia and then dialyze

PREVENTION/AVOIDANCE
• Avoid nephrotoxic drugs when possible (especially iodinated contrast, NSAID's)
• Treat all disorders known to lead to chronic renal failure
• Many drugs require dosage reduction to prevent toxicity
• Avoid volume depletion

POSSIBLE COMPLICATIONS
• Anemia
• Changes in calcium and phosphorous metabolism
• Lipid disorders
• Pericarditis-tamponade
• Serositis
• Increased magnesium
• Platelet dysfunction
• Pseudogout
• Hypothyroidism
• Infections
• Hyperkalemia
• Acidosis
• Hyponatremia
• Gout
• Accelerated hypertension
• Metabolic calcification
• Spontaneous abortion
• Infertility
• Impotence
• Bleeding
• GI mucosal ulcerations
• GI A-V malformations
• Seizures
• Fractures
• Fluid overload

EXPECTED COURSE/PROGNOSIS
Serious, chronic, mortality > 20% despite careful attention to fluid and electrolyte balance or other treatment

MISCELLANEOUS

ASSOCIATED CONDITIONS   See conditions listed under Risk factors

AGE-RELATED FACTORS
Pediatric:
• Main causes in children include congenital renal and urinary tract malformations (signs appear before age 5), glomerular and hereditary renal diseases (signs appear between ages 5-15)
• Medical management much more difficult in children
• When it develops in infancy, growth impairment more profound than when disease develops in an otherwise healthy teenager

Geriatric:
• Highest incidence, highest morbidity, highest mortality. Renal disease is secondary to many age-dependent illnesses.
• Rule out such potentially reversible causes as urinary tract obstruction (particularly in men), renal arterial occlusion, hypercalcemia, use of nephrotoxic agents
• Older patients may tolerate dialysis quite well
Others: N/A

PREGNANCY   Pregnancy to term less common in CRF. Fertility and libido disturbed in CRF.

SYNONYMS
• Uremia
• CRF
• End stage renal disease
• CRI

ICD-9-CM   585 Chronic renal failure

SEE ALSO
• Renal failure, acute (ARF)
• Hydronephrosis
• Nephrotic syndrome
• Polycystic kidney disease

OTHER NOTES   N/A

ABBREVIATIONS
CRF = chronic renal failure
ESRD = end-stage renal disease

REFERENCES
• Obrador G, Arora P, Kausz A. et al: Pre ESRD care in the U.S.: a state of disrepair. J Am Soc Nephrol 1998;9:544-554
• Glassock RJ, Cohen AH: The primary glomerulopathies. Disease-A-Month 1996;42:329-383
• Levy AS, Adler S, Caggiula AW, et al: Effects of dietary protein restriction on the progression of advanced renal disease. Am J Kid Dis 1996;27:652-663
• Maschio G, Alberti D, Janin G, et al: Effect of ACE inhibitor benazepril on the progression of chronic renal insufficiency. NEJM 1996;334:939-945
• Ruggenenti P, Perna A. Gherardi G, et al: Renal function and requirement for dialysis in chronic nephropathy patients on ramipril. Lancet 1998;352:1252-1256
• Townsend RR, Cirigliano M: Hypertension in renal failure. Disease-A-Month 1998;44:243-253
• Kobrin SM: Diabetic nephropathy. Disease-A-Month 1998;44:214-234
Illustrations: 3 available on CD-ROM
Internet references: http://www.5mcc.com

Author(s)
Jonathan Maks, MD
Gregory W. Rutecki, MD

Renal tubular acidosis (RTA)

BASICS

DESCRIPTION
A group of disorders characterized by an abnormality of renal tubular acidification, which results in hyperchloremic acidosis and a normal anion gap. Patients are not uremic. Several types have been identified:
- Classic distal RTA (type I): usually secondary to impaired ability to secrete hydrogen ions into the distal tubule or collecting duct. Urine pH > 5.5.
- Proximal RTA (type II): due to impaired bicarbonate reabsorption in the proximal tubule. Bicarbonate spills into the urine at lower than normal plasma bicarbonate concentrations. If the plasma bicarbonate level is low enough (typically between 15-18), the urine may be acidified (pH < 5.5), in contrast to type I.
- Type III: no longer considered a distinct entity
- Distal hyperkalemic RTA (type IV): several subtypes are recognized but all are characterized by aldosterone resistance or deficiency. This leads to hyperkalemia (not seen in types 1 or 2) along with acidosis. The urine pH may be < 5.5.

System(s) affected: Renal/Urologic, Endocrine/Metabolic

Genetics:
- Type I RTA: Often autosomal dominant. May occur in association with other genetic diseases such as Ehlers-Danlos syndrome, hereditary elliptocytosis, or sickle-cell nephropathy. Autosomal recessive form associated with sensorineural deafness.
- Type II RTA: occurs in Fanconi's syndrome, which is associated with several genetic diseases (Wilson's disease, tyrosinemia, hereditary fructose intolerance, Lowe syndrome, galactosemia, cystinosis, glycogen storage disease, metachromatic leukodystrophy)
- Type IV RTA: some cases familial

Incidence/Prevalence in USA: N/A

Predominant age: occurs at all ages

Predominant sex: Male = Female

SIGNS AND SYMPTOMS
- Failure to thrive in children
- Anorexia, nausea
- Vomiting
- Weakness due to potassium loss
- Polyuria due to potassium loss
- Rickets in children
- Osteomalacia in adults

CAUSES
- Type I
  ◊ Genetic – autosomal dominant
  ◊ Genetic – autosomal recessive associated with sensorineural deafness
  ◊ Sporadic
  ◊ Ehlers-Danlos syndrome
  ◊ Hematologic diseases: sickle cell disease, hereditary elliptocytosis
  ◊ Carbonic anhydrase 1 deficiency
  ◊ Hypercalciuria
  ◊ Vitamin D intoxication
  ◊ Medullary cystic disease
  ◊ Glycogenosis type III
  ◊ Autoimmune disease

  ◊ Diseases causing nephrocalcinosis
  ◊ Fabry's disease
  ◊ Wilson's disease
  ◊ Drug induced (amphotericin B, lithium, analgesics)
  ◊ Toxin induced (toluene, glue)
  ◊ Hypergammaglobulinemic syndrome
  ◊ Obstructive uropathy
  ◊ Chronic pyelonephritis
  ◊ Renal transplantation
  ◊ Leprosy
  ◊ Hepatic cirrhosis
  ◊ Malnutrition
- Type II
  ◊ Diseases associated with Franconi's syndrome (see Genetics)
  ◊ Sporadic
  ◊ Multiple myeloma and other dysproteinemic states
  ◊ Heavy metal poisoning (cadmium, lead, mercury)
  ◊ Medications: acetazolamide, sulfanilamide, outdated tetracycline)
  ◊ Autoimmune disease
  ◊ Amyloidosis
  ◊ Interstitial renal disease
  ◊ Nephrotic syndrome
  ◊ Congenital heart disease
  ◊ Defects in calcium metabolism (hyperparathyroidism)
- Type IV
  ◊ Lupus nephropathy
  ◊ Diabetic nephropathy
  ◊ Obstructive nephropathy
  ◊ Nephrosclerosis due to hypertension
  ◊ Tubulo-interstitial nephropathies
  ◊ Addison's disease
  ◊ Acute adrenal insufficiency
  ◊ Pseudohypoaldosteronism (end organ resistance to aldosterone)
  ◊ Gordon syndrome

RISK FACTORS N/A

DIAGNOSIS

DIFFERENTIAL DIAGNOSIS
- Anion gap must be normal. If not, look for causes of metabolic acidosis other than RTA. (As in mnemonic MUDPILES: Metabolic disease or methanol ingestion, uremia, diabetic ketoacidosis, paraldehyde ingestion, isoniazid ingestion, lactic acidosis, ethylene glycol ingestion, salicylate ingestion.)
- Diarrhea with bicarbonate loss in stools
- Acidosis of chronic renal failure
- Urinary diversion (ureterosigmoidostomy, ileal conduit)
- Ingestion of hydrochloric acid, ammonium chloride, lysine HCL, excess calcium or magnesium chloride
- Small bowel, pancreatic or biliary fistulas

LABORATORY
- Electrolytes reveal hyperchloremic metabolic acidosis
- Plasma anion gap normal (anion gap=(plasma Na-(Cl+CO2)). Normal values: neonates <18; infants and children <16; adolescents and adults <14)
- Hypokalemia or nomokalemia
  ◊ Type I
  ◊ Type II
- Hyperkalemia – type IV
- BUN and creatinine normal (rules out renal failure as cause of acidosis)
- Urine pH – not acidified (pH >5.5) despite metabolic acidosis in type I
- Urine culture – rule out UTI with urea splitting organism (may elevate pH) and chronic infection
- Urine anion gap, an estimate of urine ammonium excretion (urine Na+K-Cl on spot urine). Measure before treatment
  ◊ Negative in type II
  ◊ Negative in bicarbonate losses secondary to diarrhea
  ◊ Negative in UTI due to urea splitting organism
  ◊ Positive in type I
  ◊ Positive in type IV
- Urine calcium
  ◊ Typically normal in type II
  ◊ High in type II

Drugs that may alter lab results:
- Diuretics
- Sodium bicarbonate
- Cholestyramine

Disorders that may alter lab results: N/A

PATHOLOGICAL FINDINGS
- Nephrocalcinosis, nephrolithiasis
- Rickets, osteomalacia
- Findings of underlying disease causing RTA

SPECIAL TESTS
- May be helpful to measure urine pH with pH meter for increased accuracy instead of dipstick. Place oil over urine to avoid loss of carbon dioxide if pH cannot be measured quickly.
- Urine ammonium excretion (anion gap is indirect measurement of this, but is not as accurate)
- Ammonium chloride (NH4+) loading to evaluate acid excretion
- Bicarbonate titration curves

IMAGING
Not needed except to rule out underlying conditions or complications as indicated

DIAGNOSTIC PROCEDURES N/A

Renal tubular acidosis (RTA)

TREATMENT

APPROPRIATE HEALTH CARE
• Outpatient
• Inpatient if acidosis severe, patient unreliable, persistent emesis, infant with severe failure to thrive

GENERAL MEASURES Treatment with appropriate medications to correct acidosis

SURGICAL MEASURES N/A

ACTIVITY As tolerated

DIET Varies with type of acidosis

PATIENT EDUCATION
• National Kidney & Urologic Diseases Information Clearinghouse, Box NKUDIC, Bethesda, MD 20893, (301)468-6345; http://www.niddk.nih.gov/health/kidney/.
• National Kidney Foundation; http://www.kidney.org

MEDICATIONS

DRUG(S) OF CHOICE
Provide oral alkali to raise serum bicarbonate to normal. Start at a low dose and increase until serum bicarbonate is normal. Give as sodium bicarbonate or citrate mixtures (1 mEq citrate = 1 mEq HCO3) such as Bicitra (1 mEq Na, 1 mEq Citrate/mL, no K) or Polycitra (1 mEq Na, 1 mEq K, 2 mEq citrate/mL) depending on need for potassium. Sodium bicarbonate tablets available (7.7 mEq HCO3/tab)
• Type I: typical doses 1-4 mEq/kg/day oral alkali divided bid-tid, unless bicarbonate wasting present, in which case much larger doses required. May require potassium supplementation if serum potassium low.
• Type II: typical doses 5-10 mEq/kg/day alkali. May be difficult to control and require doses divided 4-6 doses/day. May require potassium supplementation if serum potassium low.
• Type IV: 1-5 mEq/kg/day alkali divided bid-tid. Avoid potassium. In some cases furosemide used to lower potassium levels, but avoid if patient wastes salt. Sodium polystyrene sulfonate (Kayexalate) enemas rarely for hyperkalemia. Fludrocortisone – 0.1-0.3 mg/day, if mineralocorticoid deficient.
Contraindications: Refer to manufacturer's literature
Precautions: Sodium bicarbonate may cause flatulence as carbon dioxide is formed, whereas citrate mixtures are metabolized to bicarbonate in the liver, thereby avoiding gas production.
Significant possible interactions: N/A

ALTERNATIVE DRUGS
• Hydrochlorothiazide an adjunct in type II after maximal alkali replacement

FOLLOWUP

PATIENT MONITORING
• Varies with patient response. Suggested: electrolytes every 2-4 weeks at onset of therapy, every 2 weeks for one or two months once bicarbonate concentration normal, then monthly for several months
• Monitor underlying disease as indicated

PREVENTION/AVOIDANCE
• Careful use or avoidance of causative agents listed above

POSSIBLE COMPLICATIONS
• Nephrocalcinosis
• Hyper- or hypokalemia
• Nephrolithiasis
• Rickets
• Osteomalacia
• Hypercalciuria

EXPECTED COURSE/PROGNOSIS
• Prognosis dependent on the associated disease, otherwise good with therapy
• Transient forms of all types of RTA may occur

MISCELLANEOUS

ASSOCIATED CONDITIONS
• Type I in children - hypercalciuria leading to rickets, nephrocalcinosis, and nephrolithiasis
• Type I in adults - autoimmune diseases such as Sjögren's disease
• Type II - Fanconi's syndrome: A generalized tubular defect with bicarbonaturia, aminoaciduria, glycosuria, phosphaturia
• Distal hyperkalemic: obstructive uropathy and renal insufficiency

AGE-RELATED FACTORS
Pediatric: N/A
Geriatric: N/A
Others: N/A

PREGNANCY N/A

SYNONYMS N/A

ICD-9-CM
588.8 Other specified disorder resulting from impaired renal function
270.0 Disorder of amino acid transport (Fanconi's syndrome)

SEE ALSO
• Sjögren's syndrome
• Fanconi's syndrome
• Wilson's disease
• Hyperkalemia

OTHER NOTES N/A

ABBREVIATIONS N/A

REFERENCES
• Morris RC, Ives HE: In: Brenner BM, ed: Brenner & Rector's: The Kidney. 5th Ed. Philadelphia, WB Saunders Co., 1996:1779-84
• Chesney RW: In: Bennett, ed: Cecil Textbook of Medicine. 20th Ed. Philadelphia, WB Saunders Co., 1996:594-9
• Chiang M, Hill LL: Renal tubular acidosis. In: Oski FA, ed: Principles and Practices of Pediatrics. 2nd Ed. Philadelphia, JB Lippincott, 1994:1810-8
• Carey CF, Hans L, eds: Washington Manual of Medical Therapeutics. 29th ed. Philadelphia, Lippincott Williams & Wilkins 1998:55-9
Illustrations: N/A
Internet references: http://www.5mcc.com

Author(s)
David E. Hall, MD

Respiratory distress syndrome, adult

BASICS

DESCRIPTION   A patient with previously normal lungs who suffers a catastrophic pulmonary or nonpulmonary event followed by a cascade of events that occur at the alveolar-arteriolar capillary membrane. Reduction in functional residual capacity and lung compliance are hallmarks.
• Hypoxemia, decreased pulmonary compliance, and an increasing shunt forms as the proteinaceous material collects in the interstitium and alveoli. Hypoxemic respiratory failure secondary to noncardiogenic pulmonary edema almost always requires mechanical ventilation

System(s) affected: Pulmonary
Genetics: N/A
Incidence/Prevalence in USA: 150,000/year
Predominant age: All ages
Predominant sex: Male = Female

SIGNS AND SYMPTOMS   Most patients demonstrate similar clinical and pathologic features regardless of the cause of the acute lung injury.
• There are 4 phases:
  ◊ Phase 1: Acute injury - normal physical exam, normal chest x-ray, tachypnea, tachycardia, and respiratory alkalosis
  ◊ Phase 2: Latent phase - 6-48 hours after injury: Hyperventilation, hypocapnia, increase in work of breathing, widening alveolar-arterial oxygen gradient
  ◊ Phase 3: Acute respiratory failure, tachypnea and dyspnea, decreased lung compliance, diffuse infiltrates on chest roentgenogram, high-pitched diffusely scattered crackles
  ◊ Phase 4: Severe abnormalities, severe hypoxemia unresponsive to therapy, increased intrapulmonary shunting, metabolic and respiratory acidosis
• Signs and symptoms common to all 4 phases:
  ◊ Tachypnea and tachycardia during the first 12 to 24 hours
  ◊ Moist and cyanotic skin
  ◊ Breathing difficulty with intercostal and accessory respiratory muscles
  ◊ Dramatic increase in work of breathing
  ◊ High-pitched end-expiratory crackles are heard throughout all lung fields
  ◊ Increased agitation
  ◊ Lethargy, then obtundation
  ◊ Hypoxemia may be present long before clinical signs

CAUSES
• Recent studies have revealed a number of mediators are involved in the initiation and perpetuation of ARDS
  ◊ Cytokines (tumor necrosis factor, interleukin 1, interleukin 6)
  ◊ Complement activation
  ◊ Coagulation activation
  ◊ Platelet - activating factor
  ◊ Oxygen radicals
  ◊ Lipoxygenase pathways (Leukotrienes C4, D4 and E4)
  ◊ Neutrophil proteases
  ◊ Nitric oxide - may be deleterious or advantageous
  ◊ Endotoxin
  ◊ Cyclooxygenase pathway products (thromboxane A2, prostacyclin)
• All of the following causes can initiate a systemic inflammatory response with activation of the previous mediators
  ◊ Aspiration
  ◊ Pulmonary and systemic infections (bacterial, fungal, viral and protozoan)
  ◊ Sepsis (gram negative, gram positive, fungi, tuberculous, pneumocystis pneumonia)
  ◊ Pulmonary contusion
  ◊ Near-drowning
  ◊ Multiple fractures, especially long bones (fat embolism)
  ◊ Multiple transfusions
  ◊ Pancreatitis, severe
  ◊ Head injury
  ◊ Inhalation of toxic gases (oxygen, smoke, NH3, chlorine, plastics, phosgene, cadmium)
  ◊ Burns
  ◊ Shock (hemorrhage, cardiogenic, septic, anaphylactic)
  ◊ Eclampsia
  ◊ Carcinomatosis
  ◊ Leukoagglutinin reaction
  ◊ Air or amniotic fluid emboli

RISK FACTORS
• Systemic sepsis
• Pulmonary contusion
• Aspiration
• Inhalation of toxic substances
• Diffuse pneumonia
• Multiple emergency blood transfusions

DIAGNOSIS

DIFFERENTIAL DIAGNOSIS   Cardiogenic pulmonary edema

LABORATORY
• PaO2 < 50 mm Hg with FiO2 > 0.6
• Overall compliance < 50 mL/cm water (usually 20-30 mL/cm water)
• Increased shunt fraction Q's/Q't and dead space ventilation VD/VT
Drugs that may alter lab results: N/A
Disorders that may alter lab results:
• Multiple pulmonary embolism
• Cardiogenic pulmonary edema
• Severe chronic obstructive pulmonary disease
• Severe pneumonia

PATHOLOGICAL FINDINGS
• Lungs show exudative phase, early proliferative phase or late proliferative phase
• Interstitial and alveolar edema
• Inflammatory cells and erythrocytes spill into interstitium and the alveolus
• Type I cells are destroyed, leaving a denuded basement membrane
• Protein-rich fluid fills the alveoli
• Type II alveolar cells appear unaltered initially
• Type II cells begin to proliferate within 72 hours of initial insult
• The type II cells cover the denuded basement membrane
• Aggregates of plasma proteins, cellular debris, fibrin and surfactant remnants form hyaline membranes
• Over next 3-10 days, alveolar septum thickens by proliferating fibroblasts, leukocytes and plasma cells
• Capillary injury begins to occur
• Hyaline membranes begin to reorganize
• Fibrosis becomes apparent in respiratory ducts and bronchioles

SPECIAL TESTS
• Pulmonary artery catheter
• Measure pulmonary edema fluid content

IMAGING   Chest roentgenogram

DIAGNOSTIC PROCEDURES
• Pulmonary artery catheterization to demonstrate:
  ◊ Normal pulmonary arterial occlusion pressure (PAOP)
  ◊ Note: The main point of this study is to determine if the PAOP is inconsistent with cardiogenic pulmonary edema. A low PAOP with low serum albumin may lead to cardiogenic etiology. The patient with chronic congestive heart failure may have high wedge, but still develop adult respiratory distress syndrome.

TREATMENT

APPROPRIATE HEALTH CARE
Intensive care unit

GENERAL MEASURES
• Treat underlying etiology as appropriate
• Corticosteroids have theoretical, but not proven, benefit. This is still controversial. Do not use if occult infection exists.
• Support ventilation mechanically as necessary
• Support oxygenation with positive end-expiratory pressure (PEEP) with an amount that allows adequate hemoglobin saturation (90-95%) with an FiO2 of ≤ 60%. PaO2 is less important than oxygen delivery.
• Maintain oxygen delivery:
  ◊ Increase O2 content with packed red blood cell transfusion as necessary
  ◊ Optimize cardiac output with fluid or inotropes. Measure CO with each PEEP change. If CO decreases, give fluids to regain adequate CO and allow additional PEEP adjustments if necessary.
• Avoid over-ventilation
• Avoid large tidal volumes (> 10 cc/kg) if peak airway pressures are high
• A pulmonary artery catheter may be helpful in assessing left ventricular function, CO, oxygen delivery and consumption. It is necessary if high levels of PEEP are used.
• Be aware of possible respiratory superinfection
• Deep vein thrombosis prophylaxis is essential
• Consider paralyzing agents (to improve compliance and decrease barotrauma) if patient is fighting ventilator. (Initiate anxiolytics when instituting treatment with paralytics.)
• Ulcer prophylaxis
• Extraordinary management
  ◊ 1. Extracorporeal membrane oxygenation (ECMO) is conceivable in children
  ◊ 2. High-frequency ventilation - it achieves adequate gas exchange; however, there is no improvement on outcome
  ◊ 3. Pressure controlled inverse ratio ventilation (PCIRV)
  ◊ 4 Extracorporeal CO2 removal with low frequency ventilation. (Used in Europe and Salt Lake City on NIH trial.)

SURGICAL MEASURES N/A

ACTIVITY Bedrest

DIET Nutritional support - avoid excess carbohydrates (could increase respiratory quotient)

PATIENT EDUCATION N/A

MEDICATIONS

DRUG(S) OF CHOICE
• Inotropic agents - dobutamine to maintain adequate cardiac output
• Vasodilators - nitroprusside, ACE inhibitors, hydralazine. (Only if BP is adequate.)
• Corticosteroids (controversial)
• Anxiolytics
• Heparin 5000 units q12h for deep-vein thrombosis prophylaxis
• Ulcer prophylaxis with H2 blockers or sucralfate
Contraindications: See manufacturer's profile of each drug
Precautions: See manufacturer's profile of each drug
Significant possible interactions: See manufacturer's profile of each drug

ALTERNATIVE DRUGS
• Specific mediator inhibitors: Are being evaluated in animal models and humans
  ◊ Xanthine oxidase inhibitors (early in burn patients)
  ◊ Monoclonal derived antibodies to released monokines, i.e., tumor necrosis factor
  ◊ NSAID's, i.e., ibuprofen
  ◊ High-dose corticosteroids are still being studied and reviewed
  ◊ Pentoxifylline - has shown to be of some benefit
  ◊ Maximizing gut barrier function by using early enteral feeds
  ◊ Surfactant replacement is being reviewed
  ◊ Ventilator management by using permissive hypercapnia with low tidal volumes to prevent extensive barotrauma from mechanical ventilation

FOLLOWUP

PATIENT MONITORING
• Vital capacity and static lung compliance are important measures of mechanics
• Daily labs until no longer critical
• Chest x-rays to assess - endotracheal tube placement; the possible development of barotrauma; the presence of infiltrates; PA cath migration
• Swan-Ganz catheter - to help assess 02 delivery and consumption; monitor cardiac output

PREVENTION/AVOIDANCE N/A

POSSIBLE COMPLICATIONS
• Multiple organ dysfunction syndrome (MODS)
• Death
• Permanent lung disease
• Oxygen toxicity
• Barotrauma
• Superinfection

EXPECTED COURSE/PROGNOSIS
• 50% mortality rate; the syndrome is heterogeneous and mortality runs from 15-90%, depending on multiple factors; mainly, underlying cause, age of patient, number of failed organs.
• There is a decrease in diffusing capacity due to fibrosis and restrictive lung disease. Many people will have abnormal pulmonary function tests up to 6 months after illness. Most who survive will reveal abnormalities only with sensitive function testing, such as pulmonary exercise tests.

MISCELLANEOUS

ASSOCIATED CONDITIONS See Causes

AGE-RELATED FACTORS N/A
Pediatric: N/A
Geriatric: Increasing mortality with increasing age
Others: N/A

PREGNANCY N/A

SYNONYMS
• Shock lung
• Wet lung
• Noncardiac pulmonary edema

ICD-9-CM
786.09 Dyspnea and respiratory abnormalities
518.5 Respiratory distress following surgery or trauma
518.82 Adult respiratory distress syndrome associated with other conditions

SEE ALSO N/A

OTHER NOTES N/A

ABBREVIATIONS
PEEP = positive end-expiratory pressure

REFERENCES
• Civetta JM: Critical Care. Philadelphia, J.B. Lippincott, 1988
• Matthay MA: Critical Care Medicines. JAMA 1991;265(23):3109-3110
• Murray JF, Matthay MA, et al: Amer Review Resp Disease 1988;138:720-723
• Bennett JC, Plum F, eds: Cecil Textbook of Medicine. 20th Ed. Philadelphia, W.B. Saunders Co., 1996
• Demling R: Adult respiratory distress syndrome: Current concepts. New Horizons 1993;1(3):388-401
Illustrations: N/A
Internet references: http://www.5mcc.com

Author(s)
Michael Ferrebee, MD
Darell E. Heiselman, DO, FCCM, FACP, FACC, FCCP

Respiratory distress syndrome, neonatal

BASICS

DESCRIPTION Serious disorder of prematurity, with clinical manifestation of respiratory distress. Pulmonary surfactants that are deficient at birth cause diffuse lung atelectasis. Must differentiate from pneumonia, sepsis.
System(s) affected: Pulmonary
Genetics: No known genetic pattern
Incidence/Prevalence in USA: Common
Predominant age: Neonatal
Predominant sex: Male = Female, although usually more severe in males

SIGNS AND SYMPTOMS
• Onset within few hours after birth
• Delayed, weak cry
• Expiratory grunt
• Frothing at lips
• Intercostal, sternal retractions
• Nasal flaring
• Rapid respiratory rate
• Respiratory excursions decreased
• Rales
• Cyanosis
• Peripheral edema
• Oliguria

CAUSES
• Prematurity
• Deficient pulmonary surfactants in the neonatal period
• Possible pulmonary ischemia

RISK FACTORS
• Premature infants born prior to 37 weeks gestation
• Infants born of diabetic mothers
• More common and more severe with greater prematurity
• Fetal asphyxia
• Multiple births

DIAGNOSIS

DIFFERENTIAL DIAGNOSIS
• Early group B streptococcal pneumonia
• Transient tachypnea of newborn
• Meconium aspiration pneumonia
• Sepsis with group B streptococcus pneumonia

LABORATORY
• Amniotic fluid:
  ◊ Lecithin:sphingomyelin ratio (L:S ratio < 2)
  ◊ Absence of phosphatidyl glycerol
  ◊ Surfactant production deficient
• Features of respiratory, metabolic acidosis
• Arterial blood gases - hypoxemia and hypercarbia
Drugs that may alter lab results: Artificial or human surfactant; betamethasone
Disorders that may alter lab results: N/A

PATHOLOGICAL FINDINGS
• Voluminous, noncrepitant, purplish red lungs
• Dilatation right heart and vena cava
• Possible patent ductus
• Extensive resorptive atelectasis
• Hyaline membranes

SPECIAL TESTS
• Monitor arterial blood gases

IMAGING
• X-ray - reticulogranular appearance of lung fields demonstrating:
  ◊ Diffuse atelectasis
  ◊ Air bronchograms

DIAGNOSTIC PROCEDURES   N/A

TREATMENT

APPROPRIATE HEALTH CARE
Inpatient - intensive care

GENERAL MEASURES
• Warm, humidified, oxygen enriched gases by hood
• CPAP
• Positive pressure ventilation
• Monitor respiratory and circulatory status carefully
• Umbilical artery catheter placed for monitoring blood pressure and sampling arterial blood gases
• Transcutaneous monitors to measure O2 and CO2 tension
• Pulse oximetry
• Radiant infant warmer
• Tube feedings or hyperalimentation
• High-frequency ventilation. Choices include conventional ventilation at faster-than-normal rates; high-frequency jet ventilation; high-frequency oscillation.
• Relationship between using surfactant and high-frequency ventilation still being studied
• Extracorporeal membrane oxygenation (ECMO) measure of last resort. Its use is still uncommon and there are risks associated. Not available for infants under 2 kg.

SURGICAL MEASURES   N/A

ACTIVITY   None; may require sedation or paralysis while on ventilator

DIET   Special premature formula or parenteral alimentation

PATIENT EDUCATION   For patient education materials favorably reviewed on this topic, contact: American Lung Association, 1740 Broadway, New York, NY 10019, (212)315-8700

MEDICATIONS

DRUG(S) OF CHOICE
• Beractant (Survanta): bovine surfactant. Dose: 2.6-8.0 mL depending on patient's weight (see Manufacturer's Dosing Table) Prophylaxis: as soon as possible after birth. Therapeutic: when signs and symptoms of RDS appear.
Contraindications: Refer to manufacturer's literature
Precautions: Do not administer beractant into a mainstem bronchus. Check endotracheal tube placement before administration. Be prepared for rapidly changing lung compliance; peak ventilator pressures may need to be reduced immediately.
Significant possible interactions: Refer to manufacturer's literature

ALTERNATIVE DRUGS   N/A

FOLLOWUP

PATIENT MONITORING   Continuous monitoring in an intensive care nursery

PREVENTION/AVOIDANCE
• Prevention of premature birth
• Systemic betamethasone given to mother when fetal lung profile is immature; at least 24 hours before delivery

POSSIBLE COMPLICATIONS
• Intraventricular hemorrhage
• Intracranial pathology
• Tension pneumothorax
• Retinopathy of prematurity
• Apnea
• Chronic lung disease - bronchopulmonary dysplasia (BPD)

EXPECTED COURSE/PROGNOSIS
• Course
  ◊ Acute, possibly fatal within 48 hours in 20-30%, increasing with lower birth weights, especially < 1,000 grams.
  ◊ In larger prematures, course may be brief and uncomplicated, with recovery in 1 week
• Prognosis
  ◊ Successful outcome expected in tertiary care centers in children older than 28 weeks gestation
  ◊ Chronic lung disease, bronchopulmonary dysplasia (BPD), frequent in severe cases, especially after prolonged artificial ventilation

MISCELLANEOUS

ASSOCIATED CONDITIONS   N/A

AGE-RELATED FACTORS
Pediatric: A disorder of the neonatal period
Geriatric: N/A
Others: N/A

PREGNANCY   N/A

SYNONYMS
• Hyaline membrane disease
• RDS
• Surfactant deficiency

ICD-9-CM
770.8 Other respiratory problems after birth

SEE ALSO   N/A

OTHER NOTES   N/A

ABBREVIATIONS
CPAP = continuous positive airway pressure

REFERENCES
• Avery, Fletcher, MacDonald. Neonatology 4th ed. JP Lippincott Co, 1994
• Hageman JR (ed): Neonatal update. Pediatr Clin of NA 1998;June
Illustrations: N/A
Internet references: http://www.5mcc.com

Author(s)
Kurt J. Wegner, MD

Respiratory syncytial virus (RSV) infection

BASICS

DESCRIPTION
• RSV causes respiratory illness
  ◊ Adults: URI's
  ◊ Infants and children: bronchitis, bronchiolitis, pneumonia
  ◊ Leading cause of pediatric admissions for respiratory illness

System(s) affected: Pulmonary
Genetics: None known
Incidence/Prevalence in USA: Common in winter. Almost all persons infected one or more times during lifetime.
Predominant Age: Birth to age 2
Predominant Sex:
• Males = females as outpatients
• 2:1 males/females in hospital

SIGNS AND SYMPTOMS
• Cold signs and symptoms (mild disease)
  ◊ Fever
  ◊ Cough
  ◊ Coryza
  ◊ Congestion
  ◊ Otitis media
  ◊ Malaise
• Bronchitis/bronchiolitis/pneumonia
  ◊ Cough
  ◊ Chest congestion, rales/rhonchi
  ◊ Wheezing
  ◊ Dyspnea
  ◊ Hypoxia
  ◊ Cyanosis
• Vomiting

CAUSES Infection with RSV

RISK FACTORS
• Impaired immunity
  ◊ AIDS
  ◊ Chemotherapy
  ◊ Other types of impaired immunity
• Occupational exposure
  ◊ Day care workers
  ◊ Pediatric hospital staff
  ◊ School teachers
• Neonatal/congenital conditions
  ◊ Congenital cardiac anomalies
  ◊ Respiratory distress syndrome
• Low socio-economic status
• More common in urban vs. rural areas

DIAGNOSIS

DIFFERENTIAL DIAGNOSIS
• Mild illness/upper respiratory tract
  ◊ Colds (non RSV)
  ◊ Allergic rhinitis
  ◊ Sinusitis
  ◊ Croup
• Severe illness/lower respiratory tract
  ◊ Asthma
  ◊ Bronchitis
  ◊ Bronchiolitis
  ◊ Pneumonia

LABORATORY
• WBC may be normal to elevated
• Positive RSV antigen test on nasal washings
Drugs that may alter lab results: None
Disorders that may alter lab results: None

PATHOLOGICAL FINDINGS
Lymphocytic peribronchiole infiltrates (autopsy)

SPECIAL TESTS N/A

IMAGING
• Chest x-ray
  ◊ Hyperinflation - most common, characteristic finding
  ◊ Interstitial infiltrates - fairly common
  ◊ Segmental or lobar consolidation in pneumonia
  ◊ Pleural fluid

DIAGNOSTIC PROCEDURES None

TREATMENT

APPROPRIATE HEALTH CARE
Outpatient for mild cases; inpatient for severe disease or for those with underlying disorders

GENERAL MEASURES
• Outpatient
  ◊ Rest/supportive care
  ◊ Bronchodilators - albuterol nebulizer/inhaler
  ◊ Monitor oxygenation-pulse oximeter
• Inpatient
  ◊ Oxygen
  ◊ Bronchodilators - albuterol nebulizer q4h
  ◊ Respiratory isolation
  ◊ Ribavirin
  ◊ Antibiotics for secondary bacterial pneumonia
  ◊ Monitor arterial blood gases/pulse oximeter
• Avoid exposing others
  ◊ Remove from day care/school until well
  ◊ Good hand washing practices
  ◊ Respiratory isolation in hospital

SURGICAL MEASURES N/A

ACTIVITY Decreased household activity/rest

DIET
• Maintain nutrition
• Avoid over-hydration (may increase lung congestion)

PATIENT EDUCATION Printed patient information available from: ICN Pharmaceuticals, Inc., ICN Plaza, 3300 Hyland Ave., Costa Mesa, CA 92626 "All about RSV: a guide for parents."

MEDICATIONS

DRUG(S) OF CHOICE
• Ribavirin 20 mg/mL mist 12-18 hours/day for 3-7 days. (Can shorten duration and severity of illness.)
• Bronchodilators - albuterol nebulizer q4h (dose appropriate for age)
• Antibiotics for secondary bacterial infections/pneumonia
　◊ Appropriate to particular pathogen
　◊ Prophylactic use of antibiotics controversial
• Potential use of RSV immune globulin in high risk infants
Contraindications: See specific drug related information
Precautions: Avoid exposure of pregnant/potentially pregnant women to ribavirin
Significant possible interactions: See specific drug information

ALTERNATIVE DRUGS
• Antibiotic appropriate to identified or suspected bacterial pathogen
• Theophylline use all right, but not recommended

FOLLOWUP

PATIENT MONITORING
• Uneventful resolution is the norm
• No special monitoring is needed as illness resolves
• May want to educate parents about SIDS - avoid prone sleeping in infants

PREVENTION/AVOIDANCE
• Avoid exposure to those ill with RSV
• Good hand washing practices (since hand-nose and hand-eye transmission is common)
• Avoid rubbing the eyes (common RSV inoculation route)

POSSIBLE COMPLICATIONS
• Pneumonia
• Sudden infant death
• Death from severe lower respiratory tract infections
• Possible residual lung damage

EXPECTED COURSE/PROGNOSIS
• Usually resolves within two weeks without sequelae
• Hospitalization rate of children ill with RSV varies from 1:50 to 1:200 (children < 2 years old)

MISCELLANEOUS

ASSOCIATED CONDITIONS
• Asthma is worse with RSV and vice versa
• SIDS may be a sequelae of RSV

AGE-RELATED FACTORS
Pediatric: Most common under age 2
Geriatric: N/A
Others: Increasing immunity with subsequent infections by RSV usually results in less serious illness

PREGNANCY Avoid ribavirin therapy in pregnancy

SYNONYMS N/A

ICD-9-CM
480.1 Pneumonia due to respiratory syncytial virus

SEE ALSO
• Bronchiolitis
• Pneumonia, bacterial
• Pneumonia, viral
• Bronchitis, acute

OTHER NOTES N/A

ABBREVIATIONS
• RSV = respiratory syncytial virus
• SIDS = sudden infant death syndrome
• URI = upper respiratory infection

REFERENCES
• Mandell GL, ed: Principles and Practice of Infectious Diseases. 4th Ed. New York, Churchill Livingstone, 1995
• Rudolph AM, ed: Rudolph's Pediatrics 19th Ed. Norwalk, CT, Appleton & Lange, 1991
• Gilchrist S, et al: National surveillance for RSV, U.S., 1985-1990. J Inf Dis 1994;170:986-990
• Levin MJ: Treatment & prevention options for RSV infections. J Pediatr 1994;124:322-325
• Groothuis J, et al: Prophylactic administration of RSV immune globulin to high risk infants and young children. New Engl J Med 1993;329:1524-1530
Illustrations: N/A
Internet references: http://www.5mcc.com

Author(s)
Joseph G. Ewing, MD

Restless leg syndrome

BASICS

DESCRIPTION
• Restless leg syndrome (RLS) and periodic limb movement disorder (PLMS) are separate and distinct but related entities classified as intrinsic disorders of sleep.
• Restless leg syndrome is characterized by vague dysesthesia, to pain in the legs, causing an irresistible urge to move the legs while awake. Symptoms are most intense at rest.
• Periodic limb movements are brief rhythmic and repetitive brief dystonic limb movements of 0.5 to 5 seconds duration occurring in clusters during the sleep period. They are most likely to occur in the first half of the night and with a predominant frequency of 5-90 seconds. Dorsiflexion at the ankle occur; or, the knee may also show flexion; and hip flexion as well may be seen in severe cases. Can occur in the upper extremities. PLMS occur in more than 80% of cases of RLS, but can occur independently from RLS.
System(s) affected: Nervous, Musculoskeletal
Genetics: N/A
Incidence/Prevalence in USA:
• 20-30% of patients seen in sleep centers will have PLMS
• Population prevalence is poorly documented
Predominant age:
• Mostly seen past age 30, and increases with age
• Rarely occur in childhood and adolescence
Predominant Sex: N/A

SIGNS AND SYMPTOMS
• PLMS patients are unaware of their movements during sleep. Their most frequent symptoms are daytime tiredness and fatigue.
• RLS patients have an inability to sit still or remain immobile due to dysesthesia or pain. These symptoms are usually worse in the evening or night.

CAUSES
Unknown; hereditary factors are involved in some patients

RISK FACTORS
• Chemical agents
   ◊ Caffeine and antidepressants will cause or aggravate PLMS and RLS (trazodone and nefazodone are exceptions)
   ◊ Dopamine antagonists (antipsychotics), metoclopramide, calcium channel blockers, theophylline, and adrenergics are among those agents reported to aggravate symptoms
   ◊ Withdrawal from sedatives/narcotics can augment symptoms.

• Diseases
   ◊ Primary neurological disorders should be considered. Among most common are peripheral neuropathies, radiculopathies, neurodegenerative disease, or, another movement disorder such as Parkinson's disease.
   ◊ Metabolic disorders
      - Diabetics have a much higher incidence of PLMS/RLS
      - Electrolyte deficiencies which may involve K, Ca, or Mg. (low normal values may indicate a low tissue level)
      - Anemia (low tissue iron or low serum ferritin)
      - Uremic/renal failure patients will have a high percentage of PLMS/RLS symptoms

DIAGNOSIS

DIFFERENTIAL DIAGNOSIS
RLS
• Akathisia produced by dopamine receptor blockers
• Painful legs and moving toes, usually caused by direct trauma
• Fasciculations from upper motor neuron disease
• Leg cramps
PLMS
• Sleep jerks or hypnic jerks are normal and occur more frequently in sleep deprived individuals
• Myoclonic epilepsy disappears in sleep

LABORATORY
• Fasting glucose
• Electrolytes Na, K, Ca, Mg
• Ferritin
• B12, folate levels
• BUN, creatinine
Drugs that may alter lab results: N/A
Disorders that may alter lab results: N/A

PATHOLOGICAL FINDINGS   N/A

SPECIAL TESTS   Nocturnal polysomnography (NPSG)

IMAGING   N/A

DIAGNOSTIC PROCEDURES
• RLS is diagnosed by history alone, though excessive leg movements will be seen with nocturnal polysomnography
• PLMS: affected individuals are often unaware and diagnosis by NPSG is appropriate

TREATMENT

APPROPRIATE HEALTH CARE
Outpatient

GENERAL MEASURES
• Eliminate aggravating factors
   ◊ Diet and drugs
      - Removal of caffeine containing foods, beverages, and OTC drugs can often result in improvement
      - Avoidance of most antidepressants (serzone and trazodone excepted)
      - Avoidance of dopamine blocker antipsychotics, metoclopramide (Reglan), and calcium channel blockers.
• Treatment of primary neurological and medical disorders
   ◊ Supplement essential minerals: K, Ca, Mg, if indicated - being careful not to overtreat (especially in presence of K-sparing diuretics)
   ◊ Ferrous sulfate in individuals with a ferritin level of 50 mcg/ml or less
• Good sleep hygiene
   ◊ Regular sleep habit with adequate 7 1/2-8 hrs sleep time
   ◊ Mild to moderate regular exercise is particularly helpful to RLS/PLMS patients

SURGICAL MEASURES   N/A

ACTIVITY
• Regular mild to moderate exercise

DIET   N/A

PATIENT EDUCATION
• The Restless Legs Syndrome Foundation Inc. publishes the "Nightwalkers Newsletter" and provides useful information and identifies support groups. Address is 4410 19th St. NW, Suite 201, Rochester MN 55901-662; http://www.rls.org
• Sleep Thief by Virginia Wilson is recommended reading. Contact Galaxy Books Inc., P.O. Box 1421 Orange Park FL 32067

MEDICATIONS

DRUG(S) OF CHOICE
Three major classes of drugs are used:
• Dopaminergic agonists are the treatment of choice.
◊ Usually carbidopa-levodopa 25/100 given 30-60 min. before hs and may be repeated once if necessary. Pergolide, pramipexole, bromocriptine, etc. are reserved for the more difficult cases.
• Benzodiazepines do not suppress movements in most patients but allow greater sleep continuity.
◊ Clonazepam 0.5-2.0 mg most frequently used, but diazepam and most shorter acting agents are effective.
• Opiates and synthetic narcotics actually reduce the number of movements
◊ Hydrocodone 5 mg before hs can be quite effective. Propoxyphene, codeine, oxycodone, pentazocine, methadone, etc. are effective in equivalent doses.
Contraindications: Refer to manufacturer's literature
Precautions: Refer to manufacturer's literature
Significant possible interactions: Refer to manufacturer's literature

ALTERNATIVE DRUGS
• Agents reported to be effective in selected individuals or subgroups include:
◊ Mineral supplements (when indicated)
◊ Quinine - circulatory
◊ Carbamazepine, valproic acid (Depakote), gabapentin, propranolol, clonidine - uremia
◊ Baclofen - motor neuron disease
◊ Gamma-hydroxybutyrate, 5-hydroxytryptophan, vitamin B12 and folate - anemia
◊ Paradoxically, tricyclics - painful neuropathy

FOLLOWUP

PATIENT MONITORING
Visits at 2 week intervals until stable; then at 6-12 months.

PREVENTION/AVOIDANCE N/A

POSSIBLE COMPLICATIONS
• Tolerance may develop to medications after months to years and necessitate change to another agent
• Augmentation of RLS into daytime symptoms may develop particularly with use of carbidopa/levodopa in which case it should be reduced while adding another agent in increments
• Side effects may occur with any medication and are usually dose related
• Electrolyte and iron supplementation in excess can have serious consequences

EXPECTED COURSE/PROGNOSIS
• Periods of spontaneous remission may occur
• RLS and PLMS tend to worsen with age

MISCELLANEOUS

ASSOCIATED CONDITIONS
• Sleep deprivation

AGE-RELATED FACTORS
Pediatric: RLS may be misdiagnosed as growing pains or ADHD in younger patients
Geriatric: N/A
Others: RLS/PLMS may occur at any age but usually after age 30.

PREGNANCY
PLMS often occur during pregnancy and resolve afterward.

SYNONYMS N/A

ICD-9-CM
333.99 Other extrapyramidal diseases

SEE ALSO
• Parkinson's disease

OTHER NOTES
Extremely rare, RLS symptoms in the torso have been reported

ABBREVIATIONS
RLS = restless leg syndrome
PLMS = periodic limb movement disorder
NPSG = nocturnal polysomnography

REFERENCES
• Allen RP. Advances in diagnosis and treatment of the restless legs syndrome and periodic limb movements in sleep. 1997, 11th Annual APSS Meeting
• Becker PM, Jamieson AO, DeLaCueva L, Cotton J, Thompson C. Restlessness evaluation scale-Texas version: Preliminary assessment of the circadian variation in restless legs syndrome. Sleep Research 1993;22:232
• Kryger MH, Roth T, Dement W. Principles and Practice of Sleep Medicine, 2nd Ed. Philadelphia: W. B. Saunders Co., 1994
• Lin SC, Kaplan J. Burger CD, Fredrickson PA. Effect of pramipexole in treatment of resistant restless legs syndrome. Mayo Clinic Proceedings 1998;73:497-500
• Uphold CR, Graham MV. Clinical Guidelines in Family Practice. Gainesville, FL, Barmarrae Books, 1993
• Wilson V N. Sleep Thief; Restless Legs Syndrome. Orange Park, FL: Galaxy Books, Inc, 1996
• The International Classification of Sleep Disorders: Diagnostic and Coding Manual
Illustrations: N/A
Internet references: http://www.5mcc.com

Author(s)
Marshall Bradshaw, MD
John R. Burk, MD
Edgar A. Lucus, PhD, ACP

Retinal detachment

BASICS

DESCRIPTION Separation of the sensory retina from the underlying retinal pigment epithelium.
• Rhegmatogenous retinal detachment (RRD): Is the most common type. It occurs when the fluid vitreous gains access to the subretinal space through a break in the retina (Greek rhegma, rent).
• Exudative or serous detachment: Occurs in the absence of a retinal break, usually in association with inflammation or a tumor.
• Traction detachment: Vitreoretinal adhesions mechanically pull the retina from the retinal pigment epithelium. The most common cause is proliferative diabetic retinopathy.
System(s) affected: Nervous
Genetics: Most cases are sporadic
Incidence/Prevalence in USA:
• 1/10,000 per year in patients who have not had cataract surgery
• 1-3% of patients after cataract surgery will develop a retinal detachment
Predominant age: The incidence increases with age.
Predominant sex: Male>Female (3:2)

SIGNS AND SYMPTOMS
• Flashes (photopsia)
• Floaters
• Visual field loss
• Pigmented cells within the vitreous "tobacco dust"
• Central vision will be preserved if the macula is not detached
• Poor visual acuity (20/200 or worse) with loss of central vision when macula is detached.
• Elevation of retina associated with one or more retinal tears in RRD or elevation of the retina without tears in exudative detachment
• In 3-10% of patients with presumed RRD, no definite retinal break is found
• Tenting of the retina without retinal tears in traction detachment

CAUSES
• Traction from a posterior vitreous detachment (PVD) cause most retinal tears. With aging, vitreous gel liquefies leading to the separation of the vitreous from the retina. The vitreous gel remains attached at the vitreous base, in the retinal periphery, resulting in vitreous traction producing tears in the retinal periphery.
• PVD associated with vitreous hemorrhage has a high incidence of retinal tears
• Exudative detachment:
  ◊ Tumors
  ◊ Inflammatory diseases (Harada's, posterior scleritis)
  ◊ Miscellaneous (central serous retinopathy, uveal effusion, malignant hypertension)
• Traction detachment:
  ◊ Proliferative diabetic retinopathy
  ◊ Cicatricial retinopathy of prematurity
  ◊ Proliferative sickle cell retinopathy
  ◊ Penetrating trauma

RISK FACTORS
• Myopia (greater than 5 diopters)
• Aphakia or pseudophakia
• PVD and associated conditions (aphakia, inflammatory disease and trauma)
• Trauma
• Retinal detachment in fellow eye
• Lattice degeneration. Lattice degeneration is a vitreoretinal abnormality found in 6-10% of the general population
• Glaucoma. 4-7% of patients with retinal detachment have chronic open angle glaucoma
• Vitreoretinal tufts. Peripheral retinal tufts are caused by focal areas of vitreous traction.
• Meridional folds. Redundant retina usually found in the supranasal quadrant

DIAGNOSIS

DIFFERENTIAL DIAGNOSIS
Retinoschisis (splitting of the retina). Vitreous cell or vitreous hemorrhage are rarely found in the vitreous with retinoschisis, whereas they are commonly seen in RRD. Retinoschisis usually has a smooth surface and is dome shaped; whereas, RRD often has a corrugated, irregular surface.

LABORATORY N/A
Drugs that may alter lab results: N/A
Disorders that may alter lab results: N/A

PATHOLOGICAL FINDINGS Elevation of the neurosensory retina from the underlying retinal pigment epithelium.

SPECIAL TESTS
• Visual field testing. Differentiate between a RRD and retinoschisis. An absolute scotoma is seen in retinoschisis whereas a RRD causes a relative scotoma.
• Ultrasonography can demonstrate a detached retina and may be helpful when the retina can not be visualized directly (cataracts, etc).

IMAGING Fluorescein dye leakage can be seen in exudative retinal detachment caused by central serous retinopathy and other inflammatory conditions

DIAGNOSTIC PROCEDURES
• Slit lamp examination
• Dilated fundus examination with binocular indirect ophthalmoscopy

TREATMENT

APPROPRIATE HEALTH CARE Referral to an ophthalmologist for examination and treatment, if indicated

GENERAL MEASURES
• Not all retinal tears or breaks need to be treated. Flap tears or horseshoe tears in symptomatic patients (that is patients with flashes or floaters) frequently are treated. Operculated holes in symptomatic patients are sometimes treated. Atrophic holes in symptomatic patients are rarely treated.
• Lattice degeneration with or without holes within the lattice in an asymptomatic patient with prior retinal detachment in the fellow eye may be prophylactically treated.
• Flap retinal tears in asymptomatic patients are frequently treated prophylactically
• Exudative detachments are usually managed by treatment of the underlying disorder
• Traction detachments usually managed by observation. If the fovea is involved, then a vitrectomy is needed

SURGICAL MEASURES
• Timing of repairs
  ◊ Macula attached: within 24 hours. If the detachment is peripheral and does not have features suggestive for rapid progression (such as large and/or superior tears) then repair can be performed within a few days.
  ◊ Macula recently detached: within one week of development of a macula-off retinal detachment
  ◊ Old macular detachment: elective repair within 2 weeks
• If a retinal break has lead to the development of a retinal detachment, then surgery will be needed. Surgical options (and combinations) include:
  ◊ Pneumatic retinopexy. Head positioning is required postoperatively.
  ◊ Scleral buckle.
  ◊ Vitrectomy.
  ◊ Perfluorocarbon liquids for giant tears (circumferential tears 90° or larger)
  ◊ Silicone oil for complex repairs
• Anesthesia. Usually with local anesthesia.
• RRD may have more than one break. If any retinal break is not closed at the time of surgery, the surgery will fail.
• Additional surgery may be required if the retina redetaches secondary to a new retinal break or due to proliferative vitreoretinopathy (PVR).

ACTIVITY Bedrest prior to surgery. Postoperatively, if an intraocular gas has been used, the patient may need specific head positioning and should not travel to high altitudes.

DIET NPO if surgery is imminent

PATIENT EDUCATION American Academy of Ophthalmology, 655 E. Beach Street, San Francisco, California 94109-1336

MEDICATIONS

DRUG(S) OF CHOICE
• Intraocular gases
 ◊ Air
 ◊ Perfluoropropane (C3F8)
 ◊ Sulfur hexafluoride (SF6)
• Perfluorocarbon liquids
• Silicone oil

Contraindications: Patients with poorly controlled glaucoma.

Precautions: Expanding intraocular gas bubble increases intraocular pressure, therefore, avoid higher altitudes

Significant possible interactions: Nitrous oxide used in general anesthesia can expand an intraocular gas bubble

ALTERNATIVE DRUGS
Steroids can cause worsening of central serous retinopathy

FOLLOWUP

PATIENT MONITORING
• Alert ophthalmologist immediately:
 ◊ Symptoms of PVD and detachment (new onset of floaters or flashes, increase in floaters or flashes, sudden shower of floaters, curtain or shadow in the peripheral visual field, or reduced vision)
• Patients with an acute symptomatic PVD associated with mild vitreous hemorrhage should be reexamined in 3-4 weeks by the ophthalmologist. The development of a retinal detachment is unlikely if no retinal tears are present on reexamination in 3-4 weeks.
• A patient with an acute symptomatic PVD, even in the absence of vitreous hemorrhage, vitreous pigment or detectable retinal break, may need to be reexamined in 3-4 weeks by the ophthalmologist, depending on clinical circumstances such as aphakia or myopia, because retinal breaks may develop over time.
• If an acute symptomatic PVD is associated with gross vitreous hemorrhage which interferes with complete visualization of the retinal periphery by indirect ophthalmoscopy, then a patient should be reexamined at short intervals with indirect ophthalmoscopy until the entire retinal periphery can be observed.
• If the examiner is not certain that the retina is detached in the presence of opaque media, ultrasonography should be performed

PREVENTION/AVOIDANCE
• Patients at risk for a retinal detachment should have regular ophthalmologic examination

POSSIBLE COMPLICATIONS
• PVR is the most common cause of failed retinal detachment repair. 10-15% of patients, whose retinas reattach initially after retinal surgery, will subsequently re-detach; usually within 6 weeks due to cellular proliferation and contraction on the retinal surface.
• Partial or total loss of vision due to macular detachment and/or PVR
• Moderate to severe forms of PVR are usually treated with pars plana vitrectomy and fluid-gas exchange. If a segmental scleral buckle was placed at the initial procedure, then this will need to be revised.
• Scleral buckles may erode the overlying conjunctiva and lead to an infection

EXPECTED COURSE/PROGNOSIS
• RRD:
 ◊ 90% of retinal detachments can be reattached successfully after one or more surgical procedures. Postoperative visual acuity depends primarily on the status of the macula preoperatively. Also important is the length of time between the detachment and the repair (75% of macular detachments of less than one week will obtain a final visual acuity of 20/70 or better).
 ◊ 87% of eyes with a retinal detachment not involving the macula attain a visual acuity of 20/50 or better postoperatively. 37% of eyes with a detached macula preoperatively attain 20/50 or better vision postoperatively.
 ◊ In 10-15% of successfully repaired retinal detachments not involving the macula preoperatively, visual acuity does not return to the preoperative level. This decrease is secondary to complications such as macular edema or macular pucker.
• Tractional retinal detachment:
 ◊ When not involving the fovea, the patient can usually be observed since it is uncommon for these to extend into the fovea.
• Exudative retinal detachment:
 ◊ Management is usually nonsurgical
 ◊ The presence of shifting fluid is highly suggestive of an exudative retinal detachment. Fixed retinal folds which are indicative of PVR are rarely seen in exudative retinal detachment. If the underlying condition is treated the prognosis is generally good.

MISCELLANEOUS

ASSOCIATED CONDITIONS
• Lattice degeneration
• High myopia
• Cataract surgery
• Glaucoma
• History of retinal detachment in the fellow eye
• Trauma

AGE-RELATED FACTORS
Pediatric: Usually associated with underlying vitreoretinal disorders and/or retinopathy of prematurity
Geriatric:
• Posterior vitreous detachment
• Cataract surgery
Others: N/A

PREGNANCY Pre-eclampsia/eclampsia may be associated with exudative retinal detachment. No intervention is indicated, provided hypertension is controlled, prognosis is usually good.

SYNONYMS N/A

ICD-9-CM
361.00 Rhegmatogenous retinal detachment
379.21 Posterior vitreous detachment
361.2 Serous (nonrhegmatogenous) detachment
361.81 Tractional detachment
362.63 Lattice degeneration of retina
361.30 Retinal break without detachment

SEE ALSO
• Retinopathy, diabetic

OTHER NOTES N/A

ABBREVIATIONS
RRD = rhegmatogenous retinal detachment
PVD = posterior vitreous detachment
PVR = proliferative vitreoretinopathy

REFERENCES
• Tani P, Robertson, DM, Langworthy A: Prognosis for Central Vision and Anatomic Reattachment in Rhegmatogenous Retinal Detachment with Macula Detached. Am J Ophthalmol 1981;92:611-620
• The American Academy of Ophthalmol. Ophthalmic Procedure Assessment: The Repair of Rhegmatogenous Retinal Detachments. Ophthalmology 1996;103:1313-1324
• The American Academy of Ophthalmol. Preferred Practice Pattern: Retinal Detachment 1990: 1-17
• The American Academy of Ophthalmol: Preferred Practice Pattern: Management of Posterior Vitreous Detachment, Retinal Breaks, and Lattice Degeneration 1998:1-24
• Regillo CD, Benson WE: Retinal Detachment Diagnosis and Management. 3rd ed. Philadelphia, J.B. Lippincott Co., 1998
• Vitrectomy with Silicone Oil or Perfluoropropane Gas in Eyes with Severe Proliferative Vitreoretinopathy: Results of a Randomized Clinical Trial. Silicone Study Report 2. Arch Ophthalmol 1992;110:780-792
• Ross WH, Kozy DW: Visual recovery in macula-off rhegmatogenous retinal detachments. Ophthalmol 1998;105:2149-2153
Illustrations: 6 available on CD-ROM
Internet references: http://www.5mcc.com

Author(s)
Richard W. Allinson, MD

Retinitis pigmentosa

BASICS

DESCRIPTION Retinitis pigmentosa is characterized by poor night vision, constricted visual fields, bone spicule-like pigmentation of the fundus, and electroretinographic evidence of photoreceptor cell dysfunction.

System(s) affected: Nervous

Genetics:
- Autosomal dominant - 20%
- Autosomal recessive - 37%
- X-linked recessive - 4.5%
- Sporadic - 38.5%

Incidence/Prevalence in USA: RP affects approximately 1 in 4,000 people in the US

Predominant age:
- X-linked RP has the earliest onset of the major hereditary types and many X-linked patients are legally blind by age 30
- Autosomal dominant RP has a later onset than autosomal recessive or X-linked recessive RP
- Leber's congenital amaurosis which is a variant of RP presents at birth
- Late onset RP typically is asymptomatic and unrecognized until age 40 or 50

Predominant sex: Male > female

SIGNS AND SYMPTOMS
- Headache and light flashes are the most common initial complaints
- Night blindness (nyctalopia)
- Bone spicule pigmentation in the retina
- Retinal arteriolar narrowing
- Optic nerve head pallor, "waxy pallor"
- Progressive visual field loss
- Central visual acuity is usually preserved until the end stages of retinitis pigmentosa
- Most patients are myopic
- Posterior subcapsular cataracts are common in all forms of retinitis pigmentosa
- Cystoid macular edema
- Optic nerve head drusen
- Electroretinogram (ERG) changes
- Retinal neovascularization
- RP associated with an exudative retinal vasculopathy. Fundus findings would include serous retinal detachment, lipid deposition in the retina and telangiectatic vascular anomalies.
- Variants of RP exists with unusual or regional distribution including:
- Sectorial RP
- Pigmented paravenous atrophy
- Unilateral RP

CAUSES
- The genetic mutations responsible for RP have been identified in some families with RP, primarily those with the autosomal dominant form
- Mutations in the rhodopsin gene account for about 30% of cases with autosomal dominant RP
- Another 4-6% of autosomal dominant RP is due to a mutation in the gene for a photoreceptor protein, peripherin/RDS

RISK FACTORS Family history

DIAGNOSIS

DIFFERENTIAL DIAGNOSIS
Bone spicule-like retinal pigmentation and retinal atrophy are nonspecific findings and can result from conditions other than retinitis pigmentosa
- Infections
- Syphilis
- Rubella
- Inflammation (severe uveitis)
- Choroidal vascular occlusion
- Toxicity (chloroquine or thioridazine)
- Choroideremia
- Gyrate atrophy of choroid and retina (10 to 20 fold elevation of plasma ornithine levels)
- Systemic metabolic disorders such as Refsum's disease and abetalipoproteinemia
- Kearns-Sayre syndrome. Usually presents in adolescents. It is characterized by progressive external ophthalmoplegia, the first sign usually being ptosis, pigmentary degeneration of the retina and a cardiac conduction defect which may cause complete heart block.
- Cone-rod dystrophy. Characterized by bilateral and symmetric loss of cone function in the presence of reduced rod function.
- Cone dystrophy characterized by marked abnormality in cone function with some or no rod involvement.
- Congenital stationery night blindness
- Oguchi's disease
- Fundus albipunctatus
- Trauma

LABORATORY
- Elevated plasma levels of phytanic acid in Refsum's disease
- Acanthocytosis of red blood cells in peripheral blood smear in abetalipoproteinemia. This is an autosomal recessive disorder in which abetalipoprotein B is not synthesized, leading to fat malabsorption and deficiencies of fat soluble vitamins. Therapy with vitamin A and E can improve retinal function.
- Syphilic neuroretinitis can be diagnosed by performing a FTA-ABS or MHA-Tp
- Elevated plasma ornithine levels in gyrate atrophy of the choroid and retina. Usually a 10-20 fold elevation of plasma ornithine levels.

Drugs that may alter lab results: N/A
Disorders that may alter lab results: N/A

PATHOLOGICAL FINDINGS
- Disappearance of the rods, cones and outer nuclear layers in the retina.
- Bone spicule formation in the retina is secondary to the migration of retinal pigment epithelial cells into the overlying retina

SPECIAL TESTS
- Electroretinography (ERG). Photoreceptors generate reduced amplitude a- and b-waves in RP. Rod and cone responses may be undetectable in advanced RP.

- Visual field testing. A ring scotoma in the mid periphery may be identified. The ring scotomas generally starts as a group of isolated scotomas in the area 20-25° from fixation. Long after the entire peripheral field is gone, there remains a small island of intact central visual field.
- Fluorescein angiography can demonstrate cystoid macular edema.
- Fundus photography to document the status of the retina.
- Hearing tests in patients complaining of hearing loss such as patients with Usher's syndrome (RP with hearing loss).

IMAGING N/A

DIAGNOSTIC PROCEDURES N/A

TREATMENT

APPROPRIATE HEALTH CARE
Outpatient

GENERAL MEASURES
- Supportive
- Genetic counseling
- Low vision aids
- Educating the patient

SURGICAL MEASURES
- The efficacy of the "Cuban" therapy, which is electric stimulation, autotransfused ozonated blood, and ocular surgery has not been proven to be of benefit
- Macular grid laser photocoagulation may be of benefit for patients with cystoid macular edema secondary to RP
- Research is being done on photoreceptor transplantation, gene therapy, and implantation of a visual prosthesis. The inner retinal neurons may be preserved after death of photoreceptors in RP, which could make some of these experimental procedures feasible one day.

ACTIVITY
Full activity. Caution should be exercised because of the reduced peripheral vision and poor night vision.

DIET
No special diet

PATIENT EDUCATION
- Counsel patients to help them understand RP and its genetics
- RP is a slowly progressive, chronic disease; patients do not go blind rapidly and total blindness is not a frequent end-point of this disease
- RP Foundation Fighting Blindness, Executive Plaza One, Suite 800, 11350 McCormick Road, Hunt Valley, MD 21031-1014, (800)683-5555
- The American Academy of Ophthalmology, 655 E. Beach Street, San Francisco, CA 94109-1336, (415)561-8540

Retinitis pigmentosa

MEDICATIONS

DRUG(S) OF CHOICE
• Vitamin A 15,000 IU q day (retinal degeneration slowed as measured by ERG/visual fields). [Note: beta-carotene not a suitable substitute; not studied in patients under age 18]
• Vitamin E 400 IU q day results in faster retinal degeneration and is not recommended
• Acetazolamide may be of benefit in the treatment of cystoid macular edema which may occur in RP. 500 mg/day in a sustained release capsule was found to be more effective than 250 mg/day.
Contraindications: Women who are pregnant or considering pregnancy should not take more than 8,000 IU of vitamin A per day. There is an increased incidence of birth defects in babies born to women who ingest higher dosages of vitamin A during pregnancy. Women should consult their obstetrician.
Precautions: Avoid vitamin A supplement dosages >15,000 IU per day as higher dosages can cause liver damage
Significant possible interactions: N/A

ALTERNATIVE DRUGS   N/A

FOLLOWUP

PATIENT MONITORING
• Ophthalmic examinations every 1-2 years
• Check for complications (cataracts, etc.)

PREVENTION/AVOIDANCE
• Genetic counseling
• There is no conclusive evidence that demonstrates that the amount of light modifies the course of RP. A study in which one eye was covered with an opaque lens did not show any difference in disease progression compared to the fellow eye.
• Ultraviolet-absorbing sunglasses and brimmed hats are recommended when patients are at the beach or in the snow.

POSSIBLE COMPLICATIONS
• Cataract
• Cystoid macular edema
• Loss of visual field
• Poor night vision
• Blindness

EXPECTED COURSE/PROGNOSIS
• Reassurance about the slow course of RP
• Most of the deafness in Usher's syndrome is congenital. It is unlikely that an RP patient who is not born deaf will go deaf later in his life.
• RP severity varies with inheritance pattern
• Autosomal recessive form has an early age of onset and may have severely constricted visual fields by age 20. Tends toward more rapid progression as compared to autosomal dominant RP; also increased incidence of cataracts.
• X-linked RP is similar in clinical presentation to autosomal recessive RP
• Autosomal dominant RP generally has less severe findings initially than autosomal recessive RP; symptoms may not occur until 30 years of age
• Good central vision usually preserved. If the central visual field radius is >30°, >90% of patients will have visual acuities of 20/40 or better. If the central visual field radius is smaller than 10°, 30% of patients will have a visual acuity of 20/40 or better.

MISCELLANEOUS

ASSOCIATED CONDITIONS
• With systemic disorders:
◊ Usher's syndrome. RP and congenital sensorineural hearing impairment.
◊ Laurence-Moon-Biedl syndrome (also called the Bardet-Biedl syndrome) is an autosomal recessive disorder associated with retinal dystrophy, mental retardation, obesity, hypogonadism, and postaxial polydactyly.
◊ Cockayne syndrome. This is an autosomal recessive disorder in which children at the age of one or two years present with retinal dystrophy, sensorineural deafness, cerebellar dysfunction, dementia, and ultraviolet light photosensitivity.

AGE-RELATED FACTORS
Pediatric: Leber's congenital amaurosis is characterized by severely reduced vision from birth and impaired ERG responses from both cones and rods. Most cases are autosomal recessive.
Geriatric: Late onset RP is asymptomatic; generally unrecognized until age >40
Others: N/A

PREGNANCY   Remember risk of teratogenicity of high intake vitamin A during pregnancy

SYNONYMS
• Rod-cone dystrophy
• Retinal dystrophy

ICD-9-CM
362.74 Retinitis pigmentosa

SEE ALSO
• Laurence-Moon-Biedl syndrome
• Cataract

OTHER NOTES   N/A

ABBREVIATIONS
RP = Retinitis Pigmentosa
ERG = Electroretinogram

REFERENCES
• Berson EL, Remulla JFC, Rosner B, et al: Evaluation of patients with retinitis pigmentosa receiving electric stimulation, ozonated blood, and ocular surgery in Cuba. Arch Ophthalmol 1996;114:560-563
• Pagon RA: Retinitis pigmentosa. Surv Ophthalmol 1988;33:137-177
• Madreperla SA, et al: Visual acuity loss and retinitis pigmentosa. relationship to visual field loss. Arch Ophthalmol 1990;108:358-364
• Rothman KJ, Moore LL, Singer MR, et al: Teratogenicity of high vitamin A intake. NEJM 1995;333:1369-1373
• Berson EL, Rosner B, Sandberg MA, et al: A randomized trial of vitamin A and vitamin E supplements for retinitis pigmentosa. Arch Ophthalmol 1993;111:751-772
• Fishman GA, Gilbert LD, Fisella RG, et al: Acetazolamide for treatment of chronic cystoid macular edema in retinitis pigmentosa. Arch Ophthalmol 1989;107:1445-1452
• Santos A, Humayun M, de Juan E, et al: Preservation of the inner retina in retinitis pigmentosa: a morphometric analysis. Arch Ophthalmol 1997;115:511-515
4 additional references available at web site
Internet references: http://www.5mcc.com
Illustrations: 1 available on CD-ROM

Author(s)
Richard W. Allinson, MD

Retinopathy of prematurity

BASICS

DESCRIPTION Retinopathy of prematurity (ROP) is a proliferative disorder of the retinal blood vessels in premature infants. The normal retinal vascularization occurs nasally at approximately 36 weeks of gestation and temporally at approximately 40 weeks of gestation.
System(s) affected: Nervous
Genetics: Black infants appear less susceptible
Incidence/Prevalence in USA:
• One third of infants weighing < 1500 grams at birth may show evidence of retinopathy of prematurity
• 65.8% of infants weighing less than 1251 grams at birth, and 81.6% of those weighing less than 1000 grams
• Babies with a birth weight of 1001-1500 grams, 2.2% will develop cicatricial changes as a complication of ROP and 0.5% of them will be blind
Predominant age: Premature infants
Predominant sex: Male = Female

SIGNS AND SYMPTOMS
Acute ROP is classified as follows:
• Location:
◊ Zone I: posterior retina within a 60 degree circle centered on the optic nerve
◊ Zone II: extends from the edge of Zone I to the nasal ora anteriorly
◊ Zone III: is the residual temporal crescent of retina anterior to Zone II
• Extent: number of clock hours involved
• Degree of abnormal vascular response observed:
◊ Stage 1: the development of a demarcation line between the vascularized and nonvascularized retina
◊ Stage 2: the presence of a demarcation line that extends out of the plane of the retina (ridge)
◊ Stage 3: a ridge with extraretinal fibrovascular proliferation
◊ Stage 4: subtotal retinal detachment
◊ Stage 5: total retinal detachment
• "Plus" disease is characterized by the tortuosity of the retinal vasculature in the posterior fundus

CAUSES
Oxidative processes, influenced by high levels of arterial oxygen, in immature retina, may be an important causative factor

RISK FACTORS
• Low birth weight
• Prematurity
• Supplemental oxygen. Once the retina becomes fully vascularized, oxygen will not affect the retina.

DIAGNOSIS

DIFFERENTIAL DIAGNOSIS
• Retinoblastoma
• Congenital cataracts
• Norrie's disease
• Incontinentia pigmenti
• Familial exudative vitreoretinopathy
• Ocular toxocariasis
• Coat's disease
• Persistent hyperplastic primary vitreous
• X-linked retinoschisis

LABORATORY N/A
Drugs that may alter lab results: N/A
Disorders that may alter lab results: N/A

PATHOLOGICAL FINDINGS
• Peripheral retinal nonperfusion
• Retinal neovascularization
• Retinal hemorrhages
• Retinal detachment

SPECIAL TESTS N/A

IMAGING N/A

DIAGNOSTIC PROCEDURES
• An ophthalmologist skilled in the detection of this disorder should examine all infants with a birth weight ≤ 1500 grams or with a gestational age of 28 weeks or less
• Infants with a birth weight over 1500 grams and who are clinically unstable and are felt to be at high risk by their pediatrician or neonatologist should have an ophthalmologic exam to detect ROP
• The initial eye exam should be performed between 4-6 weeks of chronological age or between 31-33 weeks postconceptional age (gestational age at birth plus chronological age)
• Follow-up exams are performed until the retina is fully vascularized

TREATMENT

APPROPRIATE HEALTH CARE
Treatment usually is performed in the neonatal intensive care unit or as an outpatient or inpatient as the child grows older

GENERAL MEASURES
• The multicenter trial of cryotherapy demonstrated a favorable outcome for eyes treated at threshold (Stage 3+ retinopathy of prematurity) versus control eyes
• Stage 3 retinopathy defined as a ridge of extraretinal fibrovascular proliferation
• A plus sign is added to the ROP stage number when retinal vascular tortuosity is noted in the posterior fundus

• Threshold disease was defined as at least 5 contiguous or 8 cumulative clock hours of Stage 3 associated with retinal vascular tortuosity in the posterior segment of the eye ("plus" disease)
• When threshold disease is detected in infants, ablative therapy should be considered in at least one eye within 72 hours of diagnosis
• Using Teller Acuity Card assessment an unfavorable outcome was noted in 35.0% of the treated eyes compared with 56.3% of the control eyes, at one year in the multicenter trial of cryotherapy
• The development of ROP is not influenced by reducing ambient light exposure for a short period of time in premature babies

SURGICAL MEASURES
• Transscleral cryotherapy to the avascular retina when applied to high risk eyes can reduce the incidence of sight threatening complications. The multicenter trial of cryotherapy has shown that treatment of high risk eyes reduces the incidence of unfavorable outcomes by 46%.
• The multicenter trial of cryotherapy demonstrated an unfavorable outcome, defined as posterior retinal detachment, retinal fold involving the macula, or retrolental tissue, was significantly less frequent in eyes undergoing cryotherapy
• The results at one year from the multicenter trial of cryotherapy demonstrated an unfavorable outcome in 25.7% of eyes that received cryotherapy compared with 47.4% of control eyes
• Laser treatment applied to the avascular retina in high risk eyes can reduce the incidence of sight-threatening complications; cataract formation is a possible complication
• Diode laser treatment of ROP is as effective as conventional cryotherapy. Diode laser treatment may be better tolerated than cryotherapy and is becoming the primary treatment modality.
• Scleral buckling can reduce progression from stage 4 to 5 ROP. The encircling 240 band can be divided at 3 months after surgery if it is felt the retina will remain attached.
• Vitrectomy and/or scleral buckling can be used to treat retinal detachment associated with ROP. Emphasis should be placed on prevention of retinal detachment in premature infants, because of the poor visual outcome after a lensectomy-vitrectomy procedure for retinal detachment due to ROP.

ACTIVITY N/A

DIET N/A

PATIENT EDUCATION
• Expectant mothers should avoid behavioral and environmental risk factors associated with low birth weight. These include smoking, alcohol and other substance abuse, and poor nutrition.
• American Academy of Ophthalmology, 655 Beach St., San Francisco, CA 94109-1336

Retinopathy of prematurity

MEDICATIONS

DRUG(S) OF CHOICE
• Vitamin E prophylaxis is controversial; it may reduce the severity, but not the incidence of ROP
• Extremely low birth weight infants receiving prophylactic treatment with calf lung surfactant extract have a lower incidence of any stage when compared with control infants
Contraindications: N/A
Precautions: N/A
Significant possible interactions: N/A

ALTERNATIVE DRUGS N/A

FOLLOWUP

PATIENT MONITORING
• Close follow-up of patients with ROP is required
• Follow-up exams after the initial examination are performed every 2-4 weeks until the retina is fully vascularized or until the ROP regresses
• Follow-up exams are performed every 1-2 weeks if "prethreshold" disease is present. Prethreshold disease is characterized by the following:
  ◊ Zone I, any stage
  ◊ Zone II, Stage 2 (ridge) with "plus" disease
  ◊ Zone II, Stage 3 (ridge) with extraretinal fibrovascular proliferation
• Exam infants with zone I ROP at least weekly until involution of ROP occurs and normal vascularization proceeds to zone II.
• In some cases of regressed ROP, cicatrization can develop and is associated with variable degrees of fibrosis. This can lead to vitreoretinal traction and subsequent retinal detachment from formation of a retinal hole.
• Retinal detachment secondary to cicatricial ROP can occur during the midteens; long term follow-up of ROP cicatricial cases is indicated

PREVENTION/AVOIDANCE See Patient Education

POSSIBLE COMPLICATIONS
• Retinal detachment
• Retinal fold involving the macula
• Vitreous hemorrhage
• Angle closure glaucoma
• Amblyopia
• Strabismus
• Myopia

EXPECTED COURSE/PROGNOSIS
• Spontaneous regression occurs over a period of weeks or months in most cases. Spontaneous regression occurs in approximately 85% of eyes.
• The earliest sign of regression is the growth of blood vessels beyond the demarcation line into previously avascular retina
• Some cases of ROP do not regress spontaneously without sequela, but progress. A gradual transition then occurs from active ROP to cicatricial ROP which is associated with varying degrees of fibrosis and vitreoretinal traction which can lead to retinal detachment.

MISCELLANEOUS

ASSOCIATED CONDITIONS Neonatal respiratory distress syndrome

AGE-RELATED FACTORS
Pediatric: N/A
Geriatric: N/A
Others: N/A

PREGNANCY N/A

SYNONYMS
• ROP
• Retrolental fibroplasia

ICD-9-CM
362.21 Retinopathy of prematurity

SEE ALSO N/A

OTHER NOTES N/A

ABBREVIATIONS
• ROP = retinopathy of prematurity
• RLF = retrolental fibroplasia

REFERENCES
• Cryotherapy for retinopathy of prematurity cooperative group. Multicenter trial of cryotherapy for retinopathy of prematurity: one year outcome - structure and function. Arch Ophthalmology. 108:1408-1416, 1990
• Ben-Sir I., Nissenkorn I, Kremer I: Retinopathy of Prematurity. Surv Ophthalmol 1988;33:1-16
• Cryotherapy for retinopathy of prematurity cooperative group. Multicenter trial of cryotherapy for retinopathy of prematurity. Preliminary results. Arch Ophthalmology 1988;106:471-479
• The committee for the classification of retinopathy of prematurity: An international classification of retinopathy of prematurity. Arch Ophthalmology 1984;102:1130-1134
• Screening examination of premature infants for retinopathy of prematurity: a joint statement of the American Academy of Pediatrics, the American Association for Pediatric Ophthalmology and Strabismus, and the American Academy of Ophthalmology. 1997;104:888-889
• Quinn GE, Dobson V, Barr CC, et al: Visual acuity of eyes after vitrectomy for retinopathy of prematurity: follow-up at 5 1/2 years. Ophthalmology 1996;103:595-600
• Trese M: Scleral buckling for retinopathy of prematurity. Ophthalmology 1994;101:23-26
• White JE, Repka MX: Randomized comparison of diode laser photocoagulation versus cryotherapy for threshold retinopathy of prematurity: 3-year outcome. J Pediatr Ophthamol Strabismus 1997;34:83-87
• Reynolds JD, Hardy RJ, Kennedy KA, et al: Lack of efficacy of light reduction in preventing retinopathy of prematurity. NEJM 1998;338:1572-1576
Illustrations: N/A
Internet references: http://www.5mcc.com

Author(s)
Richard W. Allinson, MD

Retinopathy, diabetic

BASICS

DESCRIPTION Noninflammatory retinal disorder characterized by retinal capillary closure and microaneurysms. Retinal ischemia leads to release of a vasoproliferative factor stimulating neovascularization on the retina, optic nerve, or iris.
• Most patients with diabetes mellitus will develop diabetic retinopathy. It is the leading cause of new cases of legal blindness among Americans between the ages of 20-64.
• Diabetic retinopathy can be divided into three stages:
    ◊ Background diabetic retinopathy
    ◊ Preproliferative diabetic retinopathy
    ◊ Proliferative diabetic retinopathy

System(s) affected: Nervous

Genetics: N/A

Incidence/Prevalence in USA:
• Approximately 6.6% of the population between ages 20-74 has diabetes
• Approximately 25% of the diabetic population has some form of diabetic retinopathy
• Diabetic retinopathy accounts for approximately 10% of new cases of blindness each year

Predominant age:
• Peak incidence of Type I, juvenile onset diabetes mellitus, is between the ages of 12-15
• Peak incidence of Type II, adult onset, between the ages of 50-70
• The incidence of diabetic retinopathy is directly related to the duration of diabetes
• In children less than 10 years of age, it is unusual to see diabetic retinopathy, regardless of the duration of diabetes
• The risk of developing diabetic retinopathy increases after puberty
• Almost all diabetics will develop background retinopathy if they have had diabetes for at least 20 years
• Two-thirds of juvenile-onset diabetics who have had diabetes for at least 35 years will develop proliferative diabetic retinopathy, and one-third will develop macular edema. The proportions are reversed for adult-onset diabetes.

Predominant sex:
• Male = Female - juvenile onset diabetes mellitus
• Female > Male: non-insulin-dependent diabetes mellitus

SIGNS AND SYMPTOMS
• Background diabetic retinopathy
    ◊ Microaneurysms
    ◊ Intraretinal hemorrhage
    ◊ Macular edema
    ◊ Lipid deposits
• Preproliferative diabetic retinopathy
    ◊ Nerve fiber layer infarctions (cotton wool spots)
    ◊ Venous beading
    ◊ Venous dilation
    ◊ Intraretinal microvascular abnormalities (IRMA)
    ◊ Extensive retinal hemorrhage
• Proliferative diabetic retinopathy
    ◊ New blood vessel proliferation (neovascularization) on the retinal surface, optic nerve, and iris

CAUSES Related to the development of diabetic microaneurysms and microvascular abnormalities.

RISK FACTORS
• Duration of diabetes mellitus (usually over 10 years)
• Poor glycemic control
• Pregnancy
• Renal disease
• Systemic hypertension
• Smoking
• Elevated serum lipid levels are associated with an increased risk of retinal lipid deposits (hard exudates)
• Proteinuria

DIAGNOSIS

DIFFERENTIAL DIAGNOSIS Other causes of retinopathy, e.g., radiation retinopathy, retinal venous obstruction, and hypertensive retinopathy.

LABORATORY N/A

Drugs that may alter lab results: N/A

Disorders that may alter lab results: N/A

PATHOLOGICAL FINDINGS
• Increased capillary permeability
• Microaneurysms
• Hemorrhages in retina
• Exudates in retina
• Capillary nonperfusion

SPECIAL TESTS Fluorescein angiography: Demonstrates retinal nonperfusion, retinal leakage, and proliferative diabetic retinopathy

IMAGING N/A

DIAGNOSTIC PROCEDURES
Eye examination: Measurement of visual acuity and documentation of the status of the iris, lens, vitreous and fundus

TREATMENT

APPROPRIATE HEALTH CARE
Inpatient or outpatient surgery for vitrectomy; outpatient for laser treatment

GENERAL MEASURES
• The Early Treatment Diabetic Retinopathy Study demonstrated that systemic aspirin did not prevent the development of proliferative diabetic retinopathy, or reduce the risk of visual loss associated with diabetic retinopathy
• Microvascular complications, including proliferative diabetic retinopathy are significantly increased when blood-sugar levels are equal to or greater than 200 mg/dL
• Poor glycemic control is associated with an increased risk, both for developing diabetic retinopathy and with its progression, regardless of the type of diabetes, insulin-dependent or non-insulin dependent
• Cataracts are more common among diabetics. Try to delay cataract surgery in diabetics with retinopathy until the symptoms are more severe than in non-diabetics; cataract surgery can cause retinopathy to worsen

SURGICAL MEASURES
• Laser treatment: Recommended for patients with proliferative diabetic retinopathy and for patients with clinically significant macular edema
• The Diabetic Retinopathy Study demonstrated panretinal photocoagulation overall reduced the rate of severe visual loss from 15.9% in untreated eyes to 6.4% in treated eyes. In certain subgroups of eyes with proliferative diabetic retinopathy, the incidence of severe visual loss in untreated eyes was as high as 36.9% with a follow-up of 2 years.
• The Early Treatment Diabetic Retinopathy Study (ETDRS) demonstrated that eyes with clinically significant diabetic macular edema benefited from focal laser treatment. Clinical significant diabetic macular edema is defined as the following:
    ◊ 1. Thickening of the retina within 500 microns of the center of the macula
    ◊ 2. Hard exudates within 500 microns of the center of the macula associated with thickening of the adjacent retina
    ◊ 3. A zone of retinal thickening 1 disc area or larger within 1 disc diameter of the center of the macula
• Patients with clinically significant diabetic macular edema (CSDME) and high risk proliferative disease can have simultaneous focal and panretinal photocoagulation without adversely affecting the visual outcome
• Cryoretinopexy can be used instead of laser treatment in certain cases to decrease the neovascular stimulus and treat proliferative diabetic retinopathy
• Vitrectomy: Recommended for patients with severe proliferative diabetic retinopathy, traction retinal detachment involving the macula, and nonclearing vitreous hemorrhage. In eyes undergoing vitrectomy for severe proliferative diabetic retinopathy, the percentage of eyes with a visual acuity of 10/20 or better was greater in the group that underwent early vitrectomy versus conventional management.
• Vitrectomy can be considered after 1 month for a vitreous hemorrhage decreasing the vision to the 5/200 level or worse

Retinopathy, diabetic

ACTIVITY As tolerated

DIET Follow prescribed diabetic diet

PATIENT EDUCATION
• Patient information available from the American Diabetes Association - (800)232-3472 or local office
• American Academy of Ophthalmology, 655 Beach St., San Francisco, CA 94109-1336
• Stress importance of strict blood glucose control through diet, exercise, drugs/insulin and monitoring of blood glucose

MEDICATIONS

DRUG(S) OF CHOICE
• None are specific for retinopathy. See Other Notes. Lisinopril, an angiotensin-converting enzyme (ACE) inhibitor was found to slow the progression of retinopathy in insulin dependent diabetes.
• An oral therapy for diabetic retinopathy is being tested. PKC-beta is an enzyme activated by hyperglycemia and is associated with the development of vascular dysfunction. Inhibition of PKC-beta could help reduce the retinal vascular complications from diabetes.
• Nutritional antioxidant intake of vitamins C, E and beta-carotene has no protective effect on diabetic retinopathy.
Contraindications: N/A
Precautions: N/A
Significant possible interactions: N/A

ALTERNATIVE DRUGS N/A

FOLLOWUP

PATIENT MONITORING
• Scheduled eye examinations by an ophthalmologist:
   ◊ The diabetic patient with no diabetic retinopathy should be followed yearly
   ◊ Patients with background diabetic retinopathy should be followed at least every six months
   ◊ Patients with preproliferative diabetic retinopathy should be followed at least every three to four months
   ◊ Patients with active proliferative diabetic retinopathy should be followed at least every two to three months

PREVENTION/AVOIDANCE
• Careful monitoring and control of blood glucose
• Routine visits to an ophthalmologist

POSSIBLE COMPLICATIONS
Blindness

EXPECTED COURSE/PROGNOSIS If
treated early, outlook good. If treatment delayed, blindness may result.

MISCELLANEOUS

ASSOCIATED CONDITIONS
• Glaucoma
• Cataracts
• Retinal detachment
• Vitreous hemorrhage
• Disc edema (diabetic papillopathy); can occur in type I or type II diabetes

AGE-RELATED FACTORS
Pediatric: N/A
Geriatric: Prevalence will increase as population ages and diabetic patients live longer
Others: N/A

PREGNANCY
• Pregnancy can exacerbate diabetic retinopathy
• Any woman with diabetes who becomes pregnant should be examined in the first trimester. She should be examined at least every three months until parturition.

SYNONYMS N/A

ICD-9-CM
362.01 Retinopathy, diabetic, background
362.02 Retinopathy, diabetic, proliferative

SEE ALSO
• Diabetes mellitus, Type 1
• Diabetes mellitus, Type 2

OTHER NOTES
• The Diabetes Control and Complications Trial (DCCT) recommends that for most patients with insulin-dependent diabetes mellitus, blood glucose levels should be as close to the nondiabetic range as is safe to do so, to reduce the risk and rate of progression of the diabetic retinopathy
• In the DCCT, insulin-dependent diabetics were randomly assigned into either conventional or intensive insulin treatment. Conventional treatment consisted of one or two daily insulin injections, with daily self-monitoring of urine or blood glucose. Intensive treatment consisted of insulin administered three or more times daily by injection or an external pump, with self-monitored blood glucose levels measured at least four times per day.
• The DCCT demonstrated intensive insulin therapy reduced the risk of macular edema and retinal neovascularization
• In the DCCT, intensive insulin therapy was more effective in reducing the risk of progression of diabetic retinopathy in the less advanced stages. However, advanced diabetic retinopathy also benefited from the intensive insulin.
• The DCCT demonstrated improvement in diabetic retinopathy was more likely to occur with intensive insulin therapy in insulin-dependent diabetes

ABBREVIATIONS
• BDR = background diabetic retinopathy
• PPDR = preproliferative diabetic retinopathy
• PDR = proliferative diabetic retinopathy
• CSDME = clinically significant diabetic macular edema

REFERENCES
• Diabetic Retinopathy Study Research Group: Indications for photocoagulation treatment of diabetic retinopathy. DRS Report No. 14. Int Ophthal Clin, 1987, 27:239-253
• Early Treatment Diabetic Retinopathy Study Research Group: Photocoagulation for Diabetic Macular Edema. ETDRS Report No. 1. Arch Ophthalmol, 1985; 103:1796-1806
• Early vitrectomy for severe proliferative diabetic retinopathy in eyes with useful vision: Results of a randomized trial diabetic retinopathy vitrectomy study. Report No. 3. The Diabetic Retinopathy Vitrectomy Study Research Group. Ophthalmol 1988;95:1307-1320
• The Diabetes Control and Complications Trial Research Group: The effect of intensive diabetes treatment on the progression of diabetic retinopathy in insulin-dependent diabetes mellitus. Arch Ophthalmol 1995;113:36-51
• Diabetic Retinopathy Vitrectomy Study Research Group: Early vitrectomy for severe vitreous hemorrhage in diabetic retinopathy: Two year results of a randomized trial. Diabetic retinopathy Vitrectomy Study Report 2. Arch Ophthalmol 1985;103:1644-1651
• Regillo CD, Brown GC, Savino PJ, et al: Diabetic papillopathy: Patient characteristics and fundus findings. Arch Ophthalmol 1995;113:889-895
• Browning DJ, Zhang Z, Benfield M, et al: The effect of patient characteristics on response to focal laser treatment for diabetic macular edema. Ophthalmol 1997;104:466-472
• Klein R, Klein BEK, Moss SE, et al: The Wisconsin epidemiologic study of diabetic retinopathy XVII. The 14-year incidence and progression of diabetic retinopathy and associated risk factors in type 1 diabetes. Ophthalmol 1998;1801-1815
• Mayer-Davis EJ, Bell RA, Reboussin BA, et al: Antioxidant nutrient intake and diabetic retinopathy: The San Luis Valley Diabetic Study. Ophthalmol 1998;2264-2270
Illustrations: 5 available on CD-ROM
Internet references: http://www.5mcc.com

Author(s)
Richard W. Allinson, MD

Reye's syndrome

BASICS

DESCRIPTION Acute encephalopathy with cerebral edema and fatty infiltration of the liver. Occurs in previously healthy children, often associated with an antecedent viral infection such as varicella or influenza. Markedly decreased in incidence since late 1970's when association with aspirin use and Reye's syndrome made. Most cases currently seen are "Reye-like syndrome" (RLS) caused by inborn error of metabolism or toxin (see Differential Diagnosis).
System(s) affected: Nervous, Gastrointestinal
Genetics: No known genetic pattern
Incidence/Prevalence in USA: Currently very rare
Predominant age: Infants, children, adolescents. Peak incidence at 6 years of age. Most cases between 4-12 years of age.
Predominant Sex: Male = Female

SIGNS AND SYMPTOMS
• Symptoms reflected in clinical staging system
  ◊ I: Vomiting, sleepy, lethargic
  ◊ II: Confusion, delirium, hyperpnea, irritability, combative, hyperreflexia, altered muscle tone
  ◊ III: Obtunded, light coma and seizures, decorticate rigidity, loss of oculocephalic reflexes, intact pupillary reflex
  ◊ IV: Coma, decerebrate posturing spontaneously or in response to painful stimuli, seizures, fixed pupils
  ◊ V: Coma, flaccid paralysis, loss of deep tendon reflexes, seizures, respiratory arrest, isoelectric EEG

CAUSES Unknown - mitochondrion is major site of injury

RISK FACTORS
• Pediatric age group
• Viral illness, especially varicella, influenza A
• Use of preparations containing aspirin, salicylates, and/or salicylamides
• More common in rural and suburban areas

DIAGNOSIS

DIFFERENTIAL DIAGNOSIS
• Acute encephalopathy without hepatic abnormalities
  ◊ Encephalitis, meningitis, diabetes mellitus, drug overdose, poisoning, psychiatric illness
• Acute toxic encephalopathy with hepatic abnormalities (Reye-like syndrome)
  ◊ Inherited metabolic disorders
    - Organic acidurias with defects in hepatic fatty acid oxidation
    - Fatty acid metabolism defects: Acyl-CoA dehydrogenase, carnitine deficiency
    - Urea cycle defects: carbamyl phosphate synthetase, ornithine transcarbamylase
    -Fructosemia
  ◊ Drug ingestions
    -Valproate, aspirin
  ◊ Toxin ingestion (produce Reye-like syndrome)
    -Margosa oil, hepantenate, aflatoxin, hypoglycin (akee fruit), Jamaican vomiting sickness

LABORATORY
• Usually severe elevations of AST (SGOT) and ALT (SGPT)
• Hypoglycemia
• Normal or slightly elevated bilirubin or alkaline phosphatase
• Elevated ammonia
• Prolonged prothrombin time - often not responsive to Vitamin K
• Increased CSF pressure without pleocytosis (< 8 leukocytes per cubic millimeter)
• Mixed respiratory alkalosis and metabolic acidosis
• Hyperaminoacidemia (glutamine, alanine, lysine)
Drugs that may alter lab results: N/A
Disorders that may alter lab results: N/A

PATHOLOGICAL FINDINGS
• Slightly enlarged, firm, yellow liver with fat droplets throughout
• Characteristic liver biopsy with foamy cytoplasm with microvesicular fat - may need special preparation
• Uniformly severe mitochondrial injury

SPECIAL TESTS   EEG

IMAGING   N/A

DIAGNOSTIC PROCEDURES
• Liver biopsy
• CSF pressure measurement

TREATMENT

APPROPRIATE HEALTH CARE
Medical emergency requiring immediate hospitalization

GENERAL MEASURES
• Supportive depending on severity of illness
• IV glucose and close monitoring of blood or serum glucose (to prevent severe hypoglycemia)
• Hyperventilation, mannitol, barbiturates to reduce intracranial pressure
• Minimize noise and other CNS stimulation (to prevent increases in intracranial pressure)
• Vitamin K, fresh frozen plasma, platelets as needed
• Mechanical ventilation
• Dialysis to reduce high ammonia levels and/or residual salicylate

SURGICAL MEASURES
• Decompression craniotomy may be necessary

ACTIVITY   Complete bedrest

DIET   Nothing by mouth

PATIENT EDUCATION   Printed material from the National Reye's Syndrome Foundation, P.O. Box 829, Byron, OH 43506-0829, (800)233-7393

MEDICATIONS

DRUG(S) OF CHOICE
All treatment is supportive.
- 10-15% glucose IV
- Vitamin K
- For increased intracranial pressure, for example:
    ◊ Mannitol 0.5-1.0 gm/kg IV, as long as there is urine output
    ◊ Dexamethasone 0.5 mg/kg/day
    ◊ Barbiturates

Contraindications: Mannitol - do not use if patient has no renal output
Precautions: Mannitol and poor renal output may result in vascular overload and pulmonary edema
Significant possible interactions: Refer to manufacturer's literature

ALTERNATIVE DRUGS   N/A

FOLLOWUP

PATIENT MONITORING   Will depend on specific residual effects; may require care of physicians, nurses, psychologists, physical, occupational and/or speech therapists

PREVENTION/AVOIDANCE
- Avoidance of salicylates in children with viral illness
- Recognition of early symptoms of the disease

POSSIBLE COMPLICATIONS
See Signs and Symptoms also.
- Aspiration pneumonia
- Respiratory failure
- Cardiac dysrhythmia/arrest
- Inappropriate vasopressin excretion
- Diabetes insipidus
- Cerebral edema
- Seizures

EXPECTED COURSE/PROGNOSIS
- Majority will have mild illness without progression. Prognosis related to degree of cerebral edema and ammonia level on admission.
- Possible neurologic sequelae include problems with attention, concentration, speech, language, fine and gross motor skills - more common with higher stages

MISCELLANEOUS

ASSOCIATED CONDITIONS   N/A

AGE-RELATED FACTORS
Pediatric: Especially in infants under age 2, essential to make correct diagnosis; rule out other causes of Reye-like syndrome (see Differential Diagnosis section)
Geriatric: N/A
Others: N/A

PREGNANCY   N/A

SYNONYMS   White liver disease

ICD-9-CM
331.81 Reye's syndrome

SEE ALSO
- Encephalitis, viral
- Hepatic encephalopathy

OTHER NOTES   N/A

ABBREVIATIONS   N/A

REFERENCES
- Balistreri W: Reye syndrome and "Reye-like" diseases in Behrman, RE, Kliegman RM, Arvin A, eds: Nelson Textbook of Pediatrics. Philadelphia, WB Saunders Co. 1996:1144-5
- Green A, Hall S: Investigation of metabolic disorders resembling Reye's syndrome. Arch Dis Child 1992;67:1313-7
- Salmona M, Tacconi MT: Reyes and Reye-like syndrome, Drug related diseases? Drug Met Rev 1995;27:517-39
- Belay E, Bresee J, Holman R, et al: Reye's syndrome in the United States from 1981 through 1997. NEJM 1999;340:1377-1382
- Monto J: The disappearance of Reye's syndrome - a health triumph. NEJM 1999;340:1423-1424
Illustrations: N/A
Internet references: http://www.5mcc.com

Author(s)
William A. Primack, MD

Rh incompatibility

BASICS

DESCRIPTION Antibody-mediated destruction of red blood cells that bear Rh surface antigens by individuals who lack the antigens and have become isoimmunized ("sensitized") to them. Can occur with transfusion of incompatible blood. More commonly seen in the Rh-positive fetus or infant of an Rh-negative mother.
System(s) affected:
Hemic/Lymphatic/Immunologic
Genetics: Complex autosomal inheritance of polypeptide Rh antigens. At least three closely-linked loci on chromosome 2 carry an assortment of alleles: Dd, Cd, Ee. Individuals who express the D antigen (also called Rho or Rho[D]) are considered Rh positive, as are those expressing the weak D (Du) variant. Individuals lacking the D antigen are Rh negative. Antibodies may be produced to C, c, D, E, or e in individuals lacking the specific antigen; only D is strongly immunogenic. Isoimmunization to Rh antigens is not inherited.
Incidence/Prevalence in USA:
• 15% of Caucasian population and smaller fractions of other races are Rh negative
• Risk of isoimmunization during or after an Rh-positive pregnancy is about 15%
• Only 1-2% of isoimmunizations occur antepartum
• With Rho(D) immune globulin prophylaxis, risk of sensitization is reduced to less than 1% of susceptible pregnancies
Predominant age: Childbearing
Predominant sex: Female only

SIGNS AND SYMPTOMS
• Hemolytic transfusion reaction in recipient of Rh-incompatible blood
• Jaundice of newborn
• Kernicterus
• Congenital or fetal anemia
• Fetal hydrops
• Fetal death in utero

CAUSES
• Transfusion of Rh-positive blood to Rh-negative recipient
• Maternal exposure to fetal Rh antigens, either antepartum or intrapartum

RISK FACTORS
• Any Rh-positive pregnancy in Rh-negative woman
• Induced abortion
• Spontaneous abortion
• Ectopic pregnancy
• Amniocentesis, chorionic villus sampling
• Fetomaternal hemorrhage (fetal death in utero)
• Fetal manipulation, external version
• Cesarean delivery
• Maternal trauma
• Placental abruption
• Placenta previa
• Manual placental removal

DIAGNOSIS

DIFFERENTIAL DIAGNOSIS
• ABO incompatibility
• Other blood group (non-Rh) isoimmunization
• Nonimmune fetal hydrops
• Hereditary spherocytosis
• Red cell enzyme defects

LABORATORY Positive indirect Coombs' test (antibody screen) during pregnancy
Drugs that may alter lab results: Prior administration of D immune globulin may lead to weakly (false) positive indirect Coombs' test in mother and direct Coombs' test in infant
Disorders that may alter lab results: N/A

PATHOLOGICAL FINDINGS N/A

SPECIAL TESTS
• Paternal blood typing
• Kleihauer-Betke test to quantify an acute feto-maternal bleed

IMAGING N/A

DIAGNOSTIC PROCEDURES N/A

TREATMENT

APPROPRIATE HEALTH CARE
Outpatient, ambulatory management in most cases. Because of the specialized, somewhat hazardous treatment measures involved, pregnancies usually managed at tertiary care level.

GENERAL MEASURES
• See Patient Monitoring also
• Depending on severity of involvement, treatment of newborn or fetus may include:
   ◊ Phototherapy
   ◊ Transfusion after delivery
   ◊ Exchange transfusion
   ◊ Diuretics and digoxin for hydrops
   ◊ Early delivery
   ◊ Intrauterine transfusion

SURGICAL MEASURES N/A

ACTIVITY N/A

DIET N/A

PATIENT EDUCATION Griffith: Instructions for Patients; Philadelphia, 1994 W.B. Saunders Co.

Rh incompatibility

MEDICATIONS

DRUG(S) OF CHOICE
- For prophylaxis:
Rho(D) immune globulin (RhIG, RhoGAM, Gamulin Rh) given to unsensitized, Rh-negative women following:
  ◊ Spontaneous abortion
  ◊ Induced abortion
  ◊ Ectopic pregnancy
  ◊ Antepartum hemorrhage
  ◊ Amniocentesis
  ◊ Chorionic villus sampling
  ◊ Routinely at 28 weeks
  ◊ Within 72 hours after delivery of Rh-positive infant
- Dose:
  ◊ 50 mcg dose for events up to 12 weeks gestation
  ◊ 300 mcg dose for events after 12 weeks
  ◊ Higher doses may be required in the event of a large fetal - maternal hemorrhage (> 30 mL whole blood)

Contraindications: Patient with known severe reaction to human globulin. Refer to manufacturer's profile.
Precautions: Refer to manufacturer's profile
Significant possible interactions: N/A

ALTERNATIVE DRUGS   N/A

FOLLOWUP

PATIENT MONITORING
- Antibody titer measured every few weeks during pregnancy. A titer of 1:16 or greater indicates need for further testing.
- Amniocentesis for amniotic fluid bilirubin levels
- Umbilical blood sampling (cordocentesis) for fetal blood type, hematocrit, reticulocyte count, presence of erythroblasts
- Fetal heart rate testing/ultrasonography to assess fetal status
- Amniocentesis for fetal lung maturity

PREVENTION/AVOIDANCE
- Blood typing (ABO and Rh) on all pregnant women
- Antibody screening early in pregnancy
- Rh immune globulin prevents only sensitization to the D antigen
- Follow prophylaxis routine listed in Medications for unsensitized, Rh-negative women

POSSIBLE COMPLICATIONS
- Pregnancy loss from umbilical blood sampling
- Pregnancy loss from intrauterine transfusion
- Fetal distress requiring emergent delivery

EXPECTED COURSE/PROGNOSIS
- With appropriate monitoring and treatment, infants born of severely affected pregnancies have a survival rate of greater than 80%
- Hydropic fetuses have poor salvage rate
- Disease is likely to be more severe in affected subsequent pregnancies

MISCELLANEOUS

ASSOCIATED CONDITIONS
- Hemolytic disease of newborn
- Hydrops fetalis
- Neonatal jaundice
- Kernicterus

AGE-RELATED FACTORS
Pediatric: N/A
Geriatric: N/A
Others: N/A

PREGNANCY   N/A

SYNONYMS
- Rh isoimmunization
- Rh alloimmunization
- Rh sensitization

ICD-9-CM
656.10-656.13 Rh isoimmunization in pregnancy
656.20-656.23 Other isoimmunization in pregnancy
773.0 Rh hemolytic disease in fetus or newborn
773.1 ABO hemolytic disease in fetus or newborn
773.2 Other hemolytic disease in fetus or newborn
773.3 Isoimmune hydrops fetalis
773.4 Isoimmune kernicterus
773.5 Isoimmune late anemia

SEE ALSO
- Jaundice
- Anemia, hemolytic
- Erythroblastosis fetalis

OTHER NOTES   N/A

ABBREVIATIONS   N/A

REFERENCES
- Perkins JT: Hemolytic Disease of the Newborn. In: Gleicher N, ed. Principles and Practice of Medical Therapy in Pregnancy. 2nd Ed. Norwalk, CT, Appleton & Lange, 1992
- Socol ML: Management of Blood Group Isoimmunization. In: Gleicher N, ed. Principles and Practice of Medical Therapy in Pregnancy. 2nd Ed. Norwalk, CT, Appleton & Lange, 1992
- Management of Isoimmunization in Pregnancy. ACOG Technical Bulletin, 148, Oct 1990
- Prevention of D Isoimmunization. ACOG Technical Bulletin, 147, Oct 1990
- Giblett ER: Blood Groups and Blood Transfusion. In: Braunwald E, et al, eds. Harrison's Principles of Internal Medicine. 12th Ed. New York, McGraw-Hill Inc., 1991
- Agre P, Cartron J: Molecular Biology of the Rh Antigens. Blood 1991;78(3):551-63
Illustrations: N/A
Internet references: http://www.5mcc.com

Author(s)
Donald A. F. Nelson, MD

Rhabdomyolysis

BASICS

DESCRIPTION A syndrome resulting from damage to skeletal muscle with the resultant appearance of free myoglobin in the circulation. Myoglobin is then filtered by the glomerulus and appears in the urine. Elevated urinary levels of myoglobin can lead to acute renal failure.
System(s) affected: Renal/Urologic, Musculoskeletal, Cardiovascular, Nervous, Gastrointestinal
Genetics: Certain inherited disorders of fatty acid metabolism (Carnitine Palmityltransferase deficiency - autosomal recessive) and glycogen storage diseases (phosphofructokinase deficiency autosomal recessive; phosphoglycerate kinase deficiency is the only of these categories which is X-linked recessive) are inherited and lead to muscle injury with exercise which may eventuate rhabdomyolysis and acute renal failure.
Incidence/Prevalence in USA: Unknown (estimate: at Harborview Medical Center, a Seattle municipal hospital, rhabdomyolysis accounts for approximately 10-15% of ARF cases, per Zager RA)
Predominant age: Depends on the etiology for rhabdomyolysis, i.e., inherited disorders lead to rhabdomyolysis at a younger age but other etiologies may occur at any time - trauma or rhabdomyolysis secondary to infection.
Predominant sex: M > F; because of greater incidence of trauma in males

SIGNS AND SYMPTOMS
Rhabdomyolysis may present with obvious muscle injury and swelling on examination, e.g., crush injury, compartment syndrome; or muscle exam may be completely negative despite severe rhabdomyolysis/myoglobinuria. The signs and symptoms with renal failure are the same as those for acute tubular necrosis (ATN) from other etiologies.

CAUSES
• Metabolic, electrolytes - hypokalemia, hypophosphatemia, myopathies, inherited disorders of fatty acid metabolism (i.e., acyl-CoA dehydrogenase deficiency), glycogen storage diseases (e.g., phosphorylase b-kinase deficiency) and others (lactate dehydrogenase A deficiency)
• Polymyositis
• Dermatomyositis
• Malignant hyperthermia
• Neuroleptic malignant syndrome (anesthesia, phenothiazines, MAO inhibitors)
• Muscle exertion (physical, secondary to convulsions or to heat injury)
• Trauma-crush syndromes and pseudo-crush syndrome
• Muscle ischemia secondary to arterial occlusion or insufficiency
• Burns
• Repetitive muscle injury (bongo drumming, torture)
• Status epilepticus
• Hyperosmolality
• Head injury

• Infections
  ◊ Viral (influenza A, Epstein-Barr virus, measles, varicella, etc.)
  ◊ Bacterial - Legionnaires
  ◊ Septicemia
  ◊ Parasites (malaria)
• Toxic muscle injury
  ◊ Alcohol induced
  ◊ Tetanus
  ◊ Snake venom (viper bite) and rattlesnake
  ◊ Carbon monoxide exposure
• Drug induced
  ◊ Crack-cocaine, heroin, amphetamine abuse, "ecstasy"
• Drug overdoses
  ◊ Theophylline and INH
  ◊ Lipid lowering agents (clofibrate, gemfibrozil in combination with HMG CoA reductase inhibitors, HMG CoA reductase inhibitors and cyclosporine or itraconazole, possibly cyclosporine alone)
  ◊ Any drug that leads to neuroleptic malignant syndrome
• Carcinoma - acute necrotizing myopathy of carcinoma
• Diabetes mellitus; ketoacidosis
• Extreme lithotomy position for extended periods
• Extended periods of muscle pressure
  ◊ After allogenic bone marrow transplant
  ◊ Hyponatremia or correction thereof
  ◊ Hypothyroidism
  ◊ Water intoxication
  ◊ Hypokalemia

RISK FACTORS   See Causes

DIAGNOSIS

DIFFERENTIAL DIAGNOSIS
• For acute renal failure with rhabdomyolysis - any disease that causes acute tubular necrosis can be confused with rhabdomyolysis
• Renal pigment injury from hemoglobin resembles pigment injury from myoglobin

LABORATORY
• Muscle enzyme elevations (creatinine kinase, aldolase, and lactic dehydrogenase)
• Marked elevations of potassium and phosphorus from muscle injury
• Hypocalcemia during oliguria with hypercalcemia occasionally during the recovery phase from acute tubular necrosis (in fact, hypercalcemia during recovery from ATN is almost diagnostic of rhabdomyolysis and myoglobulin tubular injury)
• Urinalysis - dipstick positive for blood without red cells in sediment is very suggestive of pigment injury from either hemoglobin or myoglobin; coarsely granular, pigmented casts
• Urine or serum myoglobin levels may be helpful, but normal levels do not rule out pigment injury
• Extreme hyperuricemia may be present and actually can cause acute uric acid nephropathy in the setting of rhabdomyolysis

• When measured, vitamin D levels are decreased in the oliguric phase of rhabdomyolysis
• Reversible hepatic dysfunction occurs
Drugs that may alter lab results: None
Disorders that may alter lab results: Hemoglobin may be confused with myoglobin on dipstick

PATHOLOGICAL FINDINGS Muscle necrosis; kidney-myoglobin renal injury looks like ATN from other causes

SPECIAL TESTS
• Hypocalcemia during the oliguric phase helps but is not diagnostic of rhabdomyolysis
• Extreme hyperkalemia, hyperphosphatemia and hyperuricemia is very suggestive of rhabdomyolysis

IMAGING Any renal imaging is similar as for other etiologies of ATN

DIAGNOSTIC PROCEDURES A good index of clinical suspicion with evidence of muscle damage on exam or by lab tests make the diagnosis likely

TREATMENT:

APPROPRIATE HEALTH CARE
Inpatient

GENERAL MEASURES
(See also topic on acute renal failure)
• Dialysis will be necessary for severe renal failure
• Caution: Diagnose muscle entrapment or compartment syndromes (anterior compartment rhabdomyolysis may require surgical intervention and relief of pressure to stop rhabdomyolysis - anterior tibial, soleus, lateral thigh or gluteus maximus)
• Severe hypocalcemia with symptoms (Chvostek's and Trousseau's) during the oliguric phase would benefit from intravenous calcium gluconate and intravenous vitamin D (Calcijex). Symptomatic hypocalcemia is rare.

SURGICAL MEASURES Relief of compartment syndrome by fasciotomy to preserve muscle viability and nerve function

ACTIVITY Physical exertion can lead to rhabdomyolysis and less exertion is tolerated in people with metabolic myopathies mentioned above. (See Genetics and Causes.)

DIET When acute renal failure occurs from rhabdomyolysis, protein restriction to lower BUN, potassium restriction to lower potassium and volume restriction with anuria are essential

PATIENT EDUCATION Specific for possible causes

Rhabdomyolysis

MEDICATIONS

DRUG(S) OF CHOICE
• When rhabdomyolysis is identified, appropriate intervention may prevent renal failure
◊ Volume expansion attempt to increase urine output to approximately 150 cc/hr (3 mL/kg/hr), strong support for aggressive and early fluid-replacement
◊ IV mannitol as a bolus - 12.5 to 25 grams (0.25-0.5 g/kg); not to exceed approximately 50 grams in 24 hours; or as a constant infusion of 20% mannitol to a total of 25-50 g in 24 hours
◊ Alkalinization of the urine decreases myoglobin tubular injury (sodium bicarbonate to increase urine pH above 6.5)
• When renal failure supervenes from rhabdomyolysis, severe hyperkalemia may be life threatening. Treatment is based on EKG changes (tall, thin T waves; P-R prolongation; QRS widening; P wave flattening).
◊ Calcium gluconate IV 1-2 amps (0.5 mL of 10% calcium gluconate = 4 mg elemental calcium; give 4 mg/kg/hr x 4 hrs). Remember that bicarbonate administration may lead to alkalosis and worsening hypocalcemia.
◊ If acidosis is present 1-2 amps (2-3 mL/kg) sodium bicarbonate IV
◊ If tolerated oral sodium polystyrene sulfonate (Kayexalate) as much as 20 grams (1 gm/kg)
◊ insulin and glucose; tall peaked T waves-treatment resembles wide QRS.
◊ Dialysis may then become necessary to remove potassium.
• Vitamin D and calcium were mentioned above

Contraindications: See manufacturer's literature
Precautions: See Causes, especially drug combinations
Significant possible interactions: N/A

ALTERNATIVE DRUGS N/A

FOLLOWUP

PATIENT MONITORING
• Contingent on primary disease. Some cases (crush injury) are accidental and will not occur again.
• Contingent on disease - essential for metabolic myopathies
• There have been reports of interstitial nephritis many years after rhabdomyolysis from heat stroke and exertion

PREVENTION/AVOIDANCE
• Avoidance of situations leading to rhabdomyolysis (see Causes) prevent the injury
• Avoidance of metabolic states (hypokalemia) and drug combinations that lead to rhabdomyolysis (gemfibrozil and HMG CoA reductase inhibitors) are necessary

POSSIBLE COMPLICATIONS Death especially from hyperkalemia or renal failure. With dialysis and supportive care, prognosis much better.

EXPECTED COURSE/PROGNOSIS
Contingent on primary cause of rhabdomyolysis and contingent on recovery from acute renal failure without complications (infection, GI bleeding, cardiac standstill from hyperkalemia)

MISCELLANEOUS

ASSOCIATED CONDITIONS See Causes

AGE-RELATED FACTORS
Pediatric: Inherited myopathies and trauma more common
Geriatric: N/A
Others: N/A

PREGNANCY N/A

SYNONYMS Myoglobinuria with renal failure

ICD-9-CM
728.89 Idiopathic rhabdomyolysis

SEE ALSO
• Renal failure, acute (ARF)
• Polymyositis/dermatomyositis

OTHER NOTES N/A

ABBREVIATIONS
• ATN = acute tubular necrosis
• MAO = monoamine oxidase

REFERENCES
• Homis E: Prophylaxis of acute renal failure in patients with rhabdomyolysis. Ren Fail 1997;19:283-285
• Lampley EC, Williams S, Myers SA: Cocaine-associated rhabdomyolysis causing renal failure in pregnancy. Obstet & Gynecol 1996;87:804-806
• Zager RA: Rhabdomyolysis and myohemoglobinuria acute renal failure. Kid Int 1996;49:314-326
• Singh U, Schels WM: Infectious etiologies of rhabdomyolysis: three case reports and review. CID 1996;22:642-649
• Knochel JP: in Current Therapy in Nephrology and Hypertension. Glassock RJ, ed. St Louis, Mosby, 1998
• Rutecki GW, Ognibene AJ, Geib JD: Rhabdomyolysis in antiquity: from ancient descriptions to scientific explications. The Pharos of AOA 1998;61:18-22
• Slater MS, Mullins RJ: Rhabdomyolysis and myoglobinuric failure in trauma and surgical parients: a review. J Amer Coll Surg 1998;186(6)693-716
• Szewczyk D, Ovadia P, Abdullah F, et al: Pressure-induced rhabdomyolysis and acute renal failure. J of trauma 1998;44(2):384-388
Illustrations: N/A
Internet references: http://www.5mcc.com

Author(s)
Michael Youtsey, MD
Gregory W. Rutecki, MD

Rheumatic fever

BASICS

DESCRIPTION Rheumatic fever is an inflammatory disease, possibly autoimmune in nature. Rheumatic fever involves many tissues, including the heart, joints, skin, and central nervous system. Preceding infection of the upper respiratory tract with group A Streptococcus is a prerequisite to the development of acute rheumatic fever.
• Rheumatic fever can cause permanent cardiac valvular disease as well as acute cardiac decompensation.
• Recurrences are common if not prevented with "prophylactic" antibiotic treatment. In recent years there have been multiple reports of recurrences in adults as well as children.
System(s) affected: Cardiovascular, Hemic/Lymphatic/Immunologic, Nervous, Musculoskeletal, Skin/Exocrine
Genetics: A specific genetic marker that correlates with susceptibility to rheumatic fever has not been found, but the disease is known to occur in families
Incidence/Prevalence in USA:
• The incidence of rheumatic fever in the United States has been showing an overall decline for decades. In the 1970's it was a rare disease with an incidence of 0.5-1.88 cases per 100,000. However, since the mid-1980's there has been a resurgence of cases with multiple "outbreaks" having been reported in the U. S.
• The incidence calculated based on recent outbreaks has been as high as 18.1 per 100,000 in children aged 5-17 years
Predominant age: Most common in children ages 5-15. Recurrences can be seen in adulthood.
Predominant sex: Male = Female

SIGNS AND SYMPTOMS
• Joint symptoms ranging from arthralgias to frank arthritis (75%)
• Joints involved are medium to large, e.g., ankles, knees, wrists
• Joint involvement is classically migratory
• Joint symptoms usually disappear in 3-4 weeks without permanent deformities
• Carditis (65%), mild or severe with murmurs
• Cardiac involvement may include pericarditis, myocarditis, and/or valvular insufficiency. Appears within 2 weeks and lasts 6 weeks to 6 months.
• Valvular damage may be permanent
• P-R prolongation on ECG
• Erythema marginatum (classic rash) < 5%
• Subcutaneous nodules (painless, hard swellings overlying bony prominences) 5-10%
• Chorea is often a late finding but may be a presenting complaint. It occurs in 10-15% of patients, and its duration is not altered by treatment.
• Fever 101-104°F (38.3-40.0°C)
• Abdominal pain is common. It may be severe.
• Epistaxis (historically important, but rarely seen in acute rheumatic fever)
• Facial tics
• Facial grimace

CAUSES
• Autoimmune mechanisms
• A preceding upper respiratory infection with group A Streptococcus is a prerequisite

RISK FACTORS
• Crowded living, school or working conditions
• Tendency to upper respiratory infections

DIAGNOSIS

DIFFERENTIAL DIAGNOSIS Lupus, juvenile rheumatoid arthritis, infectious arthritis, viral myocarditis, innocent murmurs, Tourette's syndrome, Kawasaki syndrome

LABORATORY
• Increased acute phase reactants, including sedimentation rate (ESR) and C-reactive protein (CRP)
• Bacteriological or serological evidence of group A streptococcal infection, antistreptolysin O (ASO), Streptozyme, or anti-deoxyribonuclease B (DNase)
• Anemia
Drugs that may alter lab results: Prior treatment with aspirin or steroids
Disorders that may alter lab results: N/A

PATHOLOGICAL FINDINGS
• Subcutaneous nodules have a characteristic histological appearance
• Pericardial effusion
• Fibrinous pericardium

SPECIAL TESTS N/A

IMAGING
• Chest x-ray
• Echocardiogram (reveals pericardial effusion and documents valvular disease)

DIAGNOSTIC PROCEDURES
• Throat cultures for beta-hemolytic streptococci
• Diagnosis is dependent on fulfilling the modified Jones criteria of two major manifestations or one major and two minor manifestations. In either case, there must be evidence of preceding group A streptococcal infection. The five major criteria are carditis, arthritis, chorea, erythema marginatum, subcutaneous nodules. The minor criteria include fever, arthralgia (cannot use if arthritis was used as a major criteria), previous rheumatic fever, acute phase labs, prolonged P-R interval on EKG.

TREATMENT

APPROPRIATE HEALTH CARE
• Outpatient
• Initial hospitalization may be helpful to diagnose and establish stability of the patient

GENERAL MEASURES
• Mainstay of therapy is anti-inflammatory
• Patients with arthritis - therapy for relief of pain
• Patients with carditis - suppress inflammation
• Patients with arrhythmias - treat with appropriate agents

SURGICAL MEASURES N/A

ACTIVITY
• Initial bedrest with activity increasing gradually as tolerated
• Advance activity cautiously if there is evidence of carditis

DIET Regular; low sodium initially if the patient has carditis

PATIENT EDUCATION Information available from the American Heart Association

MEDICATIONS

DRUG(S) OF CHOICE
• If patient has carditis with cardiomegaly, start prednisone, 2 mg/kg/day (maximum 60 mg) for two weeks then taper over two weeks. Start aspirin at beginning of steroid taper. Continue aspirin for 6 weeks.
• If no cardiomegaly, start aspirin 60 mg/kg/day (to maintain salicylate level of 20-25µg/mL), 75-100 mg/kg/day for children, for 4-6 weeks
• Treat initially with penicillin as if active streptococcal infection is present, then begin prophylaxis. See Followup.
• Chorea may require treatment with haloperidol
Contraindications: Specific drug allergies
Precautions:
• Usual steroid side effects
• Extrapyramidal effects can occur with haloperidol
Significant possible interactions: Refer to manufacturer's profile of each drug

ALTERNATIVE DRUGS
Sulfadiazine may be used for prophylaxis in penicillin allergic patients. Patients who take sulfadiazine should take at least 2 liters of fluid daily to guard against sulfadiazine crystalluria.

FOLLOWUP

PATIENT MONITORING
Each week initially, then every 6 months

PREVENTION/AVOIDANCE
• Patients will need to be on prophylactic penicillin throughout childhood and possibly indefinitely during adulthood. Monthly injections of 1.2 million units of benzathine penicillin intramuscularly is the preferred treatment.
• Adults should be treated for a minimum of five years after an attack. Some treat adults indefinitely if there has been valvular disease. Oral penicillin V-K, 125 mg twice daily is an alternative to monthly injections. In the event of penicillin allergy, Sulfadiazine, 500 mg daily for children weighing less than 30 kg or 1 gr daily for all. Others may be used.
• If patients have valvular damage from acute rheumatic fever, they will require bacterial endocarditis prophylaxis for dental and other high risk procedures

POSSIBLE COMPLICATIONS
• Subsequent attacks of acute rheumatic fever secondary to streptococcal reinfection
• Carditis
• Mitral stenosis
• Congestive heart failure

EXPECTED COURSE/PROGNOSIS
Sequelae limited to the heart and dependent of severity of carditis during an acute attack

MISCELLANEOUS

ASSOCIATED CONDITIONS N/A

AGE-RELATED FACTORS
Pediatric: More common in children
Geriatric: N/A
Others: N/A

PREGNANCY
Residual valvular disease may be exacerbated by pregnancy. Refer pregnant patient to cardiologist for assistance in management.

SYNONYMS N/A

ICD-9-CM
390 Rheumatic fever without mention of heart involvement

SEE ALSO N/A

OTHER NOTES N/A

ABBREVIATIONS N/A

REFERENCES
• Vaughn VC, McKay RJ, eds: Nelson's Textbook of Pediatrics. Philadelphia, W.B. Saunders Co., 1992
• Ferrieri P: AJDC 1987;141 (7):125-7
• Quinn RW: Review Infect Dis 1989;11:128-153
• daSilva NA: Acute rheumatic fever. Still a challenge. Rheumatol Dis Clin NA 1997;23(3)545-68
Illustrations: N/A
Internet references: http://www.5mcc.com

Author(s)
H. Gratin Smith, MD, FAAP

Rhinitis, allergic

BASICS

DESCRIPTION Immediate and delayed reactions to airborne allergens, beginning with the generation and presence of specific antigen-responsive IgE antibody receptors on mast cells of the nasal mucosa
• An antigen-antibody chemical union initiates a cascade of events in the mast cell culminating in its degranulation and production of a melange of inflammatory mediators including histamine, heparin, leukotrienes, prostaglandins, proteases and platelet activating factor
• An immediate symptomatic response occurs followed by a more prolonged, persistent late phase reaction. This involves the infiltration into the reactive region of eosinophils, neutrophils, basophils and mononuclear cells
• May be seasonal or perennial depending on climate and individual response and the offending antigens
• Seasonal responses usually to grasses, trees and weeds
• Perennial responses exampled by house dust mites, mold antigens and animal body products
System(s) affected: Pulmonary, Skin/Exocrine, Hemic/Lymphatic/Immunologic
Genetics: Complex, but strong genetic determination present
Incidence/Prevalence in USA: 8-12% of the population affected
Predominant Age:
• Onset usually before the age of 30 with tendency to diminish with time
• Mean age onset approximately 10 years
Predominant sex: Male = Female

SIGNS AND SYMPTOMS
• Nasal stuffiness and congestion
• Pale, boggy mucous membranes
• Nasal polyps
• Sneezing, often paroxysmal
• Watery eyes
• Dark circles under eyes, "allergic shiners"
• Long eye lashes often associated
• Sensation of plugged ears
• Symptom associated sleeping difficulties
• Fatigue
• Mouth breathing
• Scratchy throat
• Voice change
• Irritating cough
• Postnasal drip
• Loss or alteration of smell
• Itchy nose, eyes, ears and palate
• Transverse nasal crease from rubbing nose upwards
• Dull facies

CAUSES
• Animal and plant proteins: Pollens, molds, mite dust, animal danders, dried saliva and urine
• Insect debris: Cockroach, locusts, fish food (thirps)

RISK FACTORS
• Family history
• Repeated exposure to offending antigen
• Exposure to multiple offending allergens
• Presence of other allergies, e.g., atopic dermatitis, asthma, urticaria
• Non-compliance to appropriate therapeutic measures

DIAGNOSIS

DIFFERENTIAL DIAGNOSIS
• Nonallergic rhinitis with eosinophilia syndrome (NARES)
• Vasomotor rhinitis
• Chronic sinusitis
• IgA deficiency with recurrent sinusitis
• Nasal polyps and tumor
• Reactive rhinitis of recumbency
• Cribriform plate defect with cerebrospinal fluid leakage (rule out by testing watery discharge for sugar)
• Foreign body
• Medications
    ◊ Rebound effect associated with continued use of topical decongestant drops and sprays
    ◊ Aldosterone converting enzyme inhibitors
    ◊ Chronic aspirin use
• Septal/anatomical obstruction
• Chronic rhinitis digitorum

LABORATORY
• CBC with differential. May have slight increase in eosinophils but often normal with uncomplicated rhinitis.
• Nasal probe smear with cytologic exam for eosinophils
• Increase IgE level. May do RAST determinations for specific suspected allergens.
Drugs that may alter lab results:
• Corticosteroids will ablate eosinophilia
Disorders that may alter lab results:
• Secondary infections may alter differential and decrease nasal eosinophils
• Parasitic infestations with more marked eosinophilia

PATHOLOGICAL FINDINGS
• Nasal washing/scraping
    ◊ Eosinophils predominate
    ◊ Basophils
    ◊ May see mast cells
• Nasal mucosa
    ◊ Submucosal edema but intact without evidence of destruction
    ◊ Eosinophilic infiltration
    ◊ Granulocytes to lesser extent
    ◊ Increased amount of tissue water with poor staining of ground substance
    ◊ Congested mucous glands and goblet cells

SPECIAL TESTS
• Skin tests using suspected antigens
Either technique manifests a positive reaction by inducing an expanding wheal and flare reaction. Special training recommended and available treatment for anaphylaxis mandatory
    ◊ Scratch or prick: a superficial injury to the epidermis with application of diluted test antigen
    ◊ Intradermal: Introduction of diluted material between layers of skin raising a 4 mm wheal using a 25 or 27 gauge needle
• Radioallergosorbent test (RAST)
    ◊ More expensive and used especially in cases where skin testing not practical, e.g., in atopic dermatitis and dermatographia
• Audiometry
    ◊ For deficits and base line evaluation
    ◊ Rhinoscopy (optional) - excellent visual advantages.

IMAGING Sinus film when indicated. Check for complete opacity, fluid level and mucosal thickening.

DIAGNOSTIC PROCEDURES See special lab tests. Appropriate diagnostic prick test kits available.

TREATMENT

APPROPRIATE HEALTH CARE
Outpatient

GENERAL MEASURES
• Patient education, assurance and understanding important
• Limit exposure to offending allergen
• Try to establish specific cause(s) - history and appropriate skin testing
• Intensity of treatment determined by severity of disease
• Immunotherapy:
    ◊ Usually reserved for seasonal allergies uncontrollable with drugs and not responding to environmental adjustment.
    ◊ Specific allergen extract is injected subcutaneously in increasing doses to patient tolerance as determined by local reaction
    ◊ Patient response should be evaluated each season or year

SURGICAL MEASURES Septoplasty when deviation significant enough to interfere with benefits of medication.

ACTIVITY No specific restrictions. Emphasize avoiding activity in areas of allergen exposure.

DIET No special diet unless concomitant food reactions suspected and evaluated

PATIENT EDUCATION Printed material available from many sources including: Asthma & Allergy Foundation of America. 1717 Massachusetts Ave., Suite 305, Washington, DC 20036, (800)7-ASTHMA

MEDICATIONS

DRUG(S) OF CHOICE
Most patients present because of inability to control symptoms and improve life style with avoidance of allergens or with over the counter medications.
- Antihistamines:
  ◊ Classification charts available. Five major classes:
    - Ethanolamines - diphenhydramine (Benadryl), clemastine (Tavist)
    - Alkylamine - chlorpheniramine, brompheniramine
    - Ethylenediamines - tripelennamine (PBZ)
    - Piperazines - hydroxyzine (Atarax)
    - Phenothiazines - promethazine (Phenergan), methdilazine (Tacaryl).
  ◊ Those with sedating side effects cheaper and often nonprescription. May start using at bedtime. Drowsiness often lessens with continued, regular dosage.
  ◊ Nonsedating type, e.g., Fexofenadine (Allegra)
- Decongestants
  ◊ Oral, e.g., pseudoephedrine
  ◊ Topical drops or sprays, e.g., phenylephrine
  ◊ Topical ophthalmic vasoconstrictors for annoying conjunctival itching
- Nasal sprays
  ◊ Physiologic saline solution
  ◊ Cromolyn (Nasalcrom)
  ◊ Beclomethasone (Beconase AQ, Vancenase AQ), flunisolide (Nasalide, AeroBid), triamcinolone (Nasacort), budesonide (Rhinocort).
- Systemic steroids
  ◊ Only in urgent, selected cases and only for short-term use.

Contraindications:
- Antihistamines may precipitate urinary retention in males with prostatism and/or hypertrophy
- Decongestants if congestion is a "rebound" phenomenon
- Discourage decongestants if hypertension a problem
- Non-sedating antihistamines (Seldane and Hismanal) should not be used in patients with liver disease or in situations in which potassium channeling is a problem

Precautions: The elderly often require less aggressive treatment and will more frequently present with non-allergic rhinitis

Significant possible interactions:
- Refer carefully to manufacturer's literature for interactions
- Always mention antihistamine associated somnolence
- Terfenadine or astemizole
  ◊ Ketoconazole, macrolides, quinidine: may precipitate ventricular arrhythmias

ALTERNATIVE DRUGS Combinations with decongestants

FOLLOWUP

PATIENT MONITORING
- Emphasize that you wish to do the most for, but the least to the patient
- Initiate patient education, supplementing with available videotapes and/or literature

PREVENTION/AVOIDANCE
- Avoidance - most patients with inhalant allergy have problems controlling their symptoms totally with allergen avoidance
- Air conditioning and limited outside exposure during season helpful
- Instructions as to the best housekeeping tactics and control for dust mites in patients sensitive to this allergen helpful
- Exposure to all animal contacts minimized. Discourage house pets.
- Avoid environmental irritants, e.g., smoke and fumes
- Air cleaners
- Use of allergy control covers especially on mattresses and pillows

POSSIBLE COMPLICATIONS
- Secondary infection
- Otitis media
- Sinusitis
- Epistaxis
- Nasopharyngeal lymphoid hyperplasia
- Decreased pulmonary function
- Continue to suspect effects of medications
- Facial changes (see Signs and Symptoms)

EXPECTED COURSE/PROGNOSIS
- Maximal, beneficially acceptable control of symptoms should be the goal
- Treatment tailored to each individual case.
- Immune system changes over time often associated with lessening of symptoms of allergic rhinitis. Therefore early, adequate control important.

MISCELLANEOUS

ASSOCIATED CONDITIONS
- Other IgE mediated conditions, e.g., asthma and atopic dermatitis

AGE-RELATED FACTORS
Pediatric:
- Consider allergy as principle cause of persistent rhinitis
- Family understanding and involvement important
- Environmental control requires a cooperative effort and may include carpet and drape removal, removal of house plants, pet control, etc.

Geriatric:
- Increased medication side effects
- Number and specific types of allergens causing symptoms may change
- Symptoms may decrease by 4th-5th decade (not a hard rule)

Others: N/A

PREGNANCY Physiological changes of pregnancy may aggravate all types of rhinitis including allergic, vasomotor, nonallergic rhinitis with eosinophilia and chronic irritable airways

SYNONYMS
- Hay fever
- Pollinosis
- IgE mediated rhinitis

ICD-9-CM 477 Allergic rhinitis

SEE ALSO Conjunctivitis

OTHER NOTES N/A

ABBREVIATIONS N/A

REFERENCES
- Middleton E Jr, Reed CE, Ellis EF: Allergy Principles and Practice. 4th Ed. St. Louis, C.V. Mosby Co, 1993
- JAMA. Primer on Allergic and Immunologic Diseases. 1992
- Baraniuk JA: Pathogenesis of allergic rhinitis. J of Allergy and Clinical Immunology 1997;99(2):S763-S772
Illustrations: N/A
Internet references: http://www.5mcc.com

Author(s)
J. Harlan Dix, MD, FACP

Rocky Mountain spotted fever

 BASICS

DESCRIPTION Rocky Mountain spotted fever (RMSF) is an acute, potentially fatal febrile illness caused by Rickettsia rickettsii and transmitted by tick bite. The primary pathology is a vasculitis due to direct endothelial cell invasion by rickettsiae. The cardinal clinical features are headache, fever, and a centripetal rash which is often petechial.
System(s) affected: Cardiovascular, Skin/Exocrine, Musculoskeletal, Nervous
Genetics: N/A
Incidence/Prevalence in USA: About 600 new cases are reported each year in the USA. There is considerable geographic variability; most cases are reported from south Atlantic and south central states. Peak incidence is in late spring and summer.
Predominant age: Highest incidences occur among children and young adults, primarily due to environmental exposure patterns. All ages are susceptible.
Predominant sex: Male > Female (due to greater male outdoor activity)

SIGNS AND SYMPTOMS
- Fever (100%)
- Rash (macular, maculopapular, petechial) (90-100%)
- Headache (65%)
- Rash (petechial) (50%)
- Headache, fever, rash (50-60%)
- Other neuropsychiatric symptoms (40-50%)
- Nausea, vomiting (30-50%)
- Headache, fever, petechial rash (33%)
- Abdominal pain (30%)
- Myalgias (30%)
- Hepatosplenomegaly (30%)
- Lymphadenopathy (25%)
- Arthralgias (10%)
- Cough (15%)
- Central nervous system dysfunction (stupor, confusion, coma, focal abnormalities) (10-30%)

CAUSES RMSF is caused by Rickettsia rickettsii which is transmitted by the bite of ticks (Dermacentor andersoni, Dermacentor variabilis). Rarely by direct inoculation of tick blood into open wounds or conjunctivae.

RISK FACTORS
- Outdoor activity during warm months
- Contact with dogs

 DIAGNOSIS

DIFFERENTIAL DIAGNOSIS
- Viral exanthems (measles, rubella, etc.)
- Meningoencephalitis (viral meningitis or encephalitis, bacterial meningitis)
- Typhus, rickettsialpox
- Ehrlichiosis
- Lyme disease
- Meningococcemia
- Leptospirosis

LABORATORY
- Nonspecific laboratory changes
  ◊ Thrombocytopenia
  ◊ WBC normal, increased, or decreased
  ◊ Anemia (mild)
  ◊ Hyponatremia (usually mild)
  ◊ CSF protein and WBC modestly elevated (lymphocytic predominance), glucose usually normal
  ◊ Prolonged PT, PTT; decreased fibrinogen; elevated fibrin degradation products (FDP) (uncommon)
- Specific laboratory diagnosis
  ◊ Serum Proteus Ox-19 antibody; fourfold increase (acute and convalescent) or solitary titer > 1:320 (relatively specific)
  ◊ Serum complement fixation (CF) antibody: fourfold increase or solitary titer > 1:16
  ◊ Serum indirect fluorescent antibody (IFA): fourfold increase or solitary titer > 1:64
  ◊ Direct fluorescent antibody (DFA) test on skin biopsy (not widely available)
Drugs that may alter lab results: N/A
Disorders that may alter lab results: Early treatment may blunt antibody response

PATHOLOGICAL FINDINGS
- The principal pathological abnormality is a systemic vasculitis
- Rickettsiae may be demonstrated within endothelial cells by DFA or electron microscopy
- Petechiae due to the vasculitis may be seen on various organ surfaces (e.g., liver, brain, epicardium)
- Secondary thromboses and tissue necrosis may be seen

SPECIAL TESTS N/A

IMAGING Other than nonspecific pneumonic infiltrates which may be seen on routine chest x-ray, imaging procedures are rarely helpful

DIAGNOSTIC PROCEDURES
- Tissue (primarily skin) biopsy can be helpful if rapid DFA or electron microscopy are available
- Diagnosis is usually presumptive, based upon a compatible syndrome in a patient with exposure history in an endemic area; confirmation is obtained by subsequent serology
- Polymerase chain reaction currently unreliable

 TREATMENT

APPROPRIATE HEALTH CARE
- Patients with the full clinical presentation or who are moderately ill should usually be hospitalized
- Patients with mild disease are treated presumptively as outpatients. Close followup is important in identifying complications.

GENERAL MEASURES
- Oxygen therapy and assisted ventilation for pulmonary complications, if necessary
- Good mouth care
- Blood transfusions for anemia
- Turning bed-confined patient frequently
- Watch patient closely for signs of renal failure

SURGICAL MEASURES N/A

ACTIVITY Bed rest until symptoms subside

DIET Critically ill patients may require IV nutrition. In others, small frequent meals may be necessary to maintain nutritional levels.

PATIENT EDUCATION See information in Prevention/Avoidance

Rocky Mountain spotted fever

MEDICATIONS

DRUG(S) OF CHOICE
• For adults (choose one of the following)
◊ Doxycycline (Vibramycin) 200 mg po initially, followed by 100 mg po bid for 7-10 days; same dosage IV; 100 mg q24h in renal failure (see Contraindications)
◊ Tetracycline 500 mg po q6h for 7-10 days; should not be used in renal failure (see Contraindications)
◊ Chloramphenicol 20 mg/kg IV q6h (4 gm per day maximum); same dose in renal failure (oral chloramphenicol is not available in the U.S.)
• For children (choose one of the following)
◊ Chloramphenicol 20 mg/kg IV q6h
◊ Doxycycline (Vibramycin) 2.0-2.5 mg/kg po q12h for 7-10 days; 4.4 mg/kg IV initially, followed by 2.2 mg per kg IV q12h (see Precautions)
◊ Tetracycline 10 mg per kg po q6h for 7-10 days (see Contraindications)
Contraindications:
• Pregnant women - doxycycline and tetracyclines are contraindicated because they may cause severe hepatic disease in the mother and retarded bone growth in the fetus
Precautions:
• Patients taking doxycycline or tetracyclines should minimize sun exposure to avoid photosensitization
• Infants or children with liver disease taking chloramphenicol should have serum drug levels monitored
• Chloramphenicol may rarely cause idiosyncratic, non-reversible, aplastic anemia
• Doxycycline and tetracycline may cause staining of permanent teeth when given to children less than 9 years old. This risk appears to be minimal if no more than 5 courses of therapy are administered prior to age 9.
Significant possible interactions:
Absorption of tetracyclines may be inhibited if they are ingested with milk products, iron preparations, or antacids containing aluminum or magnesium

ALTERNATIVE DRUGS   There are no currently available or adequately studied alternative drugs

FOLLOWUP

PATIENT MONITORING
• If patients are not hospitalized, they should be seen every 2-3 days until symptoms have fully resolved
• CBC, creatinine, electrolytes should be monitored

PREVENTION/AVOIDANCE
• People who go into tick-infested areas can take measures to prevent infection
◊ Occlusive clothing should be worn and insect repellants applied
◊ After possible exposure, all body areas should be carefully inspected for ticks, especially legs, groin, external genitalia, belt lines. Likelihood of infection increases with the duration of tick attachment.
◊ Ticks should be removed from humans or animals with caution; gloves should be worn or instruments used to minimize direct contact. Place a drop of oil, alcohol, gasoline or kerosene on the tick first. Hands should be washed thoroughly afterwards.

POSSIBLE COMPLICATIONS
• Encephalopathy, usually transient (30-40%)
• Seizures, focal neurologic signs (10%)
• Renal insufficiency (10%)
• Hepatitis (10%)
• Congestive heart failure (5%)
• Respiratory failure (5%)

EXPECTED COURSE/PROGNOSIS
• When treated promptly, the usual prognosis is excellent with resolution of symptoms over several days and no sequelae
• Mortality is rare with prompt institution of appropriate therapy
• If complications develop (see above), the course may be more severe and long-term sequelae may be present, particularly neurologic sequelae

MISCELLANEOUS

ASSOCIATED CONDITIONS   N/A

AGE-RELATED FACTORS
Pediatric: N/A
Geriatric: Mortality risk higher
Others: N/A

PREGNANCY   N/A

SYNONYMS   Tick typhus

ICD-9-CM
082.0 Rocky Mountain spotted fever

SEE ALSO
• Ehrlichiosis

OTHER NOTES   Treatment should be initiated on the basis of clinical diagnosis or skin biopsy. Treatment should not be delayed for serologic confirmation.

ABBREVIATIONS   N/A

REFERENCES
• Kirk JL, Fine DP, Sexton, DJ, Muchmore HG: Rocky Mountain spotted fever. A clinical review based on 48 confirmed cases, 1943-1986. Medicine 1990;69:35-45
• Melnick CG, Bernard KW, D'Angelo L: Rocky Mountain spotted fever: Clinical, laboratory, and epidemiological features of 262 cases. J Infect Dis 1984;150:480-488
• Archibald LK, Sexton DJ: Long-term sequelae of Rocky Mountain spotted fever. Clin Infect Dis 1995;20:1122-1125
• Grossman ER, Walchek A, Freedman H: Tetracycline and permanent teeth: the relationship between dose and tooth color. Pediatr 1971; 47:567-570
• Abramson JS, Givner LB: Should tetracycline be contraindicated for therapy of presumed Rocky Mountain spotted fever in children less than 9 years of age? Pediatr 1990; 86:123-124
• Cale DF, McCarthy MW: Treatment of Rocky Mountain spotted fever in children. Ann Pharmacother 1997; 31:492-494
Illustrations: N/A
Internet references: http://www.5mcc.com

Author(s)
Douglas P. Fine, MD
Ronald A. Greenfield, MD

Roseola

BASICS

DESCRIPTION An acute disease of infants or very young children with an incubation period of about 5-15 days. Characteristically, it causes first a high fever, followed by the appearance of an eruption (whose appearance is similar to that of measles) simultaneously with, or following defervescence. Transmission now believed to be via contact of salivary secretions from adults shedding HHV-6.
System(s) affected: Endocrine/Metabolic, Skin/Exocrine
Genetics: No known genetic pattern
Incidence/Prevalence in USA:
• Estimated that 30% of all children
• More likely to occur in spring and fall
Predominant age: Infants and very young children (6 months to 3 years)
Predominant sex: Male = Female

SIGNS AND SYMPTOMS
• Abrupt fever without apparent cause (103-105°F [39.4-40.5°C]) for 3-5 days
• Sudden drop of fever. As fever disappears, skin rash begins (lasts hours to days).
• Anorexia
• Irritability
• Listlessness
• Does not appear seriously ill
• Maculopapular, nonpruritic rash, first appearing on the trunk, that blanches on pressure
• Rash appears as very slightly elevated, rose-pink papules that appear profusely on trunk, arms and neck; mild on face and legs
• Rash fades within a few hours to 2 days
• Febrile convulsions during height of fever (uncommon)
• Lymphadenopathy in cervical and posterior auricular regions
• Spleen enlarged (uncommon)

CAUSES A communicable virus, human herpesvirus-6B (HHV-6B)

RISK FACTORS
• Day care center
• Exposure to infected infant

DIAGNOSIS

DIFFERENTIAL DIAGNOSIS
• Sepsis
• UTI
• Measles
• Rubella
• Fifth disease
• Enterovirus infection
• Otitis media
• Meningitis
• Bacterial pneumonia
• Drug eruption

LABORATORY
• Blood culture for HHV-6
• Urinalysis
• CBC - leukopenia with relative lymphocytosis
• IgM, IgG for human herpesvirus-6 (HHV-6)
• PCR (serum) for HHV-6
Drugs that may alter lab results: N/A
Disorders that may alter lab results: N/A

PATHOLOGICAL FINDINGS None

SPECIAL TESTS N/A

IMAGING Chest x-ray negative

DIAGNOSTIC PROCEDURES Careful physical examination. Roseola should be suspected if it is known to be in the community and the child presents with a high temperature. IgM - diagnostic for acute infection.

TREATMENT

APPROPRIATE HEALTH CARE
Outpatient

GENERAL MEASURES
• Symptomatic
• Tap water baths to cool excess temperature elevation
• Lightweight clothing
• Maintain normal room temperature

SURGICAL MEASURES N/A

ACTIVITY Rest until rash appears and fever breaks

DIET Encourage fluids

PATIENT EDUCATION
• Infection is self-limiting
• If seizures occur, they will not cause brain damage and will cease after fever subsides

Roseola

MEDICATIONS

DRUG(S) OF CHOICE
• Antipyretics for excessively high fever. Avoid aspirin. Instead use acetaminophen, 10-15 mg/kg/q4h to a maximum of 2.6 g/24h. (Aspirin may enhance the risk of Reye's syndrome.)
• Phenobarbital if needed for seizure
Contraindications: N/A
Precautions: N/A
Significant possible interactions: N/A

ALTERNATIVE DRUGS
No clinical trials to date evaluating antiviral agents, but in-vitro data does exist

FOLLOWUP

PATIENT MONITORING
None after typical rash appears

PREVENTION/AVOIDANCE
None

POSSIBLE COMPLICATIONS
• Febrile seizures
• Encephalitis (rare)
• Meningitis
• Hepatitis

EXPECTED COURSE/PROGNOSIS
• Course - acute, benign, complete recovery without sequelae
• One attack usually confers permanent immunity
• Reactivation in immunocompromised patients is possible

MISCELLANEOUS

ASSOCIATED CONDITIONS
N/A

AGE-RELATED FACTORS
Pediatric: A disease of infants and very young children
Geriatric: N/A
Others: N/A

PREGNANCY
N/A

SYNONYMS
• Exanthem subitum
• Pseudorubella
• Sixth disease

ICD-9-CM
056.9 Roseola
056.8 Roseola complicated

SEE ALSO
N/A

OTHER NOTES
N/A

ABBREVIATIONS
N/A

REFERENCES
• Asano Y, Yoshikawa T, Suga S, Kobayashi I, et al: Clinical features of infants with primary human herpesvirus 6 (roseola infantum). Pediatrics 1994;93:104-108
• Kimberlin DW: Human herpesvirus 6 and 7: identification of newly recognized viral pathogens and their association with human disease. Pediatr Infect Dis 1998;17:59-68
• Fegin RD, Cherry JD: Textbook of Pediatric Infectious Diseases. 4th Ed. Philadelphia, WB Saunders Co, 1998
• Dockrell DH, et al: Human herpesvirus 6. Mayo Clin Proc 1999;74:163-170
Illustrations: N/A
Internet references: http://www.5mcc.com

Author(s)
Jeffery T. Kirchner, DO, FAAFP

Roundworms, intestinal

BASICS

DESCRIPTION Intestinal roundworms (nematodes) have adult stages infecting the intestinal tract of man. Larval stages may exist elsewhere in the body. Except for Trichinella spiralis, which is encysted in muscle; egg and/or larval stages can be isolated from the intestinal canal.
• Nematodes parasitizing the intestinal tract of man:
◊ Enterobius vermicularis (pinworm)
◊ Trichuris trichiura (whipworm)
◊ Ascaris lumbricoides (large roundworm of man)
◊ Necator americanus (hookworm)
◊ Ancylostoma duodenale (hookworm)
◊ Strongyloides stercoralis
◊ Trichostrongylus
◊ Trichinella spiralis (trichinosis)
System(s) affected: Gastrointestinal, Cardiovascular, Pulmonary, Nervous, Renal/Urologic, Musculoskeletal
Genetics: N/A
Incidence/Prevalence in USA:
• Up to 40% of children may have pinworms
• Trichinella 4-20%
• Others mostly in Southern regions
• Incidence of intestinal obstruction with ascaris is 2/1000
• Incidence of ascaris reportedly decreasing in the US, presumably due to improved sanitation
Predominant age: All ages; pinworm infestations more common in children
Predominant sex: Male = Female

SIGNS AND SYMPTOMS
• Lung Invasion:
◊ Fever
◊ Cough
◊ Blood-tinged sputum
◊ Wheezing
◊ Rales
◊ Dyspnea
◊ Substernal pain
◊ Pulmonary consolidations
◊ Eosinophilia
◊ Urticaria
◊ Asthma
◊ Angioneurotic edema
◊ Brain, kidney, eye, spinal cord, etc. (rare)
• Intestinal invasion:
◊ May be asymptomatic (small number)
◊ Abdominal pain (usually vague)
◊ Abdominal cramps/colic
◊ Diarrhea
◊ Rarely vomiting
◊ Occasionally constipation

• Muscle and other tissue invasion: (Trichinosis)
◊ Myalgias
◊ Fever
◊ Edema and spasm
◊ Periorbital and facial edema
◊ Photophobia
◊ Sweating
◊ Conjunctivitis
◊ Weakness or prostration
◊ Pain on swallowing
◊ Subconjunctival, retinal and nail hemorrhages
◊ Rashes and formication
◊ Encephalitis, myocarditis, nephritis
◊ Pneumonia, meningitis, neuropathy

CAUSES
• Ingestion of mature eggs in fecally contaminated food or drink
• Larval penetration of skin (hookworm)

RISK FACTORS
• Low standard of hygiene
• Poor sanitation
• Human feces fertilizer

DIAGNOSIS

DIFFERENTIAL DIAGNOSIS
• Pulmonary ascariasis with eosinophilia - consider asthma, Löffler's syndrome, eosinophilic pneumonia, systemic lupus erythematosus, Hodgkin's disease, and other parasitic causes (tropical pulmonary eosinophilia, toxocariasis, strongyloidiasis, hookworm, paragonimiasis)
• Worm-induced GI diseases - consider other causes of pancreatitis, appendicitis, diverticulitis, duodenitis, esophagitis, cholecystitis
• Anemia/hypoproteinemia (hookworm) - consider other etiology
• Neurohelminthiases - consider other causes of CNS infection or mass lesion

LABORATORY
• Based on characteristics of eggs or larvae in stool or adult worm, if passed
• Cellophane-tape impression for pinworms
• Eosinophilia
• Larvae in sputum or adult worms seen on radiologic studies (uncommon)
Drugs that may alter lab results: N/A
Disorders that may alter lab results: N/A

PATHOLOGICAL FINDINGS Characteristic eggs/worms

SPECIAL TESTS Serologic tests not useful

IMAGING Ultrasound is useful in the diagnosis of ascariasis as cause of biliary tract disease

DIAGNOSTIC PROCEDURES
• Stool exams
• Cellophane-tape impression

TREATMENT

APPROPRIATE HEALTH CARE
Outpatient

GENERAL MEASURES None other than medications to eradicate the worms

SURGICAL MEASURES N/A

ACTIVITY No restrictions

DIET No special diet

PATIENT EDUCATION Avoid fecally contaminated food, water, and soil

Roundworms, intestinal

MEDICATIONS

DRUG(S) OF CHOICE
• Enterobius vermicularis (pinworm) - mebendazole (Vermox) 100 mg single dose, or albendazole 400 mg once, or pyrantel pamoate 11 mg/kg once (maximum of 1 g), repeat after 2 weeks (all dosages for adult and pediatrics)
• Trichuris trichiura (whipworm) - mebendazole 100 mg bid x 3 days or 500 mg once (all dosages for adults and children)
• Ascaris lumbricoides (large roundworm of man), mebendazole 100 mg bid x 3 days or 500 mg once or pyrantel pamoate 11 mg/kg once (maximum of 1 g) (all dosages for adult and pediatrics), or albendazole 400 mg once
• Necator americanus (hookworm), Ancylostoma duodenale (hookworm) - mebendazole 100 mg bid x 3 days or pyrantel pamoate 11 mg/kg (maximum of 1 g) x 3 days (all dosages for adult and pediatrics), or albendazole 400 mg once
• Trichostrongylus - pyrantel pamoate 11 mg/kg once (maximum of 1 g) or mebendazole 100 mg bid x 3 day (all dosages for adult and pediatrics)
• Trichinella spiralis - mebendazole 200-400 mg tid x 3 days, then 400-500 mg tid x 10 days (adult dosage) plus steroids if severe symptoms
• Strongyloides stercoralis - thiabendazole 50 mg/kg/d in 2 doses (maximum of 3 g a day) for 2 days (adult and pediatric), or ivermectin 200 mcg/kg/day x 1-2 days (also effective against co-existing ascaris, trichuris, enterobius). Superior to benzimidazoles for this indication.
• Note: FDA may consider certain uses of above drugs investigational, consult Medical Letter or appropriate drug reference
Contraindications: Refer to manufacturer's profile of each drug
Precautions: Refer to manufacturer's profile of each drug
Significant possible interactions: Refer to manufacturer's profile of each drug

ALTERNATIVE DRUGS
• Trichuris trichiura (whipworm) - albendazole 400 mg once (adults and children). Note - albendazole investigational for this purpose
• Strongyloides stercoralis - albendazole 400 mg daily x 3 days

FOLLOWUP

PATIENT MONITORING Followup stool studies at 2 weeks and retreat if necessary

PREVENTION/AVOIDANCE Good hygiene and sanitation

POSSIBLE COMPLICATIONS
• Vomiting worms
• Cholangitis - migration to common bile duct
• Pancreatitis - migration to pancreatic duct
• Appendicitis - migration to appendix
• Diverticulitis - migration to diverticuli
• Liver abscess
• Intestinal obstruction
• Volvulus
• Intussusception
• Bowel penetration
• Anemia (hookworm)
• Hypoproteinemia (hookworm)
• CNS infection (Strongyloides)

EXPECTED COURSE/PROGNOSIS
Good for light to moderate infections. Ascariasis should always be treated due to the risk of migrating adult worms.

MISCELLANEOUS

ASSOCIATED CONDITIONS N/A

AGE-RELATED FACTORS Affects all ages
Pediatric: Children commonly infected
Geriatric: N/A
Others: N/A

PREGNANCY Benzimidazoles (mebendazole, albendazole, thiabendazole) should not be used; ivermectin has shown little teratogenic potential, and has provided an effective therapy though benefits should clearly outweigh risks

SYNONYMS N/A

ICD-9-CM 127 Other intestinal helminthiases

SEE ALSO
• Roundworms, tissue
• Intestinal parasites
• Pinworms

OTHER NOTES HIV infected patients have a higher risk of dissemination (e.g., strongyloides) and "standard" treatment failure therefore they may require prolonged, repeated, or alternative therapies

ABBREVIATIONS N/A

REFERENCES
• Steffen: Travel Medicine and Health. Ontario, Canada. BC Decker, 1997
• Markell EK, Voge M, John DT: Medical Parasitology. 6th Ed. Philadelphia, W.B. Saunders Co., 1986
• Schroeder SA, Krupp MA, Tierney LM, McPhee SJ, eds: Current Medical Diagnosis and Treatment. Norwalk, CT, Appleton & Lange, 1989
• Strickland GT: Hunter's Tropical Medicine. 6th Ed. Philadelphia, W.B. Saunders Co., 1984
• Drugs for Parasitic Infections. The Medical Letter. Vol 40 (issue 1071) Jan 2, 1998
• Tietze PE, Tietze PH: Roundworms, Ascaris Lumbricoides. Primary Care; Clinics in Office Practice 1991;16(1):25-41
• Gomez NA, et al: Ultrasound in the diagnosis of roundworms in gallbladder and common bile duct. Surgical Endoscopy 1993;7(4):339-342
• Jensenius M: Hookworm disease: A differential diagnosis in iron deficiency anemia. Tidsskrift for den Norske Laegeforening 1995;115(3):367-369
• Lessnau KD, et al: Disseminated Strongyloides stercoralis in HIV infected patients. Chest 1993;104(1):119-122
• Goodman, Gilman: The Pharmacological Basis of Therapeutics. 9th Ed. New York, McGraw-Hill, 1996
Illustrations: N/A
Internet references: http://www.5mcc.com

Author(s)
Robert L. Weston, MD

Roundworms, tissue

BASICS

DESCRIPTION Tissue roundworms (nematodes) affect man when the adults or larval stages infect certain tissues. Infective larval stages are transmitted to man by arthropod vectors or from the soil. Once in human tissue, worms mature over 6-12 months and survive as long as 15 years. Symptoms depend on tissue infected.
- Filarial infections
  ◊ Wuchereria bancrofti (bancroftian filariasis)
  ◊ Brugia malayi (Malayan filariasis)
  ◊ Brugia timori (Timorian filariasis)
  ◊ Loa loa (eye worm)
  ◊ Onchocerca volvulus (river blindness, onchocerciasis)
  ◊ Mansonella perstans
  ◊ Mansonella ozzardi (Ozzard's filariasis)
  ◊ Mansonella streptocerca
- Other tissue nematode infections
  ◊ Dracunculus medinensis (guinea worm, dracunculosis)
  ◊ Ancylostoma braziliense (cutaneous larva migrans, creeping eruption)
  ◊ Toxocara canis or cati (visceral larva migrans, toxocariasis)
- Distribution
  ◊ Over 300 million people are exposed to lymphatic filariasis in India and SE Asia; 30 million to onchocerciasis
  ◊ W. bancrofti: Tropics worldwide
  ◊ B. malayi: Southeast Asia
  ◊ B. timori: Indonesia
  ◊ L. loa: Africa
  ◊ O. volvulus: Africa, Central and South America
  ◊ M. perstans: Africa, South America
  ◊ M. ozzardi: Africa
  ◊ M. streptocerca: Central and South America
  ◊ D. medinensis: Africa, Asia
  ◊ A. braziliense: Tropics and Subtropics worldwide
  ◊ T. canis/cati: Over 50 countries worldwide, especially warmer tropical and subtropical regions

System(s) affected: Skin/Exocrine, Nervous, Gastrointestinal, Musculoskeletal, Hemic/Lymphatic/Immunologic, Cardiovascular, Renal/Urologic
Genetics: N/A
Incidence/Prevalence in USA:
- Visceral larva migrans - 4-30% seroprevalence has been reported, highest in southeastern United States
- Others - unknown
Predominant age: All ages, but children more commonly infected
Predominant sex: Male = Female

SIGNS AND SYMPTOMS
- Lymphatic filariasis (W. bancrofti, B. malayi, B. timori)
  ◊ Inflammatory signs - pain, tenderness, swelling, erythema
  ◊ Filarial adenolymphangitis
  ◊ Filarial orchitis
  ◊ Funiculitis and epididymitis
  ◊ "Filarial" and "Elephantoid" fever
  ◊ Filarial abscess
  ◊ Obstructive signs - lymph varices, lymph scrotum, hydrocele
  ◊ Lymphedema and elephantiasis
  ◊ Chyluria
  ◊ Filarial hypereosinophilia (tropical pulmonary eosinophilia)
- Loiasis (L. loa)
  ◊ Calabar swellings - recurrent subcutaneous inflammation/swelling
  ◊ Eye worm - adult or larvae migrate under conjunctiva
  ◊ Eosinophilia (may exceed 70%)
  ◊ Fever, irritability, urticaria and pruritus
- Onchocerciasis (O. volvulus)
  ◊ Dermatitis
  ◊ Nodules
  ◊ Lymphadenitis
  ◊ Ocular changes - intraocular microfilariae, punctate keratitis, sclerosing keratitis, anterior uveitis chorioretinitis, optic neuritis, optic atrophy, glaucoma, blindness (river blindness)
- Other filarial syndromes (M. ozzardi, M. perstans, M. streptocerca)
  ◊ Headaches, coldness, pruritus, and articular swelling/arthritis
  ◊ Eosinophilia and vague allergic signs
  ◊ Chronic dermatitis and macules can be confused with leprosy
  ◊ Lymphadenopathy
- Dracunculiasis (D. medinensis, guinea worm disease)
  ◊ Allergic manifestations - erythema, urticaria, pruritus, nausea, vomiting, giddiness, syncope, and occasional fever)
  ◊ Local lesions - papule, sterile blister, ulceration, abscesses
  ◊ Worm protrusion
- Toxocariasis (T. canis/cati, visceral or ocular larva migrans)
  ◊ Eosinophilia
  ◊ Visceral larva migrans
  ◊ Ocular larva migrans
- Cutaneous larva migrans (A. braziliense, creeping eruption)
  ◊ Itching and red papules
  ◊ Serpiginous track
  ◊ Edema and acute inflammation
  ◊ Scars
  ◊ Secondary infection

CAUSES Larvae introduced into human host by arthropod vector or infected soil

RISK FACTORS
- Geographic exposure to arthropod vectors
- Fishermen or women washing clothes have increased risk of 'river blindness'
- Contact with infected soil in cutaneous larva migrans (hence plumber's itch, sandworm, duckhunter's itch)

DIAGNOSIS

DIFFERENTIAL DIAGNOSIS
- Other causes of tissue inflammation (i.e., lymphangitis, epididymitis, dermatitis, conjunctivitis, blisters, pleuritis, peritonitis, pericarditis, encephalitis, nephropathy, cardiomyopathy, etc.)
- Nonfilarial causes of lymphangitis:
  ◊ Acute bacterial lymphangitis
  ◊ Phlebitis
  ◊ Unusual - plague, anthrax, TB, lymphogranuloma inguinale
- Nonfilarial causes of lymphedema, chyluria, and elephantiasis:
  ◊ Infiltrative or granulomatous process: Tumor, fungus, TB, leprosy
  ◊ Chronic venostasis or phlebitis
  ◊ Cardiac insufficiency
  ◊ Nutritional deficiencies
  ◊ Hereditary (Milroy's disease)
  ◊ Lateritious soil obstructing lymphatics

LABORATORY Examination of larvae or adult worms taken from the tissue; characteristic microfilariae on blood smear; eosinophilia. Distinction of species by larval exam is challenging and may require expert examination. Onchocerciasis is identified by skin snip/biopsy showing larval.
Drugs that may alter lab results: N/A
Disorders that may alter lab results: N/A

PATHOLOGICAL FINDINGS
Characteristic eggs/worms/larvae in tissue

SPECIAL TESTS Skin snip, nodulectomy, slit-lamp exam, and Mazzotti, test may be helpful in onchocerciasis

IMAGING Occasional worms seen on x-ray

DIAGNOSTIC PROCEDURES
Microfilariae on blood smear or other body fluids; clinical observations; serologies (e.g., ELISA)

TREATMENT

APPROPRIATE HEALTH CARE
Outpatient

GENERAL MEASURES
- Identify cause and treat accordingly
- Best treatment - direct removal of worm from tissue with caution not to break the worm
- Treat secondary infections

Roundworms, tissue

SURGICAL MEASURES Long-standing lymphatic filariasis due to W. bancrofti and B. malayi may require surgical intervention to increase lymphatic drainage. This is unusual, and likely seen in long-term residents of endemic areas, subjected to extensive exposure to parasite.

ACTIVITY No restrictions. If edema a problem, may want to elevate legs while sitting.

DIET No special diet

PATIENT EDUCATION
• Avoid bites by arthropod vectors, insect repellants and other protective measures, e.g., proper clothing
• Avoid rivers and streams and soils known to be infected

MEDICATIONS

DRUG(S) OF CHOICE
• Visceral larva migrans (Toxocara): diethylcarbamazine (DEC) 6 mg/kg/d in 3 doses x7-10 days for adult and pediatric
• Cutaneous larva migrans (Ancylostoma braziliense): thiabendazole topical and/or albendazole 400 mg qday x3 days for adults and children. Topical 15% thiabendazole in a water soluble cream base is the treatment of choice given low toxicity and high cure rate (98%). Ivermectin 150-200 mcg/kg once is effective.
• Filariasis (W. bancrofti, B. malayi):
  ◊ Diethylcarbamazine: Adult: day 1) 50 mg po after meals; day 2) 50 mg tid; day 3) 100 mg tid; days 4-14) 6 mg/kg/d in 3 doses. Children: day 1) 1 mg/kg po after meals; day 2) 1 mg/kg tid; day 3) 1-2 mg/kg tid; days 4-14) 6 mg/kg/d in 3 doses.
• Loa, loa
  ◊ Diethylcarbamazine: as above except days 4-21: 9mg/kg/day in 3 doses (adults and children)
  ◊ Antihistamines and steroids: may be useful to reduce allergic response to disintegration of microfilaria
• Onchocerciasis: ivermectin (Mectizan) 150 µg/kg po once, repeated every 6-12 months for adults and children can prevent blindness. Treatment with ivermectin only kills the larval worms, responsible for pathology, not the adult worms producing the larvae. Thus, treatment must be continued over a period of years until the adult worms die.
• Mansonella ozzardi: ivermectin 6 mg in single dose has been effective. Diethycarbamazine is not effective.
• Mansonella perstans: mebendazole 100 mg bid x 30 days (approved drug, but considered investigational for this condition)
• Guinea worm (Dracunculus): metronidazole 250 mg tid x 10 days for adult; 25 mg/kg/d (max 750 mg/d) in 3 doses x 10 days for children. Metronidazole does not cure the infection, but rather decreases the reaction to worm products. Cure is achieved only through physical removal of the adult worm.

• Note: FDA may consider certain uses of above drugs investigational and some may not be available in USA. Contact Parasitic Disease Drug Service, Parasitic Diseases Branch, Center for Disease Control, Atlanta 30333, (404)488-4240.
Contraindications: Refer to manufacturer's information
Precautions: Children, pregnancy, lactation
Significant possible interactions: Refer to manufacturer's profile of each drug

ALTERNATIVE DRUGS
• Visceral larva migrans (Toxocara): albendazole 400 mg bid x3-5 days for adults and children or mebendazole 100-200 mg bid x5 days for adults and children
• Filariasis (W. bancrofti, B. malayi): Ivermectin (available from the CDC Drug Services 404-639-3670) 150 mcg/kg as a single dose is highly effective against microfilaria but does not kill adult worms. More effective when combined with albendazole 400 mg.
• Onchocerciasis: DEC has been used, but causes bad reactions, likely due to rapid killing of the larval worms with sudden release of large amounts of worm antigens. DEC is obsolete for this indication. Suramin, a drug used in the treatment of trypanosomiasis, is effective at killing the adult worms, but severe side effects prevent its use for onchocerciasis.

FOLLOWUP

PATIENT MONITORING N/A

PREVENTION/AVOIDANCE
• Avoid sources of infection (arthropod bites, rivers/streams, or contaminated soils)
• Diethylcarbamazine (DEC) 300 mg once weekly has been used successfully in Peace Corps' workers for prophylaxis against L. loa
• Prophylaxis with ivermectin is under investigation
• Public health activities such as vector control

POSSIBLE COMPLICATIONS
• Depends upon type of worm
• Onchocerciasis - blindness
• Visceral worms - hepatitis, splenomegaly, pleuritis, peritonitis, eosinophilic granuloma or other organ damage as larvae migrate for up to 6 months
• Filariasis - lymphatic destruction leading to severe edema (elephantiasis)
• Neurohelminthiasis: CNS migrations and infection

EXPECTED COURSE/PROGNOSIS
• Good for light to moderate infections; depends on organ infected and extent of infection
• Long-term DEC treatment and immunomonitoring of filaria patients are essential in endemic areas to arrest and prevent pathology

MISCELLANEOUS

ASSOCIATED CONDITIONS N/A

AGE-RELATED FACTORS
Pediatric: Children commonly infected
Geriatric: N/A
Others: Presence of onchocerciasis increases with age

PREGNANCY N/A

SYNONYMS
• Nematodes

ICD-9-CM
127.0 Other intestinal helminthiases

SEE ALSO Roundworms, intestinal

OTHER NOTES N/A

ABBREVIATIONS N/A

REFERENCES
• Markell EK, Voge M, John DT: Medical Parasitology. 6th Ed. Philadelphia, W.B. Saunders Co., 1986
• Schroeder SA, Krupp MA, Tierney LM, McPhee SJ, eds: Current Medical Diagnosis and Treatment. Norwalk, CT, Appleton & Lange, 1989
• Strickland GT: Hunter's Tropical Medicine. 7th Ed. Philadelphia, W.B. Saunders Co., 1991
• Warren KS, Mahmoud AAF: Tropical and Geographic Medicine. New York, McGraw-Hill, 1990
• Drugs for Parasitic Infections. Medical Letter. New Rochelle, NY, Medical Letter, Inc Jan 2, 1998;Vol 40 (1017)
• Steffen: Travel Medicine & health. Ontario, Canada; BC Decker, 1997.
• Padrigel UM, et al: Immunomonitoring of filarial patients during DEC therapy in an endemic area: A seven year followup. Jour Tropical Med & Hygiene 1995;98(1):52-56
• Cook: Manson's Tropical Diseases. 20th ed, Saunders, 1996;1334.
Illustrations: 1 available on CD-ROM
Internet references: http://www.5mcc.com

Author(s)
Robert L. Weston, MD

Salicylate poisoning

BASICS

DESCRIPTION A systemic disorder caused by acute and/or chronic intoxication from salicylate containing medications.
• Following accidental or intentional exposure, toxic actions of salicylates include:
◊ Stimulation of the CNS respiratory center
◊ Uncoupling of oxidative phosphorylation
◊ Inhibition of Krebs cycle dehydrogenases
◊ Stimulation of gluconeogenesis
◊ Increased lipolysis and lipid metabolism
◊ Inhibition of aminotransferases
◊ Cyclooxygenase inhibition and decreased production of clotting factors
◊ Irritation of the gastric mucosa and stimulation of the CNS chemoreceptor trigger zone.
• These actions cause sequential and progressively severe physiologic abnormalities with increasing doses of salicylates, time following exposure, duration of chronic exposure, extremes of age, and presence of concurrent medical conditions; abnormalities include:
◊ Respiratory alkalosis accompanied by progressive metabolic acidosis
◊ Hyperpyrexia
◊ Gastrointestinal, renal, pulmonary, and skin losses of body fluids and electrolytes
◊ Initial hyperglycemia followed by hypoglycemia, particularly CNS hypoglycemia
◊ Abnormal hemostasis and coagulation.
• The clinical presentation of patients with salicylate toxicity can range from minor symptoms to a syndrome initially indistinguishable from septic shock with multiple organ failure, including encephalopathy and adult respiratory distress syndrome (ARDS). The very young and elderly are particularly prone to develop severe toxicity, as are those with chronic intoxication. Also, conditions causing concurrent acidosis may increase tissue concentrations of salicylate and result in greater morbidity and mortality.
System(s) affected: Nervous, Hemic/Lymphatic/Immunologic, Gastrointestinal, Pulmonary, Renal/Urologic, Cardiovascular, Musculoskeletal, Skin/Exocrine, Endocrine/Metabolic
Genetics: N/A
Incidence/Prevalence in USA:
• > 18,000 ingestions of salicylate containing medications reported to poison control centers in 1997
• 48 deaths in 1997, none in children < 6
Predominant age: Occurs in children and adults at any age; over 70% of cases are in children > 6 and adults
Predominant sex: Male = Female

SIGNS AND SYMPTOMS

• Acute intoxication
◊ Symptoms vary with the amount ingested, usually begin within 3-8 hours of ingestion, and progress more rapidly in children:
  - < 150 mg/kg, minimal symptoms
  - 150-300 mg/kg, moderate symptoms
  - 300-500 mg/kg, severe symptoms
  - > 500 mg/kg, potentially fatal
◊ Nausea and vomiting
◊ Hyperpnea
◊ Tachypnea
◊ Hyperpyrexia
◊ Tinnitus
◊ Disorientation
◊ Coma
◊ Convulsions
◊ Cardiac arrhythmias
◊ Hypotension
◊ Pulmonary edema
• Chronic intoxication
◊ Signs and symptoms similar to acute intoxication may occur
◊ Onset of symptoms is usually gradual
◊ Signs and symptoms may be advanced at diagnosis and include severe hypotension and ARDS
◊ Neurologic symptoms often predominate, particularly in the elderly, and include agitation, confusion, stupor, hyperactivity, paranoia, bizarre behavior, dysarthria, restlessness

CAUSES

• Accidental or intentional ingestion of salicylates or salicylate containing medications
• Percutaneous absorption of dermatologic medications containing salicylate
• Breast feeding by mothers ingesting salicylate containing medications
• Teething gels containing salicylates

RISK FACTORS

• Dehydration
• Conditions causing metabolic or respiratory acidosis
• Extremes of age - the very young and elderly
• Psychiatric illness
• History of previous toxic ingestions or suicide attempts
• Concurrent oral poisoning with other substances
• Concurrent use of acetazolamide (Diamox)

DIAGNOSIS

DIFFERENTIAL DIAGNOSIS

• All ages: infection, sepsis, DKA, other causes of metabolic acidosis
• In the elderly: delirium, CVA, myocardial infarction, ethyl alcohol (ETOH) intoxication, congestive heart failure

LABORATORY

• Serum salicylate levels initially on all patients to confirm the diagnosis. Following acute ingestions, check levels 6 or more hours after ingestion and repeat q2h until levels are declining and the patient's condition has stabilized.
• Acid-base abnormalities common; usually respiratory alkalosis or mixed respiratory alkalosis and metabolic acidosis. Metabolic acidosis often predominates in chronic or severe acute poisonings and in poisonings in young children.
• Increased anion gap, esp. in acute poisonings and salicylate-only poisonings
• Initial hyperglycemia may be followed by hypoglycemia
• Electrolyte abnormalities such as hyper- or hyponatremia, and hypokalemia common
• Findings consistent with dehydration are common including an increased BUN/Cr ratio
• PT may be increased
• Liver function abnormalities may be present
• Proteinuria, renal function abnormalities may be present
• Stool hemoccult testing may be positive
• Occasional hypouricemia
Drugs that may alter lab results:
• Diflunisal (Dolobid) may cross react with assay of salicylate concentration
• Medications affecting similar organ systems including oral anticoagulants and hypoglycemic agents
Disorders that may alter lab results:
Concurrent medical conditions involving similar organ systems

PATHOLOGICAL FINDINGS None specific for salicylate intoxication; associated findings include:
• Gastrointestinal = antral and prepyloric ulcers; small bowel ulcerations with enteric coated salicylates
• Renal = interstitial nephritis, acute tubular necrosis, minimal change nephrotic syndrome
• Pulmonary = noncardiogenic pulmonary edema

SPECIAL TESTS N/A

IMAGING

• Chest X-ray: noncardiogenic pulmonary edema; variable severity, from mild to ARDS
• Abdominal plain film: nonspecific bowel gas pattern with retained contrast in chronic bismuth subsalicylate ingestion

DIAGNOSTIC PROCEDURES None, other than correlating serum salicylate concentration with the clinical presentation.
• Following acute ingestions, the significance of the serum salicylate level can be estimated by using the Done nomogram. The nomogram may underestimate the severity of poisonings in patients with:
◊ Illnesses accompanied by dehydration and/or acidosis
◊ Chronic exposure to salicylates
◊ Ingestion of enteric coated or sustained release medications
◊ Unknown time of ingestion

Salicylate poisoning

TREATMENT

APPROPRIATE HEALTH CARE
Evaluate all patients at a healthcare facility; outpatient for non-toxic accidental ingestions; inpatient for toxic and intentional ingestions

GENERAL MEASURES
• Prevent further absorption:
◊ Gastric lavage, within 2-4 hours of ingestion. Ipecac if unable to be seen in a healthcare facility within 1 hour of ingestion.
◊ Activated charcoal after gastric emptying
• Fluid/electrolyte balance: IV fluids to restore intravascular volume and prevent hypoglycemia. With hypotension give isotonic fluid until orthostatic changes no longer present; the fluids should contain at least 5% dextrose unless hyperglycemia is a problem. Normal saline or a mixture of .45% NaCl with 1 ampule of sodium bicarbonate (50 mEq NaHCO3) may be administered at 10-15 mL/kg/hr for 1-2 hours, depending on the degree of acidosis. When blood pressure stable, fluid management is directed toward alkalinizing the urine to enhance salicylate excretion, preventing CNS hypoglycemia, and treating fluid and electrolyte abnormalities.
• Enhance elimination:
◊ Alkaline diuresis (urine pH 7-8) and prevention of hypoglycemia can usually be maintained with fluids containing approximately 40 mEq/L Na+, 35 mEq/L K+, 50 mEq/L Cl-, 20 mEq/L HCO3- and 5-10% dextrose, run at 4-8 mL/kg/hr until the salicylate level decreases into the therapeutic range. Additional bicarbonate may be needed for severe or persistent acidosis. Fluids should be run slower in patients with cardiovascular compromise. Thereafter, maintenance fluids with added bicarbonate as needed can be run at 2-3 mL/kg/hr until toxicity resolves.
◊ Hemodialysis should be considered in poisonings with markedly elevated salicylate levels (> 100 mg/dL in acute poisonings, > 40-60 mg/dL in chronic poisonings), acidosis unresponsive to alkalinization and diuresis, renal and/or hepatic dysfunction with impaired salicylate clearance, noncardiac pulmonary edema, and persistent, severe CNS symptoms.

SURGICAL MEASURES N/A

ACTIVITY Bedrest initially

DIET No special diet

PATIENT EDUCATION
• Education of parents/caregivers during well child visits
• Education of patients on chronic salicylate therapy
• Anticipatory guidance for caregivers, family, and cohabitants of potentially suicidal patients
• Patient brochure: Child Safety: How to keep your home safe for your baby. American Academy of Family Physicians, 8880 Ward Parkway, Kansas City, MO 64114 2797

MEDICATIONS

DRUG(S) OF CHOICE
• At home
◊ Give ipecac syrup if patient is alert and unable to be evaluated at a health care facility within 1 hour. Dose: 6 months-1 year: 5 mL; 1-12 years: 15 mL; > 12 years: 30 mL. Give with 240 mL (8oz) of water when possible; may repeat in 30 min if emesis has not occurred.
• Emergency facility/hospital:
◊ Patients evaluated within 4 hours of ingestion should have their stomachs evacuated. Gastric lavage is the preferred method
◊ Repeat activated charcoal every 4 hours (1 g/kg each dose) until passage of a charcoal stool
◊ Bicarbonate is used to alkalinize the urine (pH 7-8) and, when appropriate, to correct severe systemic acidosis (for pH < 7.1)
◊ Give dextrose-containing IV solution to prevent hypoglycemia; CNS hypoglycemia may be present despite a normal serum glucose

Contraindications:
• Ipecac syrup should not be given to patients with decreased responsiveness
• Medication allergies

Precautions:
• If ipecac has been given, activated charcoal should be given at least 30 minutes to 1 hour afterwards to avoid risks of decreased effectiveness and aspiration
• Intravascular overload may result from injudicious use of sodium bicarbonate, particularly in patients with cardiovascular compromise
• Dextrose should not be given to patients with severe hyperglycemia

Significant possible interactions: N/A

ALTERNATIVE DRUGS N/A

FOLLOWUP

PATIENT MONITORING
• Fluid, acid base, blood glucose, and electrolyte status until stable; urine pH (to enhance elimination of salicylate)
• Psychiatric followup after intentional ingestions

PREVENTION/AVOIDANCE
• Patient and parent/caregiver education essential. See Patient Education.
• Ipecac syrup at home
• Emergency telephone numbers

POSSIBLE COMPLICATIONS
• Noncardiogenic pulmonary edema, including development of ARDS
• Rare following recovery from poisoning

EXPECTED COURSE/PROGNOSIS
• Complete recovery with early therapy
• Clinical course and prognosis are worse in the very young and elderly, chronic intoxications, and in patients with concurrent conditions which cause dehydration and/or acidosis

MISCELLANEOUS

ASSOCIATED CONDITIONS Reye's syndrome with salicylate use and varicella or influenza viral infection

AGE-RELATED FACTORS
Pediatric: Acidosis is often more severe in the very young, particularly in chronic or repeated therapeutic dose poisonings
Geriatric:
• Increased risk for chronic toxicity because of decreased renal function
• Increased risk for bleeding or perforated gastric ulcers in patients over 70 years
Others: N/A

PREGNANCY
• No teratogenic effect in humans
• Salicylates may cause premature closure of ductus arteriosus in fetus
• Increased risk of ante and intrapartum hemorrhage

SYNONYMS N/A

ICD-9-CM 965.1 Poisoning by salicylates (aspirin)

SEE ALSO N/A

OTHER NOTES N/A

ABBREVIATIONS N/A

REFERENCES
• Yip L, Dart RC, Gabow A: Concepts and controversies in salicylate toxicity. Emerg Clin N Amer 1994;12:351-364
• Litovitz TL, Klein-Schwartz W, Dyer KS, Shannon M, Lee S, Powers M: 1997 Annual report of the American Association of Poison Control Centers Toxic Exposure Surveillance System. Am J Emerg Med 1998;16:443-97
Illustrations: N/A
Internet references: http://www.5mcc.com

Author(s)
Lars C. Larsen, MD

Salivary gland calculi

BASICS

DESCRIPTION The formation of stones in intraglandular or extraglandular ducts of submandibular, parotid, sublingual, or minor salivary glands.
System(s) affected: Gastrointestinal
Genetics: No known genetic pattern
Incidence/Prevalence in USA: Not uncommon, but reliable incidence figures not available; 1% in autopsy series, most of these asymptomatic
Predominant age: Middle to old age; uncommon in children
Predominant sex: Male > Female (slight predominance)

SIGNS AND SYMPTOMS
• Initial symptoms, consistent with partial duct obstruction:
  ◊ Episodic or variable unilateral swelling and tenderness of the affected gland,
  ◊ Worse just before meals, then tapering off till the next meal
• Symptoms of complete duct obstruction:
  ◊ Persistent swelling and pain
• Symptoms of commonly associated sialadenitis:
  ◊ Fever, sweats, chills
  ◊ Acute and severe worsening of localized pain and swelling
  ◊ Acute general malaise
• Signs when not associated with sialadenitis:
  ◊ Unilateral localized swelling
  ◊ Boggy tender mass associated with affected gland in acute obstruction
  ◊ Firm to hard mass associated with gland fibrosis in chronic obstruction
  ◊ Palpable and/or visible stone in distal duct (in 1/2 to 1/3 of cases, and more often with submandibular stones than parotid stones)
  ◊ No saliva expressed, or scant, cloudy, thick, mucinous saliva expressed on milking duct
• Signs in association with sialadenitis:
  ◊ Fever, tachycardia
  ◊ Generalized toxicity
  ◊ Diffuse, tender, hot swelling associated with affected gland
  ◊ Otherwise palpable stone now obscured by swelling and acute pain

CAUSES
• Submandibular gland/ducts are involved in more than 80% of cases, thought to be due to:
  ◊ Tortuous course of these ducts
  ◊ Flow of saliva in these ducts is "up hill"
  ◊ Submandibular saliva has higher concentration of calcium and is more viscous
• General causes of salivary gland stones:
  ◊ Any mechanical hindrances to normal flow of saliva
    - Acute or chronic inflammation in or around duct
    - Scarring or stenosis of duct (trauma, surgery, past stone damage)
    - Altered or tortuous duct path (from extrinsic masses, surgery or previous obstruction)
    - Presence of food particles or organic debris in duct as an obstruction and/or nidus of stone formation

  ◊ Alteration of saliva quality
    - Dehydration
    - Anticholinergic medications (including those with anticholinergic side effects such as tricyclic antidepressants and phenothiazines)
    - Chronic parotitis, Sjögren's syndrome, cystic fibrosis

RISK FACTORS
• Sources for alterations in gland function and duct anatomy, as mentioned above
• Previous stone formation
• Local irradiation
• Chronic, debilitating illness
• Poor oral hygiene

DIAGNOSIS

DIFFERENTIAL DIAGNOSIS
• Sialadenitis
• Lymphadenitis
• Salivary neoplasms (80% benign in parotid, 50% benign in submandibular gland)
• Foreign body in duct or soft tissue
• Neoplasms of adjacent oral or neck tissues
• Other facial/dental soft tissue infections (eg dissecting dental abscess)

LABORATORY
• WBC, acute phase reactants, and serum amylase may be elevated if associated with sialadenitis
Drugs that may alter lab results: N/A
Disorders that may alter lab results: N/A

PATHOLOGICAL FINDINGS
• Submandibular glands/ducts involved in 80% of cases, parotid in 15%, and remainder in sublingual and minor salivary glands
• In acute cases without sialadenitis:
  ◊ Acute ductal and glandular inflammation
• In chronic cases:
  ◊ Ductal ectasia, stenosis, scarring, thickening
  ◊ Metaplasia of duct lining
  ◊ Periductal chronic inflammation
  ◊ Glandular fibrosis and atrophy
  ◊ Multiple stones in intra- and extra-glandular ducts
• Stones vary size from <1 mm to >10 mm and show alternating layers of mineralization (predominantly calcium salts) and organic material (mucinous material, lipids, cellular debris)

SPECIAL TESTS   N/A

IMAGING
• Due to differences in mineralization, 80% of SMG stones are radiopaque, but 80% of parotid stones are radiolucent
• Plain head and neck radiographs
• Dental occlusive films
• Xerography
• Ultrasound (particularly useful in acute parotid sialadenitis with swelling and pain)
• CT - "CT reconstruction" most sensitive technique, showing presence of stones or differentiating multiple stones when other imaging methods fail

DIAGNOSTIC PROCEDURES
• Fine needle aspiration if glandular neoplasm is high in the differential diagnosis
• Surgical excision may be needed to differentiate chronic ductal squamous metaplasia from low-grade mucoepidermoid carcinoma

TREATMENT

APPROPRIATE HEALTH CARE
• Outpatient for conservative treatment or minor surgical procedures
• Inpatient for salivary gland excision or for treating associated severe sialadenitis

GENERAL MEASURES
• Small stones close to the ductal orifice are often removed with a conservative approach:
  ◊ Sialagogues (eg hard sour candy) to stimulate salivary flow
  ◊ Gentle ductal massage, from gland to ductal orifice
  ◊ Ductal dilatation (lacrimal probe and/or lacrimal punctum dilator)
  ◊ Incision of ductal papilla if stone is hung up just inside the orifice
  ◊ For more proximal SMG stones still within 1.25 cm from orifice (Wharton's duct) the duct may be incised longitudinally from the orifice and the stone expressed by massage
  ◊ Penicillinase-resistant staphylococcal antibiotic coverage, particularly if duct instrumented or incised
• In setting of acute sialadenitis:
  ◊ Hydration
  ◊ Sialagogues
  ◊ Local heat
  ◊ Release of a distal obstructing stone as above, if palpable
  ◊ Attempted proximal-to-distal expression of pus after release of obstruction
  ◊ Full course of penicillinase-resistant staph coverage (IV therapy in hospital for severely ill or elderly)
  ◊ Extracorporeal shock-wave lithotripsy (ECSWL) has been effective in treating >50% of the parotid stones not cleared with conservative measures

SURGICAL MEASURES
• A more extensive procedure by a surgical specialist, such as proximal duct dissection or gland excision, is appropriate for:
  ◊ Any but most distal parotid stones, particularly if ECSWL not available or ineffective
  ◊ Proximal stone with high grade obstruction
  ◊ Chronic sialolithiasis with glandular fibrosis and/or ductal scarring and stenosis
  ◊ Multiple stones
  ◊ Neoplasm is a consideration

ACTIVITY   No restrictions

DIET Until specific therapy initiated
- Liberal oral water intake for hydration
- Reduce other oral intake to reduce pain
- Particularly avoid Sialagogues to reduce pain
- No specific dietary measures required after therapy

PATIENT EDUCATION
- General management principles and diet as above
- Avoid OTC anticholinergic medications as discussed below
- Bring early signs of recurrence to medical attention

MEDICATIONS

DRUG(S) OF CHOICE
- Antibiotics, if infection present
  ◊ Erythromycin 250mg QID
  ◊ Amoxicillin-clavulanate (Augmentin) 500mg TID
  ◊ Cefuroxime (Ceftin)
- Analgesic: codeine, NSAID, etc

Contraindications: Hypersensitivity to drugs chosen

Precautions:
- Refer to manufacturer's literature for drugs chosen
- Prescribed or OTC anticholinergics may predispose to, or accelerate stone formation

Significant possible interactions: Refer to manufacturer's literature

ALTERNATIVE DRUGS
Penicillin V (Pen VK) 250-500mg QID

FOLLOWUP

PATIENT MONITORING
- Close post-procedure or post-surgical surveillance for infection
- Close follow-up during treatment of sialadenitis to ensure resolution of infection
- Patient education to seek early medical attention for symptoms of recurrence

PREVENTION/AVOIDANCE
- Treat any associated conditions
- Avoid anticholinergics
- Good hydration
- Good oral hygiene

POSSIBLE COMPLICATIONS
- Ductal scarring after stone passage, after instrumentation or surgery
- Infection associated with stone itself or with surgical procedures
- Salivary gland fibrosis and atrophy from duct obstruction or infection
- Salivary fistula after surgical procedure

EXPECTED COURSE/PROGNOSIS
- The majority of patients with uncomplicated stones who are successfully treated early in the process do not have recurrences
- A previous stone may damage the duct, setting up conditions for more stones
- Recurrence, particularly with multiple proximal stones, may warrant gland excision

MISCELLANEOUS

ASSOCIATED CONDITIONS
- Sialadenitis
- Chronic anticholinergics
- Poor oral hygiene
- Sjögren's syndrome
- Cystic fibrosis
- Oral trauma

AGE-RELATED FACTORS
Pediatric: N/A
Geriatric: Multiple chronic illnesses, multiple anticholinergics, dehydration
Others: N/A

PREGNANCY N/A

SYNONYMS Sialolithiasis

ICD-9-CM
527.5 Sialolithiasis

SEE ALSO
- Sialadenitis
- Sjögren's syndrome

OTHER NOTES Multiple stones in 20% of cases. In past, stones were felt to be secondary to altered calcium metabolism, but this has not been demonstrated.

ABBREVIATIONS N/A

REFERENCES
- Pollack CV, Severance HW. Sialolithiasis: case studies and review. J Emerg Med 1990;8:561-5
- McKenna JP, Bostock DJ, McMenamin PG. Sialolithiasis. Am Fam Physician 1987;36:119-25
- McGurk M, Escudier M. Removing salivary gland stones. Br J Hosp Med 1995;54:184-5
- Avrahami E, Englender M, Chen E, et al. CT of submandibular gland sialolithiasis. Neuroradiology 1996;38:287-90
- Raymond AK, Batsakis JG. Angiolithiasis and sialolithiasis in the head and neck. Ann Otol Rhinol Laryngol 1992;101:455-7
- Iro H, Zenk J, Waldfahrer F, et al. Extracorporeal shock wave lithotripsy of parotid stones. Ann Otol Rhinol Laryngol 1998;107:860-4
- Stanley MW, Bardales RH, Beneke J, et al. Sialolithiasis: differential diagnostic problems in fine-needle aspiration cytology. Am J Clin Pathol 1996;106:229-33

Illustrations: 1 available on CD-ROM
Internet references: http://www.5mcc.com

Author(s)
Douglas C. Woolley, MD

Salivary gland tumors

BASICS

DESCRIPTION Neoplasms benign or malignant of the major (parotid, submaxillary, sublingual) salivary glands or the minor (intra-oral, pharyngeal, nasal) salivary glands. Most tumors are discrete masses although some may manifest as diffuse enlargement of the gland or submucosal intraoral swelling. Malignant tumors are characterized by local recurrence and perineural spread (adenoid cystic), or local recurrence and lymph node metastases (mucoepidermoid, adenocarcinoma, squamous cell carcinoma).
- Types
  ◊ Pleomorphic adenoma (most common tumor) - 45% overall
  ◊ Monomorphic adenoma - 12% overall
  ◊ Mucoepidermoid carcinoma - 12% overall
  ◊ Adenoid cystic - 6% overall
  ◊ Less frequent lesions are - adenocarcinoma, squamous cell carcinoma, acinic cell carcinoma, oxyphilic adenomas, Warthin's tumor
- Distribution of neoplasms
  ◊ Parotid (80% benign, 20% malignant) - 70% are pleomorphic adenoma; 10% are monomorphic adenoma; 12% are mucoepidermoid carcinoma; 5% are adenoid cystic
  ◊ Submandibular (60% benign, 40% malignant) - 40% are pleomorphic adenoma; 10% are mucoepidermoid carcinoma; 20% are adenoid cystic carcinoma
  ◊ Minor salivary glands (40% benign, 60% malignant) - 40% are pleomorphic adenoma; 25% are mucoepidermoid carcinoma; 25% are adenoid cystic carcinoma
System(s) affected: Nervous, Gastrointestinal
Genetics: Increased incidence of adenocarcinoma of parotid in Eskimos, otherwise no known genetic pattern
Incidence/Prevalence in USA: 3% of new tumors; 6% of head and neck neoplasms
Predominant age: Malignant - age 55; benign - age 45
Predominant sex:
- Pleomorphic adenoma: Female > Male
- Other adenomas: Male = Female

SIGNS AND SYMPTOMS
- Discrete mass in anatomic area - 96% (malignant)
- Elevation of earlobe
- Pain 12-25% (malignant); 2.5% (benign)
- Trigeminal paresthesias
- Facial nerve palsy or dysfunction 8-26% (malignant)
- Fixation to masseter and pterygoids 17% (malignant)
- Skin ulceration 9% (malignant)
- Cervical lymph node metastases 20% (malignant)
- Pharyngeal mass (representing deep lobe tumors of the parotid gland)

CAUSES
- Unknown
- Possible ionizing radiation

RISK FACTORS None known

DIAGNOSIS

DIFFERENTIAL DIAGNOSIS
- Inflammatory masses
- Parotid and submandibular lymph nodes
- Mikulicz's syndrome
- Salivary gland stones
- Torus palatinus (minor)
- Necrotizing sialometaplasia (minor)
- Cervical lymph nodes
- Sjögren's syndrome
- Lymphadenopathy with AIDS

LABORATORY
- Autoimmune studies
- Fractionated amylase (inflammation)
Drugs that may alter lab results: None known
Disorders that may alter lab results: None known

PATHOLOGICAL FINDINGS Of 100 parotid masses, 70 will be non-neoplastic, 21 will be benign neoplasms, and 9 will be malignant neoplasms

SPECIAL TESTS
- Technetium-99 (Warthin's tumor)
- Ultrasound (inflammatory or malignant)
- Sialography (for calculi or chronic parotitis)

IMAGING
- CT/MRI. Both provide anatomic detail and diagnostic information.
- Chest x-ray - Sjögren's, metastases

DIAGNOSTIC PROCEDURES
- Fine needle aspiration (some authors would not utilize this procedure in fear of disseminating a malignant tumor)
- Superficial lobectomy

TREATMENT

APPROPRIATE HEALTH CARE
Inpatient

GENERAL MEASURES
- Inpatient procedures with usual nursing care
- Drain parotid bed
- Usually 1-2 day hospitalization

SURGICAL MEASURES
- Benign tumors - superficial or total conservative (nerve-sparing) parotidectomy depending on site of tumor
- Malignant tumors - total parotidectomy, or sialadenectomy with adjuvant radiotherapy to parotid base of skull with/without neck depending on histology. Preservation of facial nerve unless involved by tumor.
- Cervical lymphadenectomy if palpable nodes or elective neck dissection in squamous cell carcinoma, high grade mucoepidermoid carcinoma or high grade adenocarcinoma
- Elevate head of bed postoperative
- Suction drainage x 1-2 days
- Suture line care with antibiotic ointment

ACTIVITY Moderate restriction for 1 day

DIET Non-stimulating liquid

PATIENT EDUCATION
- Basic cancer followup
- Recurrent masses
- Trigeminal nerve symptoms
- Frey's syndrome (gustatory sweating)
- Facial nerve symptoms (paresis)

MEDICATIONS

DRUG(S) OF CHOICE N/A
Contraindications: N/A
Precautions: N/A
Significant possible interactions: N/A

ALTERNATIVE DRUGS N/A

FOLLOWUP

PATIENT MONITORING
• For malignancy - once every 4 months the first year, once every six months subsequent 3 years, once per year subsequently
• For benign tumors - once per year for five years

PREVENTION/AVOIDANCE No known etiologic agents

POSSIBLE COMPLICATIONS
• Frey's syndrome (gustatory sweating) occurs symptomatically in about 20% of patients undergoing parotidectomy
• Facial neurapraxia from surgery should resolve within six months, even with use of adjuvant radiotherapy
• Cosmetic deformity of moderate facial flattening on side of parotidectomy
• Injury to hypoglossal or lingual nerve during submandibular resection
• Pleomorphic adenoma may recur, if inadequately excised, since it has pseudopods throughout the lobe

EXPECTED COURSE/PROGNOSIS
• Parotid pleomorphic adenoma untreated will demonstrate malignant degeneration in 2-10% over 20 years. Treated adequately, parotid pleomorphic adenoma has 1.5% recurrence rate. Malignancy prognosis depends on stage.
• Adenoid cystic - parotid 5 year survival 73%, 15 year 21%; submandibular 5 year 50%, 15 year 0%; palate 5 year 80%, 15 year 38%
• Adenocarcinoma - 5 year survival 78%, 20 year 41%
• Mucoepidermoid - low grade 5 year survival 81%, 15 year 48%, high grade 5 year survival 46%, 15 year 25%

MISCELLANEOUS

ASSOCIATED CONDITIONS None known

AGE-RELATED FACTORS
Pediatric: Hemangioma is the most common benign tumor in pediatric population followed by pleomorphic adenoma. Mucoepidermoid most common malignant.
Geriatric: N/A
Others: N/A

PREGNANCY Not affected

SYNONYMS N/A

ICD-9-CM
142-142.9 malignant neoplasm of major salivary glands

SEE ALSO
• Sjögren's syndrome

OTHER NOTES N/A

ABBREVIATIONS N/A

REFERENCES
• Coleman JJ: Salivary gland disorders. In: Jurkiewicz MJ, Krizek TJ, Mathews SJ, Ariyan S, eds. Fundamentals of Plastic Surgery. St. Louis, C.V. Mosby Co., 1990
• Rankow RM, Polayes IM: Diseases of the Salivary Glands, Philadelphia, W.B. Saunders, 1976
• Batsakis JG: Tumors of the head and neck. Clinical and Pathological Considerations. 2nd Ed. Baltimore, Williams and Wilkins, 1979
Illustrations: 1 available on CD-ROM
Internet references: http://www.5mcc.com

Author(s)
John J. Coleman, MD

Salmonella infection

BASICS

DESCRIPTION Disease caused by any serotype of the genus Salmonella. Clinical syndromes include enterocolitis (75%), bacteremia (10%), enteric fever (10%) (see Typhoid fever), localized infection outside gastrointestinal tract (5%) and an asymptomatic carrier state (< 1%). Organisms invade gut mucosa, producing inflammatory, cytotoxic response. Organisms can then disseminate into systemic circulation via lymphatics. Infective dose and host defenses dictate extent of disease.

System(s) affected: Gastrointestinal

Genetics: A condition similar to Reiter's syndrome may follow Salmonella enterocolitis in patients with the HLA-B27 histocompatibility antigen

Incidence/Prevalence in USA:
• 800 cases/100,000 population/year. Peak frequency July-November. Salmonella isolations represent only 1-10% of actual yearly incidence. Second only to campylobacter as cause of bacterial diarrheal illness. Each year, an average of 55 outbreaks of salmonella infections are reported to CDC.
• Infants: 130/100,000
• Adults: 6/100,000
• Multidrug resistant strains from the United Kingdom pose a risk of new outbreaks in the USA

Predominant age:
• High prevalence in persons > 70 or < 20
• Highest in infants < 1 year

Predominant sex: Male = Female

SIGNS AND SYMPTOMS
• Acute uncomplicated illness
  ◊ Nausea, vomiting, diarrhea
  ◊ Abdominal cramps
  ◊ Headache, myalgias
  ◊ Fever to 102°F (39°C)
• Protracted disease
  ◊ Persistent fever
  ◊ Arthritis, reactive or septic
  ◊ Osteomyelitis
  ◊ Sacroiliitis
  ◊ Wound infection, soft tissue abscesses
  ◊ Meningitis
  ◊ Arteritis
  ◊ Endocarditis, pericarditis
  ◊ Pneumonia, lung abscess, empyema
  ◊ Hypovolemia
  ◊ Splenic (abscess)
  ◊ Hepatic (abscess)
  ◊ Urogenital tract infection

CAUSES
• Ingestion of contaminated food - (poultry, meat, eggs, dairy products) or water
• Person-to-person and/or fecal-oral spread
• Contact with animal reservoirs - poultry, cows, pigs, birds, sheep, seals, donkeys, lizards, snakes, pets (turtles, cats, dogs, mice, guinea pigs, hamsters)
• Iatrogenic contamination - blood transfusion, endoscopy
• Contact with asymptomatic chronic carrier
• Achlorhydria - gastroduodenal surgery, idiopathic
• Ulcerative colitis
• Systemic lupus erythematosus

• Schistosomiasis
• Cholelithiasis
• Nephrolithiasis
• Drugs - antibiotics, purgatives, opiates
• Intentional contamination of restaurant food through criminal mischief has been reported

RISK FACTORS
• Impaired gastric acidity—H2 blockers, antacids, gastrectomy, achlorhydria
• Hemolytic anemias - sickle-cell, malaria, bartonellosis
• Malignancy - lymphoma, leukemia, disseminated carcinoma
• Immunosuppression - AIDS, steroids, other immunosuppressants, chemotherapy, radiation
• Pets with high fecal carriage rates for salmonella, especially reptiles (snakes, iguanas)
  ◊ Antibiotic treatment of the animal is not recommended, due to temporary effect only

DIAGNOSIS

DIFFERENTIAL DIAGNOSIS
• Viral gastroenteritis
• Other bacterial enteritises (e.g., shigellosis, cholera)
• Other bacterial sources or systemic and localized sepsis (e.g., meningococci, staphylococci)
• Pseudomembranous colitis
• Inflammatory or granulomatous bowel disease
• Appendicitis
• Cholecystitis
• Perforated viscus

LABORATORY
• Enterocolitis
  ◊ Fecal leukocytes positive
  ◊ Stool culture positive for Salmonella species
  ◊ WBC normal or decreased
  ◊ Blood cultures negative
• Bacteremia
  ◊ Blood cultures positive
  ◊ Stool cultures negative
• Local infections
  ◊ Polymorphonuclear leukocytosis
  ◊ Tissue site culture positive
• Asymptomatic carrier state
  ◊ Stool culture positive for more than 1 year
  ◊ Urine culture may be positive with certain serotypes

Drugs that may alter lab results:
Antibiotics used early may lead to false-negative cultures and blunted immunologic response

Disorders that may alter lab results: N/A

PATHOLOGICAL FINDINGS
• Mucosal ulceration, hemorrhage and necrosis
• Reticuloendothelial hyperplasia and hypertrophy
• Focal organ and soft tissues abscesses

SPECIAL TESTS Serologic tests identify particular clinical syndromes and serve as epidemiologic markers

IMAGING Angiography in patients over 50 with bacteremia. To rule out presence of infected aneurysm, particularly of aorto-iliac vessels.

DIAGNOSTIC PROCEDURES N/A

TREATMENT

APPROPRIATE HEALTH CARE
• Outpatient for uncomplicated enterocolitis and carrier state
• Inpatient for bacteremia and extra-intestinal infection (11% hospitalization rate)
• Do not wait for stool culture results before initiating important therapeutic decisions

GENERAL MEASURES
• Correct fluid and electrolyte deficits
• Control symptoms (pain, nausea, vomiting)

SURGICAL MEASURES
• Surgical drainage and vascular bypass procedures for infected tissue sites
• When biliary tract disease is present, the best results are obtained with the combination of cholecystectomy and a 10-14 day course of parenteral antibiotics (see Drug(s) of Choice - bacteremia) initiated before surgery

ACTIVITY As tolerated

DIET Oral rehydration solution during diarrhea phase; advance to normal diet as tolerated

PATIENT EDUCATION Food Safety and Inspection Service, Office of Public Awareness, Dept. of Agriculture, Rm. 1165-S, Washington, DC 20205, (202)447-9351

MEDICATIONS

DRUG(S) OF CHOICE
- Enterocolitis uncomplicated:
  ◊ None recommended
- Enterocolitis complicated: (by age extremes, immunosuppression, underlying cardiovascular abnormalities, prosthetic orthopedic devices, hemolytic anemia)
  ◊ Ciprofloxacin (Cipro) po for 3-7 days--no pediatric dose; adult dose 500 mg q12h, or
  ◊ Ampicillin po for 10-14 days - pediatric dose 50-100 mg/kg/day in 4 divided doses; adult dose 500 mg qid, or
  ◊ Trimethoprim-sulfamethoxazole (Bactrim, Septra) po for 14 days - pediatric dose 10 mg/kg/day trimethoprim, 50 mg/kg/day sulfamethoxazole in 2 divided doses (maximum 320 mg/day trimethoprim; 1600 mg/day sulfamethoxazole); adult dose 1 double strength tablet q12h
- Bacteremia:
  ◊ Ampicillin IV for 10-14 days - pediatric dose 200-300 mg/kg/day in 4 divided doses; adult dose 1-2 gm q4h; or
  ◊ Chloramphenicol IV for 14 days - pediatric dose = adult dose, 50-100 mg/kg/24 hours in 4 divided doses; maximum dose 4 g/24 hours
  ◊ Cefotaxime (Claforan) IV for 14 days - pediatric dose 200 mg/kg/day q8h; adult dose 1-2 gm q8hr, maximum 12 gm/day; or ciprofloxacin (Cipro) 500 mg po or norfloxacin 400 mg po q12h for 7 days (adults only)
- Localized infection:
  ◊ Same as for bacteremia
  ◊ In sustained bacteremia or prolonged local infection, antibiotics can be given po for 4-6 weeks (substitute trimethoprim-sulfamethoxazole for cefotaxime, using 2-4 double strength (DS) tablets given 3 times a day)
- Chronic carrier state:
  ◊ Ampicillin 2-4 gm/day plus probenecid 1-2 gm/day, both divided into 4 oral doses, for 6 weeks; or
  ◊ 40-160 mg/day trimethoprim and 200-800 mg/day sulfamethoxazole divided into 2 doses for 6 weeks
  ◊ Consider ciprofloxacin 500 mg po bid for 4 weeks, or norfloxacin (Noroxin) 400 mg po bid for 4 weeks, if gallstones are present

Contraindications: Known drug allergy

Precautions:
- Use bowel motility inhibitors (Lomotil, Imodium) with caution, if at all
- Monitor blood levels of chloramphenicol in neonates and infants
- Ampicillin-resistant strains increasing; now at 15-30% in US

Significant possible interactions:
Ampicillin failure rate is 75% in chronic carriers with gallbladder disease

ALTERNATIVE DRUGS
Fluoroquinolones - ciprofloxacin (Cipro), ofloxacin (Floxin) gaining favor in management of gastroenteritis, osteomyelitis and carrier state. Use is restricted to nonpregnant adults only. For gastroenteritis in children > 1 year, consider furazolidone (Furoxone) 2.5 mg/kg po qid for 5 days.

FOLLOWUP

PATIENT MONITORING
Repeat stool culture at 5 months (40% of children negative, 90% of adults negative) and at 1 year (> 99% of all patients negative)

PREVENTION/AVOIDANCE
- Proper hygiene in production, transport and storage of food
- Control of animal reservoir, especially by avoiding contact with animal feces
- Hand washing emphasized
- No vaccine available to oppose salmonellosis
- The US Dept of Agriculture endorses a program to spray newly hatched chicks with benign bacterial species in order to prevent gut colonization with Salmonella

POSSIBLE COMPLICATIONS
- Toxic megacolon
- Hypovolemic shock
- Metastatic abscess formation
- Acute or chronic hydrocephalus

EXPECTED COURSE/PROGNOSIS
- Prognosis for enterocolitis is excellent. Exceptions - in the very young (7.0% fatal), the very old (8.7% fatal) and the debilitated and/or institutionalized (2.3% fatal).
- Prognosis for meningitis or endocarditis is poor, unless effective treatment given early

MISCELLANEOUS

ASSOCIATED CONDITIONS N/A

AGE-RELATED FACTORS
Pediatric: Children, especially neonates, more likely to become chronic carriers
Geriatric: Patients over 60 also have high carrier rate presumably due to biliary sequestration of organisms
Others: Contaminated marijuana is important source of infection, particularly in young adults

PREGNANCY Consult obstetrician regarding antibiotics. Keep a low threshold for hospital admission.

SYNONYMS N/A

ICD-9-CM 003.0 Salmonella gastroenteritis

SEE ALSO
- Typhoid fever
- Gastroenteritis, viral
- Diarrhea, acute

OTHER NOTES If one member of a household becomes infected with salmonellosis, the chance of at least one other member becoming infected is 60%

ABBREVIATIONS N/A

REFERENCES
- Sanford JP, Gilbert DN, Moellering RC, Sande MA: The Sanford Guide to Antimicrobial Therapy. 28th Ed. Dallas, Antimicrobial Therapy, inc., 1997
- Feldman M, Scharschmidt BF, Sleisenger MH (eds) : Sleisenger & Fordtran's Gastrointestinal & Liver Disease. 6th Ed. Philadelphia, W.B. Saunders Company, 1998
- Gorbach SL, Bartlett JG, Blacklow NR (eds) : Infectious Diseases. 2nd Ed. Philadelphia, W.B. Saunders Company, 1998
- Glynn MK, Bopp C, Dewitt W, Dabney P, et al: Emergence of multidrug-resistant Salmonella enteritica serotype typhimurium DT104 infections in the United States. N Engl J Med 1998;338:13331338
Illustrations: N/A
Internet references: http://www.5mcc.com

Author(s)
Richard Viken, MD

Sarcoidosis

BASICS

DESCRIPTION Non-infectious multisystem disease of unknown cause, commonly affecting young and middle-age adults. Frequently presents with bilateral hilar adenopathy, pulmonary infiltrates, ocular and skin lesions. Other organs may be involved, including liver, spleen, lymph nodes, heart, and central nervous system.

System(s) affected:
Hemic/Lymphatic/Immunologic, Pulmonary, Cardiovascular, Gastrointestinal

Genetics: Although world-wide in distribution, increased prevalence found in Scandinavians, Japanese, Irish females, and African American women

Incidence/Prevalence in USA: 30-80 per 100,000

Predominant age: 20-60 years

Predominant sex: Female > Male

SIGNS AND SYMPTOMS
• Patients may be asymptomatic
• Cough
• Shortness of breath
• Skin (new lesions)
• Pain or irritation of eyes
• General fatigue, malaise
• Fever
• Night sweats
• Bell's palsy

CAUSES Unknown

RISK FACTORS None known

DIAGNOSIS

DIFFERENTIAL DIAGNOSIS
• Infectious granulomatous disease such as tuberculosis and fungal infections
• Foreign body reactions
• Lymphoma
• Other malignancies associated with lymphadenopathy
• Berylliosis

LABORATORY
• Lymphopenia, anemia, or leukopenia can be seen in over half of the patients
• Abnormal liver function, especially increased alkaline phosphatase is frequently encountered
• Hypercalciuria occurs in up to 10% of patients, with hypercalcemia less frequent

Drugs that may alter lab results:
Prednisone will lower serum-angiotensin converting enzyme and normalize Gallium scan. ACE inhibitors will lower serum ACE level.

Disorders that may alter lab results:
Hyperthyroidism and diabetes will increase serum angiotensin converting enzyme level

PATHOLOGICAL FINDINGS
Noncaseating epithelioid granulomas without evidence of fungal or mycobacterial infection

SPECIAL TESTS
• Serum angiotensin converting enzyme (ACE) is elevated in over 60% of patients
• Gallium scan uptake in chest, lymph nodes, and parotids may be seen in active disease
• Characteristically in active disease, bronchoalveolar lavage (BAL) fluid has an increased percentage of lymphocytes, specifically CD4 positive (T-helper/inducer lymphocytes)
• Ophthalmologic exam

IMAGING
• Routine chest roentgenograms are staged using Scadding's classification:
  ◊ Stage 0 = normal
  ◊ Stage 1 = hilar adenopathy alone
  ◊ Stage 2 = hilar adenopathy plus parenchymal infiltrates
  ◊ Stage 3 = parenchymal infiltrates alone
  ◊ Stage 4 = pulmonary fibrosis
• Gallium scan will be positive in areas of acute disease
• Computerized tomography may enhance appreciation of lymph nodes and high resolution CT scan shows peribronchial disease

DIAGNOSTIC PROCEDURES
• Bronchoscopy with transbronchial biopsy and bronchoalveolar lavage is often performed to diagnose lung disease
• Mediastinoscopy, skin or lymph node biopsy (if needed to establish diagnosis)
• When available, Kveim-Siltzbach skin test can be performed. This test is fairly sensitive (approximately 80%) and highly specific (> 95%). Unfortunately, the antigen is not generally available.

TREATMENT

APPROPRIATE HEALTH CARE
Outpatient

GENERAL MEASURES
• The disease may require no specific therapy in the asymptomatic individual or may treat for specific indications, such as cardiac, central nervous system, ocular, or hypercalcemia
• Treatment of pulmonary and skin manifestations usually done on the basis of impairment

SURGICAL MEASURES N/A

ACTIVITY Generally no limitations

DIET
• Avoid high calcium diets
• In patients on corticosteroids, avoid high salt foods

PATIENT EDUCATION Generally stress the benign nature of the disease and the fact that it is not contagious to others and is not malignant

MEDICATIONS

DRUG(S) OF CHOICE
• Systemic corticosteroids in the symptomatic individual, usually prednisone initially 40 mg every day or every other day. Treatment with tapering doses of prednisone for at least one year.
• In patients with skin or ocular disease, topical steroids may be effective
Contraindications: Patients with known problems with corticosteroids
Precautions: Careful monitoring in patients with diabetes mellitus and/or hypertension
Significant possible interactions: Refer to manufacturer's profile of each drug

ALTERNATIVE DRUGS
Methotrexate 10 mg per week, hydroxychloroquine (Plaquenil) 100-200 mg per day, azathioprine 50-100 mg per day and chlorambucil 0.1-0.2 mg/kg. May increase risk of carcinogenicity. Use of immunosuppressants such as methotrexate, azathioprine or chlorambucil will require careful, regular monitoring of complete blood count.

FOLLOWUP

PATIENT MONITORING
• Patients on prednisone for symptoms should be seen every month or two while on therapy
• Patients not requiring therapy should be seen regularly (every three months) for at least the first two years after diagnosis
• Chest roentgenograms and pulmonary function tests are useful for monitoring for pulmonary changes
• Serum angiotensin converting enzyme level is used by some to follow disease activity. In patients with an initially elevated ACE level, it should fall towards normal while on therapy or when the disease resolves.

PREVENTION/AVOIDANCE   None known

POSSIBLE COMPLICATIONS
• Patients may develop significant respiratory involvement including cor pulmonale
• Other organs, especially the heart (congestive heart failure, arrhythmias), eyes (rarely blindness) and central nervous system can be involved with serious consequences. Fortunately, cardiac, ocular, and CNS involvement usually manifests itself early on in patients with these manifestations of the disease.

EXPECTED COURSE/PROGNOSIS
• 80% of patients will have spontaneous resolution within two years
• 10% will have significant fibrosis but no further worsening of disease after two years
• 10% (higher in some populations, including African Americans) will have chronic disease

MISCELLANEOUS

ASSOCIATED CONDITIONS   None known

AGE-RELATED FACTORS
Pediatric: Rare
Geriatric: Less than 5% of patients with active disease are 60 years or older
Others: Sarcoidosis is a disease of youth to middle age

PREGNANCY   No increased incidence

SYNONYMS
• Loeffgren's syndrome (erythema nodosum, hilar adenopathy plus uveitis)
• Besnier-Boeck disease
• Boeck's sarcoid
• Schaumann's disease

ICD-9-CM   135 Sarcoidosis

SEE ALSO   N/A

OTHER NOTES   N/A

ABBREVIATIONS   N/A

REFERENCES
• Thomas PD, Hunninghake GW: Current concepts of the pathogenesis of sarcoidosis. Am Rev Respir Dis 1987;135:747-760
• Sharma OP: Sarcoidosis. Dis Month 1990;36:469-535.3
• Baughman RP, Lower EE, Lynch JP: Treatment modalities for sarcoidosis. Clin Pulm Med 1995;1:223-231
• Lower LL, Baughman RP: Prolonged use of methotrexate for sarcoidosis. Arch Int Med 1995;155:846-851
• Baughman RP, Lower EE: Steroid-sparing alternatives for sarcoidosis. Clin Chest Med 1997;18:853-864
Illustrations: 4 available on CD-ROM
Internet references: http://www.5mcc.com

Author(s)
Robert P. Baughman, MD

Scabies

BASICS

DESCRIPTION A contagious disease caused by infestation of the skin by the mite Sarcoptes scabiei, var. hominis
System(s) affected: Skin/Exocrine
Genetics: N/A
Incidence/Prevalence in USA: Common, although number of cases per year is declining as the epidemic, which began in 1971, passed its peak (1986). Worldwide incidence is 300 million cases per year.
Predominant age: Children and young adults
Predominant sex: Male = Female

SIGNS AND SYMPTOMS
• Generalized itching (often severe)
• Nocturnal pruritus
• Burrows in finger webs, wrists, hands, feet, penis, scrotum, buttocks, waistline
• Vesicles and papules (discrete)
• Secondary erosions or excoriations
• Pustules (if secondarily infected)
• Scaling
• Erythema
• Nodules in covered areas (buttocks, groin, axillae)
• Atypical infestations in immunosuppressed patients

CAUSES
• Sarcoptes scabiei, var. hominis

RISK FACTORS
• Personal skin-to-skin contact, e.g., sexual promiscuity, crowding, poverty, nosocomial infection
• Immunocompromised patients including HIV/AIDS
• Atopic eczema

DIAGNOSIS

DIFFERENTIAL DIAGNOSIS
• Atopic dermatitis
• Dermatitis herpetiformis
• Eczema
• Insect bites
• Papular urticaria
• Pityriasis rosea
• Prurigo
• Pyoderma
• Seborrheic dermatitis
• Syphilis

LABORATORY N/A
Drugs that may alter lab results: N/A
Disorders that may alter lab results: N/A

PATHOLOGICAL FINDINGS Skin biopsy of a nodule (although rarely performed) will reveal portions of the mite in the corneal layer

SPECIAL TESTS N/A

IMAGING N/A

DIAGNOSTIC PROCEDURES
• Examination of skin with magnifying lens - look for typical burrows in finger webs, on flexor aspects of the wrists, and penis. Look for a dark point at the end of the burrow (the mite). The mite can be extracted with a 25 gauge needle and examined microscopically.
• Mineral oil mounts - place a drop of mineral oil over a suspected lesion. Non-excoriated papules or vesicles may also be sampled. Scrape the lesion with a #15 surgical blade. Examine under a microscope for mites, eggs, egg casings or feces. Scraping from under fingernails may often be positive.
• Potassium hydroxide (KOH) wet mount - transfer skin scrapings directly to a glass slide, add a drop of KOH, and apply a cover slip. Examine the slide for diagnostic material. If none is evident, heat slide gently to separate squamous cells and reexamine.
• Burrow ink test - if burrows are not obvious, apply blue black ink to an area of rash. Wash off the ink with alcohol. A burrow should remain stained and become more evident. Then apply mineral oil, scrape and observe microscopically as previously noted.

TREATMENT

APPROPRIATE HEALTH CARE
Outpatient

GENERAL MEASURES
• Treat all intimate contacts and close household and family members
• Wash all clothing, bed linen, and towels in a normal wash cycle

SURGICAL MEASURES N/A

ACTIVITY Full activity

DIET No special diet

PATIENT EDUCATION
• Patient instruction sheet "Scabies" in Epstein: Common Skin Disorders (see References)
• Griffiths: Instructions for Patients, Philadelphia, W.B. Saunders Co.
• Schmitt: Instructions for Pediatric Patients, Philadelphia, W.B. Saunders Co.

Scabies

MEDICATIONS

DRUG(S) OF CHOICE
• Permethrin (Elimite) 5% cream: considered by many to be the drug of choice for scabies. Cream is applied into the skin from the head to the soles of the feet and left on for 8 to 14 hours, then thoroughly washed off. Thirty grams is usually adequate for an adult. A second application 1 week later is sometimes recommended.
• Lindane (Kwell, Scabene) 1%: available in lotion, cream and shampoo. The cream or lotion should be applied to all skin surfaces from the neck down and washed off 8 to 12 hours later. Two applications 1 week apart are recommended.
• Crotamiton (Eurax) 10%: cream is applied into the skin from the head to the soles of the feet and left on for 8 to 14 hours, then thoroughly washed off. It is felt to be less toxic than lindane, but perhaps slightly less effective, therefore, application 2 nights in a row is advised.
Contraindications: Lindane should be avoided in children who are premature, malnourished or emaciated and those with severe underlying skin disease or a history of seizure disorders.
Precautions:
• Patients should be cautioned not to overuse the medication when applying it to the skin
• For medications other than permethrin, patients should use a second application only when specifically advised to do so by their physician
Significant possible interactions: N/A

ALTERNATIVE DRUGS
• Precipitated sulfur 6% in petroleum: applied to the entire body from the neck down. It is malodorous and messy, but is thought to be safer than lindane, especially in infants under age 6 months and safer than permethrin in infants under age 2 months
• Ivermectin 200 mg/kg in combination with topical scabicide for HIV-positive patients

FOLLOWUP

PATIENT MONITORING Recheck patient at weekly intervals only if rash or itching persists. Rescrape new lesions and retreat if mite or products found.

PREVENTION/AVOIDANCE N/A

POSSIBLE COMPLICATIONS
• Eczema
• Pyoderma
• Postscabetic pruritus
• Nodular scabies

EXPECTED COURSE/PROGNOSIS
• Lesions begin to regress in 1 to 2 days along with the worst itching
• Some itching and dermatitis commonly persists for 10 to 14 days and can be treated with antihistamines and/or topical or oral corticosteroids
• Nodular lesions may persist for several weeks, perhaps necessitating intralesional or systemic steroids
• Some instances of lindane resistant scabies have now been reported. These do respond to permethrin.

MISCELLANEOUS

ASSOCIATED CONDITIONS N/A

AGE-RELATED FACTORS
Pediatric: Infants often have more widespread involvement. They are occasionally infested on the face and scalp (rare for adults). Vesicular lesions on the palms and soles are also more commonly seen. When treating infants with permethrin, the entire body should be treated.
Geriatric: The elderly often itch more severely, despite fewer cutaneous lesions. Elderly at risk for extensive infestations, perhaps related to a decline in cell-mediated immunity.
Others: N/A

PREGNANCY Permethrin and lindane are category B drugs. Until more information is available precipitated sulfar appears to be the safest treatment in pregnant or lactating women.

SYNONYMS N/A

ICD-9-CM
133.0 scabies

SEE ALSO
• Insect bites & stings

OTHER NOTES N/A

ABBREVIATIONS N/A

REFERENCES
• Goldstein A, Goldstein B: Practical Dermatology. 2nd Ed. St Louis, Mosby, 1997
• Habif T: Clinical Dermatology. 3rd Ed. St. Louis, CV Mosby, 1996
• Weston WL, et al: Color Textbook of Pediatric Dermatology. 2nd Ed. St Louis, CV Mosby, 1996
• Freedberg IM, et al: Fitzpatrick's Dermatology in General Medicine, 5th ed. New York, McGraw Hill, 1999.
Illustrations: 5 available on CD-ROM
Internet references: http://www.5mcc.com

Author(s)
Gary J. Silko, MD

Scarlet fever

 BASICS

DESCRIPTION "Streptococcal sore throat with a rash." A childhood disease characterized by high fever, pharyngitis, and rash caused by Group A beta-hemolytic streptococci (GAS) pyogenes that produce erythrogenic toxin. Incubation period 1-7 days, duration of illness 4-10 days.
System(s) affected: Gastrointestinal, Skin/Exocrine
Genetics: N/A
Incidence/Prevalence in USA: Up to 10% of GAS pharyngitis
Predominant age: 6-12 years
Predominant sex: Male = Female

SIGNS AND SYMPTOMS
• Prodrome 1-2 days
  ◊ Sore throat
  ◊ Headache
  ◊ Vomiting
  ◊ Abdominal pain (may mimic acute abdomen)
  ◊ Fever (up to 40°C or 103.6°F)
• Oral exam
  ◊ "Beefy red" tonsils and pharynx with or without exudate
  ◊ Petechiae on palate
  ◊ White coating on tongue "White strawberry tongue" appears on days 1-2. This sheds by day 4-5 leaving a "Red strawberry tongue" - shiny, red with prominent papillae.
• Exanthem (appears within 1-5 days)
  ◊ Orange-red punctate skin eruption with sandpaper-like texture - "sunburn with goose pimples"
  ◊ Initially, chest and axillae, then spreads to abdomen and extremities; prominent in skin folds (axillae, groin, buttocks)
  ◊ Flushed face with circumoral pallor
  ◊ Transverse red streaks in skin folds of abdomen, antecubital space, and axillae: "Pastia's lines"
  ◊ Desquamation begins on face after 7-10 days and proceeds over trunk to hands and feet; may persist for 6 weeks
  ◊ In severe cases, small vesicular lesions (miliary sudamina) may appear on abdomen, hands, feet

CAUSES
• Hypersensitivity to erythrogenic toxins produced by GAS
• Site of GAS infection: Usually tonsils, may occur with skin infection
• Staphylococcus aureus may also produce erythrogenic toxin - "staphylococcal scarlet fever." May be mild form of toxic shock syndrome or scalded skin syndrome.

RISK FACTORS
• Winter/spring seasons
• Age - school age children - by age 10, 80% have antibodies to erythrogenic toxin
• Contact with infected individual
• Crowded living conditions, eg, lower socioeconomic status, military, child care

 DIAGNOSIS

DIFFERENTIAL DIAGNOSIS
• Measles
• Rubella
• Infectious mononucleosis
• Roseola
• Severe sunburn
• Secondary syphilis
• Arcanobacterium haemolyticum
• Toxic shock syndrome
• Staphylococcal scalded skin syndrome
• Kawasaki disease
• Drug hypersensitivity
• Mycoplasma pneumonia
• Viral exanthem

LABORATORY
• Throat culture definitive diagnosis
• Rapid Strep antigen tests - diagnostic if positive, but sensitivity only 50-90%, so must do throat culture if negative result
• Serologic tests (includes anti-streptolysin O titer and streptozyme tests) - confirm recent GAS infection; not helpful for diagnosis of acute disease
Drugs that may alter lab results:
• Prior antibiotic therapy may result in negative throat culture
• Penicillin within 5 days of symptoms can delay/abolish anti-streptolysin O response
Disorders that may alter lab results: N/A

PATHOLOGICAL FINDINGS N/A

SPECIAL TESTS N/A

IMAGING N/A

DIAGNOSTIC PROCEDURES N/A

 TREATMENT

APPROPRIATE HEALTH CARE
Outpatient except for severe suppurative complications

GENERAL MEASURES Supportive care

SURGICAL MEASURES tonsillectomy may be recommended with recurrent bouts of pharyngitis

ACTIVITY Fully active

DIET No special diet

PATIENT EDUCATION Must take antibiotics for full course; brief delay in initiating treatment awaiting throat culture results does not increase the risk of rheumatic fever.

MEDICATIONS

DRUG(S) OF CHOICE
• Penicillin (oral; penicillin V and others) for 10 days
 ◊ 125 mg po tid for under 60 lb/27 kg; 250 mg tid for others; bid dosing may also be effective.
 ◊ If compliance questionable, use penicillin, benzathine (Bicillin LA): single IM dose 600,000 units for under 60 lb/27 kg; 1,200,000 million units for others
• Acetaminophen for fever and comfort
Contraindications: Penicillin allergy
Precautions: Refer to manufacturer's profile of each drug
Significant possible interactions: Refer to manufacturer's profile of each drug

ALTERNATIVE DRUGS
• Erythromycin estolate (20-40 mg/kg/day divided tid or qid) or erythromycin ethyl succinate (40-50 mg/kg/day divided tid or qid) for 10 days. Maximum dose: 1 gm/day.
• Newer macrolides
 ◊ Azithromycin (Zithromax, Z pak): Adults - 500 mg the first day, then 250 mg qd for 4 days; Children over 2 years - 12 mg/kg/day (maximum of 500 mg) for 5 days
 ◊ Clarithromycin (Biaxin): Adults - 250 mg bid for 10 days; Children over 6 months - 7.5 mg/kg bid for 10 days
• Oral cephalosporins; many are effective, but first generation are less expensive.
 ◊ Cephalexin 40 mg/kg/day divided tid. Maximum: 250 mg tid for 10 days.
 ◊ Cefadroxil 30 mg/kg/day divided bid. Maximum: 500 mg bid for 10 days.
• Clindamycin 20 mg/kg/day divided tid for 10 days
• Tetracyclines and sulfonamides should not be used

FOLLOWUP

PATIENT MONITORING
• Routine follow-up throat cultures not needed unless patient is symptomatic.
• Since GAS uniformly susceptible to penicillin; bacteriologic treatment failures possibly due to:
 ◊ Poor compliance
 ◊ Beta-lactamase oral flora hydrolyzing penicillin
 ◊ GAS carrier state and concurrent viral rash (require no treatment)

PREVENTION/AVOIDANCE
• GAS spread by contact with respiratory secretions. Avoid if possible.
• Children should not return to school or day care until after 24 hours of antibiotic therapy
• Prophylactic penicillin not recommended after exposure to scarlet fever

POSSIBLE COMPLICATIONS
• Suppurative
 ◊ Sinusitis
 ◊ Otitis media/mastoiditis
 ◊ Cervical adenitis
 ◊ Peritonsillar abscess/retropharyngeal abscess
 ◊ Pneumonia
 ◊ Septicemia/meningitis/osteomyelitis/septic arthritis
• Non-suppurative
 ◊ Rheumatic fever (penicillin prevents RF when started as long as 10 days after onset of acute GAS infection)
 ◊ Glomerulonephritis (prevention even after adequate treatment of GAS is less certain)
 ◊ "Streptococcal toxic shock syndrome": Fever, hypotension, disseminated intravascular coagulation (DIC); cardiac, liver, kidney dysfunction.

EXPECTED COURSE/PROGNOSIS
• With penicillin, course may be shortened by 12-24 hours
• Can have recurrent attacks

MISCELLANEOUS

ASSOCIATED CONDITIONS
• Pharyngitis
• Impetigo
• Puerperal sepsis

AGE-RELATED FACTORS
Pediatric: Rare in infancy
Geriatric: N/A
Others: N/A

PREGNANCY N/A

SYNONYMS Scarlatina

ICD-9-CM 034.1 Scarlet fever

SEE ALSO
• Pharyngitis
• Impetigo

OTHER NOTES N/A

ABBREVIATIONS
GAS = Group A beta-hemolytic streptococci

REFERENCES
• Committee on Infectious Diseases of Amer Acad Ped. (Red Book). 483-94, 1997
• Krugman S, Katz S, Gershon A, Wilfert C: Infectious Diseases of Children. 9th ed. New York, C.V. Mosby, 1990
• Behrman R, Kliegman R, Arvin A: Nelson's Textbook of Pediatrics. 15th Ed. Philadelphia, WB Saunders Co., 1996
• Bisno AL, Gerber MA, Gwaltney JM, Kaplan EL, Schwartz RN: Diagnosis and management of group A streptococcal pharyngitis: a practice guideline. Clin Inf Dis 1997;25:574-583
Illustrations: 1 available on CD-ROM
Internet references: http://www.5mcc.com

Author(s)
Mitchell S. King, MD
Jory A. Natkin, DO

Schizophrenia

BASICS

DESCRIPTION Major psychiatric disorder with prodrome, active and residual symptoms involving disturbances (lasting at least 6 months) in:
• Appearance (deteriorational)
• Speech (loosened association)
• Behavior (stereotyped)
• Perception (hallucinations)
• Thinking (delusions)
System(s) affected: Nervous
Genetics: Genetic predisposition necessary for development
Incidence/Prevalence in USA: Lifetime (1%). Highest prevalence in lower socioeconomic classes.
Predominant age: Onset typically before age 45
Predominant sex: Male = Female; onset earlier in males (15-24) than females (25-34)

SIGNS AND SYMPTOMS
• Withdrawal from reality
• Delusions (fixed false unreal beliefs - paranoid (people persecuting or after you)
• Reference (people or things have unusual significance)
• Others can hear your thoughts, put thoughts into you or control you; grandiose or religious delusions
• Hallucinations - usually auditory
• Affect - flat or inappropriate emotion
• Thought processes - loose associations (thoughts don't follow)
• Much speech but convey little information
• Extremes of gross overactivity to stupor with mutism

CAUSES
Unknown - not initiated or maintained by an organic factor. Probably a complex interaction between inherited and environmental factors.

RISK FACTORS
Biologic relative with schizophrenia (if first degree relative, risk is 8%)

DIAGNOSIS

DIFFERENTIAL DIAGNOSIS
• Organic mental disorder - characterized by JOMAC (a mnemonic that stands for impaired Judgment, Orientation, Memory, Affect and Concentration). Disorientation, in particular indicates organicity. Organic mental disorders may be due to trauma, infection, tumor, metabolic, endocrine, intoxication (psychoactive substance use), epilepsy, neurological disorders, etc.
• Organic delusional syndrome - secondary to substance use/abuse (e.g., amphetamines, LSD, or phencyclidine) may have identical symptoms
• Mood disorders - especially bipolar disorder (manic depressive disorder); schizoaffective disorder; mood disorders with psychotic features
• Cultural belief system

LABORATORY
• No test available to indicate schizophrenia
• Laboratory tests needed to rule out organicity - may include CBC, blood chemistries, thyroid screen, urinalysis, vitamins (B12, folate, thiamine), blood and urine for drugs and alcohol
• Others for: heavy metals - ceruloplasmin, urine porphobilinogen
Drugs that may alter lab results: N/A
Disorders that may alter lab results: N/A

PATHOLOGICAL FINDINGS N/A

SPECIAL TESTS
• Psychological - Bender Gestalt, intelligence testing (WAIS-R), MMPI-2; neuropsychological testing
• EEG - to rule out seizure disorder, brain damage, etc.
• Glucose tolerance

IMAGING
CT and MRI to rule out organicity

DIAGNOSTIC PROCEDURES
Lumbar puncture

TREATMENT

APPROPRIATE HEALTH CARE
• Usually hospitalize initially for organic workup and for treatment of psychotic symptoms
• Outpatient if not dangerous to self or others, able to cooperate with treatment, and supportive family: community treatment and case management
• Family intervention: psycho-education

GENERAL MEASURES
Ensure safety of patient and others - may act on delusional thinking

SURGICAL MEASURES N/A

ACTIVITY
Establish safe hospital environment

DIET
No special diet

PATIENT EDUCATION
Education and support groups for patient and family available from National Alliance for the Mentally Ill (NAMI), 2101 Wilson Blvd., Suite 302, Arlington, VA 22201, (703)524-7600

Schizophrenia

MEDICATIONS

DRUG(S) OF CHOICE
• Neuroleptic and/or benzodiazepines
• While evaluating for organicity, may treat agitation with benzodiazepines - lorazepam (Ativan) 1, 2 or 4 mg po or IM every 2-6 hrs up to 10 mg/day
• If violent or severely disruptive - rapid neuroleptization - haloperidol 5 mg IM every 4-8 hrs up to 30 mg/day or chlorpromazine 10-25 mg IM test dose (check for hypotension in one hour) then 25 mg IM every 4 hr up to 150 mg day for low dose
• After stable - change to oral medicines and titrate dosage
• After 6 months in remission, may withdraw from neuroleptics. If relapse, reinstitute medications.
Contraindications: Refer to manufacturer's profile of each drug
Precautions:
• For acute side effects of neuroleptic - dystonic reaction (especially of head and neck) - diphenhydramine (Benadryl) 25-50 mg IM
• For pseudoparkinsonism reaction - trihexyphenidyl (Artane) 2 mg bid (may be increased to 15 mg/day if needed) or benztropine (Cogentin) 0.5 bid (range: 1-4 mg/day)
• Neuroleptic malignant syndrome-hyperthermia, severe extrapyramidal effect and autonomic dysfunction (hypertension, tachycardia, diaphoresis and incontinence)
Significant possible interactions: Refer to manufacturer's profile of each drug

ALTERNATIVE DRUGS
• Thioridazine (Mellaril) - only by mouth. Do not exceed 800 mg/day
• Trifluoperazine (Stelazine) 4-30 mg/day for maintenance
• Thiothixene (Navane) 8-30 mg/day for maintenance
• Clozapine (Clozaril) 25 mg qd or bid
  ◊ Increase slowly to dose of 300-400 mg given tid; do not exceed 900 mg/day
  ◊ Serious toxicity of agranulocytosis mandates weekly CBC; obtain WBC before initiating therapy; withhold clozapine if < 3,500; if < 2,000, discontinue immediately; reserve for therapy resistant patients.
• Risperidone (Risperdal) - optimal dose 3-6 mg/day; possibly less extrapyramidal symptoms due to serotonergic blockade

FOLLOWUP

PATIENT MONITORING   Continue
neuroleptic as well as psychiatric therapies (individual, group, family), vocational rehabilitation, social skills training, day treatment

PREVENTION/AVOIDANCE   N/A

POSSIBLE COMPLICATIONS
• Side effects of neuroleptics especially risk of tardive dyskinesia with chronic use
• Self-inflicted trauma
• Combative behavior toward others

EXPECTED COURSE/PROGNOSIS
• Chronic course - remission and exacerbations
• Guarded prognosis, although 30% recover completely
• The negative symptoms (consisting of decreased ambition, energy, emotional responsiveness and social withdrawal) are often most difficult to treat

MISCELLANEOUS

ASSOCIATED CONDITIONS   N/A

AGE-RELATED FACTORS
Pediatric: Unusual before puberty
Geriatric: Those who survive enter into a chronic phase
Others: Onset in 30's - more paranoid type

PREGNANCY   Complications of being on neuroleptic medication

SYNONYMS   N/A

ICD-9-CM   295 Schizophrenic disorders

SEE ALSO   N/A

OTHER NOTES   Schizophrenic patients occupy about half the beds in mental hospitals and 1/4 of all hospital beds

ABBREVIATIONS   N/A

REFERENCES
• Kaplan HI, Sadock BJ (eds). Comprehensive Textbook of Psychiatry. 6th Ed. Baltimore, Williams & Wilkins, 1995
• American Psychiatric Association: Diagnostic and Statistical Manual of Mental Disorders (DSM-IV-R). 4th Ed. Washington, DC, 1994
• Blin O. A comparative review of new antipsychotics. Can J Psychiatry 1999;44(3):235-44.
• Lehman AF, Steinwachs, DM. At issue: Translating research into practice: The schizophrenia patient outcomes research team (PORT) treatment recommendations. Schizophr Bull 1998;24(I):1 10
• Mojtabai R, Nicholson RA, Carpenter BN. Role of psychosocial treatments in management of schizophrenia: a meta-analytic review of controlled outcome studies. Schizophr Bull 1998; 24(4):569-87
• Clark AF, Lewis SW. Treatment of schizophrenia in childhood and adolescence. J Child Psychol Psychiatry 1998;39(8):1071-8 1
Illustrations: N/A
Internet references: http://www.5mcc.com

Author(s)
Doug Post, PhD

Schönlein-Henoch purpura

BASICS

DESCRIPTION A vasculitis of small vessels characterized by nonthrombocytopenic, usually dependent, palpable purpura, arthritis, abdominal pain and nephritis
System(s) affected: Skin/Exocrine, musculoskeletal, gastrointestinal, renal/urologic
Genetics: N/A
Incidence/Prevalence in USA: Incidence 14/100,000 in 2-14 year old age range. Seasonal variation - more common in winter.
Predominant age: Most occur between 2-8 years old, but can occur at any age
Predominant race: N/A
Predominant sex: Male > Female (2:1)

SIGNS AND SYMPTOMS
• Onset can be acute or gradual
• 50% of patients have malaise and low grade fever
• 100% of patients have skin lesions:
  ◊ Lesions appear on lower extremities and buttocks but may involve face, trunk and upper extremities
  ◊ Begin as small wheals or erythematous maculopapular
  ◊ Lesions blanch on pressure but later become petechial or purpuric
  ◊ Lesions appear in crops
  ◊ Angioedema of scalp, lips, eyelids, ears, dorsa of hands and feet, back, scrotum and perineum may be seen
• 70% of patients experience arthritis:
  ◊ Large joints (knees and ankles) are most commonly involved
• 35% of patients experience GI symptoms:
  ◊ Colicky abdominal pain associated with vomiting is most common
  ◊ Occult or gross blood in stool
  ◊ Hematemesis
  ◊ Intussusception, obstruction or infarction rarely occurs
  ◊ Pancreatitis
• 20% of patient have renal involvement:
  ◊ Hematuria, with or without casts or proteinuria
• Other manifestations
  ◊ Seizures, neuropathies
  ◊ Hepatosplenomegaly
  ◊ Lymphadenopathy
  ◊ Cardiac involvement
  ◊ Pulmonary hemorrhage
  ◊ Rheumatoid-like nodules
  ◊ Orchitis
• Infantile HSP
  ◊ Children < 2 years old
  ◊ Rare
  ◊ Edema and diffuse purpura of face and ears
  ◊ Fewer GI and renal symptoms

CAUSES Multiple infectious agents, drugs and toxins have been investigated, with no firm link found. *Helicobacter pylori* infection has been implicated.

RISK FACTORS N/A

DIAGNOSIS

DIFFERENTIAL DIAGNOSIS
• Hemorrhagic diathesis
• Septicemia
• Intussusception
• Acute appendicitis
• Acute glomerulonephritis
• Familial IgA nephropathy
• Polyarteritis nodosa
• Systemic lupus erythematosus
• Inflammatory bowel disease
• Subacute bacterial endocarditis
• Rocky Mountain spotted fever
• Thrombocytopenic purpura

LABORATORY
• Not diagnostic
• Sedimentation rate, white blood cell count may be elevated
• Coagulation studies, platelet count and complement determinations are normal
• Serum IgA elevated in 50%
• Urinalysis shows protein, red blood cells, white blood cells if renal involvement
Drugs that may alter lab results: N/A
Disorders that may alter lab results: N/A

PATHOLOGICAL FINDINGS
• Renal
  ◊ Focal and segmental increases in mesangial cells and matrix
  ◊ IgA deposition in glomerular basement membrane
  ◊ A minority show generalized mesangial changes
  ◊ Rarely, diffuse necrotizing glomerulonephritis with crescent formation
• Skin
  ◊ Small vessels are surrounded by an acute leukocytoclastic inflammatory reaction of neutrophils and round cells, with IgA deposition

SPECIAL TESTS N/A

IMAGING
• Abdominal x-rays may show ileus and segmental narrowing due to submucosal edema and hemorrhage
• Barium studies acutely may show large filling defects in the bowel wall, mimicking Crohn's disease or neoplasm

DIAGNOSTIC PROCEDURES
• Clinical diagnosis
• Renal biopsy rarely indicated except in cases of decreased renal function or development of nephrotic syndrome

TREATMENT

APPROPRIATE HEALTH CARE
• Outpatient
• Inpatient if hypertension, severe abdominal pain, renal insufficiency, or other major complication

GENERAL MEASURES
• Generally supportive

SURGICAL MEASURES N/A

ACTIVITY No restrictions in uncomplicated cases

DIET Usually no restrictions; NPO for severe gastrointestinal disease

PATIENT EDUCATION N/A

MEDICATIONS

DRUG(S) OF CHOICE
• Anti-inflammatory agents may be used for arthritis and fever
• Corticosteroids (prednisone 1-2 mg/kg/day) for severe GI symptoms and/or painful angioedema. Corticosteroids do not alter the progression of the lesions.
Contraindications: N/A
Precautions: N/A
Significant possible interactions: N/A

ALTERNATIVE DRUGS
Azathioprine, cyclophosphamide, plasmapheresis, factor XIII have been used in severe cases

FOLLOWUP

PATIENT MONITORING Urinalysis in follow-up, even if normal initially

PREVENTION/AVOIDANCE N/A

POSSIBLE COMPLICATIONS
• Hypertension
• Renal failure (but renal involvement usually has a benign course)
• Intestinal hemorrhage
• Bowel obstruction or perforation
• Death very rare

EXPECTED COURSE/PROGNOSIS
• Disease may last for a few days with transient arthritis; however, in many cases, the average duration is 4-6 weeks
• Occasionally recurrent
• 25% of patients with initial renal involvement will have persistently abnormal urine sediment

MISCELLANEOUS

ASSOCIATED CONDITIONS
• Possible association:
◊ Duodenal ulcer
◊ *Helicobacter pylori* infection

AGE-RELATED FACTORS
Pediatric: More common in children
Geriatric: N/A
Others: N/A

PREGNANCY Rare reports only

SYNONYMS
• Henoch-Schönlein purpura
• Anaphylactoid purpura

ICD-9-CM
287.0 Allergic purpura

SEE ALSO N/A

OTHER NOTES N/A

ABBREVIATIONS
HSP = Henoch-Schönlein purpura

REFERENCES
• Amitai Y, et al: Henoch-Schonlein purpura in infants. Pediatrics 1993;92:865
• Tapson KMP: Henoch-Schonlein purpura. Amer Fam Phys 1993;47:633
• Martin SR, et al: Henoch-Schonlein syndrome. In: Oski FA, et al. Principles and Practice of Pediatrics. 2nd Ed. Philadelphia, J.B. Lippincott Co., 1994
• Gasbarrini A, Franceschi F. Autoimmune diseases and Helicobacter pylori infection. Biomed Pharmacother 1999 Jun;53(5-6):223-6
• Sticca M, Barca S, Spallino L, Livio L, Longhi R. [Schonlein-Henoch syndrome: clinical-epidemiological analysis of 98 cases]. Peditr med Chir 1999 jan-Feb;21(1):9-12
• Cecchi R, Torelli E. Schonlein-Henoch purpura in association with duodenal ulcer and gastric Helicobacter pylori infection. J Dermatol 1998 Jul;25(7):482-4
Illustrations: N/A
Internet references: http://www.5mcc.com

Author(s)
Mark R. Dambro, MD, FAAFP

Scleritis

BASICS

DESCRIPTION Scleritis is an inflammation of the scleral outer coat of the eye
System(s) affected: Nervous
Genetics: None
Incidence/Prevalence in USA: Scleritis is uncommon
Predominant age: None
Predominant sex: Male = Female

SIGNS AND SYMPTOMS
• Redness and inflammation of the sclera
• Pain ranging from mild discomfort to extreme localized tenderness

CAUSES The most common cause of scleritis is in association with collagen vascular diseases such as rheumatoid arthritis

RISK FACTORS Individuals with autoimmune disorders, and chronic rheumatoid arthritis are most at risk

DIAGNOSIS

DIFFERENTIAL DIAGNOSIS
• Conjunctivitis
• Episcleritis
• "Pink eye"
• Iritis
• Trauma

LABORATORY
• Rheumatoid factor
• ANA, and HLA serotyping may help aid in the diagnosis
• Elevated sedimentation rate
Drugs that may alter lab results: None
Disorders that may alter lab results: None

PATHOLOGICAL FINDINGS
• Nodules can form on the sclera which demonstrate fibrinoid necrosis of the sclera
• There may or may not be adjacent inflammation
• The scleritis may be diffuse, nodular, or necrotizing
• If the posterior region of the globe is involved, adjacent swelling of orbital tissues may occur

SPECIAL TESTS N/A

IMAGING CT scan of the orbit may help differentiate the extensiveness and location of scleritis

DIAGNOSTIC PROCEDURES History and physical examination

TREATMENT

APPROPRIATE HEALTH CARE
Outpatient

GENERAL MEASURES
• Treatment of the inflammation usually with systemic steroids is required
• All of the immunosuppressants and antimetabolites used for autoimmune and collagen vascular disorders may be of help in active scleritis

SURGICAL MEASURES N/A

ACTIVITY No restrictions

DIET No special diet

PATIENT EDUCATION N/A

MEDICATIONS

DRUG(S) OF CHOICE Prednisone is the mainstay of treatment including both topical, periocular, and systemic administration
Contraindications: None
Precautions: Scleritis can progress to ocular perforation which may be hastened with periocular steroid injection
Significant possible interactions: Refer to manufacturer's literature

ALTERNATIVE DRUGS Nonsteroidal anti-inflammatory medications

FOLLOWUP

PATIENT MONITORING The patient should be followed very closely in the active stage of inflammation to assess the effectiveness of therapy

PREVENTION/AVOIDANCE None

POSSIBLE COMPLICATIONS
• Increased intraocular pressure
• Cataract and glaucoma can result as a result of treatment
• Ocular perforation can occur in severe stages

EXPECTED COURSE/PROGNOSIS
• Scleritis is indolent, chronic, and often times progressive
• Recurrent bouts of inflammation occur

MISCELLANEOUS

ASSOCIATED CONDITIONS
• Sjögren's syndrome
• Pseudo tumor

AGE-RELATED FACTORS
Pediatric: N/A
Geriatric: N/A
Others: N/A

PREGNANCY N/A

SYNONYMS N/A

ICD-9-CM
379.0 Scleritis and episcleritis

SEE ALSO
• Sjögren's syndrome

OTHER NOTES N/A

ABBREVIATIONS N/A

REFERENCES Merrill GM: Diseases of The Cornea. Boston, Little, Brown, 1990
Illustrations: N/A
Internet references: http://www.5mcc.com

Author(s)
Robert M. Kershner, MD, FACS

Scleroderma

BASICS

DESCRIPTION Scleroderma (systemic sclerosis [SSc]) is a chronic disease of unknown etiology, characterized by diffuse fibrosis, degenerative changes, and vascular abnormalities in the skin, articular structures and other organs (kidneys, lung, heart, gastrointestinal and skeletal muscles). The majority of manifestations have vascular features (e.g., Raynaud's phenomenon), but frank vasculitis is rarely seen. It can range from a mild disease, affecting the skin, to a systemic disease that can cause death in a few months.
System(s) affected: Skin/Exocrine, Renal/Urologic, Cardiovascular, Gastrointestinal, Musculoskeletal, Pulmonary
Genetics: Familial clustering is rare, but has been seen
Incidence/Prevalence in USA: 1/100,000
Predominant age:
• Young adult (16-40 years); middle age (40-75 years)
• Symptoms usually appear in the 3rd to 5th decade
Predominant sex: Female > Male (4:1)

SIGNS AND SYMPTOMS
• CREST syndrome (calcinosis, Raynaud's phenomenon, esophageal dysmobility, sclerodactyly, telangiectasia)
• Digital ulcerations
• Dry crackles at lung bases
• Dysphagia
• Dyspnea
• Finger tightness, swelling, thickening
• Flexion contractures
• Friction rub on tendon movement
• Hand swelling
• Hyperpigmentation, hypopigmentation
• Hypertension
• Joint stiffness
• Malabsorptive diarrhea
• Narrowed oral aperture
• Nausea and vomiting
• Peripheral neuropathy
• Polyarthralgia
• Proximal muscle weakness
• Pruritus
• Raynaud's phenomenon
• Scaling of skin
• Sclerodactyly
• Subcutaneous calcinosis
• Substernal fullness
• Telangiectasia
• Trigeminal neuropathy
• Weakness
• Weight loss
• Xerostomia

CAUSES
• Unknown
• Possible alterations in immune response
• Possibly some association with quartz mining, quarrying, vinyl chloride, hydrocarbons, toxin exposure, rape seed oil
• Treatment with bleomycin has caused a scleroderma-like syndrome

RISK FACTORS Unknown

DIAGNOSIS

DIFFERENTIAL DIAGNOSIS
• Sclerodermatomyositis
• Mixed connective tissue disease
• Toxic oil syndrome (Madrid, 1981, affecting 20,000 people)
• Eosinophilia-myalgia syndrome
• Diffuse fasciitis with eosinophilia
• Scleredema of Buschke's

LABORATORY
• Increased ESR
• Normocytic anemia
• Normochromic anemia
• Positive ANA
• Anti-centromere antibody
• Anti-Scl-70 (topoisomerase antibody)
• Positive nucleolar immunofluorescence
• Albuminuria
• Microscopic hematuria
• Eosinophilia
• Hemolysis
• Hypergammaglobulinemia
• Decreased maximum breathing capacity
• Increased residual volume
• Diffusion defect
• Positive rheumatoid factor test (33%)
Drugs that may alter lab results: N/A
Disorders that may alter lab results: N/A

PATHOLOGICAL FINDINGS
• Skin - edema
• Lymphocytic infiltrate around sweat glands
• Loss of capillaries
• Endothelial proliferation
• Hair follicle atrophy
• Subcutaneous tissue replaced by thick collagen bundles
• Synovium - pannus formation, fibrin deposits in tendons
• Kidney - small kidneys, intimal proliferation in interlobular arteries
• Heart - endocardial thickening, myocardial interstitial fibrosis
• Enlarged heart
• Cardiac hypertrophy
• Lung - interstitial pneumonitis, cyst formation
• Interstitial fibrosis
• Bronchiectasis
• Esophagus - esophageal atrophy, fibrosis

SPECIAL TESTS
• ECG - low voltage; possibly nonspecific abnormalities
• Lung function tests - decreased diffusion and vital capacity
• Skin biopsy - marked thickening of the dermis, occlusive vessel changes
• Nail fold capillary loop abnormalities

IMAGING
• Hand x-ray - absorption of tufts from terminal phalanges, soft tissue atrophy, subcutaneous calcinosis
• Upper GI - distal esophageal dilatation, atonic esophagus
• Barium enema - colonic diverticula, megacolon
• Chest x-ray - diffuse reticular pattern, bilateral basilar pulmonary fibrosis
• Gallium-67 lung scan - can be positive in early interstitial disease
• High resolution CT scan for detecting alveolitis - giving a "ground glass" appearance

DIAGNOSTIC PROCEDURES N/A

TREATMENT

APPROPRIATE HEALTH CARE
Outpatient. Inpatient possibly for some surgical procedures.

GENERAL MEASURES
• Treatment is symptomatic and supportive
• Esophageal dilatation
• Avoid cold, dress appropriately for the weather
• Avoid smoking (crucial)
• For chronic digital ulcerations - débridement after soaking in half-strength hydrogen peroxide solution, digital plaster to immobilize
• Physical therapy to maintain function and promote strength
• Avoid finger sticks (e.g., blood tests)
• Be wary of air conditioning
• Heat therapy to relieve joint stiffness
• Elevation of the head of the bed during sleep may help relieve gastrointestinal symptoms
• Skin - use softening lotions, ointments, bath oils to help prevent dryness and cracking
• Dialysis may be necessary as disease progresses

SURGICAL MEASURES Some success with gastroplasty for correction of gastroesophageal reflux

ACTIVITY Stay as active as possible, but avoid fatigue

DIET
• Soft, bland diet with frequent small meals
• Drink plenty of fluids with meals

PATIENT EDUCATION
• Printed patient information available from: Scleroderma Federation, 1725 York Avenue, No. 29F, New York, NY 10128, (212)427-7040
• Advise patient to report any abnormal bruising or non-healing abrasions
• Assist patient in smoking cessation, if needed

Scleroderma

MEDICATIONS

DRUG(S) OF CHOICE
• There are no drug therapies of proven value, except for ACE inhibitors for hypertensive renal crisis
• Corticosteroids - for disabling myositis, pulmonary alveolitis or mixed connective tissue disease
• NSAID's - for joint or tendon symptoms
• Antibiotics - for secondary infections in bowel
• Antacids or cimetidine - for gastric reflux
• Dipyridamole (Persantine) or aspirin - antiplatelet therapy
• Hydrophilic skin ointments - skin therapy
• Topical clindamycin or erythromycin or silver sulfadiazine (Silvadene) cream - may prevent recurrent infectious cutaneous ulcers; use systemic antibiotic therapy for active infections
• Consider immunosuppressives - used alone or with plasmapheresis for treatment of life-threatening or potentially crippling scleroderma
• Vasoactive agents and antihypertensives - for Raynaud's phenomenon
• Penicillamine (d-penicillamine) - reduce skin thickening and delay the rate of new visceral involvement
• Angiotensin-converting enzyme (captopril) - for kidney disease
Contraindications: Refer to manufacturer's literature
Precautions: Refer to manufacturer's literature
Significant possible interactions: Refer to manufacturer's literature

ALTERNATIVE DRUGS Many other drugs are currently under investigation, but no evidence of real benefits as yet

FOLLOWUP

PATIENT MONITORING Frequent to monitor medications and offer encouragement

PREVENTION/AVOIDANCE None

POSSIBLE COMPLICATIONS
• Renal failure
• Respiratory failure
• Flexion contractures
• Disability
• Esophageal dysmotility
• Reflux esophagitis
• Arrhythmia
• Megacolon
• Pneumatosis intestinalis
• Obstructive bowel
• Death

EXPECTED COURSE/PROGNOSIS
• Variable
• Possible improvement, but incurable
• Prognosis is poor if cardiac, pulmonary or renal manifestations present early

MISCELLANEOUS

ASSOCIATED CONDITIONS
• Rheumatoid arthritis
• Systemic lupus erythematosus
• Polymyositis

AGE-RELATED FACTORS
Pediatric: Rare in this age group
Geriatric: Not rare until after age 75
Others: N/A

PREGNANCY N/A

SYNONYMS
• Progressive systemic sclerosis
• Morphea
• PSS

ICD-9-CM 710.1 Systemic sclerosis

SEE ALSO N/A

OTHER NOTES N/A

ABBREVIATIONS N/A

REFERENCES
• Kelley WN, Harris ED, Ruddy S, Sledge CB, eds: Textbook of Rheumatology. 5th Ed. Philadelphia, W.B. Saunders, 1997
• Koopman WJ, eds: Arthritis and Allied Disorders. 13th Ed. Philadelphia, Lea & Febiger, 1997
• Kippel JH, Dippe PR, eds: Rheumatology, St. Louis, Mosby, 1994
Illustrations: 9 available on CD-ROM
Internet references: http://www.5mcc.com

Author(s)
Michael Tutt

Seizure disorders

BASICS

DESCRIPTION A sudden alteration of behavior, characterized by a sensory perception or motor activity without or with change in awareness or consciousness, due to aberrant cortical electrical activity
• Classification of seizures
◊ I. Partial seizures (seizures begin locally) - (A) without impairment of consciousness, (B) with complex symptoms (with impairment of consciousness)
◊ II. Generalized seizures (bilaterally symmetrical and without local onset)
◊ III. Unclassified epileptic seizures
System(s) affected: Nervous
Genetics: Three times the prevalence of seizures in close relatives of seizure patients
Incidence/Prevalence in USA:
• 1.5 million for epilepsy
• Annual incidence is 1.2/1000 for all types of seizures and 0.54/1000 for recurrent seizures
• The age adjusted prevalence is 0.625% or 6.25/1000; isolated seizures may occur in 10% of the general population
• 10-20% of all patients have intractable epilepsy
Predominant age: All ages
Predominant sex: Male = Female

SIGNS AND SYMPTOMS
• General
◊ Fever - indicative of infectious etiology
◊ Focal neurologic finding - may indicate tumor or localized injury to the brain
◊ Papilledema - suggestive of increased intracranial pressure
◊ Hemorrhagic eye grounds - suggests underlying hypertension
◊ Meningismus - may be present with meningitis
◊ Headache - sometimes associated with infectious or hemorrhagic causes of seizures
• Generalized seizures
◊ Absence - loss of consciousness or posture
◊ Myoclonic - repetitive muscle contractions
◊ Tonic-clonic - sustained contraction followed by rhythmic contractions of all four extremities
• Partial seizures
◊ Simple - Focal seizures without alteration of awareness/consciousness
◊ Complex - Focal seizures with alteration of awareness/consciousness
• Febrile seizures (see separate chapter on febrile seizures)
◊ Occurs between three months and five years of age
◊ Fever without evidence of any other defined cause for seizures
◊ If febrile seizures occur in the first year, the recurrence rate is 51%.
◊ If febrile seizures occur in the 2nd year, the recurrence rate is 25%.
◊ 88% of all recurrences of febrile seizures occur in the first 2 years
◊ The earlier the age of onset, the more likely repetitive febrile seizures will occur
◊ Recurrent febrile seizures probably do not increase the risk of epilepsy

• Status epilepticus (see separate chapter)
◊ Repetitive generalized seizures without return to consciousness between seizures
◊ Considered a neurological emergency

CAUSES
• Brain tumor
• Cerebral hypoxia (breath holding, carbon monoxide poisoning, anesthesia)
• Cerebrovascular accident (infarct or hemorrhage)
• Convulsive or toxic agents (lead, alcohol, picrotoxin, strychnine)
• Eclampsia
• Exogenous factors (sound, light, cutaneous stimulation)
• Fever (see chapter on febrile seizures)
• Head injury
• Heat stroke
• Infection
• Metabolic disturbances
• Withdrawal from, or hereditary intolerance of, alcohol

RISK FACTORS
• Susceptibility to seizures determined by a complex interplay between genetic factors and acquired brain disorders
• Children delivered breech have a prevalence rate of 3.8% compared with 2.2% in children delivered vertex

DIAGNOSIS

DIFFERENTIAL DIAGNOSIS
• Infancy (0-2)
◊ Perinatal hypoxia
◊ Birth injury
◊ Metabolic - hypoglycemia, hypocalcemia, hypomagnesemia, vitamin B6 deficiency, phenylketonuria
◊ Acute infection
• Childhood (2-10)
◊ Febrile seizure
◊ Idiopathic
◊ Acute infection
◊ Trauma
• Adolescent (10-18)
◊ Idiopathic
◊ Trauma
◊ Drug and alcohol withdrawal
◊ Arteriovenous malformations
• Early adulthood (18-25)
◊ Idiopathic
◊ Drug and alcohol withdrawal
◊ Trauma
• Middle age (25-60)
◊ Drug and alcohol withdrawal
◊ Trauma
◊ Tumor
◊ Vascular disease
• Late adulthood (over 60)
◊ Vascular disease
◊ Tumor
◊ Degenerative disease
◊ Metabolic - hypoglycemia, uremia, hepatic failure, electrolyte abnormality

LABORATORY
• Serum tests - glucose, sodium, potassium, calcium, phosphorus, magnesium, BUN, ammonia
• Anticonvulsant levels - inadequate level of anticonvulsant medication is the most common cause of recurrent seizures in children, and many adults
• Drug and toxic screens - include alcohol
• Complete blood count - helpful in evaluating infection
Drugs that may alter lab results:
• Anticonvulsant therapy may dramatically affect the EEG results
• Levels of anticonvulsants may be altered by a variety of common medications such as erythromycin, sulfonamides, warfarin, and cimetidine, as well as alcohol
Disorders that may alter lab results:
Pregnancy decreases serum concentration. Frequent monitoring and dosage adjustments are necessary.

PATHOLOGICAL FINDINGS None

SPECIAL TESTS
• Electroencephalogram (EEG). A negative EEG does not rule out a seizure disorder. Sensitivity, specificity and predictive value of the test depends on the underlying cause and anatomic location of the seizure focus.
• 24-hour ambulatory EEG - allows for continuous monitoring of cortical activity during regular activities
• Video-monitoring - useful in conjunction with simultaneous EEG monitoring in separating true events from pseudoseizures

IMAGING
• MRI of brain - superior in evaluation of the temporal lobes
• CT scan of brain - indicated routinely in work-up of tonic-clonic seizures

DIAGNOSTIC PROCEDURES None

TREATMENT

APPROPRIATE HEALTH CARE
Outpatient therapy except for status epilepticus

GENERAL MEASURES Protect the patient's airway

SURGICAL MEASURES N/A

ACTIVITY As tolerated

DIET Regular

PATIENT EDUCATION
• Stress the importance of compliance with anticonvulsant therapy
• Printed patient information available from: Epilepsy Foundation of America, 4351 Garden City Drive, Landover, MD 20785-2267, (800)EFA-1000

MEDICATIONS

DRUG(S) OF CHOICE
• To avoid a particular side effect, one drug may be preferred within one of the seizure groups listed below
• Generalized seizures - tonic clonic
◊ Phenytoin (Dilantin): 200-400 mg/day in 1-3 doses; therapeutic range: 10-20 µg/mL
◊ Phenobarbital: 100-200 mg/day in 1-2 doses; therapeutic range: 10-30 µg/mL
◊ Carbamazepine (Tegretol): 600-1200 mg/day in 2-4 doses; therapeutic range: 4-12 µg/mL
◊ Valproic acid (Depakene): 750-3000 mg/day in 1-3 doses (begin at 15 mg/kg/day; increase in one week by 5-10 mg/kg/day; split at 250 mg; maximum 60 mg/kg/day); therapeutic range 50-150 µg/mL
• Generalized seizures - absence
◊ Ethosuximide (Zarontin): 250-1500 mg/day in 1-3 doses; therapeutic range: 40-100 µg/mL
◊ Valproic acid: dose noted above; therapeutic range: 50-100 µg/mL
◊ Clonazepam (Klonopin): 0.01-0.3 mg/kg/day in 2-3 doses (maximum 20 mg/day); therapeutic range: 20-80 ng/mL (63-254 nmol/L)
• Partial seizures
◊ Phenytoin (Dilantin)
◊ Carbamazepine (Tegretol)
◊ Phenobarbital
Contraindications: Refer to manufacturer's profile of each drug
Precautions: Doses should be individualized according to the patient's age and weight. Refer to manufacturer's profile of each drug.
Significant possible interactions: Refer to manufacturer's profile of each drug

ALTERNATIVE DRUGS
• Felbamate (Felbatol)
• Gabapentin (Neurontin) 300mg hs, then BID, then TID. Adjust to maximum of 2400 mg/day.
• Lamotrigine (Lamictal)
• Primidone (Mysoline)
• Topiramate (Topamax)
• Several additional drugs awaiting FDA approval

FOLLOWUP

PATIENT MONITORING
• Regular monitoring of anticonvulsant levels
• CBC as indicated
• Monitor medication side effects and adverse reactions

PREVENTION/AVOIDANCE   Maintain
adequate epileptic drug therapy. Patient education on compliance.

POSSIBLE COMPLICATIONS   Drug
toxicity

EXPECTED COURSE/PROGNOSIS
• Depends on the pathophysiology of seizure within particular patient
• Seizure activity may become quiescent. If a patient has been seizure-free for two years, withdrawal of therapy may be considered. Relapse rate after three years of being off medications is 33%.

MISCELLANEOUS

ASSOCIATED CONDITIONS
• Infections
• Tumors
• Drug abuse
• Metabolic disorders

AGE-RELATED FACTORS
Pediatric: Breastfeeding is not contraindicated in mothers receiving epileptic medication, although drug concentration in the infant may require monitoring if problems such as sedation occur
Geriatric: N/A
Others: N/A

PREGNANCY   Serum levels of
anticonvulsants may decline, frequent monitoring recommended. There is a two-fold increased risk of congenital malformation in mothers taking anticonvulsant medication

SYNONYMS
• Convulsions
• Epilepsy
• Fits
• Spells

ICD-9-CM
780.3 Convulsions (excludes epileptic and newborn)

SEE ALSO
• Seizures, febrile
• Status epilepticus

OTHER NOTES   Jacksonian epilepsy -
characterized by unilateral clonic movements that start in one group of muscles and spread systematically to adjacent groups, reflecting the march of epileptic activity through the motor cortex. Usual course - chronic; recurrent; intermittent.

ABBREVIATIONS   N/A

REFERENCES
• Beignat JL: Getting a handle on an adult's first seizure. Emergency Med 1989;20:20-28,
• Schewer ML, Pedley TA: The evaluation and treatment of seizures. New Engl J Med 1990;323(21):1468-1474
• Applegate MS, Lo W: Febrile seizures: current concepts concerning prognosis and clinical management. Journal of Fam Prac 1989;299(4):422-428
• Freeman J, Vinny E: Decision making and the child with afebrile seizure. Pediatrics in Review 1992;13(8):305-310
Illustrations: N/A
Internet references: http://www.5mcc.com

Author(s)
William L. Toffler, MD
Scott A. Fields, MD

Seizures, febrile

BASICS

DESCRIPTION Seizure occurring with fever in infancy or childhood without evidence of other underlying cause. Seizures secondary to other CNS events like meningitis, tumor, or afebrile convulsive history excluded from this topic.
• Simple febrile seizure - single episode in 24 hours, lasting less than 15 minutes and generalized tonic-clonic activity. Accounts for 85% of febrile seizures.
• Complex febrile seizure - multiple episodes in 24 hours with focalizing findings and lasting more than 15 minutes. Accounts for 15% of febrile seizures.
System(s) affected: Nervous
Genetics: Uncertain but may be autosomal dominant with variable expression and incomplete penetrance
Incidence/Prevalence in USA:
Approximately 2500/100,000. 2-5% of all children, comprising 30% of all childhood seizures.
Predominant age: 95% occur by 5 years; peak at 2 years
Predominant sex: Male > Female (slightly)

SIGNS AND SYMPTOMS
• Fever usually 39°C (102.2°F) or greater
• Tonic-clonic convulsive activity
  ◊ Generalized with simple seizure or focal with complex event
  ◊ Usually occurs within hours of fever onset
  ◊ The seizure is the initial sign of illness in 25% of patients
  ◊ Duration is less than 15 minutes with simple seizures; longer with complex episodes
  ◊ Average frequency is once in 24 hours with simple; more with complex

CAUSES
• Fever may lower seizure threshold in susceptible children
• Temperature usually greater than 39°C (102.2°F), but rate of change may be more important than temperature
• Viral illnesses: Upper respiratory infections, roseola infantum, influenza A, gastroenteritis
• Bacterial infections: Shigella, salmonella, otitis media
• Mumps, measles, rubella immunization (MMR) within prior 7-10 days or diphtheria, pertussis, tetanus immunization (DPT) within prior 48 hours

RISK FACTORS Febrile seizure in sibling raises risk 2-3 times

DIAGNOSIS

DIFFERENTIAL DIAGNOSIS
• Febrile delirium
• Febrile shivering with pallor and peri-oral cyanosis
• Breath holding spell during fever event
• Afebrile seizure occurring during fever event
• Acute meningitis presenting with seizure
• Head injury and fever
• Drug induced seizures
• Sudden discontinuance of anticonvulsants

LABORATORY
• First episode: CBC, calcium, glucose, magnesium, electrolytes (especially sodium), urinalysis, blood culture, BUN, creatinine
• A toxologic screen may be indicated in unclear cases
• First episode or under 1 year old, consider a lumbar puncture to rule out meningitis
Drugs that may alter lab results: N/A
Disorders that may alter lab results: Infections

PATHOLOGICAL FINDINGS   N/A

SPECIAL TESTS EEG may be indicated: If recurrent frequent febrile seizures, those with focal findings, complex type, underlying neurological disorder, family history of afebrile seizures, delayed awakening after event, or if this is first event after age 3. Perform EEG 2-4 weeks after event. EEG not indicated for simple febrile seizure when there is a ready explanation for fever and recovery is quick.

IMAGING CT scan of brain for complex types, focal findings, underlying neurological disorder, or prolonged recovery phase

DIAGNOSTIC PROCEDURES Lumbar puncture

TREATMENT

APPROPRIATE HEALTH CARE
Emergency room or extended observation based on clinical situation, seizure type and whether first or subsequent event

GENERAL MEASURES
• Supportive care
• If seizure ended and simple type with recovery progressing, determine fever source so underlying cause can be treated
• Tepid sponge bath to lower temperature
• If seizure less than 10 minutes, supportive measures with laying on side, protecting from injury, maintaining airway, low flow oxygen

SURGICAL MEASURES   N/A

ACTIVITY Bedrest during observation interval

DIET Nothing by mouth until status clarified

PATIENT EDUCATION
• Parents need much support
• Febrile seizures do not cause developmental delay
• Febrile seizures do not cause retardation
• Febrile seizures do not cause behavioral abnormalities
• Febrile seizures do not cause death
• Recurrence risk 33%, with 95% occurring within next 1 year

MEDICATIONS

DRUG(S) OF CHOICE
• Rectal or oral acetaminophen for fever 10-15 mg/kg/dose or ibuprofen 10 mg/kg/dose
• Anticonvulsants rarely indicated. See topic Status epilepticus for treatment of prolonged seizures.
• Oxygen
Contraindications: Allergy to drug
Precautions: Respiratory compromise needing support or intubation
Significant possible interactions: N/A

ALTERNATIVE DRUGS
• Phenobarbital 10-15 mg/kg IV, slower onset of action and may cause respiratory depression and hypotension
• Phenytoin 10-15 mg/kg IV, slower onset of action and may cause cardiac arrhythmias and hypotension
• Valproic acid 40-60 mg/kg in equal parts water - 5 cm rectally is longer acting but may cause hepatotoxicity in under 2 year age group, slower onset of action
• Paraldehyde - 0.2 ml/kg up to 2 ml at one site IM, but slower onset of action, or paraldehyde in rectal dosage form - 0.3 cc (300 mg)/kg/dose in 1:1 dilution with cottonseed oil or olive oil (maximum dose 5 mL)

FOLLOWUP

PATIENT MONITORING
Based on the site, severity, and origin of the fever.

PREVENTION/AVOIDANCE
• Acetaminophen 10 mg/kg orally or rectally or ibuprofen 10 mg/kg - temperature greater than 38°C (100.5°F) rectal
• May use intermittent prophylactic rectal diazepam for fever greater than 38.5°C (101.3°F); 5 mg if under 3 years or 7.5 mg 3 to 6 years or 0.5 mg/kg (up to 15 mg), repeated every 12 hours for 4 doses total
• Continuous prophylaxis is controversial; may consider for high risk child with strong family history, multiple recurrences, complex events, or underlying neurological abnormalities until 1 year after last seizure. Phenobarbital 3-5 mg/kg/day may be used but often causes behavioral problems; valproic acid 30-40 mg/kg/day may be tried but may cause severe hepatotoxicity

POSSIBLE COMPLICATIONS
• Febrile seizures do not cause death, retardation, behavioral problems nor developmental delays
• Children with febrile seizures are at greater than average risk to develop epilepsy later in life

EXPECTED COURSE/PROGNOSIS
• 33% develop recurrent febrile seizures, 50% if first episode before 12 months, 45% if two involved siblings
• 95% of recurrences occur within 1 year
• Epilepsy occurs in 0.5% of general population but 3-4% of population with prior febrile seizure
• Risks for epilepsy include: Complex initial event with risk climbing with each complex feature independently, age at first episode under 6 months, three or more recurrences, pre-seizure neurological abnormalities, and family history of epilepsy

MISCELLANEOUS

ASSOCIATED CONDITIONS
• Examine child for port wine stain over trigeminal nerve with Sturge-Weber syndrome, adenoma sebaceum and hypopigmented skin of tuberous sclerosis, and café-au-lait spots and subcutaneous nodules of neurofibromatosis
• 13-18% of meningitis cases present with seizures

AGE-RELATED FACTORS
Pediatric: Range 3 months to 5 years with 95% by age 5 and peak incidence at age 2 years
Geriatric: N/A
Others: N/A

PREGNANCY   N/A

SYNONYMS
• Febrile convulsions
• Febrile fits

ICD-9-CM
780.31 Seizures, convulsions, febrile

SEE ALSO
• Seizure disorders
• Status epilepticus

OTHER NOTES
• Intermittent phenobarbital prophylaxis not recommended
• Phenytoin and carbamazepine are ineffective for prophylaxis
• No evidence that preventing recurrent febrile seizures prevents epilepsy
• Critical to distinguish between simple and complex events
• Post-ictal sleepiness is common; if marked may indicate underlying pathology

ABBREVIATIONS   N/A

REFERENCES
• Leung AKC: Febrile Convulsions: How dangerous are they? Postgraduate Medicine 1991;89(5):217-224
• Applegate MS, Lo W: Febrile Seizures: Current Concepts Concerning Prognosis and Clinical Management. Journal of Family Practice 1989;29(4):422-428
• Sexton ME: Childhood Seizures. AAFP Home Study Audio Series, Sept. 1991
Illustrations: N/A
Internet references: http://www.5mcc.com

Author(s)
Barbara J. Moront, MD

Sepsis

BASICS

DESCRIPTION
The systemic response to infection; it encompasses a broad array of clinical manifestations and overlaps with inflammatory reactions to other clinical insults (e.g., severe trauma or burn)
• Bacteremia: Bacteria in the blood; may have no accompanying symptoms
• Systemic inflammatory response syndrome (SIRS): inflammatory reaction to different clinical insults manifest by two of the following: (1) temperature >38°C or < 36°C, (2) heart rate > 90/min; (3) respiratory rate >20/min or PaCO2 < 32 mm Hg, and (4) WBC count > 12,000/mm3, < 4,000/mm3 or > 10% immature forms (bends)
• Sepsis: SIRS with documented infection (typically bacterial)
• Septic shock: Sepsis induced hypotension (systolic BP < 90 mmHg or ≥ 40 mmHg drop from baseline) despite adequate fluid resuscitation plus hypoperfusion abnormalities (oliguria, lactic acidosis, acute change in mental status)
• Multiple organ dysfunction syndrome (MODS): altered organ function in an acutely ill patient - requires intervention to maintain homeostasis
System(s) affected: Cardiovascular, Endocrine/Metabolic, Hemic/Lymphatic/Immunologic, Renal/Urologic, Nervous, Pulmonary, Gastrointestinal
Genetics: N/A
Incidence/Prevalence in USA: 176/100,000 persons/year
Predominant age: All ages
Predominant sex: Male = Female

SIGNS AND SYMPTOMS
• Fever
• Chills, rigors
• Myalgias
• Changes in mental status - restlessness, agitation, confusion, delirium, lethargy, stupor, coma
• Tachycardia
• Tachypnea
• Hypotension
• Skin lesions - erythema, petechiae, ecthyma gangrenosum, embolic lesions
• Signs and symptoms related to site of primary infection:
  ◊ Respiratory tract - cough, sputum production, dyspnea, chest pain
  ◊ Urinary tract - dysuria, flank pain, frequency, urgency
  ◊ Intra-abdominal source - nausea, vomiting, diarrhea, constipation, abdominal pain
  ◊ Central nervous system - stiff neck, headache, photophobia, focal neurologic signs
• Signs and symptoms related to end organ failure:
  ◊ Pulmonary - cyanosis
  ◊ Renal - oliguria, anuria
  ◊ Hepatic - jaundice
  ◊ Cardiac - congestive heart failure

CAUSES
• Specific etiologic agents include:
  ◊ Gram positive organisms - most commonly Staphylococcus sp, Streptococcus sp, Enterococcus sp
  ◊ Gram negative organisms - most commonly Escherichia coli, Klebsiella sp, Proteus sp, Pseudomonas sp
  ◊ Fungi - most commonly Candida sp
  ◊ Other agents - anaerobes. Also, see Differential diagnosis.
• Common sources of septicemia include:
  ◊ Lungs
  ◊ Urinary tract
  ◊ Intra-abdominal focus - biliary tree, abscess, peritonitis
  ◊ Intravascular catheters
  ◊ Skin - cellulitis, decubitus ulcer, gangrene
  ◊ Heart valves

RISK FACTORS
• Age extremes (very old and very young)
• Impaired host (see associated conditions)
• Indwelling catheters - intravascular, urinary, biliary, etc.
• Complicated labor and delivery - premature and/or prolonged rupture of membranes, etc.
• Certain surgical procedures

DIAGNOSIS

DIFFERENTIAL DIAGNOSIS
• Viral diseases (influenza, dengue and other hemorrhagic viruses, Coxsackie B virus)
• Rickettsial diseases (Rocky Mountain spotted fever, endemic typhus)
• Spirochetal diseases (leptospirosis, relapsing fever [Borrelia sp], Jarisch-Herxheimer reaction in syphilis)
• Protozoal diseases (Toxoplasma gondii, Trypanosoma cruzi, Pneumocystis carinii, Plasmodium falciparum)
• Collagen vascular diseases, vasculitides, myocardial infarction, pulmonary embolus, thrombotic thrombocytopenic purpura/hemolytic-uremic syndrome, thyrotoxicosis, adrenal insufficiency (Addison's disease), dissecting aortic aneurysm, multiple trauma, third-degree burn

LABORATORY
• Positive blood cultures
• Positive cultures from other sites (sputum, urine, cerebrospinal fluid [CSF], etc.)
• Gram stain of clinical specimens (sputum, urine, CSF, etc.)
• Common:
  ◊ Leukocytosis
  ◊ Proteinuria
  ◊ Hypoxemia
  ◊ Eosinopenia
  ◊ Hypoferremia
  ◊ Hyperglycemia
  ◊ Hypocalcemia
  ◊ Mild hyperbilirubinemia
• Less common:
  ◊ Lactic acidosis
  ◊ Leukopenia
  ◊ Azotemia
  ◊ Thrombocytopenia
  ◊ Prolonged prothrombin time
  ◊ Anemia
  ◊ Hypoglycemia

Drugs that may alter lab results: Prior antibiotic use
Disorders that may alter lab results: N/A

PATHOLOGICAL FINDINGS
• Inflammation at primary site of infection
• Disseminated intravascular coagulation
• Noncardiogenic pulmonary edema

SPECIAL TESTS
• Antigen detection systems - counterimmune electrophoresis (CIE) and latex agglutination tests (pneumococcus, H. influenzae type B, group B streptococcus, meningococcus)
• Gram stain of buffy coat smears occasionally useful

IMAGING
• X-rays (e.g., chest)
• Ultrasound, CT scan, or MRI may be useful in delineating sites of infection

DIAGNOSTIC PROCEDURES
• Aspiration of potentially infected body fluids (pleural, peritoneal, CSF) when appropriate
• Biopsy, drainage of potentially infected tissues (abscess, biliary tree, etc.) when appropriate

TREATMENT

APPROPRIATE HEALTH CARE
• Hospitalization
• Intensive care treatment of patients with shock, respiratory failure

GENERAL MEASURES
• Removal or drainage of septic foci
• Correction of metabolic abnormalities (hypoxemia, hyperglycemia, hypoglycemia, severe acidemia [pH < 7.10])
• Mechanical ventilation for respiratory failure
• Transfusion of RBC, platelets, and/or fresh frozen plasma for bleeding
• Volume replacement followed by pressors for hypotension
• Stress ulcer and deep venous thrombosis prophylatic measures

SURGICAL MEASURES
Drainage of infected sites, débridement of necrotic tissues

ACTIVITY
Bedrest

DIET
NPO initially; intravenous hyperalimentation appropriate in some severely malnourished patients and in patients who will be unable to receive enteral alimentation within the week

PATIENT EDUCATION
N/A

Sepsis

MEDICATIONS

DRUG(S) OF CHOICE
- Antibiotic coverage should be broad initially and directed against organisms associated with identified septic foci. After culture results are available, treatment should be more organism-specific. Knowledge of the antibiotic susceptibility patterns of local pathogens extremely important.
- Neonatal (< 7 days old) sepsis - ampicillin 300 mg/kg/d in 3 divided doses and gentamicin (Garamycin) 5 mg/kg/d in 2 divided doses
- Non-immunocompromised child - cefotaxime (Claforan) 200 mg/kg/d in 4 divided doses
- Non-immunocompromised adult - cefotaxime (Claforan) 1-2 gm q8-12 or ticarcillin-clavulanate (Timentin) 3.1 g q6h plus gentamicin 5 mg/kg/day in 1-3 divided doses
- Neutropenic host - ceftazidime (Fortaz) 1-2 gm q8-12h, and gentamicin (Garamycin) or tobramycin 3-5 mg/kg/day in 2-3 divided doses; vancomycin (Vancocin) is added when there is an obvious catheter-related infection or a known gram positive bacteremia or if there is an increased likelihood of infection with resistant gram positive organisms.

Contraindications: History of anaphylaxis or other allergic reaction to the antibiotic
Precautions: Dose adjustments required in renal failure
Significant possible interactions:
- Aminoglycosides - increased nephrotoxicity with enflurane, cisplatin and possibly vancomycin; increased ototoxicity with loop diuretics; increased paralysis with neuromuscular blocking agents
- Ampicillin - increased frequency of rash with allopurinol

ALTERNATIVE DRUGS
- Antibodies against gram negative cell wall antigens may reduce mortality
- Many other drug combinations are possible to get adequate coverage
- Antifungals
- Antimicrobials for anaerobic infections
- Antipseudomonals

FOLLOWUP

PATIENT MONITORING
- Depends upon source of infection, underlying disease(s)
- Peak and trough drug levels for aminoglycosides, vancomycin
- BUN, creatinine, electrolytes and complete blood counts at least twice weekly; more frequently if unstable

PREVENTION/AVOIDANCE
- Vaccination - pneumococcal (geriatric patients, patients with certain chronic diseases), Hemophilus influenzae type B (infants, young children)
- Gamma globulin (for hypo- or agammaglobulinemic patients)
- Hand washing by hospital personnel, appropriate catheter care, etc., for hospitalized patients

POSSIBLE COMPLICATIONS
- Death
- Adult respiratory distress syndrome (ARDS)
- Multi-organ failure (cardiac, pulmonary, renal, hepatic)
- Disseminated intravascular coagulation (DIC)
- Gastrointestinal hemorrhage

EXPECTED COURSE/PROGNOSIS
Even with optimal care, mortality will be 10-50% overall; this is increased in patients with neutropenia, diabetes, alcoholism, renal failure, respiratory failure, hypogammaglobulinemia, certain etiologic agents (e.g., Pseudomonas aeruginosa), a delay in appropriate antimicrobial therapy, and those patients at the age extremes

MISCELLANEOUS

ASSOCIATED CONDITIONS
- Neutropenia
- Diabetes mellitus
- Alcoholism
- Leukemia, lymphoma, and solid tumors
- Cirrhosis
- Burns
- Multiple trauma
- Intravenous drug abuse
- Malnutrition
- Complement deficiencies
- Hypo- or agammaglobulinemia
- Splenectomy
- HIV infection

AGE-RELATED FACTORS
Pediatric: Screen newborns for infection due to prolonged rupture of membranes (> 24 h), maternal fever, prematurity
Geriatric:
- Often more difficult to diagnose clinically in the elderly
- Change in mental status/behavior may be only early manifestation
Others: N/A

PREGNANCY Beta lactam antibiotics, aminoglycosides, erythromycin are considered safe

SYNONYMS
- Septicemia
- Sepsis neonatorum

ICD-9-CM 038 Septicemia

SEE ALSO
- Pneumonia, bacterial
- Pyelonephritis
- Meningitis, bacterial
- Endocarditis, infective (part 1)
- Toxic shock syndrome
- Rocky Mountain spotted fever
- Candidiasis
- Listeriosis
- Tularemia

OTHER NOTES High dose steroids of no benefit

ABBREVIATIONS N/A

REFERENCES
- Bone RC, et al: Definitions for sepsis and organ failure and guidelines for the use of innovative therapies in sepsis. Chest 1992;101:1644-1655
- Task Force of the American College of Critical Care Medicine, Society of Critical Care Medicine: Practice parameters for hemodynamic support of sepsis in adult patients in sepsis. Crit Care Med 1999;27:639-660
- Wheeler AP, Bernard GR: Current concepts: treating patients with severe sepsis. NEJM 1999;340:207-214
Illustrations: N/A
Internet references: http://www.5mcc.com

Author(s)
Robert L. Atmar, MD

Serum sickness

BASICS

DESCRIPTION Allergic reaction to foreign serum or drugs, usually appearing 5-14 days after administration of the allergen. Characterized by fever, arthralgias, skin rash and lymphadenopathy.
System(s) affected: Musculoskeletal, Gastrointestinal, Skin/Exocrine, Hemic/Lymphatic/Immunologic, Cardiovascular
Genetics: N/A
Incidence/Prevalence in USA: Common
Predominant age: All ages
Predominant sex: Male = Female

SIGNS AND SYMPTOMS
• History of antibiotic therapy (especially penicillin and related drugs)
• History of injection of horse serum or other species serum
• Fever
• Arthralgias (particularly TM joint)
• Malaise
• Pruritus
• Nausea
• Vomiting
• Abdominal pain
• Splenomegaly
• Myalgias
• Extremity weakness
• Sneezing
• Coughing
• Dyspnea
• Melena
• Cutaneous eruptions
• Facial swelling
• Lymphadenopathy
• Urticaria
• Joint effusion
• Myocarditis (rare)

CAUSES
• IgG antibodies that form soluble complexes with the antigen to cause an immune complex (type III) reaction
• Drugs (penicillin, cephalosporins, sulfonamides, thiouracils, iodinated dyes, streptomycin)
• Tetanus toxoid
• Rabies antiserum
• Release of vasoactive substance
• Rabbit antiserum
• Crotalidae antivenin

RISK FACTORS
Previous exposure to injection of foreign protein (reaction usually occurs sooner than the expected 5-14 days)

DIAGNOSIS

DIFFERENTIAL DIAGNOSIS
• Periarteritis nodosa
• Anaphylaxis
• Drug hypersensitivity

LABORATORY
• Proteinuria
• Decreased C3
• Decreased C4
• Increased ESR
• Mixed IgG-IgM cryoprecipitates
Drugs that may alter lab results: N/A
Disorders that may alter lab results: N/A

PATHOLOGICAL FINDINGS
Nodular lesions in segments of arteries resembling periarteritis nodosa

SPECIAL TESTS
Test all persons prior to administering a foreign serum (see Prevention/avoidance)

IMAGING N/A

DIAGNOSTIC PROCEDURES N/A

TREATMENT

APPROPRIATE HEALTH CARE
Inpatient, if severe; outpatient for mild cases

GENERAL MEASURES
Treat symptomatically. Usually self-limited.

SURGICAL MEASURES N/A

ACTIVITY
Bed rest during acute illness

DIET
No special diet

PATIENT EDUCATION N/A

MEDICATIONS

DRUG(S) OF CHOICE
• Antihistamine of choice for urticaria and generalized pruritus
• Aspirin 0.6-1.5 grams orally q 4h
Contraindications: Refer to manufacturer's literature
Precautions: Refer to manufacturer's literature
Significant possible interactions: Refer to manufacturer's literature

ALTERNATIVE DRUGS
Prednisone - 40 mg/day orally if simpler medicines do not bring symptomatic relief. Prednisone also used if peripheral neuritis or myocarditis (rare) develops.

FOLLOWUP

PATIENT MONITORING
During acute illness, monitor closely for signs of myocarditis or peripheral neuritis

PREVENTION/AVOIDANCE
• Special caution in patients who need foreign serum if they have history of asthma, hay fever, urticaria or other allergic symptoms
• Testing in patients with no previous exposure or allergic history: Before administering a foreign protein - prick test with 1:10 dilution. If this is negative, 0.02 mL of 1:10 dilution given intracutaneously.
• Testing in patients with previous exposure or allergic history: Test first with 1:1000 dilution
• If skin test is positive and serum treatment is essential, then desensitization is necessary

POSSIBLE COMPLICATIONS
• Vasculitis
• Neuropathy
• Glomerulonephritis (rare)
• Anaphylaxis
• Shock
• Death

EXPECTED COURSE/PROGNOSIS
Favorable; self-limiting with 2-3 weeks for recovery

MISCELLANEOUS

ASSOCIATED CONDITIONS
Drug hypersensitivity

AGE-RELATED FACTORS
Pediatric: N/A
Geriatric: N/A
Others: N/A

PREGNANCY
N/A

SYNONYMS
• Inoculation reaction
• Protein sickness

ICD-9-CM
999.5 Other serum reaction

SEE ALSO
N/A

OTHER NOTES
Horse antiserum still used in treatment of botulism, diphtheria, venomous snake bites, spider bites. Antilymphocyte or antilymphocyte serum is used to suppress immune reactions to transplanted organs.

ABBREVIATIONS
N/A

REFERENCES
• Isselbacker KJ, et al, eds: Harrison's Principles of Internal Medicine. 14th Ed. New York, McGraw-Hill Inc., 1998
• Virella G: Hypersensitivity reactions. Immunology Series 1993;58:329
Illustrations: N/A
Internet references: http://www.5mcc.com

Author(s)
Brian J. Murray, MD

Sexual dysfunction in women

BASICS

DESCRIPTION Difficulty getting or staying sexually aroused, reaching orgasm too quickly, difficulty or inability to reach orgasm, inability to relax, lack of interest in sex, distaste or revulsion with sex, too little foreplay, too little tenderness after intercourse.
• Most women who have orgasms do not do so invariably during intercourse, and some mistakenly think this is dysfunction
• Four major types:
  ◊ Disorder of desire - both hypo- and hyper- (initiation and response), global desire disorder, couple desire discrepancy, situational desire disorder - these must be evaluated in the context of the relationship overall
  ◊ Disorder of arousal
  ◊ Dyspareunia, vaginismus
  ◊ Orgasmic disorders - primary and secondary, during masturbation or coitus, situational or partner specific

System(s) affected: Reproductive, Nervous
Genetics: N/A
Incidence/Prevalence in USA:
• 1 in 5 women is sexually dissatisfied, and two thirds of women report some degree of sexual dysfunction. Only one third of anorgasmic women in general think it is a problem.
• Overall prevalence for dysfunction is 15-30% of all women. Desire disorders are complaint of 30-55% of individual patients presenting to clinics, and 31% of couples; arousal disorders present in about 14-48% in community studies. Orgasmic disorders probably the most common; about 10% primary, and up to 65-80% secondary in community studies.
• There are many barriers to seeking help, so data for prevalence incomplete; barriers include stigma of exposing sexual inadequacy, fear of unknown therapy, e.g., of having to perform before a therapist.
Predominant age: Can occur in post-pubertal age group; women's ability to experience orgasm increases gradually from puberty; in later teens nearly half have not had orgasm; by mid-thirties, about 10% have not
Predominant sex: Female (heterosexual, homosexual, and bisexual women)

SIGNS AND SYMPTOMS
• Complaint to health care provider (if the clinician inquires, over twice as many are revealed than if clinician waits for patient to mention)
• Infertility
• Marital conflict
• Family dysfunction

CAUSES
• Interrelational difficulties and conflict regarding intimacy
• Anxiety
• Survivor of sexual abuse, including incest
• Alcohol
• Drug use, including prescription medications (e.g., MAO inhibitors, tricyclic antidepressants, beta-blockers, especially SSRI antidepressants [Prozac, Paxil, Zoloft, etc.])
• Proximity of other people in household (mother-in-law)
• Anorgasmia can be due to diabetes
• Spinal cord damage
• Hormonal imbalance?
• Thyroid disease
• Sexual frequency myths
• Control issues in the relationships
• Dyspareunia, including vaginal dryness causing interference with lubrication, secondary to infection or endocrine
• There is little endocrine data on women with sexual dysfunction

RISK FACTORS Couple discrepancies in - expectations, cultural backgrounds, attitudes toward sexuality in family of origin, previous sexual trauma, low self-esteem

DIAGNOSIS

DIFFERENTIAL DIAGNOSIS
• Medications including psychotropics (monoamine oxidase inhibitors, tricyclic and other antidepressants)
• Marital dysfunction including domestic violence
• Decreased sensation secondary to back or nerve disease
• Multiple sclerosis
• Abdominal surgery (can interfere with pelvic innervation)
• Depression
• Vaginitis
• Decreased vaginal lubrication secondary to hormonal imbalance
• Pregnancy
• Anatomic or congenital abnormalities
• Pseudodyspareunia (use of complaint of pain to distance from partner)

LABORATORY As needed to identify infections and other medical causes
Drugs that may alter lab results: N/A
Disorders that may alter lab results: N/A

PATHOLOGICAL FINDINGS Varied if any

SPECIAL TESTS May need life experiences or some other psychological inventory to evaluate couple. (Alcohol, marijuana or other illicit drug use may make these evaluations unreliable.)

IMAGING N/A

DIAGNOSTIC PROCEDURES N/A

TREATMENT

APPROPRIATE HEALTH CARE
Outpatient

GENERAL MEASURES
• For childhood trauma - scripting, psychotherapy, cognitive restructuring
• For anorgasmia - directed masturbation and "homework" with partners
• For prescription drug causes - reduced dosages, or change to different medication
• Other - family therapy, sensate conditioning; referral to specialized sex therapy

SURGICAL MEASURES N/A

ACTIVITY Varies with couple

DIET Weight reduction if needed for either partner

PATIENT EDUCATION Information about normal sexual function and human reproductive anatomy and function and changes expected with aging

MEDICATIONS

DRUG(S) OF CHOICE These are usually multifactorial psychosocial conditions. Using medications doesn't address the cause of the problem and can make it worse.
Contraindications: N/A
Precautions: N/A
Significant possible interactions: N/A

ALTERNATIVE DRUGS Adding testosterone to hormone replacement therapy may increase sexual desire in postmenopausal women

FOLLOWUP

PATIENT MONITORING Varies with patient

PREVENTION/AVOIDANCE Sex education starting in elementary years, early intervention in dysfunctional family or incest

POSSIBLE COMPLICATIONS Marital or family stress, breakup and divorce

EXPECTED COURSE/PROGNOSIS
Lack of desire is the most difficult to treat (less than 50% successful by patient report), and success is sometimes less optimal than patient's initial wish. Best predictors are desire to change and overall healthy relationship.

MISCELLANEOUS

ASSOCIATED CONDITIONS Marital stress

AGE-RELATED FACTORS
Pediatric: N/A
Geriatric:
• Societal expectations about geriatric sexuality, (especially the myth older women aren't sexually active) can cause distress if patient has sexual desires or sexual experience
• Normal physiologic changes in aging are misinterpreted as dysfunction
Others: Sex role stereotypes

PREGNANCY Often affects but the effect varies depending on the patient and couple's beliefs about pregnancy and the problem

SYNONYMS
• Hypoactive sexual desire disorder
• Sexual aversion disorder
• Female sexual arousal disorder
• Inhibited female orgasm

ICD-9-CM
302.70 Psychosexual dysfunction, unspecified
302.72 Psychosexual dysfunction with inhibited sexual excitement
302.73 Psychosexual dysfunction with inhibited female orgasm
302.76 Psychosexual dysfunction with inhibited functional dyspareunia

SEE ALSO
• Vaginismus
• Dyspareunia

OTHER NOTES
• Women must feel safe in order to let go and lose some control to experience orgasm
• Performance anxiety makes males ejaculate prematurely, while it inhibits orgasm in women
• Simple lack of knowledge about anatomy and physiology of sex can lead to problems

ABBREVIATIONS N/A

REFERENCES
• Leiblum SR, Rosen RC: Principles and Practice of Sex Therapy: Update for the 1990's. New York, The Guilford Press, 1989
• Wincze JP, Carey MP: Sexual Dysfunction: A Guide for Assessment and Treatment. New York, The Guilford Press, 1991
• Bancroft J: Human Sexuality and Its Problems. 2nd Ed. New York, Churchill Livingstone, 1989
Illustrations: N/A
Internet references: http://www.5mcc.com

Author(s)
S. Shevaun Duiker, MD

Shock, circulatory

BASICS

DESCRIPTION Inadequate perfusion (oxygen supply) of tissues which results in organ dysfunction, cellular and organ damage and, if not corrected quickly, death of the patient. Classification of shock:
• Hypovolemic shock - cardiac output is severely reduced due to loss of intravascular volume which results in reduced return of venous blood to the heart. Most often caused by blood loss.
• Cardiogenic shock - cardiac output is severely reduced due to a loss of myocardial muscle function, valvular dysfunction or arrhythmia. Most often caused by large myocardial infarctions.
• Obstructive shock - cardiac output is severely reduced by vascular obstruction to venous return to the heart (vena cava syndrome), compression of the heart, (pericardial tamponade, tension pneumothorax) or outflow from the heart (aortic dissection, pulmonary embolism)
• Distributive shock - maldistribution of blood flow
• Venous pooling (most often due to spinal shock or drug overdose) behaves much like hypovolemic shock, cardiac output severely reduced because blood is pooled in peripheral veins rather than being returned to the heart
• High output or vasodilating shock (most often due to sepsis or septic like states such as toxic shock) is unique in that cardiac output is normal or elevated, but not distributed appropriately, resulting in over perfusion of some tissues and underperfusion (to the point of critical ischemia) of other tissues.
System(s) affected: Cardiovascular
Genetics: Unknown
Incidence/Prevalence in USA: N/A
Predominant age: All ages. Determined by underlying diseases causing shock. More frequent and less well tolerated in the elderly.
Predominant sex: Male = Female

SIGNS AND SYMPTOMS
• Underlying disease:
  ◊ Upper gastrointestinal (UGI) bleeding (ulcer pain, hematemesis, melena)
  ◊ Sepsis (fever, chills, dysuria and/or costovertebral angle [CVA] tenderness with urinary tract infection)
  ◊ Myocardial infarction (chest pain, diaphoresis, nausea, vomiting, S4 or S3 gallop, new heart murmur, rales due to pulmonary edema)
• Underperfusion of organ systems:
  ◊ Brain: confusion, anxiety, agitation, coma only if severe
  ◊ Kidney: oliguria
  ◊ Skin: peripheral cyanosis, sluggish capillary refill, mottling, coolness, may be overperfused (flushed) in high output (septic) shock
  ◊ GI: absence of bowel sounds

◊ Circulation: thready pulses, tachycardia, hypotension (mean arterial pressure < 60 torr or systolic pressure < 90 torr or blood pressure > 40 torr less than usual blood pressure in chronic hypertension), secondary cardiac ischemia (ST depression) or heart failure may occur due to underperfusion of the heart during shock. Jugular-venous distention (JVD), pulsus paradoxus in pericardial tamponade.

CAUSES
• Hypovolemic shock
  ◊ Blood loss due to trauma or gastrointestinal bleeding
  ◊ Third space loss of plasma volume (pancreatitis, bowel obstruction, infarction, anaphylaxis)
  ◊ Diarrhea (e.g., in cholera like states)
  ◊ Burns
• Cardiogenic shock
  ◊ Acute myocardial infarction (> 40% of LV mass)
  ◊ Arrhythmia (heart block, ventricular tachycardia, atrial fibrillation with rapid ventricular response, etc.)
  ◊ Acute valvular dysfunction (mitral valve due to papillary muscle rupture following inferior MI's or chordal rupture) aortic or mitral valve due to bacterial endocarditis
  ◊ Ventricular septal rupture following anterior/septal MI's
• Obstructive shock
  ◊ Pericardial tamponade
  ◊ Inferior/superior vena caval obstruction usually due to neoplasms
  ◊ Aortic dissection
  ◊ Massive pulmonary embolism
• Distributive shock
  ◊ Venous pooling is due to a loss of venous tone caused by loss of sympathetic nervous system activity due to acute spinal injury, general or spinal anesthesia or overdose of sedative drugs
  ◊ High output shock is due to sepsis, toxic shock or anaphylaxis (once plasma volume normalized)

RISK FACTORS   Included with Causes

DIAGNOSIS

DIFFERENTIAL DIAGNOSIS   N/A

LABORATORY
• Specific to shock
  ◊ Elevated lactate (> 2 mmol/L) indicates anaerobic metabolism due to underperfusion of tissues
  ◊ Reduced mixed venous P02 (< 28 mm Hg) (< 3.7 kPa) obtained from the pulmonary artery indicates vigorous extraction of oxygen from tissues due to underperfusion
• Underlying diseases responsible to shock
  ◊ ECG, CPK (serial)
  ◊ Chest x-ray
  ◊ Arterial blood gases
  ◊ Gram stain and culture of infected sites
  ◊ Blood cultures
  ◊ CBC (serial determination of Hgb/Hct in bleeding patients)

Drugs that may alter lab results: N/A
Disorders that may alter lab results: N/A

PATHOLOGICAL FINDINGS   N/A

SPECIAL TESTS
• Certain tests are essential to making correct and prompt diagnosis in order to dictate specific therapy of disease states producing shock. For example:
• Endoscopy/Radioisotope bleeding scans enable localization of ongoing bleeding which may direct surgical intervention. The endoscopist may intervene directly via the endoscope. (e.g., injection of sclerosants into varices or ulcers).
• Echocardiograms may detect and/or quantify pericardial effusions in shock due to pericardial tamponade. Pericardiocentesis can then be performed under echocardiographic guidance. Also useful for detection of valvular failure.
• Lung scans and/or pulmonary arteriography for the detection of massive pulmonary embolism
• Pulmonary artery (Swan-Ganz) catheterization for serial measurement of cardiac output, central venous, pulmonary arterial and pulmonary arterial occlusion pressures (left atrial pressure) and vascular resistance. Mixed venous blood gases can be drawn from the catheter. Indicated when the etiology of shock is uncertain, in cardiogenic and septic shock, or when initial therapy of shock fails to provide for rapid correction of perfusion failure.

IMAGING   See Special Tests

DIAGNOSTIC PROCEDURES
See Special Tests

TREATMENT

APPROPRIATE HEALTH CARE
• Emergency room or intensive or coronary care unit
• Continuous electrocardiographic monitoring with frequent assessment of blood pressure, respiratory status, and urine output

GENERAL MEASURES
• Therapy must proceed quickly before extensive damage to vital organs occur. Therapy is directed simultaneously to correct both the deficit in tissue perfusion and the underlying disease causing shock (see Associated conditions).
• Maintain SaO2 > 95% with supplemental oxygen. Intubate and mechanically ventilate patient if patient cannot be oxygenated with 100% oxygen or has markedly increased breathing effort (excessive oxygen cost of breathing).
• Maintain pH above 7.3 (but less than 7.5) to preserve vascular responsiveness to endogenous or exogenous catecholamines.

• Correct plasma volume deficits rapidly by volume expanders consisting of isotonic saline (.9Ns or Ringer's lactate) with or without colloid (albumin 5% or hydroxyethyl starch 6%)
• Packed red blood cell transfusion to correct or prevent anemia. HB maintained at or above 10 grams/dl.
• Administer coagulation factors (fresh frozen plasma, cryoprecipitate) and platelets if coagulopathy (prolonged PT, PTT or platelet count < 50,000) is present in a patient who is bleeding
• Tachyrrhythmias (other than sinus tachycardia) should be promptly corrected by electrocardioversion. Transvenous pacemakers should be placed to correct bradyrhythmias.
• Vasopressors (see Medications) to correct hypotension or low cardiac output due to myocardial failure or hypotension due to low vascular resistance
• End points of resuscitation: adequate blood pressure (> 60 mm Hg [8.0 kPa] mean or > 90 mm Hg [12.0 kPa] systolic or within 40 mm Hg [5.32 kPa] of patient's normal blood pressure). Patient is awake/alert, urine output adequate, heart rate < 100, warm skin with brisk capillary refill, bowel sounds present. Lactate < 2 mmol/L, mixed venous PO2 > 30 mm Hg.

SURGICAL MEASURES N/A

ACTIVITY None

DIET N/A

PATIENT EDUCATION N/A

MEDICATIONS

DRUG(S) OF CHOICE
• Dopamine, low dose, 1-4 µg/kg/min augments contractility and cardiac output (beta-1) and increases heart rate. This provides increased blood flow to kidneys and gut. Also acts directly on dopaminergic receptors in the renal vasculature to enhance renal blood flow.
• Dopamine > 4 µg/kg/min: augments contractility, and cardiac output (beta-1) and increased heart rate. Increases blood pressure by a combination of increased cardiac output and vasoconstriction (alpha).
• Norepinephrine 2-12 µg/min: augments blood pressure by increased vascular resistance (alpha). Reduced blood flow to splanchnic bed can be reversed by low dose dopamine.
• Phenylephrine 20-200 µg/min: see norepinephrine
• Dobutamine 5-10 µg/kg/min augments contractility and cardiac output (beta-1). Has both vasoconstrictive (alpha) and vasodilator (beta-2) properties. These effects have a minimal effect on systemic vasculature.
Contraindications: Refer to manufacturer's profile of each drug

Precautions:
• Myocardial oxygen consumption is increased by increased heart rate, afterload, and contractility
• Pressors can increase myocardial ischemia if present
• May precipitate or worsen tachyarrhythmias
• Should be used in lowest possible dose for as limited period of time as possible
Significant possible interactions: Refer to manufacturer's profile of each drug

ALTERNATIVE DRUGS N/A

FOLLOWUP

PATIENT MONITORING Careful monitoring of all life functions in intensive care

PREVENTION/AVOIDANCE Shock is best avoided by prompt recognition and treatment of underlying diseases which cause shock (e.g., early antibiotic therapy for infections)

POSSIBLE COMPLICATIONS
• Multiple organs may be damaged by underperfusion during shock
• Acute tubular necrosis
• Ischemic hepatitis
• Ischemic bowel
• Disseminated intravascular coagulopathy
• Adult respiratory distress syndrome (ARDS)
• Encephalopathy and/or cerebrovascular accident

EXPECTED COURSE/PROGNOSIS
• Mortality is determined by a complex interaction of primary disease causing shock, age, coexisting chronic disease and shock severity as marked by the number of acute organ system failures that follow shock
• Best outcome (> 90% survival) in young patient with transient shock due to trauma or gastrointestinal blood loss without chronic irreversible illnesses
• Poor outcome (> 90% mortality) in elderly patient with septic shock, underlying chronic liver disease, who develops acute renal failure, ARDS, and coagulopathy

MISCELLANEOUS

ASSOCIATED CONDITIONS
• Gastrointestinal blood loss: may require endoscopic or surgical intervention if bleeding doesn't spontaneously cease, e.g., electrocoagulation or injecting sclerosant for bleeding peptic ulcers, sclerotherapy in esophageal varices

• Sepsis: empiric antibiotic therapy, antibodies against gram negative antigens
• Cardiogenic shock: therapy should help reduce cardiac ischemia (oxygen, nitrates) and accomplish rapid reperfusion of injured, but potentially viable, myocardium (thrombolysis with fibrinolytic agents, balloon angioplasty of stenotic vessels or surgical bypass grafting) A balloon pump may temporize by providing improved coronary blood flow during and following diagnostic testing and revascularization therapy. If shock is due to acute failure of the mitral or aortic valve, surgical valve replacement may be lifesaving.
• Pulmonary embolism
• Cardiac tamponade

AGE-RELATED FACTORS
Pediatric: N/A
Geriatric: N/A
Others: N/A

PREGNANCY N/A

SYNONYMS N/A

ICD-9-CM
785.50 Shock, unspecified
785.51 Cardiogenic shock
785.59 Other shock (endotoxic, septic, hypovolemic)

SEE ALSO
• Anaphylaxis
• Cardiac tamponade
• Myocardial infarction
• Pulmonary embolism
• Peptic ulcer disease
• Sepsis

OTHER NOTES N/A

ABBREVIATIONS N/A

REFERENCES
• Parillo JE: Shock. In: Braunwald E, et al. Harrison's Principles of Internal Medicine. 12th Ed. New York, McGraw-Hill, Inc, 1991
• Schuster DP, Lefrah SS: Shock. In: Civetta JF, et al. Critical Care. Philadelphia, J.B. Lippincott Corp, 1988:891-908
Illustrations: N/A
Internet references: http://www.5mcc.com

Author(s)
Sheldon M. Traeger, MD

Sialadenitis

BASICS

DESCRIPTION Inflammation of the salivary glands from nonspecific bacterial infection or inflammation most often arises in the excretory duct. The parotid is the most commonly affected gland with invasion of bacteria from the oral cavity. Inflammation may also follow trauma, spread of infection from adjoining tissues, and via hematogenous routes during bacteremia. Inflammation may lead to stone formation (sialolithiasis) or an obstructed duct may lead to inflammation of the gland. Stones are more commonly associated with the submaxillary glands. Recurrent infections or other chronic inflammatory processes can lead to decreased gland function with resulting xerostomia.

System(s) affected: Skin/Exocrine, Gastrointestinal
Genetics: Unknown
Incidence/Prevalence in USA: N/A
Predominant age: N/A
Predominant sex: N/A

SIGNS AND SYMPTOMS
- Enlarged, painful salivary gland
- Purulent discharge from duct orifice
- Red, painful duct orifice
- Fever
- Xerostomia
- Decreased salivary secretion (aptyalism)

CAUSES
- Bacteria from the oral cavity are the most common infectious cause of sialadenitis.
- The causative agents of the following diseases may also infect a salivary gland to cause sialadenitis:
  ◊ Mumps
  ◊ Actinomycosis
  ◊ Tuberculosis
  ◊ Syphilis
  ◊ CMV
  ◊ Cat-scratch disease

RISK FACTORS
- Dehydration
- Fever
- Hypercalcemia

DIAGNOSIS

DIFFERENTIAL DIAGNOSIS
Decreased salivary secretion is associated with:
- Drugs:
  ◊ Tricyclic antidepressants (amitriptyline, etc.)
  ◊ Phenothiazines (chlorpromazine, fluphenazine, thioridazine, prochlorperazine, etc.)
  ◊ Anticholinergics
- Myxedema
- Plummer-Vinson disease
- Pernicious anemia
- Febrile diseases
- Neuropsychiatric disorders
- Mikulicz's disease (benign lymphoepithelial lesion)
Enlarged glands may be the result of a variety of neoplasms including:
- Pleomorphic adenoma
- Mucoepidermoid carcinoma
- Other tumor types can also occur very rarely (lipoma, neurofibroma, fibrosarcoma, melanoma, lymphocytoma, Hodgkin's, etc.)
Also, obesity results in what appears to be enlarged parotids, but the bilateral nature and non-progressive course should help differentiate this from malignant neoplasms.

LABORATORY N/A
Drugs that may alter lab results: N/A
Disorders that may alter lab results: N/A

PATHOLOGICAL FINDINGS
With chronic infection of the gland:
- Enlarged gland
- Ductal dilatation with retention of saliva
- Acinar atrophy or dilated and filled with mucus
- Purulent/seropurulent exudate within the duct
- Glandular replacement by fibrotic tissue
- Infiltration with leukocytes

SPECIAL TESTS N/A

IMAGING Radiographs may reveal a stone in sialolithiasis

DIAGNOSTIC PROCEDURES
- Digital manipulation of the duct may express pus from the ductal orifice

TREATMENT

APPROPRIATE HEALTH CARE
Outpatient

GENERAL MEASURES Heating pad and/or cool compresses may be comforting

SURGICAL MEASURES
- Superficial parotidectomy in patients with chronic non-specific sialadenitis. Complications include temporary (or permanent) facial nerve weakness, neuromas, but a reduction in symptoms can be expected.

ACTIVITY Unrestricted

DIET Avoid pain-producing sialagogues (lemon, etc.) during an acute episode

PATIENT EDUCATION N/A

MEDICATIONS

DRUG(S) OF CHOICE
• Antibiotics
  ◊ Penicillin V (Pen VK) 250-500mg QID
  ◊ Erythromycin 250mg QID
  ◊ Amoxicillin-clavulanate (Augmentin) 500mg TID
  ◊ Cefuroxime (Ceftin)
• Analgesic: codeine, hydrocodone, NSAIDs, etc
Contraindications: N/A
Precautions: N/A
Significant possible interactions: N/A

ALTERNATIVE DRUGS   N/A

FOLLOWUP

PATIENT MONITORING   N/A

PREVENTION/AVOIDANCE   N/A

POSSIBLE COMPLICATIONS
Occasional loss of salivary function

EXPECTED COURSE/PROGNOSIS
Complete recovery and good prognosis

MISCELLANEOUS

ASSOCIATED CONDITIONS
• Rheumatoid arthritis (Sjögren's syndrome)
• Sarcoidosis (Herrfordt's syndrome)

AGE-RELATED FACTORS
Pediatric: Rare in children
Geriatric: N/A
Others: N/A

PREGNANCY   N/A

SYNONYMS
• Sialadenosis

ICD-9-CM
527.2 sialadenitis

SEE ALSO
• Sjögren's syndrome
• Salivary gland calculi

OTHER NOTES   N/A

ABBREVIATIONS
CMV = cytomegalovirus

REFERENCES
• Cotran RS, et al, eds: Robbins Pathological Basis of Disease, 4th Ed. Philadelphia, W.B. Saunders Co., 1989
• Bhatty MA, Piggot RA, Soames JV, McLean NR. Chronic non-specific parotid sialadenitis. Br J Plast Surg 1998 Oct;51(7):517-21
Illustrations: N/A
Internet references: http://www.5mcc.com

Author(s)
Mark R. Dambro, MD, FAAFP

Silicosis

BASICS

DESCRIPTION Pneumoconiosis (fibrogenic) caused by inhaling silica dust (in the form of quartz, cristobalite, or tridymite)
• Chronic (classical) silicosis can be simple or complicated
• Chronic simple silicosis (sim sil) is asymptomatic, non-progressive once exposure ends, and consists solely of small round radiographic pulmonary opacities
• Chronic complicated silicosis (comp sil) has progressively worsening symptoms and enlarging pulmonary opacities, even after exposure ends.
• Subacute silicosis (sub sil) develops after 3-6 years of high exposure, and resembles chronic complicated silicosis
• Acute silicosis (ac sil) develops within a couple years of massive exposure and is clinically distinct from the other forms
System(s) affected: Pulmonary
Genetics: No known genetic pattern
Incidence/Prevalence in USA: Unknown
Predominant age: 40-75
Predominant sex: Male > Female

SIGNS AND SYMPTOMS
• Sim sil
  ◊ Asymptomatic
  ◊ Cough and mild dyspnea typically accompany, and are due to smoking or occupational bronchitis
• Comp sil; sub sil
  ◊ Chest tightness
  ◊ Cough
  ◊ Dyspnea
  ◊ Expectoration
  ◊ Signs and symptoms of right heart failure as cor pulmonale develops
• Ac sil
  ◊ Dry cough
  ◊ Fever
  ◊ Severe dyspnea

CAUSES
• Sim sil: 10-12 years of exposure to silica dust
• Comp sil: > 20 years of exposure
• Sub sil: 3-6 years of heavy exposure
• Ac sil: < 2 years of massive exposure

RISK FACTORS
• Industrial activities that involve cutting, polishing, or shearing rock, or involve the use of sand, including:
  ◊ Metal mining (copper, silver, gold, lead, hard coal)
  ◊ Foundries
  ◊ Pottery making
  ◊ Sandstone cutting
  ◊ Granite cutting

DIAGNOSIS

DIFFERENTIAL DIAGNOSIS
• Sim sil
  ◊ Sarcoidosis
  ◊ Radiographic egg shell calcifications also seen in sarcoidosis and Hodgkin's disease
• Comp sil, sub sil
  ◊ Coal worker's pneumoconiosis
  ◊ Consider especially when consolidations are rapidly progressive, unilateral, or cavitating - tuberculosis, neoplasia, fungal pneumonia
• Ac sil
  ◊ Alveolar proteinosis

LABORATORY
• Hypoxemia
• Hypercarbia
Drugs that may alter lab results: N/A
Disorders that may alter lab results: N/A

PATHOLOGICAL FINDINGS
• Lung
  ◊ Pleural adhesions
  ◊ Pleural thickening
  ◊ Gray-black subpleural nodules
  ◊ Blackened lung
  ◊ Leathery lung
  ◊ Concentric layers of dense connective tissue
  ◊ Cellular infiltrate
  ◊ Ischemic degeneration of central nodule
  ◊ Metachromatic silica particles

SPECIAL TESTS
• Pulmonary function testing is normal in simple silicosis. Other forms show decreased pulmonary compliance, decreased lung volumes, decreased diffusing capacity.
• International Labor Office (ILO) classification system for quantification of chest radiograph abnormalities.
• Yearly PPD

IMAGING
Chest x-ray:
• Sim sil
  ◊ Egg shell calcification in hilar and mediastinal lymph nodes
  ◊ Small round opacities, initially in upper lobes
• Comp sil, sub sil
  ◊ Pulmonary opacities > 1 cm
  ◊ Opacities form bilateral conglomerate shadows (progressive massive fibrosis)
  ◊ Opacities initially peripheral, later migrate towards hilum.
  ◊ Opacities may cavitate (rule out tuberculosis!)
CT:
• May be helpful in identifying nodules

DIAGNOSTIC PROCEDURES
• Bronchoscopy
• Detailed occupational history
• Open lung biopsy

TREATMENT

APPROPRIATE HEALTH CARE
Prevention - respiratory protective devices for unavoidable short-term exposure

GENERAL MEASURES
• No known effective treatment
• Postural drainage
• Mist inhalation
• Chest physical therapy
• Breathing exercises

SURGICAL MEASURES
• Lung transplantation
• Whole lung lavage remains investigational

ACTIVITY Maintain regular exercise program

DIET
• No special diet
• Increase fluid intake

PATIENT EDUCATION Printed patient information available from: American Lung Association, 1740 Broadway, New York, NY 10019, (212)315-8700

MEDICATIONS

DRUG(S) OF CHOICE
• None specific for silicosis
• Isoniazid, 300 mg/d for one year, if tuberculin skin test is positive
• Silicotuberculosis requires at least 3 anti-tuberculous drugs initially, including rifampin

Contraindications: Avoid sedatives and hypnotics

Precautions: Refer to manufacturer's literature

Significant possible interactions: Refer to manufacturer's literature

ALTERNATIVE DRUGS Antifibrinogenic agents remain investigational

FOLLOWUP

PATIENT MONITORING
• Monitor for heart failure and hypoxemia
• Treat intercurrent infections aggressively

PREVENTION/AVOIDANCE Avoid dust exposure; substitute other materials for silica

POSSIBLE COMPLICATIONS
• Progressive massive fibrosis
• Respiratory infection
• Pneumothorax
• Emphysema
• Cor pulmonale
• Right heart failure
• Mycobacterial infections
• Fungal infections

EXPECTED COURSE/PROGNOSIS
• Sim sil - remains asymptomatic and does not progress if exposure ends
• Comp sil; sub sil - progressive pulmonary fibrosis with cor pulmonale and right heart failure, even after exposure ends.

MISCELLANEOUS

ASSOCIATED CONDITIONS
• Tuberculosis
• Caplan's syndrome

AGE-RELATED FACTORS
Pediatric: Unusual
Geriatric: Symptoms and complications more severe
Others: N/A

PREGNANCY N/A

SYNONYMS N/A

ICD-9-CM 502 Silicosis

SEE ALSO
• Tuberculosis
• Chronic obstructive pulmonary disease & emphysema
• Pneumothorax
• Cor pulmonale

OTHER NOTES Silica - formula for calculating the threshold limit value (TLV) for respirable dust: TLV (threshold limit value) = (10 mg per cu meter/% SiO2) + 2

ABBREVIATIONS
Ac sil = Acute silicosis
Comp sil = Chronic complicated silicosis
Sim sil = Chronic simple silicosis
Sub sil = Subacute silicosis

REFERENCES
• Silicosis and Silicate Disease Committee. Diseases associated with exposure to silica and non-fibrous silicate materials. Arch Pathol Lab Med 1988;112:673
• Banks DE, et al: Strategies for the treatment of pneumoniosis. Occ Med 1993;8(1):205-232
Illustrations: N/A
Internet references: http://www.5mcc.com

Author(s)
Robert Dolin, MD

Sinusitis

BASICS

DESCRIPTION Acute sinusitis is a symptomatic inflammation of the paranasal sinuses of less than 8 weeks duration occuring as a result of impaired drainage and retained secretions. Allergies are not thought to play a major role in the pathogenesis of sinusitis.
System(s) affected: Pulmonary
Genetics: No known genetic pattern
Incidence/Prevalence in USA:
• 16% of US population annual diagnosis of sinusitis
• Fifth leading reason for antibiotic prescriptions in USA
• Approximately 5% of office visits for young adults
Predominant age: All ages
Predominant sex: Both sexes equally

SIGNS AND SYMPTOMS
• Symptoms predictive of acute infection:
  ◊ Preceding URI symptoms, particularly if seemed to be spontaneously resolving with acute return of symptoms ("double-sickening")
  ◊ History of colored nasal discharge
  ◊ Unilateral facial pain which is worse with bending forward or with cough or sneezing
  ◊ Maxillary toothache
  ◊ Poor response to antibiotics
  ◊ In young children, URI symptoms, clear or purulent nasal discharge and persistent cough, persisting > 10-days
• Other Associated Symptoms:
  ◊ Headache
  ◊ Retroorbital pain
  ◊ Otalgia
  ◊ Hyposomia
  ◊ Halitosis
  ◊ Chronic cough
• Symptoms indicating urgency:
  ◊ Orbital pain
  ◊ Visual disturbances, especially diplopia
  ◊ Periorbital swelling or erythema
  ◊ Facial swelling or erythema
• Predictive physical examination findings:
  ◊ Purulent rhinorrhea
  ◊ Abnormal transillumination
• Other associated signs
  ◊ Edematous nasal mucosa
  ◊ Nasal obstruction/polyps
• Signs indicating urgency or complications:
  ◊ Visual changes
  ◊ Abnormal extraocular movements
  ◊ Periorbital edema or erythema

CAUSES
• Infectious
  ◊ Bacteria (Strep. pneumoniae, H. influenzae, Branhamella [Moraxella] catarrhalis)
  ◊ Viral
  ◊ Fungal (Aspirgillus most common)

RISK FACTORS
• Viral upper respiratory infection
• Age < 10 or > 50
• Anatomical abnormalities
  ◊ Tonsillar and adenoid hypertrophy
  ◊ Deviated septum
  ◊ Nasal polyps
  ◊ Cleft palate
• Nasotracheal intubation
• Barotrauma
• Dental infections and procedures
• Trauma
• Immunodeficiency & HIV disease

DIAGNOSIS

DIFFERENTIAL DIAGNOSIS
• Viral URI
• Dental disease
• Nasal foreign body
• Migraine, cluster or tension headache
• Temporal arteritis
• TMJ disorders
• Wegener's granulomatosis

LABORATORY
• Sedimentation rate > 10 mm/hr
• C-reactive protein greater than 10 mg/L
Drugs that may alter lab results: N/A
Disorders that may alter lab results: N/A

PATHOLOGICAL FINDINGS
• Inflammation
• Edema
• Thickened mucosa
• Impaired ciliary function
• Inflammatory metaplasia to ciliated columnar cells
• Relative acidosis and hypoxia within sinuses

SPECIAL TESTS
• Nasolaryngoscopy
• Maxillary sinuscopy

IMAGING
• Plain sinus radiographs (single Waters view may be sufficient)
  ◊ May be helpful when only 2-3 associated signs and symptoms are present
  ◊ Look for air-fluid levels, sinus opacity, mucosal thickening (> 6-mm in children or >8 mm in adults)
  ◊ Negative predictive value about 90%; Positive predictive value about 80% or higher
• Limited coronal CT of sinuses
  ◊ Most useful in evaluation of chronic sinusitis (3-4 annual episodes or failure to respond to medical therapy)

DIAGNOSTIC PROCEDURES
• History and physical exam sufficient for majority of cases of acute disease; 4 or more associated symptoms and signs listed above has high likelihood of diagnostic accuracy.
• Maxillary antrum aspiration and culture gold standard, but generally performed by ENT only in selected cases

TREATMENT

APPROPRIATE HEALTH CARE
• Outpatient
• Hospitalization for complications (meningitis, abscess)

GENERAL MEASURES
• Adequate hydration (8-10 glasses water daily)
• Steam inhalation 20-30 minutes tid or use of facial steamer
• Saline irrigation or saline nose drops
• Sleep with head of bed elevated
• Avoid exposure to cigarette/cigar/pipe smoke, fumes

SURGICAL MEASURES
• If medical therapy fails, irrigation of sinuses can be performed to wash out the inspissated material
• Functional endoscopic sinus surgery less invasive and associated with fewer adverse effects than the traditional Caldwell-Luc procedure
• Absolute surgical indications:
  ◊ Massive nasal polyposis
  ◊ Acute complications: subperiosteal or orbital abscess, frontal soft tissue spread of infection)
  ◊ Mucocele or mycopyocele
  ◊ Invasive or allergic fungal sinusitis
  ◊ Suspected obstructing tumor
  ◊ CSF rhinorrhea

ACTIVITY
• Adequate rest, otherwise no restrictions

DIET
• No special diet

PATIENT EDUCATION
• Call back if no significant improvement in symptoms within one week, or if symptoms should worsen, progression of symptoms such as headache, neck stiffness, visual changes, nausea or vomiting
• Educate patient on potential major side effects of selected medications
• For patient education materials favorably reviewed on this topic, contact:
  ◊ American College of Allergy, Asthma & Immunology, 85 West Algonquin Road, Suite 550, Arlington Heights, IL 60005, 1-847-427-1200
  ◊ Smoots E. American Family Physician 1998; 58(5):1805-6 (available on Am Fam Phys Web site)

Sinusitis

MEDICATIONS

DRUG(S) OF CHOICE
• Antibiotics. Several recent randomized controlled trials and meta-analyses suggest in vast majority of cases of sinusitis or those with mild disease, antibiotics may have no significant effect. First-line therapy for moderate or severe disease: amoxicillin or trimethoprim-sulfamethoxazole; a macrolide can be use if the patient is allergic to both penicillin or sulfa-moieties.
  ◊ Amoxicillin 250-500 mg tid for 10-days in adults; 20-40 mg/kg/d in children
  ◊ Trimethoprim-sulfamethoxazole (SMX-TMP) double-strength bid for 10 days; 8 mg TMP/kg/day in children
  ◊ Azithromycin 500 mg 1st day, then 250 mg daily for 4 days or clarithromycin 500 mg bid for 10 days
  ◊ For partial response (some resolution of symptoms), if used 250 mg of amoxicillin, increase dose to 500 mg and treat for additional 10-14 days; TMP-SMX double-strength tab bid for additional 10-14 days
  ◊ For treatment failure (no resolution of symptoms), if first used amoxicillin, now use TMP as above for 10-14 days; if first used TMP-SMX, use amoxicillin-clavulanate (Augmentin) 875-mg bid in adults or 45 mg/kg/d divided bid in children for 10-14 days; if allergic to both amoxicillin/TMP-SMX, azithromycin or clarithromycin can be used as above.
  ◊ Lack of response to three weeks of antibiotics, consider: Waters view film, limited coronal CT scan or ENT referral.
• Decongestants. Useful for first 3-5 days
  ◊ Pseudoephedrine HCL 60 mg q 4-6 hours, not to exceed 4 doses in 24 hours (avoid or monitor closely in patients with hypertension)
  ◊ Phenylephrine 2-3 sprays in each nostril q 4-6 hours; for 2-3 days
  ◊ Oxymetazoline (Afrin)
• Analgesics: acetaminophen, aspirin, NSAIDS, acetaminophen-codeine
Contraindications:
• Refer to manufacturer's literature for drug contraindications
Precautions:
• Decongestants can exacerbate hypertension
• Prolonged use of topical decongestants (> 4-days) may precipitate rhinitis medicamentosa
• Major side effect of sulfonamides is Steven-Johnson's syndrome: inform patients to report any mucous membrane ulcerations
Significant possible interactions:
• Warfarin (Coumadin): Increased effect of warfarin with TMP-SMX resulting in marked increase in INR and PT. Similar effect can also be seen with use of macrolides.

ALTERNATIVE DRUGS
• Causal role of allergy controversial; some patients may report benefits from use of antihistamine agents or nasal steroids [fluticasone (Flonase), beclomethasone (Beconase AQ, Vancenase AQ)] with underlying asthma or allergies; use established if underlying history of asthma

• Antihistamines
  ◊ Loratadine (Claritin) 10 mg/day for all patients over age 6
  ◊ Fexofenadine (Allegra) 60 mg bid in adults
  ◊ Chlorpheniramine (Chlor-Trimeton) 0.35 mg/kg/day divided q6h or 8 mg tid in adults
• Alternative antibiotics include ceftibuten (Cedax) 400 mg/d for adults or 9mg/kg/d for children, cefuroxime 250 mg bid in adults or 30mg/kg/d in children divided bid; levofloxacin 500 mg/d in adults-DO NOT USE IN CHILDREN

FOLLOWUP

PATIENT MONITORING
• Return if no improvement after completion of first course of antibiotics
• Report skin rash during use of antibiotics

PREVENTION/AVOIDANCE
• No documented evidence for prevention measures

POSSIBLE COMPLICATIONS
• Brain abscess
• Cavernous sinus thrombosis
• Meningitis
• Osteomyelitis
• Orbital cellulitis
• Subdural empyema

EXPECTED COURSE/PROGNOSIS
• Alleviation of symptoms within 72 hours with complete resolution within 10 days

MISCELLANEOUS

ASSOCIATED CONDITIONS
• Allergic Rhinitis
• Asthma
• Bronchitis
• Otitis Media
• Pharyngitis

AGE-RELATED FACTORS
Pediatric:
• Average 6-8 colds per year; more frequent may indicate or place at risk for sinusitis
• Incidence of both acute and chronic sinusitis increases in the latter part of childhood
• May be more prevalent in children who have had tonsils and adenoids removed
• Chronic sinusitis indicates a need to search for underlying cause, eg., nasal deformities, or infected and hypertrophied adenoids
Geriatric:
• Incidence increases up to age 75 and then decreases
• More difficult to heal when it occurs in this age group
Others: N/A

PREGNANCY
• TMP-SMX carries labeling of Category B and during term Category D; can be used during lactation except for premature infants, those with hyperbilirunbinemia and those with G-6-PD deficiency; avoid in children < 2, those with severe asthma or allergies; hemolytic anemia may occur in patients with G-6-PD deficiency
• Azithromycin labeled as Category B; clarithromycin listed as Category C
• Penicillins listed as Category B; they are excreted in low concentrations into breast milk and can cause symptoms

SYNONYMS Rhinosinusitis

ICD-9-CM
473.9 Sinusitis (chronic)
473.0 Chronic maxillary sinusitis
461.9 Sinusitis (acute)
461.2 Ethmoidal
461.1 Frontal
461.0 Maxillary
461.3 Sphenoidal
461.8 Other acute sinusitis (pansinusitis)
117.9 Sinusitis (fungal)

SEE ALSO
• Asthma
• Common cold
• Rhinitis, allergic
• Temporomandibular joint (TMJ) syndrome
• Wegener's granulomatosis

OTHER NOTES N/A

ABBREVIATIONS
CSF = cerebrospinal fluid
TMP-SMX = trimethoprim-sulfamethoxazole
URI = upper respiratory infection

REFERENCES
• Osguthorpe JD and Hadley JA. Rhinosinusitis: Current concepts in evaluation and management. Med Clin N Am 1999;83(1):27-41
• Fagnan LF. Acute sinusitis: a cost-effective approach to diagnosis and treatment. Am Fam Phys 1998; 58(8):1795-1802
• Slack R and Bates G. Functional Endoscopic Sinus Surgery. Am Fam Phys 1998; 58(3):707-718
• Lindboek M, Hjortdahl P, Johnsen U. Use of symptoms, signs, and blood tests to diagnose acute sinusitis infections in primary care: comparison with computed tomography. Family Practice 1996; 28:183-8.
• Hansen JG, Schmidt H, Rosborg J, Lund E. Predicting acute maxillary sinusitis in a general practice population. BMJ 1995;311:233-6
• Williams JW, Simel DL, Roberts L, Samsa GP. Does this patient have sinusitis? Clinical evaluation for sinusitis: making the diagnosis by history and physical examination. Ann Int Med 1992;117:705-710
Illustrations: N/A
Internet references: http://www.5mcc.com

Author(s)
A. Peter Catinella, MD

Sleep apnea, obstructive

BASICS

DESCRIPTION Repetitive episodes of upper airway occlusion during sleep, often with oxygen desaturation. Nearly always associated with snoring. Apneas often terminate with a snort or gasp. Repetitive apneas produce sleep disruption, leading to excessive daytime sleepiness (EDS). Usual course is chronic.
System(s) affected: Pulmonary, Nervous
Genetics: Hereditary factors unknown. Familial patterns sometimes seen.
Incidence/Prevalence in USA: 4% of middle-age and older males; 2% middle-age and older females
Predominant age: Middle-age
Predominant sex: Males > Females

SIGNS AND SYMPTOMS
• Cardinal symptom is excessive daytime sleepiness (EDS)
• Loud snoring
• Complaints of disrupted sleep
• Repetitive awakenings with transient sensation of shortness of breath or for unclear reasons
• Tired and unrefreshed upon A.M. awakening
• Witnessed apneas at night
• Complaints of poor concentration, memory problems, irritability
• Morning headaches
• Short-tempered
• Decreased libido is also common
• Depression
• Systemic and pulmonary hypertension

CAUSES Upper airway narrowing may be due to obesity, enlarged tonsils or uvula, low soft palate, redundant tissue in soft palate or tonsillar pillars, large or posteriorly located tongue or craniofacial abnormalities. Anatomical narrowing superimposed upon a coexistent abnormality of neurological control of upper airway muscle tone or ventilatory control during sleep.

RISK FACTORS
• Obesity
• Nasal obstruction (due to polyps, rhinitis or deviated septum)
• Hypothyroidism
• Macroglossia
• Micrognathia (retrognathia)
• Acromegaly
• Persons with hypertension, cardiovascular or arteriovascular disease or alveolar hypoventilation have a much higher risk of obstructive sleep apnea (OSA)

DIAGNOSIS

DIFFERENTIAL DIAGNOSIS
• Other causes of EDS such as narcolepsy, idiopathic daytime hypersomnolence, inadequate sleep, depressive episodes with EDS, periodic limb movements of sleep
• Respiratory disorders with nocturnal awakenings such as asthma, COPD, CHF
• Central sleep apnea may mimic OSA
• Sudden nocturnal awakenings due to panic attacks
• Sleep-related choking or laryngospasm
• Gastroesophageal reflux may also present with similar symptoms
• Sleep associated seizures (temporal lobe epilepsy)

LABORATORY
• Polycythemia (occasional) reflects the degree of nocturnal hypoxemia due to OSA
• Thyroid function should be evaluated to rule out concomitant hypothyroidism
• Daytime hypercapnia occasionally seen
Drugs that may alter lab results: Benzodiazepines or other sedatives can accentuate the severity of apnea seen on sleep study
Disorders that may alter lab results: N/A

PATHOLOGICAL FINDINGS
• Anatomically small upper airway common
• CNS abnormalities rare

SPECIAL TESTS
• Echocardiography may demonstrate right and/or left ventricular enlargement or pulmonary hypertension
• Polysomnogram (nighttime sleep study) including O2 saturation, CO2
• Multiple sleep latency testing (MSLT) provides an objective measurement of daytime sleepiness

IMAGING
• Cephalometric measurements from lateral head and neck x-rays are occasionally useful if surgery is contemplated
• MRI, CT scans or fiberoptic evaluation of upper airway occasionally helpful

DIAGNOSTIC PROCEDURES
• Nighttime sleep study (polysomnogram)
  ◊ Shows repetitive episodes of cessation or marked reduction in airflow despite continued respiratory efforts
  ◊ These apneic episodes must last at least 10 seconds and occur 10-15 times per hour to be considered clinically significant
  ◊ Polysomnogram demonstrates severity of hypoxemia, sleep disruption and cardiac arrhythmias associated with OSA and elevated end tidal CO2

TREATMENT

APPROPRIATE HEALTH CARE
Outpatient for treatment or sleep study; inpatient for surgery

GENERAL MEASURES
• For patients with significant EDS and 15-20 apneas per hour or more, CPAP is probably the best treatment
• If OSA present only when supine - keep patient off the back (e.g., tennis ball sewn on nightshirt or fanny-pack with tennis balls worn at back)
• Mild to moderate OSA - surgery (tonsillectomy or uvulopalatopharyngoplasty [UPPP]), dental appliances or nasal continuous positive airway pressure (CPAP)
• Moderate to severe OSA - CPAP or BiPAP (biphasic positive airway pressure) is the standard therapy
• Avoid driving if EDS significant
• No alcohol within 6 hours of bedtime
• Avoid sedatives and sleeping pills

SURGICAL MEASURES
Severe OSA that is not controllable with nasal CPAP or UPPP - tracheostomy or craniofacial surgery (mandibular advancement)

ACTIVITY
Significantly sleepy patients should not drive motor vehicle or operate equipment with risk for injury until treated

DIET
Obese patients must lose weight. All patients must avoid weight gain and alcohol.

PATIENT EDUCATION
• Stress the fact that obesity can be the cause of OSA and weight loss may "cure" the condition
• Necessity to avoid alcohol and sedatives
• Stress the dangers of driving while suffering EDS

MEDICATIONS

DRUG(S) OF CHOICE Protriptyline 10-30 mg/d or fluoxetine 20-60 mg can occasionally be useful adjunct in the management of OSA (especially OSA in REM sleep) and to improve EDS
Contraindications: None
Precautions: May cause or exacerbate narrow angle glaucoma or urinary retention. Use with caution in patients with supraventricular tachycardia.
Significant possible interactions: See manufacturer's profile of each drug

ALTERNATIVE DRUGS
• Medroxyprogesterone is helpful in Pickwickian patients with both daytime alveolar hypoventilation and OSA
• Acetazolamide (Diamox) may increase central respiratory drive by acidifying blood/CSF. Used in central sleep apnea only.

FOLLOWUP

PATIENT MONITORING Physician followup improves compliance with CPAP therapy. Observe for return of snoring, EDS, or sleep disruption which may indicate inadequate control of apneas.

PREVENTION/AVOIDANCE See Patient Education

POSSIBLE COMPLICATIONS
• Untreated OSA can be associated with development of pulmonary hypertension, ventricular arrhythmias, cor pulmonale, CHF
• Significant morbidity and mortality due to accidents caused by EDS and inattentiveness
• Acute blood pressure elevations

EXPECTED COURSE/PROGNOSIS
• With appropriate control of apneas, EDS dramatically improves quickly
• All therapeutic measures other than surgery and aggressive weight loss in obese patients are methods of apnea control, rather than cure. Lifelong compliance with weight loss or nasal CPAP are necessary for therapy of OSA.
• Untreated, OSA appears to progress in severity
• Death due to OSA usually secondary to arrhythmias, cardiac ischemia or hypertensive complications, or motor vehicle accidents

MISCELLANEOUS

ASSOCIATED CONDITIONS
• Hypertension
• Arteriosclerotic vascular disease
• Coronary arterial disease
• Diabetes
• Obesity
• Nasal obstructive problems
• Acromegaly
• Hypothyroidism

AGE-RELATED FACTORS
Pediatric:
• OSA not as common in pediatric age group. If present, often due to tonsillar enlargement, craniofacial abnormalities. Response to tonsillectomy often good.
• Seen commonly in children with neuromuscular diseases, such as cerebral palsy, spinal muscular atrophy
Geriatric: OSA appears to increase in frequency after middle age and after the menopause in women. Often coexists with other health problems in the elderly.
Others: N/A

PREGNANCY Rare

SYNONYMS
• Pickwickian syndrome
• Sleep apnea syndrome
• Nocturnal upper airway occlusion

ICD-9-CM 306.1 Psychogenic apnea

OTHER NOTES OSA rare in premenopausal women unless there is coexistent morbid obesity or neurologic/craniofacial abnormalities

SEE ALSO N/A

OTHER NOTES N/A

ABBREVIATIONS
• CPAP = continuous positive airway pressure
• BiPAP = bilevel positive airway pressure
• UPPP = uvulopalatopharyngoplasty
• EDS = excessive daytime sleepiness
• OSA = obstructive sleep apnea

REFERENCES
• Kryger MH: Principles and Practice of Sleep Medicine. Philadelphia, W.B. Saunders Co., 1989
• Thorpy MJ: Handbook of Sleep Disorders. New York, Marcel Dekker Inc., 1990
Illustrations: N/A
Internet references: http://www.5mcc.com

Author(s)
Mary E. Klink, MD

Snake envenomations: Crotalidae

BASICS

DESCRIPTION Symptom complex occurring following human envenomation by a snake of the family Crotalidae (pit vipers)
• These include those of the genus Crotalus (rattlesnakes), Agkistrodon (moccasins) and Sistrurus (pygmy rattlesnakes). Occurs most commonly in southeastern and southwestern US.
• These snakes characteristically have triangular-shaped heads, eyes with elliptical pupils, and small heat-sensing facial pits located between the nostril and the eye
System(s) affected: Cardiovascular, Skin/Exocrine, Nervous, Hemic/Lymphatic/Immunologic
Genetics: N/A
Incidence/Prevalence in USA: 3.2/100,000. 8,000 bites/year (20-25% of bites do not result in envenomation)
Predominant age: 19-30 years
Predominant sex: Male > Female

SIGNS AND SYMPTOMS
• These vary by species; prevalence as stated refers to family as whole
• Fang marks (may be two or only one) (>90%)
• Pain out of proportion to puncture wound (>50%)
• Edema of site, progressing proximally up extremity (>50%)
• Weakness, dizziness (>50%)
• Numbness/tingling in extremity, in mouth, tongue (>50%)
• Ecchymosis of skin, vesiculations around bite (>50%)
• Tachycardia (>50%)
• Nausea/vomiting (<50%)
• Hypo/Hypertension (<50%)
• Muscle fasciculations (<50%)
• Mental status changes including coma (<25%)
• Elevated creatine kinase (CK)

CAUSES Pit viper venom is a complex mixture which contains cytotoxins, hemotoxins, neurotoxins, and cardiotoxins

RISK FACTORS
• Risk taking behaviors
• Acute ethanol intoxication or intoxication with other drugs which impair judgment

DIAGNOSIS

DIFFERENTIAL DIAGNOSIS Bite of non-venomous snake, bite of venomous species other than from Crotalidae family

LABORATORY
• CBC (Hgb/Hct decreased in < 50%)
• PT/PTT (prolonged in > 50%)
• Fibrinogen (decreased in < 50%), fibrin degradation products (increased in < 50%)
• Urinalysis - glycosuria (< 50%), proteinuria (< 25%), hematuria (< 25%)
• Decrease in blood platelets (< 50%)
• Type and crossmatch "to hold" in severe envenomations
• Electrolytes, blood urea nitrogen, creatinine
• Creatine kinase in severe envenomations
• Serum ethanol level if suspicious
Drugs that may alter lab results:
Anticoagulants
Disorders that may alter lab results: N/A

PATHOLOGICAL FINDINGS N/A

SPECIAL TESTS N/A

IMAGING N/A

DIAGNOSTIC PROCEDURES If suspicious of developing compartment syndrome, measure compartment pressures (rarely needed)

TREATMENT

APPROPRIATE HEALTH CARE
Patients with true envenomations and resulting signs/symptoms need emergency department evaluation with admission if necessary

GENERAL MEASURES
• Support vital signs
• Reassurance
• Remove rings and constrictive items proximal to site of envenomation
• Place affected injured part at level of heart
• Evaluate all pre-hospital care. If tourniquet has been placed in pre-hospital setting, sudden removal could "bolus" patient with venom.
• Obtain toxicology consultation by contacting American Association of Poison Centers (AAPCC) Regional Poison Information Center for your area
• Level 1:
  ◊ If local signs of edema are confined to area of bite without any other symptom of envenomation, place intravenous line of crystalloid at maintenance rates (if no history of renal or heart disease requiring fluid restriction) and draw laboratory studies
  ◊ Place reference marks for measuring circumference of extremity at 10 cm and 20 cm proximal to site of envenomation
  ◊ Measure every 15 minutes and trace leading edge of swelling
  ◊ Give tetanus toxoid
  ◊ Pain relief with opiate or acetaminophen (avoid aspirin)
  ◊ Repeat laboratory studies in six hours. If all remain normal and swelling does not progress, observe 8-12 hours then follow as outpatient.
  ◊ If swelling progresses or systemic signs and symptoms appear will need admission and further therapy (progresses to Level 2)
• Level 2:
  ◊ If edema, vesiculations, erythema progress beyond the immediate bite area and there are associated systemic signs/symptoms or laboratory abnormalities (as above), all therapy as in Level 1 above plus intravenous antivenom
  ◊ Intensive care monitoring may be necessary in most institutions
  ◊ Repeat laboratory evaluations every 6 hours initially until stable, then less frequently
  ◊ Continue to monitor vital signs and circumference of affected part

SURGICAL MEASURES N/A

ACTIVITY Bedrest with extremity elevated to level of atria

DIET Nothing by mouth initially

PATIENT EDUCATION Snake bite prevention and first aid

MEDICATIONS

DRUG(S) OF CHOICE
• Polyvalent Crotalidae antivenin
◊ First administer skin test according to product brochure. If negative, prepare five vials of antivenin in 250 mL normal saline IV fluid.
◊ Begin infusion at 3-5 mL/hr and, if no systemic reaction occurs, increase until a rate of 180-240 mL/hr is achieved (one vial every 15-20 minutes)
◊ Give by continuous infusion, not IV push
◊ If signs/symptoms continue to progress rapidly following the first 5 vials, repeat dose of 5 vials. Severe envenomations may require up to 30 vials.

Contraindications:
• History of allergy to horse serum product
• If skin test positive, and antivenin is necessary to save life or limb, contact Poison Information Center. Pretreatment with antihistamines, steroids, etc., in ICU setting may make antivenin administration possible.

Precautions:
• Have equipment and medications readily at hand to treat anaphylaxis
• Avoid aspirin or other anticoagulants
Significant possible interactions: N/A

ALTERNATIVE DRUGS
• Blood products only necessary for coagulopathies with clinical bleeding, not for treatment of laboratory abnormalities
• Steroid use is controversial.

FOLLOWUP

PATIENT MONITORING
• First return visit within 48 hours, then as clinically indicated
• Physical therapy referral should be made early for optimal outpatient intervention

PREVENTION/AVOIDANCE
• Use of preventive measures if handling snakes
• In snake-infested areas
◊ Wear protective shoes and clothing when walking
◊ Do not insert hands or feet into cracks or crevices or hollow logs
◊ Carry a flashlight if walking at night

POSSIBLE COMPLICATIONS
• Serum sickness from antivenom therapy (perhaps in > 50%)
• Local wound infection

EXPECTED COURSE/PROGNOSIS   If properly treated, mortality is very rare. Morbidity rare.

MISCELLANEOUS

ASSOCIATED CONDITIONS   Underlying health of patient

AGE-RELATED FACTORS
Pediatric: Course may be more severe
Geriatric: Course may be more severe
Others: N/A

PREGNANCY   N/A

SYNONYMS
• Snakebite
• Venomous snakebite
• Pit viper snake bite

ICD-9-CM   989.5 Venomous snake bite

SEE ALSO   Snake envenomations: Elapidae

OTHER NOTES   N/A

ABBREVIATIONS   N/A

REFERENCES
• Ellenhorn MJ, Barceloux DG: Medical Toxicology: Diagnosis and Treatment of Human Poisoning. New York, Elsevier 1988;1113-1126
• Russell FE: Snake Venom Poisoning. Philadelphia, J.B. Lippincott, 1980
• Kurecki BA, Brownlee HJ: Venomous snakebites in the United States. J Fam Prac 1987;25(4):386-392
Illustrations: N/A
Internet references: http://www.5mcc.com

Author(s)
Gregory G. Gaar, MD, FAAP, FACEP

Snake envenomations: Elapidae

BASICS

DESCRIPTION Symptom complex occurring following human envenomation by a snake of the family Elapidae
• In the US these include the genera Micrurus and Micruroides, commonly called "Coral Snakes." The Sonoran or Arizona coral snake is found mainly in Arizona (Micruroides euryxanthus), the Texas coral snake (Micrurus fulvius tenere) in Texas, Arkansas, and Louisiana, and the eastern coral snake (Micrurus fulvius fulvius) throughout the Southeastern US.
• The snakes have a characteristic rounded head with round pupils. Coloration is important in that in the U.S. broad rings of red and black are separated by narrow rings of yellow. ("Red on yellow, kill a fellow; red on black, venom lack.")
• Unlike Crotalidae envenomations, local signs and symptoms are mild in envenomation of Elapidae, even those which prove to be severe envenomations. Neurologic symptoms may be delayed; they have been reported to develop up to 12 or more hours after the envenomation.
System(s) affected: Nervous, Skin/Exocrine
Genetics: N/A
Incidence/Prevalence in USA: Unknown
Predominant age: 19-30 years
Predominant sex: Male > Female

SIGNS AND SYMPTOMS
• Fang marks; may be shallow or appear as scratch (> 75%)
• Local swelling (<50%)
• Numbness/change in sensation (< 50%)
• Nausea/vomiting (< 50%)
• Weakness (< 25%)
• Dizziness (< 15%)
• Diplopia (< 15%)
• Muscle fasciculations (< 15%)

CAUSES Venom is primarily a neurotoxin. Little or no cytotoxin to cause local tissue reaction.

RISK FACTORS Coral snakes are nocturnal and timid. Therefore they rarely bite humans. They must be deliberately provoked to bite.

DIAGNOSIS

DIFFERENTIAL DIAGNOSIS
• Bite of other venomous snake (Crotalidae) without envenomation ("dry bite")
• Bite of a non-venomous snake

LABORATORY
• Creatine kinase (CPK) often elevated
• Blood ethanol level often elevated
• Laboratory not diagnostic
Drugs that may alter lab results: N/A
Disorders that may alter lab results: N/A

PATHOLOGICAL FINDINGS N/A

SPECIAL TESTS None

IMAGING N/A

DIAGNOSTIC PROCEDURES N/A

TREATMENT

APPROPRIATE HEALTH CARE All patients with suspected coral snake envenomation need Emergency Department evaluation

GENERAL MEASURES
• All patients who have (1) confirmed bite by a snake identified as a coral snake, (2) history of the snake's having chewed on the person, and, (3) visible fang marks which pierce the epidermis, should be admitted to hospital for intensive care monitoring
• In this group of patients, perform a skin test for horse serum sensitivity. If negative, antivenom to Micrurus fulvius should be given early, even if there are no neurologic signs or symptoms present.
• If skin test is positive, and neurological symptoms are rapidly progressing, admission to ICU is indicated
• Pretreatment with IV diphenhydramine, steroids, and other antihistamines may allow for infusion of antivenom, although it is not clear from the literature if antivenom should be administered in light of a positive skin test. In this instance, obtain toxicology consultation from the American Association of Poison Control Centers (AAPCC) certified Poison Information Center for your area.
• Support vital signs, intubation may be necessary if respiratory compromise ensues
• Good supportive care with cardiac, respiratory, neurological monitoring
• Reassurance
• Immobilize extremity and keep at level of atria
• Contact AAPCC Regional Center for your area

SURGICAL MEASURES N/A

ACTIVITY Bedrest initially. May need physical therapy in severe cases of envenomation.

DIET Nothing by mouth initially

PATIENT EDUCATION N/A

MEDICATIONS

DRUG(S) OF CHOICE
• There is no antivenom available for Micruroides euryxanthus
• Tetanus booster if necessary
• Antivenom to the North American coral snake (Micrurus fulvius antivenin)
◊ Is available commercially. It is a horse serum product and is effective only for the envenomation of the Texas and eastern coral snakes (Micrurus fulvius tenere and Micrurus fulvius fulvius).
◊ If patients meet the criteria above (see General Measures), skin test should be performed according to directions taken from package insert. If negative, 4-6 vials of the antivenom should be reconstituted and diluted into 250 mL of normal saline. Begin infusion at 3-5 mL/hr and, if no systemic reaction occurs, increase until a rate of 1 diluted vial is being given every thirty minutes.
◊ Envenomations with more severe sequelae or prolonged sequelae may require larger doses of antivenom. Unfortunately it is impossible to specify dosage more specifically.
Contraindications: History of allergy to horse serum
Precautions: Have equipment and medications readily at hand to treat anaphylaxis
Significant possible interactions: N/A

ALTERNATIVE DRUGS Steroid use is controversial.

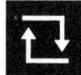

FOLLOWUP

PATIENT MONITORING First return visit within 48 hours, then as clinically indicated

PREVENTION/AVOIDANCE
• Use of preventive measures if handling snakes
• In snake-infested areas:
◊ Wear protective shoes and clothing when walking
◊ Do not insert hands or feet into cracks or crevices or hollow logs
◊ Carry a flashlight if walking at night

POSSIBLE COMPLICATIONS
• Serum sickness from antivenom therapy (perhaps in 10% or more)
• Local wound infection
• Aspiration pneumonia

EXPECTED COURSE/PROGNOSIS
• Neurologic deterioration may progress despite antivenom administration. Complete paralysis can occur.
• Early, elective intubation during progression of paralysis may help to prevent aspiration pneumonia
• Discharge should not occur until the patient has made neurologic recovery to the point that there is no concern of respiratory failure
• Muscle strength may not return to normal for 4-6 weeks
• Long-term morbidity rare
• Mortality does occur even with antivenom therapy

MISCELLANEOUS

ASSOCIATED CONDITIONS N/A

AGE-RELATED FACTORS
Pediatric: Not well described
Geriatric: Morbidity and danger of mortality is greater
Others: N/A

PREGNANCY N/A

SYNONYMS
• Neurotoxic snake bite
• Snakebite

ICD-9-CM 989.5 Venomous snake bite

SEE ALSO Snake envenomations: Crotalidae

OTHER NOTES N/A

ABBREVIATIONS N/A

REFERENCES
• Kitchens CS, Van Mierop LHS: Envenomation by the eastern coral snake (Micrurus fulvius fulvius). JAMA 1987;258(12):1615-1618
• Russell FE: Snake Venom Poisoning. Philadelphia, J.B. Lippincott, 1980
• Ellenhorn MJ, Barceloux DG: Medical Toxicology: Diagnosis and Treatment of Human Poisoning. New York, Elsevier, 1988:1127-1128
Illustrations: N/A
Internet references: http://www.5mcc.com

Author(s)
Gregory G. Gaar, MD, FAAP, FACEP

Sporotrichosis

BASICS

DESCRIPTION Subacute or chronic fungal infection occurring in 4 forms: cutaneous or lymphocutaneous, pulmonary, osteo-articular, or disseminated; and rarely musculoskeletal (joint and tendon by puncture wounds). Most likely to occur in farmers, horticulturists, gardeners. Cutaneous lesions occur 20-90 days after cutaneous inoculation.
System(s) affected: Skin/Exocrine, Hemic/Lymphatic/Immunologic, Musculoskeletal
Genetics: No known genetic pattern
Incidence/Prevalence in USA: N/A
Predominant age: Adults
Predominant sex: Male > Female (mostly due to occupational exposure)

SIGNS AND SYMPTOMS
• Cutaneous or lymphocutaneous:
  ◊ Characteristic skin lesions, beginning as an inoculation chancre, or erythematous plaque with satellite, small papule, painless, movable, subcutaneous nodules in a linear distribution. Lesions progress to larger nodules which may ulcerate and drain. Affects primarily upper extremities.
  ◊ Additional lesions spread proximally along lymphatics
• Pulmonary
  ◊ Cough, occasionally productive
  ◊ Cavitary lung disease
  ◊ Hilar adenopathy
  ◊ Signs and symptoms indistinguishable from other chronic pneumonias
• Osteo-articular
  ◊ Subacute or chronic inflammatory arthritis, often monoarticular, may persist for many years
  ◊ Signs and symptoms of osteomyelitis
  ◊ Generally afebrile
• Disseminated
  ◊ Multifocal skin lesions
  ◊ Polyarticular arthritis
  ◊ Weight loss
  ◊ Chronic lymphocytic meningitis

CAUSES
Infection with Sporothrix schenckii, a fungus found in soil, sphagnum peat moss, and decaying vegetation. Infection acquired by direct inoculation (usual) or inhalation (rare).

RISK FACTORS
• Gardening - contact with mulch, sphagnum moss, hay, timber, thorny bushes
• Occupations handling gardening materials, such as nursery workers, landscapers, florists, carpenters
• Animal handlers (transmission from animals, especially cats, to humans has been documented)
• Immunocompromised (drugs or HIV infection)
• Alcoholism (pulmonary and disseminated)

DIAGNOSIS

DIFFERENTIAL DIAGNOSIS
• Cutaneous or lymphocutaneous
  ◊ Sporotrichoid nocardiosis
  ◊ Leishmaniasis
  ◊ Chromomycosis
  ◊ Atypical mycobacterial infection (M. marinum, M. chelonei, M. kansasii)
  ◊ Tularemia
  ◊ Plague
• Pulmonary
  ◊ Tuberculosis
  ◊ Sarcoidosis
  ◊ Chronic fungal pneumonia
  ◊ Neoplasm
• Osteo-articular
  ◊ Rheumatoid arthritis
  ◊ Bacterial arthritis/osteomyelitis

LABORATORY
• Culture of S. schenckii in sputum, pus, synovial fluid or bone drainage
• Organism found with difficulty with PAS and Gomori stains of skin or other biopsied lesions
• Serum antibody tests may be useful for extracutaneous disease
Drugs that may alter lab results:
Antifungal drugs
Disorders that may alter lab results: N/A

PATHOLOGICAL FINDINGS
Granulomas with central necrosis

SPECIAL TESTS
Immunohistochemical staining of biopsy specimens

IMAGING
Chest and skeletal x-rays

DIAGNOSTIC PROCEDURES
• Careful history and physical
• Culture of draining lesions
• Culture of inflammatory joint effusions or sputum
• Biopsy if diagnosis not confirmed

TREATMENT

APPROPRIATE HEALTH CARE
• Many patients can be managed on outpatient basis
• Hospitalization for adjunctive surgical procedures or initiation of amphotericin B therapy

GENERAL MEASURES
• Local heat application useful for cutaneous and lymphocutaneous disease
• Keep cutaneous lesions clean
• Repeated drainage of infected joints may be indicated

SURGICAL MEASURES
• Synovectomy of infected joints may be indicated
• Surgical débridement of osteomyelitis usually indicated

ACTIVITY
No restrictions

DIET
No special diet

PATIENT EDUCATION
Patients should be advised of the nature of the infection, the toxicities associated with therapy, and the need for sustained therapy

Sporotrichosis

MEDICATIONS

DRUG(S) OF CHOICE
• Cutaneous or lymphocutaneous disease:
◊ Itraconazole 200 mg per day orally for 3-12 months is a preferred treatment
◊ Potassium iodide saturated solution (SSKI) is an alternative treatment. Initially 10 drops orally tid increased by 1 drop each dose to maximum tolerated dose or 120 drops/day. Dilute in a beverage to disguise taste. Continue for 1-2 months after all lesions have healed.
• Extracutaneous disease:
◊ Itraconazole 400 mg per day orally is a preferred treatment. Therapy should be continued for 12-18 months.
◊ IV amphotericin B, 1.5-2.5 g total dose is alternative treatment
Contraindications: SSKI contraindicated in tuberculosis
Precautions:
• Amphotericin B can cause fever, chills, nausea and vomiting. Dosage varies for sex and age groups. Refer to manufacturer's literature for precautions, adverse effects and interactions.
• SSKI requires extra care if patient also has tuberculosis, kidney disease, renal dysfunction or hyperthyroidism. Can cause folliculitis and tender, swollen salivary glands.
Significant possible interactions: SSKI taken concurrently with amiloride, spironolactone or triamterene may result in hyperkalemia

ALTERNATIVE DRUGS
• Ketoconazole 400 mg orally daily may be effective alternative therapy in immunocompetent hosts
• Fluconazole 800 mg per day orally is an alternative therapy in patients unable to receive itraconazole therapy

FOLLOWUP

PATIENT MONITORING
Check for compliance with long-term drugs (SSKI should be continued for 1-2 months after lesions heal)

PREVENTION/AVOIDANCE
• Avoid endemic areas
• Wear gloves when working in soil

POSSIBLE COMPLICATIONS
• Secondary bacterial infection
• Bone and joint deformities from osteo-articular disease

EXPECTED COURSE/PROGNOSIS
• Prognosis is excellent for complete recovery from cutaneous or lymphocutaneous infections
• Other disease forms demonstrate a chronic indolent course and are variably responsive to therapy

MISCELLANEOUS

ASSOCIATED CONDITIONS
See Risk Factors

AGE-RELATED FACTORS
Pediatric: Rare
Geriatric: N/A
Others: N/A

PREGNANCY
N/A

SYNONYMS
• Schenck's disease
• Beurmann's disease
• Rose gardener's disease

ICD-9-CM
117.1 Sporotrichosis

SEE ALSO
N/A

OTHER NOTES
Rare ocular disease due to direct inoculation

ABBREVIATIONS
N/A

REFERENCES
• Winn RE: Sporotrichosis. Infect Dis Clinic North Am 1988;2:899
• Mandell GL, ed: Principles and Practice of Infectious Diseases. 4th Ed. New York, Churchill Livingstone, 1995
• Sharkey-Mathis PK, Kauffman CA, Graybill JR, Stevens DA, Hostetler JS, Cloud G, Dismukes WE & other members of the NIAID Mycoses Study Group: Treatment of sporotrichosis with itraconazole. Am J Med 1993;95:279
• Kauffman CA, Pappos PG, McKinsey DS, Greenfield RA, Perfect JR, Cloud GA, et al: Treatment of Lymphocutaneous and Visceral Sporotrichosis with Fluconazole. Clin Infect Dis 1996;22:46
Illustrations: N/A
Internet references: http://www.5mcc.com

Author(s)
E. Nan Scott, PhD
Ronald A. Greenfield, MD
Douglas P. Fine, MD

Sprains & strains

 BASICS

DESCRIPTION
• Sprain: complete or partial ligamentous injury, either within the body of the ligament or at the site of attachment to bone. It may be classified as Grade I, II, or III. Grades I and II are incomplete tears and differ in severity; Grade III is complete dissolution of the ligamentous connection. Physical exam is key to the diagnosis. Usually secondary to trauma (falls, twisting injuries or motor vehicle accidents).
• Strain: partial or complete disruption of the muscle or tendon, usually associated with overuse injuries.
System(s) affected: Musculoskeletal
Genetics: N/A
Incidence/Prevalence in USA:
• Total incidence including spine, upper and lower extremities probably occurs in close to 80% of all athletes sometime in their career
• Prevalence - approximately 30,000
Predominant age:
• Sprains- any age where patient is physically active
• Strains - usually 15-40
Predominant sex: Male > Female

SIGNS AND SYMPTOMS
• Swelling
• Pain
• Erythema and/or ecchymosis
• Tenderness
• Gait disturbances if severe
• Decreased range of motion of joint and joint instability

CAUSES
• Falls
• Motor vehicle accident
• Trauma
• Excessive exercise or inadequate warm-up and stretching prior to activity
• Poor conditioning

RISK FACTORS
• Change in or improper shoe gear, protective gear, or environment (e.g., surface)
• Inappropriate increase in training schedule

 DIAGNOSIS

DIFFERENTIAL DIAGNOSIS
• Sprains (ligament tears) must be differentiated from strains (muscle-tendon unit tears), although this is difficult and often the diagnosis is strain/sprain
• Tendonitis
• Bursitis
• Bony injuries
• Rarely, muscle hematomas account for some of the signs and symptoms of strains

LABORATORY   N/A
Drugs that may alter lab results: N/A
Disorders that may alter lab results: N/A

PATHOLOGICAL FINDINGS   N/A

SPECIAL TESTS
• Exam under anesthesia
• Arthroscopy in some cases
• For ankle, anterior drawer test, which tests the integrity of the anterior talofibular ligament

IMAGING
• Ankle films - only required if there is pain in malleolar zone and
1. Bone tenderness posterior edge or tip of lateral malleolus
or
2. Bone tenderness posterior edge or tip of medial malleolus
or
3. Unable to bear weight, both immediately and in emergency department
• Foot films - only required if there is midfoot zone pain and
1. Bone tenderness at base of 5th metatarsal
or
2. Bone tenderness at navicular
or
3. unable to bear weight, both immediately and in emergency department
• X-rays to rule out bony injury. Stress views may be helpful.
• CT scan of the affected area
• MRI
• Exam under anesthesia in difficult cases

DIAGNOSTIC PROCEDURES
• Sprains/strains
  ◊ Grade I - pain/tenderness without loss of motion
  ◊ Grade II - pain/tenderness; ecchymosis with some loss of range of motion
  ◊ Grade III - pain/tenderness; swelling and ecchymosis and complete loss of range of motion

 TREATMENT

APPROPRIATE HEALTH CARE
Outpatient

GENERAL MEASURES
History and physical exam along with treatment of the worst possible suspected injury
• Acutely
  ◊ RICE therapy - Rest, Ice, Compression, Elevation
    - Elastic bandage wrap (Ace) is comfortable
    - Jone's dressing for more severe injuries
  ◊ Orthosis (splint) for pain relief and stability; "Air Cast" type devices provide effective stability and pain relief
  ◊ Crutches and crutch gait training

SURGICAL MEASURES
• Casting and surgery reserved for select Grade III injuries

ACTIVITY
• Bed rest for acute injuries
• Physical therapy for more severe injuries
• Elevate joint while sleeping

DIET   Weight loss if obesity etiologic

PATIENT EDUCATION
• Instructions on how to wrap with elastic bandage
• Prevention of injury

MEDICATIONS

DRUG(S) OF CHOICE
• NSAIDs: ibuprofen 200-800mg TID, naproxen 375-500mg BID, indomethacin 25-50mg TID
• Narcotics for severe pain, e.g., hydrocodone-acetaminophen (Vicodin)
Contraindications: Refer to manufacturer's profile of each drug
Precautions: Refer to manufacturer's profile of each drug
Significant possible interactions: Refer to manufacturer's profile of each drug

ALTERNATIVE DRUGS
• Analgesic balms
• Capsaicin (Dolorac, Zostrix) cream 0.025% or capsaicin (Zostrix-HP) cream 0.075%: apply qid

FOLLOWUP

PATIENT MONITORING
After initial treatment, consider rehabilitation. Direct emphasis towards limiting swelling and providing a pain-free full range of motion.

PREVENTION/AVOIDANCE
• Maintaining a reasonable level of physical fitness
• Avoidance of excessive physical stresses and wearing of proper exercise gear (particularly shoes). Using proper equipment for the activity.
• Knowledge of the risks associated with the intended activity
• Appropriate conditioning, warm-up and cool-down exercises

POSSIBLE COMPLICATIONS
• Chronic joint instability
• Arthritis

EXPECTED COURSE/PROGNOSIS
With appropriate treatment and rest, 6-8 weeks or longer for recovery, depending on severity of injury

MISCELLANEOUS

ASSOCIATED CONDITIONS
Hemarthrosis, stress, avulsion, or other fractures, syndesmotic injuries, contusions, wounds, dislocations

AGE-RELATED FACTORS
Pediatric: Sprains and strains accounted for 24% of injuries in an analysis of 1,124 sports injuries of children in a study done in West Germany, 1980-82
Geriatric: More likely to see associated bony injuries due to decreased joint flexibility and prevalence of osteoporosis and osteopenia
Others: N/A

PREGNANCY N/A

SYNONYMS N/A

ICD-9-CM
848.9 Sprain and strain, site unspecified

SEE ALSO
• Tendinitis

OTHER NOTES N/A

ABBREVIATIONS
NSAID = nonsteroidal anti-inflammatory drug

REFERENCES
• Kvist M, Kujala VM, Heinonen OJ, Vuori IV, Aho AJ, Pajulo O, Hintsa A, Parvinen T: Sports related injuries in children. IJSM 1989;10(2):81-86
• Strong WB, Stanitski EL, Smith RE, Wilmore JH: Diagnosis and treatment of ankle sprains. AJDC 1990;144:809-814
• Ruda S: Sports Nursing. In Nursing Clinics of North America. Philadelphia, W.B. Saunders Co., Mar, 1991
• Stiell I.G, McKnight D, Greenberg GH, et al: Implementation of the Ottawa ankle rules. JAMA 1994;271(11):827-832
Illustrations: N/A
Internet references: http://www.5mcc.com

Author(s)
Timothy Robinson, DO

Status epilepticus

BASICS

DESCRIPTION Epileptic seizure longer than 30 minutes or absence of full recovery of consciousness between seizures. Tonic-clonic (grand mal) status epilepticus (SEp) is the most common and most serious form. SEp is a life-threatening emergency; begin treatment if seizure >10 min.
System(s) affected: Nervous
Genetics: Unknown
Incidence/Prevalence in USA: More than 60,000 cases per year; 1/3 as unprovoked first seizure, 1/6 in patients with known epilepsy, 1/2 secondary to acute CNS insult
Predominant age: > 50% of new cases of SEp occur in young children. Risk is also increased in those over age 60.
Predominant sex: Male = Female

SIGNS AND SYMPTOMS
• Depend on the duration and type of seizure
• Recurrent tonic-clonic convulsions: May be preceded by aura. Tonic phase (stiffening) for 30 to 45 seconds. Clonic phase (rhythmic jerking) for 2-5 minutes. No intervening consciousness before seizure recurs. (For additional seizure types see Other Notes.)
• Associated autonomic phenomena: Excess catecholamine secretion resulting in glandular hypersecretion, piloerection, cyclic pupillary dilation, and prolonged apnea (may lead to cyanosis)
• Metabolic changes: Lactic acidosis, carbon dioxide narcosis, hyperkalemia, hyperglycemia - followed by hypoglycemia
• Cardiac changes: Hypertension (may be followed by hypotension), arrhythmias, high output failure
• Respiratory changes: Increased secretions, lax tongue, possible airway obstruction, pulmonary edema, aspiration
• Renal complications: Acute tubular necrosis from myoglobinuria after rhabdomyolysis
• Cerebrovascular changes: Loss of autoregulation, focal ischemia, cerebral edema
• Postictal findings: Fever, tachycardia, mydriasis, conjugate deviation of eyes, decreased corneal reflex, positive Babinski's sign, fecal and urinary incontinence and tongue, cheek, or lip lacerations

CAUSES
• Febrile convulsions (especially in children)
• Acute CNS injury - trauma, infection, mass/ vascular lesion, metabolic disorder or anticonvulsant withdrawal/noncompliance
• Idiopathic
• Intoxication - cocaine, tricyclic antidepressants
• Chronic CNS injury - previous trauma, stroke, infection, encephalopathy (hypoxic or other chronic or degenerative type)

RISK FACTORS
• Known seizure disorder plus any precipitating insult. Prior history of SEp (recurrence rate is 17% in children; 50% in those with neurologic abnormality).
• Porphyria

DIAGNOSIS

DIFFERENTIAL DIAGNOSIS
• Pseudostatus may occur with pseudoseizures; avoid dangerous therapy
• While tonic/clonic status is usually apparent, paralyzed patients and other forms of status require neurologic exam and EEG
• Primary diagnostic problem is identification of the underlying pathology

LABORATORY Glucose, electrolytes, CBC, calcium, magnesium and osmolarity; arterial blood gases; toxicology screen; anticonvulsants serum levels; liver/renal function.
Drugs that may alter lab results: N/A
Disorders that may alter lab results: N/A

PATHOLOGICAL FINDINGS Variable

SPECIAL TESTS EEG will differentiate pseudoseizures and prolonged seizures not recognized as status.

IMAGING CT scan, MRI

DIAGNOSTIC PROCEDURES
Lumbar puncture. CAUTION - intracranial pressure may be increased.

TREATMENT

APPROPRIATE HEALTH CARE Tonic-clonic SEp is an emergency; treat if a seizure lasts >10 min.

GENERAL MEASURES
• Manage airway, breathing and circulation (ABCs). Monitor pulse oximetry, end-tidal CO_2, blood pressure, ECG and temperature. Give oxygen. Ventilate and intubate if hypoventilation, hypoxia and/or hypercarbia occur or if aspiration is a concern.
• Observe and confirm the fit is SEp
• Pursue available drug history
• Establish IV (or intraosseous line for a child); obtain initial lab studies (above)
• Determine blood glucose and treat with dextrose and thiamine if indicated
• Initiate anticonvulsant therapy to end seizure; then add maintenance therapy
• Use muscle relaxant if seizures impair ventilation or lactic acidosis develops

SURGICAL MEASURES N/A

ACTIVITY Protect the patient from injury. Place on side. Clear airway secretions. Prevent tongue laceration.

DIET NPO

PATIENT EDUCATION Epilepsy Foundation (800)EFA-1000

MEDICATIONS

DRUG(S) OF CHOICE Depend on the type of seizure. Tonic-clonic SEp is the most serious and may be approached as follows. (For other types, see Other Notes.)
• Stabilization: Continue "ABC" assessment and monitoring. Intubate if needed. Prevent hypotension with vasopressors (e.g., dopamine).
  ◊ Thiamine: 100 mg IV or IM (adults only)
  ◊ 50% dextrose - if blood sugar is low or cannot be measured; give 50 mL IV (for child - use D25W; give 2 mL/kg slowly)
  ◊ Naloxone (Narcan): if pupils are myotic or drug overdose suspected; give 2 mg IV (for child - 0.1 mg/kg IV, up to 2 mg slowly)
• To stop seizures (IV available):
Give BOTH a benzodiazepine and fosphenytoin. As each drug is added - watch for hypoventilation, hypotension and ECG changes.
  ◊ Lorazepam (Ativan): 0.05-0.15 mg/kg IV at 1-2 mg/min to maximum of 10 mg (for child 0.05-0.1 mg/kg IV at <2 mg/min to maximum of 4 mg). May repeat q10min x 2 (some prefer diazepam [see below]).
PLUS
  ◊ Fosphenytoin (Cerebyx), prodrug of phenytoin: 15-20 mg phenytoin equivalents (PE)/kg IV at < 150 mgPE/min. Maintenance 4-6 mg/kg/day IV or IM. For child, fosphenytoin safety not established; for phenytoin in child < 50 kg, load with 20 mg/kg at < 1 mg/kg/min (see Precautions). May repeat 5 mg/kg q30min to total of 30 mg/kg.
• To stop seizures (IV not available):
  ◊ Intraosseous infusion in small children for benzodiazepines, phenytoin and phenobarbital - doses are the same as IV
  ◊ Rectal diazepam: 0.5-1.0 mg/kg (child - 20 mg maximum) use the IV solution (less respiratory depression)
  ◊ Sublingual lorazepam: use IV dose
  ◊ IM fosphenytoin: dose same as IV (slow)
  ◊ Midazolam (Versed): 0.2 mg/kg IM or 0.5 mg/kg intranasal (onset 5-10 min, brief duration)
• If seizures persist (refractory status):
  ◊ Induce drug coma (anesthesia) with a short acting barbiturate or benzodiazepine to obtain a burst suppression (BSup) pattern EEG. Requires intubation, continuous respiratory support, cardiovascular and EEG monitoring, and (often) blood pressure support.
    - Thiopental: induction 3-6 mg/kg in divided doses, then add 50 mg IV q 2-5 min to produce EEG BSup. Maintain with IV drip of 0.2% solution; start at 2 mg/kg/min and adjust to keep EEG at BSup.
    - Pentobarbital induction dose 5 mg/kg IV then add 1 mg/kg IV until EEG is at BSup. Maintain with IV drip of 1-3 mg/kg/min adjusted to keep EEG at BSup.
    - Diazepam: 4-8 mg/hr IV drip
Contraindications:
• Review current package inserts
• Benzodiazepines (diazepam, lorazepam, midazolam) - in acute narrow-angle glaucoma
• Barbiturates - in acute intermittent porphyria

Precautions:
- Reduce dosage of depressants in patients with shock, coma or alcohol intoxication
- Most drugs listed may exacerbate porphyria; exceptions are lorazepam, midazolam and propofol
- Benzodiazepines - apnea may occur with rapid IV injection, especially with barbiturates. Reduce dose in the chronic pulmonary patient, the elderly and hepatic insufficiency.
- Diazepam - venous thrombosis/phlebitis
- Phenobarbital - caution in pulmonary insufficiency, hepatic disease and pregnancy. Withdrawal seizures may occur following abrupt termination of high doses. Increase the dosing interval in renal failure. Reduce dose in severe liver disease.
- Phenytoin - monitor ECG for arrhythmias, prolonged QT interval, and hypotension. If these occur, decrease the rate of administration. Use with caution in pregnancy (increased risk of malformations), liver disease, hyperglycemia, and elderly patients. Abrupt withdrawal may precipitate status. Use in normal or half normal saline to prevent precipitation that occurs in dextrose solutions. Overdose may cause paradoxical inefficacy.
- Fosphenytoin (phenytoin prodrug) - similar to phenytoin but less toxicity and cardiovascular suppression
- Carbamazepine - reduce dose in liver disease. Caution in pregnancy and breast feeding.

Significant possible interactions:
CNS depressants: depression enhanced
- Phenobarbital: reduced efficacy of quinidine and warfarin; induces metabolism of phenytoin
- Phenytoin: increased serum levels and toxicity of warfarin, disulfiram, phenylbutazone, and isoniazid. Decrease dose with renal insufficiency; monitor free levels if possible.
- Carbamazepine - may reduce effects of warfarin, phenytoin/fosphenytoin, and ethosuximide; avoid with MAO inhibitors

ALTERNATIVE DRUGS
- Alternate benzodiazepines:
  ◊ Medium acting/convenient: diazepam (Valium) 0.2-0.5 mg/kg IV at 5 mg/min up to a dose of 30 mg (for child 0.3 mg/kg at <2 mg/min up to 10 mg). Repeat q 5 min x 3.
  ◊ Faster/shorter acting: midazolam (Versed) 0.125-0.5 mg/kg IV (sedative to anesthetic dose) plus titrated infusion of 0.5-10 µg/kg/min
- Second line drugs:
  ◊ Phenobarbital (Luminal): 10-20 mg/kg IV (in saline) at a rate of <100 mg/min (use lower rate for old age or cardiac history); may repeat dose of 4-6 mg/kg IV until no seizures or total dose of 1-2 grams. (For child - 20 mg/kg IV at 1 mg/kg/min, maximum 30 mg/kg
  ◊ Lidocaine (Xylocaine): 1 to 3 mg/kg IV bolus; if effective, drip 3-10 mg/kg/hr IV
  ◊ Valproic acid: 500 mg via nasogastric tube or 500 mg with 300 mL water via rectal tube (clamp for 15 minutes)
  ◊ Carbamazepine - 400 mg in 2 divided doses via NG or PR. For child age 6-12 - 100 mg bid; child age < 6 - 100 mg via NG tube

- Investigational drugs:
Isoflurane, desflurane by inhalation; propofol by continuous IV and bolus; etomidate by continuous IV infusion; chlormethiazole by IV infusion; IV valproic acid; ketamine, NMDA antagonist–IV as neuroprotectants

FOLLOWUP

PATIENT MONITORING
Therapeutic blood levels of anticonvulsants

PREVENTION/AVOIDANCE
Establish maintenance regimen of anticonvulsants

POSSIBLE COMPLICATIONS
- Morbidity/mortality related to the acute CNS insult, stress, injury from repeated seizures
- Causes of death - cardiopulmonary arrest, renal failure, hyperthermia, aspiration pneumonia, the underlying pathology or the treatment instituted
- Anticonvulsants cause respiratory and cardiovascular depression

EXPECTED COURSE/PROGNOSIS
Mortality is 6-18% (3-6% in children) and is improving. Usually related to the underlying cause. Prolonged seizures (> 30 min) may cause neurologic injury or death. Seizure >4 hr, mortality = 50%; >12 hr = 80%.

MISCELLANEOUS

ASSOCIATED CONDITIONS
Etiology or underlying pathology associated with SEp varies significantly by age group. In adults, usually related to a known condition, e.g., established epilepsy, alcohol withdrawal or acquired CNS lesion (especially frontal).

AGE-RELATED FACTORS
Pediatric: Lower mortality rate. More likely present in SEp as their first seizure due to febrile seizure; new onset epilepsy (idiopathic); CNS infection; metabolic derangement.
Geriatric: More likely to have SEp secondary to a change in drug therapy (noncompliance, drug interaction or toxicity); tend to have localized (often frontal lobe) CNS lesions.
Others: Neonatal status is most often related to meningitis or metabolic disorders (deficiencies of calcium, magnesium, or pyridoxine); needs careful workup for cause

PREGNANCY
- Phenytoin - use with caution (increased risk of malformations in first trimester)
- Phenobarbital - use with caution
- Valproate - increased risk of neural tube defects

SYNONYMS
Status convulsivus

ICD-9-CM
345.3 grand mal status and status epilepticus
345.7 Epilepsia partialis continua, psychomotor status and temporal lobe status

SEE ALSO
- Seizure disorders
- Seizures, febrile

OTHER NOTES
- Additional forms of status include:
  ◊ Focal motor status - starts distally with clonic jerking in ascending pattern; eyes and head deviate to side opposite the focus; may progress to generalized status; underlying CNS pathology is common. Treat like tonic-clonic SEp. May respond to carbamazepine.
  ◊ Epilepsia partialis continua - rapid focal jerking; no loss of consciousness; worsened by voluntary movements; may persist for hours to days; poor response to therapy; often associated with underlying pathology. Pentobarbital and lorazepam recommended.
  ◊ Myoclonic status - sudden spasmodic contraction of limbs; usually secondary to widespread neurologic or metabolic dysfunction; consciousness usually maintained. Treat with lorazepam.
  ◊ Complex partial status (psychomotor status) - short seizures with automatisms (e.g., lip smacking, random eye movements, chewing, staring); followed by post ictal confusion. May respond to carbamazepine. With status, treat like tonic-clonic SEp.
  ◊ Absence status - varies from mild lethargy to severe confusion, 10 second duration, no aura, eyes flutter and turn upward, with irregular myoclonic jerks, automatisms, no post ictal confusion; may progress to generalized status. If so, treat as tonic-clonic status.
  ◊ Neonatal status epilepticus - subtle multifocal, clonic, tonic, and myoclonic features; risk of intracerebral hemorrhage; meningitis and metabolic disorders (deficiencies of calcium, magnesium, pyridoxine) more common. Begin with phenobarbital and diazepam.

ABBREVIATIONS
SEp = status epilepticus
BSup = burst suppression

REFERENCES
5 additional references available at web site
Internet references: http://www.5mcc.com
Illustrations: N/A

Author(s)
Jeff Ray Gibson, Jr., MD

Stevens-Johnson syndrome

BASICS

DESCRIPTION
Until recently Stevens-Johnson syndrome (SJS) was considered to be the same as erythema multiforme major, a severe form of erythema multiforme in which more than one mucosal surface was involved. Now it is thought that erythema multiforme spectrum is a single entity. The milder form, also known as erythema multiforme-Hebra, either has no mucous membrane involvement, or may involve one mucous membrane. The more severe form is erythema multiforme major, involving more than one mucus membrane. In both these variants, it is a self limited hypersensitivity reaction, usually to a preceding viral infection, and has an excellent prognosis. SJS is a generalized hypersensitivity reaction, usually to a drug, in which the skin and mucus membrane lesions are early manifestation. It may progress to its more severe form, toxic epidermal necrolysis which has a high morbidity and up to 40% mortality.
System(s) affected: Skin/exocrine, Nervous, Cardiovascular, Renal/Urologic, Hemic/Lymphatic/Immunologic
Genetics: Possibly associated with HLA-B15
Incidence/prevalence in USA: Difficult to estimate because of confusion with erythema multiforme major, perhaps 0.1/100,000, or less.
Predominant age: More common in children and young adults
Predominant sex: Males > Females (2:1)

SIGNS AND SYMPTOMS
• There is usually a preceding illness for which medication was given
• Sudden onset with rapid progressive pleomorphic rash which includes petechiae, vesicles, bullae
• The condition is classified as SJS if epidermal detachment affects less than 10% of the skin, as toxic epidermal necrolysis (TEN) if epidermal detachment exceeds 30%, or if it exceeds 10% in the absence of discrete skin lesions. Cases with discrete skin lesions and between 10% and 30% epidermal detachment are in the overlap between SJS and TEN.
• Vesicles and ulcers on the mucous membranes, especially of the mouth and throat
Burning sensation of the skin and sometimes of the mucous membranes
• Usually no pruritis
• Fever 39-40°C (102-104°F)
• Headache
• Malaise
• Arthralgias
• Epistaxis
• Crusted nares
• Conjunctivitis
• Corneal ulcerations
• Erosive vulvovaginitis or balanitis
• Cough productive of thick purulent sputum
• Tachypnea/respiratory distress
• Albuminuria/hematuria
• Arrhythmias
• Pericarditis
• Congestive heart failure

• Mental status changes
• Electrolyte disturbance
• Seizures
• Coma
• Sepsis

CAUSES
• Often unknown
• Medications - especially sulfonamides, penicillins, anticonvulsants, salicylates, nonsteroidal anti-inflammatory drugs, methazolamide, carvedilol (3,4)
• Vaccines - diphtheria/typhoid, bacillus Calmette Guerin (BCG), oral polio vaccine (OPV)
• Mycoplasma pneumonia virus infection

RISK FACTORS
• Patients with HIV infection appear to be predisposed to developing SJS in response to their medications
• Previous history of SJS
• Male sex

DIAGNOSIS

DIFFERENTIAL DIAGNOSIS
• Exfoliative dermatitis
• Staphylococcal scalded skin syndrome
• Acute generalized exanthematic pustulosis
• Pemphigus (paraneoplastic)
• Generalized fixed drug eruption
• Erythema multiforme major
• Burns
• Pressure blisters (coma, barbiturates)

LABORATORY
Culture or serological tests for suspected sources of infection
Drugs that may alter lab results: N/A
Disorders that may alter lab results: N/A

PATHOLOGICAL FINDINGS
Compared with the mainly inflammatory changes in erythema multiforme, necrotic changes predominate in SJS and TEN. There is a cell poor infiltrate in which macrophages and dendrocytes predominate with a strong immunoreactivity for TNF-alpha.

SPECIAL TESTS
None

IMAGING
N/A

DIAGNOSTIC PROCEDURES
Skin biopsy

TREATMENT

APPROPRIATE HEALTH CARE
Since this disease can progress quickly, all patients should be admitted. If the sloughed skin exceeds 10% of the body surface, consideration should be given to transferring the patient to a burns unit. Bronchiolitis, adult respiratory distress syndrome or multi-organ damage may require care in an intensive care unit.

GENERAL MEASURES
• Withdrawal of any suspected medication, and treatment of any underlying disease
• Meticulous care of damaged skin
• Reverse isolation when epidermal loss is extensive
• Maintenance of fluid, electrolyte and protein balance
• Adequate calorie intake, parenteral nutrition if necessary
• Oral hygiene with mouthwashes of warm saline, or solution of diphenhydramine, lidocaine, and kaolin suspension
• Ophthalmological consultation and monitoring for corneal damage

SURGICAL MEASURES
Sterile débridement of areas of extensive epidermal loss. Application of biosynthetic dressings such as Biobrane to denuded areas (13) Long term damage to the vulva or vagina or to the cornea or may need surgical repair.

ACTIVITY
Bed rest until clinically stabilized

DIET
As tolerated. Increased fluid intake is recommended. Intravenous nutritional support may be needed.

PATIENT EDUCATION
• The patient should be kept informed of the progress of the disease, and the treatment options available
• Recurrences are possible. Etiologic agents should be identified if possible, and avoided indefinitely.

MEDICATIONS

DRUG(S) OF CHOICE Administration of steroids is controversial. If there is no clear benefit within a few days, they should be withdrawn. Experimental treatments that appear to have been useful include recombinant granulocyte colony stimulating factor, plasmapheresis, cyclophosphamide, cyclosporine, and, in HIV positive patients, IV immune globulin. Empiric use of antibiotics is not recommended.
Contraindications: Particularly avoid steroids in diabetic or immunosuppressed patients or those with chronic infections.
Precautions: Refer to the manufacturer's profile for each drug
Significant possible interactions: Refer to manufacturer's profile of each drug

ALTERNATIVE DRUGS Treat herpetic infections with acyclovir; mycoplasma infections with erythromycin or related antibiotic

FOLLOWUP

PATIENT MONITORING
• Secondary or intercurrent infections
• Dehydration
• Electrolyte imbalance
• Malnutrition
• End-organ damage

PREVENTION/AVOIDANCE
• It is rarely possible to anticipate a first attack
• Avoid reexposure to the presumed cause

POSSIBLE COMPLICATIONS
• Secondary infections
• Sepsis
• Pneumonia
• Adult respiratory distress syndrome
• Bronchiolitis obliterans in children
• Dehydration/electrolyte disturbance
• Acute tubular necrosis
• Corneal ulceration or iritis
• Arrhythmias
• Death in about 15% of untreated cases of SJS, and up to 40% of TEN

EXPECTED COURSE/PROGNOSIS
• Disease may have a rapid onset, or may evolve slowly over 1-2 weeks, with resolution over 4 to 6 weeks
• There may be scarring of the skin or mucous membranes, especially of the vulva
• There may be blindness or corneal opacities in 7-20% of patients
• Risk of recurrence may be a s high as 37%
• Death occurs in 5-15% of patients with SJS, and up to 40% of patients with TEN

MISCELLANEOUS

ASSOCIATED CONDITIONS
• Stevens-Johnson syndrome and toxic epidermal necrolysis are associated conditions
• Mycoplasma pneumonia has been described as a viral precursor

AGE-RELATED FACTORS
Pediatric: Rare under 3 years. More common in children and young adults
Geriatric: TEN has a greater mortality in older patients
Others: N/A

PREGNANCY Reported as a possible predisposing condition

SYNONYMS
• Ectodermosis erosiva pluriorificialis
• Febrile mucocutaneous syndrome
• Herpes iris
• Erythema polymorphe

ICD-9-CM 695.1 Stevens-Johnson syndrome and toxic epidermal necrolysis

SEE ALSO
• Erythema multiforme
• Pemphigus vulgaris
• Pemphigoid, bullous
• Serum sickness

OTHER NOTES N/A

ABBREVIATIONS N/A

REFERENCES
• Saunders Electronic Atlas of Dermatology. Philadelphia, WB Saunders Co, 1996
• Mockenhaupt M, Schopf E: Epidemiology of drug-induced severe skin reactions. Seminars in Cutaneous Medicine and Surgery 1996;15(4):236-243
• Shirato S, et al: Stevens-Johnson syndrome induced by methazolamide treatment. Archives of Ophthalmology 1997;115(4):550-553
• Kowalski BJ, Cody RJ: Stevens-Johnson syndrome associated with carvedilol therapy. American Journal of Cardiology 1997;80(5):669-670
• Tay YK, et al: Mycoplasma pneumonia infection is associated with Stevens-Johnson Syndrome, not erythema multiforme (von Hebra). Journal of the American Academy of Dermatology 1996;35(5pt1):757-760
• Revuz JE, Roujeau JC: Advances in toxic epidermal necrolysis. Seminars in Cutaneous Medicine & Surgery 1966;15(4):258-266
• Paquet P, Pierard GE: Erythema multiforme and toxic epidermal necrolysis: a comparative study. American Journal of Dermatopathology 1997;19(2):127-132
• Criton S, et al: Toxic epidermal necrolysis - a retrospective study. International Journal of Dermatology 1997;36(12):923-925
• Engelhardt SL, et al: Toxic epidermal necrolysis: an analysis of referral patients and steroid usage. Journal of Burn Care and Rehabilitation 1997;18(6):520-524
• Yarbrough DR 3rd: Treatment of toxic epidermal necrolysis in a burn center. Journal South Carolina Medical Association 1997;93(9):347-350
• Khoo AK, Foo CL: Toxic epidermal necrolysis in a burns center. Burns 1996;22(4):275-278
• Wallis C, McClymont W: Toxic epidermal necrolysis with adult respiratory distress syndrome. Anaesthesia 1995;50(9):801-803
• Bradley T, et al: Toxic epidermal necrolysis: a review and report of the successful use of Biobrane for early wound coverage. Annals of Plastic Surgery 1995;35(2)124-132
• Kakourou T, et al: Corticosteroid treatment of erythema multiforme major (Stevens-Johnson syndrome in children. European Journal of Pediatrics 1997;156(2):90-93
• Murphy JT, et al: Toxic epidermal necrolysis. Journal of Burn Care & Rehabilitation 1997;18(5):417-420
• Jarret P, et al: Toxic epidermal necrolysis treated with cyclosporin and granulocyte colony stimulating factor. Clinical and Experimental Dermatology 1997;22(3):146-147
• Chaidemenos GC, et al: Plasmapheresis in toxic epidermal necrolysis. International Journal of Dermatology 1997;36(3):218-221
• Goulden V, Goodfield MJ: Recombinant granulocyte colony stimulating factor in the management of toxic epidermal necrolysis. British Journal of Dermatology 1996;135(2):305-306
• Frangogiannis NG, et al: Cyclophosphamide in the treatment of toxic epidermal necrolysis. Southern Medical Journal 1996;89(10):1001-1003
• Kim MJ, Lee KY: Bronchiolitis obliterans in children with Stevens-Johnson syndrome: follow-up with high resolution CT. Pediatric Radiology 1996;26(1):22-25
Illustrations: 2 available on CD-ROM
Internet references: http://www.5mcc.com

Author(s)
Lewis C. Rose, MD

Stokes-Adams attacks

BASICS

DESCRIPTION Syncope due to transient complete heart block and resulting severe bradycardia or asystole with hypotension
System(s) affected: Cardiovascular, Nervous
Genetics: No known genetic pattern
Incidence/Prevalence in USA: Undocumented
Predominant age: Most commonly, greater than 40 years of age
Predominant sex: Male = Female

SIGNS AND SYMPTOMS
• Acute bradycardia
• Hypotension
• Paleness
• Altered sensorium or loss of consciousness, unrelated to position or exertion
• Acute onset of syncopal or near syncopal symptoms (with or without palpitations)

CAUSES
• Medications:
  ◊ Calcium channel blockers
  ◊ Beta blockers
  ◊ Sotolol
  ◊ Digoxin
  ◊ Clonidine
• Other causes:
  ◊ Myocardial ischemia involving the AV node
  ◊ Infiltrative or fibrosing diseases involving the heart and its conduction system
  ◊ Degeneration of the AV node secondary to aging
  ◊ Neuromuscular diseases (e.g., myotonic muscular dystrophy or Kearns-Sayre syndrome)

RISK FACTORS
• Use of the above mentioned medications
• Coronary artery disease
• History of previous AV nodal dysfunction
• Acute myocardial infarction (especially acute right coronary artery occlusion)
• Amyloidosis
• Chagas' disease
• Connective tissue diseases involving the heart (e.g., systemic lupus erythematosus, rheumatoid arthritis)

DIAGNOSIS

DIFFERENTIAL DIAGNOSIS
• Seizures
• Transient ischemia attacks
• Orthostatic hypotension
• Vasovagal attacks
• Neurocardiogenic syncope
• Cardiac arrhythmias
  ◊ Ventricular tachycardia
  ◊ Supraventricular tachycardia
  ◊ Re-entrant tachycardia
  ◊ Wolff-Parkinson-White syndrome
  ◊ Sinus arrest
  ◊ Sinus exit block
  ◊ "Sick-sinus syndrome"
  ◊ Transition from normal sinus rhythm to atrial fibrillation or from atrial fibrillation to normal sinus rhythm

LABORATORY
• Serum digoxin level
• Cardiac enzymes
Drugs that may alter lab results: None
Disorders that may alter lab results: Transient or long-standing renal failure may falsely elevate cardiac enzymes (creatine kinase)

PATHOLOGICAL FINDINGS N/A

SPECIAL TESTS N/A

IMAGING Transthoracic cardiac 2d-echo if infiltrative disease is suspected

DIAGNOSTIC PROCEDURES
• Cardiac coronary catheterization to rule out coronary ischemia
• Electrophysiologic testing to assess status of AV nodal conduction
• Myocardial biopsy if infiltrative disease is suspected
• ECG, event monitor or Holter monitor demonstrating (transient) complete heart block with slow or no ventricular escape

TREATMENT

APPROPRIATE HEALTH CARE
• Inpatient assessment in a monitored setting
• Continuing treatment - ambulatory

GENERAL MEASURES
• Cardiac monitoring
• Trans-thoracic pacer availability
• Atropine by the bedside

SURGICAL MEASURES
• Consider temporary pacemaker placement
• Permanent pacemaker placement, if etiology of transient complete heart block not reversible

ACTIVITY As tolerated after assessment

DIET Regular

PATIENT EDUCATION Once the diagnosis has been made and pacemaker has been implanted (if indicated) patient should be instructed in pacemaker guidelines

MEDICATIONS

DRUG(S) OF CHOICE
• For symptomatic bradyarrhythmias:
◊ For acute bradyarrhythmias - atropine, 1 mg IV push to be given during the complete heart block with hypotension; may be repeated once for a total dosage of 2 mg
◊ Epinephrine, 1 mg 1:10,000 IV push to be given during the complete heart block if associated with asystole; may be repeated every 5 minutes
◊ Isoproterenol drip,1 mg in 250 cc D5W or normal saline to be started at 5 micrograms per minute if patient maintains bradycardia and hypotensive after atropine given; may titrate drip as necessary
Contraindications: Use of epinephrine in bradycardia patient with a normal blood pressure may precipitate hypertensive crisis
Precautions: Possible tachycardiac response to the above mentioned medications
Significant possible interactions: None

ALTERNATIVE DRUGS   N/A

FOLLOWUP

PATIENT MONITORING
• Routine pacemaker checks, if permanent pacemaker implanted
• Followup Holter and/or event, monitor within two weeks after causal medications have been discontinued
• Discontinuation of driving, heavy machinery operation and being at unprotected heights pending normal followup

PREVENTION/AVOIDANCE   Avoidance
of taking any drug similar to those causing the complete heart block

POSSIBLE COMPLICATIONS
• Protracted bradycardia with hypotension leading to end-organ damage or death
• Loss of consciousness while operating machinery or at unprotected heights

EXPECTED COURSE/PROGNOSIS
Once diagnosis is made and appropriate treatment is implemented (e.g., pacemaker insertion), prognosis is excellent and further difficulty not expected

MISCELLANEOUS

ASSOCIATED CONDITIONS
• Myocardial ischemia
• Acute myocardial infarction
• Systemic manifestations of connective tissue disease
• Unreliable self-administration of medications
• Neuromuscular disease

AGE-RELATED FACTORS
Pediatric: N/A
Geriatric: More common problem in this age group
Others: N/A

PREGNANCY   Rare during pregnancy

SYNONYMS   Drop attacks

ICD-9-CM
426.9 Stokes-Adams syndrome

SEE ALSO
• Seizure disorders
• Sinus bradycardia
• Complete heart block
• Myocardial infarction
• Amyloidosis

OTHER NOTES   N/A

ABBREVIATIONS   N/A

REFERENCES
• Brandenburg RO, Fuster V, Giuliani ER, McGoon DC: Cardiology: Fundamentals and Practice. Chicago, Year Book Medical Publishers, 1987
• Braunwald E, ed: Heart Disease: A Textbook of Cardiovascular Medicine. 4th Ed. Philadelphia, W.B. Saunders Co., 1992
Illustrations: N/A
Internet references: http://www.5mcc.com

Author(s)
David J. Framm, MD, FACC

Stomatitis

BASICS

DESCRIPTION Generalized inflammation of the oral mucosa of many possible etiologies
System(s) affected: Skin/Exocrine
Genetics: N/A
Incidence/Prevalence in USA:
• Herpetic stomatitis, hand-foot-and-mouth disease, and recurrent aphthous stomatitis are very common
• Herpangina is fairly common as are nicotinic and denture related stomatitis. The remaining causes are uncommon or rare.
Predominant age:
• Herpetic-primary infections - children
• Hand-foot-and-mouth disease - children
• Vincent's stomatitis - teenagers and young adults
• Behçet's disease - young adults
• Herpangina - children
• Others - N/A
Predominant sex: Male = Female

SIGNS AND SYMPTOMS
• General:
  ◊ Depends on etiology
  ◊ Varies from minimal to severe pain
  ◊ Many have multiple intraoral ulcers from 1 mm to several centimeters in diameter
  ◊ Some with constitutional symptoms - fever, malaise, headache
• Allergic stomatitis:
  ◊ Intense shiny erythema
  ◊ Slight swelling
  ◊ Itching
  ◊ Dryness
  ◊ Burning
• Vincent's infection:
  ◊ Necrotic ulceration of interdental papillae and mucous membrane
• Thrush (candidiasis):
  ◊ White patches, slightly raised (resembling milk curds)
  ◊ Distribution - tongue, buccal mucosa, palate, gums, tonsils, larynx, pharynx, GI tract, skin; commonly seen in infants, immunocompromised patients; patients on long-term antibiotics, corticosteroids, and anti-neoplastic treatment
• Pseudomembraneous stomatitis:
  ◊ Membrane-like exudate
• Mucous lesions accompanying systemic disease:
  ◊ Mucous patches (syphilis)
  ◊ Strawberry (measles)
  ◊ Koplik's spots (measles)
  ◊ Ulcers (erythema multiforme)
  ◊ Smooth, fire-red, painful (pellagra)

CAUSES
• Allergy - foods, drugs, contact (some erythema multiforme)
• Vitamin deficiency - riboflavin (angular stomatitis)
• Viral - herpes simplex I and II (herpetic stomatitis), Coxsackie A (herpangina and hand-foot-and-mouth disease)
• Smoking (nicotinic stomatitis)
• Hormonal (possibly recurrent ulcerative stomatitis)
• Uncertain (recurrent aphthous stomatitis, Vincent's stomatitis, recurrent scarifying stomatitis, Behçet's disease, angular stomatitis, gangrenous stomatitis, erythema multiforme)
• Bacterial (scarlatina)
• Uremic (uremic/nephritic)
• Dentures

RISK FACTORS Listed with Causes

DIAGNOSIS

DIFFERENTIAL DIAGNOSIS
• Squamous cell cancer
• Herpetic stomatitis
• Hand-foot-and-mouth disease
• Recurrent aphthous stomatitis
• Vincent's stomatitis
• Nicotinic stomatitis
• Denture related stomatitis
• Erythema multiforme/Stevens-Johnson syndrome
• Recurrent ulcerative stomatitis
• Recurrent scarifying stomatitis
• Behçet's disease
• Angular stomatitis
• Noma (gangrenous stomatitis)
• Scarlatina (scarlet fever)
• Herpangina
• Uremic
• Pemphigus/pemphigoid

LABORATORY
• Hematologic profile
• Tzanck test of historic interest only
• Serologic test for syphilis
Drugs that may alter lab results: N/A
Disorders that may alter lab results: N/A

PATHOLOGICAL FINDINGS Biopsy suspicious lesions or lesions that fail to heal or chronically recur to rule out cancer or vasculitis

SPECIAL TESTS N/A

IMAGING N/A

DIAGNOSTIC PROCEDURES Biopsy if persistent/recurrent/suspicious

TREATMENT

APPROPRIATE HEALTH CARE
Outpatient, unless severe

GENERAL MEASURES
• In most cases treatment is symptomatic only
• Severe cases may require parenteral fluids, particularly in children
• Topical anesthesia
• Analgesics
• Oral rinses such as 1/2 strength hydrogen peroxide
• Mycostatin, if superinfected with candida
• Stop smoking

SURGICAL MEASURES N/A

ACTIVITY As tolerated by patient

DIET May need to avoid spicy, sharp, hard, and dry foods

PATIENT EDUCATION Griffith: Instructions for Patients; Philadelphia, W.B. Saunders Co.

MEDICATIONS

DRUG(S) OF CHOICE
• Steroids and cytotoxic drugs for Behçet's disease
• 2% viscous lidocaine (Xylocaine) for local discomfort
• Liquid diphenhydramine (Benadryl) po, or swish and spit
• Antibiotics for gangrenous stomatitis
• Antifungal ointment, e.g., nystatin (Mycostatin) for candida complicating angular stomatitis
• For candidiasis - nystatin oral suspension 400,000 units (4 mL) qid for 10 days. Use as oral rinse, then swallow.
• Acyclovir - 200-800 mg 5 times a day for 7-14 days for herpetic stomatitis
• Sucralfate (Carafate) - suspension 1 tsp swish in mouth or place on ulcers 4 times a day (is helpful)
Contraindications: Allergy to specific medication
Precautions: Toxic dose of topical lidocaine uncertain, but likely only 25-33% of infiltration dose - may have significant absorption from open ulcers or mucous membrane
Significant possible interactions: Refer to manufacturer's literature

ALTERNATIVE DRUGS
Steroid oral rinses or topical preparations for aphthous ulcers

FOLLOWUP

PATIENT MONITORING
Lesions need to be followed until resolved. If they fail to resolve, continuously recur, or appear suspicious, biopsy may be needed to establish a diagnosis.

PREVENTION/AVOIDANCE
Avoid causative factors

POSSIBLE COMPLICATIONS
• Recurrent scarifying stomatitis may result in intraoral scarring with restriction of oral mobility
• Behçet's disease may result in visual loss, pneumonia, colitis, vasculitis, large artery aneurysms, thrombophlebitis, or encephalitis
• Gangrenous stomatitis may lead to death
• Scarlet fever may result in cardiac disease
• Herpetic stomatitis may be complicated by ocular or CNS involvement

EXPECTED COURSE/PROGNOSIS
• Herpetic - self-limited with resolution in 7-14 days
• Hand-foot-and-mouth disease - same as herpetic
• Recurrent aphthous - 7-14 day course per episode
• Vincent's - may progress to fascial space infection with airway compromise or sepsis
• Nicotinic - will resolve with cessation of smoking
• Denture - will resolve with careful oral hygiene and daytime denture wear only
• Erythema multiforme - resolution in 2-3 weeks
• Stevens-Johnson: resolution in about 6 weeks with adequate supportive care
• Recurrent ulcerative - as the name implies, these recur over time, but the overall prognosis is good
• Recurrent scarifying - occasional patients suffer continuous ulcers, others recur with eventual scarring. The prognosis is otherwise good.
• Behçet's disease - may recur for several years. Prognosis for vision is poor. Overall prognosis is related to other aspects of the disease.
• Angular - after correction of mechanical problems, allergic disorders, and nutritional deficiencies the prognosis is good
• Gangrenous - this is the most serious stomatitis, requiring aggressive treatment with IV antibiotics and débridement to avoid death
• Scarlatina - the prognosis is related to other manifestations of the disease
• Herpangina - 7-14 day course with total resolution
• Uremic - depends on the underlying renal disease

MISCELLANEOUS

ASSOCIATED CONDITIONS
AIDS - associated with severe lesions

AGE-RELATED FACTORS
Pediatric: Certain etiologies more likely in the pediatric population: Herpetic-primary, hand-foot-and-mouth disease, herpangina
Geriatric: Certain etiologies more likely in the geriatric population, e.g., dentures
Others: N/A

PREGNANCY
May bring on recurrent ulcerative stomatitis

SYNONYMS
N/A

ICD-9-CM
528.0 Stomatitis
054.2 Herpetic stomatitis
528.2 Aphthous stomatitis
101 Vincent's stomatitis

SEE ALSO
N/A

OTHER NOTES
N/A

ABBREVIATIONS
N/A

REFERENCES
• Moran WJ: Diseases of the mouth. In: Rakel E, ed. Conn's Current Therapy, Philadelphia, W.B. Saunders Co., 1990
• Teele DW: Inflammatory diseases of the mouth and pharynx. In: Paparella MM, Shumrick DA, eds. Otolaryngology. Philadelphia, W.B. Saunders Co., 1980:974-1017
Illustrations: 11 available on CD-ROM
Internet references: http://www.5mcc.com

Author(s)
Douglas M. Hoy, MD

Stroke (Brain attack)

BASICS

DESCRIPTION The sudden onset of a focal neurological deficit resulting from either infarction or hemorrhage within the brain
System(s) affected: Nervous, Cardiovascular
Genetics: Inheritance is polygenic with a tendency to clustering of risk factors within families
Incidence/Prevalence in USA: Overall incidence 160/100,000 (age 50-65, 1000/100,000; > 80, 3000/100,000). Prevalence 135/100,000.
Predominant age: Risk increases over age 45 and is highest in the seventh and eighth decades
Predominant sex: Male > Female (3:1), but equalizes after menopause

SIGNS AND SYMPTOMS
• Carotid circulation (hemispheric): Hemiplegia, hemianesthesia, neglect, aphasia, visual field defects; less often headaches, seizures, amnesia, confusion
• Vertebrobasilar (brainstem or cerebellar): Diplopia, vertigo, ataxia, facial paresis, Horner's syndrome, dysphagia, dysarthria
• Impaired level of consciousness
• Cerebellar lesion in patients with headache, nausea, vomiting and ataxia

CAUSES
• Ischemic: Carotid atherosclerotic disease with artery-to-artery thromboembolism
• Cardiac: Cardioembolism secondary to valvular (mitral valve) pathology; mural hypokinesias or akinesias with thrombosis (acute anterior myocardial infarctions or congestive cardiomyopathies); cardiac arrhythmia (atrial fibrillation)
• Hypercoagulable states: Antiphospholipid antibodies, deficiency of protein S, protein C; presence of antithrombin 3, oral contraceptives
• Other causes: Spontaneous and post-traumatic (i.e., chiropractic manipulation) artery dissection, fibromuscular dysplasia, vasculitis, drugs (cocaine, amphetamines)
• Hemorrhagic
• Hypertension: may cause damage to putamen, internal capsule, cerebellum, brainstem, corona radiata
• Amyloid (congophylic) angiopathy: Lobar (cortical) hemorrhages in the elderly
• Vascular malformations: Arteriovenous malformation, cavernous angioma, venous angioma and capillary angioma

RISK FACTORS
• Age
• Hypertension
• Cardiac disease
• Smoking
• Diabetes
• Antiphospholipid antibodies
• Family history

DIAGNOSIS

DIFFERENTIAL DIAGNOSIS
• Migraine
• Focal seizure
• Tumor
• Subdural hematoma
• Hypoglycemia

LABORATORY   N/A
Drugs that may alter lab results: N/A
Disorders that may alter lab results: N/A

PATHOLOGICAL FINDINGS   N/A

SPECIAL TESTS
• Duplex carotid ultrasonography
• Cerebral angiography
• ECG
• Transthoracic echocardiogram (TTE); if normal and a cardiac source is suspected, followup with transesophageal echocardiogram
• Holter monitoring
• EEG for suspected seizure
• International normalized ratio (INR) and partial thromboplastin time (PTT). Coumadin prolongs PT.
• Antiphospholipid antibodies

IMAGING   Acute phase: CT of head to rule out hemorrhage

DIAGNOSTIC PROCEDURES   N/A

TREATMENT

APPROPRIATE HEALTH CARE
• Acute phase: Inpatient care, preferably in a stroke unit, IV tissue plasminogen activator (tPA) 0.9/kg in highly selected cases within 3 hours of ischemic stroke
• Surgical therapy: In medically fit patients with non-disabling stroke, carotid endarterectomy is indicated for stenosis of > 70% on side ipsilateral to stroke; medical therapy for < 50% stenosis, 50-69% depends on risk factors

GENERAL MEASURES
• Maintain oxygenation
• Monitor cardiac rhythm for 48 hours
• Control hyperglycemia (keep glucose < 220 mg/dL [12.1 mmol/L])
• Control of hypertension pressure if > 200/100 mm Hg (26.6/13.3 kPa)
• Prevent hyperthermia
• Early introduction of physiotherapy and ambulation
• Subcutaneous heparin 5,000 units subcutaneously every 12 hours

SURGICAL MEASURES   N/A

ACTIVITY   Ambulate as soon as possible

DIET
• Alert with no dysphagia: Diet as tolerated (no added salt if hypertensive)
• Alert with dysphagia: Pureed dysphagia diet or nasogastric feeding tube if indicated

PATIENT EDUCATION   National Stroke Association, 300 East Hampden Ave., Suite 240, Englewood, CO 80110-2622

Stroke (Brain attack)

MEDICATIONS

DRUG(S) OF CHOICE
• Enteric coated aspirin (EC ASA) 325-1300 mg/day
or
• Ticlopidine (Ticlid) 250 mg po bid
• Clopidogrel (Plavix)75 mg/day is ticlopidine's descendent, has fewer side effects, but shows an only slight advantage over ASA
Contraindications:
• EC ASA - active peptic ulcer disease, hypersensitivity to aspirin, patients who had bronchospastic reaction to ASA or other nonsteroidal anti-inflammatory drugs
• Ticlopidine - known hypersensitivity to the drug, presence of hematopoietic disorders, presence of a hemostatic disorder, conditions associated with active bleeding, severe liver dysfunction
Precautions:
• EC ASA - may aggravate pre-existing peptic ulcer disease, may worsen symptoms in some patients with asthma
• Ticlopidine - 2.4% of patients develop neutropenia (0.8% severe neutropenia) which is reversible with cessation of drug; monitor blood counts every 2 weeks for the first 3 months
Significant possible interactions:
• EC ASA - may potentiate effects of anticoagulants and sulfonylurea, hypoglycemic agents
• Ticlopidine - digoxin plasma levels decreased 15%, theophylline half-life increased from 8.6 to 12.2 hours

ALTERNATIVE DRUGS
• Dipyridamole (Persantine) alone or in combination with ASA of possible benefit
• Sulfinpyrazone (Anturane) of no proven benefit

FOLLOWUP

PATIENT MONITORING   Follow every 3 months for first year then yearly

PREVENTION/AVOIDANCE
• Stop smoking
• Control blood pressure, diabetes, hyperlipidemia
• EC ASA 650 mg bid or ticlopidine 250 mg po bid for patients with prior transient ischemic attack
• Use alcohol in moderation, if at all
• Regular exercise
• Maintain positive psychological outlook
• Maintain weight control

POSSIBLE COMPLICATIONS
• Shoulder subluxation
• Hyperextension knee injury
• Depression
• Sympathetic dystrophy

EXPECTED COURSE/PROGNOSIS
• Variable depending on severity of stroke
• Posterior circulation strokes have a higher acute mortality rate but generally make a better functional recovery than hemispheric strokes

MISCELLANEOUS

ASSOCIATED CONDITIONS   Major cause of death in first five years after a stroke is cardiac disease

AGE-RELATED FACTORS
Pediatric:
• Cardiac (especially developmental abnormalities)
• Metabolic: Homocystinuria, Fabry's disease
Geriatric: Amyloid (congophylic) angiopathy is most prevalent in elderly, especially if patient also has dementia
Others: Adults < 45 years old most likely to have a cardiac source of embolism

PREGNANCY
• Parturition may increase risk of rupture for aneurysm; amniotic fluid embolism may cause stroke at time of delivery
• Postpartum period associated with increased risk for cerebral venous thrombosis

SYNONYMS
• Cerebrovascular accident
• CVA
• Reversible ischemic neurological accident
• RIND

ICD-9-CM
431 Intracerebral hemorrhage
434.11 Cerebral embolism with cerebral infarction
436 Acute, ill-defined cerebrovascular disease (stroke)

SEE ALSO
• Transient ischemic attack (TIA)
• Stroke rehabilitation

OTHER NOTES   N/A

ABBREVIATIONS
EC ASA = enteric-coated aspirin

REFERENCES
• Hachinski V (ed): Stroke. Lancet 1998;352:(suppl III):1-30
• Hachinski V: Brain Attack: The Clinical Handbook. Meducom International,1999
Illustrations: N/A
Internet references: http://www.5mcc.com

Author(s)
Bart Demaerschalk, MD, FRCPC
Vladimir Hachinski, MD, DSc, FRCPC

Stroke rehabilitation

BASICS

DESCRIPTION Stroke rehabilitation involves restoration of function after medical and neurologic stability have been achieved
• Cerebrovascular diseases and/or disorders that affect central nervous system function by compromising delivery of blood or by hemorrhage resulting in ischemia, necrosis and gliosis
• Anterior lesions in the cerebrovascular system affect the arteries that supply the cerebral hemispheres and cause thrombotic strokes
• Posterior lesions affect arteries that supply the brain stem and yield crossed motor and/or sensory signs and symptoms of hemorrhagic strokes
• Both anterior and posterior lesions can cause sudden death, but the lower in the central nervous system the lesion, or the more incomplete the lesion, or the more hemorrhagic the lesion, the higher the chance for neurologic return and also for second, etc., strokes
System(s) affected: Nervous, Cardiovascular
Genetics: Similar to the probability of developing hypertension or coronary artery disease
Incidence/Prevalence in USA: 459/100,000
Predominant age: Over 45
Predominant sex: Male > Female

SIGNS AND SYMPTOMS
• Variable - depends upon the arterial system affected
• Hemiparesis
• Hemianesthesia
• Unilateral central facial palsy
• Homonymous hemianopsia
• Aphasia, apraxia (if the dominant cerebral hemisphere is involved)

CAUSES
• Coronary artery disease
• Hypertension
• Cerebral arteriosclerosis
• Cardiac thrombus embolus
• Foreign body embolus
• Frequently, the combination of gout, diabetes, hypertension has been untreated for some 5-10 years before the onset of the stroke disorder
• aneurysms and arteriovenous malformations

RISK FACTORS
• Many are lifestyle oriented and preventable. Factors include coffee ingestion, cigarette smoking, obesity, inactivity, hyperactivity to the point of exhaustion, emotional lability, sexual hyperactivity, starvation, antidepressant or diet reduction medication, alcohol or recreational drug habituation, unusual stress states.
• Ethnicity may be a risk factor but relationships to factors above first must be clarified

DIAGNOSIS

DIFFERENTIAL DIAGNOSIS
• Infection, tumor, bleeding disorders, endocrinologic, metabolic, gastrointestinal, toxic, etc.
• Different types of stroke disorders can occur in one patient
• Liver failure with/without transplantation can be associated with cognitive deficits that persist even after transplantation
• Brain tumors often present as stroke syndromes with significant personality and/or aphasic disorders and relatively less obvious weakness or spasticity upon examination

LABORATORY
• CBC
• Spinal fluid for routine studies (only if indicated)
• Urinalysis
• RPR
• ANA for collagen vascular disorders
• Consider quantitative immunoelectrophoresis with the combination of stroke disorders, anemia, hypertension
• Carotid flow studies
Drugs that may alter lab results: N/A
Disorders that may alter lab results: N/A

PATHOLOGICAL FINDINGS
Thrombotic, hemorrhagic, mixed, combinations can be present

SPECIAL TESTS
• Somatosensory, auditory, and visual evoked potential technology can monitor neurologic recovery.
• EEG sometimes useful in evaluating seizure disorders

IMAGING
• Scanning - CT, MRI and PET scanning give good data about anatomy, blood flow, and metabolic activity
• Serial exams can delineate the course of this disease and reveal hydrocephalus or brain tumors

DIAGNOSTIC PROCEDURES
• Spinal taps, myelography, pneumoencephalography, angiography all have special indications and contraindications at this time. None are routinely used.
• Electrodiagnosis for neuritis, radiculitis in specialized centers if available
• Endovascular procedures have great diagnostic implications.

TREATMENT

APPROPRIATE HEALTH CARE
Referral to a full service rehabilitation center - a rehabilitation medicine team can make the difference between independence and dependency. Refer when medically and neurologically stable.

GENERAL MEASURES
• Full service rehabilitation center characteristics: Comparison with national standards for admission, process, discharge, and followup care; closed units; regular team meetings to discuss long and short term objectives; quality assurance system in place; accreditation by Commission on Accreditation of Rehabilitation Facilities.
• Use deep heat (e.g., ultrasound, prolonged hydrotherapy) with caution in patients with reduced sensation and/or taking anticoagulants
• Use hydrotherapy and/or isometric exercise cautiously in patients with limited cardiopulmonary reserve
• In patients able to respond to the protocols after surgery, restorative, tendon transplant, or nerve transplants may be of value
• Cardiac precautions and a CPR team may be required during exercise programs since obese, hypertensive, or patients with coronary artery disease are at increased risk. Real-time monitoring might be required.
• Open units, especially in investor owned rehabilitation centers, need to be closely monitored for outcome and cost/benefit ratio type productivity quality
• Inpatient rehab in acute rehab units for 15-21 days after first uncomplicated strokes

SURGICAL MEASURES
• Microcatheter and microsurgical technology have been used to clip, embolize or reset aneurysms and other lesions.
• Applied cardioangiographic technology has generated new endovascular treatment procedures.

ACTIVITY
• Physical therapy, occupational therapy, speech pathology, psychology, nursing therapy should be delivered to the patient for at least three hours/day throughout the inpatient stay.
• The patient must be able to tolerate this vigorous activity level. If the patient becomes medically or neurologically unstable during the inpatient stay, a 48 hour leeway is usually built into the system. After that period, therapy must resume or the patient must be returned to an acute hospital bed. Most stroke acute rehabilitation units are usually able to deliver this type of functional return within one month of inpatient stay, although length of stay is individually determined.
• While most rehabilitative efforts take place within a very short time after ictus, successful rehabilitative efforts have taken place as long as five years later

DIET Depends upon other medical conditions

Syphilis

TREATMENT

APPROPRIATE HEALTH CARE
Outpatient, except for initiating IV penicillin or desensitization

GENERAL MEASURES
• Baseline serologies prior to treatment to monitor its success
• Prompt institution of antibiotics
• Symptomatic treatment of the chancres and rash of secondary syphilis (for patient's comfort only) includes baths, antihistamines, etc. Chancres require only routine cleansing with water and mild soap.

SURGICAL MEASURES N/A

ACTIVITY
• Full activity, but no sexual contacts until declared cured

DIET No special diet

PATIENT EDUCATION
• Need to trace and treat all sexual contacts of the patient
• Keep followup appointments to monitor success of therapy
• Advise patient to avoid intercourse until treatment is complete
• Local health department can provide literature and contact tracing

MEDICATIONS

DRUG(S) OF CHOICE
• Primary, secondary and latent less than one year: benzathine penicillin G, 2.4 million units IM for 1 dose
• Latent > 1 year: benzathine penicillin G, 2.4 million units IM weekly for 3 doses
• Neurosyphilis: aqueous procaine penicillin G (APPG) 2-4 million units IM daily for 10-14 days with probenecid 500 mg q6h, or 2-4 million units penicillin G IV every 4 hours for at least 10 days. Follow each therapy with benzathine penicillin G 2.4 million units IM weekly for 3 doses.
• Congenital: with abnormal CSF, 50,000 units/kg of aqueous procaine penicillin G (APPG) IM for at least 10 days. With negative CSF serologies, 50,000 units/kg benzathine penicillin G in one IM injection.
• Epidemiologic treatment for contacts without symptoms, treat as primary after baseline serologies are obtained
Contraindications: Allergy to penicillin
Precautions:
• HIV infected and pregnant patients may show poor response to recommended IM doses. Use IV therapy for all treatment failures in these patients.
• Do NOT give benzathine or procaine penicillins IV

Significant possible interactions: See manufacturers literature

ALTERNATIVE DRUGS
• Erythromycin, tetracyclines, ceftriaxone (Rocephin) may be used. However, in penicillin allergic patients, desensitization is easily accomplished and is recommended for HIV infected and pregnant patients so that penicillin can be used.
• Standard treatment with ceftriaxone and tetracycline used for gonorrhea is usually therapeutic for incubating syphilis

FOLLOWUP

PATIENT MONITORING Repeat serologies at 6, 12, and 24 months. Do serological studies more frequently in HIV infected patients.

PREVENTION/AVOIDANCE
• Discuss safe sex
• Use of condoms

POSSIBLE COMPLICATIONS
• Cardiovascular disease
• Central nervous system disease
• Membranous glomerulonephritis
• Paroxysmal cold hemoglobinemia
• Organ damage that cannot be reversed
• Jarisch-Herxheimer reaction, marked by fever, chills, headache, myalgias, new rash is common on starting treatment (of primary or secondary disease; less common with tertiary) due to the lysis of treponemes and should not be confused with a reaction to antibiotics. It is managed with antihistamines and antipyretics.

EXPECTED COURSE/PROGNOSIS
Excellent in all cases except late syphilis complications and a few HIV infected patients

MISCELLANEOUS

ASSOCIATED CONDITIONS
• Other sexually transmitted diseases
• HIV infection and hepatitis B (strongly urge patients treated for syphilis to obtain screenings for both)

AGE-RELATED FACTORS
Pediatric: In non-congenital cases, must consider possible child abuse
Geriatric: N/A
Others: N/A

PREGNANCY Early detection is imperative, all expectant mothers should have serologies as part of routine prenatal care in the first trimester. If high exposure risk, repeat in second trimester and at delivery.

SYNONYMS
• Lues
• The Great Imitator

ICD-9-CM 090.0-097 Syphilis

SEE ALSO
• Chlamydial sexually transmitted diseases
• Pelvic inflammatory disease (PID)
• Gonococcal infections

OTHER NOTES Many experts urge more aggressive treatment than standard regimens in all patients and strongly advocate the use of penicillin rather than any alternative antibiotic

ABBREVIATIONS
• CSF = cerebrospinal fluid
• FTA-ABS = fluorescent treponemal antibody absorption
• MHA-TP = microhemagglutination treponema pallidum
• VDRL = Venereal Disease Research Laboratory
• RPR = rapid plasma reagin

REFERENCES
• Centers for Disease control: Sexually transmitted diseases: Treatment guidelines 1998. MMWR Morb Mortal Wkly Rep 1998, 47 (RR-1), 1-118.
• Drugs for Sexually Transmitted Diseases. Medical Letter, 37:964, Dec 1995.
• Elimination of syphilis in the U.S. Science Vol 281;17 July 1998, p.353-354.
Illustrations: 3 available on CD-ROM
Internet references: http://www.5mcc.com

Author(s)
Kevin M. Hepler, MD, MBA

Systemic lupus erythematosus (SLE)

BASICS

DESCRIPTION A multi-system, autoimmune inflammatory condition characterized by a fluctuating, chronic course. Varies from mild to severe and may be lethal (CNS and renal forms).
System(s) affected: Hemic/Lymphatic/Immunologic, Nervous, Renal/Urologic, Endocrine/Metabolic, Skin/Exocrine, Gastrointestinal, Musculoskeletal
Genetics: Markers: HLA-B8; HLA-DR2; HLA-DR3
Incidence/Prevalence in USA: 20/100,000
Predominant age: All ages, but 30-50 are most common
Predominant sex: Female > Male (10:1)

SIGNS AND SYMPTOMS
- Arthritis
- Fever
- Anorexia
- Malaise
- Weight loss
- Skin lesions
- Oral ulcers
- Eye pain and/or redness
- Chest pain and/or shortness of breath
- Pallor
- Nausea, vomiting, diarrhea
- Muscles - tenderness, aching and stiffness
- Headaches and visual problems
- Psychosis/delirium

CAUSES
- Most cases are idiopathic
- Drugs - drug induced lupus is clinically different from idiopathic SLE

RISK FACTORS
- Race - blacks, Hispanics, Asians, and Native Americans have higher prevalence than whites.
- Genetic markers - HLA-B8, HLA-DR2, HLA-DR3.
- Hereditary complement deficiency especially C1q. C1r. C1s, C4 and C2
- Polymorphisms in the Fc gammaRIIa + Fc gammaRIIIa gene may be important risk factor in SLE

DIAGNOSIS

DIFFERENTIAL DIAGNOSIS
- SLE mimics numerous systemic conditions, especially those involving inflammation
- Many other disorders mimic SLE - rheumatoid arthritis, mixed connective tissue disease (MCTD), scleroderma, metastatic malignancy, fever of unknown origin, psychogenic rheumatism and many cutaneous rashes. No one test or biopsy is pathognomonic.

LABORATORY
- Positive antinuclear antibody (ANA)
- Anti-double standard DNA (dsDNA), anti-Sm, false-positive VDRL, or positive LE preparation. These tests have either high sensitivity (ANA, false-positive VDRL) or specificity (anti-dsDNA, anti-Sm and LE preparation) and are included as American Rheumatology Association (ARA) criteria for the diagnosis of SLE along with the clinical features.
- Sedimentation rate is nonspecific, but valuable in assessing activity of SLE
- Anemia
- Anticardiolipis antibody
- Leukopenia
- Lymphopenia
- Abnormal urinary sediment
- Proteinuria
- Increased prothrombin time
- Hypoalbuminuria
- Thrombocytopenia
- Increased serum creatinine
- Positive Coombs test
Drugs that may alter lab results: N/A
Disorders that may alter lab results: N/A

PATHOLOGICAL FINDINGS
Connective tissue disorders affecting skin, blood vessels, serous and synovial membranes
- Collagenous swelling
- Fibrinoid change
- Cellular necrosis
- Periarterial sclerosis
- Granulomatous reaction
- Infiltration of polymorphonuclear leukocytes, plasma cells, lymphocytes in walls of small vessels, arterioles of skin, spleen, glomeruli, endocardium pericardium, brain
- Hematoxylin bodies resembling those in LE cells
- Vegetation on heart valves

SPECIAL TESTS
- Complement levels, immune complex assays (cryoglobulins, Raji cell test, C1q precipitins)
- Coagulation studies (lupus anticoagulant)
- Biopsy of skin, kidney and peripheral nerves may reveal typical histopathology

IMAGING
- Cerebral angiography in CNS lupus
- Chest x-ray for pulmonary infiltration, pleural effusion
- MRI to detect CNS lupus
- Echocardiogram for pericardial effusion

DIAGNOSTIC PROCEDURES
- American Rheumatology Association (ARA) criteria are a combination of any 4 manifestations of the 11 listed
  ◊ Malar (butterfly) rash
  ◊ Discoid rash
  ◊ Photosensitivity
  ◊ Oral/nasopharyngeal ulcers
  ◊ Nonerosive arthritis
  ◊ Pleuritis or pericarditis
  ◊ Renal disorder - proteinuria or cylindruria
  ◊ Neurologic disorder - psychosis or seizures
  ◊ Hematologic disorder - hemolytic anemia, leukopenia (less than 4,000), lymphopenia (less than 1,500), thrombocytopenia (less than 100,000)
  ◊ Immunologic disorder
  ◊ Positive antinuclear antibody (ANA) in absence of drugs known to cause positive ANA
  Note: While the above criteria are required for proper epidemiologic classification of SLE, in practical situations, the combination of a multi-system inflammatory illness, positive antinuclear antibody (ANA) and absence of a better diagnosis often represents the most practical way to make a clinical diagnosis

✚ TREATMENT

APPROPRIATE HEALTH CARE
Outpatient with regular monitoring

GENERAL MEASURES
- Avoidance of or protection from ultraviolet light by using sunscreens, hats, etc.
- Early intervention when infections occur
- Energy conservation
- Stress avoidance/management

SURGICAL MEASURES N/A

ACTIVITY
- As active as possible
- Those with arthritis may be limited by their pain, but active exercises are to be encouraged

DIET
No special diet unless for complications such as renal failure

PATIENT EDUCATION
Printed materials available on lupus from the Arthritis Foundation, 1314 Spring Street N.W., Atlanta, GA 30309, (404)872-7100; and from the Lupus Foundation of America, 1717 Massachusetts Avenue, NW, Suite 203, Washington, DC 20036, (800)558-0121

Systemic lupus erythematosus (SLE)

MEDICATIONS

DRUG(S) OF CHOICE
No one drug of choice available. Treatment is symptomatic with certain exceptions. Use of local steroids for cutaneous manifestations, NSAIDs for minor arthritis symptoms, low dose steroids for minor discomfort and high dose steroids for major inflammatory disease.
• Immunosuppressants are indicated for renal disease and severe disease in other organs
• NSAIDs: minor arthritis
• Sunscreen and topical steroids for cutaneous lupus
• Hydroxychloroquine 310 mg (400 mg of the sulfate salt) qd for more significant arthritis or dermal lupus
• Prednisone 30-60 mg qd for major symptoms in one or more organ systems
• Cyclophosphamide 0.5 gm/m2 IV monthly together with prednisone 60 mg po qd tapering to 10 mg every other day after 4 months for glomerulonephritis
• Methotrexate 5-25 mg oral or subcutaneous, weekly in 1 single dose has been effective as a "steroid sparer" for arthritis, rash, serositis or fever
• IV immune globulin (IVIG) pulse has been effective in the temporary treatment of SLE thrombocytopenia
• Heparin or warfarin (Coumadin) in obvious thrombotic disease and/or CNS symptoms, when associated with a positive "lupus anticoagulant" test or anticardiolipin antibody
Contraindications: Refer to manufacturer's profile of each drug
Precautions: Ensure good hydration when administering cyclophosphamide due to possibility of hemorrhagic cystitis
Significant possible interactions: Refer to manufacturer's profile of each drug

ALTERNATIVE DRUGS N/A

FOLLOWUP

PATIENT MONITORING
• Follow acute flares frequently, (weekly to monthly) for adjustment of medication based on clinical impression. Laboratory parameters are of limited value. CBC useful in hematologic lupus. Serum creatinine or renal clearance tests of value in renal lupus. Sedimentation rate often helps determine adequate suppression of symptoms or development of a remission.
• The confirming tests for lupus (ANA titers, anti-DNA titers, complement levels, etc.) are usually not helpful in follow-up assessment
• Use of continuing medication depends upon symptoms. Exception is in the case of renal lupus for which it has been shown that a defined course of monthly IV cyclophosphamide has been of value.
• Baseline ophthalmological exam and yearly exam while on hydroxychloroquine

PREVENTION/AVOIDANCE
• Avoiding sun exposure is only necessary for approximately one sixth of SLE patients (those who self report such sensitivity)
• Routine vaccinations are safe and appropriate for SLE patients
• Drugs known to induce SLE in normal individuals are not necessarily contraindicated in patients who have idiopathic SLE

POSSIBLE COMPLICATIONS Fever, vasculitis, panniculitis, myositis, avascular necrosis of bone, endocarditis, pulmonary fibrosis, renal failure, organic brain syndromes, peripheral neuropathy, stroke syndromes, pancreatitis and elevated liver enzymes, infertility, ascites, venous thrombosis, seizures

EXPECTED COURSE/PROGNOSIS
• Most patients with lupus follow a course of remissions and exacerbations. Many experience spontaneous permanent remission.
• Treatment of renal lupus (the most serious form) with immunosuppressors, renal dialysis, and renal transplantation, has increased the five year life expectancy to over 90%. For those patients surviving the first two years of disease, life expectancy is essentially normal.
• In patients with drug-induced lupus, symptoms should gradually decrease upon discontinuation of the suspected agent.

MISCELLANEOUS

ASSOCIATED CONDITIONS Other autoimmune diseases - rheumatoid arthritis, hypothyroidism, diabetes

AGE-RELATED FACTORS
Pediatric: Stroke syndromes frequently seen in children
Geriatric:
• Higher percentage of males involved among the elderly
• Since "false-positive ANA" reaches 15% in the elderly, caution in interpretation is required in this age group
Others: N/A

PREGNANCY
• Onset of lupus and lupus flares are more common during pregnancy
• Fetal loss is increased for mothers with lupus
• Newborns of mothers who have lupus are more likely to have cardiac arrhythmias
• Specialists' collaboration during pregnancy is indicated

SYNONYMS
• SLE
• Disseminated lupus erythematosus

ICD-9-CM 710.0 Systemic lupus erythematosus

SEE ALSO
• Anemia, autoimmune hemolytic
• Glomerulonephritis, membranous

OTHER NOTES N/A

ABBREVIATIONS N/A

REFERENCES
• Kelley WN, Harris ED, Ruddy S, Sledge CB: Textbook of Rheumatology. 4th Ed. Philadelphia, W.B. Saunders Co., 1993
• Kippel JH, Dippe PA, eds: Rheumatology, St. Louis, Mosby, 1994
• Tan FK, Arnett FC: The genetics of lupus. Curr Opin in Rheumatol 1998;10(4):399-408
• Godfrey T, et al: Therapeutic advances in SLE. Curr Opin in Rheumatol 1998;10(4):435-41
Illustrations: 5 available on CD-ROM
Internet references: http://www.5mcc.com

Author(s)
Michael Tutt

Tapeworm infestation

BASICS

DESCRIPTION Tapeworms, which can be parasitic in humans, are cestodes which in their adult phase are segmented flatworms that may reside in the gastrointestinal tract. Adult worms consist of a head (scolex), which is where it attaches to the host; the neck (germinal region); and a segmented body (strobila), with each individual segment (proglottid) containing sets of male and female reproductive organs that produce eggs. The life cycle of all but one tapeworm (Hymenolepis nana) requires an intermediate host, where they grow as larval forms in tissue that is then ingested by the final host such as humans, where it subsequently develops as an adult. Hymenolepis nana can complete all stages of development in humans, helping to make it the most common tapeworm in humans. Most tapeworm infections are confined to the gastrointestinal tract, however somatic disease can occur with Taenia Solium eggs being ingested (Cysticercosis), or with Echinococcus infections, making infections with these more serious. Neurocysticercosis is the most common inpatient disorder due to parasite infection. Tapeworms/their usual intermediate host/and type of infection in humans/description include:
• Taenia saginata/beef/intestinal worm/ Takes 2-4 months after ingestion to become adult tapeworm. 3-10 meters long. Usually single tapeworm. Proglottids are motile and can crawl out of anus. May live 30 years.
• Taenia solium/pork/a.) intestinal worm, b.) Cysticercosis, a somatic infection/2-4 months to become adult worm. 3 meters long, occasionally multiple. Proglottids not motile. May live up to 25 years. Ingestion of encysted larvae (cysticerci) cause intestinal tapeworm. Ingestion of T.solium eggs causes Cysticercosis. Eggs look identical to T. saginata eggs.
• Diphyllobothrium latum and other species/fresh water fish/intestinal worm/longest adult tapeworm - up to 25 meters. Matures to adult in 3-5 weeks.
• Hymenolepis nana/rodent, insects, or even the human themselves/intestinal worm/ Mature to adult worms in 10-12 days. Seldom exceeds 40 mm long. Proglottids rarely seen in stool. Eggs can autoinfect individual, or occasionally insects (especially meal worms). Fecal oral transmission possible. Lifespan 4-10 weeks, but autoinfection can perpetuate infection. Usually self cleared by adolescence.
• Echinococcus a.) granulosis, b.)multilocularis/humans, sheep, cattle are intermediate hosts with dogs the definitive hosts for granulosis and rodents for multilocularis/Somatic infections: a.) hydatid disease of liver, spleen, etc., b.) alveolar hydatid disease/Adult worm lives in dogs (or rodents), human ingests eggs, larvae hatch and are carried through circulation to various organs such as liver and lungs where develop into hydatid cysts which enlarge causing symptoms perhaps 5-20 years later.

• Hymenolepis diminuta/rodents and insects/intestinal worm/90 cm long. Humans rare accidental host by swallowing contaminated mealworms or grain beetles in grain.
• Dipylidium caninum/dogs and cats and flea/intestinal worm/10-70 cm long. Motile proglottids, shape of cucumber seeds, can crawl out anus. Rare accidental infection of humans from ingesting infected flea that came from dogs or cats.
System(s) affected: Gastrointestinal, Nervous
Genetics: N/A
Incidence/Prevalence in USA: Occurs infrequently in USA. More often associated with immigrant population and ethnic groups with certain cultural eating habits. Can be endemic in other parts of the world, where fecal contamination can get into water or food source.
Predominant age: All ages affected. Hymenolepis nana and diminuta more common in children.
Predominant sex: Male = Female

SIGNS AND SYMPTOMS
• Taenia saginata (beef tapeworm): Generally asymptomatic. Often noted by passing eggs or proglottids, which can occasionally be felt crawling out of anus. Mild gastrointestinal symptoms may occur (one third) - nausea, abdominal pain, change in appetite, weakness, weight loss, allergic symptoms urticaria, pruritis.
• Taenia solium (pork tapeworm):
  ◊ Intestinal worm - generally asymptomatic, noted passing eggs or proglottids (which are not motile). Occasional minor abdominal complaints similar to T. saginata.
  ◊ Larval migration - Cysticercosis - most common to brain and skeletal muscle. Neurologic manifestations such as new onset of seizures, focal neurologic deficits, hydrocephalus, headache, vomiting, visual changes, dizziness.
• Diphyllobothrium latum (fish tapeworm): Generally asymptomatic, noted passing eggs, vomiting segment of worm, or occasionally passing proglottid segments. Occasionally mild abdominal discomfort, weight loss. Worm has marked affinity for vitamin B12, 40% decreased B12 levels, 2% megaloblastic anemia with glossitis, rare B12 associated neurologic symptoms.
• Hymenolepis nana (dwarf tapeworm): Usually asymptomatic. If heavy infection: anorexia, abdominal pain, and diarrhea.
• Echinococcosis (hydatid disease): Symptoms related to growth of cyst. Liver cysts - abdominal pain, RUQ mass, obstructive jaundice. Cyst rupture - fever, urticaria, pruritis, anaphylaxis. Pulmonary cyst, cough, chest pain, hemoptysis. Other organs possible - bone with pathologic fractures, CNS - space-occupying lesions, heart - conduction defects, pericarditis.
• Hymenolepis diminuta (rodent tapeworm): Most asymptomatic. Pass eggs in stool, proglottids disintegrate. Headache, mild GI symptoms - anorexia, nausea, cramps diarrhea.

• Dipylidium caninum (dog tapeworm): Most asymptomatic. Occasionally abdominal pain, diarrhea, anal pruritis, urticaria. May observe proglottid in diaper or stool.

CAUSES Eating the infective form of the parasite either by eating contaminated food such as undercooked beef, pork, fish, or infected insects that may be in cereals or grains, or through fecal-oral contamination.

RISK FACTORS
• Taenia's: Eating raw or undercooked beef or pork, particularly in Africa, Latin America, Middle East, Central Asia, India
• Cysticercosis: Presence of a tapeworm carrier in close environment. Water contaminated with sewage
• Diphyllobothrium: Eating raw or undercooked fish, particularly in northern Europe
• Hymenolepis nana: More frequent in children, institutionalized, malnourished, immunodeficient
• Echinococcus: Keeping dogs around sheep and goats highest risk for hydatid cyst disease

DIAGNOSIS

DIFFERENTIAL DIAGNOSIS When diagnosed by passing egg or proglottid must differentiate from other parasitic diseases. Possible to present as gastroenteritis, irritable bowel syndrome, intestinal obstruction, cholecystitis, or biliary obstruction. Cysts disease, depending upon location of cysts, may resemble other mass lesions in similar locations. Neurocysticercosis can be common cause of new onset of seizures. Diphyllobothrium may present as pernicious anemia.

LABORATORY
• May have mild to moderate eosinophilia, increased IgE
• Microscopic analysis of eggs or proglottids
Drugs that may alter lab results: N/A
Disorders that may alter lab results: N/A

PATHOLOGICAL FINDINGS
• Intestinal tapeworms generally no pathological findings
• Cysticercosis: Cysts, 5-10 mm in soft tissue. Calcified cysts in CNS, muscle
• Echinococcus: Hydatid cyst in liver, lung, other tissues
• Diphyllobothrium: Macrocytic megaloblastic anemia in 2%

SPECIAL TESTS
- Stool evaluation of O&P
- Microscopic evaluation of proglottid collected in water or saline
- Antibody testing by ELISA to differentiate T. saginata eggs from T. solium
- Immunoblot assay for certain parasites
- DNA probes for T. saginata or T. solium
- Consider serologic testing if identify tinea solium eggs or proglotids (as autoinfection possible)

IMAGING
- Intestinal tapeworms occasionally seen by small bowel enteroclysis
- Cysticercosis best diagnosed by CT or MRI. Possibly by plain films.
- Echinococcus cysts may be seen on CT, ultrasound, liver scan, plain films

DIAGNOSTIC PROCEDURES
- Occasional excisional biopsy of cysticercosis cyst.
- CT guided aspiration of hydatid cysts, with instillation of ethanol after aspiration and pretreatment for 1 month with albendazole.

TREATMENT

APPROPRIATE HEALTH CARE
Outpatient unless complications from cysts

GENERAL MEASURES
- Treatment of large percentage of population in endemic area can help
- General supportive care during treatment
- Good hygienic measures should be employed
- Asymptomatic cysticercosis may resolve spontaneously without treatment. Treatment may induce an inflammatory response and symptoms.

SURGICAL MEASURES
Cysticercosis cysts and hydatid cysts have been removed surgically, with care not to leak fluid.

ACTIVITY
As tolerated

DIET
As tolerated

PATIENT EDUCATION
- Proper cooking of beef, pork, fish
- Proper freezing of meat or fish
- Fecal-oral precautions with good hand washing
- Treatment of infected dogs, and preventing fleas

MEDICATIONS

DRUG(S) OF CHOICE
- Praziquantel:
  ◊ Single dose of 5-10 mg/kg for taeniasis, diphyllobothriasis, and most other intestinal cestodes (cure rate > 95%)
  ◊ Single dose of 25 mg/kg for H. nana (cure rate >95%)
  ◊ 50 mg/kg/day divided tid x 14 days for children and adults for Cysticercosis
- Niclosamide: Single dose of 2 gm for adult or 1 gm for children (cure rate 90% for taeniasis and slightly less for Diphyllobothriasis)
- Albendazole:
  ◊ For Echinococcus hydatid cysts. Adults 400 mg bid x 28 days. May need several courses. Children > 2 years, use adult dose. Children 1-2 years, 200 mg/day.
  ◊ For Neurocysticercosis, 15 mg/kg tid x 8-15 days
- Steroids and anticonvulsants for neurocysticercosis

Contraindications: Prior sensitivity

Precautions:
- Niclosamide: Occasional nausea and abdominal pain, diarrhea, drowsiness, dizziness
- Praziquantel: Mild but frequent dizziness, myalgias, nausea, diarrhea, abdominal pain
- Albendazole: Occasional diarrhea and abdominal pain. Rare leukopenia, increased serum transaminase levels.

Significant possible interactions:
Phenytoin and carbamazepine can induce metabolism of praziquantel by cytochrome P-450 causing treatment failures. Cimetadine can increase concentration of praziquantel and albendazole enhancing their effects.

ALTERNATIVE DRUGS Niclosamide: 2 gm, then 1 gm qd X 5 more days for H. nana.

FOLLOWUP

PATIENT MONITORING
Examine several stool specimens for O&P at sufficient interval to allow regrowth of worms: 3 months for Taenia species and 1 month for others. May follow neurocysticercosis with subsequent CT to see if resolved.

PREVENTION/AVOIDANCE
- Treatment of infected animals, populations and screening household contacts, immigrants
- Improved sewage treatment
- See Patient Education

POSSIBLE COMPLICATIONS
- Larval form of T. solium can cause systemwide cysticercosis, including neurocysticercosis, which can be etiology of up to 25% of cases of new-onset seizures in indigenous areas
- Echinococcus hydatid cysts may occur causing abnormalities in the organ involved. Cyst rupture can cause spread of disease and anaphylaxis.
- B12 deficiency with D. latum
- Proglottid of T. saginata can rarely obstruct appendix, pancreatic and bile ducts
- D. latum can occasionally cause intestinal obstruction, cholangitis, cholecystitis

EXPECTED COURSE/PROGNOSIS
- Cure of > 95% of intestinal tapeworms with medications, occasionally requiring a second treatment
- H. nana often self cured by adolescence
- E. multilocularis often severe and even fatal
- Prognosis of systemic cysts influenced by their location

MISCELLANEOUS

ASSOCIATED CONDITIONS N/A

AGE-RELATED FACTORS
Pediatric: H. nana, highest among children with fecal-oral spread. H. diminuta, and Dipylidium caninum more common in children, as more likely to accidentally ingest insects.
Geriatric: N/A
Others: N/A

PREGNANCY N/A

SYNONYMS N/A

ICD-9-CM
122 Echinococcus (4th digit specifies location of disease)
123 Other cestode infection. (specific organisms coded separately)

SEE ALSO N/A

OTHER NOTES N/A

ABBREVIATIONS
O&P = Ova and Parasites

REFERENCES
- Isselbacher KJ, et al (eds): Harrison's Principles of Internal Medicine 13th Edition, New York, McGraw-Hill, 1994
- Liu LX, Weller PF: Antiparasitic Drugs. New England Journal of Medicine 1996 May 2; 334(18): 1178-1184
- Miranda A: Neurocysticercosis. Amer Fam Phys 1993;47(5):1193-1197
- Schantz PM: Tapeworms (cestodiasis). Gastroenterology Clinics of North America 1996;25(3):637-653
- Wyngaarden JB, Smith LH, Bennett JC (eds): Cecil Textbook of Medicine. 19th Ed. Philadelphia, W.B. Saunders Co., 1992
Illustrations: N/A
Internet references: http://www.5mcc.com

Author(s)
Kenton Voorhees, MD

Teething

BASICS

DESCRIPTION Teething is the eruption of the deciduous teeth which most children experience without difficulty. It is a natural, gradual and predictable process but the timetable varies from baby to baby.
- Deciduous teeth
  ◊ Most deciduous teeth begin to erupt at 5-7 months of age and teething is completed by 2-3 years
  ◊ The mandibular central incisors erupt first, then the two or four maxillary incisors followed by the lower lateral incisors
  ◊ After a few months, the four molars appear (lower ones at 12 months, the upper ones at 14 months)
  ◊ After the cuspid teeth appear at 16-18 months of age the second molars erupt at 25-33 months
  ◊ About 25% normal babies may have delayed eruption of teeth until 4 or 6 teeth simultaneously appear after their first birthday
  ◊ Premature babies erupt teeth according to their gestational age rather than chronological age. If teething seems particularly delayed, refer patient to a pediatric dentist.
- Teeth in neonates
  ◊ One in 2000 neonates are born with a tooth (appears to be familial)
  ◊ These neonatal teeth may be loose but most are the normal deciduous lower central incisors and can persist
  ◊ Mild ulceration in the sublingual area has been reported in 18% of these babies
  ◊ Because of the potential for aspiration there is some controversy about elective removal of the loose teeth (most pediatric dentists would remove these teeth if they are loose)

System(s) affected: Gastrointestinal
Genetics: N/A
Incidence/Prevalence in USA: N/A
Predominant age: Birth to 2 1/2 years
Predominant sex: N/A

SIGNS AND SYMPTOMS
- A large percent of babies have no signs or symptoms of teething
- Excessive drooling and chewing on fingers begins at 3-4 months of age. This is also the time that normal hand-mouth stimulation increases salivation.
- A small red or white spot may appear over the swollen gum just prior to tooth eruption
- Local inflammation, swelling and occasional hemorrhage can be found on the involved gums
- Discomfort may be noted more with the eruption of the first tooth, the molars and/or with the simultaneous eruption of multiple teeth
- Restlessness, irritability, disturbed sleep, changes in feeding patterns, nasal discharge, mild cough, chin rash, fever, diarrhea, pulling of ear and rubbing of the cheeks have been reported by parents. It is impossible to document that these are caused by teething, so parents and health providers should consider other possible etiologies so as not to miss or delay diagnosing an illness.

CAUSES   N/A

RISK FACTORS   N/A

DIAGNOSIS

DIFFERENTIAL DIAGNOSIS
Herpetic gingivostomatitis - infants with fever, irritability, sleeplessness and difficulty feeding may have underlying infection caused by herpes simplex virus. Some of these infants with positive culture may not have evidence of inflammation or ulceration expected in gingivitis.

LABORATORY   N/A
Drugs that may alter lab results: N/A
Disorders that may alter lab results: N/A

PATHOLOGICAL FINDINGS   N/A

SPECIAL TESTS   N/A

IMAGING   N/A

DIAGNOSTIC PROCEDURES   N/A

TREATMENT

APPROPRIATE HEALTH CARE
Outpatient

GENERAL MEASURES
- Treatment for teething include reassurance for the parents and symptomatic relief, if needed
- Provide the infant with a safe, one piece teething ring, clean cloth or pacifier for gumming
- Rub the involved swollen gums if the baby appears to be comforted
- Cool fluids may be offered but avoid frozen foods or objects. These could cause thermal damage to the tissues.
- Toast, cookies, bagels and crackers are offered by some parents for teething, but parents must observe carefully to prevent choking
- Avoid over-the-counter preparations for teething such as Xylocaine 2%, Baby Ora-Gel, Num-zit Gel, Num-zit Liquid, Ambesol. Misuse, overuse and sensitivity have been reported.
- Avoid the use of alcohol
- For the infant with low grade fever, irritability and/or inflamed gums (where other comforting measures have not been of help) - acetaminophen, in proper doses (10-15 mg/kg/dose every 4 hours prn), can be used intermittently
- Gum hematomas that erupt appear as a blue cyst. Most do not require medical intervention. Be sure there are no other signs of a bleeding disorder.
- Breast feeding babies may attempt to chew on the nipple at the end of sucking while teething but can be taught not to bite. Breast feeding can continue after teeth are present.
- Advise parents to avoid: Sugared pacifiers, painted furniture which may contain lead, tying teething ring with cord around the infant's neck, and imported fluid-filled teething rings

SURGICAL MEASURES   N/A

ACTIVITY   No restrictions

DIET   No special diet

PATIENT EDUCATION
- Parents should be cautioned not to misinterpret teething as the cause of any systemic manifestation. The health provider should be consulted for any systemic complaints.
- The ABC's of Teething, Am Academy of Pediatric Dentistry, Public Relations Manual

MEDICATIONS

DRUG(S) OF CHOICE N/A
Contraindications: N/A
Precautions: N/A
Significant possible interactions: N/A

ALTERNATIVE DRUGS N/A

FOLLOWUP

PATIENT MONITORING N/A

PREVENTION/AVOIDANCE N/A

POSSIBLE COMPLICATIONS N/A

EXPECTED COURSE/PROGNOSIS
Normal progression through the teething process without illness

MISCELLANEOUS

ASSOCIATED CONDITIONS N/A

AGE-RELATED FACTORS
Pediatric: N/A
Geriatric: N/A
Others: N/A

PREGNANCY N/A

SYNONYMS N/A

ICD-9-CM N/A

SEE ALSO N/A

OTHER NOTES N/A

ABBREVIATIONS N/A

REFERENCES
• King NM, Lee A: Prematurely erupted teeth in the newborn infant. J Ped, 1989;114:807
• Gardiner J: Erupted teeth in the newborn. Proc Roy Soc Med, 1961;4:504
• Falkner F: Deciduous tooth eruption. Archives Disease of Childhood, 1957;32:386-391
• Seward M: General disturbances attributed to the eruption of human primary dentition. J of Dent for Children, 1972;39(3):178-183
• Golden N, Takieddine F, Hirsch V: Teething age - prematurely born infants. Am J of Dis of Child, 1981;135:903-904
• McDonald RE: Eruption of the teeth, local, systematic and congenital factors that influence the process. In: Dentistry for the Child and Adolescent. 5th Ed. St. Louis, C.V. Mosby Co., 1987:189-196
• King DL, Steinhauer W, Garcia-Godoy F, Elkins CO: Herpetic gingivostomatitis and teething difficulty in infants. Pediatric Dentistry 1992;14:82-85
Illustrations: N/A
Internet references: http://www.5mcc.com

Author(s)
Dan Doss, DDS

Temporomandibular joint (TMJ) syndrome

 BASICS

DESCRIPTION Syndrome characterized by pain and tenderness in the jaw muscles, sound and/or pain over the temporomandibular joint (TMJ), with limitation of mandibular movement
System(s) affected: Musculoskeletal
Genetics: N/A
Incidence/Prevalence in USA: Symptoms or signs of TMJ dysfunction are present in up to one half of the population but only 5-25% seek treatment
Predominant age: Symptoms more common age 30-50
Predominant sex: Female > Male (3:1)

SIGNS AND SYMPTOMS
- Facial and/or TMJ pain
- Locking or catching of the jaw
- TMJ noises - clicking, grinding, popping
- Headache
- Earache
- Neck pain

CAUSES
- TMJ synovitis
- TMJ disc derangement
- Hyper- or hypomobile TMJ
- Occluso-muscular dysfunction (bruxism)
- Masticatory muscle spasm
- Trauma
- Poorly fitting dentures

RISK FACTORS
- Chronic oral habits such as clenching or grinding of the teeth
- Osteoarthritis, rheumatoid arthritis
- Dental malocclusion
- Fibrositis
- Psychosocial stress

 DIAGNOSIS

DIFFERENTIAL DIAGNOSIS
- Condylar fracture/dislocation
- Trigeminal neuralgia
- Dental or periodontal conditions
- TMJ neoplasm

LABORATORY N/A
Drugs that may alter lab results: N/A
Disorders that may alter lab results: N/A

PATHOLOGICAL FINDINGS
- Condylar head displacement
- Anterior disc displacement
- Posterior capsulitis
- Loosening of disc and capsular attachments
- Chondroid metaplasia of disc leading to disc perforation and degeneration

SPECIAL TESTS Jaw range of motion (opening, closing, lateral, protrusive) and masticatory muscle strength

IMAGING
- Single-contrast videoarthrography demonstrates joint dynamics and disc movement
- Panoramic dental radiographs
- MRI - noninvasive study for disc position. Information gained helps in deciding conservative versus surgical management.

DIAGNOSTIC PROCEDURES
Arthroscopy

 TREATMENT

APPROPRIATE HEALTH CARE
Outpatient treatment

GENERAL MEASURES
- Jaw rest
- Local heat therapy
- Anti-inflammatory medications
- Muscle relaxants
- Analgesics
- Correction of malocclusion with orthodontic appliance
- Stress reduction
- Behavior modification to eliminate tension-relieving oral habits
- Buccal separator orthodontic appliance

SURGICAL MEASURES N/A

ACTIVITY Jaw rest

DIET Soft diet to reduce chewing

PATIENT EDUCATION
- Be aware of any teeth-clenching or grinding habits, and relax the jaw by disengaging the teeth
- Avoid wide uncontrolled opening such as yawning
- Management of stress. Behavioral modification counseling may be helpful.

MEDICATIONS

DRUG(S) OF CHOICE Nonsteroidal anti-inflammatory drugs (NSAID's) - no single drug more efficacious than another
Contraindications:
• History of anaphylaxis to aspirin
• Peptic ulcer disease
• Renal insufficiency
Precautions:
• Peptic ulcers, gastritis or GI bleeding may occur with chronic use
• May cause acute interstitial nephritis
• Drug accumulation with renal insufficiency
• Liver function abnormalities in up to 15% of patients
Significant possible interactions:
• Albumin-bound drugs - displacement of either drug
• Warfarin - increased prothrombin time
• Lithium - increased lithium plasma level
• Furosemide - decreased natriuretic effect
• Propranolol - decreased anti-hypertensive effect

ALTERNATIVE DRUGS Analgesic agents; muscle relaxants

FOLLOWUP

PATIENT MONITORING
• Ongoing assessment of clinical response to conservative therapies (NSAID's, behavior modification, occlusal splints) is necessary
• A surgical procedure to correct disc displacement or replace a damaged disc may be indicated only if the patient has not responded to conservative treatment

PREVENTION/AVOIDANCE Elimination of tension-relieving oral habits and reducing overall muscle tension

POSSIBLE COMPLICATIONS
• Secondary degenerative joint disease
• Chronic TMJ dislocation
• Loss of joint range of motion
• Depression and chronic pain syndromes

EXPECTED COURSE/PROGNOSIS
• With conservative therapy, symptoms resolve in 3/4 of the cases within three months
• Patients benefit the most from a comprehensive treatment approach including correction of occlusal discrepancies, restoration of normal muscle function, pain control, stress management and behavior modification

MISCELLANEOUS

ASSOCIATED CONDITIONS
Cranio-mandibular disorders

AGE-RELATED FACTORS
Pediatric: N/A
Geriatric: N/A
Others: N/A

PREGNANCY No association

SYNONYMS
• Myofascial pain-dysfunction (MPD) syndrome

ICD-9-CM
524.60 Temporomandibular joint disorders, unspecified (TMJ)

SEE ALSO
• Bruxism

OTHER NOTES N/A

ABBREVIATIONS N/A

REFERENCES
• Dolwick MF, Dimitroulis G: Is there a role for temperomandibular joint surgery? British Jour of Oral and Maxillofacial Surg 1994;32(5): 307-313
• Wright EF, Schiffman EL: Treatment alternatives for patients with masticatory myofacial pain. J ADA 1995;126(7):1030-1039
• dosSantos J: Supportive conservative therapies for temporomandibular disorders. Dental Clin NA 1995;39(2):459-477
• Laskin DM: Putting order into temperomandibular disorders. J Oral Maxillofac Surg 1998;56(2):121
• Kumar KL, Cooney TG: Temporomandibular disorders. J Gen Intern Med 1994;9(2):106-112
Illustrations: N/A
Internet references: http://www.5mcc.com

Author(s)
Scott A. Fields, MD

Tendinitis

BASICS

DESCRIPTION Inflammation of tendon occurring usually at its point of insertion into bone or at the point of muscular origin. The inflammation can extend to adjacent bursal tissue.
System(s) affected: Musculoskeletal
Genetics: N/A
Incidence/Prevalence in USA: Common
Predominant age: None
Predominant sex: Male > Female (slightly)

SIGNS AND SYMPTOMS
• Pain overlying the point of inflammation. This is usually worsened by active motion, but can be present at rest.
• Tenderness over the affected tendon
• Mild erythema and increased heat of overlying skin, especially if the tendon is superficial as in the case of the tendo Achilles

CAUSES Usually related to repetitive activity or trauma, but can be without obvious cause

RISK FACTORS Professional athletes and manual laborers are especially prone to tendinitis due to repetitive use

DIAGNOSIS

DIFFERENTIAL DIAGNOSIS
• Avulsion of the tendon - may occur with loss of function of the affected muscle. X-rays may show a portion of bone avulsed with the tendon, though this is not constant.
• Bursitis - can be impossible to differentiate, especially since the two conditions may coexist
• Infectious tenosynovitis - this occurs largely in the hand. The tenderness and swelling are located along the synovial lines proximally, instead of the insertion. Pain is more marked as is swelling and erythema. The sedimentation rate and white count will usually be elevated.
• Arthritis - the joint may be swollen. Tenderness and pain are in the joint proper in contrast to tendinitis which will be localized to the side of the joint where tendon insertion occurs.

LABORATORY Normal
Drugs that may alter lab results: N/A
Disorders that may alter lab results: N/A

PATHOLOGICAL FINDINGS Tendinitis is usually associated with some degenerative changes in the tendon under microscopic examinations with presence of fibrinoid, mucoid or hyaline degeneration of the connective tissue

SPECIAL TESTS Sonogram - this can be an accurate examination when done with real-time machines. Dynamics of the tendon during contraction may be obtained. Exert care that the ultrasound beam does not cross the tendon obliquely.

IMAGING The CT scan and MRI have replaced even arthrography of the shoulder in most instances. In case where diagnosis is in doubt, especially as regards tendon integrity, an MRI can be obtained and this will usually identify tears, partial tears, inflammation, or tumors. MRI cannot show irregularities of the tendon sheath itself however, and will not diagnose stenosing tenosynovitis or minimal tenosynovitis, unless fluid is present.

DIAGNOSTIC PROCEDURES N/A

TREATMENT

APPROPRIATE HEALTH CARE
Outpatient

GENERAL MEASURES Treatment goals are to relieve pain, reduce inflammation, rest the joint

SURGICAL MEASURES N/A

ACTIVITY
• In acute phases the involved muscle and tendon should be put at rest. Use slings and splints for the upper extremity. Use braces, canes and/or crutches for the lower limbs.
• Physical therapy, once patient is free of pain

DIET No special diet

PATIENT EDUCATION
• Explanation of the problem
• Instructions for use of supportive devices (e.g., crutches, slings)

MEDICATIONS

DRUG(S) OF CHOICE
• Anti-inflammatory drugs:
◊ NSAID's - all have about the same efficacy and the one which is most familiar to the prescriber can be used e.g., piroxicam (Feldene) 10 mg daily or indomethacin (Indocin) 25 or 50 mg tid after meals. Ibuprofen is a low-cost NSAID available over-the-counter.
◊ Corticosteroids - injectable, 40 mg of methylprednisolone (Depo-Medrol) accompanied by 4-6 cc of 1% or 2% lidocaine (Xylocaine) often results in dramatic relief. Never inject tendon, only into tendon sheath or surrounding bursa. (Careful preparation of the skin using Betadine or similar surgical prep is mandatory to prevent infection.)
Contraindications: A tendon should never be injected with a local anesthetic and/or cortisone to allow participation in an athletic event. This can result in complete rupture of the tendon.
Precautions: See manufacturer's profile of each drug
Significant possible interactions: See manufacturer's profile of each drug

ALTERNATIVE DRUGS N/A

FOLLOWUP

PATIENT MONITORING Symptoms will usually subside within a few days after treatment

PREVENTION/AVOIDANCE After adequate rest and treatment, prevention of recurrences is important. Splints such as circular bands for forearm extension tendinitis or patella tendinitis may be useful.

POSSIBLE COMPLICATIONS
• Tendon rupture or avulsion fractures may occur
• Repeated exacerbations of pain. This is probably the most common indication for MRI to confirm the diagnosis and determine the extent of attenuation of the tendon.

EXPECTED COURSE/PROGNOSIS
The great majority subside without complications

MISCELLANEOUS

ASSOCIATED CONDITIONS Bursitis, arthritis - osteophytes may be a factor in traumatizing tendons if located adjacent to a tendon

AGE-RELATED FACTORS
Pediatric: A prevalent form of tendinitis is patellar tendinitis associated with inflammation of the tibial apophysis. Known as Osgood-Schlatter disease, it is seen in adolescents especially during a growth spurt. Splinting with a patella band and restricted activity usually alleviate symptoms. However, some are recalcitrant and may require steroid injections and even surgery with splitting of the patella tendon.
Geriatric: N/A
Others: N/A

PREGNANCY N/A

SYNONYMS N/A

ICD-9-CM
726.90 Enthesopathy, unspecified site

SEE ALSO Osgood-Schlatter disease

OTHER NOTES N/A

ABBREVIATIONS N/A

REFERENCES
• Fornage BD, Rifkin MD: Ultrasonic examinations of tendons. Radiologic Clinics of North America 1988;26(1):87-107
• Baker KS, Gilula LA: Current Role of tenography and bursography. American Journal of Roentgenography 1990;154(7):129-137
• Lawrence BD, et al: Recent advances in magnetic resonance imaging of the knee. Radiologic Clinics of North America 1990;28(1)
Illustrations: N/A
Internet references: http://www.5mcc.com

Author(s)
Furnie W. Johnston, MD
R. Bruce Hall, MD

Testicular malignancies

BASICS

DESCRIPTION Primary testicular neoplasms may arise from any testicular or adnexal cell component. They are divided into germinal (90-95%) and non-germinal tumors. The germinal tumors, discussed here, are further divided into seminomatous and non-seminomatous types (embryonal, teratoma, choriocarcinomas, yolk sac).
• Clinical staging - Skinner/Walter Reed
  ◊ A: tumor limited to testis and cord
  ◊ B: tumor of testis and retroperitoneal nodes
  ◊ B1: <6 nodes all less than 2 cm
  ◊ B2: > 6 nodes > 2 cm in diameter
  ◊ B3: positive retroperitoneal nodes > 5 cm in diameter (bulky)
  ◊ C: metastases above diaphragm or involving abdominal solid organs
System(s) affected: Reproductive
Genetics: Weak influence
Incidence/Prevalence in USA:
• 1-2% of all neoplasms in male
• 2.3-6.3 cases/year per 100,000 men (less common in African-Americans - 0.9 cases/year per 100,000)
• In adults, germ cell types comprise 90-95% of testicular cancers; in children, they represent only 60-75%
Predominant age: Peak incidence - age 20-40; smaller peaks between age 0-10 years and > 60
Predominant sex: Male only

SIGNS AND SYMPTOMS
• In adults
  ◊ Testicular nodule or swelling most common
  ◊ Sensation of fullness or heaviness of scrotum, may be interpreted as "pain"
  ◊ Previously "small" testicle enlarging to size of "normal" contralateral one
  ◊ Firm, non-tender mass within confines of tunica albuginea usually palpably distinct from cord structures
  ◊ Acute or chronic epididymitis/epididymo-orchitis resulting in delay of diagnosis (10%)
  ◊ Manifestations due to metastasis e.g., neck mass (supraclavicular node), respiratory symptoms (lung metastasis), low back pain (nerve root or psoas irritation), uni- or bilateral lower extremity swelling (iliac or caval thrombosis or obstruction) palpable abdominal mass.
  ◊ Hydrocele (10-20%)
  ◊ Gynecomastia (may or may not be due to elevated hormones) (5%)
  ◊ Rapid tumor growth resulting in hemorrhage and necrosis
• In children
  ◊ Non-tender, non-painful scrotal mass
  ◊ Non-transilluminable, large, non-tender testicle
  ◊ Hydrocele (15-20%)
  ◊ With hormonally active tumors, the scrotal exam may be unrevealing

CAUSES No real clear cause and effect relations identified

RISK FACTORS
• Caucasian race; especially Scandinavian background
• Higher social status
• Unmarried
• Rural resident
• History of cryptorchism (even if previously repaired) - only undisputed risk factor
• Positive HIV
• Weak associations
  ◊ Maternal ingestion of hormones during 1st trimester
  ◊ Intersex disorders in genotypic male with dysgenetic gonad, trauma (no hard evidence of significant risk factor)
  ◊ Atrophy of any cause

DIAGNOSIS:

DIFFERENTIAL DIAGNOSIS
• Hernia
• Hydrocele
• Hematoma
• Spermatocele
• Syphilitic gumma
• Varicocele
• In children - epidermoid/dermoid cyst, para-testicular rhabdomyosarcoma, macro-orchidism, torsion
• Epididymitis

LABORATORY
Serum markers should be performed pre and post-operatively
• Alpha fetoprotein (AFP) - serum half life is 5-7 days; levels elevated by pure embryonal carcinoma, teratocarcinoma, yolk sac tumor or combinations of these three, but not by pure choriocarcinoma or seminoma
• Beta human chorionic gonadotropin (beta-HCG) - serum half life is 24-36 hours; elevated by all choriocarcinoma, 40-60% embryonal carcinoma; 5-10% pure seminomas have detectable levels of beta-HCG (usually < 500 ng/mL)
• Placental alkaline phosphatase (PLAP) - may be marker of choice for seminoma. 70-90% patients with recurrent or disseminated seminomas have elevated PLAP.
• Lactate dehydrogenase (LDH) - too ubiquitous to be specific. May be direct relationship between elevated LDH levels and tumor burden. Elevated LDH may be sole biochemical abnormality in 10% of patients with persistent or recurrent non-seminomatous tumors.

Drugs that may alter lab results: N/A
Disorders that may alter lab results:
• AFP alterations may be caused by - benign liver disease; telangiectasia and tyrosinemia; malignancies of the liver, pancreas, stomach and lung; heavy marijuana smoking
• PLAP may be elevated by heavy tobacco smoking
• Beta-HCG - pancreatic, stomach, kidney, breast and bladder cancers

PATHOLOGICAL FINDINGS Basically, two different groups based on germinal vs. non-germinal and seminomatous vs. non-seminomatous types

SPECIAL TESTS N/A

IMAGING
• Scrotal ultrasound - see mass clearly originating within testis with echotexture pattern (hypoechoic) distinct from surrounding normal testicular tissue. Echotexture may be mixed.
• For staging:
  ◊ Chest x-ray - good PA and lateral
  ◊ CT scan - very accurate; able to define pelvic retroperitoneal and mediastinal lymphadenopathy as well as to detect abdominal visceral and lung metastases
  ◊ Pedal lymphangiography (LAG) - is sensitive in picking up lymph node involvement intra-abdominally but not as accurate as CT scan in picking up upper para aortic nodes or visceral involvement
  ◊ MRI - still largely experimental

DIAGNOSTIC PROCEDURES
• Transinguinal scrotal exploration with biopsy and/or radical orchiectomy (testicle and spermatic cord excised) makes definite diagnosis, helps stage, and debulks the tumor
• Transscrotal open or percutaneous biopsy or transscrotal orchiectomy contraindicated secondary to anatomical trespassing into different lymph drainage system

Testicular malignancies

TREATMENT

APPROPRIATE HEALTH CARE
Inpatient and outpatient

GENERAL MEASURES
Radical orchiectomy and adjuvant measures:
• Both seminomatous and non-seminomatous tumors are chemo-sensitive and have good chemotherapeutic response. Seminomas are extremely radiosensitive.
• Treatment for seminomas by stage:
◊ A: irradiation, 2500 R to ipsilateral inguinal, iliac chains and bilateral periaortic/pericaval nodes to level of diaphragm versus observation (experimental)
◊ B2: same as A, with irradiation using 600-1000 R to positive nodes
◊ B3: chemotherapy - if post-chemotherapy lymph nodes persists more than 3 cm in diameter, then a retroperitoneal lymph node biopsy is added (43% of cases have viable tumor present) and further chemotherapy given if viable tumor found. If < 3 cm, observe.
◊ C: primary chemotherapy
• Treatment for non-seminomatous germ cell tumor by stage:
◊ A: nerve sparing staging and therapeutic retroperitoneal lymph node dissection (RPLND) alone versus observation (careful followup protocol)
◊ B1 (microscopic metastasis in 1-6 nodes, < 2 cm): observation if serum markers negative
◊ B2 (microscopic metastases in > 6 nodes or grossly positive nodes, 2-6 cm): observation or two courses of chemotherapy
◊ B3 (nodes > 6 cm or tumor extension outside nodes): initially 4 courses of chemotherapy. If complete response based on CT scan, serum markers, and no teratoma seen in original specimen, then observe. If partial response, do retroperitoneal lymph node dissection and tumor excision plus 2 more courses of chemotherapy. If tumor cannot all be excised, salvage chemotherapy.
• Children: radical orchiectomy plus initial AFP level
◊ If age ≤ 1 year and AFP rapidly normalizes, no metastases: observe for 2 years with AFP and CxR
◊ If AFP doesn't normalize or CT shows suspicious lymph nodes and CxR negative: do RPLND
◊ If lymph nodes are positive and chest x-ray negative: chemotherapy; if CxR positive for solitary lesion, add surgery
◊ If CxR shows several lesions - give radiation
◊ If age > 1 year: chemotherapy

SURGICAL MEASURES
• All patients receive radical orchiectomy for diagnosis and excellent local control

ACTIVITY   As tolerated

DIET   No special diet

PATIENT EDUCATION
• Discuss patient's concerns about sterility, impotence, testicular prostheses, hormone supplements
• Patient education material available from American Cancer Society

MEDICATIONS

DRUG(S) OF CHOICE
• Commonly used chemotherapeutic agents include cisplatin + etoposide ± bleomycin, paclitaxel (taxol)
• Salvage chemotherapy includes cyclophosphamide (Cytoxan), ifosfamide [with mesna to protect against hemorrhagic cystitis], carboplatin, chemo intensification with granulocyte colony stimulating factor (G-CSF) or autologous bone marrow transplant (BMT)
• In children - vincristine, dactinomycin (actinomycin-D), cyclophosphamide, doxorubicin (Adriamycin)
Contraindications: N/A
Precautions:
• Cisplatin - nephrotoxicity, ototoxicity, neurotoxicity
• Etoposide - marrow suppression, leukemia
• Cyclophosphamide/ifosfamide - hemorrhagic cystitis
• Bleomycin - pulmonary fibrosis
• Adriamycin - marrow suppression
• Vincristine - marrow suppression, neuromuscular toxicity
• Carboplatin - ototoxicity
• Taxol - neuropathy
Significant possible interactions: Refer to manufacturer's literature

ALTERNATIVE DRUGS
• Ondansetron (Zofran), dronabinol (Marinol), metoclopramide (Reglan), and others for nausea control

FOLLOWUP

PATIENT MONITORING
• First year - markers and chest x-ray every month, physical exam (emphasizing nodes) every 2 months
• After 1 year - markers and chest x-ray every 2 months and physical exam every 4 months
• After 2 years - markers and chest x-ray and physical exam every 6-12 months
• If patient had teratoma at diagnosis, need to followup for at least 5 years and get CT scan every year for 3 years
• Annual ultrasound of remaining testicle

PREVENTION/AVOIDANCE   N/A

POSSIBLE COMPLICATIONS
• RPLND treatment - loss of seminal emission (prevented by using nerve-sparing RPLND), atelectasis, hypoalbuminemia
• Radiation treatment - radiation nephritis, enteritis

• Non-seminomatous tumors are more likely to have metastatic disease than seminomas (50-70% vs. 25%, respectively)

EXPECTED COURSE/PROGNOSIS
Usually complete cure in patients with limited disease, 70-80% cure in patients with advanced disease

MISCELLANEOUS

ASSOCIATED CONDITIONS   N/A

AGE-RELATED FACTORS
Pediatric: Rare in childhood (only 2% of all solid tumors in childhood)
Geriatric: N/A
Others: N/A

PREGNANCY   N/A

SYNONYMS   N/A

ICD-9-CM
186 Malignant neoplasm of testis

SEE ALSO   N/A

OTHER NOTES   N/A

ABBREVIATIONS
AFP = alpha fetoprotein
Beta-HCG = beta human chorionic gonadotropin
LDH = lactate dehydrogenase
PLAP = placental alkaline phosphatase
RPLND = retroperitoneal lymph node dissection
G-CSF = granulocyte cell stimulating factor
BMT = bone marrow transplant

REFERENCES
• Lleibovitch I: Annual ultrasound screening of remaining testicle following radical orchiectomy for testicular cancer. Multi-center trial proceedings of 94th annual American Urological Association Meeting, Dallas, 1999
• Skinner EC: In: Walsh PC, et al, eds. Campbell's Urology. Philadelphia, W.B. Saunders Co., 1998
• Klein EA: Tumor Markers in Testis Cancer. The Urologic Clinics of North America 1993;20(1):67
• Motzer RJ, Bosl GJ: Role of adjuvant chemotherapy in patients with Stage II, non-seminomatiour germ cell tumors. The Urologic Clinics of North America 1993;20(1):111
Illustrations: N/A
Internet references: http://www.5mcc.com

Author(s)
Charles Jennings, MD, FACS

Testicular torsion

BASICS

DESCRIPTION Twisting of testis and spermatic cord resulting in acute ischemia.
• Intravaginal torsion: occurs within tunica vaginalis
• Extravaginal torsion: involves twisting of testis, cord and processus vaginalis (especially in newborns) and in undescended testes
System(s) affected: Reproductive
Genetics: Unknown
Incidence/Prevalence in USA: 1:160 males
Predominant age: Occurs from newborn period to 7th decade; 2/3 of cases occur in 2nd decade, with peak at age 14 years; 2nd peak in neonates
Predominant sex: Males only

SIGNS AND SYMPTOMS
• Scrotum is enlarged, red, and edematous
• First symptom is pain (sudden or gradual onset, increasing in severity)
• Nausea and vomiting are common
• Fever may occur
• Testicle exquisitely tender
• Testis may be high in scrotum with a transverse lie
• Absence of cremasteric reflex

CAUSES
• Torsion is usually spontaneous and idiopathic
• History of trauma in 20% of patients
• 1/3 have had prior episodic testicular pain
• Contraction of cremasteric muscle or dartos may play a role and is stimulated by trauma, exercise, cold, sexual stimulation
• Possible alterations in testosterone levels during nocturnal sex response cycle; possible elevated testosterone levels in neonates
• Testis must have inadequate, incomplete or absent fixation within scrotum

RISK FACTORS
• May be more common in winter
• Paraplegia

DIAGNOSIS

DIFFERENTIAL DIAGNOSIS
• Epididymo-orchitis
• Incarcerated/strangulated inguinal hernia
• Acute hydrocele
• Traumatic hematoma
• Idiopathic scrotal edema
• Torsion appendix testis
• Acute varicocele
• Testicular tumor
• Henoch-Schönlein purpura
• Scrotal abscess
• Leukemic infiltrate

LABORATORY Urinalysis may be helpful (usually not)
Drugs that may alter lab results: N/A
Disorders that may alter lab results: N/A

PATHOLOGICAL FINDINGS
• Venous thrombosis
• Tissue edema and necrosis
• Arterial thrombosis

SPECIAL TESTS N/A

IMAGING CT scan or ultrasound may confirm testicular swelling, but are rarely indicated

DIAGNOSTIC PROCEDURES
• Doppler ultrasonic flow detection demonstrates absent or reduced pulse with torsion, increased flow with inflammatory process (only reliable in 1st 12 hrs.)
• Radionuclide testicular scintigraphy with technetium 99m. pertechnetate demonstrates absent/decreased vascularity in torsion, increased vascularity with inflammatory processes (including torsion of appendix testes)

TREATMENT

APPROPRIATE HEALTH CARE
• Manual reduction - may be successful, facilitated by Lidocaine 1% (plain) injection at level of external ring. Must always be followed by orchidopexy.
• Surgical exploration via scrotal approach with detorsion, evaluation of testicular viability, orchidopexy of viable testicle, orchiectomy of non-viable testicle.

GENERAL MEASURES N/A

SURGICAL MEASURES
• Bilateral testicular fixation is recommended
• At least 3-4 point fixation with non-absorbable sutures
• Excision of window of tunica albuginea with suture to dartos fascia
• Any testis that is not clearly viable (and obvious) should be removed.

ACTIVITY As tolerated

DIET Regular

PATIENT EDUCATION Possibility of testicular atrophy in salvaged testis with depressed sperm counts

MEDICATIONS

DRUG(S) OF CHOICE N/A
Contraindications: N/A
Precautions: N/A
Significant possible interactions: N/A

ALTERNATIVE DRUGS N/A

FOLLOWUP

PATIENT MONITORING
• Postoperative visit at 1-2 weeks
• Yearly visits until puberty to evaluate for atrophy

PREVENTION/AVOIDANCE N/A

POSSIBLE COMPLICATIONS
• Possible testicular atrophy
• Abnormal spermatogenesis
• Infertility

EXPECTED COURSE/PROGNOSIS
• Testicular salvage directly related to duration of torsion (85-97% if less than 6 hours, less than 10% if greater than 24 hrs)
• 80-94% may have depressed spermatogenesis related to duration of ischemic injury (possibly related to autoimmune - mediated injury)
• As many as 2/3 of salvaged testicles may atrophy in first 2-3 years post torsion

MISCELLANEOUS

ASSOCIATED CONDITIONS N/A

AGE-RELATED FACTORS N/A
Pediatric: Most common at age 14
Geriatric: Rare in this age group
Others: N/A

PREGNANCY N/A

SYNONYMS N/A

ICD-9-CM
608.2 Torsion of testis

SEE ALSO
• Epididymitis

OTHER NOTES N/A

ABBREVIATIONS N/A

REFERENCES
• Ashcraft KW: Pediatric Urology. Philadelphia, W.B. Saunders Co, 1990.
• Ashcraft KW, Holder TM: Pediatric Surgery. 2nd Ed. Philadelphia, W.B. Saunders Co., 1993.
• Kelalis PP, King LR, Belman AB: Clinical Pediatric Urology. 3rd Ed. Philadelphia, W.B. Saunders Co, 1992.
Illustrations: N/A
Internet references: http://www.5mcc.com

Author(s)
Timothy L. Black, MD, FACS, FAAP

Tetanus

 BASICS

DESCRIPTION
Severe illness characterized by intermittent tonic spasms of voluntary muscles. Toxin enters the central nervous system along the peripheral nerves or is blood borne. Tetanospasmin binds at synapses and blocks inhibitors. Usual course is acute.

System(s) affected: Nervous
Genetics: N/A
Incidence/Prevalence in USA: Rare
Predominant age: Over 70% of cases in persons > 50 years of age
Predominant sex: Male = Female

SIGNS AND SYMPTOMS
- Arrhythmias
- Asphyxia
- Convulsions
- Cyanosis
- Drooling
- Dysphagia
- Fluctuating hypertension
- Hydrophobia
- Hyperhidrosis
- Hyperpyrexia
- Hyperreflexia
- Hypotension
- Irritability
- Low-grade fever
- Muscular rigidity
- Muscular spasticity
- Nuchal rigidity
- Opisthotonos
- Pain at wound site
- Painful tonic convulsions
- Risus sardonicus (fixed smile)
- Stiffness of the jaw
- Sudden bradycardia
- Sudden cardiac arrest
- Tachycardia
- Tingling at wound site
- Trismus
- Wound history (may be absent)

CAUSES
- Infection with Clostridium tetani
- Neurotoxin produced by Clostridium tetani
- Tetanospasmin (an exotoxin)

RISK FACTORS
- Burns
- Drug addiction (parenteral)
- Ear infection (with tympanic membrane perforation)
- Early postpartum with an infected uterus
- Exposure of open wounds to soil and animal feces
- Frostbite
- Newborn (umbilicus stump entry)
- Skin ulcers
- Surgical wounds
- Age > 50 years
- Traumatic wound

 DIAGNOSIS

DIFFERENTIAL DIAGNOSIS
- Dental abscess
- Subarachnoid hemorrhage
- Seizure disorder
- Meningoencephalitis
- Peritonsillar abscess
- Dystonic reaction to phenothiazines
- Hypocalcemic tetany
- Strychnine poisoning
- Alcohol withdrawal

LABORATORY
- Polymorphonuclear leukocytosis
- Culture of Clostridium tetani from wound (may not be positive even if tetanus is the problem)

Drugs that may alter lab results: N/A
Disorders that may alter lab results: N/A

PATHOLOGICAL FINDINGS   N/A

SPECIAL TESTS
- ECG - supraventricular tachycardia
- Multifocal ventricular ectopia
- Bradycardia
- EEG sleeping pattern
- Culture of wound infrequently recover C. tetani

IMAGING   N/A

DIAGNOSTIC PROCEDURES   N/A

 TREATMENT

APPROPRIATE HEALTH CARE
Intensive care

GENERAL MEASURES
- Wound excision
- Quiet observation
- Intubation
- IV hydration
- Catheterize the bladder
- Prevent jarring of bed or drafts

SURGICAL MEASURES   Tracheostomy if needed

ACTIVITY   Absolute bedrest with sedation

DIET   Nothing by mouth until well

PATIENT EDUCATION   Griffith: Instructions for Patients. Philadelphia, W.B. Saunders Co.,1994

MEDICATIONS

DRUG(S) OF CHOICE
- Anticonvulsants
- Diazepam for muscle rigidity
- Pancuronium bromide (administered by anesthesiologist) plus ventilation
- Tetanus toxoid in a previously immunized patient
- Tetanus immune globulin (TIG) 3000 units to 6000 units IM. May infiltrate the area around the wound with a portion of the dose.
- Penicillin G - 2 million units IV q6h. In a penicillin allergic patient, use doxycycline 100 mg q12h, or clindamycin 150-300 mg IV q6h.

Contraindications: Refer to manufacturer's literature

Precautions: Refer to manufacturer's literature. Do not use tetanus immune globulin intravenously.

Significant possible interactions: Refer to manufacturer's literature

ALTERNATIVE DRUGS
Equine tetanus antitoxin 50,000 units IM - only if tetanus immune globulin (human) is not available

FOLLOWUP

PATIENT MONITORING
Careful observation in intensive care

PREVENTION/AVOIDANCE
Active immunization with tetanus toxoid; wound débridement; passive immunization with tetanus immune globulin; benzathine penicillin; penicillin G; erythromycin

POSSIBLE COMPLICATIONS
- Respiratory arrest
- Cardiac failure
- Pulmonary emboli
- Bacterial infection
- Dehydration
- Vertebral fractures
- Airway obstruction
- Anoxia
- Urinary retention
- Constipation
- Pneumonia
- Rhabdomyolysis

EXPECTED COURSE/PROGNOSIS
- 25-50% mortality
- Poor prognostic factors:
  ◊ Form of tetanus
  ◊ Incubation period
  ◊ Onset period
  ◊ Patient's age
  ◊ Severity of symptoms
  ◊ Heart wound
- Recovery is complete if patient survives

MISCELLANEOUS

ASSOCIATED CONDITIONS N/A

AGE-RELATED FACTORS
Pediatric:
- Mortality high in young
- Infection may enter through umbilical cord

Geriatric: Mortality high in elderly and may not have adequate immunizations.

Others: N/A

PREGNANCY
- Must treat vigorously despite pregnancy
- Infection may enter uterus postpartum
- Tetanus toxoid probably safe, but few data available

SYNONYMS Lockjaw

ICD-9-CM 037 Tetanus

SEE ALSO
- Meningitis, bacterial
- Immunizations
- Anaerobic & necrotizing infections

OTHER NOTES N/A

ABBREVIATIONS N/A

REFERENCES
- von Behring E, Kitasato S: Uber das Zustandelkommen der Diphtherie-Immunität und der Tetanus-Immunität bei Thieren. Dtsch Med Wochenschr 1890;16:1113
- Centers for Disease Control, Tetanus: United States 1981-1984. MMWR, 1985;34:602
- Mandell GL, ed: Principles and Practice of Infectious Diseases. 4th Ed. New York, Churchill Livingstone, 1995

Illustrations: N/A

Internet references: http://www.5mcc.com

Author(s)
Abdulrazak Abyad, MD, MPH, AGSF

Tetralogy of Fallot

BASICS

DESCRIPTION Large ventricular septal defect (VSD) associated with right ventricular outflow obstruction (infundibular and/or valvular pulmonic stenosis), right ventricular (RV) hypertrophy and an overriding aorta
• Pathophysiology dependent primarily on severity of right ventricular outflow tract obstruction
• Right and left ventricular pressures are generally equal (VSD is proximal to level of RV obstruction, therefore, RV pressures are elevated)
• Right to left shunting is typical
System(s) affected: Cardiovascular, Pulmonary
Genetics: Familial occurrence, components indicating dominant hereditary
Incidence/Prevalence in USA:
• 5-10% of all congenital heart disease. Most common cardiac cyanotic anomaly after age 1.
• 40 per 100,000 live births
Predominant age: Newborn
Predominant sex: Male > Female (slightly)

SIGNS AND SYMPTOMS
• With mild RV outflow tract obstruction a left to right shunt predominates, and the patient is acyanotic = ("Pink" tetralogy of Fallot)
• Cyanosis with severe RV outflow tract obstruction (generally recognized early)
• Exertional dyspnea, poor exercise tolerance
• Lower birth weight, retarded growth
• Clubbing and polycythemia commonly in children
• Squatting position, typical following exertion (allows increased systemic vascular resistance, lessening right to left shunting)
• No typical facies
• Scoliosis is common
• Normal arterial and jugular venous pulses
• Systolic thrill along the left sternal border
• Early systolic ejection sound (aortic)
• Single S2 (decreased P2)
• Systolic ejection murmur due to flow across narrowed RV outflow tract
• May auscultate the continuous diminished murmur of bronchial collateral vessels
• Right aortic arch in 30%
• Atrial septal defect (ASD) in 15%
• Anomalous coronary arteries in 2-10%
• Retinal engorgement
• Hemoptysis
• Aortic ejection click

CAUSES Unknown

RISK FACTORS
• Documented increased incidence with increased maternal age
• Occasional familial occurrence

DIAGNOSIS

DIFFERENTIAL DIAGNOSIS
• Fallot's tetralogy with absent pulmonic valve
• Fallot's tetralogy with absent pulmonary artery
• Pseudotruncus arteriosus

LABORATORY N/A
Drugs that may alter lab results: N/A
Disorders that may alter lab results: N/A

PATHOLOGICAL FINDINGS
• Anterior deviation of the infundibular septum, resulting in malalignment with the muscular septum, creating a ventricular septal defect
• Malposition of the infundibular septum, which encroaches on the right ventricular outflow tract, resulting in an increased aortic root size
• Aortic root rotated into overriding position

SPECIAL TESTS
• ECG
  ◊ Right axis deviation, right ventricular hypertrophy, subsequent right ventricular conduction abnormality
  ◊ Sinus rhythm in general, however, some may develop atrial fibrillation or flutter

IMAGING
• Chest x-ray
  ◊ In children, typically a small boot-shaped heart (coeur en sabot) with diminished pulmonary blood flow
  ◊ Prominent right ventricle
  ◊ Possibly a right sided aortic arch and knob
  ◊ Normal (or perhaps decreased) pulmonary vascularity in approximately 50% adults
• 2D echocardiogram/Doppler echocardiogram
  ◊ 2D images demonstrate the VSD, overriding aorta, extent and location of the infundibular obstruction, assessment of pulmonic valve, right ventricular hypertrophy, and coronary anatomy, additional ventricular septal defects, and peripheral branch pulmonic arteries
  ◊ Doppler echocardiogram allows quantification of the outflow gradient
  ◊ Colorflow Doppler provides assessment of the VSD
  ◊ Coronary anatomy

DIAGNOSTIC PROCEDURES
• Cardiac catheterization
  ◊ Assesses pulmonary annulus size and pulmonary arteries
  ◊ Assesses severity of right ventricular outflow obstruction
  ◊ Locates position of VSD and its size
  ◊ Rules out possible coronary artery anomalies

TREATMENT

APPROPRIATE HEALTH CARE
Inpatient for diagnosis and surgery

GENERAL MEASURES
• Good dental hygiene
• Endocarditis prophylaxis

SURGICAL MEASURES
• Palliative surgical therapy
  ◊ It is important to emphasize that complete repair is the preferable modality of treatment
  ◊ Blalock-Taussig shunt or modified shunt (subclavian to pulmonary artery)
  ◊ Pott's procedure (descending aorta to pulmonary artery)
  ◊ Waterston's shunt (ascending aorta to pulmonary artery)
• Total correction surgical therapy
  ◊ Includes patch closure of VSD and relief of right ventricular outflow obstruction

ACTIVITY As tolerated

DIET Salt restriction

PATIENT EDUCATION American Heart Association, 7320 Greenville Avenue, Dallas, TX 75231, (214)373-6300

Tetralogy of Fallot

MEDICATIONS

DRUG(S) OF CHOICE No specific drug therapy in the absence of heart failure
Contraindications: N/A
Precautions: N/A
Significant possible interactions: N/A

ALTERNATIVE DRUGS N/A

FOLLOWUP

PATIENT MONITORING
• Postoperative (or post-balloon valvotomy) Doppler ultrasound suggested at approximately 1 year from procedure
• Post-valvotomy SBE prophylaxis still required
• Regular followup assessment for patients not undergoing surgical correction

PREVENTION/AVOIDANCE N/A

POSSIBLE COMPLICATIONS
• Erythrocytosis may develop secondary to chronic hypoxemia (risk for thrombosis, thrombotic CVA and paradoxical emboli)
• Increased risk for brain abscess, acute gouty arthritis
• Infective endocarditis
• Cerebrovascular thrombosis
• Delayed puberty
• Postoperatively
  ◊ Residual right ventricular outflow obstruction
  ◊ Residual VSD
  ◊ Pulmonic regurgitation
  ◊ Ventricular arrhythmias
  ◊ Right bundle branch block quite common
  ◊ Left anterior hemiblock
  ◊ Infective bacterial endocarditis

EXPECTED COURSE/PROGNOSIS
Fatal if not surgically corrected

MISCELLANEOUS

ASSOCIATED CONDITIONS
• Stenotic pulmonary artery
• Patent ductus arteriosus
• Atrial septal defect
• Iron deficiency anemia

AGE-RELATED FACTORS
Pediatric: Congenital disorder
Geriatric: N/A
Others: N/A

PREGNANCY Well tolerated after total surgical correction

SYNONYMS N/A

ICD-9-CM
745.2 Tetralogy of Fallot

SEE ALSO N/A

OTHER NOTES N/A

ABBREVIATIONS
• VSD = ventricular septal defect
• RV = right ventricle

REFERENCES
• Braunwald E, ed: Heart Disease: A Textbook of Cardiovascular Medicine. 4th Ed. Philadelphia, W.B. Saunders Co., 1992
• Liberthson R: Congenital Heart Disease: Diagnosis & Management in Children and Adults. Boston, Little Brown, 1989
• Perloff J: Clinical Recognition of Congenital Heart Disease. 4th Ed. Philadelphia, W.B. Saunders Co., 1994
Illustrations: N/A
Internet references: http://www.5mcc.com

Author(s)
Sylvia A. Mamby, MD

Thalassemia

 BASICS

DESCRIPTION
A group of inherited disorders that affect the synthesis of hemoglobin. In beta-thalassemia, there is deficient synthesis of beta globin, while in alpha-thalassemia, there is deficient synthesis of alpha globin. This leads to deficient hemoglobin accumulation, resulting in hypochromic and microcytic red cells. Abnormality of the red cells is the most characteristic feature of the thalassemias. Thalassemia is prevalent in the Mediterranean region, Middle East and Southeast Asia, and among ethnic groups originating from these areas
• Types
  ◊ Beta-thalassemia major (Cooley's anemia) - severe anemia, growth retardation, hepatosplenomegaly, bone marrow expansion and bone deformities. Transfusion therapy necessary to sustain life.
  ◊ Thalassemia intermedia - milder form. Transfusion therapy may not be needed.
  ◊ Thalassemia trait (alpha or beta) - mild anemia with microcytosis and hypochromia. No transfusion therapy needed.
• Varieties unique to Southeast Asians include hemoglobin H disease (a more severe form of alpha thalassemia) and hemoglobin E/beta thalassemia which often mimics Beta thalassemia major in its severity. Both alpha and beta thalassemia trait (minor) are frequent in African-Americans but symptomatic thalassemia is very rare.
System(s) affected:
Hemic/Lymphatic/Immunologic
Genetics:
• Inherited in an autosomal recessive pattern
• Inheritance of one defective gene = milder type of thalassemia, two defective genes = severe type of thalassemia
Incidence/Prevalence in USA:
• Approximately 1000 patients with severe thalassemia
• The incidence of thalassemia trait within the ethnic groups involved ranges from 3-5%
Predominant age: Symptoms start to appear 3-6 months after birth
Predominant sex: Male = Female

SIGNS AND SYMPTOMS
(Thalassemia trait has no signs or symptoms)
• Pallor
• Poor growth
• Inadequate food intake
• Fatigue
• Shortness of breath
• Splenomegaly
• Jaundice
• Maxillary hyperplasia
• Dental malocclusion
• Cholelithiasis
• Pathologic fractures

CAUSES   Genetic

RISK FACTORS   Family history

 DIAGNOSIS

DIFFERENTIAL DIAGNOSIS
• Iron deficiency
• Other hemoglobinopathies
• Other hemolytic anemias

LABORATORY
• Hemoglobin
  ◊ Elevated Hb A2 levels in beta-thalassemia trait
  ◊ Elevated Hb A2, elevated Hb F, reduced or absent Hb A1 in beta-thalassemia major or intermedia
• Peripheral blood
  ◊ Pronounced microcytosis
  ◊ Anisocytosis
  ◊ Hypochromia
  ◊ Punctate basophilic stippling
  ◊ High percentage of target cells
  ◊ Reticulocyte count elevated
• Hematocrit
  ◊ 28-40% in alpha-thalassemia trait and beta-thalassemia trait
  ◊ May fall to less than 10% in beta-thalassemia major
Drugs that may alter lab results: N/A
Disorders that may alter lab results:
Parvovirus B19 infection may produce "aplastic crisis" and severe reticulocytopenia

PATHOLOGICAL FINDINGS
• Bone marrow hyperactivity
• Iron deposits in heart muscle
• Hepatic siderosis

SPECIAL TESTS
Bone marrow aspiration

IMAGING
Skull x-ray: thickened diploë of skull, osteoporosis

DIAGNOSTIC PROCEDURES
Family history

 TREATMENT

APPROPRIATE HEALTH CARE
Outpatient for mild cases. Inpatient for transfusion therapy.

GENERAL MEASURES
• Mild cases require no therapy
• Thalassemia intermedia - normally no therapy necessary unless hemoglobin levels fall to a dangerous level, then may need transfusion therapy
• Patients with severe thalassemia
  ◊ Maintain the mean hemoglobin level of at least 9.3 g/dL (1.4 mmol/L) with a regular transfusion schedule (transfusions of about 15 mL per kg at 3-5 week intervals)
  ◊ Folate supplementation
  ◊ Treat infections promptly
• Iron overload
  ◊ Patients receiving transfusion therapy increase total body iron 4 times over the normal amount
  ◊ Therapy is iron chelation

SURGICAL MEASURES
• Splenectomy
  ◊ May be needed if hypersplenism causes a marked increase in the transfusion requirement
  ◊ Recommendation is to defer surgery until patient is 4-6 years of age (due to increased infection risk)
  ◊ Administer polyvalent pneumococcal vaccine one month prior to splenectomy
  ◊ Prophylaxis with a daily regimen of penicillin
• Bone marrow transplantation
  ◊ Available for selected patients with a matched sibling or unrelated donor
  ◊ Cures the disease, but may be associated with significant mortality and morbidity

ACTIVITY
• Avoid strenuous activities (e.g., football, soccer)
• Acceptable activity levels will need to be determined on an individual basis depending on severity of disorder

DIET
• Avoid iron-rich foods (meats such as liver, and some cereals)
• Drinking tea may possibly help reduce iron

PATIENT EDUCATION
• Genetic counseling
• Teach parents signs of hepatitis, iron overload
• Printed patient information available from: Cooley's Anemia Foundation, 105 E. 22nd St., Suite 911, New York, NY 10010, (212)598-0911

MEDICATIONS

DRUG(S) OF CHOICE
• Antibiotics for infection
• Folic acid supplements
• Iron chelation with deferoxamine (Desferal). Continuous subcutaneous or intravenous infusion with a small infusion pump 40 mg per kg per day (about a 10 hour period). Usually started before 5-8 years of age.
Contraindications: Refer to manufacturer's literature
Precautions: Refer to manufacturer's literature
Significant possible interactions: Refer to manufacturer's literature

ALTERNATIVE DRUGS N/A

FOLLOWUP

PATIENT MONITORING Life-long monitoring necessary because both the therapy and disease progression have numerous possible complications

PREVENTION/AVOIDANCE
• Prenatal information
    ◊ Genetic counseling
    ◊ Prenatal diagnosis - study of beta globin genes performed on fetal cell DNA obtained by amniocentesis after 14 weeks
• Complication prevention
    ◊ Evaluation for thalassemia by 1 year of age for offspring of adult thalassemia patients
    ◊ Avoidance of infections
    ◊ Prompt treatment of infections (after splenectomy, patients should maintain a supply of ampicillin to take if symptoms of infection appear)
    ◊ Periodic dental checkups
    ◊ Avoidance of activities that could result in bone fractures

POSSIBLE COMPLICATIONS
• Chronic hemolysis
• Susceptibility to infections after splenectomy
• Infections from blood transfusion
• Intercurrent infections
• Worsening of anemia during infections
• Jaundice
• Leg ulcers
• Cholelithiasis
• Pathologic fractures
• Impaired growth rate
• Delayed or absent puberty
• Hepatic siderosis
• Hemolytic anemia
• Splenomegaly
• Cardiac disease from iron overload
• Aplastic and megaloblastic crises

EXPECTED COURSE/PROGNOSIS
• Outlook varies depending on type
• Thalassemia major patients live an average of 17 years, some into their mid-twenties. Effective iron chelation is improving longevity.
• Thalassemia minor patients live a normal life span

MISCELLANEOUS

ASSOCIATED CONDITIONS See Possible complications

AGE-RELATED FACTORS
Pediatric: A disorder of childhood
Geriatric: N/A
Others: N/A

PREGNANCY Genetic counseling - advised for parents or other relatives of a child with thalassemia and for any individual with beta-thalassemia minor

SYNONYMS
• Mediterranean anemia
• Hereditary leptocytosis
• Thalassemia major and minor
• Cooley's anemia

ICD-9-CM
282.4 Thalassemia

SEE ALSO N/A

OTHER NOTES N/A

ABBREVIATIONS N/A

REFERENCES
• Nathan DG, Oski F, eds: Hematology of Infancy and Childhood. Philadelphia, W.B. Saunders Co., 1997
• Fosburg MT, Nathan DG: Treatment of Cooley's anemia. Blood 1990;76:435
Illustrations: N/A
Internet references: http://www.5mcc.com

Author(s)
W. Paul Bowman, MD

Thoracic outlet syndrome

BASICS

DESCRIPTION A constellation of symptoms that affect the head, neck, shoulders and upper extremities caused by compression of the neurovascular structures (viz. cords of brachial plexus and subclavian artery and vein) at the thoracic outlet
• May be due to congenital bony muscular or tendonous anomalies; post traumatic, following clavicular or cervical spine injures; or idiopathic, without discernible cause
System(s) affected: Nervous, Musculoskeletal, Cardiovascular
Genetics: N/A
Incidence/Prevalence in USA: Unknown
Predominant age:
• Neurologic type (95%) - 20-60 years
• Venous type (4%) - 20-35 years
• Arterial type (1%) (atherosclerosis) - young adult or older than 50
Predominant sex:
• Neurologic type - Female > Male (3.5:1)
• Venous type - Male > Female
• Arterial type - Male = Female

SIGNS AND SYMPTOMS
• General symptoms
◊ Positive costoclavicular maneuver
◊ Positive hyperabduction maneuver
◊ Positive Adson's maneuver(head rotation to the affected side with slight cervical extension)
◊ Positive elevated arm stress test
◊ Tenderness to percussion or palpation of supraclavicular area
◊ Worsening of symptoms with elevation of arm, overhead extension of arms, or with arms extended forward (e.g., driving a car, typing, carrying objects). Prompt disappearance of symptoms with arm returning to neutral position.
◊ Supraventricular bruit
• Neurologic type, upper plexus (C4-C7)
◊ Pain and paresthesias in head, neck, mandible, face, temporal area, upper back/chest, outer arm & hand in a radial nerve distribution
◊ Occipital and orbital headache
• Neurologic type, lower plexus (C8-T1)
◊ Pain and paresthesias in axilla, inner arm and hand in an ulnar nerve distribution, often nocturnal
◊ Hypothenar and interosseous muscle atrophy
• Venous type
◊ Arm claudication
◊ Cyanosis
◊ Swelling
◊ Distended arm veins
• Arterial type
◊ Digital vasospasm
◊ Thrombosis/embolism
◊ Aneurysm
◊ Gangrene

CAUSES
• Upper thoracic neurovascular bundle compression
• Cervical rib
• Taut anomalous scalene muscles
• Elongated C7 transverse process
• Poor posture

• Pancoast's tumor
• Atherosclerotic plaques within vessels
• Subclavian muscle
• Fibrous and ligamentous bands
• Costocoracoid tendon
• Callous bone formation from fractured clavicle or first rib
• Aberrant tissue

RISK FACTORS
• Exuberant callus after fracture of clavicle or first rib
• Exostosis of clavicle or first rib
• Postural abnormalities (e.g., drooping of shoulders, scoliosis)
• Body building, with increased muscular bulk in thoracic outlet area
• Rapid weight loss combined with vigorous physical exertion and/or exercise

DIAGNOSIS

DIFFERENTIAL DIAGNOSIS
• Cervical disk syndrome
• Carpal tunnel syndrome
• Orthopedic shoulder problems (shoulder strain, rotator cuff injury, tendinitis)
• Cervical spondylitis
• Ulnar nerve compression at the elbow
• Multiple sclerosis
• Spinal cord tumor or disease
• Angina pectoris
• Migraine
• Reflex sympathetic dystrophy

LABORATORY N/A
Drugs that may alter lab results: N/A
Disorders that may alter lab results: N/A

PATHOLOGICAL FINDINGS
• Bony abnormalities (cervical rib, anomalous first thoracic rib)
• Abnormal muscles
• Congenital fibromuscular bands

SPECIAL TESTS
• Plethysmography with previously mentioned maneuvers
• Doppler and duplex ultrasound if venous obstruct suspected
• Nerve conduction studies (< 70 m/sec is abnormal)
• Venogram if presents with endematous changes in upper extremity

IMAGING
• X-ray (chest x-ray, oblique C-spine)
• Arteriogram - if arterial obstruction, aneurysm or emboli are suspected
• Phlebogram - if signs of venous obstruction
• CT scan - if cord compressive lesions (disc and/or tumor) are suspected

DIAGNOSTIC PROCEDURES
• Thoracic outlet syndrome (TOS) is a clinical diagnosis
• Anterior scalene muscle injections are useful in confirming the diagnosis and in determining which patients may respond favorably to surgery

TREATMENT

APPROPRIATE HEALTH CARE
• Outpatient for conservative treatment
• Inpatient if surgery required

GENERAL MEASURES
• Conservative
◊ If no vascular involvement is present and/or if no loss of function or lifestyle is present due to severity of symptoms, conservative therapy may be undertaken for 2-3 months
◊ Improvement can be expected in 60% of patients
◊ Exercise program to promote shoulder muscle function
◊ Physical therapy for postural faults
◊ Cervical collar, traction
◊ Weight loss if axillary folds are causing compression

SURGICAL MEASURES
• Operative - if vascular involvement is present and/or if there is loss of function or lifestyle secondary to severity of symptoms and if conservative therapy fails after 2-3 months
• Resection of first rib or cervical ribs (transaxillary, supraclavicular, posterior approaches)
• Excision of adhesive bands
• Anterior scalenectomy

ACTIVITY
• Light activity with arm and hand encouraged
• No straining or heavy activity for 3 months

DIET N/A

PATIENT EDUCATION Physical therapy following surgery

Thoracic outlet syndrome

MEDICATIONS

DRUG(S) OF CHOICE
- Analgesics
- Muscle relaxants
- Antispasmodics

Contraindications: Refer to manufacturer's profile of each drug
Precautions: Refer to manufacturer's profile of each drug
Significant possible interactions: Refer to manufacturer's profile of each drug

ALTERNATIVE DRUGS N/A

FOLLOWUP

PATIENT MONITORING Office follow-up visits e.g., q3 weeks x 2

PREVENTION/AVOIDANCE N/A

POSSIBLE COMPLICATIONS
- Postoperative shoulder, arm, hand pain and paresthesias in 10%, usually responds to physiotherapy
- 1.5-2% of patients will have symptomatic recurrences 1 month to 7 years postoperatively (usually within 3 months)
- 0.5-1% of patients have brachial plexus injury, probably due to intraoperative traction
- Re-operation indicated for symptomatic recurrence with long posterior remnant of first rib (posterior approach) or with disrupted fibrous adhesions (transaxillary approach)
- Venous obstruction or arterial emboli; usually responds to thrombolytics

EXPECTED COURSE/PROGNOSIS
- 60% improve with appropriate physiotherapy program
- 90% have excellent or good early results with surgery
- 70-80% have no recurrence at 5 years and 10 years

MISCELLANEOUS

ASSOCIATED CONDITIONS N/A

AGE-RELATED FACTORS N/A
Pediatric: N/A
Geriatric: N/A
Others: N/A

PREGNANCY Generalized tissue fluid accumulations and postural changes could aggravate symptoms

SYNONYMS
- Scalenus anticus syndrome
- Cervical rib syndrome
- Costoclavicular syndrome
- TOS

ICD-9-CM 353.0 Thoracic outlet syndrome

SEE ALSO N/A

OTHER NOTES 2-3 months trial of physiotherapy always indicated except in presence of obvious bony abnormality

ABBREVIATIONS N/A

REFERENCES
- Ursche HC, Rassuk MA: Thoracic Outlet Syndromes. In: Sabiston DC, Spencer FC, eds. Surgery of the Chest. 5th Ed. Philadelphia, W.B. Saunders Co.,1990
- Roos DB: Thoracic Outlet Nerve Compression. In: Ruthford RB, ed. Vascular Surgery. 3rd Ed. Philadelphia, W.B. Saunders Co.,1989
- Dale WQ: Thoracic outlet compression syndrome. Arch Surg 1982;117:1437
- Stallworth JM: Thoracic Outlet Compression Syndromes. In: Haimoviei H, ed. Vascular Surgery. 3rd Ed. Norwalk, Appleton & Lange,1989
- Novak CB, Mackinnon SE: Thoracic outlet syndrome. Orthopedic Clinics of NA 1996;27:747-762
- Oates SD, Daley RA: Thoracic outlet syndrome. Hand Clinics 1996;12:705-728
- Jordan SE: Diagnosis of thoracic outlet syndrome using electrophysiologically guided scalene blocker. Am Vasc Surg 1998;12:260-264
- Functional anatomy of the thoracic outlet: evaluarion with spinal CT. Thoracic Radiology 1997;295:843-851
Illustrations: N/A
Internet references: http://www.5mcc.com

Author(s)
Violet Siwik, MD

Thromboangiitis obliterans (Buerger's disease)

BASICS

DESCRIPTION Occlusion of small and medium sized arteries and veins caused by inflammatory changes in these vessels. It primarily occurs in men who smoke.
System(s) affected: Cardiovascular
Genetics: Greater prevalence of HLA-A54, HLA-A9 and HLA-B5. Familial cases reported rarely.
Incidence/Prevalence in USA: 13/100,000
Predominant age: 20 to 40 years
Predominant sex: Male > Female (3:1). Increasing numbers of women are being diagnosed, presumably due to increased smoking.

SIGNS AND SYMPTOMS
Symptoms tend to wax and wane in early disease and are often asymmetric. Symptoms may be gradual or have a sudden onset related to impaired vasculature.
• Ulceration of digits; pain may be disabling
• Coldness in feet and/or fingers
• Cold sensitivity
• Paresthesias (numbness, tingling, burning, hypoesthesia) of feet and/or fingers
• Intermittent claudication in arch of foot or leg (rarely hand, forearm)
• Persistent extremity pain (may be worse at rest)
• Paroxysmal "electric shock" pain of ischemic neuropathy
• Raynaud's phenomenon
• Postural color changes (pallor on elevation; rubor on dependency)
• "Buerger's color" - cyanosis of hands and feet
• Migratory superficial phlebitis
• Tender skin nodules on extremities
• Impaired distal pulses; proximal pulses normal
• Foot edema
• Gangrene

CAUSES
(Postulated)
• Smoking
• Genetic factors
• Autoimmune disorder with cell mediated sensitivity to types I and III human collagens (both are constituents of blood vessels)
• Impaired peripheral endothelium-dependent vasodilation

RISK FACTORS
• Smoking tobacco
• Incidence higher in Israel, Eastern Europe, Japan, India, Far East

DIAGNOSIS

DIFFERENTIAL DIAGNOSIS
• Peripheral neuropathy
• Peripheral atherosclerotic disease
• Arterial embolus and thrombosis
• Idiopathic peripheral thrombosis
• Other causes of vasculitis
• Scleroderma
• Occupational trauma
• Cervical rib
• Livedo reticularis
• Raynaud's disease
• Acrocyanosis
• Ergotism
• Frostbite
• Neurotrophic ulcers
• Reflex sympathetic dystrophy
• Metatarsalgia
• Gout
• Periarteritis nodosa
• Juvenile temporal arteritis with eosinophilia
• Polyarteritis
• Carpal tunnel syndrome
• Takayasu's arteritis (Japanese young women)

LABORATORY
Routine laboratory studies show no changes characteristic of this disorder. Auto-antibodies to collagen and circulating immune complexes may be present, but are considered a research tool only.
Drugs that may alter lab results: N/A
Disorders that may alter lab results: N/A

PATHOLOGICAL FINDINGS
• Segmental nonsuppurative panarteritis or panphlebitis with thrombosis
• Histologic findings may vary between acute, subacute, and chronic stages of the disease
• Histologic sine qua non - granulomas with collections of neutrophils in the organizing thrombus. Inflammation reaction permeates the entire thickness of the vessel wall.
• Chronic lesions show recanalized thrombus and perivascular fibrosis.

SPECIAL TESTS
• Doppler ultrasound (not specific)
• Point scoring systems may help clarify clinical diagnosis

IMAGING
• Arteriogram or digital-subtraction angiography (DSA)
  ◊ Multiple areas of segmental occlusion of small to medium arteries of arms and legs
  ◊ "Skip" areas may be demonstrated
  ◊ Numerous collateral vessels around occluded segments may give a characteristic "cork screw" appearance
  ◊ Larger arteries are spared

DIAGNOSTIC PROCEDURES
• History and physical examination
• Studies of nerve conduction velocity (to exclude neuropathy)

TREATMENT

APPROPRIATE HEALTH CARE
• Outpatient
• Inpatient if surgery needed for gangrene
• Inpatient for dorsal or lumbar sympathectomy if indicated

GENERAL MEASURES
• Stop smoking (mandatory)
• Protect against trauma (poor fitting shoes)
• Protect against infections
• Protect against vasoconstriction from cold or drugs
• Eliminate exposure to thermal damage
• Eliminate exposure to chemical damage (iodine, carbolic acid, salicylic acid)
• Thrombolytic therapy of occlusive thrombus and angioplasty are experimental

SURGICAL MEASURES
• Amputation for non-healing ulcers, gangrene or intractable pain. Should preserve as much limb as possible. Rarely required.
• Omental autotransplantation has been successful in treating ulcers
• In severe disease, a lumbar sympathectomy to increase blood supply to the skin
• Direct revascularization of distal arteries is not practical unless coexistent atherosclerotic disease or patients stop smoking

ACTIVITY
Restricted by symptoms. Use a bed cradle (non-heated) to prevent pressure from bed linens.

DIET
No restrictions

PATIENT EDUCATION
• Must stop smoking
• Remove possibilities of exposure to others in the environment who smoke
• Use heel pads or foam rubber boots
• See General Measures

Thromboangiitis obliterans (Buerger's disease)

MEDICATIONS

DRUG(S) OF CHOICE
- Medications are not a substitute for discontinuance of smoking
- Antibiotics for infected digital ulcers and osteomyelitis
- Iloprost, a prostacyclin analogue, promotes ulcer healing
- Urokinase selectively infused into occluded artery
- No form of medical treatment has been shown to be effective (including steroids, calcium channel blockers, reserpine, pentoxifylline, vasodilators, antiplatelet drugs, anticoagulants)

Contraindications: Refer to manufacturer's literature
Precautions: Refer to manufacturer's literature
Significant possible interactions: Refer to manufacturer's literature

ALTERNATIVE DRUGS
Calcium channel blocking agents such as nifedipine may allow vasodilatation, but have not been proven effective.

FOLLOWUP

PATIENT MONITORING Frequent history and physical examinations

PREVENTION/AVOIDANCE Never smoke

POSSIBLE COMPLICATIONS
- Ulcerations
- Gangrene
- Need for amputation
- Rare occlusion of cerebral, coronary, renal, splenic or mesenteric arteries

EXPECTED COURSE/PROGNOSIS
- Occasional remissions
- Unremitting progression if patient continues to smoke
- Death rare; normal survival curve

MISCELLANEOUS

ASSOCIATED CONDITIONS N/A

AGE-RELATED FACTORS
Pediatric: Not a problem in this age group
Geriatric: Not common in this age group, but diagnosis in the elderly is increasing
Others: N/A

PREGNANCY N/A

SYNONYMS
- Buerger's disease
- TAO

ICD-9-CM 443.1 Thromboangiitis obliterans (Buerger's disease)

SEE ALSO N/A

OTHER NOTES May be difficult to differentiate from some types of atherosclerosis, systemic emboli or idiopathic peripheral thromboses

ABBREVIATIONS N/A

REFERENCES
- Hurst JW, et al: The Heart. 7th Ed. New York, McGraw-Hill, 1998
- Case records of the Mass. General Hospital. Weekly clinicopathological exercises. case 16-1989. A 36 year-old man with peripheral vascular disease. New Eng J Med 1989;20;320(16):1068-76
- Olin JW, et al: The changing clinical spectrum of thromboangiitis obliterans (Buerger's disease). Circulation Supplement IV 1990;82(5)
- Dale DC, Federman DD. eds: Scientific American Medicine. New York, Scientific American, Inc 1998

Illustrations: N/A
Internet references: http://www.5mcc.com

Author(s)
Rick Kellerman, MD

Thrombophlebitis, superficial

BASICS

DESCRIPTION Superficial thrombophlebitis is an inflammatory condition of the veins with secondary thrombosis.
- Septic (suppurative) thrombophlebitis types:
  ◊ Iatrogenic
  ◊ Infectious, mainly syphilis and psittacosis
- Aseptic thrombophlebitis types:
  ◊ Primary hypercoagulable states - disorders with measurable defects in the proteins of the coagulation and/or fibrinolytic systems
  ◊ Secondary hypercoagulable states - clinical conditions with a risk of thrombosis
System(s) affected: Cardiovascular
Genetics:
- Septic - no known genetic pattern
- Antithrombin III deficiencies - autosomal dominant
- Proteins C and S deficiency - autosomal dominant with variable penetrance
- Disorders of fibrinolytic system - congenital defects inheritance variable
- Dysfibrinogenemia - autosomal dominant
- Factor XII deficiency - autosomal recessive
Incidence/Prevalence in USA:
- Septic
  ◊ Up to 10% of all nosocomial infections
  ◊ Incidence of catheter-related thrombophlebitis is 88/100,000
  ◊ Develops in 4-8% if cut down is performed
- Aseptic primary hypercoagulable state
  ◊ Antithrombin III and heparin cofactor II deficiency incidence is 50/100,000
- Aseptic secondary hypercoagulable state
  ◊ Trousseau incidence in malignancy 5-15%
  ◊ Trousseau in pancreatic carcinoma 50%
  ◊ In pregnancy 49-fold increased incidence of phlebitis
  ◊ Superficial migratory thrombophlebitis in 27% of patients with thromboangiitis obliterans
Predominant age:
- Septic
  ◊ More common in childhood
- Aseptic primary hypercoagulable state
  ◊ Antithrombin III and heparin cofactor II deficiency - neonatal period, but first episode usually at age 20-30 years
  ◊ Proteins C and S - before age 30
- Aseptic secondary hypercoagulable state
  ◊ Mondor's disease: women, ages 21-55 years
  ◊ Thromboangiitis obliterans onset: 20-50 years
Predominant sex:
- Suppurative:
  ◊ Male = Female
- Aseptic
  ◊ Mondor's - Female > Male (2:1)
  ◊ Thromboangiitis obliterans - Female > Male (1-19% of clinical cases)

SIGNS AND SYMPTOMS
- Swelling, tenderness, redness along the course of the veins
- May look like cellulitis or erythema nodosa
- Fever in 70% of patients
- Warmth, erythema, tenderness, or lymphangitis in 32%
- Sign of systemic sepsis in 84% in suppurative
- Red, tender cord
- Pain

CAUSES
- Septic
  ◊ Staphylococcus aureus in 65-78%
  ◊ Enterobacteriaceae, especially Klebsiella
  ◊ Multiple organisms in 14%
  ◊ Anaerobic isolate rare
  ◊ Candida spp.
  ◊ Cytomegalovirus in AIDS patients
- Aseptic primary hypercoagulable state
  ◊ Antithrombin III and heparin II deficiency
  ◊ Protein C and protein S deficiency
  ◊ Disorder of tissue plasminogen activator
  ◊ Abnormal plasminogen and co-plasminogen
  ◊ Dysfibrinogenemia
  ◊ Factor XII deficiency
  ◊ Lupus anticoagulant and anticardiolipin antibody syndrome
- Aseptic secondary hypercoagulable states
  ◊ Malignancy (Trousseau syndrome: Recurrent migratory thrombophlebitis). Most commonly seen in - metastatic mucin or adenocarcinomas of the GI tract (pancreas, stomach, colon and gall bladder); lung, prostate, ovary.
  ◊ Pregnancy
  ◊ Oral contraceptive
  ◊ Infusion of prothrombin complex concentrates
  ◊ Behçet's disease
  ◊ Buerger's disease
  ◊ Mondor's disease

RISK FACTORS
- Nonspecific
  ◊ Immobilization
  ◊ Obesity
  ◊ Advanced age
  ◊ Postoperative states
- Septic
  ◊ Intravenous catheter
  ◊ Duration of intravenous catheterization (68% of cannulae have been left in place for 2 days)
  ◊ Cutdowns
  ◊ Cancer, debilitating diseases
  ◊ Steroid
  ◊ Incidence is 40 times higher with plastic cannula (8%) than with steel or scalp cannulas (0.2%)
  ◊ Thrombosis
  ◊ Dermal infection
  ◊ Burned patients
  ◊ Lower extremities intravenous catheter
  ◊ Intravenous antibiotics
  ◊ AIDS
  ◊ Varicose veins
- Antithrombin II and heparin cofactor II deficiency
  ◊ Pregnancy
  ◊ Oral contraceptives
  ◊ Surgery; trauma; infection

- In pregnancy
  ◊ Increased age
  ◊ Hypertension
  ◊ Eclampsia
  ◊ Increased parity
- Thromboangiitis obliterans
  ◊ Persistent smoking
- Mondor's disease
  ◊ Breast abscess
  ◊ Antecedent breast surgery
  ◊ Breast augmentation
  ◊ Reduction mammoplasty

DIAGNOSIS

DIFFERENTIAL DIAGNOSIS
- Cellulitis
- Erythema nodosa
- Cutaneous polyarteritis nodosa
- Sarcoid
- Kaposi's sarcoma
- Hyperalgesic pseudothrombophlebitis

LABORATORY
- Septic
  ◊ Bacteremia in 80-90%
  ◊ Culture of IV fluid bag
  ◊ Leukocytosis
- Aseptic
  ◊ Acute phase reactant
  ◊ Factor levels
  ◊ Thrombin activity
  ◊ Platelet function test
Drugs that may alter lab results: In septic, broad spectrum antibiotics
Disorders that may alter lab results: N/A

PATHOLOGICAL FINDINGS
- The affected vein is enlarged, tortuous, and thickened
- Associated perivascular suppuration and/or hemorrhage
- Vein lumen may contain pus and thrombus
- Endothelial damage, fibrinoid necrosis and thickening of the vein wall

SPECIAL TESTS Leukocyte imaging

IMAGING
- Septic and aseptic
  ◊ Ultrasound of veins reveal an increase in the diameter of the lumen
  ◊ Chest x-ray - multiple peripheral densities or a pleural effusion consistent with pulmonary embolism, abscess, or empyema
  ◊ Bone and gallium scan - for associated subperiosteal abscess in septic thrombophlebitis
  ◊ Evaluation of complications (deep vein thrombosis and others)

DIAGNOSTIC PROCEDURES Skin biopsy

TREATMENT

APPROPRIATE HEALTH CARE
• Septic - inpatient
• Aseptic - outpatient

GENERAL MEASURES
• Heat application
• Extremity elevation

SURGICAL MEASURES
• Septic
◊ Excision of the involved vein segment and all involved tributaries
◊ Excision from ankle to groin may be required in some burn patients
◊ If systemic symptoms persist after vein excision, re-exploration is necessary with removal of all involved veins
◊ Drainage of contiguous abscesses
◊ Remove all cannulae
• Aseptic
◊ Mondor's disease, consider surgical transection of the phlebitic cord
◊ Management of underlying conditions

ACTIVITY Bedrest

DIET No restrictions

PATIENT EDUCATION
• Avoid trauma
• Be alert to change in skin color
• Be alert to tenderness over extremities

MEDICATIONS

DRUG(S) OF CHOICE
• Septic
◊ Initially: semisynthetic penicillin (e.g., nafcillin 2 g IV q6h) plus an aminoglycoside (e.g., gentamicin, 1.0-1.7 mg/kg IV)
◊ Duration of therapy is empiric
◊ If due to Candida albicans, consider a short course of amphotericin B, approximately 200 mg cumulative dose
◊ If osteomyelitis documented, antibiotic therapy for at least 6 weeks
• Aseptic general
◊ Nonsteroidal anti-inflammatories
◊ Oral anticoagulant warfarin
◊ Systemic anticoagulant heparin
• Antithrombin III and heparin cofactor II deficiency
◊ IV heparin
◊ Antithrombin III concentrate
◊ Prophylaxis: warfarin, oxymetholone
• Proteins C and S
◊ Long-term warfarin, lower dose, no loading
• Disorder of tissue plasminogen activator
◊ Phenformin and ethylestrenol
◊ Stanozolol and phenformin
◊ Stanozolol alone
◊ Ethylestrenol alone

• Dysfibrinogemia
◊ Acute attack - anticoagulation
◊ Prophylaxis - stanozolol
• Abnormal plasminogen and plasminogenemia
◊ Acute attack - anticoagulation
◊ Prophylaxis - warfarin
• Factor XII deficiency
◊ Standard therapy
• Lupus anticardiolipin
◊ Prophylaxis - warfarin
• Trousseau's syndrome
◊ Heparin
• For pregnancy
◊ Heparin
• Behçet's disease
◊ Phenformin
◊ Ethylestrenol
◊ Stanozolol
• Thromboangiitis obliterans
◊ Stop smoking
◊ Pentoxifylline

Contraindications: Refer to manufacturer's literature
Precautions: Refer to manufacturer's literature
Significant possible interactions:
Refer to manufacturer's literature

ALTERNATIVE DRUGS
• Factor XII deficiency - streptokinase or alteplase (tissue plasminogen activator, TPA)
• Behcet's - oral anticoagulants plus cyclosporine
• Thromboangiitis obliterans - corticosteroid, antiplatelets and vasodilating drugs

FOLLOWUP

PATIENT MONITORING
• Septic
◊ Routine WBC and differential and culture
◊ Repeat culture from the phlebitic vein
• Aseptic
◊ Clinical followup to rule out secondary complications
◊ Repeat of blood studies for fibrinolytic system, platelets and factors

PREVENTION/AVOIDANCE
• Use of scalp vein cannulae
• Avoidance of lower extremity cannulations
• Insertion under aseptic conditions
• Secure anchoring of the cannulae
• Replacement of cannulae, connecting tubing, and IV fluid every 48-72 hrs
• Neomycin-polymyxin B-bacitracin ointment in cutdown

POSSIBLE COMPLICATIONS
• Septic: Systemic sepsis, bacteremia (84%); septic pulmonary emboli (44%); metastatic abscess formation; pneumonia (44%); subperiosteal abscess of adjacent long bones in children
• Aseptic: Deep vein thrombosis; thromboembolic phenomena

EXPECTED COURSE/PROGNOSIS
• Septic high mortality (50%), if untreated
• Aseptic
◊ Usually benign course; recovery 7-10 days
◊ Antithrombin III and heparin cofactor deficiency; recurrence rate is 60%
◊ Proteins C and S, recurrence rate 70%
◊ Prognosis depends on development of DVT and early detections of complications
◊ Aseptic thrombophlebitis can be isolated, recurrent or migratory

MISCELLANEOUS

ASSOCIATED CONDITIONS Varicose
veins, manifestation of systemic disease, hypercoagulable states, surgery, trauma, burns, obesity, pregnancy

AGE-RELATED FACTORS
Pediatric: Subperiosteal abscesses of adjacent long bone may complicate
Geriatric: Septic thrombophlebitis is more common, prognosis poorer
Others: N/A

PREGNANCY
• Associated with increased risk of aseptic superficial thrombophlebitis
• Warfarin and NSAID's are contraindicated

SYNONYMS
• Phlebitis
• Phlebothrombosis

ICD-9-CM
451 Phlebitis and thrombophlebitis -
451.0 Phlebitis and thrombophlebitis of superficial vessels of lower extremities
451.1 Phlebitis and thrombophlebitis of deep vessels of lower extremities

SEE ALSO
• Thrombosis, deep vein (DVT)
• Cellulitis

OTHER NOTES N/A

ABBREVIATIONS DVT = deep vein
thrombosis

REFERENCES
• Samlaskie CP, James WD: Superficial thrombophlebitis II. Secondary hypercoagulable states. J Am Acad Dermato 1990;23(1)1-18
• Samlaskie CP, James WD: Superficial thrombophlebitis I. Primary hypercoagulable states. J Am Acad Dermatol 1990;22:975-89
• Mandell GL, ed: Principles and Practice of Infectious Diseases. 4th Ed. New York, Churchill Livingstone, 1995
Illustrations: N/A
Internet references: http://www.5mcc.com

Author(s)
Abdulrazak Abyad, MD, MPH, AGSF

Thrombosis, deep vein (DVT)

BASICS

DESCRIPTION Development of single or multiple blood clots within the deep veins of the extremities or pelvis, usually accompanied by inflammation of the vessel wall. The major clinical consequence is embolization, usually to the lung, that is frequently life-threatening.
System(s) affected: Cardiovascular
Genetics: N/A
Incidence/Prevalence in USA: Common (approximately 2 million cases per year)
Predominant age: Usually over 40
Predominant sex: Female > Male (1.2:1)

SIGNS AND SYMPTOMS

• Many cases are completely asymptomatic, diagnosed retrospectively after embolization
• Limb pain (common)
• Limb swelling (common)
• Leg pain on dorsiflexion of the foot (Homan's sign; common)
• Palpable tender cord in affected limb (uncommon)
• Warmth of skin over area of thrombosis (uncommon)
• Redness of skin over area or thrombosis (uncommon)
• Fever (uncommon, except in septic thrombophlebitis)
• Non-tender swelling of collateral superficial veins (uncommon)
• Massive edema with cyanosis and ischemia (Phlegmasia cerulea dolens, rare)

CAUSES

• Venous stasis
• Injury to vessel wall
• Abnormalities of coagulation

RISK FACTORS

• Clinical risk factors:
  ◊ Trauma, especially long bone fractures or crush injuries
  ◊ Surgery, particularly hip and knee surgery
  ◊ Prolonged immobility
  ◊ Pregnancy, especially the puerperium
  ◊ Indwelling central venous catheters
  ◊ Estrogen use (risk is confined to current usage and is proportional to estrogen content)
  ◊ Extreme high altitude (> 14,000 feet)
• Pathological risk factors:
  ◊ Carcinoma
  ◊ Deficiencies of protein C, protein S, antithrombin III, all endogenous anticoagulants
  ◊ Presence of anti-phospholipid antibodies (also known as lupus anticoagulant or anti-cardiolipin antibodies)
  ◊ Nephrotic syndrome
  ◊ Polycythemia vera
  ◊ Homocystinuria (rare)
  ◊ Campylobacter jejuni bacteremia (very rare)
  ◊ Mutation on Factor V conferring resistance to activated protein C (most common risk factor for idiopathic DVT)

DIAGNOSIS

DIFFERENTIAL DIAGNOSIS

• Cellulitis
• Ruptured synovial cyst (Baker's cyst)
• Lymphedema
• Extrinsic compression of vein by tumor or enlarged lymph nodes
• Pulled, strained, or torn muscle

LABORATORY

• No specific laboratory test is available for DVT
• Protein C, protein S, antithrombin III and anti-phospholipid antibodies can be measured in some laboratories. But as these are rare causes of DVT they are not routinely indicated and should be ordered only when the clinical circumstances suggest such a disorder.
Drugs that may alter lab results:
• Heparin, estrogens may lower antithrombin III levels
• Coumadin affects protein C and protein S function so may interfere with functional assays of these proteins
Disorders that may alter lab results:
• Thrombosis itself lowers antithrombin III levels so any workup for antithrombin III deficiency must be performed after patient has completed therapy
• Syphilis and systemic lupus erythematosus are associated with increased anti-phospholipid antibodies

PATHOLOGICAL FINDINGS

• Clot consisting predominantly of red blood cells, with some platelets and fibrin attached to vessel wall at one end with proximal end floating free in the lumen. Varying degrees of inflammation of the vessel wall are present.
• Biochemical abnormalities such as proteins S, C or antithrombin III deficiency, anti-phospholipid antibody or homocystinuria are found in only a small minority of cases
• Mutant Factor V conferring resistance to protein C ("Factor V Leiden") is a common abnormality, but routine clinical tests for the mutation are not yet in widespread use

SPECIAL TESTS N/A

IMAGING

• Imaging studies are necessary to diagnose or rule out suspected DVT
• Contrast venography is the gold standard test (i.e., most sensitive and specific). Disadvantages include discomfort, technical difficulty and small risk of morbidity.
• B-mode ultrasound combined with Doppler flow detection (duplex ultrasound); noninvasive, highly sensitive and specific for popliteal and femoral thrombi. Disadvantages include poor ability to detect calf vein thrombi; it is a highly operator-dependent technique; and its inability to reliably distinguish extrinsic compression of the vein from intrinsic clot.
• Impedance plethysmography (IPG); probably as accurate as duplex ultrasound, less operator dependency, but poor at detecting calf vein thrombi
• 125 I-fibrinogen scan; detects only active clot formation; very good at detecting ongoing calf thrombi. Major disadvantage is that it takes 4 hours for results. This test has generally been supplanted by duplex ultrasound and IPG.

DIAGNOSTIC PROCEDURES N/A

TREATMENT

APPROPRIATE HEALTH CARE

Patients with DVT confined to the calf (i.e., distal to the popliteal system) can be managed conservatively as outpatients. All others should be admitted.

GENERAL MEASURES For hospitalized patient - intravenous anticoagulation, a brief period of bedrest, and close observation for embolic events

SURGICAL MEASURES Non-drug therapy - if anticoagulants and thrombolytics are contraindicated, filtering devices ("umbrellas") can he inserted into the vena cava to "trap" emboli before reaching the lungs

ACTIVITY Bedrest for 1-2 days, then gradual resumption of normal activity, with avoidance of prolonged immobility

DIET No special diet

PATIENT EDUCATION

• Advise women taking estrogen of the risks, and the common symptoms of thromboembolic disease
• Discourage prolonged immobility

MEDICATIONS

DRUG(S) OF CHOICE
• Immediate therapy: Heparin 80 units/kg intravenous bolus followed by continuous IV infusion starting at 18 units/kg/hr. Adjust dosage based on activated partial thromboplastin time (APTT) to achieve APTT of approximately 3 x control value.
• Maintenance therapy: warfarin (Coumadin) beginning 1-3 days after starting heparin, in a single daily dose starting at 5-10 mg daily and adjusting based on prothrombin time (PT) with a target value of PT of 1.5-2x control value. Patient should remain on heparin until target PT level is achieved. Physicians should use international normalized ratio (INR), if available, to guide therapy. Aim for INR 2.0-3.0.

Contraindications:
• Absolute contraindications: Severe active bleeding, recent neurosurgical procedure (within 30 days), pregnancy (warfarin only), previous adverse reaction to the drug (other than bleeding, which is a known side effect)
• Relative contraindications: Recent severe hemorrhage, recent surgical procedure other than neurosurgery, history of significant peptic ulcer disease, recent non-embolic stroke

Precautions:
• Observe patient carefully for signs of embolization, further thrombosis or bleeding
• While on anticoagulant therapy avoid intramuscular injections. Periodically check stool and urine for occult blood, monitor complete blood counts including platelets.
• Heparin - other possible but rare adverse reactions include thrombocytopenia and/or paradoxical thrombosis with thrombocytopenia
• Warfarin - necrotic lesions of the skin (Warfarin necrosis) occasionally result from treatment

Significant possible interactions:
• Agents that may prolong or intensify the response to oral anticoagulants: Alcohol, allopurinol, amiodarone, anabolic steroids, androgens, many antimicrobials, cimetidine chloral hydrate, disulfiram, all nonsteroidal anti-inflammatory drugs (NSAID's), sulfinpyrazone, tamoxifen, thyroid hormone, vitamin E, ranitidine, salicylates, acetaminophen
• Agents that may diminish the response to anticoagulants: Aminoglutethimide, antacids, barbiturates, carbamazepine, cholestyramine, diuretics, griseofulvin, rifampin, oral contraceptives

ALTERNATIVE DRUGS
• Thrombolytic agents (urokinase, streptokinase, alteplase [tissue plasminogen activator]) are effective in dissolving clots and are currently investigational for treatment of DVT. In current clinical practice they should he reserved for massive thromboembolic disease. The same contraindications apply as to anticoagulants.
• Low molecular weight heparin enoxaparin (Lovenox) 1 mg/kg/dose bid SC, may be as effective as IV heparin in treatment of uncomplicated DVT

• If warfarin (Coumadin) is contraindicated, heparin can be given in the ambulatory setting by intermittent subcutaneous self-injection (see Pregnancy)

FOLLOWUP

PATIENT MONITORING
• APTT must be monitored several times a day while on IV heparin until dose stabilizes. Platelets should also be monitored and heparin discontinued if platelets fall below 75,000
• While on warfarin, PT must be monitored daily until target achieved, then weekly for several weeks, then (if stable) monthly as long as patient is on the drug
• For first episode of DVT patients should be treated for 3-6 months. Subsequent episodes should be treated for at least a year.
• Significant bleeding such as hematuria or gastrointestinal hemorrhage should be thoroughly investigated since anticoagulant therapy frequently unmasks a pre-existing lesion such as cancer, peptic ulcer disease, or arteriovenous malformation

PREVENTION/AVOIDANCE
• General preventive measures such as avoiding prolonged immobility and using low-estrogen birth control pills when possible
• Surgical patients need active prophylaxis: Low dose subcutaneous heparin with dosage adjusted to slightly prolong the APTT, low dose Coumadin, enoxaparin (low molecular weight heparin) and intermittent mechanical compression of the legs have all been effective in reducing the risks of DVT following various types of surgery.

POSSIBLE COMPLICATIONS
• Pulmonary embolism (fatal in 10-20% of cases)
• Systemic embolism ("paradoxical embolization") in cases where there is arteriovenous shunting (rare)
• Chronic venous insufficiency
• Post-phlebitic syndrome, i.e., pain and swelling in affected limb without new clot formation
• Treatment induced hemorrhage
• Soft tissue ischemia associated with massive clot and very high venous pressures - phlegmasia cerulea dolens (very rare but should be considered a surgical emergency)

EXPECTED COURSE/PROGNOSIS
• About 20% of untreated proximal (i.e., above the calf) DVT's progress to pulmonary emboli and 10-20% of those are fatal. With aggressive anticoagulant therapy the mortality is decreased five to tenfold.
• DVT confined to the calf virtually never causes clinically significant emboli so does not require anticoagulation. However calf DVT's do sometimes propagate into the proximal system so known or suspected calf DVT's should be followed with IPG or duplex ultrasound every 3-5 days for 10 days and treated aggressively if they propagate into the popliteal or femoral system.

MISCELLANEOUS

ASSOCIATED CONDITIONS
• Budd-Chiari syndrome (hepatic vein thrombosis)
• Renal vein thrombosis
• Homocystinuria
• Anti-phospholipid antibody syndrome

AGE-RELATED FACTORS
Pediatric: In this age group patients with DVT, in absence of preceding trauma, should be worked up for congenital coagulopathy
Geriatric: More common because predisposing conditions are more common
Others: N/A

PREGNANCY
• Warfarin (Coumadin) is a known teratogen so is contraindicated in pregnancy. Treat pregnant women with DVT with full dose heparin initially followed by subcutaneous heparin starting at 15,000 units twice daily with target APTT of 1.5-2 x control value.
• Septic thrombophlebitis, usually associated with childbirth, requires antibiotic therapy as well as anticoagulation

SYNONYMS Deep venous thrombophlebitis

ICD-9-CM 451.19 Phlebitis and thrombophlebitis, of deep vessels of lower extremities, other

SEE ALSO
• Pulmonary embolism

OTHER NOTES N/A

ABBREVIATIONS
• DVT = deep vein thrombophlebitis
• IPG = impedance plethysmography
• INR = international normalized ratio

REFERENCES
• Hirsh J: Venous thromboembolism. In: Rubenstein E, Federman DD, eds. Scientific American Medicine. New York, Scientific American, 1994
• Kontos HA: Vascular Diseases of the Limbs. In: Wyngaarden JB, Smith LH, eds. Cecil Textbook of Medicine. Philadelphia, W.B. Saunders Co., 1992
• Weinman EE, Salzman EW: Deep-vein thrombosis. New Engl J Med 1994;331:1630-1641
Illustrations: N/A
Internet references: http://www.5mcc.com

Author(s)
Robert J. Sliman, MD

Thyroglossal duct cyst

BASICS

DESCRIPTION   Cystic remnant of thyroid descent in the neck
System(s) affected: Endocrine/Metabolic, Skin/Exocrine
Genetics: N/A
Incidence/Prevalence in USA: N/A
Predominant age: 50% less than 10 years, 65% less than 20 years of age
Predominant sex: Male = Female

SIGNS AND SYMPTOMS
• Midline neck mass
• Non-tender, unless infected
• Rises in the neck with tongue protrusion
• 80% juxtaposed to the hyoid bone

CAUSES   Failure of obliteration of the thyroglossal duct following descent of the thyroid in the 6th week of fetal life

RISK FACTORS   None

DIAGNOSIS

DIFFERENTIAL DIAGNOSIS
• Ectopic midline thyroid
• Dermoid cyst
• Thyroid adenoma of isthmus or pyramidal lobe
• Lymphadenitis

LABORATORY   None
Drugs that may alter lab results: N/A
Disorders that may alter lab results: N/A

PATHOLOGICAL FINDINGS   Cyst lined with stratified squamous or pseudostratified ciliated columnar epithelium. Thyroid tissue seen in 10-45% of cysts.

SPECIAL TESTS   N/A

IMAGING
• Ultrasound
• Thyroid scan if midline ectopic thyroid or thyroid nodule is suspected

DIAGNOSTIC PROCEDURES   N/A

TREATMENT

APPROPRIATE HEALTH CARE
Outpatient surgery

GENERAL MEASURES   N/A

SURGICAL MEASURES
• Once diagnosed, the excision can be done with Sistrunk procedure. This requires removal of the center portion of the hyoid bone to minimize recurrence.
• If the cyst is infected, it should be initially treated (antibiotics and local heat) or drained. After resolution of the inflammation, excision should be performed.

ACTIVITY   Unrestricted

DIET   Unrestricted

PATIENT EDUCATION
• Reassurance to family about absence of malignancy
• Patient may require thyroid medication for life, if ectopic, midline thyroid mistakenly removed

MEDICATIONS

DRUG(S) OF CHOICE None. All thyroglossal duct cysts should be surgically removed.
Contraindications: N/A
Precautions: N/A
Significant possible interactions: N/A

ALTERNATIVE DRUGS N/A

FOLLOWUP

PATIENT MONITORING 1-2 weeks after drainage or resection

PREVENTION/AVOIDANCE N/A

POSSIBLE COMPLICATIONS Infection and malignant degeneration if not excised

EXPECTED COURSE/PROGNOSIS Resolution with resection (less than 5% recurrence using the Sistrunk procedure)

MISCELLANEOUS

ASSOCIATED CONDITIONS None

AGE-RELATED FACTORS
Pediatric: N/A
Geriatric: N/A
Others: N/A

PREGNANCY N/A

SYNONYMS N/A

ICD-9-CM
759.2 Anomalies of other endocrine glands

SEE ALSO N/A

OTHER NOTES N/A

ABBREVIATIONS N/A

REFERENCES Welch KJ, Randolph JG, Ravitch MM, et al, eds: Pediatric Surgery. 4th Ed. New York, Year Book Medical Publishers, 1986
Illustrations: N/A
Internet references: http://www.5mcc.com

Author(s)
James P. Miller, MD, FACS, FAAP
Timothy L. Black, MD, FACS, FAAP

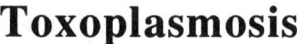

TREATMENT

APPROPRIATE HEALTH CARE
• Outpatient for acquired disease in immunocompetent host and ocular toxoplasmosis
• Inpatient initially for CNS toxoplasmosis and acute disease in immunocompromised host

GENERAL MEASURES
• Usually no treatment in asymptomatic hosts except in child under 5
• Symptomatic patients should be treated until immunity is assured

SURGICAL MEASURES N/A

ACTIVITY Level of activity dependent on severity of disease and organ systems involved

DIET No special diet

PATIENT EDUCATION
• Infected mother must be completely informed of potential consequences to fetus
• Explain prevention methods, e.g., protecting children's play area from cat litter
• Additional materials available from:
• National Institute of Allergy and Infectious Disease, Dept. of Health and Human Services, Bldg. 31, Rm 7A-32, 9000 Rockville Pike, Bethesda, MD 20892, (301)496-5717

MEDICATIONS

DRUG(S) OF CHOICE
• Acute toxoplasmosis in immunodeficient host:
  ◊ Sulfadiazine (Microsulfon) 100 mg/kg/day up to 8 grams/day plus pyrimethamine (Daraprim) 200 mg the first day, then 25-50 mg/day plus leucovorin (folinic acid) 10 mg/day for several weeks followed by maintenance therapy with the same drugs at lower dosage for several months
• Ocular toxoplasmosis: Above regimen for 1-2 months
• Acute toxoplasmosis in pregnant women: Above regimen may be used after the 16th week of pregnancy
• Congenital toxoplasmosis: Sulfadiazine 100 mg/kg/day plus pyrimethamine I mg/kg every 2 days plus leucovorin (folinic acid) 5 mg every 2 days

Contraindications:
• Pyrimethamine should not be used in first trimester of pregnancy
• Known hypersensitivity to pyrimethamine or sulfadiazine (Note: many HIV positive patients have a sulfa sensitivity)

Precautions:
• Bone marrow toxicity an important problem while treating toxoplasmosis
• Use with caution in patients with possible folate deficiency
• Use with caution in patients with renal or hepatic dysfunction
• Sulfonamides may increase anticoagulant effect of coumadin
• Sulfonamides may increase phenytoin (Dilantin) levels
• Sulfonamides may increase hypoglycemic effect of oral hypoglycemic agents
• Adequate hydration is essential since sulfadiazine is poorly soluble and may crystallize in the urine

Significant possible interactions:
Sulfonamides may interact with phenytoin, coumadin and oral hypoglycemic agents

ALTERNATIVE DRUGS
• In pregnancy - Spiramycin 3 g/day for 3 weeks, then 2 weeks off, then repeat 5 week cycles throughout pregnancy. Drug not yet FDA approved in U.S. Contact manufacturer - Rhone-Poulenc, Inc., CN5266, Princeton, NJ 08543-5266.
• Clindamycin 900-1200 mg tid IV has been used for ocular and CNS toxoplasmosis alone and in combination with pyrimethamine. May be as effective as the sulfa/pyrimethamine combination, but with fewer adverse effects.
• Corticosteroids (prednisone 1-2 mg/kg/day) may be added for macular chorioretinitis or CNS infection
• Atovaquone (Mepron), azithromycin (Zithromax) and clarithromycin (Biaxin) - promising new agents for CNS toxoplasmosis

FOLLOWUP

PATIENT MONITORING
• Followup visits every 2 weeks until stable, then monthly during therapy
• CBC weekly for first month, then every 2 weeks
• Renal and liver function tests monthly

PREVENTION/AVOIDANCE Prevention is important in seronegative pregnant women and immunodeficient patients. Avoid eating raw meat, unpasteurized milk, uncooked eggs and avoid contact with cat feces.

POSSIBLE COMPLICATIONS
• Seizure disorder or focal neurologic deficits in CNS toxoplasmosis
• Partial or complete blindness with ocular toxoplasmosis
• Multiple complications may occur with congenital toxoplasmosis including mental retardation, seizures, deafness and blindness

EXPECTED COURSE/PROGNOSIS
• Immunodeficient patients often relapse if treatment is stopped
• Treatment may prevent the development of untoward sequelae in both symptomatic and asymptomatic infants with congenital toxoplasmosis

MISCELLANEOUS

ASSOCIATED CONDITIONS Cellular immune compromised patients, especially those with AIDS, have a higher incidence of toxoplasmosis

AGE-RELATED FACTORS
Pediatric: With acute congenital toxoplasmosis, children often die in the first month of life. Subacute congenital disease may not be observed until some time after birth, when symptoms start to appear.
Geriatric: Acquired infection. Often reactivation disease more likely.
Others: None

PREGNANCY
• Have serum examined for Toxoplasma antibodies. Those with negative titers should take extra precautions to avoid contact with cats, not to eat raw meat and wash all fruits and vegetables carefully.
• For toxoplasmosis infection during pregnancy, refer patient to specialist

SYNONYMS N/A

ICD-9-CM
130.9 Toxoplasmosis, unspecified
771.2 Other congenital infections

SEE ALSO N/A

OTHER NOTES N/A

ABBREVIATIONS N/A

REFERENCES
• Mandell G, ed: Principles and Practice of Infectious Diseases. 4th Ed. New York, Churchill Livingstone, 1995
• Katkama C, et al: Pyrimethamine-clindamycin vs. pyrimethamine-sulfadiazine in acute and lon term therapy for toxoplasmic encephalitis in patients with AIDS. Clin Infect Dis 1996;22(2):268-75
Illustrations: 2 available on CD-ROM
Internet references: http://www.5mcc.com

Author(s)
William G. Gardner, MD

Tracheitis, bacterial

BASICS

DESCRIPTION
• Severe, potentially life-threatening infraglottic infection; relatively rare, caused by a secondary bacterial infection following a primary viral infection, usually H. parainfluenzae or H. influenzae
• Also called pseudomembranous croup or membranous tracheitis was described by C.L. Jackson as "an acute infection of the larynx, trachea, and bronchi characterized by toxemia, edema of the larynx and subglottic regions, and a thick, viscid, obstructive, often crusting exudate in the tracheobronchial tree."
System(s) affected: Pulmonary
Genetics: No known genetic predisposition
Incidence/prevalence in USA: True incidence is unknown; was a fairly common childhood illness in the pre-antibiotic era; a resurgence of cases has been noted since 1979; fall/winter predominance; in one series, 2% of all children hospitalized with "croup" had bacterial tracheitis
Predominant age: Mean age 54 months; range 3 weeks to 13 years; infections in adolescents have been reported
Predominant sex: Male > Female (1.8: 1); no gender predominance seen in other studies

SIGNS AND SYMPTOMS
• Barking, "brassy" cough
• Inspiratory stridor
• Variable degree of respiratory distress
• Child is usually lying flat
• Fever > 38°C (100.4°F)
• Toxic-appearing
• There is a gradual progression of mild upper airway symptoms over 1 hour to six days to an acute, febrile phase of rapid respiratory decompensation
• Voice and cry are usually normal
• Absence of drooling and dysphagia help distinguish it from epiglottitis
• Does not respond to aerosolized epinephrine (unlike patients with croup)
• Subglottic edema

CAUSES
• Staphylococcal aureus
• H. influenzae
• Streptococcus pneumoniae
• Moraxella catarrhalis
• Klebsiella
• Streptococci (group A)
• Neisseria

RISK FACTORS   Periods of increased seasonal activity of respiratory viruses

DIAGNOSIS

DIFFERENTIAL DIAGNOSIS
• Laryngotracheomalacia
• Epiglottitis
• Foreign body
• Retropharyngeal abscess
• Pneumonia
• Asthma
• Spasmodic croup
• Diphtheritic laryngitis

LABORATORY   Elevated WBC count with predominance of PMN's and some bands present; blood cultures are usually negative
Drugs that may alter lab results: N/A
Disorders that may alter lab results: N/A

PATHOLOGICAL FINDINGS
• Mucosal destruction and/or local immunodeficiency caused by viral infection may predispose to bacterial infection
• Intense inflammation, sloughing of subglottic epithelium, and profuse mucopurulent secretions which compromise the airway and which make airway management very difficult

SPECIAL TESTS   Rapid antigen tests are available for bacteria and viruses in some centers

IMAGING
• AP and lateral neck radiographs show subglottic and tracheal narrowing with haziness and radiopaque linear or particulate densities (crusts)
• In patients with risk of acute respiratory obstruction, either do not obtain radiographs or monitor carefully
• Often see pneumonic infiltrates

DIAGNOSTIC PROCEDURES
• Endoscopy is diagnostic and demonstrates severe inflammation of the subglottic region and trachea with copious mucopurulent secretions and sloughed epithelium that separates from the tracheal wall in sheets
• Obtain Gram stain and culture of tracheal secretions

TREATMENT

APPROPRIATE HEALTH CARE   ICU care

GENERAL MEASURES
• Constitutes a true pediatric emergency
• Maintain airway – this is often very difficult due to copious secretions
• Hydration, humidification, antibiotics
• Endotracheal or nasotracheal intubation
• Does not respond to epinephrine

SURGICAL MEASURES   Tracheotomy may be necessary

ACTIVITY   Complete bed rest

DIET   Peripheral venous nutrition

PATIENT EDUCATION   Usually requires 3-13 days intubation with complete recovery expected

MEDICATIONS

DRUG(S) OF CHOICE
- Nafcillin 150 mg/kg/day divided QID plus cefotaxime 150 mg/kg/day in 4-6 divided doses; maximum of 2 grams q6h
or
- Cefuroxime 75 mg/kg/day divided QID
- Does not respond to epinephrine
- Narrow the antibiotic regimen when pathogens and sensitivities available

Contraindications: Refer to manufacturer's literature

Precautions: Refer to manufacturer's literature

Significant possible interactions: See manufacturer's literature

ALTERNATIVE DRUGS
For patients with penicillin allergy: Clindamycin 40 mg/kg/day divided QID plus chloramphenicol 75 mg/kg/day divided QID

FOLLOWUP

PATIENT MONITORING ICU care with cardiopulmonary monitoring

PREVENTION/AVOIDANCE N/A

POSSIBLE COMPLICATIONS
- Postintubation subglottic stenosis
- Cardiopulmonary arrest
- Pneumonia
- Toxic shock syndrome secondary to enterotoxin-producing staphylococci

EXPECTED COURSE/PROGNOSIS
- With vigorous airway management and intubation for up to 13 days, complete recovery is expected
- Cardiopulmonary arrest and death have occurred.

MISCELLANEOUS

ASSOCIATED CONDITIONS Consider anatomic abnormalities or foreign body

AGE-RELATED FACTORS
Pediatric: Typically affects children below the age of three
Geriatric: N/A
Others: N/A

PREGNANCY No more contagious than the common cold; scrupulous handwashing is recommended

SYNONYMS
- Pseudomembranous croup
- Membranous tracheitis

ICD-9-CM
464.1 Acute tracheitis
464.2 Acute laryngotracheitis

SEE ALSO
- Common cold
- Epiglottitis
- Bronchiolitis
- Laryngotracheobronchitis

OTHER NOTES N/A

ABBREVIATIONS
- ED = emergency department
- LTB = laryngotracheobronchitis

REFERENCES
- Cunningham MJ: The old and new of acute laryngotracheal infections. Clinical Pediatrics 1992;31(1): 56-64
- Donnelly BW, McMillan JA, Weiner LB: Bacterial tracheitis: report of eight new cases and review. Reviews of Infectious Diseases 1990;12(5):729-735
- Jackson CL: Acute infective laryngotracheobronchitis. In Mitchell-Nelson Textbook of Pediatrics. 4th Ed. Philadelphia, W.B. Saunders Co, 1945
- Kasian GF, Bingham WT, Steinberg, et al: Bacterial tracheitis in children. Canadian Medical Association Journal 1989;140(1):46-50
- Klassen TP, Feldman ME, et al: Nebulized budesonide for children with mild-to-moderate croup. New Engl J Med 1994;331:285-89
- Rabie I, McShane D, Warde D: Bacterial tracheitis. Journal of Laryngology & Otology 1989;103(11):1059-1062
- Walker P, Crysdale WS: Croup, epiglottitis, retropharyngeal abscess, and bacterial tracheitis: evolving patterns of occurrence and care. International Anesthesiology Clinics 1992;30(4):57-70
Illustrations: N/A
Internet references: http://www.5mcc.com

Author(s)
Barcey T. Levy, PhD, MD

Transfusion reaction, hemolytic

BASICS

DESCRIPTION A cytotoxic, hemolytic reaction that occurs after administration of blood or blood components, resulting in hemolysis of donor's or recipient's RBC's (usually the latter). Reactions may be immune or nonimmune, and can vary from a mild to a fatal consequence. (Infection risks outweigh immune risks.)
System(s) affected:
Hemic/Lymphatic/Immunologic, Cardiovascular
Genetics: No known genetic pattern
Incidence/Prevalence in USA: Uncommon
Predominant age: All ages
Predominant sex: Female > Male

SIGNS AND SYMPTOMS
• Immediate (intravascular) hemolytic transfusion reaction:
  ◊ Anxiety
  ◊ Flushing
  ◊ Tachycardia
  ◊ Hypotension
  ◊ Chest or back pain
  ◊ Dyspnea
  ◊ Fever
  ◊ Chills
  ◊ Note: symptoms are masked in anesthetized patient
• Delayed (extravascular) hemolytic transfusion reaction:
  ◊ Fever
  ◊ Anemia (2-14 days after transfusion)
  ◊ Jaundice

CAUSES
• Immune reactions - incompatibility within ABO system
• A nonhemolytic febrile reaction due to immune sensitivity to leukocytes, platelets, plasma constituents
• Hemolytic reactions:
  ◊ Transfusion of mismatched blood
  ◊ Destruction of donor erythrocytes by recipient incompatible isoantibodies
  ◊ Isosensitization by repeated transfusions
  ◊ Isosensitization by prior pregnancies
  ◊ Universal blood donor type considered dangerous unless thoroughly checked for agglutination titer
  ◊ Acquisition of B antigen by Group A individuals with colon cancer

RISK FACTORS
• Multiple blood transfusions
• Rh negative mother
• Multiple pregnancies

DIAGNOSIS

DIFFERENTIAL DIAGNOSIS
• Other causes of acute hemolysis
  ◊ Autoimmune diseases
  ◊ Hemoglobinopathies
  ◊ Red blood cell enzyme defects
  ◊ Bacterial contamination of stored blood

LABORATORY
• Positive direct antiglobulin test (Coomb's)
• Plasma obtained 2-4 hours after lysis is red or pink, indicating free hemoglobin
• Increased BUN, creatinine
• Elevated serum bilirubin (mild)
• Wine-colored urine indicating hemoglobinuria
• Reduced serum haptoglobin
Drugs that may alter lab results: N/A
Disorders that may alter lab results: N/A

PATHOLOGICAL FINDINGS N/A

SPECIAL TESTS Blood bank evaluation for immune reactions

IMAGING N/A

DIAGNOSTIC PROCEDURES N/A

TREATMENT

APPROPRIATE HEALTH CARE
Inpatient

GENERAL MEASURES
• Stop transfusion immediately upon first sign of reaction
• Substitute infusion with normal saline at 150-300 mL per hour
• Check paperwork for any clerical error (usual cause of an ABO-incompatible transfusion)
• Monitor vital signs
• Maintain urine flow at 100 mL/hr for 6-8 hours or until hemoglobinuria clears
• Recognize and treat disseminated intravascular coagulation if it occurs
• Posttransfusion blood sample and discontinued blood to blood bank for investigation
• Maintain systolic blood pressure above 100 mm Hg

SURGICAL MEASURES N/A

ACTIVITY Bedrest

DIET As tolerated

PATIENT EDUCATION N/A

MEDICATIONS

DRUG(S) OF CHOICE
• Oxygen as needed
• Epinephrine for wheezing and/or dyspnea
• Corticosteroids to reduce inflammation
• Adequate colloid or crystalloid (may need 1000 mL/hr normal saline for 2-3 hours) to maintain systolic blood pressure above 100 mm Hg
• Mannitol not of proven value
• Dopamine effective against hypotension and impaired renal perfusion
• Heparinization, at moderate doses, is indicated if DIC present
• Diuretic: furosemide 80-120 mg IV or ethacrynic acid 50 mg IV

Contraindications: Refer to manufacturer's literature

Precautions: Refer to manufacturer's literature

Significant possible interactions: Refer to manufacturer's literature

ALTERNATIVE DRUGS
Diphenhydramine to combat cellular histamine release from mast cells

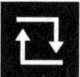
FOLLOWUP

PATIENT MONITORING
Until hemolytic signs are gone

PREVENTION/AVOIDANCE
• History of patient's responses to previous transfusions
• Risk/benefit of any transfusion needs to favor benefit
• Autologous transfusion
• Careful typing and crossmatch, double-check all data available
• Identity of unit of blood is carefully checked before administered
• Close observation of the patient during the transfusion
• Consider leukocyte depleted blood in people with history of recurrent febrile reactions
• Avoid prophylactic antipyretics
• Use of genotype specific RBCs in sickle cell anemia

POSSIBLE COMPLICATIONS
• Uremia, oliguria, anuria
• Right heart failure

EXPECTED COURSE/PROGNOSIS
• Usual course - acute
• Usually no harm if transfusion is stopped at onset of manifestations
• Severe - mortality 50%

MISCELLANEOUS

ASSOCIATED CONDITIONS
• Disseminated intravascular coagulation
• Acute renal failure

AGE-RELATED FACTORS
Pediatric: Reaction greater and outlook poorer in the very young
Geriatric: Outlook more grave in the elderly
Others: N/A

PREGNANCY N/A

SYNONYMS N/A

ICD-9-CM 999.8 Other transfusion reaction

SEE ALSO
• Renal failure, acute (ARF)
• Disseminated intravascular coagulation (DIC)
• Anemia, sickle cell
• Anemia, autoimmune hemolytic
• Anemia, hemolytic

OTHER NOTES N/A

ABBREVIATIONS N/A

REFERENCES
• Lee RG, Bithell TC, et al: Wintrobe's Clinical Hematology. 9th Ed. Philadelphia, Lea & Febiger, 1993
• Huestis DW, Bove JR, Case S: Practical Blood Transfusion. 4th Ed. Boston, Little, Brown and Co., 1988
Illustrations: N/A
Internet references: http://www.5mcc.com

Author(s)
Bruce G. Bellamy, MD

Transient ischemic attack (TIA)

BASICS

DESCRIPTION The sudden onset of a focal and transient (< 24 hours) neurological deficit due to brain ischemia

System(s) affected: Nervous

Genetics: Inheritance is polygenic with a tendency to clustering of risk factors within families

Incidence/Prevalence in USA: Incidence 160/100,000; prevalence 135 per 100,000

Predominant age: Risk increases over age 45 and is highest in the seventh and eighth decades

Predominant sex: Male > Female (3:1)

SIGNS AND SYMPTOMS

• Carotid circulation (hemispheric) - monocular visual loss, hemiplegia, hemianesthesia, neglect, aphasia, visual field defects; less often headaches, seizures, amnesia, confusion
• Vertebrobasilar (brainstem or cerebellar) - bilateral visual obscuration, diplopia, vertigo, ataxia, facial paresis, Horner's syndrome, dysphagia, dysarthria
• Cerebellar or brainstem lesion in patients with headache, nausea, vomiting and ataxia

CAUSES

• Carotid atherosclerotic disease with artery to artery thromboembolism
• Small, deep, vessel disease associated with hypertension
• Cardiac - cardioembolism secondary to valvular (mitral valve) pathology; mural hypo- or akinesias with thrombosis (acute anterior myocardial infarctions or congestive cardiomyopathies); cardiac arrhythmia (atrial fibrillation)
• Hypercoagulable states - antiphospholipid antibodies, deficiency of protein S, protein C. Presence of antithrombin 3, oral contraceptives.
• Other causes - spontaneous and post-traumatic (i.e., chiropractic manipulation) arterial dissection, fibromuscular dysplasia

RISK FACTORS

• Age
• Hypertension
• Cardiac disease
• Smoking
• Diabetes
• Antiphospholipid antibodies
• Family History

DIAGNOSIS

DIFFERENTIAL DIAGNOSIS

• Migraine (hemiplegic)
• Focal seizure (Todd's paralysis)
• Hypoglycemia
• Todd's paralysis

LABORATORY N/A

Drugs that may alter lab results: N/A

Disorders that may alter lab results: N/A

PATHOLOGICAL FINDINGS N/A

SPECIAL TESTS

• Duplex carotid ultrasonography
• Cerebral angiography
• ECG
• Transthoracic echocardiogram (TTE); if normal and a cardiac source is suspected, follow with transesophageal echocardiogram
• Holter monitoring
• EEG for suspected seizure
• INR and partial thromboplastin time (PTT) (Coumadin prolongs INR)
• Antiphospholipid antibodies

IMAGING

• Acute phase - CT of head to rule out hemorrhage
• Angiography - carotid arterial stenosis
• Digital substraction - stenosis

DIAGNOSTIC PROCEDURES N/A

TREATMENT

APPROPRIATE HEALTH CARE

• Acute phase: Outpatient for investigations; inpatient for surgery

GENERAL MEASURES

• Strict control of medical risk factors, e.g., diabetes, hypertension, hyperlipidemia, cardiac disease
• Counseling towards cessation of smoking

SURGICAL MEASURES
In medically fit patients with non-disabling stroke, carotid endarterectomy (CEA) is indicated for stenosis of 70-99% on side ipsilateral to stroke; CEA is of modest benefit for carotid stenosis 0f 50-69% and depends on risk factors. The North American Symptomatic Carotid Endarterectomy Trial (NASCET) showed no benefit of CEA above medical therapy alone in stenosis of <50%.

ACTIVITY No restrictions

DIET
As appropriate to underlying medical problems (diabetic diet, low fat diet, low salt diet etc.)

PATIENT EDUCATION National Stroke Association, 300 East Hampden Ave., Suite 240, Engle Wood, CO 80110-2622

MEDICATIONS

DRUG(S) OF CHOICE
• Enteric coated aspirin (EC ASA) 325-1300 mg/day,
or
• Ticlopidine (Ticlid)250 mg po bid
Contraindications:
• EC ASA - active peptic ulcer disease, hypersensitivity to aspirin, patients who had bronchospastic reaction to ASA or other nonsteroidal anti-inflammatory drugs
• Ticlopidine - known hypersensitivity to the drug, presence of hematopoietic disorders, presence of a hemostatic disorder, conditions associated with active bleeding, severe liver dysfunction
Precautions:
• EC ASA - may aggravate pre-existing peptic ulcer disease , may worsen symptoms in some patients with asthma
• Ticlopidine - 2.4% of patients develop neutropenia (0.8% severe neutropenia) which is reversible with cessation of drug. Monitor blood counts every 2 weeks for the first 3 months.
Significant possible interactions:
• EC ASA - may potentiate effects of anticoagulants and sulfonylurea, hypoglycemic agents
• Ticlopidine - digoxin plasma levels decreased 15%, theophylline half-life increased from 8.6 to 12.2 hours

ALTERNATIVE DRUGS
• Dipyridamole (Persantine) alone or in combination with ASA of possible benefit
• Sulfinpyrazone (Anturane) of no proven benefit
• Clopidogrel (Plavix) 75 mg daily; ticlopidine's descendent has fewer side effects, but shows only a slight advantage over ASA

FOLLOWUP

PATIENT MONITORING
Followup every 3 months for first year then yearly

PREVENTION/AVOIDANCE
• Stop smoking
• Control blood pressure, diabetes, hyperlipidemia
• EC ASA 650 mg bid or ticlopidine 250 mg po bid for patients with prior transient ischemic attack

POSSIBLE COMPLICATIONS
• Stroke
• Seizure
• Trauma if patient experiences sudden fall due to weakness

EXPECTED COURSE/PROGNOSIS
5-20% risk of stroke on ipsilateral side within one year and cumulative thereafter. Frequency increases with addition of multiple risk factors and severity of carotid stenosis.

MISCELLANEOUS

ASSOCIATED CONDITIONS
• Atrial fibrillation
• Major cause of death in first five years after a TIA is cardiac disease

AGE-RELATED FACTORS
Pediatric:
• Cardiac (especially developmental abnormalities)
• Metabolic - homocystinuria, Fabry's disease
Geriatric: Atrial fibrillation is a frequent cause of TIA among the elderly
Others: Adults < 45 years old most likely to have a cardiac source of embolism

PREGNANCY
A hypercoagulable state is associated with pregnancy and parturition

SYNONYMS
• Mini-stroke

ICD-9-CM
435.9 Transient cerebral ischemia, unspecified

SEE ALSO
• Stroke (Brain attack)

OTHER NOTES
N/A

ABBREVIATIONS
EC ASA = enteric coated aspirin
INR = international normalized ratio

REFERENCES
• Hachinski V, ed: Stroke. Lancet 1998;352(suppl3):1-30
• Hachinski V: Brain attack: The Clinical Handbook. Meducom International, 1999
Illustrations: N/A
Internet references: http://www.5mcc.com

Author(s)
Bart Demaerschalk, MD, FRCPC
Vladimir Hachinski, MD, DSc, FRCPC

Trichinosis

BASICS

DESCRIPTION
• Trichinosis is a parasitic disease that develops after ingesting infected pork or other meat containing viable cysts of Trichinella spiralis, a nematode, with rarer cases attributable to several different species of Trichinella. The cysts remain viable and can cause disease when the infected meat is undercooked. Most common outbreaks are attributable to undercooked pork, wild boar meat, homemade and commercial sausage, bear, walrus and other wild animal meats.
• Enteric phase, phase I: Cysts are broken down by digestive acid and pepsin in the stomach freeing larvae which develop into mature adult worms in the upper to middle small intestine, taking about one week after ingestion and may last 3 to 5 weeks
• Systemic phase, phase II: Female worms then release newborn larvae that migrate through blood vessels and lymphatics to multiple organ systems, occurring 2 to 3 weeks after ingestion and may last for 2 months
• Muscular encystment phase, phase III: Larvae become encysted in striated skeletal and sometimes cardiac muscle and can remain viable for years
System(s) affected: Gastrointestinal, Musculoskeletal
Genetics: N/A
Incidence/Prevalence in USA: 50 to 100 cases are reported annually in the United States, but most mild cases probably are undiagnosed, based on autopsy studies.
Predominant age: Cases have been reported from all age groups. It occurs most frequently in ages 20-49.
Predominant sex: Male = Female

SIGNS AND SYMPTOMS
Signs and symptoms begin within one week of ingesting infected meat.
• Common symptoms:
  ◊ Diarrhea (mostly phase I)
  ◊ Abdominal Cramping (mostly phase I)
  ◊ Fever (mostly phase II and III)
  ◊ Myalgias (mostly phase II and III)
  ◊ Eosinophilia (mostly phase II and III)
  ◊ Periorbital edema (mostly phase II and III)
  ◊ Weakness (mostly phase II and III)
• Clinical symptoms depend on the number of ingested infective larvae, and the phase of the parasitic invasion. Most light infections with <10 larvae per gram of muscle are asymptomatic. Skeletal muscle is the most frequent site of symptoms due to larval migration, however in severe cases there can be myocardial damage, pulmonary infiltration and focal neurologic damage. Most common muscles involved include the gastrocnemius, masseter, diaphragm, biceps, lower back, extraocular muscles, jaw and neck. Heavy infections with > 50 larvae per gram of muscle can be life threatening. Symptoms from the various phases can occur concurrently.

• Less common symptoms (mostly phase II and III):
  ◊ Conjunctivitis
  ◊ Subconjunctival hemorrhage
  ◊ Retinal hemorrhages
  ◊ Maculopapular rash
  ◊ Splinter hemorrhages
  ◊ Headache
  ◊ Photophobia
  ◊ Pneumonitis
  ◊ Tachycardia
  ◊ Heart failure
  ◊ CNS involvement

CAUSES
Eating undercooked meat that is infected with viable Trichinella cysts.

RISK FACTORS
• Access to wild game, homemade pork products, noncommercial sources of meat
• Eating pigs that were fed uncooked garbage
• Under cooking pork
• Eating wild game inadequately cooked or frozen
• Ethnic groups from Southeast Asia raising their own pork or favoring partially cooked pork products.
• Higher incidence in Alaska and northeastern United States.

DIAGNOSIS

DIFFERENTIAL DIAGNOSIS
• Acute rheumatic fever
• Arthritis, angioedema
• Botulism
• Collagen vascular disease
• Dermatomyositis
• Encephalitis
• Eosinophilia-myalgia syndrome
• Gastroenteritis
• Idiopathic hypereosinophilic syndrome
• Idiopathic polymyositis
• Influenza
• Meningitis
• Pneumonitis
• Polyarteritis nodosa
• Polymyositis
• Typhoid fever
• Tuberculosis

LABORATORY
• Eosinophilia (>600/cubic millimeter), with leukocytosis
• Increased creatine phosphate kinase (CPK)
• Increased lactate dehydrogenase (LDH)
• Hypergammaglobulinemia
• Elevated erythrocyte sedimentation rate (several weeks)
Drugs that may alter lab results: Rare increases in SGOT with thiabendazole
Disorders that may alter lab results: N/A

PATHOLOGICAL FINDINGS
Larvae on muscle biopsy (often gastrocnemius), however absence of larvae does not exclude diagnosis. Rarely find worm in stool.

SPECIAL TESTS
• Serologic tests for T. spiralis, IgM and IgG
• ELISA (enzyme linked immunosorbent assay) IgM and IgG
• Bentonite flocculation after 3rd week for parasite specific antibody
• Indirect immunoflourescence
• Complement fixation
• DNA testing [RAPD (random amplified polymorphic DNA), PCR (polymerase chain reaction)]
• Antibody levels are often not detectable until 3-5 weeks post infection

IMAGING
• CT may help see calcified muscle cysts
• MRI may help in evaluation of neurologic complications
• Chest x-ray may detect patchy infiltrates

DIAGNOSTIC PROCEDURES
Muscle biopsy of gastrocnemius or deltoid with at least 1 gram of muscle, including examination between compressed slides (higher detection rate)

TREATMENT

APPROPRIATE HEALTH CARE
• Outpatient unless complications such as cardiac, pulmonary, or neurological
• May call CDC for appropriate diagnostic tests (404-639-3311).

GENERAL MEASURES
Bedrest, antipyretics and analgesics.

SURGICAL MEASURES
Pacemaker has been required on occasion for severe myocarditis

ACTIVITY
As tolerated. Bedrest may help muscular pain.

DIET
As tolerated

PATIENT EDUCATION
• Manage complications as appropriate
• Measures at prevention
• Cook potentially contaminated meat such as pork to 170°F (77°C), no longer pink
• Freeze at -15°C for 21 days (longer if meat is >15 cm thick), however Trichinella larvae in wild game may be resistant to freezing
• Do not feed hogs uncooked garbage

MEDICATIONS

DRUG(S) OF CHOICE
• For early intestinal phase (presenting in 1st 1 to 2 weeks), to treat adult worms:
  ◊ Albendazole 400 mg bid x 15 days
  ◊ Mebendazole may be used 200-400 mg tid x 3 days, then 400-500 mg tid for 10 days
• No drugs are very effective against larvae once encysted in muscle, however they may halt further dissemination
• Call CDC for current dosage and recommendation (404)639-3311
• Corticosteroids such as prednisone 40 to 60 mg/day for 3-5 days and then tapered as symptoms subside may be helpful in severe cases, particularly to help decrease inflammation when signs of myocarditis, neurologic disease, pulmonary insufficiency, or severe myositis

Contraindications: Corticosteroids have been reported to be contraindicated in the intestinal phase, as they could prolong this phase

Precautions: Minimal experience exists with the use of medications in small children and in pregnancy. Mebendazole should not be given in the first trimester, and any medications should only be used if felt absolutely necessary.

Significant possible interactions: Carbamazepine or alcohol may decrease the effect of mebendazole. Cimetidine may increase the level of mebendazole.

ALTERNATIVE DRUGS
Thiabendazole, which used to be the drug of choice at 25 mg/kg bid x 1 week, maximum dose 1.5 gm, has been replaced by the above drugs because they have fewer side effects, and are equally effective.

FOLLOWUP

PATIENT MONITORING
Monitor for signs and symptoms of complications such as cardiac, neurological and pulmonary

PREVENTION/AVOIDANCE
Avoid eating undercooked pork and game meat. Prolonged freezing may also be effective, but less so for wild game meat.

POSSIBLE COMPLICATIONS
• Meningitis
• Subcortical infarcts
• Encephalitis
• Myocarditis with congestive heart failure
• Nephritis
• Glomerulonephritis
• Sinusitis
• Pneumonitis

EXPECTED COURSE/PROGNOSIS
• Most infections are asymptomatic, short-lived and generally have uneventful recovery without medication
• Encysted larvae remain viable for several years
• Prognosis is good in most cases, although 5-10% of cases can be severe
• There is no clear evidence that chronic trichinosis exists
• Less than 1% of cases can be fatal, generally around the 4th-8th week, and a result of cardiac failure or pneumonia

MISCELLANEOUS

ASSOCIATED CONDITIONS N/A

AGE-RELATED FACTORS
Pediatric: N/A
Geriatric: N/A
Others: N/A

PREGNANCY
Although not much information, there is one case of a woman 16 weeks pregnant who delivered a normal child without complications or evidence of problems

SYNONYMS
Trichinellosis
Trichinelliasis

ICD-9-CM   124 Trichinosis

SEE ALSO N/A

OTHER NOTES N/A

ABBREVIATIONS N/A

REFERENCES
• Bailey T, Schantz P: Trends in the Incidence and Transmission Patterns of Trichinosis in Humans in the United States: Comparisons of the Periods 1975-1981 and 1982-1986. Reviews of Infectious Diseases 1990:12(1):5-11
• Clausen MR, et al: Trichinella infection and clinical disease. QJ Med 1996;89(8)631-636
• McAuley JB et al: Trichinosis surveillance, United States, 1987-1990. Morbidity and Mortality Weekly Report CDC Surveillance Summary 1992:40:35-42
• Stack PS: Trichinosis, Still a public health threat. Postgraduate Medicine 1995;97(6):137-139/143-144
Illustrations: N/A
Internet references: http://www.5mcc.com

Author(s)
Kenton Voorhees, MD

Trichomoniasis

BASICS

DESCRIPTION Trichomonas is a protozoan parasite found in men and women at genitourinary sites
System(s) affected: Reproductive, Renal/Urologic
Genetics: N/A
Incidence/Prevalence in USA:
• Makes up 10-25% of vaginal infections
• 300/100,000 women/year for first time diagnosis of trichomoniasis; 600/100,000 women/year for any diagnosis for trichomoniasis
• In sexually active adult women: 2,000/100,000 in a family planning clinic; 35,000/100,000 in a STD clinic
Predominant age:
• Young and middle aged adults
• Rare until onset of sexual activity
• Not uncommon in postmenopausal women
Predominant sex: Both affected, but women more commonly symptomatic

SIGNS AND SYMPTOMS
• Female
  ◊ 40% can be asymptomatic at time of diagnosis
  ◊ Symptoms typically begin or worsen at time of menstrual period
  ◊ Vaginal discharge (75%, usually copious, watery and pooling, can be frothy)
  ◊ Vulvovaginal irritation (50%)
  ◊ Dysuria (50%)
  ◊ Vaginal odor (10%)
  ◊ A "strawberry cervix" from punctate hemorrhages (5% of cases)
  ◊ Vaginal hyperemia
  ◊ Dyspareunia
  ◊ Suprapubic discomfort
  ◊ Cervical erosion
• Male
  ◊ Most are asymptomatic
  ◊ Symptomatic (20%)
  - Urethral discharge
  - Dysuria
  - Epididymitis (rare)

CAUSES
• Trichomonas vaginalis is a pear shaped protozoan which is a facultative anaerobe. It is usually sexually transmitted although a non-venereal route is possible as the organism survives for several hours in a moist environment.
• Transmission is rarely seen in female children of infected women
• Incubation period is 3-28 days

RISK FACTORS Multiple sexual partners

DIAGNOSIS

DIFFERENTIAL DIAGNOSIS
• Female - vaginal candidiasis, bacterial vaginosis. Cervical inflammation can lead to the mistaken diagnosis of cervicitis.
• Male - chlamydia urethritis

LABORATORY
• Female
  ◊ Wet prep is 60-70% sensitive and highly specific. Sensitivity is reduced with loss of motility due to cooling, low inoculum size and rapid scanning of the slide. Specificity is about 100%.
  ◊ Vaginal pH is > 4.5 in 90% of women
  ◊ Wet prep usually shows many more PMN's than epithelial cells
• Male
  ◊ A wet prep and culture of urethral discharge after prostatic exam is 50-80% sensitive
Drugs that may alter lab results: N/A
Disorders that may alter lab results: N/A

PATHOLOGICAL FINDINGS N/A

SPECIAL TESTS
• Culture has a sensitivity of greater than 95% but takes 4-7 days
• ELISA and direct fluorescent antibody tests are available and are 80-90% sensitive
• Pap smear has a 60% sensitivity and 99% specificity
• Rapid diagnostic kits using DNA probes have sensitivity of 90% and specificity of 99.8%

IMAGING N/A

DIAGNOSTIC PROCEDURES N/A

TREATMENT

APPROPRIATE HEALTH CARE
Outpatient

GENERAL MEASURES Education about the venereal aspect of the infection

SURGICAL MEASURES N/A

ACTIVITY Sexual activity should not be resumed until patient and partner are both treated

DIET Should abstain from alcohol if metronidazole used for therapy

PATIENT EDUCATION
• Vaginitis, Questions and Answers Planned Parenthood Federation of America, Inc., (212)541-7800
• Roses Have Thorns, RAJ Publications, P.O. Box 150720, Lakewood, CO 80215
• American College of Obstetricians & Gynecologists (ACOG), 409 12th St., SW, Washington, DC 20024-2188, (800)762-ACOG

MEDICATIONS

DRUG(S) OF CHOICE
• Metronidazole: adult dose 2 grams at one time, or 250 mg tid for 7 days, or 500 mg bid for 7 days. The routines are effective in women but the one time dose has a higher failure rate in men. All sexual partners need treatment.
Contraindications: First trimester pregnancy or allergy to the antibiotic
Precautions: Avoid metronidazole or reduce the dosage in patients with liver failure
Significant possible interactions: Ethanol, warfarin, disulfiram, phenobarbital

ALTERNATIVE DRUGS
• Clotrimazole: 100 mg vaginal tablets qhs for 14 days. Cure rate is 20-25% but symptoms will be reduced in most women.
• Alternatively, saline or vinegar douching can be tried

FOLLOWUP

PATIENT MONITORING
Monitor target symptoms. No followup is needed if symptoms resolve with treatment.

PREVENTION/AVOIDANCE
Practice safe sex by using condoms. Trichomonas can be identified in 30-40% of the male sexual partners of infected women.

POSSIBLE COMPLICATIONS
Recurrent infections

EXPECTED COURSE/PROGNOSIS
Prognosis is good but recurrent infection raises possibility of non-compliance with therapy, re-infection, or infection with a resistant organism. If resistance is suspected, try metronidazole 500 mg tid for 7 days along with vaginal 0.75% metronidazole gel.

MISCELLANEOUS

ASSOCIATED CONDITIONS
Other sexually transmitted diseases

AGE-RELATED FACTORS
Pediatric: Very uncommon in prepuberty (confirmed diagnosis should raise concern of sexual abuse)
Geriatric: Older people remain at risk for Trichomonas
Others: N/A

PREGNANCY
Do not use metronidazole in the first trimester

SYNONYMS
• Trick
• Trichomonal urethritis

ICD-9-CM
131.9 Trichomoniasis, unspecified
131.01 Vulva or vagina
131.00 Urogenitalis

SEE ALSO
• Vulvovaginitis, bacterial
• Abnormal Pap smear

OTHER NOTES   N/A

ABBREVIATIONS   N/A

REFERENCES
• Lossick JG, Kent H: Trichomoniasis: trends in diagnosis and management. Am J Obstet & Gyno 1991165;1217-22
• Krieger JN: Clinical manifestations of trichomoniasis in men. Ann Int Med 1993;118:844-849
• CDC: 1993 Sexually transmitted disease treatment guidelines. MMWR 1993;42:RR-14
• Heine P, McGregor JA: Trichomonas vaginalis: A reemerging pathogen. Clin OB Gyn 1993;36:137-142
• Schweke JR: Metronidazole utilization in the obstetric gynecologic patient. Sex Trans Dis 1995;22:370-376
• Sobel JK: Vaginitis. NEJM 1997;337:1896-1903
Illustrations: N/A
Internet references: http://www.5mcc.com

Author(s)
George R. Bergus, MD

Trigeminal neuralgia

BASICS

DESCRIPTION A disorder of the sensory nucleus of the 5th cranial nerve (trigeminal nerve), producing episodic, paroxysmal, severe lancinating pain lasting seconds to minutes followed by a pain free period in the distribution of one or more of its divisions. Often precipitated by stimulation of well-defined, ipsilateral trigger zones, usually perioral, perinasal, occasionally intraoral (eg washing, shaving).
System(s) affected: Nervous
Genetics: N/A
Incidence/Prevalence in USA: 16/100,000
Predominant age: Over age 50, peak age 60, rare before age 35
Predominant sex: Female > Male (2:1)

SIGNS AND SYMPTOMS
• Unilateral (< 4% bilateral, rarely at the same time; bilateral mostly in MS), symptoms rarely present at night
• Excruciating lip pain
• Excruciating gum pain
• Excruciating cheek pain
• Paroxysmal facial pain
• Wincing
• Pain elicited by tickle or touch
• Flushing
• Lacrimation
• Salivation
• Pain "bursts" several seconds to minutes with refractory period after
• Right > left side preference
• 2nd > 3rd >> 1st (less than 5%) division trigeminal nerve most commonly affected

CAUSES
• When present, most commonly compression of the trigeminal nerve by anomalous arteries or veins of the posterior fossa, usually the superior cerebral artery compressing the trigeminal root.
• Etiology classification
  ◊ Idiopathic
  ◊ Secondary - disseminated sclerosis; cerebellopontine angle tumors, e.g., meningioma; tumors of the 5th nerve, e.g., neuroma, vascular malformations

RISK FACTORS Unknown

DIAGNOSIS

DIFFERENTIAL DIAGNOSIS
• Other forms of neuralgia usually have sensory loss. The presence of sensory loss nearly excludes the diagnosis of trigeminal neuralgia (if younger patient frequently is MS).
• Neoplasia in the cerebellopontine angle
• Vascular malformation of the brain stem
• Demyelinating lesion (of all patients with MS, 10% have facial pain first, other MS symptoms may not appear for 6 years)
• Vascular insult
• Migraine
• Chronic meningitis
• Acute polyneuropathy

LABORATORY N/A
Drugs that may alter lab results: N/A
Disorders that may alter lab results: N/A

PATHOLOGICAL FINDINGS
• Semilunar ganglion - inflammatory changes
• Degenerative changes

SPECIAL TESTS N/A

IMAGING N/A

DIAGNOSTIC PROCEDURES MRI or CT scan - neoplasm in cerebellopontine angle must be ruled out. Special MRA technique of collapsed MRA superimposed on routine spin echo T-1 weighted images.

TREATMENT

APPROPRIATE HEALTH CARE
Outpatient

GENERAL MEASURES
• Drug treatment is first approach. Invasive procedures for patients who cannot tolerate, or fail to respond to, drug treatment.
• Avoidance of stimulation (air, heat, cold) of trigger zones (lips, cheeks, gums)
• Alcohol block or glycerol injection into the trigeminal cistern
• 4% tetracaine dissolved in 0.5% bupivacaine nerve block (only a few case reports to date)
• 25-50% of TN patients eventually fail medical treatment

SURGICAL MEASURES
• Microvascular decompression of the 5th cranial nerve at its entrance to (or exit from) the brainstem (70-90% effective)
• Partial sensory rhizotomy
• Peripheral block or section of 5th nerve proximal to the Gasserian ganglion
• Gamma knife radiosurgery (minimally invasive, 77% significant relief)
• Balloon compression of the Gasserian ganglion (especially effective for 1st division TN pain)
• Peripheral nerve ablation
  ◊ Neurectomy
  ◊ Cryotherapy
  ◊ Radiofrequency thermocoagulation
(possibly 90-97% partial or complete relief; recurrence rate is unknown)

ACTIVITY Full activity

DIET No special diet

PATIENT EDUCATION Instruct regarding medication dosage and side effects

MEDICATIONS

DRUG(S) OF CHOICE Carbamazepine (Tegretol) starting dose 100-200 mg bid; effective dose usually 200 mg qid; 1200 mg/day maximum. By 3 years, 30% no longer helped. Most common side effect is sedation.
Contraindications: MAO inhibitors taken concurrently
Precautions: Use with caution in presence of liver disease
Significant possible interactions:
Macrolide antibiotics with Carbamazepine. Oral anticoagulants, anticonvulsants, tricyclics, oral contraceptives, steroids, digitalis, INH, MAO inhibitors, methyprylon nabilone, nizatidine, other H2 blockers, phenytoin, propoxyphene, benzodiazepines, calcium, channel blockers.

ALTERNATIVE DRUGS
• Phenytoin (Dilantin) 300-400 mg/day (synergistic with carbamazepine)
• Baclofen (Atrofen, Lioresal) 10-80 mg/day; start at 5-10 mg tid with food (as adjunct with phenytoin or carbamazepine): drowsiness, weakness, nausea, vomiting
• Chlorphenesin carbamate (Maolate) 800-2400 mg/day: drowsiness, (as adjunct with phenytoin and/or carbamazepine)
• Ozcarbazepine (Trileptal) - derivative of carbamazepine also similar to gabapentin. Faster with less drowsiness. Decreases serum sodium. Not available in U.S. yet.
• Antidepressants, especially used with anticonvulsants. Particularly effective for atypical forms of TN - amitriptyline, fluoxetine, trazodone.
• Clonazepam (Klonopin): frequently causes drowsiness and ataxia
• Mexiletine (Mexitil). Experimental for this condition.
• Capsaicin cream (not standard therapy; anecdotal evidence)
• Pimozide (Orap) superior to carbamazepine in one study of 48 patients, but it is an antipsychotic drug with extrapyramidal affects, dystonia and tardive dyskinesia. High side effect profile.
• Valproic acid (Depakene, Depakote)

FOLLOWUP

PATIENT MONITORING
• Carbamazepine and/or phenytoin serum levels
• If carbamazepine is prescribed: CBC and platelets at baseline then weekly for a month, then monthly for 4 months, then every 6-12 months if dose stable (regimens for monitoring vary)
• CBC as needed

PREVENTION/AVOIDANCE Reduce drugs after 4-6 weeks to determine if condition is in remission, resume at previous dose if pain recurs. Withdraw drugs slowly after several months again to check for remission or if lower dose of drugs can be tolerated.

POSSIBLE COMPLICATIONS Mental and physical sluggishness, dizziness with carbamazepine

EXPECTED COURSE/PROGNOSIS
Exacerbations in fall and spring; otherwise good

MISCELLANEOUS

ASSOCIATED CONDITIONS
• Sjögren's syndrom
• Rheumatoid arthritis
• Chronic meningitis
• Facial migraine
• Acute polyneuropathy
• Multiple sclerosis
• Hemifacial spasm
• Pretrigeminal neuralgia

AGE-RELATED FACTORS
Pediatric: Unusual in childhood
Geriatric: N/A
Others: N/A

PREGNANCY N/A

SYNONYMS
• Tic douloureux
• Fothergill's neuralgia
• Trifacial neuralgia

ICD-9-CM
350.1 Trigeminal neuralgia

SEE ALSO
• Migraine
• Headache, cluster
• Sjögren's syndrome

OTHER NOTES N/A

ABBREVIATIONS N/A

REFERENCES
• Bell WE: Orofacial Pain. 4th Ed. Chicago, Year Book Medical Publishers, 1989
• Adams RD, Victor M: Principles of Neurology. 5th Ed. New York, McGraw-Hill, 1993
• Sweet WH: The treatment of trigeminal neuralgia (tic douloureux). New Engl J Med 1986;174-177
• Moller AR: The cranial nerve vascular compression syndrome: A review of treatment. Acta Neurochirurgica 1991;113:18-23
• Merrill R, Graff-Radford SB: Trigeminal neuralgia: How to rule out the wrong treatment. JADA 1992;123:63-68
• Smith LH Jr, Bennett C: Trigeminal neuralgia. In: Wyngaarden JB, ed. Cecil Textbook of Medicine. Philadelphia, W.B. Saunders Co., 1992
• Fields HL: Treatment of trigeminal neuralgia (editorial). NEJM 1996;334(17):1125-1126
Illustrations: N/A
Internet references: http://www.5mcc.com

Author(s)
Paul J. Jaster, MD

Tropical sprue

BASICS

DESCRIPTION Malabsorption syndrome of unknown etiology that occurs primarily in the tropics and subtropics. Characteristics include protein malnutrition and folic acid anemia. Usual course - relapsing without treatment. Symptoms may appear years after leaving an endemic area.
• Endemic areas - tropical regions only, Far East, India, Caribbean and the Middle East. Distribution is sporadic.
• The presence of normal jejunal biopsy nearly excludes this diagnosis
System(s) affected: Gastrointestinal, Hemic/Lymphatic/Immunologic
Genetics: N/A
Incidence/Prevalence in USA: Unknown
Predominant age: None
Predominant sex: Male = Female

SIGNS AND SYMPTOMS
• Fatigue
• Asthenia
• Weight loss, pallor
• Diarrhea
• Abdominal cramps
• Borborygmus
• Night blindness
• Stomatitis
• Glossitis
• Cheilosis
• Anorexia
• Steatorrhea
• Hyperkeratosis
• Edema
• Abdominal distension
• Hyperpigmentation
• Koilonychia

CAUSES
• Unknown
• Possible dietary deficiency
• Possible infectious agent
• Vitamin deficiency (folate), B12
• Food toxins (rancid fats)
• Toxigenic strains of coliform bacteria

RISK FACTORS Parasitic infestation

DIAGNOSIS

DIFFERENTIAL DIAGNOSIS
• Other causes of megaloblastic anemia
• Other malabsorption syndromes
• Celiac disease
• Inflammatory bowel disease
• Giardiasis
• Strongylosis
• Other infectious causes:
  ◊ Coccidial isospora
  ◊ Capillaria philippinensis
  ◊ Cryptosporidium

LABORATORY
• Megaloblastic anemia in 60% of cases
• Steatorrhea
• Decreased D-xylose
• Decreased serum iron
• Decreased calcium
• Decreased folic acid
• Decreased serum vitamin B12
• Decreased serum carotene
• Decreased cholesterol, albumin
• Deficiency of magnesium
• Deficiency of alpha-tocopherol
Drugs that may alter lab results: N/A
Disorders that may alter lab results: N/A

PATHOLOGICAL FINDINGS Jejunal biopsy - mild villous atrophy, increased villous crypts, mononuclear cell infiltration

SPECIAL TESTS Serum vitamin B12

IMAGING
• Mild jejunal dilatation
• Jejunal fold coarsening
• Flocculation and segmentation of Barium meal

DIAGNOSTIC PROCEDURES
• Jejunal biopsy - not specific
• Malabsorption of at least two nutrients is considered essential for diagnosis
• D- Xylose, fat and radiolabeled vitamin B12 are used to test for absorptive capacity
• Stool microscopy
• Imaging - not specific

TREATMENT

APPROPRIATE HEALTH CARE
Outpatient

GENERAL MEASURES
• Replace deficiencies, such as vitamin B12 and folic acid
• Control of diarrhea
• Fluid and blood replacement

SURGICAL MEASURES N/A

ACTIVITY No restrictions

DIET No special diet (gluten-free diets do not improve this disease)

PATIENT EDUCATION Written patient information available from:
National Digestive Diseases Information Clearinghouse
Box NDDIC
Bethesda, MD 20892
(301)654-3810

MEDICATIONS

DRUG(S) OF CHOICE
• Vitamin B12 1000 mcg SC for several days, then monthly thereafter for 6 months
• Folic acid 5 mg po daily
• Tetracycline 250 mg qid for 1-2 months, then half doses for up to 6 months. Occasionally, longer course is required.
• Combination folic acid and B12 plus tetracycline or sulfonamide
Contraindications: Allergy to tetracycline or oxytetracycline
Precautions:
• Use with caution in patients with lupus, myasthenia gravis, kidney or liver disease
• Don't take with milk, antacids or iron preparations
• Don't use during pregnancy
• Don't use in children under age 8
Significant possible interactions:
• Antacids, anticoagulants, bismuth subsalicylate
• Oral contraceptives
• Lithium

ALTERNATIVE DRUGS
• Oxytetracycline
• Nonabsorbable sulfonamides

FOLLOWUP

PATIENT MONITORING   As needed for symptoms

PREVENTION/AVOIDANCE   N/A

POSSIBLE COMPLICATIONS
• Malabsorption
• Relapse if medication regimen is stopped too soon

EXPECTED COURSE/PROGNOSIS
• Good with appropriate treatment
• Recurrences can happen in native residents treated in the tropics

MISCELLANEOUS

ASSOCIATED CONDITIONS   N/A

AGE-RELATED FACTORS
Pediatric: Don't treat with tetracycline
Geriatric: N/A
Others: N/A

PREGNANCY   Don't treat with tetracycline during pregnancy

SYNONYMS   N/A

ICD-9-CM
579.1 Tropical sprue

SEE ALSO
• Whipple's disease
• Diarrhea, chronic
• Celiac disease
• Anemia, pernicious

OTHER NOTES   N/A

ABBREVIATIONS   N/A

REFERENCES
• Sleisenger MH, Fordtran JS, eds: Gastrointestinal Disease: Pathophysiology, Diagnosis, Management. 5th Ed. Philadelphia, W.B. Saunders Co., 1994
• Mandell GL, ed: Principles and Practice of Infectious Diseases. 4th Ed. New York, Churchill Livingstone, 1995
Illustrations: N/A
Internet references: http://www.5mcc.com

Author(s)
Abdulrazak Abyad, MD, MPH, AGSF

Tuberculosis

BASICS

DESCRIPTION A common disease transmitted by inhaling airborne bacilli from a person with active tuberculosis (TB). The bacilli multiply in the alveolus and are carried by macrophages, lymphatics and blood to distant sites (eg., lung pleura, brain, kidney and bone). Tissue hypersensitivity usually halts infection within 10 weeks.
• Infected persons: are asymptomatic, are not infectious, and usually have a positive tuberculin skin test
• TB: active disease - occurs in 10% of infected individuals without preventive therapy. Chance of disease increases with immunosuppression and is highest for all individuals within 2 years after infection - 85% of cases are pulmonary which is infectious.
• Primary TB: disease resulting from the initial pulmonary infection which the immune system is unable to control
• Recrudescent TB: active disease occurring after a period of latent asymptomatic infection
• Miliary TB: disseminated disease
System(s) affected: Pulmonary, Hemic/Lymphatic/Immunologic, Renal/Urologic, Gastrointestinal, Nervous, Endocrine/Metabolic, Musculoskeletal
Genetics: N/A
Incidence/Prevalence in USA: Overall 7.4/100,0000, but varies greatly, may be 32-100/100,000 among high risk
Predominant age:
• Primary infection - any age, especially pediatric
• Recrudescent disease - adults and elderly
Predominant Sex: Male > Female

SIGNS AND SYMPTOMS
• Cough
• Hemoptysis
• Fever and night sweats
• Weight loss
• Malaise
• Adenopathy
• Pleuritic chest pain
• Hepatosplenomegaly
• Renal, bone or CNS disease are late findings

CAUSES Mycobacterium tuberculosis, Mycobacterium bovis, and Mycobacterium africanum

RISK FACTORS
• For infection: Urban, homeless, minority, migrant workers; institutional (eg, prison, nursing home); close contact with infected individual; foreign born (Asia, Africa, Latin America); healthcare workers
• For disease: HIV; recent infection; IV drug abuse; lymphoma; diabetes mellitus; chronic renal failure; malnutrition; steroids; immunosuppressive drugs; silicosis

DIAGNOSIS

DIFFERENTIAL DIAGNOSIS
• Other pneumonias
• Lymphomas
• Fungal infections, especially other atypical Mycobacteria or Nocardia

LABORATORY
• Tine test: not recommended for screening
• PPD [5 units (.1cc) intermediate strength, 0.1 cc volar forearm; measure induration at 72 hrs]
  ◊ > 5 mm - positive if HIV infection (or suspected), immunosuppressed, exposed household contact, clinical evidence of disease
  ◊ > 10 mm - positive if other risk factor or < 4 years old
  ◊ > 15 mm - positive if older than 4 years and no risk factors
  ◊ Two step testing if: no recent PPD, age > 55 years, nursing home, prison or healthcare worker
• Nonspecific laboratory includes anemia, monocytosis, thrombocytosis, hypergammaglobulinemia, SIADH and sterile pyuria
Drugs that may alter lab results:
• BCG: false-positive skin test
• Inactive vaccine or improper placement: false-negative skin test
• Steroids: false-negative skin test
Disorders that may alter lab results:
Recent viral infections, new (<10 weeks) infection, severe malnutrition, HIV, anergy, age < 6 months. overwhelming TB: false-negative skin test

PATHOLOGICAL FINDINGS
• Granulomas with foci of caseating necrosis surrounded by epithelioid histiocytes and giant cells, in turn surrounded by lymphocytes
• AFB stains positive

SPECIAL TESTS
• Persons with TB should be tested for HIV
• Lumbar puncture, if meningitis suspected
• Bone marrow and liver biopsy for culture
• Polymerase chain reaction (PCR) - rapid diagnosis of TB, costly, false positives occur, does not replace standard tests

IMAGING
• CXR with primary disease: may show infiltrate with or without effusion atelectasis or adenopathy
• With recrudescent TB: cavitary lesions and upper lobe disease with hilar adenopathy common. Diffuse miliary pattern possible with appearance of "millet seeds".
• HIV: atypical findings with primary infection - right upper lobe atelectasis
• CXR useful to rule out TB in asymptomatic infected persons
• CT chest - good sensitivity

DIAGNOSTIC PROCEDURES
• AFB stain can give a presumptive diagnosis
• Culture confirms diagnosis; 4-6 weeks on solid media or 2 weeks on Bactec broth system
• For suspected pulmonary TB, obtain at least 3 morning sputum samples for AFB stain and culture - use aerosol induction, gastric aspirate (children) or bronchoalveolar lavage if needed
• Other specimens: bone marrow, urine, tissue, CSF, peritoneal/pleural fluids
• Culture and sensitivity guide treatment

TREATMENT

APPROPRIATE HEALTH CARE
• Prophylaxis for positive PPD at any age if: HIV, close contact, recent converter (< 2 years), IV drug use, abnormal CXR, high risk medical condition or if age < 35 in other high risk group. Use INH (or rifampin if resistant) in usual daily dose for minimum 6 months, 12 months if HIV. Consider twice a week DOT if adherence not assured.
• For active disease, use minimum of 3 drugs for 2 months, then 2 drugs to complete 6 months - start with 4 drugs if resistance possible. Several regimen options available using DOT.
• If HIV infected, treat at least 6 months after culture negative

GENERAL MEASURES Careful reevaluation required. Only change to twice weekly dosing if using DOT.

SURGICAL MEASURES For extra pulmonary complications (spinal cord compression, constrictive pericarditis)

ACTIVITY
• As tolerated - respiratory isolation for infectious pulmonary TB
• Children without cough and negative sputum smears: no isolation required after treatment started

DIET Regular. Consider pyridoxine (10-50 mg/day) supplement.

PATIENT EDUCATION
• Teach pathogenesis, emphasize importance of drug therapy, warn of effects and/or interactions, find contacts
• Inform local health department

MEDICATIONS

DRUG(S) OF CHOICE
• Isoniazid (INH) - scored tabs 100 mg, 300 mg or syrup 10 mg/mL
  ◊ Daily dose - adult 300 mg; pediatric 10-15 mg/kg (maximum 300 mg)
  ◊ Twice weekly - adult 15 mg/kg; pediatric 20-30 mg/kg (maximum 900 mg)
  ◊ Consider pyridoxine

• Rifampin (RIF) capsules (150/300 or syrup 10 mg/mL)
◊ Daily dose - adult 600 mg; pediatric dose 10-20 mg/kg (maximum 600 mg)
◊ Twice weekly - adult 600 mg; pediatric 10-20 mg/kg (maximum 600 mg)
• Pyrazinamide (PZA), scored 500 mg
◊ Daily dose - adult 20-35 mg/kg (maximum 1-3 gm); pediatric 20-40 mg/kg (maximum 2 gm)
◊ Twice weekly - adult 50-70 mg/kg; pediatric 50 mg/kg (maximum 4 gm)
• Streptomycin (SM) IM only, vials 1,4 gm
◊ Daily dose - 20-40 mg/kg (maximum 1 gm); pediatric 20-40 mg/kg (maximum 1 gm)
◊ Twice weekly - 25 mg/kg; pediatric 20-40 mg/kg (maximum 1.5 gm)
• Ethambutol (EMB) - tablets 100/400 mg bacteriostatic
◊ Daily dose 15-25 mg/kg, with maximum of 2.5 gm a week or twice weekly dose 50 mg/kg, with maximum of 2.5 gm

Contraindications:
• Streptomycin: avoid use longer than 12 weeks secondary to ototoxicity
• Ethambutol: because of optic neuritis, never use ethambutol unless patient old enough to cooperate for visual acuity and color testing.

Precautions:
• INH, RIF or PZA may cause hepatitis
• Follow liver function if the patient has history of liver dysfunction or new signs develop
• RIF - colors urine, tears and secretions orange. Can permanently stain contact lenses.
• INH - peripheral neuritis and hypersensitivity possible. Consider pyridoxine.
• PZA - may increase uric acid
• EMB - may cause optic neuritis; follow monthly vision and color tests
• SM - ototoxicity and nephrotoxic

Significant possible interactions: RIF alters the level of Dilantin and other drugs metabolized by the liver and may inactivate birth control pills (recommend a barrier method)

ALTERNATIVE DRUGS
• Steroids - use only with concurrent anti-TB therapy. Consider for meningitis, effusions, severe miliary disease or endobronchial disease.
• Other antituberculous drugs may be useful for multidrug resistant TB (MDRTB)
• Combination tablets to enhance adherence

FOLLOWUP

PATIENT MONITORING
• During preventive therapy - monthly visits to assess adherence to regimen and monitor for hepatitis and neuropathy
• If age > 35 or symptoms, check liver enzymes, modify drugs if needed
• During TB therapy - obtain sputum culture monthly until negative and at completion of therapy
• If culture positive after 2 months of therapy, reassess drug sensitivity and initiate DOT
• CXR at 3 months and at completion of therapy

PREVENTION/AVOIDANCE
• PPD screening
• Identify and treat contagious persons. Notify public health department and hospital infection control if admitted
• Inpatient - use personal sealed respirators, negative pressure ventilation, ultraviolet
• Ambulatory patients use mask and tissues
• Not infectious if: favorable clinical response after 2-3 weeks of therapy and 3 AFB smears are negative.

POSSIBLE COMPLICATIONS
• Cavitary lesions can be secondarily infected
• Spread to susceptible persons of all ages
• Drug resistance - suspect if immigrant, drug resistant source or noncompliant

EXPECTED COURSE/PROGNOSIS
Generally few complications and full resolution if drugs taken for full course as prescribed

MISCELLANEOUS

ASSOCIATED CONDITIONS HIV infection

AGE-RELATED FACTORS
Pediatric:
• Caution with ethambutol
• Children on medication may attend school
• Disseminated TB more common in infants; prompt treatment with 4 drugs if TB suspected
• Congenital infection may occur with miliary TB of maternal bacillemia, endometritis or amniotic aspiration. If suspected, get PPD, CXR, LP, culture placenta and infant, then start treatment promptly
• Protocol for newborn with mother/household member with infection or disease
◊ Member with positive PPD, but no disease: no special evaluation or treatment. Skin test all household members; prophylaxis if infected.
◊ Member has abnormal CXR: separate infant until infectious status known; if not contagious, monitor infant PPD
◊ Member with disease and possibly contagious: evaluate infant for congenital TB and test for HIV; separate newborn until member is noninfectious
◊ If congenital TB suspected, treat as above
◊ If no congenital disease, INH for 3-4 months, then repeat PPD: if positive, reassess for infant disease. If negative, finish 6 months INH. If repeat PPD negative and source not infectious, stop INH and monitor infant.
• Consider BCG
Geriatric:
• Symptoms may be more subtle and may be attributed to associated conditions or to aging
• Should have a PPD prior to entering a chronic-care facility using two step protocol
• Side effects of INH more pronounced
Others: N/A

PREGNANCY
• Treat pregnant woman with INH, rifampin (and ethambutol, if resistance suspected); add pyridoxine
• Avoid streptomycin and pyrazinamide
• Prophylaxis - postpone INH until delivery unless recent contact
• Breast feeding okay while taking TB drugs

SYNONYMS
• Consumption

ICD-9-CM
011.9 Pulmonary tuberculosis, unspecified

SEE ALSO N/A

OTHER NOTES
• BCG vaccine, live attenuated Mycobacterium bovis
◊ 50% efficacy for pediatric pulmonary TB
◊ In USA, consider BCG for children with negative PPD and HIV tests with unavoidable high risk and for health care workers at high risk for drug resistant infection
◊ Abscess, ulceration and regional lymphadenitis occur in 1-2%, osteitis and fatal infection can occur in immunosuppressed
◊ Used more commonly in developing countries to prevent complications of TB

ABBREVIATIONS
PPD = purified protein derivative
BCG = Bacillus Calmette-Guérin
DOT = directly observed treatment

REFERENCES
• Centers for Disease Control; Screening for tuberculosis and tuberculosis infection in high risk populations. MMWR, 39:1-12, 1990
• American Thoracic Society: Treatment of tuberculosis and tuberculosis infections in adults and children. Am J Respir Crit Care Med 1994;149:1359-1374
• Report of the Committee on Infectious Diseases (Red Book). Elk Grove Village, Ill, American Academy of Pediatrics, 1997
• Centers for Disease Control: Core curriculum on tuberculosis-what the clinician should know, 1994
• Dutt AK: Tuberculosis. Part 1 and 2. Disease-A-Month 1997;43(3 & 4)
Illustrations: N/A
Internet references: http://www.5mcc.com

Author(s)
Gregory Snyder, MD

Tuberous sclerosis

BASICS

DESCRIPTION One of the neurocutaneous syndromes (phakomatoses). A genetic developmental disorder with variable presentations, a broad clinical spectrum and multi-organ involvement. Organ systems may be few and subtle, but can encompass multiple types of cutaneous lesions and tumor formation in the central nervous system, skin, retina, heart lung, viscera, liver, kidney, bone, teeth and nails. Other phakomatoses include neurofibromatosis, Sturge-Weber disease, von Hippel-Lindau syndrome, and ataxia-telangiectasia.

System(s) affected: Skin/Exocrine, Nervous, Cardiovascular, Pulmonary, Renal/Urologic, Musculoskeletal

Genetics:
- Autosomal dominant with variable penetrance
- Two thirds are sporadic
- Two chromosomal foci are mapped (9q34 and 16p13)

Incidence/prevalence in USA: Reported to affect 1 in 10,000 in the general population

Predominant age: Clinical expression is variable, and diagnosis may be delayed. Usually diagnosed during the first decade.

Predominant sex: Male = Female (but autism more common in males)

SIGNS AND SYMPTOMS
- Most cases have more than one of the following: Angiofibromata (labeled as adenoma sebaceum and ranging from 0.1-1.0 cm) and often present as facial lesions in a "butterfly" distribution (80%)
  ◊ Hypopigmented areas mainly on trunk and extremities often the first sign (ash-leaf spots). Present at birth or shortly after (50%).
  ◊ Seizure disorders including myoclonic (90%)
  ◊ Renal cysts (50-80%)
  ◊ Pulmonary lymphangiomatosis (<10%)
  ◊ Periventricular calcifications (50-80%)
  ◊ Retinal astrocytomas and hamartomas (50-80%)
  ◊ Cardiac rhabdomyomas (50%)
  ◊ Mental retardation (60-70%)
  ◊ Ungual fibromas, multiple (20%)
  ◊ Dental pits
  ◊ Liver hamartomas (10%)

CAUSES Congenital

RISK FACTORS Family history

DIAGNOSIS

DIFFERENTIAL DIAGNOSIS
- Polycystic kidney disease
- Other causes of seizure disorders, mental retardation, autistic behavior, traumatic ungual fibromata
- Other neurocutaneous syndromes (phakomatoses)

LABORATORY
- Present day diagnostic criteria mainly confined to clinical evaluations
- Abnormal electroencephalogram
- Search for reliable molecular marker and gene appears fruitful

Drugs that may alter lab results: N/A
Disorders that may alter lab results: N/A

PATHOLOGICAL FINDINGS
- Nodular lesions made up largely of irregular groups of glial fibrils, ganglion cells and atypical cells seeming to result from faults in developing tissue combinations as in hamartomas
- Lesions may be sparse at birth
- Calcification of subependymal lesions may not occur until several months after birth
- Facial angiofibromas, ungual fibromas, renal angiomyolipomas are quite specific lesions which may develop months after birth
- 1% present with tuberous sclerosis and lymphangioleiomyomatosis and are almost always women of reproductive age
- Not practical to have age specific criteria. Periodic reassessment in at-risk families necessary.

SPECIAL TESTS Must rely on clinical diagnostic criteria pending development of reliable molecular marker

IMAGING
- Magnetic resonance imaging (MRI) has become a major diagnostic technique
- With gadolinium enhancement, MRI provides more detailed imaging of characteristic subependymal nodules and cortical white matter tubers

DIAGNOSTIC PROCEDURES
- Woods lamp evaluation for ash-leaf spots.
- EEG
- Biopsy of indeterminate lesions
- MRI with gadolinium contrast
- Renal and cardiac ultrasound
- Lab analysis for genetic marker

TREATMENT

APPROPRIATE HEALTH CARE
Outpatient care, except for complications for severely involved manifestations or uncontrolled seizures

GENERAL MEASURES
- Team approach with neurological, orthopedic, surgical and radiological involvement
- Physical, occupational and speech therapy
- Social work for home care, and vocational training support
- Periodic reassessment in at-risk families
- Genetic counseling for patient and family
- Neurosurgical consideration for uncontrollable seizures

SURGICAL MEASURES Surgical excision of tumors where and when appropriate

ACTIVITY Determined by degree and complexity of involvement

DIET No restrictions. A ketogenic diet has been used for seizure control.

PATIENT EDUCATION
- Precautions related to seizures
- Updated information available from: National Tuberous Sclerosis Association, Inc., 8181 Professional Place, Suite 110, Landover, MD 20785 (800) 225-6872, E-mail ntsa@ntsa.org, Web site www.ntsa.org

MEDICATIONS

DRUG(S) OF CHOICE
• Anticonvulsants for seizure control
• Antibiotic prophylaxis for surgery if indicated
Contraindications: N/A
Precautions: Refer to manufacturer's profile of each drug
Significant possible interactions:
• Knowledge of anticonvulsant used is necessary to avoid drug interactions especially with antibiotics
• Refer to manufacturer's profile of each drug

ALTERNATIVE DRUGS   N/A

FOLLOWUP

PATIENT MONITORING
• Clinical features of proband periodically reviewed and updated
• Periodic reassessment of at-risk individuals

PREVENTION/AVOIDANCE   Genetic counseling

POSSIBLE COMPLICATIONS   See Signs and Symptoms

EXPECTED COURSE/PROGNOSIS
Variable; decreased longevity compared to general population

MISCELLANEOUS

ASSOCIATED CONDITIONS   N/A

AGE-RELATED FACTORS
Pediatric: N/A
Geriatric: N/A
Others: Stigmata may be present at, or shortly after birth or may become apparent in late childhood or adulthood

PREGNANCY   Genetic counseling

SYNONYMS   Bourneville disease

ICD-9-CM   759.5 Tuberous sclerosis

SEE ALSO
• Ataxia-telangiectasia
• Von Hippel-Lindau disease
• Neurofibromatosis
• Sturge-Weber disease

OTHER NOTES   N/A

ABBREVIATIONS
• TS = tuberous sclerosis
• TSC = tuberous sclerosis complex

REFERENCES
• Aicardi, J., Tuberous Sclerosis. International Pediatrics 1993;8:2:171-175
• Perspective Newsletter, National Tuberous Sclerosis Association, Inc., Spring/Summer/Fall/ Winter Publications
Illustrations: N/A
Internet references: http://www.5mcc.com

Author(s)
Nuhad D. Dinno, MD

Tularemia

BASICS

DESCRIPTION   Acute infection with Francisella tularensis. Incubation averages 3-4 days. May be ulceroglandular, glandular, typhoidal, oculoglandular, or oropharyngeal.
System(s) affected: Skin/Exocrine, Pulmonary, Cardiovascular, Hemic/Lymphatic/Immunologic
Genetics: N/A
Incidence/Prevalence in USA: (Incidence) 0.1 per 100,000
Predominant age: All ages
Predominant sex: Male > Female

SIGNS AND SYMPTOMS
• Nearly all cases have fever, chills, fatigue, malaise
• Ulceroglandular (3/4 of cases)
  ◊ Non-healing ulcer
  ◊ Regional adenopathy
  ◊ Failure of cephalosporin treatment
• Glandular
  ◊ Localized adenopathy
  ◊ No ulcer
• Typhoidal
  ◊ Systemic febrile illness
  ◊ Fulminating sepsis
  ◊ Pleuropulmonary disease
  ◊ No ulcer
• Oropharyngeal
  ◊ Exudative pharyngitis
  ◊ Membranous pharyngitis
  ◊ Cervical adenopathy
• Oculoglandular
  ◊ Purulent conjunctivitis
  ◊ Preauricular adenopathy
  ◊ Cervical adenopathy

CAUSES
• Inoculation of F. tularensis via:
  ◊ Tick bite
  ◊ Deer fly bite
  ◊ Cat bite
  ◊ Aerosol inhalation
  ◊ Contact with infected carcass (can penetrate unbroken skin)
  ◊ Ingestion

RISK FACTORS
• Location in endemic area (> 50% cases in AR, MO, OK, TN, TX)
• Outdoor work
• Rural residence
• Game handling
• Laboratory work

DIAGNOSIS

DIFFERENTIAL DIAGNOSIS
• Ulceroglandular/glandular
  ◊ Staphylococcal infections
  ◊ Streptococcal infections
  ◊ Cat-scratch disease
  ◊ Pasteurella infections
  ◊ Lymphogranuloma venereum
  ◊ Sporotrichosis
  ◊ Plague
  ◊ Toxoplasmosis
• Typhoidal
  ◊ Legionellosis
  ◊ Rocky Mountain spotted fever
  ◊ Ehrlichiosis
  ◊ Borreliosis (including Lyme disease)
  ◊ Infectious mononucleosis
  ◊ Non-typhoid salmonellosis
  ◊ Typhoid fever
  ◊ Brucellosis
  ◊ Q fever
  ◊ Psittacosis
  ◊ Tick-borne typhus
  ◊ Viral pneumonia
• Oropharyngeal
  ◊ Streptococcal pharyngitis
  ◊ Viral pharyngitis
  ◊ Diphtheric pharyngitis
  ◊ Infectious mononucleosis

LABORATORY
• Fourfold rise in antibody titer (peak in 4-8 weeks)
• Convalescent titer of 160 or greater
• Delayed growth on specific media or blood culture
• Elevated ESR
• Normal WBC, left shift
• PCR, investigational
Drugs that may alter lab results: N/A
Disorders that may alter lab results: Brucella antibodies may cross-react

PATHOLOGICAL FINDINGS
• Necrotic areas in liver, spleen, other organs
• Caseating granulomata
• Microscopic foci with PMN's, macrophages, giant cells

SPECIAL TESTS
• Referral to specialized lab
• Pleomorphic Gram-negative coccobacilli
• Metabolic profile of isolate
• Specific immunofluorescent stain
• Culture ulcer

IMAGING   Chest x-ray may show ill-defined infiltrates, lobar consolidation, or pleural effusion

DIAGNOSTIC PROCEDURES
• Lymph node aspiration
• Thoracentesis
• Thorough history of patient's contact with wild rodents or exposure to arthropod vectors

TREATMENT

APPROPRIATE HEALTH CARE
Inpatient or outpatient depending on severity.

GENERAL MEASURES
• Isolation not needed for patient, but handle secretions carefully
• Hydration, fever control, antibiotics
• Wet saline dressings for skin lesions
• Recovery requires intact cell-mediated immunity

SURGICAL MEASURES   Incision and drainage of abscesses

ACTIVITY   As tolerated

DIET   As tolerated, high caloric, easily digestible

PATIENT EDUCATION
• Person-to-person transmission not documented
• See Prevention/Avoidance
• Vaccine for high-risk persons; contact CDC

MEDICATIONS

DRUG(S) OF CHOICE
• Streptomycin 15-20 mg/kg IM per day, divided bid for 7-14 days (may be difficult to obtain)
• Gentamicin

Contraindications: Known hypersensitivity, pregnancy

Precautions:
• Long-term therapy may produce eighth nerve damage
• Reduce dose in renal dysfunction
• Long-term therapy may produce renal dysfunction
• Use with care post-anesthesia (respiratory paralysis), and in patients with myasthenia gravis

Significant possible interactions: Other aminoglycosides, cephaloridine, polymyxin B, amphotericin B, colistin, muscle relaxants, paralyzing anesthetic agents

ALTERNATIVE DRUGS
• Ciprofloxacin - successful treatment reports increasing
• Chloramphenicol - may be difficult to obtain
• Tetracyclines - associated with higher relapse rate
• 3rd generation cephalosporins - high relapse rate or failure rate

FOLLOWUP

PATIENT MONITORING
• Monitor eighth nerve function in long-term therapy
• Monitor renal function in long-term therapy

PREVENTION/AVOIDANCE
• Tick repellents
• Remove tick by grasping near mouthparts
• Avoid squeezing body of embedded tick
• Wear gloves while dressing game
• Avoid contact if game appeared ill
• Lab workers - vaccine possibly protective. Wear protective hoods.
• Cook wild game thoroughly

POSSIBLE COMPLICATIONS
• Lung abscess
• Adult respiratory distress syndrome
• Hepatic dysfunction
• Rhabdomyolysis
• Renal failure
• Osteomyelitis, meningitis, endocarditis, pericarditis, peritonitis
• Mediastinitis

EXPECTED COURSE/PROGNOSIS
• Cure complete if treated early and vigorously
• Immunity is lifelong
• Mortality is 1-3%, higher in typhoidal-type disease

MISCELLANEOUS

ASSOCIATED CONDITIONS
• Other arthropod-borne diseases
• Tularemic conjunctivitis
• Bacteremia
• Atypical pneumonia

AGE-RELATED FACTORS
Pediatric: Often affected
Geriatric: Complications more likely, mortality rate higher
Others: More likely to occur in outdoor-type, young adult males

PREGNANCY
Streptomycin may cause fetal 8th nerve damage

SYNONYMS
• Rabbit fever
• Deer-fly fever
• Pasteurella tularensis
• Bacterium tularense
• Tick fever
• Ohara's disease
• Francis' disease
• Parvovirus B19 infection

ICD-9-CM 021.0-021.9 Tularemia

SEE ALSO
• Bartonella infections
• Diphtheria
• Ehrlichiosis
• Lymphogranuloma venereum
• Plague
• Psittacosis
• Q fever
• Rocky Mountain spotted fever
• Toxoplasmosis
• Typhus fevers

OTHER NOTES Incidence higher in summer and fall. Has received mention as a bioweapon.

ABBREVIATIONS N/A

REFERENCES
• Mandell GL, Bennett JE, Dolin R, eds: Principles and Practice of Infectious Diseases. 4th Ed. New York, Churchill Livingstone, 1995
• Feigin RD, Cherry JD: Textbook of Pediatric Infectious Disease. 3rd Ed. Philadelphia, W.B. Saunders Co., 1992
• Sjostedt A, et al: Detection of Francisella tularensis in ulcers by PCR. J Clin Microbiology 1997;35(5):1045-1048
Illustrations: N/A
Internet references: http://www.5mcc.com

Author(s)
Greg Elders, MD

Turner's syndrome

 BASICS

DESCRIPTION Edema of hands and feet and excess skin of the neck (webbing) are presenting features during infancy. As children, girls are short and may have left sided heart or aortic abnormalities. Primary amenorrhea or delayed onset of puberty with short stature are important clues during adolescence.
System(s) affected: Nervous, Reproductive, Endocrine/Metabolic, Cardiovascular, Musculoskeletal, Renal/Urologic
Genetics: usually sporadic
Incidence/Prevalence in USA: 40 per 100,000 female births
Predominant age: All ages
Predominant sex: Female only

SIGNS AND SYMPTOMS
Frequencies are for classic 45,X and vary with other chromosomal abnormalities associated with Turner's syndrome
- Short stature (98%)
- Gonadal dysgenesis (95%)
- Lymphedema (70%)
- Broad chest (75%)
- Hypoplastic, wide-spaced nipples (78%)
- Prominent, anomalous ears (70%)
- High palate (82%)
- Short neck (80%)
- Webbing of neck (65%)
- Low hairline (80%)
- Cubitus valgus (75%)
- Short fourth metacarpal (65%)
- Nail hypoplasia (75%)
- Excess nevi (70%)
- Renal anomalies (60%)
- Heart malformations (30%)
- Hearing impairment (70%)

CAUSES Monosomy for all or part of the X chromosome can result in symptoms consistent with Turner's syndrome

RISK FACTORS Familial chromosome translocations involving the X chromosome increase the risk of conceiving a child with Turner's syndrome

 DIAGNOSIS

DIFFERENTIAL DIAGNOSIS
- Short stature
  ◊ Noonans syndrome
  ◊ Hypothyroidism
  ◊ Familial short stature
  ◊ Léri-Weil syndrome
  ◊ Brachydactyly E
  ◊ Growth hormone deficiency
  ◊ Glucocorticoid excess
  ◊ Klippel-Feil anomaly
  ◊ Short stature due to chronic disease
- Amenorrhea or delayed puberty
  ◊ Pure gonadal dysgenesis
  ◊ Stein-Leventhal syndrome
  ◊ Primary/secondary amenorrhea
- Lymphedema
  ◊ Hereditary congenital lymphedema
  ◊ Milroy's disease
  ◊ Lymphedema with recurrent cholestasis
  ◊ Lymphedema with intestinal lymphangiectasia
- Other
  ◊ Multiple pterygium syndrome
  ◊ Pseudohypoparathyroid

LABORATORY
- Chromosome analysis (a buccal smear is not adequate to rule out Turner's)
- At puberty FSH and LH levels may approach castration levels. FSH may be transiently high in infancy
Drugs that may alter lab results: N/A
Disorders that may alter lab results: N/A

PATHOLOGICAL FINDINGS
- Ovarian dysgenesis (> 90%)
- Renal: horseshoe kidney, double collecting system (60%)
- Cardiac: bicuspid aortic valve, coarctation of aorta, valvular aortic stenosis (70% with heart defects also have coarctation)
- Bone dysplasia (> 50%)
- Gonadoblastomas in X/XY mosaics

SPECIAL TESTS
- Upper/lower extremity blood pressures
- ECG

IMAGING
- Renal ultrasound
- Cardiac ultrasound

DIAGNOSTIC PROCEDURES N/A

 TREATMENT

APPROPRIATE HEALTH CARE
Outpatient

GENERAL MEASURES
Once diagnosis is confirmed by karyotype, the following measures are appropriate:
- Cardiology evaluation to include upper and lower extremity blood pressures, and echocardiography. If an abnormality exists, prophylactic antibiotics may be indicated (e.g., dental procedures).
- Renal ultrasound or intravenous pyelography
- Thyroid function test and antithyroid antibodies
- Routine hearing examination
- Treat gonadal failure in girls who do not enter puberty spontaneously
  ◊ Replacement therapy: begin with one to two years of low dose estrogen followed by larger dose estrogens cycled with progesterone
  ◊ Maintenace therapy: Birth control pills, after menses and secondary sexual characteristics are established. Continue into the late forties.
  ◊ Routine gynecologic evaluation indicated
  ◊ Infertility is the general rule, but alternatives such as in vitro fertilization and embryo transfer may options
- Growth retardation has been managed with sex hormone replacement, anabolic agents, and human recombinant growth hormone (hrGH). Some patients increase final height attainment with hrGH treatment. Start hrGH therapy (0.05 mg/kg SC qDay) before significant growth deceleration occurs (between 3-10 years of age).
- Intelligence is usually normal. Problems may exist in non-verbal areas such as imagining objects in relationship to one another. If concerns about school performance arise, they should be evaluated and treated.
- Regular physician visits are recommended. Be aware of the social and emotional problems associated with issues such as short stature and infertility.

SURGICAL MEASURES
• Removal of gonads in X/XY individuals
• Physical appearance may be enhanced by plastic surgery for inner canthal folds, protruding auricles and webbed neck.

ACTIVITY Normal other than limitations that may be placed on individuals with similar cardiac or renal abnormalities.

DIET Normal, but there is a tendency toward obesity

PATIENT EDUCATION
• Families and patients need a thorough explanation of the condition and its management, especially in regards to sexual development and growth. Jones/Smith suggest advising patient between age 8 and adolescence that she will probably not bear children.
• Excellent patient educational materials include:
  ◊ Plumridge D: Good things come in small packages: the whys and hows of Turner's Syndrome. Crippled Children's Division, University of Oregon Health Sciences Center, Portland, OR 97203.
  ◊ Rieser PA, Underwood LE: Turner's syndrome: a guide for families. Turner's Syndrome Society, York University, ASB 006, 4700 Keele St., Downsview, Ontario, Canada, M3J 1P3, (416)667-3773 or Turner's Syndrome Society, 3539 Tonkawood Rd., Minnetonka, MN 55345, (612)938-3118

MEDICATIONS

DRUG(S) OF CHOICE N/A
Contraindications: N/A
Precautions: N/A
Significant possible interactions: N/A

ALTERNATIVE DRUGS N/A

FOLLOWUP

PATIENT MONITORING
• Regular measurement of growth parameters
• Regular blood pressure checks
• Annual urinalysis if renal abnormality is present
• Monitor for signs of hypothyroidism
• Regular hearing testing
• Regular eye exams
• Consider screening for occult blood loss

PREVENTION/AVOIDANCE Prenatal
detection is available for high risk couples (who carry chromosomal translocations or who have had an affected child). There is no in utero treatment, but pregnancy termination is an option if a fetus with Turner's syndrome is identified

POSSIBLE COMPLICATIONS
Complications are related to associated abnormalities

EXPECTED COURSE/PROGNOSIS
Most girls with Turner's syndrome can be expected to lead reasonably normal lives with appropriate medical management

MISCELLANEOUS

ASSOCIATED CONDITIONS
• Hashimoto's thyroiditis
• Hypothyroidism
• Alopecia
• Vitiligo
• Gastrointestinal vascular malformations
• Gastrointestinal disorders
• Carbohydrate intolerance

AGE-RELATED FACTORS
Pediatric: N/A
Geriatric: N/A
Others: N/A

PREGNANCY N/A

SYNONYMS
• Ullrich-Turner syndrome
• Bonnevie-Ullrich
• XO syndrome
• Monosomy X
• Short stature-sexual infantilism
• Gonadal dysgenesis

ICD-9-CM 758.6 Gonadal dysgenesis

SEE ALSO
• Amenorrhea
• Coarctation of the aorta
• Hypothyroidism, adult
• Thyroiditis

OTHER NOTES N/A

ABBREVIATIONS N/A

REFERENCES
• Buyse ML, ed: Birth Defects Encyclopedia. Cambridge, Massachusetts, Blackwell Scientific Publications, 1990
• Hall JG, Gilchrist DM: Turner's Syndrome and Its Variants. Pediatr Clinics NA 1990;37(6):1421-1440
• Jones KL: Smith's Recognizable Patterns of Human Malformation. Philadelphia, W.B. Saunders Co., 1997
• American Academy of Pediatrics Committee on Genetics. Health Supervision for Children with Turner Syndrome. Pediatrics 1995;96:1166-73
Illustrations: N/A
Internet references: http://www.5mcc.com

Author(s)
John R. Waterson, MD, PhD

Typhoid fever

BASICS

DESCRIPTION Typhoid fever is an acute systemic illness unique to humans caused by Salmonella typhi. It is a classic example of enteric fever caused by the Salmonella family of bacteria.
• It is endemic in some developing nations where sanitation is suboptimal. Majority of cases in North America are acquired after travel to endemic areas.
• Mode of transmission is fecal-oral through ingestion of contaminated food (commonly poultry), water and milk. Incubation period varies from 7 to 21 days.
System(s) affected: Gastrointestinal, Pulmonary, Skin/Exocrine
Genetics: N/A
Incidence/Prevalence in USA: 300-500 cases per year
Predominant age: All ages
Predominant sex: Male = Female

SIGNS AND SYMPTOMS
• Fever
• Headache
• Malaise
• Abdominal discomfort/bloating/constipation
• Diarrhea (less common)
• Dry cough
• Confusion/lethargy
• Rose spot (transient erythematous maculopapular rash in anterior thorax or upper abdomen)
• Splenomegaly
• Hepatomegaly
• Cervical adenopathy
• Relative bradycardia
• Conjunctivitis

CAUSES Salmonella typhi

RISK FACTORS Must be considered in any patient presenting with fever after tropical travel or exposed to chronic carrier

DIAGNOSIS

DIFFERENTIAL DIAGNOSIS
• Malaria
• "Enteric fever-like" syndrome caused by Yersinia enterocolitica, Yersinia pseudotuberculosis, and Campylobacter sp.
• Enteric fever caused by non-typhi Salmonella
• Infectious hepatitis
• Atypical pneumonia
• Infectious mononucleosis
• Subacute bacterial endocarditis
• Tuberculosis
• Brucellosis
• Q fever

LABORATORY
• Definitive diagnosis by isolation of S. typhi from blood. Isolation of S. typhi in sputum, urine or stool is presumptive diagnosis in typical clinical presentation.
• Serology is nonspecific and usually not useful
• If multiple blood cultures are negative or in patients with prior antibiotic therapy, diagnostic yield is better with bone marrow culture
• Anemia, leukopenia (neutropenia), thrombocytopenia or evidence of DIC (disseminated intravascular coagulopathy) are supportive evidence. Elevated liver enzymes are commonly seen.
Drugs that may alter lab results:
• Prior antibiotic therapy
• Vaccination
Disorders that may alter lab results: N/A

PATHOLOGICAL FINDINGS
Classically, mononuclear proliferation involving lymphoid tissue of intestinal tract especially Peyer's patch in terminal ileum

SPECIAL TESTS N/A

IMAGING Consider serial plain abdominal films for evidence of intestinal perforation

DIAGNOSTIC PROCEDURES Bone marrow aspirate for culture is rarely indicated

TREATMENT

APPROPRIATE HEALTH CARE
• Inpatient if acutely ill
• Outpatient for less ill patient or for carrier

GENERAL MEASURES
• Fluid and electrolyte support
• Strict isolation of patient's linen, stool and urine
• Monitor clinically and consider serial plain abdominal films for evidence of perforation, usually in the third to fourth week of illness
• Indication for treatment must be determined on an individual basis. Factors to be considered are age, public health (food handler, chronic care facilities, medical personnel), intolerance to antibiotics, and evidence of biliary tract disease.
• For hemorrhage - need blood transfusion and shock management

SURGICAL MEASURES
Cholecystectomy may be warranted in carriers with cholelithiasis, relapse after therapy, or intolerance to antimicrobial therapy

ACTIVITY Bedrest initially, then as tolerated

DIET If abdominal symptoms severe, nothing by mouth. With improvement, normal low-residue diet, possibly enriched in calories.

PATIENT EDUCATION
• Discussion of chronic carrier state and its complications
• For family members, travelers or workers at risk, provide hygiene education, possibly vaccination

MEDICATIONS

DRUG(S) OF CHOICE
• Chloramphenicol: Children - 50 mg/kg/d po qid x 2 weeks; adult dose - 50 mg/kg per day, divided q6h x 2 weeks,
or
• Ampicillin: Children - 100 mg/kg/d qid po x 2 weeks; adults - 500 mg q6h x 2 weeks,
or
• Ciprofloxacin 500 mg po bid x 2 weeks, indicated in MDR-T, has been successfully and safely used in children
or
• Ceftriaxone 1-2 gm IV qd x 2 weeks,
or
• Furazolidone 7.5 mg/kg/d po x 10 days; in uncomplicated MDR-T; safe in children; efficacy > 85% cure
• Chronic carrier state
◊ Is treated with ampicillin 4-5 gram/day plus probenecid 2 grams/day qid x 6 weeks (for patients with normal functioning gallbladder without evidence of cholelithiasis)
◊ Ciprofloxacin 500 mg po bid x 4-6 weeks is also efficacious
Note: Chloramphenicol resistance - reported in Mexico, South America, Central America, Southeast Asia, India, Pakistan, Middle East and Africa
Contraindications: Refer to manufacturer's profile of each drug
Precautions: Rarely, Jarisch-Herxheimer reaction post antimicrobial therapy
Significant possible interactions: Refer to manufacturer's profile of each drug

ALTERNATIVE DRUGS
Trimethoprim-sulfamethoxazole

FOLLOWUP

PATIENT MONITORING   See General Measures

PREVENTION/AVOIDANCE
• For travel to an endemic area, consider vaccination for typhoid, parenterally (phenol-killed or Vi vaccines) or live oral vaccine (Ty21a)
• Avoid tap water, salad/raw vegetables, unpeeled fruits, dairy products in tropical travel
• Avoid poultry or poultry products left unrefrigerated for prolonged period of time

POSSIBLE COMPLICATIONS
• Intestinal hemorrhage and perforation in distal ileum
• Patient may become chronic carrier state (up to 3%) defined as persistent stool excretor for longer than 1 year
• Predilection for seeding in the biliary tract exists and may become a focus for relapse of typhoid fever. Most common in female and the elderly (> 50 years old).
• Osteomyelitis especially in sickle cell anemia, systemic lupus erythematosus, hematologic neoplasms and immunosuppressed hosts
• Endovascular infection in the elderly and in patients with history of by-pass operation or aneurysm
• Rarely, endocarditis or meningitis

EXPECTED COURSE/PROGNOSIS
Overall prognosis good with therapy. < 2% mortality rate; 15% relapse rate with some antibiotic treatments; 3% bowel perforation

MISCELLANEOUS

ASSOCIATED CONDITIONS   N/A

AGE-RELATED FACTORS
Pediatric: Disease more critical in infants, but may be milder in children
Geriatric: Disease more serious in elderly
Others: N/A

PREGNANCY   Ciprofloxacin relative contraindicated in pregnancy

SYNONYMS
• Typhoid
• Typhus abdominalis
• Enteric fever

ICD-9-CM   002.0 Typhoid and paratyphoid fevers

SEE ALSO   N/A

OTHER NOTES   N/A

ABBREVIATIONS   N/A

REFERENCES   Mandell GL, ed: Principles and Practice of Infectious Diseases. 4th Ed. New York, Churchill Livingstone, 1995
Illustrations: N/A
Internet references: http://www.5mcc.com

Author(s)
D. W. MacPherson, MD, MSc (CTM), FRCPC

Typhus fevers

BASICS

DESCRIPTION Acute infectious diseases caused by three species of rickettsiae
• Epidemic typhus - human to human transmission by body louse. Primarily in circumstances such as refugee camps, war, famine and disaster. Recrudescent disease, occurring years after initial infection can be source of human outbreak. Flying squirrels also reservoir.
• Endemic (murine) typhus - infection of rodents. To humans by rat flea.
• Scrub typhus - infection of chiggers and of rodents. To humans by the chigger. Primarily in Asia and the Western Pacific.
System(s) affected: Endocrine/Metabolic, Pulmonary, Skin/Exocrine, Hemic/Lymphatic/Immunologic
Genetics: N/A
Incidence/Prevalence in USA:
• Epidemic typhus - rare
• Endemic typhus - fewer than 100 cases annually, primarily in gulf states, especially South Texas, under-reporting suspected
• Scrub typhus - travelers returning from endemic areas, only (rare)
Predominant age: N/A
Predominant sex: N/A

SIGNS AND SYMPTOMS
• General
 ◊ Acute onset
 ◊ Fever
 ◊ Chills
 ◊ Headache
 ◊ Myalgia
 ◊ Malaise
 ◊ Diffuse organ involvement, e.g., intestine, liver, heart, kidneys, brain
• Epidemic typhus
 ◊ Incubation period about 1 week
 ◊ Macular or maculopapular rash beginning on trunk about fifth day of illness
 ◊ Nonproductive cough
 ◊ Pulmonary infiltrates
• Endemic typhus
 ◊ Incubation period 1-2 weeks
 ◊ Macular or maculopapular rash beginning on trunk third to fifth day of illness
• Scrub typhus
 ◊ Incubation period 1-3 weeks
 ◊ Eschar at bite site
 ◊ Regional lymphadenopathy
 ◊ Generalized lymphadenopathy
 ◊ Splenomegaly
 ◊ Macular or maculopapular rash beginning on trunk about the fifth day of illness
 ◊ Relative bradycardia early in disease
 ◊ Ocular pain
 ◊ Conjunctival injection

CAUSES
• Epidemic typhus by Rickettsia prowazekii
• Endemic typhus by R. typhi
• Scrub typhus by R. tsutsugamushi

RISK FACTORS
• Exposure to vectors, e.g., travel to certain countries
• Elderly may have more severe disease
• Laboratory worker

DIAGNOSIS

DIFFERENTIAL DIAGNOSIS
• Any acute febrile disease
• Rocky Mountain spotted fever
• Meningococcemia
• Bacterial meningitis
• Boutonneuse fever (R. conorii)
• Measles
• Rubella
• Toxoplasmosis
• Leptospirosis
• Typhoid fever
• Dengue
• Relapsing fever
• Secondary syphilis
• Infectious mononucleosis

LABORATORY
• WBC usually normal
• Abnormalities reflecting the particular organs affected
• Weil-Felix serological reaction may be positive; test limited to mid-illness or after, and by low sensitivity and non-specificity. Epidemic and endemic typhus, fourfold titer rise or titer > 1/320 to OX-19. Scrub typhus, fourfold rise in titer to OX-K.
• Hyponatremia in severe cases
• Hypoalbuminemia in severe cases
Drugs that may alter lab results: Prior antibiotic use
Disorders that may alter lab results: N/A

PATHOLOGICAL FINDINGS Diffuse vasculitis

SPECIAL TESTS Specific serological test showing a rising antibody titer. Isolation of rickettsia should be undertaken only in special laboratories to minimize risk of laboratory acquired infection.

IMAGING N/A

DIAGNOSTIC PROCEDURES N/A

TREATMENT

APPROPRIATE HEALTH CARE
Outpatient unless severely ill

GENERAL MEASURES
• Protect agitated patient from injury
• Skin and mouth care
• Supportive care for the severely ill, directed to the complications

SURGICAL MEASURES N/A

ACTIVITY Bedrest during acute stages, otherwise as tolerated

DIET As tolerated

PATIENT EDUCATION
• Prevention information to travelers
• Vaccination information

MEDICATIONS

DRUG(S) OF CHOICE
• Treatment should begin when diagnosis is reasonably likely and continue until improved and afebrile for a minimum of 48 hours
• Children over 8 years and adults:
  ◊ Tetracycline , or a congener, orally 25 mg per kg initially, and then 25 mg per kg daily in equally divided doses every 6 hours
  ◊ If severely ill, may use doxycycline IV, adults 100 mg every 12 hours, children >8 years 5 mg per kg in 24 hours (maximum of 200 mg/24 hrs)
• Children under 8 years, pregnant women or if typhoid fever is possible cause of illness:
  ◊ Chloramphenicol orally 50 mg per kg initially, and then 50 mg per kg daily in equally divided doses every 6 hours
  ◊ If severely ill, chloramphenicol sodium succinate intravenously 20 mg per kg initially infused in 30-45 minutes, and then 50 mg per kg daily infused in equally divided doses every 6 hours until orally tolerable.
Contraindications: N/A
Precautions: Refer to manufacturer's profile of each drug
Significant possible interactions: Refer to manufacturer's profile of each drug

ALTERNATIVE DRUGS
• Doxycycline single oral dose of 100 or 200 mg in refugee camps, disasters or limited medical services
• Isolated reports indicate that erythromycin and ciprofloxacin are effective

FOLLOWUP

PATIENT MONITORING   Severely ill patients should be observed regularly in hospital. Outpatients checked periodically as improvement is evident.

PREVENTION/AVOIDANCE
• Avoid vectors for each disease, e.g., scrub typhus; wear protective clothing and use insect repellents, endemic typhus; practice ectoparasite and rodent control, and epidemic typhus; delousing and cleaning of clothing
• Epidemic typhus vaccine considered for persons at high risk of exposure

POSSIBLE COMPLICATIONS
• Consequences of specific organ system involvement in the second week, e.g., azotemia, meningoencephalitis, seizures, delirium, coma, myocardial failure, hyponatremia, hypoalbuminemia, hypovolemia, and shock
• Death

EXPECTED COURSE/PROGNOSIS
• Recovery expected if treatment is instituted before complications
• Relapses may follow treatment, especially if initiated within 48 hours of onset (this is not an indication to delay treatment). Relapses treated same as primary disease.
• Without treatment the mortality is 40-60% in epidemic, 1-2% in endemic, and up to 30% in scrub typhus. Mortality higher among the elderly.

MISCELLANEOUS

ASSOCIATED CONDITIONS   N/A

AGE-RELATED FACTORS
Pediatric: N/A
Geriatric: N/A
Others: N/A

PREGNANCY   N/A

SYNONYMS
• Louse-borne typhus
• Brill-Zinsser disease
• Murine typhus

ICD-9-CM
080 Louse-born [epidemic] typhus
081.0 Murine [endemic] typhus
081.1 Brill's disease

SEE ALSO   N/A

OTHER NOTES
• Severe headache often intractable and not eased by the usual drugs
• Report case to Health Department

ABBREVIATIONS   N/A

REFERENCES
• Dumlev JS, Taylor JP, Walker DH: Clinical and laboratory features of murine typhus in south Texas, 1980 through 1987. JAMA 1991;266:1365-1370
• Walker DH, et al: Emerging bacterial zoonotic and vector-borne diseases: ecological and epidemiological factors. JAMA 1996;275:463-469
Illustrations: N/A
Internet references: http://www.5mcc.com

Author(s)
D. W. MacPherson, MD, MSc (CTM), FRCPC

Ulcerative colitis

BASICS

DESCRIPTION One of a group of inflammatory bowel diseases of unknown etiology characterized by intermittent bouts of inflammation of all or portions of the colon. Manifested by recurrences of rectal bleeding and various constitutional symptoms.
System(s) affected: Gastrointestinal
Genetics: Family aggregates common, positive family history in 8-11%. More likely vertical than horizontal. More common in Jews.
Incidence/Prevalence in USA: 70-150 per 100,000. Incidence 6-8 new cases per 100,000 population.
Predominant age: Between ages of 15 and 35 years. There is a second and smaller peak in the 7th decade.
Predominant sex: Male = Female

SIGNS AND SYMPTOMS
- Bloody diarrhea
- Abdominal pain
- Fever
- Weight loss
- Arthralgias and arthritis (15-20%)
- Spondylitis (3-6%)
- Ocular complications (4-10%) includes episcleritis, uveitis, cataracts, keratopathy, marginal corneal ulceration, and central serous retinopathy
- Erythema nodosum
- Pyoderma gangrenosum
- Aphthous ulcers of mouth (5-10%)
- Asymptomatic fatty liver common - occasional hepatomegaly
- Pericholangitis (uncommon)
- Primary sclerosing cholangitis (1-4%)
- Cirrhosis of liver (1-5%)
- Bile duct carcinoma
- Thromboembolic disease (1-6%)
- Pericarditis (rare)
- Amyloidosis (rare)

CAUSES Unknown (genetic, infectious, immunologic, and psychological factors have all been suggested)

RISK FACTORS
- None known
- Higher incidence in Jews and those with positive family history
- Negative association with smoking

DIAGNOSIS

DIFFERENTIAL DIAGNOSIS
- Other sources of rectal bleeding including hemorrhoids, neoplasms, colonic diverticuli, A-V malformation, Crohn's disease
- Infectious causes of diarrhea including bacteria (Enterotoxigenic E. coli, E. coli 0157:H7, Salmonella, Shigella, Aeromonas, Plesiomonas), parasitic (Entamoeba histolytica)
- "Gay bowel" syndrome causes (*Herpes simplex, Chlamydia trachomatis, Cryptosporidium, Isospora belli,* cytomegalovirus, and other infectious causes as listed above)
- Antibiotic associated diarrhea
- Radiation proctitis
- Ischemic proctitis

LABORATORY
- Nonspecific. Usually reflects the degree of severity of the bleeding and inflammation.
- Anemia may reflect chronic disease as well as iron deficiency from blood loss
- Leukocytosis during exacerbation
- Elevated sedimentation rate
- Electrolyte abnormalities, especially hypokalemia
- Hypoalbuminemia
- Elevated liver function tests (if there is associated hepatobiliary disease)
Drugs that may alter lab results: N/A
Disorders that may alter lab results: N/A

PATHOLOGICAL FINDINGS
Inflammation of the colonic mucosa with ulcerations. These appear hyperemic and hemorrhagic. Rectum involved 95% of time. The inflammation extends proximally in a continuous fashion, but for a variable distance. May affect terminal ileum - referred to as "backwash ileitis."

SPECIAL TESTS None

IMAGING Air contrast barium enema

DIAGNOSTIC PROCEDURES
- Sigmoidoscopy, may include biopsy
- Colonoscopy, may include biopsy for evaluation for premalignant features; also used to differentiate from Crohn's disease, and to investigate abnormalities that appear on radiography, such as stricture or mass lesions. Colonoscopy useful to define the extent of involvement and specific segments involved as this has bearing on therapy and prognosis.

TREATMENT

APPROPRIATE HEALTH CARE
Outpatient, except for severe exacerbations which may require hospitalization

GENERAL MEASURES Goal is to control
inflammation, prevent complications, replace nutritional losses and blood volume

SURGICAL MEASURES Complications or
refractory disease may require surgical intervention

ACTIVITY Full activity as tolerated

DIET No specific diet; milk products not
withheld unless an associated lactase deficiency exists

PATIENT EDUCATION
- Close doctor/patient relationship encouraged
- Self-help organizations such as: National Foundation for Ileitis and Colitis 444 Park Avenue S., 11th Floor, New York, NY 10016-7374, (800)343-3637

MEDICATIONS

DRUG(S) OF CHOICE
- Sulfasalazine is treatment of choice both for mild flare-ups and for the chronic treatment used to decrease the frequency of relapses (dosage range 1-4 grams daily)
- Disease limited to the rectum (proctitis) or to the left side of the colon and rectum (proctosigmoiditis) may be treated topically with steroid enemas or mesalamine (5-aminosalicylic acid, 5-ASA) enemas and suppositories
- Oral or parenteral corticosteroids are used for more severe flare-ups (e.g., prednisone 40-60 mg qd, gradually tapered off over two months)
- Approximately 10% of patients have chronic disease activity and require continuous low - moderate steroid doses
- Newer agents include oral 5-ASA derivatives. Topical use of sodium cromoglycate and sucralfate being studied.
- Immunomodulators such as azathioprine, mercaptopurine (6-mercaptopurine), methotrexate, levamisole, and cyclosporine are controversial in a disease potentially curable by colectomy. However, have been shown to be effective in patients who either refuse surgery or are poor surgical candidates.
- Antimicrobial agents (anti-mycobacteriums and metronidazole) sometimes useful in Crohn's disease but not in ulcerative colitis
- Antidiarrheal agents, diphenoxylate-atropine and loperamide may be used to help control diarrhea, but require careful monitoring since they may precipitate toxic megacolon

Contraindications:
- Allergy to any of above agents
- Refer to manufacturer's profile of each drug

Precautions: Use of antidiarrheal agents in severe disease could precipitate toxic megacolon

Significant possible interactions: Refer to manufacturer's profile of each drug

ALTERNATIVE DRUGS   Included in Drug(s) of Choice

FOLLOWUP

PATIENT MONITORING   Regularly scheduled appointments are important to evaluate for disease activity, appearance of complications, and the psychological and social well being of the patient

PREVENTION/AVOIDANCE
Colonoscopic evaluation for cancer surveillance with biopsy evaluation of the mucosa for evidence of dysplasia must be performed every 1-2 years after the disease has been present for 7-8 years. This is particularly important in pancolitis. Low grade dysplasia warrants more frequent evaluation (e.g., every 3-6 months) and high grade dysplasia (or low grade dysplasia within a mass) warrant consideration of colectomy.
- Annual liver tests
- Cholangiography for cholestasis

POSSIBLE COMPLICATIONS
- Perforation
- Toxic megacolon
- Liver disease
- Stricture formation (less than Crohn's disease)
- Colon cancer (may occur in as many as 30% of those with pancolitis for 25 years). Incidence of cancer is cumulative and begins after 7-8 years of disease; risk may be considerably less in left sided disease.

EXPECTED COURSE/PROGNOSIS
- Course extremely variable; mortality for initial attack approximately 5%. Approximately 75-85% of patients experience relapse, and up to 20% in some studies eventually require colectomy.
- Colon cancer risk is the single most important risk factor affecting long-term prognosis
- Left-sided colitis and ulcerative proctitis have very favorable prognosis with probable normal life span

MISCELLANEOUS

ASSOCIATED CONDITIONS   Ankylosing spondylitis

AGE-RELATED FACTORS
Pediatric:
- Approximately 20% of patients are 21 years or younger
- Cancer surveillance is important since occurrence of cancer relates to the duration and extent of disease, whether frequently symptomatic or not

Geriatric: Increased mortality with initial attack in patients over 60

Others: N/A

PREGNANCY
- Outcome of pregnancy similar to general population. One study showed 30% of those with inactive disease at onset of pregnancy relapsed and 14% did so in first trimester.
- Treatment with sulfasalazine does not seem to affect outcome of pregnancy
- Recommend patient delay pregnancy until time when disease is inactive

SYNONYMS   Idiopathic proctocolitis

ICD-9-CM   556 Idiopathic proctocolitis

SEE ALSO
- Crohn's disease
- Diarrhea, acute
- Diarrhea, chronic
- Intestinal parasites

OTHER NOTES   N/A

ABBREVIATIONS   N/A

REFERENCES
- Isselbacher KJ, et al,eds: Harrison's Principles of Internal Medicine. 13th Ed. New York, McGraw-Hill, 1994
- Farmer RG: Inflammatory Bowel Disease. Medical Clinics Issue, Volume 74/number 1. Philadelphia, W.B. Saunders Co., January 1990

Illustrations: 3 available on CD-ROM
Internet references: http://www.5mcc.com

Author(s)
Mark Eric Worshtil, MD

Urethritis

BASICS

DESCRIPTION Syndrome of urethral inflammation marked by painful urination and discharge. Usually a sexually transmitted disease (STD); other causes not uncommon. Two types: Gonorrhea (GC) found usually in males, rarely in women, and nongonococcal urethritis (NGU).
• In males - gonorrhea marked by a yellow purulent discharge, abrupt onset of symptoms 3 to 5 days after exposure to *Neisseria gonorrhea*. Nongonococcal urethritis marked by clear to white scanty discharge developing gradually at least a week after exposure, waxing and waning in intensity from a variety of other organisms, most commonly *Chlamydia trachomatis*
• In females, classic urethral syndrome present when patient complains of dysuria, urinalysis is clear, urine cultures are negative and patient fails to respond to regimens for simple cystitis. However, females with GC or other infections which cause simple urethritis in males will often have symptoms besides dysuria, including vaginal discharge and suprapubic pain.
• Untreated cases will gradually resolve, but complications, especially urethral stricture in males or pelvic inflammatory disease (PID) in women, may then ensue
System(s) affected: Renal/Urologic
Genetics: N/A
Incidence/Prevalence in USA: Very common - annually 2 million cases of gonorrhea, probably many more cases of Chlamydia. Highest incidence in urban, non-white populations.
Predominant age: Sexually active, postpubertal
Predominant sex: Classic symptoms more commonly reported by males; incidence in females probably equal

SIGNS AND SYMPTOMS
• Both sexes may be asymptomatic carriers of the causative organisms
• Dysuria - pain throughout urination
• Urethral discharge - may be profuse and purulent in acute GC, or scanty, evident only with milking of the urethra in NGU
• Suprapubic discomfort
• Urethral itching or tenderness
• Tenderness, edema and inflammation of the urethral meatus, especially in women
• Dyspareunia
• Vaginitis, cystitis, cervicitis in women
• Proctitis, pharyngitis, conjunctivitis may also be present (sexual history is important)
• Lymphadenopathy or fever are not part of the syndrome and suggest another diagnosis
• Bloody discharge - rarely seen and suggests another diagnosis

CAUSES Sexual contact with carrier of causative organisms. Most common are N. gonorrhea, C. trachomatis, Ureaplasma urealyticum, Trichomonas vaginalis, viruses (including herpes, cytomegalovirus [CMV], human papilloma virus), many other bacteria, rarely fungi

RISK FACTORS
• Multiple sexual partners
• History of other STD's

DIAGNOSIS

DIFFERENTIAL DIAGNOSIS
• Postgonococcal urethritis (PGU) - following adequate treatment of acute GC, patient continues to have symptoms, due to a second organism resistant to original medication (see Treatment)
• Other urinary tract infections - cystitis, epididymitis, prostatitis, etc.
• Trauma - frequent milking of the urethra in males, caused by concern about possible infection may lead to dysuria and a clear discharge. Young girls may occasionally develop symptoms from external irritation.
• Atrophy, especially in postmenopausal women
• Intraurethral foreign bodies or growths, e.g., venereal warts, congenital polyps
• Allergic or sensitivity reactions - vaginal douches and lubricants, foods, other medications (rare)
• Substance abuse - frequent heavy users of amphetamines or other stimulants may develop a scant, clear discharge without white cells and mild dysuria
• Stevens-Johnson syndrome
• Reiter's syndrome - probably an immunological reaction to Chlamydial infection

LABORATORY
• Gram stain of discharge: Polymorphic neutrophils with intracellular gram-negative diplococci strongly indicates GC; sheets of polymorphonuclear leukocytes without organisms suggests NGU; few to no polymorphonuclear leukocytes suggests other etiologies
• Discharge cultures or slide reagins for GC: False-negatives can occur, so treatment should be directed by physical exam and Gram stain results and should not wait for culture results. Conjunctiva, pharynx, rectum cultured as indicated by history and symptoms. Labs should test positives for drug resistances.
• Cultures or reagin detection for Chlamydia: Negatives may be false results or indicate another infecting organism

• Urinalysis: If indicated, sample discharge before patient voids, usually normal in cases of simple urethritis
• Urine culture: Performed only if Gram stain of discharge is unremarkable or unobtainable
• Wet prep of discharge: may reveal Trichomonas, unusual to demonstrate trichomoniasis in infected males
• Syphilis, HIV serology as indicated to rule out concomitant STD's
Drugs that may alter lab results: Previous recent treatment with antibiotics may lead to false negative results
Disorders that may alter lab results: N/A

PATHOLOGICAL FINDINGS Urethral strictures (untreated GC), intraurethral lesions (venereal warts, congenital anomalies)

SPECIAL TESTS Viral cultures if typical lesions are present

IMAGING Urethrogram for persistent symptoms, rarely indicated

DIAGNOSTIC PROCEDURES Urethrocystoscopy for persistent cases with suspected foreign body, intraurethral warts

TREATMENT

APPROPRIATE HEALTH CARE All cases can be treated as outpatients except females with severe symptoms of PID

GENERAL MEASURES Identification and treatment of sexual partners

SURGICAL MEASURES N/A

ACTIVITY Full activity, except no sexual intercourse until treatment is completed

DIET No special diet

PATIENT EDUCATION
• Many handouts available from local health departments on avoidance, causes and treatments
• Most important to emphasize need for compliance with therapy and treatment of sexual partners. Also, patients should be urged to undergoing screening for other STD's.

MEDICATIONS

DRUG(S) OF CHOICE
• Note: There is an ever-increasing incidence of multiple drug resistances
• Gonorrhea - ceftriaxone (Rocephin) 250 mg IM x 1 dose. All cases of GC need to be treated additionally with a regimen specific for Chlamydia due to the high incidence of mixed infections.
• Chlamydia - doxycycline 100 mg po bid for at least 7 days. Patients who continue with symptoms after treatment (and their sexual partners) should be retreated with erythromycin.
• NGU (especially U. urealyticum) - doxycycline 100 mg po bid for at least 7 days
• Trichomonas - 2 grams metronidazole (Flagyl) po for 1 dose or 250 mg tid for 7 days

Contraindications: Sensitivity to any of the indicated medications. Pregnant patients should not receive tetracyclines

Precautions: Patients taking tetracyclines need to be told of the possibility of increased sensitivity to sunlight

Significant possible interactions:
Tetracyclines should not be taken with milk products or antacids. Oral contraceptives may be rendered ineffective by oral antibiotics. Patients and partners should use a back-up method of birth control for remainder of the cycle.

ALTERNATIVE DRUGS
• Gonorrhea
  ◊ Spectinomycin 2 grams IM once
  ◊ Ciprofloxacin (Cipro) 500 mg po once
  ◊ Ofloxacin (Floxin) 400 mg po once
  ◊ Amoxicillin 3 grams with 1 gram probenecid (Benemid) po once
• Chlamydia
  ◊ Erythromycin 500 mg po qid x 7 days
  ◊ Azithromycin (Zithromax)1 g po once
  ◊ Ofloxacin (Floxin) 300 mg po q12h x 7 days

FOLLOWUP

PATIENT MONITORING
• Patients with positive cultures should have cultures repeated several days after completing treatment as a test of cure
• Ensure that sexual partners were treated

PREVENTION/AVOIDANCE
Safer sex protection techniques, urinating immediately after intercourse, treatment of all sexual partners

POSSIBLE COMPLICATIONS
• Stricture formation in untreated patients, PID in women
• When urethritis is accompanied by suprapubic discomfort, consider prostatitis in males, PID in females

EXPECTED COURSE/PROGNOSIS
If diagnosis is firmly established, appropriate medications prescribed and patient is compliant with treatment, there will be relief of symptoms within 24 hours and the problem will resolve without sequelae

MISCELLANEOUS

ASSOCIATED CONDITIONS
Other STD's - patients should be strongly urged to undergo testing for syphilis and HIV

AGE-RELATED FACTORS
Pediatric: Proven cases of GC or Chlamydia, trichomoniasis should raise the question of sexual abuse
Geriatric: N/A
Others: None

PREGNANCY
Tetracyclines are contraindicated. Use erythromycin instead but not the estolate form because of an increased risk of cholestatic jaundice.

SYNONYMS N/A

ICD-9-CM
098.0 gonorrhea
099.4 nongonococcal urethritis
131.02 trichomonas infections
99.3 Reiter's syndrome

SEE ALSO
• Gonococcal infections
• Chlamydial sexually transmitted diseases
• Pelvic inflammatory disease (PID)
• Vulvovaginitis, bacterial
• Vulvovaginitis, candidal
• Urinary tract infection in men
• Urinary tract infection in women
• Prostatitis
• Epididymitis

OTHER NOTES
For patients who present without symptoms stating that a sexual partner was treated for this problem: Obtain specimens for lab tests, but treat this patient before the results are available (due to the high prevalence of the illness and the possibility of false-negative test results). Use any of the regimens discussed in Medications section.

ABBREVIATIONS
• STD = sexually transmitted disease
• GC = gonococcus infection
• NGU = nongonococcal urethritis
• PGU = postgonococcal urethritis

REFERENCES
• Centers for Disease control: Sexually transmitted diseases: Treatment guidelines 1989. MMWR Morb Mortal Wkly Rep 1989;38 (Suppl 8):1
• Drugs for Sexually transmitted Diseases. Medical Letter, Vol. 36, Issue 913, Jan. 7, 1994
Illustrations: N/A
Internet references: http://www.5mcc.com

Author(s)
Kevin M. Hepler, MD, MBA

Urinary incontinence

BASICS

DESCRIPTION Urinary incontinence is the involuntary loss of urine from the bladder. It can occur while asleep or awake. The amount of urine lost can vary greatly. The condition comes to medical attention when it is perceived to be a social and/or health problem by the patient or family.
System(s) affected: Renal/Urologic
Genetics: Unknown
Incidence/Prevalence in USA:
• 11-55% in community-dwelling elderly (over age 65)
• 13 million in U.S.
• Up to 50% in nursing home populations
Predominant age: Geriatric populations. Increases with age.
Predominant sex: Female > Male

SIGNS AND SYMPTOMS
• Involuntary loss of urine
• Urinary urgency

CAUSES
• Pelvic floor muscle weakness
• Post TURP
• Urethral sphincter weakness
• Bladder irritation (cystitis, tumors, stones, diverticula)
• Detrusor motor/sensory instability (stroke, dementia, parkinsonism)
• Anatomic obstruction (prostate, stricture, cystocele)
• Neurogenic bladder (diabetes, spinal cord injury, multiple sclerosis)
• Loss of central nervous system control (severe dementia)
• Fecal impaction
• Drugs (cyclophosphamide, caffeine, beta blockers, cholinergic agents, alcohol, alpha agonist)

RISK FACTORS
• Increasing age
• Female sex/estrogen deficiency
• Prostatic hypertrophy (males)
• Multiparity (females)
• Dementia
• Diabetes
• Spinal cord injury
• Multiple sclerosis
• General debilitated condition
• Stroke

DIAGNOSIS

DIFFERENTIAL DIAGNOSIS
• Urinary tract infection
• Vaginal discharge (women)
• Urethral discharge (men)
• Medication effect (diuretics, alcohol, caffeine)
• Polyuria (diabetes, excessive H2O intake)

LABORATORY
• Urinalysis - generally normal. May show glycosuria (diabetes), proteinuria (glomerular disease), white blood cells (infection), red blood cells (tumor), or bacteria (infection).
• Urine culture - will be positive in urinary tract infection
Drugs that may alter lab results:
• Diuretics (low urine specific gravity)
• Antibiotics (negative urine culture)
Disorders that may alter lab results: Not applicable. Disorders producing abnormal lab results generally contribute to the problem of incontinence.

PATHOLOGICAL FINDINGS
• Relate to the primary cause of incontinence
• Urinary sphincter incompetence
• Prostatic hypertrophy
• Neurogenic bladder
• Bladder tumors
• Urinary tract infection
• Fecal impaction

SPECIAL TESTS
• Voiding cystourethrogram - may show bladder and/or urethral pathology
• Cystometrograms - may show abnormal sphincter pressure or bladder physiology
• Post-voiding residual measurement - may show increased residual urine (normally less than 50 cc)

IMAGING
• Renal ultrasound - may show renal pathology
• IVP - may show renal pathology

DIAGNOSTIC PROCEDURES
• The diagnosis is generally made by history
• Physical examination of men should include palpation of abdomen (for distended bladder), digital rectal exam (for prostatic hypertrophy), and neurological exam
• Physical exam of women should include palpation of abdomen (for distended bladder), vaginal speculum and bimanual pelvic exam (for genitourinary pathology), and neurologic exam
• Both men and women should be examined for fecal impaction
• It is sometimes helpful to ask the patient to reproduce the activities (e.g., coughing, sneezing, laughing) which result in loss of urine
• Office cystometry - using a catheter and 60 cc Asepto syringe (without plunger)

TREATMENT

APPROPRIATE HEALTH CARE
Outpatient

GENERAL MEASURES
• All primary conditions relating to urinary incontinence should be identified and treated specifically (e.g., urinary tract infection, bladder tumors, prostatic hypertrophy, diabetes)
• Good perineal hygiene
• Pelvic floor (Kegel) exercises
• Biofeedback/behavioral training
• Intermittent catheterization (selected patients)
• Impress Soft Patch (Uro Med Corp.)
• Incontinence pads
• Indwelling catheterization (selected patients)
• Condom catheters (male patients)
• Treatment for fecal impaction
• Electrical stimulation (selected patients)

SURGICAL MEASURES
• Some patients with overflow incontinence secondary to prostatic hypertrophy may benefit from transurethral resection of the prostate (TURP)
• Some patients with stress incontinence may benefit from bladder suspension procedures
• Some patients with poor urethral tone may benefit from periurethral collagen injections or sphincter implants

ACTIVITY Full activities should be encouraged

DIET
• No special diet
• In situations where access to bathroom facilities is limited, may want to avoid high volume fluid intake and reduce intake of caffeine or alcohol-containing beverages

PATIENT EDUCATION
• Should be directed at the general problem, as well as any underlying diseases
• Should include instructions regarding good general nutrition and exercise practices
• Rational toileting schedule, based on the patient's pattern of incontinence
• Easy access to toilet facilities
• Pelvic floor (Kegel) exercises
• Bladder training - timed voiding, increasing slowly to 3 hours
• Examples of specific instructions can be found in Clinics in Geriatric Medicine, November, 1986, pages 841-855

MEDICATIONS

DRUG(S) OF CHOICE
* Detrusor instability
  ◊ Oxybutynin (Ditropan) 2.5-5 mg qid
  ◊ Propantheline (Pro-Banthine) 15-30 mg tid
  ◊ Flavoxate (Urispas) 100-200 mg tid
  ◊ Imipramine (Tofranil) 25-50 mg tid
* Sphincter incompetence
  ◊ Pseudoephedrine (Sudafed) 30-60 mg tid
  ◊ Phenylpropanolamine (Ornade) 75 mg bid
  ◊ Imipramine (Tofranil) 25-50 mg tid
* Overflow/atonic bladder
  ◊ Bethanechol (Urecholine) 10-30 mg tid
* Overflow/prostatic enlargement
  ◊ Cardura 1-8 mg qd
  ◊ Finasteride (Proscar) 5 mg q day
  ◊ Tamsulosin (Flomax) 0.4-0.8 mg q day
* Urge incontinence (could be part of detrusor instability) tolterodine (Detrol) 2 mg bid

Contraindications:
* Should be reviewed for each specific medication prior to initiating
* Anticholinergic agents are contraindicated in patients with glaucoma or prostatic hypertrophy

Precautions:
* Use smallest dose possible in elderly patients
* Common side effects include: Dry mouth, blurred vision, constipation, postural hypotension, mental confusion

Significant possible interactions: Will vary for each of the drugs listed

ALTERNATIVE DRUGS
* Oral or topical estrogens for stress incontinence associated with atrophic vaginitis
* Prostaglandin inhibitors (investigational)
* Calcium antagonists (investigational)
* Desmopressin (DDAVP) nasal spray (nocturnal enuresis)
* Herbal remedies Huang qi, Cypress and Horsetail (dosage recommendations vary)

 (FOLLOWUP icon)

FOLLOWUP

PATIENT MONITORING
* Biweekly at first (while exercises are being learned and medication dosage is being adjusted)
* Quarterly, once incontinence is under control and medication doses are stable
* Ask about side effects of medication
* Check for orthostatic hypotension
* Consider measuring intraocular pressure in high risk patients
* Periodic urinalysis to detect early urinary tract infection

PREVENTION/AVOIDANCE
* Instruct women in routine use of Kegel exercises after birth of children
* Regular pelvic examination of female patients to detect pelvic pathology
* Regular rectal examination in male patients to pick up early prostatic pathology. Treatment for hypertrophy.

POSSIBLE COMPLICATIONS
* Urinary tract infection
* Hydronephrosis (with atonic bladder or outlet obstruction)
* Renal failure (with obstructive hydronephrosis)
* Adverse drug reactions

EXPECTED COURSE/PROGNOSIS
* Prognosis is generally good. Most patients can achieve an increase in bladder control with appropriate medical management
* Some feel that sphinctor incompetence is best treated surgically

MISCELLANEOUS

ASSOCIATED CONDITIONS N/A

AGE-RELATED FACTORS
Pediatric: N/A
Geriatric: This problem is most commonly seen in the aging population
Others: N/A

PREGNANCY Stress incontinence can occur during pregnancy

SYNONYMS
* Transient incontinence
* Urge incontinence
* Overflow incontinence
* Stress incontinence

ICD-9-CM 788.3 Incontinence of urine

SEE ALSO
* Urethritis
* Urinary tract infection in males
* Urinary tract infection in females
* Prostatic hyperplasia, benign (BPH)
* Vulvovaginitis, estrogen deficient

OTHER NOTES N/A

ABBREVIATIONS N/A

REFERENCES
* Hazard W, et al, eds: Principles of Geriatric Medicine and Gerontology. 2nd Ed. New York, McGraw-Hill Co, 1990
* Brocklehurst JC, ed: Gerontology; 36/52/90. Basel, Switzerland, S. Karger Publisher, September, 1990
* Houston KA: Clinics in Geriatric Medicine 1993;9(1):157-171
* Davila GW: Urinary incontinence in women: How to help patients regain bladder control. Postgrad Med 1994;96(2):103-109
* Fantl JA, et al: Estrogen therapy in the management of urinary incontinence in postmenopausal women; a meta-analysis. Obstet- Gynecol 1994;83:12-18
* Ramsey SD, et al: Estimated costs of treating stress urinary incontinence in elderly women according to the AHCPR Clinical Practice Guidelines. Am J Manag Care 1996;2(2):147-154
* Mold JW: Pharmacotherapy of urinary incontinence. Am Fam Phys 1996;54(2):673-680
* Ody P: The Complete Medicinal Herbal. New York, Darling Kindersley, 1993.
* Thom D: Variations in estimates of urinary incontinence in the community. Jour Am Ger Soc 1998;46:473-480
Illustrations: N/A
Internet references: http://www.5mcc.com

Author(s)
Jon A. Elias, MD

Urinary tract infection in females

BASICS

DESCRIPTION Inflammation of the bladder mucosa caused by bacterial infection. This topic refers primarily to infectious cystitis. Other urinary tract infections are discussed elsewhere.
System(s) affected: Renal/Urologic
Genetics: N/A
Incidence/Prevalence in USA: 3-8% of women have bacteriuria at any given time. 30% of females have at least one UTI; 7 million doctor visits a year
Predominant age: Young adults and older
Predominant sex: Female

SIGNS AND SYMPTOMS
Note: Any or all may be present
• Burning during urination
• Pain during urination
• Urgency (sensation of need to urinate frequently)
• Frequency
• Sensation of incomplete bladder emptying
• Blood in urine
• Lower abdominal pain or cramping
• Offensive odor of urine
• Nocturia

CAUSES Acute infection, usually with gram negative bacteria (E. coli in >90% of uncomplicated cystitis).

RISK FACTORS
• Previous urinary tract infection
• Diabetes mellitus
• Pregnancy
• More frequent or vigorous sexual activity than usual
• Use of spermicides or diaphragm
• Underlying abnormalities of the urinary tract such as tumors, calculi, strictures, incomplete bladder emptying, etc.

DIAGNOSIS

DIFFERENTIAL DIAGNOSIS
• Vaginitis
• Sexually transmitted diseases causing urethritis or pyuria
• Hematuria from causes other than infection (e.g., neoplasia, calculi)
• Psychological dysfunction

LABORATORY
• Urinalysis demonstrating pyuria (more than 10 neutrophils per high power field on microscopic exam). Leukocyte esterase dipsticks also useful for detecting pyuria but fail to detect pyuria in up to 20% of patients, and false positives occur from vaginal leukocytes.
• Urinalysis demonstrating bacteriuria (any amount on unspun urine, or 10 rod-shaped bacteria per high power field on centrifuged urine). Nitrite dipsticks also useful (and 94% specific), but fail to detect bacteriuria in 30-50% of patients. Nitrite dipsticks will be negative in patients who do not eat meat.
• Urine culture demonstrating growth of single species of bacteria. Suspect contaminated specimen when culture shows multiple types of bacteria.
Drugs that may alter lab results: N/A
Disorders that may alter lab results: N/A

PATHOLOGICAL FINDINGS N/A

SPECIAL TESTS N/A

IMAGING
• For all infants and may be indicated for older patients with recurrent infections:
  ◊ Radiographic, ultrasound, and/or endoscopic imaging of upper and lower urinary tract
  ◊ For infants and children, obtain ultrasound and if ureteral dilation detected, obtain either voiding cystourethrogram or isotope cystogram to detect reflux

DIAGNOSTIC PROCEDURES
• Suprapubic bladder aspiration or urethral catheterization to obtain urine specimen from infants
• Urethral catheterization to obtain urine specimen from children and adults if voided urine suspected of being contaminated
• Classic symptoms in non-pregnant young adult female with first episode of UTI require no urine culture for diagnosis. Obtain urinalysis and culture in other age groups, if repeat episode, if pregnant, or if symptoms not classic.
• Some recent research suggests the most cost-effective approach is empiric treatment without lab tests in non-pregnant premenopausal women with symptoms of UTI and no risks for complicated infection

TREATMENT

APPROPRIATE HEALTH CARE
Outpatient, except for complicated or upper tract infections

GENERAL MEASURES
• Maintain good hydration
• One-fourth of women with simple UTI experience a second UTI within six months, and half at some time during lifetime. Patients with multiple recurrent UTI and no underlying urinary tract abnormality may receive long-term prophylactic antibiotic treatment. Trimethoprim-sulfamethoxazole and nitrofurantoin commonly used.
• Patients with chronic indwelling urinary catheters always have infections that should not be treated unless symptomatic with fever, sepsis, or other systemic symptoms.
• Vaccinium macrocarpon (Cranberry Juice) may help prevent and treat UTIs by inhibiting bacterial adherence to bladder epithelium

SURGICAL MEASURES N/A

ACTIVITY Avoid sexual intercourse when symptoms present

DIET No special diet

PATIENT EDUCATION
• Take antibiotic as directed
• Return if symptoms not resolved or markedly improved within 48 hours
• Return if fever, chills, or flank pain develop
• If taking prophylactic antibiotics, take at bedtime

Urinary tract infection in females

MEDICATIONS

DRUG(S) OF CHOICE
• First, rare, or infrequent UTI in adolescents and adults who are non-pregnant, non-diabetic, afebrile, non-immunocompromised and have no abnormality of the urinary tract (i.e., uncomplicated)
◊ 3 day treatment with trimethoprim-sulfamethoxazole (TMP-SMX) or fluoroquinolone. Increasing resistance being reported to TMP-SMX. Use local sensitivity patterns to dictate first-choice antibiotic.
• Postcoital
◊ Single-dose TMP/SMX or cephalexin may reduce frequency of UTI in sexually active women
• Pregnant patients
◊ 10-14 day or longer treatment with pregnancy-safe antibiotic chosen based on culture/sensitivity results. May begin with cephalosporin, amoxicillin, or other antibiotic while awaiting culture/sensitivity results.
• All other patients
◊ 10-14 day treatment with antibiotic chosen based on culture/sensitivity results. May begin with fluoroquinolone, TMP/SMX, cephalosporin or other antibiotic while awaiting culture/sensitivity results.
Contraindications: Refer to manufacturer's literature. Fluoroquinolones not safe during pregnancy. TMP/SMX use in pregnancy not desirable, but appropriate is some circumstances.
Precautions: Refer to manufacturer's literature
Significant possible interactions: Refer to manufacturer's literature

ALTERNATIVE DRUGS   Change antibiotic if indicated by culture/sensitivity results

FOLLOWUP

PATIENT MONITORING
• First or rare UTI: In young or middle-age, non pregnant adult female requires no followup if patient cured after 3 day therapy. If not resolved within two to three days, obtain culture/sensitivity and change antibiotic accordingly.
• All other patients should have post-treatment urine culture to document eradication of infection

PREVENTION/AVOIDANCE
• Maintain good hydration
• Women with frequent or intercourse-related UTI should empty bladder immediately before and following intercourse and consider postcoital antibiotic treatment
• Take showers instead of tub baths
• Avoid feminine hygiene sprays and scented douches
• Wipe urethra from front to back

POSSIBLE COMPLICATIONS
• Pyelonephritis
• Renal abscess

EXPECTED COURSE/PROGNOSIS
Symptoms resolve within 2-3 days after starting treatment in almost all patients

MISCELLANEOUS

ASSOCIATED CONDITIONS   Described under Risk Factors

AGE-RELATED FACTORS
Pediatric: Infants and young children at higher risk of pyelonephritis
Geriatric:
• Elderly may have bacteriuria without symptoms; generally does not require treatment if urinary tract otherwise normal
• Elderly more apt to have underlying urinary tract abnormality
• Acute UTI often associated with incontinence in the elderly
Others: N/A

PREGNANCY   UTI during pregnancy always requires culture/sensitivity and usually requires 10-14 day treatment. Limited data suggest that single dose or three-day treatment may be effective in some women. Following treatment of acute infection, pregnant women often receive prophylactic antibiotics for the remainder of pregnancy.

SYNONYMS   Cystitis

ICD-9-CM
595 Cystitis
595.1 Acute cystitis
595.2 Chronic cystitis

SEE ALSO
• Pyelonephritis

OTHER NOTES   N/A

ABBREVIATIONS
TMP/SMX = trimethoprim-sulfamethoxazole

REFERENCES
• Barry HG, Ebell MH, Hickner J: Evaluation of suspected urinary tract infection in ambulatory women: a cost-utility analysis of office-based strategies. J of Fam Prac 1997;44:49-60
• Ebell MH, Barry NC: Urinary tract infection. In: Weiss BD, ed. 20 Common Problems in Primary Care. New York, McGraw-Hill, 1999
• Gupta K, Scholes D, Stamm WE. Increasing prevalence of antimicrobial resistance among uropathogens causing acute uncomplicated cystitis in women. JAMA 1999;281:736-738
• Stamm WE, Hooton T: Management of urinary tract infections in adults. New Eng J Med 1993;329:1328-1334
Illustrations: N/A
Internet references: http://www.5mcc.com

Author(s)
Barry D. Weiss, MD

Urinary tract infection in males

BASICS

DESCRIPTION Cystitis is an infection of the lower urinary tract, usually resulting from a single gram-negative enteric bacteria. (See separate chapters for information on prostatitis, pyelonephritis, and non-gonococcal urethritis.)
System(s) affected: Renal/Urologic
Genetics: No specific genetic pattern
Incidence/Prevalence in USA: Not common
Predominant age: Increases with age. Uncommon in men under 50. 8 infections/10,000 men, ages 21-50.
Predominant sex: Male only (for this discussion)

SIGNS AND SYMPTOMS
• Urinary frequency
• Urinary urgency
• Dysuria
• Hesitancy
• Slow urinary stream
• Dribbling of urine
• Nocturia
• Suprapubic discomfort
• Low back pain
• Hematuria
• Systemic symptoms (chills, fever) present with concomitant pyelonephritis or prostatitis

CAUSES
• Escherichia coli (80% of infections)
• Klebsiella
• Enterobacter
• Proteus
• Pseudomonas
• Serratia
• Streptococcus faecalis and Staphylococcus

RISK FACTORS
• Benign prostatic hypertrophy
• Cognitive impairment
• Fecal incontinence
• Urinary incontinence
• Anal intercourse
• Recent urologic surgery, catheterization
• Infection of the prostate or kidney
• Urinary tract instrumentation
• Immunocompromised host
• Outlet obstruction

DIAGNOSIS

DIFFERENTIAL DIAGNOSIS
• Anatomic or functional pathology
• Urethritis
• Infections in other sites of the genitourinary tract (e.g., epididymis)

LABORATORY
• Pyuria
• Bacteriuria
• Urine dipstick leukocyte esterase (75-90%, sensitivity, 95% specificity), and nitrate (35-85% sensitivity, 70% specificity)
• Urine culture - 10/high power colonies of pathogens (or counts > 100,000 bacteria/mL of urine) confirms diagnosis (Escherichia coli, Klebsiella, Pseudomonas, other agents). Lower counts can also be indicative of infection, especially in presence of pyuria.
• Segmented bacteriologic localization cultures
  ◊ VB1 - collect 5-10 mL of urine of patient's initial voiding
  ◊ VB2 - then a sample of sterile midstream urine is obtained
  ◊ EPS - prostatic massage performed, and expressed prostatic secretion is collected from the meatus
  ◊ VB3 - patient completes voiding and 4th sample is collected
  ◊ Cultures and sensitivity collected from each specimen
Drugs that may alter lab results:
Antibiotics prior to culture
Disorders that may alter lab results: N/A

PATHOLOGICAL FINDINGS Depends on site of infection

SPECIAL TESTS Urologic investigations necessary to rule out other disorders

IMAGING Intravenous pyelography, cystoscopy, ultrasound

DIAGNOSTIC PROCEDURES Careful history and physical

TREATMENT

APPROPRIATE HEALTH CARE
Outpatient, except for acute illness with toxicity or kidney failure

GENERAL MEASURES
• Hydration and analgesia if required
• Discontinue sexual activity until cured
• Patient with indwelling catheters
  ◊ If asymptomatic bacterial colonization - no need to treat (sterilization of urine not possible and resistant organisms can take up residence)
  ◊ If symptomatic of acute infection - institute treatment

SURGICAL MEASURES N/A

ACTIVITY Activity as tolerated.

DIET No special diet

PATIENT EDUCATION For patient education materials favorably reviewed on this topic, contact: National Kidney Foundation, 30 E. 33rd Street, Suite 1100, New York, NY 10016, (212)889-2210

MEDICATIONS

DRUG(S) OF CHOICE
• Acute UTI , first infection, no risk factors for treatment: 7-10 days of oral antibiotics either empirically or based on cultures and sensitivity results. For empiric therapy, trimethoprim-sulfamethoxazole (SMX-TMP) bid will usually treat the most likely pathogens.
• Complicated or recurrent UTI: 14-21 days of antibiotics based on antimicrobial sensitivities with repeat urine check after treatment
Contraindications: Refer to manufacturer's information
Precautions: Refer to manufacturer's information
Significant possible interactions: Refer to manufacturer's information

ALTERNATIVE DRUGS According to culture and sensitivity results and patient's history

FOLLOWUP

PATIENT MONITORING Close followup until clinically well and repeat urinalysis after treatment

PREVENTION/AVOIDANCE
• Prompt treatment of predisposing factors
• Catheter use only when necessary. If needed, use aseptic technique and closed system, with removal as soon as possible.

POSSIBLE COMPLICATIONS
• Pyelonephritis
• Ascending infection
• Recurrent infection

EXPECTED COURSE/PROGNOSIS
Clearing of infections with appropriate antibiotic treatment

MISCELLANEOUS

ASSOCIATED CONDITIONS
• Acute bacterial pyelonephritis
• Chronic bacterial pyelonephritis
• Urethritis
• Prostatitis
• Prostatic hypertrophy
• Prostate cancer

AGE-RELATED FACTORS
Pediatric: Usually associated with obstruction to normal flow of urine, such as vesicoureteral reflux
Geriatric: Bacteriuria is common in the elderly, appears related to functional status and is usually transient. If asymptomatic bacteriuria is noted, no treatment is needed.
Others: N/A

PREGNANCY N/A

SYNONYMS
• UTI
• Cystitis

ICD-9-CM
595 Cystitis
595.1 Acute cystitis
595.2 Chronic cystitis

SEE ALSO
• Prostatic cancer
• Prostatitis
• Prostatic hyperplasia, benign (BPH)
• Pyelonephritis
• Urethritis

OTHER NOTES N/A

ABBREVIATIONS N/A

REFERENCES
• Lipsky BA: Urinary tract infections in men. Epidemiology, pathophysiology, diagnosis, and treatment. Ann Intern Med 1989;110:138-150
• Finn SD: Urinary tract infections - diagnosis and treatment in women and men. Consultant 1992;10:43-58
• Hooton TM, Stamm WE: Management of acute uncomplicated urinary tract infection in adults. Med Clin of North Am 1991;75(2); 339-57
• Khan AJ, Schaffer HA, Evans H: Urinary tract infections in adolescent boys. J Nat Med A 1996;88(1):25-26
• Hutton J, Hughes M, Raymond CH: Management of bacterial urinary tract infections in adults. Ann Pharm 1994;28(11): 1264-1272
Illustrations: N/A
Internet references: http://www.5mcc.com

Author(s)
Scott A. Fields, MD

Urolithiasis

BASICS

DESCRIPTION The state describing the presence of calculi within the urinary system. Commonly known as kidney stones.
System(s) affected: Renal/Urologic
Genetics: Familial tendency
Incidence/Prevalence in USA: 70-210 in 100,000 population. 2%-5% of population in lifetime.
Predominant age: Peak 20-30. Range 20-60.
Predominant sex: Male > Female (4:1)

SIGNS AND SYMPTOMS
- Usually sudden onset
- Severe agonizing pain, costovertebral angle to groin depending on stone location
- Patient in constant motion, no comfort
- Nausea with or without vomiting
- Diaphoresis
- Tachycardia
- Intestinal ileus
- Abdominal guarding and rebound (rare)
- Tenderness to deep abdominal palpation, usually at CVA
- Lower tract stone with frequency, urgency, dysuria
- Fever, with infection
- Hematuria
- Pyuria, with infection
- May be asymptomatic if stone stays within kidney

CAUSES
- Calcium oxalate/calcium phosphate 65%-85%
  ◊ Supersaturation from any cause
  ◊ Dehydration
  ◊ Increased absorption
  ◊ Increased calcium excretion - familial
  ◊ Renal tubular acidosis
  ◊ Hyperparathyroidism
  ◊ Chronic bowel disease with absorptive disorders
  ◊ Poor GI citrate absorption
  ◊ Excessive oral vitamin D or C
  ◊ Alkaline urinary pH
  ◊ Chronic use of calcium antacids
  ◊ Diet high in calcium or oxalate
  ◊ Malignancy
  ◊ Hyperthyroidism
  ◊ Chronic steroid therapy
  ◊ Thiazide diuretics
- Struvite (staghorn calculus) 15%-20%
  ◊ Infection
  ◊ Alkaline urine
- Uric acid 5%
  ◊ Hereditary
  ◊ Gout
  ◊ Chronic bowel disease
  ◊ High purine diet
  ◊ Acidic urine, very low pH
  ◊ Malignancy with chemotherapy
- Cystine 1%-3%
  ◊ Hereditary homocystinuria

RISK FACTORS
- Family history
- Climate, hot
- Work in hot environment
- Poor fluid consumption
- Diet high in oxalate, purine, calcium
- Excessive vitamins
- Malignancy
- Sarcoidosis
- Gout
- Thiazide diuretics
- Bowel or kidney disease

DIAGNOSIS

DIFFERENTIAL DIAGNOSIS
- Pyelonephritis
- Clot or sloughed papillae (secondary to diabetes, infection, analgesic abuse)
- Drug-seeking addiction
- Acute abdomen
- Gynecological problems
- Diverticulitis

LABORATORY
- Urinalysis: Hematuria nearly 100%; if pH < 5.5 means uric acid, if pH > 7.5 means struvite
- Chemistries: Calcium, phosphorus, electrolytes, uric acid, creatinine, magnesium
- Parathyroid hormone: If serum calcium high
- Urine cystine: If stone not visible on plain x-ray
- Urine culture: If pyuria or fever
Drugs that may alter lab results: Pyridium may alter urinalysis
Disorders that may alter lab results: See Causes and Risk Factors

PATHOLOGICAL FINDINGS Stone analysis: 60-80% calcium base, 15-20% struvite, 5% uric acid, 1-3% cystine

SPECIAL TESTS Stone analysis

IMAGING
- Plain kidney, ureter and bladder (KUB) x-ray: 80%-90% visible with some calcium
- Intravenous pyelogram (IVP): Primary study for urolithiasis
- Ultrasound: Technique varies, if good has equal sensitivity and specificity to IVP

DIAGNOSTIC PROCEDURES
Retrograde pyelogram, if necessary for high grade obstruction or poor visualization on IVP

TREATMENT

APPROPRIATE HEALTH CARE
- 80% outpatient only, most pass in 48 hrs
- 20% hospitalization and urology referral
- Stone size and liklihood of passing spontaneously
  ◊ < 4 mm - 80%
  ◊ 4-6 mm - 59%
  ◊ > 6 mm - 21%

GENERAL MEASURES
- Reassurance
- Strain urine
- Hydration
- Pain control
- Refer to urologist for: Intractable pain, obstruction, size > 6 mm, infection, dehydration, failure to progress, stone growth, single kidney, persistent gross hematuria, pregnancy, severe renal disease
- Hospitalize for:
  ◊ Pain - intractable - parenteral medications
  ◊ Persistent vomiting
  ◊ High grade fever
  ◊ Obstruction with infection
  ◊ Solitary kidney with obstruction

SURGICAL MEASURES
- Extracorporeal shock wave lithotripsy: Stone in renal pelvis or upper 2/3 ureter, size < 2 cm, noninfected, no coagulopathy
- Urethroscopy: Lower 1/3 ureter, normal anatomy present. Newer graspers available for upper ureter.
- Percutaneous nephrolithotomy: Renal collecting system or upper 2/3 ureter, size > 2 cm, ureter stricture, cystine or uric acid stones, struvite, infection, obesity - may be used with intracorporeal lithotripsy
- Open surgery: Less than 5% of patients, complex anatomy, obstruction, large infected struvite stone
- Urethroscopy with lithotripsy available for lower 1/3 ureter
- Stenting for upper 1/3 or lower 1/3 ureter

ACTIVITY Bedrest, if necessary during acute phase. No restrictions after stone passes.

DIET
- Normal diet, 8 oz. water every 1 hour while awake, and if possible every 2 hours during sleep hours
- If uric acid stones, less protein in diet and take sodium bicarbonate to alkalinize urine

PATIENT EDUCATION
- Instructions on urine straining, dietary advice
- See Patient Care, August 15, 1990, p.42

MEDICATIONS

DRUG(S) OF CHOICE

• Acute therapy:
  ◊ Pain control (in office) - IM meperidine (Demerol) or morphine or buprenorphine (Buprenex), etc.
  ◊ 3 day supply pain control - oxycodone-acetaminophen (Percocet), pentazocine (Talwin), hydrocodone-acetaminophen (Vicodin), etc.
  ◊ Uric acid stone - potassium citrate (Urocit-K), 60-80 mEq/d (30-40 mmol/d) to keep urine pH 6.5-7.0. Check urine pH qid.
  ◊ Cystine stone - penicillamine (Cuprimine, Depen) 1-4 g/d, K-citrate (Urocit-K) 60 mEq/d (30 mmol/d)
  ◊ Infected stones - antibiotics for complicated pyelonephritis
• Maintenance therapy:
  ◊ Hypercalciuria - sodium cellulose phosphate 10-15 g/d (2.5-5.0 grams with each meal), hydrochlorothiazide (HCTZ) 50 mg bid, K-citrate 15-20 mEq (7.5-10 mmol) bid
  ◊ Uric acid - allopurinol (Zyloprim) 300 mg/d, K-citrate 20-30 mEq bid
  ◊ Cystine - K-citrate 30 mEq (15 mmol) bid, penicillamine 1-4 g/d

Contraindications:
• Penicillamine with pregnancy, renal failure, aplastic anemia, hypersensitivity reaction
• Avoid potassiumcitrate with renal insufficiency

Precautions: Penicillamine requires regular CBC with differential counts, urinalysis, liver function tests

Significant possible interactions: Refer to manufacturer's profile of each drug

ALTERNATIVE DRUGS Individualize to any underlying metabolic etiology found

FOLLOWUP

PATIENT MONITORING

• Acute urolithiasis:
  ◊ Strain urine until stone or 72 hours after symptoms cease
  ◊ Repeat urinalysis 2-3 days
  ◊ Repeat KUB x-ray and or IVP/ultrasound if no stone passed
  ◊ Stone analysis
  ◊ KUB x-ray at 3-6 months and at 1 year, if no new stone, then no further followup needed
• Recurrent urolithiasis:
  ◊ 24 hour urine: volume, pH, calcium, phosphorus, sodium, uric acid, oxalate, citrate, creatinine clearance
  ◊ Measure parathyroid hormone (PTH)
  ◊ Calcium restricted diet test for urine calcium level

PREVENTION/AVOIDANCE Hydration
with urine > 2 liters a day (including nocturia once nightly). Dietary calcium < 1 g/d.

POSSIBLE COMPLICATIONS

• Hydronephrosis or kidney damage
• Infection and sepsis

EXPECTED COURSE/PROGNOSIS

• 80% will pass in 48-72 hours with outpatient therapy
• Recurrence - 10% 1 year, 35% 5 years, 50% 10 years

MISCELLANEOUS

ASSOCIATED CONDITIONS See
Causes section

AGE-RELATED FACTORS
Pediatric: Homocystinuria or other hereditary disorder
Geriatric: N/A
Others: N/A

PREGNANCY Urology referral

SYNONYMS
• Nephrolithiasis
• Kidney stone
• Renal colic

ICD-9-CM
592.9 Urinary calculus, unspecified

SEE ALSO Renal calculi

OTHER NOTES N/A

ABBREVIATIONS
KUB = kidney, ureter and bladder
IVP = intravenous pyelogram
HCTZ = hydrochlorothiazide

REFERENCES
• Coe FL, Parks JH, Asplin JR: The pathogenis and treatment of kidney stones. New Eng J Med 1992;327(46):1141-1152
• Resnick MI, ed: The Urologic Clinics of North America: urolithiasis. Philadelphia, WB Saunders Co, 1997;2:1-185
• Rakel RE, ed: Conn's Current Therapy. Philadelphia, WB Saunders Co., 1997:727-732
Illustrations: N/A
Internet references: http://www.5mcc.com

Author(s)
William H. Billica, MD

Urticaria

BASICS

DESCRIPTION Itchy rash. Single or multiple superficial raised pale macules with red halo. Subside rapidly; no scars or change in pigmentation. May be recurrent.
- Acute urticaria
  ◊ Response to many stimuli
  ◊ IgE-mediated histamine release from mast cells
  ◊ Sometimes idiosyncratic response to drug exposure
  ◊ Subsides over several hours
- Chronic urticaria: Persists > 6 weeks (30% of cases). Not mediated by IgE. Multiple types:
  ◊ Cold urticaria - from cooling, rewarming. Can be fatal (cold immersion with massive histamine release). Also a familial form with fever, chills, arthralgia, myalgia, headache, lymphocytosis.
  ◊ Cholinergic urticaria - heat urticaria. Small (5-10 mm) wheals on upper trunk from overheating, hot shower
  ◊ Exercise-induced urticaria - from extreme exercise; presents as cholinergic urticaria, angioedema, wheezing, hypotension. Often associated with eating food to which patient is allergic.
  ◊ Dermatographism - linear wheal and flare resulting from scratching the skin
  ◊ Solar urticaria - result of exposure to sunlight. Several types, by wavelength of light which induces reaction. Majority react to ultraviolet. Onset in minutes; subsides in 1-2 hours.
  ◊ Delayed pressure urticaria - occurs 4-6 hours after pressure to skin (elastic, shoes, etc.)
  ◊ Aquagenic urticaria - rare. Small wheals after contact with water at any temperature.
- Idiopathic urticaria
  ◊ Acute or chronic

System(s) affected: Skin/Exocrine
Genetics: No consistent genetic pattern known
Incidence/Prevalence in USA: 1 in 1000. Affects 15-20% of population at some time during life.
Predominant age: All ages. Acute form mainly in children, young adults.
Predominant sex: Male = Female (chronic forms more often in older women)

SIGNS AND SYMPTOMS
- Seen alone or with angioedema
- May occur with generalized anaphylactic reaction, potentially fatal
- Single or multiple raised, blanched, central wheals surrounded by red flare
- Intensely pruritic
- May occur anywhere on body
- Variably sized, 1-2 mm to 15-20 cm or larger; sometimes confluent
- Rapid onset, resolves spontaneously in less than 48 hours

CAUSES
- Allergic or non-allergic; massive histamine release from mast cells in superficial dermis
- Drug reaction (any drug) either from allergy or idiosyncrasy
- Aspirin, NSAID's seem to trigger by inhibiting cyclo-oxygenase, without IgE
- Food or food additive allergy
- Allergy to peanuts and/or tree nuts a leading cause of severe (sometimes fatal) food-induced allergic reactions. Affects 1% of the general population. Other foods that cause hives are chocolate, fish, tomatoes, eggs, fresh berries, milk. Also food additives and preservatives.
- Inhalant, contact, or ingestant allergy
- Transfusion reaction
- Insect bite, sting
- Infection - viral upper respiratory infections (esp. in children) and infectious mononucleosis, viral hepatitis; bacterial (strep throat, sinusitis, dental abscess, otitis); vaginitis; fungal (tineas); helminthic; protozoan. Helicobacter pylori has been increasingly associated with, and its eradication may stop, chronic urticaria.
- Collagen vascular disease (cutaneous vasculitis, serum sickness, lupus)
- Thyroid autoimmunity often associated. Administering thyroid hormone may alleviate chronic urticaria in hypothyroid patients with autoantibodies.
- Physical trauma (heat, cold, sunlight, etc.)
- Emotional stress (reported; little supporting evidence)
- Histamine-releasing autoantibodies have been identified in some cases of chronic idiopathic urticaria

RISK FACTORS   Listed with Causes

DIAGNOSIS

DIFFERENTIAL DIAGNOSIS
- Insect bites
- Morbilliform drug eruptions
- Erythema multiforme
- Vasculitis and polyarteritis
- Systemic lupus erythematosus
- Urticaria pigmentosa (mastocytosis). Pink lesions urticate when scratched (Darier's sign).
- Bullous pemphigoid (urticarial stage)

LABORATORY
- More likely to discover the cause of acute than of chronic urticaria. Routine lab screening not helpful in diagnosing chronic urticaria.
- Cause found in only 10-25% of chronic cases
- Food and drug reactions - elimination diets, challenges with suspected agents
- Inhalant allergens - skin tests, radioallergosorbent (RAST)
- Idiopathic for > 6 weeks - CBC, skin biopsy, ESR, urinalysis, ANA
- 50% of patients with chronic urticaria have a cutaneous autoimmune disorder mediated by autoantibodies to the IgE receptor on mast cells.

Drugs that may alter lab results: Antihistamines, H2-blockers, tricyclic antidepressants
Disorders that may alter lab results: N/A

PATHOLOGICAL FINDINGS Edema, vasculitis and/or perivasculitis involving only superficial dermis

SPECIAL TESTS
- Cold urticaria - ice cube test (place ice cube on skin 5 minutes, observe 10-15 minutes)
- Cholinergic or exercise-induced: exercise challenge; methacholine skin test (local reaction to 0.01 mg in 0.05 ml saline intradermally. 50% false negatives).
- Dermatographism - scratch skin with piece of tongue blade, observe
- Solar - expose to defined wavelengths of light. Must rule out erythropoietic protoporphyria.
- Delayed pressure: apply 5-10 pound sandbag for 3 hours, observe
- Aquagenic - apply tap water at different temperatures
- Vibratory: apply vibration 4-5 minutes with a lab mixing device, observe
- Infection - pharyngeal culture, antistreptolysin (ASO) titer, rapid plasma reagin (RPR), parasitology, liver function tests, mononucleosis test
- Autoimmune - antinuclear antibody (ANA), rheumatoid arthritis (RA), complement, cryoglobulins, serum protein electrophoresis

IMAGING N/A

DIAGNOSTIC PROCEDURES Skin biopsy (correlates poorly with clinical picture)

TREATMENT

APPROPRIATE HEALTH CARE Don't work up acute cases (results usually inconclusive)

GENERAL MEASURES Cool moist compresses help to control itching

SURGICAL MEASURES N/A

ACTIVITY As desired. Avoid overheating.

DIET As desired. Avoid foods implicated as possible etiologic agents.

PATIENT EDUCATION Avoidance if etiology is apparent. Antihistamines if accidentally re-exposed.

Urticaria

MEDICATIONS

DRUG(S) OF CHOICE
• First generation antihistamines
  ◊ Older children and adults: hydroxyzine or diphenhydramine, 25-50 mg q6h
  ◊ Children under six: diphenhydramine 12.5 mg (elixir) q6-8h (5 mg/kg/day)
• Second generation H1 blockers are more expensive, about as effective as older antihistamines, but are less sedating (14% of patients, still less than 1st generation drugs), because they do not cross the blood-brain barrier.
  ◊ Fexofenadine (Allegra) 60 mg bid
  ◊ Loratadine (Claritin) 10 mg daily
  ◊ Acrivastine (Semprex) 8 mg tid
  ◊ Cetirizine (Zyrtec) 10 mg daily. More sedating than others in this class.
Contraindications: Danazol not for use in childhood, pregnancy.
Precautions:
• Drowsiness with first generation drugs
• Second generation H1 blockers should be used with caution in pregnancy and the elderly
Significant possible interactions: Refer to manufacturer's profile of each drug

ALTERNATIVE DRUGS
• Doxepin (Sinequan), tricyclic antidepressant with strong H1 and H2 blocking properties; very effective for urticaria (10 to 25 mg at bedtime).
• H2-blockers (cimetidine, ranitidine, etc.) may be helpful in chronic urticaria
• Corticosteroids for unresponsive cases (not acutely), e.g., prednisone 40 mg daily for 5-7 days, followed by taper as antihistamines are introduced.

FOLLOWUP

PATIENT MONITORING
No followup for initial episode. Evaluate if symptoms persist or recur.

PREVENTION/AVOIDANCE
If etiology identified, avoidance is best solution

POSSIBLE COMPLICATIONS
Severe systemic allergic reaction (bronchospasm, anaphylaxis)

EXPECTED COURSE/PROGNOSIS
70% better in < 72 hours. 30% chronic. 20% have attacks for > 20 years. Becomes chronic in 75% of patients with both urticaria and angioedema.

MISCELLANEOUS

ASSOCIATED CONDITIONS
Angioedema, anaphylaxis

AGE-RELATED FACTORS
Pediatric: Acute isolated incidents are more frequent, chronic urticaria is rare
Geriatric: Less likely to occur in this age group
Others: N/A

PREGNANCY
Chronic urticaria

SYNONYMS
Hives

ICD-9-CM
708.8 Other specified urticaria

SEE ALSO
• Anaphylaxis
• Angioedema

OTHER NOTES
Same pathophysiology for urticaria and angioedema - localized anaphylaxis causes vasodilatation, vascular permeability of skin (urticaria) or subcutaneous tissue (angioedema)

ABBREVIATIONS
N/A

REFERENCES
• Lockey RF, Bukantz SC: Principles of Immunology and Allergy. Philadelphia, W.B. Saunders Co., 1987
• Cooper KD: Urticaria and angioedema: Diagnosis and evaluation. J Am Acad Dermatol 1991;25(1):166
• Monroe EW: Nonsedating H1 antihistamines in chronic urticaria. Ann Allergy 1993;71:585-91
• Woosley R, Darrow WR: Analysis of potential adverse drug reactions - a case of mistaken identity. Amer J Cardiol 1994;74:208-209
• Heymann WR: Chronic urticaria and angioedema associated with thyroid autoimmunity; review and therapeutic implications. J Am Acad Dermatol 1999;40(2pt1):229-232
• Kozel MM, et al: The effectiveness of a history-based diagnostic approach in chronic urticaria and angioedema. Arch Dermatol 1998;134(12):1575-80
• Kumar SA, Martin BL: Urticaria and angioedema: diagnostic and treatment considerations. J Am Osteopath Assoc 1999;99(3suppl):s1-4
• Mortureux P, et al: Acute urticaria in infancy and early childhood: a prospective study. Arch Dermatol 1998;134(3):319-23
• Sabroe RA, et al: Chronic idiopathic urticaria: comparison of the clinical features of patients with and without anti-FcepsilonRI or anti-IgE autoantibodies. J Am Acad Dermatol 1999;40(3):443-50
• Sicherer SH, et al: Clinical features of acute allergic reactions to peanut and tree nuts in children. Pediatrics 1998;102(1):e6
• Wedi B, et al: Prevalence of helicobacter pylori-associated gastritis in chronic urticaria. Int Arch Allergy Immunol 1998;116(4):288-94
Illustrations: 8 available on CD-ROM
Internet references: http://www.5mcc.com

Author(s)
John E. Perchalski, MD, FAAFP

Uterine corpus malignancy

BASICS

DESCRIPTION
• Endometrial cancer: Malignancy of the endometrial lining of the uterus. Tumor grade - low, moderate, high. Cell types - adenocarcinoma, adenosquamous (benign or malignant squamous elements), clear cell, papillary serous.
• Sarcomas:
◊ Mixed müllerian sarcoma - heterologous elements not native to the müllerian systems, such as cartilage or bone; homologous elements native to the mullerian system
◊ Endometrial stromal sarcoma develops from the stromal component of the endometrium
◊ Leiomyosarcoma develops in the myometrium or in a myoma (fibroid)
System(s) affected: Reproductive
Genetics: Unknown
Incidence/Prevalence in USA: Most common gynecologic malignancy, 35,000 new cases per year
Predominant age:
• Endometrial cancer - postmenopausal (mid fifties to mid sixties). Also can occur in young women in their twenties and thirties with polycystic ovarian disease or chronic anovulation.
• Sarcomas - forties to sixties
Predominant sex: Female only

SIGNS AND SYMPTOMS
• Endometrial cancer:
◊ Postmenopausal bleeding is the most frequent sign. Any spotting should lead to evaluation.
◊ Pap smear is rarely positive
◊ Occasionally a patient will pass tissue that will render a diagnosis
• Sarcoma:
◊ Mixed müllerian sarcoma - bleeding and prolapsing tissue
◊ Leiomyosarcoma - increasing size of presumed uterine myomas
◊ D&C rarely diagnostic

CAUSES
• Unopposed estrogen due to:
◊ Polycystic ovarian disease
◊ Obesity
◊ Chronic anovulation
◊ Estrogen replacement therapy. (Estrogen replacement without concomitant progesterone increases the risk 70 times. When progesterone is added the risk does not decrease to zero but decreases to that of the population in general).
• Tamoxifen. Increases risk similar to that for unopposed estrogen.
• Sarcomas:
◊ Etiology unknown

RISK FACTORS
• Early menarche
• Late menopause
• Nulliparity
• Hypertension and diabetes are probably associated with underlying obesity

DIAGNOSIS

DIFFERENTIAL DIAGNOSIS
• Atypical complex hyperplasia (a premalignant lesion of the endometrium)
• Bleeding from cervical cancer
• Ovarian cancer invading the uterus
• Adenocarcinoma of the cervix
• Endometriosis

LABORATORY
• Liver function tests
• CA-125 can be elevated when intra-abdominal disease is present
Drugs that may alter lab results: N/A
Disorders that may alter lab results: A biopsy of a pregnant uterus can produce tissue which has a hyperplastic or premalignant appearance

PATHOLOGICAL FINDINGS
• Stage I
◊ A. Confined to endometrium
◊ B. Less than 50% myometrial invasion
◊ C. More than 50% myometrial invasion
• Stage II
◊ A. Endocervical involvement (microscopic)
◊ B. Cervical stromal invasion (macroscopic)
• Stage III
◊ A. Uterine serosal/adnexal involvement/positive peritoneal cytology
◊ B. Vaginal metastases
◊ C. Involved pelvic/para aortic lymph nodes
• Stage IV
◊ A. Extension to involve the mucosa of the bladder or rectum
◊ B. Distant metastatic disease or inguinal node involvement
• Stages are also subgrouped according to histologic grade:
◊ GI - Well differentiated
◊ G2 - Moderately differentiated
◊ G3 - Poorly differentiated

SPECIAL TESTS
Any that may be indicated preoperatively

IMAGING
• Chest x-ray - the most common site of metastases is the lungs. Rarely does this malignancy go to the bone or the liver except in advanced disease.
• CT scan, bone scan, liver spleen scan - not part of the routine evaluation, but may be needed occasionally
• Mammogram (endometrial cancer is associated with breast cancer)
• Barium enema (endometrial cancer is associated with colon cancer)
• MRI has been reported to accurately show the depth of myometrial penetration, but this is not always cost-effective
• Vaginal ultrasound can show increased endometrial echoes prior to D & C which will lead to the diagnosis

DIAGNOSTIC PROCEDURES
• Office endometrial biopsy (90% accurate). If this is negative, a D & C is necessary. Endometrial stromal sarcoma and leiomyosarcoma are rarely diagnosed preoperatively.
• D & C (99% accurate)

TREATMENT

APPROPRIATE HEALTH CARE
Inpatient surgery

GENERAL MEASURES
• Radiation is used to prevent the recurrence of tumor at the vaginal cuff
• When distant metastatic disease occurs, progesterone produces a 30% response rate. Active chemotherapeutic agents are cisplatin and Adriamycin.

SURGICAL MEASURES
• Surgical procedure is abdominal exploration with extrafascial total abdominal hysterectomy, bilateral salpingo-oophorectomy, cytology, pelvic and para-aortic node sampling
• Surgery is followed by radiation therapy in high-risk patients who have Stage 1B disease or greater, or for patients with poorly differentiated tumors regardless of stage. There is no adjuvant therapy that has been shown to be effective after surgery and radiation.

ACTIVITY
Patients are usually ambulatory and able to resume full activity by six weeks after surgery

DIET
Unrestricted unless they are undergoing radiation

PATIENT EDUCATION
• The American Cancer Society in the local community
• American College of Obstetricians & Gynecologists (ACOG), 409 12th St., SW, Washington, DC 20024-2188, (800)762-ACOG

MEDICATIONS

DRUG(S) OF CHOICE
• There are no drugs as adjuvant therapy
• Premalignant lesions in young women or in patients unsuitable for hysterectomy can be treated with megestrol (Megace), 160 mg qd x 3 months. This is followed by repeat D & C to ascertain whether the hyperplasia has resolved.
• Metastatic disease is treated with high dose progesterone, or doxorubicin (Adriamycin) or cisplatin

Contraindications:
• Progestational agents can cause significant fluid retention in 5-10% of patients
• Patients with congestive heart failure must be observed closely

Precautions: Usual precautions with chemotherapeutic agents. Refer to manufacturer's profile of each drug.

Significant possible interactions: Refer to manufacturer's profile of each drug

ALTERNATIVE DRUGS
• Ondansetron (Zofran), dronabinol (Marinol), metoclopramide (Reglan), and others for nausea control

FOLLOWUP

PATIENT MONITORING
• Pap smear every 3 months for two years, then every 6 months for 3 years
• Chest x-ray once a year

PREVENTION/AVOIDANCE
• In young women who are obese or anovulatory, endometrial cancer can be reduced by cyclic progesterone to prevent unopposed estrogen or by taking birth control pills
• Estrogen replacement therapy should always include progestational agents unless the woman has undergone hysterectomy

POSSIBLE COMPLICATIONS Those attendant upon major abdominal surgery

EXPECTED COURSE/PROGNOSIS
Five year survival is based on stage and tumor grade

```
Grade      5 yr survival (%)
-----------------------------
IAG1        98
IBG2        85
ICG3        60
IIA/B       60
III         40
IV          15
-----------------------------
```

MISCELLANEOUS

ASSOCIATED CONDITIONS
• Obese patients with endometrial cancer should be screened annually because of increased risk of breast and colon cancer
• Patients who have breast or colon cancer are at increased risk for endometrial cancer. Granulosa cell tumors of the ovary produce estrogen and these patients will have an increased risk of endometrial cancer.

AGE-RELATED FACTORS
Pediatric: N/A
Geriatric: Older (especially obese) patients may be at high risk for surgery. Alternative radiation therapy can be considered.
Others: If preserving fertility is desired - young anovulatory women, polycystic ovarian patients with atypical complex hyperplasia, or patients with well differentiated endometrial cancer can be treated with progestational agents x 3 months followed by D&C

PREGNANCY This malignancy is not associated with pregnancy

SYNONYMS
• Uterine cancer
• Endometrial cancer
• Corpus cancer

ICD-9-CM
182.0 Malignant neoplasm of body of uterus, corpus uteri, except isthmus
182.8 Malignant neoplasm of body of uterus, other specified sites of body of uterus
182.1 Malignant neoplasm of body of uterus, isthmus
180.0 Malignant neoplasm of body of cervix uteri, endocervix

SEE ALSO
Cervical malignancy

OTHER NOTES N/A

ABBREVIATIONS N/A

REFERENCES Hopkins MP: Benign and Malignant Diseases of the Uterus. In: Willson JR, ed. Obstetrics and Gynecology. St. Louis, Mosby Year Book, 1991
Illustrations: N/A
Internet references: http://www.5mcc.com

Author(s)
Michael P. Hopkins, MD
Eric L. Jenison, MD

Uterine myomas

BASICS

DESCRIPTION Uterine leiomyomas are well circumscribed, pseudo-encapsulated benign tumors composed mainly of smooth muscle but with varying amounts of fibrous connective tissue
• Three major types:
  ◊ Submucous: 5% of total, susceptible to abnormal uterine bleeding, infection and occasionally protrude from cervix
  ◊ Subserous: Common, may become pedunculated and rarely parasitic
  ◊ Intramural: Common, may cause marked uterine enlargement
System(s) affected: Reproductive
Genetics: N/A
Incidence/Prevalence in USA: 4-11% of all women, 20% of all women over 35 years of age and 40% of women over 50 years of age
Predominant age: Fourth and fifth decades
Predominant sex: Female only

SIGNS AND SYMPTOMS
• Majority are asymptomatic and are only suspected from pelvic examination
• Most common symptom is abnormal uterine bleeding. Hypermenorrhea most common. Secondary anemia with associated symptomatology may result.
• Pressure on bladder may result in suprapubic discomfort, urinary frequency
• Pressure on rectosigmoid may result in low back pain
• Edema and varicosities of the lower extremities may result from large tumors
• Pain may result from twisted, pedunculated myomas or degenerating, hemorrhagic or infected myomas
• Sterility may result from submucous myomas or with distortion of uterine cavity
• Rapid growth particularly in perimenopausal or postmenopausal may indicate sarcoma

CAUSES
• May arise from totipotential cells normally giving rise to muscle and connective tissue cells
• May arise from small immature smooth muscle cell nests
• Positive correlation with estrogen stimulation, i.e., not seen before menarche, may grow rapidly during pregnancy, with use of oral estrogen, and with estrogen producing tumors. Myomas regress following pregnancy and after menopause.

RISK FACTORS
• Later reproductive and perimenopausal age groups
• 3-9 times higher among African-Americans

DIAGNOSIS

DIFFERENTIAL DIAGNOSIS
• Intrauterine pregnancy
• Ovarian tumor
• Cecal or sigmoid tumor
• Appendiceal abscess
• Diverticulitis
• Pelvic kidney
• Urachal cyst

LABORATORY
• Pregnancy test
• CBC, differential count
• SED rate
• CA-125 - may be slightly elevated in some cases of uterine myomas, but generally is more useful in differentiating myomas from various gynecologic adenocarcinomas
Drugs that may alter lab results: N/A
Disorders that may alter lab results: N/A

PATHOLOGICAL FINDINGS
• Myomas are usually multiple and vary in size and location. Have been reported up to 100 pounds (45 kg).
• Gross pathology reveals firm tumors with characteristic whorl-like trabeculated appearance. A thin psuedocapsular layer is present.
• Microscopic appearance reveals bundles of smooth muscle mixed with varying amounts of connective tissue elements running in different directions
• Cellular variant has a preponderance of muscle cells. Mitoses are rare.
• May undergo various types of degeneration:
  ◊ I - Hyaline degeneration. Very common, eventually results in liquefaction and cyst formation.
  ◊ II - Calcification. Late result of circulatory impairment to myomas.
  ◊ III - Infection and suppuration. Submucous myomas most prone to infection and may lead to sepsis.
  ◊ IV - Necrosis. Pedunculated subserous fibroids most prone to necrosis secondary to torsion.
  ◊ V - Sarcomatous change. Incidence ranges from 1.0 to 0.1% of clinically apparent myomas.

SPECIAL TESTS   N/A

IMAGING
• Ultrasonography shows characteristic hypoechoic appearance
• Saline infusion hystersonography may help to distinguish submucous myomas
• CT scan, MRI may help to differentiate complex cases
• Intravenous pyelogram (IVP)
• Barium enema

DIAGNOSTIC PROCEDURES
• Presumptive diagnosis by abdominal and pelvic examination: Firm, smooth nodules or masses arising from uterus. Masses are mobile without pain.
• Fractional D & C aids in ruling out cervical, uterine carcinomas
• Hysteroscopy may help diagnose submucous myomas
• Laparoscopy may be useful in complex cases and in ruling out other pelvic pathology

TREATMENT

APPROPRIATE HEALTH CARE
Outpatient usually; inpatient for some surgical procedures

GENERAL MEASURES
• Treatment must be individualized
• Patients with minimal symptoms may be managed with iron preparations and analgesics
• Conservative management: Asymptomatic myomas of less than 14 weeks' size gestation should be closely observed with pelvic examinations and ultrasonography at 3-6 month intervals, as long as size stable. Usually regress after menopause.
• Nonsurgical therapies
  ◊ Luteinizing hormone releasing hormone (LHRH) agonists induce an abrupt artificial menopause with cessation of bleeding and shrinkage of myomas. Not recommended for more than six months. May be useful in perimenopausal patients or as an adjunct in preparation for surgery.
  ◊ Myolysis by needle cautery or cryotherapy. Long term outcome is unknown
  ◊ Uterine artery embolization average 50% shrinkage; painful

SURGICAL MEASURES
• Surgical management is indicated in the following situations:
  ◊ Excessive uterine size (> 14 weeks gestation) or excessive rate of growth (except during pregnancy)
  ◊ Submucous location if associated with hypermenorrhea
  ◊ Pedunculated myomas may undergo torsion, pain, necrosis and hemorrhage
  ◊ Symptomatic from pressure on bladder or rectum
  ◊ If differentiation from ovarian mass is not possible
  ◊ If there is associated pelvic disease, i.e., endometriosis, pelvic inflammatory disease, etc.
  ◊ If infertility or habitual abortion is likely due to the anatomic location of the myoma
• Surgical procedures:
  ◊ Hysteroscopic or laparoscopic cautery or laser myoma resection can be performed in selected cases
  ◊ Myomectomies may be performed in younger women desiring to maintain fertility
  ◊ Hysterectomy, either vaginal or abdominal, is procedure of choice for symptomatic women no longer desiring fertility
  ◊ Preliminary Pap smear and endometrial sampling or D & C must be performed to rule out malignant or premalignant conditions

ACTIVITY
• Following hysteroscopic or laparoscopic myoma resection, bedrest 24 hours, no sexual intercourse for two weeks
• Following laparotomy for myomectomy or hysterectomy, 3-5 days hospital, followed by limited activity and no sexual intercourse for one month

DIET No restrictions

PATIENT EDUCATION ACOG (American College of Obstetricians and Gynecologists) pamphlet entitled "Uterine Fibroids," ACOG p-074

MEDICATIONS

DRUG(S) OF CHOICE
• Luteinizing hormone releasing hormone (LHRH) agonists such as nafarelin (Synarel Nasal Spray), goserelin (Zoladex Depot), leuprolide (Lupron Depot)
  ◊ Induce abrupt, artificial menopause and render patients asymptomatic
  ◊ Induce atrophy of myomas by 40-60% within 2-3 months
  ◊ May be valuable as a preoperative adjunct to myomectomy or hysterectomy by allowing recovery of anemia, donation of autologous blood and possibly converting abdominal to vaginal hysterectomy, thereby decreasing postoperative pain, hospitalization, and morbidity. Generally used two to three months prior to surgery.
  ◊ Not recommended for use longer than six months
  ◊ Following discontinuation, myomas return within 60 days to pretherapy size
• Patients with minimal symptoms
  ◊ May be managed conservatively with iron preparations and analgesics
  ◊ Progestins such as norethindrone, 10 mg daily, or medroxyprogesterone (Depo-Provera) 200 mg IM, once monthly, may reduce the amount of blood flow. They do not reduce myoma size.
Contraindications:
• Progestins - history of thromboembolic phenomenon
• LHRH agonists - history of osteoporosis
Precautions: LHRH agonists induce acute menopausal symptoms: hot flashes, night sweats, insomnia, emotional lability, and osteoporosis
Significant possible interactions: Refer to manufacturer's profile of each drug

ALTERNATIVE DRUGS N/A

FOLLOWUP

PATIENT MONITORING
• Newly diagnosed uterine myoma, if symptomatic or excessive size, 2-3 months with pelvic exam and ultrasonography
• Consider CA-125 antigen
• Monitor hemoglobin and hematocrit, if uterine bleeding excessive
• If uterine size and symptoms stable, monitor every 6 months

PREVENTION/AVOIDANCE
Excessive growth during estrogen stimulation, i.e., birth control pills, postmenopausal estrogen replacement therapy and pregnancy

POSSIBLE COMPLICATIONS
• Complications during pregnancy include abortion; premature labor; second trimester rapid myoma growth leading to degeneration and pain; third-trimester fetal dystocia during labor and delivery
• Previous myomectomy patients in labor may develop uterine rupture. C-section is recommended if entered endometrial cavity during myomectomy.
• May mask other gynecologic malignancies, i.e., uterine sarcoma, ovarian cancer

EXPECTED COURSE/PROGNOSIS
• Following myomectomy, 40% pregnancy rate in patients previously infertile
• At least 10% myomas recur following myomectomy

MISCELLANEOUS

ASSOCIATED CONDITIONS
Endometrial carcinoma also associated with high unopposed estrogen stimulation

AGE-RELATED FACTORS
Pediatric: N/A
Geriatric: In postmenopausal patients with newly diagnosed uterine myoma or enlarging uterine myomas, highly suspect uterine sarcoma or other gynecologic malignancy
Others:
• Not seen in premenarchal females
• Incidence increases with each decade during reproductive years and is highest in perimenopausal age group

PREGNANCY See associations above

SYNONYMS
• Fibroids
• Myoma
• Fibromyoma
• Myofibroma
• Fibroleiomyoma

ICD-9-CM 218 (4th digit 0-9) Submucous leiomyoma of uterus

SEE ALSO N/A

OTHER NOTES N/A

ABBREVIATIONS N/A

REFERENCES
• Zacur HA, Murray AA, Tulandi T, Verkauf BS: Myomas: advances in diagnosis and treatment. Contem OB/Gyn 1999;44(2):84-108
• Cunningham FG, MacDonald PC, Gant NF, eds: Williams' Obstetrics. 20th Ed. Norwalk, CT, Appleton and Lange, 1997
• Ryan KJ, Berkowitz R, Barbieri RL: Kistners' Gynecology: Principles & Practice. 6th Ed. Chicago, Year Book Publishers, 1995
• Jones HW III, Wentz AC, Burnett LS: Novak's Textbook of Gynecology. 12th Ed. Baltimore, Williams and Wilkins, 1996
• ACOG (American College of Obstetricians and Gynecologists) pamphlet entitled "Uterine Fibroids," ACOG p-074
• Rock JA, Thompson JD: Leiomyomata uteri and myomectomy. In: Thompson JD, Rock JA (eds): Telinde's Operative Gynecology. 8th ed. Philadelphia, Lippincott-Raven, 1997
• Verkauf BS: Myomectomy as a fertility-promoting procedure. Infertil & Reprod Med Clin NA 1996;1:69-89
• Goodwin SC, Vedantham S, McLucas B, et al: Preliminary experience with uterine artery embolization for uterine fibroids. J Vasc Interv Radiol 1997;8:517-526
Illustrations: N/A
Internet references: http://www.5mcc.com

Author(s)
Eric L. Jenison, MD
Michael P. Hopkins, MD

Uterine prolapse

BASICS

DESCRIPTION Uterine prolapse occurs when the integrity of supporting structures is lost. This allows the uterus to descend into the vagina. In advanced cases, complete protrusion with inversion of the vagina occurs.
• Prior to menopause, the degree and severity of prolapse is usually related to the number of children and the difficulty of childbirth. After menopause, atrophy and loss of tissue integrity further leads to prolapse.
System(s) affected: Reproductive, Renal/Urologic, Renal/Urologic, Gastrointestinal
Genetics:
• Common among Caucasian races
• Less common among Orientals and African Americans and particularly uncommon in South African Bantus and West Africans
Incidence/Prevalence in USA:
Approximately 1 in 10 women will experience some degree of prolapse
Predominant age: Peri- and postmenopausal female
Predominant sex: Female only

SIGNS AND SYMPTOMS
• Pelvic pressure and low back pain
• As prolapse progresses, eventually a bulging is noticed as a result of protrusion
• Dyspareunia
• Difficulty with urination or defecation

CAUSES
• Advancing age and vaginal childbirth are the most important factors
• The incidence of prolapse increases with the frequency and difficulty of vaginal deliveries. Less than 2% of prolapse occurs in nulliparous women.
• Other causes of prolapse include connective tissue disorders with lax tissue, i.e., Marfan's syndrome and neurogenic disorders, i.e., multiple sclerosis, cloacal agenesis, chronic constipation, pelvic tumors or ascites and chronic coughing from chronic lung disease
• Patients who have undergone radical vulvectomy with loss of the external supporting structures have a higher rate of prolapse

RISK FACTORS
• Childbirth, particularly multiple parity
• Advancing age
• Caucasian race
• Various connective tissue and neurogenic disorders
• Conditions resulting in increased intra-abdominal pressure, such as obesity, abdominal or pelvic tumors, pulmonary disease with chronic coughing, chronic constipation
• Occupations requiring heavy lifting

DIAGNOSIS

DIFFERENTIAL DIAGNOSIS Diagnosis is by physical and pelvic examination. With coughing and straining, the cervix will prolapse toward introitus or beyond. The patient may need to be examined in the standing as well as lying position for diagnosis. Herniations of the bladder (cystocele or urethrocele), rectum (rectocele) and small bowel (enterocele) are associated conditions that may be simultaneously diagnosed.

LABORATORY
• Evaluation of renal function to rule out ureteral obstruction
• Urinalysis to rule out urinary tract infection
Drugs that may alter lab results: N/A
Disorders that may alter lab results: N/A

PATHOLOGICAL FINDINGS
• Hyperkeratosis of the cervical and vaginal tissues occur with prolapse beyond the introitus due to chronic irritation and drying. As the irritation becomes more pronounced, bleeding and ulceration occur.
• Degrees of prolapse:
  ◊ First degree prolapse - to the ischial spine
  ◊ Second degree prolapse - to the introitus
  ◊ Third degree prolapse - just beyond the introitus
  ◊ Fourth degree prolapse - complete uterine and vaginal inversion involving bladder and bowel

SPECIAL TESTS   N/A

IMAGING
• Intravenous pyelogram to rule out ureteral obstruction in complete uterine prolapse (optional)
• Pelvic ultrasound or CT scan to rule out other pelvic pathology, if suspected (optional)

DIAGNOSTIC PROCEDURES
• If ulceration or bleeding is present, Pap smears and appropriate cervical and endometrial biopsies should be done to rule out concomitant malignancies

TREATMENT

APPROPRIATE HEALTH CARE
• Outpatient
• Inpatient when surgery is necessary

GENERAL MEASURES
• Treatment depends on multiple variables including the severity of prolapse, age, sexual activity, associated pelvic pathology and desire for future fertility
• Treatment of first and second degree prolapse is expectant unless patient is symptomatic
• Mildly symptomatic patients and poor surgical candidates - can be treated nonoperatively with perineal (Kegel) exercises, estrogen replacement and vaginal pessaries. Estrogen replacement restores healthy vaginal mucosa and promotes healing.

SURGICAL MEASURES
• Surgically able patients without additional pelvic pathology - vaginal hysterectomy with or without enterocele, cystocele, rectocele repair and vaginal vault suspension
• For patients who desire to maintain reproductive function - uterine suspension with vaginal reapir is an option
• Elderly, non-sexually active women - can be treated with a colpocleisis or vaginal obliteration procedure

ACTIVITY Heavy lifting or significant increases in intra-abdominal pressure will lead to worsening of prolapse or recurrence after surgical correction. Lifting should therefore be restricted.

DIET Unlimited. Avoid constipation.

PATIENT EDUCATION
• Kegel exercises when applicable
• American College of Obstetricians & Gynecologists (ACOG), 409 12th St., SW, Washington, DC 20024-2188, (800)762-ACOG

MEDICATIONS

DRUG(S) OF CHOICE Estrogen replacement therapy (oral or vaginal cream) can increase the blood supply to the vaginal tissues and in mild cases increase supporting tissue strength to a point where surgery or pessary use may be avoided
Contraindications: Those associated with the use of estrogen. Refer to manufacturer's literature.
Precautions: If estrogen therapy is utilized and the uterus is present, progesterone should be utilized to offset the potential of endometrial carcinoma
Significant possible interactions: Refer to manufacturer's literature

ALTERNATIVE DRUGS None

FOLLOWUP

PATIENT MONITORING
• Expectant management is appropriate with periodic follow-up examinations
• If a pessary is placed, it should be removed, cleaned and replaced each month or more often

PREVENTION/AVOIDANCE
• Kegel exercises will increase the strength of the pelvic diaphragm muscles and may provide some pelvic support
• Weight loss and proper management of conditions that would increase abdominal pressure help to prevent prolapse

POSSIBLE COMPLICATIONS
• Ureteral obstruction and renal failure
• Incarceration of bowel herniations
• Pessary use - may not always be effective, and may cause discomfort, ulcers, infection

EXPECTED COURSE/PROGNOSIS
• It is expected that as patients age, the incidence and severity of prolapse will increase
• Surgical correction usually successful

MISCELLANEOUS

ASSOCIATED CONDITIONS Cystocele, rectocele, enterocele and vaginal vault prolapse are often associated with uterine prolapse

AGE-RELATED FACTORS
Pediatric: Prolapse in newborn has been reported, but is rare and usually associated with congenital disorders and neuropathies
Geriatric: This is largely a disease of aging and will be much higher as the population ages
Others: N/A

PREGNANCY This disorder in large part results from vaginal childbirth and the distention and distortion of supporting tissues with childbirth

SYNONYMS
• Uterine prolapse
• Genital prolapse
• Genital relaxation
• Uterine descensus
• Total or partial procidentia
• Dropped uterus

ICD-9-CM 618. Genital prolapse (fourth digits 1-9)

SEE ALSO N/A

OTHER NOTES N/A

ABBREVIATIONS N/A

REFERENCES
• Nichols DH, Randall CL: Vaginal Surgery. 4th Ed. Baltimore, Williams & Wilkins, 1996
• Ryan KJ, Berkowitz R, Barbieri RL: Kistner's Gynecology: Principles and Practice. 6th Ed. Chicago, Year Book Medical Publishers, Inc., 1995
• American College of Obstetricians & Gynecologists (ACOG), 409 12th St., SW, Washington, DC 20024-2188, (800)762-ACOG
• Nichols DH: Gynecologic and Obstetric Surgery. 1st ed. St Louis, MO, CV Mosby, 1993
• Thompson JD, Rock JA: Telinde's Operative Gynecology. 8th ed. Philadelphia, Lippincott-raven, 1997
• Mishell DR, Stenchever MA, et al: Comprehensive Gynecology. 3rd ed. St Louis, CV Mosby, 1997
• Mann WJ, Stovall TG: Gynecologic Surgery. 1st ed. New York, Churchill Livingstone, 1996
Illustrations: N/A
Internet references: http://www.5mcc.com

Author(s)
Eric L. Jenison, MD
Michael P. Hopkins, MD

Uveitis

BASICS

DESCRIPTION Uveitis is a nonspecific term used to describe any intraocular inflammatory disorder. Symptoms vary depending on depth of involvement and associated conditions.
• Anterior uveitis - refers to ocular inflammation limited to the iris (iritis) alone or iris and ciliary body (iridocyclitis)
• Intermediate uveitis - refers to inflammation of the structures just posterior to the lens (pars planitis or peripheral uveitis)
• Posterior uveitis - refers to inflammation of the choroid (choroiditis), retina (retinitis), or vitreous near the optic nerve and macula
System(s) affected: Nervous
Genetics: No specific pattern for uveitis in general; iritis: 50-70% of patients are HLA-B27 positive
Incidence/Prevalence in USA:
• Anterior uveitis most common (8.2 cases/100,000 annual incidence)
• Iritis is 4 times more prevalent than posterior uveitis
Predominant age: All ages
Predominant sex: Male = Female (except for HLA-B27 anterior uveitis male > female (2.5:1))

SIGNS AND SYMPTOMS
• Anterior uveitis (approximately 80% of patients with uveitis)
  ◊ Decreased visual acuity
  ◊ Generally acute in onset
  ◊ Deep eye pain
  ◊ Photophobia (consensual)
  ◊ Conjunctival vessel dilation
  ◊ Perilimbal (circumcorneal) dilation of episcleral and scleral vessels (ciliary flush)
  ◊ Small pupillary size of affected eye
  ◊ Frequently unilateral (95% of HLA-B27 associated cases)
  ◊ Bilateral involvement and systemic symptoms (fever, fatigue, abdominal pain) may be associated with interstitial nephritis
  ◊ Systemic disease is most likely to be associated with anterior uveitis (53% of patients found to have systemic disease in one study)
• Intermediate and posterior uveitis
  ◊ Decreased visual acuity
  ◊ Generally insidious in onset
  ◊ More commonly bilateral
  ◊ Posterior inflammation will generally cause minimal pain or redness unless associated with an iritis

CAUSES
• Infectious - may result from viral, bacterial, parasitic, or fungal etiologies
• Suspected immune-mediated - possible autoimmune or immune-complex mediated mechanism postulated in association with systemic (especially rheumatologic) disorders
• Isolated eye disease
• Idiopathic (approximately 25%)
• Masquerade syndromes - diseases such as malignancies that may be mistaken for inflammation of the eye

RISK FACTORS No specific risk factors. Higher incidence seen with specific associated conditions.

DIAGNOSIS

DIFFERENTIAL DIAGNOSIS
• Conjunctivitis
• Episcleritis
• Scleritis
• Keratitis
• Acute angle-closure glaucoma

LABORATORY
• No specific test for the diagnosis of uveitis. Tests for etiologic factors or associated conditions should be based on history and physical examination.
• CBC, BUN, creatinine (interstitial nephritis)
• HLA-B27 typing (ankylosing spondylitis, Reiter's syndrome)
• ANA, ESR (SLE, Sjögren's syndrome)
• VDRL, FTA (syphilis)
• PPD (tuberculosis)
• Lyme serology (Lyme disease)
Drugs that may alter lab results: N/A
Disorders that may alter lab results: Immune deficiency

PATHOLOGICAL FINDINGS Keratic precipitates, inflammatory cells in anterior chamber or vitreous, synechiae (fibrous tissue scarring between iris and lens), macular edema, perivasculitis of retinal vessels

SPECIAL TESTS Slit lamp examination and indirect ophthalmoscopy are necessary for precise diagnosis

IMAGING
• Chest x-ray (sarcoidosis, histoplasmosis, tuberculosis, lymphoma)
• Sacroiliac x-ray (ankylosing spondylitis)

DIAGNOSTIC PROCEDURES Slit lamp examination

TREATMENT

APPROPRIATE HEALTH CARE
Outpatient with urgent ophthalmologic consultation

GENERAL MEASURES
• Medical therapy best initiated following full ophthalmologic evaluation
• Treatment of underlying cause, if identified
• Cycloplegia
• Anti-inflammatory therapy

SURGICAL MEASURES N/A

ACTIVITY Full activity

DIET No special diet

PATIENT EDUCATION
• Instructions on proper method for instilling eye drops
• Wear dark glasses, if photophobia a problem
• Medication side effects to watch for and report

MEDICATIONS

DRUG(S) OF CHOICE
• Homatropine hydrobromide (Isopto) 2% ophthalmic solution - 2 gtts to the affected eye bid, or as often as every 3 hours if necessary, plus
• Prednisolone acetate 1% ophthalmic suspension - 2 gtts to the affected eye every 1 hour initially, tapering to qid with improvement
Contraindications:
• Hypersensitivity to the medication or component of the preparation
• Cycloplegia is contraindicated in patients known to have, or predisposed to, glaucoma
• Topical corticosteroid therapy is contraindicated in uveitis secondary to infectious etiologies
Precautions:
• Homatropine hydrobromide may produce adverse systemic antimuscarinic effects. Use extreme caution in infants and young children because of increased susceptibility to systemic effects.
• Topical corticosteroids may increase intraocular pressure. Prolonged use may cause cataract formation and exacerbate existing herpetic keratitis which may masquerade as iritis.
Significant possible interactions: Refer to manufacturer's profile of each drug

ALTERNATIVE DRUGS
• Cycloplegia - scopolamine hydrobromide 0.25% (Isopto Hyoscine) up to 3 times daily, or cyclopentolate hydrochloride 1% (Cyclogyl)
• Anti-inflammatory - prednisolone sodium phosphate 1% (Ocu-Pred Forte), dexamethasone sodium phosphate 0.1% (Ocu-Dex), and dexamethasone suspension
• Systemic nonsteroidal anti-inflammatory agents may provide some benefit

FOLLOWUP

PATIENT MONITORING
• Ophthalmologic followup as recommended by consultant
• Schedule for complete history and physical to evaluate for associated systemic disease

PREVENTION/AVOIDANCE N/A

POSSIBLE COMPLICATIONS
• Loss of vision as a result of the following:
  ◊ Keratic precipitate deposition on the corneal or lens surfaces
  ◊ Increased intraocular pressure, acute angle-closure glaucoma
  ◊ Formation of synechiae
  ◊ Cataract formation
  ◊ Vasculitis with vascular occlusion, retinal infarction
  ◊ Macular edema
  ◊ Optic nerve damage

EXPECTED COURSE/PROGNOSIS
• Dependent upon the presence of causal diseases, or associated conditions
• Uveitis resulting from infections (systemic or local) tend to resolve with eradication of the underlying infection
• Uveitis associated with seronegative arthropathies tend to be acute (lasting less than 3 months) and frequently recurrent

MISCELLANEOUS

ASSOCIATED CONDITIONS
• Viral infections: HIV, herpes simplex, herpes zoster, cytomegalovirus
• Bacterial infections: Tuberculosis, leprosy, Propionibacterium, syphilis, leptospirosis, brucellosis, Lyme disease, Whipple's disease
• Parasitic infections: Toxoplasmosis, acanthamebiasis, toxocariasis, cysticercosis, onchocerciasis
• Fungal infections: Histoplasmosis, coccidioidomycosis, candidiasis, aspergillosis, sporotrichosis, blastomycosis, cryptococcosis
• Suspected immune-mediated: Ankylosing spondylitis, Behçet's disease, Crohn's disease, drug or hypersensitivity reaction, interstitial nephritis, juvenile rheumatoid arthritis, Kawasaki disease, multiple sclerosis, psoriatic arthritis, Reiter's syndrome, relapsing polychondritis, sarcoidosis, Sjögren's syndrome, systemic lupus erythematosus, ulcerative colitis, vasculitis, vitiligo, Vogt-Koyanagi (Harada's) syndrome
• Isolated eye disease: Acute multifocal placoid pigmentary epitheliopathy, acute retinal necrosis, bird-shot choroidopathy, Fuch's heterochromatic cyclitis, glaucomatocyclitic crisis, lens-induced uveitis, multifocal choroiditis, pars planitis, serpiginous choroiditis, sympathetic ophthalmia, trauma
• Masquerade syndromes: Leukemia, lymphoma, retinitis pigmentosa, retinoblastoma

AGE-RELATED FACTORS
Pediatric: Infection should be the primary consideration. Allergies and psychological factors (depression, stress) may serve as a trigger factor.
Geriatric: The inflammatory response to systemic disease may be suppressed
Others: N/A

PREGNANCY May be of importance in the selection of medications

SYNONYMS
• Iritis
• Iridocyclitis
• Choroiditis
• Retinochoroiditis
• Chorioretinitis
• Anterior uveitis
• Posterior uveitis
• Pars planitis
• Panuveitis

ICD-9-CM
364.3 Uveitis nos

SEE ALSO
• Conjunctivitis
• Scleritis
• Keratitis, superficial punctate
• Glaucoma, primary angle-closure
• Sjögren's syndrome

OTHER NOTES
• Synonyms are anatomic descriptions of the focus of the uveal inflammation
• Severe or unresponsive uveitis may require therapy including periocular injection of corticosteroids, systemic corticosteroids, cytotoxic agents (azathioprine, cyclophosphamide, chlorambucil and methotrexate), or immunosuppressive agents (cyclosporine)

ABBREVIATIONS
gtt = drop

REFERENCES
• Rosenbaum JT: Uveitis: an internist's view. Arch Intern Med 1989;149(5):1173-6
• Rosenbaum JT: An algorithm for the systemic evaluation of patients with uveitis: guidelines for the consultant. Semin Arthritis Rheum 1990;19(4):248-57
• Herman DC: Endogenous uveitis: current concepts of treatment. Mayo Clin Proc 1990;65(5):671-83
Illustrations: N/A
Internet references: http://www.5mcc.com

Author(s)
Dana W. Peterson, MD
William L. Toffler, MD

Vaginal adenosis

BASICS

DESCRIPTION Adenosis is a term used to describe non-epithelialized columnar glandular epithelium in the vagina. At approximately the 15th week of embryological development, the müllerian system, which forms the upper two-thirds of the vagina, fuses with the invaginating cloaca, which forms the lower vagina. Squamous metaplasia from the cloacal region then produces a squamous epithelium through the vagina. Adenosis occurs when this squamous epithelium fails to completely epithelialize the vagina.
System(s) affected: Reproductive
Genetics: Unknown
Incidence/Prevalence in USA: Adenosis is relatively common, affecting 10-20% of young females studied. As maturation progresses with puberty, epithelialization occurs.
Predominant age:
• Teenage years. From puberty to approximately age twenty, epithelialization occurs.
• By age thirty, it is extremely rare to have adenosis present
Predominant sex: Female only

SIGNS AND SYMPTOMS A clear, watery vaginal discharge which is the glandular epithelium producing a small amount of mucus

CAUSES
• In the vast majority of young females, the etiology is incomplete squamous metaplasia. This occurs as a natural phenomenon and resolves with age.
• In diethylstilbestrol (DES) exposed females, the incidence of adenosis is higher and the etiology presumably is from the effect of the DES on the developing embryological system

RISK FACTORS Diethylstilbestrol (DES) exposed females

DIAGNOSIS

DIFFERENTIAL DIAGNOSIS A thorough evaluation for adenocarcinoma of the vagina arising in adenosis should be done. A biopsy may be necessary to ensure that the process represents only benign adenosis. Colposcopy of the upper vagina aids in choosing the areas for biopsy. On visual inspection, adenosis appears as a fine, raised, reddened, granular type tissue.

LABORATORY
• When extensive adenosis is present
  ◊ Four-quadrant Pap smear of the vagina should be obtained
    ◊ Initial colposcopy performed
    ◊ Once squamous metaplasia is complete, four quadrant pap smear need not be performed
Drugs that may alter lab results: N/A
Disorders that may alter lab results: N/A

PATHOLOGICAL FINDINGS Biopsy will show benign glandular epithelium, which has not yet undergone squamous metaplasia. Biopsies in the areas of ongoing squamous metaplasia will be typical for this process.

SPECIAL TESTS N/A

IMAGING N/A

DIAGNOSTIC PROCEDURES
• Four quadrant Pap smear should be liberally utilized to isolate quadrants of the vagina which may contain abnormalities. This can be followed by colposcopy and biopsy.
• Colposcopy should be used to outline areas of adenosis and insure that no malignancy is present

TREATMENT

APPROPRIATE HEALTH CARE
Outpatient

GENERAL MEASURES
• Unless malignancy is present, conservative treatment is indicated
• In the vast majority of young females with this condition, it will resolve with expectant management

SURGICAL MEASURES Aggressive therapy such as laser or surgical excision is only necessary if premalignant or malignant changes arise

ACTIVITY
• No limitations
• It is not necessary to avoid intercourse or placing objects in the vagina

DIET No special diet

PATIENT EDUCATION The patient should be educated that in the vast majority of situations this is benign and expectant management is all that is necessary
• American College of Obstetricians & Gynecologists (ACOG), 409 12th St., SW, Washington, DC 20024-2188, (800)762-ACOG

MEDICATIONS

DRUG(S) OF CHOICE N/A
Contraindications: N/A
Precautions: N/A
Significant possible interactions: N/A

ALTERNATIVE DRUGS N/A

FOLLOWUP

PATIENT MONITORING
• Initial evaluation consists of four-quadrant vaginal Pap smear, cervical Pap smear and colposcopy of the upper vagina and cervix
• If the initial colposcopy is normal, a yearly four-quadrant Pap smear of the vagina and Pap smear of the cervix is all that is necessary

PREVENTION/AVOIDANCE N/A

POSSIBLE COMPLICATIONS N/A

EXPECTED COURSE/PROGNOSIS
• It is expected that the vast majority of patients will have squamous metaplasia with complete resolution of the adenosis
• The rare patient, 1:1,000 to 1:10,000, may develop adenocarcinoma in the adenosis and will require definitive therapy as for vaginal cancer

MISCELLANEOUS

ASSOCIATED CONDITIONS
• DES exposure
  ◊ Adenosis from DES exposure should lead to an evaluation of other DES related abnormalities
  ◊ The greatest risk to the patient is from müllerian tract anomalies of the reproductive tract. These include cervical abnormalities with cervical hood, ridges, shortened cervix and incompetent cervix.
  ◊ Patients with a known DES exposure should have the reproductive tract evaluated prior to conception
  ◊ The vast majority of patients with adenosis have not been DES exposed and do not require evaluation of the reproductive system
  ◊ DES was last used to prevent spontaneous abortion in approximately 1970. This is a problem of decreasing importance.

AGE-RELATED FACTORS
Pediatric: N/A
Geriatric:
• Adenosis is a disorder of the young female. By the time of menopause the vagina and cervix should be completely epithelialized.
• The presence of glandular epithelium in the postmenopausal patient is an indication for excision and close evaluation for the possibility of a well-differentiated adenocarcinoma
Others: N/A

PREGNANCY Pregnancy produces a wide eversion of the transformation zone of the cervix. This will occasionally become so widely everted that it will extend onto the vaginal fornices leading to the impression of adenosis. This will resolve after the pregnancy is completed.

SYNONYMS N/A

ICD-9-CM 752.49 other anomalies of cervix, vagina, and external female genitalia

SEE ALSO N/A

OTHER NOTES N/A

ABBREVIATIONS N/A

REFERENCES
• Sandberg EC: The incidence and distribution of occult vaginal adenosis. Am J Obstet Gynecol 1968;101:322-34
• Hopkins MP: Vaginal Neoplasms. In: Copeland LJ, ed. Textbook of Gynecology. Philadelphia, W.B. Saunders Co., 1993
Illustrations: N/A
Internet references: http://www.5mcc.com

Author(s)
Michael P. Hopkins, MD
Eric L. Jenison, MD

Vaginal bleeding during pregnancy

 BASICS

DESCRIPTION Vaginal bleeding during pregnancy has many etiologies and ranges in severity from mild (with normal pregnancy outcome) to life-threatening for both infant and mother. The bleeding can vary from scant to excessive, from brown to bright red, and can be painless or painful. The different causes can be divided into vaginal, cervical and uterine factors. The differential diagnosis is guided by the gestational age of the pregnancy.
System(s) affected: Reproductive, Cardiovascular
Genetics: No known genetic pattern
Incidence/Prevalence in USA: Common
Predominant age: Childbearing
Predominant sex: Female only

SIGNS AND SYMPTOMS
• Bleeding can vary from scant to excessive
• Color of blood varies from brown to bright red
• May be painless or painful

CAUSES
• Vaginal infection or trauma
• Cervicitis
• Cervical polyp
• Cervical neoplasia
• Hyperemia of cervix
• Postcoital bleeding
• Ectopic pregnancy
• Molar pregnancy
• Implantation bleeding
• Spontaneous abortion
• Placenta previa
• Placental abruptio
• Bloody show
• Unknown - 50% of first trimester bleeding, no cause ever found

RISK FACTORS Varies, based on individual causes

 DIAGNOSIS

DIFFERENTIAL DIAGNOSIS
• Vaginal or cervical causes can occur throughout the pregnancy
• First trimester bleeding - ectopic pregnancy, molar pregnancy, or spontaneous abortion
• Second or third trimester bleeding - placenta previa, placental abruptio, or bloody show

LABORATORY
• CBC
• Quantitative beta human chorionic gonadotropin (HCG) - in early pregnancy bleeding; follow serially every couple of days. Levels fall in spontaneous abortion, are extremely high in molar pregnancy, and rise gradually in ectopic or intrauterine pregnancy.
• Blood type and screen - Rh negative patients need Rho(D) immune globulin (RhoGAM). If bleeding profuse, a transfusion may be required.
• Coagulation studies (fibrinogen, fibrin split products, platelets) - useful in late pregnancy bleeding and missed abortion
Drugs that may alter lab results: N/A
Disorders that may alter lab results: N/A

PATHOLOGICAL FINDINGS Depends on cause

SPECIAL TESTS N/A

IMAGING
• Ultrasound - gestational sac seen at 5-6 weeks, fetal heart tones at 8-9 weeks. Diagnostic of molar pregnancy with 98% accuracy, locates placenta, may show degree of placental separation in abruptio.
• Serial ultrasound may be required in early pregnancy to make diagnosis

DIAGNOSTIC PROCEDURES
• In first trimester bleeding - pelvic exam, culdocentesis, laparoscopy, laparotomy
• In second or third trimester bleeding - locate placenta by ultrasound prior to pelvic exam. If placenta previa, do not perform bimanual or speculum exam unless set up for immediate cesarean delivery.

 TREATMENT

APPROPRIATE HEALTH CARE
• In first trimester bleeding most patients can be managed as outpatient
• In late pregnancy bleeding, most patients need inpatient monitoring

GENERAL MEASURES
• In late pregnancy bleeding, the amount of bleeding and presence of maternal or fetal compromise indicates whether emergent cesarean section is performed or whether conservative measures are appropriate until greater fetal maturity can be obtained
• Threatened abortion: Bedrest and nothing per vagina. If bleeding is severe, hospitalization and close observation. Type and screen for possible transfusion

SURGICAL MEASURES
• If ectopic or molar pregnancy is diagnosed immediate surgical treatment is appropriate
• Inevitable or incomplete abortion: D&C (usually suction)
• If completeness of abortion is in doubt, then D&C and removal of retained products

ACTIVITY Bedrest, no coitus, no douching

DIET No restrictions

PATIENT EDUCATION
• Patient should be instructed to report any increase in the amount and frequency of bleeding and should seek immediate care if experiencing abdominal pain or sudden increased bleeding. She should bring for examination any tissue passed vaginally.
• Grief counseling is appropriate if pregnancy loss is inevitable
• American College of Obstetricians & Gynecologists (ACOG), 409 12th St., SW, Washington, DC 20024-2188, (800)762-ACOG

MEDICATIONS

DRUG(S) OF CHOICE   None
Contraindications: N/A
Precautions: N/A
Significant possible interactions: N/A

ALTERNATIVE DRUGS
• Tocolytics in suspected premature labor

FOLLOWUP

PATIENT MONITORING   Daily to weekly depending on diagnosis and severity of bleeding

PREVENTION/AVOIDANCE   N/A

POSSIBLE COMPLICATIONS
• Anemia
• Shock
• Fetal or maternal death
• Infection
• Choriocarcinoma or invasive mole in the case of hydatidiform mole
• Premature delivery of infant with associated complications
• Coagulopathy

EXPECTED COURSE/PROGNOSIS
Depends on the cause of vaginal bleeding, the severity of bleeding and the rapidity of diagnosis. Maternal mortality is 1 in 826 of ectopic pregnancies.

MISCELLANEOUS

ASSOCIATED CONDITIONS   Depends on cause of vaginal bleeding

AGE-RELATED FACTORS
Pediatric: N/A
Geriatric: N/A
Others: N/A

PREGNANCY   A complication of pregnancy

SYNONYMS   N/A

ICD-9-CM
630 Molar pregnancy
633.9 Ectopic pregnancy
634.9 Spontaneous abortion
641.1 Placenta previa
641.2 Placental abruptio

SEE ALSO
• Abortion, spontaneous
• Abruptio placentae
• Cervical malignancy
• Cervical dysplasia
• Cervical polyps
• Cervicitis
• Cervicitis, ectropion & true erosion
• Chlamydial sexually transmitted diseases
• Ectopic pregnancy
• Placenta previa
• Premature labor
• Vaginal malignancy
• Vulvovaginitis, bacterial
• Vulvovaginitis, candidal

OTHER NOTES   N/A

ABBREVIATIONS   N/A

REFERENCES
• American College of Emergency Physicains: Clinical policy for the initial approach to patients presenting with a chief complaint of vaginal bleeding. Ann Emerg Med 1997;29(3):435-458
• Signore CC: Second trimester vaginal bleeding: correlation of ultrasonographic findings with perinatal outcome. Am J Ob Gyn 1998:179(2):336-40
• Cunningham FG, MacDonald PC, Gant NF, eds: Williams' Obstetrics. 19th Ed. Norwalk, CT, Appleton and Lange, 1993
• Danforth DM, Scott JR., et al, eds: Obstetrics and Gynecology. 6th Ed. Philadelphia, J.B. Lippincott, 1990
Illustrations: N/A
Internet references: http://www.5mcc.com

Author(s)
Kimberle Vore, MD

Vaginal malignancy

BASICS

DESCRIPTION
• Vaginal intraepithelial neoplasia (carcinoma in situ): A premalignant phase with full thickness neoplastic changes in the superficial epithelium. However there is no invasion through the basement membrane.
• Invasive malignancies: Vaginal malignancies are squamous cell in 90% of the patients and the remaining 10% are adenocarcinomas, sarcomas and melanomas. The clear cell carcinoma is a subtype of adenocarcinoma.
• To be classified as a vaginal malignancy, only the vagina can be involved. If the cervix or the vulva is involved, then the tumor is classified as a primary cancer arising from the cervix or the vulva.
System(s) affected: Reproductive
Genetics: No known genetic pattern
Incidence/Prevalence in USA: This is the rarest of all gynecological malignancies
Predominant age:
• Carcinoma in situ - mid-forties to sixties
• Invasive squamous cell malignancy - mid-sixties to seventies
• Adenocarcinoma - any age range, fifties is mean age
• Mixed müllerian sarcomas and leiomyosarcomas in the adult population - mean age sixty
• Sarcoma botryoides and embryonal sarcomas - occur in the pediatric population
Predominant sex: Female only

SIGNS AND SYMPTOMS
• Abnormal bleeding is the most common symptom. This results from a fungating tumor present in the vagina.
• Dyspareunia
• Postcoital bleeding can result from direct trauma to the tumor
• Pain along with symptoms and signs of hydroureter are late findings when tumor has spread into the paravaginal tissues and extends to the pelvic side wall
• In the pediatric population, sarcomas can present either as a mass protruding from the vagina or as abnormal genital bleeding

CAUSES
• Women with a history of cervical malignancy have a higher probability of developing squamous cell malignancy in the vagina after hysterectomy
• The human papilloma virus (HPV) has been associated with vulvovaginal, cervical, adenocarcinoma and squamous cell carcinoma
• Smokers have a higher incidence
• Clear cell adenocarcinoma of the vagina in young women has been associated with diethylstilbestrol (DES) exposure. The incidence, however, is exceedingly rare estimated at 1:1,000 to 1:10,000 DES exposed females.
• Metastatic lesions can involve the vagina from the other gynecologic organs
• Renal cell carcinoma and breast cancer can metastasize to the vagina (rarely)

RISK FACTORS
• History of squamous cell cancer of the cervix or vulva
• Smoking
• Multiple sex partners

DIAGNOSIS

DIFFERENTIAL DIAGNOSIS
• Vaginal intraepithelial neoplasia (VAIN) involves premalignant changes that do not infiltrate beyond the basement membrane
• Adequate biopsies ensure that invasive lesions are not overlooked. Invasive lesions penetrate the basement membrane and cannot be treated conservatively. Other malignancies such as endometrial, cervix, bladder or colon cancer can invade directly into the vagina or metastasize to the vagina.
• In the childbearing age, female trophoblastic disease should be considered. The vagina is a common site of metastases. Biopsy will usually provide a clue to the primary site.

LABORATORY
Cytology will usually be positive when an obvious lesion is present
Drugs that may alter lab results: N/A
Disorders that may alter lab results: N/A

PATHOLOGICAL FINDINGS
• Stage 0 - carcinoma in situ
• Stage I - infiltrative tumor not involving the paravaginal tissues
• Stage II - paravaginal extension but not to the side wall
• Stage III - paravaginal extension to the side wall
• Stage IVA - tumor involving the bladder or the rectum
• Stage IVB - distant metastatic disease

SPECIAL TESTS   N/A

IMAGING
• Chest x-ray - lung metastases are a late finding.
• IVP - to evaluate for ureteral obstruction
• CAT scan to evaluate the retroperitoneum and especially the lymph nodes in the pelvic and periaortic area
• Lymphangiography is also useful for evaluation of the lymph node status
• Barium enema to rule out rectal invasion

DIAGNOSTIC PROCEDURES
• Colposcopy with directed biopsies for small lesions
• Wide excision under anesthesia of superficial disease may be necessary to insure that invasive cancer is not present
• Cystoscopy to rule out bladder invasion
• Sigmoidoscopy to rule out rectal invasion

TREATMENT

APPROPRIATE HEALTH CARE
Outpatient or inpatient depending on treatment

GENERAL MEASURES
• Carcinoma in situ can be treated by a variety of methods: Laser vaporization under microscopic guidance; fluorouracil (Efudex) intravaginal cream; partial vaginectomy
• There is no effective chemotherapy for squamous cell malignancy of the vagina
• In all tumor types, metastatic disease from the vagina to other sites is only minimally responsive to chemotherapy

SURGICAL MEASURES
• Whenever there is a doubt as to the presence or absence of invasive disease, vaginectomy must be performed
• Invasive lesions are usually treated by radiation therapy, however, stage I lesions can be treated with radical hysterectomy, radical vaginectomy with pelvic lymph node dissection
• If the lesion involves the lower vagina, inguinal node dissection must also be done as cancer involving the lower vagina can metastasize to the groin region
• Sarcomas are treated by radiation therapy followed by pelvic exenteration if persistent disease is present
• Childhood sarcomas are treated with chemotherapy followed by local resection. Childhood sarcomas are responsive to multiagent combination chemotherapies.

ACTIVITY
• The patients are usually ambulatory and able to resume full activity by six weeks after surgery
• Most patients are fully active while receiving radiation therapy

DIET
Unrestricted unless they are undergoing radiation

PATIENT EDUCATION
• This is a rare malignancy and these patients should be treated by a physician familiar and experienced with this malignancy
• Printed patient information available from: American College of Obstetricians & Gynecologists, 409 12th St., SW, Washington, DC 20024-2188, (800)762-ACOG

MEDICATIONS

DRUG(S) OF CHOICE
• With one exception, there are no chemotherapeutic agents to which this tumor is responsive. The exception is the childhood sarcomas, which have been treated with combinations of:
  ◊ Vincristine
  ◊ Dactinomycin (actinomycin-D)
  ◊ Cyclophosphamide (Cytoxan)
  ◊ Cisplatin
  ◊ Etoposide (VP-16)
• Adjuvant chemotherapy has no proven benefit in squamous cell or adenocarcinoma of the vagina
• Carcinoma in situ can be eradicated in 90% of patients with fluorouracil (Efudex) cream 5% applied bid x 2 hours x 7 days, then qd x 7 days, repeated in six weeks

Contraindications:
• Prior to treatment the diagnosis must be established with certainty
• If there is any doubt that a process beyond in situ disease exists, vaginectomy must be performed. Because these patients are often elderly, aggressive therapy is limited by the patient's performance status and ability to tolerate radical surgery, chemotherapy or radiation.

Precautions: Refer to manufacturer's literature

Significant possible interactions: Refer to manufacturer's literature

ALTERNATIVE DRUGS
• Ondansetron (Zofran), dronabinol (Marinol), metoclopramide (Reglan), and others for nausea control

FOLLOWUP

PATIENT MONITORING
• Pelvic examination and Pap smear every 3 months for 2 years and then every 6 months for subsequent 3 years
• Chest x-ray once a year

PREVENTION/AVOIDANCE
• A Pap smear should be performed for all women on a yearly basis, even after hysterectomy
• Premalignant changes discovered on Pap smear screening should be followed up with colposcopy, biopsy and treatment. This needs to be undertaken by a physician well trained in the diagnosis and treatment of vaginal disease.
• Patients with a history of in situ or invasive disease of the cervix and/or the vulva should be followed at close intervals for development of disease in the vagina

POSSIBLE COMPLICATIONS Those
associated with major abdominal surgery or radiation therapy

EXPECTED COURSE/PROGNOSIS
• Stage and 5 year survival
  ◊ I - 60%
  ◊ II - 40%
  ◊ III - 20%
  ◊ IVA - 5%
  ◊ IVB - 0%

MISCELLANEOUS

ASSOCIATED CONDITIONS Due to the
field effect, patients with vaginal cancer are more likely to develop malignancy in the cervix or vulva and should be followed closely

AGE-RELATED FACTORS
Pediatric: Childhood sarcomas can be treated in a conservative fashion with multi-modality therapy. This avoids the loss of the young child's bladder and/or rectum.
Geriatric: Older patients, many with a long smoking history are at a higher risk for surgery
Others:
• Younger patients, who have not completed their family, can occasionally be treated with limited resection and localized radiation to the area
• Premenopausal women, who desire to retain ovarian function, are better candidates for radical surgery for early stage disease

PREGNANCY This malignancy is not
associated with pregnancy

SYNONYMS
• Bowen's disease
• Vaginal intraepithelial neoplasia (VAIN)

ICD-9-CM
184.0 Malignant neoplasm of the vagina

SEE ALSO N/A

OTHER NOTES N/A

ABBREVIATIONS N/A

REFERENCES
• Hopkins MP: Vaginal Neoplasms. In: Copeland LJ, ed. Textbook of Gynecology. Philadelphia, W.B. Saunders Co., 1993
• Peters WA, Kumar NB, Morley GW: Carcinoma of the vagina: Factors influencing treatment outcome. Cancer 1985;55(4):892-97
Illustrations: N/A
Internet references: http://www.5mcc.com

Author(s)
Michael P. Hopkins, MD
Eric L. Jenison, MD

Vaginismus

BASICS

DESCRIPTION Involuntary painful contraction of perineal muscles prior to or during vaginal intercourse. The experience of or even the anticipation of pain on vaginal entry causes theses muscles to contract, occluding the vaginal opening and causing further pain when penetration is attempted.
System(s) affected: Reproductive
Genetics: N/A
Incidence/Prevalence in USA: 6-8% of women in some studies report complete vaginismus and up to 30% some degree of vaginismus
Predominant age: Postpubertal
Predominant sex: Female

SIGNS AND SYMPTOMS
• Inability to allow entry for vaginal sexual intercourse secondary to involuntary muscle spasms
• Reluctance or avoidance of pelvic examination
• Relationship discord or difficulty
• Infertility
• Sexual satisfaction may be independent of sexual function!

CAUSES
• Primary: Often multifactorial
  ◊ Negative messages about sex and sexual relations in upbringing may cause phobic reaction
  ◊ Poor body image of genital area
  ◊ History of sexual trauma, although rates of vaginismus appear to be similar in sexually abused and non-abused populations of women (studies show incidence of sexual abuse of women to be from 12-40%)
• Secondary
  ◊ New onset of infection
  ◊ Surgical or post delivery scarring
  ◊ Endometriosis
  ◊ Inadequate vaginal lubrication

RISK FACTORS
• Previous sexual trauma, but rates appear to be similar in abused and non-abused women
• Often associated with other sexual dysfunctions

DIAGNOSIS

DIFFERENTIAL DIAGNOSIS
• Dyspareunia

LABORATORY N/A
Drugs that may alter lab results: N/A
Disorders that may alter lab results: N/A

PATHOLOGICAL FINDINGS Rarely found in primary vaginismus, but may be varied such as endometriosis or scarring in secondary vaginismus

SPECIAL TESTS Psychiatric consultation if not responsive to primary physician's therapy or if primary provider not comfortable with caring for sexual problems

IMAGING N/A

DIAGNOSTIC PROCEDURES
• General and sexual history
• At some point, a careful pelvic examination to rule out medical cause

TREATMENT

APPROPRIATE HEALTH CARE
Outpatient care

GENERAL MEASURES
• Can often treat vaginismus successfully without defining/treating its etiologies!!
• No published controlled studies on success of psychotherapy for vaginismus
• Patient education as noted below on pelvic anatomy and sexual function
• Kegel's exercises to control perineal muscles
• Stepwise vaginal desensitization exercises:
  ◊ A) with vaginal dilators (patient inserts/controls), or
  ◊ B) with woman's own finger(s) (promotes sexual self-awareness)
• Valsalva can help with vaginal entry
• Advance to husband's fingers with patient's control
• Coitus after achieving largest vaginal dilator or 3 fingers; important to begin with sensate focused exercises/sensual caressing without necessarily a demand for coitus
  ◊ A) Female superior at first; passive (non-thrusting); female directed
  ◊ B) Later, thrusting may be okay

SURGICAL MEASURES Contraindicated

ACTIVITY Simple techniques of gentle, progressive, patient-controlled vaginal dilation

DIET No special diet

PATIENT EDUCATION
• Education about pelvic anatomy, nature of the vaginal spasms, normal adult sexual function
• Hand held mirror can help the woman visually learn to tighten and loosen perineal muscles
• Important to teach the partners that the spasms are not under conscious control and are not a reflection on the relationship or a woman's feelings about her partner
• Instruction in techniques for vaginal dilation
• Resources
  ◊ American College of Obstetricians & Gynecologists (ACOG), 409 12th St., SW, Washington, DC 20024-2188, (800)762-ACOG
  ◊ Valins L. When a Woman's Body Says No to Sex: Understanding and Overcoming Vaginismus. New York: Penguin, 1992.

MEDICATIONS

DRUG(S) OF CHOICE N/A
Contraindications: Anxiolytics, especially benzodiazepines
Precautions: N/A
Significant Possible interactions: N/A

ALTERNATIVE DRUGS N/A

FOLLOWUP

PATIENT MONITORING General preventive health care

PREVENTION/AVOIDANCE

POSSIBLE COMPLICATIONS
Precipitation of memory of incest prior to patient's readiness to deal with it

EXPECTED COURSE/PROGNOSIS
• Some studies show high degrees of success (58-70%) with behavioral interventions
• History of sexual abuse does not predict outcome negatively or positively

MISCELLANEOUS

ASSOCIATED CONDITIONS
• Marital stress, family dysfunction
• Dyspareunia

AGE-RELATED FACTORS Vaginismus is generally primary, e.g. happens with first attempt at intercourse
Pediatric: N/A
Geriatric: N/A
Others: N/A

PREGNANCY Pregnancy can occur in patients with vaginismus via perineal ejaculation

SYNONYMS N/A

ICD-9-CM 306.51 Psychogenic vaginismus

SEE ALSO
• Sexual dysfunction in women
• Dyspareunia

OTHER NOTES N/A

ABBREVIATIONS N/A

REFERENCES
• Biswas A: Vaginismus and outcome of treatment: Human Sexuality and Sexual Dysfunction 1995;24:755-758
• Heiman JR: Evaluating sexual dysfunctions: Primary Care of Women. Norwalk, CT, Appleson and Lange, 1995
• Read S, King M, Watson J: Sexual dysfunction in primary medical care. Journal of Public Health Medicine, Oxford University Press 1997;19(4):387-391
• Sarwer D, Durlak J: A field trial of the effectiveness of behavioral treatment for sexual dysfunctions. Journal of Sex and Marital Therapy 1997;23(2):87-97
Illustrations: N/A
Internet references: http://www.5mcc.com

Author(s)
Kay A. Bauman, MD, MPH

Varicose veins

BASICS

DESCRIPTION Elongated, dilated, tortuous superficial veins with congenitally absent valves, or valves that have become incompetent. Affects legs where reverse flow occurs when dependent.
System(s) affected: Cardiovascular, Skin/Exocrine
Genetics: Familial, dominant, x-linked
Incidence/Prevalence in USA: About 20% of adults
Predominant age: Middle age
Predominant sex: Female > Male (5:1)

SIGNS AND SYMPTOMS
• Sometimes asymptomatic
• Leg muscular cramp
• Dilatation, tortuosity of superficial veins chiefly in the lower extremities
• Edema of affected limb
• Leg aching
• Fatigue
• Symptoms worse during menses
• Pain if varicose ulcer develops

CAUSES
• Faulty valves in one or more perforator veins in the lower leg causing secondary incompetence at the saphenofemoral junction
• Deep thrombophlebitis
• Increased venous pressure from any cause
• In many individuals, no cause or precipitating factor found

RISK FACTORS
• Pregnancy
• Occupations requiring prolonged standing, restrictive clothing (e.g., very tight girdles)

DIAGNOSIS

DIFFERENTIAL DIAGNOSIS
• Nerve root compression
• Arthritis
• Peripheral neuritis

LABORATORY None helpful
Drugs that may alter lab results: N/A
Disorders that may alter lab results: N/A

PATHOLOGICAL FINDINGS
• Elongation and tortuosity of veins
• Medial fibrosis of veins
• Disappearance or atrophy of valves

SPECIAL TESTS Trendelenburg's test

IMAGING N/A

DIAGNOSTIC PROCEDURES Clinical inspection

TREATMENT

APPROPRIATE HEALTH CARE
Outpatient

GENERAL MEASURES
• Conservative methods
  ◊ Frequent rest periods with legs elevated
  ◊ Lightweight, elastic compression hosiery. Best put on before getting out of bed.
  ◊ Avoid girdles and other restrictive clothing
  ◊ If stasis ulcers present, use warm, wet dressings
• Spider veins (idiopathic telangiectases)
  ◊ Fine intracutaneous angiectasis
  ◊ May be extensive/unsightly
  ◊ Eliminate with intracapillary injections of 1% solution of sodium tetradecyl sulfate (or hypertonic saline 23.4%) using a fine-bore needle
  ◊ Subsequent treatments may be required until optimal results attained

SURGICAL MEASURES
• Surgical and other methods
  ◊ If there is pain, recurrent phlebitis, skin changes, or for cosmetic improvement for severe cases
  ◊ Ligation and stripping of the saphenous vein
  ◊ Injection of sclerosing solution
  ◊ Stab evulsion phlebectomy - newer procedure with shorter recovery time
  ◊ For extensive fibrosis - excision of the entire area, followed by skin graft may be necessary

ACTIVITY
• Avoid long periods of standing
• Appropriate exercise routine as part of conservative treatment
• Walking regimen after sclerotherapy is important to help promote healing
• Apply elastic stockings before lowering legs from the bed
• Never sit with legs hanging down

DIET
• No special diet
• Weight loss diet recommended, if obesity a problem

PATIENT EDUCATION
• Inform patients that the surgery or sclerotherapy may not prevent development of varicosities and that the procedure may need to be repeated in later years
• For patient education materials favorably reviewed on this topic, contact: National Heart, Lung & Blood Institute, Communications & Public Information Branch, National Institutes of Health, Building 31, Room 41-21, 9000 Rockville Pike, Bethesda, MD 20892, (301)496-4236

MEDICATIONS

DRUG(S) OF CHOICE Injection sclerotherapy with compression to totally obliterate the vein by fibrosis. Sclerosant is sodium tetradecyl sulfate 1-3% solution. Bandages remain 3 weeks or longer.
Contraindications: Refer to manufacturer's literature
Precautions: No oral contraceptives for at least 6 weeks prior to sclerotherapy because of their thrombogenic effect
Significant possible interactions: Refer to manufacturer's literature

ALTERNATIVE DRUGS Antibiotics for infected varicose ulcers

FOLLOWUP

PATIENT MONITORING Until surgery or conservative therapy brings maximal benefit

PREVENTION/AVOIDANCE N/A

POSSIBLE COMPLICATIONS
• Petechial hemorrhages
• Chronic edema
• Superimposed infection
• Varicose ulcers
• Pigmentation
• Eczema
• Recurrence after surgical treatment
• Scarring or nerve damage from stripping technique

EXPECTED COURSE/PROGNOSIS
• Usual course - chronic
• Prognosis - favorable with appropriate treatment

MISCELLANEOUS

ASSOCIATED CONDITIONS
• Stasis dermatitis
• Stasis ulcer

AGE-RELATED FACTORS
Pediatric: Unlikely in this age group
Geriatric:
• More common, usually valvular degeneration, but may be secondary to chronic venous deficiency
• Recommended therapy - elastic support hose and frequent rests with legs elevated rather than ligation and stripping
Others: N/A

PREGNANCY Frequent problem. Use of elastic stockings recommended for individuals who have a history of varicosities or when activities involve a great deal of standing.

SYNONYMS N/A

ICD-9-CM
454.1 Varicose veins of lower extremities with inflammation

SEE ALSO Dermatitis, stasis

OTHER NOTES N/A

ABBREVIATIONS N/A

REFERENCES Berkow R, et al, eds: Merck Manual. 16th Ed. Rahway, NJ, Merck Sharp & Dohme, 1992
Illustrations: N/A
Internet references: http://www.5mcc.com

Author(s)
Joseph A. Florence, MD

Ventricular septal defect (VSD)

BASICS

DESCRIPTION Congenital or acquired defect of the interventricular septum that allows communication of blood between the left and right ventricles. Other than bicuspid aortic valve, this is the most common congenital heart malformation reported in infants and children. It also occurs as a complication of acute myocardial infarctions (MI). Blood flow across the defect is typically left to right and depends on the size of the defect and the pulmonary vascular resistance (PVR). Prolonged shunting of blood can lead to pulmonary hypertension and eventually reversal of flow across the defect, and to cyanosis (Eisenmenger's complex).
System(s) affected: Cardiovascular
Genetics: Multifactorial etiology; autosomal dominant and recessive transmission have been reported
Incidence/Prevalence in USA:
• Congenital - 100-500 of 100,000 live births
• Acute myocardial infarctions - estimated to complicate 1-3%
Predominant age: Infants and children
Predominant sex: Male = Female (male > female if secondary to myocardial infarction)

SIGNS AND SYMPTOMS
• Depend on the degree of shunting across the defect
• Respiratory distress, tachypnea
• Forceful apical impulse
• Thrill along the left lower or midsternal borders
• High-frequency holosystolic murmur
• S3
• Increased intensity of P2
• Elevated jugular venous pressure
• Diastolic murmur of pulmonic insufficiency
• Diastolic rumble due to increased flow across the mitral valve
• If pulmonary hypertension exist: cyanosis with exertion
• If Eisenmenger's complex is present: cyanosis and clubbing

CAUSES
• Congenital
• In adults, secondary to myocardial infarction

RISK FACTORS
• Congenital
  ◊ 4.2% risk of sibling being affected
  ◊ 4.0% of offspring being affected
• Post-acute myocardial infarctions
  ◊ First MI
  ◊ Limited coronary artery disease
  ◊ Hypertension
  ◊ Most frequent within first week after myocardial infarction (MI)
  ◊ Occur in 1-2% of MI, most commonly after anterior MI

DIAGNOSIS

DIFFERENTIAL DIAGNOSIS
• Any disease with left-to-right shunt, such as large patent ductus arteriosus or atrial septal defect
• Children - Tetralogy of Fallot
• Adults - acute mitral regurgitation

LABORATORY None specific
Drugs that may alter lab results: N/A
Disorders that may alter lab results: N/A

PATHOLOGICAL FINDINGS
• Congenital VSD's (4 major anatomical types):
  ◊ Membranous (75%)
  ◊ Muscular (10%)
  ◊ Atrioventricular canal type (10%)
  ◊ Supracristal (5%; higher percent in Oriental population)
• Postmyocardial infarction VSD's
  ◊ Involve predominantly the muscular septum

SPECIAL TESTS
• ECG may suggest severity of VSD. Initially, left ventricular hypertrophy and left atrial enlargement may be evident. With pulmonary hypertension, right ventricular hypertrophy and right atrial enlargement may be seen.
• After surgical repair, right bundle branch block and left anterior hemi-block are common

IMAGING
• Chest x-ray may demonstrate increased pulmonary vascularity and/or cardiomegaly
• Two-dimensional echocardiogram for visualization
• Color-flow Doppler, for detection of ventricular septal defect jet

DIAGNOSTIC PROCEDURES
• Cardiac catheterization (left and right heart) can establish the diagnosis
• Demonstration of an oxygen saturation step-up (> 8 mm Hg) (1.1 kPa) from the right atrium to the distal pulmonary artery with Swan-Ganz catheter

TREATMENT

APPROPRIATE HEALTH CARE
• Outpatient, until surgical repair is indicated
• Inpatient in setting of acute MI
• Inpatient for treatment of severe congestive heart failure

GENERAL MEASURES N/A

SURGICAL MEASURES
• Surgical closure is indicated if the pulmonic to systemic flow is > 1.5:1
• Congenital VSD surgery is usually performed before the child enters school or earlier, if hemodynamically indicated
• In the post-MI setting, afterload reduction, inotropic support and intra-aortic balloon pump may be used to stabilize the patient prior to surgery

ACTIVITY As tolerated

DIET Low sodium

PATIENT EDUCATION
• Endocarditis prophylaxis
• Parents need support and instructions for prevention of complications until the child is ready for surgery

Ventricular septal defect (VSD)

MEDICATIONS

DRUG(S) OF CHOICE
- Antibiotic prophylaxis
- Pediatric
  - ◊ Nitroglycerin 0.5-5 µg/kg/min IV (max 60 µg/kg/min)
  - ◊ Hydralazine 0.5 mg/kg/day po q6-8h (max 200 mg/day)
  - ◊ Captopril 0.1-0.4 mg/kg/dose po given q6-24h. (max 6 mg/kg/24h)
  - ◊ Nitroprusside 0.5-8 µg/kg/min IV
  - ◊ Prazosin first dose 5 µg/kg po (max 25 µg/kg/dose q6h)
- Adult
  - ◊ Nitroglycerin drip beginning at 5 µg/kg/min and increasing by 5 µg/kg/min every few minutes, then by up to 20 µg/kg/min and titrate effect blood pressure, cardiac output, etc.
  - ◊ Nitroprusside beginning at 10 µg/min and increasing by 5-10 µg/min every few minutes, titrating to blood pressure, cardiac output, etc.
  - ◊ Angiotensin converting enzyme (ACE) inhibitors (e.g., captopril 6.25-25 mg po tid or lisinopril 2.5-20 mg po qd or enalapril 2.5-15 mg po qd or bid)
  - ◊ Hydralazine 10-100 mg po qid
  - ◊ Dobutamine 2.5-10 µg/kg/min titrating to cardiac output and systemic resistance (SVR)
  - ◊ Dopamine 5-10 µg/kg/min titrating to cardiac output and SVR

Contraindications: Drugs that increase peripheral vascular resistance may increase right-to-left shunting

Precautions: Hypotension

Significant possible interactions: Refer to manufacturer's profile of each drug

ALTERNATIVE DRUGS
Diuretics and digoxin may also be beneficial in certain circumstances

FOLLOWUP

PATIENT MONITORING
Close followup (at least every 6 months) of a congenital VSD is necessary until primary intracardiac repair is performed to ensure that significant pulmonary hypertension does not develop

PREVENTION/AVOIDANCE
- For adults, avoid risk factors for myocardial infarction and obtain evaluation before pregnancy

POSSIBLE COMPLICATIONS
- Congestive heart failure
- Infective endocarditis
- Sudden death
- Hemoptysis
- Chest pain
- Cerebral abscess
- Paradoxical emboli
- Cardiogenic shock
- Heart block may rarely accompany surgical closure
- Pulmonary hypertension

EXPECTED COURSE/PROGNOSIS
- Congenital
  - ◊ 25-45% of VSD will close spontaneously by age 3
  - ◊ Course is variable depending on the size of the VSD
  - ◊ 4% of patients with VSD develop infective endocarditis by the third or fourth decade of life
  - ◊ Progressive pulmonary vascular disease and pulmonary hypertension are the most feared complications of VSD caused by left-to-right shunting, and may eventually lead to reversal of the shunt (Eisenmenger's complex)
  - ◊ Death usually occurs in the fourth decade of life if untreated
- Postmyocardial infarction
  - ◊ 80-90% mortality in the first two weeks with medical management alone
  - ◊ Prognosis worse with inferior MI compared to anterior MI

MISCELLANEOUS:

ASSOCIATED CONDITIONS
- Congenital
  - ◊ Tetralogy of Fallot
  - ◊ Aortic valvular deformities, especially aortic insufficiency
  - ◊ Down's syndrome (Trisomy 21)
  - ◊ Transposition of the great arteries
  - ◊ Tricuspid atresia
  - ◊ Truncus arteriosus
  - ◊ Patent ductus arteriosus
  - ◊ Atrial septal defect
  - ◊ Pulmonic stenosis
  - ◊ Subaortic stenosis
- Adult
  - ◊ Coronary artery disease

AGE-RELATED FACTORS
Pediatric: Congenital
Geriatric: Almost entirely associated with myocardial infarction
Others: N/A

PREGNANCY
- May exacerbate symptoms and signs with a congenital VSD
- Tolerated during pregnancy if the septal defect is small

SYNONYMS N/A

ICD-9-CM
745.4 Ventricular septal defect

SEE ALSO
- Down syndrome
- Myocardial infarction
- Tetralogy of Fallot

OTHER NOTES N/A

ABBREVIATIONS N/A

REFERENCES
- Friedman WF, Perloff JK: Congenital heart disease in infancy and childhood. In: Braunwald E, ed. Heart Disease. 4th Ed. Philadelphia, W.B. Saunders Co., 1992
- Hillis DL, Lange RA, Winniford MD, Page RL: Manual of Clinical Problems in Cardiology. New York, Little, Brown and Co., 1995
- Radford MJ, et al: Ventricular septal rupture: a review of clinical and physiologic features and an analysis of survival. Circulation 1981;64(3)
Illustrations: N/A
Internet references: http://www.5mcc.com

Author(s)
Karil Bellah, MD

Vitamin deficiency

BASICS

DESCRIPTION
Vitamin deficiency syndromes develop slowly and are difficult to diagnose. Vitamins can not be synthesized by humans and therefore must be supplied by diet vitamins are required for maintenance of optimal health and prevention of chronic diseases. Multiple deficiencies of vitamins occur more frequently than a deficiency in a single vitamin. Vitamin classification follows:
• Fat-soluble
◊ Vitamin A (retinol)
◊ Vitamin D (vitamin D2 = ergocalciferol; vitamin D3 = cholecalciferol)
◊ Vitamin E
◊ Vitamin K (K1 = phytomenadione; K2 = menaquinone; K3 = menadione)
• Water-soluble
◊ Vitamin B1 (thiamine)
◊ Vitamin B2 (riboflavin)
◊ Vitamin B3 (niacin, nicotinic acid, niacinamide)
◊ Vitamin B6 (pyridoxine)
◊ Vitamin B12 (cobalamin)
◊ Vitamin C (ascorbic acid)

System(s) affected: Endocrine/Metabolic
Genetics:
• Hereditary vitamin D-dependent rickets - autosomal recessive syndrome
• Thiamine-dependent beriberi - rare hereditary metabolic disorder
• Pernicious anemia

Incidence/Prevalence in USA: Unknown
Predominant age: Elderly
Predominant sex: Male = Female

SIGNS AND SYMPTOMS
• Vitamin (A) (retinol)
◊ Early - dryness of conjunctiva (xerosis)
◊ Bitot's spots (small whites spots on conjunctiva)
◊ Loss of appetite, growth retardation and anemia commonly found in children
◊ Late - keratomalacia (ulceration & necrosis of cornea), endophthalmitis, blindness
• Vitamin B 1 (thiamine)
◊ Infantile beriberi - occur in infants breast-fed by thiamine deficient mothers
◊ "Wet beriberi" - cardiovascular symptoms - peripheral vasodilation, high output failure and dyspnea tachycardia
◊ "Dry beriberi" - neurological symptoms symmetrical motor and sensory peripheral neuropathy with, paresthesias, loss of reflexes
◊ Wernicke's encephalopathy - nystagmus, ophthalmoplegia, truncal ataxia, confusion
◊ Korsakoff syndrome - amnesia, impaired learning, confabulation
• Vitamin B3 (niacin [nicotinic acid] niacinamide)
◊ Anorexia, weakness, irritability, mouth soreness, glossitis, stomatitis, weight loss
◊ Dermatitis seen symmetrically in sun exposed areas, skin is dry dark and scaly
◊ Dementia, insomnia, irritability, apathy, confusion, memory loss, psychosis, hallucination
◊ Diarrhea
◊ Death
• Vitamin B12 (cobalamin)
◊ Anorexia, diarrhea, glossitis
◊ Peripheral nerves - paresthesias

◊ Posterior column - difficulty with balance
◊ Confusion, memory loss, disorientation
◊ Dementia
• Vitamin C (ascorbic acid)
◊ Scurvy - develops in children between 6-24 months
◊ Early - weakness, malaise
◊ Late - perifollicular hemorrhage and hyperkeratotic papules, petechia, purpura, splinter hemorrhages, bleeding gums, hematomas, subperiosteal hemorrhages
◊ Terminal - edema, oliguria, neuropathy, intracranial, hemorrhage, death
• Vitamin E (alpha-tocopherol)
◊ RBC hemolysis, creatinurias ceroid deposition in muscle
◊ Areflexia, gait disturbances ophthalmoplegia
• Vitamin K (K1 - phytomenadione; K2 - menaquinone; K3 - menadione)
◊ Early - hemolytic disease of newborn (HDN) seen within first 24 hours of birth
◊ Classic - seen within 7-14 days of birth - bleeding from skin gut, circumcision site
◊ Late - seen 2-12 weeks after birth, intracranial hemorrhage

CAUSES
• Inadequate dietary intake
• Impaired absorption or storage

RISK FACTORS
• Social and psychological - social isolation, depression, alcohol abuse, elder abuse and neglect, institutionalization, poverty, inadequate assistance with eating, eating disorders (anorexia/bulimia), loss of spouse/caretaker
• Physical - chronic disease (eg cancer), poorly fitting/missing dentures, reduced calorie intake with advanced age, impaired mobility, memory and attention disorders, neurological impairment of chewing/swallowing
• Others
◊ Parenteral nutrition, malabsorption, bile deficiency, dialysis, chronic protein-calorie undernutrition, drug interactions, infants, elderly, laxative abuse, genetic disorder (abetalipoproteinemia) (vitamin E), intestinal parasites, food faddism, gastro intestinal surgery
◊ Increase physiological demand pregnancy, hemolytic anemia, and exfoliative skin diseases

DIAGNOSIS

DIFFERENTIAL DIAGNOSIS
• Vitamin A deficiency - retinitis pigmentosa
• Vitamin B1 deficiency - polyneuropathy
• Vitamin B2 deficiency - other causes of seborrheic dermatitis and ocular lesions
• Vitamin D - infantile scurvy; congenital syphilis; chondrodystrophy; readily distinguishable disorders (creatinism, hydrocephalus, poliomyelitis, etc.); convulsions due to other causes
• Vitamin K - liver damage, anticoagulant or salicylate therapy, other disorders that produce hemorrhagic symptoms (scurvy,

allergic purpura, leukemia, thrombocytopenia)
• Niacin - other causes of stomatitis, glossitis, diarrhea, dementia
• Vitamin B12 - other causes of myelodysplasia

LABORATORY
• Vitamin A - serum levels below normal
• Vitamin BI - elevated blood pyruvate
◊ Decreased urinary thiamin excretion
◊ Erythrocyte transketolase activity > 15-20%
• Vitamin B2
◊ Erythrocyte glutathione reductase coefficient >1.2 - 1.3
◊ Lower serum levels of plasma and red cell plasma
◊ Lower urinary excretion of riboflaxin
• Vitamin B3 (niacin)
◊ Lower levels of N-methylnicotinamide
◊ Lower levels of serum and Red cell NAD and NADP
• Vitamin B6 - lower levels of pyridoxal in blood (normal - 50 ng/ml)
• Vitamin B 12
◊ Serum levels <150 pg/ml
◊ MCV 110-140 fl, ovalocytes, hypersegmented neutrophils, decreased reticulocyte count, pancytopenia
◊ Bone marrow - erythroid hyperplasia
◊ Increased LDH - increased indirect bilirubin
◊ Schilling test
• Vitamin C - levels <0.1 mg/dl
• Vitamin D - plasma calcium level < 7.5 mg/dL (1.88 mmol/L); low plasma vitamin D sterolsinorganic phosphate serum levels < 3 mg/dL (0.97 mmol/L); serum citrate levels, 2.5 mg/dL; alkaline phosphate < 4 Bodansky units/100 mL
• Vitamin E - serum levels < 0.8 mg/dL (18.5 µmol/L) (adults)
• Vitamin K - prothrombin time 25% longer than normal range (diagnostic for vitamin deficiency after ruling out other disorders), PIUKA II test

Drugs that may alter lab results: Refer to laboratory test reference
Disorders that may alter lab results: Refer to laboratory test reference

PATHOLOGICAL FINDINGS   N/A

SPECIAL TESTS   N/A

IMAGING   N/A

DIAGNOSTIC PROCEDURES   History and physical

TREATMENT

APPROPRIATE HEALTH CARE
Outpatient usually. Inpatient in severe cases.

GENERAL MEASURES
• Treatment of any underlying causes
• Oral or parenteral vitamin therapeutic replacement
• Maintenance vitamin supplement as required
• For vitamin D deficiency - adequate exposure to sunlight

SURGICAL MEASURES N/A

ACTIVITY As tolerated

DIET
• For dietary deficiencies - provide nutritional counseling with emphasis on appropriate foods and the proper methods for their preparation
• Abstain from alcohol

PATIENT EDUCATION
• Refer patients to appropriate social service agencies if socioeconomic factors contribute to deficient diet
• Emphasis on compliance with vitamin supplementation regimens
• Help with alcohol or smoking cessation

MEDICATIONS

DRUG(S) OF CHOICE
• Vitamin A: retinol, carotene, or beta-carotene. Acute deficiencies require aqueous vitamin A solution IM.
• Vitamin B1: oral thiamine 5-30 mg tid depending on deficiency. Acute symptoms: 100 mg IV q day. Maintenance: supplemental B complex vitamin.
• Vitamin B2: oral riboflavin 10-30 mg/day in divided doses until patient response is evident, then decrease to 2-4 mg/day until recovered. May be given IM 5-20 mg/day.
• Vitamin B3: confirmed deficiencies require niacinamide 300-500 mg/day in divided doses by mouth or IV. Supplemental B complex vitamins and dietary increase in foods high in niacin.
• Vitamin B6: oral or parenteral replacement for confirmed deficiency. Prophylactic doses for epileptic children. Women on oral contraceptives may need supplement, pyridoxine 2.5-10 mg po.
• Vitamin B12
  ◊ 100 mg IM - qd x one week
  ◊ 100 mg IM - qd x one month
  ◊ 100 mg IM - qd x lifetime
• Vitamin C (ascorbic acid): daily doses of 100-200 mg in synthetic form or in orange juice for mild scurvy, doses up to 500 mg/day in severe disease
• Vitamin D (cholecalciferol, ergocalciferol): oral doses. For rickets refractory to vitamin D, include 25-hydroxycholecalciferol, active form of vitamin D.
• Vitamin E: oral or parenteral replacement with a water soluble vitamin E supplement, 60-70 units/day for adult, 1 unit/kg/day for children
• Vitamin K1: 10 mg (adult dose) phytonadione (Mephyton) for hypoprothrombinemia given subcutaneously or IM. For non-emergency, give oral dose 5-20 mg. A single dose of 0.5-1 mg IM or SC for newborns.
Contraindications: Refer to manufacturer's literature
Precautions: Refer to manufacturer's literature
Significant possible interactions: Refer to manufacturer's literature

ALTERNATIVE DRUGS
• In Vitamin D deficiency: Calcitriol (Rocaltrol) 0.25 mcg q day, increasing weekly to maintenance of 1 mcg q day (1 mg - 40,000 units)

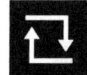

FOLLOWUP

PATIENT MONITORING As needed depending on severity of problem

PREVENTION/AVOIDANCE
• Proper nutrition
• Supplemental vitamins if needed
• Reduce risk factors that lead to deficiency where possible
• Vitamin D deficiency - adequate exposure to sunlight (30 minutes several times a week)
• Postoperative vitamin K for patients are NPO
• Neonates - should receive vitamin K1 IM, subcutaneously or orally to prevent hemolytic disease of the newborn

POSSIBLE COMPLICATIONS
• Vitamin A deficiency - mortality high in advanced cases; eye lesions are a threat to vision
• Vitamin B1 (thiamine) deficiency - cardiac beriberi and Wernicke-Korsakoff syndrome may be fatal if left untreated
• Vitamin B6 chronic deficiency - may increase risk of kidney stone formation
• Vitamin D deficiency - skeletal deformities, greenstick fractures, bone pain
• Excessive synthetic vitamin K may lead to hemolytic anemia and kernicterus in infants

EXPECTED COURSE/PROGNOSIS
With proper diagnosis and adequate therapy, expect full recovery without complications

MISCELLANEOUS

ASSOCIATED CONDITIONS N/A

AGE-RELATED FACTORS
Pediatric:
• Vitamin D deficiency rickets is now rare in the U.S., but may occur in breast-fed infants who do not receive a vitamin D supplement, or in infants fed a formula with a nonfortified milk base
• Vitamin E deficiency in infants usually results from formulas high in polyunsaturated fatty acids that are fortified with iron but not vitamin E
• Vitamin E - seen with severe malabsorption, genetic disorder of abetalipoproteinemias, children with cholestatic liver disease, biliary atresia or cystic fibrosis
• Vitamin K deficiency - common among newborns
Geriatric: More likely to have multiple risk factors that can lead to vitamin deficiencies
Others: N/A

PREGNANCY Women should take a supplemental multivitamin tablet that contains at least 60 mg of elemental iron and 1.0 mg of folic acid

SYNONYMS N/A

ICD-9-CM
269.2 Multiple deficiency
264.9 Vitamin A deficiency
266.9 Vitamin B complex
265.1 Vitamin B1
266.0 Vitamin B2
266.1 Vitamin B6
266.2 Vitamin B12
267 Vitamin C
268.9 Vitamin D
269.1 Vitamin E
269.0 Vitamin K
776.0 Vitamin K deficiency, newborn

SEE ALSO N/A

OTHER NOTES Alcohol withdrawal - initial therapy of alcohol withdrawal should include B vitamins, especially thiamine to avoid causing neurological complications

ABBREVIATIONS N/A

REFERENCES
• Machlin LJ, ed: Handbook of Vitamins. 2nd Ed. New York, Marcel Dekker, 1990
• Shils ME, Young VR, eds: Modern Nutrition in Health and Disease. 7th Ed. Philadelphia, Lea & Febiger, 1988
• Konis AB: Vitamin deficiency in the elderly. NY State Dent J;1991
• Tierney LM, et al: Current Medical Diagnosis & Treatment. 38th Ed. New York, Appleton & Lange, 1999
• Rakel RE: Conn's Current Therapy. Philadelphia, WB Saunders Co, 1997
• Champe PC: Lippincott's Illustrated Review: Biochemistry. 2nd Ed. 1994, Philadelphia, Lippincott Williams & Wilkins
Illustrations: N/A
Internet references: http://www.5mcc.com

Author(s)
Chandramohan Batra, MD

Vitiligo

BASICS

DESCRIPTION An acquired, slowly progressive depigmenting condition in small or large areas of the skin due to the disappearance of previously active melanocytes
• Type A is non-dermatomal and widespread. It represents 75% of cases
• Type B is dermatomal or segmental. It represents the remaining 25% of cases
System(s) affected: Skin/Exocrine
Genetics: Autosomal dominant with variable expression and incomplete penetrance. Positive family history in 30% of cases.
Incidence/Prevalence in USA:
1000-2000/100,000
Predominant age: All ages: 50% begin between ages 10 and 30
Predominant sex: Male = Female

SIGNS AND SYMPTOMS
• Loss of pigment
• Locally increased sunburning
• Predilection for acral areas and around orifices such as eyes, mouth, anus
• Pruritus (10%)
• Premature graying (35%)
• Koebner's phenomenon (aggravation by trauma)

CAUSES Etiology is unclear, but is thought to be an autoimmune reaction to preexisting melanocytes

RISK FACTORS
• Positive family history
• Autoimmune disorders including hemolytic anemia and adrenal insufficiency

DIAGNOSIS

DIFFERENTIAL DIAGNOSIS Any condition that causes acquired hypomelanosis, including tinea versicolor, leprosy, lupus erythematosus, pityriasis alba, atopic dermatitis, albinism, alopecia areata, chemical exposure (phenols, arsenic, chloroquine, hydroquinone) steroid exposure, retinoic acid use, tuberous sclerosis, neurofibromatosis, melanocytic nevi (halo nevi), tumor regression of malignant melanoma, piebaldism, hypopituitarism, hyperthyroidism

LABORATORY Routine blood and urine studies are usually normal in the absence of associated diseases in adults. In children screen for autoimmune diseases with TSH, CBC, and fasting glucose.
Drugs that may alter lab results: N/A
Disorders that may alter lab results: N/A

PATHOLOGICAL FINDINGS Complete absence of melanocytes in skin biopsy. At the margins one may see a few lymphocytes and large melanocytes with abnormal melanosomes.

SPECIAL TESTS N/A

IMAGING N/A

DIAGNOSTIC PROCEDURES
• Examination under Wood's light accentuates the hypopigmented areas, especially in light-skinned individuals
• Skin scraping and a potassium hydroxide (KOH) preparation can be examined microscopically to rule out tinea versicolor

TREATMENT

APPROPRIATE HEALTH CARE
Outpatient except in rare cases of surgical skin-grafting or transplantation

GENERAL MEASURES
• Sun exposure can accentuate the difference between normal and abnormal skin, so for cosmetic reasons patients may wish to avoid this
• Skin dyes and cosmetics may be used as cover-ups (Dermablend or Covermark)

SURGICAL MEASURES N/A

ACTIVITY Full activity

DIET No special diet

PATIENT EDUCATION
• Reassure patient that in absence of associated autoimmune illness the problem is purely cosmetic. Successful cosmetic cover-up is usually quite simple. Some areas offer vitiligo support groups.
• Information available through National Vitiligo Foundation, P.O. Box 6337, Tyler TX 75711; (903)531-0074

Vitiligo

MEDICATIONS

DRUG(S) OF CHOICE
• Localized vitiligo: Begin with a mid-potency steroid cream applied daily for 3-4 months. If no response, advance to high potency steroids. Clobetasol propionate (Temovate) cream applied qd for 2 months (qod on the face). Treatment may be resumed following a 1 to 4 month respite. Alternatively topical psoralens applied in a 1% solution followed in 90 minutes by ultraviolet exposure (UVA). Caution for subsequent exposure to light (sunburn).
• Widespread vitiligo: Oral systemic steroids, e.g., betamethasone 5 mg given 2 days in a row, then held the remainder of the week. This pattern continued for 2-4 months minimizes side effects and is effective in arresting the disease in many patients. Oral trimethylpsoralen or 8-methoxypsoralen (methoxsalen) (Oxsoralen-Ultra) and UVA over a 12-24 month period. Alternatively depigmenting the remaining normal skin with hydroquinone (Benoquin) 20% cream may be elected.
Contraindications:
• Absolute contraindications to use of psoralen compounds: Idiosyncratic reaction to psoralens, photosensitive disease (e.g., systemic lupus erythematosus, albinism, porphyria), invasive squamous cell carcinoma, melanoma, aphakia
• Relative contraindications to use of psoralen compounds: Cardiac disease, hepatic dysfunction, multiple basal cell carcinomas, prior radiation therapy, prior arsenic therapy
Precautions:
• Watch for skin atrophy and telangiectasias when using topical steroids, especially on the face
• Watch for photosensitizers with UVA treatment
• Severe burns possible with topical psoralens. Partially avoided with - 1:10 or 1:50 dilution of psoralens.
• Psoralen plus UVA (PUVA) cannot be used for children less than 12 years of age due to immaturity of the ocular lens
• Patients undergoing PUVA therapy should have a screening ophthalmologic examination to rule out subclinical retinal pigmentary disease that is frequently associated with vitiligo
Significant possible interactions: Other photosensitizers, e.g., tetracyclines and retinoic acid

ALTERNATIVE DRUGS
Patients with unresponsive localized vitiligo may be candidates for minigrafting with or without PUVA therapy

FOLLOWUP

PATIENT MONITORING
• With PUVA therapy, CBC, liver, renal function tests, and an ANA should be done every 6 months.
• With topical steroids, follow at monthly intervals to avoid steroid-atrophy of the skin.

PREVENTION/AVOIDANCE
• While undergoing all therapies, avoid excessive sun exposure

POSSIBLE COMPLICATIONS
• Phototoxic reactions ranging from mild to severe with PUVA
• Skin atrophy and telangiectasias with topical steroids
• Contact dermatitis can occur with use of depigmenting agents and cosmetic covers

EXPECTED COURSE/PROGNOSIS
• Only 5% spontaneously repigment
• Best results are with PUVA therapy where 70% have repigmentation of head and neck area, less in other body areas. Lower percentages respond to topical therapy
• There is no response in at least 20% of cases, especially long-standing cases
• Once repigmentation occurs it usually persists.

MISCELLANEOUS

ASSOCIATED CONDITIONS
• Addison's disease
• Alopecia areata
• Chronic mucocutaneous candidiasis
• Diabetes mellitus
• Hypoparathyroidism
• Melanoma
• Pernicious anemia
• Polyglandular autoimmune syndrome
• Thyroid disorders (hyper- and hypothyroidism) - 30% of patients with vitiligo
• Uveitis
• Halo nevi

AGE-RELATED FACTORS
Pediatric: Childhood vitiligo is a distinct subset of vitiligo. Higher incidence of Type B (segmental) vitiligo. Also higher incidence of autoimmune and endocrine disease. Response is poor to topical PUVA therapy, but can be tried. Topical steroids may be prescribed, e.g., desonide 0.05% cream qDay for 4 months
Geriatric: NA
Others: N/A

PREGNANCY
• Treatment with topical or oral psoralens is contraindicated

SYNONYMS
• Hypomelanosis
• Depigmentation

ICD-9-CM
709.0 Dyschromia

SEE ALSO
• Arsenic poisoning
• Pityriasis alba
• Hyperthyroidism
• Hypothyroidism, adult
• Tinea versicolor

OTHER NOTES
If PUVA therapy considered, dermatologic consultation should be considered

ABBREVIATIONS
CBC = complete blood count

REFERENCES
• Habif T: Clinical Dermatology. 3rd Ed. St Louis, Mosby, 1996
• Fitzpatrick TB, et al: Color Atlas and Synopsis of Clinical Dermatology. 3rd Ed. New York, McGraw-Hill, 1997
• Goldstein A, Goldstein B: Practical Dermatology. 2nd ed. St. Louis, Mosby, 1997.
Illustrations: 5 available on CD-ROM
Internet references: http://www.5mcc.com

Author(s)
Gary J. Silko, MD

Vulvar malignancy

BASICS

DESCRIPTION
• Carcinoma in situ (Bowen's disease). Premalignant changes involving the squamous epithelium of the vulva.
• Squamous cell carcinoma - invasive squamous cell carcinoma is the most common malignancy involving the vulva in 85% of the patients. The malignancy can be well, moderately or poorly differentiated.
• Other invasive cell types include melanoma, Paget's disease, adenocarcinoma, adenocystic carcinoma, small cell carcinoma and sarcomas. Sarcomas are usually leiomyosarcoma and probably arise at the insertion of the round ligament in the labium majus.
System(s) affected: Reproductive
Genetics: No known genetic pattern
Incidence/Prevalence in USA: Invasive vulvar malignancy is a rare gynecologic malignancy accounting for approximately 2,000 new cases per year in the USA
Predominant age:
• In situ disease - mean age, forties
• Invasive malignancy - mean age, sixties with a range of twenties to nineties
Predominant sex: Female only

SIGNS AND SYMPTOMS
• In situ disease - a small raised area associated with pruritus
• Invasive malignancy - an ulcerated, non-healing area; as lesions become large, bleeding occurs with associated pain and foul smelling discharge
• In far advanced diseases - the patients can develop rectal bleeding or urethral obstruction
• Large involved inguinal lymph nodes are also associated with advanced disease

CAUSES
• Patients with cervical cancer are more likely to develop vulvar cancer at a later date. This is due to the so-called field effect with a carcinogen involving the lower genital tract.
• Human papilloma virus (HPV) has been associated with squamous cell abnormalities of the cervix, vagina and the vulva but has not been proven to be the causative agent
• Smoking is associated with squamous cell disease of the vulva possibly from direct irritation of the vulva by the transfer of tars and nicotine on the patient's hands

RISK FACTORS
• Old age. Invasive disease is rarely seen before age forty and the majority of the patients are elderly.
• In situ disease can occur at any age but is rarely seen before the age of twenty-five

DIAGNOSIS

DIFFERENTIAL DIAGNOSIS
• The definitive diagnosis for vulvar lesions is made by biopsy. Infectious processes can present as ulcerative lesions and include syphilis, lymphogranuloma venereum and granuloma inguinale.
• Crohn's disease can present as an ulcerative area on the vulva
• Rarely, lesions can metastasize to the vulva

LABORATORY
• Squamous cell antigen can be elevated with invasive disease
• Hypercalcemia can occur when metastatic disease is present
Drugs that may alter lab results: N/A
Disorders that may alter lab results: N/A

PATHOLOGICAL FINDINGS
• A surgical staging system is used for vulva cancer - TNM Classification = tumor, node, and metastases:
  ◊ T1 - tumor less than or equal to 2.0 cm
  ◊ T2 - tumor greater than 2.0 cm
  ◊ T3 - lower urethra or vagina involved
  ◊ T4 - upper urethra, bladder, or rectum involved
  ◊ N0 - nodes negative
  ◊ N1 - unilateral positive lymph nodes
  ◊ N2 - bilateral positive lymph nodes
  ◊ M0 - no metastatic disease
  ◊ M1 - distant metastatic disease, positive pelvic lymphs node
• International Federation of Obstetrics and Gynecology Classification using TNM:
  ◊ Stage I - T1, N0, M0
  ◊ Stage II - T2, N0, M0
  ◊ Stage III - T1-3, N1, M0; T3, N0-I, M0
  ◊ Stage IVA - T1-3, N2, M0
  ◊ Stage IVB - any T, any N, any M

SPECIAL TESTS   N/A

IMAGING
• Chest x-ray to evaluate for metastatic disease to lungs
• CAT scan to evaluate pelvic lymph node status and periaortic lymph node status

DIAGNOSTIC PROCEDURES
• Office vulvar biopsy; vulvar punch biopsy should be done to establish the diagnosis
• Wide excision can be performed for carcinoma in situ and any lesion where there is doubt should be further excised for definitive diagnosis to insure that invasive disease is not coexistent with the carcinoma in situ
• Cystoscopy and sigmoidoscopy should be performed if there is a question of invasion into the urethra, bladder or rectum

TREATMENT

APPROPRIATE HEALTH CARE
Inpatient for treatment

GENERAL MEASURES
• Radiation therapy is used as adjuvant therapy for patients with positive inguinal lymph nodes
• In advanced malignancy involving the urethra and rectum, concomitant cisplatin/5-FU chemotherapy with radiation produces significant decrease in size of the primary tumor, usually obviating the need for pelvic exenteration

SURGICAL MEASURES
• In situ disease can be treated with wide excision or laser vaporization of the affected area. Laser vaporization is preferable in the younger patient while wide excision is preferable in the elderly patient where the risk of invasive disease is also higher.
• Invasive disease is treated primarily by radical vulvectomy and bilateral groin node dissection
• In selected patients, pelvic lymphadenectomy can be performed. If the pelvic lymph nodes are negative, radiation therapy can be avoided.
• Pelvic exenteration provides effective therapy for advanced or recurrent malignancies involving the bladder or rectum after radiation
• Radical vulvectomy and bilateral groin node dissection can be performed through three separate incisions
• Unilateral lesions can be treated with radical hemivulvectomy and unilateral groin node dissection. These modified techniques provide fewer complications and better cosmetic results.

ACTIVITY   The patients are usually ambulatory and able to resume full activities by six weeks after surgery unless wound breakdown occurs

DIET   Unrestricted, unless undergoing radiation

PATIENT EDUCATION   Two complications are common with radical vulvectomy and bilateral groin node dissection, which is the usual treatment of this disease. In the immediate postoperative period, approximately 50% of patients will experience breakdown of the wound. This requires aggressive wound care by visiting nurses approximately twice a day. The wounds usually will granulate and heal over a period of six to ten weeks. Approximately 15-20% of the patients experience some form of mild to moderate lymphedema after the groin node dissection. The patients should be instructed in use of leg elevation and support hose. Less than 1% of the patients will experience severe debilitating lymphedema.
• American College of Obstetricians & Gynecologists (ACOG), 409 12th St., SW, Washington, DC 20024-2188, (800)762-ACOG

Vulvar malignancy

 MEDICATIONS

DRUG(S) OF CHOICE
• There are no curative drugs
• As an adjuvant therapy, fluorouracil (Efudex) cream for in situ disease can produce occasional results, but the regimen is not well tolerated because of the excoriation and irritation of the vulva. Adjuvant chemotherapy has not proven to be effective in this disease.
• Metastatic disease, especially in the subcutaneous tissues of the leg or abdomen will produce hypercalcemia, which is treated in the usual medical fashion for hypercalcemia
Contraindications: Elderly patients - if chemotherapeutic agents are used, pay close attention to the patient's performance status and ability to tolerate aggressive chemotherapy
Precautions: The usual precautions for chemotherapy agents. Refer to manufacturer's literature.
Significant possible interactions: Refer to manufacturer's literature

ALTERNATIVE DRUGS N/A

 FOLLOWUP

PATIENT MONITORING
• Clinical examination of the groin nodes and vulvar area every 3 months for 2 years, then every 6 months for 3 years
• Chest x-ray should be obtained once a year

PREVENTION/AVOIDANCE
• Any woman complaining of symptoms related to the vulva should have a close examination and biopsies made of appropriate areas
• The vulva can be washed with 3% acetic acid to highlight areas. Areas of white raised epithelium should be biopsied.
• Patients with new onset of pruritus should be biopsied in the area of pruritus
• Liberal biopsy must be used to diagnose in situ disease prior to invasion and to diagnose early invasive disease
• The patient should not be treated for presumed benign conditions of the vulva without full examination and biopsy
• When symptoms persist, reexamination and rebiopsy should be undertaken
• The treatment of benign condyloma of the vulva has not been shown to decrease the eventual incidence of in situ or invasive disease of the vulva

POSSIBLE COMPLICATIONS The major complications from radical vulvectomy and groin node dissection are wound breakdown, lymphedema and urinary stress incontinence

EXPECTED COURSE/PROGNOSIS
• The five year survival is based on stage:
  ◊ Stage I 90%
  ◊ Stage II 85%
  ◊ Stage III 70%
  ◊ Stage IVA 25%
  ◊ Stage IVB 5%

MISCELLANEOUS

ASSOCIATED CONDITIONS
• The patients with invasive vulvar cancer are often times elderly and have associated medical conditions
• High rate of other gynecologic malignancies. Patients should be evaluated for these.

AGE-RELATED FACTORS
Pediatric: N/A
Geriatric:
• Older patients with associated medical problems are at high risk for radical surgery. The surgery, however, is external, usually well-tolerated and is the treatment of choice.
• In the very elderly, palliative vulvectomy provides relief of symptoms for ulcerating symptomatic advanced disease
Others:
• More limited surgery
  ◊ Has been undertaken for invasive lesions especially in young patients to preserve the clitoris and sexual function
  ◊ Radical vulvectomy with groin node dissection through separate incisions provides better cosmetic results than the en bloc technique
  ◊ Radical hemivulvectomy can also be utilized for smaller lesions

PREGNANCY This malignancy is not associated with pregnancy

SYNONYMS
• Bowen's disease
• Vulvar cancer

ICD-9-CM
184.4 Malignant neoplasm of vulva, unspecified

SEE ALSO N/A

OTHER NOTES N/A

ABBREVIATIONS N/A

REFERENCES
• Hopkins MP: Disease of the vulva. In: Willson JR, ed. Obstetrics & Gynecology. St. Louis, C.V. Mosby Co., 1991
• Hopkins MP, Reid GC, Vettrano I, Morley GW: Squamous cell carcinoma of the vulva: Prognostic factors influencing survival. Gynecol Oncol 1991;43:113-7
Illustrations: N/A
Internet references: http://www.5mcc.com

Author(s)
Michael P. Hopkins, MD
Eric L. Jenison, MD

Vulvovaginitis, bacterial

BASICS

DESCRIPTION Infectious disease affecting the vagina, only rarely affecting the vulva
System(s) affected: Reproductive
Genetics: N/A
Incidence/Prevalence in USA: As low as 4% in unselected populations; up to 33% in STD clinics; up to 44% in patients with vaginitis
Predominant age: N/A
Predominant sex: Female

SIGNS AND SYMPTOMS
• Unpleasant vaginal odor, musty or fishy, exacerbated immediately after intercourse
• Thin gray-white vaginal discharge, mildly adherent to vaginal walls
• 10-30% with vaginal/vulvar irritation
• 10% with frothy discharge.

CAUSES
• Polymicrobial; Gardnerella vaginalis, Mobiluncus species, Mycoplasma hominis, Peptostreptococcus, other various anaerobes, including Prevotella, Bacteroides, and Fusobacterium
• There is a shift from a healthy lactobacilli based endogenous flora to an anaerobically based endogenous flora
• Rectal reservoir of organisms leading to autoinfection

RISK FACTORS
• Controversial regarding multiple sexual partners
• IUD

DIAGNOSIS

DIFFERENTIAL DIAGNOSIS
• Gonorrhea
• Chlamydial infection
• Trichomoniasis
• *E. coli* vaginitis
• Staphylococci vaginitis
• Fungal vaginitis
• Trophic vaginitis

LABORATORY
• Affirm VP microprobe
• PH paper (pH > 4.5)
• Wet prep - clue cells in > 10-20% of epithelial cells, fewer WBC's than epithelial cells
• 10% KOH - "whiff test" transient amine or fishy odor
• Gram stain indicating absence of lactobacilli
• May be seen on cytology
• Culture difficult for mycoplasma, not useful
Drugs that may alter lab results: Recent douching
Disorders that may alter lab results: N/A

PATHOLOGICAL FINDINGS Biopsies demonstrate no histologic evidence of inflammation

SPECIAL TESTS N/A

IMAGING N/A

DIAGNOSTIC PROCEDURES N/A

TREATMENT

APPROPRIATE HEALTH CARE
Outpatient

GENERAL MEASURES Consider repletion of lactobacilli

SURGICAL MEASURES N/A

ACTIVITY No restrictions

DIET No restrictions

PATIENT EDUCATION N/A

MEDICATIONS

DRUG(S) OF CHOICE
• Metronidazole 500 mg po bid for 7 days (95% cure) or vaginal gel 5 gm bid for 5 days
• Clindamycin 300 mg bid for 7 days or 2% vaginal cream 5 gm for 7 days
Contraindications: Refer to manufacturer's literature
Precautions: Refer to manufacturer's literature
Significant possible interactions: Metronidazole and alcohol

ALTERNATIVE DRUGS
• Amoxicillin-clavulanate (Augmentin) 500 mg q8h for 7 days
• Cephradine 500 mg q6h for 7 days
• Less effective - ampicillin 500 mg q6h (66% cure rate)
• Consider treating partner, especially in recurrent cases
• Reported in vitro susceptibility to penicillin, erythromycin, chloramphenicol and trimethoprim

FOLLOWUP

PATIENT MONITORING None indicated

PREVENTION/AVOIDANCE
• Good hygiene
• Use of condoms for sexual intercourse

POSSIBLE COMPLICATIONS
• Uncommon but include
  ◊ Adnexal tenderness
  ◊ PID
  ◊ Intrauterine infections
  ◊ Chorioamnionitis
  ◊ Post abortion PID
  ◊ Postpartum endometritis
  ◊ Pelvic abscesses
  ◊ Vaginitis emphysematous
  ◊ Rare extravaginal disease
  ◊ Pre-term labor
  ◊ Premature rupture of membranes
  ◊ Chorioamnionitis
  ◊ Newborn infections, including scalp electrode sites, abscesses, and 1 reported case of meningitis
  ◊ Fetal loss
• Post-hysterectomy infection, septicemia, gaseous crepitation in wound

EXPECTED COURSE/PROGNOSIS
Relapses fairly common, can be decreased by increased colonization of lactobacilli

MISCELLANEOUS

ASSOCIATED CONDITIONS N/A

AGE-RELATED FACTORS
Pediatric: N/A
Geriatric: N/A
Others: N/A

PREGNANCY N/A

SYNONYMS
• Gardnerella vaginosis
• Bacterial vaginosis
• Nonspecific vaginitis
• Haemophilus vaginitis
• Corynebacterium vaginitis

ICD-9-CM
616.10 Vaginitis and vulvovaginitis, unspecified

SEE ALSO
• Abnormal Pap smear

OTHER NOTES N/A

ABBREVIATIONS N/A

REFERENCES
• Ray A, et al: Non-specific vaginitis vis-a-vis Gardnerella vaginalis. J of Communicable Dis 1990;22(4)
• Herbst A, Mishell D Jr, Stenchever A, Droegueller W: Comprehensive Gynecology. 2nd Ed. C.V. Mosby Yearbook, 1992
• Caitlin BW: Garderella vaginalis: Characteristics, clinical considerations and controversies. Clinical Microbiology Review 1992;5(3):213-217
• Kharsany AB, Hosen AA, Vanden Ende J: Antimicrobial susceptibility of Gardnerella vaginalis. Antimicrobial Agents and Chemotherapeutics 1993;37(12):2733-2735
• Reed B, Eyler A: Vaginal infections: Diagnosis and management. Amer Fam Phys 1993;47(8)
• Briselden AM, Hillier SL: Evaluation of affirm VP microbial identification test for Gardnerella vaginalis and trichomonas vaginalis. J Clin Microbiology 1994;32(1):148-152
• Curry SL, Barclay: Benign disorders of the vulva-vagina. In: DeCherry & Perroll, eds. Current Obstetric & Gynecologic Diagnosis & Treatment. 8th Ed. Norwalk, Appleton & Lang, 1994
• Majerone BA: Bacterial vaginosis: An update. American Family Physician 1998;57(6)
Illustrations: N/A
Internet references: http://www.5mcc.com

Author(s)
Elizabeth I McCord, MD, MS

Vulvovaginitis, candidal

BASICS

DESCRIPTION Vulvar pruritus and/or burning, often with abnormal vaginal discharge
System(s) affected: Reproductive, Skin/Exocrine
Genetics: N/A
Incidence/Prevalence in USA:
• 40% of vulvovaginitis is caused by Candida
• 16% of non-pregnant premenopausal women are asymptomatic carriers
Predominant Age: Menarche to menopause
Predominant sex: Female only

SIGNS AND SYMPTOMS
• Intense vulvar itching
• Thick curd-like vaginal discharge
• Dyspareunia at times
• Erythema of vulva
• Erythema, pain and pruritus of crural and perineal area
• Thick white patches appear attached to vaginal mucosa
• Inflamed vulvar skin

CAUSES
Overgrowth of Candida species (C. albicans, C. glabrata, C. tropicalis) in vagina

RISK FACTORS
• Pregnancy
• Diabetes mellitus
• Antibiotic therapy
• Corticosteroid therapy
• Immunosuppressed states
• HIV infection
• Occlusive synthetic underpants and undergarments
• Hypothyroidism
• Oral contraceptive medications (low dose usually not a cause of increased infection risk)
• Anemia
• Zinc deficiency

DIAGNOSIS

DIFFERENTIAL DIAGNOSIS
• Trichomonas vaginitis
• Gonorrheal vaginitis - in prepubertal girls
• Pinworm vaginitis
• Contact dermatitis/vaginitis

LABORATORY
• Yeast, spores, and/or pseudohyphae on smear with 10% KOH solution
• Culture findings on Nickerson's or Sabouraud's media; usually only indicated for recurrent infections
• Vaginal pH < 4.5
Drugs that may alter lab results: N/A
Disorders that may alter lab results: N/A

PATHOLOGICAL FINDINGS N/A

SPECIAL TESTS N/A

IMAGING N/A

DIAGNOSTIC PROCEDURES
• Smear of discharge with 10% KOH solution
• Pap smear

TREATMENT

APPROPRIATE HEALTH CARE
Outpatient

GENERAL MEASURES
• Remove foreign body if one present
• Consider providone iodine douche 15 to 30 mL/L (2 tbsp/qt) of water for symptomatic relief until specific therapy is effective
• If urination causes burning, have the patient
  ◊ Urinate through a tubular device such as a toilet-paper roll or plastic cup with the end cut out
  ◊ Pour warm water over vaginal area while urinating
• Insist on strict diabetic control if patient is diabetic

SURGICAL MEASURES N/A

ACTIVITY
• Avoid overexertion, heat, and excessive sweating
• Delay sexual relations until symptoms clear

DIET Limit sweets (sucrose) and dairy products (lactose) in recurrent infections

PATIENT EDUCATION
• Keep the genital area clean. Use plain unscented soap.
• Take showers rather than tub baths
• Wear cotton underpants with a cotton crotch. Avoid clothing made from non-ventilating materials, including most synthetic underclothing. Avoid tight-fitting jeans or slacks
• Sleep in loose gown without underpants
• Don't sit around in wet clothing - especially a wet bathing suit
• Avoid frequent douches
• Avoid broad-spectrum antibiotics when possible
• After urinating or bowel movements, cleanse by wiping or washing from front to back (vagina toward anus)
• Lose weight, if obese
• American College of Obstetricians & Gynecologists (ACOG), 409 12th St., SW, Washington, DC 20024-2188, (800)762-ACOG

Vulvovaginitis, candidal

MEDICATIONS

DRUG(S) OF CHOICE
• Fluconazole (Diflucan): 150 mg po once
• Miconazole nitrate (Monistat): one suppository q night x 3, or miconazole vaginal cream q night x 7, or
• Butoconazole nitrate (Femstat): vaginal cream q night x 3, or
• Terconazole (Terazol): one suppository or vaginal cream q night x 3, or
• Clotrimazole (Gyne-Lotrimin): two 100 mg tablets intravaginally x 3 days or cream each night x 7 days
Contraindications: N/A
Precautions: Refer to manufacturer's profile of each drug
Significant possible interactions: Refer to manufacturer's profile of each drug

ALTERNATIVE DRUGS
• Retreat with different agent, if recurrence
• Course of oral nystatin; 100,000 units tid for 2 weeks
• Topical gentian violet 1% aqueous solution painted onto vagina weekly until infection resolves (usually 2-3 weeks)
• Boric acid 600 mg in gelatin capsule inserted vaginally daily for 2 weeks.

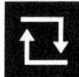

FOLLOWUP

PATIENT MONITORING
Generally no specific followup needed. If symptoms persist, then repeat pelvic exam and culture.

PREVENTION/AVOIDANCE
• Follow instructions under patient education
• For recurrences consider re-infection from sexual partner(s). Examine and treat sex partner for Candida balanitis and oral Candida if vaginitis recurs.
• Review Risk Factors

POSSIBLE COMPLICATIONS
Secondary bacterial infections of the vagina or vulva

EXPECTED COURSE/PROGNOSIS
• Complete cure with vigorous treatment
• Recurrences are common

MISCELLANEOUS

ASSOCIATED CONDITIONS Sexually transmitted diseases

AGE-RELATED FACTORS
Pediatric: Less common before puberty
Geriatric: N/A
Others: N/A

PREGNANCY Common

SYNONYMS
• Monilial vulvovaginitis

ICD-9-CM
112.1 Candidiasis of vulva and vagina

SEE ALSO N/A

OTHER NOTES N/A

ABBREVIATIONS N/A

REFERENCES
• Jones HW, Wentz-Colston A, eds: Novak's Textbook of Gynecology. 11th Ed. Baltimore, Williams & Wilkins Co., 1988
• Kaufman RH, Faro S, (eds: Benign Diseases of the Vulva and Vagina. 4th Ed. St. Louis, Mosby-Year Book, 1994
Illustrations: N/A
Internet references: http://www.5mcc.com

Author(s)
Albert T. Shiu, MD, FACOG

Vulvovaginitis, estrogen deficient

BASICS

DESCRIPTION Decreased blood flow with a thinning and atrophy of the female genital tissue. Changes from estrogen deficiency occur throughout the body. The genital tissues are hormone responsive. Estrogen deficient vulvovaginitis is frequently associated with urinary incontinence.
System(s) affected: Reproductive
Genetics: No known genetic pattern
Incidence/Prevalence in USA: This disorder will affect all women, to some degree, unless estrogen replacement therapy is provided
Predominant age: This is predominantly a problem of the postmenopausal female. The average age of menopause in the United States is 52.5 years.
Predominant sex: Female only

SIGNS AND SYMPTOMS
• Vaginal dryness
• Decreased vaginal secretions
• Dyspareunia
• Vulva undergoes a thinning of the epidermis along with decreased integrity of the supporting structures. The thinning and atrophy often produces pruritus.

CAUSES
• Estrogen deficiency
  ◊ Menopause (surgical or natural)
  ◊ Ovariectomy
  ◊ Radiation of the pelvis

RISK FACTORS
• Estrogen deficient states accompanying metabolic disorders
• Vaginal infections with bacteria and fungi

DIAGNOSIS

DIFFERENTIAL DIAGNOSIS
• Malignancy
• Vulvar dystrophies

LABORATORY
• Cytology for maturation index will show a low maturation index, signifying a decreased turnover of the cells from the decreased estrogen effect
• In the perimenopausal or menopausal female, follicle stimulating hormone (FSH) will be elevated and estradiol will be decreased
Drugs that may alter lab results:
• Estrogen therapy will alter the maturation index
• Digoxin has estrogen-like properties
• Tamoxifen (Nolvadex) can produce menopausal type symptoms but also can act on genital tissues as a weak estrogen agonist. Symptoms can vary.
• Drugs used to treat endometriosis or uterine bleeding such as progestins, Danazol or gonadotropin releasing hormone (GnRH) agonists can produce a pseudomenopause which is reversible
Disorders that may alter lab results: N/A

PATHOLOGICAL FINDINGS Thinning of the cornified squamous layer of both the vulva and the vagina

SPECIAL TESTS N/A

IMAGING N/A

DIAGNOSTIC PROCEDURES
• Examination of the vagina and the vulva for maturation index
• FSH level to confirm menopause
• Estradiol level to evaluate circulating estrogen level

TREATMENT

APPROPRIATE HEALTH CARE
Outpatient

GENERAL MEASURES
• Estrogen replacement therapy (ERT) will alleviate and reverse the symptoms and the thinning of the squamous epithelial layer. Replacement therapy leads to an increased blood supply to the genital tissues.
• Symptomatic relief, if needed, e.g., cool baths or compresses

SURGICAL MEASURES N/A

ACTIVITY No restriction

DIET No special diet

PATIENT EDUCATION
• American College of Obstetricians & Gynecologists (ACOG), 409 12th St., SW, Washington, DC 20024-2188, (800)762-ACOG

Vulvovaginitis, estrogen deficient

MEDICATIONS

DRUG(S) OF CHOICE
• A wide variety of preparations are available:
  ◊ Estrogen, conjugated (Premarin) 0.625 mg daily
  ◊ Estradiol (Estrace) 1 mg daily
  ◊ Estradiol (Estraderm) patch 0.05 mg, changed twice weekly
  ◊ If the uterus is not removed, progesterone should be considered. This can be added as medroxyprogesterone (Provera) 2.5 mg daily or 10 mg for 10 days of each month.
  ◊ Conjugated estrogen vaginal cream (2-4 g/day intravaginally)
Contraindications:
• Estrogen therapy is contraindicated in patients with a history of breast cancer or estrogen positive tumor receptors
• A history of uterine malignancy is a relative contraindication
Precautions: Refer to manufacturer's literature
Significant possible interactions: Refer to manufacturer's literature

ALTERNATIVE DRUGS   N/A

FOLLOWUP

PATIENT MONITORING   The patient should be instructed that symptoms should resolve within 30-60 days. If they do not, reevaluation and reexamination for other causes should be undertaken.

PREVENTION/AVOIDANCE   N/A

POSSIBLE COMPLICATIONS   Those associated with estrogen replacement - postmenopausal bleeding, nausea, headache, libido changes, thrombophlebitis

EXPECTED COURSE/PROGNOSIS
Excellent. The vast majority of symptoms will be relieved with estrogen replacement therapy.

MISCELLANEOUS

ASSOCIATED CONDITIONS   None

AGE-RELATED FACTORS
Pediatric: N/A
Geriatric: N/A
Others: N/A

PREGNANCY   The lactating postpartum woman with high levels of prolactin are in a hypo-estrogenic state. These women should be instructed to use lubrication for symptoms of dyspareunia. The symptoms will resolve when breast-feeding is stopped.

SYNONYMS   N/A

ICD-9-CM
616.10 Vaginitis and vulvovaginitis, unspecified

SEE ALSO   N/A

OTHER NOTES   The obese patient, especially those weighing more than 100 pounds (45 kg) over the ideal body weight, have higher levels of circulating estrogen and thus may have fewer symptoms. (Androstenedione is converted to estrone in peripheral adipose tissue and when there is an abundance of adipose, higher estrone levels are present.)

ABBREVIATIONS   N/A

REFERENCES
• Cunningham FG, MacDonald PC, Gant NF, eds: Williams Obstetrics. 19th Ed. Norwalk CT, Appleton & Lange, 1993
• Novak ER, et al, eds: Novak's Textbook of Gynecology. 11th Ed. Baltimore, Williams & Wilkins, 1988
Illustrations: N/A
Internet references: http://www.5mcc.com

Author(s)
Michael P. Hopkins, MD
Eric L. Jenison, MD

Vulvovaginitis, prepubescent

BASICS

DESCRIPTION Irritation and/or inflammation of the vulva and/or vagina frequently associated with vaginal discharge
System(s) affected: Reproductive, Skin/Exocrine
Genetics: Not well studied
Incidence/Prevalence in USA: Common
Predominant age: Toddlers to menarche
Predominant sex: Female only

SIGNS AND SYMPTOMS
• Irritation and erythema of vulva
• Vaginal discharge
• Offensive odor
• Itching
• Excoriation
• Bleeding

CAUSES
• Most often due to:
  ◊ Poor hygiene
  ◊ Secondary infection elsewhere, e.g., otitis media, pharyngitis
• Most common specific organisms:
  ◊ Group A beta-hemolytic streptococci; Streptococcus pyogenes, Streptococcus pneumoniae
  ◊ E. coli
  ◊ Staphylococcus aureus
  ◊ Hemophilus influenzae
• Less common specific organisms:
  ◊ Pinworms
• Systemic illnesses:
  ◊ Measles
  ◊ Chickenpox
  ◊ Stevens-Johnson syndrome
• Localized vulvar disease:
  ◊ Seborrheic dermatitis
  ◊ Psoriasis
  ◊ Atopic dermatitis
  ◊ Contact dermatitis
  ◊ Lichen sclerosus et atrophicus
• Other:
  ◊ Sexual abuse
  ◊ Other trauma
  ◊ Foreign body
  ◊ Tumors or polyps
  ◊ Masturbation
  ◊ Genital tract malformations

RISK FACTORS
• Co-existing pharyngitis or other systemic conditions
• Faulty hygiene
• Trauma

DIAGNOSIS

DIFFERENTIAL DIAGNOSIS
• Contact dermatitis
• Eczema
• Psoriasis

LABORATORY
• Culture for bacteria, fungi or viruses
• Gram stain
• Tape examination for pinworms
• Potassium hydroxide and saline smears
Drugs that may alter lab results: N/A
Disorders that may alter lab results: N/A

PATHOLOGICAL FINDINGS   N/A

SPECIAL TESTS   Exploration of vagina for foreign body may be necessary in long-standing vaginal discharge

IMAGING   N/A

DIAGNOSTIC PROCEDURES
Visualization of the vagina may be necessary using a nasal speculum or infant laryngoscope. If blood or foul-smelling discharge is present, visualization is mandatory. Place child in knee-chest position for best result. Hold buttocks apart and slightly upward.

TREATMENT

APPROPRIATE HEALTH CARE
Outpatient (except where systemic illness requires hospital care)

GENERAL MEASURES
• Hygiene:
  ◊ Wipe front-to-back after elimination
  ◊ Avoid bubble baths and other irritating products
  ◊ Clean daily with mild soap and water, drying thoroughly with soft towel
  ◊ Apply bland ointments for protection of the skin, if necessary

SURGICAL MEASURES   N/A

ACTIVITY   Normal

DIET   N/A

PATIENT EDUCATION   As noted above under General measures

MEDICATIONS

DRUG(S) OF CHOICE
• For empiric treatment, amoxicillin 20 mg/kg/day for 7 days; in areas of high prevalence of resistant H. flu, amoxicillin-clavulanate (Augmentin) 20 mg/kg/day
• Estrogen deficiency with labial adhesion/agglutination - estrogen, conjugated cream to fused area nightly for two weeks
• Specific organisms on culture:
  ◊ Group A beta-Streptococcus, Streptococcus pneumoniae - penicillin V (Pen Vee K) 25-50 mg/kg/day, maximum of 3 gm/day, divided qid x 10 days
  ◊ H. influenzae - amoxicillin 20-40 mg/kg/day x 7 days; amoxicillin-clavulanate 20 mg/kg/day
  ◊ Staphylococcus aureus - cephalexin 25-50 mg/kg/day, divided qid x 7-10 days or dicloxacillin 12.5-25 mg/kg/day x 7-10 days
  ◊ Candida spp - topical nystatin (Mycostatin), miconazole, clotrimazole or terconazole
Contraindications: Allergy to proposed treatment
Precautions: Avoid potential allergens/topical sensitizers if possible
Significant possible interactions: See manufacturer's profile of each drug

ALTERNATIVE DRUGS Topical corticosteroids for pruritus

FOLLOWUP

PATIENT MONITORING Only if symptoms do not respond to treatment

PREVENTION/AVOIDANCE
• Perineal hygiene
• Avoidance of irritants and tight or occlusive, non-breathable clothing
• White, unscented toilet paper

POSSIBLE COMPLICATIONS Labial agglutination or adhesions

EXPECTED COURSE/PROGNOSIS
Usually clears with appropriate treatment with no permanent sequelae (if not due to underlying disease such as psoriasis, etc.)

MISCELLANEOUS

ASSOCIATED CONDITIONS N/A

AGE-RELATED FACTORS
Pediatric:
• Usual adult vulvitis/vaginitis organisms are rare in the prepubertal child
• Lack of estrogen causing thin vaginal mucosa which is more susceptible to trauma and infection
Geriatric: N/A
Others: N/A

PREGNANCY N/A

SYNONYMS Vaginitis, vulvitis

ICD-9-CM
616.10 Vaginitis and vulvovaginitis, unspecified

SEE ALSO N/A

OTHER NOTES N/A

ABBREVIATIONS N/A

REFERENCES
• Vandeven AM, Emans SJ: Vulvovaginitis in the child and adolescent. Pediatric Rev 1993;14:141
• Pierce AM, Hart CA: Vulvovaginitis: causes and management. Arch Dis Child 1992;67:509-512
• Jones R: Childhood vulvovaginitis and vaginal discharge in general practice. Family Practice 1996;13(4):369-372
Illustrations: N/A
Internet references: http://www.5mcc.com

Author(s)
Janice E. Daugherty, MD

Warts

BASICS

DESCRIPTION Warts are painless, benign skin tumors characterized by an area of well circumscribed epithelial thickening. The DNA papillomavirus is causative and is passed by direct contact with an infected person or from recently shed virus kept intact in a moist, warm environment. Five types of warts are caused by specific genotypes of HPV:
• Common wart (verruca vulgaris)
• Plantar wart (verruca plantaris)
• Flat wart (verruca plana)
• Venereal wart (condyloma acuminatum)
• Epidermodysplasia verruciformis
System(s) affected: Skin/Exocrine
Genetics: N/A
Incidence/Prevalence in USA: 7-10% of the population
Predominant age: Young adults and children
Predominant sex: Female > Male

SIGNS AND SYMPTOMS
• Verruca vulgaris: Rough surfaced, raised, skin-colored papules 5-10 mm in diameter. They may coalesce into a mosaic 1-3 cm in diameter. Most frequently seen on hands.
• Verruca plantaris: Rough surfaced (although smoother than the common wart), flat, skin-colored papules not infrequently attaining 2-3 cm in diameter
• Verruca plana: Slightly elevated, flat-topped, skin-colored papules 1-3 mm in diameter sometimes in a linear arrangement often on hands and face
• Condyloma acuminatum: thin, flexible, tall, papules sometimes demonstrating a confluent growth resembling cauliflower. They do not have the visible or palpable keratin of the previous warts. In infants, laryngeal papillomatosis may occur if condyloma is transmitted during vaginal delivery.
• Epidermodysplasia verruciformis: Flat, reddish lesions on the hands and shoulders presenting in childhood with lifelong persistence

CAUSES Human papillomavirus (HPV)

RISK FACTORS
• AIDS and other immunosuppressive diseases (e.g., lymphomas)
• Immunosuppressive drug use
• Atopic dermatitis
• Locker room use
• Skin trauma

DIAGNOSIS

DIFFERENTIAL DIAGNOSIS
• Corns (on paring, a single "eye" of keratin is observed, whereas a wart shows hemorrhagic spots or "roots")
• Scar tissue
• Molluscum contagiosum (central umbilication and, after curettage, the characteristic pearl)
• Condyloma lata (flat warts of syphilis)
• Seborrheic keratoses

LABORATORY HPV cannot be cultured
Drugs that may alter lab results: N/A
Disorders that may alter lab results: N/A

PATHOLOGICAL FINDINGS
• Papillomavirus found in the nuclei and nucleoli of the stratum granulosum and keratin layers of the epidermis.
• Plantar warts have rete pegs (a downward proliferation of epidermal ridges).
• Thrombosed dermal capillaries

SPECIAL TESTS
Definitive diagnosis can be achieved with the following, but are not clinically relevant for most presentations:
• Electron microscopy
• Immunohistochemical study
• Nucleic acid hybridization

IMAGING N/A

DIAGNOSTIC PROCEDURES Paring or débridement and simple visualization will be diagnostic in most cases.

TREATMENT

APPROPRIATE HEALTH CARE
Outpatient

GENERAL MEASURES Spontaneous remissions are common, probably related to a host immune response. Conservative, non-scarring treatments are preferred. Each treatment is associated with a 60-70% cure rate. Cure is achieved when skin lines are restored to a normal pattern.

SURGICAL MEASURES
• Pretreat with anesthetic cream such as EMLA
• Cryotherapy - often preferred because scar formation is minimized. Freezing periungual warts may result in nail deformation.
• Excision with electrocautery, laser ablation, curettage (the virus may be found in smoke so masks should be worn)
• Disfiguring scars and wart recurrence are problems

ACTIVITY If plantar warts are on weight-bearing surface, they may cause significant discomfort and subsequent decrease in activity

DIET N/A

PATIENT EDUCATION Infectious nature should be discussed; keep warts covered while under treatment to avoid auto-inoculation and transmission to others.

MEDICATIONS

DRUG(S) OF CHOICE
• Benign neglect - safe cost effective treatment option except when warts are extensive, spreading, symptomatic
• Hyperthermia - safe and inexpensive approach; immerse affected area into 45°C water bath for 30 minutes three times per week
• Chemotherapy - all treatments begin by paring the wart, then soaking the area in warm water to moisten the wart
  ◊ Topical retinoids: tretinoin (retinoic acid, Retin-A) for flat warts, less scarring than cryotherapy or surgical approaches; may be best for warts on the face. Apply bid for 4-6 weeks.
  ◊ Lactic-salicylic acid (Duofilm): daily treatment for about 3 months
  ◊ Salicylic acid (Trans-Ver-Sal) in a transdermal delivery system : daily treatment for about 6 weeks
  ◊ Keralyt (salicylic acid in propylene glycol); rub into warts each night
  ◊ Combination cantharidin; 30% salicylic acid, 2% podophyllin, and 19% cantharidin in flexible collodian: apply thin coat, occlude 4-6 hours (or less if painful), then wash off; blisters when form require roof to be removed, base to be debrided, and antibiotic cream applied: multiple applications at 2-4 week intervals
  ◊ Induction of delayed type hypersensitivity with dinitrochlorobenzene or diphencyclopropene, or squaric acid dibutylester: apply 2% solution to light shielded area every 2-3 weeks until sensitivity reaction occurs; then apply lower concentration to affected areas
  ◊ Occlusion - the easiest and least expensive; cover the wart with a waterproof tape and leave on for a week. Remove and leave open for 12 hours then re-tape if wart is still present. The environment under the tape does not foster viral growth. May be the best for periungual warts.
Contraindications: See specific treatments. Vascular insufficiency is a relative contraindication to some treatments.
Precautions: Avoid normal skin when using the topical chemicals
Significant possible interactions: N/A

ALTERNATIVE DRUGS
• Chemotherapy
  ◊ Benzoyl peroxide: apply bid for 4-6 weeks
  ◊ Bleomycin - intradermal injection, is expensive and causes severe pain, but has a 75% cure rate
  ◊ Cimetidine - 30-40 mg/kg divided tid for 3 months. 86% of patients will have partial or complete regression.
  ◊ 24% podophyllin applied weekly to anogenital warts, or 5% podofilox (Condylox) self-applied twice daily for 3 days each week for 1 month
  ◊ Others - dichloroacetic acid, trichloroacetic acid, podophyllin, 5-fluorouracil, silver nitrate, idoxuridine (Herplex Liquifilm), formaldehyde, glutaraldehyde
• Immunotherapy
  ◊ Dinitrochlorobenzene (DNCB) - should be considered a last resort because of side effects and possible mutagenicity
  ◊ Interferon - intralesional for urogenital warts
  ◊ Interferon alpha - systemic for genital warts
  ◊ Interferon beta or gamma - systemic for disseminated verruca vulgaris

FOLLOWUP

PATIENT MONITORING
One third of the warts of epidermodysplasia may become malignant

PREVENTION/AVOIDANCE
• Cover warts under treatment. Avoid the wound fluid after cryotherapy.
• Use personal footwear in locker room settings

POSSIBLE COMPLICATIONS
• Auto-inoculation
• Scar formation
• Chronic pain after plantar wart removal and scar formation
• Nail deformity after injury to nail matrix

EXPECTED COURSE/PROGNOSIS
Good; complete resolution with or without treatment

MISCELLANEOUS

ASSOCIATED CONDITIONS
• Acquired immunodeficiency syndrome
• Renal transplantation
• Other conditions with immunosuppression
• Lewandowsky-Lutz disease (associated with epidermodysplasia)

AGE-RELATED FACTORS
Pediatric: Generally more prevalent in children
Geriatric: Less common in non-immunocompromised adults
Others: N/A

PREGNANCY Podophyllin is contraindicated

SYNONYMS N/A

ICD-9-CM
078.1 viral warts
078.10 Warts, all sites

SEE ALSO
• Condyloma acuminata
• Warts, plantar

OTHER NOTES N/A

ABBREVIATIONS
HPV = Human papillomavirus

REFERENCES
• Bolton RA: Warts. Am Fam Phys 1991;43(6):2049-2056
• Lynch PJ: Dermatology for the House Officer. 3rd Ed. Baltimore, Williams & Wilkins, 1994
• Sams W, et al: Principles and Practices of Dermatology. 2nd Ed. New York, Churchill Livingston, 1996
• Ordoukhanian E: Warts and molluscum contagiosum; beware of treatments worse than the disease. Postgrad Med 1997;2:223-235
• Siegfried EC: Warts on children: an approach to therapy. Ped Annuals 1996;2:79-90
• Gaspari AA, et al: Successful treatment of a generalized human papillomavirus infection with granulocyte-macrophage colony-stimulating factor and interferon gamma immunotherapy in a patient with a primary immunodeficiency and cyclic neutropenia. Arch of Dermatol 1997;133(4):491-96
Illustrations: 12 available on CD-ROM
Internet references: http://www.5mcc.com

Author(s)
Barbara J. Moront, MD
Jeffrey B. Kessler, MD

Warts, plantar

BASICS

DESCRIPTION Discrete or grouped firm keratotic masses on the sole of the foot initiated by a viral infection of keratinocytes
System(s) affected: Skin/Exocrine
Genetics: Unknown
Incidence/Prevalence in USA: Widespread; 2000/100,000
Predominant age: Any age, although more common in children and young adults
Predominant sex: Female > Male (slightly)

SIGNS AND SYMPTOMS
• Foot pain
• Discrete or grouped masses on sole of foot with disruption of normal skin markings
• Rough, hyperkeratotic surface with brown-black dots (thrombosed capillaries)
• Callus formation
• Leg or back pain (distortion of posture)

CAUSES Human papillomaviruses, types 1, 2 and 4

RISK FACTORS
• AIDS
• Atopic dermatitis
• Lymphomas
• Patient taking immunosuppressive drugs

DIAGNOSIS

DIFFERENTIAL DIAGNOSIS
• Corns (clavi)
• Calluses
• Black heel (ruptured capillaries)

LABORATORY N/A
Drugs that may alter lab results: N/A
Disorders that may alter lab results: N/A

PATHOLOGICAL FINDINGS Acanthotic epidermis with hyperkeratosis, papillomatosis, and parakeratosis

SPECIAL TESTS N/A

IMAGING N/A

DIAGNOSTIC PROCEDURES
• Inspection usually confirms the diagnosis
• If cannot distinguish between callus and wart, can examine with a magnifying lens. The wart should demonstrate a highly organized mosaic pattern.

TREATMENT

APPROPRIATE HEALTH CARE
• Outpatient cryotherapy at weekly intervals
• Repeated parings at weekly intervals with or without use of a keratolytic is also an option. Most successful appears to be curettage and chemical cautery (with phenol or trichloroacetic acid) or light electrocautery. (Note: extreme care must be exercised with this procedure because excessive cautery or curettage can cause a painful scar.)

GENERAL MEASURES
• If warts are asymptomatic, no treatment is necessary. However patient may be at risk for spread of warts.
• Warm soaks followed by patient's paring of the top layer of skin on repeated occasions may speed disappearance
• Patient may use pumice stone, emery board or a blade
• Over-the-counter keratolytics containing salicylic acid may help. The advised procedure is paring of skin followed by warm soaks, and finally application of a few drops of keratolytic.
• Hyperthermia - hot water immersion (113°F) 1/2-3/4 hour 2-3 times per week for 16 treatments is effective for some patients
• Other measures include use of a heel bar or appropriate padding to relieve pressure points where warts tend to aggregate

SURGICAL MEASURES
• Cryotherapy - application of liquid nitrogen is often effective. It usually requires at least 4 applications at weekly or biweekly intervals. Aggressive cryotherapy may cause blistering or even scarring, so light applications are preferred.
• Blunt dissection - a simple surgical procedure is effective and usually nonscarring. It requires inserting a blunt dissector between the wart and normal skin and separating the wart using short, firm stroke.
• CO_2 laser surgery - used for recalcitrant warts

ACTIVITY Ambulatory unless warts or treatment is painful

DIET No special diet

PATIENT EDUCATION
• In Epsteln: Common Skin Disorders, patient instructions, pages 123 (see References)
• Griffith: Instructions for Patients, Philadelphia, W.B. Saunders Co.
• American Academy of Dermatology (708)330-0230

MEDICATIONS

DRUG(S) OF CHOICE
No effective antiviral wart medications currently exist. Keratolytics (over-the-counter or prescription) and a variety of chemotherapeutic acids may be used.
- Salicylic acid - see General Measures for instructions
- 40% salicylic acid plasters - available as Mediplast. It is supplied in 3 by 4 inch sheets which are cut to the size of the wart and the sticky surface applied to the wart. They are removed every 1 to 2 days, the white keratin peeled and a fresh plaster applied.
- Chemotherapy, dichloroacetic acid and trichloroacetic acid kits are available. Callus is pared and the surrounding skin is protected by a ring of petrolatum. The wart(s) are coated with acid which is then worked into the wart with a sharp toothpick. Procedure should be repeated at weekly intervals.
- Transdermal salicylates (Trans-Plantar)
- Vesicants containing cantharidin (Cantharone, Verrusol)

Contraindications: Infection, vascular insufficiency

Precautions:
- If the dermis is damaged with any of the above procedures, a scar may result which can be permanently painful
- Care should be taken to avoid excessive contact with normal skin when using keratolytics or chemotherapy
- Avoid bleomycin treatment during pregnancy

Significant possible interactions: N/A

ALTERNATIVE DRUGS
- Bleomycin injected intralesionally q 2 weeks

FOLLOWUP

PATIENT MONITORING
With any treatment modality, followup weekly

PREVENTION/AVOIDANCE
Use rubber footwear in communal shower areas

POSSIBLE COMPLICATIONS
- Scarring with overly aggressive treatment
- A rare type of verrucous carcinoma, epithilioma cuniculatum, is thought to arise from these warts

EXPECTED COURSE/PROGNOSIS
The course of plantar warts is like that of other varieties of warts, i.e., highly variable. Most resolve spontaneously in weeks to months.

MISCELLANEOUS

ASSOCIATED CONDITIONS N/A

AGE-RELATED FACTORS
Pediatric: Duration of warts is generally shorter in children than in adults
Geriatric: N/A
Others: N/A

PREGNANCY
- Avoid beomycin treatments

SYNONYMS Verruca plantaris

ICD-9-CM
078.19 Viral warts, other specified

SEE ALSO
- Warts
- Condyloma acuminata

OTHER NOTES N/A

ABBREVIATIONS N/A

REFERENCES
- Epstein E: Common Skin Disorders. 4th Ed. Philadelphia, W.B. Saunders Co., 1994
- Fitzpatrick T, et al: Color Atlas and Synopsis of Clinical Dermatology. 3rd Ed. New York, McGraw-Hill, 1997
- Habif T: Clinical Dermatology. 3rd Ed. St Louis, Mosby, 1996

Illustrations: 2 available on CD-ROM
Internet references: http://www.5mcc.com

Author(s)
Gary J. Silko, MD

Wegener's granulomatosis

BASICS

DESCRIPTION A multisystem disease characterized by granulomatous vasculitis involving multiple organs. The characteristic "triad" of involvement includes the upper airway (otitis, sinusitis, nasal mucosa), lung, and kidney. Other organ systems involved include skin, joints, nervous system (peripheral or central).
• As the condition progresses untreated, upper airway erosions, necrotic pulmonary nodules, and renal failure are common, and, without treatment, mortality rate is high
System(s) affected: Cardiovascular, Pulmonary, Renal/Urologic, Gastrointestinal, Nervous, Skin/Exocrine
Genetics:
• Increased presence in HLA-B8
• Increased presence in HLA-DR2
Incidence/Prevalence in USA: Incidence estimated at approximately 0.4/100,000; prevalence 3/100,000
Predominant age: Mean age of onset in mid-40's, but has been described in all age groups
Predominant sex: Male > Female (3:2)

SIGNS AND SYMPTOMS
• Pulmonary infiltrates (71%)
• Sinusitis (67%)
• Arthralgia/arthritis (44%)
• Fever (34%)
• Cough (34%)
• Otitis (25%)
• Rhinitis (22%)
• Hemoptysis (18%)
• Ocular inflammation (16%)
• Weight loss (16%)
• Skin rash (13%)
• Epistaxis (11%)
• Renal failure (11%)
• Chest pain, anorexia, proptosis, dyspnea, oral ulcers, hearing loss, headache (all < 10%)

CAUSES No known etiology. Autoimmune phenomena and immune complex deposition in arterial walls are implicated as pathogenetic factors. Triggering infectious agents, yet unidentified, may be involved.

RISK FACTORS None identified

DIAGNOSIS

DIFFERENTIAL DIAGNOSIS
• Infectious otitis and sinusitis (bacterial or fungal)
• Midline granuloma or other upper airway malignancy
• Relapsing polychondritis
• Fungal or tuberculous pulmonary infections, (Goodpasture's syndrome)
• Other vasculitic syndromes (including polyarteritis nodosa, lymphomatoid granulomatosis, Churg-Strauss vasculitis, and overlap vasculitis syndromes)
• Any disease associated with necrotizing and crescentic glomerulonephritis, sarcoidosis

LABORATORY
• Anemia, leukocytosis, and thrombocytosis common during active phases of disease
• Erythrocyte sedimentation rate (ESR) usually markedly elevated (75%)
• Rheumatoid factor present in low to moderate titer in up to 50%
• Hematuria and/or cellular casts with moderate range proteinuria
• Renal insufficiency, mild to moderate at first, but frequently progresses to end-stage renal disease
Drugs that may alter lab results: Corticosteroids and cytotoxic drugs, used to treat the disease, may cause normalization of most abnormal laboratory findings
Disorders that may alter lab results: See disorders listed under Differential Diagnosis

PATHOLOGICAL FINDINGS
• Upper airways: Granulomatous inflammation frequently seen, although not specific unless showing actual vasculitis
• Lung: Granulomatous arteritis involving vessels of all sizes, classically medium-sized arteries
• Kidney: Necrotizing and crescentic glomerulonephritis without immunofluorescent staining (pauci-immune) is common, granulomatous vasculitis rarely seen
• Skin: Vasculitic lesions, from leukocytoclastic vasculitis of small vessels; granulomatous arteritis seen occasionally

SPECIAL TESTS
Antibodies to neutrophilic cytoplasmic antigens with a cytoplasmic pattern of staining (c-ANCA) are detected in a majority (60-90%) of patients. Such pattern of staining is highly specific (90+%) for this diagnosis. A similar finding, with perinuclear staining (p-ANCA), is nonspecific, but frequently seen in patients with other vasculitic syndromes or isolated necrotizing glomerulonephritis.

IMAGING
• Upper airways: Chronic otitis and sinusitis, often with evidence of erosion into bony structures - seen on plain x-rays
• CT scans of sinuses useful in demonstrating mucosal and bony involvement
• Lungs: X-rays show nodular pulmonary densities, often with central necrosis and cavitation. Local infiltrates, or more diffuse interstitial involvement also described, as are radiographic findings of pulmonary hemorrhage.

DIAGNOSTIC PROCEDURES
• Renal biopsy may give findings consistent with diagnosis, although not always definitive
• Sinus or upper airway mucosal biopsy often helpful, although findings are often nonspecific
• Open lung biopsy most likely to confirm granulomatous arteritis
• Diagnosis best made by demonstration of granulomatous arteritis of involved organ, although compatible renal lesion in setting of chronic destructive sinusitis and/or pulmonary nodules can be used to make a presumptive diagnosis
• A positive serologic test for c-ANCA in proper clinical setting felt to be diagnostic by many

TREATMENT

APPROPRIATE HEALTH CARE
• Patients are usually ill enough with fever, sinus or pulmonary involvement, or renal disease to require hospitalization for diagnostic tests (to rule out infectious causes) and appropriate biopsies
• An occasional patient can be managed as an outpatient

GENERAL MEASURES Careful attention to upper airway drainage, and supportive measures for pulmonary, renal, or neurologic involvement

SURGICAL MEASURES N/A

ACTIVITY No specific restrictions. Fatigue, fever, and weight loss usually limit activity.

DIET Vigorous nutritional support may be needed early in illness

PATIENT EDUCATION Nutritional and drug counseling when patient is able to return home

MEDICATIONS

DRUG(S) OF CHOICE
• Prednisone - given initially in high doses (60-100 mg/day). After initial 2-4 weeks may be tapered to alternate-day regimen. Then gradually discontinued over 2-6 months in most patients, depending on clinical course.
• Cyclophosphamide - in critically ill patient, may be given initially at a dose of 4 mg/kg/day IV for 2-3 days, then continued at 2 mg/kg/day orally. In stable patient, may be started at 2 mg/kg/day orally. Dosage may need to be adjusted, based on patient response and toxicity (usually bone marrow suppression). Usually continued for 1-2 years after patient felt to be in remission, and tapered slowly, with careful monitoring for re-activation of disease.

Contraindications: No absolute contraindications, although diabetes, hypertension, metabolic bone disease are relative contraindications to prednisone

Precautions:
• Careful monitoring if taking corticosteroids
• Consider reducing dose of cyclophosphamide in patient with baseline leukopenia, renal insufficiency

Significant possible interactions:
• Prednisone may interfere with hypoglycemics, anti-hypertensives
• Cyclophosphamide may increase risk of other drugs with potential for bone marrow toxicity

ALTERNATIVE DRUGS
• Azathioprine: in patients with history of severe bone marrow toxicity or hemorrhagic cystitis from cyclophosphamide
• Trimethoprim-sulfamethoxazole (TMP-SMX) has been used alone with success in some patients with limited (usually upper airway) disease, and has some potential as adjunctive therapy with prednisone and cyclophosphamide
• Methotrexate: in some patients without renal involvement and may be useful in maintaining remission in patients with stable disease, as an alternative to chronic cyclophosphamide therapy

FOLLOWUP

PATIENT MONITORING
• Early, careful monitoring of upper airway, pulmonary, and renal manifestations for response to therapy
• Monitor blood pressure, glucose, potassium for steroid effects
• Frequent (every 2-4 weeks) CBC with differential to monitor for bone marrow toxicity from cyclophosphamide. Leukopenia most common. Dose needs to be reduced if peripheral WBC < 3000/ mm3.
• Monitor urinalysis for potential of hemorrhagic cystitis from cyclophosphamide. Consider cystoscopy for persistent or recurrent hematuria, especially later in course of treatment.

PREVENTION/AVOIDANCE
• Calorie and salt reduction in patients on prednisone
• High fluid intake to prevent hemorrhagic cystitis from cyclophosphamide
• Give cyclophosphamide dose in morning to decrease amount of drug present overnight in bladder.

POSSIBLE COMPLICATIONS
• Disease related
◊ Destructive nasal lesions with "saddle nose" deformity
◊ Deafness from refractory otitis
◊ Necrotic pulmonary nodules with hemoptysis
◊ Interstitial lung disease
◊ Renal failure
◊ Foot drop from peripheral nerve disease
◊ Skin ulcers, digital and limb gangrene from peripheral vascular involvement
• Drug related
◊ Prednisone - weight gain, hyperglycemia, hypertension, hypokalemia, skin thinning and bruising, infection, osteoporosis
◊ Cyclophosphamide - bone marrow suppression (especially leukopenia, neutropenia), alopecia, hemorrhagic cystitis, mucosal membrane irritation, sterility and premature gonadal failure, secondary malignancies (especially leukemias) with long term therapy. Risk of bladder cancer is 5% (10 years) and 16% (15 years) after first treatment, and is related to previous cystitis.

EXPECTED COURSE/PROGNOSIS
• Without treatment, almost uniformly fatal with 10% 2 year survival and mean survival of 5 months
• With aggressive treatment, survival improved to 75-90% at 5 years
• Treatment-related toxicity is significant, especially from long-term cyclophosphamide. After 1-2 years of disease-free interval, cyclophosphamide is usually tapered, although some patients demonstrate disease re-activation during this phase.

MISCELLANEOUS

ASSOCIATED CONDITIONS None

AGE-RELATED FACTORS
Pediatric: N/A
Geriatric: N/A
Others: N/A

PREGNANCY
• Rarely reported. Pregnancy should be considered only when patient is disease-free and off therapy.
• Cyclophosphamide often causes sterility and is potentially teratogenic

SYNONYMS N/A

ICD-9-CM 446.4 Wegener's granulomatosis

SEE ALSO
• Polyarteritis nodosa
• Goodpasture's syndrome, pulmonary component
• Goodpasture's syndrome, renal component

OTHER NOTES N/A

ABBREVIATIONS
• c-ANCA = antibodies to neutrophilic cytoplasmic antigens with cytoplasmic staining pattern
• p-ANCA = antibodies to neutrophilic cytoplasmic antigens with perinuclear staining pattern

REFERENCES
• Hoffman GS, et al: Wegener's granulomatosis: an analysis of 158 patients. Ann of Intern Med 1992;115:488-498
• Hoffman GS: Editorial-Treatment of Wegener's granulomatosis: time to change the standard of care? Arthritis Rheum 1997;40:2099-2104
• Nolle B, et al: Anticytoplasmic autoantibodies: Their immunodiagnostic value in Wegener's granulomatosis. Ann Intern Med 1989;111:28
• Lieberman KV, Churg A: Wegener's granulomatosis. In: Churg A, Churg J, eds. Systemic Vasculitides. New York, Igaku-Shoin, 1991
• Rao JK, et al: The role of antineutrophil cytoplasmic antibody (c-ANCA) testing in the diagnosis of Wegener's granulomatosis. Ann Int Med 1995;123:925-932
Illustrations: 1 available on CD-ROM
Internet references: http://www.5mcc.com

Author(s)
Christopher M. Wise, MD

Williams syndrome

BASICS

DESCRIPTION
Williams syndrome is an unusual multisystem neurodevelopmental disorder typified by characteristic craniofacial features, mild microcephaly, mild to moderate mental retardation with a distinctive cognitive-behavioral profile, connective tissue abnormalities, growth retardation, supravalvular aortic stenosis, peripheral pulmonary stenosis, renal artery stenosis, limited joint movement and transient hypercalcemia. Its occurrence is sporadic, although familial autosomal dominant cases have been infrequently reported. The phenotypic expression is somewhat varied and associated with a hemizygous microdeletion of 114-250 kb in the 7q11.23 region which includes the elastin (ELN) and LIM-kinase (LIMK) gene.

System(s) affected: Musculoskeletal, Nervous, Renal/Urologic, Cardiovascular, Endocrine/Metabolic

Genetics: The pattern of occurrence is nearly always sporadic and observed in both sexes, although there are several reported cases of familial transmission as an autosomal dominant mutation.

Incidence/Prevalence in USA: Affected individuals have been estimated at 1:20,000 live births

Predominant age: Life-long condition

Predominant sex: Male=Females

SIGNS AND SYMPTOMS
• The signs and symptoms observed in the classic case of WS may be diagnostic but the clinical presentation is somewhat varied
• Early childhood: Global developmental delay albeit with seemingly normal speech and expressive language
◊ Hyperacusis
◊ Characteristic craniofacial features
- Elfin-like facial appearance
- Medial eyebrow flare and stellate irises
- Wide mouth
- Long flat philtrum
- Upturned nose with a flat nasal bridge
- Dental anomalies
◊ Characteristic clinical features
- Supravalvar aortic stenosis
- Peripheral pulmonary stenosis
- Renal artery stenosis
- Infantile hypercalcemia
- Growth retardation and short stature
- Slender limbs and trunk
◊ Characteristic cognitive/behavioral features
- Weakness in abstract/visual reasoning
- Highly developed expressive language skills
- Low levels of daily living skills
• Postpubertal males and females
◊ Characteristic clinical features
- Hypertension
- Lordosis and/or limited joint movement
◊ Characteristic behavioral features
- Anxiety
- Depression and suicidal ideation

CAUSES
Microdeletion in the 7q11.23 region

RISK FACTORS
Possible familial transmission as an autosomal dominant mutation

DIAGNOSIS

DIFFERENTIAL DIAGNOSIS
• Infantile hypercalcemia
• Supravalvar aortic stenosis and/or peripheral pulmonary stenosis
• Elfin-like craniofacial features
• Growth retardation
• Developmental delay
• Mild microcephaly

LABORATORY
Molecular-genetic (DNA) evaluation is the diagnostic test of choice and can determine the size of the deletion
Drugs that may alter lab results: N/A
Disorders that may alter lab results: N/A

PATHOLOGICAL FINDINGS
N/A

SPECIAL TESTS
Affected individuals require cognitive, behavioral, psychological and educational evaluations to develop individual education programs

IMAGING
N/A

DIAGNOSTIC PROCEDURES
N/A

TREATMENT

APPROPRIATE HEALTH CARE
Affected individuals will generally need life-long adult supervision. Early intensive educational intervention and behavior modification should be implemented.

GENERAL MEASURES
• Early detection will permit early intervention and intensive behavioral training
• Treatment for hypercalcemia by controlling dietary intake of calcium and vitamin D
• Ophthalmological evaluations are recommended for visual acuity
• Preventive dentistry to reduce risk of malocclusion
• Continual monitoring of cardiovascular anomalies and for hypertension
• Filtered ear protection for hyperacusis

SURGICAL MEASURES
Treatment for aortic, pulmonary or renal artery stenoses if needed

ACTIVITY
Full activity unless cardiovascular stenoses are problematic

DIET
For hypercalcemia, control intake of calcium and vitamin D

PATIENT EDUCATION
• The patient and family should receive genetic evaluation and counseling
• Patient and family should contact the WSA Office, Box 297, Clawson, MI 48017, (248) 541-3630, or e-mail tmonkaba@aol.com

MEDICATIONS

DRUG(S) OF CHOICE Medication for hypertension and for hyperparathyroidism.
Contraindications: N/A
Precautions: N/A
Significant possible interactions: N/A

ALTERNATIVE DRUGS N/A

FOLLOWUP

PATIENT MONITORING Regular pediatric care and general health maintenance with particular attention to endocrine, renal and cardiovascular function

PREVENTION/AVOIDANCE Genetic counseling and evaluation, especially among high-functioning patients, about pregnancies. Prenatal diagnosis is available.

POSSIBLE COMPLICATIONS
• Learning problems, especially in abstract/visual reasoning
• Behavioral problems concerning indifference to personal safety
• Post-pubescent anxiety and depression
• Risk of cardiovascular disease and/or renal dysfunction

EXPECTED COURSE/PROGNOSIS
• Individuals may need life-long supervision
• Life span may be affected by renal dysfunction; or, hypertension resulting from supravalvar stenosis and/or peripheral pulmonary stenosis

MISCELLANEOUS

ASSOCIATED CONDITIONS
• Developmental delay
• Growth retardation
• Cardiovascular dysfunction
• Renal dysfunction
• Attention deficit disorder (ADD)
  ◊ Frequently associated with neuropsychological dysfunction
  ◊ Treatment for ADD is similar to methods used in the general population

AGE-RELATED FACTORS
Pediatric: Infantile hypercalcemia
Geriatric: N/A
Others: N/A

PREGNANCY Patient and family should receive genetic evaluation and counseling as prenatal diagnosis is available

SYNONYMS
• Williams-Beuren syndrome
• Fanconi type idiopathic infantile hypercalcemia

ICD-9-CM
758.9 conditions due to anomaly of unspecified chromosome

SEE ALSO
• Hyperparathyroidism
• Hypertension, essential
• Mental retardation
• Down syndrome
• Fragile X syndrome
• Attention deficit hyperactivity disorder

OTHER NOTES N/A

ABBREVIATIONS
ADD = attention deficit disorder

REFERENCES
• Anderson PE, Rourke BP: Williams Syndrome. In: White BP (ed): Syndrome of Nonverbal Learning Disabilities. New York, Guilford Press, 1995
• Bellugi U, Wang PP, Jernigan TL: Williams Syndrome: An Unusual Neuropsychological Profile. In Broman SH, Grafman J (eds.) Atypical Cognitive Deficits in Developmental Disorders: Implication for Brain Function. Hillsdale NJ, Lawrence Earlbaum Associates, 1994
Illustrations: N/A
Internet references: http://www.5mcc.com

Author(s)
Gene S. Fisch, PhD

Wilms' tumor

BASICS

DESCRIPTION An embryonal renal neoplasm containing blastema, stromal or epithelial cell types usually affecting children before the 5th year.

System(s) affected: Renal/urologic

Genetics: Several congenital anomalies are known to be associated with Wilms' tumor. A two stage mutational model has been proposed: occurrence in either hereditary form or sporadic form. Patients with aniridia have a deletion of the short arm of chromosome 11 (11p13).

Incidence/Prevalence in USA: 0.69/100,000 people in the U.S. 8 cases/100,000 children under 15 year of age.

Predominant age: Median age of 36.5 months

Predominant sex: Female > Male (1.1 : 1)

SIGNS AND SYMPTOMS
- Usually asymptomatic
- Palpable upper abdominal mass
- Abdominal pain
- Fever
- Anemia
- Rarely, signs of acute abdomen with free intraperitoneal rupture
- Cardiac murmur
- Hepatosplenomegaly
- Ascites
- Prominent abdominal wall veins
- Varicocele
- Gonadal metastases

CAUSES
- Hereditary or sporadic forms of genetic mutation
- Familial form: autosomal dominant trait with incomplete penetrance (1%)
- Potential of paternal occupational exposure (machinists, welders, motor vehicle mechanics, autobody repairmen)

RISK FACTORS
- Aniridia (600 times greater than normal risk)
- Hemihypertrophy (100 times greater than normal risk)
- Cryptorchidism
- Hypospadias
- Duplicated renal collecting systems
- Wiedemann-Beckwith syndrome
- Drash's syndrome
- Klippel-Trenaunay syndrome
- Familial occurrence
- Paternal occupation (see Causes)

DIAGNOSIS

DIFFERENTIAL DIAGNOSIS
- Neuroblastoma
- Hepatic tumors
- Sarcoma
- Rhabdoid tumors

LABORATORY
- Urinalysis (occasional hematuria)
- CBC (anemia)
- LDH
- Plasma renin (rarely helpful)
- Urine catecholamines

Drugs that may alter lab results: N/A
Disorders that may alter lab results: N/A

PATHOLOGICAL FINDINGS
- Favorable findings (mortality of 7%)
  - ◊ Bulky lesion, well-encapsulated
  - ◊ Focal areas of hemorrhage and necrosis
  - ◊ Absence of anaplasia and sarcomatous cell types
  - ◊ Presence of blastema, stomal and epithelial elements
- Unfavorable histology (mortality rate of 57%)
  - ◊ Anaplasia - markedly enlarged and multipolar mitotic figures 3-fold enlargement of nuclei in comparison with adjacent similar nuclei, hyperchromasia of enlarge nuclei. Anaplasia may be diffuse or focal.
  - ◊ Sarcomatous changes - are now considered to be separate from Wilms, not subtypes. (Mortality of 64%)
- Nephroblastomatosis
  - ◊ Considered premalignant

SPECIAL TESTS N/A

IMAGING
- Chest x-ray
- KUB (presence of linear calcifications)
- Abdominal ultrasound - gives best information about extension into IVC
- CT (with IV and oral contrast) of chest and abdomen
- IVP rarely helpful

DIAGNOSTIC PROCEDURES
Occasionally bone marrow aspiration necessary to distinguish from neuroblastoma

TREATMENT

APPROPRIATE HEALTH CARE
- In-patient work-up and treatment until stable postoperative and induction chemotherapy completed

GENERAL MEASURES
- Chemotherapy
- Radiation therapy in Stage II, unfavorable histology, Stage II and Stage IV

SURGICAL MEASURES
- Examination (visual and manual) of contralateral kidney
- Radical nephroureterectomy and biopsies as needed to provide precise staging information
- Sampling of any enlarged lymph nodes
- Identification of any retained tumor with titanium clips.
- Tumor should be given to pathologist fresh, not on formalin
- Vertical midline incision if tumor extension to right atrium present (possible use of cardiopulmonary bypass)
- With bilateral Wilms' tumors, biopsy, then chemotherapy and 2nd look operation 6 weeks to 6 month later for partial bilateral nephrectomy if possible

ACTIVITY As tolerated

DIET No special diet

PATIENT EDUCATION
- Patient and family teaching regarding long-term outlook
- Possibility of second malignancy
- Side effects of chemotherapy, radiation therapy

Wilms' tumor

MEDICATIONS

DRUG(S) OF CHOICE
- Dactinomycin (actinomycin-D)
- Vincristine
- Doxorubicin
- Cyclophosphamide (Cytoxan)

Contraindications: Refer to manufacturer's literature
Precautions: Refer to manufacturer's literature
Significant possible interactions: Refer to manufacturer's literature

ALTERNATIVE DRUGS
- Doxorubicin (Adriamycin)
- Cyclophosphamide

FOLLOWUP

PATIENT MONITORING
- Multidrug chemotherapy every 3-4 weeks for 16 weeks - 15 months depending on stage
- Every 4 months for 1 year, every 6 months for 2nd - 3rd year, yearly after that
- CBC, CT chest and abdomen with each visit

PREVENTION/AVOIDANCE   N/A

POSSIBLE COMPLICATIONS
- 1-2% will develop second malignant neoplasms (leukemia, lymphoma, hepatocellular carcinoma, soft tissue sarcoma)
- High risk of low birth weight infants, perinatal mortality in offspring of female survivors of Wilms' tumor
- Chest is usual site of recurrence

EXPECTED COURSE/PROGNOSIS
- With favorable histology, 91% survival
- With diffuse anaplasia, 20% survival
- With focal anaplasia, 64% survival
- Staging
  ◊ I - tumor limited to kidney, completely excised
  ◊ II - Tumor extends beyond kidney, completely excised
  ◊ III - Residual non-hematogenous tumor confined to abdomen (lymph nodes positive, spillage of tumor, peritoneal implants, extension beyond resection region)
  ◊ IV - Hematogenous metastases
  ◊ V - Bilateral renal involvement

MISCELLANEOUS

ASSOCIATED CONDITIONS   See risk factors

AGE-RELATED FACTORS   Occurs only in children
Pediatric: N/A
Geriatric: N/A
Others: N/A

PREGNANCY   N/A

SYNONYMS
- Nephroblastoma

ICD-9-CM
189.0 Malignant neoplasm of kidney

SEE ALSO   N/A

OTHER NOTES
- Mesoblastic nephroma - distinguished only by histology. Age usually under 6 months. Essentially benign although metastases have been reported; tends to be locally invasive. Operative spillage may lead to recurrence. No chemotherapy or radiotherapy needed with complete excision.
- Nephroblastomatosis - considered premalignant; may present as nodularity as one or both kidneys; treated with biopsy and local excision (renal tissue sparing)

ABBREVIATIONS   N/A

REFERENCES
- Ashcraft KW, Holder TM: Pediatric Surgery. 2nd Ed. Philadelphia, W.B. Saunders Co., 1993
- Shochat SJ: Wilms' Tumor: Diagnosis and Treatment in the 1990's. Seminars in Pediatric Surgery 1993;2(1):59-68
- O'Neill JA, Rowe MI, Grosfeld JL, et al: Pediatric Surgery. 5th ed., St Louis, Mosby, 1998

Illustrations: N/A
Internet references: http://www.5mcc.com

Author(s)
Timothy L. Black, MD, FACS, FAAP

Wiskott-Aldrich syndrome

BASICS

DESCRIPTION Males affected by this rare x-linked genetic disorder display combined immunodeficiency, microcytic thrombocytosis and eczema leading to life threatening infections and bleeding complications. Average life span is 11 years. The syndrome has variable expression. XLT is a related but milder form with mostly platelet defects.
System(s) affected:
Hemic/Lymphatic/Immunologic, Skin/Exocrine
Genetics:
• Family history in >60%
• X-Linked recessive trait
• WASP and XLT genes located at X/11.22
  ◊ Codes for cytoplasmic protein that signals cell membrane structure changes required for activation of blood cells
Incidence/Prevalence in USA: 1 in 4 million live male births
Predominant age: Onset at birth, most diagnosed by 24 months
Predominant sex: Male > Female
• Rarely females develop WAS
  ◊ Some carriers express disease
  ◊ Other have different but related gene defect

SIGNS AND SYMPTOMS
• Neonatal:
  ◊ Excessive bleeding from circumcision
  ◊ Bloody diarrhea
  ◊ Petechiae and purpura
• Childhood:
  ◊ Eczema with secondary skin infections
  ◊ Recurrent bacterial infections
  ◊ Viral infections
  ◊ Hepatosplenomegaly
  ◊ Autoimmune vasculitis and hemolytic anemia

CAUSES
• Hematopoietic cells express WASP
  ◊ Defective WASP fails to organize membrane activation
  ◊ Membranes don't form normal actin cytoskeletons
  ◊ Altered motility and inability to change cell shapes inhibits normal functions
• Platelets are intrinsically abnormal
  ◊ Accelerated destruction, sequestered in spleen
• T cells show decreased responsiveness to antigens
• B cells show abnormal antibody production

RISK FACTORS
• Family history of WAS
• History of congenital defects

DIAGNOSIS

DIFFERENTIAL DIAGNOSIS May be difficult in infancy before immune changes present
• ITP other causes of TCP
• Severe Atopic Disease
• Acute lymphoblastic anemia
• Other causes of immunodeficiency
  ◊ SCID, HIV
• Leukemias or marrow aplasias

LABORATORY
• Platelets abnormal at birth
  ◊ <30,000, MPV 2/3 normal
• B cell and T cell changes over time
  ◊ WBC count fall by age 6
  ◊ Low IgM, Normal IgG, High IgA and IgE
  ◊ Decreased response to capsular antigens
  ◊ Low CD 8 counts in 61%
  ◊ Decreased delayed hypersensitivity responses
  ◊ Decreased mitogenic responses
Drugs that may alter lab results:
Antibiotics
Disorders that may alter lab results:
Infections

PATHOLOGICAL FINDINGS
• Hyperplasia of lymphoreticular system
• Vasculitic changes with multiple thromboses of small arterioles of kidney, lung, pancreas, brain

SPECIAL TESTS
• Genetic testing for WASP
• Carrier identification

IMAGING Not helpful

DIAGNOSTIC PROCEDURES Bone marrow aspiration to exclude leukemia and aplastic conditions and to HLA type for bone marrow transplantation.

TREATMENT

APPROPRIATE HEALTH CARE
• Inpatient for acute infections
• No live virus vaccination

GENERAL MEASURES
• HLA typed bone marrow transplant restores all abnormalities with an 85% cure rate
• Crossmatched platelets
• Irradiated, CMV negative blood products
• Aggressive antibiotic therapy for infections
• Prophylactic antibiotics

SURGICAL MEASURES
• Splenectomy can transiently improve TCP but increases the risk of infection

ACTIVITY
• Plan activities to help normal development
• Avoid contact sports and prevent head injuries
• Avoid crowds

DIET No special diet

PATIENT EDUCATION
• Patient/parent counseling to cope with disease and outcome
• Genetic testing and counseling for family

MEDICATIONS

DRUG(S) OF CHOICE
- Immunoglobulin infusions
- Prophylactic penicillin after splenectomy
- Antibiotics as indicated by culture
- Topical steroids for eczema
- Parenteral steroids, vincristine or plasmapheresis for autoimmune complications

Contraindications: Refer to manufacturer's literature

Precautions: Corticosteroids in immunosuppressed patients. Refer to manufacturer's literature

Significant possible interactions: Refer to manufacturer's literature

ALTERNATIVE DRUGS N/A

FOLLOWUP

PATIENT MONITORING As needed for therapy, monitor for infections, for progression of disease, complications

PREVENTION/AVOIDANCE
- Genetics counseling
  ◊ Identify carriers
  ◊ Prenatal diagnosis

POSSIBLE COMPLICATIONS
- Severe infections especially after splenectomy
- Hemorrhage, cerebral common
- Malignancies (lymphoreticular, leukemia, Kaposi's)
- Nephropathy
- Autoimmune disease in 40% can be aggressive
- Malabsorption syndrome

EXPECTED COURSE/PROGNOSIS
- Usual course is acute and chronic infections with progressive decrease in immune status.
- Average life expectancy is 11 years with more living past twenty with bone marrow transplant. Transplant therapy can restore all abnormalities. Causes of death have been infection (50%), bleeding (27%), malignancies (12%).

MISCELLANEOUS

ASSOCIATED CONDITIONS
- Lymphomas, brain is primary site in 50%, nephropathy, other lymphoreticular tumors

AGE-RELATED FACTORS
Pediatric:
- Onset at birth
- First year infections with encapsulated bacteria: respiratory, meningitis, sepsis
- Later infections occur with opportunistic organisms and virus

Geriatric: None have survived this long

Others: N/A

PREGNANCY N/A

SYNONYMS
- Aldrich syndrome
- Eczema-TCP
- Immunodeficiency-2

ICD-9-CM
279.12 Wiskott-Aldrich syndrome

SEE ALSO
Idiopathic thrombocytopenic purpura
Leukemia
Immunodeficiency diseases

OTHER NOTES N/A

ABBREVIATIONS
- WAS = Wiskott-Aldrich syndrome
- XLT = x linked thrombocytopenia
- WASP =Wiskott-Aldrich syndrome protein
- TCP = thrombocytopenia
- SCID = severe combined Immunodeficiency

REFERENCES
- Ochs HD: The Wiskott-Aldrich Syndrome. Seminars In Hematology 1998;35(4):332-45
- Brickell PM, Katz DR, Thrasher AJ: Wiskott-Aldrich syndrome: current research concepts. British J of Haematol 1998;101(4):603-08
- Mamlok RJ: Primary immunodeficiency disorders. Allergy and Immunology 1998;25(4):739-58.
- Kuska B: Wiskott-Aldrich syndrome is a "wonderful mystery". J National Cancer Institute 1996;88(18):1258-61
- Litzman J, Jones A, Hann I, Chaper H, Strobel S,Morgan G: Intraveneous immunoglobulin, splenectomy, and antibiotic prophylaxis in Wiskott-Aldrich syndrome. Archives of Dis in Childhood 1996;75(5):436-39

Illustrations: N/A

Internet references: http://www.5mcc.com

Author(s)
Patricia Borman, MD

Zinc deficiency

BASICS

DESCRIPTION Constellation of growth retardation, hypogonadism, cell mediated immune dysfunction, and skin changes related to decreased zinc
System(s) affected: Endocrine/Metabolic, Skin/Exocrine, Nervous
Genetics: Usually acquired, but rarely acrodermatitis enteropathica (autosomal recessive) and associated with sickle cell anemia (autosomal recessive)
Incidence/Prevalence in USA: Unknown
Predominant age: All ages, most often adolescent
Predominant sex: Male = Female

SIGNS AND SYMPTOMS
• Mild deficiency
 ◊ Hypogeusia
 ◊ Decreased dark adaptation
 ◊ Decreased lean body mass
• Moderate deficiency
 ◊ All of the above
 ◊ Diarrhea
 ◊ Growth retardation
 ◊ Hypogonadism (especially male)
 ◊ Mental lethargy
 ◊ Anergy
 ◊ Rough skin
 ◊ Delayed wound healing
 ◊ Glucose intolerance
 ◊ Impaired cell mediated immunity
• Severe deficiency
 ◊ All of the above
 ◊ Bullous pustular dermatitis
 ◊ Weight loss
 ◊ Dwarfism
 ◊ Emotional instability
 ◊ Tremors
 ◊ Ataxia
 ◊ Alopecia
 ◊ Death

CAUSES
• Increased requirements
 ◊ Pregnancy
 ◊ Lactation
 ◊ Rapid growth phase of childhood
 ◊ Burns
 ◊ Major trauma
• Increased losses
 ◊ Diabetes
 ◊ Cirrhosis
 ◊ Renal disease
 ◊ Malabsorption states, e.g., inflammatory bowel diseases
 ◊ Sickle cell anemia
• Decreased absorption
 ◊ Acrodermatitis enteropathica, an autosomal recessive deficiency in the enzyme required for intestinal absorption
 ◊ Geophagia
 ◊ Chelating agents
 ◊ Parasitism
 ◊ Diet high in phytates

• Insufficient dietary intake
 ◊ Vegetarianism
 ◊ Parenteral hyperalimentation without supplementation
 ◊ Breast feeding
 ◊ Suboptimal zinc conditions in diet (rare)
 ◊ Alcoholism

RISK FACTORS
• High milk consumption
• Low socioeconomic status

DIAGNOSIS

DIFFERENTIAL DIAGNOSIS
• Congenital dwarfism
• Failure to thrive in infants
• Primary hypogonadism
• Mental retardation

LABORATORY
• Plasma zinc levels decreased (in moderate to severe zinc deficiency)
• Erythrocyte or leukocyte zinc levels more adequately assess tissue stores, but these are more costly and not widely available
• Hair or fingernail zinc levels not useful
Drugs that may alter lab results: N/A
Disorders that may alter lab results: N/A

PATHOLOGICAL FINDINGS N/A

SPECIAL TESTS N/A

IMAGING N/A

DIAGNOSTIC PROCEDURES N/A

TREATMENT

APPROPRIATE HEALTH CARE
Outpatient

GENERAL MEASURES N/A

SURGICAL MEASURES N/A

ACTIVITY Full activity

DIET
• Balanced omnivorous diet
• Avoid excessive intake of foods with high phytate content, (e.g., cereals)

PATIENT EDUCATION Dietary consultation

MEDICATIONS

DRUG(S) OF CHOICE
• Zinc gluconate or zinc sulfate 25-50 mg po qd for 6-9 months
• 4-6 mg of elemental zinc qd added to hyperalimentation in adult patient, may increase to 12 mg qd if suspect ongoing heavy zinc losses, e.g., burns or major trauma
• In pediatric patients, 0.02-0.04 mg zinc/kg/day in hyperalimentation
• Prenatal vitamins with minerals during pregnancy and lactation to prevent deficiency
Contraindications: None
Precautions: Avoid large (> 20 mg elemental zinc) parenteral doses
Significant possible interactions: N/A

ALTERNATIVE DRUGS   N/A

FOLLOWUP

PATIENT MONITORING   Clinical status such as improved outlook, weight gain, resolution of symptoms

PREVENTION/AVOIDANCE
• Adequate diet
• Supplementation when indicated (see Medications)

POSSIBLE COMPLICATIONS   N/A

EXPECTED COURSE/PROGNOSIS
Immediate improvement in clinical status. Full resolution of signs and symptoms.

MISCELLANEOUS

ASSOCIATED CONDITIONS
• Sickle cell anemia
• Pregnancy and lactation
• Alcoholism
• Malabsorption
• Parenteral hyperalimentation
• In the older patient, diabetes, cirrhosis, those taking diuretics

AGE-RELATED FACTORS
Pediatric: Zinc deficiency may cause failure to thrive, impair growth and development of secondary sexual characteristics
Geriatric:
• Zinc deficiency may cause poor night vision leading to falls; poor wound healing or chronic skin ulcer; loss of taste which may cause worsening nutrition
• Elderly persons living in institutions may have low zinc intake
Others: N/A

PREGNANCY   Requirements increase; deficiency may cause spontaneous abortion, inadequate weight gain

SYNONYMS   N/A

ICD-9-CM
269.3 Mineral deficiency, NEC
686.8 acrodermatitis enteropathica

SEE ALSO
• Alcoholism
• Acrodermatitis enteropathica
• Failure to thrive (FTT)
• Anemia, sickle cell

OTHER NOTES   N/A

ABBREVIATIONS   N/A

REFERENCES
• Tasman-Jones C: Disturbances of trace mineral metabolism. In: Wyngaarden JB, et al, eds. Cecil Textbook of Medicine. 19th Ed. Philadelphia, W.B. Saunders Co., 1992
• Ronaghy H: World Review Nutr. Diet 1987:54
Illustrations: 3 available on CD-ROM
Internet references: http://www.5mcc.com

Author(s)
Clyde L. Harris, MD

Zollinger-Ellison syndrome

BASICS

DESCRIPTION
- A triad of
  ◊ Marked elevated gastric acid secretion
  ◊ Peptic ulcer disease
  ◊ A gastrinoma or non-beta islet cell tumor of the pancreas or duodenal wall which produces gastrin
- Gastrinomas (at time of diagnosis) may be single or multiple (1/2-2/3), large or small, benign or malignant (2/3), sporadic (70-75%) or associated with multiple endocrine neoplasia (MEN 1)(25-30%)

System(s) affected: Gastrointestinal, Endocrine/Metabolic

Genetics: 25-30% occur in association with the MEN 1 syndrome

Incidence/Prevalence in USA: 1 per million per year

Predominant age: Middle age (30-65)

Predominant sex: Male>Female (3:2)

SIGNS AND SYMPTOMS
- Abdominal pain >80%
- Epigastric pain
- Reflux esophagitis
- Vomiting unresponsive to standard therapy
- Diarrhea including while fasting 40-70%
- Peptic ulcer disease
- Weight loss
- Hepatomegaly with metastasis
- Steatorrhea
- Endoscopic findings including esophagitis, duodenal ulceration with multiple ulcers and prominent gastric and duodenal folds
- Complications of severe peptic ulcer disease including hemorrhage, perforation and obstruction
- Signs of MEN 1 including those of hypercalcemia hyperparathyroidism and Cushing's syndrome.

CAUSES
Gastrinoma equally distributed between the head of the pancreas and the first or second portion of the duodenum. May also be found rarely in the mesentery, peritoneum, spleen, skin or mediastinum (possibly metastasis with primary not identified).

RISK FACTORS
- MEN 1
- Family history of ulcer disease

DIAGNOSIS

DIFFERENTIAL DIAGNOSIS
- Elevated serum gastrin with hypochlorhydria/achlorhydria
  ◊ Atrophic gastritis
  ◊ Drug induced
  ◊ Gastric cancer
  ◊ Pernicious anemia
  ◊ Postvagotomy

- Elevated serum gastrin with normal or increased gastric acid
  ◊ Antral G-cell hyperfunction
  ◊ Chronic renal failure
  ◊ H. pylori infection
  ◊ Gastric outlet obstruction
  ◊ Retained gastric antrum
- Consider gastrinoma in all patients with:
  ◊ Recurrent or refractory ulcer disease
  ◊ Gastric hypertrophy and ulcers
  ◊ Duodenal and jejunal ulcers
  ◊ Ulcers and diarrhea
  ◊ Ulcers and kidney stones
  ◊ Hypercalcemia and ulcers
  ◊ Pituitary disease
  ◊ Family history of ulcer disease or endocrine tumors suggestive of MEN 1

LABORATORY
- Elevated serum gastrin-fasting (>1000 pg/mL with ulcers diagnostic, >200 pg/mL with ulcers suggestive)
- Elevated basal gastric acid output >15 mEq/hr (>15 mmol/hr)
- Elevated maximal acid output >150 mEq/hr
- Gastric pH <2.0 with elevated gastrin
- Check serum calcium, phosphorous, cortisol and prolactin (to R/O MEN 1)

Drugs that may alter lab results: H2 blockers and proton pump inhibitors may increase gastric pH

Disorders that may alter lab results: N/A

PATHOLOGICAL FINDINGS
- 90% of gastrinomas found in gastric triangle (borders are bile duct, junction of 2nd and 3rd portion of duodenum, junction of head and body of pancreas)
- Almost 50% in head of pancreas
- Almost 50% in wall of 1st or 2nd portion of duodenum (more likely to be small, solitary)
- 2/3 malignant in both sites (defined by behavior not histology)
- 50% of gastrinomas stain positive for ACTH, VIP, insulin or neurotensin (in decreasing order of incidence)
- 1/3 of patients have metastasis on presentation with regional nodes>liver>bone. More rarely seen metastasis to peritoneum, spleen, skin and mediastinum.
- Duodenal, jejunal and gastric ulcers which are often multiple
- Gastric and duodenal mucosal fold thickening
- Hyperplasia of antral gastrin producing cells
- Histology similar in appearance to carcinoid

SPECIAL TESTS
- Preferred test is secretion stimulation test-gastrin level increases > 200 pg/mL (>200 ng/L)
- Gastric secretory studies - basal and maximal acid outputs (after pentagastrin)
- Alternative test is calcium infusion test-gastrin level increases > 400 pg/mL (test less specific and is more dangerous because of IV calcium infusion)

IMAGING
- Used to localize tumor for possible resection
- Abdominal CT scan (finds 30-38% of primaries and 42-70% of liver metastases)
- Abdominal ultrasound (finds 20% of primaries and 46% of liver metastases)
- Abdominal angiography (finds 40-50% of primaries)

- Selective venous sampling of gastrin from portal venous tributaries (28% of primaries and 62% of liver metastases)- sensitivity increased by administering secretin before sampling
- Abdominal MRI (finds 30-45% of primaries and 70-90% of liver metastases)
- Somatostatin receptor scintigraphy (finds 70% of primaries and 92% of liver metastases)
- Somatostatin receptor scintigraphy is most sensitive, combining with CT or MRI and angiography will find around 75% of primaries
- Sella turcica imaging can help if MEN 1 suspected to look for pituitary tumors

DIAGNOSTIC PROCEDURES
Endoscopy may see tumors in duodenal wall, multiple ulcers including jejunal ulcers and prominent gastric and duodenal folds.

TREATMENT

APPROPRIATE HEALTH CARE
- Advise daily care based on symptoms
- Appropriate surveillance of basal gastric acid output to monitor anti acid secretory therapy
- Appropriate surveillance postoperatively to look for metastasis

GENERAL MEASURES
- Advanced imaging initially to assess for possible resection
- Surgical removal when primary can be identified and as an adjunct for symptom control
- Medical treatment for symptom control when primary not found or metastasis present on diagnosis

SURGICAL MEASURES
- Laparotomy to search for resectable tumors unless have liver metastasis on presentation or MEN 1
- Definitive therapy-removal of gastrinomas when found (surgery finds 95% of tumors, 5 year cure 30% when all can be removed)
- Total gastrectomy was formerly used to stop acid production before pharmacologic therapy available, now seldom done
- Vagotomy in some patients will reduce acid secretion and improve therapeutic effect of medication. May allow decrease dose of medication.
- In MEN 1 parathyroidectomy by lowering calcium may decrease acid production and decrease antisecretory drug use. Gastrinomas generally benign but multiple and not usually cured by surgery.

ACTIVITY
As tolerated

DIET
Restrict foods whioch aggravate symptoms

PATIENT EDUCATION
Inform as to nature of disease and prognosis

MEDICATIONS

DRUG(S) OF CHOICE
• General guidelines
◊ Heal 80-85% of ulcers
◊ While medications heal ulcers, they nearly always recur. While doses may be adjusted, need to plan on life long medication use.
◊ Dosages frequently exceed usual doses for treatment of ulcers by 4-8 fold. Start at lower recommended dose below and titrate up to resolution of symptoms or maximum listed below.
◊ If hyperparathyroidism present because of MEN 1, must correct hypercalcemia.
◊ Proton pump inhibitors first line treatment. May need to add H2 blockers.
• Proton pump inhibitors
◊ Omeprazole 60-120 mg/d
◊ Lansoprazole 60-180 mg/d (doses>120 mg need to be divided bid)
• H2 blockers
◊ Cimetidine 300 mg q6h, up to 1.25-5.0 gm/day
◊ Ranitidine 150 mg q 12 hrs, up to 6 gm/day
◊ Famotidine 20 mg at bedtime up to 800 mg/day
Contraindications:
• Known hypersensitivity to the drug
• H2-blockers-androgen effects, drug interactions due to Cytochrome P-450 stimulation
• Omeprazole-none
• Lansoprazole-none
Precautions:
• Adjust doses for renal and geriatric patients depending on drug
• Gynecomastia reported with high dose cimetidine (>2.4 gm/d)
Significant possible interactions: Refer to the drug manufacturer's literature.

ALTERNATIVE DRUGS
• Chemotherapy regimes of streptozocin, 5-fluorouracil and doxorubicin show only limited response
• Interferon and octreotide show even more limited response

FOLLOWUP

PATIENT MONITORING
• Usual close follow-up necessary after any surgery, in addition need to monitor over time for evidence of metastasis
• Careful dose titration needed of medical therapy to control symptoms
• Gastric acid analysis to maintain basal gastric acid output to <10 mEq/hr (<2 mEq/hr if have complications such as perforation or esophagitis)

PREVENTION/AVOIDANCE Screen first degree relatives of patients with MEN 1

POSSIBLE COMPLICATIONS
• Complications of peptic ulcer disease (bleeding, perforation, obstruction)
• 2/3 of gastrinomas are malignant with metastasis
• Other substances may be produced by the tumor such as ACTH (5-8% of patients) with resulting Cushing's syndrome

EXPECTED COURSE/PROGNOSIS
• Overall survival rate- 5 year=62-75%, 10 year=47-53%
• Prognosis improves if complete surgical removal of tumor possible
• If liver metastasis present on initial surgery, 5 year survival 30-40%, 10 year 25%

MISCELLANEOUS

ASSOCIATED CONDITIONS
• MEN 1: hyperparathyroidism, prolactinomas, other pituitary tumors
• Insulinoma
• Carcinoid tumors

AGE-RELATED FACTORS
Pediatric: There are cases reported in teenagers which are very aggressive.
Geriatric: Consider diagnosis in patient with persistent or recurring peptic ulcer disease. Is less aggressive disease if appears after 65 years.
Others: N/A

PREGNANCY Cases reported. Influences medication choices and surgical timing.

SYNONYMS
• Z-E syndrome
• Pancreatic ulcerogenic tumor syndrome
• Multiple endocrine neoplasia, partial
• Ulcerogenic islet cell tumor

ICD-9-CM
251.5 Zollinger-Ellison syndrome (other codes based on related diagnosis)

SEE ALSO N/A

OTHER NOTES N/A

ABBREVIATIONS
• MEN = multiple endocrine neoplasia
• ACTH = adrenocorticotropic hormone
• VIP = vasoactive intestinal polypeptide

REFERENCES
• Friedman LS, Peterson WL: Zollinger-Ellison syndrome (Gastrinoma). In: Fauci AS, Braunwald E, Isselbacher KJ, Wilson JD, et al (eds0: Harrison's Principles of Internal Medicine 14th Ed. Vol.2. New York, McGraw-Hill, Inc., 1998:1613-1615
• Alexander H, Fraker, et al: Prospective study of somatostatin receptor scintigraphy and its effect on operative outcome in patients with Zollinger-Ellison syndrome. Annuls of Surgery 1998;228:2 228-38
• Termanini B, Gibril F, et al: Value of somatostatin receptor scintigraphy: a prospective study in gastrinoma of its effect on clinical management. Gastroenterology 1997;112(2):335-47
• Feldman M: Peptic ulcer disease. In Dale DC, Federman DD (eds): Scientific American Medicine. New York, Scientific American, Inc., 1997;4:II:3,8
• Jensen RT: Zollinger-Ellison syndrome. In Bennett JC, Plum F, eds. Cecil Textbook of Medicine. 20th Ed. Philadelphia, W.B. Saunders Co,. 1996:674-676
Illustrations: N/A
Internet references: http://www.5mcc.com

Author(s)
Douglas S. Parks, MD

Short
Topics

Acanthosis nigricans

DESCRIPTION A circumscribed melanosis consisting of a brown pigmented velvety verrucosity or fine papillomatosis appearing in the axillae and other body folds. Occurs in association with endocrine disorders, underlying malignancy, administration of certain drugs, or as in inherited disorder. Usual course - chronic.

CAUSES
• congenital
• associated with malignant disease
• obesity
• idiopathic

TREATMENT
• treat underlying cause
• malignancy workup

ICD-9-CM
701.2 acquired acanthosis nigricans

 Acoustic neuroma

DESCRIPTION A tumor arising from Schwann cells of the 8th cranial nerve (most often the vestibular division, rather than the acoustic division). Neurofibromatosis type II strongly predisposes patients to acoustic neuromas. Symptoms include unilateral hearing loss and other neurologic findings when the tumor compresses the cerebellum, pons, or facial nerve.

SYNONYMS
• Acoustic schwannoma

CAUSES
• Unknown

TREATMENT
• Surgical excision

ICD-9-CM
225.1 (M9560/0) Benign neoplasm of cranial nerves

 Acquired adrenogenital syndrome

DESCRIPTION A condition of adults that is acquired or congenital in which excessive output of adrenal androgenic hormones causes virilization. The effects depend on age. Usual course - chronic; progressive.

CAUSES
• androgen producing tumors
• adrenal adenoma
• adrenal adenocarcinoma

TREATMENT
• surgery

ICD-9-CM
255.2 adrenogenital disorders

 Acrodermatitis enteropathica

DESCRIPTION Previously fatal disorder resulting from malabsorption of zinc. Characteristics: psoriasiform dermatitis, hair loss, paronychia, diarrhea, and growth retardation. Symptoms begin in infants just after weaning.

SYNONYMS
• Danbolt-Closs syndrome
• Brandt syndrome

CAUSES
• zinc deficiency
• defective zinc absorption

TREATMENT
• oral elemental zinc

ICD-9-CM
686.8 acrodermatitis enteropathica

 Acromegaly

DESCRIPTION A disorder due to excessive secretion of pituitary growth hormone, characterized by progressive enlargement of the head and face, hands and feet, and thorax. Usual course - progressive.

SYNONYMS
• Acromegalia
• Eosinophilic adenoma syndrome

CAUSES
• growth hormone excess from pituitary adenoma

TREATMENT
• transsphenoidal resection
• heavy particle irradiation
• radiotherapy
• bromocriptine

ICD-9-CM
253.0 acromegaly and gigantism

 Actinomycosis of the kidney

DESCRIPTION Infectious bacterial disease that appears in 4 clinical forms - abdominal, cervicofacial, thoracic, and generalized. The generalized form can involve the kidneys as well as other organs. Characteristics - back pain, lethargy, weight loss, fever, hematuria. Usual course - acute.

CAUSES
• retrograde infection by actinomyces israelii

TREATMENT
• antibiotics
• drainage

ICD-9-CM
039.2 abdominal actinomycotic infection

 Actinomycosis of the thorax

DESCRIPTION Infectious bacterial disease affecting the thorax and lungs. It also occurs in three other forms that include abdominal, cervicofacial and generalized. Usual course - progressive.

CAUSES
• actinomyces infection
• oral commensal
• aspiration of infected material
• impaired consciousness
• alcoholism

TREATMENT
• prolonged antibiotic therapy
• surgical drainage of suppurative lesions

ICD-9-CM
039.1 actinomycosis, thoracic

 Adenocarcinoma of the bladder

DESCRIPTION Malignant growth in the bladder with characteristic hematuria, dysuria, urinary frequency, weight loss and suprapubic mass. Usual course - progressive.

CAUSES
• cystitis glandularis
• exstrophy of the bladder

TREATMENT
• segmental bladder resection
• total cystectomy

ICD-9-CM
188.9 malignant neoplasm of bladder, part unspecified

 Adenocarcinoma of the colon

DESCRIPTION The colon and rectum account for more new cases of cancer each year than any other site, exclusive of the lung. The incidence increases with age and peaks at 60-75. Characteristics - melena, diarrhea, rectal mass, iron deficiency anemia. Usual course - progressive.

CAUSES
• familial polyposis
• chronic ulcerative colitis
• possibly low fiber, high fat diet
• granulomatous colitis

TREATMENT
• surgery
• radiotherapy
• palliative chemotherapy

ICD-9-CM
153.9 malignant neoplasm of colon, unspecified

Hyperbilirubinemia, physiologic neonatal

DESCRIPTION A mild, transient physiological hyperbilirubinemia of unconjugated (indirect) type occurring in the normal neonate.

SYNONYMS
• icterus neonatorum
• hyperbilirubinemia in the newborn

CAUSES
• fetal hemolysis
• inadequate bilirubin conjugation
• prematurity

TREATMENT
• phototherapy

ICD-9-CM
774.6 transient neonatal jaundice

 Hyperhidrosis

DESCRIPTION Excessive perspiration due to over-activity of the sweat glands. Distribution - general or confined to palms, soles, axillas, inframammary region, groin. Symptoms include skin maceration, fissuring, scaling. A bad odor may be produced by decomposition of sweat and cellular debris resulting from yeast and bacteria infection.

CAUSES
• various skin diseases, such as pyogenic or fungal infections, contact dermatitis, fever, hyperthyroidism, central nervous system disorders, psychogenic

TREATMENT
• bromhidrosis (malodorous exudate). Treat with soap containing chlorhexidine. Apply aluminum chlorhydroxy complex after bathing.
• treat any uncovered underlying cause
• localized hyperhidrosis - treat with nighttime applications of aluminum chloride in absolute ethyl alcohol. Cover with polyethylene films if possible. Wash applications away next morning.

ICD-9-CM
780.8 hyperhidrosis

 Hyperthermia, malignant

DESCRIPTION Autosomal inherited condition occurring in patients undergoing general anesthesia. Characteristics - sudden, rapid temperature rise, tachycardia, tachypnea, sweating, cyanosis, muscle rigidity. Usual course - acute.

SYNONYMS
• fulminating hyperpyrexia
• malignant hyperpyrexia

CAUSES
• general anesthesia
• sukamethonium
• succinylcholine
• halothane
• duchenne muscular dystrophy

TREATMENT
• cooling
• cessation of anesthesia
• correct acidosis
• dantrolene
• mannitol

ICD-9-CM
995.89 hyperpyrexia, malignant, due to anesthetic

 Hyphema

DESCRIPTION Hemorrhage within the anterior chamber of the eye. Usual course - acute; recurrent.

CAUSES
• traumatized iris roof
• traumatized stromal vessels
• spontaneous bleeding

TREATMENT
• strict bed rest
• keep upright
• binocular patching
• mydriatics
• miotics
• antifibrinolytic agents
• surgery
• sedation
• ocular hypotensives

ICD-9-CM
364.41 hyphema of iris and ciliary body

 Hypocalcemia

DESCRIPTION Calcium level of 8.5 mg/dL (2.13 mmol/L) or less (with a normal albumin)
• Characteristics - symptoms include neuromuscular irritability, weakness, weight loss, diarrhea, abdominal cramping, bone pain, paresthesias, headache, seizures, dry skin. Signs include Chvostek's sign and Trousseau's sign.

CAUSES
• Surgically induced hyperparathyroidism, Addison's disease, candidiasis, carcinoma of the thyroid, chronic liver disease, hyperphosphatemia, idiopathic, malabsorption, malnutrition, nephrosis, pancreatitis, pernicious anemia, pseudohypoparathyroidism, renal disease, rickets and osteomalacia

TREATMENT
• treat any discovered underlying disorder
• carefully replace calcium

ICD-9-CM
275.4 hypocalcemia

 Hypohidrotic ectodermal dysplasia syndrome

DESCRIPTION Inherited, ectodermal hypoplasia disorder characterized by decreased or no sweating, hairlessness, thin skin, anodontia, mental deficiency, hyperthermia. Usual course - chronic.

CAUSES
• ectodermal hypoplasia

TREATMENT
• cool climate
• water cooling
• dentures
• wig

ICD-9-CM
757.31 congenital ectodermal dysplasia

 Hypophosphatasia

DESCRIPTION Genetic metabolic disorder resulting from serum and bone alkaline phosphatase deficiency leading to ethanolamine phosphaturia and ethanolamine phosphatemia. Clinical characteristics include severe skeletal defects resembling rickets, failure of the calvarium to calcify, dyspnea, cyanosis, and gastrointestinal symptoms, renal calcinosis, failure to thrive. Usual course - chronic; progressive.

SYNONYMS
• juvenile Paget's disease
• hyperostosis corticalis juvenilis deformans
• Rathbun's syndrome

CAUSES
• unknown

TREATMENT
• symptomatic
• sodium fluoride
• calcitonin
• corticosteroids

ICD-9-CM
275.3 hypophosphatasia

 Hypoprothrombinemia

DESCRIPTION Deficiency of prothrombin (coagulation Factor II) in the blood. Characteristics - epistaxis, gingival bleeding, hematuria, melena, excessive bleeding with injury. Usual course - chronic.

SYNONYMS
• prothrombin deficiency
• factor II deficiency

CAUSES
• genetic deficiency
• vitamin K deficiency

TREATMENT
• fresh frozen plasma
• vitamin K

ICD-9-CM
286.3 hypoprothrombinemia

 Hypospadias

DESCRIPTION A congenital anomaly, occurring in 0.5% of males. The urethra exits at an abnormal position along the ventral midline of the penis.

CAUSES
• Thought to be secondary to an unknown defect in androgen action
• Maternal ingestion of progestational agents in early pregnancy

TREATMENT
Surgical repair.

ICD-9-CM
752.61 Hypospadias (male)

Ichthyosis

DESCRIPTION   A symptom in several rare hereditary syndromes - ichthyosis vulgaris; X-linked ichthyosis; lamellar ichthyosis (nonbullous congenital ichthyosiform erythroderma), epidermolytic hyperkeratosis (bullous congenital ichthyosiform erythroderma). Also occurs in several systemic disorders. Xeroderma, the mildest form is neither congenital nor associated with systemic disease. Characteristics - skin is dry, scaling, thick over widespread parts of the body.

SYNONYMS
• Xeroderma
• Dry skin
• Xerosis

CAUSES
• inherited, Refsum's syndrome (hereditary mental deficiency and spastic paralysis), Sjögren-Larrson syndrome, leprosy, hypothyroidism, AIDS

TREATMENT
• skin lubricants

ICD-9-CM   757.1 ichthyosis congenital

 Icterohemorrhagic leptospirosis

DESCRIPTION   A severe form of leptospirosis. Characterized by jaundice usually accompanied by azotemia, hemorrhages, anemia, continued fever, and disturbances of consciousness. Usual course - acute; biphasic.
Endemic areas: worldwide

SYNONYMS
• Weil's syndrome
• leptospiral jaundice
• spirochetal jaundice
• spirochaetosis icterohemorrhagica

CAUSES
• spirochetes of genus leptospira
• systemic infectious disease
• zoonosis
• contact with infected animal tissues
• contact with infected animal urine

TREATMENT
• supportive therapy
• antibiotics

ICD-9-CM
100.0 leptospirosis icterohemorrhagica

 Idiopathic edema

DESCRIPTION   Swellings of unknown cause affecting women, occurring intermittently over a period of years. Usually worse during premenstrual phase. Associated with increased aldosterone secretion. Usual course - intermittent; relapsing.

SYNONYMS
• cyclic edema
• periodic edema
• stress edema
• distress edema
• periodic swelling

CAUSES
• unknown
• abnormal albumin metabolism
• hormonal imbalance

TREATMENT
• DECR salt intake
• elastic stockings
• captopril
• bromocriptine
• diuretics

ICD-9-CM
782.3 edema

 IgG heavy chain disease

DESCRIPTION   A rare malignant neoplasm of lymphoplasmacytic cells consisting of monoclonal immunoglobulin heavy chains. Usual course - progressive; fatal.

SYNONYMS
• gamma chain disease
• Franklin disease

CAUSES
• secretion of free gamma immunoglobulin chains

TREATMENT
• unresponsive to chemotherapy

ICD-9-CM
273.2 heavy chain disease

 IgM heavy chain disease

DESCRIPTION   Rarest heavy chain disease. Found in patients with chronic lymphocytic leukemia. Characteristics - hepatomegaly, splenomegaly. Usual course - slowly progressive.

SYNONYMS
• mu chain disease

CAUSES
• secretion of free mu chains

TREATMENT
• no specific therapy

ICD-9-CM
273.2 heavy chain disease

 Interstitial keratitis

DESCRIPTION   Chronic, non-ulcerative infiltration of the deep layers of the cornea, rare in the USA. Characteristics - signs and symptoms include photophobia, pain, lacrimation, gradual loss of vision.

CAUSES
• congenital or acquired syphilis; tuberculosis

TREATMENT
• refer to an ophthalmologist for treatment

ICD-9-CM
090.3 interstitial keratitis

 Intrahepatic cholestasis due to pregnancy

DESCRIPTION   A benign disorder of pregnancy causing jaundice, pruritus, and hepatomegaly that clears upon delivery. Usual course - intermittent.

SYNONYMS
• cholestatic jaundice of pregnancy

CAUSES
• sensitivity to hormones normally produced in pregnancy

TREATMENT
• unnecessary
• cholestyramine for pruritus

ICD-9-CM
646.7 icterus gravis of pregnancy

 Jaundice

DESCRIPTION   A descriptive term implying deposition of bile pigment in the skin and mucous membranes with resulting yellow appearance of the patient. Yellow skin and sclerae appear whenever bilirubin reaches 3 mg/mL. Characteristics - jaundice is usually brought about by hemolysis, virus infection, alcoholism, drugs, stones in the bile ducts, cancer of the pancreas or liver.

CAUSES
• preponderance of direct (conjugated) bilirubin:
  ◊ obstruction - gallstones, common duct stones, tumors, strictures
  ◊ hepatitis
  ◊ cirrhosis
  ◊ drugs
  ◊ pregnancy (idiopathic cholestatic jaundice of pregnancy)
  ◊ hereditary
• preponderance of indirect (unconjugated) bilirubin:
  ◊ hemolysis
  ◊ neonatal
  ◊ drugs
  ◊ Gilbert's syndrome
  ◊ congestive heart failure

TREATMENT
• according to cause

ICD-9-CM
782.4 jaundice

Jaundice, breast milk

DESCRIPTION   Self-limited hyperbilirubinemia in a healthy vigorous neonate. Cause unknown. Usual course - progressive; self-limiting.

CAUSES
• unknown
• possibly maternal estrogen isomer interference with infant bilirubin conjugation

TREATMENT
• interrupt nursing as diagnostic trial

ICD-9-CM
774.3 neonatal jaundice due to delayed conjugation from other causes

Jet lag

DESCRIPTION The syndrome of jet lag results from transmeridian (east-west) travel between different time zones. (North-south travel does not cause jet lag.) It is a state of physiological desynchronization (e.g., clock shows that it is lunchtime, but the body says it is the middle of the night). The degree of severity depends on the number of time zones crossed and the direction traveled. Most people find traveling eastward and adapting to a shorter day is more difficult than traveling westward and adapting to a longer day. Resulting symptoms include: extreme fatigue, sleep disturbances, loss of concentration, malaise, disorientation, sluggishness, gastrointestinal upset and loss of appetite.

CAUSES
• disturbance in the body's physiological processes (circadian dysrhythmia) that control not only sleep and wakefulness, but also alertness, hunger, digestion, urine production, temperature and hormone secretion

TREATMENT
• no clear evidence that extensive and elaborate prevention programs to avoid jet lag are of value
• short-acting benzodiazepines (e.g., lorazepam) for sleep in transit
• plan destination activities to accommodate for time differences
• the hormone melatonin may be a promising remedy

ICD-9-CM
780.50 Sleep disturbance, unspecified

 Juvenile amaurotic familial idiocy

DESCRIPTION Neuronal ceroid lipofuscinosis. Characteristics - loss of vision, onset 5-10 years, death during late adolescence, atypical retinitis pigmentosa, cerebellar ataxia, dementia. Genetics - autosomal recessive. Usual course - progressive.

SYNONYMS
• Spielmayer-Sjogren chronic neuronal ceroid lipofuscinosis
• Spielmayer-Vogt disease
• Batten disease

CAUSES
• neuronal accumulation of ceroid
• neuronal accumulation of lipofuscin

TREATMENT
• rehabilitation as needed

ICD-9-CM
330.1 Spielmayer-Vogt disease

 Kartagener's syndrome

DESCRIPTION An inherited disorder involving a combination of situs inversus, bronchiectasis, and sinusitis. Genetics - familial; autosomal recessive; 1/70 persons of those involved are heterozygous. Usual course - chronic; variable onset.

SYNONYMS
• Kartagener triad

CAUSES
• defective mucociliary clearance

TREATMENT
• chest physiotherapy
• antibiotics
• bronchodilators

ICD-9-CM
759.3 Kartagener's syndrome

 Kearns-Sayre syndrome

DESCRIPTION Inherited disorder (autosomal dominant with onset before age 15). Characteristics - progressive ophthalmoplegia, pigmentary degeneration of the retina, ataxia, myopathy, cardiac conduction defect. Usual course - progressive; ophthalmic onset at ages 5-20; retinal onset at ages 8-40; cardiac onset at ages 10-40.

SYNONYMS
• oculocraniosomatic neuromuscular disease
• ragged red fiber disease
• ophthalmoplegia-plus
• hereditary external ophthalmoplegia

CAUSES
• unknown

TREATMENT
• folic acid
• coenzyme Q10
• pacemaker

ICD-9-CM
378.55 external ophthalmoplegia

 Keratitis, superficial punctate

DESCRIPTION Loss of epithelium from the corneal surface of one or both eyes. Often associated with trachoma, staphylococcus blepharitis, conjunctivitis, or a respiratory tract infection.
• Characteristics - symptoms include photophobia, pain, lacrimation, diminished vision, conjunctival injection

CAUSES ultraviolet light exposure, bacterial infection, viral infection

TREATMENT
• topical antibiotics after positive culture
• for gram-positive organisms: 10-30% sulfacetamide drops every 2 hours and 0.5% erythromycin or 500 u./gm bacitracin ointment tid
• gram-negative organisms: 0.3% gentamycin drops every 2 hours
• use dark glasses
• systemic analgesics for pain

ICD-9-CM
370.21 keratitis, superficial punctate

 Keratoconus

DESCRIPTION Degenerative eye disorder characterized by thinning and anterior protrusion of the cornea, usually bilateral, beginning between ages 10 and 20. More frequent in females. Signs and symptoms: blurred vision, myopia, astigmatism.

CAUSES
• transmitted as an autosomal recessive trait

TREATMENT
• hard contact lenses
• glasses with high astigmatic correction
• corneal graft or transplantation

ICD-9-CM
371.60 keratoconus

 Kernicterus

DESCRIPTION A condition characterized by high levels of nonconjugated bilirubin in the blood with biliary pigmentation of certain nuclei in the brain and spinal cord and frequently resulting in cerebral palsy, mental retardation, and hearing deficit. It is commonly a sequel to icterus gravis neonatorum. Usual course - acute; progressive; chronic.

SYNONYMS
• bilirubin encephalopathy
• nuclear jaundice

CAUSES
• isoimmunization
• erythrocyte biochemical defects
• erythrocyte structural abnormalities
• infection
• sequestered blood

TREATMENT
• physical therapy

ICD-9-CM
773.4 kernicterus due to isoimmunization
774.7 kernicterus not due to isoimmunization

 Klinefelter's syndrome

DESCRIPTION Congenital disorder. Characteristics - small testes, azoospermia, infertility, increased urinary excretion of gonadotropin, tall long legs, gynecomastia. Associated with an abnormality of the sex chromosomes. Usual course - chronic; manifestations begin at puberty.

SYNONYMS
• seminiferous tubule dysgenesis
• XXY syndrome

CAUSES
• congenital
• supernumerary X chromosome
• mosaicism
• advanced maternal age predisposes

TREATMENT
• mastectomy for disfiguring gynecomastia
• supplemental androgens for delayed secondary sexual characteristics
• supplemental androgens for impotence

ICD-9-CM
758.7 Klinefelter's syndrome

 Korsakoff's psychosis

DESCRIPTION Anterograde and retrograde amnesia with confabulation associated with alcoholic or nonalcoholic polyneuritis. Usual course - subacute; possibly acute; possibly chronic.

SYNONYMS
• alcohol amnestic syndrome

CAUSES
• alcoholism
• thiamine deficiency
• malnutrition

TREATMENT
• parenteral thiamine replacement
• vitamin supplementation

ICD-9-CM
291.1 Korsakoff's psychosis

Krabbe leukodystrophy, infantile form

DESCRIPTION Lysosomal storage disease. Characteristics - begins in infancy, fretfulness, rigidity, followed by tonic seizures, convulsions, quadriplegia, deafness, progressive mental deterioration. Usual course - progressive.

SYNONYMS
• globoid cell leukodystrophy; Krabbe's disease
• Krabbe's brain leukodystrophy
• globoid cell brain sclerosis

CAUSES
• galactocerebrosidase deficiency

TREATMENT
• none

ICD-9-CM
330.0 leukodystrophy

Kuru

DESCRIPTION Progressive nervous system disorder of melanesian tribes of central New Guinea thought to be associated with cannibalism. Usual course - progressive.

CAUSES
• Scrapie PrP (prion)

TREATMENT
• none

ICD-9-CM
046.0 Kuru

Kyasanur forest disease

DESCRIPTION Severe hemorrhagic fever. Tick-borne arbovirus infection occurring the in the Kyasanur Forest in India. Characteristics - fever, hemorrhagic manifestations and rash. Usual course - recurrent.

CAUSES
• ixodes
• haemaphysalis spinigera
• tick-borne flavivirus
• rodent hosts
• monkey hosts

TREATMENT
• symptomatic
• fluid replacement
• transfusion

ICD-9-CM
065.2 kyasanur forest disease

Lassa fever

DESCRIPTION Acute, possible fatal infectious disease occurring in West Africa. Characteristics - high fever, pharyngitis, vomiting, abdominal pain, dyspnea followed by hemorrhages and shock. Usual course - acute; gradual defervescence.

CAUSES
• lassa virus form of arenavirus found in excreta of wild rodents

TREATMENT
• supportive care
• fluid plus electrolyte therapy

ICD-9-CM
078.89 lassa fever

Lathyrism

DESCRIPTION A morbid condition resulting from eating leguminous plants (includes many kinds of peas). characteristics - spastic paraplegia, pain, hyperesthesia, paresthesia. Usual course - progressive. Endemic areas - Africa; Asia.

SYNONYMS
• neurolathyrism

CAUSES
• beta-aminopropionitrile ingestion
• sweet peas of species Lathyrus sativus

TREATMENT
• none

ICD-9-CM
988.2 lathyrism

Laurence-Moon-Biedl syndrome

DESCRIPTION A hereditary syndrome of childhood, transmitted as an autosomal recessive trait, with obesity, retinitis pigmentosa, mental retardation, polydactyly, and hypogonadism as the main features. Usual course - progressive.

SYNONYMS
• Laurence-Moon syndrome
• Bardet-Biedl syndrome

CAUSES
• genetic

TREATMENT
• supportive

ICD-9-CM
759.8 Laurence-Moon-Biedl syndrome

Left ventricular failure, acute

DESCRIPTION Left heart failure. Characteristics - dyspnea, cough, sense of suffocation, frothy sputum, cyanosis, rales, wheezing, tachycardia, Cheyne-Stokes respiration. Usual course - acute.

SYNONYMS
• ventricular failure
• left heart failure

CAUSES
• hypertension
• coronary artery disease
• incompetent mitral valve
• incompetent aortic valve
• myocardial infarction

TREATMENT
• diuretics
• vasodilators
• digitalis

ICD-9-CM
428.1 left heart failure

Leptospirosis

DESCRIPTION Infection by leptospira organisms transmitted to man from dogs, swine, and rodents or by contact with contaminated water. Characteristics - lymphocytic meningitis, hepatitis, nephritis. Weil's syndrome is severe leptospirosis with jaundice, bleeding and renal failure. Usual course - acute; abrupt; biphasic; relapsing. Endemic areas - Southern USA; tropics.

SYNONYMS
• autumnal fever
• Fort Bragg fever
• mud fever
• pea-picker's disease
• European swamp fever
• wycon fever
• Bushy Creek fever
• cane field fever
• swineherd disease

CAUSES
• leptospira interrogans
• spirochete
• contact with infected animal tissues
• contact with infected animal excrement

TREATMENT
• antibiotics, supportive care, fluid replacement, electrolyte therapy, possibly steroids if hepatic coma

ICD-9-CM
100.9 leptospirosis, unspecified

Lesch-Nyhan syndrome

DESCRIPTION An X-linked disease caused by a deficiency of an enzyme of purine metabolism, hypoxanthine-guanine phosphoribosyl transferase, and characterized by physical and mental retardation, hyperuricemia, self-mutilation, and choreoathetosis.

SYNONYMS
• hypoxanthine-guanine phosphoribosyltransferase deficiency syndrome
• HG-PRT deficiency syndrome

CAUSES
• hypoxanthine-guanine phosphoribosyltransferase deficiency

TREATMENT
• symptomatic and supportive
• protective restraint

ICD-9-CM
277.2 Lesch-Nyhan syndrome

Letterer-Siwe disease

DESCRIPTION Acute, disseminated, rapidly progressive form of Langerhans-cell histiocytosis. Genetics - Some familial predisposition. Characteristics include - hemorrhage tendency, eczematoid skin eruption, hepatosplenomegaly, progressive anemia, lymphadenopathy. Usual course - acute; fulminant; progressive; chronic.

SYNONYMS
• acute diffuse histiocytosis
• acute infantile reticuloendotheliosis
• acute reticulosis of infancy
• generalized histiocytosis
• non-lipid reticuloendotheliosis

CAUSES
• nonneoplastic proliferation of langerhans cells

TREATMENT
• irradiation, chemotherapy, steroids, vasopressin replacement, antibiotics

ICD-9-CM
202.50 Letterer-Siwe disease, unspecified site

 Leukemia, acute monocytic

DESCRIPTION Leukemia in which the predominating leukocytes are identified as monocytes. Characteristics - fever, fatigue, bleeding, lymphadenopathy, hepatosplenomegaly, anemia. Usual course - acute; possibly relapsing.

SYNONYMS
• acute monocytoid leukemia
• monoblastic leukemia
• acute monoblastic leukemia

CAUSES
• chloramphenicol, phenylbutazone, ionizing radiation, benzene, Down syndrome, alkylating agents

TREATMENT
• cytosine arabinoside
• daunorubicin
• 6-thioguanine

ICD-9-CM
206.0 monocytic leukemia, acute

 Leukemia, acute myeloblastic

DESCRIPTION An acute nonlymphoblastic leukemia occurs at all ages and is the more common leukemia among adults. Usually associated with irradiation as a causative agent and occurring as a second malignancy following cancer chemotherapy. Characteristics - bleeding, pallor, fever, headaches, vomiting, weakness, lethargy, pallor, joint pain. Usual course - acute; progressive; relapsing.

SYNONYMS
• acute granulocytic leukemia
• acute myelocytic leukemia

CAUSES
• idiopathic
• retroviral infection
• ionizing radiation
• genetic defect
• chemical poisoning

TREATMENT
• chemotherapy
• immunotherapy
• bone marrow transplantation

ICD-9-CM
205.0 myeloid leukemia, acute

 Leukemia, acute myelogenous

DESCRIPTION Leukemia arising from myeloid tissue in which the granular, polymorphonuclear leukocytes and their precursors predominate. Characteristics - fever, anorexia, bleeding, hepatosplenomegaly, anemia, lymphadenopathy. Usual course - acute; possibly relapsing.

CAUSES
• Bloom's syndrome
• Philadelphia chromosome
• chloramphenicol
• ionizing radiation
• benzene
• Down syndrome
• Fanconi's syndrome
• phenylbutazone
• alkylating agents

TREATMENT
• cytosine arabinoside, daunorubicin, 6-thioguanine, prednisone, vincristine, intrathecal methotrexate, cranial radiotherapy

ICD-9-CM
205.0 myeloid leukemia, acute

 Leukemia, chronic myelogenous

DESCRIPTION Clonal myeloproliferation caused by malignant transformation of a pluripotent cell. Characteristics - extraordinary overproduction of granulocytes. Usual course - slowly progressive.

SYNONYMS
• chronic granulocytic leukemia

CAUSES
• unknown
• possibly ionizing radiation

TREATMENT
• busulfan, allopurinol, leukophoresis, localized radiotherapy, vincristine, prednisone, cytosine arabinoside, doxorubicin

ICD-9-CM
205.1 myeloid leukemia, chronic.

 Leukemia, hairy cell

DESCRIPTION A neoplastic disease of the lymphoreticular cells which is considered to be a rare type of chronic leukemia. It is characterized by an insidious onset, splenomegaly, anemia, granulocytopenia, thrombocytopenia, little or no lymphadenopathy, and the presence of "hairy" or "flagellated" cells in the blood and bone marrow. Usual course - chronic; progressive.

SYNONYMS
• leukemic reticuloendotheliosis

CAUSES
• precise cause unknown

TREATMENT
• splenectomy
• interferon

ICD-9-CM
202.4 hairy-cell leukemia

 Lichen sclerosis of the vulva

DESCRIPTION Thickened skin and accentuated markings affecting the vulva. Characteristics - external genital itching and pain. Usual course - chronic; progressive; may have spontaneous regression.

SYNONYMS
• lichen sclerosis et atrophicus
• lichen albus
• Csillag's disease
• white spot disease
• circumscribed scleroderma

TREATMENT
• vitamin A ointment
• intralesional corticosteroids
• topical corticosteroids
• oral estrogen

ICD-9-CM
701.0 circumscribed scleroderma

 Liddle's syndrome

DESCRIPTION A rare disease resulting in enhanced sodium loses in the CCD (cortical collecting duct). This results in enhanced sodium delivery distally (along with a non-reabsorbable anion) and subsequent enhanced potassium secretion.

CAUSES Autosomal dominant condition caused by a mutation at the beta subunit of the principal apical sodium channel

TREATMENT
Sodium restriction and amiloride (which inhibits the luminal sodium channel in the CCD)

ICD-9-CM
276.8 Hypokalemia

 Lipoid nephrosis

DESCRIPTION Nephrosis characterized by edema, albuminuria, changes in lipids and proteins in the blood, accumulation of globules of cholesterol esters in the tubular epithelium of the kidney.

SYNONYMS
• minimal change disease
• foot process disease
• nil disease
• minimal change nephropathy
• minimal change glomerulopathy

CAUSES
• loss of negative charge in glomerular capillary wall

TREATMENT
• steroids
• antibiotics
• cyclophosphamide
• chlorambucil

ICD-9-CM
581.3 lipoid nephrosis

Loiasis

DESCRIPTION   A parasitic infection caused by the nematode Loa loa. The vector in the transmission of this infection is the horsefly (Tabanus) or the deerfly or mango fly (Chrysops). The larvae may be seen just beneath the skin or passing through the conjunctiva. Eye lesions are not uncommon. The disease is generally mild and painless. Usual course - chronic; progressive; 10-15 year incubation period. Endemic areas - West Africa; Central Africa.

SYNONYMS
• calabar swellings

CAUSES
• Loa loa filaria

TREATMENT
• diethylcarbamazine

ICD-9-CM
125.2 loiasis

 Ludwig's angina

DESCRIPTION   Severe form of cellulitis affecting the submandibular, submental, and sublingual spaces. Characteristics - tongue elevation, difficult eating and swallowing, edema of the glottis, fever, tachypnea, and moderate leukocytosis. Usual course - acute.

CAUSES
• oral trauma
• aerobic infection of submandibular space
• anaerobic infection of submandibular space

TREATMENT
• broad-spectrum intravenous antibiotics
• maintain airway
• tracheostomy if necessary

ICD-9-CM
528.3 Ludwig's angina

 Lupus nephritis

DESCRIPTION   Glomerulonephritis associated with systemic lupus erythematosus. Characteristics - hematuria, a fulminant or chronic progressive course. Hypertension does not occur until late in the course of the disease. Usual course - relapsing; progressive.

SYNONYMS
• focal glomerulonephritis
• lupus glomerulonephritis

CAUSES
• SLE

TREATMENT
• steroids
• renal transplantation

ICD-9-CM
710.0 lupus nephritis

 Lymphangitis

DESCRIPTION   Inflammation of a lymphatic vessel or vessels. Characteristics - painful subcutaneous streaks along the course of the vessels. Usual course - acute; relapsing.

CAUSES
• beta-hemolytic streptococci
• staphylococcus

TREATMENT
• antibiotics
• drainage
• heat
• moisture

ICD-9-CM
457.2 lymphangitis

 Lymphoma, non-Hodgkin's

DESCRIPTION   Heterogenous group of malignant lymphomas with absence of giant Reed-Sternberg cells characteristic of Hodgkin's disease. Characteristics - widespread disease, painless enlargement of one or more peripheral lymph nodes. Usual course - progressive.

CAUSES
• malignant tumors of lymphoid tissues with the exception of hodgkin's disease

TREATMENT
• radiotherapy
• chemotherapy

ICD-9-CM
202.8 non-hodgkin's lymphoma, nos

 Lymphoma, pulmonary

DESCRIPTION   Malignant disease of the lung. Characteristics - cough, weight loss, chest pain. Usual course - progressive.

CAUSES
• tumor of the immune system
• Hodgkin's lymphoma
• lymphocytic lymphoma

TREATMENT
• radiotherapy
• chemotherapy

ICD-9-CM
202.8 malignant lymphoma, nos

 Magnesium deficiency syndrome

DESCRIPTION   Abnormally low magnesium content of the blood plasma. Characteristics - neuromuscular hyperirritability. Usual course - progressive; acute; relapsing.

SYNONYMS
• hypomagnesemia

CAUSES
• dietary deficiency
• decreased absorption
• increased excretion
• alcoholism
• uremia
• diuretics
• parathyroid disease
• eclampsia

TREATMENT
• magnesium

ICD-9-CM
275.2 magnesium deficiency

 Mallory-Weiss syndrome

DESCRIPTION   Mucosal tears usually linear and confined to the esophagogastric junction but may be located in the fundus of the stomach or in the distal esophagus. Upper gastrointestinal bleeding from these lacerations is often precipitated by retching or vomiting. Usual course - acute.

SYNONYMS
• gastroesophageal laceration-hemorrhage syndrome

CAUSES
• retching after alcoholic bout
• hiatus hernia
• atrophic gastritis
• esophagitis
• straining at stool

TREATMENT
• vasopressin
• gastrotomy with sutures

ICD-9-CM
530.7 Mallory-Weiss syndrome

 Maple bark stripper's disease

DESCRIPTION   Granulomatous, interstitial pneumonitis caused by a mold found under the bark of maple logs. Usual course - acute; relapsing.

CAUSES
• hypersensitivity reaction to spores of cryptostroma corticale

TREATMENT
• eliminate etiological agent

ICD-9-CM
495.6 maple bark-strippers' lung

Maple syrup urine disease

DESCRIPTION   Familial cerebral degenerative disease caused by a defect in branched chain amino acid metabolism and characterized by severe mental and motor retardation and urine with a maple-syrup-like odor. Usual course - progressive.

SYNONYMS
• branched chain ketoaciduria

CAUSES
• deficiency of branched chain alpha-ketoacid decarboxylase

TREATMENT
• controlled intake of branched-chain amino acids
• peritoneal and/or hemodialysis

ICD-9-CM
270.3 maple syrup urine disease

Marburg virus disease

DESCRIPTION   Severe, acute often fatal viral hemorrhagic fever. Characteristics - prostration, fever, pancreatitis, hepatitis. The Marburg virus first infected laboratory workers handling infected African green monkeys. Usual course - acute. Endemic areas: Germany; Yugoslavia; Africa.

SYNONYMS
• green monkey virus disease

CAUSES
• Marburg virus

TREATMENT
• isolation
• treat dehydration
• nasogastric suction
• heparin

ICD-9-CM
078.89 Marburg virus disease

Marchiafava-Bignami syndrome

DESCRIPTION   Progressive degeneration of the corpus callosum. Characteristics - progressive intellectual degeneration, confusion, hallucinations, tremor, rigidity, and convulsions. Usual course - chronic; progressive.

SYNONYMS
• Marchiafava disease
• callosal demyelinating encephalopathy

CAUSES
• chronic alcoholism
• addiction to crude red wine

TREATMENT
• avoid alcohol

ICD-9-CM
341.8 Marchiafava-Bignami disease or syndrome

Mastocytosis

DESCRIPTION   A rare disease characterized by an abnormal increase in mast cells in various body organs and tissues. It can occur in any age group and demonstrates a slight male predominance. Various forms are identified: mastocytoma (a benign cutaneous tumor); urticaria pigmentosa (multiple, small collections of mast cells, salmon or brown color, that may become vesicular or even bullous); and systemic mastocytosis (mast cell infiltrates in the bone marrow, liver, spleen, lymph nodes, gastrointestinal tract, skin and bones). Symptoms include arthralgias, bone pain and anaphylactoid symptoms. Mast cell leukemia is a form of mastocytosis.

SYNONYMS
• cutaneous mastocytosis
• systemic mast cell disease

CAUSES
• exact cause is unknown

TREATMENT
• cutaneous mastocytosis and urticaria pigmentosa seldom require treatment
• systemic mastocytosis:
  ◊ H1 and an H2 antihistamine
  ◊ aspirin therapy (use with caution)
  ◊ oral cromolyn sodium (if GI symptoms are inadequately controlled)
  ◊ surgical excision of mast cells (rare)

ICD-9-CM
757.33 urticaria pigmentosa
202.6 mastocytosis

Meckel's diverticulum

DESCRIPTION   Sacculation or appendage of the ileum derived from an unobliterated yolk stalk. Symptoms of infection may resemble those of appendicitis. Usual course - acute; intermittent; chronic.

CAUSES
• vestigial remnant of omphalomesenteric duct

TREATMENT
• surgery

ICD-9-CM
751.0 Meckel's diverticulum

Meigs' syndrome

DESCRIPTION   Ascites and hydrothorax associated with ovarian fibroma or other pelvic tumors. Usual course - acute; relapsing.

SYNONYMS
• ovarian ascites-pleural effusion syndrome
• Demons-Meigs syndrome
• Meigs-Coss syndrome

CAUSES
• benign fibroma
• ovarian tumor
• movement of the ascitic fluid across the diaphragm

TREATMENT
• tumor excision

ICD-9-CM
789.5 ascites

Melioidosis

DESCRIPTION   A glanders-like infection of man and animals endemic in SE Asia, NE Queensland Australia, Central, West and Eastern Africa. Likely to be one of the infections seen in patients with AIDS. May be asymptomatic or symptoms can include chills; cough; bloody purulent sputum; abdominal pain; diarrhea.

SYNONYMS
• Stanton disease
• Whitmore disease
• pneumoenteritis
• pseudocholera

CAUSES
• pseudomonas pseudomallei; transmitted by direct contact with infected rodents or infected food, soil, water, excreta; person-to-person transmission possible through use of injection needle

TREATMENT
• trimethoprim-sulfamethoxazole
• ceftazidime

ICD-9-CM
025 melioidosis

Meningioma

DESCRIPTION   Hard, slow growing, vascular tumor arising along the meningeal vessels and superior longitudinal sinus. It invades the dura and skull and leads to thinning and erosion of the skull. Usual course - progressive; surgical cure.

SYNONYMS
• arachnoidal fibroblastoma
• leptomeningioma
• dural endothelioma
• meningeal fibroblastoma

CAUSES
• unknown

TREATMENT
• surgical excision
• radiotherapy for incomplete removal
• radiotherapy for recurrence

ICD-9-CM
225.2 Benign neoplasm of cerebral meninges
225.4 Benign neoplasm of spinal meninges

Mesenteric adenitis, acute

DESCRIPTION   Inflammation of lymph glands located in the mesentery. It causes a clinical picture at times that is difficult to differentiate from acute appendicitis.

SYNONYMS
• acute mesenteric lymphadenitis

CAUSES
• yersinia enterocolitica
• yersinia pseudotuberculosis
• streptococcus viridans
• giardia lamblia
• staphylococcus aureus

TREATMENT
• antibiotics

ICD-9-CM
289.2 acute mesenteric lymphadenitis

Metachromatic leukodystrophy, late infantile form

DESCRIPTION   A form of leukoencephalopathy transmitted autosomal recessive. Characteristics - accumulation of sphingolipid in neural and non-neural tissues with a diffuse loss of myelin in the central nervous system. The infantile form begins in the second year of life with blindness, motor disturbances, mental deterioration. Usual course - progressive.

SYNONYMS
• metachromatic brain leukodystrophy
• metachromatic leukoencephalopathy
• sulfatidosis
• Greenfield disease
• arylsulfatase A deficiency

CAUSES
• arylsulfatase A deficiency

TREATMENT
• none

ICD-9-CM
330.0 leukodystrophy

 Metastatic neoplasm of the liver

DESCRIPTION   Progressive form of hepatic cancer that has metastasized from malignancies arising primarily from other locations. Usual course - progressive.

CAUSES
• colon metastases
• rectal metastases
• gastric metastases
• pancreatic metastases
• breast metastases

TREATMENT
• palliative chemotherapy
• palliative radiotherapy
• surgical resection in rare cases

ICD-9-CM
197.7 secondary malignant neoplasm to the liver

 Milker's nodules

DESCRIPTION   A disease caused by paravaccinia virus, transmitted to humans during milking. Characteristics - purple nodules on fingers or adjacent areas. Lesions break down and crust and heal without scarring. It can be retransmitted to uninfected cows. Usual course - acute; relapsing. Endemic areas - dairy farms.

SYNONYMS
• pseudocowpox
• paravaccinia

CAUSES
• paravaccinia virus of poxviridae family
• transmitted through direct contact
• cutaneous disease of cow teats
• oral lesions in suckling calves

TREATMENT
• none

ICD-9-CM
051.9 paravaccinia, nos

 Millard-Gubler syndrome

DESCRIPTION   Paralysis caused by infarction of the pons involving the 6th and 7th cranial nerves and fibers of the corticospinal tract. Characteristics - crossed paralysis affecting the limbs on one side of the body and the face on the opposite side. Additionally, paralysis of outward movement of the eye. Usual course - acute; chronic; progressive.

SYNONYMS
• alternating inferior hemiplegia
• Gubler paralysis
• abducens-facial syndrome

CAUSES
• basal pontine infarction
• basal pontine tumor

TREATMENT
• supportive plus rehabilitative
• treat underlying cause of infarction

ICD-9-CM
344.8 Millard-Gubler syndrome

 Mitral regurgitation due to papillary muscle dysfunction

DESCRIPTION   Retrograde blood flow from the left ventricle in the left atrium through an incompetent mitral valve. Characteristics - fatigue, orthopnea, systolic murmur, left ventricular hypertrophy, S3 gallop. Usual course: chronic; progressive; acute (after myocardial infarction).

CAUSES
• coronary artery disease
• infiltrative diseases
• cardiac tumors

TREATMENT
• dental endocarditis prophylaxis
• surgical endocarditis prophylaxis
• nitrates
• calcium channel blockers
• diuretics
• digitalis
• inotropic agents
• afterload reducing agents
• mitral valve replacement

ICD-9-CM
394.9 other and unspecified mitral valve diseases

 Mitral regurgitation due to rheumatic fever

DESCRIPTION   Retrograde blood flow from the left ventricle into the left atrium through an incompetent mitral valve. Characteristics - history of rheumatic fever, fatigue, dyspnea, holosystolic murmur, left ventricular hypertrophy. Usual course - chronic; progressive disability.

CAUSES
• autoimmune cross reaction between streptococcal antigens and heart tissue

TREATMENT
• medical endocarditis prophylaxis
• dental endocarditis prophylaxis
• surgical endocarditis prophylaxis
• afterload reducing agents
• nitrates
• calcium channel blockers
• digitalis
• diuretics
• mitral valve replacement

ICD-9-CM
394.1 rheumatic mitral insufficiency

 Munchausen's syndrome

DESCRIPTION   A chronic disorder characterized by habitual presentation for medical care. Often requires hospitalization. The patient gives a plausible and dramatic history, all of which is factitious.
Also, Munchausen's by proxy, in which a caregiver creates a history or illness requiring frequent medical care. The caregiver often has a medical background.

SYNONYMS
• chronic factitious disorder with physical symptoms
• hospital-addiction syndrome

CAUSES
• factitious
• external incentives

TREATMENT
• psychotherapy
• behavior modification techniques

ICD-9-CM
301.51 Munchausen syndrome

 Mushroom poisoning, Amanita phalloides

DESCRIPTION   Characteristics include: nausea, vomiting, abdominal pain, diarrhea, followed by a period of improvement up to 48 hours. Then culminating in severe renal, hepatic, and central nervous system damage. Usual course - acute; progressive. Endemic areas - Western USA; Europe.

CAUSES
• cyclic octapeptide amatoxin
• hepatic cytotoxicity by interference with RNA polymerase
• renal cytotoxicity by interference with RNA polymerase

TREATMENT
• intragastric activated charcoal
• intensive supportive care
• charcoal hemoperfusion
• thiotic (alpha-lipoic acid)

ICD-9-CM
988.1 toxic effect of mushrooms eaten as food

 Mushroom-worker's disease

DESCRIPTION   Allergic respiratory disease, resembling farmer's lung, developing in persons working with moldy compost prepared for growing mushrooms. Characteristics - fever, dyspnea, dry cough, chills, malaise, myalgia, tachypnea. Usual course - acute; chronic; intermittent; progressive; relapsing.

SYNONYMS
• pulmonary granulomatosis of mushroom pickers

CAUSES
• immunological reaction to inhaled antigens
• micropolyspora faeni
• thermoactinomyces vulgaris

TREATMENT
• corticosteroids
• eliminate etiological agent

ICD-9-CM
495.5 mushroom workers' lung

Mussel poisoning

DESCRIPTION Food poisoning due to ingestion of toxin from dinoflagellate Gonyaulax. Characteristics - dysesthesias of tongue, lips, fingertips, dysphagia, abdominal cramps, ascending weakness, seizures. Usual course - acute; progressive. Endemic areas - Mid-Pacific coast from May to October; Northeastern seaboard; Western European coast.

SYNONYMS
• mytilotoxism
• paralytic shellfish poisoning

CAUSES
• alkaloid saxitoxin of dinoflagellate gonyaulax catenella
• alkaloid saxitoxin of dinoflagellate gonyaulax tamarensis
• neuromuscular blockade by preventing depolarization
• aerosolized ingestion has been reported

TREATMENT
• emergent gastrointestinal decontamination
• supportive
• mechanical ventilation

ICD-9-CM
988.0 toxic effect of fish and shellfish eaten as food

 Mycetoma

DESCRIPTION Infectious disease of the skin, subcutaneous tissues, and bone, usually affecting the lower extremeties, especially the foot. Characterized by chronicity, tumefaction and multiple sinus formation. With early diagnosis, prognosis is good; if identified late in disease, treatment response is limited and amputation may be necessary.

SYNONYMS
• maduromycosis
• madura foot

CAUSES
• allescheria boydii or actinomycetales bacteria; more than 20 species of fungi and bacteria have been implicated

TREATMENT
• penicillin
• tetracycline
• sulfonamides
• streptomycin
• itraconazole
• dapsone
• surgery

ICD-9-CM
039.4 madura foot

 Myiasis

DESCRIPTION The invasion of living tissues of man and other mammals by dipterous larvae (fly maggots). Usual course - acute. Endemic areas - tropical America; Africa; South America; Mexico; California.

SYNONYMS
• maggot infestation

CAUSES
• ingestion of fly eggs
• eggs deposited in open wounds

TREATMENT
• surgery
• local anesthesia
• mineral oil
• ether bath

ICD-9-CM
134.0 myiasis

 Myringitis, infectious

DESCRIPTION Inflammation, hemorrhage and emission of fluid into the tissue at the end of the external ear canal and the tympanic membrane. Pain is typically sudden in onset and continues for 24 to 48 hours. Bacterial otitis media is suggested if hearing loss and fever are present.

SYNONYMS
bullous myringitis

CAUSES
• bacterial or viral infection

TREATMENT
• analgesics
• antibiotics for secondary infection
• rupture of vesicles with myringotomy knife

ICD-9-CM
384.00 myringitis

 Myxedema heart disease

DESCRIPTION Heart disease associated with primary hypothyroidism. Usual course - acute; progressive.

CAUSES
• decreased thyroid hormone
• congenital developmental defect
• idiopathic
• postablative
• postradiation
• iodine deficiency

TREATMENT
• thyroid hormone replacement

ICD-9-CM
244.9 myxedema

 Necrobiosis lipoidica diabeticorum

DESCRIPTION Degenerative disease of dermal connective tissue. Characteristics - erythematous papules or nodules in the pretibial area that extend to form waxy, yellowish red plaques covered with telangiectatic vessels. The plaques have a red-violet border and depressed atrophic center. Usual course - chronic.

SYNONYMS
• Oppenheim-Urbach disease

CAUSES
• unknown

TREATMENT
• triamcinolone acetonide

ICD-9-CM
250.8 Diabetes with specified manifestation
709.3 Degenerative skin disorders

 Nephropathy, analgesic

DESCRIPTION Kidney damage due to massive intake of analgesics, particularly phenacetin. Usual course - chronic.

CAUSES
• phenacetin
• aspirin
• acetaminophen

TREATMENT
• cessation of analgesic use

ICD-9-CM
965 poisoning by analgesics, antipyretics, and antirheumatics

 Nephropathy, chronic lead

DESCRIPTION Kidney damage due to lead poisoning. Particularly present in Queensland, Australia. Usual course - chronic.

SYNONYMS
• lead related hyperuricemia
• hyperuricemic nephropathy
• saturnine gout

CAUSES
• lead poisoning
• lead paint ingestion
• lead vapor inhalation
• moonshine alcohol

TREATMENT
• EDTA

ICD-9-CM
984 toxic effect of lead and its compounds (including fumes)

 Nephrosclerosis

DESCRIPTION Hardening of the kidney due to overgrowth and contraction of interstitial connective tissue. Characteristics - edema, headache, hypertension, retinal hemorrhages. Usual course - chronic; progressive.

CAUSES
• unknown
• essential hypertension
• diabetes

TREATMENT
• antihypertensive medication

ICD-9-CM
403.9 nephrosclerosis

Neuritis/neuralgia

DESCRIPTION Degeneration of peripheral nerves
• Characteristics - insidious onset, muscle weakness with sensory loss, muscle atrophy, decreased tendon reflexes, paresthesias, hyperesthesias in hands and feet. Electromyography shows delayed action potential.

SYNONYMS
• Multiple neuritis
• Peripheral neuropathy
• Polyneuritis

CAUSES
• chronic intoxication (alcohol, arsenic, lead, other drugs)
• infections
• metabolic and inflammatory (diabetes) gout, rheumatoid arthritis, systemic lupus erythematosus
• nutritive (vitamin deficiencies, cachexia)

TREATMENT
• supportive
• physical therapy
• analgesics
• treat underlying specific disorders if possible
• drugs - amitriptyline, carbamazepine, phenytoin (uneven and unpredictable response, but helpful for some)

ICD-9-CM
729.2 neuritis/neuralgia

 Neutropenia, autoimmune

DESCRIPTION Decreased number of neutrophilic leukocytes in the blood due to an autoimmune mechanism. Usual course - acute; chronic; intermittent; progressive; relapsing.

CAUSES
• antineutrophil antibodies

TREATMENT
• antibiotics
• prednisone
• splenectomy
• supportive

ICD-9-CM
288.0 neutropenia

 Neutropenia, chronic idiopathic

DESCRIPTION An autosomal dominant, familial disorder with a chronic decrease in number of neutrophilic granulocytes. Characteristics - repeated non-life-threatening infections of skin, oral cavity, and sometimes upper respiratory tract. Usual course - chronic; relapsing.

SYNONYMS
• chronic benign neutropenia

CAUSES
• abnormal homeostasis of mitosis of granulocyte precursors

TREATMENT
• symptomatic

ICD-9-CM
288.0 neutropenia

 Neutropenia, cyclic

DESCRIPTION Autosomal dominant disorder of children and young adults characterized by cyclical neutropenia, producing fever, malaise, mouth ulcers and cervical lymphadenopathy. Usual course - relapsing; 21-day cycles.

SYNONYMS
• cyclic agranulocytosis
• periodic neutropenia
• cyclic leukopenia
• periodic myelocytic dysplasia

CAUSES
• defective regulation of hematopoietic cell proliferation

TREATMENT
• glucocorticoids
• androgens
• splenectomy
• antibiotics

ICD-9-CM
288.0 agranulocytosis

 Nevus of ota

DESCRIPTION A macular lesion on the side of the face (usually lifelong and unilateral), involving the conjunctiva and lids, as well as the adjacent facial skin, sclera, ocular muscles, and periosteum. Histological features vary from those of a mongolian spot to those of a blue nevus. Usual course - chronic.

SYNONYMS
• oculodermal melanocytosis
• nevus fusco-caeruleus ophthalmo-maxillaris

CAUSES
• unknown

TREATMENT
• cosmetic cover up

ICD-9-CM
224.3 nevus conjunctiva

 Niemann-Pick disease

DESCRIPTION Sphingolipidosis due to sphingomyelinase deficiency with sphingomyelin accumulation in the reticuloendothelial system. There are 5 types (A, B, C, D, and E) with differing ages of onset and differing amounts of CNS involvement and sphingomyelinase activity. Genetics - autosomal recessive. Usual course - acute; chronic; progressive.

SYNONYMS
• sphingomyelin lipidosis
• sphingomyelinase deficiency

CAUSES
• sphingomyelinase deficiency

TREATMENT
• supportive
• splenectomy
• bone marrow transplantation

ICD-9-CM
272.7 Niemann-Pick disease

 Nitrobenzene poisoning

DESCRIPTION Poisoning due to excessive exposure to nitrobenzene, a benzene derivative used in the manufacture of aniline. Complete recovery from pathologic changes can be expected if survival greater than 24 hours.

SYNONYMS
• nitrobenzol toxicity
• oil of mirbane toxicity

CAUSES
• direct mucous membrane irritation
• methemoglobin formation

TREATMENT
• cutaneous plus gastric decontamination
• oxygen
• 1% methylene blue
• exchange transfusion
• hemodialysis

ICD-9-CM
983.0 poisoning, nitrobenzene

 Osteopetrosis

DESCRIPTION Excessive formation of dense trabecular bone leading to pathological fractures, osteitis, splenomegaly with infarct, anemia and extramedullary hemopoiesis. Genetics: malignant form: autosomal recessive; benign form: autosomal dominant. Usual course - progressive; chronic.

SYNONYMS
• marble bone disease
• Albers-Schonberg disease
• osteosclerosis fragilis generalisata

CAUSES
• replacement of marrow space with bone
• no carbonic anhydrase II in erythrocytes
• defective osteoclast function

TREATMENT
• bone marrow transplantation
• calcitriol

ICD-9-CM
756.52 osteopetrosis

Ovarian mucinous cystadenocarcinoma

DESCRIPTION Carcinoma and cystadenoma of the ovary. Characteristics — multilocular tumor produced by the epithelial cells of the ovary having mucin-filled cavities. Symptoms include abdominal pain and distention, menstrual disturbances, weight loss, dyspareunia, ascites. Clinical findings are the same as those with ovarian serous cystadenocarcinoma.

SYNONYMS
• pseudomucinous ovarian cystadenocarcinoma

CAUSES
• unknown

TREATMENT
• hysterectomy
• stage I: bilateral salpingo-oophorectomy plus omentectomy if high grade
• stage II: add radiotherapy or chemotherapy
• stage III: surgical debulking

ICD-9-CM
183.0 malignant neoplasm of ovary

Paralysis of the recurrent laryngeal nerve

DESCRIPTION Paralysis may be unilateral or bilateral with many possible underlying causes. Characteristics — dysphagia, stridor, dyspnea, and aphonia. Usual course: acute; insidious.

CAUSES
- innominate artery aneurysm
- right subclavian artery aneurysm
- neck surgery
- thyroid goiter
- trauma
- aortic aneurysm
- left atrial enlargement
- laryngeal tuberculosis

TREATMENT
- treat underlying condition

ICD-9-CM
478.31 partial unilateral paralysis of vocal cords

 ## Parapsoriasis

DESCRIPTION A group of slowly evolving erythrodermas. common characteristics: chronicity, resistance to treatment. The group includes chronic and acute lichenoid pityriasis and large and small plaque parapsoriasis. Usual course - chronic; relapsing; benign forms; premalignant forms.

SYNONYMS
- maculopapular erythroderma

TREATMENT
- ultraviolet B light therapy

ICD-9-CM
696.2 parapsoriasis

 ## Paratyphoid

DESCRIPTION An infection due to any of the salmonella serotypes except S. typhi and salmonellosis. Characteristics — prolonged febrile illness less severe than typhoid fever, frequently follows an attack of salmonella food poisoning.

SYNONYMS
- paratyphoid fever
- enteric fever

CAUSES
- salmonella paratyphi A
- salmonella paratyphi B
- salmonella paratyphi C
- salmonella sendai
- enteric pathogens

TREATMENT
- fluid replacement
- antibiotics in elderly at greatest risk
- antibiotics in infants at greatest risk

ICD-9-CM
002.9 paratyphoid fever, nos

 ## Paroxysmal atrial tachycardia

DESCRIPTION Heart rate greater than 140 beats per minute. May increase up to 250. P waves regular but aberrant. Onset may be sudden. Symptoms include light-headedness and palpitations.

SYNONYMS
- Premature atrial tachycardia
- Paroxysmal supraventricular tachycardia

CAUSES
- abnormal AV conduction system
- physical or psychological stress
- hypokalemia, hypoxia, caffeine, marijuana, digitalis toxicity, sympathomimetics

ICD-9-CM
427.0 paroxysmal atrial tachycardia

 ## Paroxysmal cold hemoglobinuria

DESCRIPTION A rare disease in which blood hemolyzes minutes to hours after exposure to cold (atmospheric, drinking cold water, handwashing in cold water). Usually occurs following a non-specific viral type illness. Usual course - acute; progressive; relapsing.

SYNONYMS
- Donath-Landsteiner hemolytic anemia
- Dressler syndrome
- Harley syndrome

CAUSES
- immune-mediated hemolysis upon rewarming after cold exposure

TREATMENT
- supportive
- transfusion
- oxygen
- maintain adequate urine output
- alkalinize urine
- steroids

ICD-9-CM
283.2 paroxysmal cold hemoglobinuria

 ## Paroxysmal hemoglobinuria following exercise

DESCRIPTION A benign disorder characterized by red urine, hemoglobinuria, myoglobinuria and abdominal pain. Usual course - acute.

SYNONYMS
- march hemoglobinuria

CAUSES
- strenuous exercise
- running on hard ground
- poorly cushioned shoes

TREATMENT
- unnecessary

ICD-9-CM
283.2 march hemoglobinuria

Paroxysmal nocturnal hemoglobinuria

DESCRIPTION Chronic acquired blood cell dysplasia with proliferation of a clone of stem cells producing erythrocytes, platelets, and granulocytes that are abnormally susceptible to lysis by complement. Characteristics — episodic intravascular hemolysis, particularly following infections, and by various thromboses, particularly of the hepatic veins. Usual course - chronic. Genetics - genetic mutation

SYNONYMS
- Marchiafava-Micheli syndrome

CAUSES
- intrinsic erythrocyte defect
- unusual complement sensitivity

TREATMENT
- transfusion
- androgens
- corticosteroids
- anticoagulants

ICD-9-CM
283.2 paroxysmal nocturnal hemoglobinuria

 ## Pellagra

DESCRIPTION Clinical deficiency syndrome. Characteristics — dermatitis, diarrhea, dementia, inflammation of mucus membranes. Skin lesions appear in area exposed to light and/or trauma. Mental symptoms include depression, irritability, anxiety, confusion, disorientation, delusions and hallucinations. Usual course - progressive. Endemic areas - Southern USA.

SYNONYMS
- niacin deficiency disease

CAUSES
- nicotinic acid deficiency
- tryptophan deficiency
- folic acid deficiency
- carcinoma
- isoniazid

TREATMENT
- nicotinic acid

ICD-9-CM
265.2 pellagra

 ## Pemphigus, benign chronic familial

DESCRIPTION Benign, persistently recurrent bullous dermatitis (autosomal dominant; 66% positive family history). Characteristics — crops of lesions (may remain localized or become generalized), that rupture, undergo erosion and become thickly crusted. sites: sides of the neck, axillae, groin, and flexural and opposing surfaces of the body. Usual course - intermittent; spontaneous exacerbations with remissions.

SYNONYMS
- Hailey-Hailey disease

CAUSES
- defective intercellular cohesion
- defective tonofilament attachment to desmosomes
- precipitated by infection
- precipitated by trauma

TREATMENT
- antibiotics
- dapsone
- systemic steroids for severe cases
- topical steroids of limited value
- complete excision with split thickness skin graft

ICD-9-CM
694.4 pemphigus

Pemphigus, Brazilian

DESCRIPTION Progressive and sometimes fatal variant of pemphigus foliaceous endemic in south central Brazil. Most frequently in children and adolescents. Characteristics — flaccid blisters that rupture easily, forming erosions with peripheral rolls of epidermis, associated with a burning sensation. Usual course - progressive; variable. Endemic areas - South Central Brazil.

SYNONYMS
• fogo selvagem

CAUSES
• unknown
• possibly infectious agent

TREATMENT
• topical corticosteroids for localized disease
• systemic corticosteroids for generalized disease

ICD-9-CM
694.4 pemphigus

Pericholangitis

DESCRIPTION Inflammation of the tissues that surround the bile ducts. Characteristics — fever, mild icterus, hepatomegaly, mild pruritus. Usual course - progressive.

CAUSES
• unknown

TREATMENT
• none

ICD-9-CM
576.9 biliary tract disorder, nos

Perleche

DESCRIPTION Single or multiple fissures and cracks at corners of the mouth. In advanced stages may extend to lips and cheeks. Usual course - chronic; relapsing; acute.

SYNONYMS
• angulus infectiosus

CAUSES
• poorly fitting dentures
• monilia infection
• dietary deficiency

TREATMENT
• antimonilial drugs
• vitamins
• refit dentures

ICD-9-CM
686.8 perleche

Personality disorders

DESCRIPTION A group of conditions that are not forms of illnesses, but ways of behaving. They are classified depending on the predominant symptoms and their severity. Characteristics include relatively fixed, inflexible and maladaptive patterns of behavior that cause trouble with relationships, work and the law. The individuals feel their behavior patterns are "normal" and "right."
• Paranoid: shows unwarranted suspiciousness and distrust of others, defensive, oversensitive.
• Schizoid and schizotypal: cold emotionally, difficulty in forming relationships, withdrawn, shy, superstitious, socially isolated.
• Compulsive: perfectionist, rigid in habits, indecisive, need for control.
• Histrionic: dependent, immature, excitable, vain, constantly crave stimulation.
• Narcissistic: exaggerated sense of own importance, exhibitionist, preoccupied with power, lack of interest in others, demands attention,
• Avoidant: fears and overreact to rejection, low self-esteem, socially withdrawn, dependent.
• Dependent: passive, overaccepting, unable to make decisions, lack of confidence.
• Passive-aggressive: stubborn, sulking, fear of authority, procrastinates, chronic lateness, argumentative, helpless, clinging.
• Antisocial: selfish, callous, promiscuous, impulsive, reckless, unable to learn from experience, failure at school and work.
• Borderline: impulsive, has unstable and intense inter-personal relationships, inappropriate anger, fear and guilt, lacks self-control, has identity problems, is suicidal.

TREATMENT
• Long-term psychotherapy
• Antidepressants for depression or anxiety
• Clomipramine or fluoxetine for compulsive disorders
• Antipsychotic drugs for psychoses

ICD-9-CM
301.9 unspecified personality disorder

Peutz-Jeghers syndrome

DESCRIPTION Multiple pigmented (melanin) macules of the skin and mouth mucosa and multiple polyposis of the small intestine. Usual course - chronic.

SYNONYMS
• intestinal polyposis II
• intestinal polyposis-cutaneous pigmentation syndrome
• periorificial lentiginosis syndrome

CAUSES
• hereditary

TREATMENT
• surgery

ICD-9-CM
759.6 Peutz-Jeghers syndrome

Peyronie's disease

DESCRIPTION A disease of unknown etiology producing fibrosis of the sinusoidal spaces of the corpora cavernosa. Patients present with a painful plaque on the dorsum of the penis and may develop penile curvature and erectile failure. Pain generally disappears in 6-12 months.

CAUSES
• Unknown

TREATMENT
• Options which may be valuable:
  ◊ Conservative observation
  ◊ Surgical correction
• Options which may be of little value:
  ◊ p-aminobenzoic acid
  ◊ Vitamin E
• Options of little value or hampers subsequent treatments:
  ◊ Vitamin A
  ◊ Radiotherapy
  ◊ orgotein (Peroxinorm) injections
  ◊ corticosteroid injections

ICD-9-CM
607.89 Other specified disorders of corpus cavernosum or penis

Phlyctenular keratoconjunctivitis

DESCRIPTION Conjunctivitis and keratitis with discrete nodules of inflammation (phlyctenules).
• Characteristics - signs and symptoms include blepharospasm, severe lacrimation, photophobia, and pain

CAUSES
• atopic reaction of a hypersensitive conjunctiva to an unknown allergen, perhaps the protein of staphylococcal, tuberculous or other bacteria

TREATMENT
• Topical corticosteroid and antibiotic combination
• Ophthalmological referral or consultation

ICD-9-CM
370.31 Phlyctenular keratoconjunctivitis

Phosphine poisoning

DESCRIPTION Poisoning by hydrogen phosphide, PH3, a malodorous gas. Usual course - acute; progressive

CAUSES
• acid on phosphorus-contaminated metals
• water on phosphorus-contaminated metals
• acetylene to release phosphine gas
• phosphides to release phosphine gas

TREATMENT
• gastric decontamination
• irrigate eyes
• supportive
• excise sequestered jaw bone

ICD-9-CM
987.8 poisoning, phosphine

Phosphorus poisoning

DESCRIPTION Condition resulting from inhalation or ingestion of phosphorous. Characteristics — garlic breath odor, mandibular necrosis, toothache, anemia, anorexia, weakness, luminescent vomitus. Usual course - acute; progressive.

SYNONYMS
• yellow phosphorous poisoning

CAUSES
• cytotoxicity

TREATMENT
• gastric decontamination
• irrigate eyes
• supportive
• bone excision

ICD-9-CM
983.9 poisoning, phosphorus

Pick's disease

DESCRIPTION Rare progressive degenerative disease of the brain. Clinically similar to Alzheimer's with impaired reasoning, poor insight, memory loss, apathy, amnesia, aphasia, incontinence, and extrapyramidal signs. Pathologically, cortical atrophy is confined to frontal and temporal lobes. Usual course - chronic; progressive.

SYNONYMS
• lobar atrophy
• circumscribed brain atrophy
• presenile dementia

CAUSES
• degenerative disease

TREATMENT
• occupational therapy
• family counseling

ICD-9-CM
331.1 Pick's disease

 Pickwickian syndrome

DESCRIPTION Extreme obesity with polycythemia, somnolence, hypoventilation, arterial unsaturation and hypercapnia, and pulmonary hypertension. Usual course - chronic; intermittent.

SYNONYMS
• hypoventilation associated with extreme obesity

CAUSES
• marked obesity

TREATMENT
• caloric restriction
• progesterone
• tracheostomy

ICD-9-CM
278.8 pickwickian syndrome

 Pilonidal cyst

DESCRIPTION Hair-containing sacrococcygeal dermoid cyst or sinus that opens at a post anal dimple. Usual course - acute; chronic.

SYNONYMS
• pilonidal sinus
• jeep driver's disease
• coccygeal sinus
• pilliferous cyst

CAUSES
• ingrown broken hair
• stocky body build
• trauma

TREATMENT
• drainage
• excision

ICD-9-CM
685.1 pilonidal cyst without mention of abscess

 Pituitary basophilic adenoma

DESCRIPTION Small tumor of the anterior lobe whose cells stain with basic dyes and give rise to excessive secretion of ACTH resulting in Cushing's syndrome. Characteristics include truncal obesity, hypertension, visual disturbances, menstrual irregularity, impotence, muscle atrophy, osteoporosis, psychic disturbances. Usual course - chronic; progressive.

CAUSES
• unknown

TREATMENT
• transsphenoidal resection
• pituitary irradiation
• bromocriptine

ICD-9-CM
227.3 benign neoplasm of the pituitary

 Pituitary chromophobe adenoma

DESCRIPTION Anterior lobe of the pituitary gland tumor. Characteristics — hypopituitarism, headache, lassitude, visual disturbances, galactorrhea, hypogonadism. Usual course - chronic; progressive.

CAUSES
• unknown

TREATMENT
• transsphenoidal resection
• irradiation
• bromocriptine

ICD-9-CM
227.3 benign neoplasm of the pituitary

 Pituitary dwarfism

DESCRIPTION Dwarfism caused by hypofunction of the anterior pituitary gland with decreased secretion of growth hormone.

SYNONYMS
• ateliotic dwarfism
• panhypopituitary dwarfism
• hypopituitary dwarfism

CAUSES
• idiopathic
• pituitary tumor
• intrathecal methotrexate
• trauma
• CNS irradiation
• hemochromatosis
• sarcoidosis
• hypothalamic failure
• hypothalamic tumor
• CNS infection
• histiocytosis
• septo-optic dysplasia
• holoprosencephaly
• biologically inactive growth hormone
• growth hormone receptor insensitivity
• deficiency insulin-like growth factor I
• psychosocial dwarfism

TREATMENT
• exogenous growth hormone
• counseling

ICD-9-CM
253.3 pituitary dwarfism

 Pituitary eosinophilic adenoma

DESCRIPTION A tumor of the anterior lobe of the pituitary associated with acromegaly and gigantism Usual course - chronic; progressive.

SYNONYMS
• pituitary acidophilic adenoma

CAUSES
• unknown

TREATMENT
• transsphenoidal resection
• pituitary irradiation
• bromocriptine

ICD-9-CM
227.3 benign neoplasm of the pituitary

 Pituitary gigantism

DESCRIPTION Giantism due to excessive pituitary secretion occurring before puberty and before epiphyses close. May be caused by eosinophilia or chromophobe adenoma. Usual course - insidious.

CAUSES
• somatotropic cell adenoma of the pituitary
• somatotropic cell adenoma of mixed cell
• somatotropic cell adenoma of stem cell
• bronchial adenoma
• pancreatic islet cell tumor
• carcinoid tumor
• ectopic growth hormone production

TREATMENT
• surgery
• irradiation
• bromocriptine

ICD-9-CM
253.0 pituitary gigantism

 Pituitary hypothyroidism

DESCRIPTION Hypothyroidism caused by deficiency of thyrotropin secretion. Usual course - chronic.

CAUSES
• pituitary irradiation
• pituitary ablative surgery
• failure of anterior pituitary due to infarction

TREATMENT
• thyroid hormone replacement

ICD-9-CM
244.9 pituitary hypothyroidism

Placental insufficiency syndrome

DESCRIPTION Malnutrition and hypoxia of the fetus due to degenerative changes in the placenta.

CAUSES
• postterm fetus

TREATMENT
• good perinatal care

ICD-9-CM
762.2 Fetus affected by unspecified abnormality of placenta
656.5 Poor fetal growth (from placental problem) affecting management of mother

 Pleural malignant mesothelioma

DESCRIPTION Malignant tumor derived from mesothelial tissue. Characteristics — chest pain, dyspnea, weight loss, asthenia, cough, hemoptysis. Usual course - progressive; insidious onset.

CAUSES
• primary tumor of the pleura
• asbestos
• first exposure 20 to 60 years prior to diagnosis

TREATMENT
• surgery
• radiotherapy
• chemotherapy

ICD-9-CM
163.9 malignant neoplasm of the pleura

 Portal vein thrombosis

DESCRIPTION Clotting of the portal vein of the liver usually from unknown cause. Characteristics — hematemesis, melena splenomegaly, pancytopenia, encephalopathy, portal hypertension. It occurs in pregnancy (especially eclampsia) chronic heart failure, constrictive pericarditis, malignancies. Diagnosis established by angiography. Usual course - chronic; progressive.

CAUSES
• usually idiopathic
• neonatal septicemia
• omphalitis
• hepatocellular cancer
• umbilical vein catheterization for exchange transfusion

TREATMENT
• treat underlying condition
• possible shunt surgery

ICD-9-CM
452 portal vein thrombosis

 Postpoliomyelitis syndrome

DESCRIPTION A slow, progressive muscle weakness and deterioration of function in the previously affected muscles of an individual who had poliomyelitis at least 10 years earlier. The syndrome can appear 30 or more years after a partial or full recovery from the initial polio episode and is noninfectious. It usually involves those muscles most affected by the polio virus, but sometimes affects muscles that are fully recovered or never involved in the initial infection. Other symptoms include fatigue, muscle pain and fasciculations.

SYNONYMS
• polio late effects
• postpoliomyelitis progressive muscular atrophy

CAUSES
• exact cause is unknown

TREATMENT
• physical and occupational therapy
• exercise, e.g., swimming
• consider changes in braces, medication or diet
• weight loss diet, if overweight
• respiratory support, if breathing is affected

ICD-9-CM
138 late effects of acute poliomyelitis

 Prader-Willi/Angelman syndrome

DESCRIPTION A congenital disorder of unknown etiology characterized by mental retardation, muscular hypotonia, obesity, short stature, hypogonadism and frequently developing insulin-resistant diabetes. Genetics - occasional small deletion of chromosome 15; sporadic; possible autosomal recessive. Usual course - progressive. When deletion is inherited from father the expression is Angelman's syndrome; when deletion is inherited from mother, the manifestations are Prader-Willi.

CAUSES
• hypothalamic dysfunction

TREATMENT
• dietary restrictions
• testosterone
• gastric bypass
• jaw wiring
• progesterone

ICD-9-CM
759.8 prader-willi syndrome

 Premature atrial contraction (PAC)

DESCRIPTION Premature, abnormal P waves. QRS complexes follow except in very early or blocked PAC. P wave may be buried in the preceding T wave or may be identified in the preceding T wave.

CAUSES
• congestive heart failure, coronary artery disease with ischemia, acute respiratory failure, chronic obstructive pulmonary disease, digitalis toxicity, aminophylline, adrenergic drugs, anxiety, caffeine

TREATMENT
• eliminate known causes

ICD-9-CM
427.61 premature atrial contraction

 Premature ventricular contraction (PVC)

DESCRIPTION Irregular pulse. Ventricular beat occurs prematurely, followed by a compensatory pause after the premature ventricular contraction. QRS complex is wide and distorted. Most ominous when clustered, multifocal, with R wave on T pattern.

CAUSES
• multiple causes can include psychological stress, physiologic stress, drug toxicity (digitalis, aminophylline, tricyclic antidepressants, beta adrenergics (isoproterenol or dopamine)), caffeine, tobacco, electrolyte imbalances (especially hypokalemia)

TREATMENT
• lidocaine IV bolus and drip infusion
• procainamide IV if induced by digitalis toxicity
• stop digitalis. If caused by hypokalemia, give potassium chloride intravenous drip
• eliminate known causes

ICD-9-CM
427.69 premature ventricular contraction

 Primary lateral sclerosis

DESCRIPTION Degeneration of the lateral columns of the spinal cord. Characteristics — spastic paraplegia, rigidity of limbs, increased tendon reflexes, absence of nutritive and sensory disturbance. Usual course - chronic; slowly progressive.

CAUSES
• unknown
• existence as separate clinical entity questioned

TREATMENT
• none

ICD-9-CM
335.24 primary lateral sclerosis

 Prion diseases

DESCRIPTION A group of degenerative disorders of the central nervous system (and perhaps of peripheral nerves and muscles) caused by proteins, rather than by infectious agents carrying DNA and/or RNA. These disorders affect about 1 person in a million, typically around age 60; 10-15% are inherited. Recognized human disorders in this group include: Kuru, Creutzfeldt-Jakob disease, Gerstmann-Straussler-Scheinker disease, and fatal familial insomnia.

SYNONYMS
• Spongiform encephalopathies

CAUSES Prions (scrapie PrP)

TREATMENT
• None known

ICD-9-CM
046.0 Kuru
046.1 Creutzfeldt-Jacob disease

Proctalgia fugax

DESCRIPTION Abrupt, sharp or gripping-like pain in the anorectal area. The pain does not radiate. Often the pain wakes the individual in the night. Typically, relief occurs within seconds to minutes, although rare, the pain can be present for hours. The disorder is benign and there is no cure.

SYNONYMS
levator syndrome

CAUSES
• unknown; attributed to spasm of levator ani and coccygeal muscles, sometimes associated with stress or anxiety

TREATMENT
• reassuring patient of benign nature of disease is satisfactory in most cases
• warm baths
• periodic massage
• for severe pain, consider inhaled albuterol, oral clonidine, diltiazem

ICD-9-CM
564.6 anal spasm

 Progressive external ophthalmoplegia

DESCRIPTION Slowly progressive bilateral myopathy affecting the extraocular muscles. Characteristics — weakness of levators of the upper lids, ptosis, followed by total ocular paresis. Usual course - chronic; progressive.

SYNONYMS
• chronic dystrophic ophthalmoplegia

CAUSES
• unknown

TREATMENT
• none

ICD-9-CM
378.72 progressive external ophthalmoplegia

 Progressive hemiatrophy face

DESCRIPTION Atrophy of one half of the face which is usually progressive, but may eventually become stationary.

SYNONYMS
• Romberg's disease
• Parry-Romberg syndrome
• progressive hemifacial atrophy

CAUSES
• unknown
• possible lipodystrophy

TREATMENT
• plastic reconstructive surgery
• skin transplantation
• subcutaneous fat transplantation

ICD-9-CM
349.89 hemiatrophy, face, progressive.

 Progressive multifocal leukoencephalopathy

DESCRIPTION Serious, usually fatal viral disease. Characteristics — demyelination in white matter of the brain, but may be seen in the brain stem and cerebellum. It occurs secondary to lymphosarcoma and lymphatic myeloid leukemia. Usual course - progressive.

CAUSES
• latent papovavirus

TREATMENT
• cytosine arabinoside

ICD-9-CM
046.3 progressive multifocal leukoencephalopathy

 Prolactinoma

DESCRIPTION A pituitary adenoma which secretes prolactin, leading to increased serum levels of prolactin. Prolactinomas in women are presented with galactorrhea associated with amenorrhea. Though much less common for men, prolactinomas in men rarely produce galactorrhea and are later presented as larger, space-occupying tumors. Usual course - progressive.

SYNONYMS
• prolactin secreting pituitary adenoma
• PRL secreting pituitary adenoma

CAUSES
• prolactin-secreting pituitary microadenoma

TREATMENT
• transsphenoidal resection
• bromocriptine
• irradiation

ICD-9-CM
253.1 forbes-albright syndrome

 Pseudocyst pancreas

DESCRIPTION Unilocular cyst of the pancreas. Characteristics — tender mass in left upper quadrant, abdominal pain, weight loss, nausea, anorexia, jaundice. Usual course - acute; progressive.

CAUSES
• acute pancreatitis
• trauma
• pancreatic enzymes released into lesser omentum

TREATMENT
• needle aspiration
• internal drainage surgery
• external drainage

ICD-9-CM
577.2 cyst and pseudocyst of pancreas

 Pulmonary artery thrombosis

DESCRIPTION Blood clot in the pulmonary artery. Characteristics — dyspnea, weakness, chest pain, tachycardia, tachypnea.

CAUSES
• reduction in blood flow of pulmonary artery
• organization of previous embolism
• malignancy
• infection
• trauma
• intrinsic disease

TREATMENT
• anticoagulants

ICD-9-CM
415.1 pulmonary artery thrombosis

 Pulmonary hypertension, secondary

DESCRIPTION Increased pressure in the pulmonary circulation above 30 millimeters of mercury systolic, and 12 millimeters of mercury diastolic, secondary to any of the listed causes.

CAUSES
• CHF, left ventricular failure, mitral stenosis, mitral regurgitation, myxoma, pulmonary embolism, interstitial fibrosis, sarcoidosis, asbestosis, radiation, alveolar hypoventilation, chronic obstructive pulmonary disease, chronic bronchitis, emphysema, ventricular septal defect, atrial septal defect, silicosis, anthrosilicosis, tuberculosis, SLE, scleroderma, dermatomyositis, connective tissue disorder, cystic fibrosis

TREATMENT
• corticosteroids, oxygen, cardiac catheterization, nitroprusside, hydralazine, diazoxid, isoproterenol, phentolamine, prazosin, verapamil, nifedipine, captopril

ICD-9-CM
416.8 secondary pulmonary hypertension

 Pulmonary infarction

DESCRIPTION Hemorrhagic consolidation of lung parenchyma resulting from thromboembolic pulmonary arterial occlusion. Usual course - acute.

CAUSES
• stasis, vein injury, hypercoagulable state, phlebitis, phlebothrombosis, thrombus, deep vein thrombosis, burn, surgery, oral contraceptives, trauma, hip fracture, immobilization, congestive heart failure, cardiomyopathy, subacute bacterial endocarditis, atrial myxoma, polycythemia rubra vera, sickle cell anemia, pancreatic carcinoma

TREATMENT
• anticoagulation
• heparin
• coumadin
• warfarin
• thrombolytic agent
• urokinase
• streptokinase
• embolectomy
• vena cava clip

ICD-9-CM
415.1 pulmonary embolism and infarction

Pulmonary interstitial fibrosis, idiopathic

DESCRIPTION Interstitial pneumonia, "nonspecific," or "usual." The term used when etiology leading to pulmonary fibrosis cannot be defined (about 50% of cases). Usual course - chronic; progressive.

SYNONYMS
• alveolocapillary block
• fibrosing alveolitis

CAUSES
• unknown
• loss of functional alveolar-capillary units
• inflammation

TREATMENT
• corticosteroids

ICD-9-CM
516.3 diffuse interstitial pulmonary fibrosis

 Pyogenic abscess liver

DESCRIPTION Bacterial abscess of the liver. Characteristics - fever, abdominal pain, anorexia, jaundice, hepatomegaly, elevated hemidiaphragm. Usual course - acute; relapsing.

CAUSES
• portal vein bacteremia
• systemic bacteremia
• ascending cholangitis
• direct extension
• trauma

TREATMENT
• aspiration
• antibiotics
• surgical drainage

ICD-9-CM
572.0 abscess of liver

 Pyrogenic shock

DESCRIPTION Shock associated with overwhelming infection, most commonly with gram-negative bacteria. Characteristics - fever, tachycardia, chills, myalgia, confusion, tachypnea, hypotension, nausea. Usual course - acute.

SYNONYMS
• septic shock
• endotoxic shock

CAUSES
• inadequate tissue perfusion following bacteremia
• escherichia coli
• klebsiella
• pseudomonas
• serratia
• neisseria meningitidis
• staphylococci; pneumococci; streptococci; bacteroides

TREATMENT
• respiratory support
• fluid replacement
• antibiotics
• vasoactive drugs

ICD-9-CM
785.59 septic shock

 Q fever

DESCRIPTION Acute, generally self-limited rickettsial infection. Characteristics — fever, chills, headache, myalgia, malaise, rash (rarely), pneumonitis, hepatitis, and endocarditis. No vector involved. Infection by inhalation of dust or aerosols derived from infected domestic animals. Usual course - abrupt; relapsing; chronic; usually mild. Endemic areas - Western USA; Australia; Africa; England; Mediterranean countries.

SYNONYMS
• Australian Q fever
• Balkan grippe
• nine mile fever
• hiberno-vernal bronchopneumonia
• Derrick-Burnet disease
• Query fever

CAUSES
• Coxiella burnetii (rickettsia)
• Aspiration of infected material
• Contaminated raw milk ingestion
• Infected animal conceptional product exposure

TREATMENT
• antibiotics

ICD-9-CM
083.0 Q fever

 Rat-bite fever, spirillary

DESCRIPTION Infection caused by a rat or mouse bite. Characteristics — wound heals promptly; inflammation recurs at bite site after 10 or more days, accompanied by relapsing fever and regional lymphadenitis; WBC elevated; myalgia, skin rash, chills, malaise, headache. Usual course - relapsing. Endemic areas - Asia; Europe; USA.

SYNONYMS
• sodoku

CAUSES
• spirillum minor-a spirochete
• rodent bite
• rodent scratch
• rodent-ingesting animal bite

TREATMENT
• antibiotics
• rapid bite cleaning

ICD-9-CM
026.9 rat-bite fever

 Rat-bite fever, streptobacillary

DESCRIPTION Bacterial infection caused by a rat or mouse bite, although occasionally associated with ingestion of contaminated milk or with the bite of a different rodent. Characteristics (10 or more days following the bite) — abrupt illness with chills, fever, vomiting, headache, arthralgia, backache, elevated WBC, morbilliform petechial skin rash. Usual course - relapsing. Endemic areas - Asia; Europe; USA.

CAUSES
• streptobacillus moniliformis
• rodent bite
• rodent scratch
• contaminated raw milk ingestion

TREATMENT
• antibiotics
• rapid bite cleansing

ICD-9-CM
026.9 rat-bite fever

 Relapsing fever

DESCRIPTION An acute infectious disease caused by arthropod-borne spirochetes. Clinically characterized by recurrent episodes of fever typically lasting three to five days, headache, arthralgia, myalgia, diarrhea, vomiting, coughing, eye and chest pain, splenomegaly. Two forms of the disease exist: louse-borne and tick-borne. Louse-borne relapsing fever occurs primarily in developing countries and is transmitted by body lice. Tick-borne relapsing fever is less severe and is caused by several species of Borrelia. It is transmitted by soft body ticks of the genus Ornithodoros.

SYNONYMS
• recurrent fever
• tick fever
• famine fever

CAUSES
• body lice
• body ticks

TREATMENT
• tetracyclines
• erythromycin
• penicillin

ICD-9-CM
087.9 fever

 Renal artery stenosis

DESCRIPTION Occlusive disease of the renal arteries. This problem occurs in about 5% of patients with hypertension and is one form of hypertension that is surgically correctable. The disease is most often unilateral. Usual course - progressive.

CAUSES
• atherosclerosis
• fibromuscular dysplasia

TREATMENT
• surgery
• angioplasty
• antihypertensives

ICD-9-CM
440.1 renal artery stenosis

 Renal infarction

DESCRIPTION Localized area of kidney necrosis caused by either renal arterial or venous occlusion. Characteristics - steady, aching, flank pain, fever, nausea, vomiting, hypertension, leukocytosis, proteinuria, microscopic hematuria. Renal imaging confirms the diagnosis. Usual course - acute.

CAUSES
• renal artery thrombosis
• renal emboli
• arteriosclerosis
• renal artery aneurysm
• fibrous dysplasia
• aortic dissection
• periarteritis nodosa
• vasculitis
• sickle cell disease
• scleroderma
• polycythemia
• trauma
• surgery
• cardiomegaly
• subacute bacterial endocarditis
• atrial myxoma
• rheumatic heart disease

TREATMENT
• surgery
• balloon angioplasty

ICD-9-CM
593.81 renal infarction

Renal vein thrombosis

DESCRIPTION Clotting within the renal vein. Characteristics — lumbar pain; dysuria; enlarged, tender kidney. Usual course - acute; chronic.

CAUSES
• abdominal operation
• CHF
• dehydration
• renal disease
• reduction in renal blood flow
• pregnancy
• constrictive pericarditis
• morbid obesity

TREATMENT
• anticoagulants
• corticosteroids

ICD-9-CM
453.3 embolism and thrombosis of renal vein

 Reticulum cell sarcoma

DESCRIPTION Malignant histiocytic lymphoma made of a substance like embryonic connective tissue. Characteristics — fatigue, anorexia, weight loss, excessive sweating, fever, painless adenopathy, hepatosplenomegaly. Usual course - chronic; progressive; relapsing.

SYNONYMS
• reticulum cell lymphosarcoma
• diffuse histiocytic lymphoma
• reticulosarcoma

CAUSES
• unknown

TREATMENT
• chemotherapy
• radiotherapy
• surgery

ICD-9-CM
200.00 reticulosarcoma, nos

 Retinal vein occlusion

DESCRIPTION One of the causes of sudden unilateral vision loss. Characteristics — extensive retinal hemorrhages; dilated, tortuous retinal veins. Usual course - acute.

SYNONYMS
• central retinal vein occlusion
• CRVO

TREATMENT
• panretinal photocoagulation

ICD-9-CM
362.35 central retinal vein occlusion

 Retinoblastoma

DESCRIPTION Malignant congenital hereditary blastoma (autosomal dominant with high penetrance). Characteristics - appears in one or both eyes in children under 5 years of age, diagnosed initially by a bright white or yellow pupillary reflex. Usual course - progressive.

SYNONYMS
• glioma retina

CAUSES
• genetic

TREATMENT
• radiotherapy to preserve vision
• photocoagulation to preserve vision
• cryotherapy to preserve vision
• brachytherapy to preserve vision
• enucleation
• palliative radiotherapy for extraocular disease

ICD-9-CM
190.5 malignant neoplasm of the retina

 Rhabdomyosarcoma

DESCRIPTION Highly malignant tumor of striated muscle. There are 3 forms - pleomorphic affecting predominantly the extremities of adults; alveolar form, occurring primarily in adolescents and young adults affecting muscles of extremities, trunk, and orbital region; embryonal form, occurring mainly in infants and children, affecting the head and neck, lower genitourinary tract, pelvis and extremities. Usual course - progressive.

SYNONYMS
• rhabdosarcoma

CAUSES
• fetal alcohol syndrome

TREATMENT
• surgical excision
• add radiotherapy in most cases
• group 2: add chemotherapy with vincristine plus dactinomycin
• group 3: add chemotherapy with vincristine plus dactinomycin
• combination chemotherapy for advanced disease

ICD-9-CM
171.9 malignant neoplasm of connective and soft tissue

 Rheumatoid pneumoconiosis

DESCRIPTION Pneumoconiosis associated with rheumatoid arthritis. Characteristics — multiple spherical modular lesions with clearly demarcated borders found throughout both lungs. Usual course: chronic; progressive.

SYNONYMS
• Caplan syndrome
• rheumatoid lung with silicosis
• silicoarthritis

CAUSES
• unknown
• immune mechanism

TREATMENT
• manage complications

ICD-9-CM
714.81 caplan's syndrome

 Rhinosporidiosis

DESCRIPTION Chronic, localized granulomatous infection of mucocutaneous tissues, especially the nose. Characteristics — nasal polyps, tumors, papillomas, or wart-like lesions. Other (rare) areas of infection include the conjunctiva, penis, anus, vagina, ears, pharynx, larynx. Usual course - progressive. Endemic areas - India; Sri-Lanka.

SYNONYMS
• rhinosporosis

CAUSES
• rhinosporidium seeberi

TREATMENT
• surgery

ICD-9-CM
117.0 rhinosporidiosis

 Rhodococcus infections

DESCRIPTION A recognized animal pathogen which is emerging as a human pathogen, especially in immunocompromised hosts. Necrotizing pneumonia, presumed the result of inhalation inoculation, is the most common type of infection; extra-pulmonary infections usually occur as a result of bacteremic spread from the lungs, especially to the brain.

CAUSES
• Rhodococcus equi, a pleomorphic Gram-positive rod when cultured on solid media, which may also stain acid-fast. (It may have coccus morphology on primary Gram stain from clinical material.) This bacterium is found in nature most commonly in the soil of terrain habituated by grazing animals.

TREATMENT
Antibiotics: particularly erythromycin, rifampin, vancomycin, ciproflaxacin, and gentamicin. Successful therapy in immunocompromised persons almost always requires combinations of at least two antibiotics administered for a long duration, not uncommonly in conjunction with "debulking" resection of necrotic, infected tissue. Relapse is common after discontinuation of therapy, and long-term secondary prophylaxis with an oral agent should be considered. Prophylaxis against Mycobacterium avium-complex (MAC) bacteremia in AIDS patients, using rifabutin, clarithromycin, or azithromycin, may also have a prophylactic effect against Rhodococcus equi in those patients.

ICD-9-CM
482.89 Pneumonia due to specified bacteria NEC

 Riboflavin deficiency

DESCRIPTION Deficiency of vitamin B2. Deficiency characteristics — cheilosis, photophobia, sore throat, glossitis, fissure tongue, seborrheic dermatitis. Usual course - acute; progressive.

SYNONYMS
• vitamin B2 deficiency
• ariboflavinosis

CAUSES
• inadequate dietary intake
• intestinal malabsorption

TREATMENT
• riboflavin administration

ICD-9-CM
266.0 ariboflavinosis

Rickettsialpox

DESCRIPTION   Mild, self-limited disease transmitted by
a mite that is an ectoparasite of the house mouse.
Characteristics — eschar-like primary skin lesion,
generalize papulovesicular rash, headache, and backache.
Usual course - acute; incubation period 10 days to 3 weeks
after bite. Endemic areas - USA; Europe; Africa.

CAUSES
• Rickettsia akari
• bite from mite (vector) infected by rodent

TREATMENT
• tetracycline
• chloramphenicol

ICD-9-CM
083.2 rickettsialpox

Ruptured chordae tendineae

DESCRIPTION   Rupture of a tendinous chord that
connects each cusp of atrioventricular valves to
approximate papillary muscles in the heart ventricles.
Characteristics include a dramatic holosystolic apical
murmur, precordial thrill, chest pain, dyspnea. Rupture of
the chordae of the mitral valve is not uncommon. Usual
course - acute; progressive.

CAUSES
• endocarditis
• trauma
• thoracic compression
• myxomatous perforation

TREATMENT
• diuretics
• surgical repair

ICD-9-CM
429.5 rupture of chordae tendineae

Ruptured mitral papillary muscle

DESCRIPTION   Rupture of conical muscular projections
from walls of the cardiac ventricles, attached to cusps of
the mitral arterioventricular valves by the chordae tendinae.
Characteristics — pansystolic murmur, apical thrill, signs
and symptoms of congestive heart failure. Usual course -
acute; progressive.

SYNONYMS
• papillary muscle rupture

CAUSES
• myocardial infarction
• myocardial necrosis
• trauma

TREATMENT
• diuretics
• surgery

ICD-9-CM
429.6 rupture of papillary muscle

Schatzki's ring

DESCRIPTION   Ring-like narrowing of the distal
esophagus at the squamo-columnar junction. It is probably
congenital and measures 2-4 mm in the submucosa.
Characteristics — dysphagia. X-ray with barium swallow
confirms the diagnosis by displaying the annular constriction
of the lower esophagus. Usual course - chronic;
progressive.

SYNONYMS
• esophagogastric ring syndrome
• lower esophageal ring syndrome

CAUSES
• unknown

TREATMENT
• rubber dilatation of ring

ICD-9-CM
530.3 Stricture and stenosis of esophagus
750.3 Tracheoesophageal fistula, esophageal atresia and
stenosis (congenital)

Schistosomiasis haematobium

DESCRIPTION   Parasitic disease caused by blood
flukes of the genus Schistosoma haematobium. S.
Haematobium causes symptoms in the genitourinary
system or lower colon and rectum. Endemic in Africa,
India, Middle East, Indian Ocean islands. Usual course -
acute; chronic; intermittent; progressive.

SYNONYMS
• endemic hematuria
• urogenital schistosomiasis

CAUSES
• trematode Schistosoma haematobium
• fresh water snail reservoir

TREATMENT
• praziquantel
• metrifonate
• niridazole

ICD-9-CM
120.0 schistosomiasis due to Schistosoma haematobium

Schistosomiasis japonica

DESCRIPTION   Parasitic disease caused by blood
flukes of Schistosoma japonica causing disturbances in the
small intestine, colon, and rectum. Characteristics — may
be asymptomatic, melena, diarrhea, hepatosplenomegaly.
Endemic area - Africa, India, Middle East, Indian Ocean
islands. Usual course - acute; chronic; intermittent;
progressive.

SYNONYMS
• eastern schistosomiasis
• katayama disease
• Yangtze River disease

CAUSES
• trematode Schistosoma japonica
• fresh water snail reservoir

TREATMENT
• praziquantel
• niridazole
• stibocaptate

ICD-9-CM
120.2 schistosomiasis due to Schistosoma japonicum

Schistosomiasis mansoni

DESCRIPTION   Parasitic disease caused by blood flukes
of Schistosoma mansoni causing disturbances in the small
intestine, colon, and rectum. Characteristics — diarrhea,
weight loss, anorexia, melena, jaundice,
hepatosplenomegaly. Endemic areas - Africa, South
America, Caribbean, Middle East. May occur in Americans
who lived in Puerto Rico. Usual course - acute; chronic;
intermittent; progressive.

SYNONYMS
• intestinal bilharziasis
• schistosomal dysentery
• katayama fever
• Manson's schistosomiasis
• Schistosoma mansonii infection
• intestinal schistosomiasis

CAUSES
• trematode Schistosoma mansoni
• fresh water snail reservoir

TREATMENT
• praziquantel
• oxamniquine

ICD-9-CM
120.1 schistosomiasis due to Schistosoma mansoni

Schistosomiasis of the liver,
chronic

DESCRIPTION   Parasitic disease caused by blood flukes
of the genus Schistosoma that penetrate the skin and
develop in the liver, causing fever, eosinophilia, urticaria,
hepatosplenomegaly, lymphadenopathy, ascites, esophageal
varices. Endemic areas - Africa, Asia, South America,
Caribbean Islands.

SYNONYMS
• bilharziasis

CAUSES
• Schistosoma mansoni
• Schistosoma japonicum
• fresh water snails

TREATMENT
• oxamniquine
• praziquantel
• niridazole
• splenorenal anastomosis surgery

ICD-9-CM
120.9 schistosomiasis, unspecified

Schistosomiasis, cutaneous

DESCRIPTION   Parasitic disease caused by blood flukes
of the genus Schistosoma. Fresh and salt water mollusks
are intermediate hosts. Characteristics — intense pruritus,
stinging, macules, papules, and vesicles. Endemic areas -
Hawaii, Florida, Great Lakes area. Usual course - acute;
intermittent; relapsing.

SYNONYMS
• swimmer's itch
• clam digger's itch

CAUSES
• nonspecific Schistosome cercaria
• snail reservoir
• skin penetration
• abnormal host foreign body reaction

TREATMENT
• antipruritics
• antibiotics for secondary bacterial infections

ICD-9-CM
120.3 cutaneous schistosomiasis

Scleredema

DESCRIPTION Diffuse, symmetrical, wooden-like, non-pitting induration of the skin of face, head, shoulders, arms, thorax. Usually preceded by an infectious process. It occurs in association with diabetes mellitus. Resolves in 6 months to 2 years. Usual course - acute; chronic.

SYNONYMS
• scleredema adultorum of buschke

CAUSES
• unknown
• following streptococcal infection

TREATMENT
• self-limited
• unnecessary

ICD-9-CM
710.1 scleredema adultorum

 Sclerosis of the brain

DESCRIPTION Familial form of leukoencephalopathy occurring in early life and running a slowly progressive course into adolescence or adulthood. Characteristics — nystagmus, ataxia, tremor, choreoathetotic movements, dyarthria, and mental deterioration.

SYNONYMS
• Pelizaeus-Merzbacher disease
• diffuse familial cerebral sclerosis
• aplasia axialis extracorticalis congenita

CAUSES
• genetic

TREATMENT
• supportive

ICD-9-CM
330.0 leukodystrophy

 Scoliosis

DESCRIPTION A lateral curvature of the spine that may be found in the thoracic, lumbar, or thoracolumbar spinal segment. The curve may be convex to the right or to the left. Rotation of the vertebral column around its axis occurs and may cause rib cage deformity. May be associated with kyphosis (humpback) or lordosis (swayback). The most common type is idiopathic (80% of cases), usually begins about ages 8-10, is more common in girls than boys (4-5:1) and is classically asymptomatic.

CAUSES
• structural scoliosis
  ◊ idiopathic (may be transmitted as an autosomal dominant or multifactoral trait)
  ◊ congenital defects of the spine (hemivertebral or unilateral vertebral bridge)
  ◊ paralytic or musculoskeletal (due to polio, cerebral palsy, or muscular dystrophy)
• functional scoliosis
  ◊ poor posture
  ◊ uneven leg length

TREATMENT
• physical therapy and back exercises aimed at strengthening back muscles
• orthopedic back brace (sometimes worn for several years)
• if legs are of unequal length, a shoe lift for the shorter leg
• surgery to correct the deformity (severe cases only)

ICD-9-CM
737.30 scoliosis (and kyphoscoliosis), idiopathic
754.2 congenital musculoskeletal deformities of spine

 Scurvy, infantile

DESCRIPTION Nutritional disease of children caused by ascorbic acid deficiency. Characteristics — weakness, anemia, spongy gums, mucocutaneous hemorrhages, brawny induration of calves and legs.

SYNONYMS
• vitamin C deficiency
• Barlow disease
• subperiosteal hematoma syndrome

CAUSES
• ascorbic acid deficiency

TREATMENT
• ascorbic acid
• fruit juice

ICD-9-CM
267 infantile scurvy

 Seasonal affective disorder

DESCRIPTION Depression caused by dysfunction of circadian rhythms, that occurs most often in the winter months and is believed to be due to a decrease in exposure to full-spectrum light. In addition to feelings of sadness and anxiety, symptoms include hypersomnia, lethargy, carbohydrate craving and weight gain. Diagnosis usually requires a 2-3 year mood disturbance pattern, with the onset occurring in the autumn, and a remission in the spring. It occurs more commonly in women and among individuals living in the northern latitudes.

SYNONYMS
SAD

CAUSES
• exact cause is unknown; may be linked to amount of melatonin released by the pineal gland

TREATMENT
• phototherapy (light therapy) is preferential treatment
• MAO inhibitor or fluoxetine
• psychotherapy

ICD-9-CM
300.4 neurotic depression

 Second degree AV block

DESCRIPTION Two subtypes:
• Type I or Wenckebach: P-R interval becomes progressively longer with each cycle until a non-conducted atrial beat occurs. After the dropped beat the P-R interval is shorter.
• Type II: Constant P-R intervals preceding a non-conducted atrial beat.
Ventricular rate is irregular. Atrial rhythm is regular.

SYNONYMS
• Mobitz type 1
• Wenckebach's period

CAUSES
• inferior wall myocardial infarction, digitalis toxicity, vagal stimulation

TREATMENT
• discontinue digitalis
• atropine if patient is symptomatic.

ICD-9-CM
426.13 second degree heart block

 Selective IgA deficiency

DESCRIPTION The most common and mildest immunoglobulin deficiency (<15 mg/dL). IgA is the primary immunoglobulin in human saliva, nasal and bronchial fluids and intestinal secretions. It normally guards against bacterial and viral infections. The deficiency is lifelong and precautions need to be taken to prevent infections.

CAUSES
• autosomal dominant or recessive inheritance
• some drugs may cause transient IgA deficiency
• chromosome 18 abnormalities
• occurs in relatives patients with common variable immunodeficiency

TREATMENT
• no known cure
• treatment for associated diseases
• wear medical alerting identification

ICD-9-CM
279.01 selective IgA immunodeficiency

 Sheehan's syndrome

DESCRIPTION Postpartum pituitary necrosis resulting form hypovolemia and shock in the immediate peri-partem period. Characteristics — endocrine deficiency syndromes due to loss of anterior lobe pituitary function. Usual course - progressive; acute.

SYNONYMS
• postpartum panhypopituitary syndrome
• postpartum hypopituitarism

CAUSES
• intrapartum hemorrhage
• postpartum hemorrhage
• postpartum infection
• peripheral vascular collapse
• vascular spasm
• DIC

TREATMENT
• hormone replacement therapy
• new pregnancy

ICD-9-CM
253.2 Sheehan's syndrome

 Shigellosis

DESCRIPTION Acute infection of the bowel. Source of infection: excreta of infected individuals that may be indirectly spread by contaminated food. Incubation period - 1 to 4 days. Characteristics — sudden onset of fever, irritability, drowsiness, anorexia, nausea, vomiting, diarrhea, abdominal pain and distention. Stools show blood, pus and mucus.

CAUSES
• shigella ingestion

TREATMENT
• fluid replacement
• ampicillin
• tetracycline
• sulfamethoxazole-trimethoprim
• chloramphenicol

ICD-9-CM
004.9 shigellosis, unspecified

Short-bowel syndrome

DESCRIPTION   A malabsorption syndrome resulting from massive resection of small bowel. Characteristics — diarrhea, steatorrhea, malnutrition. Usual course - chronic; progressive.

SYNONYMS
• massive bowel resection syndrome

CAUSES
• excessive resection of small bowel

TREATMENT
• parenteral nutrition
• low fat diet
• trace metal replacement
• mineral replacement
• vitamin replacement
• parenteral bile-salt sequestering agent
• H-2 receptor antagonist

ICD-9-CM
579.2 short bowel syndrome

 Shoulder-hand syndrome

DESCRIPTION   Clinical disorder of the upper extremity. Characteristics — pain and stiffness in the shoulder with puffy swelling and pain in the ipsilateral hand, sometimes occurring after myocardial infarction. Usual course - chronic; acute exacerbations.

SYNONYMS
• Steinbrocker syndrome
• reflex sympathetic dystrophy syndrome
• coronary-scapular syndrome
• postinfarction sclerodactylia

CAUSES
• reflex sympathetic stimulation
• cerebral vascular accident
• myocardial infarction
• upper extremity trauma

TREATMENT
• physical therapy
• analgesics
• oral steroids
• stellate ganglion block
• steroid injections

ICD-9-CM
337.9 shoulder-hand syndrome

 Siderosis of the lung

DESCRIPTION   Pneumoconiosis due to inhalation of iron particles. X-rays are abnormal, but there is no functional impairment and there are no symptoms. Usual course - chronic; acute; progressive.

SYNONYMS
• silver polisher lung
• welder lung

CAUSES
• inhalation of iron oxide dust

TREATMENT
• unnecessary

ICD-9-CM
503 siderosis of the lung

 Silo filler disease

DESCRIPTION   Pulmonary edema caused by nitrogen dioxide intoxication, which may take place among welders or silo fillers. Symptoms may not appear for 12 hours after exposure. Usual course - progressive; acute.

SYNONYMS
• nitrogen dioxide toxicity
• silage gas poisoning
• silo filler pneumoconiosis

CAUSES
• inhalation of nitrogen dioxide

TREATMENT
• bronchodilators
• mechanical ventilation
• supplemental oxygen

ICD-9-CM
506.9 silo fillers' disease

 Silver poisoning

DESCRIPTION   Permanent ashen-gray discoloration of the skin, conjunctiva, and internal organs resulting from long over-exposure to silver. Usual course - acute; chronic.

SYNONYMS
• argyria
• argyriasis

CAUSES
• absorption through skin
• inhalation of dust fumes
• accidental ingestion
• abuse of silver nose drops
• mining
• silver plating
• handling of metallic silver

TREATMENT
• emesis
• hydration
• gastric lavage
• activated charcoal

ICD-9-CM
985.8 argyria

 Sinoatrial arrest or block

DESCRIPTION   Unexpectedly long P-P interval interrupting normal sinus rhythm. Often terminated by a junctional escape beat or return to normal sinus rhythm. QRS complexes uniform, but irregular.

SYNONYMS
• Sinus arrest

CAUSES
• digitalis toxicity, quinidine toxicity, sick sinus syndrome

TREATMENT
• atropine, 0.5 mg intravenously
• Pacemaker for repeated episodes

ICD-9-CM
426.6 sinoatrial heart block

 Sinus bradycardia

DESCRIPTION   Rate of less than 60 beats per minute. A QRS complex follows each P wave.

CAUSES
• sick sinus syndrome, hypothyroidism, mechanical ventilation, inferior myocardial infarction, increased intracranial pressure, increased vagal tone (straining at stool), vomiting, intubation, treatment with beta-blockers and sympatholytic drugs

TREATMENT
• atropine, 0.5 mg every 5 minutes to total of 2.0 mg if needed
• temporary pacemaker if atropine fails

ICD-9-CM
427.89 other rhythm disorder

 Sinus tachycardia

DESCRIPTION   Cardiac rate greater than 100 beats per minute. May rarely increase to exceed 160 beats per minute. Every QRS complex follows a P wave.

CAUSES
• cardiac response to fever, anxiety, vigorous exercise, pain, dehydration, shock, left ventricular heart failure, cardiac tamponade, anemia, hyperthyroidism, hypovolemia, pulmonary embolus, myocardial infarction

TREATMENT
• treat the underlying cause

ICD-9-CM
427.89 other rhythm disorder

Sjögren's syndrome

DESCRIPTION   An autoimmune disorder causing decreased function and progressive destruction of the salivary and lacrimal glands.

SYNONYMS
• Sicca syndrome

CAUSES
• Unknown

ICD-9-CM
710.2 Sjögren's syndrome

Smallpox

DESCRIPTION An acute infectious disease caused by pox virus. This disease is now extinct worldwide due to successful inoculation. Alastrim, a mild form of the disease is known as variola minor.

SYNONYMS
• variola
• variola major

CAUSES
• double-stranded DNA virus transmitted by inhalation
• rare family transmission

TREATMENT
• isolation, report to health department, meticulous fluid management, skin hygiene, antihistamines, antibiotics for secondary bacterial infections

ICD-9-CM
050.9 smallpox, nos

 Somatoform disorders

DESCRIPTION A group of disorders in which there are physical symptoms for which no physical cause can be found. Included in this group are somatization disorder, conversion disorder, and body dysmorphic disorder. Hypochondriasis and chronic pain disorder (somatoform pain disorder) are also classified as somatoform disorders, but are covered in separate topics.
• Somatization disorder: multiple physical symptoms that recur over a period of several years with no medical basis. The patient has usually consulted numerous doctors for treatment and medications. This disorder was previous called hysteria. The symptoms often involve neurological problems (double vision), gynecological problems (painful menstruation) or gastrointestinal problems (abdominal pain).
• Conversion disorder: loss or change of a physical function (paralysis of an arm, blindness, seizures). The symptom is not intentionally produced or faked.
• Body dysmorphic disorder: preoccupation with an imagined defect in a normal-appearing person. The defect may be very minor, but the concern is blown out of proportion. The focus is often on skin wrinkles and blemishes, facial hair, shape of the nose, mouth or jaw.

CAUSES Exact cause is unknown

TREATMENT
• Psychotherapy
• Group therapy
• Family therapy

ICD-9-CM
306.9 unspecified psychophysiological malfunction

 Sotos syndrome

DESCRIPTION A genetic disorder causing physical overgrowth with delayed motor, cognitive, and social development.

SYNONYMS
• cerebral gigantism

CAUSES Unknown

TREATMENT
• Physical therapy
• Speech therapy

ICD-9-CM
253.0 Gigantism

 Sparganosis

DESCRIPTION Infection of animals, including fish and man, with a developmental stage of Diphyllobothrium. This stage has recently been referred to as a plerocercoid but the name sparganum has persisted. Therefore, infection of fish or other animals with the plerocercoid larvae is sparganosis. Fish-eating mammals, including man, are the final hosts. Usual course - chronic.

SYNONYMS
• larval diphyllobothriasis
• sparganosis (larval diphyllobothriasis)

CAUSES
• spirometra species
• larval diphyllobothrium ingestion from undercooked flesh
• animal flesh poultices

TREATMENT
• surgical excision only

ICD-9-CM
123.5 sparganosis

 Spinal cord compression

DESCRIPTION Impingement on the spinal cord, usually by an extramedullary neoplasm. Characteristics — local back pain, hyperreflexia, Babinski's sign, weakness of lower extremities, sensory loss, loss of sphincter control. Back pain and weakness may last hours to days, but total loss of function control to the site of compression may take only minutes. Usual course - acute onset; chronic onset; often progressive primary disease.

CAUSES
• carcinoma of the lung
• breast carcinoma
• carcinoma of the prostate
• lymphoma
• neural malignancy
• herniated disk
• extradural abscess
• spinal tuberculosis
• rheumatoid arthritis
• cervical spondylosis

TREATMENT
• high dose corticosteroids
• radiotherapy
• surgery
• chemotherapy for primary tumor

ICD-9-CM
336.9 spinal cord compression, nos

 Splenic agenesis syndrome

DESCRIPTION Congenital absence of the spleen, partial situs inversus viscerum accompanied by cardiac defects (right type atria, endocardial cushion defect). This is a familial disorder that is autosomal recessive with sporadic penetrance. Usual course - acute; chronic; progressive.

SYNONYMS
• Ivemark syndrome
• asplenia

CAUSES
• failure of normal asymmetry in morphogenesis

TREATMENT
• antibiotics
• cardiac surgery
• gastrointestinal surgery

ICD-9-CM
759.0 agenesis of the spleen

 Squamous cell carcinoma, anterior tongue

DESCRIPTION Malignancy of the oral tongue that does not include the base of the tongue. Characteristics — located on lateral aspects of the undersurface of the tongue.

CAUSES
• unknown

TREATMENT
• surgery plus radiotherapy, depending on staging

ICD-9-CM
141.4 malignant neoplasm of anterior two-thirds of tongue

 Squamous cell carcinoma, anus

DESCRIPTION These malignancies comprise 3-5% of rectal and anal cancers. Characteristics — fungating anal mass, tight sphincter, perineal pain and pressure. Usual course - insidious onset; surgical cure; progressive if untreated.

CAUSES
• condylomata
• rectal fistulae
• rectal fissures
• rectal abscesses
• leukoplakia of the anus
• irradiation

TREATMENT
• surgery
• radiotherapy

ICD-9-CM
154.3 malignant neoplasm of anus

Squamous cell carcinoma, bladder

DESCRIPTION Bladder malignancy frequently associated with parasitic infection or chronic mucosal irritation. Characteristics — highly infiltrative, poor prognosis, gross hematuria, dysuria. Usual course - progressive.

SYNONYMS
• epidermoid bladder carcinoma

CAUSES
• beta-naphthylamine
• 4-aminodiphenyl
• tobacco smoking
• chronic schistosoma haematobium infection
• aniline dye

TREATMENT
• endoscopic resection
• segmental bladder resection
• total cystectomy
• methotrexate
• cis-platin
• doxorubicin
• intravesical thiotepa
• preoperative radiotherapy
• supervoltage radiotherapy
• intracavitary radium
• interstitial implantations

ICD-9-CM
188.9 malignant neoplasm of the bladder

Squamous cell carcinoma, floor of the mouth

DESCRIPTION These account for 20,000 new cases of oral cancer each year. Appears most often as a red (erythroblastic) lesion at first appearing as an inflammatory lesion. Characteristics — lump in floor of the mouth; chronic, non-healing ulcer; foul breath odor; very few are indurated or raised. Usual course - progressive if not cured.

CAUSES
• tobacco
• alcohol
• poor oral hygiene
• epstein-barr virus
• chronic oral trauma
• plummer-vinson virus
• betel nut chewing

TREATMENT
• surgery plus radiotherapy depending on stage
• surgery plus radiotherapy depending on location

ICD-9-CM
144.9 malignant neoplasm of the floor of the mouth

 Squamous cell carcinoma, lung

DESCRIPTION A type of bronchogenic carcinoma. Characteristics — cough, hemoptysis, chest pain, dyspnea, weight loss, fever. Usual course - usually progressive.

SYNONYMS
• epidermoid carcinoma of the lung

CAUSES
• tobacco smoking
• radioisotopes
• asbestos
• halogen ethers
• polycyclic aromatic hydrocarbons
• tuberculosis
• nickel
• chromium
• inorganic arsenic
• iron ore
• printing inks
• other pollutants

TREATMENT
• surgery
• radiotherapy

ICD-9-CM
162.9 malignant neoplasm of the lung

 Squamous cell carcinoma, nasopharynx

DESCRIPTION Malignancy associated with tobacco consumption and the Epstein-Barr virus. Characteristics — nasal obstruction, epistaxis, tinnitus, facial pain, painless upper neck mass, occipital and temporal headache. Usual course - relapsing; early cure.

CAUSES
• nitrosamines
• Epstein Barr virus
• salted fish

TREATMENT
• high dose external beam radiotherapy
• surgical resection in selected patients

ICD-9-CM
147.9 malignant neoplasm of the nasopharynx

 Strabismus

DESCRIPTION Deviation of one eye from parallelism with the other

SYNONYMS
• Squint
• Cross eyes
• Heterotropia

CAUSES
• paralytic (nonconcomitant) strabismus - paralysis of one or more ocular muscles. Nonparalytic (concomitant) - unequal muscle tone.

TREATMENT
• treatment before age 6 years - complete eye exam; corrective lenses or contact lenses; miotics; orthoptic training; surgical restoration of muscle balance

ICD-9-CM
378.9 Unspecified disorder of eye movement

 Strongyloidiasis

DESCRIPTION Infection with Strongyloides stercoralis occurring widely in tropical and subtropical countries. Larvae develop in the soil and penetrate the human skin on contact. They travel to the lungs via the bloodstream and thence to the trachea and esophagus and intestines. Usual course - intermittent.

CAUSES
• parasitic infection caused by strongyloides stercorous
• penetration of the skin by larvae
• contaminated food ingestion
• autoinfection

TREATMENT
• thiabendazole

ICD-9-CM
127.2 strongyloidiasis

 Sturge-Weber disease

DESCRIPTION One of the neurocutaneous syndromes. Congenital capillary hemangiomas affect the skin of the face and neck, mucous membranes, meninges, choroid and conjunctiva. Usually unilateral and in trigeminal nerve distribution, hemangiomata can involve the meninges with associated focal brain atrophy, sclerosis, and calcifications. Early onset of seizures is associated with poor outcome of intellectual performance and with neurologic deficits. Course - variable. Complications - seizures, glaucoma, mental retardation, paresis.

SYNONYMS
• Encephalotrigeminal angiomatosis

CAUSES Congenital, but genetics unknown. Occasionally other family members have hemangiomata in non-facial areas to a lesser degree.

TREATMENT
• Seizures: Anticonvulsants, neurosurgery
• Monitoring for glaucoma
• Genetic counseling for patient and family

ICD-9-CM
759.6 Other hamartoses, NEC

 Subacute combined degeneration

DESCRIPTION The neurologic manifestations of pernicious anemia. Characteristics — peripheral paresthesias, weakness, leg stiffness, unsteadiness, lethargy, fatigue. Usual course - progressive.

SYNONYMS
• subacute combined degeneration of spinal cord
• combined system disease
• posterolateral sclerosis
• ataxic paraplegia
• neuroanemic syndrome
• funicular spinal disease
• Dana syndrome
• Putnam-Dana syndrome
• Lichtheim syndrome

CAUSES
• vitamin B12 deficiency
• pernicious anemia
• no intrinsic factor in gastric secretion

TREATMENT
• intramuscular cobalamin

ICD-9-CM
336.2 subacute combined degeneration of spinal cord in diseases classified elsewhere

 Sulfur dioxide poisoning

DESCRIPTION Irritant gas poisoning as an industrial accident. Characteristics — cough, hemoptysis, wheezing, retching, dyspnea, X-ray findings of diffuse mottled infiltrates indicating pulmonary edema. Usual course - acute; chronic; progressive; relapsing.

CAUSES
• cytotoxicity due to reactions between organic compounds and nitrogen oxides
• oxidation to form sulfuric acid
• occupational exposure
• industrial cleaners

TREATMENT
• supportive
• oxygen
• bronchodilators
• eye dilution plus irrigation
• acid dilution
• analgesia
• corticosteroids
• dilute skin contact
• treat shock
• antibiotics

ICD-9-CM
987.3 poisoning, sulfur dioxide

 Sunburn

DESCRIPTION
• Characteristics - mild erythema with subsequent scaling, pain, swelling, skin tenderness, blisters, fever, chills, weakness, shock, secondary infections, miliaria-like eruptions, exfoliation

CAUSES
• exposure to sunlight (or other ultraviolet light source) following administration of phototoxicity-producing drugs
• overexposure to ultraviolet rays of UVB (2800 to 3200A); danger increases proportionately to high altitude

TREATMENT
• prophylaxis with sunscreens rated 15 or better
• avoid additional exposure until well
• use tap-water compresses
• avoid topical anesthetic lotions and ointments
• use oral corticosteroids for extensive, severe sunburn (prednisone 10 mg qid for 4-6 days).

ICD-9-CM
692.71 Sunburn

Superior sagittal sinus thrombosis

DESCRIPTION Blood clotting in the superior sagittal sinus, a single venous sinus of the dura mater beginning in front of the crista galli and extending backward in the convex border of the falx cerebri. Characteristics — fever, prostration, headache, obtundation, engorged scalp veins, seizure, aphasia, hemiplegia. Usual course - acute.

SYNONYMS
• superior longitudinal sinus thrombosis

CAUSES
• infection
• extension from osteomyelitis
• dehydration
• trauma
• tumors

TREATMENT
• antimicrobials
• drainage
• surgery

ICD-9-CM
437.6 nonpyogenic thrombosis of intracranial venous sinus

Syringomyelia

DESCRIPTION Often associated with syringobulbia. Fluid-filled cavity (syrinx) within the substance of the spinal cord or brainstem.
• Characteristics - lack of sensation for noxious stimuli in fingers (painless cut or burn). Capelike sensory defect over shoulders and back. Spasticity and weakness of the lower extremities. Muscular atrophy and fasciculations. Vertigo, nystagmus

CAUSES
• congenital (50%), intramedullary tumors

TREATMENT
• surgical drainage of the syrinx; plugging obex in 4th ventricle; section of spinal cord at filum terminale

ICD-9-CM
336.0 syringomyelia

Tabes dorsalis

DESCRIPTION Parenchymatous neurosyphilis in which there is slowly progressive degeneration of the posterior columns and roots and ganglia of the spinal cord. Occurs 15 to 20 years after initial syphilitic infection. Characteristics — lancinating lightning pains, urinary incontinence, ataxia, impaired position and vibratory sense, optic atrophy, hypotonia, hyporeflexia and trophic joint degeneration (Charcot's joints).

SYNONYMS
• tabetic neurosyphilis
• locomotor ataxia
• Duchenne's disease
• spinal cord syphilis

CAUSES
• treponema pallidum

TREATMENT
• penicillin, tetracycline, erythromycin
• anticonvulsants, carbamazepine, phenytoin
• surgery

ICD-9-CM
094.0 tabes dorsalis
094.89 other specified neurosyphilis

Takayasu syndrome

DESCRIPTION Pulseless disease. Progressive obliteration of the brachiocephalic trunk and the left subclavian and left common carotid arteries above their origin in the aortic arch. Characteristics — loss of pulse in both arms and carotids; symptoms associated with ischemia of the brain (syncope, transient hemiplegia), eyes (transient blindness), face and arms. Usual course - progressive. Endemic areas - Orient.

SYNONYMS
• pulseless disease
• reverse coarctation
• Martorell syndrome
• brachiocephalic ischemia
• aortic arch syndrome

CAUSES
• unknown; autoimmune; hypersensitivity

TREATMENT
• corticosteroids
• surgery

ICD-9-CM
446.7 takayasu's disease

Tardive dyskinesia

DESCRIPTION A neurological syndrome characterized by involuntary and abnormal movements, usually involving bucco-oral muscles (but any muscle in the body can be affected). The movements include grimacing, sticking out the tongue, smacking and sucking of the lips, and sometimes, rapid movements of the arms and legs (chorea and athetosis). Tardive dyskinesia is associated with long-term use of neuroleptic drugs, usually appears late in the course of drug therapy and may persist indefinitely after discontinuation of the medication.

CAUSES
• up-regulation of dopamine receptors caused by long-term neuroleptic drug use (3 mos to years), prescribed for psychoses, also gastrointestinal and neurologic disorders

TREATMENT
• no effective treatment is available
• when possible, consider discontinuing the neuroleptic drug; some patients may prefer the movements to the possibility of relapse; also, discontinuance of the drug may not reverse tardive dyskinesia

ICD-9-CM
332.82 orofacial dyskinesia

Thallium poisoning

DESCRIPTION Poisoning due to ingestion of thallium compounds. Characteristics — vomiting, alopecia, neurologic and psychic symptoms, (ataxia, restlessness, delirium, hallucinations, semicoma, blindness), liver and kidney damage. Thallium is commonly found in ant, rat, and roach poisons. Symptoms usually begin approximately 3 weeks after poisoning. Usual course - acute; progressive.

CAUSES
• thallium ingestion

TREATMENT
• gastric decontamination
• potassium ferric hexacyanoferrate
• skin decontamination
• forced diuresis
• hemoperfusion
• hemodialysis
• urine output maintenance
• supportive

ICD-9-CM
985.8 poisoning, thallium

Thrombocythemia (adult), idiopathic

DESCRIPTION Hemorrhagic thrombocythemia (one of the myeloproliferative syndromes). Characteristics — repeated spontaneous hemorrhages, either external or into the tissues and an extraordinary increase in the number of circulating platelets. Usual course - chronic; progressive.

SYNONYMS
• primary thrombocythemia
• essential thrombocythemia
• primary hemorrhagic thrombocythemia
• essential thrombocytosis
• primary thrombohemorrhagic thrombocytosis

CAUSES
• clonal megakaryocytic disorder

TREATMENT
• chemotherapy
• radiotherapy
• iron replacement
• plateletpheresis
• platelet anti-aggregating agents

ICD-9-CM
238.7 idiopathic thrombocythemia

Thymoma, malignant

DESCRIPTION Tumor derived from the epithelial or lymphoid elements of the thymus. Characteristics — cough, dyspnea, dysphagia, chest pain, weakness. Usual course - possibly acute; otherwise progressive.

CAUSES
• unknown

TREATMENT
• surgical thymectomy
• radiotherapy for invasive thymoma
• corticosteroids if radiotherapy fails
• chemotherapy for advanced disease

ICD-9-CM
164.0 malignant neoplasm of the thymus

Thyrotoxic heart disease

DESCRIPTION Heart disease associated with hyperthyroidism. Characteristics — atrial fibrillation, cardiac enlargement, congestive heart failure. Usual course - progressive; relapsing.

SYNONYMS
• hyperthyroid heart disease

CAUSES
• hyperthyroidism

TREATMENT
• treat underlying hyperthyroidism
• radioactive iodine
• surgery
• beta-adrenergic blockers

ICD-9-CM
242.9 Thyrotoxicosis without mention of goiter or other cause
425.7 Nutritional and metabolic cardiomyopathy

Thyrotoxic storm

DESCRIPTION Severe thyrotoxicosis accompanied by organ system decompensation. Characteristics — fever, severe tachycardia, dehydration, mental status abnormalities representing dysfunction of the cardiovascular and central nervous systems. Usual course - acute.

SYNONYMS
- thyrotoxicosis
- thyrotoxic crisis
- basedow crisis

CAUSES
- exacerbation of hyperthyroidism
- thyroid surgery
- infection
- trauma

TREATMENT
- fluids
- propylthiouracil
- iodine
- hydrocortisone
- external cooling
- beta-adrenergic blockers
- oxygen
- treat precipitating factors

ICD-9-CM
242.91 thyrotoxicosis without mention of goiter or other cause, with mention of thyrotoxic crisis or storm

 Tick paralysis

DESCRIPTION A progressive, ascending paralysis caused by a neurotoxin secreted by a tick who has fed for several days on the host.

CAUSES Neurotoxin in saliva of ticks

TREATMENT
Removal of the tick, including any mouth parts retained in the skin. Complete recovery occurs in about 2 days.

ICD-9-CM
989.5 Tick paralysis

 Tinea barbae

DESCRIPTION Fungal infection involving the bearded area of the face and neck. Characteristics — kerion-like swellings and nodular swellings with marked crusting. Usual course - acute; chronic.

SYNONYMS
- tinea sycosis
- barber's itch
- beard ringworm

CAUSES
- fungal infection of coarse facial hair
- zoophilic dermatophytes

TREATMENT
- systemic antifungal agents
- systemic steroid added in severe inflammatory infections

ICD-9-CM
110.0 tinea barbae

 Tinnitus

DESCRIPTION A very common condition typified by the perception of sound in the absence of an acoustic stimulus. The sound may be of a buzzing, ringing, roaring, whistling or hissing quality or may involve more complex sounds that vary over time. It may be intermittent, continuous or pulsatile (synchronous with the heartbeat).

CAUSES
- damage to inner ear or cochlea
- middle ear infection or result from just about any ear disorder
- aneurysm's
- hardening of the arteries
- several medications

TREATMENT
- treat the underlying cause
- background music
- tinnitus masking device
- hearing aid for associated deafness

ICD-9-CM
388.3 tinnitus

 Toluene poisoning

DESCRIPTION A form of poisoning from toluene, a colorless liquid obtainable from coal tar. Toluene is an organic solvent used in rubber, plastic cements, paint removers, etc. Poisoning may result from inhalation or ingestion. Usual course - acute; chronic; progressive.

SYNONYMS
- toluol poisoning
- methylbenzene poisoning
- methylbenzol poisoning
- phenylmethane poisoning

CAUSES
- cytotoxicity

TREATMENT
- supportive; oxygen; bicarbonate
- CPR; gastric decontamination; skin decontamination; eye irrigation
- epinephrine contraindicated

ICD-9-CM
982.0 poisoning, toluene

 Toxaphene poisoning

DESCRIPTION Poisoning among agricultural workers using DDT. Characteristics — vomiting, paresthesias, malaise, course tremors, convulsions, pulmonary edema, ventricular fibrillation, respiratory failure. Usual course - acute; chronic; progressive.

SYNONYMS
- chlorinated camphene poisoning

CAUSES
- direct cytotoxicity
- diffuse neuronal excitation

TREATMENT
- gastric decontamination
- skin decontamination
- oxygen
- anticonvulsants
- avoid sympathomimetics
- supportive

ICD-9-CM
989.2 poisoning, toxaphene

 Trachoma

DESCRIPTION Chronic infectious disease of the conjunctiva and cornea. Characteristics — photophobia, pain, lacrimation. The organism is a bacterium, *Chlamydia trachomatis*. Usual course - acute; progressive. Endemic areas - Africa; Middle East; Asia; Central America.

SYNONYMS
- granular conjunctivitis
- Egyptian ophthalmia

CAUSES
- Chlamydia trachomatis
- transmission through birth canal

TREATMENT
- tetracyclines
- erythromycin
- sulfonamides

ICD-9-CM
076 trachoma
076.0 trachoma, initial stage
076.9 trachoma, unspecified

 Transposition of the great vessels

DESCRIPTION A congenital heart defect where the great arteries are reversed - the aorta arises from the right ventricle and the pulmonary artery from the left ventricle. This produces two noncommunicating circulatory systems (pulmonary and systemic). It often coexists with other congenital anomalies and affects boys 2 to 3 times more than females. Usual course - acute.

SYNONYMS
- complete dextrotransposition of the great arteries

CAUSES
- abnormal embryogenesis

TREATMENT
- balloon septostomy
- surgical redirection

ICD-9-CM
745.10 complete transposition of the great vessels

 Trench fever

DESCRIPTION Louse-borne disease occurring sporadically in Eastern Europe, Asia, North Africa and Mexico and producing multiple symptoms: fever, weakness, dizziness, severe leg and back pain.

SYNONYMS
- Wolhynia fever
- shin bone fever
- His-werner disease
- quintana fever

CAUSES
- Rochalimaea quintana transmitted by body lice

TREATMENT
- analgesics
- antipyretics
- delousing

ICD-9-CM
083.1 trench fever

Trichloroethylene poisoning

DESCRIPTION Trichloroethylene is a widely used industrial solvent and formerly used as an inhalation anesthetic. Poisoning characteristics: dizziness, headache, delirium, vomiting, abdominal pain, jaundice, flush. Usual course - acute; chronic; progressive.

CAUSES
• decomposition to dichloroethylene
• decomposition to phosgene
• decomposition to carbon monoxide
• hepatotoxicity
• renal toxicity

TREATMENT
• supportive
• gastric decontamination
• remove contaminated clothing
• epinephrine contraindicated
• volume expanders
• diuretics for urine output maintenance

ICD-9-CM
982.3 poisoning, trichloroethylene

 Trichostrongyliasis

DESCRIPTION Infection by nematodes of the genus Trichostrongylus whose eggs are frequently mistaken for hookworms. Endemic areas - Middle East; Far East; Iran. Usually asymptomatic but may cause cramps and diarrhea. Usual course - acute.

SYNONYMS
• trichostrongyloidiasis

CAUSES
• trichostrongylus larvae ingestion

TREATMENT
• thiabendazole
• pyrantel pamoate

ICD-9-CM
127.6 trichostrongyliasis

 Tricuspid atresia

DESCRIPTION Absence of the orifice between the right atrium and ventricle. Circulation made possible by presence of an atrial septal defect, allowing blood to pass from the right to left atrium and then to the left ventricle and aorta. Intra-atrial communication due to anomalous embryonal development.
• Signs and symptoms include marked underdevelopment, severe cyanosis, clubbing of fingers, prominent jugular A wave, apical heave, pulmonic second sound absent, systolic murmur, enlarged liver, presystolic pulsation. EKG shows left axis deviation, left ventricular hypertrophy, tall P waves. Transposition of great vessels, patent foramen ovale and ventricular septal defect all may accompany tricuspid atresia.

CAUSES
• unknown

TREATMENT
• anticongestive therapy
• surgery to correct condition

ICD-9-CM
746.1 tricuspid valve atresia

 Tricuspid regurgitation

DESCRIPTION Retrograde blood flow from the right ventricle to the right atrium due to inadequate apposition of the tricuspid valves. Characteristics — low output symptoms plus pulsations in the neck due to high jugular regurgitant waves from the transmitted right ventricular pressure. Usual course - acute; chronic.

SYNONYMS
• tricuspid valve insufficiency

CAUSES
• marked dilatation of right ventricle
• right ventricular failure
• rheumatic heart disease
• cor pulmonale
• congenital heart disease

TREATMENT
• treat underlying condition
• surgery
• tricuspid annuloplasty
• tricuspid valve replacement

ICD-9-CM
424.2 tricuspid valve insufficiency (nonrheumatic)

 Tricuspid stenosis

DESCRIPTION Narrowing of the tricuspid orifice obstructing blood flow from the right atrium to the right ventricle. Characteristics — fatigue, enlarged liver, fluttering discomfort in the neck caused by giant A waves in the jugular pulse. Usual course - chronic; progressive.

SYNONYMS
• tricuspid valve stenosis

CAUSES
• rheumatic fever
• bacterial vegetations
• atrial thrombi
• tumors
• carcinoid heart disease
• fibroelastosis

TREATMENT
• sodium restriction
• digitalization
• diuretics
• surgery
• valvulotomy

ICD-9-CM
397.0 disease of tricuspid valve
424.2 tricuspid valve disorders, specified as nonrheumatic
746.1 tricuspid atresia and stenosis, congenital

 Tropical eosinophilia

DESCRIPTION Subacute or chronic form of filariasis. Characteristics — episodic nocturnal wheezing and coughing, strikingly elevated eosinophilia and lung infiltrations. Usual course - chronic; progressive.

CAUSES
• adult wuchereria bancrofti worms
• adult brugia malayi worms

TREATMENT
• diethylcarbamazine

ICD-9-CM
518.3 tropical eosinophilia

 Truncus arteriosus

DESCRIPTION Congenital anomaly in which there is a single arterial trunk arising from the heart, receiving blood from both ventricles and supplying blood to the coronary, pulmonary, and systemic circulations. Frequently co-exists with malformations of other organ systems.
• Characteristics - signs and symptoms begin during the first week of life and include poor development, minimal or absent cyanosis, marked hypertrophy of the heart, loud and clear second sound, harsh systolic murmur at the base and along the left sternal border, continuous bruit over the upper sternum, thrill with maximum intensity over base of the heart, dyspnea, wide pulse pressure.

CAUSES
• unknown

TREATMENT
• surgery
• anticongestive therapy

ICD-9-CM
745.0 truncus arteriosus

 Trypanosomiasis, East African

DESCRIPTION Acute, severe, sometimes fatal form of African trypanosomiasis, transmitted by bites of tsetse flies. Usual course - acute; progressive; lethal within 1 year. Endemic areas - tropical East Africa.

SYNONYMS
• sleeping sickness
• Rhodesian sleeping sickness

CAUSES
• Trypanosoma brucei rhodesiense
• tsetse fly bites
• bushbuck antelope reservoir of infection

TREATMENT
• suramin prior to CNS involvement
• pentamidine prior to CNS involvement
• melarsoprol plus suramin pretreatment for CNS disease

ICD-9-CM
086.4 Rhodesian trypanosomiasis

Trypanosomiasis, West African

DESCRIPTION Chronic, less severe form of African trypanosomiasis. Disease persists for several months or years with central nervous system involvement late in its course. Usual course - chronic; intermittent; relapsing; progressive; delayed onset; successive bouts; intervening latent periods; may persist many years. Endemic areas - tropical West Africa; Central Africa.

SYNONYMS
• sleeping sickness
• Gambian sleeping sickness

CAUSES
• Trypanosoma brucei gambiense
• tsetse fly bites
• transplacental transmission
• human reservoir

TREATMENT
• suramin prior to CNS involvement
• pentamidine prior to CNS involvement
• melarsoprol plus suramin pretreatment for CNS disease

ICD-9-CM
086.3 Gambian trypanosomiasis

Tubular necrosis, acute

DESCRIPTION Acute renal tubular necrosis is a syndrome with multiple causes accounting for 70% of renal failure patients. Types include - stage 1: onset azotemia; stage 2: oliguria; stage 3: diuresis; stage 4: resolving diuresis
Usual course - acute; reversible;

SYNONYMS
• lower nephron nephrosis
• vasomotor nephropathy

CAUSES
• ischemia
• disseminated intravascular coagulation
• nephrotoxins
• trauma
• dehydration
• circulatory insufficiency

TREATMENT
• hemodialysis
• maintain renal perfusion
• maintain euvolemia
• diuretics
• vasopressors
• alkalinization

ICD-9-CM
584.5 acute renal failure with lesion of tubular necrosis

 Uterine bleeding postmenopausal

DESCRIPTION Bleeding from female genital tract beginning one or more years following menopause. Characteristics - may occur from any part of the reproductive tract including uterus, cervix, vagina, vulva; bleeding may be heavy or light.

CAUSES
• Iatrogenic as a result of estrogen replacement therapy
• Infection, atrophy, tumors (benign or malignant), polyps, adnexal pathology. Endometrial carcinoma is the cause of 1/3 of all cases of postmenopausal bleeding.

TREATMENT
• D&C
• discontinue all exogenous estrogens, including creams, etc.
• definitive treatment depends on finding and treating underlying cause

ICD-9-CM
627.1 postclimacteric bleeding

 Ventricular fibrillation

DESCRIPTION Ventricular rhythm rapid and chaotic. QRS complexes wide and irregular.

CAUSES
• myocardial infarction or ischemia, untreated ventricular tachycardia, electrolyte imbalances, digitalis or quinidine toxicity, electric shock, hypothermia

TREATMENT
• if pulse is absent, follow protocol using defibrillation, epinephrine, lidocaine, bretylium. Pronestyl, and sodium bicarbonate as indicated.

ICD-9-CM
427.41 ventricular fibrillation

 Ventricular standstill

DESCRIPTION No QRS complexes. Symptoms include loss of consciousness. No peripheral pulses, blood pressure or respirations. Death.

SYNONYMS
• Asystole

CAUSES
• myocardial infarction or ischemia, untreated ventricular tachycardia, electrolyte imbalances, digitalis or quinidine toxicity, electric shock, hypothermia

TREATMENT
• follow protocol using epinephrine, defibrillation, lidocaine, bretylium. Pronestyl, and sodium bicarbonate as indicated.

ICD-9-CM
427.5 Asystole

 Ventricular tachycardia (VT)

DESCRIPTION Symptoms include chest pain, anxiety, palpitations, dyspnea, shock, coma, death. Ventricular rate usually regular at 140-220 beats per minute. QRS complexes are wide and bizarre.

CAUSES
• myocardial ischemia, infarction, or aneurysm, ventricular catheters, drug toxicity (digitalis or quinidine), hypokalemia, hypercalcemia, anxiety

TREATMENT
• lidocaine bolus if pulse is present. If pulse is absent, follow protocol using defibrillation, epinephrine, lidocaine, bretylium, Pronestyl, and sodium bicarbonate as indicated.

ICD-9-CM
427.1 ventricular tachycardia

 Vernal keratoconjunctivitis

DESCRIPTION Bilateral conjunctivitis associated with corneal epithelial changes. Most likely to occur in spring and fall in males aged 5-20.
• Characteristics - signs and symptoms include tearing; intense itching; redness of the conjunctiva; and a tenacious, mucoid discharge containing numerous eosinophils. Symptoms usually disappear during cold months.

CAUSES
• allergies (probably)

TREATMENT
• topical corticosteroid drops, (e.g., 0.1% dexamethasone drops q 2 h) with supplemental small oral doses if needed
• long-term maintenance treatment with 0.25 prednisolone acetate applied bid
• remember to check ocular pressure if steroids are needed for more than a few weeks

ICD-9-CM
372.13 vernal conjunctivitis

 Von Gierke's disease

DESCRIPTION An autosomal recessive glycogen storage disease, (Type Ia) Glucose-6-phosphatase deficiency affecting liver and kidneys. Characteristics — hepatomegaly, hypoglycemia, hyperuricaemia, xanthomas, bleeding, adiposity. Patients live into adulthood. May lead to symptomatic hypoglycemia. Patients needed added precautions when taking many drugs. Usual course - chronic; progressive.

SYNONYMS
• glucose-6-phosphatase deficiency type Ia
• hepatorenal glycogen storage disease

CAUSES
• genetic enzyme deficiency

TREATMENT
• frequent feeding
• allopurinol

ICD-9-CM
271.0 Von Gierke's disease

 Von Hippel-Lindau disease

DESCRIPTION One of the neurocutaneous syndromes (phakomatoses). A familial cancer syndrome with predisposition to ocular and CNS hemangioblastomas, renal cell carcinoma, and pheochromocytomas. Prognosis is variable.

SYNONYMS
• Angioblastomatosis
• Cerebelloretinal hemangioblastomatosis
• Angiophakomatosis retinae et cerebelli

CAUSES
• Autosomal dominant with gene locus at chromosome region 3p25-3p26

TREATMENT
• Surgery and radiation therapy as indicated
• Genetic counseling of patient and family
• Supportive measures

ICD-9-CM
759.6 Von Hippel-Lindau disease

 Von Willebrand's disease

DESCRIPTION Group of hemorrhagic disorders in which the von Willebrand factor is either quantitatively or qualitatively abnormal. Usually inherited as an autosomal dominant trait though rare kindreds are autosomal recessive. Symptoms vary depending on severity and disease type but may include prolonged bleeding time, deficiency of factor VIII, and impaired platelet adhesion. Usual course - chronic.

SYNONYMS
• pseudohemophilia
• vascular hemophilia
• angiohemophilia

CAUSES
• no factor VIII associated proteins
• decreased factor VIII associated proteins activity

TREATMENT
• factor VIII replacement
• epsilon-aminocaproic acid
• DDAVP
• oral contraceptives to suppress menses

ICD-9-CM
286.4 von Willebrand's disease

Waldenstrom's macroglobulinemia

DESCRIPTION Malignant neoplasm of cells with lymphocytic, plasmacytic or intermediate morphology which secrete an IgM M component. Usual course - slowly progressive; death 3-10 years. Genetics - slight increased familial incidence.

CAUSES
• IgM M-component secretion

TREATMENT
• chlorambucil
• plasmapheresis for hyperviscosity
• prednisone

ICD-9-CM
273.3 Waldenstrom's macroglobulinemia

 Werner's syndrome

DESCRIPTION Premature senility in an adult. Characteristics — early graying and some hair loss, cataracts, hyperkeratinization, and scleroderma-like changes in the skin of the lower extremities. Usual course - chronic.

SYNONYMS
• adult progeria
• progeria adultorum

CAUSES
• altered glycosaminoglycan turnover
• chromosomal instability

TREATMENT
• symptomatic

ICD-9-CM
259.8 Werner's disease or syndrome

 Wernicke's encephalopathy

DESCRIPTION Acute, subacute, or chronic neurological disorder. Characteristics — confusion, apathy, drowsiness, atoxic, nystagmus, ophthalmoplegia. Most commonly results from chronic alcohol abuse and accompanied by organic amnesia and other nutritional polyneuropathies. Usual course - acute; subacute; chronic.

SYNONYMS
• Wernicke syndrome
• Wernicke's disease
• Gayet-Wernicke syndrome

CAUSES
• thiamine deficiency

TREATMENT
• intravenous thiamine supplementation
• supportive measures

ICD-9-CM
265.1 Wernicke's encephalopathy

 Whipple's disease

DESCRIPTION A malabsorption disorder. Characteristics — diarrhea, steatorrhea, skin pigmentation, arthralgia, arthritis, lymphadenopathy, and central nervous system lesions. Usual course - progressive; curative with treatment.

SYNONYMS
• lipophagic intestinal granulomatosis
• intestinal lipodystrophy
• secondary nontropical sprue

CAUSES
• probable bacterial infection

TREATMENT
• penicillin G
• ampicillin
• tetracycline
• corticosteroids

ICD-9-CM
040.2 Whipple's disease

 Wilson's disease

DESCRIPTION An inherited metabolic disorder characterized by excessive amounts of copper in the liver, brain, kidneys, and corneas. It can lead to tissue necrosis and fibrosis, which in turn can cause hepatic disease and neurologic changes. Without treatment, it leads to fatal hepatic failure. Usual course - chronic.

SYNONYMS
• progressive lenticular degeneration
• Westphal-Struempell pseudosclerosis

CAUSES
• genetic

TREATMENT
• avoid copper-rich foods
• penicillamine, potassium sulfide, pyridoxine, zinc acetate as alternative to penicillamine

ICD-9-CM
275.1 Wilson's disease

 Wolff-Parkinson-White syndrome

DESCRIPTION A form of pre-excitation characterized by a short PR interval and long QRS interval with a delta wave associated with paroxysmal tachycardia (or atrial fibrillation). Usual course - intermittent.

SYNONYMS
• preexcitation syndrome
• anomalous atrioventricular excitation

CAUSES
• accessory atrioventricular pathway
• circus movement conduction due to AV reentrant tachycardia

TREATMENT
• vagal maneuvers
• antiarrhythmic agents
• cardioversion
• electrical pacing
• surgical ablation

ICD-9-CM
426.7 Wolff-Parkinson-White syndrome

 Yaws

DESCRIPTION Non-venereal, infectious, tropical disease usually affecting persons under the age of 15. Spread by direct contact. Characteristics — painless papule that grows into a papilloma. The papule heals, leaving a scar. Late manifestations: deforming lesions of bones, joints, and skin. Usual course - chronic; progressive. Endemic areas - tropical regions.

SYNONYMS
• frambesia
• buba
• pian

CAUSES
• skin contact
• treponema pertenue

TREATMENT
• penicillin

ICD-9-CM
102.9 yaws

 Yellow fever

DESCRIPTION An acute infectious disease primarily of the tropics, caused by a virus and transmitted to man by mosquitoes of the genus Aedes and Haemagogus. A live virus vaccine (with few side effects) is effective and should be administered every 10 years. Usual course - acute. Endemic areas - Africa; South America.

CAUSES
• flavivirus
• mosquito bite
• Aedes aegypti

TREATMENT
• fluid replacement
• supportive therapy
• treatment for complications

ICD-9-CM
060.9 yellow fever

 Yersinia enterocolitica infection

DESCRIPTION Gram negative, facultatively anaerobic bacteria causing acute gastroenteritis and mesenteric lymphadenitis in children, and arthritis, septicemia, and erythema nodosum in adults. Transmitted through food, water, and person-to-person contact. Usual course - acute.

SYNONYMS
• yersinosis
• pasteurella pseudotuberculosis infection

CAUSES
• contaminated food ingestion

TREATMENT
• streptomycin
• gentamycin
• tetracycline
• chloramphenicol
• sulfamethoxazole-trimethoprim
• fluid replacement

ICD-9-CM
027.2 pasteurellosis

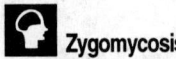 **Zygomycosis**

DESCRIPTION Fungal infection typically seen in immunocompromised or debilitated patients. In healthy individuals, the organisms seldom cause infection. Several forms exist - gastrointestinal, rhinocerebral, disseminated mucormycosis, pulmonary, cutaneous, central nervous system. Prognosis is guarded.

SYNONYMS
• phycomycosis
• mucormycosis

CAUSES
• fungi of the class Zygomycetes

TREATMENT
• amphoterecin B
• surgical removal of necrotic tissue

ICD-9-CM
117.7 zygomycosis

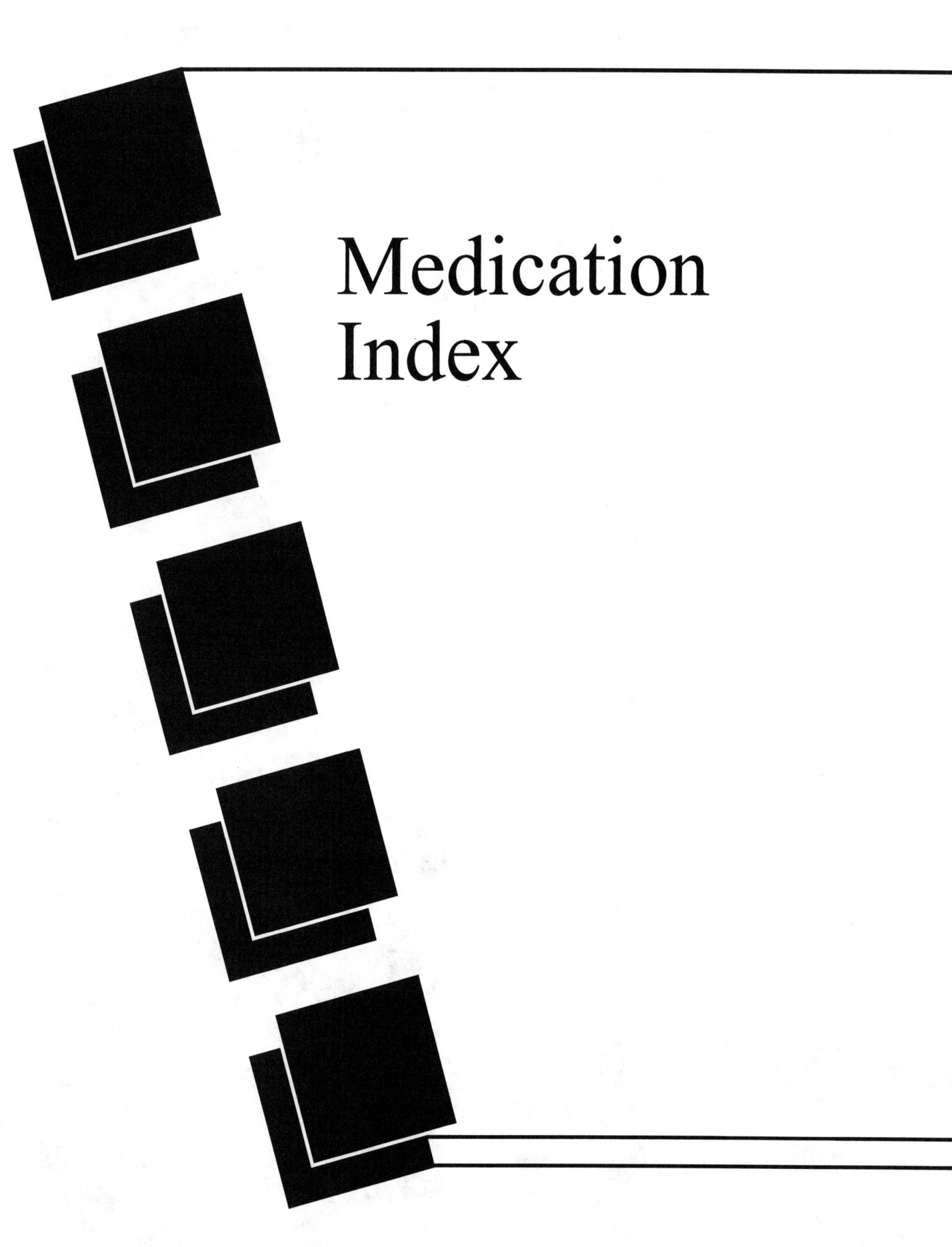

Medication
Index

Medication Index

haloperidol
- Dementia
- Dissociative disorders
- Hiccups
- Huntington's disease
- Multiple sclerosis
- Rheumatic fever
- Schizophrenia
- Suicide
- Tourette's syndrome

haloprogin
- Onychomycosis
- Pressure ulcer

Halotex, see haloprogin

Havrix, see hepatitis A vaccine

HCG, see chorionic gonadotropin

HCQ, see hydroxychloroquine

HCTZ, see hydrochlorothiazide

HDCV, see rabies vaccine, human diploid cell

Hemabate, see carboprost

hemin
- Porphyria

heparin
- Angina
- Arterial embolus & thrombosis
- Atrial fibrillation
- Cryptococcosis
- Disseminated intravascular coagulation (DIC)
- Interstitial cystitis
- Kawasaki syndrome
- Myocardial infarction
- Nephrotic syndrome
- Primary pulmonary hypertension
- Puerperal infection
- Pulmonary embolism
- Respiratory distress syndrome, adult
- Systemic lupus erythematosus (SLE)
- Thrombophlebitis, superficial
- Thrombosis, deep vein (DVT)

hepatitis A vaccine
- Hepatitis, viral

hepatitis B human immune globulin
- Hepatitis, viral

hepatitis B immune globulin
- Immunizations

hepatitis B vaccine
- Hepatitis, viral
- Immunizations
- Polyarteritis nodosa

Herplex Liquifilm, see idoxuridine

hexachlorophene
- Hearing loss

hexamethylmelamine
- Ovarian cancer

hib vaccine
- Immunizations

hibTITER, see hib vaccine

Hivid, see zalcitabine

homatropine hydrobromide
- Uveitis

hrGH, see human recombinant growth hormone

Humalog, see insulin

human recombinant growth hormone
- Turner's syndrome

Humatin, see paromomycin

Humegon, see menotropins

Humulin, see insulin

hydralazine
- Cardiomyopathy, end stage
- Complete atrioventricular (AV) canal
- Congestive heart failure
- Cor pulmonale
- Glomerulonephritis, acute
- Hypertension, essential
- Hypertensive emergencies
- Preeclampsia
- Primary pulmonary hypertension
- Respiratory distress syndrome, adult
- Ventricular septal defect (VSD)

hydrochlorothiazide
- Diabetes insipidus
- Hydronephrosis
- Hypertension, essential
- Pulmonary edema
- Renal calculi
- Renal tubular acidosis (RTA)
- Urolithiasis

hydrocodone
- Dysmenorrhea
- Restless leg syndrome

hydrocodone-acetaminophen
- Pancreatitis
- Sprains & strains
- Urolithiasis

hydrocortisone
- Addison's disease
- Anaphylaxis
- Chronic obstructive pulmonary disease & emphysema
- Crohn's disease
- Cryptococcosis
- Dermatitis, atopic
- Dermatitis, diaper
- Hemorrhoids
- Hypopituitarism
- Insect bites & stings
- Leukemia, acute lymphoblastic in adults (ALL)

Medication Index

Medication Index

Medication Index

Medication Index

Maltsupex, see malt soup extract
mannitol
    Brain injury, traumatic
    Burns
    Glaucoma, primary angle-closure
    Hypokalemic periodic paralysis
    Ocular chemical burns
    Renal failure, acute (ARF)
    Reye's syndrome
    Rhabdomyolysis
    Subdural hematoma
Maolate, see chlorphenesin carbamate
maprotiline
    Depression
    Post-traumatic stress disorder (PTSD)
Marinol, see dronabinol
Maxair, see pirbuterol
Maxalt, see rizatriptan
mazindol
    Obesity
measles, mumps and rubella
    Immunizations
measles, mumps, and rubella vaccine
    Immunizations
mebendazole
    Intestinal parasites
    Pinworms
    Roundworms, intestinal
    Roundworms, tissue
    Trichinosis
mechlorethamine
    Cutaneous T cell lymphoma
    Hodgkin's disease
meclizine
    Hyperemesis gravidarum
    Labyrinthitis
    Ménière's disease
    Motion sickness
Mectizan, see ivermectin
medroxyprogesterone
    Amenorrhea
    Contraception
    Dysfunctional uterine bleeding (DUB)
    Endometriosis
    Herpes eye infections
    Hirsutism
    Menopause
    Menorrhagia
    Polycystic ovarian disease
    Sleep apnea, obstructive
    Uterine myomas
    Vulvovaginitis, estrogen deficient
mefenamic acid
    Dysfunctional uterine bleeding (DUB)
    Menorrhagia
mefloquine
    Malaria
Mefoxin, see cefoxitin
Megace, see megestrol
megestrol
    Endometriosis
    Menorrhagia
    Uterine corpus malignancy
meglumine antimoniate
    Leishmaniasis
melatonin
    Insomnia
    Jet lag
Mellaril, see thioridazine
melphalan
    Amyloidosis
    Multiple myeloma
    Neuroblastoma
    Ovarian cancer
menotropins
    Artificial insemination
    Polycystic ovarian disease
Mentax, see butenafine
meperidine
    Anemia, sickle cell
    Blastomycosis
    Diverticular disease
    Epstein-Barr virus infections
    Insect bites & stings
    Pancreatitis
    Peritonitis, acute
    Renal calculi
    Urolithiasis
Mepron, see atovaquone
mercaptopurine
    Crohn's disease
    Leukemia
    Leukemia, acute lymphoblastic in adults (ALL)
    Ulcerative colitis
mesalamine
    Crohn's disease
    Ulcerative colitis
mesna
    Bone tumor, primary malignant
    Neuroblastoma
    Testicular malignancies
mestranol
    Contraception
Metamucil, see psyllium
metaproterenol
    Chronic obstructive pulmonary disease & emphysema

Medication Index

Medication Index

Medication Index

Medication Index

Medication Index

Medication Index

phentolamine
- Erectile dysfunction
- Hypertensive emergencies
- Pheochromocytoma
- Primary pulmonary hypertension

phenylbutazone
- Pericarditis

phenylephrine
- Barotitis media
- Epistaxis
- Priapism
- Rhinitis, allergic
- Shock, circulatory
- Sinusitis

phenylephrine - phenylpropanolamine - guaifenesin
- Hearing loss

phenylpropanolamine
- Barotitis media
- Obesity
- Urinary incontinence

phenytoin
- Brain abscess
- Brain injury, traumatic
- Complex regional pain syndrome
- Digitalis toxicity
- Eclampsia (toxemia of pregnancy)
- Hiccups
- Insulinoma
- Seizure disorders
- Seizures, febrile
- Status epilepticus
- Subdural hematoma
- Trigeminal neuralgia

pHisoHex, see hexachlorophene

phosphate of soda
- Constipation

physostigmine
- Glaucoma, chronic open-angle

pilocarpine
- Glaucoma, chronic open-angle
- Glaucoma, primary angle-closure

pimozide
- Tourette's syndrome
- Trigeminal neuralgia

pindolol
- Hypertension, essential

piperacillin
- Cellulitis, periorbital & orbital
- Osteomyelitis
- Pneumonia, bacterial
- Puerperal infection

piperacillin-tazobactam
- Osteomyelitis

piperazine
- Eosinophilic pneumonias
- Intestinal parasites

pirbuterol
- Chronic obstructive pulmonary disease & emphysema

piroxicam
- Cervical spondylosis
- Tendinitis

Pitocin, see oxytocin

Plaquenil, see hydroxychloroquine

Plavix, see clopidogrel

plicamycin
- Hypercalcemia associated with malignancy
- Osteitis deformans

pneumococcal vaccine
- Immunizations

podofilox
- Condyloma acuminata
- Warts

podophyllin
- Abnormal Pap smear
- Condyloma acuminata
- Molluscum contagiosum
- Warts

polycarbophil
- Constipation
- Encopresis

polyethylene glycol
- Constipation
- Encopresis
- Immunodeficiency diseases
- Iron toxicity, acute

polymyxin-gramicidin
- Conjunctivitis

Polysporin, see bacitracin-polymyxin B

polyvalent Crotalidae antivenin
- Snake envenomations: Crotalidae

potassium
- Complete atrioventricular (AV) canal

potassium bicarbonate
- Hypokalemia

potassium chloride
- Cardiomyopathy, end stage
- Diabetic ketoacidosis (DKA)
- Hypokalemia
- Hypokalemic periodic paralysis
- Inappropriate secretion of antidiuretic hormone

potassium citrate
- Renal calculi
- Urolithiasis

potassium citrate-citric acid
- Nephropathy, urate

potassium iodide

Medication Index

Medication Index

Medication Index

Medication Index

Labyrinthitis
Ménière's disease
Motion sickness
Ocular chemical burns
Uveitis
Sebulex, see sulfur-salicylic acid
secnidazole
Diarrhea, acute
Seldane, see terfenadine
selegiline
Alzheimer's disease
Dementia
Narcolepsy
Parkinson's disease
selenium sulfide
Tinea versicolor
Semprex, see acrivastine
senna
Constipation
Laxative abuse
Senokot, see senna
Septra-DS, see trimethoprim-sulfamethoxazole
Septra, see trimethoprim-sulfamethoxazole
serenoa repens
Hirsutism
Prostatic hyperplasia, benign (BPH)
Serevent, see salmeterol
sertraline
Anxiety
Autism
Dementia
Depression
Obsessive compulsive disorder
Post-traumatic stress disorder (PTSD)
Premenstrual syndrome (PMS)
Stroke rehabilitation
Suicide
Serzone, see nefazodone
SF6, see sulfur hexafluoride
sibutramine
Obesity
sigma-aminocaproic acid
Anaphylaxis
sildenafil
Erectile dysfunction
silicone oil
Retinal detachment
Silvadene, see silver sulfadiazine
silver nitrate
Burns
Interstitial cystitis
Molluscum contagiosum
Onychomycosis

Warts
silver sulfadiazine
Burns
Herpes zoster
Pressure ulcer
simethicone
Colic, infantile
Irritable bowel syndrome
simvastatin
Arteriosclerotic heart disease
Hypercholesterolemia
Hypertriglyceridemia
Sinemet, see levodopa-carbidopa
Sinequan, see doxepin
Skelid, see tiludronate
SM, see streptomycin
SMX-TMP, see trimethoprim-sulfamethoxazole
sodium antimony gluconate
Leishmaniasis
sodium bicarbonate
Cardiac arrest
Diabetic ketoacidosis (DKA)
Glossitis
Hydronephrosis
Hyperkalemia
Hypernatremia
Hypothermia
Near drowning
Nephropathy, urate
Renal tubular acidosis (RTA)
Rhabdomyolysis
sodium cellulose phosphate
Urolithiasis
sodium chloride
Inappropriate secretion of antidiuretic hormone
Milk-alkali syndrome
sodium fluoride
Osteoporosis
Otosclerosis (otospongiosis)
sodium iodide131 I
Hyperthyroidism
sodium phosphate
Encopresis
sodium polystyrene sulfonate
Glomerulonephritis, acute
Hyperkalemia
Renal tubular acidosis (RTA)
sodium tetradecyl sulfate
Varicose veins
Solatene, see beta-carotene
Solu-Medrol, see methylprednisolone
somatostatin
Colorectal malignancy

Medication Index

Medication Index

Medication Index

Medication Index

Medication Index

Medication Index

vitamin C
- Common cold
- Furunculosis
- Ocular chemical burns
- Pressure ulcer
- Vitamin deficiency

vitamin D
- Celiac disease
- Hypoparathyroidism
- Nephrotic syndrome
- Osteomalacia & rickets
- Osteoporosis
- Otosclerosis (otospongiosis)
- Polymyositis/dermatomyositis
- Renal failure, chronic
- Rhabdomyolysis
- Vitamin deficiency

vitamin E
- Alzheimer's disease
- Dementia
- Fibrocystic breast disease
- Glossitis
- Mastalgia
- Premenstrual syndrome (PMS)
- Vitamin deficiency

vitamin K
- Reye's syndrome

vitamin K1
- Vitamin deficiency

Vitrasert, see ganciclovir
Vivactil, see protriptyline
Vivelle, see estradiol
Voltaren, see diclofenac
Vontrol, see diphenidol
VP-16, see etoposide
VZIG, see varicella-zoster immune globulin

warfarin
- Atrial fibrillation
- Hip fracture
- Kawasaki syndrome
- Mitral stenosis
- Mitral valve prolapse
- Nephrotic syndrome
- Primary pulmonary hypertension
- Pulmonary embolism
- Systemic lupus erythematosus (SLE)
- Thrombophlebitis, superficial
- Thrombosis, deep vein (DVT)

Wellbutrin, see bupropion

whitfield's ointment
- Onychomycosis

Xalatan, see latanoprost
Xanax, see alprazolam

Xenical, see orlistat
Xylocaine, see lidocaine

xylometazoline
- Epistaxis

Yutopar, see ritodrine
Z pak, see azithromycin

zafirlukast
- Asthma

zalcitabine
- HIV infection & AIDS

Zantac, see ranitidine
Zarontin, see ethosuximide
Zaroxolyn, see metolazone
Zebeta, see bisoprolol
Zerit, see stavudine
Ziagen, see abacavir

zidovudine
- HIV infection & AIDS
- Immunodeficiency diseases

zinc chloride
- Common cold

zinc gluconate
- Zinc deficiency

zinc oxide
- Dermatitis, contact

zinc sulfate
- Macular degeneration, age-related (ARMD)
- Pressure ulcer
- Zinc deficiency

Zithromax, see azithromycin
Zocor, see simvastatin
Zofran, see ondansetron
Zoladex Depot, see goserelin
Zoladex, see goserelin

zolmitriptan
- Migraine

Zoloft, see sertraline

zolpidem
- Alzheimer's disease
- Dementia
- Fibromyalgia
- Insomnia

Zomig, see zolmitriptan
Zostrix, see capsaicin
Zovirax, see acyclovir
Zyloprim, see allopurinol
Zyprexa, see olanzapine
Zyrtec, see cetirizine

13-cis retinoic acid
- Myelodysplastic syndromes (MDS)

131-I Lipiodol
- Hepatoma

131-I-antiferritin

Medication Index

Hepatoma
2-CDA, see cladribine
3TC, see lamivudine
5-aminosalicylic acid, see mesalamine
5-ASA, see mesalamine
5-azacitidine
    Myelodysplastic syndromes (MDS)
5-dimethyltriazenoimidazole-4-carboxamine, see
dacarbazine
5-fluorocytosine, see flucytosine
5-fluorouracil
    Ovarian cancer
    Paget's disease of the breast
    Zollinger-Ellison syndrome
5-FU, see fluorouracil
5-hydroxytryptophan
    Restless leg syndrome
6-mercaptopurine, see mercaptopurine
6-thioguanine, see thioguanine

Topic
Index

Index

Index

Index

Index

-I-

-J-

Index

-M-

Index

-N-

Index

-P-

Index

Index

Index

Index

Index

-Q-

-R-

-S-

Index

Index

Index

Index

Index

Index

Index

Index

-X-

-W-

Index